Culture Boxes

Nutrition Concepts

INTRODUCTION TO MEDICAL-SURGICAL NURSING

THIRD EDITION

Adrianne Dill Linton, PhD, RN
Associate Professor
The University of Texas Health Science Center at San Antonio
School of Nursing
San Antonio, Texas

Nancy K. Maebius, PhD, RN
Instructor
The Health Institute of San Antonio
San Antonio, Texas

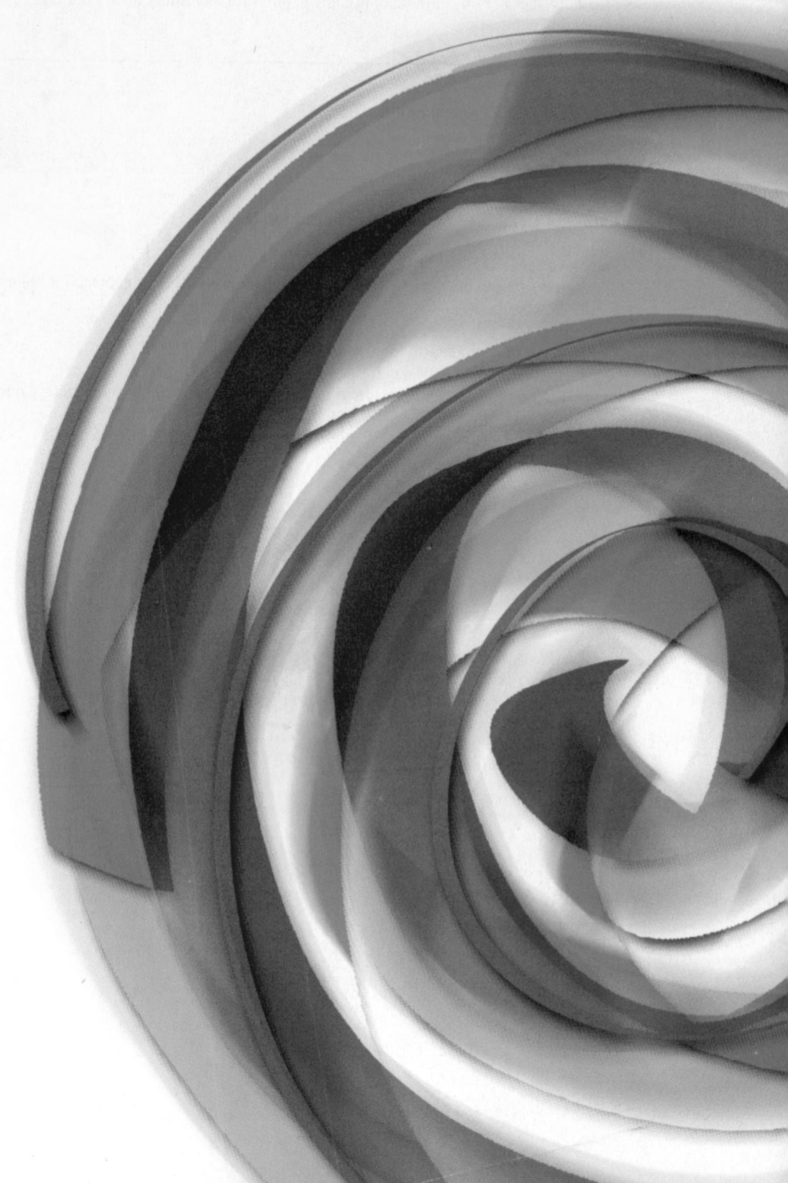

SAUNDERS
An Imprint of Elsevier

SAUNDERS
An Imprint of Elsevier

The Curtis Center
Independence Square West
Philadelphia, Pennsylvania 19106

Notice

Nursing is an ever-changing field. Standard safety precautions must be followed, but as new research and clinical experience broaden our knowledge, changes in treatment and drug therapy become necessary or appropriate. Readers are advised to check the product information provided by the manufacturer of each drug to be administered to verify the recommended dose, the method and duration of administration, and the contraindications. It is the responsibility of the treating licensed prescriber, relying on experience and knowledge of the patient, to determine dosages and the best treatment for each individual patient. Neither the Publisher nor the editor assumes any liability for any injury and/or damage to persons or property arising from this publication.

The Publisher

First Edition 1995. Second Edition 2000.

Library of Congress Cataloging in Publication Data

Linton, Adrianne Dill.
Introduction to medical-surgical nursing / Adrianne Dill Linton, Nancy K. Maebius.—3rd ed.
p. ; cm
Rev. ed. of: Introductory nursing care of adults. 2nd ed. 2000.
ISBN 0-7216-9527-2
1. Nursing. 2. Surgical nursing. I. Linton, Adrianne Dill. Introductory nursing care of adults. II. Maebius, Nancy K. III. Title.
[DNLM: 1. Nursing Care. 2. Nursing Process. WY 100 L761ia 2003]
RT41.L735 2003
610.73—dc21 2002030489

Vice President, Publishing Director: Sally Schrefer
Senior Editor: Terri Wood
Associate Developmental Editor: Teena Ferroni
Publishing Services Manager: Linda McKinley
Project Manager: Julie Eddy
Designer: Amy Buxton

TOP/KPT

Printed in China

Last digit is the print number: 9 8 7 6 5 4

Dedicated to our nursing students who motivate and inspire us.
Thank you for exploring this path of learning with us.

ADRIANNE DILL LINTON
NANCY K. MAEBIUS

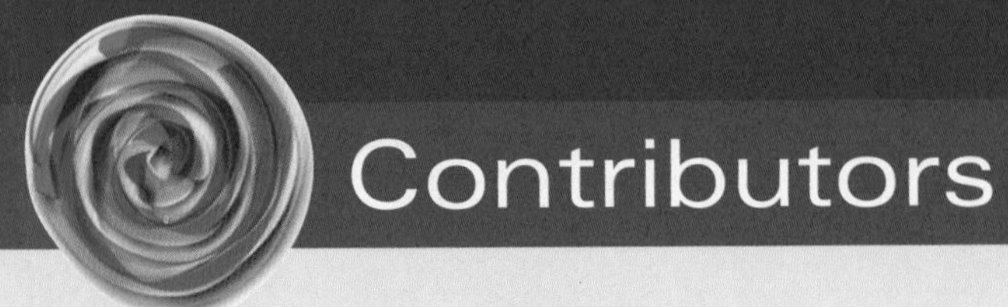

Contributors

LESLIE GODDARD, PhD, RN, CNRN
Clinical Nurse Specialist, Neuroscience
Methodist Healthcare System
San Antonio, Texas

MARY L. HEYE, BSN, MSN, PhD
Associate Professor
University of Texas Health Science Center at San Antonio
San Antonio, Texas

JANEAN W. JENKINS, MSN, CNS
Clinical Nurse Specialist
Southwest Texas Methodist Hospital
San Antonio, Texas
Clinical Faculty Associate
University of Texas Health Science Center at San Antonio
San Antonio, Texas

LOUIS K. LINTON, BS, RRT, CPFT
Instructor of Respiratory Therapy
U. S. Army: Respiratory Specialist Program
Brooke Army Medical Center
Ft. Sam Houston, Texas

JUDY L. MALTAS, MSN, CCRN
Clinical Assistant Professor
University of Texas Health Science Center at San Antonio
San Antonio, Texas

KATHLEEN A. REEVES, MSN, RN, C
Clinical Assistant Professor
University of Texas Health Science Center at San Antonio
San Antonio, Texas

VIRGINIA SHAW, MSN, RN
Clinical Instructor
University of Texas Health Science Center at San Antonio
San Antonio, Texas

LAURIE J. SINGEL, MSN, RN, C
Instructor/Clinical, School of Nursing, Department of Chronic Nursing Care
University of Texas Health Science Center at San Antonio
San Antonio, Texas

MARK D. SOUCY, MS, APRN, BC
Assistant Professor/Clinical
University of Texas Health Science Center at San Antonio
San Antonio, Texas

CHERYL ROSS STAATS, MSN, RN, CS
Associate Professor/Clinical
University of Texas Health Science Center at San Antonio
San Antonio, Texas

STACEY YOUNG-MCCAUGHAN, RN, PhD, AOCN
Deputy Director
Congressionally Directed Medical Research Programs
Fort Detrick, Maryland

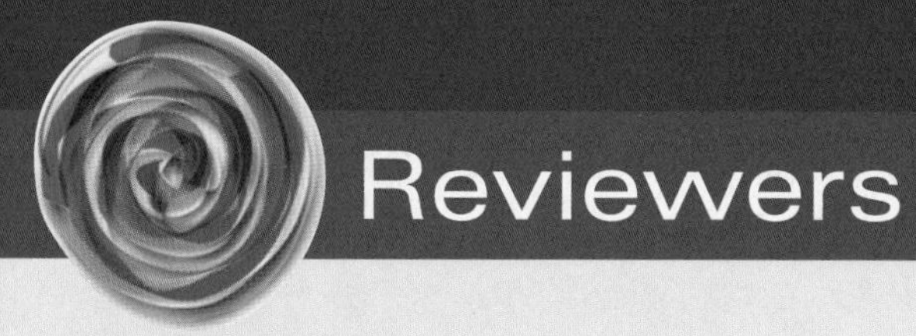

Reviewers

LINDA C. ARNOLD, RN, BSN
Ivy Tech State College
Bloomington, Indiana

JO-ANN DEAN, RN, BSN, MS
New England Technical Institute
New Britain, Connecticut

SHARON M. ERBE, RN, BSN
Washington-Saratoga-Warren-Hamilton-Essex Board of Cooperative Education Services
Southern Adirondack Education Center Career & Technical School
Hudson Falls, New York

BARBARA C. FAIR, MA, RN
St. Clair County Community College
Port Huron, Michigan

DARLENE D. GATTENS, RN, MN
Alvernia School of Practical Nursing at St. Francis Medical Center
Pittsburgh, Pennsylvania

M. SUSAN GRINSLADE, RN, MSN, PhD Candidate
Assistant Professor
University of Texas Health Science Center at San Antonio
San Antonio, Texas

KAREN KATHRYN HAAGENSEN, RNC
Howard College
San Angelo, Texas

BEVERLY F. HALTER, RN, BSN, MSN
Consultant
North Central Baptist Hospital
San Antonio, Texas

PAMELA ROCHELLE HINCKLEY, RN, MSN
Redlands Adult School
Redlands, California

PATRICIA A. KNECHT, MSN, RN
Center for Arts and Technology
Coatesville, Pennsylvania

FRANK LAUREANO, MSN, RN, CNOR
Assistant Professor/Clinical
University of Texas Health Science Center at San Antonio
San Antonio, Texas

VALERIE I. LEEK, MS, RN, CS
Cumberland County Technical-Education Center
Bridgeton, New Jersey

YVONNE B. MEINKET, RN, BS, MEd
Charlotte Vocational Technical Center
Port Charlotte, Florida

LISA D. MORLAN, BSN, RN
Gordon Cooper Technology Center
Shawnee, Oklahoma

LORI MOSELEY, RN
Hill College
Cleburne, Texas

SALLIE NOTO, RN, MS
Career Technology Center School of Practical Nursing
Scranton, Pennsylvania

TONI L. PRITCHARD, ADN, RN, LPN
Louisiana Technical College, Lamar Salter Campus
Leesville, Louisiana

JULIE S. VERNON, BSN
Tri County Technical College
Pendleton, South Carolina

KAY YANNACCONE, RN, BS
Central Susquehanna LPN Career Center
Washingtonville, Pennsylvania

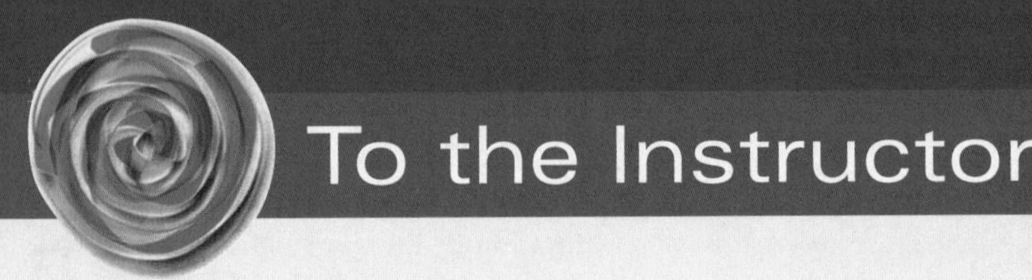

To the Instructor

The first two editions, titled *Introductory Nursing Care of Adults,* were designed to provide practical and vocational nursing students with comprehensive coverage of the nursing care of adults with disorders requiring medical, surgical, and psychiatric management. The needs of older adults and residents of long-term care facilities received special attention. The third edition, now titled *Introduction to Medical-Surgical Nursing,* maintains that focus, but with some very exciting changes and new features in response to feedback from instructors and students.

ORGANIZATION

Unit I explores patient care concepts, including the health care system, patient care settings, leadership, the nurse-patient relationship, cultural aspects of nursing care, the nurse and the family, health and illness, nutrition, developmental processes, the older patient, and the nursing process and critical thinking. **Unit II** focuses on physiologic responses common to many disorders: inflammation, infection, and immunity; fluid and electrolyte disorders; and pain. **Unit III** covers first aid and emergency care, general care of the surgical patient, and intravenous therapy. New to this edition is a separate chapter on care of the patient in shock. The in-depth coverage of topics in Units II and III provides both a foundation for understanding many disorders and a scientific basis for many aspects of nursing care. This approach is efficient because conditions such as specific fluid and electrolyte imbalances need not be explained repeatedly in the many situations where they occur.

Acknowledging the important role the LPN plays in the care of older adults, **Unit IV** provides comprehensive coverage of four clinical problems, as well as end-of-life care. The last of the introductory units, **Unit V,** presents an overview of nursing care of patients with cancer and patients with ostomies. This overview creates a foundation for the student to access when studying a variety of systems and disorders.

Units VI through **XVI** follow a systems approach to medical-surgical disorders. For each system, a thorough nursing assessment, age-related considerations, diagnostic tests and procedures, and common therapeutic measures are discussed. These common therapeutic measures are not intended to replace a fundamentals text, but to provide a limited summary or review of key aspects of nursing care. Specific conditions are covered, including pathophysiology, signs and symptoms, complications, diagnosis, medical treatment, and nursing care.

Nursing care is the heart of this text, which is organized using the steps of the *nursing process.* For each major disorder covered, nursing diagnoses, goals and outcome criteria, and interventions are presented. Sample *nursing care plans* illustrate how the text translates into a bedside tool for patient care. Patient and family teaching are emphasized throughout, with teaching plans presented in a special format. The *patient teaching plans* are not intended to be complete, but rather to give the student some critical points to emphasize.

Each chapter dealing with a particular body system contains a table detailing nursing interventions with specific *diagnostic tests and procedures* and a table that presents common *drug therapies. Pharmacology capsules* alert the student to important precautions, interactions, and adverse effects. *Nutrition concepts* emphasize the role nutrition plays in disease and nursing care. *Key points* summarize important information at the end of every chapter.

Unit XVII consists of three chapters that address psychosocial responses to illness, psychiatric disorders, and substance abuse. This material can eliminate the need for a separate mental health nursing textbook.

USING THIS TEXT

In general, the first five units provide a foundation for later chapters and the reader is referred to these units periodically. Therefore the text is best approached by studying these chapters first. Subsequent units are independent so that they can be studied in any order.

Each body system unit begins with assessment, age-related changes, diagnostic tests and procedures, and common therapeutic measures that are related to the body system that is being studied. Specific disorders and nursing care are then discussed. Nursing care is spelled out in detail except for conditions that are rare, generally treated on an out-patient basis, or require highly specialized care.

NEW TO THE THIRD EDITION

The third edition has been completely updated to include the latest developments in patient care. We have continued to use direct language rather than the cumbersome third person. We have also worked to improve consistency and to standardize and lower the reading level throughout the text. To reduce repetition, certain chapters have been condensed. In response to faculty requests, a chapter devoted to care of the patient in shock has been added.

In addition to a new, **full color design and art program,** specific changes to the third edition include:

- An Introduction to **critical thinking** and characteristics of a critical thinker in the context of nursing added to Chapter 11, *Nursing Process and Critical Thinking.* Exercises, called *Put on your Thinking Cap!!,* appear throughout the book. Discussion points for these exercises are included in the Instructor's Manual. In addition, critical thinking exercises have been added to each chapter in the Study Guide.

- **Key terms** are provided to aid readers in assessing their reading comprehension, and **phonetic pronunciations**—reviewed by an English as a Second Language (ESL) specialist—are provided for select terms. The terms that were assigned simple phonetic pronunciations were selected because they are either (1) difficult medical, nursing, or scientific terms or (2) other words that may be difficult for students to pronounce. The goal is to help the student reader with limited proficiency in English to develop a greater command of the pronunciation of scientific and nonscientific English terminology. It is hoped that a more general competency in the understanding and use of medical and scientific language may result. All key terms appear in color in the text as they are defined and used.
- **Cultural considerations** are presented in a separate chapter (5), and a new boxed feature called *What Does Culture Have to do with . . . ?* is presented throughout the text. In addition, culture questions have been added to corresponding chapters in the Study Guide.
- New **multiple-choice review questions** are included at the end of each chapter and allow for immediate reinforcement of the chapter content. Answers are provided on the inside back cover of the book.
- A new chapter (18) on **Shock** is included.
- New **complementary and alternative therapies boxes,** called *Consider the Alternative!,* appear as appropriate throughout the book. The boxes summarize what nurses need to know about complementary and alternative medicine as it relates to medical-surgical nursing. Questions related to this content have been added to corresponding chapters in the Study Guide.
- **NIC, NOC, and NANDA** are introduced in Chapter 11, *The Nursing Process and Critical Thinking.*
- Expanded coverage of **management skills,** including conflict management.
- Enhanced coverage of **nursing practice in nonacute care settings.**
- Additional **patient and family teaching plans.**
- Many **improved illustrations,** simplified to increase the emphasis on the most important components.
- An **upgraded and expanded ancillary package.**

TEACHING AND LEARNING PACKAGE

The **Study Guide** to accompany *Introduction to Medical-Surgical Nursing,* third edition, reviews important content and allows self-evaluation with matching, labeling, completion, and multiple-choice questions derived from the text. The Study Guide includes text page number references, and a complete answer key for the Study Guide appears in the Instructor's Resource.

The **Instructor's Resource (CD-ROM),** available free to adopters of the textbook, also includes (1) an **Instructor's Manual** with one open-book quiz for each textbook chapter; (2) an expanded **Computerized Test Bank** with over 1,300 NCLEX-style multiple-choice questions with topic, step of the nursing process, objective, cognitive level, NCLEX category of client need, correct answer, rationale, and text page reference; and (3) **PowerPoint** presentations for each text chapter. Contact your local Saunders sales representative to obtain a copy of the Instructor's Resource.

We welcome suggestions or other feedback that you may have concerning *Introduction to Medical-Surgical Nursing,* third edition, and its ancillaries. Please address your comments to the Nursing Editorial Department, Elsevier Science, The Curtis Center, Independence Square West, Philadelphia, PA 19106-3399.

ADRIANNE DILL LINTON
NANCY K. MAEBIUS

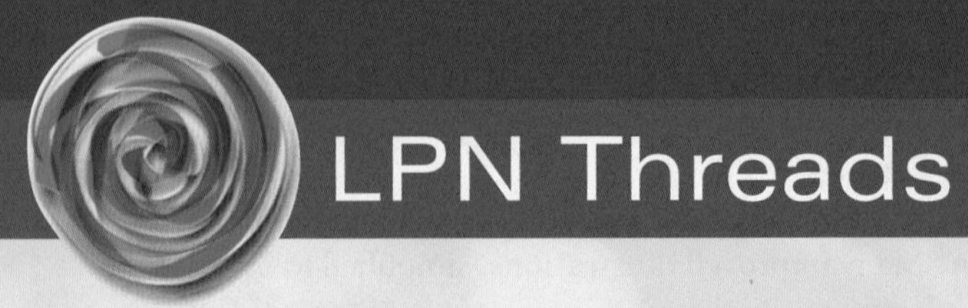

LPN Threads

Introduction to Medical-Surgical Nursing, third edition, shares some features and design elements with other LPN titles on the Mosby and Saunders lists. The purpose of these "LPN Threads" is to make it easier for students and instructors to incorporate multiple books into the fast-paced and demanding LPN curriculum.

The shared features in *Introduction to Medical-Surgical Nursing,* third edition, include:

- A **reading level evaluation** was performed on every manuscript chapter during the book's development.
- Cover and internal **design similarities.**
- Numbered lists of **Objectives** that begin each chapter.
- **Key Terms** with phonetic pronunciations and page number references at the beginning of each chapter. The key terms are in color the first time they appear in the chapter. An ESL (English as a Second Language) consultant reviewed all pronunciations.
- **Critical Thinking Questions** throughout the text. Answers to the critical thinking questions are provided in the Instructor's Manual component of the Instructor's Resource CD-ROM.
- Bulleted lists of **Key Points** at the end of each chapter.
- **Multiple-Choice Review Questions** at the end of each chapter. Answers are provided on the inside back cover of the text, for easy access.
- A **Complete Bibliography and Reader References** list at the end of the text.
- A **Glossary** at the end of the text.
- A **Computerized Test Bank** with the following categories of information: Topic, Step of the Nursing Process, Objective, Cognitive Level, NCLEX Category of Client Need, Correct Answer, Rationale, and Text Page Reference.
- A **PowerPoint slide presentation** in the Instructor's Resource CD-ROM.
- **Open-Book Quizzes** in the Instructor's Manual.
- **Study Guide answer keys** in the Instructor's Manual. The Study Guide itself contains text page number references where students can find the answers.
- **Tips for teaching English as a Second Language (ESL) students** in the Instructor's Manual.
- **Study Hints for English as a Second Language (ESL) students** in the Study Guide.

In addition to content and design threads, these LPN textbooks benefit from the advice and input of the Mosby & Saunders LPN Advisory Board.

LPN Advisory Board

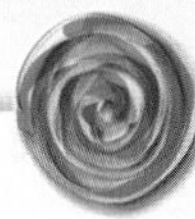

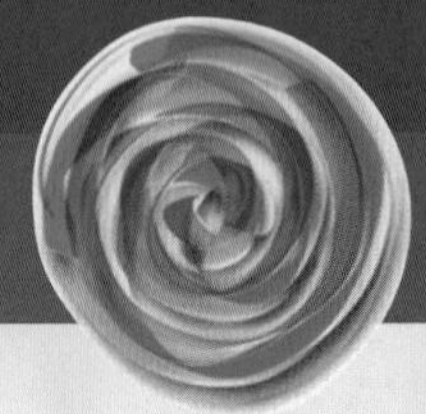

To the Student

KEY FEATURES

This book was designed to help you learn all the basic medical-surgical concepts and skills in a visually appealing and easy-to-use format. The writing is clear and engaging and hundreds of full-color drawings and photographs complement the text. In addition, there are numerous special features included to help you learn, understand, and apply the material. Here are some of the features of this book:

Objectives provide an overview of what will be learned from the chapter content.

Key Terms with **phonetic pronunciations** and page number references emphasize and clarify essential terminology.

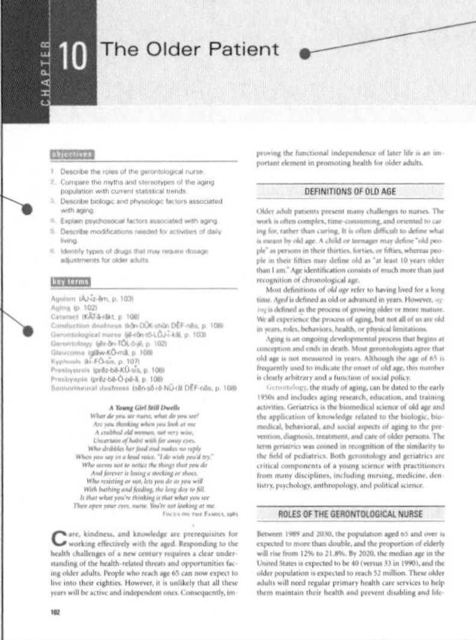

CHAPTER 10 The Older Patient

objectives

key terms

A Young Girl Still Dwells

DEFINITIONS OF OLD AGE

ROLES OF THE GERONTOLOGICAL NURSE

Care of the Elderly Patient provides basis for care of the elderly in acute long-term care and home settings.

Full-Color Design and Illustrations increase effectiveness of key concepts.

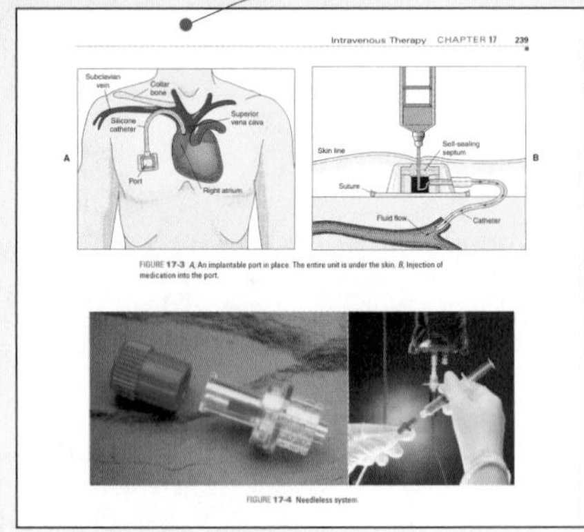

Intravenous Therapy CHAPTER 17 239

FIGURE 17-3 *A,* An implantable port in place. The entire unit is under the skin. *B,* Injection of medication into the port.

FIGURE 17-4 Needleless system.

Chapter 11 introduces **NIC**, **NOC**, **NANDA**, and their roles in clinical practice.

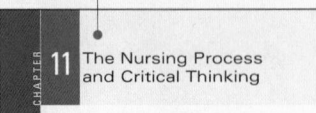

CHAPTER 11 The Nursing Process and Critical Thinking

Consider the Alternative introduces nontraditional approaches to health care.

Shock Chapter, now its own chapter with increased content.

CHAPTER 18 Shock

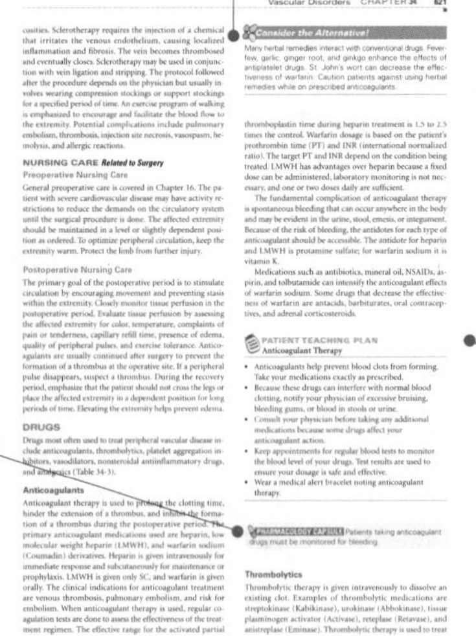

Vascular Disorders CHAPTER 34 821

Consider the Alternative

NURSING CARE Related to Surgery

PATIENT TEACHING PLAN Anticoagulant Therapy

DRUGS

PHARMACOLOGY CAPSULE Patients taking anticoagulant drugs must be monitored for bleeding.

Pharmacology Capsules alert students to important precautions, interactions, and adverse effects of medications.

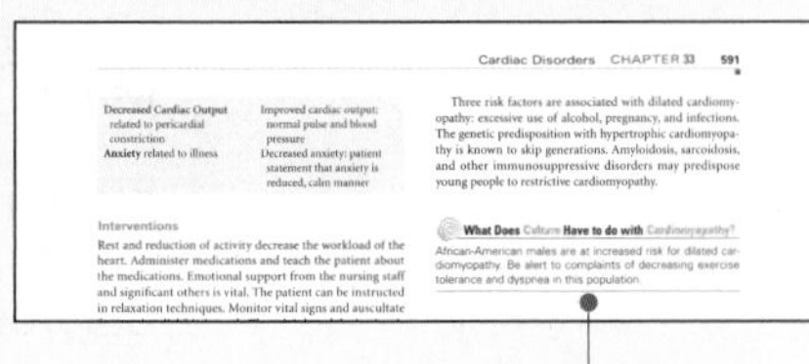

Cardiac Disorders CHAPTER 33 591

What Does Culture Have to do with Cardiomyopathy?

Cultural Considerations provide essential knowledge to ensure individualized care for patients.

Patient Teaching Plans illustrate examples of individualized patient care using the nursing process.

Drug Therapy tables in each systems chapter provide quick references to relevant drugs.

Diagnostic Tests and Procedures tables provide quick references to relevant tests.

Complementary & Alternative Therapies tables increase awareness of nontraditional approaches in today's health care settings and summarize what nurses need to know about CAM as it relates to medical-surgical disorders.

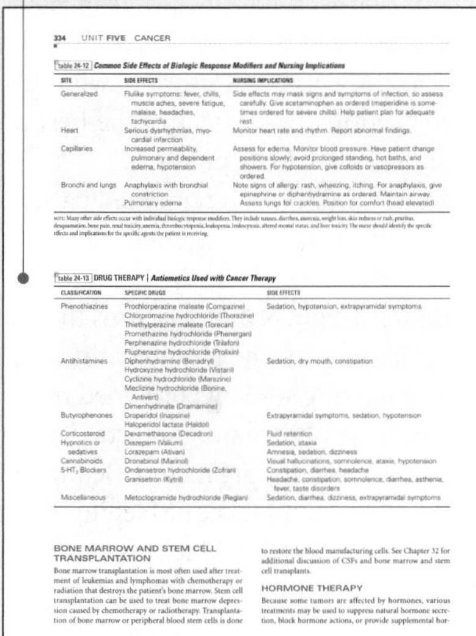

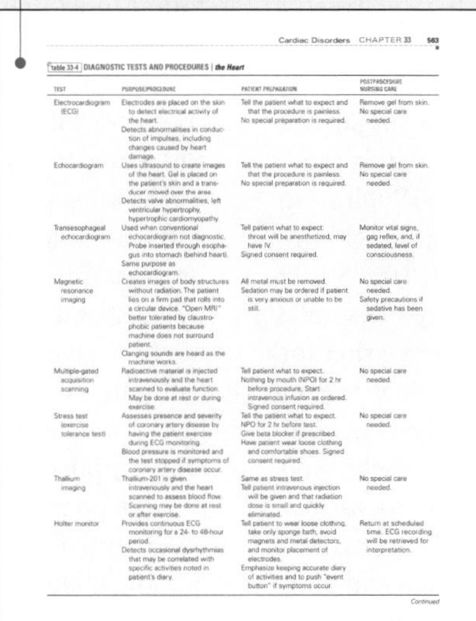

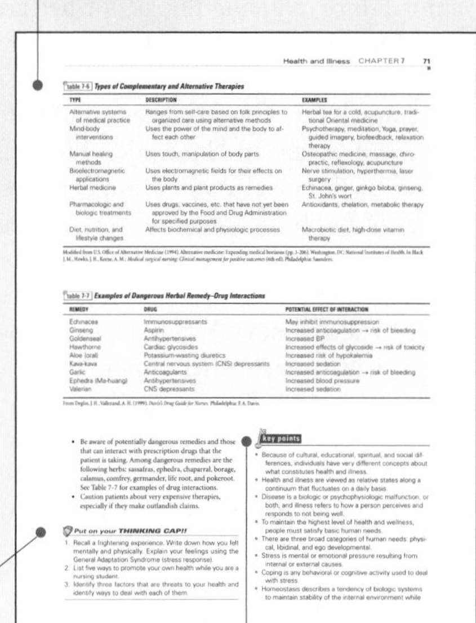

Put on your Thinking Cap encourages analysis of content for application to clinical situations.

Nutrition Concepts emphasize the role nutrition plays in disease and nursing care.

Key Points reinforce important information in each chapter.

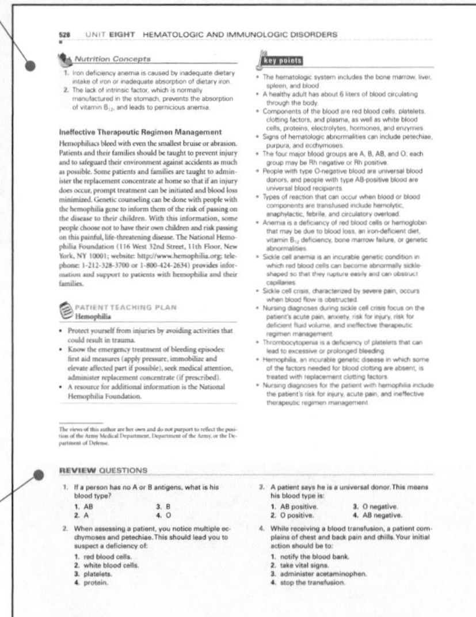

Complete Bibliography appears at the end of the book and provides additional sources of information.

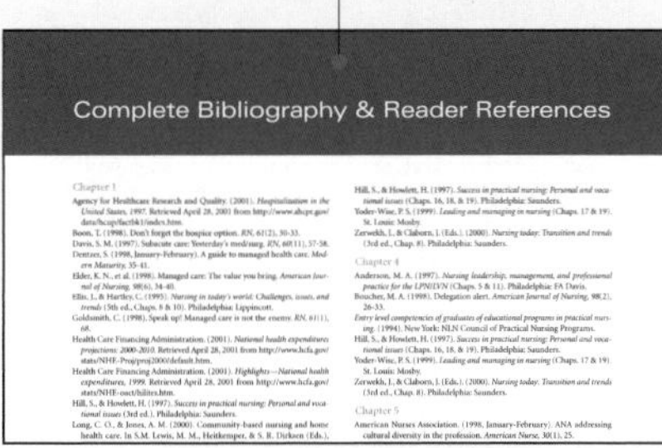
Complete Bibliography & Reader References

Multiple-Choice Review Questions test knowledge of the chapter content and help prepare for NCLEX-PN.

NEW STUDY GUIDE

Study guide provides detailed, clear methods to identify the most important material for more efficient learning.

Acknowledgments

Writing, editing, illustrating, publishing, and revising *Introduction to Medical-Surgical Nursing* have involved the combined efforts of many outstanding individuals. Grateful thanks to the staff at Elsevier Science, especially Terri Wood, Senior Editor, Nursing Books, for her great effort in seeing this edition through to completion. Other Elsevier supporters include Catherine Ott, Senior Editorial Assistant; Linda Morris, Senior Marketing Manager; Linda McKinley, Publishing Services Manager; and Julie Eddy, Project Manager. Lisa Hernandez of Editorial Production Services typeset the Study Guide, and Bob Browne produced the Instructor's Resource CD-ROM. Dr. Shirley Pisarek joined us as the item writer for the Test Bank, and Cindy Wesso created the PowerPoint slides. In addition, we would like to recognize the contributions of Ilze Rader, former Senior Editor, Nursing Books, who got this textbook off the ground, and Marie Thomas, former Senior Editorial Assistant, who was a wonderful support.

We appreciate the patience and skill of the artists and photographers who produced the fine illustrations. They, along with other reviewers, assured readability, accuracy, and timeliness of the manuscript. Over the past decade, students who have used our text have offered suggestions that we have found most helpful. Their feedback has always been most welcome.

We miss our colleague, Dr. Mary Ann Matteson, who was co-author of the first two editions. We wish her the best as she retires to enjoy her family and artistic pursuits.

We must not overlook our families who remained patient and encouraging during the time we were immersed in this process. Adrianne Linton wishes to express appreciation to her husband Ken and daughter Leigh. Nancy Maebius thanks her friends, students, and colleagues at The Health Institute of San Antonio. The vocational nursing students provided many ideas for inclusion of content. Family, friends, and colleagues who supplied encouragement and support include Jed Maebius, Stephen, Maria, Allison, Sarah and Jessica Maebius, Elizabeth and Tom Brady, Brian and Justine Maebius, Andrew Maebius, Donna Albee, Collette Moreno, Michael Pleuger, Peggy Richardson, and Eileen Mayo.

ADRIANNE DILL LINTON
NANCY K. MAEBIUS

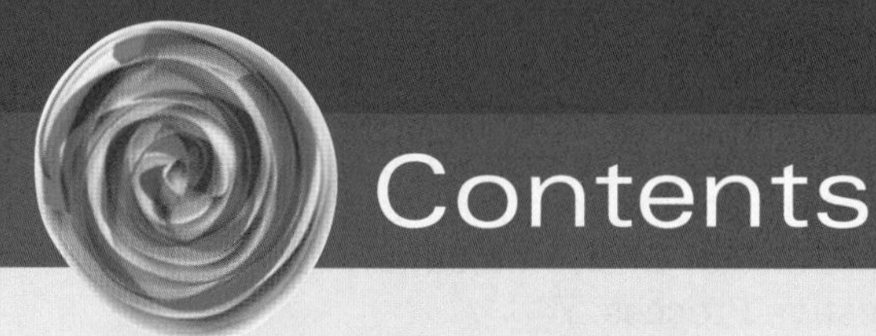

Contents

UNIT FIVE CANCER

UNIT SIX NEUROLOGIC DISORDERS

INTRODUCTION TO MEDICAL-SURGICAL NURSING

UNIT **ONE** PATIENT CARE CONCEPTS

CHAPTER 1

The Health Care System

objectives

1. Describe the organization of the health care system in the United States.
2. Describe the focus of public health services.
3. Define the three levels of prevention.
4. Discuss financing of health care in the United States, including Medicare and Medicaid programs.
5. Describe the components of the health care system that provide both outpatient and inpatient care and the types of service each provides.
6. Describe the impact of cost-containment measures on the delivery of care.

key terms

Capitation (p. 2)
Diagnosis-related group (DRG) (p. 3)
Extended care (p. 10)
Fee-for-service (p. 2)
Health maintenance organization (HMO) (p. 1)
Long-term care facility (p. 9)
Managed health care (p. 1)
Medicaid (p. 3)
Medicare (p. 3)
Older Americans Act (p. 8)
Preferred provider organization (PPO) (p. 1)
Primary prevention (p. 2)
Public health service (p. 1)
Secondary prevention (p. 2)
Skilled nursing facility (p. 10)
Tertiary prevention (TĚR-shē-ĕr-ē, p. 2)

The health care system in the United States today is very complex. With an increase in the elderly population and a resulting increase in the incidence of chronic illness, costs have risen alarmingly. Government officials, health care providers, and consumers now face the hard issues of deciding who is to receive care and how to pay for it. Health care reform is a major issue for government officials and the American people, all of whom are interested in the provision of equitable health care to all Americans.

ORGANIZATION OF THE HEALTH CARE SYSTEM

The health care system is made up of the patient, the patient's family, the community, governmental agencies, health care providers, and insurance companies. Many of the health-related services available to individuals are funded with financial assistance from government or private agencies. Unfortunately, not all citizens of the United States are eligible for government funds, and some are unable or unwilling to obtain private insurance. In addition, government funding and private insurance frequently do not cover all the costs of health care. Therefore, many people are unable to pay for care and may not receive the services they need. In the United States, about 17% of the population is uninsured.

In addition to the problem of inadequate financing, there is no overall philosophy or plan for health care. Critical care and the treatment of illness receive more attention than health promotion and disease prevention. Standards to ensure quality of care are inadequate, and there is little consumer participation in decision making. There is a lack of coordination of services, and communication among service providers is poor.

The health care system is now dominated by managed care. **Managed care** is intended to provide comprehensive health care at a reasonable cost through enrollment in a **health maintenance organization (HMO), preferred provider organization (PPO),** or similar plan that includes incentives to save costs. Managed care has stimulated increased interest in wellness and prevention, increased outpatient and home health care, and increased cost sharing.

ADMINISTRATION

In 1953, the Department of Health, Education and Welfare was established to organize the various health and welfare agencies of the U.S. government. The department became known as the Department of Health and Human Services (DHHS) in 1980, when education became a separate department. The four primary branches of DHHS are the Office of Human Development Services, the Social Security Administration, the **Public Health Service,** and the Centers for **Medicare** and **Medicaid** Services.

The Office of Human Development Services is responsible for activities related to health prevention and welfare. The Public Health Service and the Centers for Medicare and Medicaid

Services are of major concern to nursing because their purpose is to provide better health services for the American people. The major activities of the Public Health Service include (1) reviewing health care, particularly in relation to Medicare and Medicaid; (2) providing grants and conducting research to study health problems; (3) raising public awareness of serious health problems; (4) operating hospitals for national health problems, such as drug addiction, tuberculosis, and mental illness; (5) providing health science training grants to educational institutions; and (6) publishing vital statistics related to public health programs. The major agencies that carry out the activities of the Public Health Service are the National Institutes of Health, the Food and Drug Administration, the Health Services Administration, the Centers for Disease Control and Prevention, the Health Resources Administration, and the Alcohol, Drug Abuse, and Mental Health Administration.

Public Health Service

The focus of public health is the improvement of the health of communities and aggregates (collections of people). The main goals of public health intervention are to protect and improve the health of populations at risk in the community and to prevent disease and disability.

The focus of pubic health is usually directed to the three levels of prevention: primary, secondary, and tertiary (Table 1-1). See Chapter 7 for prevention behaviors.

Primary Prevention

The aim of primary prevention is to improve health and prevent disease and injury. Examples of health promotion activities include exercise programs to increase strength and cardiovascular fitness. Campaigns in schools to prevent children from smoking and efforts to educate people to wear seat belts are examples of primary prevention.

Secondary Prevention

The focus of secondary prevention is early detection and treatment of disease to improve patient outcomes. Papanicolaou's smears and reduced-cost mammograms are examples of secondary prevention activities.

Tertiary Prevention

Tertiary prevention is aimed at the prevention of disease recurrences or complications. The use of physical therapy to prevent contractures in a stroke patient and teaching a diabetic patient proper diet and foot care are examples of this third level of prevention activities.

table 1-1 ***Levels of Prevention***

PRIMARY PREVENTION
Health promotion: e.g., exercise, diet
Prevention: e.g., smoking cessation, seat belt use
SECONDARY PREVENTION
Early diagnosis and treatment: e.g., Papanicolaou's smears
TERTIARY PREVENTION
Rehabilitation: e.g., physical therapy after cerebrovascular accident

FINANCING

An overview of health care financing is essential in light of the astronomical rise in expenditures. In 1999, 13% of our gross domestic product was spent on health care, compared with 5% in 1960. In 1999, over $1.2 trillion was spent on health care. The Centers for Medicare and Medicaid Services has projected that total health care expenditures will total $2.6 trillion in 2010 and will account for 15.9% of the gross domestic product. It has become obvious that measures must be taken to control what is spent on health care. In an effort to contain the rapidly rising costs of health care, the government has established rules and regulations aimed at decreasing costs. *Cost containment* occurs when the rate of increase is controlled rather than costs being reduced. As a result, private spending for health care is growing rapidly. Prescription drugs account for 9.4% of the privately paid costs.

Many different approaches to financing health care are used in the United States. HMOs, PPOs, and governmental agencies all affect the way in which health care is delivered. For the most part, health care systems have operated on a fee-for-service basis. This means that the patient pays a fee to the provider for specific services, after which the patient may seek reimbursement from an insurance company. Although this traditional system of payment is changing, there are still some private-pay insurance options that support fee-for-service activities. Such coverage tends to be costly, typically requires deductions and copayments, and has limits that may not cover actual costs. However, it permits the patient to choose care providers, rather than being assigned to them. Many employers provide group health care insurance for employees. A type of coverage that blends multiple options is the point-of-service (POS) arrangement. Point-of-service includes a variety of options including HMO and PPO participation. Each option has advantages and disadvantages. Enrollees select which option they want to use. When health insurance pays for the health care expenses of members enrolled in health care plans, the payments are called third-party reimbursements.

Capitation is a strategy designed to control costs. With capitation, HMOs pay physicians a fixed amount of money each month for each member (patient) enrolled in the plan, regardless of whether or not the physician sees the patient that month. If physician costs are below the payment amount, the physician keeps the difference. However, if costs exceed the payment amount, the physician does not receive additional payment. There are a variety of HMOs that receive capitated payments from enrollees to cover a variety of services, such as preventive care and acute care.

Most health care agencies are funded through government funds or private insurance. Others are funded through out-of-pocket fees-for-service. The major means of government funding are Medicare and Medicaid (Table 1-2). Increasingly, other components of the health care system in addition to HMOs are moving toward capitation. With hospitals offer-

table 1-2 ***Comparisons Between Medicare and Medicaid***

MEDICARE	MEDICAID
FUNDING	
Monthly premium from paycheck; funds matched by federal government	Federal, state, and local taxes
ELIGIBILITY	
All persons older than 65 years, anyone with permanent kidney failure, plus disabled persons younger than 65 who qualify for Social Security benefits	Needy, low-income, and disabled persons younger than 65 years and their dependent children
HOW ADMINISTERED	
Federal government	Both federal and state governments
BENEFITS	
Physician services, hospital expenses, home health care, and outpatient services; geared toward acute, short-term care	Same health benefits as Medicare, plus nursing home care

ing capitation contracts, new budget-cutting procedures have been implemented.

Medicare

Established in 1965, Medicare is a health insurance program administered by the U.S. government (the Centers for Medicare and Medicaid Services) as part of the Social Security Act. It helps to pay for health care for anyone aged 65 and older, persons of any age with permanent kidney failure, and individuals younger than 65 who qualify for Social Security disability benefits. In 1999, Medicare spending represented 17.6% of every dollar spent on health care.

A monthly premium is deducted from each worker's paycheck, and the funds are matched by the federal government. Medicare insurance provides two types of coverage. Part A, hospital insurance, helps pay for inpatient care in a hospital or a skilled nursing facility, and certain home health services. Part B, medical insurance, helps pay for physician services and other services not covered by Part A. The list of services covered varies from time to time, depending on changing government regulations. Medicare benefits are geared toward acute, short-term care. Coverage in a skilled care facility is usually limited to a period of 100 days, and patient eligibility is based on the need for skilled care services on a daily basis. Medicare does not cover long-term care, such as nursing home care, over an extended period of time.

Changes in hospital funding in the early 1980s caused hospitals to discharge patients more quickly than ever before. Up to that time, hospitals had billed Medicare for their costs after they were incurred, a process referred to as *retrospective* payment. That system offered little incentive to save money. The system changed in 1983, and since that time hospitals have been advised in advance how much they would be reimbursed for treatment of a patient with a certain condition. This is referred to as *prospective* payment. Under the prospective payment system, patients are grouped according to diagnoses that account for similar amounts of resources, or diagnosis-related groups (DRGs). Under this system, hospitals are reimbursed a flat fee for a specified number of days based on a predetermined fee schedule for a diagnosis. If the patient gets better faster, the hospital makes money. If the patient requires a longer stay, the hospital loses money. This abrupt change in Medicare financing has caused the early discharge of thousands of patients and stimulated interest in transitional and community-based health care services.

The prospective payment system was originally developed by the federal government for Medicare patients, but it has been adopted by other insurers as well because it rewards cost-effective management of patients. A method for reimbursing hospice care was included in the 1982 revision.

Medicaid

Like Medicare, Medicaid was established in 1965 as part of the Social Security Act. It is the government insurance program for persons of very low income. Whereas Medicaid is funded by federal, state, and local taxes, and is administered by both federal and state governments on a partnership basis, Medicare is administered only by the federal government. States develop and operate the Medicaid programs within federal guidelines. Thus, benefits vary from state to state.

Medicaid benefits are provided for needy, low-income, disabled individuals under age 65 and their dependent children. Individuals older than 65 who are below a specified income level may also receive benefits, including services that Medicare does not cover. Services covered by Medicaid include inpatient and outpatient care, maternal and child health care, skilled nursing home care, physicians' fees, medications, laboratory work, radiographs, equipment, and home health care. Medicaid is more likely to cover long-term care than Medicare.

Many problems have developed related to Medicare and Medicaid because costs have risen much more quickly than anticipated. Some instances of fraud and abuse related to these programs have been reported. The goals of providing comprehensive health care for those over 65 and for the indigent have not yet been achieved.

COMPONENTS OF THE HEALTH CARE SYSTEM

Components of the health care system can be categorized into outpatient (ambulatory) care and inpatient care. Outpatient care is provided for patients who do not need hospitalization. It may involve health promotion and disease prevention, the diagnosis of disease, or the treatment and follow-up of disease processes. Outpatient care settings include physicians' offices, clinics, day surgery centers, adult day care centers for the handicapped or disabled, patients' homes, and hospices.

Inpatient settings include acute care hospitals, transitional and subacute hospitals, emergency rooms, psychiatric hospitals, rehabilitation centers, and long-term care facilities. The number of persons in inpatient settings is decreasing as the length of hospitalizations is reduced and as services are shifted to outpatient settings.

Over the past decade, cost-containment measures have resulted in a shift from inpatient care so that more services are offered in outpatient settings. The term *community based care* is sometimes used to describe the variety of services, both inpatient and outpatient, provided to meet the changing needs of patients in various states of health. The term also implies the provision of services based on the needs of individual communities.

OUTPATIENT CARE

Physicians' Offices

Many people, especially the elderly, receive their primary medical care in physicians' offices. Older people have more office visits per year than younger people, especially since the enactment of Medicare and Medicaid. The cost of visits to physicians' offices is covered in part by some forms of private health insurance and by Medicare, Part B. Physicians may practice in individual or group settings. Many group practices now are made up of various medical specialties, so that clients may have all of their health care needs dealt with in one location. The focus of care has traditionally been on the diagnosis and treatment of specific illnesses rather than on health promotion and preventive services. That may change as medical education begins to place greater emphasis on health maintenance.

Clinics

Outpatient clinics may be associated with community hospitals, teaching hospitals, or public health departments (Fig. 1-1). They usually focus on care for people with chronic illnesses, such as diabetes or heart disease, but people with acute illnesses also may be seen. The goal of care in clinics is to diagnose and treat the current illness.

Clinics offer many services, including physician services, nursing services, rehabilitative services, prenatal care, well-baby checkups, immunizations, preventive dental and eye care, and laboratory and diagnostic services. In large hospitals, clinics are usually organized according to medical subspecialties, such as urology, neurology, and orthopedics. For many people, especially the elderly, specialty clinics can be a problem because the elderly have many chronic illnesses and are seen in many different clinics. This makes the coordination of care more difficult than if the patient were seen in a facility with one set of health care providers.

Health Maintenance Organizations

HMOs provide health care and services through group practice. The principles on which HMOs are based include group

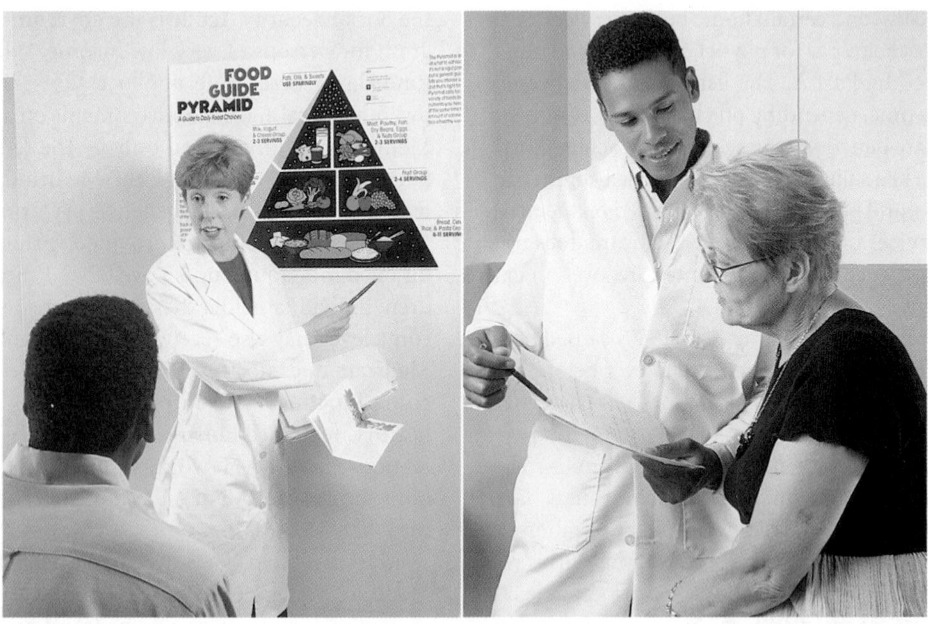

FIGURE **1-1** Outpatient clinics serve many people in the community.

practice with prepayment, voluntary enrollment, a combination of hospital and outpatient facilities, an emphasis on health promotion and prevention of illness, and physician responsibility for direction of patient care. The membership fee covers all health care services. Depending on the plan, there may be an additional small charge, called a copayment, for services. The copayment is paid at each visit.

Because HMOs collect only a set fee from clients, they are interested in promoting health and maintaining wellness. Healthy clients do not need as many services as sick ones and therefore are less expensive to treat. HMOs employ physicians, nurses, and other health care providers and also have a broad group of specialists available for referral. Clients are required to use only the services of the health care providers and hospitals associated with the HMO.

In 1973, the federal government enacted the Health Maintenance Organization Act. Its purpose was to help private agencies develop new methods of health care delivery in an effort to control the accessibility, quality, and cost of health care. This act helped stimulate the development of HMOs throughout the United States. The original HMO in the United States was the Kaiser-Permanente Medical Care Program.

HMOs are considered to be one way to stop rising health care costs and have become very popular in the United States. These organizations are able to provide both inpatient and outpatient care to persons at about the same cost that commercial insurance companies charge for inpatient care only. Costs have been contained as a result of utilization reviews conducted by the HMO, discharge planning, and home or "step-down" care. Utilization review entails looking at how resources are used and how health care money is spent. It is the process of reviewing resource utilization based on an external standard. Utilization reviews have resulted in decreased rates of hospitalization, shorter lengths of stay (by up to 45%), and the promotion of preventive care and wellness.

Ambulatory Surgery Centers (Outpatient or Day Surgery)

An alternative to inpatient surgery is outpatient or day surgery. Increasingly, surgical procedures are being done in ambulatory settings. Ambulatory surgery centers may be located in hospitals, freestanding clinics, health care centers, and physicians' offices. Many procedures such as cataract extraction, hernia repair, tonsillectomy, and the removal of foreign objects that once required hospitalization are now often done in outpatient facilities. Most forms of insurance cover the expenses. In addition, urgent care centers provide 24-hour service for patients with minor injuries or illnesses such as lacerations or influenza.

Ambulatory surgery is less costly and allows people to recover in the familiar surroundings of their own homes. Preoperative assessments and laboratory tests are usually performed on an outpatient basis several days ahead of the procedure, and then the patient reports to the setting early on the morning of surgery. Following recovery from anesthesia, the patient is discharged home, usually the same day.

The primary criticism of outpatient surgery is concern that patients may be at greater risk for postoperative complications in the absence of professional monitoring. This makes the role of the nurse in patient and family teaching a critical one. It also requires that the patient have appropriate support at home.

Home Health Agencies

History of Home Health Care

Home health nursing has a long and distinguished history that began when St. Vincent de Paul organized the Daughters of Charity in 1617. Members went from house to house, bringing food, education, and health care to the sick in their homes. This was one of the first organized groups to provide health education to the poor and to help people help themselves.

In the mid-1800s, William Rathbone, a wealthy English businessman, was impressed with the skill of the nurses who cared for his dying mother at home. Convinced that visiting nurses could help the poor and ill of Liverpool, he organized the first district nursing organization. This experiment was so successful that he opened the first training school for visiting nurses in 1859. Because he was the first to employ the district nursing concept, he is often called the Father of the Visiting Nurses Association.

In the United States, Lillian Wald is considered to be the forerunner of the modern public health nurse. She came from a wealthy family and studied nursing at New York Hospital in 1891. Her experiences teaching bedside nursing to women in the poor sections of New York City had a profound impact on her and led to the founding of the Henry Street Settlement House in 1893. The facility was a place where the poor could come for care and was supported by funds from the wealthy. Lillian Wald believed that all people had the right to direct access to the services of a nurse. She also maintained that nurses should live in the area where their patients lived to gain insight into the complexity of health care problems and their probable causes. Many of Lillian Wald's beliefs about people and nursing find expression today in Nursing's Agenda for Health Care Reform, in which community-based services and access to care are key issues.

Focus of Home Health Care

Home health services are provided to individuals and families in their homes or in assisted living centers to promote, maintain, or restore health or to minimize the effects of illness and disability (Fig. 1-2). As hospitals strive to reduce inpatient days, the demand for professional home health care is rising in all age groups. One of the fastest growing fields of nursing is home health care. Fewer people are being admitted to hospitals, and they are being discharged sooner with more needs for special care. The necessary services may include medical and dental care, nursing care, physical and occupational therapy, speech therapy, enterostomal therapy, social work, nutrition counseling, transportation, laboratory services, provision of medical equipment and supplies, and the assistance of home health aides and homemakers. Home health care is provided by hospitals, private profit-making and nonprofit agencies, and public agencies, such as public health and social service departments.

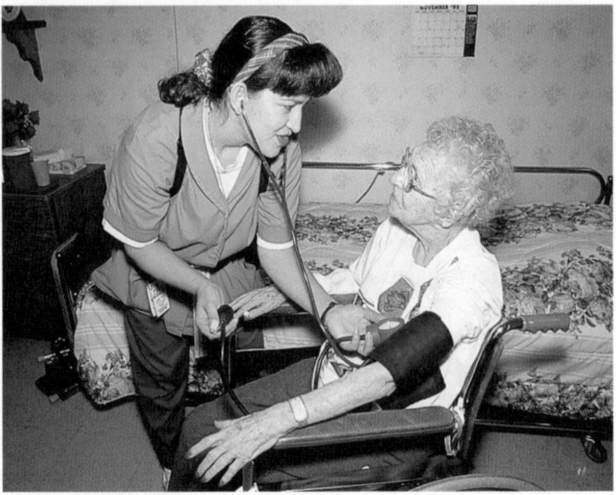

FIGURE **1-2** A nurse takes the blood pressure of a resident in an extended care facility.

Funding of Home Care Services

Home care services may be short term, long term, or intermittent. Services are funded by individual payment, by private insurance, by Medicare, and by Medicaid. To be covered by Medicare, the agencies must adhere to regulations put forth by the federal government. Most nursing services that are paid for by Medicare must be skilled care, with strict governmental guidelines defining the skilled care that must be provided. Regulations vary from state to state but are generally patterned after federal governmental regulations. The registered nurse is the case manager of services provided by health care workers in the home. Federal Medicare regulations for home care identify standard duties of the licensed practical nurse, which include furnishing health services, preparing progress notes, assisting the registered nurse in special procedures, and assisting the patient in learning self-care techniques.

Types of Home Care Agencies

There are several types of home care agencies: voluntary, official, proprietary, and hospital-based agencies. Some agencies specialize in specific care such as intravenous therapy or ventilator management. These include hospital-based, private for-profit, nonprofit, and Medicare-certified agencies.

Voluntary agencies. Voluntary agencies were the first to deliver nursing care in the home. They were financed by wealthy philanthropists in the community, and their mission was to care for the sick poor. Today the Visiting Nurses Associations are the most common examples of voluntary agencies. These associations are usually governed by a community board of directors that determines service delivery policies and assists with fund-raising. Because board members are drawn from different areas and social strata within the community, services often reflect community needs. Funding for voluntary agencies usually comes from a variety of sources, including Medicare, Medicaid, the United Way, private insurance, endowments, donations, and patients themselves. Once the primary provider of home care services, Visiting Nurses Associations saw their share of the home care market dwindle with the growth of proprietary (for-profit) agencies during the 1990s. However, the 1997 Balanced Budget Act put a limit on the amount of money spent on a patient's home health care regardless of diagnosis or needs. This payment limitation has been a factor in the closing of many home health agencies.

Official agencies. Official agencies are those supported by tax dollars and are authorized by law to deliver services to a defined area or community. Traditionally, state, regional, and local health departments have been assigned the responsibility of providing health promotion and disease prevention services as well as communicable disease investigation and environmental health protection. The nursing divisions of state, regional, and local health departments are usually tasked with delivering nursing services to populations at risk. In most states, this includes maternal and child services, sexually transmitted disease clinics, tuberculosis surveillance and treatment, and other health services as funds permit.

Thirty years ago, home health services were often delivered by local health departments as well as by voluntary agencies. As the concept of public health became more defined, caring for the sick in the home was no longer seen as a public health role. Gradually, more and more health departments dropped home health services. By the 1980s, competition from proprietary and hospital home health agencies had reduced the number of official home health agencies to a handful.

Proprietary agencies. Proprietary agencies are organized to make a profit on their operation. They may or may not participate in Medicare, but most do. Proprietary agencies may be owned by individuals or by corporate chains. Often their sources of revenue are private insurance, private-pay clients, Medicare, and Medicaid.

The prospective payment system contributed substantially to the growth of home health care. Much of this growth was in the number of proprietary and hospital-based home health agencies. As noted earlier, the limitations imposed by the Balanced Budget Act (1997) affected the profitability of proprietary agencies, and many have closed.

Hospital-based agencies. Institution-based home health agencies also increased in number during the 1990s. Hospitals that were losing money under the prospective payment system saw the opportunity to recoup lost profits by opening home health agencies. These agencies are usually governed by the hospital's board of directors. The hospital-based agency usually gets most of its referrals from the hospital itself. Philosophy and policies are usually consistent with those of the parent institution. Some hospital-based agencies closed when profits declined.

Home Health Care Services

There are three primary skilled services in home health care: (1) nursing, (2) physical therapy, and (3) speech therapy. Secondary services include occupational therapy (which may be primary under certain conditions), social work services, and home health aide services. The role of the nurse in home health is discussed in detail in Chapter 2. An overview of other services is provided here.

Physical therapy. Home health patients recovering from health problems affecting mobility, such as hip fractures and strokes, are common candidates for physical therapy. Physical therapists assess the need for assistive devices such as walkers, wheelchairs, and grab bars and work with patients and their families on therapies to regain strength and mobility. To receive these services in the home, it is necessary for the patient to be homebound.

Speech therapy. Speech therapists work with patients who have speech or swallowing disorders. A common indication for speech therapy is aphasia. As with all home health services, to receive speech therapy in the home that is reimbursed by Medicare, it is necessary to meet all of the criteria for Medicare.

Occupational therapy. Patients who have conditions impairing movement of the upper extremities are prime candidates for occupational therapy. People with arthritis or strokes may benefit from assistive devices for dressing and other daily personal care and household activities. Occupational therapists also provide muscle reeducation, splinting, and improved control of fine motor movement. Timely occupational therapy interventions can help the patient become safer and more independent in the home setting.

Social work services. Social workers can provide valuable assistance to families trying to manage chronic illness in the home. Typically, social workers work with families to identify problems that arise in managing illness at home and recommend referrals to community resources. They may also provide information about financial assistance and help families with applications for community services such as Meals on Wheels and respite care.

Home health aide services. The home health aide is a valuable member of the home care team. Home health aides provide personal care for the patient in the home, such as bathing, ambulating, transferring, skin care, and oral hygiene. They may also measure and record vital signs and do other basic, nonskilled tasks. Incidental homemaking such as making the bed and straightening the client's room are also common home health aide tasks. General housecleaning, shopping, and laundry are inappropriate for home health aides. Patients qualify for home health services if they already receive one of the three primary skilled services.

Homemaker services. Homemakers are usually provided by families or state and local assistance programs. Their duties include common household chores such as cooking, light housekeeping, laundry, shopping, and picking up medications.

Enterostomal therapy. Enterostomal therapists are employed in many large home health agencies. They are specialists in the care of all types of wounds, such as pressure ulcers, surgical wounds, and ostomies. They provide care to patients and consultation to nurses on how to manage wounds. They also have extensive knowledge of skin care products and ostomy appliances.

Other home health care services. Dietitians, nurse practitioners, or psychologists may deliver services in the home.

Specialty Home Care Services

Prospective payment systems and the use of DRGs have provided a stimulus for the development of specialty home care, especially for pediatric, psychiatric, and terminally ill patients. In addition, insurance companies, faced with the rising costs of intravenous and ventilator therapies in the hospital setting, have recognized the potential cost savings of delivering these therapies in the home. In the past few years, the use of high technology in the home has increased dramatically. Patients using these technologies most commonly are those needing intravenous therapy or those who are ventilator dependent. Pediatric home care and mental health home care are also specialties.

Pediatric home care. Since the late 1980s there has been an increase in the number of sick children cared for in the home. This increase is largely the result of advances in technology that have enabled the medical community to save many newborn infants who otherwise would not have survived. These same technological advances have produced the equipment necessary to provide adequate care in the home environment. Small, compact pumps, ventilators, and monitors have enabled children with cancer, respiratory disease, and cerebral palsy to live more normal lives at home.

Pediatric home care provides a better quality of life for young patients, but it also contributes to strain and role overload for parents and other caregivers. Many pediatric home care services are funded by Medicaid and state children's services. Private insurance companies are becoming more interested in funding pediatric home care because of the potential cost savings over hospital treatment.

Mental health home care. Another growing area of home health care is the delivery of mental health services in the home. Nurses in this role have advanced training in psychiatric disorders; they provide medication monitoring and teaching and perform mental status examinations and suicide assessments. They often provide consultation to other home care nurses on mental health problems that arise in patients with nonpsychiatric problems.

Hospices

The hospice concept is a concept of caring that originated in fifteenth-century Europe as the provision of respite and comfort for travelers. Later, this concept was extended to the dying in both hospitals and home settings. Families and hospital personnel collaborated to provide palliative care to dying family members.

During the early part of the twentieth century, the dying experience in the United States gradually shifted from the home to the hospital. Instead of being surrounded by family and friends in familiar settings, the dying found themselves in unfamiliar settings and being largely cared for by strangers. The first hospice in America was established in Connecticut in 1974 and provided both home care and inpatient care. Today, many more freestanding and hospital-based hospices all over the country deliver around-the-clock services to the dying.

Hospice services may be delivered in the home, acute care hospital, or extended care facility. Requirements for admission to hospice care include:

- A diagnosis of a terminal illness
- A prognosis of less than 6 months to live
- Informed consent by the patient to elect hospice care
- A physician's order

Hospices provide care for terminally ill patients in the home and other specified facilities. Their purpose is to enable terminally ill patients to live as full a life as possible, with skilled personnel managing the pain, discomfort, and other symptoms associated with the illness. In addition, hospices assist families during the bereavement process. Some hospices are associated with hospitals, whereas others are associated with home health agencies. Most are independent organizations in the community.

Hospice services are provided by the Medicare statute. Under law, hospice services are granted for a total of 210 days. If the patient elects hospice services, he or she must waive the traditional home health services. All the criteria for the home health care benefit must be met except for the homebound requirement. In return, the patient is eligible for the following services:

- Nursing, home health aide, social worker, and therapist visits as determined by the team
- Other services, including pastoral care, dietary counseling, and respite care
- Prescription drugs related to symptom management and pain control
- Durable medical equipment as required

Hospice care is a worthwhile alternative for the terminally ill that provides a more natural and humane approach to the dying process. The team method is used to meet a variety of physical, psychological, social, and spiritual problems encountered by the terminally ill and their families. A multidisciplinary team of professionals and volunteers contributes collective efforts to provide a better quality of life for the dying and their families.

Adult Day Care Centers

Day care is a structured program designed to provide activities related to health and socialization for selected populations. The activities are most often directed toward the elderly and the mentally ill. Day care centers may be associated with hospitals or nursing homes, or they may function independently. Older people benefit from day care services because they can continue to live in the community and have supervision during the day while family members work. The centers provide all kinds of health-related services, health promotion programs, nutritional meals, and social activities. Most services are provided on a sliding scale fee basis or without charge.

Many of the services provided at day care centers are funded through the Older Americans Act, which was originally passed in 1965. The goals of the Older Americans Act are to ensure that elderly persons have adequate income and suitable housing, physical and mental health services, community services, and the opportunity to pursue meaningful activities.

Mental health services are also offered through day care. People who need counseling, follow-up care after hospitalization, and rehabilitation related to chemical dependence may benefit from day care programs. Most are covered by private insurance for a limited period of time.

INPATIENT CARE

Hospitals

Hospitals vary greatly in size, shape, and organization throughout the United States. Some are small, 20-bed rural hospitals, some are intermediate-sized community hospitals, and others are large urban university medical centers. Some hospitals are public and financed by the local, state, or federal government; others are private and owned by churches, businesses, corporations, or charitable organizations. Hospital care accounts for about 40% of personal health care expenditures in the United States. The average hospital stay is about 5 days and costs over $11,000. The predominant sources of payment for hospital services to the elderly are Medicare and private insurance. Medicare and Medicaid are billed for over half of all hospital stays.

The five most frequent reasons for hospitalization are infant delivery, coronary atherosclerosis, pneumonia, congestive heart failure, and acute myocardial infarction. Hospitals are major providers of health and related services to the elderly. People age 65 and older, while comprising only 13% of the U.S. population, account for 36% of all hospital stays. In addition, older people tend to have longer hospital stays than younger people (Fig. 1-3).

The DRG system has had a great impact on hospital care and length of stay for patients. Because hospitals receive only a fixed amount of money, physicians are now discharging patients as early as possible to reduce costs. As a result, admissions to nursing homes and the use of home health agencies are increasing to care for people who are not leaving the hospital as fully recovered as those who have had longer hospital stays. Therefore, the demand for high-technology services such as respiratory therapy and intravenous therapy at home and in nursing homes is increasing. In addition, many health care providers feel there is now a "revolving door syndrome" with clients: patients return to the hospital for care after discharge because they did not fully recover at home.

Transitional and subacute facilities are intended to provide intermediate levels of care when needed following hospital discharge. Transitional hospitals receive patients with

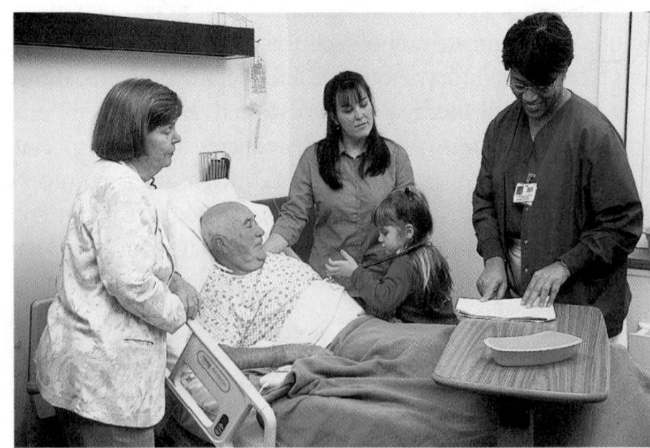

FIGURE 1-3 A large number of patients in the hospital setting are older adults.

acute but stable conditions who will need a lengthy minimum stay (often 25 days). Examples of patients who might need such a service are those with spinal cord injuries, patients with severe diabetes who have had amputations, and patients who are ventilator dependent. DRG requirements for Medicare patients are waived for transitional care. Some transitional hospitals lease space in acute care hospitals and contract for some of the acute care facility's services, such as laboratory and radiology services.

Subacute care units provide care for patients who need more intensive care than what is usually provided in a skilled nursing facility, but who no longer need acute care. When DRG days are used up, patients may be transferred from acute care hospitals to subacute units.

Psychiatric Hospitals

Psychiatric patients may be treated in specialty areas of regular acute care hospitals, or separate hospitals may be designated specifically for mentally ill patients. These facilities provide inpatient and outpatient treatment for individuals with acute psychiatric illnesses, with a focus on helping clients control their behavior or restore their behavior to what it was before entering the hospital.

Psychiatric hospitals may be private, nonprofit organizations that are sponsored by organized churches or may be operated by the local, state, or federal governments. The cost of care is covered by most private insurance companies, but only for 30 to 60 days.

Rehabilitation Centers

The aim of rehabilitation is either to restore individuals to their former level of functioning or to maintain or maximize remaining function (Fig. 1-4). Rehabilitation can and should be carried out in all health care settings by a variety of health care professionals with the active involvement of patients and their families. Most formal rehabilitation centers are located either within the hospital or nursing home or in a freestanding residential institution.

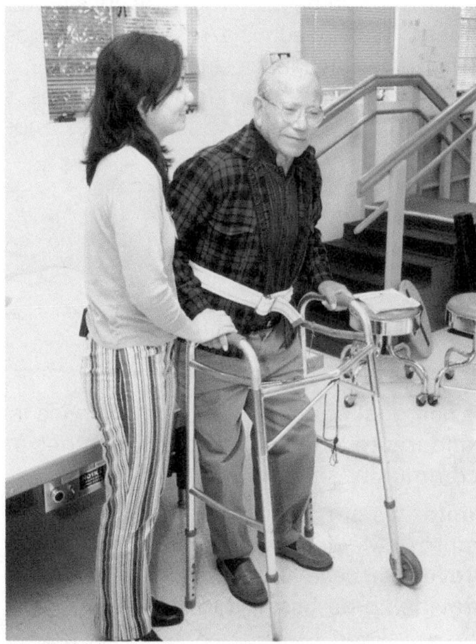

FIGURE **1-4** A patient is assisted with ambulation in a rehabilitation center.

Rehabilitation may focus on physical problems, such as those caused by stroke, spinal cord injury, or amputation, or on mental health problems, such as drug dependency or mental illness. To restore affected persons to their highest level of functioning, the rehabilitation process attempts to meet psychological, social, and physical needs. Therefore, the rehabilitation team includes many health professionals, including physicians, nurses, social workers, physical and occupational therapists, and speech therapists. It is very difficult to conduct a rehabilitation program without a team effort.

Long-Term Care Facilities

The term long-term care facility was originally used to describe institutions that were attached to hospitals for the purpose of recovery from acute illness. The term is now used to describe several different kinds of institutions, such as nursing homes, convalescent homes, and some residential institutions, whose primary purpose is to care for people with chronic illnesses and physical impairments. The focus of care is on those who do not need hospitalization but who are unable to care for themselves.

Modern long-term care for the elderly and disabled had its beginnings in nursing home care, which dates back at least to the turn of the twentieth century. The ill and elderly who had no families to care for them were housed in publicly funded homes or boarding homes. The care provided was largely custodial and included housing, food, and personal care. These homes were not licensed, and standards were few. Quality depended on the good graces of those providing the care. Later, nursing home care became tied to the medical care system, and the nursing home increasingly became a place for patients needing skilled nursing and social services.

The range of services now available for people requiring some level of assistance is expanding to provide a variety of options. Examples include independent living retirement centers, boarding and personal care homes, assisted living facilities, special care units for dementia patients, intermediate-care nursing homes, and skilled nursing homes. Independent living retirement centers commonly offer levels of care that permit the resident to access the level of care needed at a given point in time. Boarding and personal care homes typically provide a room and meals and, in some cases, minimal assistance and supervision. Residents of these facilities usually come and go as they please. Assisted-living facilities permit a high degree of independence but usually have limited access to nursing care. Help with medications and some treatments may be provided. Although residents often have kitchens, some group meals are typically provided. The intermediate-care skilled nursing facility provides care from a licensed nursing staff, including rehabilitative care for people who have the potential to regain function. Services include medical and nursing care; physical rehabilitation; long-term ventilator care; wound care; pharmaceutical, dietary, and social services; dental care; and activities. Federal regulations require a registered nurse to serve as director of nursing and a licensed nurse to be on duty at least 8 hours a day in an intermediate-care facility. This level of care is also referred to as extended care.

To be admitted to a skilled nursing facility, residents must be in need of nursing care that consists of observation during an acute or unstable phase of an illness, administration of enteral (tube) feedings or intravenous fluids, bowel and bladder retraining (for a limited period of time), administration of intramuscular or intravenous medications, or changing of sterile dressings. Persons who do not fit into any of these categories are deemed to be in need of custodial care and thus are ineligible for skilled nursing care benefits under Medicare. These facilities must have skilled health professionals available around the clock. The care of patients in these settings requires physician supervision and the services of a registered nurse, physical therapist, or speech therapist.

Put on your THINKING CAP!!

You have a friend who has limited income and no health insurance. She is a single mother with two small children. She has been advised to apply for Medicaid, and she asks you to help her. Find out the qualifications for Medicaid and how to make an application. Obtain an application form and complete it. Discuss the implications of the application process for persons with low reading levels, poor vision, poor hearing, no personal transportation, and/or no telephone.

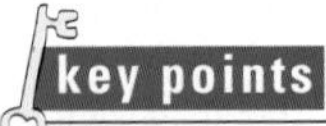

- The health care system is made up of patients, families, the community, governmental agencies, health care providers, and insurance companies.
- Despite a complex health care system, some people in the United States still do not receive the services they need.
- One effect of managed health care is an increasing focus on wellness and prevention.
- The Department of Health and Human Services is charged with organizing the various health and welfare agencies in the federal government.
- The purpose of the Public Health Service is to provide better health services by reviewing health care, providing grants and conducting research, raising public awareness of health problems, operating hospitals for national health problems, providing health science training grants, and publishing vital statistics.
- Financing of health care is a complex system made up of insurance companies, health maintenance organizations, preferred provider organizations, and governmental systems.
- Medicare is a federal health insurance program that is geared toward acute, short-term care for people aged 65 and older and for disabled people of any age, including those with permanent kidney failure.
- Medicaid provides health care benefits for needy, low-income, and disabled people and their children.
- Cost increases have created stresses in the health care system and have resulted in a variety of approaches to contain costs.
- The health care system includes outpatient and inpatient services.
- Increasingly, more health care, including surgery, is being carried out in ambulatory settings, and the number and length of hospitalizations are decreasing.
- Outpatient services are provided in physicians' offices, clinics, ambulatory (day) surgery facilities, and day care centers.
- Hospice services may be delivered to terminally ill patients who meet certain criteria in their homes, in acute settings, or in extended care facilities.
- Inpatient services are provided in acute care hospitals, in psychiatric hospitals, in rehabilitation centers, and in long-term care facilities.
- Home health care grew rapidly through the 1990s as fewer people were admitted to hospitals and those admitted were being discharged sooner with special needs for health care services.
- The Balanced Budget Act of 1997, which limited the total amount that could be spent on a patient's home health care regardless of diagnosis, resulted in the closure of many home health agencies.
- Long-term care facilities include nursing homes, skilled nursing facilities, and intermediate-care (extended care) facilities.

REVIEW QUESTIONS

1. One outcome of managed care has been:
   1. decreased cost sharing.
   2. increased emphasis on inpatient care.
   3. decreased use of home health care.
   4. increased focus on wellness.
2. The main goal of the Public Health Service is to protect and improve the health of populations at risk in the community and to:
   1. control health care costs.
   2. improve Medicare services.
   3. prevent disease and disability.
   4. provide home-based nursing care.

3. Medicare coverage includes:
    1. inpatient care in a hospital or skilled nursing facility.
    2. unlimited nursing home care.
    3. no eligibility requirements for skilled nursing care.
    4. private nursing care when needed.

4. Criteria for admission to hospice care includes:
    1. a prognosis of less than 1 year to live.
    2. a diagnosis of a terminal illness.
    3. cooperation of the patient's family.
    4. inability to pay for care in a hospital.

5. Which of the following has most directly resulted in earlier discharge of patients from hospitals?
    1. Decreased Medicare/Medicaid funding
    2. Balanced Budget Act of 1997
    3. The implementation of DRGs
    4. Improved medical and surgical care

CHAPTER 2

Patient Care Settings

objectives

1. Describe the role of the nurse in community and home health, rehabilitation, and long-term care settings.
2. Differentiate community health and community-based nursing.
3. Describe the types of specialty care that nurses may provide in home health care.
4. Describe the principles of rehabilitation.
5. List the four levels of disability.
6. Discuss legislation passed to protect the rights of the disabled.
7. Identify the goals of rehabilitation.
8. Name the members of the rehabilitation team.
9. List the types of extended care facilities.
10. Discuss the effects of institutionalization on the elderly person.
11. Describe the principles of nursing home care.

key terms

Disability (p. 16)
Handicap (p. 16)
Impairment (p. 16)
Rehabilitation (p. 16)

Chapter 1 briefly introduced the most common settings in which health care is delivered. Throughout this book, the care of patients in acute care settings is covered in detail. As the health care system changes, however, licensed practical nurses are finding a variety of opportunities for employment in community, rehabilitation, and long-term care settings. This chapter provides a more complete description of nursing in those settings.

COMMUNITY AND HOME HEALTH NURSING

Community health nursing and home health nursing are specialized areas of nursing practice that are often thought of as being similar. This probably comes from defining community health nursing as anything that occurs outside the hospital setting. These two practice areas, although sharing common historic roots, have significant differences.

COMMUNITY HEALTH NURSING

For both humane and economic reasons, it is better to keep people healthy than to treat them after disease or disability occurs. Traditional community health nursing focuses on (1) improving the health status of communities or groups of people (called *aggregates*) through public education, (2) screening for early detection of disease, and (3) providing services for people who need care outside the acute care setting.

Community Health Nursing Roles

The following example demonstrates typical community health nursing roles.

> A community health nurse notices a rise in blood pressure, an increase in weight, and a general lack of fitness in members of a senior citizen high-rise in her district. Her assessment shows that there are no recreational facilities nearby, the meals served at the high-rise tend to be high in fat, and there is a general lack of social activity at the facility. On the positive side, a residents' organization exists, although it has never been very active. By working with the residents' organization and a local church, the nurse initiates a group exercise program to improve the strength, cardiovascular fitness, and weight control of the elderly residents. By working with the management of the high-rise and the residents' association, the nurse gets the building manager to serve low-fat, low-cholesterol meals. The nurse also asks a local school of nursing to hold a monthly blood pressure and health education clinic for the residents.

In this example, the community health nurse not only gave direct service to individual clients but also worked with three existing community groups to provide a number of services designed to increase the health of the senior citizen group. Community health nurses often work with many different individuals and groups to create or modify systems of care to improve the health of a defined group. This function requires the nurse to assume a number of roles to accomplish care goals. The roles listed in the example include case finder, care manager, teacher, advocate, and coalition builder. Table 2-1 lists many of the roles assumed by the community health nurse. Most of these roles require at least a bachelor's degree in nursing to perform all aspects of the role; however, the LPN is increasingly visible in community health settings.

table 2-1 Community Health Nursing Roles

Advocate	Group leader
Caregiver	Health planner
Care manager	Home visitor
Case finder	Occupational health nurse
Clinic nurse	Researcher
Coalition builder	School nurse
Counselor	Supervisor
Epidemiologist	Teacher

Community-Based Nursing

The term *community-based nursing* has been used in several contexts but should not be confused with community health nursing. Community-based nursing may be described as deriving health care services based on identified community needs and providing various types of care that meet the needs of citizens at various levels of wellness and illness. In a more general sense, the term is sometimes used to describe the provision of various levels of care in traditional and nontraditional community settings

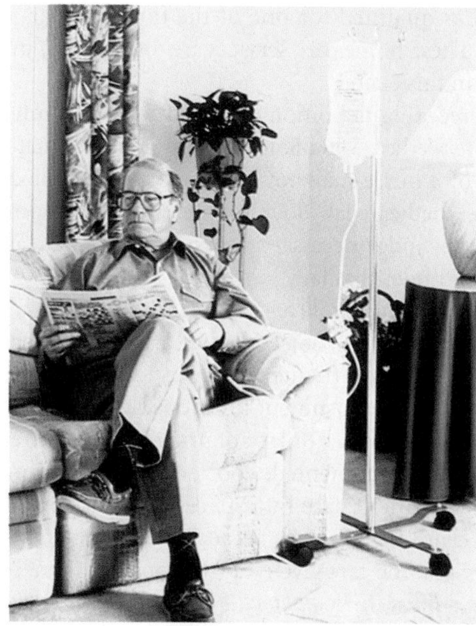

FIGURE 2-1 Home health agencies deliver the services of a variety of professionals.

HOME HEALTH NURSING

Home health nursing blends direct nursing care and community health nursing. The main difference between home health nursing and traditional public health nursing is that home health nursing provides more direct care to patients. The main difference between home health nursing and nursing in an institution is the increased emphasis on the family and the environment in the home.

Home health nursing requires careful consideration of the family and its role in the care of the ill member. Although giving direct care to an individual is an important part of home health care, a more important nursing role is to teach the patient and family to care for themselves (Fig. 2-1). This important role is similar to that of the rehabilitation nurse, for whom the goal is the independent functioning of the patient and family.

The environment in which home health nursing is practiced is very different from the hospital practice environment. Homes often have only a fraction of the resources of the hospital. Small bedrooms, low beds, inadequate climate control, and lack of space are common. Often families are overwhelmed by the task of caring for loved ones. They need instruction not only in the care of the patient but also in how to perform the care within the context of daily family activities in a home that was not designed for that purpose.

Home health nurses must assess the patient, the family, and the environment and use that information to plan care. Ongoing assessments are critical because the home health nurse often sees the patient more frequently than other care providers and can detect problems early. For example, the observation of weight gain and ankle edema alerts the nurse to possible heart failure in the cardiac patient. Prompt intervention may prevent serious consequences.

To illustrate the importance of assessing the family and the environment, consider the patient who requires wound care. In the home setting decisions to make include: Who can do the care? What does that person need to know? What supplies are needed and where can they be obtained? How should the patient dispose of soiled dressings? Questions like these require the home health nurse to be resourceful, knowledgeable, skillful, and creative.

Implications of Reimbursement Realities in Home Health Nursing

Medicare, though not the sole source of home health care funding, is probably the most important. Reimbursement by the Medicare program depends on documentation in the patient record that five basic criteria have been met: (1) the care must be skilled; (2) the care must be reasonable and necessary; (3) the patient must be homebound; (4) the physician must authorize a plan of care; and (5) the care must be intermittent.

Care Must Be Skilled

Medicare reimburses nursing care in the home provided that the care given is "skilled." This means that the care delivered must be the kind that only a nurse trained in that care could be expected to do it. However, not all the care done by a nurse qualifies as skilled care. Skilled nursing care is discussed further with the types of home health services.

Nursing is one of three primary home health care services considered to be skilled. The others are physical therapy and speech therapy. Occupational therapy may be considered skilled, depending on the complexity of the patient's problems. Social work and home health aide services are not considered skilled in themselves but may be reimbursed if the patient has qualified for one of the three primary skilled services. These home care services are discussed in more detail later in this chapter.

The preceding definition of skilled care is an interpretation of the Medicare law. Some nursing activities that require the skill of a nurse may not be recognized as skilled under Medicare. Medicare law does not prevent nurses from giving the care they judge necessary. It only defines what care is *reimbursable* under that law.

Care Must Be Reasonable and Necessary

To meet this criterion, objective clinical evidence clearly justifying the type and frequency of services is required. The nurse must clearly document functional losses and goals for care. Ongoing progress or lack of progress toward treatment goals must be documented. Poor documentation not only jeopardizes patient care but often results in denial of the agency's claim for payment because the documentation did not prove that the care given was "reasonable and necessary."

The Patient Must Be Homebound

This criterion does not mean that the patient must be bedridden. It does mean, however, that the patient must exert considerable effort to leave the home. Medicare also requires that absences from home be infrequent and of short duration. According to Medicare regulations, if patients are well enough to leave home frequently, they are able to visit a physician's office for treatment and therefore are not in need of home care.

The Physician Must Authorize a Plan of Care

All home care treatment must be authorized by a physician. A plan of care must include pertinent diagnoses, mental status evaluations, identification of the types of services needed, the supplies and equipment ordered, frequency of visits, prognosis, rehabilitation potential, functional limitations, nutritional requirements, medications, and treatments. This plan must also include safety measures to protect against injury and plans for discharge from home care.

In practice, the initial referral usually includes the patient's name, address, and telephone number, the major diagnoses, and a list of medications and treatments—not unlike physician's orders in a hospital. On the first visit, the admitting nurse usually formulates the plan of care, adding all other required elements. This plan is sent to the physician for review and signature. Because the care provided in the home is predominately *nursing* care, it is not surprising that the nurse has a major role in developing the plan of care.

Care Must Be Intermittent

The fifth criterion for Medicare reimbursement requires that the visits be intermittent in nature. This means that visits occur periodically and usually do not exceed 28 hours per week. Under normal circumstances, the patient is not seen daily. Situations exist, however, in which daily visits are justified. In these situations, there is usually the need for family members to be trained in daily procedures such as diabetic care or dressing changes. Under these circumstances, Medicare will reimburse daily visits for 2 or 3 weeks. These are considered special cases, and reimbursement depends on clear and accurate documentation of the need for daily visits. Otherwise, visiting frequency can range from three to four times per week to monthly.

Types of Home Health Services

The primary skilled services in home health care are (1) nursing, (2) physical therapy, and (3) speech therapy. Secondary services include occupational therapy (which may be primary under certain conditions), social work services, and home health aide services.

Skilled Nursing

According to Medicare regulations, skilled nursing includes skilled observation and assessment, teaching, and performing skilled procedures.

Skilled observation and assessment. The phrase "skilled observation and assessment" implies that the skills of a nurse are required to observe a patient's progress, to assess the importance of signs and symptoms, and to decide on a course of action. For example, good assessment and judgment skills are needed to detect the signs and symptoms of congestive heart failure early enough to prevent rehospitalization.

Teaching. Teaching is considered a skilled task because to do it effectively the nurse must identify the patient's and family's current level of knowledge, discern their learning style, relay information at a pace they can handle, and evaluate the results of the teaching.

Teaching is the most important skill in home care. Much of what is done in the home must be done by the patient and caregiver. Good patient teaching begins in the hospital setting, but newly arrived home care patients may need considerable teaching to manage their care at home. When high-technology therapies are involved, teaching is doubly important.

Families often have difficulty understanding high-technology concepts and are easily intimidated by technology when answers to their questions are not readily available. Skilled nurses understand this problem and ensure that their teaching is thorough and addresses precisely what the family needs to know to care successfully for their loved one at home. To do this, the nurse must identify the exact nature of the problem. A family member's difficulty in administering an injection may arise from a lack of knowledge of the procedure, a fear of needles, an inability to read the markings on the syringe, or a denial of the disease process. Identifying the specific learning need is critical to successful patient teaching. In teaching high-technology care, it is especially important to keep instructions as simple and specific as possible. Each step in the procedure should be written down and reviewed with the patient. The skill should be demonstrated several times, asking the family caregiver to cue the nurse for each step. After this is done a few times, the caregiver should perform a return demonstration of the skill.

Family caregivers must understand exactly what should be done in an emergency. Any questions about the family's ability to manage their portion of the care should be immediately referred to the home care nurse responsible for establishing the care plan and managing the case.

Performing skilled procedures. Skilled procedures include dressing changes, Foley catheter insertions, and venipunctures. However, after certain nursing procedures are taught to the family, they are no longer considered skilled procedures and are not reimbursable under Medicare. For example, injecting insulin is not considered skilled because most diabetics can inject insulin themselves. Teaching how to draw up the insulin and inject it properly, however, is considered skilled because teaching is considered a skilled activity. Once the injection skill is learned, the injection itself is no longer a skilled activity according to the Medicare definition. Also, procedures such as enema administration, unsterile dressing changes, care of small wounds, and administration of eyedrops usually are not considered skilled because they can be performed safely by most people.

Specialty Home Care

In the past few years, the number of high-technology cases in the home has increased dramatically. Most often patients need intravenous therapy or are ventilator dependent.

Intravenous Therapy

Rising hospital costs and the development of reliable intravenous pumps have stimulated the growth of intravenous therapy in the home. The most common intravenous therapies provided in the home are hydration, antibiotics, pain control, total parenteral nutrition, and chemotherapy. Many different types of lines may be used. Nurses should be familiar with the devices commonly used in their area. Chemotherapy drugs are almost always given through central lines.

High-technology therapies add to the complexity of home health care. Home use may be more cost-effective than a hospital stay, but it also significantly increases the risk to the client and the liability of the home health agency. Agency policies and procedures should be current and specific enough to guide the nurse in managing the provision of intravenous therapy in the home. These policies protect not only the agency and the patient but also the nurse.

The successful provision of any high-technology therapy in the home depends on the commitment of everyone involved. Families must be capable of understanding what is required and have the time to participate fully in the patient's care. Nurses delivering this type of care must be thoroughly trained in the procedures and use of equipment involved in these therapies. Agencies must have appropriate staff to provide care at any time if needed, including days, evenings, nights, and weekends. The pharmacy or intravenous therapy company must provide high-quality products and support to both the nurse and the family. Finally, physicians must be closely involved and available to the nurse and family to respond to emergency problems.

The nurse's role in the delivery of high-technology care in the home includes skilled observation and assessment, the ability to perform skilled procedures, and teaching. Skilled observation and assessment in the delivery of intravenous therapy includes determining the adequacy of the home environment and the patient's and family's knowledge regarding care procedures. The intravenous access site must be assessed for signs of swelling and redness. Any side effects of the treatment should be noted, along with the family's level of comfort with performing specific procedures.

Skilled procedures include changing access site dressings and performing venipunctures. Because home care nurses are not instantly available 24 hours a day, some procedures must be taught to the family.

Ventilator Therapy

Ventilator-dependent patients are increasingly being cared for in the home setting. This type of care is complex and should be provided only by nurses and caregivers specifically trained in the use of necessary equipment and procedures. Often the care of ventilator-dependent patients in the home is coordinated by the respiratory therapist. The home care nurse seeing the patient should be aware of policies and procedures followed by the respiratory therapy company, be familiar with respiratory therapy equipment, and be certified in cardiopulmonary resuscitation.

Initial assessment of the home environment includes an assessment of all the factors important in other high-technology therapies, with the addition of an assessment of the electrical and structural condition of the home. This is important to ensure proper functioning of the equipment and necessary backup systems. As with intravenous therapy, committed family members or other caregivers must be available. In this case, the commitment is for around-the-clock observation. Physicians and respiratory therapists must be on call for any problems.

Communication Between Home Health Care Team Members

The importance of the team approach in home health care cannot be overemphasized. Quality home care is the result of the collaboration of several disciplines. Because these disciplines may provide their services in the home at different times, interdisciplinary communication is necessary if effective collaboration is to occur. Interdisciplinary communication is accomplished through clear, detailed documentation and case conferences.

Documentation

In any interdisciplinary work, the actions of one discipline often depend on the actions of another. A nursing discovery of an unused walker in the corner of a room may prompt the physical therapist to recommend strengthening exercises and gait training. A social worker's attempts to find funding for a patient's medications may reveal that the patient is fearful of taking pain medications, which can be addressed by the nurse. If these concerns are not communicated, however, they will not be addressed. Most quality-of-care problems in home health care can be attributed to failure to communicate patient care problems. Most of the time, the failure lies with either incomplete documentation or failure to keep the nursing case manager informed.

As mentioned earlier, reimbursement for home health nursing visits depends on clear documentation of the patient's homebound status, the skilled nature of the services provided, and the medical need for the services. Failure to provide such documentation often results in denial of reimbursement by the Medicare fiscal intermediary. Denials of reimbursement have serious consequences for the home health agency and, when excessive, have resulted in agencies going out of business.

Case Conferences

Clear documentation of interdisciplinary case conferences can go a long way toward preventing reimbursement denials based on lack of medical necessity. These conferences often provide detailed information about the complexity of problems that justifies increased visits.

Usually, a home health nurse must report to a patient's case manager who is responsible for admitting the patient, establishing the plan of care, including visit frequencies, and coordinating the efforts of other disciplines. The case manager schedules periodic, formal case conferences in which all disciplines work together to solve clinical problems. The details of these conferences are recorded in the patient's record.

In addition to these regularly scheduled conferences, it is important to keep the case manager informed of any changes in the response of the patient or family to the plan of care. Changes in vital signs, weight, and wound parameters are important physiologic indications for a call to the case manager. A change in the home environment such as an absence of family caregivers, deterioration in sanitation, or signs of patient neglect or abuse should also prompt a call to the case manager.

Communication by the case manager also is important. Field nurses have the right to expect clear and current information regarding recent changes in physicians' orders, current laboratory information, and the availability of documentation by other nurses and disciplines. High-quality patient care cannot be accomplished without meticulous communication from all disciplines involved in the care of the patient.

REHABILITATION

The acute phase of many illnesses is often followed by a prolonged chronic phase. This phase may last from days to years and usually involves the delivery of a number of health care services in a variety of settings, such as rehabilitation centers, long-term care facilities, outpatient facilities, group residential homes, and, increasingly, the patient's own home. Rehabilitation focuses on restoring maximum possible function following illness or injury.

REHABILITATION CONCEPTS

Rehabilitation Is a Process of Restoration

Rehabilitation is the process of restoring an individual to the best possible health and functioning following a physical or mental impairment. The type of assistance provided allows people to care for themselves as much as possible. Inherent in this process is a commitment by the caregiver to provide the care and support that foster the client's independence.

Impairment Is a Disturbance in Functioning

Impairment refers to a disturbance in functioning that may be either physical or psychological. An example of physical impairment is paralysis of an arm or leg as the result of a stroke. Mental impairment such as loss of memory may occur as a result of Alzheimer's disease. In either case there is a loss of function.

Disability Is a Measurable Loss of Function

The term *disability* generally refers to a measurable loss of function and is usually delineated to indicate a diminished capacity for work. For example, individuals with an injured back may be classified as 50% disabled, meaning that they are incapable of doing 50% of their job. This type of measurable loss of function allows for specific reductions in work responsibility or may indicate how much compensation a worker may be entitled to.

Handicap Is an Inability to Perform Daily Activities

The term *handicap* means that an individual is not able to perform one or more normal activities of daily living (ADL) because of a mental or physical disability. For example, the person who experienced a stroke may be handicapped in driving a car because of the paralysis.

Remember that disability and handicap are not the same thing. A person can be moderately disabled but still manage to perform routine daily activities. People who were born without arms are often able to perform all essential ADLs by using their feet and certain assistive devices. It can be said that, although these people are disabled, they are not handicapped. Impairments and their resulting disabilities may not be reversible, but handicaps often can be prevented or reduced with modifications of the environment and a community attitude that seeks to promote the abilities of the disabled.

LEVELS OF DISABILITY

A disability is often classified by level to determine its impact on an individual's quality of life and appropriate levels of compensation:

Level I: Slight limitation in one or more ADL, usually able to work

Level II: Moderate limitation in one or more ADL, able to work but workplace may need modifications

Level III: Severe limitation in one or more ADL, unable to work

Level IV: Total disability characterized by nearly complete dependence on others for assistance with ADL, unable to work

GOALS OF REHABILITATION

The goals of rehabilitation are to return the disabled individual to a maximum state of functioning and to prevent further disability.

Return of Function

The goal of return of function includes the restoration of as much function as possible in the traditional ADLs, such as bathing, dressing, eating, toileting, and walking. Ideal functioning includes independence in the instrumental activities of daily living (IADL) as well, such as preparing meals, shopping, doing laundry, and using the telephone. The ultimate goal of rehabilitation is to live independently. Full independence implies a return to employment status.

Prevention of Further Disability

Rehabilitation also involves the prevention of further disability (secondary disability) that may potentially be caused by the patient's primary disability. Examples include prevention of problems in stroke patients such as pneumonia, decubitus ulcers, and limb contractures, which are often caused by lack of mobility. The nurse plays an important role in the prevention of secondary disability.

Rehabilitation is a long-term process requiring the commitment of both the patient and the family. The process is often difficult and marked by periods of progress followed by occasional relapses in functional disability. These relapses can be frustrating to everyone involved and require determination on the part of the family as well as patience and understanding by the nurse. The rehabilitation process can place additional burdens on family members when roles once filled by the disabled family member must be filled by other members. Attention is frequently focused on the disabled member, leaving other family members feeling neglected. Ongoing family problems may intensify during this time, making the rehabilitation process even more difficult.

It is important when caring for a disabled patient to be aware of the attitudes and behaviors of all family members. Often families can be assisted in adjusting to role changes that occur during the rehabilitation process. The more consistently patients and family are involved in the process, the more likely it is success will occur. Involvement in goal setting and a clear explanation of patient and family roles in daily rehabilitation activities help families understand better the challenges of the process. This gives a sense of control and increases family strength.

LEGISLATION

Public attitudes toward people with disabilities play a significant role in the degree of handicap experienced by the disabled. Lack of knowledge about a disability often causes the public to react negatively to people who appear disabled. Individuals who are blind are sometimes treated as though they are deaf as well. People with conditions such as cerebral palsy that affect speech and muscle control are often treated as though they have decreased intelligence. Employers are reluctant to hire disabled workers, fearing an increase in insurance rates or negative reactions from their customers.

The federal government has passed laws over the years to protect the rights of the disabled. The first law passed to aid the rehabilitation of World War I servicemen was the Vocational Rehabilitation Act of 1920. This law provided job training for injured veterans. The Social Security Act of 1935 provided additional aid to states for both direct relief and vocational rehabilitation. It was the Rehabilitation Act of 1973, however, that provided a comprehensive approach to problems experienced by the disabled. The act not only expanded available resources for vocational training but also defined services to be included in rehabilitation programs. It also began affirmative action programs to assist in the employment of the disabled and prohibited discrimination against the disabled in programs receiving federal funds. In 1990, the Americans With Disabilities Act was passed. This law extended the protection given to the disabled in the public sector by the Rehabilitation Act of 1973 to the private sector as well. It was designed to give the disabled full access to housing, employment, transportation, and communications. As a result of this law, any business endeavor designed to serve the public must ensure that its services are accessible to the disabled. In many cases, this involves the installation of wheelchair ramps, the construction of restrooms that can accommodate wheelchairs, and the provision for communication services for the hearing and speech impaired. Public transportation authorities must ensure that buses, train cars, and concession shops are all accessible to the disabled. Businesses with fewer than 15 employees are currently exempt from many of the law's provisions. This law has prompted significant progress toward improving the quality of life of many disabled people.

THE REHABILITATION TEAM

Nurses who care for disabled clients must consider the whole patient when planning interventions. Difficulties in physical functioning may affect many aspects of a person's life and require the coordinated services of a number of health care professionals in order for the individual to stay well and avoid complications or injuries.

The case of Mr. Thompson, who has had a recent stroke and resulting right-sided paralysis, provides a good example of the kinds of expertise and the number of services that may be required during rehabilitation.

> Mr. Thompson, age 72, suffered a left-sided brain hemorrhage 3 weeks earlier. Because of this, he was unable to speak or use his right arm or leg. He was also incontinent of urine and exhibited some right-sided facial paralysis. After 5 days in the hospital, it was determined that Mr. Thompson's condition had stabilized, and he was transferred to a rehabilitation facility to continue the rehabilitation process. At this time, his speech had returned but was slurred and halting. He had minimal movement in his right arm and leg but was still unable to walk or feed himself. The incontinence of urine persisted, and he had several reddened areas on his right hip and coccyx. Before his injury Mr. Thompson had been living with only his wife of 50 years, who also was in poor health. They had no family living in the state, and she was quite concerned about how she would care for him once he was sent home.

When trying to comprehend all that is involved in helping Mr. Thompson return to full functioning (if that is possible), it is helpful first to imagine a typical day in the Thompson household and to identify all the ADL and IADL competencies required to get through the day. Next, the types of people and services that may be necessary to prevent further injury and to increase functioning should be considered. At a minimum, the rehabilitation team will consist of the patient's wife, personal physician, rehabilitation physician, and rehabilitation nurse. Other likely members include the physical therapist, who assists the patient in all aspects of mobility from regaining strength and function in the extremities to the use of assistive devices such as crutches and walkers; the occupational therapist, who assists the patient with regaining fine motor skills necessary for dressing, eating, and grooming; the speech therapist, who assists the patient in regaining swallowing or speaking functions; and the social worker, who may assist with coordinating resources for placement in the home or a convalescent facility after discharge. Other members of the team may include a clinical nurse specialist in rehabilitation nursing, a psychologist, a recreational therapist, and a vocational counselor.

The nurse's concern at this time should be that of becoming an effective member of the rehabilitation team. The successful resolution of rehabilitation problems often depends on the ability of health care workers to consider how the individual functions within the family and to work closely with other health professionals toward a common goal. If this goal is to be successful, good communication skills are essential. These entail clear, specific documentation of the patient's functional deficits and abilities and active participation in multidisciplinary conferences to resolve patient problems.

APPROACHES TO REHABILITATION

Perhaps the most important goal of successful rehabilitation of a disabled person is independence. This fact is sometimes forgotten when a caregiver sees the slow, agonizing attempts to move an arm or a leg. The tendency is to do for patients what is difficult for them to accomplish on their own. There are times when patients should be helped to complete a task, especially when they become increasingly frustrated. However, caregivers who intervene too soon encourage dependence and delay rehabilitation. Rehabilitation patients should be cheerfully encouraged to do as much as possible for themselves. Praise for accomplishing a task should be given promptly, and caregivers should reflect continuing optimism about the patient's progress.

Health professionals frequently plan comprehensive programs of rehabilitation without much thought as to how the program will be implemented once the patient returns home. To be effective, the program should commence immediately after an injury and should involve of the patient and family from the outset. Failure to involve the family in establishing goals and strategies often produces family dependence, just as doing too many things for the patient produces individual dependence.

Rehabilitation nurses undertake a number of roles, all designed to assist the patient and family in returning to a high level of functioning. These roles include care planner, teacher, caregiver, counselor, coordinator, and advocate.

In the home setting, nurses can best assist patients and families by helping them adjust their activities to accommodate the disability (Fig. 2-2). Even though families may have been taught care routines in a previous setting, routines must often be adapted to the new setting and prioritized differently. In this role, the nurse is an expert caregiver and teacher. Problem-solving sessions often identify ways in which care routines can

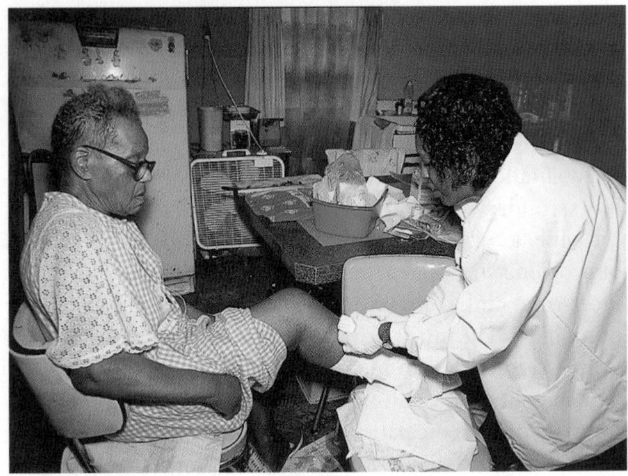

FIGURE **2-2** An important nursing role in home health care is to teach patients to care for themselves.

be adapted to the realities of the home setting. Caregivers may not have thought through changes in sleeping arrangements, how they will transport the patient for follow-up office visits, or how to plan for periodic relief from their caregiver role. Nurses can help families anticipate these predictable stress points and plan realistically for how they will handle them.

Nurses should also be prepared to handle a wide range of patient and family emotions, ranging from extreme optimism to depression. At these times, families need a great deal of support and may need the assistance of outside community support systems. Local support groups can often be very effective in helping families respond appropriately to the stresses of a disabled family member. Professional organizations such as the Association of Rehabilitation Nurses can be an invaluable resource to nurses working in the rehabilitation field.

LONG-TERM CARE

Many people think only of elderly persons in institutional settings when they think of long-term care settings. Long-term care services, however, are required by people of all ages who struggle to return to a level of independent functioning. Thus, long-term care refers to a range of services that address the health, personal care, and social needs of all people who lack some capacity for self-care.

It may be a surprise to many that only 5% of elderly persons live in institutions. Many live with extended families or by themselves. Unfortunately, a large number of elderly who live alone are poor and live in inadequate housing, often without adequate heat, ventilation, food, or telephones. Eventually, problems with mobility and mental functioning force many elderly into nursing homes.

RISKS FOR INSTITUTIONALIZATION

Government statistics indicate that only 1% of people aged 65 to 74 reside in nursing homes. This figure rises to 6% for ages 75 to 84, and to 20% for those 85 and over. The main reason for institutionalization, however, is not age. The best indicator of who will need nursing home placement is ADL dependency. Only about 12% of those with one or two ADL limitations live in nursing homes, whereas 50% of elderly persons with five or six ADL limitations reside there. These statistics highlight the fact that if home care services were available to assist the elderly in meeting more ADL needs, costly institutionalization could be delayed.

Other factors bearing on who requires nursing home placement include such things as financial resources, whether the person lives alone or with family, the presence of mental illness, the type of disease process, and the degree of social support.

LEVELS OF CARE

Modern long-term residential care consists of four levels: (1) domiciliary care, (2) sheltered housing, (3) intermediate care, and (4) skilled care. Often one type of facility will offer more than one level of care (usually skilled and intermediate); however, in most states, institutions must have approval for whatever levels of care they plan to provide.

Domiciliary Care

Facilities providing basic room, board, and supervision are sometimes called domiciliary care facilities. In this arrangement, 24-hour care is not provided. Residents usually come and go as they please.

Sheltered Housing

Similar to domiciliary care facilities, sheltered housing settings have some modification to provide care for the frail elderly and usually include community dining facilities. Twenty-four-hour care, however, is not provided.

Intermediate Care

Intermediate-care facilities provide custodial care at a level usually associated with nursing homes. Patients at this level often need assistance with two to three ADLs (Fig. 2-3). Facilities offering this level of care must have personnel available 24 hours a day. They are not considered by the government to be medical facilities and thus receive no reimbursement under Medicare. Many do, however, receive the bulk of their financing under Medicaid. Federal regulations require a registered nurse to serve as director of nursing and a licensed nurse to be on duty at least 8 hours a day.

Skilled Care

Skilled nursing facilities must have skilled health professionals present around the clock. The care of patients in skilled nursing facilities must be supervised by a physician and requires the services of a registered nurse, physical therapist, or speech therapist.

IMPACT OF RELOCATION

Relocation to a long-term care facility is rarely easy. In the best of circumstances, patients, families, and health professionals anticipate the possible future need for long-term care, set aside funds for that purpose, and make plans that are acceptable to all. When patients cannot make sound decisions for themselves, families seek help from extended family members and professionals in making decisions for long-term care placement. More commonly, however, the situation is quite different. Often a crisis situation precipitates the decision. A sole caregiver may become ill, leaving the care of the disabled elder to the hands of extended family members who may be either unable or unwilling to continue care. Patients suddenly may become physically or mentally incapable of caring for themselves or making their own decisions. Family members frequently feel guilty for considering institutional care. Few know very much about modern long-term care facilities and have not investigated potential placement.

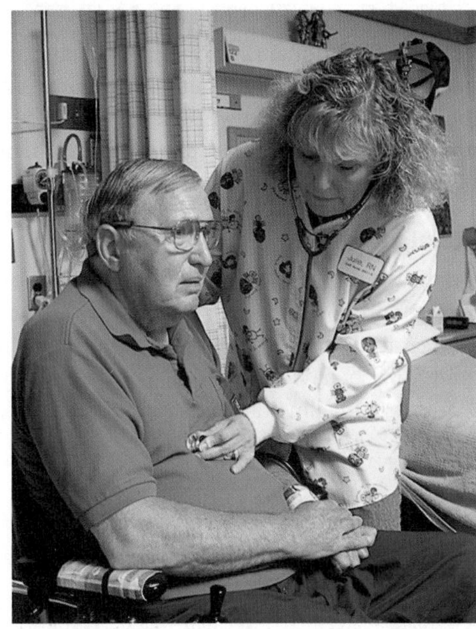

FIGURE 2-3 Patients in intermediate-care facilities often need assistance with activities of daily living.

In this situation, home health nurses, social workers, and other health professionals must work closely with the family to defuse the crisis situation and provide realistic options from which the family may choose. This is a time when families need the utmost support and acceptance. Simply clarifying the situation, affirming the family's previous caring and concern, and pointing out realistic options will often return a family to effective functioning.

If placement in a long-term care facility is the only logical choice, the patient and family must be prepared for the relocation. Research has shown that the more prepared the patient, the better is the adjustment. Preparation includes providing as much choice as possible for the patient. If possible, choices of facility, room location, types of personal belongings, and room decor are helpful, as are tours of the facility prior to entering. It is also helpful if professional staff check on the new patient frequently during the first few weeks. Questions should be encouraged. It is also helpful to introduce patients to other residents with like interests.

EFFECTS OF INSTITUTIONALIZATION

The effects of institutionalization are predictable and must be considered in helping the new nursing home resident adjust to the surroundings. Frequently observed effects include depersonalization, indignity, redefinition of "normal," regression, and social withdrawal.

Depersonalization

Depersonalization plays a major part in institutional life. Caregivers often know little of a resident's life history and therefore treat individual resident in light of their diagnosis or dysfunctional behavior patterns. The case study about Herman and Kristina illustrates this point.

CASE STUDY

I don't think I truly understood what depersonalization was until I met Herman. Herman and his wife Kristina lived alone in a small house in a northwestern city. Herman was 62 years old and had Alzheimer's disease. I met them while working as a home health nurse. I was asked to look into respite services to help relieve Kristina of the strain of caring for Herman. I remember my first impression of Herman, formed after reading his chart and talking to the staff nurse about his care problems. He was starting to neglect his personal appearance. The staff nurse said he often put soup on the stove for lunch, then went out into the garden to tend his flowers, forgetting about the soup. This and other images of his functioning created in me a picture of an incompetent and helpless old man.

Over a period of weeks, Kristina shared many stories with me about who this man was, what he cared about, how they met, and her deep devotion to her husband of 35 years. Gradually, I was able to see the distorted image I held. In his youth, Herman was an Olympic gold medal skier from Austria who came to this country as a young man. He held several jobs as a ski instructor and repaired ski equipment until he met and married Kristina and moved to the northwestern United States to become owner and manager of a small ski resort. He was tall and muscular with an easy smile and a kind word for everyone. He was admired by many in the community for his skill as a skier and his friendliness. He was a good father and family man who was known as "the rock" because all of his family and friends relied on him for advice and assistance.

Over a period of 5 years, Herman became more and more forgetful, less talkative, and often preoccupied with household tasks that he would start but not complete. He also failed to recognize many of his close friends and, at times, would wander off downtown without knowing why, or where he was going. Throughout this, Kristina remained fiercely devoted to Herman, though the strain of the caregiver role was beginning to affect her health. "He cared for us for so many years. Now it is my turn to care for him."

I was surprised at how different was my previous view of Herman. I was seeing him as dependent, helpless, and a burden to his small and frail wife—a view created by my observations of his behavior and what I knew of the Alzheimer's disease process and a view that changed radically once I knew more about Herman. I doubt I will ever minimize the importance of learning about the whole patient.

One way to help see the resident of a long-term care facility as a whole person with past relationships, accomplishments, and interests is to ask family members to bring in photographs. The photographs may have been taken on significant occasions, such as graduation or wedding days, or may be simple family pictures that depict the older person's place in the family or community. The photographs can be mounted on posterboard or placed on a bulletin board in the resident's room. This effort helps caregivers see more than a frail, weak, older person and can open up conversation that encourages reminiscing, which is a therapeutic means of dealing with one's past life and preparing for death.

Indignity

Indignity is another effect of institutionalization. Routine activities such as toileting and obtaining food and drink must be requested. Sometimes the prompt fulfillment of the request depends on the relationship between the patient and the caregiver. Residents of long-term care facilities may be exposed unnecessarily, especially when caregivers enter rooms without knocking. Simple courtesies such as using a person's title and last name, knocking before entering the room, and draping during care activities help the resident maintain dignity. It is useful to think to yourself, "How would I want to be treated if I were weak and frail and could not do the things that I can do for myself now?"

Redefinition of "Normal"

Behaviors that were considered normal at home may be labeled abnormal or be unacceptable in an institution. Watching television at 3:00 A.M., loud singing, or sexual activity may not be tolerated, depending on the residence's rules and routines. Although consideration of others is important, it is also important to give residents of long-term care facilities some flexibility and some measure of control in their daily lives.

Regression

Over a period of time, a resident's physical, mental, and social abilities may be lost because of disuse. If people are left in bed a greater part of the day, it soon becomes impossible for them to walk. If visits from friends and relatives are few, the skill of conversation may also be lost. It is important to encourage independence and social interaction as much as possible. Avoid infantilizing older patients. Although it may be necessary to simplify language and activities for those who are cognitively impaired, avoid baby talk.

Social Withdrawal

If a resident never leaves the nursing home, or if family visits are few and include little discussion of the outside world, the institution can become a barrier, cutting off interest and participation in the outside world. If this is allowed to continue, life in the facility becomes, for many patients, their entire world. They tend to withdraw into the boundaries of their own room. Nurses can help by conversing with residents about events inside and outside the nursing home. When you know your patients well, you can bring up news that you expect will be of interest to them. Discussion of current events in small groups can broaden the resident's horizons.

Put on your THINKING CAP!!

If you have a clinical experience in a long-term care facility, interview a resident there. Specifically, ask:

1. What circumstances brought you here to live?
2. What are the benefits and disadvantages of living in this type of facility?
3. What advice would you give to a new resident here?
4. What can nurses do to make it easier for you to adjust to living here?

Discuss the resident's responses in relation to the effects of institutionalization and implications for nurses.

PRINCIPLES OF LONG-TERM RESIDENTIAL CARE

Long-term residential care has been called custodial care. This term invokes passive images such as maintenance, warehousing, or waiting to die. Some people have called such facilities "heaven's waiting rooms." Publicized abuses by some nursing homes are at least partly responsible for negative stereotypes of long-term residential care. However, long-term care facilities in general have changed substantially in recent years. Although some continue to provide care of questionable quality, many excellent facilities do exist.

Modern facilities care for patients with a wide array of medical and surgical problems. In many communities, the nursing home has become a convalescent hospital for elderly patients who have recently undergone surgical procedures, such as repair of a fractured hip. These acute cases often strain already limited resources.

Not all patients are admitted for permanent stays in the facility. Many are admitted for short stays that are prompted by care demands that temporarily overwhelm the family. Illness of a family caregiver also can result in temporary admission to the facility. When the home situation has stabilized, these patients often return home. Increasingly, those admitted for long stays are elderly and suffer from mental health problems. In these cases, the family has exhausted most of its physical, emotional, and financial resources, and home care is no longer feasible.

When the patient is admitted to a long-term care facility, the care delivered is based on three principles: (1) promotion of independence, (2) maintenance of function, and (3) maintenance of autonomy.

Promotion of Independence

Successful relocation to a long-term care facility depends in part on the ability of patients to do things for themselves and on the involvement of families to keep the elderly family member in contact with the outside world. It may be tempting for institutional caregivers to feed residents rather than to spend time encouraging residents to feed themselves. When the workday is a never-ending series of tasks, doing things quickly often takes priority over promoting independence. Watch for this type of behavior and try to restructure assignments of nonprofessional personnel to reward the promotion of independence. This can be accomplished by setting specific goals for each patient that encourage independent functioning. Then explain to the nonprofessional staff members how their efforts can contribute to the goal. Involvement of staff in this way often produces results.

Maintenance of Function

Often it is loss of function that prevents an elderly person from staying at home. Health professionals who are disease oriented often concentrate on the disease process at the expense of a functional assessment. An incontinent patient may be incorrectly perceived as having a complication of the aging process. This kind of thinking fosters an emphasis on maintenance care, leading to efforts to prevent skin breakdown by frequent changes of clothing and linens. A more thorough assessment would begin with the determination of possible causes for the incontinence. A functional assessment explores factors that might be responsible for the incontinence. Immobility may be the basic problem. Questions to ask include: Is the patient normally mobile? If so, is there a light in the room allowing him or her to find the way to the bathroom? Is the patient able to manage clothing for independent toileting? Are the side rails normally up or down? Viewing this problem as a functional problem may lead to simple solutions such as placing a light in the room at night or a urinal next to the bed. Interventions, whenever possible, should focus on restoring and preserving function.

Maintenance of Autonomy

Most people value control over their lives. Successful relocation to a long-term care facility depends on preserving as much autonomy as possible. Elders who participate in selecting the facility adjust better than those who have no choice in the matter.

It is also important to allow as much flexibility as possible in establishing a routine for the new resident. Choices in activities, such as when to have a bath or how late to watch television, go a long way toward preserving the autonomy and self-esteem of the elderly resident. As much as possible, encourage the resident to assist in establishing care goals. The frequency and duration of exercise and the amount of weight to be lost or gained are all goals that require the facility resident's commitment. Mutually established goals are more likely to be achieved than those selected for the resident.

Families also have a role in maintaining autonomy in the elderly member. Autonomy depends on knowing one's place in the world and what roles one still holds in the family structure. Families who relate to their elder members by reinforcing their importance in the family and keeping them up to date on family happenings and decisions reinforce one very important idea: the elder remains a valued family member who simply resides at another address.

 ***Put on your THINKING CAP!!***

Identify one thing you can do to achieve each of the following: (1) maintain autonomy, (2) maintain function, and (3) promote independence in:

a. The long-term care facility resident
b. The hospitalized patient

OTHER PATIENT CARE SETTINGS

The settings addressed in this chapter represent many of those that traditionally employ licensed nurses. Other employment settings include clinics, physicians' offices, schools, adult day care, respite care, and prisons. Each setting presents unique experiences and challenges. The LPN may be the only licensed nursing professional on site in these settings. Therefore it is vital that the nurse's responsibilities be clearly defined and consistent with legal functions.

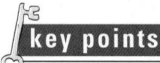

- The changing health care system has greatly increased the number and types of health care settings.
- Community health nurses work with individuals and groups to improve the health of the entire community.
- The main difference between home health care and public health nursing is that home health care is more focused on providing direct care to patients.
- A major nursing function in home health care is teaching the patient and family to care for themselves to promote independent functioning.
- Medicare is a major source of home health care funding.
- To receive Medicare reimbursement, five basic criteria must be met: (1) the care must be skilled; (2) the care must be reasonable and necessary; (3) the patient must be homebound; (4) the physician must authorize a plan of care; and (5) the care must be intermittent.
- Specialty home care services include high-technology interventions (the provision of intravenous therapy and ventilator therapy), hospice services, pediatric care, and mental health care.
- Rehabilitation is the process of restoring an individual to the best possible health and functioning following a physical or mental impairment and the prevention of further disability.
- Caring for disabled clients requires the coordinated services of a number of health care professionals to help clients stay well and avoid complications or injuries.
- As an effective member of a multidisciplinary rehabilitation team, the nurse is a care planner, teacher, caregiver, counselor, coordinator, and advocate.
- Health care workers must consider how a disabled individual functions within the family, and the patient and family should be involved from the outset in determining the plan of care.
- Government statistics indicate that only 1% of people aged 65 to 74, 6% of people aged 75 to 84, and 20% of people aged 85 and over reside in nursing homes.
- Dependence in activities of daily living is the best indicator of who will need nursing home placement.
- Modern long-term residential care exists in four levels: (1) domiciliary care, (2) sheltered housing, (3) intermediate care, and (4) skilled care.
- Care delivered in a residential facility is based on three principles: (1) promotion of independence, (2) maintenance of function, and (3) maintenance of autonomy.

REVIEW QUESTIONS

1. A home health nurse performed all the activities listed below with Medicare patients. Which one may *not* be reimbursable?
   1. Used sterile technique to clean and dress a large wound
   2. Took a frail older couple for a short walk to provide exercise
   3. Performed a venipuncture to obtain a blood sample for lab tests
   4. Taught a patient with recently diagnosed diabetes how to inject insulin

2. Which nursing activity might commonly be provided by home health nurses but not by community health nurses?
   1. Conducting health education programs in a senior citizen residence
   2. Assessing the recovery of a postoperative patient at home
   3. Arranging blood pressure screening at a community shopping center
   4. Seeing patients in a clinic to monitor problems related to chronic illness

3. The definition of the term *community-based nursing* is best reflected in which of the following activities?
   1. Meeting with residents of low-income housing to identify their health needs
   2. Telephoning patients at home after discharge from the hospital
   3. Asking nurses to identify the health services most needed in their communities
   4. Developing a hospital-based home health care service

4. Individuals who are unable to feed or dress themselves independently because of a neurological disease are most accurately described as:
   1. impaired.
   2. disabled.
   3. handicapped.
   4. disadvantaged.

5. Which legislation began affirmative action programs to protect the disabled from discrimination in employment?
   1. Social Security Act
   2. Americans with Disabilities Act
   3. Rehabilitation Act
   4. Vocational Rehabilitation Act

6. A patient who has suffered a head injury is feeding herself with considerable difficulty. From a rehabilitation perspective, what is the most appropriate nursing response?
   1. Offer to feed her so that she will not be embarrassed by her handicap
   2. Order a liquid diet so that she will not have to use eating utensils
   3. Point out that the sooner she can feed herself, the sooner she can go home.
   4. Be sure her food is accessible, and compliment her efforts at self-feeding

7. A nursing home resident has his name neatly printed on the door to his room. The interior of the room is decorated in masculine colors. One wall is covered with pictures of the resident at various occasions in his personal and professional life. In one corner is a leather recliner with a reading lamp and table. This room reflects an effort to:
   1. avoid depersonalization.
   2. maintain the resident's dignity.
   3. prevent regression.
   4. prevent social withdrawal.

CHAPTER

3 The Leadership Role of the Licensed Practical Nurse

objectives

1. Differentiate leadership from management.
2. Describe leadership styles.
3. Discuss management theories.
4. List tips for effective management.
5. Describe the role of the licensed vocational nurse as a team leader.

key terms

Assignment (p. 27)
Autocratic leadership (p. 25)
Delegation (p. 30)
Democratic leadership (p. 25)
Laissez-faire leadership (lĕs-ā-FĂR, p. 25)
Leadership (p. 24)
Management (p. 24)
Participative leadership (păr-tĭs-ĭ-PĀ-tĭv, p. 25)
Theory X (p. 26)
Theory Y (p. 26)
Theory Z (p. 26)

Licensed practical nurses (LPNs) manage the care of patients in many health care settings in addition to the hospital. Especially in long-term care settings, they typically also manage other care providers. However, the LPN of tomorrow will be expected to have additional skills not only as managers, but also as leaders.

A variety of factors are contributing to this evolution.The latest nurse shortage is upon us—a situation that often stimulates reevaluation of job responsibilities. Nurses at all levels are being called on to add new skills and functions. Cost-control measures seek to maximize the contribution of each member of the health care team. Consumers of care expect increasingly high-quality care from all care providers. The increase in long-term residential care required by the growing elderly population has increased the demand for LPNs.

Most long-term care homes are staffed primarily by LPNs and nursing assistants, who provide the bulk of the "hands-on" care. LPNs have traditionally filled leadership or management positions in long-term care homes, usually as team leaders. Because LPNs are managers of care for the patients to whom they are assigned, it is important that LPNs have a working knowledge of leadership, management, and safe health care delivery. Now LPNs are assuming more responsible positions such as charge nurses in long-term care facilities and various management roles in other settings. So, we are seeing a shift from LPNs who must manage only their assigned patients, to LPNs who must plan, organize, direct, coordinate, and control care provided by others.

LEADERSHIP VERSUS MANAGEMENT

The terms *leadership* and *management* are sometimes used interchangeably, but in fact they have different meanings. Leadership comes first, and management comes second. A leader selects the role; a manager is assigned or appointed to the role. Leadership is a difficult concept to define, but it generally means "guidance" or showing the way to others. There are formal leaders (for example, your boss) and there are informal leaders (a person without an official title to whom people go for assistance). Leaders inspire people to strive to accomplish particular goals by doing the right thing. In contrast, management is the effective use of selected methods to accomplish goals. Management provides the means to achieve the goals by doing the thing right. Managers get things organized so the leader's goals can be achieved. In other words, leadership may be thought of as the inspiration, and management may be thought of as the perspiration.

Both leaders and managers must have certain characteristics to be effective. First, they must be competent. They must have the respect of the people who work with them to accomplish their goals. Second, they must be able to communicate with others. People in leadership and management positions work with other people. Success or failure in interactions with others depends on their ability to communicate. Finally, leaders and managers must be able to motivate others. They must determine what motivates people, what other people consider important, and why they behave in certain ways. For example, some people are motivated by internal forces, such as needs or desires, and some are motivated by external forces, such as environmental or cultural influences.

Good leaders and managers seem to have certain characteristics in common, such as the ability to set realistic goals, the willingness to try out new ideas, and the ability to be pos-

table 3-1 Characteristics of Leaders and Managers

A good leader and manager:
Sets realistic goals and works to achieve them
Seeks new ideas and methods; is willing to try them
Is a positive thinker
Is accountable for actions
Is willing to make decisions even though they involve risks
Is competent in performing work
Is an effective communicator
Is assertive; refuses to be manipulated
Accepts responsibilities of leadership and delegation
Is emotionally mature; exercises self-control
Is committed to providing quality patient care
Recognizes worth of co-workers and welcomes suggestions; answers their questions
Is not selfish; is willing to share information with co-workers
Is able to use self-criticism; gives constructive criticism to others
Has a sense of humor; is able to laugh at self, never at others
Is loyal to co-workers
Is self-confident
Is never self-satisfied; recognizes the need for continued improvement
Is a facilitator

Adapted from Corona, D. F. (1982). Followership: The indispensable corollary to leadership. In Hein, E. C., & Nicholson, M. J. (Eds.), *Contemporary leadership behavior: Selected readings.* Boston: Little, Brown.

itive thinkers. Table 3-1 lists the characteristics of good leaders and managers.

LEADERSHIP STYLES

Many different leadership styles are used in various situations. The four basic types of leadership are (1) **autocratic,** (2) **democratic,** (3) **laissez-faire,** and (4) **participative.** As an LPN, you need to understand your predominant style and how to reinforce it or change it, depending on how effective it is in a given situation. You need to understand the styles and approaches of others in these roles. Leadership styles vary according to degrees of freedom and control, the identity of the decision makers, leader activity level, assumption of responsibility, output of the group, efficiency, and the situation (Table 3-2).

AUTOCRATIC LEADERSHIP

The autocratic type of leadership is also known as authoritarian, directive, or bureaucratic. Individuals who practice this type of leadership achieve their goals by setting objectives and having them carried out without input or suggestions from others on how to do so. They believe that they have complete authority that should not be questioned. Autocratic leaders do not encourage individual initiative or cooperation among members of the organization; instead, they are task oriented, making decisions independently and issuing orders to those working with them. When an autocratic leader hires an autocratic manager, a power struggle is likely to occur.

Autocratic leadership does not work well in many situations, but in some situations this type of leadership is necessary. For example, during an emergency one person must take charge because there is no time for group conferences on the best plan of action. Autocratic leadership may also be justified when the leader obviously knows more or has more experience than anyone else in the group. In this situation group members often need or want someone to tell them what to do and how to do it.

DEMOCRATIC LEADERSHIP

Democratic leaders achieve their goals through the participation of group members by focusing on the individual abilities of each member. People are encouraged to provide input into the problem-solving process, and decisions are often made through group consensus. Everyone in the group is informed of the goals and direction of the organization, so that input has a direct relationship to attaining the goals. Instead of power struggles, democratic leaders turn problems over to the group to manage.

The primary role of the leader is to keep the group headed in the right direction. Democratic leaders lead by suggestion rather than by domination. They persuade and teach rather than rule. Most people who work with a democratic leader have a feeling of satisfaction because they have a part in managing their work situation.

LAISSEZ-FAIRE LEADERSHIP

The opposite of autocratic leadership is laissez-faire leadership. A laissez-faire leader provides little or no directive leadership. Individuals working in this environment are allowed to do anything they want with no direction from administration. Often the result is that people do not know or care about what they are supposed to do, and they may lose all sense of initiative and desire for achievement. The organization then gradually disintegrates into a muddle of confusion. However, laissez-faire leadership may work well with a highly motivated, focused group.

PARTICIPATIVE LEADERSHIP

Participative leaders are crosses between autocratic and democratic leaders; they are sometimes called multicratic or situational leaders. They present their own personal views to group members, who provide criticism and comments. The participative leader analyzes feedback from the group and then makes all final decisions. Participative leaders work well within a group as well as in emergency situations when events need to be handled quickly. The response may not be as quick as it is under autocratic leadership. Group members assist the participative leader with setting goals, thereby achieving for themselves a sense of empowerment and control.

table 3-2 Comparison of Authoritarian, Democratic, Laissez-Faire, and Participative Leadership Styles

	AUTHORITARIAN	DEMOCRATIC	LAISSEZ-FAIRE	PARTICIPATIVE
Degree of freedom	Little freedom	Moderate freedom	Much freedom	Little to moderate freedom
Degree of control	High control	Moderate control	No control	Moderate to high control
Decision making	By the leader	Leader and group	By the group or by no one	By the leader with group input
Leader activity level	High	High	Minimal	High
Assumption of responsibility	Primarily by the leader	Shared	Abdicated	Primarily by the leader
Output of the group	High quantity, good quality	Creative, high quality	Variable, may be poor quality	High quality, high quantity
Efficiency	Very efficient	Less efficient than authoritarian	Inefficient	Efficient

Modified from Tappen, R. M. (1989). *Nursing leadership and management: Concepts and practice* (2nd ed.). Philadelphia: Davis.

CLASSIC MANAGEMENT THEORIES

Management theories attempt to explain what motivates people to work. Awareness of management theories helps nurses determine the best management style for their work setting. The classic management theories are labeled X, Y, and Z.

THEORY X

In 1957, Douglas McGregor developed two theories, which he labeled theory X and theory Y, to explain the nature of people and their relationship to the work environment. Theory X assumes that people in the workplace

- Find no pleasure in their work
- Dislike responsibility
- Are naturally lazy and prefer to do nothing
- Work mainly for the money
- Work only because they fear being fired
- Are basically childlike and like being told what to do
- Do not want to think for themselves
- Are not capable of making decisions for themselves

According to theory X, people have these general characteristics and therefore want to be directed and controlled. Leaders who adhere to the X theory of management usually have an autocratic style.

THEORY Y

According to theory Y, people are dynamic, flexible, and adaptive. It is assumed by believers in this theory that people

- Are active and enjoy setting their own goals
- Work for rewards other than money, such as doing the job well and working with others in the process
- Are productive because of their own personal goals rather than because of goals set for them
- Are mature and responsible
- Are self-directed
- Accept responsibility
- Care about what they are doing
- Are constantly striving to grow

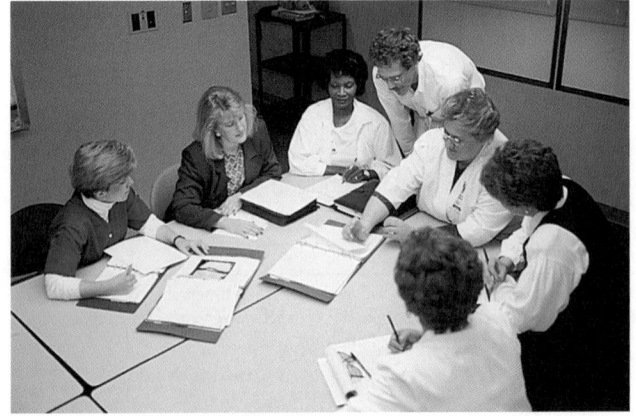

FIGURE **3-1** In the theory Z form of management, workers are involved in every phase of the operation of the organization.

According to theory Y, people are thought to like their work when they know what is expected of them and when their work gives them satisfaction. Leaders who adhere to the Y theory of management usually have a democratic style.

THEORY Z

Theory Z originated in Japan and describes an organizational philosophy and structure. It grew out of the times when most employees were related to one another and worked together for the good of the company rather than for individual gain. The focus is on participative management based on mutual trust and loyalty.

This form of management involves all workers in every phase of the operation of the company, including planning, organizing, decision making, and problem solving (Fig. 3-1). All members of the group have similar abilities and status, so they may be rotated to perform different duties. They have complete knowledge and understanding of their organizational objectives and methods of achieving them. It is thought that the theory Z form of management results in greater efficiency and satisfaction among members of the work force. Leaders with a democratic management style often are able to fit into this type of management.

FUNCTIONS IN THE MANAGEMENT PROCESS

Management is a problem-oriented process similar to the nursing process. The major functions of management are planning (what is to be done), organizing (how it is to be done), directing (who is to do it), coordinating (who is doing what), and controlling (when and how the task is done).

PLANNING

Planning is the first step in the management process. Planning entails deciding in advance what needs to be done and how to do it. To provide effective care for patients, a good plan for carrying out their care must be developed. Effective planning is as important for individual patient care as it is for a group of patients.

Two important components of planning are *decision making* and *problem solving*. Decision making is the process of selecting one course of action from alternatives. Problem solving is a part of the decision-making process.

The first step in decision making is to identify a problem. Sometimes the problem is quite obvious, but at other times underlying issues make the real problem less obvious. You should go on a "fact-finding mission" to explore all aspects of the situation to identify the real problem. Seek answers to such questions as who, how, when, and why.

Once the real problem has been identified, all possible solutions should be explored. This is a creative process that can involve other people in the health care setting. Often brainstorming sessions are held to obtain input from a variety of sources.

The next step in the decision-making process involves choosing the most desirable action for solving the problem. To select the best solution, you must consider whether the action is likely to accomplish the objectives of the organization. In addition, it is desirable to determine whether the action increases the effectiveness and efficiency of the organization and whether it is realistic to try to implement it.

After the decision has been made, it can be implemented. The decision should be communicated to other people who are involved in the organization to gain their support for carrying out the action. The communication should be expressed in such a way that other individuals become supportive of the decision rather than antagonistic toward it. Antagonism and negative feelings can be avoided in many cases when others are involved in the decision-making and problem-solving process from the beginning.

The final step in the decision-making process is to determine how the results will be evaluated. There are many ways to carry out an evaluation. Written tools such as audits or checklists may be used, as may verbal or written feedback from individuals in the organization or from patients who are receiving the care. If the solution to the problem is not satisfactory, another alternative can be selected and tried, followed by another evaluation. Table 3-3 lists the steps in the decision-making process.

table 3-3 Steps in the Decision-Making Process

PROCESS	HOW TO ACCOMPLISH
Identify a problem	Go on fact-finding mission: who, how, when, why
Explore possible solutions	Involve others: brainstorm
Choose most desirable action	Determine whether action is realistic and can achieve organization's objectives
Implement action	Communicate decision to others
Plan evaluation	Identify how results will be evaluated (audits, feedback, etc.)

ORGANIZING

Organizing is the second step in the management process. When the planning has been completed, there must be a formal structure or organization to ensure that individuals can carry out actions in the most efficient and effective manner possible. Organization also helps to develop order, promote cooperation among workers, and foster productivity.

Part of the process of organizing is developing objectives. Objectives help to guide the process of planning and organizing. Another part is establishing policies and procedures to provide guidelines for carrying out the objectives. The most qualified people should be assigned to carry out the specific activities and tasks that will best achieve the objectives. In nursing, the process of delegating responsibility for carrying out activities may involve the development of job descriptions, performance standards, and staffing patterns to provide the best patient care possible.

DIRECTING

The third step of the management process is directing. Directing involves making **assignments** and directing people to carry out the assignments. It also involves explaining what is to be done, how it is to be done, and why it is to be done.

In nursing, making assignments is related to patient care. Assignments should be made carefully so that the skills of assigned personnel match patient needs. It is important to estimate the difficulty of the task and the time needed to complete the care. Help or additional instruction should be provided whenever necessary.

Only one person should be responsible for making assignments, especially with team nursing. Assignments must be specific, easily understood, and posted where everyone can see them. Staff members should be helped to understand their assignments and the importance of each task.

Directing people to carry out their assignments requires good communication skills and assertive behavior. For directions to be effective, they must be complete and understandable. It is also helpful to give directions in a clear, logical order and to limit the number of directions given at any one time. Providing written directions increases understanding and compliance.

The manner in which directions are given is also important. Usually directions are given in the form of a request, such as "Will you help Mrs. Smith with her bath today?" Requesting that an individual carry out a task encourages cooperation and tends to ensure that more is accomplished. It implies that the individuals who are giving directions are "working with" people rather than having people "work for" them.

COORDINATING

The fourth step of the management process is coordinating. Coordinating helps to pull together various activities to achieve a goal. It ensures that all important activities are being carried out and helps to identify overlap, duplication, and omissions. In nursing, coordinating involves personnel and services. You must be sure that proper nursing care is given by the appropriate people.

The coordination process may be carried out within a specific nursing unit or among units and departments in a hospital, long-term care facility, or community agency. For example, the nurse may want to be sure that medications are being given by designated team members on a unit.

Coordinating involves skill and experience in problem solving and decision making. It also requires good communication skills and an ability to resolve conflicts within an organization. To be a good coordinator, you should be able to assess what all individuals and groups in the organization are doing and recognize that it is important for all parts of the organization to function effectively for the good of the whole.

CONTROLLING

Controlling or evaluation is the last step in the management process. It is an ongoing process in which the activities of the organization are analyzed to make sure that the plans are being carried out. Both the efficiency and the effectiveness of the organization are evaluated in the controlling process. The purposes of control in nursing service are to determine whether there are enough staff and supplies, whether the operation is economical, and whether the desired objectives have been achieved. Controlling is basically a form of evaluation.

Control has three basic steps:

1. Establishing standards and objectives
2. Measuring performance and comparing the results with the standards
3. Making corrections or adjustments to remedy the deficiencies in the caregiving operations

Continuous quality improvement (CQI) and *total quality management* (TQM) are terms that are frequently used in relation to control. The purpose of CQI is to ensure good nursing practice and quality care. The American Nurses' Association, the American Hospital Association, and the Joint Commission on Accreditation of Healthcare Organizations are organizations that set standards for nursing practice and medical care. Most agencies also have CQI committees that set standards for care. Agencies are evaluated to ensure that objectives and standards are being met, and recommendations are made for necessary change.

CONFLICT RESOLUTION

Dealing with conflict is an important part of the manager's role. Conflicts arise from differences in many factors such as beliefs, knowledge, opinions, values, personalities, and backgrounds. When a conflict occurs, it creates stress and negative feelings that can adversely affect the work situation. A conflict may be within an individual (intrapersonal conflict), between two or more people (interpersonal conflict), or between individuals and organizations (organizational conflict).

Conflict is a process with four stages:

1. Frustration: People believe their goals are being blocked; they feel frustrated. Individuals may become angry or resigned.
2. Conceptualization: Each party formulates a view of the basis for the conflict. Typically, conflicts center on perceived differences in facts, goals, how to achieve goals, and the values on which goals are based.
3. Action: The conflict leads to various behaviors that may or may not help resolve the conflict.
4. Outcomes: Outcome follows the action; may be reformulation of goals that is acceptable to all parties; one party may "win," the other "lose"; emotions may be positive or negative.

There are multiple approaches to conflict resolution. The positive and negative consequences of each are summarized in Table 3-4. Each approach has advantages and disadvantages, so the leader must select the best approach in each situation. To understand how each of these approaches works in a "real" situation, let's apply them to this scenario: You are the charge nurse on a 30-bed unit in a long-term care facility. Nursing assistants (NA) are assigned to equal numbers of residents in adjacent rooms. During report, one NA, Alice, complains that her assignment is unfair because all but two of her residents require almost total care. She says that all the other NAs have easier assignments. Using various strategies, here are possible solutions:

- Accommodation: You shift the care of two residents to other NAs.
- Collaboration: You reassess the needs of each group of assigned residents. Recognizing that Alice is correct, you work with the NAs to identify more equitable distribution of assignments to ensure good patient care.
- Compromise: You tell Alice that you will alternate NAs assigned to that group of residents.
- Competition: You tell Alice that everyone has some residents who require a lot of care, and the assignment will stand.

table 3-4 ***Modes of Conflict Resolution***

MODE	POSITIVE OUTCOMES	NEGATIVE OUTCOMES	WHEN TO USE
Accommodation	Agreement is reached	Differences are suppressed; may leave anger or resentment	You are wrong The other person really does have a better idea The issue is more important to the other party than to you You are outnumbered or outranked
Collaboration	Generates commitment to work together. Focuses on shared higher goals such as good patient care; not individual immediate needs. Builds understanding and empathy	Wastes time if used for resolution of trivial issues or issues where the outcome has already been decided	To build understanding To find creative solutions that accommodate higher common goals To address difficult issues that affect productivity
Compromise	Can produce mutually acceptable solutions Both parties have achieved something they wanted	The compromised solution may not be the best even though it "keeps the peace"	When time pressures require quick solution When each party is firmly committed to different views A compromise can produce acceptable outcomes
Avoidance	Temporarily defuses highly charged emotional disagreement Allows both parties to "cool off" until a reasonable approach can be considered	The conflict is not resolved Neither party is satisfied	To deal with trivial issues when more important issues are waiting To delay a decision until parties are calmer, more information is obtained, etc. When one party's demands cannot possibly be met When others could resolve the issue more readily
Competition	Reflects a strong stance to defend important principles, protect vulnerable parties Person in power takes responsibility for a decision	Can generate bad feelings Creates a winner and a loser. May generate behaviors that block the actions of the "winner."	When a quick decision is essential To implement unpopular, nonnegotiable actions To defend important principles, individual rights, group welfare

- Avoidance: You tell Alice that you have more important things to deal with right now and go to your office.

For each of these "solutions," think about the positive and negative outcomes. Again, realize that the best solution will vary with the situation. The art of management is to select the best approach for the situation.

TIPS FOR EFFECTIVE MANAGEMENT

Managing health care workers is a complex task. Some strategies you may use to improve your management skills include (1) taking an active approach to planning, avoiding conflict before it happens; (2) emphasizing the importance of documentation as a part of management; (3) treating other health care workers or team members as you would like to be treated yourself; (4) keeping confidential information confidential; (5) making employees accountable for their actions; and (6) seeking help and support from a variety of sources. LPNs are frequently asked to assume responsibilities for the care that other staff members give to patients. You may have nursing assistants, unlicensed assistive personnel, technicians, or other practical nurses reporting to you. Your role is not simply to tell them what to do; you must be both a leader and a manager.

THE LICENSED PRACTICAL NURSE AS A LEADER

TEAM NURSING

Team nursing was introduced during the 1950s, when there was a shortage of professional nurses and an abundance of auxiliary nursing staff. The team functions by using the skills and knowledge of the professional nurse to direct the care provided by a diverse staff through group action. All members of the team are expected to have input into the nursing care process by contributing suggestions and sharing ideas.

THE ROLE OF THE LICENSED PRACTICAL NURSE AS A TEAM LEADER

The functions of the team leader are to plan, set priorities for, supervise, and evaluate patient care. The role of the team leader traditionally was carried out by a registered nurse (RN) because it was thought that only RNs were prepared to plan nursing interventions, provide supervision, make independent decisions, and evaluate nursing care or the work of team members. However, in many cases, an LPN is assigned to the position of team leader, especially in long-term care settings. In these cases, the job description must differentiate between the practice of an RN team leader and that of an LPN team leader.

Team leaders are responsible for ongoing assessments of each patient and determination of appropriate nursing interventions. They must be sure that medical orders and plans are carried out and documented. They are also responsible for keeping care plans current and documenting the nursing care provided. In addition, team leaders are responsible for planning and conducting team conferences and reporting changes to the RN supervisor. An LPN who assumes the position of team leader can help carry out these responsibilities under the supervision and guidance of an RN.

ISSUES RELATED TO TEAM LEADERSHIP

Specific issues such as making assignments, accident prevention and safety, and accountability concern the team leader.

Making Assignments

You cannot do everything for all patients. To be effective, you must be able to assign tasks to others who are hired to perform them and make sure that those tasks are carried out. **Delegation** involves gaining the cooperation of others to carry out a specific task.

Making assignments involves identifying and delegating specific tasks of care to a specific person. You usually assign the care of several patients to each staff member. Before you can make assignments, you must know what care each patient requires and you must know the strengths and weaknesses of staff members.

Effective delegation requires delegating a clearly identified task, assessing patient needs, empowering the staff person to carry out activities to complete the task, and monitoring staff performance. Delegating tasks is specified in your job description; you are delegating some of your responsibilities, according to your state's nurse practice act. The 1994 Entry-Level Competencies Report for practical nursing school graduates states that the graduate practical nurse is accountable for nursing care delegated to unlicensed health care providers. To delegate, you must know the background skill level of the persons to whom you delegate tasks. You must find out what the unlicensed personnel know, delegate appropriately, and document the outcomes.

Essential elements of effective delegation include knowing your state nurse practice act statements on delegation and your institution's policy and procedures manual, knowing the training and background of persons to whom you delegate tasks, deciding which tasks can be safely delegated, and evaluating the patient's response. You must delegate only *tasks* to unlicensed personnel; you may not delegate *nursing processes* to unlicensed personnel.

Accident Prevention and Safety

Every health care facility must meet minimal safety regulations established by law in addition to those adopted by the agency to meet its unique needs. All staff members, particularly the team leader, should learn these regulations during orientation to the job. The team leader should know the regulations and be sure that staff members are aware of them. Everyone must understand procedures to follow in case of disasters such as fires, tornadoes, or hurricanes. In addition, everyday safety issues related to handling equipment, using proper procedures, and working with potentially dangerous drugs must constantly be addressed to be sure that knowledge and skills are up to date.

Accountability

Team leaders must demonstrate accountability for their own actions as well as the actions of the staff they are directing. Accountability means that a person is answerable for his or her actions; that is, he or she may be called on to explain or justify them. Team leaders also are legally responsible for all nursing care and documentation. The team leader must ensure that proper and accurate charting is carried out for all nursing assessments, interventions, and evaluations. If permitted by agency policy, nurses take verbal orders from physicians. In the case of both written and verbal orders, the licensed practical nurse (LPN) should verify orders with an RN or with the physician who wrote the orders.

Accountability also involves communicating patient needs to others through both oral and written interactions. A common form of communication is the report given at the end (or beginning) of every shift. The LPN is usually responsible for reporting to the RN in charge but may be only indirectly responsible for the report. Guidelines for clear and complete reporting are as follows:

1. Organize the report before beginning.
2. Give the patient's room number, name, age (if appropriate), diagnosis, and physician.
3. Provide a brief account of each patient's condition, including new or changed orders.
4. Refer to vital signs, temperature elevations, intravenous fluids, and intake and output as relevant.
5. For patients receiving pain medication, note the drug name, dosage, prescribed frequency, time of last administration, and effectiveness.
6. Cover the necessary information for preoperative patients, including the preoperative teaching done, the time of preoperative medications, completion of surgical checklists, and the like.
7. Give information about postoperative patients, including the time of arrival from the operating or recovery room,

general condition, vital signs, intravenous fluids required (e.g., kind, rate of flow, fluids to follow), dressings, voiding, diet, nature of breathing, coughing, and type, location, and patency of tubes.

The report may be given by means of a tape recording, in a one-to-one discussion with another nurse, as a summary in a group conference, or during walking rounds at the bedside. The key to good communication is to be clear, concise, and thorough.

CHARACTERISTICS OF AN EFFECTIVE TEAM LEADER

Effective team leaders must have skills in leadership, management, and supervisory techniques. They should be able to communicate effectively, both orally and in writing. Effective team leaders are able to work well with others and show that they value others' input and suggestions regarding patient care. Figure 3-2 illustrates components of effective team leadership. The leader's possession of these qualities leads to greater satisfaction among the staff and a higher quality of patient care.

To be a good team leader, you must also understand how to build an effective team. A team is more than just a group of people. It is a group of people who need to work together to achieve a goal or task, in this case, delivery of care to patients. Strategies to build an effective team include:

- **Establish a clear purpose.** All team members must understand and value their purpose.
- **Listen actively.** Active listening requires genuine interest in understanding another's message, not just waiting for your turn to speak.
- **Be compassionate.** Recognize stress and distress in team members; show genuine concern.

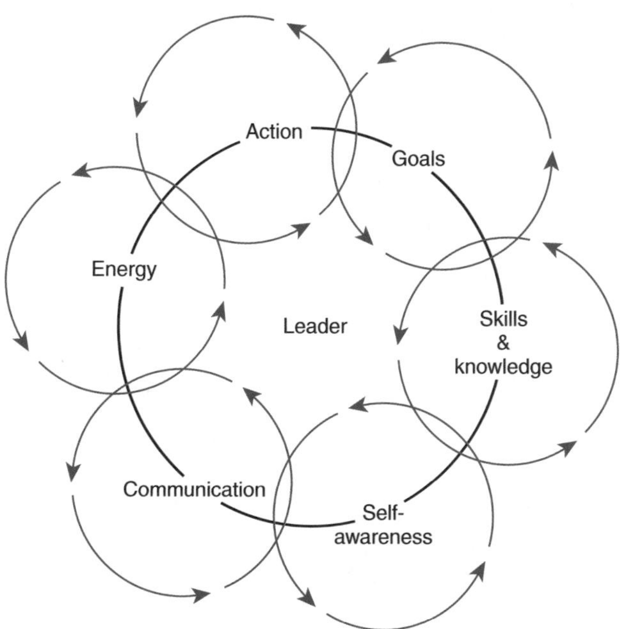

FIGURE **3-2** Components of effective team leadership.

- **Be honest.** Take ownership of your opinions and attitudes; provide constructive feedback.
- **Be flexible.** Recognize that good ideas can come from any team member; invite input and be willing consider other suggestions and viewpoints.
- **Be committed to conflict resolution.** Resolve to find creative solutions that leave all involved in agreement.

CHARACTERISTICS OF AN EFFECTIVE TEAM

Characteristics of an effective team include clear goals, good communication, a result-driven structure, competent team members, a unified commitment, a collaborative climate, standards of excellence, external support and recognition, and effective leadership.

Put on your ***THINKING CAP!!***

Situation: You are the charge nurse in a long-term care facility.

1. The nurse manager has asked you to explain the increasing use of disposable items being used on your shift.
2. Explain how you would approach this problem using each of the four management theories.

key points

- Licensed practical nurses comprise the primary staffing and management of most long-term care homes.
- Leadership is defined as guidance, or showing the way to others.
- Management is defined as the effective use of selected methods to accomplish goals.
- Leaders and managers must be competent, must have the respect of the people they work with, and must be able to motivate others.
- Four basic types of leadership are autocratic, democratic, laissez-faire, and participative.
- Autocratic leaders are authoritarian, meaning they act without input or suggestions from others.
- Democratic leaders achieve their goals through participating, encouraging others to provide input, and making decisions through group consensus.
- Laissez-faire leaders allow group members to do anything they want with no direction from administration.
- Participative leaders have a mixture of autocratic and democratic characteristics, soliciting input from group members but making the final decisions themselves.
- Leadership styles are based on leaders' assumptions about workers' motivations.
- The major functions of management are planning, organizing, coordinating, directing, and controlling.
- Planning, the first step in the management process, involves decision making and problem solving.
- Organizing provides a structure for carrying out the plan.
- Directing involves making assignments and directing people to carry out the assignments.
- Coordinating pulls various activities together to achieve a goal.

- Controlling includes establishing standards, measuring performance by the standards, and making corrections to remedy deficiencies.
- Strategies for conflict resolution include accommodation, compromise, competition, avoidance, and collaboration.
- The most appropriate strategy for conflict resolution depends on the situation.
- Team nursing was designed to use the skills and knowledge of the professional nurse to direct the care provided by a diverse staff through group action.
- Team leaders conduct ongoing assessments of patients and determine appropriate nursing interventions.
- A good team leader is skilled in leadership, management, and supervisory techniques.
- To build an effective team, the leader must establish a clear purpose; listen actively; be compassionate, honest, and flexible; and be committed to resolution of conflicts.

Put on your THINKING CAP!!

Think of a person in your class whom you consider to be a leader. Write down the characteristics that led you to this conclusion. Compare your class leader's characteristics with the identified characteristics in this chapter. Identify the person's leadership style.

REVIEW QUESTIONS

1. An LPN has been offered a position as a charge nurse in a nursing home. How can the nurse best determine the legal limits of practice in this role?
   1. Ask the nursing home administrator what the charge nurse is expected to do.
   2. Review a textbook that discusses the LPN as charge nurse.
   3. Ask other LPNs who have experience as charge nurses.
   4. Contact the state board of nursing.
2. Which leadership style is demonstrated when a charge nurse makes the following statement during report: "I don't care how you organize your work, as long as you finish your assignments on time"?
   1. Autocratic
   2. Democratic
   3. Laissez-faire
   4. Participative
3. A manager who applies the theory Y assumes that people in a work environment:
   1. Find no pleasure in their work
   2. Work mainly for the money
   3. Are mature and responsible
   4. Have similar abilities and status
4. The nursing assistants on your unit complain that the workload is unevenly distributed and ask you to try to find a better way to make assignments. The first step in your decision-making process should be to:
   1. Identify and explore the nature of the problem
   2. List potential solutions to the problem
   3. Tell the nursing assistants to work it out together
   4. Change the way you make their assignments
5. Which direction by the team leader is most likely to encourage cooperation among nursing assistants?
   1. I expect you to pitch in and help each other.
   2. Since you have finished your morning care, go help Mary catch up.
   3. Whoever finishes morning care first can take the first lunch break.
   4. Ed, would you please help Mary by taking vital signs on her newly admitted patient?
6. What is the most important factor an LPN team leader must consider when delegating a task to a nursing assistant?
   1. Institutional policies regarding nursing assistant functions
   2. The background skill level of the nursing assistant
   3. The nursing assistant's willingness to perform the task
   4. State board of nursing regulations related to nursing assistants

CHAPTER

4 The Nurse–Patient Relationship

objectives

1. Define the holistic view of nursing.
2. Define the concept of *self.*
3. Discuss the use of self in the practice of nursing.
4. Compare the meaning of the terms *patient* and *client.*
5. List commonly held expectations of patients and families.
6. Describe the meaning of the Patient's Bill of Rights.
7. Describe guidelines for nurse–patient relationships.
8. Describe basic components of communication.
9. Describe four basic principles of ethics.

key terms

Action (p. 33)
Caring (p. 33)
Client (p. 34)
Empathy (p. 38)
Empower (p. 35)
Ethics (p. 39)
Holism (p. 33)
Morals (p. 39)
Patient (p. 34)
Self (p. 33)
Therapeutic relationship (p. 33)
Understanding (p. 33)
Values (p. 34)

Nursing means caring for persons. *Caring* is a process characterized by understanding, action, and concern. *Understanding* is the ability to listen to and relate to others in order to perceive their feelings and the meaning of their words. *Action* denotes responding to others with genuineness, compassion, sensitivity, and self-disclosure to promote their well-being.

In the caring process, a therapeutic relationship develops between patients or clients and nurses. Unlike a social relationship, a **therapeutic relationship** is goal-directed and focuses on one individual (the patient). To develop therapeutic relationships, nurses must value and accept patients or clients as unique individuals. In addition, nurses must be aware of themselves as individuals. Knowing how your own attitudes, feelings, and beliefs affect others is vital to effective communication. A nonjudgmental attitude of caring is essential to the practice of nursing.

A HOLISTIC VIEW OF NURSING CARE

Holism is a way of viewing people as whole individuals. According to the holistic theory, people are complex creatures made up of many parts. Each part interacts with the others, and the sum of the parts forms a unified whole. Holistic health care is a system of comprehensive patient care that considers the physical, emotional, social, economic, and spiritual needs of individuals.

Individuals are composed of mind, body, and spirit. It is not possible to care for one part without considering how the other parts are affected. Thus, in nursing, the physiologic, psychological, sociologic, and spiritual influences on individual behaviors become integrated into a plan of care (Fig. 4-1). For example, patients who have undergone surgery have physical needs, but you also need to consider their emotional needs and their feelings about the surgery. In addition, patients may have spiritual needs as they deal with the prospect of sickness and death. Families are also included in a holistic approach to nursing care (see Chapter 6).

USE OF THE SELF IN NURSING

Many tools are used in the tasks of nursing, including stethoscopes, sphygmomanometers, and thermometers; however, there is no more important tool that you bring to each patient encounter than the use of self. *Self* is a term used to describe one's personhood: the knowledge, experience, values, beliefs, perceptions, strengths, and weaknesses that make each individual unique. As a nurse, your attitudes, beliefs, self-esteem, and feelings become a part of the patient's therapeutic environment, just as those of the patient become a part of your environment. With your assistance, individuals and their families may find meaning in their experience and may achieve a harmonious state of health.

VALUES, BELIEFS, AND ATTITUDES

Self-awareness involves knowing one's own values, beliefs, and attitudes. You should be able to answer the questions "Who am I?," "What do I believe?," and "What is important to me?" so that you can help others answer those questions. Almost every day, you will encounter situations that require value judgments. You must make certain choices related to patient care, respond to requests for help and guidance, and

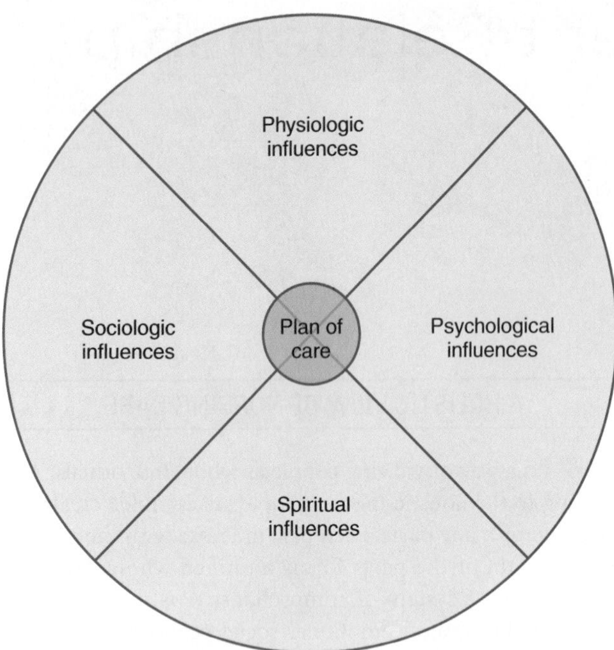

FIGURE **4-1** Physiologic, psychological, sociologic, and spiritual influences on individual behaviors become integrated into a plan of care.

provide emotional and spiritual support. Your values, attitudes, and beliefs are outwardly expressed in your behavior as you interact with patients.

Values can be defined as principles or standards shared by members of a society that determine what is desirable or worthwhile. A value is reflected in the worth you give to an idea or action. A *belief* is a conviction or opinion. *Attitudes* are reactions that flow from values and beliefs. An attitude indicates a feeling toward persons or things. Values and personal beliefs are developed in many ways. They may be acquired from religious education, from examples set by authority figures such as parents and teachers, or from peers.

Acquiring values and beliefs is a lifelong process that is affected by one's life experience. As people age, they generally have a fairly fixed set of values, but even older people are able to grow and change.

KNOWLEDGE

Knowledge is a component of self that is acquired through experience or study. The safe practice of nursing is dependent on one's knowledge base, and nursing education provides a basic introduction to the physical and social sciences. Nurses use their knowledge of biological, psychological, and social sciences to give the best care possible. This knowledge is often shared with patients, families, and the community to promote health, prevent disease, and cope with illness. Nurses also share their knowledge with colleagues on the health care team. As a nursing student, you will be expected to develop your critical thinking skills. Critical thinking enables you to think through problems in an efficient and organized manner. It requires that you seek and use information, not just recite facts. This is essential because real-life situations are seldom as "cut and dried" as they are in textbooks. Because each patient is unique, nursing care must be individualized, and that requires critical thinking.

The health care field is continually growing and changing. There is a greater emphasis on prevention of disease and promotion and maintenance of health. Nurses act as models of good health care practices. It is important to continue to learn and expand your knowledge to benefit others as well as yourself.

SKILLS

Nursing is a skill-oriented field. Nursing care involves the use of many skills that require efficiency and safety. A nurse must master the skills required to carry out nursing interventions including the technical skills needed to use sophisticated equipment. Your hands can be instruments of healing when used with compassion, competence, and gentleness. The simple act of giving a bed bath or a back rub can be the best use of self that you offer a suffering patient.

Nurses need *interpersonal skills* to communicate effectively and to establish caring relationships with patients. It is through the caring relationship that you are able to build a therapeutic relationship with the patient. Developing therapeutic nurse–patient relationships requires:

- A humanistic system of values
- Ability to instill faith and hope
- Sensitivity to one's self and to others
- Ability to develop helping, trusting relationships
- Ability to express both positive and negative feelings
- Ability to use problem-solving methods for decision making
- Ability to promote interpersonal teaching and learning
- Ability to provide a supportive, protective, and corrective mental, physical, sociocultural, and spiritual environment
- Ability to assist with the gratification of human needs
- Allowance for the uniqueness of individuals and their experiences

THE PERSPECTIVE OF THE PATIENT

The term *patients* is used to refer to individuals, families, groups, or communities. Patients may function in independent, interdependent, and dependent roles. As recipients of nursing care, patients may receive nursing interventions related to disease prevention, health promotion, health maintenance, illness, and end-of-life care.

PATIENT VERSUS CLIENT

Some nurses use the term *client* rather than *patient.* This term evolved from a general belief or attitude about the nurse–patient relationship. The word *client* denotes a feeling of partnership or working with someone. The word *patient* has a connotation of doing to or for someone; it also implies that an individual is ill. For some nurses, *client* seems to represent a more accurate view of the roles in the nurse–patient relationship, because the nurse values patients as individuals, honors their individuality, and helps them achieve the highest level of wellness possible. However, because *patient* also is used and accepted by nurses and other health care professionals, and frequently by elderly people as well, *patient* and *client* are used interchangeably. The term *patient* has been used for years and is used frequently in this text in support of the long-established tradition of the nurse–patient relationship. Depending on the context, patients may be referred to as *clients* or *consumers of nursing services.*

PATIENTS' RIGHTS

Patients, as participants in nursing care, are entitled to receive quality care in a safe, supportive, and nurturing environment. As the health consumer movement becomes more and more active, greater attention is being paid to the rights of patients. In 1973, the American Hospital Association issued a Patient's Bill of Rights (Table 4-1) that outlines the rights of hospital patients and incorporates the components of quality care. No catalogue of rights can guarantee patients the kind of treatment they have a right to expect; however, hospitals, community agencies, and nursing homes, along with health care personnel, must provide the kind of nurse–client relationship that is based on trust and mutual respect.

Part of helping patients to retain their individuality is to speak and refer to them by name at all times. Pronounce the name correctly, and introduce the patient by name to other health care providers. Never refer to patients by bed number or medical diagnosis.

Older patients, no matter what their state of mind, deserve to be treated with the same respect as younger patients. It is inappropriate for a nurse to call an older patient anything other than *Mr.* Smith or *Mrs.* Smith unless the patient has requested it. Terms such as "Pops," "Sweetie," "Gramps," or "Baby" are unprofessional and demeaning to older individuals (Fig. 4-2).

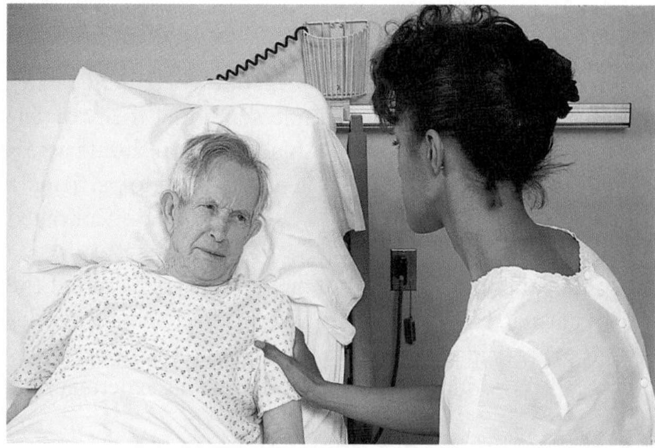

FIGURE **4-2** Older people should be treated with the same respect as younger people.

table 4-1 ***A Patient's Bill of Rights***

1. Considerate and respectful care
2. Complete and current information concerning a patient's condition and care
3. Necessary information in order to give an informed consent and the freedom to refuse treatment
4. Right to an "advance directive" (e.g., a living will) concerning treatment and the naming of a surrogate decision maker
5. Protection of privacy
6. Protection of confidentiality
7. Review of a patient's own medical records
8. Response to reasonable requests for service
9. Attainment of information regarding the hospital's relationship with other health and educational institutions
10. Knowledge of any experimentation regarding a patient's care
11. Reasonable continuity of care
12. Explanation of the hospital bill and knowledge of hospital rules and regulations that will affect a patient's care

Adapted from American Hospital Association. (1992). *A patient's bill of rights.* Reprinted with permission of the American Hospital Association, copyright 1992.

PATIENTS' EXPECTATIONS

Explanation of the Care

The experience of illness and all the changes in a person's life that it precipitates is very stressful. A method that you can use to help reduce patients' stress and anxiety levels is to *empower* them to participate in their care. To do this, patients must be given the information they need to be active participants. They want to know what is going to be done to them, when, how, and why. With so many new technological and medical advances, the worth of the patient's involvement in their own care is emphasized. Patients need to learn to make their own health care choices; they need health care information and disease prevention guidelines given to them in a way that is individualized to their own personal characteristics and lifestyles.

Patients need and are entitled to an explanation of the care to be given so that they know what to expect and what is expected of them. Patients who are knowledgeable about their care are more likely to be active participants who are better satisfied and less anxious. Explanations and teaching are often left to the nurse. Communication should take place in language that patients understand, without talking down to them. Interpreters should be utilized if needed to improve communication. Explanation of care is not only a therapeutic method to reduce the client's stress and fears but also a patient's right. Patients who are not given adequate explanations of what is to be done have been denied their rights as human beings.

Patients as Partners in Care

As a consumer of health care services, the patient no longer is willing to assume a passive role. Most patients not only want to assume more responsibility for their care but also expect to do so. Patients who see themselves as partners in their care are more likely to accept responsibility for their care. Their sense of responsibility may serve to prevent needless complications resulting from noncompliance that may otherwise prolong their care.

The patient can assume an active role from the point of admission. The initial assessment is your first opportunity to set the tone for a relationship that encourages patient participation. You can help patients understand that their participation is not only wanted but also needed. You should assess patients to determine to what extent they wish to participate in their care. The patient's family also should be encouraged to participate in the care whenever possible.

Some patients are more willing than others to accept the role of partner. Factors that may have an effect on patients' decisions to participate in their care are age, ethnicity, personality, social class, educational level, and previous experiences.

Acceptance of Patient Behaviors

It is important to patients that nurses and health care providers accept patients' behavior. Illness is a stressful event and can cause people to react in unusual ways. In many cases, individuals behave differently than they would under normal circumstances, and nurses should not take this personally.

For a nurse–patient relationship to be therapeutic, you must be able to see patients' experiences from their perspectives. Encourage patients to share thoughts and feelings freely without fear of being judged. You must be willing to accept unconditionally the patient's values, beliefs, behaviors, and attitudes. This kind of a nurse–patient relationship is a special kind of caring in which the nurse has a high regard for the whole person. It conveys a sense of worth and dignity. Avoid imposing your own values and beliefs on the patient whose values differ from yours. Nurses should provide compassionate understanding of their patients' behavior and maintain a therapeutic, accepting environment.

Safety and Security

You have a high degree of responsibility for keeping your patients both physically and psychologically safe while in your care. You must assess a situation quickly, make a decision, and act promptly to solve the problem. A patient needs to feel that a nurse can act quickly and decisively in a crisis to provide the best care possible.

Competence and consistency are two factors that can alleviate stress in patients. Nurses who appear confident and competent help patients feel more secure. In addition, performing nursing procedures consistently can help reduce anxiety and build patients' confidence in the nurse. For example, changing dressings in the same step-by-step manner every time helps patients know what to expect and reassures them of the competence of your care.

GUIDELINES FOR THE NURSE–PATIENT RELATIONSHIP

THE HELPER ROLE

A helping role occurs when one person reaches out to help another. The goal is to help another individual grow, mature, cope, and function. A helping relationship is one in which there is genuine caring and compassion.

To assume the helper role, a nurse must have certain characteristics:

- Awareness of self
- Ability to analyze own feelings
- Ability to serve as a model to others
- Desire to help others
- Strong sense of ethics and high principles
- Sense of responsibility

Nurses act as helpers by administering direct care to patients, acting as advocates on behalf of patients, giving psychosocial support, and providing health education and counseling.

The role of helper obliges the nurse to maintain a therapeutic relationship. The nurse must provide an environment of trust. Trust occurs when the client experiences safety. A feeling of safety comes from knowing that the nurse is honest and open and from confidence in the nurse's skill and knowledge.

A helper in the professional sense cannot be a friend. The term *friend* connotes intimacy or affection. You must transcend the role of friend to take on a caring role. In this way you can facilitate the health of the patient. There is mutual responsibility between patient and nurse in a partnership.

Although friendships with patients can interfere with the therapeutic process, so can strong authoritarian approaches. Therapeutic communication is an art and a skill. It takes time and practice to be able to set firm limits with genuine warmth and honesty. Self-disclosure refers to the ability to be open and honest about one's feelings. You should not disclose personal information, however, as you would do in a friendship. Table 4-2 notes some differences between a helping person and a friend.

Touch can be used to show concern, to let the patient know you are present, or to provide comfort. Giving a bedridden patient a back rub before sleep can stimulate circulation, provide a caring moment, and promote relaxation. Perceptions differ from person to person. Some people are more comfortable with touching and being touched than others. Some patients may mistake touch as an invitation to intimacy.

COMMUNICATION

Communication skills are essential for carrying out the helper role. Communication is the process of exchanging ideas, beliefs, thoughts, and feelings between two or more people. It involves a message, a sender, and a receiver. The sender gives the message to the receiver.

There are two types of communicative behavior: (1) verbal language, which conveys meanings through words, and (2) nonverbal language, which conveys meanings through symbols and actions other than words. Examples of nonverbal communication are body position, facial expression, gestures, moaning, crying, laughing, and smiling.

To communicate effectively, nurses must be able to recognize the meanings of both verbal and nonverbal language. Language is influenced by the cultural context in which it is used. To interpret the meaning of what is said or done without consideration of cultural context equals stereotyping.

table 4-2 ***Comparison Between a Nurse as a Helping Person and a Nurse as a Friend***

HELPING PERSON	FRIEND
Responsible to client	Relationship is for friendship or support
Objective of relationship is to meet client's needs	Individuals meet each other's needs
Relationship is goal directed	No plan involved
Attitude is nonjudgmental	Both individuals express feelings, attitudes, and opinions
Does not attempt to influence client to helper's way of thinking	Friends try to influence each other in discussing issues such as religion, politics, and personal philosophy
Does not keep secrets, and explains in a direct manner the need to work with the treatment team	Friends may keep secrets
Discourages any sexual overtones in relationship	Sexual overtones or a sexual relationship may develop
Interacts with clients in health care settings	
Relationship is time limited	Relationship may continue

Communication can be assertive or aggressive. Assertive communication is the ability to express yourself without violating the rights of another person. Aggressive communication does violate the rights of others. Try to express yourself without violating the rights of another person.

Two essential parts of communication are *listening* and *observation.* Listening is an active process that involves trying to understand what is being said. The listener must display genuine interest and concentration to derive meaning from the words. A good listener can provide reassurance, lighten another person's burden, and clarify misunderstandings.

Observation of nonverbal language is as important to the communication process as listening is to verbal language. Nonverbal language can indicate a person's thoughts and feelings as well as, if not better than, verbal language can. Nonverbal actions can be in conflict with the content of what is being said and thus can give clues to true feelings. For example, patients may claim that everything is all right but may be slumped over and wringing their hands. An astute nurse should recognize that something is indeed wrong even though patients deny it verbally.

Therapeutic communication is a skill that can be learned through study, observation, and practice. Remember to be open, honest, and nonjudgmental. Self-awareness should be of primary concern. Nurses must actively seek to be cognizant of their own holistic dynamics. This implies that they have had the opportunity to self-explore and assess how the following areas may affect their ability to establish a therapeutic nurse–patient relationship:

- Ethnic, cultural, and socioeconomic background
- Attitudes, values, opinions, and beliefs
- Past unresolved experiences that are still emotionally laden
- Physical and psychological strengths and weaknesses

This self-awareness facilitates the therapeutic process.

Behaviors that may help you initiate a therapeutic interaction include the following:

- Focus attention on the client.
- Listen carefully.
- Ask the client to repeat information if necessary.
- Begin a mental assessment.

Questions that you may ask of the client, or use as areas of focus, to obtain a holistic assessment of the client include the following:

1. What is the client's age?
2. What is the client's cultural background?
3. What is the client's perception of his or her illness?
4. Is the client using direct eye contact?
5. What is the client's body language? Is it relaxed or tense?
6. What is the quality of the client's voice? Is it loud or soft?
7. Does the client use gestures?
8. Does the client's emotional tone (or affect) vary or does it remain constant (e.g., does the client appear sad, happy, or angry)?
9. Is the verbal message congruent with the client's body language, or is the client smiling while speaking of what would seem to be a sad event?

Listening is an active element of therapeutic communication. You must listen and attempt to understand what the client is saying. Tips for effective listening include:

1. Make sure you hear what is said; focus on what is being said.
2. Accept your client's needs and feelings.
3. Pay attention to nonverbal communication.
4. Obtain feedback of your understanding by verifying what you have heard.

Understanding is the ability to listen to others to perceive their feelings and the meaning of their words. Some techniques used to facilitate communication are listed in Table 4-3. Other suggestions for therapeutic communication are the following:

1. Use *I statements.* These are sentences that begin with the word *I* and indicate acceptance of responsibility for one's feelings and thoughts (e.g., "I worry less when I know what to expect."). *You statements* generally are not as well accepted by the listener (e.g., "You ought to try getting more sleep.").
2. Observe the client's gestures and nonverbal behavior. All behavior has meaning. Try to find the meaning in behavior.
3. Use open-ended questions. Stay clear of questions that can be answered with a "yes" or a "no."
4. Focus the client on pertinent issues.

table 4-3 Therapeutic and Nontherapeutic Communication Techniques

TECHNIQUE	DESCRIPTION	EXAMPLE
THERAPEUTIC		
Silence	Waiting attentively while the patient speaks or thinks. Allows the patient to think and respond.	Sitting quietly and expectantly when the patient is speaking or gathering his thoughts. Resisting the urge to fill quiet periods with conversation.
Reflecting	"Mirrors" back to patients what you have heard them say. Provides opportunities for patients to confirm whether they were understood.	"You say you're feeling better since your brother has returned?"
Summarizing	Reviews the subject matter that the client has discussed. Assures common understanding between nurse and patient.	"So you have decided to have surgery, but will delay it until after Christmas."
Restating	Repeats information in your own words so the patient can confirm your interpretation.	"I hear you're concerned about your son."
Clarification	Seeks additional information so you can better understand the patient's meaning.	"Do you mean sad when you say upset?"
Open-ended statement	A question or comment that requires more than a yes or no answer. Indicates interest, but leaves specific details for client to provide.	"Tell me your reactions to your new treatment."
NONTHERAPEUTIC		
Premature advice	Offers advice without first encouraging clients to explore their feelings fully. The problem must be explored carefully and potential actions considered before the patient can make a good decision. You cannot decide what is best for the patient.	"The first thing you need to do is make your teenagers help you more."
Assuming truth of statements rather than checking them out	Accepts information without questioning or clarifying. Misunderstandings can persist.	"It's incredible that your doctor did not tell you when to take this medication."
Commanding	Directing client to do something that creates a power struggle or resistance.	"You must quit smoking immediately."
Communication cut-off	Remark that discourages patient communication. Shows lack of effort to understand.	"Try to think positively."
False reassurance	Inappropriately offers personal opinion that the patient should not be concerned about something. Minimizes the patient's feelings. Can lead to feelings of guilt and anger.	"You shouldn't worry about the new treatment."

Processing is the act of reviewing a therapeutic communication with a trusted teacher, supervisor, or colleague to evaluate content and themes as well as the techniques that are used. This tool enables the nurse to be critiqued and to learn new techniques. Communication is a complex process. "Helping" can occur regardless of one's experience if respect and authenticity are brought to each interaction.

EMPATHETIC RESPONSE

Effective communication requires an empathetic response from a nurse. ***Empathy*** is the ability to identify with and understand another person's situation, feelings, and motives. An empathetic response requires compassion, understanding, and good therapeutic communication skills. Empathy differs from *sympathy.* When people sympathize with others, they understand another's feelings, but they also become immersed in the situation. Whatever affects one affects the other. The person who sympathizes can become as distressed as the person getting the sympathy. Empathy, in contrast, is an expression of understanding of another's thoughts and feelings without becoming overly emotionally involved or distressed.

Communicating empathy can be carried out through the simple use of verbal and nonverbal language. You can communicate empathy by telling the patient what to expect, even when the patient is comatose or confused. Discussing plans for care, such as treatments or medications, and explaining laboratory studies can provide reassurance to patients who may be frightened. You should also demonstrate your concern to patients and families by sharing your feelings. By sharing feelings, nurses show that they are human and can understand the difficulties of being ill or hospitalized.

You can show sensitivity in nonverbal ways, such as by respecting confidentiality, allowing the expression of feelings, and respecting patients' privacy. The use of touch is an excellent means of communicating empathy. Holding a patient's hand during a period of anxiety or pain can provide effective relief and, in many cases, can be more effective than any verbal interaction. The judicious use of touch conveys the message that "I care what happens to you, and I will help you in every way that I can" (Fig. 4-3).

When you respond empathetically, you respond with genuineness, warmth, and sensitivity to promote well-being in the client. This is the essence of therapeutic communication.

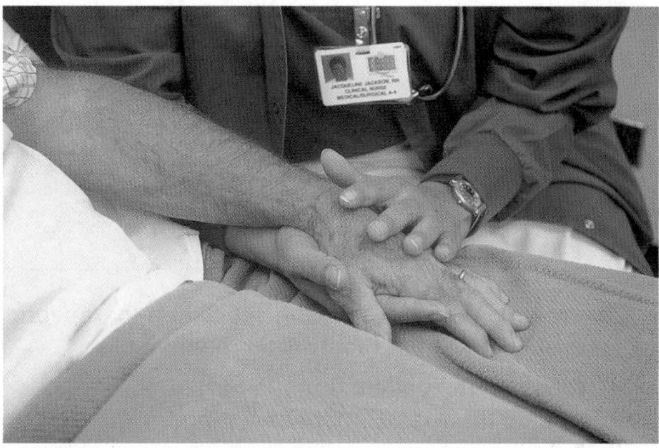

FIGURE 4-3 The judicious use of touch conveys the message that "I care what happens to you, and I will help you in every way I can."

ETHICAL CONSIDERATIONS

Ethics, which refers to the values, codes, and principles related to what is right, influence decisions. The ethical habits of an individual are described as *morals.* In addition to helping, communicating therapeutically, and providing empathetic care to patients, nurses need to consider ethical principles when establishing a nurse–patient relationship. Patients in today's health care system present a variety of ethical dilemmas. Because nurses spend so much time with the patients and their families, they are often the first ones to recognize and deal with ethical problems.

As long as patients retain decision-making ability, their wishes need to be respected. Patients are permitted to make treatment decisions based on their value systems, even when such decisions conflict with the beliefs of family or hospital personnel. The nurse is in a strategic position to identify ethical concerns regarding patient care and proposed treatments. Most nurses face ethical decisions in their practice. Knowing how to respond to ethical problems is the key to making good choices. Basic concepts involved in most ethical situations include beneficence (obligation to do good and act in the best interests of the person); nonmaleficence (do no harm); autonomy (the right to make one's own decisions); justice (obligation to be fair to everyone); fidelity (obligation to be faithful to agreements and responsibilities); and veracity (telling the truth). These concepts can be used as a way to evaluate possible decisions or actions when an ethical dilemma presents.

Practicing nursing ethically is more complex than knowing right from wrong. There may be two or more different ways of looking at the same situation. One way may place patient autonomy (the patient's right to self-determination) higher than beneficence (the professional duty to help others). Resolving ethical dilemmas depends on gathering all the facts. Ethical conflicts may arise between the good of one person and the good of many. For example, a physician may discharge a patient whom the nurse thinks could benefit from a longer stay or more treatment, but the patient's insurance has run out. After gathering facts and analyzing conflicting principles, the nurse considers the options and makes an ethical decision. Making ethical decisions helps develop a therapeutic relationship between nurses and patients. It is part of valuing and accepting patients as unique individuals.

Put on your THINKING CAP!!

1. During your next clinical experience, listen for therapeutic and nontherapeutic communication techniques used by health care providers in interactions with patients. Describe and label three examples. Discuss the impact of each statement on the interaction.
2. Identify three things you did in your last patient contact that demonstrated empathy.
3. Identify a nursing situation that you have encountered that has ethical implications. Discuss whether the resolution of the dilemma met the criteria of beneficence, nonmaleficence, fidelity, and veracity.

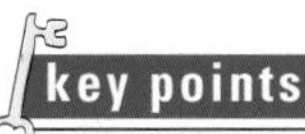

key points

- Caring is a process characterized by understanding and action.
- Action is the response to others with genuineness, warmth, sensitivity, and self-disclosure to promote their well-being.
- Holism views people as complex creatures made up of many parts that interact and form a unified whole.
- The nurse incorporates physiologic, psychological, sociologic, and spiritual influences into the plan of care.
- Nurses must have awareness of their own values, beliefs, and attitudes and be willing to accept unconditionally the client's values, beliefs, and attitudes.
- Nurses use their knowledge of physiology, psychology, and social science disciplines and their technical and interpersonal skills to give the best possible care to clients.
- Nurses can reduce clients' stress and anxiety levels by empowering them to participate in their own care and by demonstrating competence and consistency.
- Clients are the recipients of nursing care and are entitled to receive quality care, as detailed in the Patient's Bill of Rights.
- The role of a helper is to assist another to grow, mature, cope, and function.
- Communication is basic to the helper role.
- Empathy, genuineness, warmth, sensitivity, and self-disclosure are essentials of therapeutic communication.

- Empathy is the ability to identify with and understand another person's situation, feelings, and motives.
- Making ethical decisions is a part of establishing a therapeutic nurse–patient relationship.
- Ethics is a system or code of behavior, involving values, codes, and principles, related to what is right as applied to interactions within society.

REVIEW QUESTIONS

1. The main difference between social and therapeutic relationships is that therapeutic relationships:
   1. focus on the patient and the nurse.
   2. remain limited to inpatient settings.
   3. help the nurse work through personal problems.
   4. exist to meet patient-centered goals.
2. You are caring for an older adult who has been chronically ill for several years. The patient has decided not to continue life-sustaining treatment. You believe that life should be maintained at all costs. Which action best reflects acceptance of the patient in a therapeutic relationship?
   1. Ask the patient's family members to try to convince their loved one to continue treatment.
   2. Tell the patient that you believe life is sacred and it is wrong to refuse available treatment.
   3. Tell your nurse manager you cannot continue to care for the patient who refuses treatment.
   4. Plan with the patient ways to maintain quality of life for as long as possible.
3. Within a therapeutic relationship, it is appropriate for you as a nurse to:
   1. be honest about your feelings.
   2. try to influence the patient's religion.
   3. spend time with the patient in social settings.
   4. assure the patient that any information shared will be kept secret.
4. Which of the following reflects an empathetic response to a patient who is distressed?
   1. Ask the physician to order a sedative.
   2. Tell the patient that the situation could be worse.
   3. Gently touch the patient's arm.
   4. Firmly advise the patient to regain control.
5. When facing an ethical dilemma, the nurse must remember the principle of *nonmaleficence,* which means:
   1. Be fair to everyone.
   2. Act in the best interest of the patient.
   3. Tell the truth.
   4. Do no harm.
6. Which of the following is considered to be *open-ended?*
   1. "How many children do you have?"
   2. "Describe your usual day."
   3. "I see that you take thyroid replacement drugs."
   4. "Are you nervous about surgery?"
7. A patient who is scheduled for a biopsy of a lump in her breast says tearfully, "I am so afraid it will be cancer." The nurse replies, "There is no sense worrying about that until you know for sure." This is an example of:
   1. Premature advice
   2. Commanding
   3. False reassurance
   4. Assuming truth of statements

CHAPTER 5

Cultural Aspects of Nursing Care

objectives

1. Describe cultural concepts related to nursing and health care.
2. Identify traditional health habits and beliefs of major ethnic groups in the United States.
3. Explain cultural influences on the interactions of patients and families with the health care system.
4. Discuss cultural considerations in providing culturally sensitive nursing care.
5. Discuss ways in which planning and implementation of nursing interventions can be adapted to a patient's ethnicity.

key terms

Assimilation (ă-sĭm-ĭ-LĀ-shŭn, p. 50)
Cultural diversity (p. 41)
Culture (p. 41)
Enculturation (ĕn-kŭl-chĕr-Ā-shŭn, p. 41)
Ethnic group (p. 42)
Subculture (p. 41)
Transcultural nursing (p. 41)

Nurses encounter people of many different backgrounds in their practice. The differences may stem from race, ethnicity, language, or religion. Diverse backgrounds affect the ways individuals react to health and illness, hospitalization, and nursing care.

CULTURAL CONCEPTS

CHARACTERISTICS OF CULTURE

Culture is an integrated system of learned values, beliefs, and practices that guides an individual's behavior. Culture includes the arts, beliefs, customs, folk practices, habits, institutions, and all other products of human work and thought created by a people or a group at a particular time. Culture represents the ideas, beliefs, values, and attitudes that a group of people possess. These values and beliefs are the foundation for setting standards and rules of behavior that members of a society consider acceptable and proper. Culture includes learned ways of acting and thinking that are transmitted by group members and that provide solutions for problems. Dietary habits, customs, modes of communication, religion, art, and history are all aspects of culture. Not only does culture affect a person's decisions and actions, but it also affects health care practices.

Cultural diversity is a term used to describe the existence of many cultures in a society. The United States has a rich cultural diversity as a result of the large number of immigrants who have entered the country over the past 200 years. America is sometimes called a "melting pot" because many immigrants have been assimilated into their new society. Today, the term "salad bowl" is often used instead to describe the way in which new arrivals seek to maintain individual differences while acclimating to new surroundings. It is important to value and respect the differences among the various cultural groups within our society, for each group provides unique contributions to art, science, politics, and health care.

Within certain cultures are groups of individuals who share different beliefs, values, and attitudes from those of the dominant culture. These groups are called *subcultures.* Examples of subcultures in the United States are members of various ethnic groups, such as African Americans, Latinos/Hispanics, Asians, and Native Americans (Fig. 5-1); homosexuals; the military; and religious groups, such as the Amish or Mormons. Transcultural nursing is the integration of culture into all aspects of nursing care.

Similarities

All cultures share certain basic characteristics: (1) Culture is learned; (2) culture is shared; and (3) culture is based on symbols. People *learn* to be a part of a culture as they are growing up, and the learning may continue into adulthood. This process is known as *enculturation.* Cultural learning is passed down from parent to child to grandchild, affecting the personality development of each generation. People learn what is expected of them and how they should behave, dress, and interact on particular occasions. For example, important life events are celebrated differently in different cultures (Fig. 5-2). Weddings and funerals may be quiet, small occasions for introspection or they may be robust, noisy celebrations with mobs of people in attendance.

Culture also is *shared.* Cultural beliefs, values, and behaviors are shared among individuals within a particular group. Individual behavior does not reflect a particular culture unless it is manifested by other people in the cultural group. From group behavior, the behavior of individuals can then be predicted.

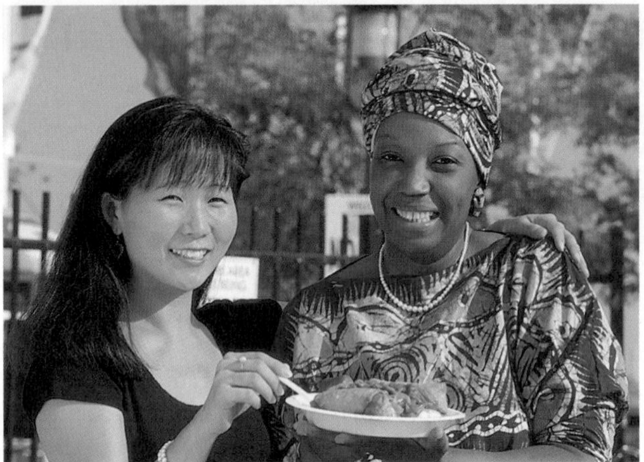

FIGURE 5-1 Many people living in the United States represent many different subcultures.

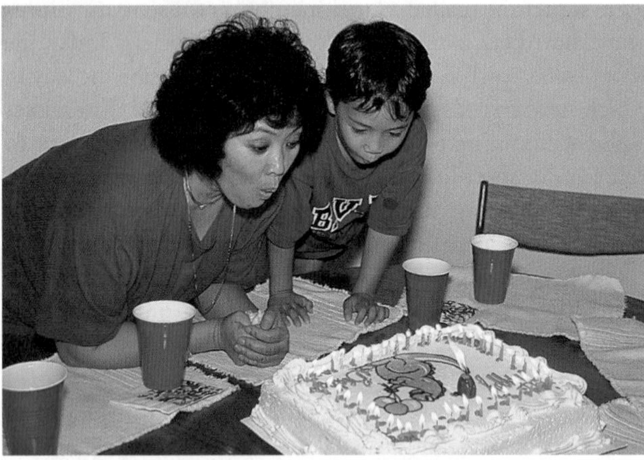

FIGURE 5-2 People of various heritages share a culture as they adopt American practices.

Culture is based on *symbols.* Symbols represent means of communication, spiritual beliefs, economic interactions, and national origins, among other things. Examples of symbols are language (words), religious artifacts (crucifix, Star of David), money (economic interactions), and flags (national origin). Symbols help to convey the beliefs, values, and behaviors of a society or culture.

Differences

Cultural differences may occur among various groups in relation to family, religion, communication, educational background, social class, and economic level. Nurses should be aware of the differences in these areas and recognize how they affect the wellness, illness, and health care practices of their patients.

Family

The family provides a major means for reproducing the population and rearing its children. The family unit is basic to every society. It is mainly through the family that cultural attitudes, values, and behaviors are transmitted.

The family structure may vary among and within cultures. The traditional nuclear family, consisting of a mother, a father, and children, is becoming less of a standard. Single-parent families make up about 20% of all households in the United States. In addition, some cultural groups continue to have extended families living under the same roof (e.g., grandparents, parents, children, and other relatives). Some families have a strong patriarchal (male, father-dominated) influence, whereas others have strong matriarchal (female, mother-dominated) tendencies.

Culture can have an influence on the attitudes and beliefs of families in relation to health care. Behaviors related to health practices, hospitalization, and placement in long-term care facilities can vary among cultures. For example, Latinos and Filipinos are thought to have strong extended family units and family ties, and when a person is hospitalized, family members visit frequently. In addition, Latinos and Filipinos tend to care for their elders in a home setting rather than placing them in residential facilities. Nurses should become acquainted with the various cultural backgrounds of families and how they influence behavior rather than being judgmental about family behaviors.

Religion

Religious beliefs are culturally determined, and how individuals fulfill their spiritual needs stems from a lifetime of experience. Religious beliefs and practices can influence perceptions of health and illness, hospitalization, and death and dying. Some patients may observe specific dietary rules, and others may have particular practices regarding dress, modesty, daily living habits, or medical interventions. Religious differences also occur in relation to the observation of the Sabbath, baptism, the sacrament of the sick, and last rites (Table 5-1).

Communication

Communication involves language. Certain cultural or ethnic groups speak different languages, making communication almost impossible without an interpreter. However, there are also subtler forms of miscommunication that can arise because of group differences. The speed with which people speak and their tone and inflections vary according to cultural background.

Nonverbal communication also is culturally based. Personal space, eye contact, gestures, displays of emotions, and the amount and meaning of touch may have different connotations in different cultures. Some cultures find emotional display more acceptable than others. Some are more comfortable with silence than others.

Educational Background and Economic Level

There are wide differences in educational backgrounds within the United States. Approximately 60 million Americans have literacy skills below the eighth grade level. That means that one out of every three people has difficulty with reading and writing.

Educational level attained is strongly tied to ethnicity and economic background. School dropout rates appear to be

Text continued on p. 50

table 5-1 ***Religious Beliefs and Practices Affecting Health Care***

RELIGIOUS GROUP	BELIEFS AND PRACTICES
WESTERN RELIGIONS	
Judaism	
Orthodox Jews and some Conservative Jewish groups	*Care of women:* A woman is considered to be in a ritual state of impurity whenever blood is coming from her uterus, such as during menstrual periods and after the birth of a child. During this time, her husband will not have physical contact with her. When this time is completed, she will bathe herself in a pool called a mikvah. Nurses need to be aware of this practice and be sensitive to the husband and wife because the husband will not touch his wife. He cannot assist her in moving in the bed, so the nurse will have to do this. An Orthodox Jewish man will not touch any women other than his wife, daughters, and mother. *Dietary rules:* (1) Kosher dietary laws include the following: No mixing of milk and meat at a meal; no consumption of food or any derivative thereof from animals not slaughtered in accordance with Jewish law; use of separate cooking utensils for milk and milk products; if a patient requires milk and meat products for a meal, the dairy foods should be served first, followed later by the meat. (2) During Yom Kippur (Day of Atonement), a 24-hour fast is required, but exceptions are made for those who cannot fast because of medical reasons. (3) During Passover, no leavened products are eaten. (4) May say benediction of thanksgiving before meals and grace at the end of the meal. Time and a quiet environment should be provided for this. *Sabbath:* Observed from sunset Friday until sunset Saturday. Orthodox law prohibits riding in a car, smoking, turning lights on and off, handling money, and using television and telephone. Nurses need to be aware of this when caring for observant Jews at home and in the hospital. Medical or surgical treatments should be postponed if possible. *Death:* Judaism defines death as occurring when respiration and circulation are irreversibly stopped and no movement is apparent. (1) Euthanasia is strictly forbidden by Orthodox Jews, who advocate the strict use of life-support measures. (2) Prior to death, Jewish faith indicates that visiting of the person by family and friends is a religious duty. The Torah and Psalms may be read and prayers recited. A witness needs to be present when a person prays for health so that if death occurs God will protect the family and the spirit will be committed to God. Extraneous talking and conversation about death are not encouraged unless initiated by the patient or visitors. In Judaism, the belief is that people should have someone with them when the soul leaves the body, so family and/or friends should be allowed to stay with the patients. After death, the body should not be left alone until buried, usually within 24 hours. (3) When death occurs, the body should be untouched for 8 to 30 minutes. Medical personnel should not touch or wash the body but allow only an Orthodox person or the Jewish Burial Society to care for the body. Handling of a corpse on the Sabbath is forbidden to Jewish persons. If need be, the nursing staff may provide routine care of the body, wearing gloves. Water in the room should be emptied, and the family may request that mirrors be covered to symbolize that a death has occurred. (4) Orthodox Jews and some Conservative Jews do not approve of autopsies. If an autopsy must be done, all body parts must remain with the body. (5) For Orthodox Jews, the body must be buried within 24 hours. No flowers are permitted. A fetus must be buried. (6) A 7-day mourning period is required by the immediate family. They must stay at home except for Sabbath worship. (7) Organs or other body parts such as amputed limbs must be made available for burial for Orthodox Jews, because they believe that all of the body must be returned to earth. *Birth control and abortion:* Artificial methods of birth control are not encouraged. Vasectomy is not allowed. Abortion may be performed only to save the mother's life. *Organ transplants:* Donor organ transplants generally are not permitted by Orthodox Jews but may be allowed with rabbinical consent. *Shaving:* The beard is regarded as a mark of piety among observant Jews. For the very Orthodox, shaving should not be done with a razor but with scissors or electric razor, because a blade should not contact the skin.

From Black, J.M., & Matassarin-Jacobs, E. (1993). *Luckmann and Sorensen's medical-surgical nursing: A psychophysiologic approach* (4th ed.). Philadelphia: Saunders. Modified from Carson, V.B. (1989). *Spiritual dimensions of nursing practice.* Philadelphia: Saunders.

Continued

table 5-1 Religious Beliefs and Practices Affecting Health Care—cont'd

RELIGIOUS GROUP	BELIEFS AND PRACTICES
WESTERN RELIGIONS—cont'd	
Judaism—cont'd	
Orthodox Jews and some Conservative Jewish groups —cont'd	*Head coverings:* Orthodox men wear skull caps at all times, and women cover their hair after marriage. Some Orthodox women wear wigs as a mark of piety. Conservative Jews cover their heads only during acts of worship and prayer. *Prayer:* Praying directly to God, including a prayer of confession, is required for Orthodox Jews. Nurses should provide quiet time for prayer.
Reform Jews	*Care of women:* Reform Jews do not observe the rules against touching. *Dietary rules:* Reform Jews usually do not observe kosher dietary restrictions. *Sabbath:* Usually worship in temples on Friday evenings. No strict rules. *Death:* Advocate use of life support without heroic measures. Allow for cremation but suggest that ashes be buried in a Jewish cemetery. *Organ transplants:* Donation or transplantation of organs allowed with permission of a rabbi. *Head coverings:* Generally pray without wearing skullcaps.
Christianity	
Roman Catholic	*Holy Eucharist:* For patients and health care givers who are to receive communion, abstinence from solid food and alcohol is required for 15 minutes (if possible) prior to reception of the consecrated wafer. Medicine, water, and nonalcoholic drinks are permitted at any time. If a patient is in danger of death, the fast is waived because the reception of the Eucharist at this time is very important. *Anointing of the sick:* The priest uses oil to anoint the forehead and hands and, if desired, the affected area. The rite may be performed on any who are ill and desire it. Patients receiving the sacrament seek complete healing and strength to endure suffering. Prior to 1963, this sacrament was given only to patients at the time of imminent death, so the nurse must be sensitive to the meaning this has for the patient. If possible, the nurse calls a priest before the patient is unconscious but may also call when there is sudden death, because the sacrament may also be give shortly after death. The nurse records on the care plan that this sacrament has been administered. *Dietary habits:* Obligatory fasting is excused during hospitalization. However, if there are no health restrictions, some Catholics may still observe the following guidelines: (1) Anyone 14 years or older must abstain from eating meat on Ash Wednesday and all Fridays during Lent. Some older Catholics may still abstain from meat on all Fridays of the year. (2) In addition to abstinence from meat, persons 21 to 59 years of age must limit themselves to one full meal and two light meals on Ash Wednesday and Good Friday. (3) Eastern Rite Catholics are stricter about fasting and fast more frequently than Western Rite Catholics, so it is important for the nurse to know if a patient is Eastern or Western Catholic. *Death:* Each Roman Catholic should participate in the anointing of the sick as well as the Eucharist and penance before death. The body should not be shrouded until after these sacraments are performed. All body parts that retain human quality must be appropriately buried or cremated. *Birth control:* Prohibited except for abstinence or natural family planning. Referral to a priest for questions about this can be of great help. Nurses can teach the techniques of natural family planning if they are familiar with them; otherwise, this should be referred to the physician or to a support group of the church that instructs couples in this method of birth control. Sterilization is prohibited unless there is an overriding medical reason. *Organ transplants:* Donation and transplantation of organs are acceptable as long as the donor is not harmed and is not deprived of life. *Religous objects:* Rosary prayers are said using rosary beads. Medals bearing the images of saints, relics, statues, and scapulars are important objects that may be pinned to a hospital gown or pillow or be at the bedside. Extreme care should be taken not to lose these objects, because they have special meaning to the patient.

From Black, J.M., & Matassarin-Jacobs, E. (1993). *Luckmann and Sorensen's medical-surgical nursing: A psychophysiologic approach* (4th ed.). Philadelphia: Saunders. Modified from Carson, V.B. (1989). *Spiritual dimensions of nursing practice.* Philadelphia: Saunders.

table 5-1 ***Religious Beliefs and Practices Affecting Health Care—cont'd***

RELIGIOUS GROUP	BELIEFS AND PRACTICES
WESTERN RELIGIONS—cont'd	
Christianity—cont'd	
Eastern Orthodox	*Holy Eucharist:* The priest is notified if the patient desires this sacrament. *Anointing of the sick:* The priest conducts this in the hospital room. *Dietary habits:* Fasting from meat and dairy products is required on Wednesday and Friday during Lent and on other holy days. Hospital patients are exempt if fasting is detrimental to health. *Special days:* Christmas is celebrated on January 7 and New Year's Day on January 14. This is important to the care of a patient who is hospitalized on these days. *Death:* Last rites are obligatory. This is handled by an ordained priest who is notified by the nurse while the patient is conscious. The Russian Orthodox Church does not encourage autopsy or organ donation. Euthanasia, even for the terminally ill, is discouraged, as is cremation. *Birth control:* This as well as abortion is not permitted.
Protestant	
Assemblies of God (Pentecostal)	*Holy Communion:* Notify clergy if the patient desires. *Anointing of the sick:* Members believe in divine healing through prayer and the laying on of hands. Clergy is notified if patient or family desires this. *Dietary habits:* Abstinence from alcohol, tobacco, and all illegal drugs is strongly encouraged. *Death:* No special practices. *Other practices:* Faith in God and in the health care providers is encouraged. Members pray for divine intervention in health matters. Nurses should encourage and allow time for prayer. Members may speak in "tongues" during prayer.
Baptist (over 27 different groups in the United States)	*Holy Communion:* Clergy should be notified if the patient desires. *Dietary habits:* Total abstinence from alcohol is expected. *Death:* No general service is provided, but the clergy does minister through counseling, prayer, and Scripture as requested by the patient or family, and the patient is encouraged to believe in Jesus Christ as Savior and Lord. *Other practices:* The Bible is held to be the word of God, so the nurse should either allow quiet time for Scripture reading or offer to read to the patient.
Christian Church (Disciples of Christ)	*Holy Communion:* Open communion is celebrated each Sunday and is a central part of worship services. The nurse notifies the clergy if the patient desires it, or the clergy may suggest it. *Death:* No special practices. *Other practices:* Church elders as well as clergy may be notified to assist with meeting the patient's spiritual needs.
Church of the Brethren	*Holy Communion:* Usually received within church, but clergy will give it in the hospital when requested. *Anointing of the sick:* Practiced for physical healing as well as spiritual uplift and held in high regard by the church. The clergy is notified if the patient or family desires. *Death:* The clergy is notified for counsel and prayer.
Church of the Nazarene	*Holy Communion:* Pastor will administer if the patient wishes. *Dietary habits:* The use of alcohol and tobacco is forbidden. *Death:* Cremation is permitted, and term stillborn infants are buried. *Other practices:* Believe in divine healing but not to the exclusion of medical treatment. Patients may desire quiet time for prayer.
Episcopal (Anglican)	*Holy Communion:* The priest is notified if the patient wishes to receive this sacrament. *Anointing of the sick:* Priest may administer this rite when death is imminent, but it is not considered mandatory. *Dietary habits:* Some patients may abstain from meat on Fridays. Others may fast before receiving the Eucharist, but fasting is not mandatory. *Death:* No special practices. *Other practices:* Confession of sins to a priest is optional; if the patient desires this, the clergy should be notified.

Continued

table 5-1 ***Religious Beliefs and Practices Affecting Health Care—cont'd***

RELIGIOUS GROUP	BELIEFS AND PRACTICES
WESTERN RELIGIONS—cont'd	
Christianity—cont'd	
Protestant—cont'd	
Lutheran (18 different branches)	*Holy Communion:* Notify the clergy if the patient desires this sacrament. Clergy may also inquire about the patient's desire. *Anointing of the sick:* The patient may request an anointing and blessing from the minister when the prognosis is poor. *Death:* A service of Commendation of the Dying is used at the patient's or family's request.
Mennonite (12 different groups)	*Holy Communion:* Served twice a year, with foot washing as part of ceremony. *Dietary habits:* Abstinence from alcohol is urged for all. *Death:* Prayer is important at time of crisis, so contacting a minister is important. *Other practices:* Women may wear head coverings during hospitalization. Anointing with oil is administered in harmony with James 5:14 when requested.
Methodist (over 20 different groups)	*Holy Communion:* Notify the clergy if a patient requests it prior to surgery or another health crisis. *Anointing of the sick:* If requested, the clergy will come to pray and sprinkle the patient with olive oil. *Death:* Scripture reading and prayer are important at this time. *Other practices:* Donation of one's body or part of the body at death is encouraged.
Presbyterian (10 different groups)	*Holy Communion:* Given when appropriate and convenient, at the hospitalized patient's request. *Death:* Notify a local pastor or elder for prayer and Scripture reading if desired by the family or patient.
Quaker (Friends)	*Holy Communion:* Because Friends have no creed, there is a diversity of personal beliefs, one of which is that outward sacraments are usually not necessary because there is the ministry of the Spirit inwardly in such areas as baptism and communion. *Death:* Believe that the present life is part of God's kingdom and generally have no ceremony as a rite of passage from this life to the next. Personal beliefs and wishes need to be ascertained, and the nurse can then act on the patient's wishes.
Salvation Army	*Holy Communion:* No particular ceremony. *Death:* Notify the local officer in charge of the Army Corps for any soldier (member) who needs assistance. *Other practices:* The Bible is seen as the only rule for one's faith, so the Scriptures should be made available to a patient. The Army has many of its own social welfare centers, with hospitals and homes where unwed mothers are cared for and outpatient services provided. No medical or surgical procedures are opposed, except for abortion on demand.
Seventh-Day Adventist	*Holy Communion:* Although this is not required of hospitalized patients, the clergy are notified if the patient desires. *Anointing of the sick:* The clergy are contacted for prayer and anointing with oil. *Dietary habits:* Because the body is viewed as the temple of the Holy Spirit, healthy living is essential. Therefore, the use of alcohol, tobacco, coffee, and tea and the promiscuous use of drugs are prohibited. Some are vegetarians, and most avoid pork. *Special days:* The Sabbath is observed on Saturday. *Death:* No special procedures. *Other practices:* Use of hypnotism is opposed by some. Persons of homosexual or lesbian orientation are ministered to in the hope of correction of these practices, which are believed to be wrong. A Bible should always be available for Scripture reading.
United Church of Christ	*Holy Communion:* Clergy are notified if the patient desires to receive this sacrament. *Death:* If the patient desires counsel or prayer, notify the clergy.

From Black, J.M., & Matassarin-Jacobs, E. (1993). *Luckmann and Sorensen's medical-surgical nursing: A psychophysiologic approach* (4th ed.). Philadelphia: Saunders. Modified from Carson, V.B. (1989). *Spiritual dimensions of nursing practice.* Philadelphia: Saunders.

table 5-1 ***Religious Beliefs and Practices Affecting Health Care—cont'd***

RELIGIOUS GROUP	BELIEFS AND PRACTICES
WESTERN RELIGIONS—cont'd	
Other	
Christian Science	*Dietary habits:* Because alcohol and tobacco are considered drugs, they are not used. Coffee and tea are often declined. *Death:* Autopsy is usually declined unless required by law. Donation of organs is unlikely but is an individual decision. *Other practices:* Christian Scientists do not normally seek medical care, because they approach health care in a different, primarily spiritual, framework. They commonly use the services of a surgeon to set a bone but decline drugs and, in general, other medical or surgical procedures. Hypnotism and psychotherapy are also declined. Family planning is left to the family. They seek exemption from vaccinations but obey legal requirements (e.g., report infectious diseases and obey public health quarantines). Nonmedical care facilities are maintained for those needing nursing assistance in the course of a healing. *The Christian Science Journal* lists available Christian Science nurses. When a Christian Science believer is in the hospital, the nurse should allow and encourage time for prayer and study. Patients may request that a Christian Science practitioner be notified to come.
Jehovah's Witnesses	*Dietary habits:* Use of alcohol and tobacco is discouraged because these harm the physical body. *Death:* Autopsy is a private matter to be decided by the persons involved. Burial and cremation are acceptable. *Birth control and abortion:* Use of birth control is a personal decision. Abortion is opposed based on Exodus 21:22-23. *Organ transplants:* Use of organ transplant is a private decision and if used must be cleansed with a nonblood solution. *Blood transfusions:* Blood transfusions violate God's laws and therefore are not allowed. Patients do respect physicians and will accept alternatives to blood transfusions. These might include use of nonblood plasma expanders, careful surgical techniques to decrease blood loss, use of autologous transfusions, and autotransfusion through use of a heart-lung machine. Nurses should check unconscious patients for Medic Alert cards that state that the person does not want a transfusion. Since Jehovah's Witnesses are prepared to die rather than break God's law, nurses need to be sensitive to the spiritual and the physical needs of the patient.
The Church of Jesus Christ of Latter-Day Saints	*Holy Communion:* A hospitalized patient may desire to have a member of the church priesthood administer this sacrament. *Anointing of the sick:* Mormons frequently are anointed and given a blessing before going to the hospital and after admission by laying on of hands. *Dietary habits:* Abstinence from the use of tobacco; beverages with caffeine such as cola, coffee, and tea; alcohol and other substances considered injurious. Mormons eat meat but encourage the intake of fruits, grains, and herbs. *Death:* Prefer burial of the body. A church elder should be notified to assist the family. If need be, the elder will assist the funeral director in dressing the body in special clothes and will give other help as needed. *Birth control and abortion:* Abortion is opposed except when the life of the mother is in danger. Only natural means of birth control are recommended. Artificial means can be used when the health of the woman is at stake (including emotional health). *Personal care:* Cleanliness is very important to Mormons. A sacred undergarment may be worn at all times by Mormons and should only be removed in emergency situations. *Other practices:* Allowing quiet time for prayer and the reading of the sacred writings is important. The church maintains a welfare system to assist those in need. Families are of great importance, so visiting should be encouraged.

Continued

table 5-1 *Religious Beliefs and Practices Affecting Health Care—cont'd*

RELIGIOUS GROUP	BELIEFS AND PRACTICES
WESTERN RELIGIONS—cont'd	
Other—cont'd	
Unitarian Universalist Association	*Death:* Cremation is often preferred to burial. *Other practices:* Use of birth control is advocated as part of responsible parenting. Strong support for a woman's right to choice regarding abortion is maintained. Unitarian Universalists advocate donation of body parts for research and transplants.
Unification Church	*Baptism:* No baptism occurs. *Special days:* Sunday mornings are used to honor Reverend and Mrs. Moon as the true parents, and members get up at 5:00 AM, bow before a picture of the Moons three times, and vow to do what is needed to help the Reverend accomplish his mission on earth. *Death:* They believe that after death one's place of destiny will depend on his or her spirit's quality of life and goodness while on earth. In the afterlife, one will have the same aspirations and feelings as before death. Hell is not a concern, because it will not be a place as heaven grows in size. Persons who leave the Unification Church are warned that Satan may try to possess them. *Other practices:* All marriages must be solemnized by Reverend Moon to be part of the perfect family and have salvation. The church supplies its faithful members with life's necessities. Members may use occult practices to have spiritual and psychic experiences.
Islam	*Dietary habits:* No pork is allowed, or alcoholic beverages. All halal (permissible) meat must be blessed and killed in a special way. This is called zabihah (correctly slaughtered). *Death:* Prior to death, family members ask to be present so that they can read the Koran and pray with the patient. An Imam may come if requested by the patient or family but is not required. Patients must face Mecca and confess their sins and beg forgiveness in the presence of their family. If the family is unavailable, any practicing Muslim can provide support to the patient. After death, Muslims prefer that the family wash, prepare, and place the body in a position facing Mecca. If necessary, the health care providers may perform these procedures as long as they wear gloves. Burial is performed as soon as possible. Cremation is forbidden. Autopsy is also prohibited except for legal reasons, and then no body part is to be removed. Donation of body parts or organs is not allowed, because according to culturally developed law, persons do not own their body. *Abortion and birth control:* Abortion is forbidden, and many conservative Muslims do not encourage the use of contraceptives because this interferes with God's purpose. Others feel that a woman should have only as many children as her husband can afford. Contraception is permitted by Islamic law. *Personal devotions:* At prayer time, washing is required, even by those who are sick. A patient on bedrest may require assistance with this task before prayer. Provision of privacy during prayer is important. *Religious objects:* The Koran must not be touched by anyone ritually unclean, and nothing should be placed on top of it. Some Muslims wear taviz, a black string on which words of the Koran are attached. These should not be removed and must remain dry. Certain items of jewelry such as bangles may have religious significance and should not be removed unnecessarily. *Care of women:* Because women are not allowed to sign consent forms or make a decision regarding family planning, the husband needs to be present. Women are very modest and frequently wear clothes that cover all of the body. During a medical examination, the woman's modesty should be respected as much as possible. Muslim women prefer female doctors. For 40 days after giving birth and also during menstruation, a woman is exempt from prayer because this is a time of cleansing for her.

From Black, J.M., & Matassarin-Jacobs, E. (1993). *Luckmann and Sorensen's medical-surgical nursing: A psychophysiologic approach* (4th ed.). Philadelphia: Saunders. Modified from Carson, V.B. (1989). *Spiritual dimensions of nursing practice.* Philadelphia: Saunders.

table 5-1 *Religious Beliefs and Practices Affecting Health Care—cont'd*

RELIGIOUS GROUP	BELIEFS AND PRACTICES
WESTERN RELIGIONS—cont'd	
Islam—cont'd	
American Muslim Mission	*Dietary habits:* In addition to refusing pork, many will not eat traditional black American foods such as corn bread and collard greens. *Death:* The family is contacted before any care of the deceased is performed. There are special procedures for washing and shrouding the body. *Other practices:* Quiet time is necessary to permit prayer. Members are encouraged to use black physicians for health care. Because these patients do not smoke, their request for a nonsmoking roommate should be honored.
EASTERN RELIGIONS	
Hinduism	*Dietary habits:* Some sects are vegetarian, believing meats and intoxicants to be too stimulating to the senses. *Belief about illness:* View illnesses as a result of misuse of the body or a consequence of sins committed in a previous life. They do not oppose medical treatment, but view its effect as transitory. Believe that praying for health is the lowest form of prayer. *Death:* See death as a union with Brahman (God) achieved through prayers, ritual, purity, self-control, detachment, truth, nonviolence, charity, and compassion toward all creatures. Following death, one will be reborn (reincarnated) into a future life based on the behavior in this life. The record of behavior is called karma. Eventually, the process of rebirth stops, which is called moksha. A priest may be called at the time of death, and may tie a thread around the neck or waist as a blessing. The family washes the body, and it is cremated. *Other practices:* Offer daily worship at a shrine in the home. Daily offering to God, and morning and evening rites. Society is organized into castes, or strata. People are born into a caste, and the caste shapes one's entire life. Hindus practice a discipline of the mind and body, called yoga, to reach god. In the highest state, a meditating yogi does not see, hear, taste, feel, or smell. Beyond good and evil, time and space, the yogi is one with God.
Buddhism	*Death:* Believe that salvation depends on one's own right living. Believe in reincarnation. Can speed the process toward Nirvana, the goal of all humanity's striving, through acts of merit. Meditation, worship, and prayer are some of the acts of merit. Buddhists may drive themselves into more and more ritual or contemplation in the hope that their last moments of consciousness may be filled with thoughts worthy enough to elevate them to a higher existence. Last rights of chanting may be performed at bedside. *Renunciation:* The most important Buddhist feasts. Young boys are taught to despise the world's vanity, and the boy spends a night in a nearby monastery.
Taoism/Confucianism	*General beliefs:* Founded on ethical principles of Confucius. God is not clearly defined as in other religions. Taoism is a mixture of magic and religion. Believe that humans and nature are inseparable, and that if heaven is upset, earth does not prosper. This relationship is described as yang and yin, which are two interplaying forces. When yang and yin are in balance, good occurs. *Death:* The dead are remembered in all festivals. The fate of the dead in the afterworld depends not only on the life they led but also on being properly honored after death. Otherwise they may become demons. Graves are mounds like those dedicated to the gifts of the soil. Graves and houses must be in harmony with the universe, otherwise evil will befall the occupants.

higher among teenagers living in poverty areas. Ethnic groups that are found in large numbers in poverty areas tend to have high dropout rates.

Educational background and economic levels affect the ways in which people perceive the world, health and illness, and the health care system. Teaching about health becomes a challenge because many with low literacy levels have difficulty reading the materials presented and understanding health care jargon. In addition, people from economically deprived backgrounds may live in crowded, unsafe housing and have inadequate diets. Such conditions make health promotion and disease prevention more difficult.

CULTURAL BELIEFS RELATED TO HEALTH AND ILLNESS

Health and illness have different meanings for different people and cultural groups. For some groups, illness is something that is expected as part of life and is out of one's own control. For others, it is believed that illness can be prevented by taking action, such as eating a proper diet, getting exercise, or scheduling regular physical examinations.

Some groups attempt to attach meaning to illness to explain why illness occurs. They have developed many beliefs regarding the onset, course, and cure of disease, as well as the process of death and dying. For example, there is a belief in divine punishment as the cause of illness. Believers in divine punishment claim that illness is a result of punishment for a sin that an individual has committed. Another belief involves an individual's balance with nature. If a person maintains a proper balance, good health results; if a person is not in harmony with the environment, illness occurs.

The "hot" and "cold" theory is an ancient belief about health and illness that still is held widely in many cultures. According to the hot and cold theory, health and illness are influenced by four humors that regulate body functions. The four humors are phlegm, blood, black bile, and yellow bile. The humors are considered either hot (blood and yellow bile) or cold (phlegm and black bile), and an imbalance between the hot and the cold areas of the body causes illness. Examples of illnesses that are thought to be caused by cold entering the body are earaches, paralysis, stomach cramps, and arthritis. Examples of illnesses thought to be caused by heat include dysentery, sore throats, abscessed teeth, and kidney disease. Illnesses are treated with herbs, potions, and food that are considered to be either hot or cold, depending on their effects on the body.

Many ethnic groups use healers who practice health care outside of the formal health care delivery system. Patients may visit a folk healer or use folk remedies along with or in place of conventional treatment. Western societies generally believe that illness has a known cause that can be treated or cured if the cause is identified. Western medicine is also focused on risk reduction and prevention. Generally, non-Western societies believe illness is due to supernatural causes, and they have a more holistic approach to illness. Traditional healers deal with forms of healing that may be secular, sacred, or both. The variety of healers depends on the number of health cultures. Examples of traditional healers are root doctors, who often practice among urban African Americans, and *curanderos,* who are consulted by Latinos. They may be sought when mainstream health care is perceived as being too expensive, inconvenient, or unable to provide relief for the problem at hand. The healers provide psychosocial support and counseling in addition to helping with physiologic problems. They use a variety of potions and plants in their practice.

TRADITIONAL HEALTH HABITS AND BELIEFS OF MAJOR ETHNIC GROUPS IN THE UNITED STATES

Although it is inappropriate to stereotype individual members of any culture or subculture, various ethnic groups in the United States tend to have unique, traditional health-culture beliefs and practices. Great variations in beliefs and practices exist not only between but also within ethnic and subcultural groups. Although individuals vary, in a given ethnic group there are generally some common ideas and practices regarding health promotion and disease prevention, attitudes and behaviors related to illness, and utilization of health care resources. One factor that affects the extent to which an individual maintains traditional practices is the extent of enculturation and assimilation into U.S. society that has occurred. First- or second-generation Americans may have more characteristics associated with their ethnic group than people who have been in the United States for several generations.

Listed next are examples of traditional health care beliefs and practices of selected ethnic groups. Remember that these examples are included to show a range of possible health customs for selected ethnic groups. They cannot be generalized to all members of the ethnic group or subculture.

WHITES (EURO-AMERICANS)

Like other racial/ethnic groups, white Americans are very homogeneous even though most descended from European roots. Nevertheless, it is useful to identify some values and beliefs common to this group of people. Whites generally believe in the work ethic, which values personal achievement, individualism, and competition. Values related to health include individual decision making, personal space, and privacy. Illness is viewed primarily as caused by germs in the environment or, in certain religious groups, by divine punishment. The risk of illness can be reduced by eating a proper diet, getting enough exercise, and allowing for adequate rest. In the treatment of illness, the mind, body, and spirit are thought of as separate. Whites look to science and technology for the treatment of illness.

White Americans often communicate directly and tend to express feelings of pain openly. Although members of this group tend to use the formal health care system for their medical and nursing needs, they may consult spiritual advisers in times of illness. Traditionally the health care provider has been seen as the manager of care.

AFRICAN AMERICANS

African Americans value family, community, religion, health, and work. In addition to an understanding about germs as a cause of illness, some traditional beliefs attribute illness to divine punishment or to an imbalance among body, mind, and spirit. Prevention of illness is thought to be achieved through eating good food, living right, and keeping the system cleaned out. Communication may be direct or indirect, and expressions of pain during illness may entail varying degrees of stoicism or vocal outcries to God for assistance. African Americans tend to attempt self-care before consulting a health care professional when they are ill. They also may use folk medicine or consult a root doctor or spiritualist for help.

LATINOS/HISPANICS

People whose heritage is rooted in various parts of South or Central America refer to themselves as Latinos or Hispanics. To reduce repetition, the term Latinos will be used in this text. Latinos, particularly those who live in the southwestern United States, are family oriented and value harmony in interpersonal relationships. Traditional beliefs about the cause of illness include magical fright, divine punishment, an imbalance of hot and cold elements in the body, and environmental hazards. Some believe that illness can be prevented through the use of charms, amulets, or crucifixes. Communication is usually indirect; however, expressions of pain are open and direct. Folk health specialists *(curanderos)* and family members may be consulted along with the formal health care system in times of illness.

ASIANS

Asians value self-respect, self-control, respect for elders, family honor, loyalty, and pride. There is an emphasis on holistic health and harmony between the self and the universe. Asians in the United States may favor health care that is provided by herbalists, acupuncturists, and other cultural healers, but many use the formal health care system in times of illness. Communication patterns tend to be indirect, and pain is endured with varying degrees of stoicism.

NATIVE AMERICANS

There is considerable diversity among tribes and groups, so it is important to use caution when making generalizations about Native Americans. However, some general characteristics may be noted. Native Americans value family, respect for elders, generosity, and cooperation with others. They attempt to live in harmony with nature and have deep respect for the environment. Communication is usually indirect, with a great emphasis on nonverbal cues. Pain is usually dealt with stoically. Traditional health practices emphasize total healing, mental and spiritual renewal, and health maintenance. Ceremonial rituals guided by a medicine man may be used for treating illnesses before structured medical care is sought.

To emphasize once again, the examples given here are intended to convey the wide scope of culturally based practices that may need to be considered when working with individuals from various cultures. The nursing assessment should include gathering information about personal health practices so that the care plan can be individualized.

Put on your THINKING CAP!!

Considering your own race/ethnicity, identify three cultural beliefs related to health that are held by your family. For example, how are you expected to respond to illness or stress? When do you seek medical care, and what kind of provider do you see? Do you use any complementary or alternative therapies? What activities are believed to promote health or prevent disease?

CULTURAL INFLUENCES ON PATIENT AND FAMILY INTERACTIONS WITH THE HEALTH CARE SYSTEM

In all health care settings, patients of different cultures may exhibit behavior that is not understood by health care providers. The culturally different patients may be labeled "complaining," "difficult," "uncooperative," or "noncompliant" when in reality they are struggling to adapt to a culture that is foreign to them. Fear of the unknown may result in these behaviors. Culturally competent care is urgently needed. With increasing cultural diversity among all people in the United States, you must consider your patients' cultures and develop culture-specific nursing care.

HOSPITAL HEALTH CARE

The hospital environment is often frightening, even to people who are familiar with it. For individuals who may speak different languages, have different eating preferences, and maintain different attitudes toward health and illness, adapting to the hospital environment is a formidable task. Admission to the hospital may seem like traveling to a foreign country where an entirely different language is spoken. Hospital personnel become authority figures, and their permission is needed to carry out the most basic activities, such as toileting, eating, and dressing. Patients are stripped of their dignity when they are told to wear hospital gowns that barely cover private parts of the body. Modesty is often ignored, causing humiliation and anxiety.

Not only do people find themselves in a totally new environment, but they must also endure separation from their family and friends. Their support systems topple when strict visiting rules are enforced. In some cultures families expect to help with the nursing care, or at least sit with sick people to keep them company and provide support. Nurses and hospital personnel often are uncomfortable with this infringement on their territory. Language barriers may complicate the process of providing care.

Culture shock associated with hospitalization occurs in three phases. During the first phase, the patient asks questions regarding the hospital routine and the hospital's expectations of the patient. In the second phase, the patient becomes disenchanted with the whole situation and is frustrated, hostile, and then depressed and withdrawn. In the final phase, the patient begins to adapt to the new environment and is even able to maintain a sense of humor during interactions with others.

COMMUNITY AND HOME HEALTH CARE

Community settings in which culturally different individuals interact with the health care system include physicians' offices, outpatient clinics, community mental health centers, home health care, hospices, and day care centers. As mentioned earlier, individuals who have different cultural backgrounds also may have their own network of health care, such as spiritualists, *curanderos,* or root doctors. A day's assignment in home health care may include visits to Jewish, Hispanic, Filipino, and Anglo-American homes. Community nursing presents examples of cultural diversity that nurses everywhere are experiencing with the expanded need for home health services.

Many ethnic or cultural minorities have difficulty getting through the maze of health care services, either because of language differences or because of negative attitudes toward health care providers based on past experiences. Minority group members whose financial resources are limited frequently are clinic patients who must wait hours for an appointment, only to receive a cursory assessment from the physician or nurse. Their questions about their condition may be left unanswered because of communication difficulties, which can affect the ability to follow directions for care. These patients may be labeled "noncompliant" or "difficult," which only perpetuates a cycle of negative attitudes among patients and health care providers alike.

When you enter a patient's home, watch for symbolic objects that may indicate cultural identity. Shrines, religious pictures or statues, and special candles are examples of symbols. Assess your patient's health beliefs and practices that are affected by culture. Patients and their families may have magical, religious, biomedical, or holistic beliefs.

If the patient speaks a different language from yours, sometimes a family member is able to translate. If there is no translator available, you may need to spend extra time demonstrating a procedure to the patient and the family.

LONG-TERM FACILITY HEALTH CARE

The majority of residents in long-term care facilities are white women. Some ethnic groups such as Latinos and Asians are extremely reluctant to admit older relatives to residential care facilities and prefer to provide care at home.

Many residents of such facilities suffer from functional impairments (impaired ability to carry out activities of daily living such as bathing and dressing). Those from different cultural groups have the added strain of communication problems and extreme changes in lifestyle and dietary practices. These differences may contribute to confusion, disability, and incontinence. For example, an older woman who speaks little English may have difficulty asking for help getting to the bathroom or using a bedpan. Because older people tend to have very little time between the urge to void and the actual voiding experience, urinary incontinence can occur when a nurse has difficulty understanding their needs.

CULTURAL EXPRESSIONS AND IMPLICATIONS FOR NURSING CARE

When caring for a patient who is from another religious or ethnic background, you should be sensitive to different cultural attitudes, beliefs, and behaviors. Cultural sensitivity and valuing alternative ways of dealing with health issues as well as spiritual beliefs allow you to individualize care. Avoid labeling patients "difficult" or "uncooperative" because you do not understand their behavior. As a practical nurse, you must be able to accept a wide diversity of beliefs, practices, and ideas about health and illness, including many that are different from your own. The more sensitive you are to cultural differences, the more effective your nursing intervention will be. Failure to provide culturally sensitive care can cause additional stress and prolong the patient's recovery time.

It is important to gather information regarding the cultural background of a patient to provide sensitive care. For example, communication patterns, including the language spoken and the use of touching and gesturing, may differ among patients. Obtain information regarding health beliefs, interpersonal relationships, the role of the family during illness, attitudes toward modesty, expressions of fear and pain, and dietary practices. Remember that reactions to pain differ among cultures; some groups are very stoic and do not complain, while other groups cry out with pain much of the time.

Sensitivity to cultural factors that affect behavior comes from cultural awareness. To develop cultural awareness, make a conscious and consistent effort to study different cultural groups and their special cultural background. It is helpful to learn the language of your patients. No matter how different your beliefs are from your patient's beliefs, you must respect each person's values and cultural beliefs and respond in a nonjudgmental way.

THERAPEUTIC RELATIONSHIP

Because all nursing care takes place in the framework of the nurse–patient relationship, an environment of acceptance and respect for the beliefs and behaviors of culturally different patients should be established. Patients can develop a feeling of trust if they feel safe, respected, and accepted.

Maintain an open and inquiring, respectful attitude regarding cultural differences. Patients of another culture initially may be quiet, polite, conforming, or shy. This behavior may reflect a guarded or cautious response because patients are not sure what is expected of them and how the interaction will go. It is a time to "size up" unfamiliar health care personnel without being too offensive or alarming. A good rule of thumb during an initial encounter with minority patients is to speak softly and in an unhurried manner to put them at ease. When nursing staff members are aggressive and demanding, patients tend to be silently angry and withdrawn.

Take the time to sit down with patients and their families, listen to their needs and concerns, and learn how they interact.

Culture serves as a guide to action and beliefs in times of crisis. Illness is a time of crisis. Therefore you need to know the patient's cultural patterns of thinking, feeling, and acting before developing a therapeutic plan of care. Once you understand the lifestyle of the patient, you can tailor the nursing care plan to help the patient get through the crisis. Involve the patient in the care plan, identifying familiar ways of coping with an illness or with any other crisis.

Conflicts between the patient's health practices and beliefs and those of the health care system may arise. However, the cultural values of patients and families must be given full consideration. Patients are not likely to change their cultural values if they do not want to.

Changes in health patterns for many patients often require some major changes in lifestyle. If a patient does not respond well to prescribed changes in health practices or lifestyle, the patient may be labeled "uncooperative." Try to understand each situation from the viewpoint of the patient, family, and community. It is only then that effective modifications in health practices can take place. As a culturally competent nurse, you can respond to diversity with respect based on accurate knowledge, an accepting attitude, and a belief in the value of each individual. Cultural competence involves knowledge about cultural differences and interpersonal skills in adapting care to these differences.

BASIC PHYSIOLOGIC NEEDS

Cultural attitudes may affect patients' perceptions of personal hygiene and the role of the nurse in assisting with caring for basic bodily needs. Some patients may not take baths routinely. Others may be extremely modest about disrobing in front of family and strangers. Show sensitivity to these feelings by knocking before entering the room and asking permission before touching the patient or assisting with personal hygiene.

During the bath, do not remove a patient's charms, crosses, medals, or other objects without permission. These objects usually have special meaning and cultural significance. Family members may assist with the bath, oral hygiene, bed making, ambulation, or other care giving. The inclusion of significant others in care giving helps to alleviate the stress and anxiety associated with entering the hospital environment and to fulfill cultural expectations for both patients and family members.

Nutrition is an aspect of care affected by culture. Diet is often culturally based, and modifications in diet, to be successful, must take culture into account. An example is recommending corn tortillas instead of flour tortillas, because corn tortillas have more nutritional value.

DRUG THERAPY

We are just beginning to understand that ethnicity influences how people react to drugs. Factors that contribute to the differing responses can be categorized as environmental, cultural, and genetic. Environmental factors related to drug absorption, metabolism, and action include diet, smoking, and alcohol use. For example, Japanese diets are typically high in salt, which makes antihypertensive drugs less effective.

Cultural factors can affect drug response by influencing the patient's expectations, adherence to prescribed drugs, and willingness to report problems to the physician. Additionally, some culturally based nontraditional remedies can interact with prescribed drugs to increase or decrease their effects.

Perhaps the greatest influence of ethnicity in relation to drug therapy is that liver enzymes are controlled by genetic factors. Liver enzymes determine the rate and extent of drug metabolism. People who metabolize drugs slowly are generally at greater risk for drug toxicity than those who metabolize drugs rapidly. To illustrate, people of Japanese and Chinese descent are more likely to be oversedated by diazepam (Valium) because they metabolize the drug more slowly than people of European descent.

There are numerous other examples of variations in drug effects related to ethnicity. In the treatment of hypertension, when compared to whites, blacks respond better to diuretics and not as well to beta blockers and angiotensin-converting enzyme inhibitors. Also, for unknown reasons, people of Asian and Hispanic descent generally respond better to lower doses of antidepressants than whites.

This information is important for the nurse to know when teaching patients about drugs and monitoring for therapeutic and adverse effects. When a patient is not responding in the way we would expect, ethnicity may explain the difference. The patient may require a change in dosage or a different medication.

PATIENT TEACHING

Communication between the nurse and patients and families of different cultures may be especially difficult in the context of teaching. Patients and their families may not be able to understand written or spoken English even if they have some command of the language. Much of the language of health and illness is confusing and complicated and contains many new words that have not been heard before.

The first approach with people of other cultures is to be warm, understanding, and patient. It is important to establish a good interpersonal relationship to develop enough trust so that people feel free to ask questions. Many patients and their families nod their heads in agreement with everything that is taught, even though little comprehension is taking place.

Using both oral and written communication can help to reinforce what has been taught. Written communication in the native language of patients and families greatly aids in their understanding. Having them demonstrate what they have learned helps to confirm that learning has taken place. It may be helpful to seek assistance from staff members who are from the same or similar ethnic backgrounds to facilitate communication. Health care facilities should have a list of interpreters available.

Consider the timing of patient and family teaching in culturally diverse populations. Many cultural groups do not work by the clock and schedules; persons from these groups may not appear for appointments or may come several hours late. Rather than characterizing such individuals as "lazy" or "undisciplined," it would be wiser to carry out patient teaching informally and spontaneously when the opportunity arises.

In addition to considerations of communication and time, other factors related to cultural uniqueness are important to assess when you are teaching patients. These factors include personal space, social organization (patterns of behavior around life events such as illness or death), environmental control, and biologic variations (such as the occurrence of specific diseases in certain ethnic groups).

COMPLEMENTARY AND ALTERNATIVE THERAPIES

Until fairly recently, Western medicine looked at many culturally based preventive and treatment agents and practices as unscientific at best and as dangerous at worst. Growing public interest in the use of "natural" remedies either to replace or to complement Western medicine has gradually forced a reevaluation of the use of such remedies. In 1998, Congress established the National Center for Complementary and Alternative Medicine to formally evaluate these methods for safety and effectiveness, and to provide a source of information for the public. Research is beginning to support the use of some "folk" treatments and to dispel the value of others. This is a rapidly growing field of study, and you are likely to see an increase in the use of these treatments, either alone or in concert with traditional Western practices.

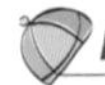

Put on your THINKING CAP!!

Consider how your family reacts to health crises. Identify your family practices related to death. Identify food preferences in your family and discuss health implications. Discuss these culturally related factors with classmates.

key points

- Culture is the integrated system of learned values, beliefs, and practices that is characteristic of a society and that guides individual behavior.
- Cultural diversity denotes the existence of many cultures in a society.
- Culture is learned, shared, and based on symbols.
- Cultural differences may occur among various groups in relation to family, religion, communication, educational background, and economic level.
- Health and illness have different meanings for different people and cultural groups; the nurse must be careful not to stereotype people on the basis of their culture.
- When caring for a patient who is from another religious or ethnic background, the nurse should be sensitive to different cultural attitudes, beliefs, and behaviors.

REVIEW QUESTIONS

1. The process of replacing or giving up values, beliefs, and practices for those of another culture is:
   1. enculturation.
   2. assimilation.
   3. immigration.
   4. diversification.
2. In the United States, Asians and Native Americans are said to be subcultures, which means that they:
   1. share beliefs, values, and attitudes that are different from those of the dominant culture.
   2. are opposed to the basic political structure in the United States.
   3. are highly unlikely to become assimilated into U.S. culture in the future.
   4. believe that their native cultures are superior to the dominant U.S. culture.
3. A patient who is a recent Vietnamese immigrant is recovering from abdominal surgery. Four hours after surgery, he has not asked for any pain medication. It would be most appropriate for you to:
   1. assume that he has a very high level of pain tolerance.
   2. consider that he may be reluctant to report pain.
   3. administer pain medication even if he does not want it.
   4. tell him that suffering is unnecessary when pain medication is ordered.
4. In Labor and Delivery, two patients are at the same stage of labor. Ms. L. is lying still with her eyes closed and her breathing controlled. Ms. G. is grasping the side rails and crying out with each contraction. The nursing assistant says, "I don't know why Ms. G. can't be quiet like Ms. L." Your best response is:
   1. "Tell Ms. G. to be quiet because she is disturbing the other patients."
   2. "There is no reason for Ms. G. to be having more pain than Ms. L."
   3. "People like Ms. G. just like to be very dramatic to get a lot of attention."
   4. "Some people believe that pain should be quietly endured; others express it freely."
5. Nurses need to understand culture because:
   1. care can be based on the patient's culture rather than on individual assessments.
   2. all members of an ethnic group have the same beliefs, values, and attitudes.
   3. culture influences beliefs about health and illness and about health practices.
   4. nurses should encourage members of subcultures to adopt the dominant culture.

CHAPTER

6 The Nurse and the Family

objectives

1. Describe the concept of family and its relationship to society.
2. Compare various family structures or lifestyles that characterize modern American families.
3. Discuss the family from a developmental perspective.
4. Describe roles and communication patterns within families.
5. Describe adaptive and maladaptive mechanisms used by families to cope with various stressors.
6. Describe the role of the nurse in dealing with families experiencing various stresses.
7. Identify community resources that may help to meet the family's needs.

key terms

Dysfunctional communication (p. 58)
Family (p. 55)
Functional communication (p. 58)
Role (p. 57)

The **family** is fundamental to human life. Families exist everywhere and have existed since humankind began. The family unit occupies a position between the individual and society, functioning to meet the needs of the individual members and the needs of the society of which it is a part. The family meets individuals' needs in several ways. For the spouse or adult members, it helps to stabilize their lives by meeting their affectional, socioeconomic, and sexual needs. For children, the family provides physical and emotional support, directs personality development, and is the main learning context for behaviors, thoughts, and feelings. Among its many functions, of prime importance is the role of providing emotional support and security to its members through love, acceptance, concern, and nurturing.

There are several definitions of a family. A general definition is "two or more persons who are joined together by bonds of sharing and emotional closeness and who identify themselves as being part of the family" (Friedman, 1997, p. 9).

TYPES OF FAMILIES

Families differ in their makeup, interactions, and relationships. Many families today vary from the traditional formula of mother, father, and children. More and more family units are composed of single parents or a combination of spouses and offspring from previous marriages. In addition, friends or partners of the same or opposite sex now are often considered family or extended family.

The major types of families are nuclear, extended, stepparent, single-parent, and nontraditional. The traditional nuclear family is made up of biological or adoptive parents—a mother and father—and their children. The extended family consists of relatives of either spouse who live with the nuclear family. This type of family arrangement was more prevalent in the late 1800s and early to mid-1900s than it is now; however, extended family living arrangements still exist, primarily to meet financial or caregiving needs. The stepparent family, or blended family, is made up of stepparents and their children, most often a mother, her biologic children, and a stepfather; however, other variations exist. The single-parent family is characterized by one head of the household, usually a mother or father. The parent may be widowed, divorced, separated, or never married. The nontraditional family takes various forms, including open marriages, communal families, cohabiting couples, group marriages, and gay and lesbian families.

The Census Bureau, in a report on living arrangements of children in the United States, revealed that 56% lived in traditional families, 5.9% lived in multigenerational families, 25% lived in single-parent families, and 16.5% lived in blended families. There also were differences according to race. Children of racial minorities were twice as likely as Anglo children to live in extended families; blended families were more common for African Americans, Native Americans, and Alaskan natives. These figures provide an estimate of the proportion of various types of families in our society, although they do not reflect families with no children.

FAMILY AND CULTURE

In the United States, there are many variations in cultural patterns among families. Within the family, cultural patterns are transmitted from parent to child. The cultural patterns are related to the ethnic background and class of the family and the attitudes of the parents toward people of other ethnic backgrounds and classes. Cultural values and attitudes influence how a family communicates and interacts, carries out activities of daily living, and views health and health care.

Cultural diversity may occur within ethnic groups and classes, so the best way to assess specific cultural patterns of a family is to get the information from the family itself. It is important to determine the family's values, beliefs, customs, and behaviors that influence health needs, health care practices, and family attitudes toward health and illness, health care providers, and health care systems.

FAMILY DEVELOPMENTAL THEORY

FAMILY LIFE CYCLE AND DEVELOPMENTAL TASKS

Every family goes through predictable stages of growth and development, just as individuals do. However, because not all families fit into the traditional nuclear family model, there is variation among stages, depending on the makeup of the family. Responsibilities for growth (developmental tasks) must be met at each developmental stage in order to meet biological needs, cultural demands, and goals. Traditionally, the five major stages of the family life cycle are beginning families, families with young children, families with adolescents, launching children and moving on, and families in later life (Table 6-1).

Beginning Families

The beginning families stage is also referred to as married couples or the stage of marriage. The marriage of a couple marks the beginning of a new family in which the couple moves from their families of origin to a new relationship. During this stage, the developmental tasks include establishing a mutually satisfying marriage, working out satisfactory relationships with each spouse's family, and making decisions about parenthood.

Families with Young Children

During the stage when families have young children, the major activities are childbearing and child rearing up to about age 12. The major developmental tasks are setting up a young family as a stable unit (including integrating a new baby into the family), developing parental roles to meet the changing needs of the children as they grow, maintaining a satisfying marital relationship, maintaining and expanding relationships with the extended family by adding parenting and grandparenting roles, socializing the children, and maintaining healthy relationships outside the family.

Families with Adolescents

The stage when families have teenagers is often the most challenging and difficult. As an adolescent moves from being dependent on and controlled by parents to independence and assumption of adult roles, conflicts and turmoil often emerge. The family developmental tasks at this stage are balancing freedom with responsibility as teenagers mature and become increasingly independent, refocusing on the marital relationship, and communicating openly between parents and children.

Launching Children and Moving On

The stage when families are launching young adults and moving on begins when the first child leaves the parental home and ends with the "empty nest," when the last child has left home. This stage can be short or long, depending on the number of children in the family, how many children remain at home after finishing high school or college, and how many children move back into the home after living independently for a while. The parents are generally middle-aged and may feel "sandwiched" between the demands of youth and the needs of their own elderly family members. It also is a time

table 6-1 ***Stages of the Family Life Cycle***

STAGE	DEVELOPMENTAL TASK
Beginning families	Establish mutually satisfying marriage. Work out satisfactory relationships with spouse's family. Make decisions about parenthood.
Families with young children	Set up young family as a stable unit. Develop parental roles to meet changing needs of children. Maintain satisfying marital relationship. Maintain and expand relationships with extended family. Maintain healthy relationships outside the family.
Families with adolescents	Balance freedom with responsibility in teenagers. Refocus on the marital relationship. Communicate openly between parents and children.
Launching children and moving on	Expand family circle to include new family members acquired by marriage of children. Continue to renew and readjust in the marital relationship. Assist aging and ill parents of the husband and wife.
Families in later life	Maintain satisfying living arrangement. Adjust to loss of a spouse. Maintain intergenerational family ties. Continue to make sense of one's existence.

when they assume the grandparenting role, which requires a change in their roles and self-image. The major family goal is the reorganization of the family into a continuing unit while releasing mature young people into lives of their own. The developmental tasks of this stage include expanding the family circle to include new family members acquired by marriage of children, continuing to renew and readjust in the marital relationship, and assisting aging and ill parents of the husband and wife.

Families in Later Life

The last stage of the family life cycle begins with the retirement of one or both spouses, continues through the loss of one spouse, and ends with the death of the other spouse. In retirement and during the aging process, role modification is necessary, and declines in income, self-esteem, status, and health may occur. The family developmental tasks for this stage are maintaining a satisfying living arrangement, adjusting to a reduced income, maintaining the marital relationship, adjusting to the loss of a spouse, maintaining intergenerational family ties, and continuing to make sense of one's existence.

At each stage, working on and maintaining the marital relationship is identified as a developmental task when the family is made up of a married couple. This type of responsibility for growth is an ongoing and never-ending process throughout life.

FAMILY ROLES AND COMMUNICATIONS

FAMILY ROLE STRUCTURE

Each member of the family has a role. A **role** is how one is expected to behave in a situation or what is expected of a person in a certain position. Culture and social class usually influence how roles are allocated to family members, although greater flexibility of roles has become apparent in recent years. Through these roles, family functions are carried out. Family roles may be performance oriented, such as breadwinner, homemaker, handyman or handywoman, or gardener, or the roles may be emotional, such as leader, nurturer, protector, healer, and rebel. Members may fill more than one role, and any member can satisfactorily fill any role in either category. A healthy family is one in which there is opportunity to shift roles easily from time to time.

In the traditional nuclear family, roles frequently are characterized as formal or informal. Formal roles consist of a limited number of positions in the family that are explicitly defined, such as wife-mother, husband-father, son-brother, and daughter-sister. There are certain role expectations with each of the formal roles, such as wage-earner, homemaker, financial manager, cook, and so on, and these roles are usually given to the person with the skills to carry them out. In smaller families, there are fewer people to take on the various roles, so individuals may play several roles at different times. If for some reason a family member is unable to fill a role or roles, another member must step in to keep the family functioning.

Whereas formal roles are explicit roles that each family role structure contains, informal roles are often not as apparent, and usually meet the emotional needs of individuals or maintain the family's equilibrium. Informal roles have different requirements that are less likely to be based on age or sex and more likely to be based on the personality attributes of individual members. Effective performance of informal roles can strengthen the performance of the formal roles. Some of the roles enhance the well-being of the family, whereas others can interfere with family functioning.

Common informal roles include encourager (praises others' contributions to the family), harmonizer (mediates differences among other members), initiator-contributor (suggests new ideas and initiates action), blocker (opposes and rejects all ideas), martyr (sacrifices everything for the sake of the family), family scapegoat (problem member of the family), family caretaker (nurtures and cares for other members in need), family go-between (the family "switchboard"—transmits and monitors communication within the family), and family coordinator (organizes and plans family activities). The scapegoat usually assumes or is assigned this role to preserve the family and maintain homeostasis. Scapegoating of a family member generally serves to divert attention from marital conflict between the spouses. The go-between is usually the mother, who monitors all communications and is in charge of settling all disputes. When the conflicts are not resolved, the go-between is often blamed. This type of interaction is sometimes considered dysfunctional because it interferes with direct communication between family members.

Family members assume informal roles through role modeling, having to fill in gaps in family roles, and being reinforced for role behaviors. Parents reward children for fulfilling certain roles, so the children gradually adopt these roles as they are growing up. The children then begin to develop a self-identity based on the roles, which may be either positive or negative, and may continue in these roles throughout their lives.

FAMILY INTERACTION

Family interaction is a unique form of social interaction based on a set of intimate and continuing relationships. It is the sum total of all the family roles being actualized within a family at a given time. Family functions and tasks are carried out through the process of interaction. One of the most important influences on family interaction is the self-esteem of each member. If adult members have adequate self-esteem, they are able to provide the love and nurturing to develop self-esteem, belonging, and acceptance necessary for the growth and development of the children. If they lack self-acceptance and self-respect, it is unlikely that they will be loving spouses or parents. In a healthy family, the members love and respect one another.

FAMILY COMMUNICATION PATTERNS

Within family interactions, certain types of communication patterns develop. Communication refers to the process of exchanging feelings, desires, needs, information, and opinions.

Just as individuals have their own distinct style of communication, families also have their unique communication style or pattern. Clear communication is a means of providing a nurturing environment in which family members function well. Conversely, unclear communications may be a major contributor to poor family functioning.

A continual exchange of communication occurs in families. This involves introducing new information, correcting misinformation, problem solving, and having and resolving misunderstandings. The information exchanged may take different routes to reach the receivers. The routes taken depend on the relationships and roles within the family, and these depend on the family power structure, the closeness of relationships, and the popularity of individual members. For example, as noted earlier, many routes of information may go through one person—the go-between—a central member who holds the power and popularity in the family.

Communication in the family may be functional or dysfunctional. However, communication patterns are not totally one way or the other. Rather, they exist on a continuum from functional to dysfunctional, with the patterns of most families falling somewhere in between the polar extremes.

Functional Communication

Functional communication is the clear transmission of a message or information that enables the receiver to understand the intent or meaning of what the sender transmits. Communication in healthy families is a dynamic, two-way process, so that both the sender and the receiver are active participants in the communication. Communication patterns in a functional family demonstrate acceptance of individual differences, openness, honesty, and recognition of the needs and emotions of one another. In addition, the acknowledgment of feelings is essential to healthy family communication. A functional family uses communication to create and maintain mutually beneficial relationships.

Functional patterns of communication include emotional and affective communication. Emotional communication deals with the expression of emotions or feelings, such as anger, hurt, sadness, happiness, affection, and tenderness. A healthy, functional family demonstrates a wide range of emotions and feelings. For family members to be able to enjoy one another, their responses to each other should be fresh and spontaneous rather than controlled, repetitious, and predictable. Affective communication involves verbal messages of caring and nonverbal, physical gestures of touching, caressing, holding, and looking. Physical expressions of affection usually predominate in early childhood and are essential in the development of normal affectional responses. As children grow older, verbal expressions of affection usually predominate.

Families with functional communication patterns value openness, a mutual respect for each other's feelings, thoughts and concerns, spontaneity, and self-disclosure. They are usually able to discuss most personal issues and concerns and resolve conflicts.

Dysfunctional Communication

Dysfunctional communication is the opposite of functional communication. It is an unclear transmission of a message or information that prohibits the receiver from understanding the intent or meaning of what the sender transmits. Low self-esteem of the family members is the prime reason for dysfunctional communications. Communications become confusing, vague, indirect, secretive, and defensive because the individuals lack the ability to appreciate individual differences, thoughts, and feelings of other family members and are unable to deal with conflict. Children growing up in this environment often are unable to recognize and interpret a variety of feelings and experiences.

Dysfunctional patterns of communication may be subtle, and the intent of the communication is not clear. For example, individuals in an interaction may constantly restate their own issues without really listening to others' points of view or acknowledging their needs. Another example is the inability to focus on one issue. Each individual in the interaction rambles from one issue to another instead of resolving any one problem. Or there are unwritten rules about subjects that are allowed for discussion; dysfunctional families have more forbidden subjects than functional families. Sometimes they avoid discussing meaningful issues or expressing feelings by using chitchat: they talk about unimportant daily occurrences rather than the meaningful issues of family life.

Remember that cultural aspects of family communication must be considered when determining whether a family is functional or dysfunctional. Some cultures are more open and communicative, whereas others are less likely to discuss various topics or to show feelings or emotions.

FAMILY COPING

Family coping refers to a positive response that families employ to resolve problems or reduce the stress produced by a problem or event. Family coping processes and strategies enable the family to maintain its necessary functions. Without effective coping and adaptation, family functions cannot be adequately managed.

STRESS AND ADAPTATION

Coping involves the processes of stress and adaptation. The definitions of stress and adaptation are the same for families as they are for individuals. Stress is the response produced by a stressor (or event causing the stress). Adaptation is the process of adjustment to change. How a family adapts to stress and change affects family health and functioning. If adaptation to stress is negative, the family functions less effectively than if the adaptation to stress is positive.

If a family is handling stress poorly or using ineffective adaptive strategies, it may be in crisis. When a family crisis occurs, the stressors are overwhelming, and the family is unable to cope and resolve problems. You may be in a position to as-

table 6-2 Internal and External Family Coping Strategies

INTERNAL FAMILY COPING STRATEGIES

1. Family group reliance: Becoming more reliant on its own resources
2. The use of humor: Relieving anxiety and tension with humor
3. Maintaining cohesiveness: Sharing feelings, thoughts, and experiences to maintain a cohesive family unit
4. Controlling the meaning of the problem: Interpreting events in a positive way
5. Joint family problem solving: All members working together to solve problems
6. Role flexibility: Changing roles as needed
7. Normalizing: Maintaining as normal a life as possible in the face of stressors

EXTERNAL FAMILY COPING STRATEGIES

1. Seeking information: Obtaining information about a situation to maintain control
2. Maintaining active linkages with the community: Participating in clubs or community organizations, using societal resources and information as an adjunct to serve family members' needs
3. Seeking social support: Using informal and formal support systems and support groups
4. Seeking spiritual support: Obtaining spiritual support for coping with stress

From Friedman, M. M. (1992). *Family nursing: Theory and practice* (3rd ed., p. 326). Norwalk, CT: Appleton & Lange.

sess whether a family is in trouble by determining whether or not the family's problem is being adequately managed by family members, if a crisis state exists, or whether the current problem is part of a chronic inability to solve problems.

The same strategies for adapting to stress in individuals are used by the family. They include defense mechanisms, coping strategies, and mastery. Defense mechanisms are usual ways of responding to stress. They are usually avoidance behaviors, meaning that people avoid facing problems or stressors. Defense mechanisms are generally considered to be negative responses. Coping strategies are behaviors or efforts used for effective problem solving and are generally considered to be positive responses. Mastery is the end result of using effective coping strategies. Problems are solved competently, and the family functions in a healthy manner.

COPING STRATEGIES

Family coping strategies are actions that families use to respond to stressors. Coping strategies change over time in response to the particular demands or stressors being experienced.

There are several types of coping responses. One effective way that families cope with stress is to deal with the situation causing the problem. It is geared toward altering or eliminating the stressor itself. For example, if a family suddenly becomes homeless because of a major disaster, the family takes steps to find temporary quarters and a new permanent residence. Another way of coping is to attach meaning to a problem. For example, one family may be devastated by becoming homeless, whereas another may find meaning in the situation by saying that at least the family is together and no one was hurt. A third way to cope with stress occurs when families help one another rather than dealing with the stressor or situation itself. For example, the family may cope by comforting one another rather than taking action to remedy the situation. The use of many coping strategies is generally more useful than using a single coping mechanism for every stressor, event, or problem.

Coping responses include internal and external coping strategies. Internal coping strategies refer to the ability of the family to pull together and respond to problems as a cohesive unit. Positive family communication patterns are crucial for successful internal coping. External coping strategies refer to the use of social support systems to solve problems. Knowledge of resources in the community and willingness to accept help from outside the family are important for successful external coping. Specific types of internal and external family coping strategies are listed in Table 6-2.

FAMILY NURSING CARE

Some general concepts can be used when assessing families and their coping strategies. First, determine what stressors are being experienced by the family, what kinds of coping mechanisms are used, and how well the family is coping with stress. Find out whether the family uses a variety of internal and external coping strategies or whether the stress is too much to cope with and puts the family in crisis. It is important to know how well the family communicates and whether it is a functional or dysfunctional unit.

When assisting families to cope, encourage all family members to be involved in the process. Support or reinforce coping patterns that are or have been successful in the past. Help families learn additional positive coping responses by referring them to resources that can assist them by providing support for both internal and external coping strategies.

ROLE OF THE NURSE

Family members frequently provide support for patients. They also may need a great deal of support themselves during a loved one's illness. Consider the needs of family members, especially in cases in which there is a serious illness or threat of death. Families often need information and reassurance. Providing information can relieve anxiety and fear of the unknown (Fig. 6-1).

It is important to assess the relationships among the patient and other family members. Families can impose a number of burdens, provide considerable emotional support, or offer a mixed blessing. You should determine whether family members are supportive or detrimental in the recovery

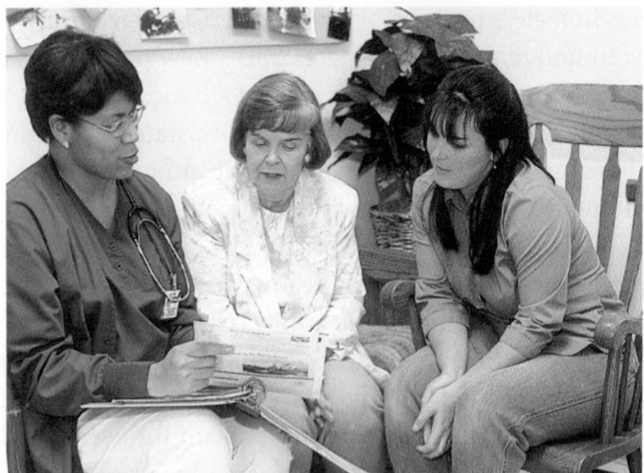

FIGURE 6-1 Family members need information and reassurance.

process. Also consider the family's influence on individual members as you assess, diagnose, plan, implement, and evaluate nursing care. The inclusion of family members in the client's care and the decision-making process helps maintain the self-esteem of both clients and families.

COMMUNITY RESOURCES

Referral to community resources can help families cope with health care problems. You should be well acquainted with both informal and formal community resources. Informal resources usually consist of family members or friends who supply long-term support, comfort, and nurturing. Formal resources include community agencies that provide ongoing services.

Information provided through books, magazines, and leaflets can help families learn about an illness or condition, learn what to expect with the disease, know that they are not alone, and deal with the situation. Information also can be provided through community groups, such as support groups, as well as health care providers and social agencies. Formal support systems help by assisting with problems such as home, institutional, and long-term care; finances; transportation; and social support. Many community agencies can help families dealing with stress or those in crisis.

*Put on your **THINKING CAP!!***

Recall a patient whose family was present when you took care of the patient. Discuss how the family member(s) and the patient interacted with each other and how the family member interacted with health care providers. What needs of family member(s) can you identify? How can nurses help to meet the needs of families?

key points

- The family unit occupies a position between the individual and society, functioning to meet the needs of the individual members and the needs of the society of which it is a part.
- A family is defined as "two or more persons who are joined together by bonds of sharing and emotional closeness and who identify themselves as being part of the family" (Friedman, 1997, p. 9).
- The major types of families are nuclear, extended, stepparent, single-parent, and nontraditional.
- Cultural values and attitudes influence how a family communicates and interacts, carries out activities of daily living, and views health and health care.
- Traditionally, the five major stages of the family life cycle are beginning families, families with young children, families with adolescents, launching children and moving on, and families in later life.
- Each family member has a role that defines expected behavior in given situations.
- Families have their own unique communication styles or patterns.
- Families, like individuals, use a variant of coping strategies to adapt to stressors.
- The inclusion of family members in a client's care and the decision-making process helps maintain the self-esteem of both clients and families.
- When working with families, the nurse assesses stressors, coping strategies, family communication, and resources.

REVIEW QUESTIONS

1. The best definition of a family is:
   1. one male and one female parent with children.
   2. two or more individuals who share bonds and emotional closeness and who consider themselves a family.
   3. at least one parent in a household with one or more children.
   4. a group of individuals related by blood and marriage who make up a single household and share financial resources.
2. The Census Bureau reveals the following living arrangements of children in the United States:
   1. Over 75% of children in the United States live in traditional families.
   2. Blended families are most common among white families.
   3. About 6% of children live in homes with more than one generation.
   4. About 50% of U.S. children live in single-parent families.

3. What function does scapegoating serve in the family?
   1. Diverts attention from conflict between spouses
   2. Brings attention to the family member who contributes the least
   3. Tests the bonds of loyalty within the family
   4. Motivates children to compete with siblings

4. After a tornado, survivors are being interviewed. A common statement made by the survivors is "We lost everything but each other. This has taught us what is really important in life." This is an example of what type of coping strategy?
   1. Dealing directly with the cause of the problem
   2. Providing comfort to each other
   3. Denying the seriousness of the situation
   4. Attaching meaning to the experience

5. The family of a critically ill patient is comforted by visits from their minister and church members. They pray often for their loved one's recovery. This is an example of a/an:
   1. Internal family coping strategy
   2. Anticipatory grieving
   3. External family coping strategy
   4. Unrealistic thinking

CHAPTER

7 Health and Illness

objectives

1. Describe the health-illness continuum.
2. Discuss traditional and current views of health and illness.
3. List Maslow's five basic human needs and explain why they constitute a hierarchy.
4. Explain the four levels of adaptability to stress.
5. Discuss concepts related to health promotion, disease prevention, and health maintenance.
6. Define acute and chronic illness.
7. Discuss illness behavior and the impact of illness on the family.
8. Describe nursing measures for health promotion, health maintenance, and illness.
9. Describe complementary and alternative therapies and the nurse's role in relation to both.

key terms

Acute illness (p. 67)
Alternative therapy (p. 63)
Chronic illness (p. 67)
Complementary therapy (p. 63)
Coping (p. 65)
Homeostasis (hō-mē-ō-STĀ-sĭs, p. 63)
Primary prevention (p. 67)
Secondary prevention (p. 67)
Stress (p. 64)
Tertiary prevention (TĔR-shē-ĕr-ē, p. 67)

Human beings are complex organisms with interacting biologic, psychological, behavioral, emotional, and spiritual systems. Systems within the human body are referred to as the internal environment. Systems outside the human body are known as the external environment. Health and illness are affected by both the internal and the external environments.

The human body, mind, and spirit are parts of a living system. Human responses to actual or potential health problems include a myriad of reactions, many of them based on thoughts, emotions, and past experiences.

Because of cultural, educational, and social differences, individuals have very different concepts about what constitutes health and illness. People define health and illness according to how they view themselves as human beings and in relation to the surrounding environment. It is important to know how people view health and illness so that you can help them achieve their personal goals for health and wellness.

THE HEALTH-ILLNESS CONTINUUM

TRADITIONAL VIEWS OF HEALTH AND ILLNESS

Traditionally, health and illness have been viewed as separate entities. Either people were healthy or they were sick. Health and illness were seen as physiologic phenomena. A typical dictionary definition of health is "soundness, especially of body or mind; freedom from disease or abnormality" (*American Heritage Dictionary,* 1992). In 1946, the World Health Organization defined health as "the state of complete physical, mental, and social well-being and not merely the absence of disease or infirmity."

Most definitions of health have not allowed for degrees of health or illness and have failed to reflect the dynamic, ever-changing nature of health. Although the World Health Organization broadened the concept of health from a strictly physiologic state to one that encompasses mental and social well-being, its definition is still seen today as a narrow view of health and illness.

CURRENT VIEWS OF HEALTH AND ILLNESS

Currently, health and illness are viewed as relative states along a continuum. Individuals have neither absolute health nor absolute illness but are in an ever-changing state of being, ranging from peak or high-level wellness to extremely poor health, with death being imminent (Fig. 7-1).

Well-being or lack of well-being for individuals fluctuates along the continuum on a daily basis. Personal and environmental factors contribute to this state of flux. Unique internal factors within each individual influence how each person responds to external forces. These responses determine how individuals fulfill their needs and reach their highest health potential.

According to Dunn, who first used the expression "high-level wellness," people must accept responsibility for their own wellness and take an active part in improving and maintaining it. Health and illness are relative terms. Each person's state of health integrates factors beyond biologic fitness. Personal, psychosocial, and spiritual values and beliefs influence how a person views health and illness.

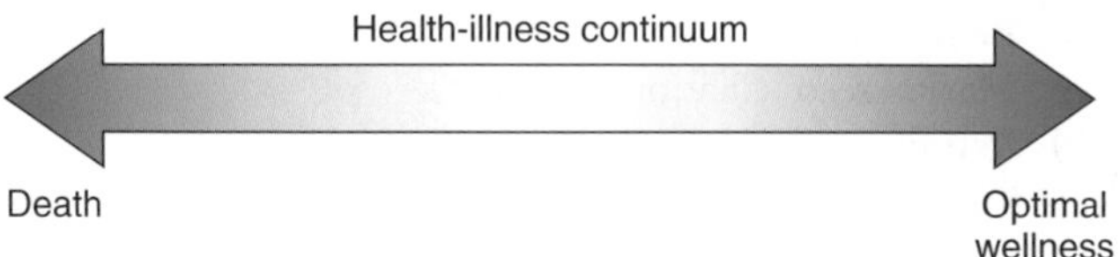

FIGURE 7-1 Common concept of health as a continuum ranging from optimal wellness at one end to illness culminating in death at the other end.

This current view of health and illness differs from the traditional view, in which health and illness were thought to be completely separate entities. An individual was considered either sick or well, with the focus of treatment on the physiologic aspects of the disease rather than on the person. The emphasis was on curing the disease or injury, not on helping individuals maintain the highest quality of life possible when diseases were not curable. Traditional health care focused on illness rather than on health promotion and disease prevention.

If we keep in mind the dynamic continuum of health and illness, health may be viewed as the ability to express the full range of one's physical and mental potential within one's environment. A healthy person maintains stability and comfort by adapting physically, mentally, emotionally, and socially to internal and external events.

In American culture, disease is regarded as a disruption of biologic and/or psychological function. Disease is a condition that can be recognized through objective findings such as fever, the presence of bacteria, or an individual's inability to perform social role tasks. Illness has a broader definition than disease as it incorporates personal, interpersonal, and cultural perceptions of and reactions to disease.

Views of health that have led to a growing use of complementary and alternative therapies are discussed later in this chapter.

BASIC HUMAN NEEDS

Key concepts in health and wellness include homeostasis, adaptation, the dynamic nature of the health-illness continuum, the influence of the internal and external environments, comfort, safety, social relationships, and prevention of disease and disability. To maintain the highest level of health and wellness, people must satisfy basic human needs.

Three broad categories of human needs must be met: (1) physical, (2) libidinal (sensual and affectional), and (3) ego developmental. Physiologic needs include oxygen, water, food, elimination, sleep, shelter, safety, and mobility. These needs must be met for individuals to survive. Libidinal needs refer to sensual-sexual and affectional-emotional needs. Sensual-sexual needs encompass the physiologic and psychological aspects of sexuality. Affectional-emotional needs are satisfied through love, security, approval, respect, support, and care. Ego developmental needs refer to needs that must be met to sustain cognitive and perceptual growth and memory development. They are satisfied through education and training and enable individuals to develop motor coordination, independence, self-identity, social skills, communication skills, problem-solving skills, and a moral view.

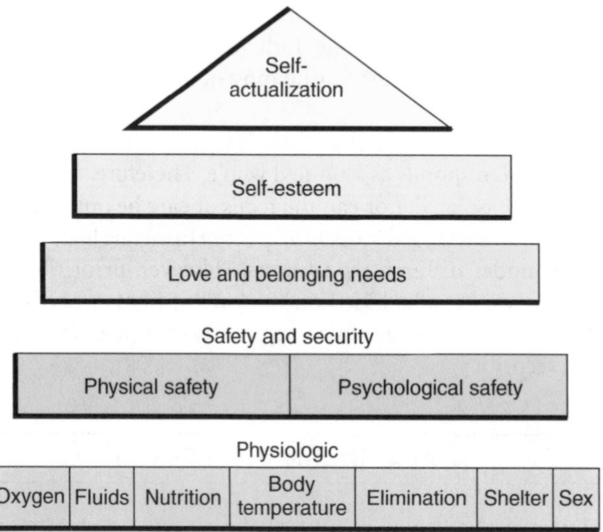

FIGURE 7-2 Maslow's Hierarchy of Needs. Needs must be met in ascending order. For example, safety and security must be achieved before love and belonging needs can be met.

Abraham Maslow, a psychologist, organized human needs into a hierarchy (Fig. 7-2). Maslow's hierarchy of human needs has five levels: (1) physiologic, (2) safety and security, (3) belonging and love, (4) self-esteem, and (5) self-actualization. A person generally progresses up the hierarchy in an attempt to satisfy needs. Physiologic needs usually must be met first to progress to the satisfaction of safety and security needs; safety and security needs must be satisfied before the needs of belonging and love can be met; and so on.

Physiologic needs include the needs for oxygen, fluids, nutrition, life-sustaining environmental temperature, elimination, shelter, rest, and sex. Physiologic needs are the most fundamental because they sustain life. Individuals cannot live without air, water, and food. Once the physical needs are satisfied, *safety needs,* such as security, protection from harm, and freedom from anxiety and fear, can be addressed. People need order and structure in their lives, and illness or disease can be very disruptive.

Love and belonging needs emerge after safety needs are met. They include feeling loved by one's family and friends and accepted by one's peers and community. Love and belonging are related to self-esteem, which is essential for carrying out health-promoting behaviors. *Self-esteem* means feeling good about oneself and feeling that others hold one in high regard. Individuals with high self-esteem feel confident about themselves and confident that they are appreciated by others. People with low self-esteem may feel helpless and inferior.

Self-actualization, or self-fulfillment, is the highest level of Maslow's hierarchy. Self-actualized people are characterized by the following traits: (1) ability to solve problems, (2) willingness to accept suggestions and criticism from others, (3) broad interests, (4) good communication skills, (5) self-confidence and high self-esteem, (6) maturity, and (7) desire for new experiences and knowledge. Individuals rarely achieve self-actualization; rather, they spend most of their lives attempting to live more fully.

Although the hierarchy of needs is arranged in levels, the individual responds as a unified whole. Therefore, the needs cannot be isolated, nor can the focus of care be only on one level. In addition, individuals may move from one level to another under different conditions. However, priorities for nursing care can be based on the level of human needs, so that the physical needs must take priority over those for safety and security.

ADAPTATION TO STRESS

Human beings cannot go through life without stress. Stress is as much a part of life as breathing and eating. Internal and external factors can trigger stress (Table 7-1). Environmental factors, life changes, and physiologic or emotional illness all contribute to stress.

Life changes that cause stress for most people include the following:

1. Death of a spouse
2. Divorce
3. Marital separation from mate
4. Detention in jail or other institution
5. Death of a close family member
6. Major personal injury or illness
7. Marriage
8. Being fired at work
9. Marital reconciliation with mate
10. Retirement from work
11. Trouble with in-laws
12. Change in schools

Life changes can be positive or negative, but they require people to expend energy to adapt to the change. Many studies have found a significant relationship between life changes and the development of physical and mental illness.

Hospitalization is a stressful event for most people. The hospital environment introduces new sights, sounds, smells, and routines into daily life. These changes challenge the patient's autonomy and control. Even people who are sick want to maintain a sense of control over their environment. When they cannot maintain control, powerlessness becomes an additional stressor. While they are sick, people seek control in relation to the following:

- Avoidance of pain and incapacitation
- The immediate hospital environment
- Treatments and procedures
- Relationships with hospital personnel
- Emotional balance
- A satisfactory self-image
- Relationships with family and friends
- Preparing for an uncertain future

THE STRESS RESPONSE

There are two types of stress response: local adaptation and general adaptation. Hans Selye called these responses to stress *syndromes.* Local adaptation syndrome is a short-term, local-

table 7-1 ***Stressors***

SOURCES	EXAMPLES
INTERNAL STRESSORS	
Physical	Overexertion or other imposed strains on body system; infections or allergens; physical trauma (e.g., surgery, accident); nutritional deficiency
Psychological	
Intrapsychic conflict	Feeling anger while fearing the consequences of expressing it
Perception of threat from events	Observing an angry person; illness of a loved one
Feelings of inadequacy, dependency, helplessness, powerlessness	Belief that life is impossible without the help and love of a significant other
Boredom	Isolated from friends and/or gratifying life experiences
EXTERNAL STRESSORS	
Interpersonal Relations	
Conflictual relations	Marital conflict; incompatibility at work
Loss of relationship	Death of a loved one
Inability to relate, or so perceived	Language barrier
Socioeconomic	
Economic inadequacies	Unemployment, poor diet, poor housing, little recreation
Climatic extremes	Rain, clouds, little sun
Noxious stimuli	Noise, odors
Sensory deprivation	Isolation from things, people
Political climate	Repressive social system
Ethnic, religious, or national difference	Prejudice based on nationality, race, or creed

From Varcarolis, E. M. (1990). *Foundations of psychiatric mental health nursing* (p. 320). Philadelphia: Saunders.

ized response to a specific stressor that restores a body region or body part to homeostasis. Examples of this syndrome are blood clotting, wound healing, pain, and inflammation.

General adaptation syndrome is a physiologic response of the whole body to stress. Because it involves primarily the autonomic nervous system and the endocrine system, it is often referred to as the neuroendocrine response. The general adaptation syndrome consists of three stages: (1) the alarm reaction, (2) the resistance stage, and (3) the exhaustion stage (Fig. 7-3). The alarm reaction causes the body to respond to stress physiologically. Hormone levels, heart rate and cardiac output, respiratory rate, oxygen intake, and mental energy are increased. The pupils are dilated to cover a larger visual field. These reactions together are called the fight-or-flight response, which helps the body defend against stressors.

After the initial alarm stage, the body stabilizes, and physiologic processes return to normal levels. The resistance stage is characterized by adaptation to the stressor. If the stressor can be overcome or the damage repaired, as in a short-term illness or injury, the body begins to heal. If the stressor is long term, such as one that accompanies a chronic physical or mental illness, an individual may enter the third stage of adaptation: exhaustion. During the exhaustion stage, the body is drained of energy and can no longer defend itself against the stressor. Death may be the ultimate outcome.

There are many signs and symptoms of stress. Among them are cold hands and feet, tensed muscles, nervous movements, excessive sweating, tooth grinding, headaches, insomnia, and subjective complaints of feeling tense or nervous. When individuals do not cope well with stressors and are unable to adapt, they may withdraw and become depressed. Signs and symptoms of withdrawal and depression are slowed speech; a lowered, hesitant speaking voice; decreased bodily movement; a hunched-over, tired posture; insomnia; and subjective complaints of feeling blue, depressed, or unable to concentrate.

COPING

Coping is any behavioral or cognitive activity used to deal with stress. People cope with stress in different ways. They may use problem-solving strategies, which involve identifying the problem, generating alternatives, choosing the best alternative, and applying it to the problem. Lazarus describes the effectiveness of coping as being related to how a person

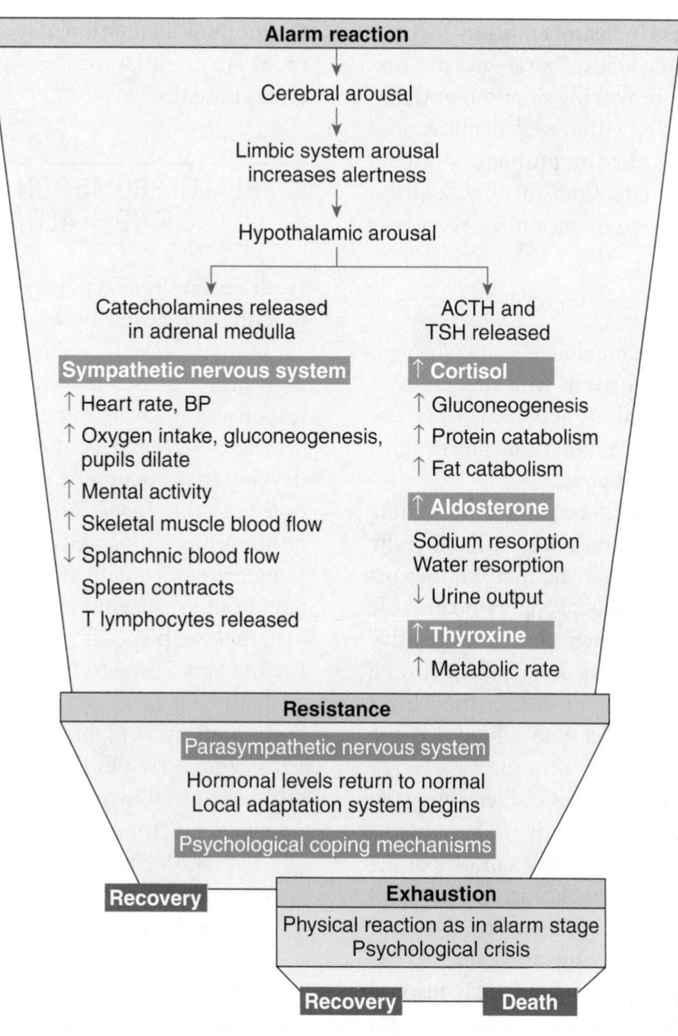

FIGURE **7-3** General adaptation syndrome.

table 7-2 Common Coping Strategies and Examples

COPING STRATEGY	EXAMPLE
Event rehearsal	Mental and verbal preparation for an event or practice of coping strategies
Confrontation	Aggressive seeking of information, anger, refusal of treatments
Distancing or denial	Unwillingness or inability to talk about events; going on as if nothing has happened
Self-control	Stoicism, showing no feelings
Social support	Seeking out family, friends, or others in similar situations
Accepting responsibility	Verbally placing responsibility for situation on self
Faith	Praying, reading religious material, seeking out of clergy or religious guidance
Problem solving	Making plans, verbally outlining what will be done next
Positive reappraisal	Speaking of how situation has fostered growth
Event review	Discussing situations or coping that has occurred

From Ignatavicius, D. D., Workman, M. L., & Mishler, M. (1999). *Medical-surgical nursing: A nursing process approach* (3rd ed., p. 100). Philadelphia: Saunders.

interprets the problem. He explains the daily hassles in life as stressors and the daily uplifts as buffers to daily hassles. For example, some hassles of daily life include "too many things to do" and misplacing things. Uplifts include feeling healthy and getting enough sleep. Hardiness is another concept that influences a person's response to stress. Hardiness encompasses concepts of control, commitment, and ability to handle challenges.

Others may cope with stress by using emotion-focused strategies. Examples of emotion-focused strategies are distancing oneself from the stress-provoking situation or denying its seriousness, self-isolation or withdrawal, blaming oneself or accepting responsibility for the problem, drawing strength from adversity, tension reduction, hostility, fatalism, social support, and faith. Common coping strategies and examples are listed in Table 7-2.

ADAPTATION

Adaptation to stress is essential to maintaining health. Through adaptation, individuals cope constructively with stressful conditions. Adaptation depends on accurate appraisal of a stressful situation and effective coping. Adaptation can result in physiologic and psychological well-being.

For reasons we do not fully understand, some people adapt better than others to life circumstances. It is generally thought that adaptability is a characteristic that is either inborn or acquired in very early childhood. People who are able to adapt to stress usually live constructively and in relative harmony with others. They view stress as a challenge to be overcome, and they have a sense of control over their lives. Adaptable people demonstrate the ability to rebound in the face of adversity.

Nurses can help patients deal with stress by identifying the patient's usual methods of coping or adapting. These methods rely on internal and external resources. Examples of internal resources are physiologic and psychological responses that occur when one is faced with a stressful situation, such as smoking, drinking alcohol, eating, crying, and exercise. External responses include getting help from family, friends, and service agencies in the community.

HOMEOSTASIS

Homeostasis is a term derived from Greek that describes a tendency of the body to maintain stability of the internal environment. The body adapts to internal and external changes in the environment, adjusts to changes, and maintains equilibrium, or homeostasis. For example, the body adjusts heart rate, blood pressure, respiration, temperature, and hormone secretions to maintain an internal steady state or balance. Continuous adaptation and change in the internal environment are essential for the organism to exist in the external environment.

HEALTH PROMOTION, DISEASE PREVENTION, AND HEALTH MAINTENANCE

Health promotion activities are directed toward maintaining or enhancing well-being as a protection against illness. Through public education, Americans have become increasingly health conscious and many are beginning to take more responsibility for maintaining healthy lifestyles.

The U.S. Department of Health and Human Services has developed a document outlining goals for the year 2010, called *Healthy People 2010. Healthy People 2010* is a national health promotion and disease prevention initiative that aims to increase the quality and years of healthy life and to eliminate health disparities. Twenty-eight focus areas are identified, each with specific objectives and strategies (Table 7-3). Factors being used to measure progress toward meeting the goals and objectives of *Healthy People 2010* are called leading health indicators (Table 7-4).

Specific activities that are generally thought to promote health are as follows:

Adequate nutrition based on the "pyramid" concept (see Chapter 8). Foods should be eaten in moderation, with an emphasis on complex carbohydrates, followed by fruits and vegetables, proteins and dairy products, and a minimum amount of fats (no more than 30% of calories consumed) and simple sugars. Approximately 20 to 30 grams of dietary fiber should be taken in daily.

table 7-3 Healthy People 2010 *Focus Areas*

1. Access to quality health services
2. Arthritis, osteoporosis, and chronic back conditions
3. Cancer
4. Chronic kidney disease
5. Diabetes
6. Disability and secondary conditions
7. Educational and community-based programs
8. Environmental health
9. Family planning
10. Food safety
11. Health communication
12. Heart disease and stroke
13. HIV
14. Immunizations and infectious diseases
15. Injury and violence prevention
16. Maternal health, infant health, and child health
17. Medical product safety
18. Mental health and mental disorders
19. Nutrition and overweight
20. Occupational health and safety
21. Oral health
22. Physical activity and fitness
23. Public health infrastructure
24. Respiratory diseases
25. Sexually transmitted diseases
26. Substance abuse
27. Tobacco use
28. Vision and hearing

From U.S. Department of Health and Human Services, Public Health Service. (2000). *Healthy people 2010.* Available at http://www.health.gov/healthypeople/ March 6, 2001.

table 7-4 Healthy People 2010 *Leading Health Indicators*

1. Physical activity
2. Overweight and obesity
3. Tobacco use
4. Substance abuse
5. Responsible sexual behavior
6. Mental health
7. Injury and violence
8. Environmental quality
9. Immunization
10. Access to health care

From U.S. Department of Health and Human Services, Public Health Service. (2000). *Healthy people 2010.* Available at http://www.health.gov/healthypeople/ March 6, 2001.

Moderate exercise on a routine schedule. Twenty minutes of walking three times per week is considered ideal.
Rest, 7 to 8 hours of sleep every 24 hours.
Healthy lifestyle, especially no smoking and limited consumption of alcohol.
Balance of work and recreation.

Disease or illness prevention behavior is action taken by individuals to decrease the potential or actual threat of illness and its harmful consequences. The three levels of prevention (primary, secondary, and tertiary) are described in Chapter 1.

THE CONCEPT OF ILLNESS

Illness is a deviation from a healthy state that may occur acutely or as a series of long-term events. Acute and chronic illnesses are experienced and viewed differently.

Acute illness is an illness or disease that has a relatively rapid onset and short duration. The condition usually responds to a specific treatment and ends in full recovery. Examples of acute illnesses are the common cold or influenza, appendicitis, and urinary tract infections.

Chronic illness usually involves permanent impairment or disability and requires long-term rehabilitation and medical or nursing treatment. Examples of chronic illnesses are coronary artery disease, endocrine disorders, and diabetes mellitus. Some chronic illnesses such as rheumatoid arthritis and asthma are characterized by periods of remission and exacerbation. During remissions, the disease seems to go away. During episodes of exacerbation, acute symptoms recur.

ILLNESS BEHAVIOR

Reactions to illness vary among individuals. Some people take action, whereas others may do nothing. Those who take action may seek the help of health care providers, such as physicians, nurses, or dentists; others may seek help from friends or family members. Among some cultures in the United States, people may seek help from folk healers or herbalists. The actions taken by individuals are influenced by the availability and affordability of health care, the individual's perception of the problem, others' perception of the problem, and the failure or success of self-prescribed treatment.

People who take no action may wait to see whether the symptoms go away by themselves. Others may deny that something is wrong and refuse to admit that they are ill. People who take no action may be influenced by the same factors that affect those who take action.

Some individuals take counteraction in response to illness. This means that they engage in activities that should be avoided just to prove to themselves that the symptoms do not exist. For example, a person with symptoms of chronic bronchitis may continue to smoke, regardless of the impaired breathing and coughing that the smoke may cause. Patients who have a history of failure to follow proper health practices or treatment regimens are referred to as "noncompliant." Such behaviors can have harmful effects on health and self-esteem and can lead to death. Because of the judgmental tone of the word "noncompliant," many people prefer to use the term "nonadherence."

The Sick Role

When people become ill, they frequently adopt a "sick role." The sick role allows individuals time to recover from their

table 7-5 Sick Role Behaviors

1. Exemption from normal activities
2. Recognition that the sick person is not responsible for causing the condition
3. Expectation that the sick person wants to get well
4. Obligation to seek competent help

disease. When they cannot get well on their own, others must care for them. They are temporarily exempt from social responsibilities so that they can concentrate on getting well. It is assumed that people who are sick want to get well and therefore should seek the help of health professionals and cooperate with prescribed health care regimens (Table 7-5). However, some people are reluctant to give up the sick role because of the attention they get or because they wish to avoid work.

IMPACT OF ILLNESS ON THE FAMILY

Illness does not affect individuals in isolation; rather, it has an impact on the entire family. An illness may affect the roles of family members, the daily activities carried out, and the family's economic stability.

Three factors influence the effect of illness on the family. The first factor is the identity of the member of the family who is ill. For example, if the head of the household and chief breadwinner is sick, the financial resources may be threatened. If the person who normally cares for the home and children becomes ill, others have to pitch in to help. If an elderly member of the family becomes ill, grown children may have to provide care. The reversal in the parent-child roles may be difficult for both parents and children.

The second factor influencing the effect of illness on the family is the seriousness and duration of the disease. An acute illness does not produce the long-term effects of a chronic disease. Family members are able to change roles temporarily to manage an acute illness, but during the long duration of a chronic illness, family relationships may become strained.

The third factor is the social and cultural customs of the family. Families of various cultures have different attitudes toward illness, caregiving, and changing family roles.

All of these factors can have an effect on family functioning. Feelings of frustration, anger, and grief must be dealt with so that all members of the family can function at their highest potential while providing care for the sick member. Chapter 6 provides more in-depth coverage of nursing care of families.

IMPLICATIONS FOR NURSING CARE

PREVENT HEALTH PROBLEMS

Nurses can help clients engage in healthier lifestyles to prevent disease. Nursing measures are geared toward helping clients make informed decisions regarding their health care practices. For example, the nurse can:

Inform clients of daily activities, such as the proper diet, exercise, and adequate sleep, that help maintain optimal health.

Inform clients about the diseases for which they are at risk.

Explain the consequences of the disease for which they are at risk.

Give clients specific information about how they can reduce their risk for the disease.

When counseling clients and their families, it is important to keep in mind that most health promotion and disease prevention measures require a change in lifestyle. Take into consideration the biophysical, psychological, sociocultural, spiritual, and environmental dimensions of family life and structure and be realistic in your expectations for change.

HELP SATISFY THE PATIENT'S UNMET BASIC HUMAN NEEDS

For people to maintain the highest levels of health and wellness, basic human needs must be met. According to Henderson, "The unique function of the nurse is to assist the individual, sick or well, in the performance of those activities contributing to health or its recovery (or to a peaceful death) that he would perform unaided if he had the necessary strength, will, or knowledge. And to do this in such a way as to help him gain independence as rapidly as possible."

Henderson identified 14 components of basic nursing care. These components include normal breathing, eating and drinking adequately, eliminating body wastes, maintaining desirable posture, sleeping and resting, selecting suitable clothing (dressing and undressing), maintaining normal body temperature, keeping the body clean, avoiding dangers in the environment, communicating with others, worshiping, working to achieve a sense of accomplishment, playing, and learning. These components of basic nursing care are closely related to Maslow's hierarchy of human needs, in that the first eight components address physiologic needs. Other components refer to safety needs, to belonging and love needs, and to self-esteem and self-actualization needs. Henderson's work provides a useful way to identify human needs that must be met for optimum health.

INCREASE ADAPTABILITY

The first step in helping clients increase their adaptability is to determine what the client perceives as stressful and how stressful it is. One way to assess the degree of stress is to ask clients to name the worst possible stressor and then compare the present stressor with that one. The second step is to assess past methods of coping with stress that have been successful for the client. It is then helpful to apply past coping strategies to new situations. To assess internal coping strategies, ask, "What kinds of things do you do when you are stressed?" "Do you eat more or less?" "Do you drink alcohol?" "Do you smoke more?" "Do you sleep more or less?" Questions that help determine external coping strategies include, "Whom do you turn to when you are feeling stressed?" "Do you talk with others or do you keep things inside?" "Do you contact any professionals such as social workers, nurses, doctors, or social agencies when you have a problem?"

Elderly persons have particular difficulty coping with stress and adapting to new situations. When any type of stressor occurs, it takes longer and is much harder to get back to their previous level of functioning. Fortunately, people who have lived a long time have experienced many stresses throughout life and generally have developed a wide range of coping mechanisms and skills for adapting to change. Help older clients use past successful coping mechanisms to deal with new stressors. Emphasize strengths rather than limitations.

During hospitalization, you can help clients and families adapt to a difficult situation by helping them cope with the stress of a new environment, illness, and uncertainty. Some clients and families benefit from detailed information about the disease and the hospital procedures; others prefer not to know. Allowing patients to have as much control as possible helps to reduce stress. Even people who are very dependent on hospital personnel need to feel that they have some control over their lives. Other measures that may help relieve stress and promote coping and adaptation are biofeedback, progressive muscle relaxation, meditation, and imagery. These strategies generally focus attention inward on the patient's own mind and body and reduce either physical or emotional tension.

FOSTER INDEPENDENCE

In acute illness, recovery is usually speedy, and people return quickly to their previous lifestyle. However, individuals with chronic illnesses must spend a lifetime managing symptoms. Many elderly persons have one or more chronic illnesses and may need some type of assistance in their daily lives. The goal is to maintain the highest level of independence possible and prevent further disability. The following tasks have been identified for chronically ill individuals: prevent and manage crises, carry out prescribed regimens, control symptoms, reorder time, adjust to changes in the course of the illness, prevent social isolation, and attempt to normalize social interactions.

Prevent and Manage Crises

When symptoms flare up, a crisis situation may arise. You can help clients and families prevent and control a crisis situation. The client and family members must learn the signs and symptoms of the onset of a crisis and make a plan for how to deal with the crisis.

Carry Out Prescribed Regimens

Chronically ill individuals may need to take many medications, eat special foods, or restrict some activities. It is very difficult to have a restricted lifestyle day in and day out, especially when symptoms are not apparent. Nursing interventions include teaching clients about the need to carry out regimens, providing moral support and encouragement, and finding ways to make carrying out regimens easier. You can increase patient compliance by forming "alliances" with patients, helping them feel that they are important participants in developing their own health regimen. Of course, when it comes to lifestyle changes, only the patient can control them.

Manage Symptoms

Chronically ill individuals must learn to manage symptoms to continue desired activities. Gear nursing interventions toward helping clients learn about the pattern of symptoms (typical onset, duration, and severity) and the limits of their ability to control symptoms. Arrange daily routines so that the highest-level activities are carried out when symptoms are lessened or absent and periods of rest are taken when symptoms are most acute.

Reorder Time

People with chronic illness may find they have either too much or too little available time. Forced retirement may increase the amount of free time; conversely, carrying out regimens to manage symptoms may be extremely time-consuming for clients and caregivers. In both situations, the chronically ill and their family members may become frustrated and depressed. The nurse can help clients and caregivers develop a daily schedule that allows time for desired activities while managing the regimens of the chronic illness.

Adjust to Changes in the Course of the Disease

Chronic illnesses often have unpredictable courses, and individuals must learn to live with the ups and downs of the disease. Chronically ill individuals need support if they are to achieve their highest potential.

Prevent Social Isolation

Chronically ill individuals and their families often become socially isolated. The ill person may withdraw from others, or others may feel uncomfortable and withdraw. Support groups are helpful for providing a social outlet with others in the same situation.

Attempt to Normalize Social Interactions

Chronically ill people need to maintain as normal a lifestyle as possible despite having to manage symptoms, adapt to changes in appearance caused by the illness, or use adaptive equipment or prostheses. Encourage them to live as independently as possible in spite of their illness.

It is important to assess the support systems for the chronically ill. Families are the major support systems for persons with chronic illnesses and often provide the day-to-day ongoing care. Formal support systems include social service agencies, health care providers, and community agencies. If family members are unavailable or unable to provide support, formal services may be needed.

HELP FAMILY MEMBERS DEAL WITH THE PATIENT'S ILLNESS

Families provide the bulk of support for the chronically ill, and the burden of caregiving is heavy for them. They must take on more physical work because of the need to assist with activities of daily living, deal with changes in the progress of the disease, cope with feeling psychologically and physically overwhelmed, and adapt to changes in their own social roles and identities as well as those of the ill family member. In some cases, a family caregiver also may have a chronic illness that must be managed, or they develop a physical illness or disability as a result of the burden of caregiving. This is especially true for elderly caregivers.

Health care providers need to assist clients and their family members in developing a collaborative plan of care. In some cases, relief or respite can be obtained to ease the caregiving responsibility. Many communities have adult day care centers for older adults or persons with particular chronic illnesses. These centers enable both the older or chronically ill individuals and their caregivers to have a more normal lifestyle, with social interaction and structure. Formal support services should be used whenever they are needed to assist families in caring for their chronically ill loved ones.

ASSIST TERMINALLY ILL PATIENTS TO A PEACEFUL DEATH

Unfortunately, everyone must die. Nurses are often the health care providers who have the most intimate relationship with people who are terminally ill. When death comes accidentally or after an acute illness, there is little or no time to prepare for death. But when disease is chronic, patients and families often need to make difficult decisions regarding death.

In today's health care system, with its sophisticated technology, terminally ill patients can be kept alive longer than was ever possible in the past. Issues related to the setting in which the terminally ill are cared for, whether machines for artificial physiologic functioning are used, and when these machines are to be turned off must be faced on a daily basis. More than anyone else, family members have to live with the memory of their loved ones and the events surrounding their death.

Nurses should be supportive of decisions made by clients and families. The dying patients and their loved ones should be informed of the options for care and their consequences. The living will and durable power of attorney for health care are legal documents called advance directives. They allow patients to designate, in advance, what treatments they would want in specific situations (living will) or to appoint one person to make treatment decisions when they are not able to make those decisions (durable power of attorney). In 1991, the federal government passed the Patient Self-Determination Act, stating that persons admitted to hospitals and nursing homes must be asked if they want to prepare an advance directive. Open communication and an acknowledgment of different attitudes toward terminal illness and death are extremely important. The nurse should have knowledge of the dying process and the needs of the dying person to provide compassionate care, promote comfort, and make the pain and physical treatment bearable. More detailed information on caring for terminally ill patients is found in Chapter 23.

COMPLEMENTARY AND ALTERNATIVE THERAPIES

This chapter has focused on the view of health and illness as defined by conventional Western medicine. However, Americans are increasingly turning to other therapies in addition to, or along with, conventional medicine. These nontraditional therapies are called *alternative* if they are used in place of conventional medicine. An example of an alternative therapy is the use of relaxation therapy or acupuncture instead of analgesics to treat pain. Nontraditional therapies that are used along with conventional therapies are called *complementary* therapies. For example, a patient with chronic pain might take analgesics but also practice guided imagery.

Conventional and nontraditional medicines are based on differing views of health and illness. Conventional medicine focuses on diseases that are treated by correcting the underlying pathological processes with drugs, surgery, diet, and physical manipulation. Health is viewed primarily as prevention of disease. Most nontraditional therapies are based on the belief that illness is caused by lack of balance or harmony within the individual or between the individual and the environment. Therapy aims to restore balance or harmony, which puts the individual in a position such that healing can occur. Many of the nontraditional therapies have long been used in folk medicine; others have been developed more recently. Examples of complementary and alternative therapies are presented in Table 7-6.

Why is the use of nontraditional therapies becoming more common in the United States? First, many can be self-taught or learned from practitioners whose fees, if any, are typically less than those of medical doctors. Botanicals and other folk remedies are available without medical prescriptions. Second, nontraditional therapies are usually noninvasive. Third, they are part of a holistic approach to health and healing rather than just focusing on the disease or injury. Fourth, many people have found these therapies to be effective. Fifth, though not always true, people generally believe nontraditional practices are safer than medical and surgical treatment. Sixth, there is a perception that anything labeled "natural" is better.

Only recently have medical and nursing publications begun to include nontraditional therapies. At this time, a relatively small number of nontraditional remedies have been scientifically studied, so we are just beginning to have scientific information to use in discussing these remedies with patients. The role of the nurse in relation to nontraditional remedies and therapies includes:

- In your nursing assessment, always ask about the use of nontraditional remedies and/or therapies: what the patient is using, why, whether it has been helpful, and any negative outcomes.
- Be open-minded about nontraditional therapies as a valid choice by some patients.
- Learn about these therapies, and try some if you feel comfortable doing so. For example, imagery and relaxation techniques are useful in many situations and have no adverse effects. However, do not attempt to use techniques with patients unless you have been properly instructed in their use. Professional education courses are a good place to learn noninvasive techniques that can be used with many types of patients.
- Teach patients about any adverse effects of nontraditional remedies.

table 7-6 ***Types of Complementary and Alternative Therapies***

TYPE	DESCRIPTION	EXAMPLES
Alternative systems of medical practice	Ranges from self-care based on folk principles to organized care using alternative methods	Herbal tea for a cold, acupuncture, traditional Oriental medicine
Mind-body interventions	Uses the power of the mind and the body to affect each other	Psychotherapy, meditation, Yoga, prayer, guided imagery, biofeedback, relaxation therapy
Manual healing methods	Uses touch, manipulation of body parts	Osteopathic medicine, massage, chiropractic, reflexology, acupuncture
Bioelectromagnetic applications	Uses electromagnetic fields for their effects on the body	Nerve stimulation, hyperthermia, laser surgery
Herbal medicine	Uses plants and plant products as remedies	Echinacea, ginger, ginkgo biloba, ginseng, St. John's wort
Pharmacologic and biologic treatments	Uses drugs, vaccines, etc. that have not yet been approved by the Food and Drug Administration for specified purposes	Antioxidants, chelation, metabolic therapy
Diet, nutrition, and lifestyle changes	Affects biochemical and physiologic processes	Macrobiotic diet, high-dose vitamin therapy

Modified from U.S. Office of Alternative Medicine (1994). Alternative medicine: Expanding medical horizons (pp. 3-206). Washington, DC: National Institutes of Health. In Black J. M., Hawks, J. H., Keene, A. M.: *Medical surgical nursing: Clinical management for positive outcomes* (6th ed). Philadelphia: Saunders.

table 7-7 ***Examples of Dangerous Herbal Remedy–Drug Interactions***

REMEDY	DRUG	POTENTIAL EFFECT OF INTERACTION
Echinacea	Immunosuppressants	May inhibit immunosuppression
Ginseng	Aspirin	Increased anticoagulation → risk of bleeding
Goldenseal	Antihypertensives	Increased BP
Hawthorne	Cardiac glycosides	Increased effects of glycoside → risk of toxicity
Aloe (oral)	Potassium-wasting diuretics	Increased risk of hypokalemia
Kava-kava	Central nervous system (CNS) depressants	Increased sedation
Garlic	Anticoagulants	Increased anticoagulation → risk of bleeding
Ephedra (Ma-huang)	Antihypertensives	Increased blood pressure
Valerian	CNS depressants	Increased sedation

From Deglin, J. H., Vallerand, A. H. (1999). *Davis's Drug Guide for Nurses.* Philadelphia: F. A. Davis.

- Be aware of potentially dangerous remedies and those that can interact with prescription drugs that the patient is taking. Among dangerous remedies are the following herbs: sassafras, ephedra, chaparral, borage, calamus, comfrey, germander, life root, and pokeroot. See Table 7-7 for examples of drug interactions.
- Caution patients about very expensive therapies, especially if they make outlandish claims.

Put on your ***THINKING CAP!!***

1. Recall a frightening experience. Write down how you felt mentally and physically. Explain your feelings using the General Adaptation Syndrome (stress response).
2. List five ways to promote your own health while you are a nursing student.
3. Identify three factors that are threats to your health and identify ways to deal with each of them.

key points

- Because of cultural, educational, spiritual, and social differences, individuals have very different concepts about what constitutes health and illness.
- Health and illness are viewed as relative states along a continuum that fluctuates on a daily basis.
- Disease is a biologic or psychophysiologic malfunction, or both, and illness refers to how a person perceives and responds to not being well.
- To maintain the highest level of health and wellness, people must satisfy basic human needs.
- There are three broad categories of human needs: physical, libidinal, and ego developmental.
- Stress is mental or emotional pressure resulting from internal or external causes.
- Coping is any behavioral or cognitive activity used to deal with stress.
- Homeostasis describes a tendency of biologic systems to maintain stability of the internal environment while

continuously adjusting to changes necessary for survival.
- Health promotion activities are directed toward maintaining or enhancing well-being as a protection against illness.
- Illness is a deviation from a healthy state that may occur in the form of an acute episode or as a series of long-term events.
- Reactions to illness vary among individuals.
- When people become ill, they often assume a "sick role" that allows them time to recover from their disease.
- The impact of illness on the family depends on which family member is ill, the seriousness of the illness, and the social and cultural customs of the family.
- Nurses help people by striving to prevent disease, helping satisfy clients' unmet basic needs, helping clients increase adaptability, fostering independence, helping family members deal with patients' illnesses, and assisting terminally ill patients to a peaceful death.
- Complementary and alternative therapies are often based on holistic beliefs about the nature of health and illness.
- Complementary therapies are employed along with conventional treatment; alternative therapies are used in place of conventional therapies.
- The nurse should be open-minded about complementary and alternative therapies and should learn about them.

REVIEW QUESTIONS

1. A cancer patient has decided to treat herself with herbal remedies instead of receiving chemotherapy and radiotherapy. The use of herbal remedies in this situation is an example of:
   1. complementary therapy.
   2. conventional therapy.
   3. alternative therapy.
   4. allopathic therapy.
2. Which statement illustrates why Maslow's basic human needs are presented as a hierarchy?
   1. The sequence in which needs are met is not important.
   2. Each level of need must be satisfied before moving to the next step.
   3. At birth, humans are self-actualized and must learn to meet other needs.
   4. A person can only move upward in a hierarchy, never downward.
3. A clinic patient cut his arm at work 3 days ago. The skin around the wound is red, warm, and swollen. The patient reports that the wound is painful. The patient's signs and symptoms are evidence of:
   1. general adaptation.
   2. defense mechanisms.
   3. local adaptation.
   4. fight-or-flight response.
4. Homeostasis is:
   1. the exhaustion stage of the stress response.
   2. the use of home remedies in treatment of illness.
   3. the ability of a living organism to remain unchanged.
   4. a tendency of the body to maintain internal stability.
5. A patient who has a chronic disease is in a period of exacerbation. This means:
   1. symptoms are recurring.
   2. the disease has been cured.
   3. symptoms will soon reappear.
   4. the terminal stage of the disease has begun.
6. Nursing interventions that can help patients adapt to stress include:
   1. Limit teaching to what the patient needs to know.
   2. Do not require that the patient make any decisions.
   3. Discourage the use of complementary and alternative therapies.
   4. Identify the patient's previously successful coping strategies.
7. After receiving a diagnosis of Parkinson's disease, a patient signed up for an educational seminar, joined a community support group, planned home adaptations, and found Internet information sites. What coping strategy is the patient using?
   1. Self-control
   2. Positive reappraisal
   3. Confrontation
   4. Denial
8. Among complementary and alternative therapies, which of the following uses the power of the mind and body to affect each other?
   1. Nerve stimulation
   2. Guided imagery
   3. Ginkgo biloba
   4. Metabolic therapy

CHAPTER

8 Nutrition

objectives

1. Explain the role of the gastrointestinal system in the digestion of food.
2. Describe how food is digested and absorbed.
3. List the functions of each of the six classes of essential nutrients.
4. Define macronutrient and micronutrient.
5. Identify the food sources of proteins, carbohydrates, and fats.
6. Identify the food sources of dietary fiber.
7. List the possible health benefits of dietary fiber.
8. Identify the food sources of each of the vitamins and minerals.
9. Describe the changes in nutrient needs as an individual ages.
10. Differentiate anorexia nervosa, bulimia, and binge eating disorder.
11. Discuss the different types of nutritional support.
12. Identify guidelines for the nutritional assessment.

key terms

Amino acids (ă-MĒ-nō ĂS-ĭds, p. 79)
Basal metabolic rate (BĀ-săl mĕt-ă-BŎL-ĭk, p. 75)
Calorie (p. 76)
Complementary proteins (p. 80)
Complete protein (p. 79)
Incomplete protein (p. 79)
Insoluble fiber (ĭn-SŎL-ū-b'l, p. 77)
Lipids (LĬ-pĭds, p. 78)
Lipoproteins (lī-pō-PRŌ-tēns, p. 78)
Macronutrients (măk-rō-NŪ-trē-ĕnts, p. 74)
Micronutrients (mīk-rō-NŪ-trē-ĕnts, p. 74)
Minerals (p. 81)
Proteins (p. 79)
Resting energy expenditure (p. 75)
Saturated fatty acids (p. 78)
Triglycerides (trī-GLĬ-sĕ-rīdz, p. 78)
Unsaturated fatty acids (p. 78)
Vitamins (p. 81)

Nutrition is the cornerstone of the healing process. To support and maintain life or fight disease, the body must be supplied with the proper nutrients.

ANATOMY AND PHYSIOLOGY OF THE GASTROINTESTINAL SYSTEM

The gastrointestinal system (GI tract or "gut") is the long, continuous tube that receives and transports food, absorbs nutrients, and eliminates waste products of digestion. The primary organs that comprise the GI tract are the mouth, pharynx, esophagus, stomach, small intestine, and large intestine. In addition, the liver, gallbladder, and pancreas are called *accessory organs* of the GI tract because they have roles in food digestion even though they are not part of the digestive tract.

DIGESTION AND ABSORPTION

Normally 92% to 97% of the mixed American diet is digested and absorbed. Most substances such as water, simple sugars, vitamins, minerals, and alcohol are absorbed in their original form. However, substances such as lipids, proteins, and complex sugars must be converted to simple forms before they are absorbed.

The digestion of food is made possible by hydrolysis, a process through which water splits complex molecules into smaller units. Enzymes along with cofactors such as bile and hydrochloric acid govern the process of hydrolysis. Enzymes help to break down food particles to their simplest form so that the nutrients can be absorbed. Enzymes are secreted throughout the intestinal tract, except in the large intestine. Because digestion and absorption already have been completed by the time the food mixture reaches the colon, only water, salt, vitamins, and minerals are absorbed there.

REGULATORS OF GASTROINTESTINAL ACTIVITY

The gastrointestinal system is regulated by (1) neural control and (2) hormone secretion. Neural control is managed by the autonomic nervous system and a nerve network in the gut wall called the enteric nervous system. The autonomic nervous system consists of sympathetic and parasympathetic nerve fibers. Parasympathetic nerves generally stimulate digestive activity, whereas sympathetic nerves inhibit activity. A parasympathetic effect that is conveyed by the vagus nerve is the stimulation of acid secretion in the stomach in response to the sight or smell of food. The enteric nervous system consists of receptors in the gastric mucosa that are sensitive to the acidity of the gastrointestinal tract and the feeling of fullness.

Hormones are secreted into the gastrointestinal tract to help regulate gastric pH, gastric motility, and appetite. They also stimulate the pancreas to secrete insulin and enzymes.

DIGESTIVE PROCESS

Digestion of food occurs in three areas of the gastrointestinal system: (1) the mouth, (2) the stomach, and (3) the small intestine. When food is placed into the mouth, the teeth grind and crush the food into small particles. The food forms into a mass that is moistened and lubricated by saliva. While food is still in the mouth, a secretion containing an enzyme known as *amylase (ptyalin)* begins to digest any starch that is present. The mass, or bolus, is then passed to the pharynx and through the esophagus by the process of swallowing. *Peristalsis* moves the food rapidly through the esophagus into the stomach.

In the stomach, the mass is mixed with gastric secretions. Active chemical digestion is accomplished by the secretion of gastric juice. The stomach produces an average of 2,000 to 2,500 ml of gastric juice daily. The juice contains hydrochloric acid, enzymes, mucus, and the gastrointestinal hormone gastrin. The juice aids in the digestive process by converting the mass to a semiliquid substance called *chyme.*

The stomach is normally emptied in 1 to 4 hours, depending on the amount and kinds of foods eaten. When eaten alone, carbohydrates leave the stomach most rapidly, followed by protein, and then by fat. However, in a mixed diet, emptying of the stomach is prolonged.

Valves (sphincters) located at the entrance (cardiac sphincter) and exit (pyloric sphincter) of the stomach prevent the backflow of the food mass from the stomach into the pharynx and from the duodenum into the stomach. The small intestine is divided into the duodenum, the jejunum, and the ileum. Most of the digestive process is completed in the duodenum, and the jejunum and ileum function mostly in the absorption of nutrients. The remaining chyme is delivered to the large intestine where water and electrolytes are absorbed, leaving a mass of wastes called *feces.* The fecal mass is stored in the rectum where it triggers the defecation reflex. When the anal sphincters relax, feces pass out of the body through the anus.

Mechanisms of Absorption

The primary organ of absorption is the small intestine. It is 22 feet long and arranged in folds. The folds are covered with finger-like projections called *villi.* The villi absorb the nutrients into the blood and lymph vessels that support them. Each day the small intestine absorbs several hundred grams of carbohydrate, 100 grams or more of fat, 50 to 100 grams of amino acids, 50 to 100 grams of ions, and 7 to 8 liters of water.

Absorption is accomplished by the combination of the processes of diffusion and active transport. *Diffusion* involves the movement of particles from an area of higher concentration to an area of lower concentration. *Active transport* requires the input of energy for the movement of particles across a membrane against an energy gradient. This movement requires a carrier protein. The best-known carrier is the *intrinsic factor,* which is responsible for the absorption of vitamin B_{12}.

NUTRIENTS

Food contains many nutrients, including carbohydrates, proteins, lipids, vitamins, minerals, and fluids. Each of these nutrients is digested and absorbed differently. Ingested plant and animal molecules that can be used by the body for energy or to synthesize carbohydrates, lipids, or proteins are called ***macronutrients.*** Other dietary essentials including vitamins and minerals are called ***micronutrients.***

Carbohydrates

Carbohydrate digestion, as discussed earlier, is begun in the mouth, where the enzyme amylase is released. When carbohydrates reach the stomach, the activity of amylase is halted when it comes in contact with hydrochloric acid. If the carbohydrates remain in the stomach long enough, the hydrochloric acid reduces most of them to their simplest form. The stomach generally empties into the small intestine before this occurs, so most of the digestion of carbohydrates occurs within the small intestine. In the small intestine, pancreatic amylase is released to continue digestion. After the carbohydrates have been broken down, they pass through the villi into the bloodstream, where they are carried by the portal vein to the liver and absorbed. Some forms of carbohydrate, particularly fiber, cannot be digested by humans and are excreted unchanged in the feces.

Protein

Digestion of protein does not begin until it reaches the stomach. There proteins are split into smaller molecules. Most protein digestion occurs in the duodenum, not in the stomach. Almost all of the protein is absorbed by the time it reaches the end of the jejunum. Only 1% of ingested protein is found in the feces.

Fat

Digestion of fat also begins in the stomach. Gastric lipase, an enzyme, breaks down the triglycerides that make up fat into fatty acids and glycerol. The major portion of fat digestion takes place in the small intestine. The peristaltic action of the small intestine, along with bile that has been secreted by the liver, breaks down the larger fat globules into smaller particles.

Fluids, Vitamins, and Minerals

Fluids, vitamins, and minerals are absorbed through the intestinal mucosa. Each day about 8 liters of fluid from the body pass back and forth across the membrane of the gut to keep the nutrients in solution. Vitamins and water pass unchanged from the small intestine into the blood by passive diffusion. Mineral absorption is a more active, complex process that takes place in several stages.

FACTORS AFFECTING DIGESTION

Factors that affect the digestion of food include psychological state, bacterial action, and food processing.

Psychological State

The look, smell, and taste of food have an impact on digestion, as does the emotional climate surrounding eating. When humans see, smell, taste, and even think of food, secretions of saliva and gastric juices increase. On the other hand, emotions such as fear, anger, and worry can inhibit peristalsis and depress gastric secretions.

Bacterial Action

The second factor that affects digestion is related to bacterial action in the gastrointestinal tract. The gut is inhabited by about 100 different species of bacteria. A healthy person is not usually disturbed by these bacteria because they dwell in the gastrointestinal tract as normal flora. Bacterial action is most intense in the large intestine. Colonic bacteria are needed to help form vitamin K, vitamin B_{12}, thiamine, and riboflavin. They also produce various gases, acids, and other toxic substances, many of which contribute to the odor of feces.

Food Processing

The last factor that affects digestion is food processing. Cooked foods generally are more digestible than raw foods. The manner in which the food was cooked can also affect digestion. Foods fried at excessive temperatures retard the flow of digestive juices, whereas foods with meat extracts added stimulate digestion. Personal characteristics or allergies may account for differences in the way various people react to certain foods, their preparation, and additives in the foods.

ENERGY

Energy is defined as the capacity to do work. In the context of nutrition, energy refers to the way in which the body makes use of the energy received through the food that is eaten.

ENERGY EXPENDITURE

To understand the concept of energy, it is important to examine energy expenditure. Energy expenditure has three components:

1. *Resting energy expenditure (REE):* the energy used to maintain vital body processes. These activities include respiration and circulation, synthesis of organic products, movement of ions across membranes, maintenance of body temperature, and movement of ions across membranes. Most of our energy (60%-75%) is expended in these activities.
2. *Energy expended in physical activity (EEPA):* the energy used to support voluntary activity
3. *Thermic effect of food (TEF):* the energy is used to digest, absorb, and metabolize nutrients, including the synthesis and storage of protein, fat, and carbohydrate.

Measurement of Energy Expenditure

Energy expenditure is measured as the *basal metabolic rate (BMR)* or the *resting energy expenditure* (REE). These rates are measured when the patient is awake but in a state of complete physical and mental rest. The test must be scheduled several hours after any strenuous exercise or activity. The temperature and environment must be comfortable. The difference between measurements of BMR and REE is that the BMR is measured in the morning after the subject awakens, 10 to 12 hours after the last meal. REE, on the other hand, is measured at any time of day, 3 to 4 hours after the last meal. Factors that can cause the metabolic rate to vary among individuals include body size and composition, periods of growth, secretion of hormones, temperature, the menstrual cycle, and pregnancy.

Body Size and Composition. In terms of body size and composition, the key factors that affect metabolic rate are body surface area and fat-free or lean body mass and body weight. A person with a large body surface area loses more heat by evaporation from the skin, thereby expending more energy. A person with a high proportion of lean body mass to adipose tissue also expends more energy because resting skeletal muscle has a high metabolic rate. Estimates of metabolic rate based on body weight are also thought to be reasonably accurate. Interestingly, even though the ratio of lean mass to fat is generally higher in males, gender does not significantly affect the estimate.

Periods of Growth. The metabolic rate is highest during the first and second years of life—a period of rapid growth. A second, lesser peak occurs during puberty and adolescence.

Hormones. The principal regulators of the metabolic rate are the endocrine hormones, particularly thyroxine and epinephrine. For example, an underactive thyroid gland does not produce sufficient thyroxine, resulting in a lower metabolic rate. Conversely, an overactive thyroid gland produces too much thyroxine, which increases the metabolic rate. Other hormones that have an effect on the BMR include cortisol, growth hormone, and insulin.

Other Factors. Other factors that affect the BMR are sleep, fever, environmental temperature, the menstrual cycle, and pregnancy. The BMR of a sleeping person is approximately 10% below that of an alert person as a result of muscle relaxation and decreased activity of the sympathetic nervous system. A fever can increase the BMR by about 7% for each degree above 98.6° F. Environmental temperature affects the metabolic rate as well. People who live in very warm climates typically have higher resting energy expenditure than people who live in temperate climates. The BMR rises and falls during the menstrual cycle and remains elevated during pregnancy.

As noted earlier, physical activity can affect the BMR. The expenditure of energy associated with exercise can vary considerably, depending on body size, level of fitness, and amount of muscle mass. Although students might disagree, it has been found that mental activity does not affect energy requirements appreciably.

Eating is another activity that can affect the BMR. The metabolism of protein increases the metabolic rate by about 25% of the total calories consumed. Compare this with the metabolism of carbohydrates and fats, which increase the metabolic rate of total calories consumed by about 5%.

Energy Measurements and Calculations

The *calorie* is the standard unit for measuring energy. A calorie is the amount of heat energy needed to increase the temperature of 1 gm of water at standard temperature by 1° C. A kilocalorie (kcal), which is equal to 1,000 calories, is the measurement used most often in nutritional guidelines. Most people refer to a kilocalorie as a Calorie (with a capital "C").

Several methods can be used to measure each component of human energy expenditure. They include direct calorimetry, indirect calorimetry, and doubly labeled water. The measurements obtained in these human studies can be used to calculate the energy required for food digestion and metabolism and for physical activity. Because actual measures require expensive procedures, many equations have been developed to estimate measurements of energy expenditure and requirements based on patient characteristics.

CARBOHYDRATES

DEFINITION AND COMPOSITION OF CARBOHYDRATES

Most of the energy we require is consumed in the form of carbohydrates. These are organic compounds consisting of carbon, hydrogen, and oxygen. All of the sugars and starches that people eat and most types of fibers are carbohydrates. The simplest sugars are monosaccharides, which cannot be hydrolyzed to a simpler form. Monosaccharides can combine to form more complex carbohydrates.

Plants manufacture and store carbohydrates as their chief source of energy. The plants gather carbon dioxide from the air and water from the soil, and with chlorophyll found inside the plant, they use the energy of sunlight to form glucose. When animals consume plants, the glucose furnishes the energy needed to live. Glucose is the main sugar in the blood and the body's basic fuel; it serves as the primary source of energy.

CLASSIFICATION AND FOOD SOURCES OF CARBOHYDRATES

Carbohydrates are classified according to the number of simple sugars or saccharides: (1) monosaccharides, (2) disaccharides, (3) oligosaccharides, and (4) polysaccharides. *Monosaccharides* (one saccharide) are the simplest form of carbohydrate. Examples of monosaccharides are glucose, fructose, and galactose. Major food sources are fruits, vegetables, and honey. *Disaccharides* (two saccharides) contain two monosaccharide molecules. Examples are sucrose, lactose, and maltose. Disaccharides are found in maple or corn syrup (sucrose), milk (lactose), and malt products (maltose). *Oligosaccharides* contain three to ten monosaccharide molecules.

Polysaccharides have 10 to 10,000 or more molecules. Some polysaccharides are soluble (digestible) whereas others are insoluble (indigestible). Starch and glycogen are soluble (digestible) polysaccharides. Starch is found in grains and vegetables, and glycogen is in meat products and seafood. Fibers such as cellulose are usually insoluble (indigestible). Major food sources of cellulose include stalks and leaves of vegetables, outer coverings of fruits and seeds, and beans. Table 8-1 shows the carbohydrate content of certain foods.

CARBOHYDRATE METABOLISM

Carbohydrates are converted primarily to glucose for immediate use by the body's cells. The serum glucose level is maintained within normal limits through the regular intake of nu-

table 8-1 ***Carbohydrate Content of Foods***

SUGAR	CARBOHYDRATE CONTENT (%)	STARCH	CARBOHYDRATE CONTENT (%)
CONCENTRATED SWEETS		**GRAIN PRODUCTS**	
Sugar: Cane, beet, powdered brown, maple	99.5	Starches: Corn, tapioca, arrowroot	86-88
Candies	70-95	Cereals (dry): Corn, wheat, oat, bran	68-85
Honey (extracted)	82	Flour: Corn, wheat (sifted)	70-80
Syrup: Table blends, molasses	55-75	Popcorn (popped)	77
Jams, jellies, marmalades	70	Cookies: Plain, assorted	71
Carbonated, sweetened beverages	10-12	Crackers, saltines	72
FRUITS		Cakes: Plain, without icing	56
Prunes, apricots, figs (cooked, unsweetened)	12-31	Bread: White, rye, whole wheat	48-52
Bananas, grapes, cherries, apples, pears	15-23	Macaroni, spaghetti, noodles, rice (cooked)	23-30
Fresh: Pineapples, grapefruits, oranges, apricots, strawberries	8-14	Cereals (cooked): Oat, wheat, grits	10-16
MILK		**VEGETABLES**	
Skim	6	Boiled: Corn, white and sweet potatoes, lima beans, dried beans, peas	15-26
Whole	5	Beets, carrots, onions, tomatoes	5-7
		Leafy: Lettuce, asparagus, cabbage, greens, spinach	3-4

From Mahan, L.K., & Escott-Stump, S. (2000). *Krause's food, nutrition, and diet therapy* (10th ed., p. 43). Philadelphia: Saunders.

trients, glycogen storage, glucogenesis, and gluconeogenesis. Normal blood glucose levels are 70 to 100 mg/100 ml under fasting conditions. After a meal, the blood glucose level may rise to 130 mg/100 ml but returns to normal within 2 to 3 hours as some glucose is metabolized and the excess is stored in the liver as glycogen. Eventually the serum glucose level falls, and glycogen in the liver is converted to glucose by the process of glycogenolysis. During long periods of fasting or prolonged exercise, glycogenolysis may not be able to provide sufficient glucose. Then amino acids are converted to glucose in the liver through the process of gluconeogenesis. This process provides additional glucose to meet metabolic demands.

A number of hormones are involved in the regulation of blood glucose levels. They include insulin, glucagon, epinephrine, glucocorticoids, and growth hormone. These hormones and their actions are summarized in Table 8-2.

DIETARY FIBER

Fiber (or roughage) is a group of polysaccharides that act differently from other carbohydrates. They are found only in plant foods and are resistant to human digestive enzymes. Their major digestive role is to help form a soft, firm stool and to aid in the process of elimination.

There are two types of fiber, insoluble and soluble. *Insoluble fibers* include cellulose, hemicellulose, and lignin. They act as sponges to absorb many times their weight in water, swelling up in the intestine. Insoluble fibers help provide a full feeling long after they have been consumed and seem to help normalize intestinal transit time (the time required for food to pass through the GI tract). *Soluble fibers* such as gums and pectin help produce a softer stool but do less to help the passage of food. Soluble fiber prevents or reduces the absorption of certain substances in the bloodstream.

Functions of Carbohydrates in the Body

Each gram of carbohydrate yields about 4 kcal of energy. The functions of carbohydrates, in the form of glucose, are to:

- Serve as a major source of energy to body tissues
- Serve as the sole source of energy for the brain
- Maintain functional integrity of nerve tissue
- Spare fats from being used for metabolism under normal circumstances
- Serve as precursors (basic building blocks) for other physiologic substances.

Lactose remains in the intestines longer than other sugars. It promotes growth of beneficial bacteria, including those that synthesize vitamin K.

Glucuronic acid is a product of glucose metabolism that combines with toxins in the liver and converts them to a form that is readily excreted.

The functions of dietary fiber are to:

- Stimulate salivation and gastric juice secretion
- Promote a sense of gastric fullness
- Slow the rate of digestion and absorption of nutrients
- Normalize transit time through the intestines
- Increase fecal bulk
- Help to lower serum cholesterol
- Promote fermentation in the colon

RECOMMENDED DIETARY ALLOWANCE

The ideal daily dietary intake for carbohydrates is not known. However, diets without at least 50 to 100 grams of carbohydrates per day are likely to lead to ketosis. *Ketosis* is a condition caused by lack of adequate glucose that causes an excessive breakdown of tissue protein, loss of sodium and other cations, and involuntary dehydration.

In addition, although many nutritionists speak about the need for fiber in the diet, no specific recommendations have been established for what amount should be consumed daily. Several groups have recommended that Americans should increase their intake of dietary fiber and that this increase should come from a wide variety of whole-grain products, fruits, vegetables, and legumes. Fiber intake should consist of a 3:1 ratio of soluble to insoluble fiber. The mean fiber intake for adults in the United States is estimated to be about 11 to 13 gm/day, or about 6 gm/1,000 kcal. Table 8-3 lists the dietary fiber content of some foods.

table 8-2 ***Hormones Involved with the Regulation of Blood Glucose***

HORMONE	SITE OR PRODUCTION	EFFECTS
Insulin	Beta cells of the islets of Langerhans in the pancreas	Increases the rate of glucose utilization for oxidation, glycogenesis, and lipogenesis
Glucagon	Alpha cells in the islets of Langerhans in the pancreas	Raises the amount of glucose in the blood by increasing glycogenolysis and gluconeogenesis; it also stimulates the release of insulin from the pancreas
Epinephrine	Adrenal gland	Causes the breakdown of liver and muscle glycogen to yield blood glucose; also decreases the release of insulin from the pancreas
Glucocorticoids	Adrenal cortex	Stimulates gluconeogenesis, reduces glucose utilization, and increases the rate at which glycogen is converted into glucose
Growth hormone	Anterior pituitary gland	Increases amino acid uptake and protein synthesis by all cells, the uptake of glucose, and the mobilization of fat for energy

table 8-3 ***Dietary Fiber Content of Foods in Commonly Served Portions***

FOOD GROUP	LOW AMOUNTS (<1 GM)	MODERATE AMOUNTS (1-4 GM)	HIGH AMOUNTS (≥4 GM)
Breads (1 slice)	Bagel, white, French	Whole wheat, bran muffin (1)	
Cereals (1 oz)	Rice Krispies, Special K, Cornflakes	Wheaties, Shredded Wheat, Most, Honey Bran	Bran Chex, 40% Bran Flakes, Raisin Bran, Corn Bran, All-Bran, Bran Buds, 100% Bran
Pasta (1 cup)		Macaroni, spaghetti, whole wheat spaghetti	Lima beans, dried peas, kidney beans, baked beans, navy beans
Rice (½ cup)	White	Brown	
Legumes		Lentils	
Vegetables (½ cup cooked unless stated)	Cucumber, lettuce (1 cup), green pepper	Asparagus, green beans, cabbage, cauliflower, potato (without skin, 1), celery, broccoli, Brussels sprouts, carrots, corn, potato (with skin, 1), spinach, peas	
Fruits (1 medium unless stated)	Grapes (20), watermelon (1 cup)	Apricots (3), grapefruit (½), peach with skin, pineapple (½ cup), apple without skin, banana, orange, apple with skin, pear with skin, raspberries (½ cup)	

From Mahan, L.K., & Escott-Stump, S. (2000). *Krause's food, nutrition, and diet therapy* (10th ed., p. 40). Philadelphia: Saunders. Adapted with permission from Slavin, J.L. (1987). Dietary fiber: Classification, chemical analyses, and food sources. *Journal of the American Dietetic Association, 87,* 1164. Copyright © The American Dietetic Association.

LIPIDS

Substances that are classified as *lipids* include fats, oils, waxes, and related compounds. Lipids may be solid or liquid forms. A characteristic of all lipids is that they are insoluble in water. Lipids are similar to carbohydrates and contain the same three elements—carbon, hydrogen, and oxygen. Fat metabolism utilizes more oxygen and releases more energy than either carbohydrate or protein metabolism. The structure of lipids also allows them to be stored compactly with little or no water. Proteins and carbohydrates generally require more space for storing the same number of calories.

Triglycerides, also called neutral fats, are the most common fat found in foods of both animal and plant origin. Triglycerides consist of three fatty acids attached to a glycerol molecule. These fatty acids vary in length and in degree of saturation of hydrogen atoms, and it is these variations that determine the properties of different fats.

All fats are combinations of *saturated* and *unsaturated fatty acids.* Fats containing mainly saturated fatty acids are described as "highly saturated," whereas fats that are primarily polyunsaturated or monounsaturated are described as "highly unsaturated." Saturated fatty acids are loaded with all the hydrogen atoms they can carry. Fats that are largely saturated come chiefly from animal sources and include butter, milk fat, and the fat in meats; two vegetable oils, coconut and palm oils, also are highly saturated. Highly saturated fats are usually solid at room temperature and keep well.

Unsaturated fatty acids do not have all the hydrogen atoms they can carry. Depending on the number of missing hydrogen atoms, these fatty acids are called either monounsaturated (olive, peanut, canola, and avocado oils are largely monounsaturated) or polyunsaturated (corn, safflower, and sesame oils). The important dietary unsaturated fats come from plants and fish. They are generally liquid at room temperature and may become rancid quickly because the absence of hydrogen makes the carbon atoms very reactive.

LIPID TRANSPORT AND STORAGE

Most dietary lipids (fats) are absorbed into the lymphatic system through the intestinal mucosa. The exception is certain fatty acids that are absorbed directly into the portal blood. For fat to be digested, it must be emulsified, or pulled into suspension with digestive juices. Bile, a secretion of the liver, is necessary to emulsify fat. Bile is stored in the gallbladder and dispensed into the duodenum when fat is present. Once emulsified, fats can be broken down and absorbed.

After absorption, lipids are transported in the bloodstream in packages of lipids wrapped in protein called *lipoproteins.* Types of lipoproteins include chylomicrons, high-density lipoproteins (HDLs), low-density lipoproteins (LDLs), and very-low-density lipoproteins (VLDLs). Of particular interest in cardiovascular disease are the HDLs and the LDLs. Both lipoproteins carry cholesterol in the bloodstream; however, it appears that the cholesterol found in the LDLs increases the risk of atherosclerosis by contributing to plaque buildup on the artery walls. In contrast, HDL cholesterol seems to have the opposite effect. It appears that the HDLs carry cholesterol from the bloodstream to the liver to be degraded and excreted. The LDLs are sometimes referred to as carrying the "lethal" cholesterol, whereas the HDLs carry the "healthy" cholesterol.

An enzyme converts the lipids into substances that are small enough to pass through the cell walls of adipose (fat) tissue. Once inside the cell, lipids are stored as triglycerides and phospholipids. These fat cells can store up to 95% of their volume as triglycerides, which provides a reserve source of energy.

Most human adipose cells are in the form of white fat, which accumulates in subcutaneous tissue (50%), around the internal organs in the abdominal cavity (45%), and in the intramuscular tissue (5%). Brown fat is much less abundant and is located primarily in the interscapular region and on the back of the neck. The amount of this fat is higher in the neonate and decreases with age, but it can increase with extended exposure to cold.

LIPID METABOLISM

Lipids are a source of energy for most body tissues except the brain, blood cells, skin, and renal medulla. Even when glucose is available, muscle tissue readily uses fatty acids for energy. When the body needs to draw on fat reserves for energy, the fat cells release glycerol and free fatty acids by the process of lipolysis. Few tissues can use glycerol, so the liver picks it up and converts it to triglycerides or glucose. Free fatty acids bind to albumin for transportation in the blood and interstitial tissue. Most lipids are carried to the liver for conversion to energy or for use in the synthesis of new triglycerides. The center for lipid metabolism is the liver, which helps to regulate lipid levels in the body by the following processes:

- Synthesis of triglycerides and other lipids from fatty acids, carbohydrates, or protein
- Desaturation of fatty acids
- Catabolism (breakdown) of triglycerides for use as energy

If the body relies too heavily on fats for energy, large quantities of fatty acids accumulate in the liver. Through a series of physiologic processes, the liver produces acetoacetic and beta-hydroxybutyric acids, leaving a by-product called *ketone bodies.* The excretion of acetoacetic and beta-hydroxybutyric acids by the kidneys results in excessive loss of bicarbonate. The net effect is lowering of body fluid pH—a condition called *ketoacidosis.*

RECOMMENDED DIETARY ALLOWANCE

Most nutritionists recommend that people limit their fat intake to 30% or less of their daily caloric intake. People also should try to eat unsaturated fats rather than saturated fats to minimize the risk of heart disease. Studies have shown that Americans tend to consume too much fat, which can contribute to the development of cardiovascular disease and diabetes mellitus. Therefore, health promotion efforts have centered on teaching people how and why to limit the dietary intake of fat, particularly saturated fat.

FOOD SOURCES OF FAT

Animal products are the major source of saturated fats in the American diet. They include beef, dairy products, and eggs. Interestingly, many manufacturers are making fat-free products such as nonfat milk, cheese, and ice cream. In addition, cattle and pigs are being bred to yield beef and pork lower in saturated fat. Sources of unsaturated fats are vegetable oils, including corn oil, cottonseed oil, and safflower oil. Fruits, vegetables, and cereal grains are relatively low in fat. Refer to Table 8-4 for more sources of dietary fat.

FUNCTIONS OF LIPIDS

The functions of lipids are to (1) store energy, (2) maintain healthy skin and hair, (3) carry fat-soluble vitamins, (4) supply essential fatty acids, and (5) promote satiety. Although carbohydrates are the body's main source of food energy, fats are the most concentrated source, supplying 9 kilocalories per gram, whereas carbohydrates and protein supply only 4 kilocalories per gram.

PROTEINS

DEFINITION AND COMPOSITION OF PROTEINS

Protein is not a single, simple substance but a multitude of thousands of chemical combinations. The basic structure of protein is actually a chain of ***amino acids*** that can form many different configurations and can combine with other substances. Like carbohydrates and fats, proteins contain carbon, hydrogen, and oxygen. However, they also contain nitrogen, sulfur, and sometimes other elements such as metals, acids, lipids, and polysaccharides. Simple proteins are those that are made of only amino acids, whereas conjugated proteins are made of amino acids in combination with other substances.

There are 22 common amino acids, and they can be bonded in a variety of ways to form different proteins. The body uses all 22 amino acids, but only nine of them are considered essential amino acids. Each amino acid has a specific, important function. The nine *essential* amino acids must be obtained from the diet. They include cysteine, proline, leucine, isoleucine, valine, tryptophan, phenylalanine, methionine, and histidine. The body can manufacture adequate amounts of the other amino acids from the essential amino acids.

Food proteins can be classified as either complete or incomplete. A ***complete protein*** contains all nine essential amino acids in sufficient quantity and ratio for the body's needs. Complete proteins are generally of animal origin and are found in foods such as meat, poultry, fish, milk, cheese, and eggs.

Incomplete proteins are lacking in one or more of the essential amino acids. Incomplete proteins are of plant origin, such as the proteins in grains, legumes, nuts, and seeds. For the body to use protein for functions other than energy, all

table 8-4 Fat Content of Some Common Foods

0 GRAMS OF FAT	4-6 GRAMS OF FAT	15 GRAMS OF FAT
Most fruits and vegetables	Low-fat yogurt, 1 cup	Hot dog, beef, 2 oz
Nonfat milk	Cheese, mozzarella, part skim, 1 oz	McDonald's Chicken McNuggets, 6 pieces
Nonfat yogurt	Chicken, roasted with skin, 3 oz	Peanut butter, 2 T
Plain pasta and rice	Egg, scrambled, 1	Pork chop, broiled, 3 oz
Angel food cake	Turkey, roasted, 3 oz	Sunflower seeds, dry roasted, ¼ cup
Popcorn, air-popped, unbuttered	Granola, 1 oz	Avocado, ½ medium
Soft drinks	Muffin, bran, 1 small	Chop suey, beef and pork, 1 cup
Jam, jelly	Pizza, cheese, ¼ of 12-inch pie	Cinnamon roll, 1
1-3 GRAMS OF FAT	Burrito, bean, 1	**20 GRAMS OF FAT**
Popcorn, oil-popped, unbuttered, 1 cup	Brownie, with nuts, 1 small	Cheesecake, ⅟₁₂ cake
Low-calorie salad dressing, 1 T	Margarine or butter, 1 tsp	Lasagna with meat, 1 medium piece
Baked beans, ½ cup	Popcorn, oil popped, buttered, 1 cup	Macaroni with cheese, homemade, 1 cup
Soup, chicken noodle, canned, 1 cup	French dressing, regular, 1 T	Peanuts, dry roasted, ¼ cup
Whole wheat bread, 1 slice	**7-10 GRAMS OF FAT**	Ground beef, broiled, 3 oz
Dinner roll, 1	Cheese, cheddar, 1 oz	**25+ GRAMS OF FAT**
Waffle, frozen, 4-inch, 1	Milk, whole, 1 cup	Polish sausage, 3 oz
Coleslaw, ½ cup	Bologna, beef, 1 slice	Cheeseburger, large
Flounder or sole, baked, 3 oz	Sausage, 1 patty	Pie, pecan, ⅛ 9-inch pie
Chicken, without skin, roasted, 3 oz	Steak, sirloin, broiled, 3 oz	Chicken pot pie, frozen, baked, 1 pie
Tuna, canned in water, 3 oz	Potatoes, French fried, 10	Quiche, bacon, ⅛ pie
Cheese, cottage, 2% fat, ½ cup	Chow mein, chicken, 1 cup	
Ice milk, soft serve, ½ cup	Chocolate candy bar, 1 oz	
	Corn chips, 1 oz	
	Doughnut, cake type, plain, 1	
	Mayonnaise, 1 T	

From Mahan, L.K., & Escott-Stump, S. (2000). *Krause's food, nutrition, and diet therapy* (10th ed., p. 44). Philadelphia: Saunders. Data from Healthy Dividends, Rosemont, Ill, National Dairy Council, 1990.
T, Tablespoon; *oz*, ounce.

nine essential amino acids must be present at the same time. When various incomplete proteins are consumed at the same time, the body can use them together to obtain a balance of the essential amino acids. Incomplete proteins consumed together are called ***complementary proteins.***

PROTEIN METABOLISM AND SYNTHESIS

When food containing protein is eaten, the protein is broken down in the small intestine to the constituent amino acids by a process called *deamination.* Deamination produces ammonia, which may be used in synthesis or transported to the liver where it is converted to urea for excretion. The amino acids are then transported by the blood to the cells, where they can be synthesized into tissue protein, processed to produce ATP, or converted into glucose.

Protein synthesis in the body is controlled by DNA in the cells. DNA essentially provides a form to link up the exact combination of amino acids needed to form a particular protein. It is important to note that if one or more of the essential amino acids are in short supply or not available at all, nonessential amino acids that may be on hand cannot be used to form a protein. That is why it is important to eat a diet that contains all of the essential amino acids, plus enough additional amino acids to allow for synthesis of the nonessential amino acids.

PROTEIN DEFICIENCY

The body cannot store protein, so it needs to be eaten in the diet each day. Nitrogen in the urine is a good indicator of protein levels in the body. If protein intake is inadequate, nitrogen will be conserved by the kidneys, causing the urine nitrogen to be low. When this adaptive process is no longer adequate, evidence of protein deficiency appears. The signs and symptoms include edema, wasting of body tissues, fatty liver, dermatosis (thickening and hardening of the skin), diminished immune response, weakness, and loss of energy.

EVALUATION OF PROTEIN QUALITY

The average American consumes considerably more than the RDA for protein. The assessment of the adequacy of one's protein should include both the quantity and the quality of the protein consumed. The protein content, by weight, of cooked meat, fish, poultry, and milk solids is between 15% and 40%. The protein content of cooked cereals, beans, and lentils ranges from 3% to 10%. Ingesting a diet high in animal protein is not necessary and may be too high in fat. Eating a mixture of foods in a meal, if the quantity is sufficient, tends to provide all of the essential amino acids.

More total protein is required in a vegetable protein diet than in a diet of mixed vegetable and animal proteins because

table 8-5 ***Protein Content of Some Foods***

0-1 GRAM	7-8 GRAMS—cont'd
Butter, margarine, 1 tsp	Cheese, 1 oz
Pear, 1 medium	Tuna, 1 oz
Cake, 1 piece	Tofu, 3½ oz
2-3 GRAMS	Milk, 1 cup
Milk chocolate, 1 oz	**9-10 GRAMS**
Cereal, refined, 1 oz	Peanuts, roasted, 1 oz
Bread, 1 slice	Macaroni and cheese, ¾ cup
Corn, canned, ½ cup	Pizza, cheese, ⅛ of a 12-inch pie
Chicken noodle soup, 1 cup	
French fries, 1 regular serving	
4-6 GRAMS	**12-15 GRAMS**
Cereal, bran, 1 oz	Taco, 1
Baked potato, 1 large	Hamburger, 1
Peas, ½ cup	Chili with meat, 1 cup
7-8 GRAMS	**22-26 GRAMS**
Navy beans, cooked, ½ cup	Meat, lean, 3 oz
Egg, 1 medium	Big Mac, 1

From Mahan, L.K., Arlin, M. (1992). *Krause's food, nutrition, and diet therapy* (8th ed., p. 67). Philadelphia: Saunders.

more of the lower-quality protein is needed to meet the minimum requirements for amino acids and nitrogen. Because of their lower digestibility values, vegetable proteins are less available. Table 8-5 gives the protein content of typical foods in the American diet.

Functions of Proteins

The roles of proteins in the body are to:

- Furnish building blocks (amino acids) to build and repair tissue
- Serve as an energy source
- Help form enzymes, hormones, and other body fluids and secretions
- Assist in the transport of fats, fat-soluble vitamins, and other substances
- Help maintain osmolarity of body fluids

VITAMINS

Vitamins are organic compounds that the body needs for normal growth and development They help regulate metabolic functions within cells; however, only tiny amounts are needed to carry out these functions. Because the body cannot manufacture vitamins, they must be obtained in the diet. As mentioned earlier, vitamins are micronutrients. Most vitamins have multiple forms called *vitamers.* For example, vitamers of vitamin A are retinol, retinal, and retinoic acid.

The use of over-the-counter vitamin supplements is very popular. It is based on the perception that modern diets and processed foods do not provide the daily vitamin requirements. It is important to educate our patients about sources of vitamins, daily needs, and the dangers of excessive vitamin intake. Although scientific evidence is lacking, many manufacturers promote "natural" vitamin supplements as being superior to other supplements. Often "natural" products cost more, but really offer no additional benefits. The use of very large doses of vitamins may be appropriate in certain conditions but generally is not thought to be beneficial and may be harmful.

Vitamins are usually designated by letters and are classified into two groups on the basis of solubility: (1) fat-soluble vitamins that can be dissolved in fat, and (2) water-soluble vitamins that can be dissolved in water.

FAT-SOLUBLE VITAMINS

Fat-soluble vitamins include vitamins A, D, E, and K. Because they are fat soluble, they are usually absorbed in the body with other lipids. Like lipids, fat-soluble vitamins need bile and pancreatic juices for absorption. After entering the body, fat-soluble vitamins attach to lipoproteins and are transported to the liver. If the amount of a vitamin taken in exceeds the amount needed, the extra amount is stored in the fat cells of the body. As stores build up, the excess vitamins can become toxic. Therefore, it is recommended that people *not* take excessive amounts of these vitamins.

WATER-SOLUBLE VITAMINS

Water-soluble vitamins include the B-complex group (thiamine, riboflavin, niacin, B_6, folate, B_{12}, pantothenic acid, and biotin) and vitamin C (ascorbic acid). Excessive intake of these vitamins is not as dangerous as high intake of fat-soluble vitamins because water-soluble vitamins are readily excreted from the body. Therefore, they do not generally accumulate and become toxic. If taken in very large doses, some can have "bad" effects, but such doses are unlikely when food is the major source of these vitamins. However, because water-soluble vitamins are readily excreted, they should be replaced daily.

Most of the water-soluble vitamins are components of essential enzyme systems. Many are involved in the reactions that support energy metabolism. They have an essential role in the metabolic processes of living cells, both plant and animal. Table 8-6 gives more information about the sources and functions of vitamins.

MINERALS

Minerals are another group of micronutrients. They are involved in enzyme regulation, maintenance of acid-base balance and osmotic pressure, and maintenance of nerve and muscular irritability. Doubtless, there are other functions that are not well understood at this time. Because excess minerals are not readily excreted from the body, there is the potential for toxicity if taken in large amounts.

Minerals are classified on the basis of the daily requirement. Macrominerals (calcium, phosphorus, magnesium, sulfur, sodium, chloride, potassium) are required in amounts

table 8-6 ***Summary of Information on Vitamins***

NAME	SOURCES	COMMENTS
FAT-SOLUBLE VITAMINS		
Vitamin A	Liver, kidney, milk fat, fortified margarine, egg yolk, yellow and dark leafy vegetables, apricots, cantaloupe, peaches.	Essential for normal growth, development, and maintenance of epithelial tissue. Essential to the integrity of night vision. Helps provide for normal bone development and influences normal tooth formation. Toxic in large quantities.
Vitamin D	Vitamin D milk, irradiated foods, some in milk fat, liver, egg yolk, salmon, tuna fish, sardines.	Essential for normal growth and development; important for formation of normal bones and teeth. Influences absorption and metabolism of phosphorus and calcium. Toxic in large quantities.
Vitamin E	Wheat germ, vegetable oils, green leafy vegetables, milk fat, egg yolk, nuts.	Is a strong antioxidant. May help prevent oxidation of unsaturated fatty acids and vitamin A in intestinal tract and body tissues. Protects red blood cells from hemolysis.
Vitamin K	Liver, soybean oil, other vegetable oils, green leafy vegetables, wheat bran. Synthesized in intestinal tract.	Aids in production of prothrombin, a compound required for normal clotting of blood. Toxic in large amounts.
WATER-SOLUBLE VITAMINS		
Thiamine	Pork, liver, organ meats, legumes, whole-grain and enriched cereals and breads, wheat germ, potatoes. Synthesized in intestinal tract.	Aids in removal of CO_2 from alpha-keto acids during oxidation of carbohydrates. Essential for growth, normal appetite, digestion, and healthy nerves.
Riboflavin	Milk and dairy foods, organ meats, green leafy vegetables, enriched cereals and breads, eggs.	Essential for growth. Plays enzymatic role in tissue respiration and acts as a transporter of hydrogen atoms.
Niacin	Fish, liver, meat, poultry, many grains, eggs, peanuts, milk, legumes, enriched grains. Synthesized by intestinal bacteria.	Aids in transfer of hydrogen and acts in metabolism of carbohydrates and amino acids. Involved in glycolysis, fat synthesis, and tissue respiration.
Vitamin B_6	Pork, glandular meats, cereal bran and germ, milk, egg yolk, oatmeal, and legumes. Synthesized by intestinal bacteria.	Aids in the synthesis and breakdown of amino acids and in the synthesis of unsaturated fatty acids from essential fatty acids. Essential for normal growth.
Folate	Green leafy vegetables, organ meats (liver), lean beef, wheat, eggs, fish, dry beans, lentils, cowpeas, asparagus, broccoli, collards, yeast. Synthesized in intestinal tract.	Essential for normal maturation of red blood cells.
Vitamin B_{12}	Liver, kidney, milk and dairy foods, meat, eggs. Vegans require supplement.	Role in metabolism of nervous tissue. Involved with folate metabolism. Related to growth.
Vitamin C (ascorbic acid)	Acerola (West Indian cherry-like fruit), citrus fruit, tomato, melon, peppers, greens, raw cabbage, guava, strawberries, pineapple, potato.	Important in immune responses, wound healing, and allergic reactions. Increases absorption of iron.
Pantothenic acid	Eggs, kidney, liver, salmon, yeast	Involved in synthesis and breakdown of many compounds; essential for metabolism.
Biotin	Liver, mushrooms, peanuts, yeast, milk, meat, egg yolk, most vegetables, banana, grapefruit, tomato, watermelon, strawberries.	Essential component of enzymes.

Adapted from Mahan, L.K., & Escott-Stump, S. (2000). *Krause's food, nutrition, and diet therapy* (10th ed., pp. 105-106). Philadelphia: Saunders.

of 100 mg/day or more. Microminerals, or trace elements, are required in amounts of less than 15 mg/day (iron, zinc, iodine). Minerals that are required in amounts measured in micrograms (selenium, chromium, copper, manganese, molybdenum, boron, cobalt) are called *ultratrace elements.* Minerals are present in the body in ionized forms (sodium, potassium, etc.) or as constituents of organic compounds (phospholipids, hemoglobin, etc.).

Minerals account for 4% to 5% of body weight. Calcium and phosphorus contribute about 75% of weight. The remaining 25% is made up of all the other minerals. Food sources and functions of minerals are presented in Table 8-7.

table 8-7 ***Minerals in Human Nutrition***

MINERAL	LOCATION IN BODY AND SOME BIOLOGICAL FUNCTIONS	FOOD SOURCES
Calcium	99% in bones and teeth. Ionic calcium in body fluids essential for ion transport across cell membranes.	Milk and milk products, sardines, clams, oysters, kale, turnip greens, mustard greens, tofu.
Phosphorus	About 80% in inorganic portion of bones and teeth. Phosphorus is a component of every cell as well as of important metabolites, including DNA, RNA, ATP (high-energy compound), and phospholipids. Important to pH regulation.	Cheese, egg yolk, milk, meat, fish, poultry, whole-grain cereals, legumes, nuts.
Magnesium	About 50% in bone. Remaining 50% is almost entirely inside body cells, with only about 1% in extracellular fluid. Ionic Mg functions as an activator of many enzymes and thus influences almost all processes.	Whole-grain cereals, tofu, nuts, meat, milk, green vegetables, legumes, chocolate.
Sodium	About 30% to 45% in bone. Major cation of extracellular fluid, with only a small amount inside cell. Regulates body fluid osmolarity, pH, and body fluid volume.	Common table salt, seafoods, animal foods, milk, eggs. Abundant in most foods except fruit.
Chloride	Major anion of extracellular fluid, functioning in combination with sodium. Serves as a buffer, enzyme activator; component of gastric hydrochloric acid. Mostly present in extracellular fluid, with less than 15% inside cells.	Common table salt, seafoods, milk, meat, eggs.
Potassium	Major cation of intracellular fluid, with only small amounts in extracellular fluid. Functions in regulating pH and osmolarity and cell membrane transfer. Iron is necessary for carbohydrate and protein metabolism.	Fruits, milk, meat, cereals, vegetables, legumes.
Sulfur	Bulk of dietary sulfur is present in sulfur-containing amino acids needed for synthesis of essential metabolites.	Protein foods such as meat, fish, poultry, eggs, milk, cheese, legumes, nuts.
Iron	About 70% is in hemoglobin; about 26% stored in liver, spleen, and bone. Iron is a component of hemoglobin, important in oxygen transfer.	Liver, meat, egg yolk, legumes, whole or enriched grains, dark green vegetables, dark molasses, shrimp, oysters.
Zinc	Present in most tissues, with higher amounts in liver, voluntary muscle, and bone. Constituent of many enzymes and insulin.	Oysters, shellfish, herring, liver, legumes, milk, wheat bran.
Copper	Found in all body tissues; larger amounts in liver, brain, heart, and kidney.	Liver, shellfish, whole grains, cherries, legumes, kidney, poultry, oysters, chocolate, nuts.
Iodine	Constituent of thyroxine and related compounds synthesized by thyroid gland. Thyroxine functions in control of reactions involving cellular energy.	Iodized table salt, seafoods, water, and vegetables in nongoitrous regions.
Manganese	Highest concentration is in bone; also relatively high concentrations in pituitary, liver, pancreas, and gastrointestinal tissue.	Beet greens, blueberries, whole grains, nuts, legumes, fruit, tea.
Fluoride	Present in bone and teeth. In optimal amounts in water and diet, reduces dental caries, and may minimize bone loss.	Drinking water (1 ppm), tea, coffee, rice, soybeans, spinach, gelatin, onions, lettuce.

Adapted from Mahan, L.K., & Escott-Stump, S. (2000). *Krause's food, nutrition, and diet therapy* (10th ed., pp. 147-148). Philadelphia: Saunders.

WATER

Water is the largest component of the body and body tissues and is essential to all life processes in the body. It provides form and structure to cells and tissues; it is essential to the digestion, absorption, and excretion of metabolic and indigestible wastes; it is a transport medium for nutrients and all body substances; it maintains physical and chemical constancy of intracellular and extracellular fluids; and it regulates body temperature through the process of evaporation of perspiration.

The intake of water is controlled by thirst. The sensation of thirst serves as a signal to seek fluids. Water is also ingested through food. The breakdown of food in the body produces water as an end product. Water is lost from the body through the kidneys as urine, through the intestines as part of feces, through the lungs with expired air, and through the skin as evaporated sweat. When an imbalance in the amount of water taken in versus the amount of water lost occurs, various organs in the body, especially the kidneys, compensate by conserving more water and excreting less. The amount of water taken in daily should be equivalent to the amount of water lost.

There is no way the body can store water. It is essential that all living things replenish water daily to maintain health and efficiency. The longest period of time that people can go without water and sustain life is approximately 4 days. Adults generally should take in about 2,500 ml, or 2 to 3 quarts, of water per day. More in-depth discussion of fluid balance is provided in Chapter 13.

AGE-RELATED CHANGES

Healthy eating is a lifelong commitment that pays particular benefits in the later years of life. Maintaining a good diet can help middle-aged and older people maintain a high level of function and reduce the risks of chronic disease. Many functional changes naturally occur in humans as they age. Table 8-8 summarizes these changes in terms of the effects on the nutritional status of the older adult.

ENERGY

Because of the normal decline in metabolism and common decrease in physical activity, energy needs are lower with age. Therefore the older person often reduces the kilocalories taken in per day. This can result in an inadequate intake of other essential nutrients. The recommended daily energy intake for light to moderately active older adults is 30 kcal/kg of body weight. This reflects a reduction of 600 kcal/day for older men and 300 kcal/day for older women. However, lifestyle and health status of older adults vary widely, and these figures may need adjustments for each individual. Nutrients previously discussed in this chapter, including proteins, carbohydrates, lipids, vitamins, minerals, and water, may need adjustment as people age (Table 8-9). For those who are less active, less than the usual recommended amounts of thiamine, riboflavin, and niacin are needed. Nevertheless, many older people take vitamin supplements believing that their diets provide insufficient vitamins and that supplements will provide energy, slow the aging process, and prevent illness.

Psychosocial factors also may lead to poor nutrition in the older person. Depression, cognitive impairment, and loneliness can affect appetite and the intake of food. The term "failure to thrive" has been applied to elders who are undernourished, depressed, and declining physically and cognitively. Failure to thrive has been attributed to organic and nonorganic factors. This phenomenon is the subject of study to determine how to identify reversible conditions, and how best to intervene.

NUTRITIONAL CARE OF THE OLDER ADULT

Dietary Planning

Dietary planning for the older adult is no different from planning for a younger adult. Meals need to be appealing, taking into consideration individual likes and dislikes, and should be tasteful and filling. Planning may be different for older adults with special needs. Many may prefer four to five small meals over three large ones. In addition, problems such as difficulty swallowing, dentures that do not fit properly, and arthritis, which makes using utensils uncomfortable, must be considered.

The diet should include all of the food groups. Severely restricted diets such as low-sodium and low-fat diets are generally not advised for elders. When food is unappetizing, the older person may simply not eat enough to obtain necessary nutrients.

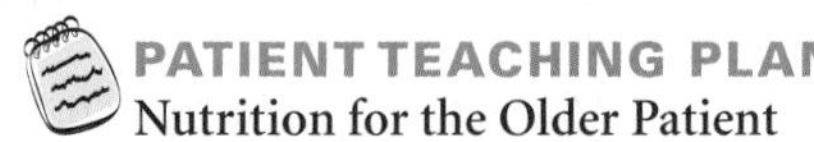

PATIENT TEACHING PLAN
Nutrition for the Older Patient

In addition to general information about nutritional requirements, you should share the following with the elderly patient:

- A normal diet typically supplies adequate vitamins.
- Megadoses (very large doses) of vitamins have not been proven beneficial and can be harmful.
- "Natural vitamins" are more expensive, and there is no evidence that they are better than synthetic vitamins.
- Vitamins do not provide more energy.

Nutrition Programs

Many community-based programs, administered by both public and private agencies, provide hot, nutritious meals to older adults. The meals are served either in a group setting or in the home. Special regulations and conditions must be met to qualify for these programs.

Nutritional Needs During Prolonged Illness

All people have increased nutritional needs during periods of illness. Older adults with chronic diseases such as emphysema and bronchitis, cancer, organic brain disease, cirrhosis, and maldigestion or malabsorption syndromes are at increased risk for protein deficiency and negative nitrogen balance. Individuals at risk need to be watched very carefully for this condition, which can be prevented by increasing nutritional support. Nasogastric tube feedings or parenteral nutrition may be required to meet these increased needs.

Nutritional Care in Institutional Settings

Good nutrition can have a dramatic effect on the physical, mental, and emotional function of your elderly patients. Nurses in long-term care and home health settings must be especially vigilant in monitoring the nutritional status of elderly patients. Age-related changes, chronic and acute conditions, cognitive and emotional disorders, medications, and situational factors can contribute to inadequate nutritional intake, digestion, or elimination. Also, patients who are obese have special needs. Excess body weight makes it more difficult to control many chronic conditions and can greatly interfere with activities of daily living. The

table 8-8 ***Nutrition-Related System Changes in the Older Adult***

SYSTEM	CHANGES
Sensory	Senses of taste, smell, sight, hearing, and touch are diminished. There is a decreased number of taste buds and a decreased sensitivity to sweet and salty tastes. Patient may experience glossodynia (pain in the tongue) and decreased olfactory sense.
Gastrointestinal	Changes in appetite response contribute to anorexia. Ill-fitting dentures and periodontal disease make eating painful. Decreased salivary secretion decreases the ability to chew and swallow foods. Decreased acid secretion causes an overgrowth of the bacteria of the gut. Lack of intrinsic factor leads to decreased absorption of vitamin B_{12}. There is an increased incidence of gallbladder disease; decreased motility of intestines leads to constipation.
Metabolic	Decreased tolerance to glucose leads to an increase in plasma glucose levels. Basal metabolic rate decreases by 20% due to decrease in lean body mass.
Cardiovascular	Blood vessels become less elastic. Total peripheral resistance increases. There is an increased risk for hypertension.
Renal	Kidney function diminishes and the acid–base response to metabolic challenges is slowed. There is increased difficulty in handling excessive amounts of protein waste products.
Musculoskeletal	Progressive replacement of lean body mass by fat and connective tissue. Body protein is decreased by 30%-40%. More fat is deposited on the trunk and around the visceral organs. Bone density is diminished, and there is shortening of the spinal column.
Immunocompetence	The immune function declines with age. There is a diminished ability to fight infection.
Psychosocial	Many experience depression as a result of a sense of loss or of loss of loved ones, productivity, a sense of worth, mobility, income, and body image.

table 8-9 ***Changes in the Nutritional Requirements for the Older Adult***

NUTRIENT	CHANGES IN NEEDS	SPECIAL PROBLEMS
Protein	Need unchanged (0.8 gm/kg) unless ill. Needs may increase with infection, altered GI function, or chronic diseases that affect metabolism.	Protein-calorie undernutrition may be a special problem for older men who live alone.
Carbohydrate	Need less sugar, more complex carbohydrates. Complex carbohydrates should contribute 55% of calorie intake.	Reduced glucose tolerance, lactose intolerance.
Lipid	Same as younger adult (not more than 30% of the total kilocalories).	Serum cholesterol levels in men tend to peak during middle age and then drop slightly; levels in women continue to rise with increasing age.
Minerals	The need for trace elements may be reduced owing to decreased lean body mass; calcium intake of 1,000-1,500 mg/day for postmenopausal women.	Hypertension is common, which results in the need to decrease sodium and increase potassium and magnesium for those taking diuretics.
Vitamins	Vitamin A is sufficient in the older adult owing to stores in the liver; may require vitamin D supplement if patient is not exposed to sunlight; some require vitamin C supplements; vitamin B_6 and folate are maintained with normal diet; vitamin B_{12} may be deficient owing to loss of intrinsic factor.	A maintenance level multivitamin and mineral supplement may be required. Patient must be monitored closely for overdose.
Water	30-35 ml/kg of ideal body weight.	Dehydration is the most common fluid and electrolyte disturbance. Patient must be monitored closely.

nutritional needs of older adults in institutional settings may change over a period of time. Therefore, periodic reassessment of nutritional status is critical to avoid imposing unnecessary diet restrictions or missing important nutritional needs.

Assisting elderly patients with meals must be a high priority. For example, how many times have you seen a meal cart with trays that have barely been touched being returned to the kitchen? You should question why patients are not eating and implement nursing measures to improve the situation.

GUIDELINES FOR DIETARY PLANNING

THE FOOD GUIDE PYRAMID

A number of guidelines have been established in the United States to help in planning for optimal nutrition. Until July 1992, the basic four food groups were considered the standard food guide. At that time, the U.S. Department of Agriculture established the food guide pyramid. The food guide pyramid expanded the basic four food groups of milk, meat, fruits and vegetables, and grains and added a fats, oils, and sweets group. This pyramid shows the ideal natural grouping for the way the American public should eat (Fig. 8-1).

RECOMMENDED DAILY ALLOWANCE

Recommended dietary allowances (RDAs) are guidelines for the amounts of nutrients that healthy people should consume daily. Nutrient requirements vary among individuals, so these recommended amounts tend to be high. The Food and Nutrition Board is in the process of revising the recommendations under the title Dietary Reference Intakes (DRIs). DRIs will include nutrient recommendations for healthy people in four categories: adequate intake (AI), estimated average intake (EAR), recommended dietary allowance (RDA), and tolerable upper intake level (UL) (Table 8-10).

Food Labeling

With the increase in public awareness of health and nutrition, people have expressed an increased need to be informed about what they are eating. Many more foods are now labeled so that the average person can make determinations about the quality and quantity of the nutrients consumed. Because of the lack of space available on a package label, the table is abbreviated to include essential information to describe the number of nutrients per serving (Fig. 8-2).

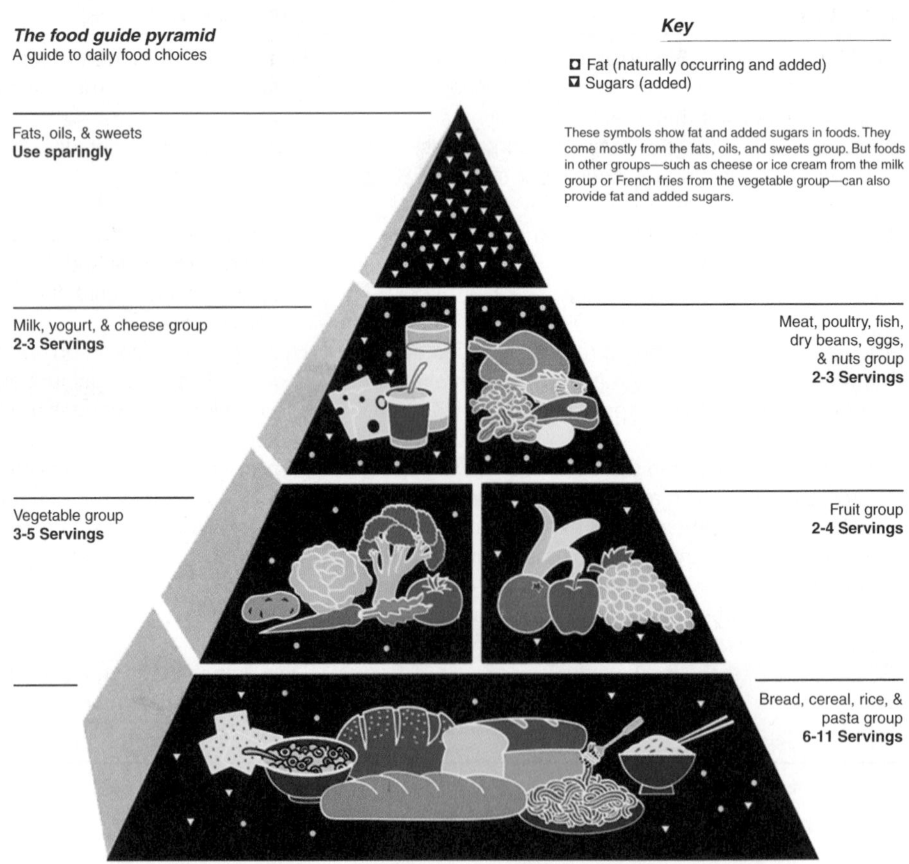

FIGURE 8-1 The Food Guide Pyramid.

table 8-10 **Dietary Reference Intakes, Recommended Dietary Allowances, and Adequate Intakes**

	MEN	WOMEN		MEN	WOMEN
Energy (kcal)	2300	1900	Vitamin B_6 (mg)	1.7	1.5
Protein (g)	63	150	Folate (μg)	400	400
Vitamin A (mcg RE)	1000	800	Vitamin B_{12} (μg)	2.4	2.4
Vitamin D (mcg)*			Calcium (mg)*	1200	1200
51-70 yrs of age	10	10	Phosphorus (mg)	700	700
>70 yrs of age	15	15	Magnesium (mg)	420	320
Vitamin E (mg α-TE)	10	8	Iron (mg)	10	10
Vitamin K (mg)	80	65	Zinc (mg)	15	12
Thiamin (mg)	1.2	1.1	Iodine (mcg)	150	150
Riboflavin (mg)	1.3	1.1	Selenium (mcg)	70	55
Niacin (mg NE)	16	14			

From Mahan, L.K., & Escott-Stump, S. (2000). *Krause's food, nutrition, and diet therapy* (10th ed., p. 295). Philadelphia: Saunders. (Reprinted with permission from Food and Nutrition Board National Research Council. Recommended Dietary Allowances, 10th ed., copyright © 1989 by the National Academy of Sciences. Published by National Academy Press; and Dietary Reference Intakes: Recommended Levels for Individual Intake. Food and Nutrition Board. Institute of Medicine, National Academy of Sciences, copyright 1998).

**RE,* Retinol equivalents; *α-TE,* alpha-tocopherol equivalents; *NE,* niacin equivalents.

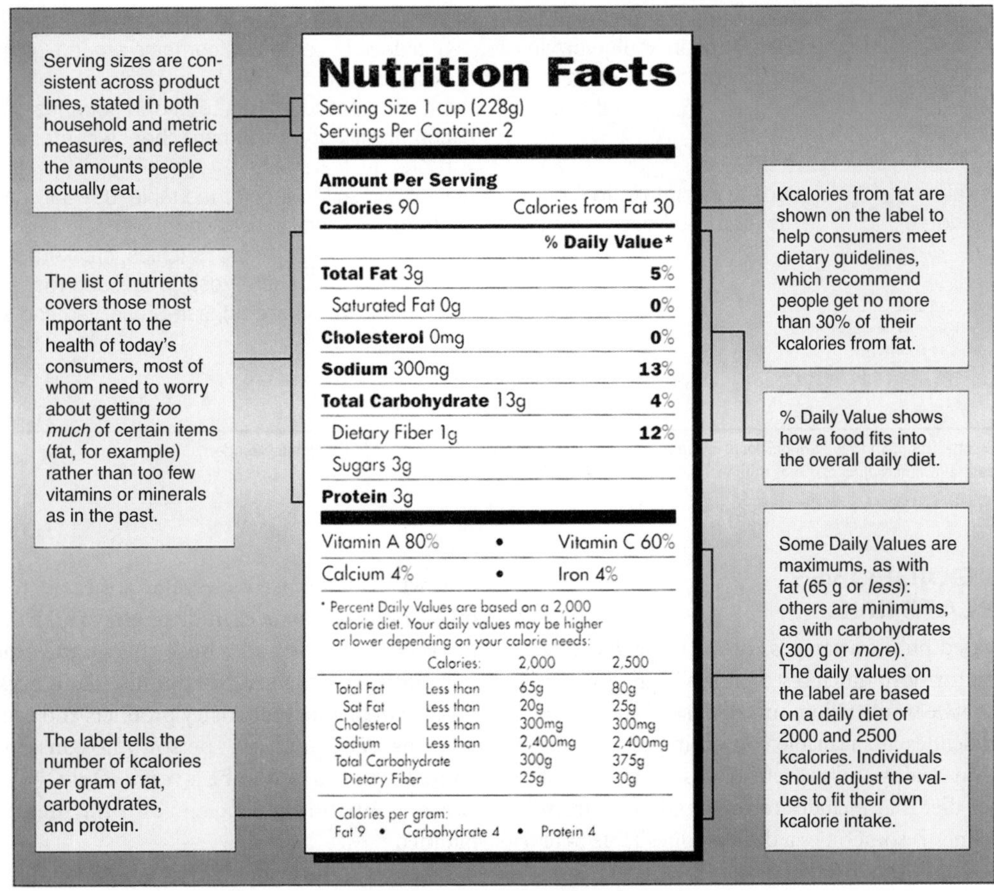

FIGURE 8-2 Example of a nutrition label.

table 8-11 ***Composite of Selected Dietary Guidelines***

GENERAL	SPECIFIC	INSTRUCTION
Reduce consumption of fat (especially saturated fat) and cholesterol.	Reduce total fat intake to 30% or less of calories. Reduce saturated fat intake to less than 10% of calories and the intake of cholesterol to less than 300 mg/day.	Substitute extra lean ("select") beef and pork, skinless chicken and turkey, fish, and shellfish (except shrimp) for high-fat meats. Eat a maximum of 7 oz of animal protein daily. Use cottage, pot, ricotta, and other low-fat cheeses in place of hard cheeses as much as possible. Maximize use of legumes, whole grains, vegetables, and fruits. Minimize use of butter, margarine, mayonnaise, salad dressings, peanut butter, rich sauces, and gravies. Use reduced-fat versions if possible. Use no more than 3-4 egg yolks per week.
Increase consumption of carbohydrates, especially complex carbohydrates and fiber.	Increase carbohydrate consumption to at least 55% of total calories. Limit intake of refined sugars to 10% of calories.	Every day, eat at least 5 servings of fruits and vegetables, including potatoes and those high in vitamins A (orange-yellow and dark green vegetables) and C. Eat at least 6 servings of whole-grain breads, cereals, or pasta each day. Eat less of sugar-rich foods (jams, jellies, syrups, candies, rich desserts, baked goods).
Maintain protein at moderate levels.	Do not exceed 2 times the RDA for protein, or approximately 100 gm for an adult woman and 125 gm for an adult man.	Eat moderate portions of high-protein foods. Limit meat servings to 7 oz/day. (A 3-oz serving is about the size of a deck of cards and contains around 20 gm of protein.) Limit dairy products to a total of 3 servings daily. One cup of milk or 1 oz of hard cheese contains 8 gm of protein.
Limit intake of salt (sodium chloride).	Limit daily salt intake to 6 gm (1 level tsp) or less.	Do not add salt to food at the table; use only small amounts during cooking and serving. Minimize use of salty foods (chips, crackers, other salted snack foods, French fries), processed foods (canned soups, frozen entrees), salt-preserved and salt-pickled foods.

From Mahan, L.K., & Escott-Stump, S. (1996). *Krause's food, nutrition, and diet therapy* (9th ed., pp. 342-343). Philadelphia: Saunders.
RDA, Recommended daily allowance; *ppm*, parts per million.

NATIONAL GUIDELINES FOR DIET PLANNING

Because of increased public awareness of the importance of health and good nutrition, much research has been done on the connection between nutrition and disease. As a result, many current guidelines are available concerning proper nutrition to maintain health and prevent disease. The task of planning a proper diet that includes recommendations from the various guidelines is sometimes a difficult one. Table 8-11 presents a composite of the dietary guidelines from the Surgeon General's Report on Nutrition and Health (1988) that can be used as a basis for dietary planning.

VEGETARIAN DIETS

Vegetarian diets are not new but have only gradually gained acceptance as a balanced nutritional option. Many Americans who call themselves vegetarians eat all foods except red meat, although some exclude poultry and fish as well. A *lactovegetarian* diet includes milk, cheese, and other dairy products but excludes meat, fish, poultry, and eggs. A *lacto-ovo-vegetarian* diet includes dairy products and eggs but excludes meat, fish, and poultry. A person who consumes no foods of animal origin is said to be a *vegan*. Only the vegan is at real risk for nutritional deficiencies if the diet is not carefully planned.

There is some evidence that vegetarian diets have distinct health benefits including reduced risks of type 2 diabetes mellitus, breast and colon cancer, and cardiovascular and gallbladder disease. Vegetarians generally consume less protein than nonvegetarians, but most still exceed the RDA for protein.

Adaptations that the vegetarian will need to be aware of include:

- Vegans are at risk for megaloblastic anemia resulting from vitamin B_{12} deficiency. Many foods, such as

table 8-11 ***Composite of Selected Dietary Guidelines—cont'd***

GENERAL	SPECIFIC	INSTRUCTION
Maintain adequate calcium intake.	Meet daily RDA, particularly for adolescents and young women up to 25 years of age (1,200 mg).	Increase daily intake of nonfat or low-fat milk or dairy products to 2 to 3 servings (1 cup milk or equivalent). Eat tofu (calcium sulfate processed), vegetable greens, broccoli, or calcium-fortified orange juice frequently.
Emphasize dietary cancer prevention.	Reduce fat consumption to 30% of calories and eat foods high in vitamins A and C (see earlier). Include cruciferous vegetables in the diet. Avoid potential dietary carcinogens.	Include broccoli, Brussels sprouts, cauliflower, cabbage, kale, turnips, and rutabagas frequently. Avoid charcoal-broiled meats or eat them infrequently. Reduce fat intake as described earlier.
Children, adolescents, and women of childbearing age should consume foods that are good sources of iron.		Eat lean red meats, fish, beans, whole-grain products, and daily servings of iron-enriched cereals.
Community water systems should contain fluoride at optimal levels for prevention of tooth decay.		Drink water containing fluoride at the level of approximately 1 ppm. When fluoridated water is not available, use supplementary fluoride.
Avoid taking dietary supplements in excess of the RDA in any 1 day.		Do not take vitamins and minerals indiscriminately just because they are available.
If you drink alcohol, do so in moderation. Pregnant women should avoid alcoholic beverages.	Limit consumption to the equivalent of less than 1 oz of pure alcohol in a single day.	Limit daily intake to 2 cans of beer or 2 small glasses of wine or 2 1½ oz jiggers of distilled spirits, each of which contains 1 oz of alcohol.
Balance food intake and physical activity to achieve and maintain appropriate body weight.	Appropriate weight is 15%-18% body fat for men and 20%-24% body fat for women. Overweight is 120% of desirable weight, or body mass index above 25.	Reduce weight slowly to appropriate level when necessary. Exercise aerobically at least 3 times per week.

fortified breakfast cereals, can provide adequate B_{12} supplements.

- Vegetarian diets must be planned to assure adequate calcium, iron, zinc, and vitamins B_{12} and D.

NURSING ASSESSMENT OF NUTRITIONAL STATUS

DIETARY HISTORY

The first step in determining the nutritional status of any person is assessment. The areas covered in a nutritional assessment include a dietary history, anthropometric data, laboratory data (if available), and physical examination data. Throughout the assessment interview, observe the patient's physical appearance for signs of malnutrition, obesity, and other factors that may indicate nutritional deficits. The well-nourished person should have shiny and healthy-looking hair, bright and clear eyes, smooth facial skin with good color, smooth lips and tongue, and healthy teeth and gums. Signs of malnutrition include dull, thin, and sparse hair; pale conjunctiva; a swollen or pale face; swollen lips and tongue; teeth with cavities or missing teeth; and bleeding or receding gums.

The diet history includes physical, psychological, social, and medical data that may have an impact on nutritional status. Table 8-12 summarizes information you should obtain in the dietary history. Commonly used tools to collect retrospective ("after the fact") data about dietary patterns include the 24-hour recall and the food frequency record. For a 24-hour recall, ask the patient to recall everything eaten during the past 24 hours, usually from the time of awakening until the next morning. Note everything that entered the mouth, including meals, snacks, drinks (especially water), and seasonings (especially salt). The food frequency record uses a list of foods from all food groups to assess how often the patient consumes specific foods. Because neither tool provides perfectly accurate data, it is probably best to use both of them.

table 8-12 Dietary History Information

ECONOMICS Income (frequency and steadiness of employment) Amount of money for food each week or month, and individual's perception of its adequacy for meeting food needs Eligibility for food stamps and cost of stamps Public aid recipient? **PHYSICAL ACTIVITY** Occupation (type, hours per week, shift, energy expenditure) Exercise (type, amount, frequency [seasonal?]) Sleep (hours per day [uninterrupted?]) Handicaps **ETHNIC OR CULTURAL BACKGROUND** Influence on eating habits Religion Education **HOME LIFE AND MEAL PATTERNS** Number in household (eat together?) Person who does shopping Person who does cooking Food storage and cooking facilities (stove, refrigerator) Type of housing (home, apartment, room, etc.) Ability to shop and prepare food **APPETITE** Good, poor; any changes? Factors that affect appetite Taste and smell perception; any changes? **ATTITUDE TOWARD FOOD AND EATING** Disinterest in food Irrational ideas about food, eating, and body weight Parental interest in child's eating	**ALLERGIES, INTOLERANCES, OR FOOD AVOIDANCES** Foods avoided and reason why Length of time of avoidance Description of problems caused by foods **DENTAL AND ORAL HEALTH** Problems with eating Foods that cannot be eaten Problems with swallowing, salivation, food sticking **GASTROINTESTINAL** Problems with heartburn, bloating, gas, diarrhea, vomiting, constipation, distention Frequency of problems Home remedies Antacid, laxative, or other drug use **CHRONIC DISEASE** Treatment Length of time of treatment Dietary modification (physician prescription?, date of modification, education, compliance with diet) **MEDICATION** Vitamin and/or mineral supplements (frequency, type, amount) Medications (type, amount, frequency, length of time on medication) **RECENT WEIGHT CHANGE** Loss or gain How many pounds, over what length of time? Intentional or nonvolitional? **DIETARY OR NUTRITIONAL PROBLEMS (AS PERCEIVED BY PATIENT)**

From Mahan, L.K., & Escott-Stump, S. (2000). *Krause's food, nutrition, and diet therapy* (10th ed., p. 367). Philadelphia: Saunders.

From these assessments, general dietary deficits and excesses can be determined.

Anthropometric Data

Anthropometric data include height, weight (including weight patterns), and body composition. Height and weight measurements should be performed correctly to complete an accurate assessment of the patient. Table 8-13 gives guidelines on the proper way to perform these measurements.

Body composition is related to the ratio of fat to lean muscle mass. Determining a person's body composition requires taking several measurements. These measurements include skinfold thickness and hydrostatic weighing. Skinfold thickness is measured by means of calipers that pinch skin over areas of the body that seem to reflect best the fat content of the subcutaneous tissue. These sites include areas over the triceps, over the biceps, below the scapula, above the iliac crest, and on the upper thigh (Fig. 8-3).

Hydrostatic weighing is done underwater. The advantage of weighing underwater is that it provides a good estimate of body density as a person is submerged, indicating the amount of adipose tissue or percentage of body fat. Body mass index (BMI) is a way to evaluate the weight of an adult. BMI is obtained by the following formula (a value of 20 to 25 is optimal):

$$\frac{\text{Patient's weight in kilograms}}{\text{Height in meters} \times \text{Height in meters}}$$

Laboratory Data

Laboratory tests that are helpful in assessing nutritional status are serum albumin, total lymphocyte count (TLC), creatinine/height index, nitrogen balance, mean corpuscular volume (MCV), and transferrin saturation:

- *Serum albumin:* There are several possible explanations for low serum albumin, including protein depletion. The normal serum albumin level is 3.5 to 5 gm/dL

table 8-13 Recommendations for the Measurement of Height and Weight

HEIGHT	WEIGHT
• Height should be measured without shoes. • Feet should be together with the heels against the wall or measuring board. • The subject should stand erect, neither slumped nor stretching, looking straight ahead, without tipping the head up or down. The top of the ear and outer corner of the eye should be in a line parallel to the floor. • A horizontal bar, a rectangular block of wood, or the top of the statiometer should be lowered to rest flat on the top of the head. • Height should be read to the nearest ¼ inch or 0.5 cm.	• Use a beam balance scale, not a spring scale, whenever possible. • Periodically calibrate the scale for accuracy, using known weights. • Weigh the subject in light clothing without shoes. • Record weight to the nearest ½ lb or 0.2 kg. Measurements above the 90th or below the 10th percentile warrant further evaluation.

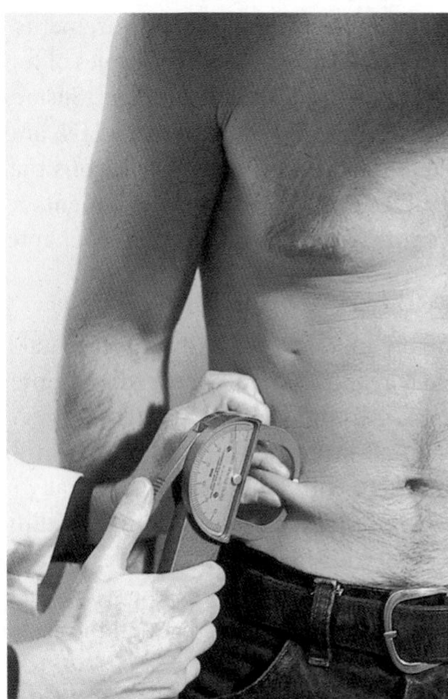

FIGURE 8-3 Skinfold calipers measure in millimeters the thickness of the subcutaneous fat tissue, which gives a rough measurement of adiposity.

- *Total lymphocyte count:* Protein and calorie deficits interfere with immune function, resulting in a low TLC. The normal lymphocyte count is 2,500 mm³. A count of less than 1,500 mm³ is consistent with protein/calorie malnutrition.
- *Urine creatinine/height index:* Expected urine creatinine is based on the patient's height. It provides an evaluation of body muscle mass.
- *Nitrogen balance:* Nitrogen balance exists when nitrogen intake and excretion are equal. A patient who is in a state of starvation will excrete more nitrogen in the urine than consumed, creating a negative nitrogen balance.
- *Mean corpuscular volume:* MCV measures the size of red blood cells (RBCs). With different types of anemia, RBC size varies. Therefore, when anemia is present, MCV helps determine the type of anemia.
- *Transferrin saturation:* Transferrin is a protein that transports iron. Transferrin saturation is normally between 30% and 50%; less than 30% indicates anemia; more than 50% indicates iron overload.

WEIGHT MANAGEMENT AND EATING DISORDERS

Many Americans today are on some form of "diet." People feel an increasing dissatisfaction with their appearance and a constant need to change that appearance. Most people view dieting as deprivation at best and punishment at worst. Changing eating patterns takes motivation, hard work, and a willingness to control behavior over a long period of time. Most adults have the ability to maintain a constant weight, but to do so, they must maintain consistent eating and exercise patterns on a daily basis.

Overweight individuals are considered obese if their weight is 20% or more above ideal body weight. Obesity is associated with coronary artery disease, lipid disorders, and type 2 diabetes mellitus (non–insulin-dependent diabetes mellitus). It is also considered a risk factor for some kinds of cancer and is associated with joint disease, gallstones, and respiratory problems.

The underweight person is one whose weight is 15% to 20% or more below accepted weight standards. This may be caused by an insufficient food intake to meet activity needs, excessive activity, poor absorption and utilization of food consumed, a wasting disease, or psychological or emotional stress.

Eating disorders are fairly common, especially among teenaged girls and young women, and may persist into adulthood. Two eating disorders, anorexia nervosa and bulimia, usually begin in adolescence or early adulthood. A third disorder, binge eating disorder, is not as well documented but represents a significant proportion of people in weight loss programs. These disorders may develop when people attempt to achieve the "perfect" body. Puberty brings with it hormonal changes and the emergence of sexual characteristics. Some teenagers, particularly girls, resist these changes and turn to inappropriate dieting. However, it is too simplistic to say that the desire to be thin is the cause of eating disorders. It is thought that multiple biologic, psychological, sociocultural, and spiritual factors influence the development of these conditions. The most common eating disorders are described here. Management of these conditions requires psychotherapy and specialized nutritional intervention that is beyond the scope of this textbook. Specialty resources should be consulted.

ANOREXIA NERVOSA

Anorexia nervosa is an eating disorder characterized by self-imposed starvation. Certain features are common in individuals with this disorder. They are generally girls in their midteens, although young adult women and men sometimes develop the disorder. Often they are high achievers from educated, middle-class families. The young person with anorexia nervosa is frequently a perfectionist who uses food and exercise as a means of controlling the body.

People with anorexia nervosa become obsessed with weight loss and soon develop a distorted body image, seeing themselves as fat even when their weight is much less than average for their height and age. They experience personality changes, depression, and apathy. Death may occur in as many as 20% of those with anorexia nervosa. Psychiatric treatment is usually recommended (see Chapter 53).

BULIMIA

Bulimia is an eating disorder characterized by periods of binge eating followed by purging. This behavior may alternate with periods of fasting as well. The cycle may go something like this: The person may binge several times a week. The episode may last 2 hours or more. The person consumes large amounts of easily ingested kilocalorie-dense foods such as ice cream, candies, cakes, breads, and pastries. The binge often is followed by self-induced vomiting or the use of laxatives, diuretics, or a combination of these.

Bulimia occurs more frequently than anorexia nervosa and is also seen most often in young women. People with bulimia are usually of normal weight or even overweight. Most are aware that their eating patterns are abnormal. They may experience fear of not being able to stop eating and depression, guilt, and remorse after a binge. Clinical signs of bulimia may include tooth erosion, callused knuckles, stomach lacerations, and esophageal infections from excessive vomiting. Electrolyte imbalances may occur, leading to abnormal heart rhythms and injury to the kidneys. Repeated infections of the bladder and kidney may lead to renal failure.

BINGE EATING DISORDER

Binge eating disorder is characterized by the intake of excessive calories at least twice a week for 6 months. The person eats very rapidly, sometimes consuming as much as 20,000 calories in one sitting. After the binge episode, the person feels guilty, embarrassed, and depressed. Binge eaters are often dieters, and many are overweight.

NUTRITIONAL SUPPORT WITH SUPPLEMENTAL FEEDINGS

The preferred method of meeting nutritional requirements is, of course, through eating a balanced diet. This is not always possible, however, and there are times when a person's nutritional needs cannot be met by oral feeding. At these times a person's needs must be met with some type of nutritional supplement. These supplements can be formulated using liquid or powdered milk, powdered whole eggs, and powdered egg albumin as concentrated protein sources. Liquid feedings can meet the nutritional requirements of patients who are unable to take solid food. Examples of formulas used for enteral feedings are Ensure, Compleat, Sustacal, Criticare HN, Pulmocare, Trauma Cal, Travasorb HN, and Travasorb Renal. Table 8-14 summarizes the situations that might require artificial feeding. Nursing care of patients receiving enteral and parenteral feedings is covered in Chapter 36.

ENTERAL TUBE FEEDINGS

Patients who are unable to take in supplemental liquid feedings orally may require enteral tube feedings. Enteral feedings bypass the mouth and deliver nutrients directly into the stomach or small intestine through inserted tubes. Conditions that interfere with taking in liquids orally include oral surgery, gastrointestinal surgery, dysphagia (difficulty swallowing), unconsciousness, anorexia, or esophageal obstruction. The tubes can be inserted into the stomach, duodenum, or jejunum through the nose or through the abdominal wall. (Fig. 8-4).

Enteral tube feedings may cause complications such as nausea or vomiting, diarrhea, gastrointestinal bleeding, aspiration pneumonia, hyperkalemia (excessive serum potassium), hyponatremia (serum sodium deficit), hyperglycemia (elevated blood glucose), or nutritional deficiencies. They are caused either by problems with the liquid supplement or by mechanical difficulties with the tube feeding, such as misplacement of the tube or too rapid administration of the feeding. Dumping syndrome may occur when hypertonic fluid enters the jejunum; water is drawn into the lumen of the intestine to dilute the fluid, causing a drop in circulating blood volume. Tube blockage can occur, most likely caused by viscous formulas with inadequate flushing, crushed medications, and incompatible medications that form clumps.

PARENTERAL NUTRITION

Another method of administering nutrients is through parenteral nutrition. The two major types of parenteral nutrition are (1) peripheral parenteral nutrition (PPN) and (2) central parenteral nutrition (CPN) or total parenteral nutrition (TPN). Peripheral parenteral nutrition is given through the pe-

table 8-14 ***Situations Requiring Artificial Feeding Techniques***

PHYSIOLOGIC PROBLEM	RECOMMENDED FEEDING	CLINICAL SITUATION OR DISORDER
Inability to ingest food	Liquid feedings: whole food or milk-based formula Route of administration: Tube Nasogastric Gastrostomy Jejunostomy Oral	Carcinoma of esophagus or stomach Dental or oral surgery Inflammatory disease of esophagus Coma
Inability to digest food	Chemically defined diet Route of administration: Oral Tube	Pancreatitis Biliary tract disease
Decreased ability or inability to absorb food	Chemically defined diet Route of administration: Oral Tube Peripheral vein nutritional support Total parenteral nutrition	Radiation therapy Sprue Inflammatory bowel disease Short-bowel syndrome Inflammatory bowel disease
Inability to handle colonic residue	Chemically defined diet Route of administration: Oral Tube Peripheral vein nutritional support Total parenteral nutrition	Presurgical preparation Ileostomy, colostomy Draining fistula
Inability to meet nutritional requirements fully with normal foods	Liquid feeding Oral supplement Tube feeding Peripheral vein nutritional support Central vein nutritional supplementation	Major surgery Burns Trauma Extended fever Anorexia of chronic illness Anorexia nervosa

From Mahan, L.K., & Escott-Stump, S. (1996). *Krause's food, nutrition, and diet therapy* (9th ed., p. 426). Philadelphia: Saunders.

ripheral veins in the arms and legs, and may employ a peripheral venous catheter or a peripherally inserted central catheter. CPN or TPN is given through a central vein, usually the superior vena cava. This method is used for nutrition only if the gastrointestinal tract cannot be used; it can be lifesaving.

Peripheral Parenteral Nutrition

Peripheral parenteral nutrition is the standard intravenous therapy, which may be composed of dextrose (5%-10%), amino acids, vitamins, minerals, and electrolytes. Fat emulsions may be administered peripherally as well. Total nutritional requirements usually are not met with PPN therapy, and at most it supplies 1,800 kcal/day. It is used primarily for short-term nutritional support.

Total Parenteral Nutrition

Central parenteral nutrition or TPN feedings are used for patients who are unable to obtain adequate nutrition enterally or with PPN. They are usually debilitated and malnourished, with a weight loss of 10% of the body weight or more. Patients with short-bowel syndrome, bowel fistulas or obstruction, inflammatory bowel disease, or hypermetabolic states in which the gastrointestinal tract is completely or partially unusable benefit from this form of nutritional support.

Total parenteral nutrition can meet the high energy and protein needs of burn patients. It can also be used for cancer patients who have become malnourished as a result of oncologic treatments. Total parenteral nutrition can supply up to 4,000 kcal/day. This is possible because the solution is administered through a Hickman or Broviac-type catheter inserted into the superior vena cava, where the hypertonic solution can be diluted rapidly by the large, fast-flowing volume of blood.

Patients who are being fed parenterally should be monitored closely for any signs of complications. Potential complications include pulmonary complications, injury to the veins and arteries surrounding the TPN catheter site, air embolism, infection, electrolyte imbalance, mineral deficiencies, hyperglycemia, and, if treatment is ended suddenly, rebound hypoglycemia.

TRANSITIONAL FEEDING

When patients are ready to be changed from one of these methods to another, they are ready for transitional feeding.

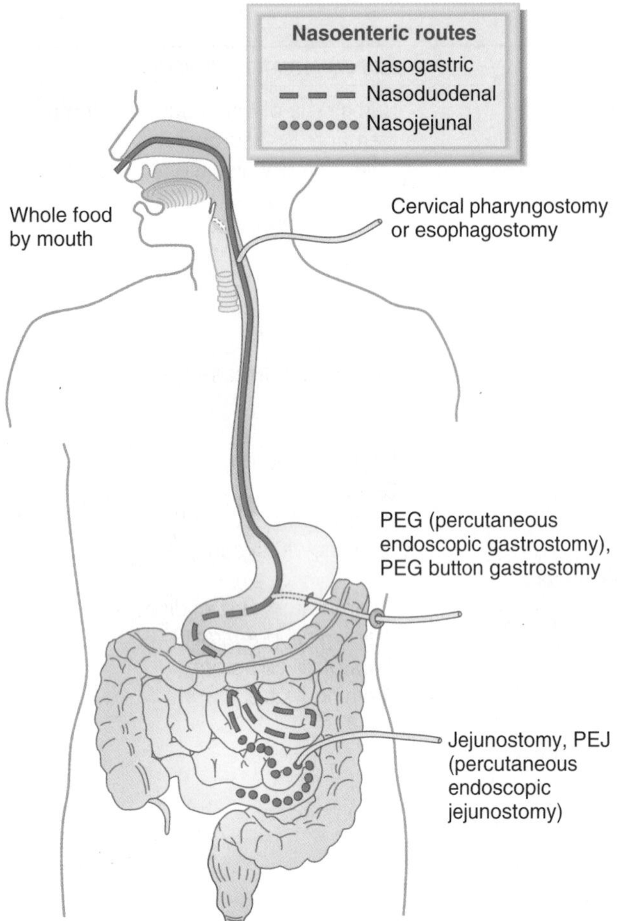

FIGURE **8-4** Diagram of the placement of enteral feeding tubes.

Transitional feeding can be from parenteral nutrition to enteral tube feeding or oral intake, from enteral tube feeding to oral formula or food, or a combination of these.

It is important that transitional feeding be done gradually and with specific principles in mind. If patients who have been without adequate food for an extended period of time are given food too quickly, they may develop nutritional recovery syndrome. This syndrome causes hypophosphatemia (deficiency of phosphates in the blood) from the shift of phosphorus from the plasma into the cells. This shift may also affect potassium as it moves into cells with the glucose during refeeding.

Refeeding of the malnourished patient disrupts the adaptive state of starvation and therefore must proceed slowly with close patient monitoring. The ideal early feeding appears to be moderate in carbohydrates, low in sodium, lactose free, and supplemented with phosphorus and potassium.

When moving from parenteral to oral or enteral feeding, it is important to continue the parenteral feeding. This allows for maintenance of adequate nutrient and fluid intake as tolerance of enteral feedings is assessed. As the patient is able to tolerate the oral or enteral feedings, the parenteral feedings can be tapered off.

When moving from enteral to oral feedings, the patient may complain of a poor appetite. In making this transition it may be helpful to change the enteral feeding from a continuous drip to an intermittent feeding. This way the patient has a chance to get hungry between feedings, and desire for food may increase.

Put on your THINKING CAP!!

Interview an older person (a patient, family member, or other acquaintance) about how their eating habits have changed with age. Identify any changes that could lead to inadequate nutrition.

key points

- Nutrition is the cornerstone of the healing process. To support and maintain life or fight disease, the body must be supplied with the proper nutrients.
- During the digestive process, enzymes help break down food particles to their simplest form so that the nutrients can be absorbed by the body.
- Regulation of the gastrointestinal system involves neural control and the secretion of hormones.
- Parasympathetic nerves generally stimulate digestive activity, and sympathetic nerves inhibit activity.
- The stomach is normally emptied in 1 to 4 hours, depending on the amount and kinds of foods eaten.
- The primary organ of absorption is the small intestine.
- Fluids, vitamins, and minerals are absorbed through the intestinal mucosa.
- The body makes use of the energy received through the food that is eaten, and the largest portion of energy expenditure occurs during rest to carry out the mechanical activities needed to sustain life processes.
- Most of the energy needed to move, perform activities, and live is consumed in the form of carbohydrates, which are converted primarily to glucose for immediate use by the body's cells.
- Although carbohydrates are the body's main source of food energy, fats are the most concentrated source, supplying 9 calories per gram, whereas carbohydrates and protein supply only 4 calories per gram.
- Lipids are a major source of energy for muscle tissue, even when glucose is available.
- People should try to limit their fat intake to 30% or less of their daily caloric intake and should try to eat unsaturated fats rather than saturated fats.
- Proteins are made of smaller units called amino acids.
- Vitamins and minerals are micronutrients; they are needed in small amounts for good health.
- Water is the largest component of the body and body tissues and is essential to all life processes in the body.
- Maintaining a good diet can help middle-aged and older adults maintain a high level of function and reduce the risks of chronic disease; however, because of the normal decline in metabolism and physical activity, energy needs lessen with age.
- Most vegetarian diets can provide all nutrients if planned properly.

- Vegans are at risk for megaloblastic anemia if adequate vitamin B_{12} is not added to the diet.
- Most adults have the ability to maintain a constant weight, but to do so, they must keep up consistent food and exercise patterns on a daily basis.
- Anorexia nervosa, bulimia, and binge eating disorder are eating disorders that often begin in adolescence.
- Eating disorders are thought to be caused by multiple biological, psychological, sociocultural, and spiritual factors.
- For the patient who cannot take oral feedings, nutritional support may be provided through enteral tube feedings, or peripheral or central catheters.

REVIEW QUESTIONS

1. Most of the absorption of nutrients occurs in the:
   1. stomach.
   2. small intestine.
   3. large intestine.
   4. liver.
2. Lipase and amylase are examples of:
   1. macronutrients.
   2. metabolic wastes.
   3. carrier proteins.
   4. digestive enzymes.
3. When is the metabolic rate highest?
   1. Infancy
   2. Puberty
   3. Adolescence
   4. Young adult
4. Excess glucose is stored in the liver as:
   1. monosaccharides.
   2. amino acids.
   3. glycogen.
   4. lactic acid.
5. The functions of dietary fiber are to:
   1. absorb excess gastric acid.
   2. increase the rates of digestion and absorption.
   3. decrease fecal bulk.
   4. promote sense of gastric fullness.
6. Nutritionists recommend that dietary fats not exceed which percentage of the daily caloric intake?
   1. 10%
   2. 20%
   3. 30%
   4. 40%
7. Which of the following is a water-soluble vitamin?
   1. Vitamin E
   2. Vitamin A
   3. Vitamin C
   4. Vitamin D
8. Factors to consider when planning meals with older adults include:
   1. Older people should eliminate all sodium from their diets.
   2. Older people who are less active need fewer calories than they did when younger.
   3. Most older people require vitamin supplements to meet basic requirements.
   4. A moderately active older woman needs 500 fewer calories daily than when younger.
9. A patient reports that she is lactovegetarian. You know that her diet includes:
   1. eggs.
   2. fish.
   3. poultry.
   4. milk.
10. Complications of total parenteral nutrition include:
    1. vomiting.
    2. air embolism.
    3. hypoglycemia.
    4. aspiration.
11. Patients must be changed *gradually* from parenteral nutrition to oral nutrition to prevent nutritional recovery syndrome, which is characterized by:
    1. hypophosphatemia.
    2. hypocalcemia.
    3. hyponatremia.
    4. hypoglycemia.

CHAPTER

9 Developmental Processes

objectives

1. List the developmental tasks for successful adulthood.
2. Identify the health problems specific to the adult age groups.
3. Discuss the health care needs of young, middle-aged, and older adults.

key terms

Biologic age (p. 99)
Psychological age (p. 99)
Social age (p. 99)

Each stage of life has specific developmental processes that must be undertaken and mastered for a person to go on to the next stage successfully. These developmental processes consist of physical, emotional, social, and psychological changes that present challenges to every living human being. In this chapter, we discuss the developmental processes associated with young adulthood, middle age, and older age.

Major changes in the stages of development in the life cycle have occurred in the past 20 years. Americans are marrying later, having fewer children, and living longer. However, certain marker events, such as marriage, childbirth, acquiring a first job, and the departure of young adults from the family home occur in various developmental stages. Despite the recent changes in the life cycle, there are still broad, general stages of adulthood with predictable movement between them. Erik Erikson developed the basis of our view of human growth and development; he introduced the idea that each stage of life is associated with specific developmental tasks (Table 9-1).

YOUNG ADULTHOOD

Young adulthood comes at a time when physical growth ends and social expectations begin. It is considered to occur during a person's 20s, 30s, and 40s; however, these decades are often divided by such terms as *young young adult* (ages 20-35) and *old young adult* (ages 35-45).

Young adulthood is a time for settling down to a job and raising a family and taking on new responsibilities. Most people in this age group are expected to leave their parents' home and establish their own home. People in their 20s and early 30s begin this process by establishing an intimate, lasting relationship with another person in which the physical satisfaction and psychological security of another are more important than their own. Without the development of an intimate relationship, the young adult can become isolated, lonely, and self-absorbed. In addition, young adults are establishing career goals.

Many young people have extended their education and have prolonged the time in which they continue to live at home; or a job loss, divorce, or other stressor may precipitate a move back home. The entire family then has to adjust to a young adult living at home by redistributing roles and responsibilities, maintaining adequate communication, and reallocating budget and space.

This may be a difficult time for parents, who had expected a new time of freedom and independence in their middle years. It is especially difficult if young grandchildren are included in the package.

DEVELOPMENTAL TASKS

The following developmental tasks must be achieved by young adults:

- Accept self and stabilize self-concept and body image.
- Establish independence from parental home and financial aid.
- Assume responsibilities and independent decision making.
- Become established in a vocation or profession that provides personal satisfaction, economic independence, and a feeling of making a worthwhile contribution to society.
- Learn to appraise and express love responsibly through more than sexual contact.
- Establish an intimate bond with another, either through marriage or with a close friend.
- Establish and maintain a home and manage a time schedule and life stresses.
- Find a congenial social and friendship group.
- Decide whether to have a family and carry out tasks of parenting.
- Formulate a meaningful philosophy of life and reassess priorities and values.
- Become involved as a citizen in the community.

It is evident that these developmental tasks focus on marriage, childbearing, and work. However, many young adults are

table 9-1 Erikson's Adult Developmental Tasks

DEVELOPMENTAL STAGE	DEVELOPMENTAL TASK	NURSING ASSESSMENT
Young adulthood	Intimacy versus isolation	Assess whether the patient has meaningful, intimate relationships. If the patient has no intimate relationships, ask whether he or she has had one or more in the past. Assess other support systems that the patient may have.
Middle adulthood	Generativity versus stagnation	Assess whether the patient is employed. Ask the patient what he or she does for leisure or recreation. If the patient is not employed or has no regular leisure activity, ask the patient what he or she does during a 24-hour day. Assess for signs of depression, such as excessive sleeping and decreased appetite.
Older adulthood	Ego integrity versus despair	Assess what the patient does each day. Ask about the patient's family and other relationships. Ask the patient if he or she feels lonely; if so, assess for signs of depression.

From Ignatavicius, D.D., Workman, M.L., & Mishler, M. (1999). *Medical-surgical nursing: A nursing process approach* (3rd ed., p. 44). Philadelphia: Saunders. Reprinted with permission.

table 9-2 Harmful Health Practices, Effects on Health in the Later Years, and Preventive Measures

HARMFUL HEALTH PRACTICE	POSSIBLE EFFECTS ON HEALTH	PREVENTIVE MEASURES
Lack of physical activity	Diabetes, osteoporosis, heart disease, cancer, obesity, stroke, depression	Increase moderate daily physical activity and reduce sedentary lifestyle.
Obesity	Heart disease, hypertension, insulin-dependent diabetes mellitus, degenerative joint disease, cancer, stroke, atherosclerosis	Maintain ideal weight; maintain low-cholesterol, low-fat (<30%), nutritious diet with plenty of vegetables, fruits, and grain products.
Cigarette smoking	Heart disease; cancers of the lung, larynx, pharynx, oral cavity, esophagus, pancreas, and bladder; chronic bronchitis and emphysema	Stop smoking or do not start smoking.
Alcohol and drug abuse	Malnutrition, cirrhosis of the liver, brain damage, mental status changes, homicides, suicides, motor vehicle fatalities	Limit alcohol intake and stop using drugs or do not start; participate in 12-step program for rehabilitation.
Stress	Stress-related conditions such as hypertension and heart disease	Recognize and modify stressors; use a stress management program, such as exercise or biofeedback.

Adapted from U.S. Department of Health and Human Services, Public Health Service. (1990). *Healthy people 2000: National health promotion and disease prevention objectives* (DHHS Publication No. [PHS] 91-50213). Washington, DC: U.S. Government Printing Office.

delaying marriage, electing to remain single, or are divorced. It should be clear that a young adult does not have to marry to be well adjusted and achieve the identified developmental tasks.

HEALTH PROBLEMS

Young adults, especially those in their twenties and early thirties, have relatively few health problems. The four major causes of death in the young adult age group do not result from illness but from accidents and violence: (1) vehicular accidents, (2) other accidents, (3) suicide, and (4) homicide. As young adults progress into their late 30s and early 40s, the primary causes of death are malignancies and heart disease, followed by accidents and infection with the human immunodeficiency virus (HIV).

Typical health problems are related to stress on the job or in social interactions, lifestyle, and childbearing. They include depression; anxiety; complications of pregnancy; cervical and breast cancer; and back, hip, and limb injuries. In the quest for meaningful social relationships and a career that will gain them independence and success, young adults may experience tension and stress and may lack the time to attend to health-promoting activities such as a proper diet and nutrition. They may work hard and party enthusiastically. Meals may be eaten on the run, and the diet may consist primarily of junk foods. The total number of calories needed is less than during adolescence, since the adult has completed physical growth. Smoking and alcohol or drug abuse are common. These practices may have a direct bearing on health in the later years (Table 9-2).

As young adults enter their 30s and early 40s, their focus is directed mainly toward raising a family and furthering their career (Fig. 9-1). It may be a time to reassess their lives and

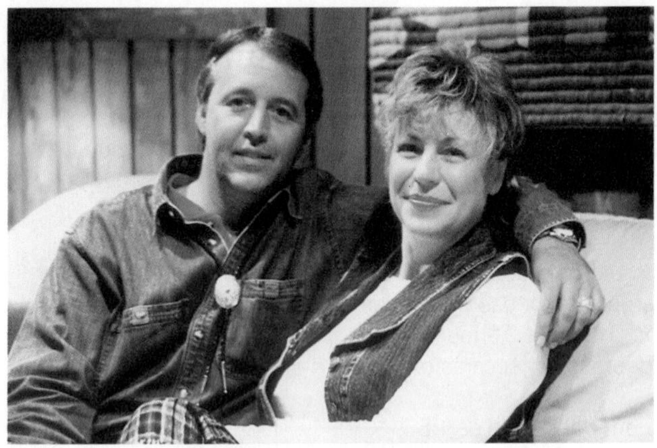

FIGURE 9-1 Middle age is a time of relatively good health, with new opportunities and personal freedom for many.

careers, and often major changes are made. Factors that contribute to health problems are stress related to work, marital problems, and stress related to managing a household. Couples who have postponed childbearing may have difficulties with conception and pregnancy.

HEALTH CARE NEEDS

Health care needs are related to promoting optimal health. It is a good idea to have at least one thorough physical examination during the 20s. A physical examination should include tests for sexually transmitted diseases, hypertension, and cholesterol level. A tetanus booster should be given if persons have not received one in the past 10 years. The hepatitis B vaccine is recommended for adults at risk of exposure to blood and body fluids. Routine dental and eye examinations should be scheduled. Young women should have a Papanicolaou's smear done every 3 years and should be taught breast self-examination. Young men should be taught to do a testicular examination.

Health counseling should focus on health-promoting behaviors. Programs may be established to include topics such as nutrition, exercise and leisure, rest and sleep, human sexuality and family planning, and the effects of smoking, drugs, and alcohol.

In the years between 30 and 45, especially after age 35, young adults should begin to think about the prevention of chronic illness, particularly cancer and heart disease. They should have periodic physical examinations, usually recommended at ages 30 and 35, and then every 3 years thereafter. The physical examination should include tests for hypertension, anemia, and cholesterol, and a cervical Papanicolaou's smear for women. Women should have a baseline mammogram at age 35. Monthly breast self-examinations for women and testicular self-examinations for men should be ongoing. It is suggested that people in this age group examine their skin and mouth periodically for precancerous lesions. Preventive dental checkups and treatment are usually recommended every 6 months to 2 years.

Health promotion and disease prevention programs have a similar focus as those for people in their 20s. Stress management, effective parenting, proper diet and nutrition, exercise, drug and alcohol awareness, and smoking cessation are appropriate topics for health teaching and counseling.

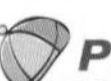

Put on your THINKING CAP!!

When a young adult is diagnosed with a serious chronic illness, how might developmental tasks be affected?

MIDDLE YEARS

The terms *middle years, middle age,* or *middle adulthood* usually refer to the ages between 45 and 65. However, other factors define middle age, particularly how a person acts and feels. Because life expectancy has increased so dramatically during the past 50 years, middle age is a relatively new concept. Previously, the majority of people did not live past their 40s, and what used to be old age is now middle age. Middle age today has been pushed into the 50s; 50 is now what 40 used to be. A woman who reaches the age of 50 today free of cancer and heart disease can expect to live until she is 91. After reaching their 50th birthday, women can expect to live 40 or more years. A healthy man who is 65 can expect to live until he is 81 (Sheehy, 1995).

More than 40 million Americans, or one fourth of the U.S. population, are considered middle-aged. They earn most of the money, pay most of the taxes, and have most of the power in business and government. Middle age is a time of relatively good health for most. People experience a new personal freedom and enjoy maximum command of themselves and influence over others.

Many people who are in their middle years belong to a group called the "sandwich generation." They may have teenagers and young adults at home and at the same time have ailing, elderly parents to care for. The fact that most middle-aged Americans today still have a living parent is a great change in family dynamics. People who delayed pregnancy and childbearing may have even younger children at home.

Many of today's middle-aged women work outside the home and have developed important careers. Work and family obligations together may require a balancing act for middle-aged women who are trying to maintain continued involvement both at work and at home. In addition to caring for children, the middle-aged woman is the most likely caregiver to elderly parents. The result can be a great deal of stress and conflict.

DEVELOPMENTAL TASKS

The following developmental tasks should be accomplished by people in their middle years:

- Discover and develop new satisfaction with a mate or significant other by enjoying mutual activities, providing mutual support, and developing a deeper sense of unity and intimacy.
- Help growing and grown children become happy and responsible adults.
- Create a pleasant, hospitable, and comfortable home, compatible with one's values, income, and resources.

- Balance work and other roles; prepare for retirement.
- Accept role reversal with aging parents; prepare emotionally for the eventual death of living parents.
- Achieve mature social and civic responsibilities and give time and resources to the community.
- Accept and adjust to the physical changes of middle age and establish and maintain a healthy lifestyle.
- Continue to formulate a philosophy of life and grow spiritually.
- Develop satisfying leisure activities.
- Recognize the inevitability of death and prepare for one's own eventual death.

Middle-aged persons who successfully master developmental tasks begin to accept their age and gradually come to value the wisdom gained from living and experience rather than the physical power and strength that accompany youth. Emotional and mental flexibility increases the ability to change and adapt to new situations and to be open to others. It is a time of "mellowing-out," of accepting what life has to offer.

HEALTH PROBLEMS

People in their middle years continue to be relatively healthy, and the same factors that contribute to the deterioration of health habits in the young adult apply to those in middle age. The major cause of death is cardiovascular disease, and the most common health problems, along with cardiovascular disease, are cancer, pulmonary disease, diabetes, obesity, alcoholism, anxiety, depression, and glaucoma. Respiratory conditions are a frequent cause for days absent from work in women; injuries are a frequent cause for men. Bone mass begins to decrease. Women lose calcium from bone tissue following menopause, leading to an increased risk of osteoporosis. Muscle mass is reduced as a result of decreased muscle fiber. In the 40s changes in vision typically begin. Age-related farsightedness, called presbyopia, develops as a result of decreasing elasticity of the lens. The clue to developing presbyopia is that the middle adult begins to hold reading material at a distance to focus on it better. Presbycusis (normal loss of hearing acuity associated with aging) may begin to appear.

HEALTH CARE NEEDS

The health care goals for middle-aged people are the same as those for younger adults. They are focused on health promotion and disease prevention to preserve and prolong the period of maximum energy and optimal mental and social activity.

During the middle years, regular assessment of health status is important for maintaining good health. Early diagnosis of illness helps prevent later complications. A complete physical examination is recommended at age 40 and every 3 years thereafter. Routine blood pressure screening and cholesterol and glucose testing are recommended.

Women should continue to conduct regular breast self-examinations and have a mammogram every 2 to 3 years during their mid-to-late 40s and every year after age 50. Women usually enter a perimenopausal period between the ages of 45 and 50. Menopause is preceded by the perimenopausal period (approximately 5 years) during which there is a gradual decrease in estrogen accompanied by a gradual decrease in menstrual flow. The permanent cessation of menstruation typically occurs between the ages of 45 and 55. During the menopausal years, women may experience symptoms such as hot flashes, dizziness, headaches, perspiration, palpitations, water retention, nausea, muscle cramps, fatigue, insomnia, or tingling of the fingers and toes. Many women take estrogen to relieve some of the symptoms of menopause.

Health-promoting activities during middle age are the same as for young adults. The focus is on proper nutrition, exercise, stress management, and the reduction or elimination of smoking, drug use, and alcohol use.

OLDER ADULTS

Age 65 is commonly thought of as the beginning of old age. However, many people in their 60s do not consider themselves old, and they continue to live healthy, productive lives. Because people are generally healthy today, people are entering old age in better condition than in the past. In America today, 8 in 10 people will live past their 65th birthday. Markers that may be more accurate than chronologic age to define older age include: (1) biologic age, (2) **psychological age**, and (3) **social age**. ***Biologic age*** focuses on the functional capabilities of various organ systems in the body. Many older people continue to function well, especially those who engage in exercise and other health-promoting activities, whereas others seem to be prematurely ill and frail. *Psychological age* refers to the behavioral capacity of the person to adapt to changing environmental demands. The older person's ability to remember, learn, and exercise behavioral control are factors that affect psychological age. *Social age* refers to the roles and habits of a person in relation to other members of society, including such aspects as the person's type of dress, language, and social relationships.

During older age, men and women are required to make many adjustments to physiologic, psychological, and social changes. Declines in bodily function, particularly in vision and hearing, and diminished physical strength and resiliency may have an effect on day-to-day functioning. Psychological changes include a decreased short-term memory, slower performance on cognitive tasks, and longer learning time. Older people retain psychological skills, but those skills usually take longer to accomplish. Social changes include retirement, a change in living conditions, and loss of spouse and significant others.

DEVELOPMENTAL TASKS

The following developmental tasks must be achieved by older adults:

- Recognize the aging process and adjust to decreasing physical strength and health changes.
- Adjust to retirement; adjust living standards to retirement income.
- Establish satisfactory living arrangements as a result of role changes.

- Maintain emotional satisfaction in relationships with spouse, children, grandchildren, and other living relatives.
- Establish an affiliation with members of own age group; maintain an interest in people outside the family and in the community.
- Maintain maximum level of health; learn to adjust to the loss of physical strength, illness, and one's own mortality.
- Cope with the death of parents, spouse, and friends.
- Learn to combine new dependency needs with the continuing need for independence.

Developmental tasks in older age focus on the redirection of energy and talents to new roles and activities, the acceptance of life with its joys and limitations, and the development of a personal view of death in preparation for this final stage of life.

HEALTH PROBLEMS

The major causes of death in older age are related to chronic illness, specifically cardiovascular disease, cancer, and diabetes mellitus. Accidents, including falls, are the fourth leading cause of death in this age group. The most common illnesses are arthritis, gastrointestinal problems (peptic ulcer and constipation), acute and chronic respiratory diseases (influenza, pneumonia, emphysema), and gallbladder disease. Benign or malignant enlargement of the prostate is common in older men; breast cancer is common in older women.

HEALTH CARE NEEDS

The health care goals in the older age group are to manage chronic illnesses and to maintain and prolong the period of optimal physical, mental, and social activity. It is important to help older adults maintain their independence as long as possible in the face of one or more chronic illnesses.

Physical examinations should be done yearly and include the same assessment as indicated for middle-aged adults. Dental examinations and treatment should also be continued into older age. As people age, periodic evaluation and treatment of the feet by a podiatrist are recommended to promote mobility. An influenza vaccination is recommended yearly for persons older than 65 years. A single dose pneumococcal vaccine is recommended with revaccination every 5 years for people with chronic illnesses.

Health-promoting activities should continue into older age. These activities can increase quality of life and, in many cases, prevent many of the chronic illnesses that accompany the later years. Proper nutrition, especially a low-fat, high-fiber diet with a large amount of complex carbohydrates, helps maintain energy, promote intestinal motility, and decrease susceptibility to some chronic illnesses. Exercise can benefit older adults, even the very old who begin an exercise program for the first time. Walking is the ideal exercise, and 20 to 30 minutes three times a week is adequate to maintain weight, blood pressure, coordination, and mobility and to create a positive outlook on life. Older people also can benefit from counseling for alcohol and drug abuse and smoking cessation. It is never too late to improve one's health habits.

Chapter 10 discusses health care issues related to the older adult in more depth.

key points

- Developmental processes are changes that present challenges that must be undertaken and mastered for a person to go on to the next stage successfully.
- Developmental tasks for young adults center on acceptance of self, independence, intimacy, home and time management, social relationships, community involvement, and formulation of a meaningful philosophy of life.
- Health problems of young adults are related to stress on the job or in social interactions, lifestyle, and childbearing.
- Developmental tasks for middle-aged adults focus on interpersonal relationships, guidance of grown children, creation of a pleasant home, balanced roles, care of aging parents, civic responsibilities, adjustment to physical changes, pursuit of satisfying leisure activities, formulation of a life philosophy, and recognition of death's inevitability.
- Health problems of middle-aged adults include cardiovascular disease, cancer, pulmonary disease, diabetes, obesity, alcoholism, anxiety, depression, and glaucoma.
- Developmental tasks for older adults include adjustment to aging and retirement, establishment of satisfactory living arrangements, maintenance of emotional satisfaction in relationships, affiliation with peers, maintenance of maximal level of health, coping with the deaths of others, and learning to combine new dependency needs with the need for independence.
- Health problems for older adults include cardiovascular disease, cancer, diabetes mellitus, accidents, arthritis, gastrointestinal problems, and respiratory diseases.

REVIEW QUESTIONS

1. An important developmental task of the young adult is to:
   1. accept role reversal with aging parents.
   2. develop satisfying leisure activities.
   3. establish an intimate bond with another.
   4. achieve mature social and civic responsibilities.
2. Which intervention is directed toward reducing the most common cause of death among young adults?
   1. Teach early warning signs of cancer
   2. Encourage cardiovascular fitness
   3. Teach principles of safe sex
   4. Promote safe driving practices

3. The term *sandwich generation* is used to describe:
   1. young adults who tend to eat on the run, primarily fast food.
   2. middle-aged adults caring for both children and parents.
   3. children who are left to care for themselves in single-parent homes.
   4. older adults who are in transition from independent to assisted living.

4. Health promotion activities designed to reduce the major cause of death for middle-aged adults include:
   1. cardiovascular fitness programs.
   2. screening for diabetes mellitus.
   3. driving instruction for older people.
   4. stress management classes.

5. A developmental task of older adults is to:
   1. maintain the pace of middle age despite physical changes.
   2. maintain emotional satisfaction in relationships with others.
   3. decrease one's involvement in social activities.
   4. remain independent regardless of physical and emotional health.

6. A leading cause of death among both young adults and older adults is:
   1. cancer.
   2. accidents.
   3. suicide.
   4. diabetes mellitus.

CHAPTER

10 The Older Patient

objectives

1. Describe the roles of the gerontological nurse.
2. Compare the myths and stereotypes of the aging population with current statistical trends.
3. Describe biologic and physiologic factors associated with aging.
4. Explain psychosocial factors associated with aging.
5. Describe modifications needed for activities of daily living.
6. Identify types of drugs that may require dosage adjustments for older adults.

key terms

Ageism (ĀJ-ĭz-ĕm, p. 103)
Aging (p. 102)
Cataract (KĂT-ă-răkt, p. 108)
Conduction deafness (kŏn-DŬK-shŭn DĔF-nĕs, p. 108)
Gerontological nurse (jĕ-rŏn-tō-LŎJ-ĭ-kăl, p. 103)
Gerontology (jĕr-ŏn-TŎL-ō-jē, p. 102)
Glaucoma (glăw-KŌ-mă, p. 108)
Kyphosis (kī-FŌ-sĭs, p. 107)
Presbycusis (prĕz-bē-KŪ-sĭs, p. 108)
Presbyopia (prĕz-bē-Ō-pē-ă, p. 108)
Sensorineural deafness (sĕn-sō-rē-NŪ-răl DĔF-nĕs, p. 108)

A Young Girl Still Dwells

What do you see nurse, what do you see?
Are you thinking when you look at me
A crabbed old woman, not very wise,
Uncertain of habit with far away eyes,
Who dribbles her food and makes no reply
When you say in a loud voice, "I do wish you'd try."
Who seems not to notice the things that you do
And forever is losing a stocking or shoes,
Who resisting or not, lets you do as you will
With bathing and feeding, the long day to fill.
Is that what you're thinking is that what you see
Then open your eyes, nurse. You're not looking at me.

Focus on the Family, 1985

Care, kindness, and knowledge are prerequisites for working effectively with the aged. Responding to the health challenges of a new century requires a clear understanding of the health-related threats and opportunities facing older adults. People who reach age 65 can now expect to live into their eighties. However, it is unlikely that all these years will be active and independent ones. Consequently, improving the functional independence of later life is an important element in promoting health for older adults.

DEFINITIONS OF OLD AGE

Older adult patients present many challenges to nurses. The work is often complex, time-consuming, and oriented to caring for, rather than curing. It is often difficult to define what is meant by old age. A child or teenager may define "old people" as persons in their thirties, forties, or fifties, whereas people in their fifties may define old as "at least 10 years older than I am." Age identification consists of much more than just recognition of chronological age.

Most definitions of *old age* refer to having lived for a long time. *Aged* is defined as old or advanced in years. However, *aging* is defined as the process of growing older or more mature. We all experience the process of aging, but not all of us are old in years, roles, behaviors, health, or physical limitations.

Aging is an ongoing developmental process that begins at conception and ends in death. Most gerontologists agree that old age is not measured in years. Although the age of 65 is frequently used to indicate the onset of old age, this number is clearly arbitrary and a function of social policy.

Gerontology, the study of aging, can be dated to the early 1950s and includes aging research, education, and training activities. Geriatrics is the biomedical science of old age and the application of knowledge related to the biologic, biomedical, behavioral, and social aspects of aging to the prevention, diagnosis, treatment, and care of older persons. The term *geriatrics* was coined in recognition of the similarity to the field of pediatrics. Both gerontology and geriatrics are critical components of a young science with practitioners from many disciplines, including nursing, medicine, dentistry, psychology, anthropology, and political science.

ROLES OF THE GERONTOLOGICAL NURSE

Between 1989 and 2030, the population aged 65 and over is expected to more than double, and the proportion of elderly will rise from 12% to 21.8%. By 2020, the median age in the United States is expected to be 40 (versus 33 in 1990), and the older population is expected to reach 52 million. These older adults will need regular primary health care services to help them maintain their health and prevent disabling and life-

table 10-1 ***Levels of Nursing Practitioners Involved in Care of the Aged***

PRACTITIONER	FUNCTION	EDUCATION PREPARATION
Nursing assistant (also known as patient care assistants [PCAs], nurses' aides [NAs])	Assist professional nurse in patient care tasks	On-the-job training, certified through taking short courses at technical colleges or through in-service training
Licensed practical nurse (LPN) or licensed vocational nurse (LVN)	Assist professional nurse in patient care tasks	Technical college or vocational high school preparation, must pass licensure examination and maintain licensure to practice
Registered nurse (RN)	Practice professional nursing with patients and families in any health care setting	Multiple levels of entry, including (1) associate degree (ADN) in 2-year program, (2) diploma (3-year hospital-based program), (3) baccalaureate degree (BSN) through 4-year university-based program, (4) nursing doctorate (ND) through 4-year program after college degree in another field; state licensure required for all levels of entry
Nurse practitioner (NP) (sometimes also qualified by specialty area, such as geriatric nurse practitioner [GNP] or family nurse practitioner [FNP])	Expanded nursing role, such as management of chronic disease, prescription of medicines, diagnosis of disease	All are RNs certified jointly by state boards of nursing and medicine. Usually have master's degree in nursing.
Clinical specialist	Advanced practitioner of nursing, clinical teacher	Individuals with master's degree (MSN, MN) who also are RNs
Nurse scientist	Nurse researcher, nurse educator, or both	Doctor of nursing science (DNSc), or doctor of philosophy (PhD) in nursing or other field (psychology, sociology, physiology, anthropology)

Matteson, M. A., McConnell, E. S., & Linton, A. D. (1997). *Gerontological nursing: Concepts and practice.* (2nd ed., p. 42). Philadelphia: Saunders.

threatening diseases and conditions. Nurses have always been involved in the care of the aged. However, many nurses need additional education to build a foundation for quality gerontological nursing care.

Formal preparation for specialized care of the elderly occurs at the master's degree level, but there are also nursing personnel who have demonstrated competencies as a result of on-the-job training. At least 11 different levels of preparation exist for those providing care to the aged (Table 10-1), and the only consistent credentialing mechanism in the United States is the state licensing examination for registered nurses and licensed vocational or practical nurses. Licensed vocational or practical nurses are in a period of transition, moving from traditional hospital-bound positions to community-based long-term care facilities and home health care positions. The shift to more community-based sites should enhance the level of care in these settings.

The term *gerontological nurse* typically refers to professional nurses and advanced-level practitioners, such as nurse practitioners, clinical specialists, and nurses holding national certification in the specialty of gerontological nursing. Laurie Gunter and Carmen Estes describe gerontological nursing as a health service that incorporates basic nursing methods and specialized knowledge about the aged to establish conditions within the patient and within the environment that (1) increase healthy behaviors in the aged; (2) minimize and compensate for health-related losses and impairments of aging; (3) provide comfort and sustenance through the distressing and debilitating events of aging, including dying and death; and (4) facilitate the diagnosis, care, and treatment of disease in the aged.

AGEISM—MYTHS AND STEREOTYPES

Are old people more or less highly valued in our society today than they were a century or more ago? This is hard to answer because we have relatively little evidence about the lives of older people in the past. Along with the lack of factual information is an abundance of myths and stereotypes about the elderly that have been accepted as reality. Nurses must be knowledgeable about aging to avoid generalizing about older adults.

Ageism is a concept introduced by a well-known gerontologist, Dr. R. N. Butler, in 1969. Ageism is the process of systematic stereotyping and discrimination against people because of their age. It is usually directed against the elderly. Older people are ridiculed and labeled senile, rigid in thought, frigid in sexuality, and old-fashioned in morality. Ageism allows for separation and denial of the older person's humanness. It also allows those who practice ageism to distance themselves from their own aging. Ageism, like all other prejudices, influences the behavior of its victims. Some older people confront the problem, whereas others deny the problem with age-inappropriate behaviors (e.g., the 69-year-old blond who attempts to dress and act young in 3-inch heels and short skirts).

Some of the myths associated with old age include nonproductivity, disengagement, inflexibility, senility, inability to learn, retirement being a cause of death, and sexlessness. Myths are a poor substitute for scientific data.

When older people are properly motivated, their intelligence does not wane. In fact, with better organizational skills born of experience, the ability to organize thoughts efficiently may increase as one ages. As a result of normal aging, the intelligence quotient does not plummet, nor do most individuals become senile. Only about 10% of persons older than 65 have dementia, with the greatest incidence after age 85. Cognitive changes in the older person are often a consequence of disease, overmedication, neglect, and despair. Most of these conditions can be reversed.

Old age, like retirement, does not kill, nor does it render elders sexless. According to researchers Masters and Johnson, sexual activity may continue well into the ninth decade. Saying that older people are not interested in sex is another way of disguising the belief that older people should not be interested in sex. Sexual activity is a healthy expression of life and vitality. However, sexual dysfunction can occur at any age and is usually evidence of some illness or disease process or a result of medication side effects. Knowledge of age-related biologic, physiologic, and psychosocial factors tends to negate many of the stereotypes of aging.

Other myths abound, but one must be shattered forever, and that is that older people are isolated, poor, ill, disabled, and living in long-term care facilities. Most older adults are members of multigenerational units and have extended family and support networks. However, some older adults appreciate being independent of children and grandchildren and enjoy their freedom. The majority of older adults are not disabled, and only about 6% of the older population live in long-term care facilities. Moreover, people older than 65 are the wealthiest age group in today's economy. This collective group leads in buying power and disposable income.

BIOLOGIC AND PHYSIOLOGIC FACTORS IN AGING

Immortality and the possibility of renewing youth have captured the imagination of humankind since time began. The ancient Greeks and Romans ascribed immortality to their gods and the few humans who they believed became gods. Magical potions to fend off death have been sought by such diverse cultures as the Chinese, the ancient Hebrews, and the Europeans of the Middle Ages.

The theme of immortality surfaces in nearly every area of human experience. Medical science has made great strides in conquering many ills, but little has been achieved in extending the life span. In modern times, the longest documented human life, recorded in Japan, was 120 years, and most experts believe that the maximal attainable age is approximately 115 to 120 years.

How and why do humans age? Why is individual aging so varied? Which of the many theories of aging are valid? Each of these questions represents a fascinating area for scientific exploration. However, despite intense interest in longevity by so many cultures, scientists do not agree on precisely why or how humans age. Much of what is now known comes from our increasing awareness of the growth in absolute numbers of older people and in the proportion of the population that is old. Knowledge of the underlying mechanisms of aging is critical for the development of a system that considers the special needs and health conditions of an aging population.

THEORIES OF AGING

Proposed theories of aging have ranged from the concept of purely genetic control of aging to the concept of environmental assaults on the organism that result in death (Table 10-2). Most experts now believe that aging is not explainable by a single theory but represents many processes working simultaneously. Therefore, several theories may be needed to explain all aging processes.

Most theories of aging can be divided into two general categories: error theories and programming theories. Error theories are based on the belief that the rate of aging is directly related to the organism's rate of living and that external events cause damage to the organism's cells. The damage from all causes accumulates over time, resulting in cellular, molecular, and organ malfunction or errors. Examples of these theories include error, catastrophe, and wear-and-tear theories.

Programming theories are based on the belief that aging is an event that is programmed into the cell itself and is internal to the organism. These theories postulate that aging, like prenatal development and menopause, is the natural and expected result of a purposeful sequence of events written internally into gene structure. Examples of these theories include programmed senescence and immunologic theory. It is important to remember that theories about aging continue

table 10-2 ***Selected Theories of Aging, 1900 to the Present***

THEORY	PROPONENT SCIENTIST (YEAR)
ERROR THEORIES	
Wear-and-tear theory	Pearl (1924)
Metabolic theory	Pearl (1928)
Somatic mutation theory	Sziliard (1959)
Error catastrophe theory	Orgel (1963)
Free radical theory	Harman (1955)
PROGRAMMING THEORIES	
Collagen theory	Verzar (1957)
Programmed senescence theory	Hayflick (1961)
Cross-linking theory	Bjorkstein (1968)
Immunologic theory	Walford (1969)

Adapted from National Institute on Aging. (1997). *Answers about aging: New pieces to an old puzzle.* Washington, DC: U.S. Department of Health and Human Services.

to evolve and that little agreement exists on any one theory of aging.

PHYSIOLOGIC CHANGES IN BODY SYSTEMS

Aging occurs slowly and is a complex and dynamic process involving many internal and external influences. It is a process that affects virtually every system, organ, and cell in the body to varying degrees. With increasing age, the ability to meet challenges and to carry out physiologic activities is reduced.

Consequently, an understanding of the age-related effects on body systems is an integral part of the scientific basis for nursing care of the aged. The effects of aging on principal systems of the body are discussed below.

NERVOUS SYSTEM

Some of the most frequently discussed changes that occur with aging focus on the neural structures. However, it is essential that nurses know that in the absence of disease, most aged people remain alert, with functional intellectual capability, sound judgment, and creativity. Only modest impairments in memory and learning are observed after age 70 in most people who are relatively free from major disease.

Brain size is generally thought to decrease with age, although evidence for this belief is not conclusive. Loss of neurons (brain cells) begins in the early thirties and continues progressively. Nevertheless, functional ability may not be affected significantly because reserve cells are able to compensate. In addition to the reduced number of neurons, other aging changes in the nervous system include decreased conduction speed and diminished activity of the enzymes associated with synaptic transmission. These changes may result in a progressive slowing of responses, impeded short-term memory, and altered learning.

Short-term memory loss is frequently a concern of the aged, although long-term memory may remain intact. Short-term memory is associated with a stimulus input into the neurons and is dependent on adequate tissue oxygenation. The aging brain may be considered to be in a chronic hypoxic state. The deficit in oxygen is related to atherosclerosis as well as decreased cellular respiration. Consequently, the aged person may experience difficulty remembering planned events for the day but may recall young adulthood experiences without difficulty. Momentary lapses in memory such as forgetting a name or misplacing an item are common examples of normal memory changes. People who have more persistent memory problems with otherwise normal cognitive function are said to have mild cognitive impairment (MCI). Forty percent of people who develop MCI will develop Alzheimer's disease within 3 years; others do not progress to more serious impairment.

Using mnemonics (stringing together known and unknown information) and rehearsal memory training (repetition) may improve memory performance for some older adults experiencing memory deficits. Further, some research indicates that long-term memory is not affected by chronic cerebral tissue hypoxia but may be attributed to permanent changes in the structure of the neuron. If this is the case, then efforts to improve memory would most likely be managed with medications to prevent permanent neuron changes.

Other neurologic features that show age-related changes include temperature regulation, pain perception, and tactile sensation. The aged individual usually has a low tolerance for extremes in temperature, which may be related to deterioration in the vascular tone as well as changes in hypothalamic temperature control. Pain and tactile sensation involve peripheral sensory receptors, a relay pathway, and cortical integration. A decrease in the number and sensitivity of sensory receptors and neurons contributes to an overall dulling of these sensations.

The neurologic changes associated with aging occur gradually; thus, the aged person is able to compensate for these changes by modifying behavior. The person may avoid temperature extremes and accomplish tasks at a slower pace. Any stressor, such as an illness or a new environmental stressor, may seriously impair the person's ability to compensate and may contribute to confusion or disorientation.

RESPIRATORY SYSTEM

Tests of pulmonary physiology have shown a number of age-related alterations. Forced vital capacity, vital capacity, and maximum breathing capacity are thought to decrease progressively with aging. These alterations are related to atrophy and weakening of the respiratory muscles and to an increase in the anteroposterior diameter of the chest as a result of kyphosis, vertebral loss of calcium, and calcification of costal cartilage.

In addition, with aging there is a loss of elastic tissue surrounding alveoli and alterations in pulmonary circulation that result in decreased diffusion across the alveolar–capillary membrane. This physiologic alteration is reflected in arterial oxygen values that decrease progressively throughout aging to approximately 70 to 80 mm Hg by the age of 70.

Pulmonary blood flow in the aged person decreases because of a reduction in cardiac output. Alterations in the pulmonary system associated with aging include a decreased number of capillaries, thickened capillary walls, and fewer capillaries surrounding the alveoli. The changes in the capillaries affect pulmonary diffusion so that gas exchange is impaired. With increasing age, alveolar dead space also occurs.

Despite the physiologic changes associated with aging, the ability of the older adult to maintain adequate oxygenation is not seriously impaired under conditions of health and moderate activity. Problems arise when increased demands are placed on the body as occurs during periods of extreme exertion or respiratory illness. Exertional dyspnea is a frequent complaint with the aged. The ability to perform prolonged strenuous work decreases with aging.

Lung disease, acute or chronic, poses a threat to the older adult, and pulmonary secretions are handled less effectively. Ciliary action, responsible for the movement of secretions, is compromised because of epithelial atrophy. The cough reflex is frequently diminished as a consequence of altered sensitivity to stimuli and decreased muscle tone. These factors, in concert with impaired gas exchange, are responsible for the devastating effects of respiratory problems in old age.

You are considered to be a patient advocate and should be concerned about environmental pollution and hazards associated with smoking. Assess baseline resting and exertional respiratory rates and pulmonary function test results, as appropriate. Deep breathing exercises and positioning to facilitate lung expansion and gas exchange are standard components of respiratory care for older adults.

CARDIOVASCULAR SYSTEM

An increase in resistance to blood flow occurs in many organs with increasing age. This increase in peripheral resistance has its greatest effect on splanchnic and renal tissues and less effect on cerebral, coronary, and skeletal tissues.

In the absence of cardiovascular disease, heart size remains unchanged or slightly decreased as a result of shrinkage or loss of myocardial fibrils. Aging results in the development of whitish patches, fibrosis, and sclerosis in the endocardium—the tissue layer that lines the inside of the heart chambers. As the heart becomes more rigid, myocardial contractility is compromised. Coronary blood flow in the aged person may be reduced by as much as 35% because of changes in the vessels. With advancing age, valvular rigidity and incomplete closure of the aortic and pulmonic valves may result in murmurs. Aging heart cells have a decreased capacity to utilize oxygen, which may help explain the aged person's reduced tolerance for physical work.

The blood vessels of the heart and the systemic circulation, particularly the arteries, undergo age-related changes that may begin as early as the teen years. Thickening and calcification of the intimal layer are evident in the coronary arteries and aorta, usually by age 20. Arterial dilation, vessel lengthening, and rigidity are in part due to changes in the structure of collagen. With aging, the pulse tends to increase in force, and the pulse pressure widens. By 70 years of age, the systolic blood pressure increases to approximately 150 mm Hg and the diastolic blood pressure to 90 mm Hg for most people. These changes are due in part to decreased baroreceptor reflexes and inelasticity of the vessel walls.

Another cardiovascular change caused by aging is a decrease in resting cardiac output, which is the amount of blood pumped by the heart each minute. Between ages 25 and 65, resting cardiac output falls 30% to 40%. This reduced cardiac output reflects a decreased heart rate and a decreased stroke volume. Despite the diminished cardiac output, cerebral blood flow is maintained. However, other body systems, such as the liver and kidneys, receive a diminished blood supply. Even with diminished blood supply, the organs maintain adequate function, partly because of reduced functional requirements.

These changes are not universal and may not be characterized as inevitable consequences of aging. It is nevertheless important that nurses be prepared to incorporate goals, plans, and actions related to nutrition, exercise, and behavior modification in providing care to older people with cardiovascular problems.

RENAL SYSTEM

The renal system of healthy older adults is functionally adequate; however, in times of injury, disease, or disability, the additional function challenge may adversely affect the aging renal system. The aging kidneys are characterized by a decrease in renal function, a decrease in cell mass, and an increase in extracellular fluid. By the seventh decade, the number of nephrons in each kidney is reduced by one half to two thirds, with corresponding changes in the glomeruli. Aging is accompanied by decreases in filtration rate, plasma flow rate, and tubular reabsorption and secretion. Blood urea nitrogen tends to increase. The renal system helps to regulate acid–base balance. However, the tubules of the aging kidneys are less able to conserve base and eliminate excess hydrogen ions.

With advancing age, the ability to concentrate or dilute urine is hindered. This is believed to be related to a decreased secretion of antidiuretic hormone by the pituitary or an overresponsiveness of the kidneys to this hormone. Additional changes brought on by aging are noted in the ureters, bladder, and urethra as a result of deterioration in muscle tone. The bladder capacity may be reduced by half, resulting in frequent trips to the bathroom. Further, response to the stretch receptors in the bladder wall that signal the need to void may be delayed until the pressure is high and the bladder almost filled to capacity. This condition results in an urgency to urinate, which may be problematic for older adults with visual and motor limitations. Urge incontinence is a major health concern for older adults. Lax muscle tone and incomplete emptying of the bladder may lead to residual urine in the bladder. This residual volume may put the older person at risk for subsequent urinary tract infections. Other types of incontinence may appear as a symptom of upper or lower urinary tract dysfunction. For several of these conditions, conservative behavioral treatment is recommended as the first level of intervention. Behavioral treatments may include scheduled or prompted voiding, environmental adaptation, and pelvic muscle exercises (Kegel exercises). Interventions for incontinence are discussed in Chapter 22.

INTEGUMENTARY SYSTEM

Skin changes caused by aging can be the most upsetting because they are so visible and readily apparent. They serve as a constant reminder that youth is fleeting. Changes related to aging of the skin include dryness, loss of elasticity, wrinkles, uneven pigmentation and brown spots, roughness, looseness, thinness, yellowing, and the development of various skin lesions.

One of the first signs of aging is the development of wrinkles. Wrinkles occur when the deep layer of the skin loses moisture and elasticity. Tiny creases and folds are formed. The extent and timing of these wrinkles are determined by genetics and sun exposure. Persons in certain ethnic groups with thicker, oilier skin wrinkle at a slower rate and tend to maintain a youthful, wrinkle-free appearance longer. The same is true of older men because of their thicker and oilier skin.

Skin that is exposed to the sun most often, such as the face, hands, and back of the neck, wrinkles quickly. Older people are encouraged to use sunscreens (SPF 15) to prevent excessive dryness and to prevent skin cancer, the third most common form of cancer in women over the age of 50.

Itching, another change caused by aging, becomes more common in later life and is due to loss of oils in the skin. Nurses might suggest to older persons that they take tepid baths, use moisturizers, and avoid overuse of antiperspirants, soaps, perfumes, and long hot baths. Furthermore, the older person needs to know that generalized itching may be a sign of illness such as diabetes, cancer, kidney disease, or liver disease. Persistent itching should be reported and appropriately assessed by the nurse and other members of the health care team.

Most older people can expect some hair loss, hair thinning, and color changes in the hair and nails. Men tend to grow bald, and women experience thinning of the hair on the head and genitalia. The number of facial and nasal hairs may increase. Gray hair is caused by a slowing of the pigment production in the hair follicles. Graying is determined by genetics and tends to be irreversible. Nails tend to become yellow and thicker. Routine visits to a podiatrist are encouraged for nail trimming and care of corns and calluses.

The most common benign lesions of aging are seborrheic dermatitis, acne, contact dermatitis, drug reactions, pressure ulcers, stasis ulcers, pruritus, herpes zoster, onychomycosis and tinea pedis, and impetigo. Routine skin assessments should be part of the comprehensive nursing assessment for older adults.

GASTROINTESTINAL SYSTEM

Changes in gastrointestinal functions occur with normal aging. Changes in the oral cavity include deterioration in the teeth and a decrease in the functional taste buds. The commonly observed decrease in the secretion of saliva is probably related to medications, inadequate hydration, and illness states rather than being a normal aging change. Saliva tends to become more alkaline as the salivary glands secrete less ptyalin and amylase. The muscles associated with chewing weaken, peristalsis is slower, and the risk of formation of intestinal diverticula increases. These changes tend to interfere with an older person's ability and desire to eat a nutritious meal.

Gastric emptying is slower in older people than in the young. The gastric glands decrease the volume and concentration of hydrochloric acid, intrinsic factor, and pepsin. The amount of calcium absorbed with advanced age is reduced. Further, some reports indicate that bile tends to be thicker and that the gallbladder empties slowly.

Collectively, the changes in the gastrointestinal system caused by aging increase the older person's risk for anorexia, bloating, indigestion, gas, diarrhea, pernicious anemia, and constipation. Constipation is one of the most frequent gastrointestinal complaints of older adults. Constipation may result from decreased intestinal motility, altered bacteria flora, a diet low in bulk and roughage, medications, and lack of physical activity.

Because digestive complaints can be signs of more serious disorders, nurses must assess them completely. Symptoms that may suggest possible illness are decreased appetite, unexplained weight loss, excessive thirst, blood in the stool, or a change in the usual pattern of bowel movements.

You can assist older adults to maintain gastrointestinal function by sharing information about the normal ranges for bowel activity. The usual frequency for a bowel movement may range from as many as three movements per day to as few as one bowel movement every 7 days. Educate elders about diet, activity, increased fluid intake, and avoidance of laxative abuse.

MUSCULOSKELETAL SYSTEM

Of the multiple changes associated with an aging musculoskeletal system, changes related to mobility are most significant. Many people begin to feel old when they wake up with stiff joints. Other age-related changes include decreases in muscle strength, endurance, range of motion of joints, coordination, density of bone, and elasticity and flexibility of connective tissue.

Arthritis is the most prevalent chronic disease in men, is more severe in women, and is the leading cause of disability in old age. Osteoarthritis, the most common form of arthritis, is caused by damage to the inside surface of the joint. Age is the most obvious risk factor for arthritis, with heredity and obesity contributing to its development. The large weight-bearing joints of the body are most affected and include the knees, hips, and spine. **Kyphosis** is the term applied to the curvature of the thoracic spine and gives rise to the bent-over appearance of some older adults.

Assess and document range of motion in all joints, signs of inflammation, and complaints of pain associated with mobility. Assess muscle strength bilaterally, and note the typical amount, type, and frequency of exercise. In addition, note a history of falls, hormonal therapy, or calcium supplementation.

Teach older adults about the benefits of weight-bearing exercises. Instruct them in the benefits of walking, bicycling, and stair climbing to help maintain bone and muscle mass (Fig. 10-1). If necessary, they should use assistive devices for

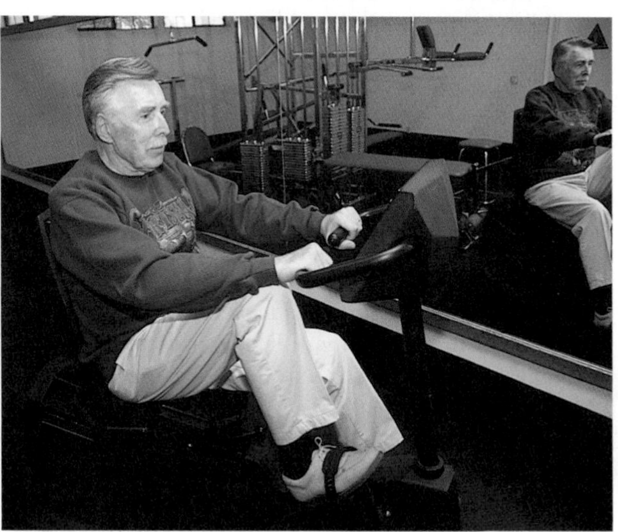

FIGURE **10-1** Regular exercise is an important part of health promotion for the older adult.

walking and preventing falls. They should avoid too much bed rest because of the detrimental effects of immobility.

SENSORY SYSTEM

Because we depend on our five senses for almost everything we do, any loss of sensory ability greatly affects our quality of life. Sensory changes in the older adult place them at risk for injury, weaken self-confidence, and can affect overall quality of life and general well-being.

Presbycusis is the term for hearing loss associated with old age. Twenty-five percent of older adults are hearing impaired. Older adults lose the ability to hear high-pitched sounds and consonants, particularly *ch, f, g, s, sh, t, th,* and *z.* Older men tend to experience greater hearing loss, but not all older adults experience this type of loss, and causes other than old age may be involved.

There are basically two types of hearing loss. Conduction deafness is a blockage of the ear canal caused by excessive wax buildup, abnormal structures, or infection. This type of loss is easily treated. The other type of hearing loss is sensorineural deafness. It results from damage to the nerve centers within the brain as a result of exposure to loud noises, disease, and certain drugs. Hearing aids may be used to correct both types of deafness.Tinnitus, an annoying ringing or buzzing in the ear, is a sensorineural disorder. Some cases of tinnitus can be caused by the use of aspirin, certain antibiotics, or diuretics or by tumors.

Failing eyesight is not an inevitable consequence of age, but several eye diseases are associated with aging. The leading cause of new cases of blindness in older people is age-related macular degeneration, a disease that affects the macula, the part of the eye that is responsible for sharp central vision. Laser surgery may be effective in preventing or delaying visual loss, and older adults should be informed of this as a treatment option.

Another serious eye disease that occurs with aging is cataract. Cataract is the development of clouding or opacity of the normal transparent lens within the eye. Cataracts are caused by changes in structural lens proteins, by damage to the lens as a result of high levels of blood sugar in people with diabetes, or by other factors.

Cataract is treated by surgical removal of the clouded lens. Surgery is highly successful, and vision is usually restored in 90% to 95% of the cases. An artificial lens is placed in the eye after cataract removal. Eyeglasses may be prescribed after surgery to further improve vision.

A less serious age-related vision change is a condition called presbyopia. Presbyopia affects the shape of the lens. The shape of the lens is controlled by muscles in the eye. By changing its shape, the lens allows us to change focus when looking from objects that are near to objects that are far. With age, the lens becomes more rigid and less able to change shape. Consequently, reading and other types of close work become difficult. Presbyopia is easily corrected by reading glasses or bifocal lenses. Further, adapting to changes in lighting is also a function of the lenses. Maintaining bright lighting in the home, particularly in hallways and around walkways, can help prevent falls and other accidents.

The leading cause of blindness in the United States is glaucoma. Glaucoma is characterized by high pressure of the fluid in the eye. The increased pressure causes damage to the optic nerve. The optic nerve carries visual impulses from the eye to the brain. Damage to the optic nerve can result in vision loss, which is characterized by "tunnel vision."

At present, glaucoma is not curable but is treatable with drugs or surgery. If glaucoma is detected early and treated effectively, the disease process can be halted or slowed and the remaining eyesight saved. Older adults should receive annual eye examinations and a test for glaucoma.

Disorders of the senses involving taste and smell are called *chemosensory disorders.* More than 10 million Americans are affected by this type of disorder. Most of these disorders occur after age 60 and involve the ability to differentiate scents. Men tend to be more affected than women, and many causes exist. Causes include nasal obstruction, allergies, and the use of certain drugs. Some scientists believe that the decline in smell is due to a decrease in olfactory nerve fibers.

A gradual loss in the number of taste buds begins around 50 to 60 years of age. In spite of this progressive loss, there is little perceptible change in taste sensitivity that can be attributed to increased age alone. Major changes in the ability to taste are most often caused by diseases or the side effects of certain drugs. Dentures, hormonal changes, medications, and changes in chemicals needed to transmit taste are all potential causes of the older person's diminished sense of taste. This loss can affect changes in appetite.

Sensory losses are more than a minor nuisance for older adults. Poor vision and hearing increase a person's risk for falls and other accidents, which are a leading cause of death and disability in people over the age of 65. Further, the inability to smell smoke, poisons, or other noxious odors endangers the lives of many older people. Decreased ability to taste food puts the older person at risk for malnutrition and food poisoning. Sensory changes greatly reduce the quality of life. The nurse must assist older adults to control, correct, or compensate for sensory losses. Assessment is, of course, the first step.

To summarize, the physiologic changes associated with aging may reflect more the presence of age-related diseases than aging itself. The interrelationship between the process of normal aging and the effects of age-related disease has not yet been defined universally. Nurse scientists are actively engaged in this process as well as in other scientific endeavors to better understand and provide care to the growing numbers of older adults. Research is rapidly expanding and changing our knowledge of aging. Conditions once thought to be the consequence of normal aging are now known to be the product of disease. Many of the conditions can be prevented or controlled by good health practices and competent nursing care.

PSYCHOSOCIAL FACTORS ASSOCIATED WITH AGING

It is important to consider psychosocial as well as biologic changes associated with aging. Older adults show cumulative developmental effects that produce unique personality styles, coping mechanisms, challenges, and growth. Family, friends, and the community are influential in the aging process and can support the individual in adapting to age-related changes (Fig. 10-2).

The fact that a person has survived to old age is one marker of successful adaptation. The survival of large numbers of relatively healthy older people is a new experience for humankind. The vast majority of older people have adapted adequately. These individuals are able to function independently and maintain a sense of well-being. Only about 15% of the aged are unable to function independently and fail to maintain or sustain a sense of well-being.

Effective adaptation requires the individual to meet environmental and functional needs and to attain some sense of well-being. The achievement of each developmental task of aging requires successful coping and adaptation to changes in the environment. Remember, environment refers to both internal and external realms.

Maturity is defined as an optimal psychological, social, and biologic adaptation achieved at some point during the midlife years, arbitrarily set between 45 and 65 years of age. The years preceding the attainment of maturity are characterized as ascending and accelerating. The years thereafter are regarded as descending and decelerating. It is thought that midlife crisis occurs, in part, when the individual in midlife becomes fully aware of his or her mortality.

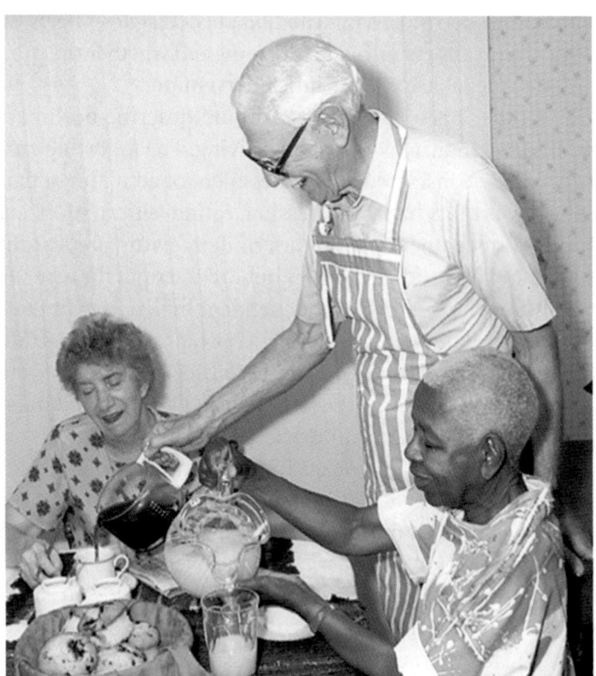

FIGURE **10-2** Most older adults are active and independent.

Erik Erikson developed one of the first developmental theories in the area of aging. He viewed the entire process of human development as a series of stages a person goes through to develop the ego fully. Erikson described eight stages of ego development from infancy to old age. Each of his stages represents a choice of crises in the ego. A complete discussion of adult developmental tasks is found in Chapter 9.

The final developmental task identified by Erikson is ego-integrity versus despair, which is the one typically associated with old age (late sixties or early seventies and older). The developmental challenge is to review life and gain a feeling of accomplishment and fulfillment. Older adults are expected to be concerned with life in the face of death and to begin to experience the wisdom that they have gained. The opposite of ego-integrity is feelings of despair, in which people feel bitter about their lack of accomplishments in life and tend to regret life as they have lived it. Many people say that they have more regrets about the things they have not done or the risks they haven't taken than the mistakes they have made.

Old age involves much more than a psychological waiting station before death. It represents an important stage of development and coping that occurs between the high points and accomplishments of the midyears and the concerns that are involved as the end of life approaches. Movement toward ego integrity is facilitated when the older person:

- Recognizes and accepts changes in physical and mental capabilities
- Gives up some roles and develops new ones
- Develops new activities that can be carried out successfully with aging
- Develops a different self-concept
- Revises life goals
- Adapts to new lifestyles

In the final stage of development elders are faced with a variety of internal and external losses that require coping and adaptation using diminished biologic, psychological, and social resources. The challenge is to maintain performance in the face of adverse circumstances.

COPING AND ADAPTATION

Old age has been described as the season of losses, including loss of roles, statuses, physical abilities, and deep personal losses through the deaths of friends and the disruption of family networks. Loss, whether real, threatened, or imaginary, is a stressor that requires adaptation, flexibility, and resiliency if a person is to cope successfully.

In most respects older people cope in much the same way as younger people. Differences are largely the result of the different types of stressors experienced. Older people tend to experience more negative and irreversible types of stressors. Given the many losses associated with old age as potential stressors, the older person may cope with these losses with positive or negative adaptation. Positive adaptation might include rational action, perseverance, positive thinking (e.g., the lost loved one is now out of pain), intellectual denial (e.g., "I don't want to think about it now"), restraint, drawing strength from adversity, and humor.

Unfortunately, in nursing and health care we are often confronted with those who are unable to cope effectively with their losses. Some older people respond to losses by losing their sense of personal identity and fulfillment and suffer from deterioration in self-esteem, an altered self-concept, and a loss of meaningfulness in life. Many older people become seriously depressed and experience additional loss. Many lose motivation for working, playing, and living. Depression resulting from loss is associated with approximately two thirds of the suicides among older people.

FAMILY

With an aging population that needs support and assistance in positive coping and adaptation, kinship networks take on added importance. Most of the aged in the United States occupy a variety of family roles and come from multigenerational units. It is not uncommon for a person at age 65 to be married, have at least one living adult child, have at least one living brother or sister, be a grandparent, and also be a great-grandparent. The person over age 65 may also be a child of a much older parent. The kinship network may also include cousins, nieces, and nephews. Of all these roles and relationships, marital relations and the relationships between parent and child seem to be most important.

In an era when the old are sometimes referred to as burdens, it is important to recognize that more financial support flows from the old to the young in the family than in the reverse direction. Although family responsibility appears to be an internalized value for most people, it is important to know that more than half of the states have legal statutes that can require children to provide financial support for needy parents. However, what is most needed and most often given is emotional support and help in times of illness and disability. Home health care for the frail elderly is most often given by a spouse or a child. Typically, the caregiver is a daughter. Three out of four caregivers are women, and almost half of these are raising children of their own simultaneously.

The combination of personal limitations, competing roles, and stresses generated by the care recipient's behavior and the physical demands created by various levels of emotional, physical, financial, and family strain places enormous stress on informal caregivers. Caregivers frequently report symptoms of depression, anxiety, helplessness, low morale, and emotional exhaustion. Try to be aware of the stressful impact of caregiving and implement actions to minimize the stresses and burdens on both the caregiver and the care recipient.

In part because of caregiver stress, more than 1 million aged persons are abused physically and psychologically or are neglected each year by their caregivers. You are in an excellent position to assess stress, depression, and abuse among caregivers and care recipients and to recommend interventions to alter these conditions. Education for learning and positive adaptive behaviors can assist both caregivers and care recipients. Caregivers who feel knowledgeable, useful, and productive are usually happier, less stressed, and less prone to be abusive. Families must be part of the holistic approach in the assessment and care of the aged.

FUNCTIONAL ASSESSMENT

Assessment has become a key word in gerontology and geriatrics because of its importance in care planning and care delivery. Functional assessment includes acquiring information about activities of daily living as well as environmental, financial, family, economic, and community resources. Functional assessment data are useful during times of health, at the onset of illness, at the beginning of treatment, and following therapeutic interventions. Comparisons across these time points help you to plot an individual's functions, which can serve to increase understanding of the aged person's problems and the effects of interventions.

Functional assessment is more than a diagnosis. A diagnosis alone cannot tell you how sick an older person is or how much care is needed. For example, a medical diagnosis of coronary artery disease does not tell you whether the older person is independent and the disease is controlled appropriately with medication or is totally dependent on care and currently needing intensive coronary care. For effective gerontological care, functional assessment is the crucial denominator in deciding care needs.

Functional status is more than a measure of activities of daily living. Knowing what activities an individual performs alone, what activities require assistance, and what activities the person is totally unable to perform or to perform safely is essential for defining care needs. This information plus a diagnosis helps you to know the cause of self-care problems and whether the problems are amenable to therapeutic intervention.

The older person's database should describe both basic and instrumental activities of daily living. The following areas are generally considered in an assessment of activities of daily living: grooming, bathing, dressing, eating, elimination, and mobility. Instrumental activities of daily living are less important in institutional settings but are essential for a person to continue or to return to independent living. Instrumental activities of daily living generally consider the older adult's ability to prepare a meal, shop for groceries, use the telephone, negotiate transportation, take medications, and maintain housekeeping and laundry tasks.

The Duke Older Americans Research and Services (OARS) Multidimensional Functional Assessment Questionnaire (MFAQ) is one example of a valid and reliable assessment guide for gathering information on the overall personal functional status and service use of adults. The OARS questionnaire has been used mainly with older adults and has two parts. The first part provides for assessment of the older adult in terms of social, economic, mental, and physical health and ability to perform activities of daily living. The second part provides for assessment of the older adult based on the need

table 10-3 Content Areas of the OARS Multidimensional Functional Assessment Questionnaire

PART A: FUNCTIONAL ASSESSMENT	
Social	**Physical**
Contact with others	Prescribed medications used
Help from family and kin	Physical conditions with impairment levels
Economic	**Activities of Daily Living**
Amount of income and adequacy	Physical and instrumental activities of daily living
Home ownership	**Demographics and Administrative**
Mental	
Mental and psychiatric status	Age, sex, race
	Location, length of interview
Mental well-being	Information source
PART B: SERVICES	
Transportation	Continuous supervision
Social or recreational	Checking
Employment	Homemaker
Sheltered employment	Meal preparation
Education	Legal and protective
Remedial training	Systematic evaluation
Mental health	Financial
Psychotropic drugs	Food, groceries
Personal care	Housing
Medical	Coordination
Supportive devices	Information
Physical therapy	Referral

Adapted from Older Americans Research and Services. (1978). *Multidimensional functional assessment questionnaire.* Durham, NC: Center for the Study of Aging and Human Development, Duke University Medical Center.

for 24 rather universal services. A content summary is provided in Table 10-3. In most instances, the nursing home Minimum Data Set incorporates all components of a quality functional assessment. This comprehensive assessment tool is valid and reliable and currently used in research.

DRUG THERAPY AND AGED ADULTS

ABSORPTION, DISTRIBUTION, METABOLISM, AND EXCRETION

Approximately 31% of all prescription drugs are given to aged adults, who make up only 12% to 13% of the population. It is projected that by the year 2005, older adults will comprise 18% of the population and consume 40% of all medications. Age-related changes influence patterns of drug use, consumption of drugs, and actions of medications on target organs (Table 10-4). The most important changes involve body composition, the cardiovascular system, the central nervous system, renal function, tissue sensitivity to drugs, and blood pressure reflex sensitivity. Age-related and disease-related changes in the elderly slow the clearance of drugs, which increases the risk of adverse effects.

table 10-4 Association Between Age-Related Physiologic Changes and Drug Effects

AGE-RELATED CHANGES	DRUG EFFECTS
Increased body fat	Increased drug storage
Decreased body water	Increased drug /active concentration
Decreased hepatic blood flow	Decreased drug clearance
Decreased lean muscle mass	Increased drug tissue concentration
Decreased renal function	Decreased drug elimination
Decreased serum albumin	Increased free drug concentration

With aging there is a reduction in body size, with a decrease in lean body mass and body water content (extracellular volume) and an increase in fat. The serum albumin concentration is lower, which tends to make more free drug available to tissues or to permit more rapid elimination of the drug. A gradual decrease in blood flow to the internal organs in the abdomen reduces drug clearance through the liver or kidney. For example, a water-soluble drug may result in higher blood concentrations of that drug. However, a highly fat-soluble drug might bind to the increased fat in the aged body and may be stored longer before excretion. For example, a 75-year-old woman was misdiagnosed as having progressive brain damage after she developed urinary incontinence, general mental deterioration, and inability to walk. She had taken 5 mg of diazepam (Valium) daily for at least 1 year. Diazepam is a fat-soluble drug that has the potential for increased distribution in tissues and for delayed elimination. After the drug was discontinued, the patient recovered in 3 days.

The liver prepares drugs for elimination in the urine or in feces. Age-related changes that have an impact on the inactivation of drugs by the liver include decreased liver size, reduced blood flow through the liver, and reduced liver enzyme activity on drugs. These changes have the overall effect of increasing drug concentrations in the blood and possibly increasing the amount of time it takes the body to get rid of the drug. Drugs that are principally eliminated in the urine may be given to older persons in reduced doses or less frequently to avoid accumulation and adverse effects.

Older persons tend to respond more vigorously to drugs that act on the central nervous system because of a greater tissue sensitivity and altered physiologic changes, as described earlier. Some of the potential adverse effects are postural imbalance, staggering, uncoordinated movements, respiratory depression, and changes in mental alertness. Drugs such as opiates, diazepam, and nifedipine may cause these effects.

ADVERSE DRUG REACTIONS

Adverse drug reactions are more common in older people because older people use more drugs. An estimated 70% of older adults take at least one prescription drug each year. In addition, older people take more over-the-counter drugs than younger people. Further, studies of hospitalized older adults revealed an average of 3 to 6 prescribed drugs per patient. Among long-term care patients, one third take 6 to 12 drugs daily. Imagine the potential for errors and drug interactions with so many medications!

The risk factors for adverse drug reactions are age, sex, race (occurring most frequently in older white females), number of drugs consumed, dosage, duration of treatment, severity of illness, and patient cooperation. Some of the common symptoms and signs of adverse drug reactions in the older person are restlessness, falls, depression, confusion, loss of memory, constipation, and urinary incontinence. Some drugs associated with adverse drug reactions are listed in Table 10-5. When patients are prescribed multiple drugs and experience unpleasant side effects, they may not follow the prescribed regimen. The use of fewer drugs at lower doses usually increases patient adherence.

Because older adults experience a greater number of drug reactions and interactions than younger people and are believed to be more sensitive to some medications, nurses must monitor their drug regimens carefully. It is helpful to assist the patient in maintaining a record of blood pressure, pulse, respiration, drug effect, and state of alertness in relation to current drug therapy. Such a record could be helpful in making necessary changes. It may be necessary to change a drug, reduce the dosage, or lengthen the intervals between doses to minimize the risk of adverse drug reactions. You are very often in the best position to minimize drug reactions. Baseline and continual assessments should include:

- The amount, frequency, and purpose of all medications taken
- The older person's ability to take medications as recommended
- The potential for drug interactions and adverse drug reactions
- The effectiveness of the medication over time
- Whether any of the drugs taken can be discontinued or decreased in dose

Assessment of drug effects and adverse reactions must be documented.

table 10-5 *Drugs Commonly Associated with Adverse Drug Reactions in Older Persons*

DRUG CLASS	EXAMPLE	PROBLEM
Analgesics	Aspirin	Bleeding
Antibiotics	Streptomycin	Nephrotoxicity
Anticoagulants	Warfarin	Hemorrhage
Antidepressants	Amitriptyline	Sedation
Antihypertensives	Verapamil	Hypotension
Antiparkinsonians	Levodopa	Extrapyramidal symptoms, dystonia
Antipsychotics	Haloperidol	Confusion
Diuretics	Diuril	Hypokalemia
Sedatives/hypnotics	Flurazepam	Drowsiness

This presentation of adverse drug reactions would not be complete without mentioning the hazards associated with potential drug interactions between over-the-counter medications and prescription medications taken by older adults. Examples might include the use of aspirin that enhances the effect of an anticoagulant or the use of large amounts of sodium bicarbonate that counteract diuretic actions. Further concern is raised in relation to the possibility of older adults mixing older prescription medications with newer ones and failing to discontinue and discard older prescriptions. Hoarding of medications may be viewed as future savings by an older adult. Nevertheless, you must learn to recognize the inherent dangers in this situation and teach elders to review all medications, prescription and over-the-counter, with their primary nurse or other health care providers.

One of the greatest challenges for those working within health care is addressing the physiologic, psychosocial, behavioral, and mental well-being of older adults. Management and care of an aging population affect every sector of the nursing profession. Nurses at all levels of preparation are encouraged to meet this mandate with care, concern, and competence.

Put on your THINKING CAP!!

1. Discuss the importance of functional assessments of older adults who receive home health care.
2. What functions would an older adult need to manage self-care in the home?
3. Recall an older adult who has been discharged from the hospital with some impairments. What instrumental activities of daily living are likely to be affected in that person?

key points

- Aging is an ongoing developmental process that begins at conception and ends at death.
- Gerontology is the study of aging.
- Geriatrics is the biomedical science of old age and the application of knowledge related to the biologic, biomedical, behavioral, and social aspects of aging to the prevention, diagnosis, treatment, and care of older persons.
- Gerontological nursing aims to increase healthy behaviors in the aged, minimize and compensate for health-related losses and impairments of aging, provide comfort and sustenance through the events of aging, and facilitate the diagnosis, care, and treatment of disease in the aged.
- Health care providers must recognize myths about the elderly and aging that result in stereotyping and discrimination against older people.
- Aging occurs slowly and is a complex and dynamic process involving many internal and external influences.
- Physiologic changes that are associated with aging may reflect more the presence of age-related diseases than the process of aging itself.

- The older adult shows cumulative developmental effects that produce unique personality styles, coping mechanisms, challenges, and growth, all of which occur in a societal context.
- Age-related changes that contribute to a decreased ability to clear drugs through the liver and renal system place the older adult at risk for adverse drug effects.

REVIEW QUESTIONS

1. Which of the following statements about aging is correct?
   1. Many older people continue to enjoy sexual activity.
   2. Older people generally lack family and other support networks.
   3. Almost 50% of people over age 65 have dementia.
   4. 25% of the older population reside in nursing homes.
2. Neurologic changes commonly found in the healthy older adult include:
   1. impaired short-term memory.
   2. inability to learn new material.
   3. decline in intellectual capability.
   4. loss of creative abilities.
3. Mr. J. had been a healthy 90-year-old man until he developed pneumonia. While acutely ill with the pneumonia, he showed signs of early heart and renal failure. He became weak, and his tolerance for physical activity declined. Even though the pneumonia resolved, it was several months before he returned to his previous level of functioning. How would you explain this?
   1. At age 90, immune function is severely impaired.
   2. He probably did not seek treatment for his pneumonia soon enough.
   3. Acute illness overwhelmed his already limited cardiac and renal function.
   4. He wanted to continue getting the attention he received when he was acutely ill.
4. When teaching a group of active older people about skin care, you would include:
   1. older skin thickens, which makes sunscreens no longer necessary.
   2. hot baths or showers followed by vigorous towel drying remove dead skin.
   3. generous use of moisturizers and minimal use of soap prevent skin drying.
   4. generalized itching is common and is insignificant for older adults.
5. You observe that an older patient's thoracic spine is curved, causing her to bend forward. Your assessment should be described as:
   1. Patient cannot stand up straight.
   2. Patient has kyphosis.
   3. Patient leans forward.
   4. Patient's spine is crooked.
6. A new patient admitted to your long-term care facility has presbycusis. What are the relevant nursing interventions?
   1. Be sure room lighting is adequate.
   2. Lower the pitch of your voice.
   3. Monitor her blood pressure.
   4. Implement body fluid precautions.
7. Which of these statements by older adults reflects movement toward ego-integrity?
   1. "Since I cannot drive now, I rarely get out or see other people."
   2. "After my children grew up and my husband died, I just wasn't needed anymore."
   3. "In my day, when you got married, you stayed married, no matter how bad it was."
   4. "I can't run marathons anymore, but I still enjoy a brisk walk around the neighborhood."
8. The home health nurse assesses an older adult's ability to carry out instrumental activities of daily living. These include:
   1. grooming.
   2. bathing.
   3. shopping.
   4. elimination.
9. An older postoperative patient is receiving pain medications that depress the central nervous system. Based on your knowledge of drug therapy and aging, what adverse effect is most likely?
   1. Respiratory depression
   2. Difficulty sleeping
   3. Vomiting and diarrhea
   4. Agitation and confusion
10. A clinic patient reports that she bruises very easily. She cut herself this morning, and the wound continues to ooze blood. An assessment of her medication history reveals that she takes the diuretic Diuril and verapamil for hypertension, Maalox for heartburn, and aspirin for arthritis pain. Which drug would you suspect is related to her bleeding?
    1. Diuril
    2. Verapamil
    3. Maalox
    4. Aspirin

CHAPTER

11 The Nursing Process and Critical Thinking

objectives

1. Describe the five components of the nursing process.
2. Describe the formats for North American Nursing Diagnosis Association (NANDA) diagnoses, Nursing Interventions Classification (NIC) interventions, and Nursing Outcome Classification (NOC) outcomes.
2. Explain the role of the licensed practical nurse in the nursing process.
3. Describe the proper documentation of the nursing process using a problem-oriented medical record format, nurses' notes, and flow sheets.
4. Explain the relationship between the nursing process and critical thinking.
5. Describe the characteristics of a critical thinker.
6. Describe how critical thinking skills are used in clinical practice.

key terms

Assessment (p. 114)
Auscultation (ăw-skŭl-TĀ-shŭn, p. 118)
Inspection (p. 117)
Nursing diagnosis (p. 119)
Nursing process (p. 114)
Objective data (p. 115)
Palpation (păl-PĀ-shŭn, p. 117)
Percussion (pĕr-KŬ-shŭn, p. 117)
Physical assessment (p. 117)
Problem-oriented medical record (POMR) (p. 126)
Subjective data (p. 115)

The **nursing process** is a systematic method of providing care to patients. It is a problem-solving approach that enables the nurse to provide care in an organized, scientific manner. The goal of the nursing process is to alleviate, minimize, or prevent actual or potential health problems. It enables the nurse to provide care in the areas of health maintenance and promotion, management of acute or chronic illness, and rehabilitation.

The nursing process can be applied in any interaction that involves a nurse and a patient or client. (As noted earlier, the terms *patient* and *client* are used interchangeably in this text.) The patient or client can be defined as an individual, a family, a group, a community, or a society. The process can take place in a variety of settings, including a hospital, community setting, private home, or long-term care facility.

COMPONENTS OF THE NURSING PROCESS

The five components or steps in the nursing process are: (1) assessment (the systematic collection of data relating to patients and their problems), (2) nursing diagnosis (interpretation of the data for problem identification), (3) planning (goals and selected interventions), (4) implementation (putting the plan into action), and (5) evaluation (assessing the achievement of goals and changing the plan as indicated by current needs). Sometimes these steps are called *phases* or *stages.* Initially, the steps are followed in sequence—data collection and assessment first, then identification of the problems or nursing diagnoses, then planning care, and so forth. However, after the process has begun, it becomes continuous or cyclic. Each phase of the nursing process is dependent on the others, and there is a continuous interaction among the stages as information about the status of the patient changes. Evaluation and revision of the plan of care occur constantly. As problems are alleviated, new problems may arise, requiring new plans and actions.

The American Nurses Association has developed standards of care for nurses for each phase of the nursing process (Table 11-1). Although the registered nurse has responsibility for developing the nursing process, the licensed practical nurse makes an important contribution. Most licensed practical nurses work in settings in which the nursing process is used to achieve goals related to recovery from acute illness, health maintenance in chronic illness, or rehabilitation. Suggested roles for LVNs in relation to the nursing process are (1) to contribute to an assessment database for patients by collecting information using a standardized form, performing basic psychosocial assessment, and taking objective measurements of body functions; (2) to assist with the development of nursing care plans and the implementation of the established plan of care; (3) to perform basic therapeutic and preventive nursing measures; and (4) to participate in the evaluation of the care given by reporting observed outcomes and making necessary changes according to the results of the evaluation.

ASSESSMENT

The **assessment** phase of the nursing process involves collecting data about the health status of the patient. The word

table 11-1 ***American Nurses Association Standards of Care***

STANDARD I: ASSESSMENT

The nurse collects client health data.

Measurement Criteria

1. The priority of data collection is determined by the client's immediate condition or needs.
2. Pertinent data are collected using appropriate assessment techniques.
3. Data collection involves the client, significant others, and health care providers when appropriate.
4. The data collection process is systematic and ongoing.
5. Relevant data are documented in a retrievable form.

STANDARD II: DIAGNOSIS

The nurse analyzes the assessment data in determining diagnoses.

Measurement Criteria

1. Diagnoses are derived from the assessment data.
2. Diagnoses are validated with the client, significant others, and health care providers, when possible.
3. Diagnoses are documented in a manner that facilitates the determination of expected outcomes and plan of care.

STANDARD III: OUTCOME IDENTIFICATION

The nurse identifies expected outcomes individualized to the client.

Measurement Criteria

1. Outcomes are derived from the diagnoses.
2. Outcomes are documented as measurable goals.
3. Outcomes are mutually formulated with the client and health care providers, when possible.
4. Outcomes are realistic in relation to the client's present and potential capabilities.
5. Outcomes are attainable in relation to resources available to the client.
6. Outcomes include a time estimate for attainment.
7. Outcomes provide direction for continuity of care.

STANDARD IV: PLANNING

The nurse develops a plan of care that prescribes interventions to attain expected outcomes.

Measurement Criteria

1. The plan is individualized to the client's condition or needs.
2. The plan is developed with the client, significant others, and health care providers, when appropriate.
3. The plan reflects current nursing practice.
4. The plan is documented.
5. The plan provides for continuity of care.

STANDARD V: IMPLEMENTATION

The nurse implements the interventions identified in the plan of care.

Measurement Criteria

1. Interventions are consistent with the established plan of care.
2. Interventions are implemented in a safe and appropriate manner.
3. Interventions are documented.

STANDARD VI: EVALUATION

The nurse evaluates the client's progress toward attainment of outcomes.

Measurement Criteria

1. Evaluation is systematic and ongoing.
2. The client's responses to interventions are documented.
3. The effectiveness of interventions is evaluated in relation to outcomes.
4. Ongoing assessment data are used to revise diagnoses, outcomes, and the plan of care, as needed.
5. Revisions in diagnoses, outcomes, and the plan of care are documented.
6. The client, significant others, and health care providers are involved in the evaluation process, when appropriate.

From American Nurses Association. (1991). *Standards of clinical practice.* Washington, DC: American Nurses Association.

data is the plural of *datum* and means information, especially information organized for analysis or decision making. There are two types of data, subjective and objective. *Subjective data* consist of information that is reported by the patient and family members in a health history in response to direct questioning or in spontaneous statements. Subjective data are usually documented in the patient's own words and include information such as previous experiences and sensations or emotions that only the patient can describe. *Objective data* are those that the nurse or other members of the health care team obtain through observation, physical examination, or diagnostic testing. Objective data can be seen or measured; for example, heart rate, wound condition, and laboratory values. Sources of subjective and objective data are the patient, the family and significant others, medical records, and other health care team members.

Health History

The health history consists of subjective data gathered by interviewing the patient or family members or both. The manner in which the interview is conducted directly affects the accuracy and completeness of the information gained. Communication should be goal directed, orderly, and systematic. Open-ended questions will allow patients to express their thoughts and feelings. Allowing expression of feelings helps establish a better working relationship with patients and families.

To obtain the health history, you should conduct the interview in a quiet, private area to ensure comfort and confidentiality. Explain the purpose of the interview to the patient and family members with the assurance that they can refuse to answer any questions and can add any pertinent information that is helpful. Usually the interview takes no longer than 20 to 30 minutes. Older patients, who may have a complex health history, may require additional time. Also, older patients may tire more easily than younger patients, so that several short interviews may be necessary.

Usually a nurse assessment form is used for the interview so that the nursing database is as complete as possible. The health history consists of the following components:

1. Biographical data
2. Reason for seeking care, or "chief complaint"
3. Present health or history of present illness
4. Medical history
5. Family history
6. Review of systems
7. Functional assessment of activities of daily living

Table 11-2 briefly describes each of these components.

When the interview is complete, summarize the data with the patient or family members to be sure the information gathered is correct. The process of summarizing the data further strengthens the nurse-patient relationship because it demonstrates your interest in the patient and the patient's needs. As the level of trust increases between you and the patient, the patient may also think of additional information that may have been omitted earlier. Subjective data are usually charted as "Patient states . . ." . For example, subjective data collected from a patient with pain could be recorded: "The patient states 'I have a shooting pain in my left arm.' "

Objective Data

Objective data are gained through physical assessment, diagnostic tests, and patient records. Observation is one of the most important means through which information is obtained. Use the senses of sight, hearing, smell, and touch to collect objective data. For example, a patient's disheveled appearance (sight) on admission may indicate an inability to carry out self-care activities at home. A patient's noisy and labored breathing (hearing) may suggest respiratory problems. A fruity mouth odor (smell) may be a sign of diabetic acidosis. Cold and clammy skin (touch) may signal that a patient is in shock.

table 11-2 ***The Health History***

BIOGRAPHICAL DATA

Name, address, phone number, age, birth date, birthplace, sex, marital status, race, ethnic origin, occupation, educational level

SOURCE OF HISTORY

Who furnishes information (patient, family); estimate of reliability of information

REASON FOR SEEKING CARE

Chief complaint (put in patient's own words)

HISTORY OF PRESENT ILLNESS

Events leading up to chief complaint or reason for seeking care:
Location of symptoms (e.g., pain in the chest radiating to the left arm)
Character or quality (e.g., burning, sharp, or dull pain; sticky, dark, or coffee grounds–colored emesis)
Quantity or severity (severity of pain interrupts normal daily activities)
Timing (onset, duration, frequency); when symptoms appeared; how long they lasted; how often they occurred
Setting (what was happening when symptoms occurred; what brought it on)
Aggravating or relieving factors (what makes symptoms worse; what makes them better)
Associated factors (what other symptoms are related, e.g., urinary frequency and burning associated with fever or chills)
Client's perception (meaning of symptoms to client; how they affect daily activities)

PAST HEALTH

Childhood illnesses
Accidents or injuries

PAST HEALTH—cont'd

Serious or chronic illnesses
Hospitalizations
Operations
Obstetric history
Immunizations
Last examination date
Allergies
Current medications

FAMILY HISTORY

Age, health, and cause of death of blood relatives
Family history of heart disease, high blood pressure, stroke, diabetes, blood disorders, cancer, sickle cell anemia, arthritis, allergies, obesity, alcoholism, mental illness, seizure disorders, kidney disease, and tuberculosis

REVIEW OF SYSTEMS

Evaluate past and present health state of each body system:
General overall health state (present weight, weight gain or loss, fatigue, weakness, fever, chills, night sweats)
Skin (history of skin disease; change in color, pigment, or mole; excessive dryness or moisture; itching; excessive bruising; rash or lesion)
Hair (recent loss, change in texture; change in shape, color, or brittleness of nails)
Head (history of head injury, headache, dizziness, or vertigo)
Eyes (difficulty with vision, including decreased acuity, blurring, blind spots; eye pain; double vision; redness or swelling; watering or discharge; glaucoma or cataracts)
Ears (earaches, infections, discharge, tinnitus or ringing in the ears)

Adapted from Jarvis, C. (1999). *Physical examination and health assessment,* (3rd ed., pp. 79-84). Philadelphia: Saunders.

When recording observational data, write exactly what is observed. Avoid words such as good, bad, better, or worse. For example, "The skin is warm and dry" is preferable to "The skin looks good."

Physical Assessment

Physical assessment or examination is a systematic, thorough way of obtaining objective data. Sometimes a complete head-to-toe examination is conducted, whereas at other times only one or two systems may be examined, as warranted by the patient' symptoms. For example, when a patient is in acute respiratory distress, only the respiratory and cardiovascular systems might be assessed initially. A complete assessment would be delayed until the patient's breathing improves. Although some aspects of the physical examination require advanced training, the complete physical examination process is presented here.

There are four methods of examination: (1) inspection, (2) palpation, (3) percussion, and (4) auscultation.

Inspection. *Inspection* is purposeful observation or scrutiny of the person as a whole and then systematically from head to toe (Fig. 11-1). The observation begins as soon as you meet the patient and continues throughout the examination.

Palpation. *Palpation* uses the sense of touch to assess various parts of the body and helps to confirm findings that are noted on inspection. The hands, especially the fingertips, are used to assess skin texture, moisture, and temperature, or the presence of swelling, lumps, masses, tenderness, or pain (Fig. 11-2). Warm your hands before palpating the patient. Palpation should be light at first for surface characteristics and then deeper for abdominal contents. If any tender areas are noted, they should be palpated last. Deep palpation is usually done only by nurses with advanced skills.

Percussion. *Percussion* is tapping on the skin to assess the underlying tissues. The chest and abdomen are the most common areas for percussion. Short, sharp strokes elicit sounds and subtle vibrations that are characteristic of underlying organs and certain conditions. To percuss, place one hand flat on the skin over the area to be assessed. Use the tip

table 11-2 *The Health History—cont'd*

REVIEW OF SYSTEMS—cont'd

Nose and sinuses (discharge; frequent or severe colds; sinus pain; nasal obstruction; nosebleeds; allergies or hayfever; change in sense of smell)

Mouth and throat (mouth pain, frequent sore throat, bleeding gums, toothache, difficulty swallowing, hoarseness, altered taste)

Neck (pain, limitation of movement, lumps or swelling, enlarged or tender nodes, goiter)

Gastrointestinal (history of abdominal diseases, e.g., ulcer, liver or gallbladder, jaundice, appendicitis, colitis; appetite; food intolerance; difficulty swallowing; heartburn; indigestion; abdominal pain; nausea and vomiting; vomiting blood; flatulence; type and frequency of bowel movement; rectal conditions, e.g., hemorrhoids, fistula)

Breast (pain, lump, nipple discharge, rash, history of breast disease or surgery)

Axilla (tenderness, lump or swelling, rash)

Musculoskeletal system (history of arthritis, gout, back pain or disk disease; pain, stiffness or swelling of joints; deformity; limitation of motion; noise with joint motion; muscle pain, cramps, or weakness; problems with gait or coordination; back pain, stiffness or limitation of motion)

Neurologic system (history of seizure disorder, stroke, fainting, or blackouts; weakness, tic, or tremor; paralysis or coordination problems; numbness or tingling; cognitive disorder; nervousness, mood changes, depression, or history of mental illness)

Respiratory system (lung diseases, e.g., asthma, emphysema, bronchitis, pneumonia, tuberculosis; chest pain with breathing; wheezing or noisy breathing; shortness of breath; cough; sputum; hemoptysis or coughing up blood)

REVIEW OF SYSTEMS—cont'd

Cardiovascular (chest pain, heart palpitation, cyanosis, dyspnea on exertion, orthopnea, nocturia, edema, heart murmur, hypertension, coronary artery disease, anemia)

Peripheral vascular (coldness, numbness and tingling of extremities; swelling of legs; discoloration of hands or feet; varicose veins; intermittent claudication or pain in legs on exertion; thrombophlebitis; leg ulcers)

Endocrine system (history of diabetes or diabetic symptoms, or thyroid disease; intolerance to heat and cold; change in skin pigmentation or texture; excessive sweating; relationship between appetite and weight; abnormal hair distribution; nervousness; tremors)

Urinary system (history of kidney disease, kidney stones, or urinary tract infections; frequency of urination; urgency; nocturia or number of times person awakens at night to urinate, painful or difficult urination; oliguria or polyuria; color of urine, e.g., cloudy, bloody, straw-colored; incontinence; pain in the flank, groin, suprapubic region, or lower back)

Male genital system (penile or testicular pain; penile discharge; sores or lesions; lumps; hernia)

Female genital system (menstrual history, e.g., age at menarche, last menstrual period, cycle and duration, amenorrhea or absence of periods, or menometrorrhagia or bleeding between periods; premenstrual pain or dysmenorrhea or menstrual pain; vaginal itching; discharge and its characteristics; age at menopause; menopausal signs or symptoms; postmenopausal bleeding)

FUNCTIONAL ASSESSMENT

Self-care ability, including bathing, dressing, grooming, toileting, and transfer from bed to chair.

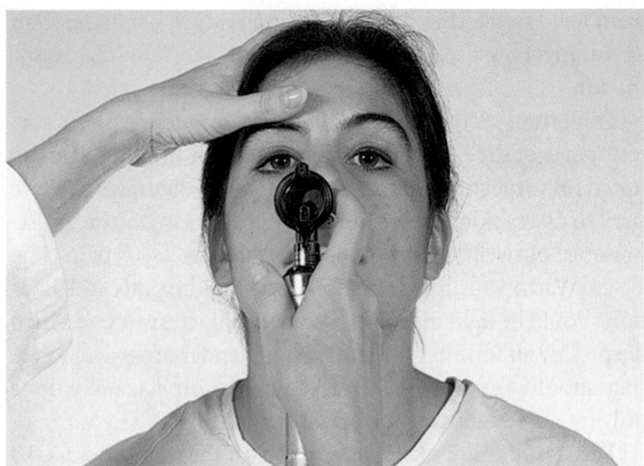

FIGURE 11-1 Inspection.

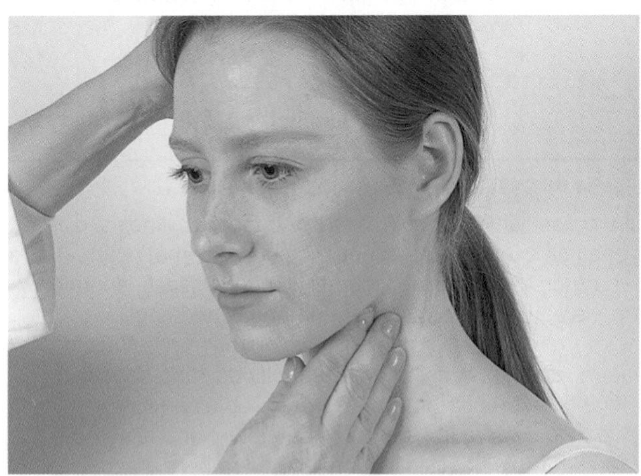

FIGURE 11-2 Palpation.

of the middle finger of your other hand to lightly tap the middle finger of the hand that rests on the patient (Figs. 11-3 and 11-4). Tap two times just behind the nail bed before moving on to the next area.

Auscultation. *Auscultation* is listening to sounds produced by the body, such as heart, lung, and intestinal sounds. Auscultation is performed with a stethoscope (Fig. 11-5). The stethoscope should have both a bell and a diaphragm. The earpieces should fit snugly and point forward to the nose. The room should be quiet so that an accurate assessment of sounds can be made. The diaphragm of the stethoscope is most frequently used for assessment. Warm the diaphragm by rubbing it against your palm, and then place it lightly over the area that is being assessed. If the area is hairy, you may hear a crackling sound. To minimize the problem, it is helpful to wet the hair before examination.

All four methods of examination require practice. Palpation, percussion, and auscultation may be awkward at first, but with time, you will master the skills.

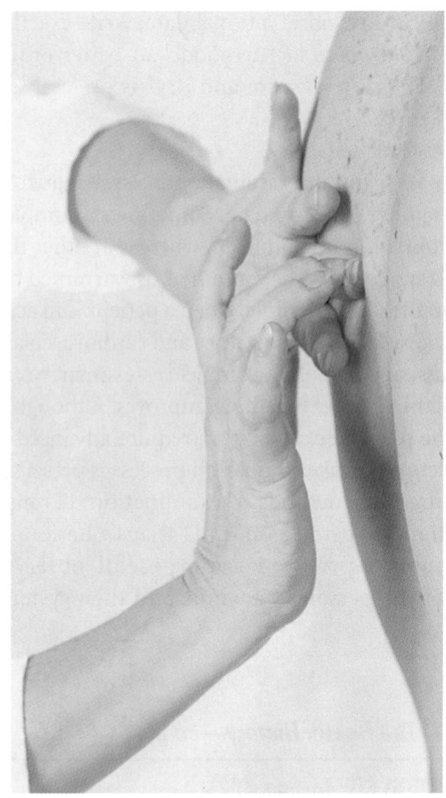

FIGURE 11-3 The stationary hand in percussion.

The physical examination includes assessment of general appearance, height and weight, vital signs, and body systems. Table 11-3 presents an overview of the content of a complete physical examination.

Diagnostic Tests

Diagnostic tests may include radiographic studies (x-rays), electrocardiograms (EKGs), magnetic resonance imaging (MRIs) scans, computed tomography (CTs) scans, ultrasound studies, laboratory blood and urine testing, and wound cultures. The information from these tests can be helpful in identifying general areas in which a patient might have a health care problem or in validating a nursing diagnosis. Common diagnostic tests are identified with each body system throughout this text.

Patient Records

Patient records provide a valuable source of information regarding the medical history and illness patterns. They can confirm the subjective data and history that the patient and family provide.

After the data are collected, organize the information into meaningful and usable clusters. When documenting data collected during the assessment phase, you should record, at the time of data collection, exactly what you heard, saw, felt, or smelled. Record patient statements very precisely. All documentation should be thorough and factual. The analysis of the data collected becomes the foundation for making the nursing diagnoses; the licensed practical nurse contributes to the for-

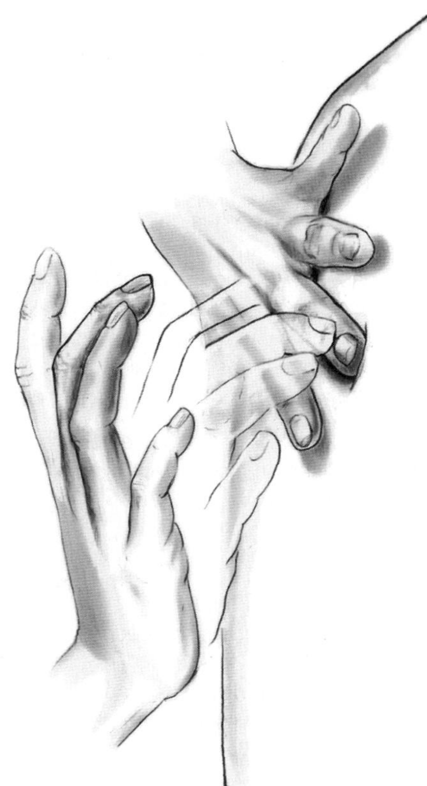

FIGURE **11-4** The striking hand in percussion.

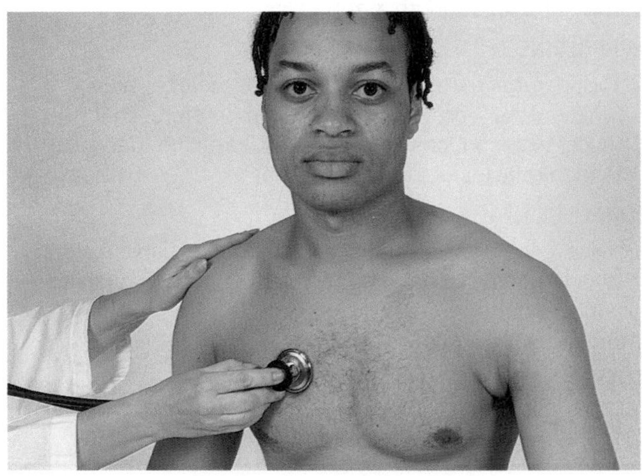

FIGURE **11-5** Auscultation.

mation of the nursing diagnosis. Baseline data also are used to assess the patient's progress or lack of progress over time.

NURSING DIAGNOSIS

The **nursing diagnosis** is derived from data gathered during the assessment. Health problems or potential health problems are identified and formulated into nursing diagnoses. Nursing diagnoses provide a basis for planning nursing interventions that can help prevent, minimize, or alleviate specific health problems.

A nursing diagnosis is different from a medical diagnosis. The medical diagnosis is used to identify the etiology (cause) of the disease. The focus of the medical diagnosis is on the function and malfunction of a specific organ system. The nursing diagnosis focuses on the response of the whole person to the health problem.

The concept of nursing diagnosis has been discussed for many years. In 1973, the National Conference Group on the Classification of Nursing Diagnosis began meeting to develop standardized nursing diagnoses to be used in all health care settings. The group, now known as the North American Nursing Diagnosis Association (NANDA), met to develop and revise nursing diagnoses. The current list (2001) of accepted nursing diagnoses is given in Table 11-4. Some of the new nursing diagnoses approved for use include: falls, risk for; powerlessness, risk for; relocation stress syndrome, risk for; self-esteem, risk for situational low; self-mutilation; suicide, risk for; and wandering. Potential nursing diagnoses are no longer stated "high risk for . . . "; instead, they are stated as "risk for . . . ."

Nursing diagnoses are written in a format, called PES, developed by NANDA. *P* stands for the *problem, E* stands for the *etiology* or cause of the problem, and *S* stands for the *signs* and *symptoms* of the problem. Only actual problems require signs and symptoms; potential problems do not list them. The PES format helps make the general nursing diagnosis fit a specific patient care problem. The following example shows the application of the general nursing diagnosis "Impaired skin integrity" to a specific patient situation. An elderly woman has developed a 2-cm pressure ulcer on her sacrum because she is bedridden and immobilized. Her specific nursing diagnosis would be written in the following manner:

> Impaired skin integrity *(P)* related to immobility *(E)* as evidenced by 2-cm pressure ulcer on sacrum *(S)*. The problem *(P)* or nursing diagnosis is "impaired skin integrity," the etiology *(E)* or cause is "immobility," and the signs or symptoms *(S)* are "2-cm pressure ulcer on sacrum."

By using all of the components of the nursing diagnosis, the problem is clearly communicated to everyone involved in the patient's care.

Although NANDA is continually working to make the structure and content of nursing diagnoses consistent, they still are not universally used and accepted. It is difficult for nursing students to work and learn in an uncertain environment, as nursing diagnoses are constantly evolving. However, nurses must work together to develop the most appropriate diagnoses to reflect current nursing practice. Some references identify collaborative problems as well as nursing diagnoses. Collaborative problems require intervention by multiple members of the health care team.

The format for nursing diagnoses in this book presents the problem and the etiology to avoid repetitious lists of signs and symptoms. In an actual patient care plan, you would include the patient's specific signs and symptoms.

table 11-3 ***The Physical Examination***

PHYSICAL APPEARANCE

Age, sex, level of consciousness, skin color, facial features, no signs of acute distress

BODY STRUCTURE

Stature, nutrition (normal weight for height and body build), symmetry, posture, body build (normal proportions), obvious physical deformities

MOBILITY

Gait, range of motion, no involuntary movement

BEHAVIOR

Facial expression, mood and affect, speech, dress, personal hygiene, hair, and makeup

MEASUREMENTS

Height, weight, vital signs

SKIN, HAIR, AND NAILS

Skin (color, general pigmentation, widespread color change, temperature, moisture, texture, thickness, edema, mobility and turgor, hygiene, vascularity or bruising, lesions)

Hair (color, texture, distribution, scalp lesions)

Nails (shape and contour, consistency, color)

HEAD AND NECK

Head (size and shape of skull, symmetry, and expression of face)

Neck (symmetry, range of motion, lymph nodes)

EYES

Central visual acuity, near and far vision, peripheral vision, extraocular muscle function (parallel alignment, nystagmus), external eye structures (eyebrows, eyelids and lashes, eyeballs, conjunctiva and sclera, lacrimal apparatus, cornea, lens, iris and pupils)

EARS

External ear (size and shape, skin condition, tenderness, the external auditory meatus), external canal, tympanic membrane, hearing acuity, vestibular apparatus

NOSE, MOUTH, AND THROAT

Nose (external nose, nasal cavity, sinus area)

Mouth (lips, teeth and gums, tongue, buccal mucosa, palate)

Throat (tonsils)

BREASTS AND REGIONAL LYMPHATICS

General appearance, skin, lymphatic drainage areas, nipple, axilla

THORAX AND LUNGS

Posterior chest (symmetric expansion, fremitus [palpable vibration], lung fields, breath sounds)

Anterior chest (shape and configuration of chest wall, level of consciousness, skin color and condition, quality of respirations, symmetric chest expansion, forced expiratory time [number of seconds to exhale])

HEART AND NECK VESSELS

Carotid artery pulse, jugular venous pulse, jugular venous pressure, anterior chest inspection, cardiac rate and rhythm, heart sounds, murmurs

ABDOMEN

Inspection (contour, symmetry, umbilicus, skin, pulsation or movement, hair distribution)

Palpation (surface and deep areas, liver edge, spleen, kidneys)

Percussion (general tympany, liver span, splenic dullness)

Auscultation (bowel sounds, vascular sounds)

PERIPHERAL VASCULAR SYSTEM

Pulses, capillary refill, skin color and temperature, edema, pain

MUSCULOSKELETAL SYSTEM

Joint (size, contour, swelling, warmth, range of motion, crepitus)

Muscles (tone, strength, size)

NEUROLOGIC SYSTEM

Cranial nerves, motor system (muscles, cerebellar function), sensory system (pain, temperature, light touch, vibration, position), reflexes (stretch or deep tendon reflexes, superficial reflexes)

FEMALE GENITALIA

External genitalia (skin color, hair distribution, labia majora, labia minoris, clitoris, urethral opening, vaginal opening, perineum)

Internal genitalia (cervix, vagina)

ANUS, RECTUM, AND PROSTATE

Perianal area, anus, rectum, stool

table 11-4 Approved Nursing Diagnoses, North American Nursing Diagnosis Association, 2001

Activity intolerance
Activity intolerance, Risk for
Adjustment, Impaired
Airway clearance, Ineffective
Allergy response, Latex
Allergy response, Risk for latex
Anxiety
Anxiety, Death
Aspiration, Risk for
Attachment, Risk for impaired parent/infant/child
Autonomic dysreflexia
Autonomic dysreflexia, Risk for
Body image, Disturbed
Body temperature, Risk for imbalanced
Bowel incontinence
Breastfeeding, Effective
Breastfeeding, Ineffective
Breastfeeding, Interrupted
Breathing patterns, Ineffective
Cardiac output, Decreased
Caregiver role strain
Caregiver role strain, Risk for
Impaired comfort
Communication, Impaired verbal
Conflict, Decisional
Confusion, Acute
Confusion, Chronic
Constipation
Constipation, Perceived
Constipation, Risk for
Coping, Ineffective
Coping, Ineffective community
Coping, Readiness for enhanced community
Coping, Defensive
Coping, Compromised family
Coping, Disabled family
Coping, Readiness for enhanced family
Denial, Ineffective
Dentition, Impaired
Development, Risk for delayed
Diarrhea
Disuse syndrome, Risk for
Diversional activity, Deficient
Energy field, Disturbed
Environmental interpretation syndrome, Impaired
Failure to thrive, Adult
Falls, Risk for
Family processes, alcoholism, Dysfunctional
Family processes, Interrupted
Fatigue
Fear
Fluid volume, Deficient
Fluid volume, Excess
Fluid volume, Risk for deficient
Fluid volume, Risk for imbalanced
Gas exchange, Impaired
Grieving
Grieving, Anticipatory
Grieving, Dysfunctional
Growth and development, Delayed
Growth, Risk for disproportionate
Health maintenance, Ineffective
Health-seeking behaviors
Home maintenance, Impaired
Hopelessness
Hyperthermia
Hypothermia
Identity, Disturbed personal
Incontinence, Functional urinary
Incontinence, Reflex urinary
Incontinence, Stress urinary
Incontinence, Total urinary
Incontinence, Urge urinary
Infant behavior, Disorganized
Infant behavior, Risk for disorganized
Infant behavior, Readiness for enhanced organized
Infant feeding pattern, Ineffective
Infection, Risk for
Injury, Risk for
Injury, Risk for perioperative-positioning
Intracranial, adaptive capacity, Decreased
Knowledge, Deficient
Loneliness, Risk for
Memory, Impaired
Mobility, Impaired bed
Mobility, Impaired physical
Mobility, Impaired wheelchair
Nausea
Neglect, Unilateral
Noncompliance
Nutrition, less than body requirements, Imbalanced
Nutrition, more than body requirements, Imbalanced
Nutrition, more than body requirements, Risk for imbalanced
Oral mucous membrane, Impaired
Pain, Acute
Pain, Chronic
Parenting, Risk for impaired
Peripheral neurovascular dysfunction, Risk for
Poisoning, Risk for
Post-trauma syndrome, Risk for
Powerlessness
Powerlessness, Risk for
Protection, Ineffective
Rape-trauma syndrome
Rape-trauma syndrome, Compound reaction
Rape-trauma syndrome, Silent reaction
Relocation stress syndrome
Relocation stress syndrome, Risk for
Role performance, Ineffective
Self-care deficit, Bathing/hygiene
Self-care deficit, Dressing/grooming
Self-care deficit, Feeding
Self-care deficit, Toileting
Self-esteem, Chronic low
Self-esteem, Situational low

From the North American Nursing Diagnosis Association. (2001). *Nursing diagnoses: Definitions and classification, 2000-2001,* Philadelphia: NANDA.

Continued

table 11-4 Approved Nursing Diagnoses, North American Nursing Diagnosis Association, 2001—cont'd

Self-esteem, Risk for situational low	Therapeutic regimen management, Effective
Self-mutilation	Therapeutic regimen management, Ineffective
Self-mutilation, Risk for	Therapeutic regimen management, Ineffective community
Sensory perception, Disturbed	Therapeutic regimen management, Ineffective family
Sexual dysfunction	Thermoregulation, Ineffective
Sexuality patterns, Ineffective	Thought processes, Disturbed
Skin integrity, Impaired	Tissue integrity, Impaired
Skin integrity, Risk for impaired	Tissue perfusion, Ineffective
Sleep deprivation	Transfer ability, Impaired
Sleep pattern, Disturbed	Trauma, Risk for
Social interaction, Impaired	Urinary elimination, Impaired
Social isolation	Urinary retention
Sorrow, Chronic	Ventilation, Impaired spontaneous
Spiritual distress	Ventilatory weaning response, Dysfunctional
Spiritual distress, Risk for	Violence, Risk for self-directed
Spiritual well-being, Readiness for enhanced	Violence, Risk for other-directed
Suffocation, Risk for	Walking, Impaired
Suicide, Risk for	Wandering
Surgical recovery, Delayed	
Swallowing, Impaired	

From the North American Nursing Diagnosis Association. (2001). *Nursing diagnoses: Definitions and classification, 2000-2001*, Philadelphia: NANDA.

PLANNING

The planning phase of the nursing process involves the development of a nursing care plan for the patient based on the nursing diagnoses. Nursing care plans are a form of communication with other health care professionals to ensure continuity of care, to prevent complications, and to provide for health teaching and discharge planning. As a licensed practical nurse, you will assist in the formation of goals of care and in the development of a plan of care.

The steps in nursing care planning are to (1) determine priorities from the list of nursing diagnoses, (2) set long-term and short-term goals to determine outcomes of care, (3) develop objectives to reach the goals, and (4) write nursing orders to direct care to meet the goals. Priorities are established according to the most immediate needs of the patient. They are usually based on Maslow's hierarchy of needs and on what the patient perceives as important. For example, you should focus on decreased cardiac output (a physiologic need) before addressing disturbed body image (a self-esteem need). Goals may be short term or long term, meaning that some may be achievable immediately whereas others will take a longer period of time.

Goals should be stated in terms of patient outcomes. To continue with our example of the patient with impaired skin integrity, the goal could be stated as "Pressure ulcer over sacrum will be healed within 2 weeks."

A new classification system for outcomes can be used. The system, called Nursing Outcome Classification (NOC), includes outcomes such as Tissue Integrity: Skin and Mucous Membranes; Wound Healing: Primary Intention; and Urinary Continence. Each of the nursing-sensitive outcomes (outcomes amenable to nursing intervention) is labeled, defined, and includes criteria for assessing the status of the outcome over time.

Nursing orders are the actions for interventions prescribed to help achieve the stated goals and objectives. Nursing orders should include a specific description (what, where, when, how much, and how long) of how the order should be carried out. For example, "Keep off sacrum to promote healing; turn side to side q 2 hr. Get OOB [out of bed] twice a day; begin ambulating as tolerated."

INTERVENTION (IMPLEMENTATION)

Implementation is the actual performance of the nursing interventions identified in the plan of care. The interventions are coordinated with other members of the health care team and include direct patient care, health teaching, or carrying out ordered medical treatments such as medications or dressing changes. Nurses provide care to achieve established goals of care and then communicate the nursing interventions by documentation and report.

Some interventions are unplanned because the nurse must respond to crises that demand immediate attention. Thus, the care plan must be flexible and reflect changes in the patient's health care needs.

The Nursing Interventions Classification (NIC) is a standardized list of nursing interventions. An NIC intervention consists of a label name, definition, specific nursing activities, and background readings. Development of NIC interventions is ongoing, and currently includes nearly 500 interventions divided into 7 domains and 30 classes. To use NIC interventions, the nurse selects the appropriate activities for a specific intervention based on individual patient data. Examples of intervention labels are: Pressure Management, Pressure Ulcer Care, Skin Surveillance, Preparation for Childbirth, Fall Prevention, and Incision Site Care. Depending on the situation, additional activities might be added. An example of a nursing care plan using NANDA, NIC, and NOC is printed here.

NURSING CARE PLAN

Plan of Care for Mrs. C

CASE STUDY

Mrs. C, a 38-year-old woman, is married and has two adult stepchildren. She maintains a healthy lifestyle and has no family history of cancer. She performs breast self-exams routinely and has never identified a lump or any unusual finding during her monthly exam. Mrs. C works full-time as a magazine publisher. One day at work as she was going down a flight of stairs, her high heel caught on the rung of the step, and she fell to the next landing. She received multiple bruises, including one in the chest area where she hit a metal railing. Ignoring her injuries because she was embarrassed about the fall, she continued to work throughout the day. That evening she told her family about her fall at work. Everyone was concerned, but she downplayed the incident since she was still more embarrassed about falling than concerned about the injuries she sustained.

Subsequently Mrs. C experienced localized pain in her left breast. The pain started out as a dull ache and did not improve over time. For several days Mrs. C was aware of the breast pain but disregarded it as simply being a bruise resulting from the accident. The pain gradually became worse, and ultimately, Mrs. C could feel a lump in her breast at the site of the pain. She finally went to a doctor 2 months after her fall. Upon examination, the doctor recommended a biopsy of the lump in her breast. The biopsy was done a week later and confirmed the presence of a malignant tumor. Mrs. C had a radical mastectomy of the left breast several days later.

Mr. C was at the hospital during the surgery but left for work after Mrs. C entered postanesthesia recovery. After work Mr. C, an alcoholic, decided to go to the bar for a few drinks. He phoned Mrs. C from the bar and told her he would call her again once he reached home. Mrs. C was concerned about her husband driving home from the bar and worried a great deal about this during the evening. Several hours later he phoned her from home. While talking to her he "passed out" on the other end, and she could not disconnect from him. This upset Mrs. C because she knew he was not dealing well with the mastectomy. She needed his support to deal with her recovery, and he needed her to help him cope with her surgery. Mrs. C relied on the nursing staff for support with accepting her body image changes and also for emotional support. The staff located Reach for Recovery, a breast cancer support group, to help Mrs. C through this difficult time in her life. The plan of care provides a summary of the information in this case showing the linkages among NANDA, NOC, and NIC.

Nursing Diagnosis	*Goals and Outcome Criteria*	*Interventions*
Disturbed Body Image	**Body Image**	**Body Image Enhancement**
Defining Characteristics	**Indicators**	**Nursing Activities**
Nonverbal response to actual or perceived change in structure and/or function; verbalization of feelings that reflect an altered view on one's body in appearance, structure, or function	Congruence between body reality, body ideal, and body presentation	Assist patient to discuss changes caused by illness or surgery
Objective: Missing body part; not touching body part; not looking at body part	Description of affected body part	Assist patient to separate physical appearance from feelings of personal worth
Subjective: Negative feelings about body; fear of rejection or of reaction by others	Willingness to touch affected body part	Assist patient to discuss stressors affecting body image after surgery
Related Factors	Satisfaction with body appearance	Monitor frequency of statements of self-criticism
Surgery; illness treatment	Adjustment to changes in physical appearance	Monitor whether patient can look at the changed body part
	Adjustment to changes in health status	Monitor for statements that identify body image perceptions concerned with body shape and body weight
	Willingness to use strategies to enhance appearance and function	Determine patient's and family's perception of the alteration in body image versus reality
		Determine if a change in body image has contributed to increased social isolation
		Assist patient to identify actions that will enhance appearance
		Facilitate contact with individuals with similar changes in body image
		Identify support groups available to patient

From Johnson, M. et al. (2001). *Nursing diagnosis, outcomes, & interventions: NANDA, NOC and NIC linkages.* St. Louis: Mosby.

table 11-5 Benefits of Clinical Pathways

PATIENT	HEALTH TEAM MEMBERS	HEALTH CARE AGENCY
Consumer involvement	Standardized, organized care	Supported by Joint Commission on Accreditation of Healthcare Organizations
Patient education	Improved communication	Supported by third-party payers
Mutual goal setting	Reflection of current practice	Integration of quality improvement, utilization management, and risk management
Increased patient satisfaction	Increased staff satisfaction, educational tool for students and new graduates	Improved communication Decreased length of stay Better competitive position Decreased costs Availability of data for evaluating care

From Ignatavicius, D. D., & Hausman, K. A. (1995). *Clinical pathways for collaborative practice* (Table 1-2, p 11). Philadelphia: Saunders.

EVALUATION

Evaluation is an ongoing process that enables you to determine what progress the patient has made in meeting the goals for care. The outcome criteria provide measures for determining outcomes of care. Using the previous example of impaired skin integrity, the outcome criteria could be "intact skin" and "absence of redness over bony prominences." Compare actual outcomes with expected outcomes of patient care and then communicate your findings. Evaluation is a way of measuring the patient's progress toward meeting goals. You are not evaluating nursing interventions. In assessing outcomes of care, determine whether the goals have been met, partially met, or not met. If the goals have not been met, reexamine the plan of care and modify it where necessary. In this text, evaluation is not discussed separately. Rather, evaluation requires that you collect data needed to see whether outcome criteria have been met. If met, the goal was achieved. If not met, the goal was not achieved and reassessment is necessary.

Evaluation helps provide data regarding the quality of care in a health care institution. Quality assurance audits are conducted by the individual health care agencies as well by as the Joint Commission on Accreditation of Healthcare Organizations, an organization that requires systematic review of hospitals and other health care organizations. Areas evaluated include the standards of nursing care used, the quality and effectiveness of nursing care, and the organization of the patient care system. Nursing audits are conducted by examining patient records as one method of gathering information to evaluate nursing performance. The American Nurses Association Standards of Care are used as a measure to determine whether nurses have carried out the nursing process as documented in the patient records.

Clinical Pathways

Clinical pathways are used in some health care facilities. They are standard care plans developed to set daily care priorities, schedule achievement of outcomes, and reduce length of hospital stays. They include patient outcomes and timelines for the sequence of interventions. Clinical pathways are collaborative and comprehensive in that they are jointly developed by all members of the health care team, and they cover many aspects of care rather than just nursing interventions. The benefits of clinical pathways for patients, health team members, and health care agencies are summarized in Table 11-5. The use of clinical pathways is controversial. There are concerns about the potential for legal liability when there are deviations from pathways (even when justified). Research is still needed to determine their value. A sample clinical pathway is presented here. However, the nursing process will be used to provide the framework for nursing care throughout this text.

NURSING PROCESS DOCUMENTATION

Documentation is an important component of the nursing process. Patient assessments and observations and all nursing interventions should be charted as a permanent part of the patient's record. Documentation helps to achieve continuity of care because it provides for communication among caregivers and is a record of the patient's progress. In addition, documentation provides a legal record of care provided and a verification of services rendered for insurance payments.

You should document the following:

1. All treatments and care given, including medications
2. Diagnostic procedures performed at the bedside, on the unit, or inside or outside the facility
3. The patient's reaction to therapeutic and diagnostic procedures
4. Observations of the patient
5. Subjective and objective signs and symptoms experienced by the patient
6. Evidence of changes in the patient's physical, psychosocial, and spiritual needs and status
7. Any unusual incidents such as falls or injuries that occur during the patient's stay in the health care facility

Documentation should be clear, concise, complete, and accurate. All sheets should have the patient's name and the date

Clinical Pathway for Hepatic Cirrhosis (Without Variceal Bleeding)

ICD-9 CODE 571.5	ELOS 3 DAYS			
NURSING DIAGNOSIS/ COLLABORATIVE PROBLEM	**EXPECTED OUTCOME (THE PATIENT IS EXPECTED TO . . .)**	**MET/ NOT MET**	**REASON**	**DATE/ INITIAL**
Fluid volume excess (ascites)	Have a decrease in extravascular and intra-abdominal fluid as evidenced by decreased abdominal girth and decreased peripheral edema.			
Potential for/actual chronic confusion	Be oriented to time, place, and person.			
Potential for major complications (esophageal varices, renal failure, advanced encephalopathy)	Not experience bleeding; have renal function tests at or near baseline; have intact neurologic function.			

ASPECT OF CARE	DATE ______ DAY 1	DATE ______ DAY 2	DATE ______ DAY 3
ASSESSMENT	Measure vital signs every 4 hr if stable. Systems assessment with focus on breath sounds, abdomen, and skin. Assess mental state every 8 hr. Observe for bruisability or frank bleeding. Measure abdominal girth daily.	Same as day 1	Same as day 2
TEACHING	Orient to hospital and unit. Review clinical pathway/plan of care with patient and family. Review diagnosis, including etiology and expected treatment.	Reinforce relationship of alcohol consumption to cirrhosis. Review discharge instructions regarding: • Drug therapy (diuretics, H_2-receptor antagonist) • Avoidance of medications other than prescribed • Diet therapy • Rest • Alcohol abstinence • Fluid restriction	Reinforce discharge instructions from day 2.
CONSULTS	Respiratory therapy Alcohol counselor Social worker	N/A	N/A
LABORATORY TESTS	Complete blood cell count, aspartate aminotransferase, alanine aminotransferase, lactate dehydrogenase, alkaline phosphatase, bilirubin, serum proteins, ammonia, prothrombin time, electrolytes Urine studies for urobilinogen Stool for urobilinogen	N/A	Transaminases, prothrombin time, complete blood cell count; ammonia
OTHER TESTS	Chest x-ray Electrocardiography Abdominal x-ray/computed tomography of abdomen	N/A	N/A

From Ignatavicius, D. D., & Hausman, K. A. (1995). *Clinical pathways for collaborative practice* (180–182). Philadelphia: Saunders. Reprinted with permission.

ICD, International classification of diseases; *ELOS*, expected length of stay; *MVI*, multivitamin; *PRN*, as needed; *IV*, intravenous; *PO*, orally; *ADL*, activities of daily living.

Continued

Clinical Pathway for Hepatic Cirrhosis (Without Variceal Bleeding)—cont'd

ICD-9 CODE 571.5	ELOS 3 DAYS		
ASPECT OF CARE	**DATE ________** **DAY 1**	**DATE ________** **DAY 2**	**DATE ________** **DAY 3**
MEDICATIONS	Diuretics as needed, such as Lasix by IV push or PO Zantac, 150 mg twice daily MVI daily Antacids PRN, such as Riopan or Amphogel Lactulose for increased ammonia levels Neomycin for increased ammonia level IV albumin if low serum albumin	Same as day 1	Same as day 2
TREATMENTS/ INTERVENTIONS	Oxygen PRN for dyspnea Paracentesis if needed for comfort Daily weight Input and output q 8 hr Fluid restriction to 1,500 ml/day Skin care for dryness and jaundice	Oxygen PRN Daily weight Input and output Fluid restriction Skin care	Same as day 2
NUTRITION	High-protein, low- to moderate-fat, high-carbohydrate diet (Low protein diet if ammonia level increased)	Same as day 1	Same as day 2
LINES/TUBES/ MONITORS	IV at 50 ml/hr, then convert to saline loc	Saline loc	D/C saline loc
MOBILITY/ SELF-CARE	Put up in chair twice daily. Keep head of bed elevated to promote breathing comfort. Keep feet elevated while patient is out of bed. Assist with ADL as needed.	Walk in room with supervision. Head of bed raised. Keep feet elevated when out of bed. Assist with ADL.	Same as day 2
DISCHARGE PLANNING	Assess home environment and available support systems. Determine need for placement in long-term care facility or other supervised environment	If discharged to home, make arrangements with home health services to follow patient. If discharged to long-term care facility or other facility, make transportation and admission arrangements, if not done.	Arrange for follow-up appointment with physician as specified.

From Ignatavicius, D. D., & Hausman, K. A. (1995). *Clinical pathways for collaborative practice* (180–182). Philadelphia: Saunders. Reprinted with permission.
ICD, International classification of diseases; *ELOS,* expected length of stay; *MVI,* multivitamin; *PRN,* as needed; *IV,* intravenous; *PO,* orally; *ADL,* activities of daily living.

and time information was entered. Writing should be legible, using proper grammar, punctuation, and spelling. Fill all spaces, leaving no empty lines. Carry out charting as soon after care is given as possible (never before care). Observations are objective and describe only what is seen, heard, felt, or smelled. Direct quotations from the patient regarding symptoms are very appropriate. Each time an entry is made, sign with your full name and title. Only permanent ink is used, and no erasures are made. If you make an error in charting, cross out the entry and write "error" or "mistaken entry," followed by your initials.

FORMATS FOR DOCUMENTATION OF PATIENT CARE

Various formats are used for the documentation of patient care, including nurses' notes, flow sheets, and **problem-oriented medical records (POMR).** Nurses' notes have traditionally consisted of pages of narrative recordings indicating the assessments, observations, and interventions carried out by the nurse. Flow sheets may be graphs of vital signs or tables in which nurses may check or initial boxes indicating activities or care provided.

Different ways of charting include focus charting (using key words such as action or response to organize charting); source-oriented charting (charting on separate sheets for different health care workers, such as physical therapy on one page and nurses on another); multidisciplinary charting (charting by different disciplines on the same page); charting by exception (CBE; charting narrative notes only when there is a change in the patient's condition); and computerized patient records (CPR; nursing notes are recorded on computers). Health care facilities may combine one or more of these methods.

The POMR is a method of record keeping that focuses on patient problems rather than on medical diagnoses. This method is popular in many clinical areas because it provides an excellent means of communication among the various disciplines that are providing care. Each health care provider involved in the care of the patient charts on the same progress notes in the same format.

The data from the history, physical examination, diagnostic tests, and medical diagnoses provide a foundation for problems formulated in the POMR. The problem list consists of active, inactive, potential, and resolved problems. The charting is done in a SOAPIER format. SOAPIER is an acronym for the components of the charting:

S *Subjective* information, or how the patient perceives the problem
O *Objective* information, or what the nurse observes about the patient
A *Assessment,* or why the patient has the problem
P *Plan,* or how the intervention is to be carried out
I *Intervention,* or what specific care is given
E *Evaluation,* or how effective was the plan or intervention
R *Revision,* or what changes should be made in the original plan of care

In many cases, the SOAPE form is used, omitting the intervention and revision sections. The intervention is closely related to the plan and can be a reiteration of the plan; a revision can be made in the plan by simply revising the original SOAPE notes.

An example of a SOAPE note using our previous example is as follows:

S Feels weak; does "not have the energy to move around"
O Does not turn self in bed; 2-cm stage 2 pressure ulcer on sacrum
A Pressure ulcer on sacrum related to immobility
P Turn from side to side q 2 hr. Get out of bed at least twice a day. Begin ambulating as tolerated.
E Turned q 2 hr. OOB twice a day, taking 6 small steps to and from bed. Pressure ulcer healing; now 1.5 cm.

Another common format is PIE charting, which includes the problem, intervention, and evaluation.

A large amount of time is spent charting and keeping records, and many facilities are transforming their record keeping into more time-saving methods of documentation, such as computerized nursing care plans and nurses' notes. Nevertheless, regardless of the format, the essential data should always be recorded systematically and must be individualized for each patient.

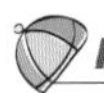
Put on your THINKING CAP!!

Ask your class or clinical group to observe 5 minutes of the local television news. Agree to do the exercise on a specific date and time and to watch a specific channel. Using objective language, document your observations of the speaker(s). Compare your description with that of classmates. If they have differences, discuss possible explanations.

CRITICAL THINKING

Critical thinking is defined as "reflective and reasonable thinking that is focused on deciding what to believe or do" (Ennis, 1985, p. 45). Although more sophisticated definitions exist, this one will suffice for our purposes. You will hear a lot about critical thinking during your nursing education. Because you spend a lot of time reading and learning facts, you may assume that critical thinking is just learning many facts. Although facts are indeed important, nursing deals with people in states of change in an environment that is constantly evolving. You will forget many of the facts you learn this year, but if you become a critical thinker, you will always have the tools to seek and apply knowledge.

This example illustrates the pitfalls of trying to use facts without thinking critically. A student assigned to a patient on the first day after abdominal surgery outlines detailed plans (from a textbook care plan) for ways to promote urination. Definitely important! However, the patient had a Foley catheter. With critical thinking skills, the student would have based plans on actual patient data so that the plan for care would have been appropriate.

RELATIONSHIP TO NURSING PROCESS

Why do you need both critical thinking and nursing process? The nursing process is a framework for developing, implementing, and evaluating a plan of care. It spells out what the patient's needs and problems are, the goals for care, interventions to achieve goals, and how goal achievement will be assessed.

If you have seen a well-written nursing process, you can see how it can be used to guide care. It tells you exactly what to do, right? Unfortunately, it's not that simple. Suppose the patient's care plan says he is to be assisted to take a shower for the first time since surgery as part of the plan to promote increasing independence in self-care. However, when you assist the patient out of bed, he becomes dizzy and nauseated. What do you do now? This is a simple situation that can be used to illustrate how critical thinking is used in nursing. Table 11-6 carries this situation through and reflects the steps of the nursing process along with the critical thinking that occurs at each step. One point to

table 11-6 ***Analysis of Critical Thinking in a Clinical Situation***

Situation: You are assigned to care for Mr. A today. It is his second postoperative day. One goal for the day is to promote independence in self-care. The nursing care plan notes that you should assist the patient with a shower.

The following table reflects a possible sequence of events when you attempt to implement the plan of care. The steps of the nursing process and the critical thinking skills are identified to illustrate how they are used and interact in a common situation.

SEQUENCE OF EVENTS	NURSING PROCESS STEPS	CRITICAL THINKING TOOLS
When you help Mr. A. stand at the bedside, he becomes dizzy and says he is nauseated. You ease him back into bed knowing that he is at risk for falling. Because Mr. A. is nauseated, you anticipate vomiting and reach for an emesis basin.	Intervention Assessment Intervention Planning Intervention	Inference: drawing conclusions Evaluation: assessing possibilities
You collect additional information immediately after Mr. A. lies down. His skin is pale, cool, and moist. His pulse is 110 and faint and his blood pressure is 90 mm Hg/60 mm Hg. When asked how he feels, he replies: "I feel better lying down."	Assessment	Interpretation: clarifying the meaning of events
Knowing that dizziness is associated with hypotension and that the supine position improves blood flow to the brain, you advise him to remain flat in bed for the time being.	Diagnosis Intervention	Inference: drawing conclusions
You reassess Mr. A. after a few minutes in the supine position. His skin is pink and warm, his pulse rate is 84 and full, and his blood pressure is 114 mm Hg/74 mm Hg.	Assessment	Interpretation: clarifying meaning of data
What do you do now? The care plan said you were supposed to get him up for a shower. You ask yourself what has just happened. You consider a drop in blood pressure r/t drug effects, immobility, or dehydration.	Planning	Inference: deriving alternatives Interpretation: clarifying meaning of events
You consider your options: Try again to get him up; give him a bedbath; let him rest for a while and see how he feels later; exercise his legs before helping him stand; notify the physician. These are all possibilities.	Planning	Inference: deriving alternatives Analysis: examining ideas
How do you choose one option? Think about the possible outcomes (positive and negative) of each action. Choose the option that would seem to be safe for the patient without delaying his recovery.	Intervention	Inference: drawing conclusions
You think the patient should remain in bed today. However, as a novice nurse, you are a bit unsure of yourself, so you explain the situation to the charge nurse and request feedback. The charge nurse suggests that you wait and try again later.		Self-regulation: recognizing need to make changes, reconsidering conclusions
After half an hour, Mr. A.'s vital signs are stable. You place a chair in the shower, exercise his legs, and then slowly get him up. He tolerates standing without dizziness. You assist him with morning care in the shower chair. You document the events.	Assessment Intervention Evaluation	Interpretation: clarifying meaning of data Inference: deriving alternatives

notice is that the nursing process does not flow smoothly from one step to the next, but often moves back and forth between steps.

This common scenario illustrates the many decision-making points that can occur in handling a fairly routine nursing situation. Notice that critical thinking was used to determine assessments needed, interventions to be implemented, and evaluation data needed. The nursing process is a sequence of steps that should be based on critical thinking. That is why your faculty may discourage you from using standardized care plans for patient care. Ready-made care plans bypass the vital experience of thinking through each step so that the care plan is specific and individualized for your patient.

CHARACTERISTICS OF A CRITICAL THINKER

In the above situation, you (the nurse) demonstrated various characteristics of a critical thinker. Those characteristics include:

- *Curiosity:* The desire, not just to know, but to understand how and why, to apply knowledge
- *Systematic thinking:* Uses an organized approach to problem solving, rather than knee-jerk responses
- *Analytical:* Applies knowledge from various disciplines, approaches a problem by examining the parts and seeing how they fit together
- *Open-minded:* Willing to consider various alternatives
- *Self-confident:* Sense of assurance that the problem-solving process produces a good conclusion/plan
- *Maturity:* Recognition that many variables are at work in patient situations, and sometimes the best plans do not work (back to the drawing board!!)
- *Truth-seeking:* Eager to know, asking questions, seeking answers, reevaluates "common knowledge"

CRITICAL THINKING TOOLS

Just as the critical thinker has certain characteristics, the critical thinker also uses specific tools. These include:

- *Interpretation:* Clarifying meaning of events, data
- *Analysis:* Examining ideas, breaking down into components
- *Evaluation:* Assessing possibilities, opinions, usual practices
- *Inference:* Deriving alternatives, drawing conclusions
- *Explanation:* Presenting arguments for views, decisions; justifying
- *Self-regulation:* Reconsidering conclusions, recognizing need to make changes

Throughout this text, you will find exercises labeled "Put on your THINKING CAP." As you encounter these, your first reaction may be to try to find the answer in the chapter. What you will find is that the content only provides the knowledge *base* to answer the question, not the answer itself. A trick question, you say. Not at all. The purpose is to help you develop the essential skills for *critical thinking.*

In closing, the nursing process is a tool—a sequence of steps that requires critical thinking to provide scientifically sound, individualized patient care. It is critical thinking that makes the nursing process scientifically sound, appropriate, flexible, and individualized.

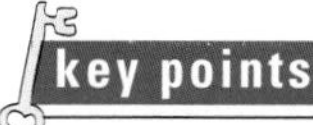

- The nursing process is a problem-solving approach that enables the nurse to provide care in an organized, scientific manner.
- The steps of the nursing process are assessment, nursing diagnosis, planning, implementation, and evaluation.
- Assessment involves collection of subjective and objective data about the client or patient from the client, family, significant others, medical records, and other care providers.
- The health history includes biographical data, chief complaint and history of present illness, medical history, family history, review of systems, and functional assessment.
- The physical examination uses inspection, auscultation, palpation, and percussion to collect objective data about the patient.
- The nursing diagnosis is a statement of an actual or potential health problem derived from the assessment.
- Nursing diagnoses differ from medical diagnoses in that nursing diagnoses focus on the response of the whole person to the medical problem.
- The parts of a NANDA diagnosis are the label, definition of the diagnosis, defining characteristics (signs and symptoms), and related (causative or associated) factors.
- The planning phase of the nursing process involves the development of a nursing care plan for the patient based on the nursing diagnoses.
- The Nursing Outcomes Classification includes standardized outcomes that serve as criteria to judge the results of nursing interventions.
- Planning includes priority setting, goal statements, and nursing interventions to achieve the goals.
- NIC interventions are standardized interventions, each including a label name, definition, list of nursing activities, and background readings.
- Implementation refers to the actual performance of the nursing interventions identified in the plan of care.
- Evaluation is an ongoing process in which the nurse uses outcome criteria to determine what progress has been made toward meeting the goals.
- The value of using systems such as NANDA, NIC, and NOC is that they standardize language that describes what nurses do.
- Documentation of assessments, interventions, and evaluation data is an essential aspect of nursing care.
- Clinical pathways are standardized, interdisciplinary plans of care that specify the sequence and timing of interventions.
- Critical thinking is defined as "reflective and reasonable thinking that is focused on deciding what to believe or do" (Ennis, 1985, p. 45).

- Critical thinking makes the nursing process appropriate, scientifically sound, flexible, and individualized.
- Critical thinking skills include interpretation, analysis, evaluation, inference, explanation, and self-regulation.
- A critical thinker is curious, open-minded, a systematic thinker, analytical, truth seeking, and has self-confidence and maturity.

REVIEW QUESTIONS

1. An example of subjective data is:
   1. Lung sounds clear to auscultation
   2. Urine clear, light yellow
   3. Heart rate 90 bpm and regular
   4. Headache and sensitivity to light
2. "Patient states pain in his neck began when he was wrestling with his brother. The pain radiates across his right shoulder and worsens with movement of the right arm." This an example of:
   1. biographical data.
   2. chief complaint.
   3. family history.
   4. review of systems.
3. Percussion is used primarily to assess the:
   1. chest.
   2. skin.
   3. joints.
   4. cranium.
4. Which of the following is a complete, correctly stated NANDA diagnosis?
   1. Disturbed body image as a result of surgical scars, as evidenced by crying and concealing scars.
   2. Decreased cardiac output related to excessive blood loss
   3. Noncompliance related to refusal to take medications as evidenced by high blood pressure.
   4. Diabetes mellitus related to obesity as evidenced by high serum glucose.
5. Which goal is most complete and measurable?
   1. Patient will correctly demonstrate clean wound dressing change before discharge.
   2. Patient will know how to care for wound before leaving the hospital.
   3. Patient will take care of wound himself when he goes home.
   4. Patient will understand the principles of medical asepsis to use during dressing changes.
6. The nurse's responsibility for documentation includes:
   1. record names of all visitors.
   2. document all medical interventions.
   3. never chart care in advance.
   4. carefully erase errors completely.
7. Which of the following skills is used in critical thinking?
   1. Copy
   2. Recite
   3. Memorize
   4. Analyze
8. A characteristic of a critical thinker is:
   1. self-controlled.
   2. self-confident.
   3. self-centered.
   4. self-righteous.
9. According to the American Nurses Association Standards of Care, the nurse evaluates the client's progress toward attainment of outcomes. What measurement criterion is used for this standard?
   1. Revisions in diagnoses, outcomes, and the plan of care are documented.
   2. Interventions are consistent with the established plan of care.
   3. Plan is developed with the client, significant others, and health care providers, when appropriate.
   4. Outcomes are realistic in relation to the client's present and potential capabilities.

CHAPTER 12 Inflammation, Infection, and Immunity

objectives

1. Describe physical and chemical barriers.
2. Describe how inflammatory changes act as bodily defense mechanisms.
3. Identify the signs and symptoms of inflammation.
4. Discuss the process of repair and healing.
5. Differentiate infection from inflammation.
6. Discuss the actions of commonly found infectious agents.
7. Describe the ways that infections are transmitted.
8. Identify the signs and symptoms of infection.
9. Compare community-acquired and nosocomial infections.
10. Discuss the nursing care of patients with infections.
11. Describe the Centers for Disease Control (CDC) standard precautions guidelines for infection control.
12. Describe the Centers for Disease Control isolation guidelines for airborne, droplet, and contact (transmission-based) precautions.
13. Describe the immune response.
14. Identify the organs involved in immunity.
15. Compare natural and acquired immunity.
16. Differentiate between humoral (antibody-mediated) and cell-mediated immunity.
17. Describe the nursing care of patients with immunodeficiency and of those with allergies.
18. Describe the process of autoimmunity.

key terms

Allergen (ĂL-ĕr-jĕn, p. 145)
Antibody (ĂN-tĭ-bŏ-dē, p. 143)
Antigen (ĂN-tĭ-jĕn, p. 143)
Autoimmunity (ăw-tō-ĭ-MŪ-nĭ-tē, p. 147)
Bacteria (p. 134)
Communicable disease (kŏ-MŪ-nĭ-kă-b'l dĭ-ZĒZ, p. 137)
Contamination (p. 136)
Fungi (FŬN-jī, p. 135)
Immunity (ĭ-Mū-nĭ-tē, p. 143)
Immunodeficiency (ĭm-ū-nō-dĕ-FĬSH-ĕn-sē, p. 144)
Infection (p. 134)
Inflammation (ĭn-flă-MĀ-shŭn, p. 132)
Medical asepsis (ā-SĔP-sĭs, p. 138)
Nosocomial infection (nō-sō-KŌ-mē-ăl ĭn-FĔK-shŭn, p. 137)
Surgical asepsis (SŬR-jĕ-kăl ā-SĔP-sĭs, p. 138)
Virus (VĪ-rŭs, p. 135)

Suppose you were being attacked. How would you defend yourself? Perhaps you would shout or in some other way sound an alarm. You might even call in reinforcements to help you fight off the attacker, telling them the most direct route to your location. You would probably surround yourself with some sort of barrier either to shield yourself from further harm or to keep the attacker in the area so that it would not escape and harm someone else. Then, after the battle was over, you would likely enlist the help of some friends to clean up the debris and return your situation to normal.

It is quite remarkable to realize that, at a cellular level, the human body is protected in much the same way. The body relies on many effective barriers to protect itself from injury and disease. However, if these barriers are compromised, several sophisticated processes are triggered to isolate and eliminate the offender. In this chapter, how the body defends itself from injury and disease, what happens when defenses fail, and how good nursing care helps the processes are described.

PHYSICAL AND CHEMICAL BARRIERS

The skin and mucous membranes are the body's first line of defense. They act as a protective covering and secrete substances that inhibit the growth of microorganisms. The sweat glands secrete lysozyme, an antimicrobial enzyme. Sebaceous glands secrete sebum, which has antimicrobial and antifungal properties. Acidic secretions from the skin and the mucosa of the gastrointestinal and genitourinary systems inhibit the growth of many pathogenic organisms. Secretions from the mammary glands and the respiratory and gastrointestinal tracts contain the antibody immunoglobulin A, as well as cleanup phagocytes. Additionally, skin and mucous membrane surfaces are colonized by "normal" bacterial flora, which prevent pathogens (disease-causing organisms) from gaining access to the body. The cilia in the respiratory tract, the motility of the gastrointestinal tract, and the sloughing of dead skin cells all work to distribute and remove microorganisms, preventing their overgrowth and invasion.

The second line of defense involves two processes: phagocytosis and inflammation. Phagocytosis helps rid the body of invading microorganisms and debris. White blood cells (leukocytes) are colorless blood cells that have the ability to phagocytose (ingest) bacteria that can invade the body and cause infection. Two types of leukocytes, neutrophils and monocytes, are especially suited for this purpose. Neutrophils fight bacterial infections. Monocytes circulate in the blood for about 1 day and then enter tissue, where they are called macrophages and ingest many foreign antigens. Eosinophils fight parasitic infections and increase during allergic reactions. Basophils initiate the inflammatory response and release histamine. Measuring the number of these cells gives an indication of the severity of infection in the body. B lymphocytes produce antibodies and T lymphocytes increase the body's immune response. Therefore, lymphocyte counts provide a measure of immune function. A more complete description of blood and components of the immune system may be found in Chapters 31 and 32 (Hematology and Immunology).

Reticuloendothelial cells are found in the blood, connective tissue, liver, spleen, bone marrow, and lymph nodes. Some reticuloendothelial cells protect the body by digesting and absorbing foreign material, such as old red blood cells, bacteria, and colloidal particles. These cells may also be called tissue macrophages.

THE INFLAMMATORY PROCESS

The inflammatory process is a series of cellular changes that signal the body's response to injury or infection. Although infection is a common cause of inflammation, this complex phenomenon may be caused by trauma from (1) physical agents (excessive sunlight, x-rays), (2) chemical stimuli (insect venom, other chemicals), and (3) biological agents (bacteria, viruses).

The word inflammation means literally "the fire within." This descriptive phrase illustrates the four classic manifestations of inflammation: (1) rubor (redness), (2) calor (heat), (3) tumor (swelling), and (4) dolor (pain). It is helpful to think about the appearance of a bee sting and recall the redness, warmth, swelling, and pain that it produces. These signs are the direct result of several related actions that occur when the inflammatory process is initiated. The actions involve hemodynamic changes, increased permeability of membranes, chemical mediators, and hormonal factors.

ACTIONS IN THE INFLAMMATORY PROCESS

Hemodynamic Changes

The first actions of the inflammatory process are the hemodynamic changes. The body initially responds to an injury or infection with dilation of the capillary bed. This dilation brings increased blood flow to the area. The increase in blood flow is responsible for the characteristic warmth and redness at the site of inflammation.

Increased Permeability

The second action is an increased capillary permeability (Fig. 12-1). After the increased blood flow brings leukocytes into the area, chemical mediators cause leukocytes to line the small blood vessel walls near the inflammatory site. This process is called pavementing. Gradually these cells pass through the vessel walls and inhabit the inflamed area. These cells, largely neutrophils and monocytes, are drawn to the site of injury or infection, where they ingest and carry away bacteria and other foreign substances (phagocytosis) (Fig. 12-2). The permeability of these vessels causes protein-rich fluid to flow through the vessel walls into the interstitial space. Some red blood cells may pass through into this area as well. This collection of fluid is responsible for the swelling that is noted when the inflammation site is close to the surface of the skin. This swelling may also produce pain.

Chemical Mediators

The hemodynamic changes and vascular permeability occur with the help of several chemical mediators, including prostaglandins, histamine, and leukotrienes. These powerful substances are found in various body tissues and are liberated during the inflammatory process. Cytokines and eicosanoids, described in Chapter 32, cause blood and blood vessel changes. The kinin system produces bradykinin, which also mediates blood vessel dilation and permeability. It also produces pain, another classic sign of inflammation. Other mediators include the complement system, which is especially important in immunologically mediated reactions involving antigen-antibody complexes. These reactions cause a massive release of histamine and other substances that produce marked vasodilation, vascular permeability, and smooth muscle contraction. These cellular changes produce the classic signs of anaphylactic shock: hypotension, swelling, and bronchoconstriction.

Anti-Inflammation

Cortisol, a hormone produced by the adrenal cortex, is an anti-inflammatory substance that slows the release of histamine, stabilizes lysosomal membranes, and prevents the influx of leukocytes. The end result of these actions is to impede the inflammatory process. Drugs (such as glucocorticoids) that mimic the action of cortisol are often used in the treatment of inflammatory conditions.

SIGNS AND SYMPTOMS OF INFLAMMATION

The signs and symptoms of inflammation vary depending on whether the reaction is local or systemic. Local inflammation generally produces the classic signs of heat, swelling, redness, pain, and loss of function, the loss of function being the result of the other four signs.

Systemic inflammation produces somewhat different reactions. Swelling, redness, and local warmth may not be visible; however, signs of the effects of the chemical mediators may be recognized in other ways. Fever is a common sign of systemic inflammation, probably caused by pyrogens (fever-producing substances) or by defense mechanisms that are liberated during phagocytosis, or by bacterial endotoxins, antigen-antibody complexes, and certain viruses. Other symptoms of systemic

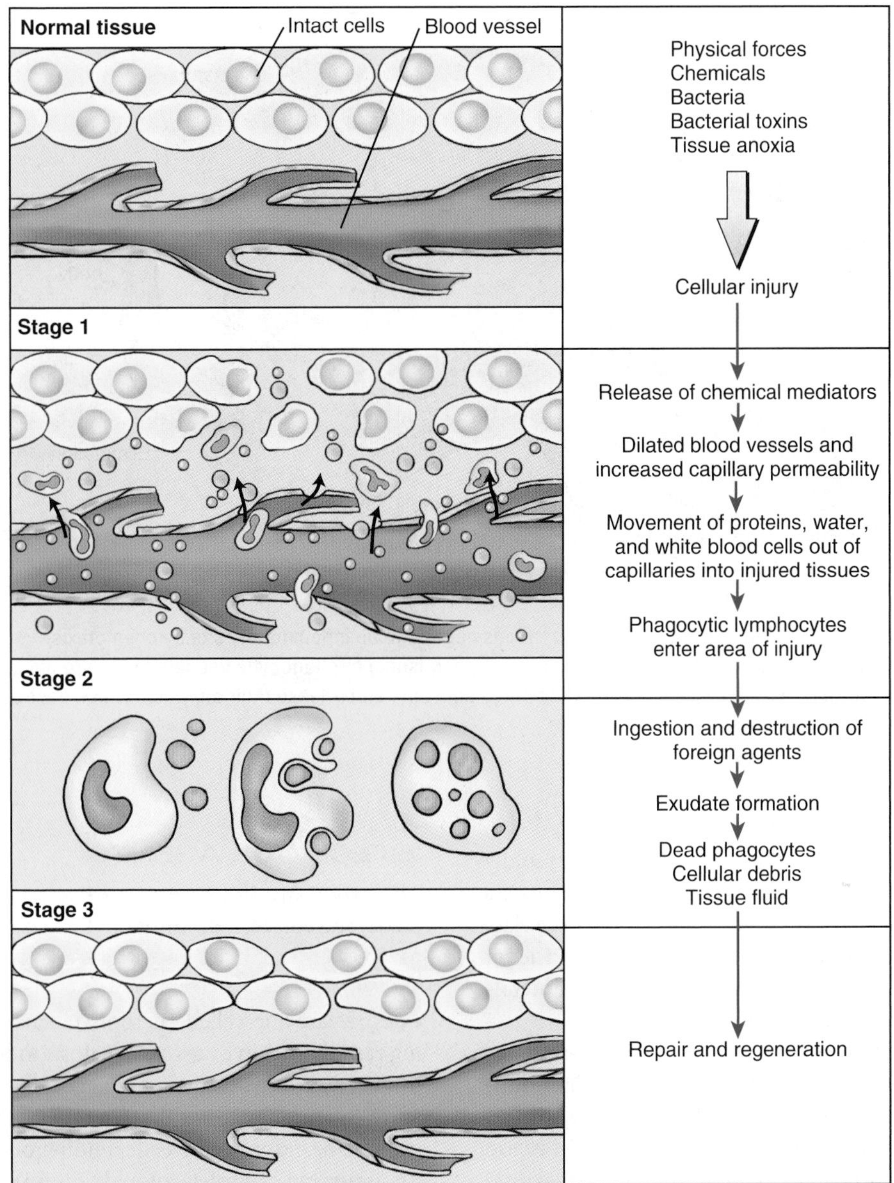

FIGURE **12-1** The anti-inflammatory response following tissue injury.

inflammation include headache, muscle aches, chills, and sweating.

Leukocytosis also is a frequent sign of systemic inflammation. This is a defensive reaction that provides abundant white blood cells for the inflammatory response. If infection is not present, inflammatory leukocytosis disappears within a few hours.

WOUND HEALING

Repair and regeneration of tissue are set in motion from the very beginning of the inflammatory process. The speed at which this process takes place depends on the type of tissue injured, the severity of the wound, the presence of infection, and the health of the host. At the outset, macrophage cells are produced to clean up inflammatory debris. Fibroblasts begin the repair process by laying down elastin and collagen at the edges of the wound; these substances gradually migrate to the base, forming granulation tissue. Epithelial cells migrate over the wound and under the scab (usually formed of dried blood and fibroblasts). After a few days, the scab falls off. Some tissue regenerates well. Regeneration means that damaged cells are replaced by new cells of their own composition. Other tissue must undergo repair, which may involve the replacement of injured cells with connective tissue and will eventually create a scar. In fact, most wounds manifest both types of tissue repair.

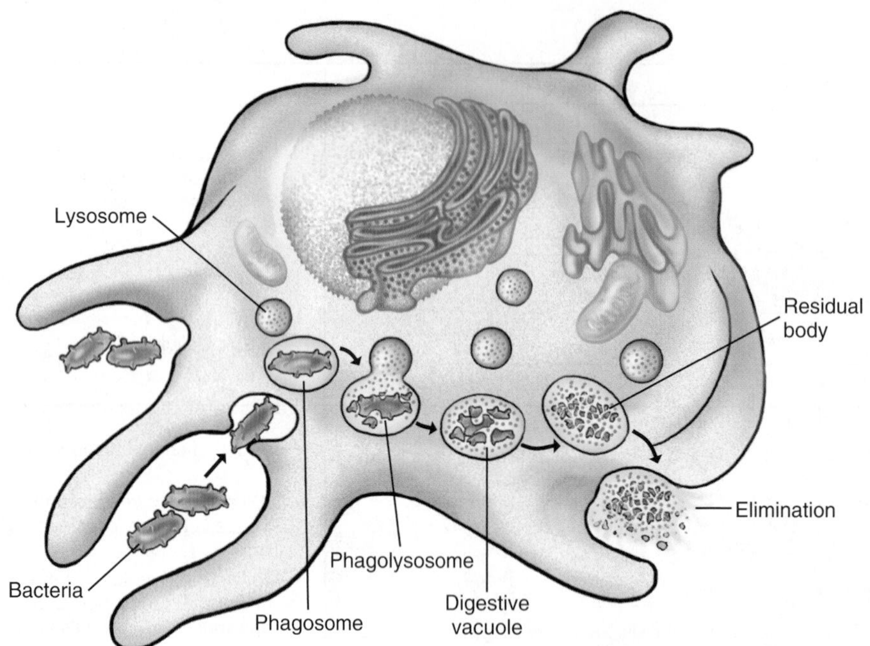

FIGURE **12-2** Phagocytosis. (1) Macrophages migrate to an inflammatory site by chemotaxis. (2) Macrophages engulf the microorganisms. A phagosome or phagocytic vacuole forms around the microorganisms. (3) Lysosomes attach to the phagosome and release their enzymes, which destroy the microorganisms.

The age and general health of the person affect how rapidly the regeneration and repair process occurs. The healing process can be delayed in the elderly as a result of decreased tissue elasticity and decreased blood supply to the tissues. Deficiencies of vitamin C, zinc, and other important vitamins and minerals can also delay the regeneration and repair process.

Occasionally a wound becomes infected or ulcerated, resulting in tissue loss. Granulation tissue and capillary buds form at the margins of the wound, and it is eventually filled with granulation tissue. Sometimes the wound bed is too large for the granulation tissue to fill. In this case the wound is cleaned and débrided in an effort to enhance healing. When infection is no longer present, the wound is sutured closed. This is called delayed primary closure.

INFECTION

Infection is a process involving the invasion of body tissues by microorganisms, the multiplication of the invading organisms, and the subsequent tissue damage. Infection is different from inflammation in that inflammation is a nonspecific reaction by the body to tissue injury, whereas infection refers to a specific process that causes tissue injury. Infection nearly always results in inflammation, but inflammation may be caused by processes other than infection. Inflammation precedes infection. Infection is usually the end result of the invasion by organisms. Infection may be caused by a wide variety of microorganisms.

INFECTIOUS AGENTS

The major infectious agents are bacteria, viruses, fungi, protozoa, rickettsiae, helminths, and mycoplasmas.

Bacteria

Bacteria are one-celled microorganisms capable of multiplying rapidly within a susceptible host. Among the factors that protect these organisms from phagocytosis are a rigid cell wall and a gelatinous capsule. Bacteria are classified as either gram positive or gram negative, depending on their ability to take up and retain a violet-colored solution called Gram stain. Gram-positive bacteria retain the stain, whereas gram-negative bacteria can be decolorized and counterstained pink.

Bacteria are also classified according to shape. Round bacteria are called *cocci;* they are further classified according to how they group or cluster together. Groups of two are called *diplococci,* and clusters of cocci are called *staphylococci.* Chains of these microorganisms are called *streptococci.*

Rod-shaped organisms, called *bacilli,* may be further subdivided into fusiform (with tapered ends) or spirochetes (spirals).

Bacteria may also be classified according to their ability to grow in the presence of oxygen. Those that do are classified as *aerobes;* those that do not are labeled *anaerobes.*

These classifications have a very important purpose. Each classification highlights a characteristic of a microorganism that is considered in the design of an antimicrobial drug to kill or retard the growth of the organism. For example, gram-positive bacteria have a thick polypeptide and peptoglycan covering that absorbs Gram stain. Antibiotics synthesized to fight these microorganisms interfere with the formation of that covering, causing the cell wall to be destroyed. Similarly, other antibiotics rely on the ability of a bacterial cell to take up oxygen to produce its effects.

The staining process aids in the identification of the organisms. The Gram stain differentiates bacteria into two major categories: gram positive and gram negative. The acid-fast stain is used to identify bacteria such as *Mycobacterium tuberculosis.* Immunofluorescent stains reveal complexes composed of various antigens (bacteria, viruses, fungi, protozoa) and antibodies when exposed to ultraviolet light.

Viruses

Viruses are very small microorganisms that cause significant morbidity in humans. Viruses cause a variety of illnesses, ranging from the common cold to acquired immunodeficiency syndrome (AIDS). Many childhood illnesses (e.g., measles, chickenpox) as well as several forms of hepatitis are caused by viruses. These microorganisms cannot be seen with ordinary microscopes but are visible with electron microscopy. They contain a strand of genetic material and are surrounded by a protein capsule, but have no cell wall. Viruses cannot replicate on their own but depend on the resources of the host cell.

Viruses produce their damage by stimulating the antigen-antibody response in the tissues that causes inflammation and cell destruction. Because replication of the virus occurs within the host cell, it is seldom possible to kill the virus without harming the host cell. This explains why there are relatively few antiviral drugs available. Prevention (immunizations, hygiene) is still the best way to combat viral illness.

Fungi

Fungi are vegetable-like organisms that exist by feeding on organic matter. Mushrooms and molds are examples of fungal organisms. A few species of fungi are capable of producing disease in humans. Ringworm (tinea corporis) and athlete's foot (tinea pedis) are two examples. Many of these infections are superficial skin infections that rarely produce serious illness. Systemic fungal infections caused by *Cryptococcus* and *Aspergillus* species, however, can be life-threatening. Patients who have conditions that affect their immune system (e.g., HIV) are at especially high risk of acquiring opportunistic fungal infections. Fungal infections are called mycoses. Because fungi tend to form spores that are resistant to many antiseptics and disinfectants, they are difficult to treat. Both systemic and topical antimycotic drugs are used to treat fungal infections.

Protozoa

Protozoa make up a large group of one-celled organisms. Ones that produce disease in humans include the *Plasmodium* species (malaria), *Entamoeba histolytica* (amoebic dysentery), *Giardia lamblia* (giardiasis, characterized by diarrhea), and *Trypanosoma gambiense* (sleeping sickness). Infections are often spread by food or water that is contaminated by human or animal feces. *Pneumocystis carinii* is another protozoal infection that was relatively rare before the onset of the HIV/AIDS epidemic. Lowered immunity with HIV infection is responsible for the dramatic rise in pneumocystic pneumonia.

Rickettsiae

Rickettsiae are microorganisms that are between bacteria and viruses in size. They may appear as rods, cocci, or pleomorphic (varied) shapes. These organisms multiply in the cells of animal hosts, such as rats and squirrels, and are transmitted to humans through the bites of fleas and ticks. Diseases produced by these microorganisms include Rocky Mountain spotted fever and typhus. Diseases caused by rickettsiae tend to be more prevalent in areas in which sanitation is poor and rodent and insect populations are not well controlled.

Helminths

Helminths are worms. These parasites are found in soil and water and are generally transmitted from hand to mouth. Infections occur commonly in the gastrointestinal tract and may produce mild abdominal pain and bloating, or they may be asymptomatic. Pinworms are most common, especially in children, and often produce rectal irritation. Tapeworms can be found in the gastrointestinal tract. Weight loss and abdominal pain and bloating may be early signs and symptoms. Hookworms often enter an individual through the soles of the feet and migrate throughout the body. Symptoms initially may be respiratory, but these parasites can also produce abdominal pain, diarrhea, and anemia.

Mycoplasmas

Mycoplasmas are gram-negative, multishaped organisms without cell walls that are responsible for several infections in humans. They are sometimes called pleuropneumonia-like organisms. Mycoplasma infections are responsible for primary atypical pneumonia and have been linked to Reiter's syndrome, a multisystem inflammatory disease that may be associated with urethritis, conjunctivitis, and pharyngitis. Infections are usually found in the upper respiratory tract and most often affect children and young adults. Mycoplasma infections respond well to erythromycin.

TRANSMISSION OF INFECTION

Infection, or the invasion of the body by microorganisms, is only possible when several factors are present. These factors must occur in sequence for human infectious disease to occur. They include (1) a causative agent, (2) a reservoir, (3) a portal of exit, (4) a mode of transfer, (5) a portal of entry, and (6) a susceptible host. This is referred to as the chain of infection.

Causative Agent

Causative agents are the microorganisms (e.g., bacteria, viruses, protozoa) that are present in sufficient number and virulence to damage human tissue.

Reservoir

Areas in which organisms can pool and reproduce are called reservoirs. Reservoirs may be human or animal tissues as well as any substance such as soil or animal feces in which microorganisms can pool and multiply. When a reservoir of microorganisms occurs in the tissues of human, the human is called a host.

Portal of Exit

Portal of exit refers to the route by which the infectious agent leaves one host and travels to another. A common route is the gastrointestinal tract, through which bacteria or viruses may escape an infected host. The nose and mouth also are common portals of exit for organisms spread by droplet contamination through sneezing or coughing. Fecal-oral transmission also occurs; hepatitis A virus is acquired by ingesting the virus in water contaminated with feces or by direct fecal-oral transmission.

Mode of Transfer

Mode of transfer refers to the means by which a microorganism is transported to a host. Person-to-person transfer may take place in either a direct or an indirect manner. Direct contact refers to the transfer of microorganisms directly, as occurs in sexually transmitted diseases. Indirect contact occurs when pathogens are spread through droplets expelled during a sneeze or a cough or through inanimate objects (such as eating utensils on which microorganisms can be transported [fomites]).

Common vehicle transmission occurs when water, food, blood, or air currents contaminated with a pathogen are shared by a number of people. Air currents, for example, are often the common vehicle for transmission of *Legionella,* the organism responsible for Legionnaire's disease. Vector transmission occurs when microorganisms are transported into a host by a living organism such as a fly or mosquito. Fomites are any items that have been touched or cross-contaminated by the host, such as bed linen, side rails, or hygiene items.

Portal of Entry

Portals of entry are the doorways or pathways into the host. Flu and cold viruses often enter the body through the mucous membranes of the nose and mouth. Other portals of entry often accessed by bacteria are the gastrointestinal tract and the urethra. Open wounds, intravenous access devices, urinary catheters, and drains also can be portals of entry for bacteria.

Susceptible Host

To produce tissue damage, microorganisms must become implanted into a susceptible host. Not all people exposed to disease-producing microorganisms become ill. Populations adequately immunized against rubella, for example, are not susceptible to measles. Similarly, individuals who have had chickenpox have developed immunity to the virus and, if exposed a second time, do not become ill.

SIGNS AND SYMPTOMS OF INFECTION

Once an individual becomes infected with a pathogen, symptoms may or may not be apparent. Often there is a period of subclinical infection or an incubation period during which there are few, if any, symptoms. During this period, asymptomatic persons may be more contagious than those who are exhibiting symptoms. This is true of people infected with such viruses as measles and many cold viruses. Persons recently infected with HIV may feel well but are highly contagious. Persons who have illnesses such as tuberculosis may remain relatively well. Still other persons may remain contagious throughout their convalescence. Asymptomatic carriers, such as patients recovering from typhoid, may go back to their communities and inadvertently infect others.

Symptoms of *localized infections,* such as bacterial infection of a wound, are essentially the symptoms of inflammation: redness, pain, warmth, and swelling. In addition, pus may form.

Patients with *generalized infections* may not show all the signs that are apparent in localized infections. Redness, for example, may not be visible. Pain may be moderate to severe, depending on the location of the infection. Swelling of infected tissues may produce symptoms ranging from mild to severe, depending on its location. Swelling in a large organ, such as the liver, may produce a dull ache, whereas swelling in a small structure, such as an infected appendix, may produce severe discomfort. Warmth is generally expressed as fever in a generalized infection as pyrogens are produced as part of the inflammatory process. Other symptoms that often are present in generalized infections include malaise, anorexia, and prostration.

In some cases, infections in the extremities such as the hands or feet exhibit a faint red line as infection extends upward along the lymphatic channels. Lymph nodes in this chain also are swollen and tender. Prompt antibiotic treatment is necessary in these cases.

TYPES OF INFECTIONS

Two types of infections are (1) community acquired and (2) hospital acquired.

Community-Acquired Infections

Community-acquired infections are acquired in day-to-day contact with the public. Many viral infections are pervasive in society and occur at predictable times of the year. Childhood illnesses are common in September when children take to school all the new viruses they were exposed to during the summer. This sharing of microorganisms is made easier when 20 to 40 children occupy the same classroom. During the fall and winter, people share more indoor activities, thus increasing the likelihood that they will share microorganisms with one another.

Poverty, low immunization rates, overcrowding, and unsanitary living conditions are at least partially responsible for the increase in infectious diseases that were once well controlled. The recent resurgence of tuberculosis is an example. This increase was attributed to poverty, the HIV/AIDS epidemic, an increase in the number of infected immigrants, declining public health resources, and the emergence of strains of bacteria that are resistant to multiple drugs. Effective treatment now requires at least two drugs to which a particular tuberculosis bacillus is susceptible.

Food-borne illness is a common community-acquired infectious disease. It is more common in the summer, when picnics and hot weather bring the possibility of food poisoning from *Staphylococcus* and *Salmonella* organisms. Periodic outbreaks of hepatitis A are possible at any time of the year and are the result of poor hygiene by food handlers.

Sexually transmitted diseases such as gonorrhea, syphilis, and HIV also are spread into the community. These diseases and many others are required to be reported to public health authorities. The reports are important because they facilitate disease control, make possible the evaluation of control programs, and keep track of emerging disease patterns.

Certain communicable diseases must be reported to state health departments. State laws vary regarding which diseases must be reported. A list of reportable diseases is given in Table 12-1.

Prevention and Control

Prevention and control of communicable diseases are possible in a number of ways. Some childhood infectious diseases can be prevented by ensuring childhood immunizations. Indifference toward childhood immunizations has resulted in the reemergence of several childhood diseases that were once well controlled. Although state laws that require certain immunizations before a child starts school have improved the picture somewhat, large groups of children from 2 to 5 years of age remain susceptible to serious illness. In addition, repeat vaccinations of older schoolchildren may be required to prevent illnesses such as measles. Adult immunizations also help prevent and control communicable diseases.

table 12-1 *Common Reportable Diseases*

Acquired immunodeficiency syndrome/ HIV infection	Meningococcal infections
Amebiasis	Mumps
Anthrax	Pertussis (whooping cough)
Aseptic meningitis	Plague
Botulism	Poliomyelitis
Brucellosis	Psittacosis
Chancroid	Rubella (German measles)
Cholera	Rabies
Diphtheria	Rheumatic fever
Encephalitis	Rocky Mountain spotted fever
Gonorrhea	Salmonellosis
Granuloma inguinale	Shigellosis
Hansen's disease (leprosy)	Syphilis
Hepatitis (all types)	Tetanus
Legionellosis	Toxic shock syndrome
Leptospirosis	Trichinosis
Lyme disease	Tuberculosis
Lymphogranuloma venereum	Tularemia
Malaria	Typhoid fever
Measles (rubeola)	Typhus
	Yellow fever

Although the solutions to this problem defy easy answers, at least part of the problem includes barriers in the health care system that result in missed opportunities to immunize those who are most susceptible. Barriers include such factors as rigid fee schedules; giving immunizations only during regular working hours, Monday through Friday; and giving immunizations only at official, fixed sites such as health departments. It is important for health professionals to take advantage of all possible opportunities to immunize. Schools, doctors' offices, shopping malls, and neighborhood health fairs are places where large numbers of children and parents may present themselves for immunization.

Transmission of infectious agents can be interrupted in a number of ways. First, education of food handlers regarding the importance of hand washing and proper food handling and refrigeration techniques decreases the spread of food-borne disease. Second, diseases such as tuberculosis can be detected through screening and treated early to prevent their spread. Isolation separates the infected individual from the public, thereby breaking the chain of infection. Other examples of measures aimed at interrupting transmission include control of vectors (spraying for mosquitos), administration of antimicrobials to children exposed to *Neisseria* meningitis, and the prompt treatment of streptococcal pharyngitis (strep throat). Sanitation of water supplies helps prevent the occurrence of water-borne diseases. Cooking meat, eggs, and poultry until well done kills bacteria that can cause serious illness and, in some cases, death.

Personal measures to control the spread of communicable disease include the use of personal barriers such as condoms and proper hygiene, especially hand washing. Deciding to stay home when symptoms of an infectious disease are present also can help break the chain of infection.

Hospital-Acquired Infections

Hospital-acquired (nosocomial) infections are an important cause of increased morbidity, prolonged hospitalization, and higher health care costs. Nosocomial infections occur within a health care facility and may affect both the patient and the health care worker. These infections are much more serious than those acquired in the community because strains of bacteria in the hospital are usually more virulent and often are resistant to antibiotics. In addition, the patient's resistance is already compromised from the disorder that led to hospitalization.

A growing number of pathogenic bacteria that are no longer susceptible to previously effective antibiotics are found in hospital patients. Vancomycin-resistant enterococcus (VRE) is one example; the incidence of vancomycin resistance in patients with nosocomial enterococcal infection is rapidly increasing. The Centers for Disease Control (CDC) has emphasized the importance of the careful use of antibiotics and infection control measures in preventing the spread of VRE. In health care agencies where the use of antibiotics has increased, an increase in bacterial resistance is also found. Antibiotics alter the body's normal flora so that resistant strains of enterococci replace susceptible strains. To prevent

VRE infection, the CDC has recommended the following guidelines for limiting patient-to-patient transmission:

- Place VRE-infected patients in a single room or in a room with other VRE patients.
- Wear gloves while in the room because organisms can extensively contaminate surfaces such as doorknobs and side rails (fomites).
- Wear a gown when you anticipate substantial contact with the patient or surfaces in the room or if the patient is incontinent or has wound drainage.
- Remove gloves and gown before leaving the patient's room and wash your hands immediately.
- After removing your gown and gloves and washing your hands, make sure that your hands and clothing do not touch surfaces, such as curtains or doorknobs, that may be contaminated.
- Use separate thermometers and stethoscopes for VRE-infected patients.
- Make sure that all patient care equipment used with VRE-infected patients is carefully disinfected.

Resistant bacterial strains develop for a number of reasons. Bacterial cells normally develop mutations. Because antibiotics suppress normal forms of the bacteria, the mutations have opportunity to grow. Chromosomal mutation also permits the bacteria to produce an enzyme that deactivates the antibiotic. Finally, mutation alters bacterial cell membranes, making antibiotic penetration more difficult. Newer antibiotics are then developed to counteract the most resistant strains. As these antibiotics in turn become more frequently used, resistance again develops and the cycle is repeated. This cycle can be slowed by the practice of culturing wound drainage fluid, collecting urine and blood for laboratory analysis, and identifying specific pathogens and their sensitivities to specific antibiotics. This practice allows more specific therapy to be administered and delays the onset of resistant strains.

Nosocomial infections are more serious for the hospitalized patient because many patients are at higher risk for infection. Patients with compromised immune systems are much more susceptible to hospital-acquired infections. These groups include patients with AIDS and cancer patients who are receiving chemotherapy. Common sites for nosocomial infections in hospitalized patients include surgical wounds, the urinary tract, and the respiratory tract. Occasionally a patient who has had a urinary catheter inserted develops a urinary tract infection because of improper technique during insertion. The risk for this infection can be reduced by using proper techniques for catheter insertion and care for indwelling catheters. Health care workers are also at higher risk for hospital-acquired infections. Hepatitis B, for example, may be transmitted through needle punctures. Small, open wounds on the upper extremities may come in contact with resistant strains of *Staphylococcus* or *Pseudomonas* and become infected. In addition, health care workers and patients have developed Legionnaire's disease when *Legionella* was spread through the facility on air currents from air conditioning systems that became contaminated with infected water.

Iatrogenic infections are caused by the treatment given the patient. For example, iatrogenic infections may be caused by giving immunosuppressive drugs to prevent rejection of a transplanted organ, resulting in an infection. Another form of iatrogenic infection can be caused by the treatment of a primary infection. Antibiotic therapy for one microorganism can cause the overgrowth of a second microorganism that can also cause illness. The term for this process is *superinfection.* It is especially common with treatment using broad-spectrum antibiotics. An example of this phenomenon is the occurrence of a bowel infection following treatment with oral broad-spectrum antibiotics. The organism *Clostridium difficile* resides in the gastrointestinal tract of many individuals. It is kept in check by the normal bacterial flora of the gastrointestinal tract. Broad-spectrum antibiotics can kill enough of the normal flora to allow *C. difficile* to grow out of control, producing severe colitis and diarrhea.

CARE OF PATIENTS WITH INFECTION

Just as controls must be instituted to stop the spread of infections acquired in the community, so must there be a process to keep hospitalized patients from acquiring a nosocomial infection. The key to preventing the spread of infection is good medical and surgical asepsis.

MEDICAL ASEPSIS

Medical asepsis means limiting the spread of microorganisms as much as possible. This is often called *clean technique* and refers to practices such as changing bed linen, sanitizing bedpans, using individual medication cups for each patient and for each medication administration, and frequent hand washing.

Hand Washing

The most basic and effective method of preventing cross-contamination is hand washing (Fig. 12-3). Soiled hands are the primary mode of transmission of nosocomial infections. Although everyone agrees in principle with the need for frequent hand washing, problems arise when nurses are busy. For example, suppose a nurse is passing medications and is asked by a patient with pulmonary secretions to hand her the box of tissues. At the same time, the patient's roommate asks the nurse to fill her water glass. After doing this, the nurse hurries out of the room to assist a physician with a dressing change. This example illustrates how a chain of infection begins. Unless the nurse interrupts the chain with good hand-washing technique, infection is easily spread from one patient to another.

Good hand-washing technique includes the use of running water, soap, and friction. The lathered hands should be rubbed together for at least 15 seconds, and longer if the nurse works in a high-risk area. The use of antimicrobial soaps is also recommended when working with patients who are more susceptible to infection, such as premature infants or immunocompromised patients.

SURGICAL ASEPSIS

Surgical asepsis, or *sterile technique,* refers to the elimination of microorganisms from any object that comes in contact with the patient. This practice includes care techniques that

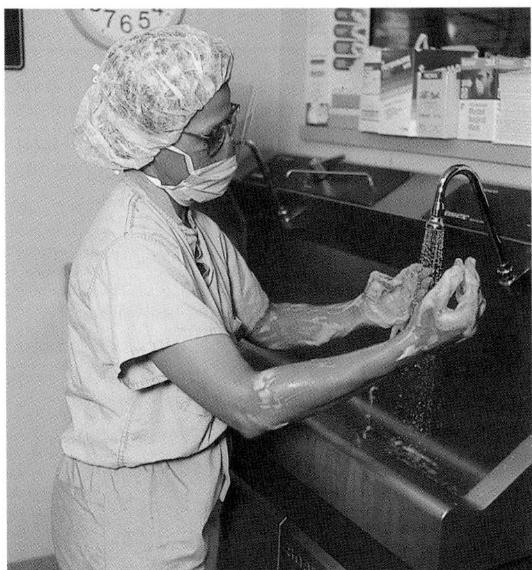

FIGURE **12-3** Hand washing is the most basic and effective way to prevent cross-contamination.

prevent unsterile surfaces from coming in contact with the patient, such as during dressing changes.

STANDARD PRECAUTIONS

A set of infection control guidelines has been developed for hospitals and other health care agencies by the Hospital Infection Control Practices Advisory Committee (HICPAC) and the CDC. Previously the terms *universal precautions, body substance isolation precautions,* and *disease-specific isolation precautions* were in use. The current guidelines, called *standard precautions,* combine the major features of universal precautions and body substance isolation precautions. Standard precautions are used for the care of all patients in hospitals regardless of their isolation status. All patients who previously required category- and disease-specific precautions are now covered under standard precautions. Another change from the previous (1983) CDC guidelines combined the old categories of isolation precautions (strict isolation, contact isolation, respiratory isolation, tuberculosis isolation, enteric precautions, and drainage/secretion precautions) and the old disease-specific precautions into *transmission-based precautions.*

Use standard precautions when you perform procedures in which you will have contact with a patient's blood, body fluids, secretions (except sweat), excretions, broken skin, and mucous membranes. In addition, use standard precautions when you have contact with materials that are soiled or contaminated with body fluids or blood. Use standard precautions with all patients, no matter what their diagnosis or infectious status may be. Guidelines for the use of standard precautions are listed in Table 12-2.

TRANSMISSION-BASED (ISOLATION) PRECAUTIONS

To prevent the spread of infection in a health care facility, infected patients are sometimes isolated from other patients. Precautions and examples of illnesses requiring transmission-based precautions are listed in Table 12-3. The extent of the isolation depends on the type of infection. Patients infected with highly virulent microorganisms that are spread easily by air or direct contact require strict precautions. Microorganisms that are less easily spread require less stringent precautions. The transmission-based precautions were developed to reduce the risk of airborne, droplet, and contact transmission in hospitals. Guidelines for using transmission-based precautions are listed in Table 12-4.

table 12-2 *Guidelines for Use of Standard Precautions*

These precautions are to be used for the care of all patients.

Hand washing should be done immediately after touching blood, body fluids, secretions, excretions, and contaminated objects, even if gloves were worn. Wash hands between tasks and procedures on the same patient to prevent cross-contamination of different body sites.

Gloves should be worn when touching blood, body fluids, secretions, excretions, and contaminated objects. Put on clean gloves before touching mucous membranes and nonintact skin.

Gloves should be changed after each patient contact, before touching noncontaminated items and environmental surfaces. If patient is allergic to latex, use only nonlatex gloves.

Masks, eye protection, or face shields should be worn to protect mucous membranes of the eyes, nose, and mouth during procedures that are likely to generate splashes of blood, body fluids, secretions, or excretions.

Gowns should be worn during procedures that are likely to result in splashes of blood, body fluids, secretions, or excretions.

Patient care equipment soiled with blood, body fluids, secretions, and excretions should be handled so that skin and mucous membrane exposures, contamination of clothing, and transfer of microorganisms to other settings are prevented.

Needles and sharp instruments should be placed in puncture-resistant containers for disposal to prevent injuries from needles or other sharp items. Needles should not be recapped, bent, or removed from the syringe.

Mouth-to-mouth resuscitation should be performed using mouthpieces or other ventilation devices.

Data from CDC isolation guidelines, 1996. (1996). Atlanta: U.S. Centers for Disease Control and Prevention.

Airborne Precautions

Use airborne precautions when caring for patients who have diseases that are spread through the air. Examples of diseases that are spread through the air are tuberculosis, varicella (chickenpox), and rubeola (measles). Respiratory protection, provided by wearing properly fitted high-efficiency particulate air (HEPA) filter respirators or N95 respirators, is indicated when entering the room of patients with tuberculosis. A private room is required. Also recommended is a ventilation

table 12-3 ***Types of Precautions and Patients With Whom Precautions Must Be Used***

STANDARD PRECAUTIONS

Use standard precautions for the care of all patients

AIRBORNE PRECAUTIONS

In addition to standard precautions, use airborne precautions for patients known or suspected to have serious illnesses transmitted by airborne droplet nuclei. Examples of such illnesses include:

- Measles
- Varicella (including disseminated zoster)
- Tuberculosis

DROPLET PRECAUTIONS

In addition to standard precautions, use droplet precautions for patients known or suspected to have serious illnesses transmitted by large-particle droplets. Examples of such illnesses include:

- Invasive *Haemophilus influenzae* type b disease, including meningitis, pneumonia, epiglottitis, and sepsis
- Invasive *Neisseria meningitidis* disease, including meningitis, pneumonia, and sepsis
- Other serious bacterial respiratory infections spread by droplet transmission, including:
  - Diphtheria (pharyngeal)
  - *Mycoplasma pneumoniae*
  - Pertussis
  - Pneumonic plague
  - Streptococcal (group A) pharyngitis, pneumonia, or scarlet fever in infants and young children
- Serious viral infections spread by droplet transmission, including:
  - Adenovirus
  - Influenza
  - Mumps
  - Parvovirus B19
  - Rubella

CONTACT PRECAUTIONS

In addition to standard precautions, use contact precautions for patients known or suspected to have serious illnesses easily transmitted by direct patient contact or by contact with items in the patient's environment. Examples of such illnesses include:

- Gastrointestinal, respiratory, skin, or wound infections or colonization with multidrug-resistant bacteria judged by the infection control program, based on current state, regional, or national recommendations, to be of special clinical and epidemiological significance
- Enteric infections with a prolonged environmental survival, including:
  - *Clostridium difficile*
  - For diapered or incontinent patients:
    - Enterohemorrhagic *Escherichia coli* O157:H7, *Shigella,* hepatitis A, or rotavirus
- Respiratory syncytial virus, parainfluenza virus, or enteroviral infections in infants and young children
- Skin infections that are highly contagious or that may occur on dry skin, including:
  - Diphtheria (cutaneous)
  - Herpes simplex virus (neonatal or mucocutaneous)
  - Impetigo
  - Major (noncontained) abscesses, cellulitis, or decubiti
  - Pediculosis
  - Scabies
  - *Staphylococcal furunculosis* in infants and young children
  - Herpes zoster (disseminated or in the immunocompromised host)
- Viral/hemorrhagic conjunctivitis
- Viral hemorrhagic infections

Data from CDC isolation guidelines, 1996 (1996). Atlanta: U.S. Centers for Disease Control and Prevention.

system that prevents contaminated air from being vented outside the room. In addition, patients with infections spread by airborne transmission must wear surgical masks when leaving their rooms. Surgical masks filter expired air; respirators such as the HEPA filter respirator and the N95 respirator filter inspired air.

Droplet Precautions

Use droplet precautions when taking care of patients with infections that are spread by droplets or dust particles containing the infectious agent. Droplets are spread primarily during coughing, sneezing, or talking, and during certain procedures such as suctioning and bronchoscopy. Because droplets usually travel only about 3 feet before falling from the air, special air handling and ventilation are not required to prevent droplet transmission, as is the case with airborne precautions. The door to the room may be left open. Diseases transmitted by droplets include rubella, mumps, diphtheria, and influenza. Patients should be placed in private rooms. Wear a surgical mask when you are within 3 feet of the patient to protect yourself from contaminated droplets.

Contact Precautions

Use contact precautions when you are caring for patients who are infected by microorganisms that are transmitted by direct (skin-to-skin) or indirect contact with contaminated equipment. Needles, dressings, stethoscopes, bed rails, and doorknobs may become contaminated. The patient is placed in a private room. Wear gloves when entering the infected patient's room; before leaving the patient's room, remove your gloves and wash your hands. Wear a gown if your clothing will come in contact with the patient, contaminated equipment, or environmental surfaces in the patient's room. A

table 12-4 ***Guidelines for Use of Transmission-Based Precautions***

AIRBORNE PRECAUTIONS

Use airborne precautions with patients who have microorganisms transmitted by droplet nuclei smaller than 5 microns. Patients with tuberculosis, measles (rubeola), and chickenpox (varicella) are in this category.

Patient Placement. Place the patient in a private room with negative air pressure of six to twelve air changes per hour. Keep the patient in the room with the door closed. When a private room is not available, place the patient in a room with a patient who has the same microorganism, but with no other infection (cohort).

Respiratory Protection. Wear respiratory protection when entering the room of patients with tuberculosis. If susceptible persons must enter the room of patients with rubeola or varicella, they should wear respiratory protection.

Patient Transport. Limit patient to essential transport only. If patient must be transported, place a surgical mask on the patient.

DROPLET PRECAUTIONS

Use droplet precautions for patients infected with microorganisms that are larger than 5 microns that are spread by coughing, sneezing, talking, or the performance of procedures. Patients with diphtheria, rubella, streptococcal pharyngitis, pneumonia, and mumps are in this category.

Patient Placement. Place the patient in a private room, or with a cohort if a private room is not available. The door may remain open, and special air handling and ventilation are not necessary.

Mask. Wear a mask when working within 3 feet of the patient; many hospitals require wearing a mask to enter the room.

DROPLET PRECAUTIONS—cont'd

Patient Transport. Limit the transport of patients to essential trips only. If transport of the patient is necessary, minimize patient spread of droplets by masking the patient.

CONTACT PRECAUTIONS

Use contact precautions for patients with microorganisms that can be transmitted by direct contact with the patient (hand or skin-to-skin contact) or indirect contact (touching) surfaces or environmental items. Patients with multidrug-resistant organisms, major wound infections, *Shigella,* herpes simplex, and scabies are in this category.

Patient Placement. Place the patient in a private room, or with a cohort.

Gloves and Hand Washing. Wear clean gloves when entering the room. Change gloves after contact with infective material. Remove gloves before leaving the patient's room and wash hands immediately.

Gown. Wear a gown into the room, if you think your clothing will have contact with the patient or environmental surfaces, or if the patient is incontinent or has diarrhea. Remove the gown before leaving the patient's room.

Patient Transport. Limit the transport of patients to essential trips only. If the patient must be transported, make sure precautions are implemented to reduce transmission of microorganisms.

Patient Care Equipment. Dedicate the use of equipment to a single patient to avoid sharing between patients. If you must use common equipment, clean and disinfect it before use for another patient.

Data from CDC isolation guidelines, 1996. (1996). Atlanta: U.S. Centers for Disease Control and Prevention.

gown is also recommended if the patient is incontinent or has wound drainage. Remove the gown before leaving the patient's room. In addition, use dedicated equipment when treating patients with multidrug-resistant organisms. Contact precautions are used for conditions such as gastrointestinal, respiratory, skin, or wound infections with multiple antimicrobial-resistant microorganisms such as VRE and methicillin-resistant *Staphylococcus aureus* (MRSA). Contagious skin diseases, such as impetigo and scabies, as well as respiratory syncytial virus represent conditions requiring contact precautions. Clinical conditions, potential pathogens, and recommended precautions are listed in Table 12-3.

IMMUNOCOMPROMISED PATIENTS

Immunocompromised patients have decreased immunity to infection and are at increased risk for bacterial, fungal, parasitic, and viral infections. Patients receiving chemotherapy and other patients with low white blood cell counts are at increased risk of infection. Leukemia and aplastic anemia are two examples of disorders that cause low white blood cell counts. The use of standard precautions for all patients and of transmission-based precautions for specific situations should reduce the risk of acquiring infections from other persons and from the environment. See Chapter 32 for a discussion of precautions to be used with immunocompromised patients.

NURSING CARE *of Patients with Infections*

Patients with generalized infections easily become dehydrated because of fever and anorexia. Urge the patient to consume adequate fluids, especially water. Fluid intake should be at least 2 liters per day to replace fluids lost through perspiration. Fluid intake is also important in the transportation of nutrients to the cells to fight infection. Nutrition is very important. Encourage patients to consume a high-protein, high-vitamin diet. Vitamin C is important in proper wound healing and in the prevention of future infections. Patients with poor appetites may benefit from a consultation with a dietician.

If a patient's infection requires isolation, remember that effective isolation techniques may also isolate the patient from normal human contact. You may be tempted to hasten your work to minimize your chance of becoming infected. Forced seclusion can cause patients, particularly children, to feel lonely, rejected, and depressed. Engage the patient in conversation while giving direct care. Discussing subjects other than the patient's disease may lessen the feeling of being unclean or rejected. Encourage the patient to move about as much as possible to increase stimulation.

Under the current CDC guidelines, some infections and conditions fall into two categories because the microorganisms are transmitted in more than one way. For example, chickenpox can spread through both the airborne and contact routes. Both airborne precautions and contact precautions are followed.

Laboratory tests used to screen patients for infection include the following:

1. White blood cell count—increased in infection
2. Erythrocyte sedimentation rate—elevated with inflammation
3. Iron level—decreased in chronic infection
4. Cultures of urine, blood, wound, sputum, and throat—infectious microorganisms present in infection are found in the culture
5. White cell differential count (neutrophils, lymphocytes, monocytes, and eosinophils)—increased; used to help differentiate causes of infection

Examples of nursing diagnoses for patients with infections or who are vulnerable to infections include risk for infection, risk for injury, impaired tissue integrity, social isolation, and disturbed body image. Ineffective therapeutic regimen management is another related nursing diagnosis. The primary goals in caring for patients with infection are recovery from the infection and prevention of the spread of infection to others.

Antibiotic drug therapy is the cornerstone of treatment for many infections. Early hospital discharges mean that patients are frequently discharged on a regimen of oral antibiotics. Many people stop taking antibiotics once they begin to feel better. This permits surviving organisms, which may be resistant, to thrive, possibly causing a recurrence of illness. Therefore, caution patients not to stop taking the medication when they start feeling better. They should continue their antibiotics until the entire course has been completed or until they are specifically ordered by their physician to stop taking the medication. The emergence of antibiotic resistance is one important reason why antibiotic therapy for bacterial infections may fail. Increasingly, bacteria are becoming resistant, often because of the widespread or inappropriate use of antibiotics, which leads to the killing of susceptible bacteria and allows more resistant strains to multiply.

Hyperbaric oxygen therapy is an intervention that is used to treat infection. Breathing 100% oxygen at higher-than-atmospheric pressure in a closed chamber increases the amount of dissolved oxygen transported in plasma. The oxygen-rich environment improves leukocyte phagocytic activity and kills anaerobic bacteria.

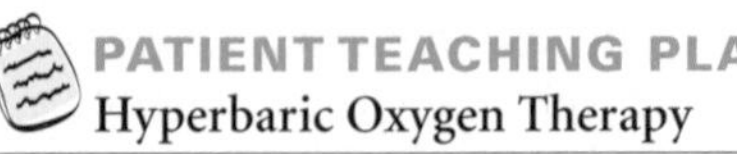

PATIENT TEACHING PLAN
Hyperbaric Oxygen Therapy

- Do not smoke for several hours before and after treatment to decrease lung irritation.
- You can prevent pressure buildup in the ears by swallowing.
- You must wear 100% cotton clothing in the hyperbaric oxygen chamber to prevent static electricity.

During hyperbaric oxygen therapy, monitor the patient for the following complications: ear or sinus pain (from pressure buildup), respiratory problems (as a result of oxygen toxicity), seizures (a central nervous system symptom of oxygen toxicity), and bradycardia (reflex response to oxygen toxicity).

Earlier hospital discharges mean that substantial therapy may continue in the home after discharge. Home health care is frequently ordered for infected patients for a number of reasons. The patient is exposed to fewer nosocomial infections, fewer opportunities arise for infection to be spread to other hospitalized patients, and patients often do better in their own surroundings. If therapy is to be continued at home, teach the patient and other family members how to manage the remaining part of the care. Close coordination between the hospital nurse and the home health nurse is important to ensure good continuity of care.

PATIENT TEACHING PLAN
Infection Control in the Home

- Infection control in the home setting is based on standard precautions. In the home, adapt the guidelines to the equipment and supplies available:
- *Equipment:* List for the family the activities that require the use of gloves, and identify the proper gloves to use. Instruct care givers to use an apron if clothing is likely to become contaminated and to wear gloves to change dressings.
- *Hand Washing:* Demonstrate good hand-washing technique to all household members. Tell family members that hand washing is the most important action they can take to prevent the spread of infection, and inform them when hand washing is appropriate.
- *Sharps Disposal:* If a sharps container is not available, tell the family to use a puncture-resistant container such as a detergent bottle or coffee can with the lid securely taped.
- *Bandages and Linens:* Instruct household members to seal soiled dressings tightly in a plastic bag and dispose of dressings in the trash bag. Clothing and linens with body fluids should be stored in a plastic bag until the laundry is done, then washed in water as hot as the fabric

in each load.

- *Spills:* Instruct household members to wash contaminated surfaces with detergent and water, then wash the surface with a freshly made solution of 1:10 household bleach. Disposable towels should be used.
- *Dishes:* Leftover portions of uneaten food should not be saved. Soiled dishes should be washed in detergent and hot water immediately after use.

IMMUNITY

The immune system is the body's defense network against infection. **Immunity** provides the body with resistance to invading organisms and enables it to fight off invaders once they have gained access. The body is constantly exposed to microorganisms capable of causing disease. If the immune system is intact and functioning properly, it is able to provide adequate protection from most infections and diseases in a healthy individual. When the immune system is not functioning properly, the potential for overwhelming infection exists. Many factors can compromise the immune system, such as disease states, congenital defects, aging, stress, and therapeutic interventions (e.g., drugs, radiation therapy). Understanding the normal immune response and common immune system disorders will help you assess patients at risk for infection and provide appropriate interventions.

Any substance that is capable of stimulating a response from the immune system is called an **antigen**. In most cases the antigen is foreign to the body, and the body recognizes the antigen because it is different from itself (nonself). Antigens can be microorganisms (bacteria, viruses, fungi, or parasites), abnormal or mutated body cells, transplanted cells (from blood transfusions or organ transplants), noninfectious substances from the environment (pollens, insect venom, foods), or foreign molecules from drugs such as penicillin. When healthy, the body protects what it recognizes as self and attempts to destroy that which is nonself. Tissue that is normally recognized as self may be seen as nonself by the immune system if the tissue undergoes change (mutation), is in an abnormal location, or changes structure. Once the body recognizes a substance as an antigen, natural and acquired defenses are put into action to destroy the invader and prevent disease.

Antibodies, also known as immunoglobulins, are proteins that are created in response to specific antigens. The formation and function of antibodies are discussed later in this chapter under Antibody-Mediated (Immediate) Immunity.

INNATE (NATURAL) VERSUS ACQUIRED IMMUNITY

Innate (natural) immunity is present in the body at birth and is not dependent on a specific immune response or previous contact with an infectious agent. It may be specific to a species, a race, or an individual. For instance, humans are not as susceptible to distemper as dogs and cats are. Factors such as nutritional status, stress, and environment may influence natural immunity. Nonspecific defense mechanisms that include physical and chemical barriers to infection, phagocytosis (the process of enveloping and destroying foreign matter), and the inflammatory process contribute to natural immunity.

An individual develops acquired immunity after birth as a result of the body's natural immune responses to antigens. Acquired immunity depends on the proper development and functioning of B and T lymphocytes, which are white blood cells that fight infection.

Active acquired immunity is developed after direct contact with an antigen through illness or vaccination. Vaccinations may be prepared by three methods: (1) using dead organisms that can no longer cause disease, as in the diphtheria and pertussis vaccines; (2) destroying bacterial toxins that act as antigens, as in the tetanus toxoid vaccine; and (3) altering the structure of live organisms so that they are unable to cause disease yet maintain their antigenic properties to prevent many viral diseases, such as measles and poliomyelitis vaccines. Once the body has been exposed to an antigen through illness or vaccination, antibodies develop and retain memory for the antigen. If the body is exposed to the same antigen later, the antibodies can react quickly to fight off disease.

When people are injected with immune globulin or antiserum (made from human or animal blood) that contains antibodies to a specific agent, such as for the emergency treatment of snakebite, rabies, or exposure to hepatitis, they receive antibodies or lymphocytes that were produced by another individual. This type of immunity, called passive acquired immunity, is temporary and is the kind of immunity newborns receive from their mothers through the placenta or through ingestion of breast milk (especially colostrum).

Both natural and acquired immunity are necessary for a healthy individual to have protection from disease. Innate and acquired immunity are discussed further in Chapter 32.

CELLS AND ORGANS INVOLVED IN IMMUNITY

A variety of cells work together to provide the body with an adequate defense against injury or disease. Leukocytes (white blood cells) play a key role in immune responses to infectious organisms and other antigens. There are two categories of white blood cells: granulocytes and nongranulocytes. Blood cells involved in immune disorders are described in Chapter 32.

Although all parts of the body work together as a whole to resist and fight off disease, several organs are vital to a functional immune system. They include the thymus, bone marrow, lymph nodes, spleen, and liver (Fig. 12-4). The thymus and bone marrow participate in the formation and maturation of immune system cells. Located throughout the body, the lymph nodes attack antigens and debris in the interstitial fluid and produce and circulate lymphocytes. The

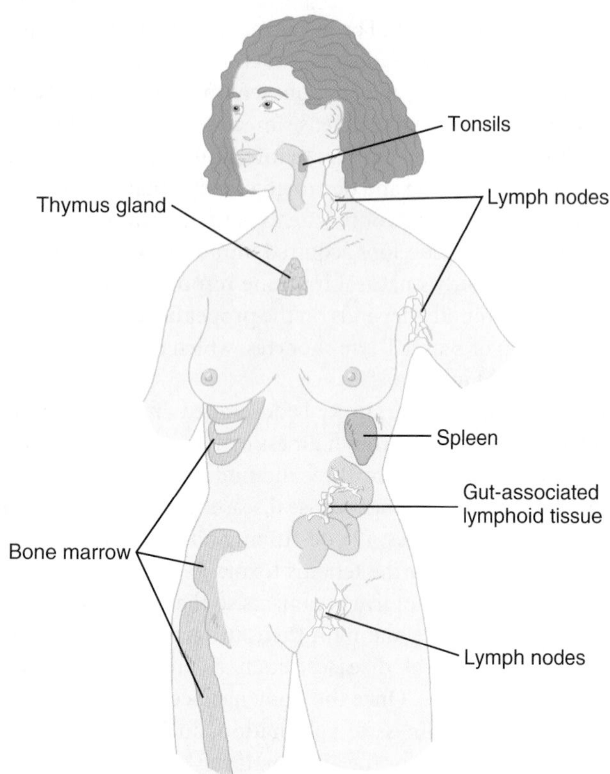

FIGURE 12-4 Organs involved in immunity.

spleen acts as a filter to remove dead cells, debris, and foreign molecules from the blood. The liver filters the blood and plays a part in the production of specific immunoglobulins and other chemicals involved in the immune response.

NONSPECIFIC DEFENSES AGAINST INFECTION

Innate (natural) immunity is present at birth and consists of physical and chemical barriers to invasion of the body as well as processes and substances that protect and repair tissues and stimulate the body to fight off disease. Physical and chemical barriers, inflammation, and phagocytosis are nonspecific defenses against infection.

Other nonspecific defenses against infection that protect the body include complement, pyrogen, and interferon. Complement is a series of proteins that enhance the inflammatory process and the immune response. Chemotaxis, phagocytosis, and the activity of antibodies are stimulated by complement. Pyrogen (an eicosanoid) is a substance released in inflammation that causes body temperature to increase. Fever is thought to inhibit the growth of pathogens and slow enzymatic reactions that occur in infectious processes. Another substance, interferon, is produced in viral infections and acts to inhibit the replication of viruses. Interferon (a cytokine) also affects the function of T lymphocytes and is used in the treatment of selected malignancies. Eicosanoids and cytokines are discussed in Chapter 32.

SPECIFIC DEFENSES AGAINST INFECTION—THE IMMUNE RESPONSE

The immune response is the process by which antigens are recognized as foreign, processed, and destroyed. The two types of immune responses, antibody-mediated (immediate or humoral) and cell-mediated, function interdependently to provide the immune response.

ANTIBODY-MEDIATED (IMMEDIATE) IMMUNITY

Antibody-mediated (humoral) immunity is immediate. This first-line defense involves B lymphocytes and the production of antibodies in response to specific antigens. The humoral immune response is initiated when an antigen binds to a special receptor on a B lymphocyte. This results in the production of antibodies that seek out and "stick to" specific antigens in the body. This combination forms antigen-antibody complexes, which are then targeted for cleanup by neutrophils and macrophages. Formation of these complexes activates complement and intensifies T-lymphocyte activity. Since circulating antibodies bind with antigens as soon as they are recognized, the chemical process is triggered immediately.

Antibodies (immunoglobulins) are divided into five classes: IgG, IgM, IgA, IgE, and IgD. IgG is the most abundant immunoglobulin; it crosses the placenta to provide passive immunity for the newborn. IgE is important in allergic reactions and in parasitic infections.

CELL-MEDIATED (DELAYED) IMMUNITY

Cell-mediated immunity is a delayed response to injury or infection. Cellular immunity is delayed because of the time needed for the migration of T cells and for the production of substances that enhance the immune response and influence the destruction of antigens.

T cells include helper cells, suppressor cells, and killer cells. Helper T cells enhance humoral immunity; suppressor T cells help "turn off" the humoral response. Disease may occur when the normal ratio of helper to suppressor cells (2:1) is altered. In AIDS, for instance, the number of helper T cells is diminished. When the number of suppressor T cells is too high, infections, allergy, or immune disease develop. Killer T cells directly destroy antigens.

Cellular immunity fights most viral or bacterial infections and hinders the growth of malignant cells. This process also launches an attack on transplanted tissue or organs in the body.

IMMUNODEFICIENCY

ETIOLOGY AND RISK FACTORS

When the body's self-defenses against foreign invasion fail to function normally, a state of immune deficiency (immunosuppression) exists. In this state, known as an immunocompromised or immunosuppressed state, the body is unable to launch an adequate immune response and is at great risk for infection. The primary clinical clue to immunodeficiency, whatever the cause, is the tendency to develop recurrent infections. Immune deficiencies can be congenital or, more commonly, acquired, and can result from problems with humoral immunity, cell-mediated immunity, vital mediators such as complement, or the process of phagocytosis.

In congenital immunodeficiencies, some part of the immune system fails to develop properly. The result is a defect in the B or T lymphocytes, phagocytes, or complement.

Acquired immunodeficiencies result from factors outside the immune system that render a previously functional immune system inadequate. Some causes of acquired deficiencies are infections, malignancies, autoimmune diseases (systemic lupus erythematosus, rheumatoid arthritis), chronic diseases (diabetes mellitus, renal disease), drugs, aging, stress, and malnutrition.

Stress, whether physical or emotional, alters the body's response to disease. Although the mechanism is not fully understood, the release of hormones plays a part. Stressors include such things as serious illness, job loss, and divorce; even noise and cold play a part.

The nutritional state of the patient also affects immunity. The malnourished patient is much more susceptible to infection, especially when a protein deficiency exists. People with chronic conditions such as diabetes and renal disease may become debilitated and unable to fully resist infection. Trauma victims, especially those with burns, have diminished immune responses. Many malignant disorders alter the functioning of the immune system. Infectious diseases also cause immunodeficiencies, especially acute viral infections.

Many treatments and interventions aimed at helping patients cause immunodeficiency. Medications often place patients at risk for infection: antibiotics (which sometimes cause superinfections), steroids, antineoplastics, and immunosuppressive drugs (used for transplant recipients) are a few.

Surgery, anesthesia, and irradiation for cancer also can alter immune function. In addition, invasive procedures such as urinary catheterization and venipuncture for intravenous therapy or blood work bypass the patient's first line of defense. In the hospitalized patient, all of these factors come into play: disease, stress, nutritional alterations, medications, and invasive procedures all set the patient up for infection.

MEDICAL TREATMENT

Congenital immunodeficiencies usually are treated with replacement therapy of the deficient immune component. Bone marrow transplants or fetal thymus tissue transplants may be used in some cases. Treating an acquired immunodeficiency entails correcting the underlying condition that is causing the problem, such as reducing stressors, correcting malnutrition, and discontinuing medications that alter immunity.

NURSING CARE *of the Immunosuppressed Patient*

The primary nursing responsibility in cases of immunodeficiency is to prevent infection. Proper hand washing by personnel and visitors is the single most important measure in prevention. In addition, teach patients to wash their hands. Vital signs should be assessed frequently.

In an immunosuppressed or immunocompromised patient, signs and symptoms of infection are often atypical, masked, or absent. Be aware that a small increase in body temperature can be significant and should be reported. Avoid rectal thermometers if possible because of the potential for damage to the rectal mucosa. Encourage adequate nutritional intake. Perform good skin, mouth, perineal, wound, and intravenous site care with continuous assessment for signs of infection. Encourage patients to turn, cough, and breathe deeply. Protective (compromised host) isolation may be necessary. Flowers or plants may be prohibited because they provide a reservoir for bacterial growth. Fresh produce may be eliminated from the diet if the white blood cell count is too low. Encourage the use of disposable equipment.

Patient education concerning the risks for and signs of infection should be reinforced. Provide a supportive listening environment, as these patients may have anxiety as well as a high stress level, and often feelings of powerlessness are overwhelming.

HYPERSENSITIVITY AND ALLERGY

ETIOLOGY AND RISK FACTORS

When a normally inoffensive foreign substance stimulates an atypical immune response, allergy or hypersensitivity occurs. Immunity is beneficial, but hypersensitivity can be harmful, sometimes producing deadly symptoms. It is estimated that 20% to 25% of the U.S. population suffers from allergies of some sort, with allergic rhinitis (hay fever) and asthma occurring most often. Other allergic disorders include allergic contact dermatitis, angioedema (localized swelling), dermatitis, anaphylaxis (severe allergic reaction), gastrointestinal allergies, and urticaria (hives) (Table 12-5). The tendency to develop an allergy is inherited, although the type of allergy may vary. Someone who is prone to allergies may be referred to as atopic. Hypersensitivity as an immune disorder is discussed in Chapter 32.

An antigen that causes a hypersensitive reaction is called an **allergen**. Any substance can act as an allergen to a susceptible person, but some of the more common ones are house dust, animal dander, pollens, molds, foods, pharmacologic agents, cigarette smoke, feathers, and insect venoms. Table 12-5 lists common allergens.

The allergic response begins with sensitization. The first encounter with a specific allergen results in only a small amount of antibody production. With subsequent exposure, however, the body steps up its defense by producing large amounts of antibodies, which circulate in the bloodstream and travel to the affected tissues. This triggers the release of histamine and other chemical agents. Neutrophils arrive at the scene to engulf and destroy the antigens. A multitude of reactions occur that produce the symptoms typical of an allergic response, although they vary according to the area affected. Local manifestations of allergic reactions include

table 12-5 ***Common Allergies and Their Causes***

ALLERGIC REACTION	STIMULUS
Asthma	Pollens, dust, molds, cigarette smoke, air pollutants, animal dander
Allergic rhinitis	Pollens, dust, molds, animal dander
Anaphylaxis	Antibiotics (penicillin) Insect venom (bee, wasp stings) Blood transfusions
Urticaria (hives)	Food, drugs
Atopic dermatitis (eczema)	Soaps, cosmetics, chemicals, fabrics
Allergic contact dermatitis	Plants (poison ivy) Metals (nickel) Chemicals, cosmetics Latex gloves
Gastrointestinal allergies	Foods, drugs

urticaria, pruritus, conjunctivitis, rhinitis, laryngeal edema, bronchospasm, dysrhythmia, gastrointestinal cramps and malabsorption, and angioedema.

MEDICAL TREATMENT

The medical treatment of allergic patients varies depending on the specific allergy. In general, antihistamines are used to reduce the symptoms caused by histamine release. Many people suffer side effects from antihistamines, such as dry mouth, nausea, blurred vision, dizziness, and drowsiness. For asthma sufferers, bronchodilators, steroids, or both may be prescribed to improve air movement and decrease inflammation in the lungs; oxygen and breathing treatments may also be ordered. Besides antihistamines, topical lotions and ointments may be prescribed to relieve itching associated with urticaria, atopic dermatitis, or allergic contact dermatitis.

Long-term medical treatment of allergies involves testing to determine specific allergens. Testing is performed by injecting small amounts of allergen under the skin (intradermally) or by pricking the surface of the patient's skin and monitoring for the degree of wheal-and-flare reaction. After the specific agents have been identified, the patient may be desensitized by injections of minute quantities of the allergen, with the dosage gradually increased over a prolonged period of time. Desensitization is aimed at increasing tolerance to the offending agent and decreasing the severity of the allergic response.

NURSING CARE *of the Patient with Allergies*

When dealing with the hospitalized allergic patient, the most important nursing intervention is to document all allergies, the symptoms they cause, and any treatment currently used. Allergies should be posted on the front of the patient's chart, on all medication records, and on the nursing care plan. Never administer any drug to which the patient reports a previous allergic reaction.

Alert the pharmacy and dietary departments to drug and food allergies. Notify the physician of any allergies that may determine which medications to avoid. For instance, a patient who is allergic to shellfish should not receive drugs containing iodine because an anaphylactic reaction may result. Make sure that patients who have been taking allergy medication, such as inhaler treatments, continue taking these medications when admitted to the hospital. A growing number of patients, as well as health care providers, are reporting latex allergies, necessitating the use of nonlatex gloves.

Patient education is important for all patients with allergies. This includes knowledge of specific allergens, limiting exposure to or avoiding allergens, the proper use of medications such as inhaled bronchodilators, and the actions and side effects of drugs. Patients who are at risk for life-threatening (anaphylactic) reactions should wear a medical alert bracelet that identifies their allergy. Individuals with insect sting allergies should obtain an emergency sting kit and be taught how to self-inject epinephrine. This kit should be kept readily available at all times.

Nurses should avoid the overuse of perfumes and scented cosmetics while working with patients. Live plants and flowers should not be allowed in the allergic patient's room.

ANAPHYLAXIS

ETIOLOGY AND RISK FACTORS

When an allergen enters the bloodstream, allergic reactions can occur throughout the body within minutes. This is anaphylaxis, a life-threatening situation that can quickly deteriorate into shock, coma, and death. Histamine released in anaphylaxis causes bronchospasm, vasodilation, and increased capillary permeability throughout the body, which causes fluid to leave the circulation and enter the tissues, causing shock from hypovolemia. Signs and symptoms of anaphylaxis include anxiety, wheezing and difficulty breathing, bluish skin color (cyanosis), hives, facial edema, joint pain (arthralgia), and low blood pressure (hypotension).

Anaphylaxis is an emergency situation, and the patient's life depends on rapid intervention. The most common cause of anaphylaxis is the use of antibiotics, especially penicillin. Other causes include the use of medicines or serum from animal sources, insect venom (especially from bees and wasps), iodinated radioactive contrast media, local anesthesia, and blood products.

MEDICAL TREATMENT

In anaphylaxis, oxygen, epinephrine, aminophylline, diphenhydramine, and corticosteroids may be administered intravenously, and other drugs such as dopamine may be necessary to raise the patient's blood pressure and relax the bronchi.

NURSING CARE *of the Patient with Anaphylaxis*

The most vital component of all nursing care is prompt recognition of the situation. Nursing interventions are aimed at minimizing the patient's anxiety, ensuring adequate hydration to combat hypovolemia, and assisting the patient with breathing and oxygenation.

The patient should be monitored for difficulty breathing, dyspnea, tachypnea, a change in respiratory rate, and cyanosis.

AUTOIMMUNE DISEASES

ETIOLOGY AND RISK FACTORS

The body's ability to determine self from nonself is called tolerance. When tolerance is disrupted, the immune system reacts against and destroys its own tissues. This breakdown in tolerance and subsequent damage to self is termed autoimmunity. An autoimmune process may be initiated when there is injury to tissues, infection, or malignancy. The exact causes and pathology of most autoimmune diseases are poorly understood, but many of these disorders cause severe illness and death.

Genetic factors appear to be involved because autoimmune diseases tend to be familial. Some autoimmune disorders have apparent causes, such as drug-induced anemia or a low platelet count (thrombocytopenia). Infection often is present before the onset of an autoimmune disease, leading to the conclusion that the disease results as a complication (sequela) of the infection. Autoimmune diseases cause injury in three ways: (1) by the effect of antibodies on cell surfaces; (2) through the deposit of antigen-antibody complexes (particularly in capillaries, joints, and renal tissue), and (3) through the action of sensitized T cells.

Autoimmunity can involve any tissue or organ system. In multiple sclerosis, the white matter of the brain and spinal cord is affected, and the myelin sheath that protects nerve fibers is destroyed. Rheumatoid arthritis affects the lining of the joints. In type 1 diabetes mellitus, the pancreatic cells that secrete insulin are attacked. Table 12-6 lists some of the more common autoimmune disorders and the tissues they affect. Probably the most familiar of the autoimmune disorders is systemic lupus erythematosus, which affects multiple organs.

table 12-6 *Autoimmune Disorders and Their Targets*

DISORDER	TISSUE AFFECTED
ENDOCRINE SYSTEM	
Hyperthyroidism (Graves' disease)	Thyroid
Autoimmune thyroiditis	Thyroid
Insulin-dependent diabetes mellitus	Pancreas
Addison's disease	Adrenal gland
CENTRAL NERVOUS SYSTEM	
Multiple sclerosis	Brain and spinal cord
Myasthenia gravis	Neuromuscular junctions
CARDIOVASCULAR SYSTEM	
Rheumatic fever	Heart
Cardiomyopathy	Heart
GASTROINTESTINAL SYSTEM	
Ulcerative colitis	Colon
Crohn's disease	Ileum
CONNECTIVE TISSUE	
Rheumatoid arthritis	Joints
Systemic lupus erythematosus	Multiple tissues
Scleroderma	Multiple tissues
HEMATOLOGIC SYSTEM	
Autoimmune hemolytic anemia	Red blood cells
Autoimmune thrombocytopenic purpura	Platelets
Idiopathic neutropenia	Neutrophils
Idiopathic lymphopenia	Lymphocytes
RESPIRATORY AND RENAL SYSTEMS	
Goodpasture's disease	Lung, kidney
SKIN	
Pemphigus vulgaris	Skin
Psoriasis	Skin

Adapted from McCance, K. L., & Huether, S. E. (1994). *Pathophysiology: The biologic basis for disease in adults and children* (2nd ed., pp. 270-271). St. Louis: Mosby.

MEDICAL TREATMENT

Medical interventions vary depending on the specific autoimmune disease and the tissues affected, as well as the symptoms. In general, corticosteroids and nonsteroidal anti-inflammatory drugs (NSAIDs) are used to treat inflammation. Immunosuppressive therapies may be tried to moderate the autoimmune response.

NURSING CARE *of the Patient with an Autoimmune Disorder*

Although nursing interventions vary according to the specific disorder, multiple nursing diagnoses may apply to any patient with an autoimmune disease. They include risk for activity intolerance, anxiety, impaired skin integrity, ineffective breathing pattern, impaired gas exchange, deficient knowledge, pain, fear, fatigue, self-care deficit, ineffective coping, risk for infection, and imbalanced nutrition: less than body requirements. Adequate rest, maintenance of optimal hydration and nutritional status, and prevention of infection are vital in preventing complications in these patients. In addition, a supportive, caring atmosphere is important to enhance the patient's coping skills and promote emotional health.

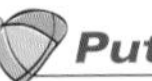

Put on your THINKING CAP!!

1. For one clinical day, note everything you did that represents use of standard precautions.
2. In your clinical site, locate everything you would need if a patient had an anaphylactic reaction to a drug. What procedure should you use to alert other personnel?

key points

- Physical and chemical barriers that shield the body from disease or injury include the skin, the mucous membranes, and various blood cells.
- Many types of leukocytes, especially neutrophils and monocytes, act as nature's cleanup mechanism by migrating to infected or inflamed areas and engulfing

and destroying antigens through a process known as phagocytosis.

- Reticuloendothelial cells, or tissue macrophages, found in the blood, connective tissue, liver, spleen, bone marrow, and lymph nodes, protect the body by digesting and absorbing foreign material such as old red blood cells, bacteria, and colloidal particles.
- The four classic signs of inflammation are rubor (redness), calor (heat), tumor (swelling), and dolor (pain).
- Wound healing begins at the same time that the inflammatory process begins.
- The process of wound healing includes the production of macrophage cells to clean up inflammatory debris, initiation of the repair process by fibroblasts, the formation of capillaries to provide circulation and nutrients to the new tissue, and the migration of epithelial cells under the scab to form a scar.
- Age and general health affect how rapidly wound healing occurs. Older adults heal more slowly as a result of a decreased blood supply to the tissues, a decrease in tissue elasticity, and poor or inadequate nutrition.
- The major infectious agents are bacteria, viruses, fungi, protozoa, rickettsiae, helminths, and mycoplasmas.
- Infection, or the invasion of the body by microorganisms, is possible only when a causative agent, a reservoir, a portal of exit, a mode of transfer, a portal of entry, and a susceptible host are present.
- Signs and symptoms of generalized infections are moderate to severe pain, swelling, fever, malaise, anorexia, and prostration.
- Two types of infections are (1) community-acquired infections, acquired through daily contact with the public, and (2) hospital-acquired, or nosocomial, infections.
- The most basic and effective method of preventing cross-contamination is hand washing with adequate friction.
- The Centers for Disease Control and Prevention recommends the use of standard precautions for all patients, especially those cared for in settings in which exposure to blood is common.
- The immune system is the body's defense network against infection; it provides the body with resistance to invading organisms and enables it to fight off invaders once they have gained access.
- Antigens are substances that stimulate a response from the immune system. Antibodies, also known as immunoglobulins, are proteins that are created in response to specific antigens.
- Innate (natural) immunity is present in the body at birth, whereas acquired immunity develops after birth as a result of the body's immune responses to antigens.
- Acquired immunity depends on the proper development of B and T lymphocytes, which are white blood cells that fight infection.
- Body organs that are vital to a functional immune system include the thymus, bone marrow, lymph nodes, spleen, and liver.
- The two types of immunity—antibody-mediated (humoral) and cell-mediated—function interdependently to provide the immune response.
- Immunodeficiency occurs when the body is unable to launch an adequate immune response, resulting in risk for infection.
- When a normally inoffensive foreign substance stimulates an atypical immune response, allergy or hypersensitivity occurs; if anaphylaxis occurs, it is a crisis situation.
- Autoimmunity occurs when the body fails to recognize itself, and the immune system reacts by destroying the body's own tissues.

REVIEW QUESTIONS

1. A condition in which the body's immune system destroys its own tissues is:
   1. immunodeficiency.
   2. nosocomial infection.
   3. autoimmunity.
   4. inflammation.
2. Bacteria that reside on the skin but do not cause infection serve what purpose?
   1. They stimulate the development of antibodies against pathogens.
   2. They prevent pathogens from gaining access to the body.
   3. They secrete sebum, which inhibits the growth of microorganisms.
   4. They phagocytose pathogenic bacteria that invade the body.
3. The classic signs of inflammation are redness, heat, swelling, and:
   1. pain.
   2. drainage.
   3. fever
   4. pus.
4. In the first phase of the inflammatory process, capillary permeability increases. What purpose does this serve?
   1. Reduces pain in the inflamed tissue by diluting bradykinin
   2. Draws excess fluid out of inflamed tissue to reduce swelling
   3. Allows monocytes and neutrophils to pass into the inflamed tissue
   4. Counteracts bronchoconstriction in antigen-antibody reactions

5. Why are there numerous antibacterial drugs, but relatively few antiviral drugs?
    1. Viruses have a more advanced ability to develop resistance to drugs.
    2. It is more profitable to make antibacterial drugs because only a few viruses exist.
    3. Very few chemicals have been developed that are capable of killing viruses.
    4. The virus lives inside the host cell, and drugs that harm viruses often harm host cells too.
6. The last factor in the chain of infection is the:
    1. portal of entry.
    2. reservoir.
    3. susceptible host.
    4. mode of transfer.
7. Characteristics of the incubation period of the infectious process include:
    1. the infected person is often very contagious.
    2. signs and symptoms are most severe.
    3. usually a high fever is present but no other symptoms.
    4. the patient is in the recovery phase of the infection.
8. An example of a hospital-borne infection is:
    1. gonorrhea.
    2. hepatitis A.
    3. tuberculosis.
    4. vancomycin-resistant *Enterococcus.*
9. Which of the following measures helps prevent the development of bacterial resistance?
    1. All infections are promptly treated with broad-spectrum antibiotics.
    2. Antibiotic selection is based on results of culture and sensitivity tests.
    3. Antibiotics are discontinued as soon as symptoms resolve.
    4. Antibiotics are prescribed only for life-threatening infections.
10. The primary mode of transmission of nosocomial infections is:
    1. soiled caregiver hands.
    2. direct contact between patients.
    3. organisms brought in by visitors.
    4. faulty sterilization procedures.
11. Which statement is true regarding the need to use standard precautions?
    1. Standard precautions are required only when caring for patients who have open wounds.
    2. You should use standard precautions any time you have contact with a patient's blood or other body fluids.
    3. You only have to use standard precautions when caring for patients with tuberculosis, hepatitis, or HIV infection.
    4. It is necessary to use standard precautions only when caring for patients who are highly susceptible to infection.
12. The advantage of using HEPA filter respirators rather than surgical masks is that:
    1. surgical masks are too expensive for routine use.
    2. HEPA filter respirators protect the care giver by filtering inspired air.
    3. surgical masks protect the care giver against tuberculosis but not other infections.
    4. HEPA filter respirators protect the patient but not the care giver.
13. Following vaccination for measles, a person will not become ill if exposed to the measles virus. The patient's ability to resist the measles virus is called:
    1. innate immunity.
    2. nonspecific defense mechanism.
    3. active acquired immunity.
    4. passive acquired immunity.
14. The rejection of transplanted organs is the result of:
    1. passive acquired immunity.
    2. antibody-mediated immunity.
    3. cell-mediated immunity.
    4. innate immunity.
15. Nursing care of the immunosuppressed patient should include:
    1. taking rectal temperatures every 4 hours to detect low-grade fever.
    2. encouraging fresh fruits and vegetables to increase vitamin intake.
    3. encouraging the family to bring in live plants to increase oxygen in the room.
    4. emphasizing the need for good hand washing by patients, visitors, and staff.

CHAPTER

13 Fluid and Electrolytes

objectives

1. Describe the extracellular and intracellular fluid compartments.
2. Describe the composition of the extracellular and intracellular body fluid compartments.
3. Discuss the mechanisms of fluid transport and fluid balance.
4. Identify the causes, signs and symptoms, and treatment of fluid imbalances.
5. Describe the major functions of all of the major electrolytes—sodium, potassium, calcium, magnesium, and chloride.
6. Identify the causes, signs and symptoms, and treatment of electrolyte imbalances.
7. List data to be collected in assessing fluid and electrolyte status.
8. Discuss the medical treatment and nursing management of persons with fluid and electrolyte imbalances.
9. Explain why the elderly are at increased risk for fluid and electrolyte imbalances.
10. List the four types of acid-base imbalances.
11. Identify the major causes of each acid-base imbalance.
12. Explain the management of acid-base imbalances.

key terms

Acid (p. 163)
Acid-base balance (p. 163)
Active transport (p. 152)
Base (p. 163)
Diffusion (dĭ-FŪ-zhŭn, p. 152)
Electrolyte (ĕ-LĔK-trō-līt, p. 151)
Extracellular fluid (ĕks-tră-SĔL-ū-lăr, p. 150)
Filtration (fĭl-TRĀ-shŭn, p. 152)
Fluid volume deficit (p. 158)
Fluid volume excess (p. 159)
Homeostasis (hō-mē-ō-STĀ-sĭs, p. 150)
Intracellular fluid (ĭn-tră-SĔL-ū-lăr, p. 150)
Osmolality (ŏz-mō-LĂL-ĭ-tē, p. 152)
Osmolarity (ŏz-mō-LĂR-ĭ-tē, p. 152)
Osmosis (ŏz-MŌ-sĭs, p. 152)
Selectively permeable membrane (sĭ-LĔK-tĭv-lē PĔR-mē-ă-b'l MĔM-brān, p. 152)

Many disease processes and medical interventions pose actual or potential threats to patients' fluid and electrolyte balances. Therefore, nurses must understand the basic principles of fluid and electrolyte balance to maintain balance and to detect and correct imbalances.

HOMEOSTASIS

Approximately 50% to 60% of the human body is composed of water. To maintain internal balance, the body must be able to regulate the fluids within it. The tendency to maintain relatively constant conditions as in the fluid compartments is called *homeostasis.* All organs and structures of the body are involved in the maintenance of homeostasis.

Homeostasis is necessary for cells to be able to carry out their work. Body fluids are in constant motion, maintaining healthy living conditions for body cells. The process of homeostasis involves the delivery of essential elements such as oxygen and glucose to the cells and the removal of wastes such as carbon dioxide from the cells. When the body does not maintain homeostasis, the cells cannot function properly, and illness results.

BODY FLUID COMPARTMENTS

Body fluids are classified as intracellular or extracellular, depending on their location. **Intracellular fluid** is fluid within a cell, and **extracellular fluid** is fluid outside the cell. Most of the body's fluids are found within the cell.

Extracellular fluids are found in the blood vessels in the form of plasma or serum (called *intravascular fluid*); in the fluid surrounding the cells (called *interstitial fluid*), including lymph fluid; and elsewhere such as in digestive secretions, sweat, and cerebrospinal fluid. Extracellular fluid is mainly responsible for the transport of nutrients and wastes throughout the body. The distribution of total body fluids varies among adult males, adult females, and infants (Table 13-1).

COMPOSITION OF BODY FLUIDS

WATER

Water makes up the largest portion of the body weight. The percentage of body weight that is water is affected by age, sex, and amount of body fat. A person's percent of body water usually decreases with advancing age. Females have a lower percentage of body water than males throughout the adult

table 13-1 Total Body Fluids

	ADULT MALE (% TBF)	ADULT FEMALE (% TBF)	INFANT (% TBF)
Intracellular	40	36	40
Extracellular	20	18	35
Total body fluids	60	54	75

TBF, Total body fluids.

years because women have more fat than men and fat cells contain less water than other cells. Obese people have a lower percentage of body water because of their increased number of fat cells.

table 13-2 Electrolyte Composition of Extracellular and Intracellular Fluids

ELECTROLYTE	EXTRACELLULAR FLUID (mEq/L)	INTRACELLULAR FLUID (mEq/L)
Sodium (Na)	130-145	14
Potassium (K)	3.5-5.1	140
Chloride (Cl)	98-107	4-6
Bicarbonate (HCO_3^-)	24	12
Calcium (Ca)	5	1-8
Magnesium (Mg)	1.5-2.5	6-30
Phosphate (HPO_4^-)	2	40-95

SOLUTES

In addition to water, body fluids contain solutes (dissolved substances) such as electrolytes and nonelectrolytes.

Electrolytes

An *electrolyte* is defined as a substance that develops an electrical charge when dissolved in water. Examples of electrolytes are sodium, potassium, calcium, chloride, bicarbonate, and magnesium. When these substances are dissolved in water, they break up into small particles called *ions,* which have either a positive (+) or a negative (−) charge. Ions that have a positive electrical charge are called *cations.* Examples of cations are sodium (Na^+), potassium (K^+), calcium (Ca^{2+}), and magnesium (Mg^{2+}). Ions that have a negative charge are called *anions.* Examples of anions are chloride (Cl^-), bicarbonate (HCO_3^-), and phosphate (HPO_4^-).

Electrolytes maintain a balance between positive and negative charges. For every positively charged cation, there is a negatively charged anion. In every fluid compartment of the body, the cations and anions combine to balance one another. This process keeps the body in homeostasis.

The concentration of an electrolyte in a solution or body fluid compartment is measured in milliequivalents per liter (mEq/L). Milliequivalents indicate the chemical activity or combining power of ions. Hydrogen is used as a standard for comparing chemical activities of electrolytes. One milliequivalent of an electrolyte has the same chemical combining power as 1 mEq of hydrogen.

Electrolytes can move from one fluid compartment to another. However, the normal concentration of specific electrolytes is different in the two compartments (Table 13-2).

Sodium

Sodium (Na^+) is the most abundant electrolyte in the body and the primary electrolyte in the extracellular fluid. It plays a major role in the regulation of body fluid volumes, muscular activity, nerve impulse conduction, and acid-base balance.

Potassium

Potassium (K^+) is found mainly in the intracellular fluid and is the major intracellular cation. Because it is so abundant within the cell, it plays an important role in maintaining fluid osmolarity and volume within the cell. Potassium is essential for normal membrane excitability—a critical factor in the transmission of nerve impulses. It also is needed for protein synthesis, for the synthesis and breakdown of glycogen, and to maintain plasma acid-base balance.

Chloride

Chloride (Cl^-) is an extracellular anion that is usually bound with other ions, especially sodium or potassium. Its major functions are to regulate osmotic pressure between fluid compartments and to assist in regulating acid-base balance.

Calcium

Calcium (Ca^{2+}) is usually combined with phosphorus to form the mineral salts of the bones and teeth. Of the total calcium in the body, 99% is concentrated in the bones and teeth, and 1% is in the extracellular fluid. Calcium is ingested through the diet and absorbed through the intestine.

In addition to maintaining strong teeth and bones, calcium promotes normal transmission of nerve impulses and helps to regulate normal muscle contraction and relaxation. Constant regulation of calcium levels takes place in the body. If the serum calcium level falls, additional calcium is absorbed in the intestine, reabsorbed through the kidneys, or taken from the bones. If more calcium is needed in the bones, it is taken from the bloodstream and also reabsorbed through the kidneys.

Magnesium

Magnesium (Mg^{2+}) is a cation that is found in bone (50% to 60%), intracellular fluid (39% to 49%), and extracellular fluid (1%). After potassium, magnesium is the most abundant cation in intracellular fluid, so it is vital to cellular function. It plays a role in the metabolism of carbohydrates and proteins, the storage and use of intracellular energy, and neural transmission. Magnesium is important in the functioning of the heart, nerves, and muscles.

About 30% to 40% of magnesium ingested through the diet is absorbed, mainly through the small intestine. Magnesium is excreted through the kidneys, and the rate of excretion is regulated by sodium and calcium excretion, extracellular fluid volume, and parathyroid hormone.

Nonelectrolytes

Although most of the solutes in the body are electrolytes, other substances are dissolved in the body fluids as well.

Examples are urea, protein, glucose, creatinine, and bilirubin. These solutes do not carry an electrical charge and are measured in milligrams per deciliter (mg/dL).

TRANSPORT OF WATER AND ELECTROLYTES

MEMBRANES

The fluid compartments of the body are separated by selectively permeable membranes that control movement of water and certain solutes. Selective permeability maintains the unique composition of each compartment of the body while allowing for the transport of nutrients and wastes to and from cells. For example, selectively permeable membranes surround cells to separate fluid in the cells from fluid in the tissues. Some solutes cross membranes more easily than others. Small molecules and water move freely across membranes, whereas larger molecules such as protein move less readily.

TRANSPORT PROCESSES

Water and solutes are transported between intracellular and extracellular fluid compartments by one or more of the following processes: (1) diffusion, (2) active transport, (3) filtration, and (4) osmosis.

Diffusion

Diffusion is the random movement of particles in all directions. The natural tendency is for a substance to move from an area of higher concentration to an area of lower concentration. One example is the movement of oxygen from the alveoli to the pulmonary capillaries. The concentration of oxygen in the alveoli is greater than in the capillaries; therefore oxygen diffuses into the capillaries and is transported through the bloodstream to other parts of the body. The term *facilitated diffusion* is used when a carrier protein transports the molecules through membranes toward an area of lower concentration.

Active Transport

Carrier proteins can transport substances from an area of lower concentration to an area of equal or greater concentration. This process, which requires expenditure of energy, is called *active transport.* Many solutes, such as sodium, potassium, glucose, and hydrogen, are actively transported across cell membranes. An example is the sodium pump. The concentration of sodium is highest in extracellular fluid. Therefore excess sodium cannot leave the cell by diffusion. Active transport "pumps" the excess sodium out of the cell into the extracellular fluid.

Filtration

Filtration is the transfer of water and solutes through a membrane from an area of high pressure to an area of low pressure. This pressure is known as *hydraulic pressure* and is a combination of pressures from the force of gravity on the fluid and the pumping action of the heart. Filtration is a necessary process for moving fluid out of the capillaries into the tissues and for filtering plasma through the kidneys.

Osmosis

Osmosis is the movement of water across a membrane from a less concentrated solution to a more concentrated solution. It involves the movement of water only, but sometimes the force of movement across the membrane carries some solutes along. If a fluid compartment has less water and more sodium, water from another compartment moves to the more concentrated compartment by osmosis to create a better fluid balance.

OSMOLALITY

Osmolality refers to the concentration of a solution determined by the number of dissolved particles per kilogram of water. A higher osmolality means that there is a higher concentration of salt, or any other solute, in the water because the solution contains less water. Osmolality controls water movement and distribution in body fluid compartments by regulating the concentration of fluid in each compartment. When solutes such as electrolytes are added to water, the volume is expanded to include both the water and the solutes.

The osmolality of intracellular fluid and extracellular fluid tends to equalize because of the constant shifting of water. A change in osmolality of intracellular fluid affects the osmolality of extracellular fluid, and vice versa. The osmolality of intracellular fluid is maintained primarily by potassium, and the osmolality of the extracellular fluid is maintained primarily by sodium. The normal range of osmolality of the body fluids is between 280 and 294 milliosmoles per kilogram (mOsm/kg). You will see the term *osmolarity* also used to refer to the concentration of particles in body water. Osmolarity refers to the concentration of particles per liter of solution. For the study of body fluids, it is more practical to measure liters of fluid than kilograms. Therefore you will see clinical studies of fluids using the term *osmolarity* rather than osmolality.

REGULATORY MECHANISMS

Regulation of fluid balance requires the constant adjustment of fluid volume, distribution, and composition. This process is accomplished by the kidneys and circulatory system, which are influenced by the sympathetic nervous system, specific hormones, and the thirst center.

KIDNEYS

The kidneys are the main regulators of fluid balance. They control extracellular fluid by adjusting the concentration of specific electrolytes, the osmolality of body fluids, the volume of extracellular fluid, blood volume, and pH. Kidney function is delicately controlled by hormones and other coordinating mechanisms (see Chapter 38 for a review of renal structure and function).

The nephron is the functioning unit of the kidney. Each nephron is made up of a glomerulus and tubules. The glomerulus is the filtering portion of the nephron, and the tubule is responsible for secretion and reabsorption. The nephrons conduct the work of the kidney through the processes of filtration, reabsorption, and secretion.

Filtration

A primary activity of the kidney is filtration. Blood plasma entering the kidney via the renal artery is delivered to the glomerulus. About 20% of the plasma is filtered into the glomerular capsule. This fluid is called *filtrate.* Most of the remaining plasma leaves the kidney through the renal vein. The filtrate then moves through the tubules, where it is transformed into urine by the processes of tubular reabsorption and secretion.

Tubular Reabsorption

Tubular reabsorption is a process by which most of the glomerular filtrate is returned to the circulation. Water and selected solutes move from the tubules into the capillaries. Waste products remain in the tubules for excretion whereas most water and sodium is reabsorbed into the bloodstream. Tubular reabsorption is important for adjusting the volume and composition of the filtrate and for preventing excessive fluid loss through the kidneys.

Tubular Secretion

Tubular secretion is the last phase in the work of the kidneys. During this phase, the filtrate is transformed into urine. Various substances, among them drugs, hydrogen ions, potassium ions, creatinine, and histamine, pass from the blood into the tubules. This process eliminates some excess substances to maintain fluid and electrolyte balance, as well as metabolic waste products.

HORMONES

Hormones that have a major effect on fluid volume and balance are renin, aldosterone, antidiuretic hormone, and atrial natriuretic factor. *Renin* is a hormone that is secreted when blood volume or blood pressure falls. Renin activates angiotensinogen, a substance secreted by the liver, to form angiotensin I. Angiotensin-converting enzyme then converts angiotensin I to angiotensin II. Angiotensin II is a potent vasoconstrictor that also stimulates the release of aldosterone with subsequent sodium and water retention.

Aldosterone is released by the adrenal glands in response to the hormone renin. Aldosterone acts on the kidney tubules to increase the reabsorption of sodium and decrease the reabsorption of potassium. Because the retention of sodium causes water retention, aldosterone acts as a volume regulator. The release of aldosterone from the adrenal gland is stimulated by many factors, including increased potassium levels and decreased sodium levels in the blood.

Antidiuretic hormone (ADH) is produced by the hypothalamus and is secreted into the general circulation by the posterior pituitary gland. It causes the capillaries to reabsorb more water, so that urine is more concentrated and less volume is excreted. An increase in plasma osmolality (plasma is more concentrated) stimulates the release of ADH into the bloodstream to replenish needed fluid in the body. Other factors that stimulate the release of ADH are related to stress situations such as hypotension, pain, surgery, and the use of certain medications.

Atrial natriuretic factor (ANF) is a hormone released by the atria in response to stretching of the atria by increased blood volume. ANF stimulates excretion of sodium and water by the kidneys, decreased synthesis of renin, decreased release of aldosterone, and vasodilation. The effect of these actions is to reduce blood volume and to lower blood pressure.

THIRST

An additional regulatory mechanism is thirst, which regulates fluid intake. Increased plasma osmolality stimulates osmoreceptors in the hypothalamus to trigger the sensation of thirst. In other words, more sodium and less water in the body make a person thirsty. Additional fluids are consumed, and the kidneys conserve water until plasma osmolality returns to normal.

FLUID GAINS AND LOSSES

In a healthy adult, the 24-hour fluid intake and output are approximately equal (Table 13-3). Fluids are gained by drinking and eating and are lost through the kidneys, skin, lungs, and gastrointestinal tract. The usual adult urine volume is between 1 and 2 liters per day (L/day), or 1 milliliter per kilogram of body weight per hour. In the kidneys, water loss varies largely with the amount of solute excreted and with the level of antidiuretic hormone.

Water and electrolyte (Na^+, Cl^-, K^+) losses through the skin occur by sweating. Water loss through the lungs occurs by evaporation at a rate of 300 to 400 ml/day. In a hot, dry environment, water loss via the skin and lungs increases. In the gastrointestinal tract, the usual loss of fluid is about 100 to 200 ml/day. The bulk of fluid secreted into the GI tract is

table 13-3 *24-Hour Intake and Output of Body Fluids*

FLUID GAINS	AMOUNT (ml)	FLUID LOSSES	AMOUNT (ml)
Liquids	1,000	Lungs	400
Food (solid)	1,200	Skin	400
H_2O of oxidation	300	Kidneys (urine)	1,500
		Intestines (feces)	200
Daily total intake	2,500	Daily total output	2,500

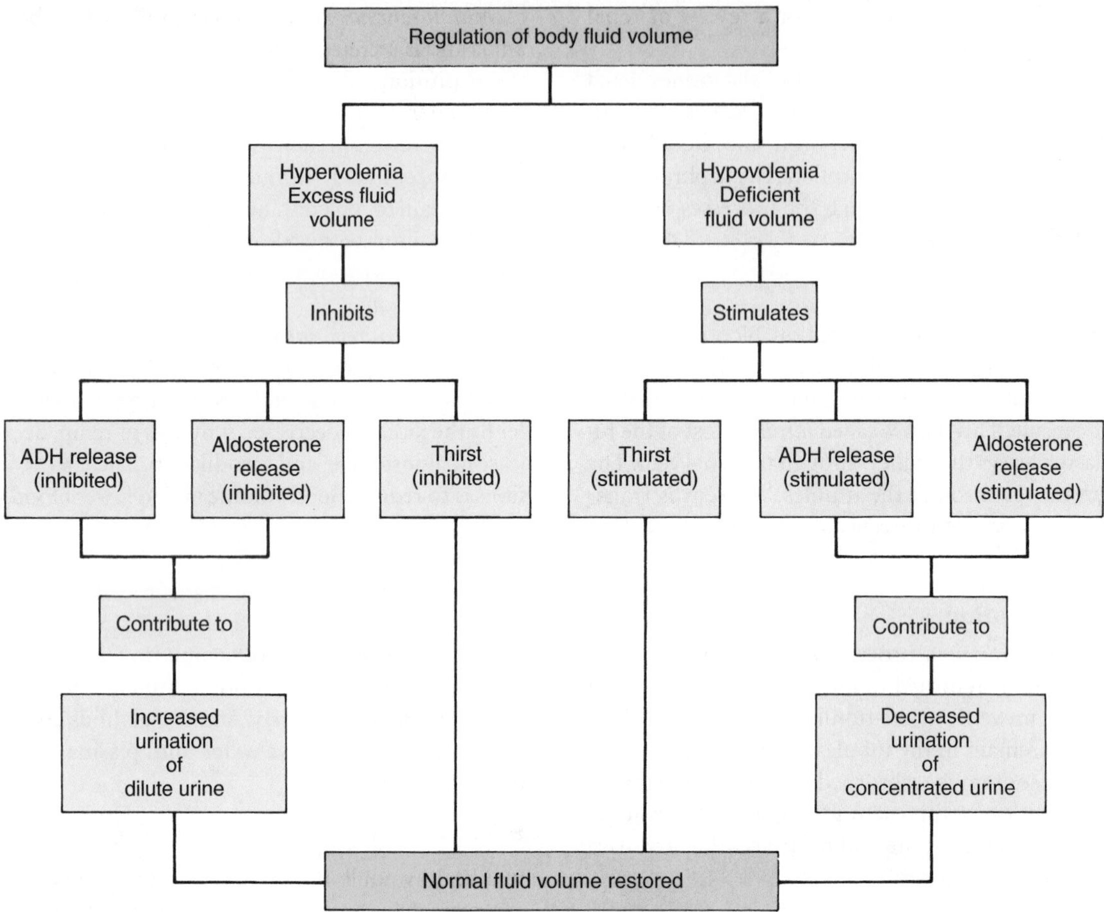

FIGURE **13-1** Regulation of body fluid volume depends on aldosterone, antidiuretic hormone (ADH), and thirst.

reabsorbed in the small intestine. Figure 13-1 diagrams the regulation of body fluid volume.

AGE-RELATED CHANGES AFFECTING FLUID BALANCE

Multiple factors place the older person at risk for fluid and electrolyte imbalances. The aging kidney is slower to adjust to changes in acid-base, fluid, and electrolyte balance. The older adult often has a reduced sense of thirst and therefore may be in a state of chronic dehydration because of inadequate fluid intake. Total body water declines with age, with the greatest loss being from the intracellular fluid compartment. Therefore an older person has limited reserves with which to maintain fluid balance when abnormal losses occur.

You must monitor fluid status in the elderly and be alert to the consequences of imbalances, including disorientation, confusion, constipation, and falls resulting from postural hypotension. The health history may reveal many chronic conditions, such as heart failure and renal insufficiency, which are more common among the elderly and place them at risk for fluid and electrolyte imbalances. Drugs such as antihypertensives, diuretics, and antacids used to treat these and other conditions can also contribute to imbalances. In addition, chronic conditions that affect mobility or mental status may interfere with adequate fluid intake. Some of the contributors to acute fluid deficits are trauma, infection, fever, flu or cold, and drug therapies (diuretics, antidepressants, sedatives). In addition to the general assessment data , it is especially important to evaluate fluid intake patterns, medications, mental status, and recent weight loss (see Table 13-7).

Components of the physical examination are described later in this chapter. Note that skin turgor is a less reliable indicator of fluid status in older persons than in younger individuals because there is normally some loss of skin elasticity with increased age. It is better to assess turgor on the sternum or forehead for better accuracy in the elderly. Serum electrolytes should be the same for all adults, so any abnormalities of such in the older person should be investigated.

Unless contraindicated, fluid requirements for older adults, based on ideal body weight, are 30 ml/kg in persons aged 55 to 65 years and 25 ml/kg in persons aged 65 years and over. Using these guidelines, a 60-year-old person who weighs 150 lb (68.1 kg) would need 2,000 ml of fluid daily. A person the same weight at age 70 would require 1,700 ml of fluid per day for adequate hydration.

ASSESSMENT OF FLUID AND ELECTROLYTE BALANCE

ASSESSMENT

Health History

Obtain a complete health history to determine whether patients have any conditions that may contribute to fluid or electrolyte imbalances. Anticipate fluid and electrolyte imbalances in patients who are at risk. Examples of conditions that have great potential for disrupting fluid balance are vomiting, diarrhea, kidney diseases, diabetes, salicylate poisoning, burns, congestive heart failure, cerebral injuries, ulcerative colitis, and hormonal imbalances. Other risk factors include the intake of drugs such as diuretics and cathartics and medical interventions such as gastric suctioning. Patient complaints of fatigue, palpitations, dizziness, edema, muscle weakness or cramps, dyspnea, and confusion are examples of signs and symptoms that may be associated with fluid imbalances. Because electrolyte disturbances produce nonspecific symptoms, they can be confirmed only with laboratory tests.

Vital Signs

Assessment of pulse, respiration, temperature, and blood pressure can detect indicators of changes in both fluid and electrolyte balance (Table 13-4). Body temperature variations can be associated with fluid volume excess or deficit. Also, fever poses a risk of water and electrolyte loss associated with sweating and an increased metabolic rate. The pulse rate and quality may change in response to blood volume alterations. Because electrolytes affect the conduction of impulses, electrolyte changes can affect heart rate and rhythm. Blood pressure is directly related to blood volume. Respirations are minimally affected by electrolyte changes. However, rapid respirations increase water loss. Also, fluid volume excess can lead to heart failure and pulmonary edema with shortness of breath. Measuring blood pressure with the patient lying, sitting, and standing can detect positional differences that may reflect inadequate blood volume.

Intake and Output

It is essential to maintain an accurate record of intake and output to be confident that the patient's intake is equal to output (Table 13-5). All fluids entering or leaving the body should be noted. A changing urine output may reflect a problem that causes fluid disturbances, or it may reflect attempts by the kidneys to maintain or restore balance. In addition to volume, urine characteristics give clues to fluid balance. Clear, pale urine in a healthy person suggests the excretion of excess water, whereas darker, concentrated urine indicates the kidneys are retaining water.

Body Weight

Measurement of body weight is a good indicator of fluid loss or retention (Table 13-6). Remember that 1 liter of fluid weighs 2.2 lb. Therefore retention of 1 liter of fluid is reflected as a weight gain of 2.2 lb (1 kg). A patient can accumulate up

table 13-4 ***Vital Sign Changes with Fluid and Electrolyte Imbalances***

PULSE

Increased pulse occurs with volume excess, sodium excess, or magnesium deficit.

Decreased pulse occurs with magnesium excess.

Weak, irregular, and rapid pulse suggests severe potassium excess or sodium deficit.

Bounding pulse occurs in volume excess, which often results in circulatory overload.

RESPIRATION

Fluid volume excess can cause pulmonary edema with dyspnea and tachypnea.

Changes in respiratory function are also noted with acid-base imbalances. Slow, shallow respirations with intermittent periods of apnea occur in severe metabolic alkalosis. Deep, rapid respirations indicate metabolic acidosis.

TEMPERATURE

Fever increases the metabolic rate, causing fluid loss. It also increases the respiratory rate, which results in loss of water vapor from the lungs.

Temperature may be subnormal with fluid volume excess.

BLOOD PRESSURE

A fall in systolic pressure of more than 20 mm Hg when the patient changes from the lying to the standing position or from the lying to the sitting position usually indicates fluid volume deficit.

Fluid volume excess that expands blood volume raises the blood pressure.

table 13-5 ***Assessment of Intake and Output***

Many serious fluid and electrolyte imbalances can be averted by carefully monitoring records of fluid intake and output.

If the total intake is substantially less than the total output, the patient is in danger of fluid volume deficit.

If the total intake is substantially more than the total output, the patient is in danger of fluid volume excess.

Intake should include all fluids taken into the body: oral fluids, foods that are liquid at room temperature, intravenous fluids, subcutaneous fluids, fluids instilled into drainage tubes or irrigants, tube feeding solutions, water given through feeding tubes, and enema solutions.

Output measures include urine, vomitus, diarrhea, drainage from fistulas, drainage from suction machines, excessive perspiration, and drainage from excisions; normal adult urine output is 40 to 80 ml/hr.

table 13-6 Assessment of Body Weight

The use of body weight as an accurate index of fluid balance is based on the assumption that the patient's dry weight remains relatively stable. Even under starvation conditions, an individual loses no more than ⅓ to ½ lb dry weight a day.

A rapid loss of body weight occurs when the total fluid intake is *less* than the total fluid output.

A rapid gain of body weight occurs when total fluid intake is *more* than the total fluid output.

	MILD	MODERATE	SEVERE
Rapid loss	2%	5%	8% = deficit
Rapid gain	2%	5%	8% = excess

Rapid gain or loss of 1 kg (2.2 lb) of body weight is approximately equivalent to the gain or loss of 1 liter of fluid.

to 10 lb (4.5 kg) of fluid before pitting edema is evident. You should weigh the patient daily on the same scale, at the same time of day, and wearing the same type of clothing.

Skin

Skin Characteristics

Skin color, moisture, turgor, and temperature all reflect fluid balance. Dry, flushed skin is associated with dehydration. Pale, cool, clammy skin is associated with the severe fluid volume deficit that occurs with shock. Moist, edematous tissue may be seen with fluid volume excess.

Facial Characteristics

The patient who is severely dehydrated usually has a pinched, drawn facial expression. Soft eyeballs and sunken eyes accompany a severe fluid volume deficit. Puffy eyelids and fuller cheeks suggest fluid volume excess.

Skin Turgor

Skin turgor is best measured by pinching the skin over the sternum, the inner aspects of the thighs, or the forehead. In patients who are dehydrated, skin flattens more slowly after the pinch is released. The term *tenting* is sometimes used to describe skin that does not flatten promptly after being gently pinched into a tent shape. The skin of older people generally has a slower return to normal, so it is inappropriate to assume a fluid deficit based only on poor skin turgor in the older person.

Edema

Edema reflects water and sodium retention, which can result from excessive reabsorption or inadequate secretion of sodium, as may occur with kidney failure. Inspect and palpate the skin for edema. Test for edema by pressing the skin that lies over the tibia, fibula, sacrum, or sternum. Edema is described as *pitting* if a depression remains in the tissue after pressure is applied with a fingertip. Pitting edema is evaluated on a four-point scale, ranging from 1+ edema (barely detectable pit) to 4+ edema (deep and persistent pit that is approximately 1 inch or 2.54 cm deep).

Edema can be so severe that pitting is not possible. The tissue becomes so full that fluid cannot be displaced. When edematous tissue feels hard, it is referred to as *brawny edema.* Following a radical mastectomy, brawny edema commonly occurs because the removal of axillary nodes causes fluid accumulation in the affected arm.

Mucous Membranes

Tongue Turgor

In a normal person the tongue has one longitudinal furrow. A person with fluid volume deficit has additional longitudinal furrows, and the tongue is smaller, as a result of fluid loss. Sodium excess causes the tongue to appear red and swollen.

Moisture of the Oral Cavity

A dry mouth may be the result of fluid volume deficit or mouth breathing. Normally, there is a pool of saliva in the area where the cheek and the gum meet. Dryness in this area usually indicates a true fluid volume deficit. However, dry mouth is a common side effect of many medications.

Veins

The appearance of the jugular veins in the neck and the veins in the hands can suggest either a fluid volume deficit or a fluid volume excess.

Neck Vein Distention

Distention of the jugular veins can indicate fluid volume excess. Inspect the neck veins for fluid volume excess by having the patient recline with the head of the bed elevated at a 30- to 45-degree angle. If the jugular veins can be seen more than 3 cm above the sternal angle, then fluid volume excess is most likely present.

Fluid volume deficit may be detected by examining the jugular neck veins with the patient lying down. If no distention occurs, then fluid volume deficit is most likely present.

Hand Veins

Observation of hand veins also can be helpful in evaluating the patient's fluid volume. First elevate the hands and then note how long it takes for the veins to empty. Veins usually empty in 3 to 5 seconds. Next place the hands in a dependent position and note how long it takes for the veins to fill. Veins usually fill in 3 to 5 seconds. If the volume is decreased, veins take longer than 3 to 5 seconds to fill. When the fluid volume is increased, veins take longer than 3 to 5 seconds to empty.

The nursing assessment of fluid and electrolyte status is summarized in Table 13-7.

DIAGNOSTIC TESTS AND PROCEDURES

A variety of laboratory tests may be performed to assess fluid and electrolyte status and to determine whether they are within the normal range (Table 13-8).

Urine Studies

Urine pH

The kidneys can change the acidity or alkalinity of the urine by excreting hydrogen (H^+) ions. Urine pH is a measure of hydrogen ions in the urine. It is useful for determining whether the kidneys are responding appropriately to meta-

table 13-7 **ASSESSMENT *of Fluid and Electrolyte Status***

HEALTH HISTORY	PHYSICAL EXAMINATION
Present Illness: Vomiting, diarrhea, burns, head injury **Past Medical History:** Renal or cardiac disease, diabetes, inflammatory bowel disease, adrenal or thyroid disease **Current Drugs:** Such as diuretics, salicylates, antacids, potassium supplements **Family History:** Diabetes, cardiac disease **Review of Systems:** Fatigue, palpitations, dizziness, edema, dyspnea, confusion **Functional Assessment:** Change in activity tolerance, mental alertness	**General Survey:** Alertness, orientation, posture **Vital Signs:** Pulse rate/rhythm; respiratory rate/pattern; blood pressure in lying, sitting, and standing positions; temperature **Weight:** Present compared to usual **Skin:** Color, moisture, turgor, temperature **Facial Characteristics:** Expression, firmness of eyeballs, edema of eyelids or cheeks **Edema:** Presence, location, pitting or brawny **Mucous Membranes:** Tongue turgor, moisture of the oral cavity **Veins:** Jugular vein distention, hand vein emptying and refilling time

table 13-8 ***Normal Values Related to Fluid and Electrolyte Balance***

URINE		BLOOD	
Urine pH	4.5-8.	Arterial blood pH	7.35-7.55
Urine specific gravity	1.010-1.025	Serum osmolality	280-294 mOsm/kg
Urine osmolality	250-900 mOsm/kg H_2O	Serum sodium	136-145 mEq/L
Urine sodium	75-200 mEq/L or 27-287 mmol/24 hr	Serum potassium	3.5-5.1 mEq/L
		Serum chloride	98-107 mEq/L
Urine potassium	25-123 mEq/24 hr	Serum phosphorus	2.7-4.5 mg/dL
Urine chloride	110-250 mEq/24 hr	Serum magnesium	1.5-2.5 mEq/L
Urine phosphorus	0.4-1.3 g/24 hr	Serum calcium	9.0-11.0 mEq/L
Urine magnesium	6.0-8.5 mEq/24 hr	Serum creatinine	0.6-1.5 mg/dL
		Serum bicarbonate	
		Arterial	21-28 mEq/L
		Venous	22-29 mEq/L

From Jaffe, M. S., & McVan, B. F. (1997). *Davis's laboratory and diagnostic handbook.* Philadelphia: Davis; Jacobs, D.S., DeMott, W. R., Grady, H. J., Horvat, R. T., Huestis, D. W., & Kasten, B. L. (1996). *Laboratory Test Handbook.* Hudson (Cleveland): Lexi-Comp, Inc.; and Heitz, U. E., & Horne, M. M. (2001) *Fluid, electrolyte, and acid-base balance.* St. Louis: Mosby.

bolic acid-base imbalances. The normal range is 4.5 to 8.0; however, fresh urine is usually acidic (about 6.0). Urine tends to be most acidic in the morning (following a fast), and more alkaline after meals. Diet is a factor in that a person who consumes large amounts of citrus fruits and vegetables tends to have alkaline urine, whereas a person who eats a lot of meat tends to have acidic urine. A urine specimen that is not tested within 4 hours of collection may become alkaline. Therefore urine pH should be measured within 1 to 2 hours of collection. If the specimen cannot be tested promptly, it should be refrigerated.

Urine Specific Gravity

Urine specific gravity (SpG) is a measure of urine concentration. In most instances, normal urine specific gravity is between 1.010 and 1.025 in adults.

Specific gravity is a good indicator of fluid balance. A high specific gravity indicates that the urine is highly concentrated, usually as a result of fluid volume deficit. A low specific gravity indicates that the urine contains a large amount of water in relation to solutes, usually as a result of fluid volume excess. The specific gravity also reflects renal function. If the kidneys are not functioning properly, they may fail to concentrate or dilute urine as needed to maintain extracellular fluid balance. The presence of x-ray dyes, glucose, or protein in the urine can cause an increased specific gravity that may be misleading; that is, the patient may not really have a fluid volume deficit. As people age, their kidneys are less efficient at conserving water by concentrating urine. Therefore the older person may produce relatively dilute urine (low or normal specific gravity) even when he or she is dehydrated.

Urine Osmolality

Osmolality measures the number of dissolved particles in a solution. This provides a more precise measurement of the kidney's ability to concentrate urine than does the specific gravity. The normal urine osmolality range is 250 to 900 mOsm/kg H_2O. For the most accurate interpretation, a serum osmolality should be done simultaneously.

Dilute urine has a low osmolality and generally reflects renal excretion of excess water. Low osmolality also is apparent when kidneys are unable to conserve water by concentrating urine. Concentrated urine has a high osmolality and generally indicates renal conservation of water. It also can be present when the kidneys are failing, because the volume of urine secreted declines.

Urine Creatinine Clearance

Urine creatinine clearance tests are used to detect glomerular damage in the kidney. A 24-hour specimen is required. The patient is instructed to void, discard the specimen, record the time, and start collecting all urine thereafter for 24 hours. The specimen must be refrigerated.

During the specimen collection period, the patient should maintain good hydration, should not engage in vigorous exercise, and should avoid high-protein foods, coffee, tea, or cola drinks. Be aware that many drugs, including cephalosporins, can alter test results. For best interpretation, serum creatinine clearance should be done as well. Also, the laboratory needs to know the patient's height, weight, and age. The normal creatinine clearance for adult males is 85 to 125 ml/min/1.73 m^2 of body surface area; for females, it is 75 to 115 ml/min/1.73 m^2 of body surface area. The range decreases with age.

Urine Sodium

Urine sodium reflects sodium intake and fluid volume status. A high sodium intake results in increased sodium excretion in the urine. When large amounts of fluids are taken in or sodium intake is restricted, the urine is more dilute, so the urine sodium falls. The urinary excretion of sodium is normally highest during the day. The normal urine sodium is 75 to 200 mEq/L. If collected over a period of 24 hours, the normal range is 27 to 287 mmol/24 hr.

Urine Potassium

Urine potassium is a measure of renal tubular function. A 24-hour specimen is most meaningful because the urinary excretion of potassium is highest at night and lowest during the day. Therefore a random sample would not truly represent function of the renal tubules. The normal value is 25 to 123 mmol/24 hr.

Blood Studies

Serum Hematocrit

The hematocrit is the percentage of blood volume that is composed of red blood cells. An increased hematocrit is seen with fluid volume deficit and dehydration because the blood is more concentrated. A low hematocrit is consistent with fluid volume excess because of dilution. The normal range for hematocrit is 40% to 54% for adult men and 38% to 47% for adult women.

Serum Creatinine

Creatinine is a metabolic waste product. The serum level is a better indicator of renal function than the blood urea nitrogen. A high level of creatinine in the blood indicates poor renal function. The normal range is 0.6 to 1.5 mg/dL. Even small changes in the serum creatinine can be significant.

Blood Urea Nitrogen

Blood urea nitrogen (BUN) provides a measure of renal function. Normal is 8 to 20 mg/dL. A high BUN is associated with fluid volume deficit and possibly impaired renal function; conversely, a low BUN is associated with fluid volume excess.

Serum Osmolality

Serum osmolality is a measure of blood concentration. High serum osmolality is related to a fluid volume deficit, and low serum osmolality is related to fluid volume excess. The normal range is 280 to 294 mOsm/kg.

Serum Albumin

Albumin is a plasma protein that helps maintain blood volume by creating colloid osmotic pressure. The normal range for serum albumin is 3.5 to 5.5 g/dL. Low serum albumin allows water to shift into the interstitial compartment, which reduces blood volume and creates edema.

Serum Electrolytes

Normal values for serum sodium, potassium, chloride, and calcium are shown in Table 13-8.

FLUID IMBALANCES

FLUID VOLUME DEFICITS

A fluid volume deficit occurs when there is less water than normal in the body. There are two types of fluid volume deficits: isotonic extracellular fluid deficit (hypovolemia) and hypertonic extracellular fluid deficit (dehydration). A fluid volume deficit may result from decreased intake, abnormal fluid losses, or both. Examples of abnormal fluid losses are the loss of water as a result of excessive bleeding, severe vomiting and diarrhea, and severe burns.

The signs and symptoms of fluid volume deficit vary depending on how suddenly the deficit develops and how severe it is. Symptoms are not as apparent with deficits that are mild and have a gradual onset, but the symptoms are quite dramatic when the loss is severe and the onset is abrupt. In general the body attempts to compensate for fluid volume deficits by decreasing urine output. The heart rate increases in an effort to maintain blood flow to body tissues. The blood pressure may fall because of the reduced blood volume.

Nursing care varies somewhat according to the cause of a fluid volume deficit and the severity of symptoms. Care should be based on appropriate nursing diagnoses, which might include:

- **Deficient Fluid Volume, Risk for Deficient Fluid Volume** related to inadequate fluid intake, excessive fluid loss, high blood glucose, inadequate antidiuretic hormone production or effect, high fever, altered capillary permeability
- **Acute Confusion** related to decreased cerebral tissue perfusion
- **Constipation** related to excessive reabsorption of water from stool in the colon
- **Fatigue** related to decreased blood volume, decreased tissue perfusion
- **Hyperthermia** related to infectious process, decreased fluid volume
- **Risk for Injury** related to decreased level of consciousness
- **Risk for Impaired Skin Integrity** related to poor tissue turgor

- **Ineffective Tissue Perfusion** related to decreased cardiac output secondary to decreased blood volume

The characteristics, causes, assessment findings, treatment, and nursing care for each type of fluid volume deficit are outlined in Table 13-9.

FLUID VOLUME EXCESSES

An increase in body water is called *fluid volume excess.* The two types of fluid volume excess are extracellular fluid excess (isotonic fluid excess) and intracellular water excess (hypotonic fluid excess). Fluid volume excess may result from renal or cardiac failure with retention of fluid, increased production of antidiuretic hormone or aldosterone, overload with isotonic intravenous fluids, or the administration of dextrose 5% in water (D_5W) after surgery or trauma. The body attempts to compensate for fluid volume excess by increasing the filtration and excretion of sodium and water by the kidneys and decreasing the production of antidiuretic hormone.

As with fluid volume deficit, the severity of the symptoms in fluid volume excess depends on how quickly the condition develops. Severe fluid volume excess can cause or aggravate heart failure and pulmonary edema.

Nursing care varies somewhat according to the cause of a fluid volume excess and the severity of symptoms. Care should be based on appropriate nursing diagnoses, which might include:

- **Excess Fluid Volume** related to fluid retention, excess or hypotonic intravenous fluid administration

table 13-9 ***Fluid Volume Deficit***

	ISOTONIC EXTRACELLULAR FLUID DEFICIT (Hypovolemia)	HYPERTONIC EXTRACELLULAR FLUID DEFICIT (Dehydration)
DEFINITION	Deficiency of both water and relative electrolytes	Deficiency of water without electrolyte deficiency
ETIOLOGY	Decreased fluid intake related to inability to obtain or ingest fluids Excessive fluid loss related to vomiting, diarrhea Shifting of fluid into interstitial space (third spacing) related to increased capillary permeability	Increased water loss related to blood glucose, as in uncontrolled diabetes mellitus, inadequate ADH production or renal response to ADH, high fever, excessive sweating Decreased fluid intake with continued intake of electrolytes, as with concentrated tube feedings
ASSESSMENT FINDINGS		
Blood pressure	Hypotension	Hypotension
Pulse	Weak, rapid	Weak, rapid
Respirations	Rapid	Rapid
Temperature	Decreased	Increased
Weight	Loss	Loss
Tissue turgor	Normal or edema	Poor
Mucous membranes	Moist	Dry
Blood cells	Hgb, Hct, RBCs increased	Hgb, Hct, RBCs increased
Urine output	Decreased	Decreased or increased
Thirst		Thirsty
TREATMENT	Correct underlying cause; replace water and electrolytes.	Correct underlying cause; replace water.
NURSING CARE	Give antiemetics, antidiarrheals as ordered. Document effects. Give oral and intravenous fluids as ordered. Protect edematous tissue with third spacing. Assist with rising and ambulating if patient is dizzy. Keep hourly records of intake and output: expect intake to exceed output at first. Be alert for fluid excess (rising pulse and blood pressure, dyspnea) caused by excessive fluid replacement.	Monitor blood glucose if patient has diabetes. Give oral and intravenous fluids as ordered. Give hypoglycemics, ADH, antipyretics as ordered. Assist with oral hygiene. Assist with rising and ambulating if patient is dizzy. Keep hourly records of intake and output: expect intake to exceed output at first. Be alert for fluid excess (rising pulse and blood pressure, dyspnea) caused by excessive fluid replacement.

ADH, Antidiuretic hormone; *Hgb*, hemoglobin; *Hct*, hematocrit; *RBCs*, red blood cells.

table 13-10 ***Fluid Volume Excess***

	EXTRACELLULAR FLUID EXCESS (Isotonic Fluid Excess)	INTRACELLULAR WATER EXCESS (Hypotonic Fluid Excess)
DESCRIPTION	Excess of both water and electrolytes. Major symptoms are due to increased blood volume.	Excess of body water without excess electrolytes. Major symptoms are due to cerebral edema.
ETIOLOGY	Retention of water and electrolytes related to kidney disease; overload with isotonic IV fluids.	Overhydration in presence of renal failure; administration of D_5W after surgery or trauma.
ASSESSMENT FINDINGS		
Blood pressure	Increased	Increased systolic
Pulse	Bounding, increased rate	Decreased rate
Respirations	Increased rate, crackles, dyspnea	Increased rate
Weight	Gain	Gain
Edema	Extremities: dependent, pitting Puffy eyelids	Cerebral
Neck veins	Distended	Normal
Mucous membranes	Moist	Moist
Blood	Hgb, Hct, RBCs decreased by dilution	Hgb, Hct, RBCs normal or decreased
Mental status	Irritability, confusion, lethargy	Irritability, confusion, lethargy
Hand vein engorgement	Present	Absent
Pupils	Sluggish response to light with cerebral edema	Sluggish response to light with cerebral edema
TREATMENT	Correct underlying cause. Restrict water and sodium intake. Give diuretics to promote fluid elimination, digitalis to improve cardiac output. Consider renal dialysis if kidney failure is a factor.	Correct underlying cause. Restrict water intake. Give intravenous oral fluids with electrolytes. Give demeclocycline (Declomycin) to decrease kidney response to ADH.
NURSING CARE	Give drugs and IV fluids as ordered. Monitor for excess diuresis. Explain and enforce fluid restriction. Offer ice chips; use small fluid containers, let patient help design plan for fluid intake. If patient not confused, allow to swish fluids in mouth and spit out without swallowing. Explain salt restriction; obtain dietary consult for teaching (Table 13-11). Protect edematous tissue: turn and reposition q2 hr. Inspect for signs of skin breakdown. If dyspneic: head of bed elevated 30 degrees or for comfort, loosen restrictive clothing, oxygen as ordered.	Give drugs and IV fluids as ordered. Explain and enforce fluid restriction. Offer ice chips, provide oral hygiene, serve only fluids allowed with meal trays, let patient design plan for fluid intake. If patient not confused, allow to swish fluids in mouth and spit out without swallowing. If confused, take safety precautions: side rails up, bed in low position, call light in reach, check often. Seizure precautions per agency policy.

IV, Intravenous; *D_5W,* dextrose 5% in water; *Hgb,* hemoglobin; *Hct,* hematocrit; *RBCs,* red blood cells.

- **Acute Confusion, Disturbed Thought Processes** related to cerebral edema
- **Activity Intolerance, Impaired Gas Exchange** related to pulmonary edema
- **Risk for Injury** related to decreased level of consciousness
- **Risk for Impaired Skin Integrity** related to edema
- **Impaired Tissue Perfusion** related to reduced cardiac output with heart failure

The causes, assessment findings, treatment, and nursing care of the patient with fluid volume excess are outlined in Table 13-10.

ELECTROLYTE IMBALANCES

The two electrolytes that cause the majority of problems when there is an imbalance are sodium (Na^+) and potassium (K^-).

HYPONATREMIA (SODIUM DEFICIT)

Hyponatremia is lower than normal sodium in the blood serum. It can be an actual deficiency of sodium or an increase in body water that dilutes the sodium excessively. Causes include excessive intake of water without sodium; excessive loss of sodium, as with vomiting, diarrhea, or diaphoresis with only water replacement; the use of distilled water to irrigate body cavities; and excessive secretion of antidiuretic hormone (ADH). Increased antidiuretic hormone secretion is associated with severe stress, some head injuries, and a condition called *syndrome of inappropriate antidiuretic hormone secretion (SIADH)*. Other disorders that put the patient at risk for hyponatremia include congestive heart failure, liver cirrhosis, and nephrotic syndrome.

Sodium normally holds water in the extracellular compartment. When serum sodium is low, water can enter cells more freely. This shift of fluids is most significant in relation to brain cells. The accumulation of fluid in brain cells produces the most important physiologic effects of hyponatremia.

Assessment

If hyponatremia is suspected or the patient is at risk, monitor for signs and symptoms, which include headache, muscle weakness, fatigue, apathy, confusion, abdominal cramps, and orthostatic hypotension. Take blood pressures with the patient lying or sitting and then standing to determine whether there is a significant drop. A drop in systolic blood pressure of more than 20 mm Hg indicates orthostatic hypotension.

Medical Treatment

The usual treatment for hyponatremia is restriction of fluids while the kidneys excrete excess water. Intravenous normal saline or Ringer's lactate may be ordered. If sodium falls below 115 mEq/L, hypertonic sodium may be ordered. The diuretic furosemide (Lasix) may be ordered because of its ability to promote water loss that exceeds the sodium loss. If the patient has SIADH, drugs such as demeclocycline and lithium that antagonize antidiuretic hormone may be ordered. A balanced diet usually provides adequate sodium, but patients with moderate or severe hyponatremia may need sodium replacement therapy.

NURSING CARE

You can help prevent hyponatremia in patients with feeding tubes by using normal saline rather than water for irrigation. For patients with hyponatremia, administer prescribed medications and intravenous fluids and monitor the response to these. Measure fluid intake and output and assess mental status. If the patient is confused, take safety measures to prevent injury. If the patient who has hyponatremia has low blood pressure or postural hypotension, assess the need for assistance with ambulation.

HYPERNATREMIA (SODIUM EXCESS)

Hypernatremia refers to a higher than normal concentration of sodium in the blood. It is a very serious imbalance that can lead to death if not corrected. Hypernatremia can occur alone or in combination with extracellular fluid volume deficit. The high level of sodium in the serum and other extracellular fluids causes water to shift out of the cells. This creates a condition of cellular dehydration. Hypernatremia occurs when there is excessive loss of water or excessive retention of sodium. Some causes of hypernatremia are vomiting, diarrhea, diaphoresis (profuse sweating), and insufficient antidiuretic hormone. Signs and symptoms of hypernatremia are thirst, a flushed skin, dry mucous membranes, a low urine output, restlessness, an increased heart rate, convulsions, and postural hypotension.

table 13-11 *Common Food Sources of Sodium*

FOODS HIGH IN SODIUM (Approximately 250 mg per Serving)	FOODS LOW IN SODIUM (Less than 50 mg per Serving)
Grains	**Fruits and Vegetables**
Cold cereal, 1 oz	Fresh fruits or canned, ½ cup
Corn chips, 14 chips	Fresh, frozen, ½ cup
Instant hot cereal, ½ cup	**Grains**
Potato chips, 14 chips	Unsalted pastas, ½ cup
Cheeses	Oatmeal, cooked, 1 cup
Natural cheese, 1 oz	Popcorn (unsalted), 1 oz
Processed cheese, 1 oz	Puffed rice, 1 cup
Creamed cheese, ½ cup	Shredded wheat, 1 biscuit
Meats	**Meats**
Sausage, 1 oz	Fresh meat, 1 oz
Luncheon meats, 1 oz	Fresh chicken, 1 oz
Frankfurters, 1 oz	Fresh fish, 1 oz
Cooked bacon, 2 slices	
Ham, 1 oz	
Convenience Foods	
Pizza, 2 to 3 slices	
Pot pies, 8 oz	
Ravioli, canned, 8 oz	
Convenience Foods—cont'd	
Soups (canned or dehydrated), 1 cup	

Data from Laquarta, I., & Gerlach, M. (1990). *Nutrition in clinical nursing*. Albany, NY: Delmar Publishers; and Burtis, G., et al. (1988). *Applied nutrition and diet therapy*. Philadelphia: Saunders. From Black, J. M., & Matassarin-Jacobs, E. (1997). *Medical-surgical nursing: Clinical management for continuity of care* (5th ed., p. 288). Philadelphia: Saunders.

Medical Treatment

Medical intervention focuses on oral or intravenous replacement of water to restore balance. The aim is to restore the fluid balance slowly to prevent cerebral edema resulting from excessive dilution of extracellular fluid. If the patient has an extracellular fluid volume deficit as well, intravenous fluids with decreasing amounts of sodium may be ordered. A low-sodium diet is often prescribed.

NURSING CARE

Encourage patients with hypernatremia to drink water for hydration. Closely monitor the infusion of intravenous fluids, especially when the patient's cardiac or renal function is abnormal. Patient education is important. Teach the patient with hypernatremia to track daily intake and output and to recognize the signs and symptoms of fluid retention or depletion. Advise patients accordingly if any dietary restrictions are part of the treatment. If a low-sodium diet is prescribed, patients should avoid foods that are high in sodium (Na^+): ketchup, monosodium glutamate (Accent), mustard, pickles, olives, ham, most canned foods, artificial sweeteners, laxatives, cough medications, and some antacids (Table 13-11). Salt substitutes can be used if potassium (K^+) intake is not restricted because salt substitutes contain significant potassium.

HYPOKALEMIA (POTASSIUM DEFICIT)

Hypokalemia is low serum potassium. Causes include vomiting, diarrhea, nasogastric suction, inadequate dietary intake of potassium, diabetic acidosis, excessive aldosterone secretion, and drugs such as potassium-wasting diuretics and corticosteroids. Because potassium is necessary for normal cellular function, deficiencies may result in gastrointestinal, renal, cardiovascular, and neurological disturbances. Most important is the effect on myocardial cells, which tends to cause abnormal, potentially fatal, heart rhythms.

Signs and symptoms of hypokalemia are anorexia, abdominal distention, vomiting, diarrhea, muscle cramps, weakness, dysrhythmias (abnormal cardiac rhythms), postural hypotension, dyspnea, shallow respirations, confusion, depression, polyuria (excessive urination), and nocturia.

Medical Treatment

Potassium replacement by the intravenous or oral route may be prescribed.

NURSING CARE

Assessment consists of monitoring at-risk patients for decreased bowel sounds, a weak and irregular pulse, decreased reflexes, and decreased muscle tone. It is especially important to monitor the heart rate and rhythm of patients taking digitalis, because hypokalemia increases the risk of digitalis toxicity. Cardiac monitors may be used to detect dysrhythmias.

Administer oral potassium supplements as prescribed. Give them with a full glass of water or fruit juice to avoid gastrointestinal irritation. Instruct patients to sip slowly. Encourage dietary sources of potassium, particularly fruits and vegetables, such as bananas and oranges or orange juice (Table 13-12).

Administer intravenous potassium as ordered. Potassium is *always* diluted and never given in concentrated form. It ideally is administered through a central venous catheter because the potassium may not be adequately diluted by blood before it reaches the heart. Monitor the infusion site because potassium salts can cause inflammation of the veins. Potassium is *never* given by intravenous push.

Check the patient's urine output before starting an intravenous infusion of potassium. When the urine output is low, intravenous fluids without potassium may be given until the urine output is acceptable, then fluids with potassium are started. If you were to administer the intravenous potassium before normal urinary output was restored, the patient could develop hyperkalemia. Urinary output should be no less than 30 ml/hr. If it is less than 30 ml/hr for 2 consecutive hours, alert the physician, who may order a stop of the infusion.

PHARMACOLOGY CAPSULE Potassium is always diluted before intravenous administration. Rapid infusion of potassium can cause cardiac arrest.

table 13-12 Common Food Sources of Potassium

FOODS HIGH IN POTASSIUM (Average 7 mEq per Serving)	FOODS LOW IN POTASSIUM (Average 3 mEq per Serving)
Vegetables (½ cup cooked or 1 cup raw)	**Vegetables**
Artichokes	Corn, ⅓ cup
Broccoli	Sweet potato, yams, ¼ cup
Brussels sprouts	Lima beans, ⅓ cup
Cabbage	French fried potatoes, 10
Carrots	**Fruit**
Celery	Apple, 1 small
Collards	Apple juice, ½ cup
Cucumber	Applesauce, ½ cup
Mushrooms	Blueberries, ¾ cup
Spinach	Cranberries, 1¼ cup
Tomatoes	**Beverages**
Fruits	Coffee, instant
Apricots, fresh, 4 medium	Cola
Apricots, canned, 4 halves	Cranberry juice cocktail, ⅓ cup
Apricots, dried, 7 halves	Ginger ale
Banana, 7 inches	Noncarbonated soft drinks
Cantaloupe, ¼ small	Root beer
Guava, 1 medium	Lemon-lime soda
Honeydew melon, ⅛ medium	
Nectarine, ½	
Orange, 1 small	
Prunes, 3 medium	
Strawberries, 1¼ cup	
Tangerines, 2 medium	
Watermelon, 1¼ cup	
Beverages	
Brewed coffee	
Tomato juice	
Vegetable juice cocktail, unsalted	

Data from Mahan, K. L., & Arlin, M. (1992). *Food, nutrition and diet therapy* (8th ed.). Philadelphia: Saunders. From Black, J. M., & Matassarin-Jacobs, E. (1997). *Medical-surgical nursing: Clinical management for continuity of care* (5th ed., p. 313). Philadelphia: Saunders.

HYPERKALEMIA (POTASSIUM EXCESS)

Hyperkalemia is high serum potassium. Potassium is plentiful in common foods, so it is easy for people on normal diets to take in adequate amounts. However, the kidneys do not readily conserve potassium, so continuous replacement is necessary. Patients at risk for hyperkalemia are those with decreased renal function, people in metabolic acidosis, and people taking potassium supplements. Also, patients who have had severe traumatic injuries may develop hyperkalemia because of the loss of potassium from damaged cells into the extracellular fluid.

Hyperkalemia is a serious imbalance because of the potential for life-threatening dysrhythmias. Elevated potassium typically causes first bradycardia, then tachycardia. There is a risk of cardiac arrest. In the gastrointestinal system, hyperkalemia can cause explosive diarrhea and vomiting. Neuromuscular effects are muscle cramps and weakness and paresthesia (a tingling sensation). Other signs and symptoms of hyperkalemia include irritability, anxiety, abdominal cramps, and decreased urine output.

Medical Treatment

Hyperkalemia is treated by correcting the underlying causes and restricting potassium intake. Polystyrene sulfonate (Kayexalate), a drug that can be given orally or rectally, promotes excretion of excess potassium through the intestinal tract. Intravenous calcium gluconate may be given to decrease the effects of potassium on the myocardium. Temporary effects may be obtained by the intravenous administration of insulin and glucose or sodium bicarbonate to promote the shifting of potassium into the cells.

NURSING CARE

Patients with low urine output or those taking potassium-sparing diuretics must be monitored carefully for signs and symptoms of hyperkalemia, because decreased renal function can cause hyperkalemia. Patients receiving potassium supplements, especially intravenously, warrant special attention. Carefully monitor the flow rate of intravenous fluids, which should not exceed 10 mEq/hr through peripheral veins. Even when extreme hypokalemia is being treated, no more than 40 mEq/hr should be given and *only* with constant cardiac monitoring. Examine the infusion site because potassium is very irritating to subcutaneous tissues. Extravasation can cause serious tissue damage.

Screen the results of laboratory studies. Because serum potassium levels greater than 5.0 mEq/L can cause cardiac arrest, immediately report the results to the physician and anticipate an order for the patient to be placed on cardiac monitoring.

Teach patients who take potassium supplements to look for signs and symptoms of abnormal potassium levels and to understand why frequent blood tests are required to monitor potassium levels.

CHLORIDE IMBALANCE

Because chloride is usually bound to other electrolytes, chloride imbalances accompany other electrolyte imbalances. High serum chloride, known as *hyperchloremia,* usually is associated with metabolic acidosis. Low serum chloride, known as *hypochloremia,* usually occurs when sodium is lost because chloride is most frequently bound with sodium. Hypochloremia may be caused by vomiting and uncontrolled diabetes.

CALCIUM IMBALANCE

Calcium in the blood is regulated by the parathyroid glands, which secrete parathyroid hormone (PTH). A low serum level of calcium (hypocalcemia) stimulates PTH secretion. PTH enhances calcium retention and phosphate excretion by the kidneys, promotes calcium absorption in the intestines, and can mobilize calcium from the bones to raise the serum level. Hypocalcemia results from diarrhea, inadequate dietary intake of calcium or vitamin D, and multiple blood transfusions (banked blood contains citrates that bind to calcium), in addition to some diseases including hypoparathyroidism. Hypercalcemia occurs with increased serum levels of calcium. Causes of hypercalcemia include a high calcium or vitamin D intake, hyperparathyroidism, and immobility that causes stores of calcium in the bones to enter the bloodstream. It is also a complication of certain types of cancer.

MAGNESIUM IMBALANCE

A lower than normal concentration of magnesium in the bloodstream is known as hypomagnesemia. Hypomagnesemia results from decreased gastrointestinal absorption or excessive gastrointestinal loss, usually from vomiting and diarrhea, or from increased urinary loss. Hypomagnesemia often is associated with hypocalcemia and hypokalemia.

A higher than normal concentration of magnesium in the bloodstream is known as hypermagnesemia. It occurs most often with the excessive use of magnesium-containing medications or intravenous solutions in patients with renal failure or preeclampsia of pregnancy.

ACID-BASE DISTURBANCES

Acid-base balance refers to homeostasis of the hydrogen ion (H^+) concentration in the body fluids. A solution containing a higher number of hydrogen ions is an *acid,* and a solution containing a lower number of hydrogen ions is an *alkaline* or *base.* The symbol used to indicate hydrogen ion concentration is pH. pH is reported on a scale of 1 to 14, with 1 to 6.9 being acidic, 7 being neutral, and 7.1 to 14 being alkaline.

The hydrogen ion concentration in extracellular fluid is indicated by the pH of the blood. The normal pH of blood is between 7.35 and 7.45, which is slightly alkaline. The normal acid-base balance is maintained by three primary, complex mechanisms: (1) buffers, (2) respiratory control of carbon dioxide (CO_2), and (3) renal regulation of bicarbonate (HCO_3^-). The principal buffers in renal tubular fluid are the carbonic acid/bicarbonate system, ammonia, and phosphate. Other substances that function as buffers are proteins and hemoglobin. Buffer systems comprise a weak acid and a salt. To maintain body fluids in the normal pH range, the blood buffers circulate throughout the body in pairs, acting as sponges to soak up hydrogen ions. One of the buffers takes away a hydrogen ion if a fluid is too acid, and one of the buffers gives an ion if the fluid is too alkaline.

The lungs and kidneys are the next line of defense after the blood buffers for maintaining acid-base balance. The lungs are primarily responsible for the regulation of carbon dioxide in the blood, which is controlled by the rate and depth of respirations. Carbonic acid in the alveolar capillaries breaks down into water and carbon dioxide, which is eliminated through exhalation. Deep, rapid breathing eliminates excess carbon dioxide, thereby reducing extracellular fluid acidity. Shallow, slow respirations reduce the loss of carbon dioxide, thereby increasing extracellular acidity. If the pH of the blood becomes too high or too low, the respiratory center in the brain sends signals to the lungs to increase or decrease respirations to "blow off" or retain the appropriate amount of carbon dioxide.

The kidneys act as the metabolic regulators of pH by excreting acids or bases as needed. Renal regulation of bicarbonate and excretion of hydrogen ions are the chief means of regulating acid-base balance through the kidneys. Bicarbonate is a major acid buffer in the blood, and it is through the kidneys that bicarbonate is reabsorbed and produced.

If the regulatory mechanisms fail, acid-base imbalances occur. The four major types of acid-base imbalances are (1) respiratory acidosis, (2) respiratory alkalosis, (3) metabolic acidosis, and (4) metabolic alkalosis.

ASSESSMENT OF ACID-BASE STATUS

Health History

Note any history of renal, endocrine, or respiratory disease. A history of diabetes mellitus is especially important because acidosis is a complication of diabetes. Assess the patient for symptoms of acid-base imbalance, which could include dyspnea, anxiety, confusion, dizziness, lightheadedness, seizures, and change in weight. List any medications the patient is taking.

Physical Examination

Observe the patient's general appearance in terms of responsiveness. Look for signs of anxiety or other distress. Take the vital signs and weigh the patient. Pay special attention to the rate, depth, and rhythm of respiration. Test muscle strength and sensory function in the extremities. Evaluate mental status.

In addition to collecting data during the nursing assessment (Table 13-13), note the results of arterial blood gas measurements (Table 13-14).

table 13-13 ASSESSMENT *of Acid-Base Balance*

HEALTH HISTORY

Signs and Symptoms: Dyspnea, anxiety, confusion, dizziness, seizures, changes in weight, muscle weakness, abnormal sensations (numbness, tingling)
Medical Conditions: Diabetes mellitus, adrenal disorders, cardiac disorders, renal failure, respiratory impairment
Current Medications

PHYSICAL EXAMINATION

Height and Weight: Compared to previous measurements
Vital Signs: Pulse rate and rhythm; respiratory rate, depth, and rhythm
Neurological Function: Muscle strength, sensation in extremities, mental status

MEASURES OF OYXGENATION

Arterial blood gases

table 13-14 *Arterial Blood Gas Values with Uncompensated Respiratory and Metabolic Acidosis and Alkalosis*

CONDITION	CAUSE	pH	HCO_3^-	Pa_{CO_2}
Respiratory acidosis	Hypoventilation	↓	Normal	↑
Respiratory alkalosis	Hyperventilation	↑	Normal	↓
Metabolic acidosis	Diabetic ketoacidosis Lactic acidosis Diarrhea Renal insufficiency	↓	↓	Normal
Metabolic alkalosis	Vomiting HCO_3^- retention Volume depletion K^+ depletion	↑	↑	Normal

RESPIRATORY ACIDOSIS

Respiratory acidosis occurs when the respiratory system fails to eliminate the appropriate amount of carbon dioxide to maintain the normal acid-base balance. Carbon dioxide is retained, with a resultant accumulation of carbonic acid and a decrease in blood pH. The body responds to respiratory acidosis by stimulating respirations to eliminate excess carbon dioxide. If that mechanism cannot restore balance, renal compensation begins. The kidneys attempt to help by reabsorbing more bicarbonate to balance the amount of carbonic acid in the blood.

Acute respiratory acidosis is caused by respiratory diseases such as pneumonia, drug overdose, head injury, chest wall injury, obesity, asphyxiation, drowning, or acute respiratory failure. People with chronic pulmonary disease may have elevated carbon dioxide levels but a normal pH as a result of renal compensation. Common clinical signs and symptoms include rapid heart rate, headache, sweating, lethargy, and confusion.

Medical Treatment

Interventions for respiratory acidosis are geared toward improving ventilation, which in turn restores the partial pressure of carbon dioxide in arterial blood (Pa_{CO_2}) to normal. Underlying respiratory conditions are treated to eliminate the cause of respiratory acidosis. Antibiotics, bronchodilators, and specific breathing treatments such as intermittent positive-pressure breathing, inspiratory and/or expiratory positive airway pressure, and continuous positive airway pressure may be prescribed. In some cases intubation and mechanical ventilation are necessary (see Chapter 29).

NURSING CARE

Assessment

The most accurate method of assessing for respiratory acidosis is the measurement of Pa_{CO_2} levels in arterial blood. The Pa_{CO_2} directly reflects the degree of respiratory dysfunction. In addition, patients should be observed for signs of respiratory distress, including restlessness, anxiety, confusion, and tachycardia. Frequently note the rate, depth, and rhythm of respirations. Respiratory rate and depth vary with the situation. For example, the patient with a head injury or drug overdose may have slow respirations that contribute to carbon dioxide retention. The patient with pneumonia may have rapid respirations in an effort to eliminate carbon dioxide that has accumulated as a result of impaired gas exchange. Assess level of consciousness, including orientation to person, place, and time, to detect changes in mental status.

Intervention

Encourage fluid intake to loosen secretions and keep mucous membranes moist. Position patients with the head elevated 30 degrees to promote comfort and ensure optimal gas exchange. Monitor confused patients frequently, and attempt to anticipate their needs. Because confused patients may fall as they try to get to the bathroom, they should be assisted to the bathroom every 2 hours, especially if fluids are increased. Constant reassurance and reorientation are helpful.

RESPIRATORY ALKALOSIS

Respiratory alkalosis is marked by low $PaCO_2$ with a resultant rise in pH. The most common cause of respiratory alkalosis is hyperventilation. Hyperventilation is characterized by rapid or deep respirations that cause excessive amounts of carbon dioxide to be eliminated through the lungs. When the body fluids become alkaline, ionized extracellular calcium decreases, and the patient has symptoms of hypocalcemia.

One cause of hyperventilation leading to respiratory alkalosis is anxiety. Other causes are conditions that result in decreased oxygen in the blood, such as pneumonia, adult respiratory distress syndrome, anemia, severe blood loss resulting from trauma, and congestive heart failure. Fever, pain, drugs (aspirin overdose), head trauma, and gram-negative septicemia also may contribute to respiratory alkalosis. The body attempts to compensate for respiratory alkalosis by eliminating excess bicarbonate through the kidneys. Clinical signs and symptoms include increased respiratory and heart rates, an anxious appearance, irritability, dizziness, lightheadedness, muscle weakness, and tingling or numbness of the fingers. In extreme respiratory alkalosis, confusion, fainting, and seizures may occur. Assessment of the rate and depth of respirations is the key observation for this condition.

Medical Treatment

The major goal of therapy is to treat the underlying cause of the condition. Sedation may be ordered for the anxious patient.

NURSING CARE

Assessment

The general assessment of patients with acid-base imbalances was described earlier in the chapter. With respiratory alkalosis, a description of respiratory status is especially important.

Intervention

In addition to giving sedatives as ordered, reassure the patient to relieve anxiety. Encourage the patient to breathe slowly, which will retain carbon dioxide in the body. Breathing slowly into a paper bag raises the $PaCO_2$ because the patient rebreathes exhaled carbon dioxide. When breathing stabilizes, allow the patient to have uninterrupted rest, because hyperventilation can result in fatigue.

METABOLIC ACIDOSIS

Metabolic acidosis occurs when the body retains too many hydrogen ions or loses too many bicarbonate ions. With too much acid and too little base, the pH of the blood falls. Metabolic acidosis leads to hyperventilation because the lungs try to compensate by blowing off carbon dioxide and lowering $PaCO_2$ levels, which raises the pH.

Causes of metabolic acidosis are starvation, dehydration, diarrhea, shock, renal failure, and diabetic ketoacidosis. Signs and symptoms vary according to the underlying cause and the severity of the acid-base disturbance. However, patients may experience changing levels of consciousness, ranging from fatigue and confusion to stupor and coma, headache, vomiting and diarrhea, anorexia, muscle weakness, and cardiac dysrhythmias.

Medical Treatment

The primary intervention for metabolic acidosis is treatment of the underlying disorder. Mechanical ventilation may be necessary, especially in patients who are comatose. Once corrective measures have been initiated, an intravenous infusion of sodium bicarbonate might be ordered, based on arterial blood gas results.

NURSING CARE

Assessment

Assessment of the patient in metabolic acidosis should focus on vital signs, mental status, and neurologic status.

Intervention

Nursing care is geared toward emergency measures to restore acid-base balance. Administer drugs and intravenous fluids as prescribed. Reassure and orient confused patients.

METABOLIC ALKALOSIS

Metabolic alkalosis is the opposite of metabolic acidosis. It results from an increase in bicarbonate levels or a loss of hydrogen ions. Loss of hydrogen ions may be caused by prolonged nasogastric suctioning, excessive vomiting, diuretics, and electrolyte disturbances. Retention of bicarbonate may result from the administration of bicarbonate or massive blood transfusions.

Clinical signs and symptoms may include headache; irritability; lethargy; changes in level of consciousness; confusion; changes in heart rate; slow, shallow respirations with periods of apnea; nausea and vomiting; hyperactive reflexes; and numbness of the extremities.

Medical Treatment

As with other acid-base imbalances, treatment depends on the underlying cause and severity of the condition.

NURSING CARE

Assessment

Take vital signs and daily weight measurements of the patient, and monitor heart rate, respirations, and fluid gains and losses. Keep accurate intake and output records, including the amount of fluid removed by suction. Assess motor function and sensation in the extremities, and monitor laboratory values, especially pH and serum bicarbonate levels.

Intervention

To prevent metabolic alkalosis, use isotonic saline solutions rather than water for irrigating nasogastric tubes because the use of water for irrigation can result in a loss of electrolytes. Provide reassurance and comfort measures to promote safety and well-being.

Put on your ***THINKING CAP!!***

1. Measure your fluid intake and output for 24 hours. If they are not equal, list possible explanations for the difference.
2. Recall a patient who either had or was at risk for fluid and electrolyte imbalances.
   a. What assessment data should have been collected?
   b. Identify factors that placed the patient at risk.
   c. Identify measures to treat or prevent the imbalances.

key points

- Approximately 50% to 60% of the human body is composed of water. To maintain homeostasis, the body must be able to regulate the fluids within it.
- The process of homeostasis involves delivery of nutrients and oxygen to the cells and removal of wastes, including carbon dioxide, from the cells.
- Body fluids are classified on the basis of location in body compartments: (1) intracellular fluid (fluid within the cell) and (2) extracellular fluid (fluid outside the cell). Most of the body's fluids are found within the cell.
- Extracellular fluid is mainly responsible for the transport of nutrients and wastes throughout the body.
- Electrolytes, which are substances that develop an electrical charge when dissolved in water, maintain a balance between positive and negative charges to keep the body in homeostasis.
- Total body water decreases in the elderly, with the greatest decline in intracellular fluid.
- The fluid compartments of the body are separated by selectively permeable membranes that control movement of water and certain solutes.
- Water and solutes move between intracellular and extracellular fluid compartments by one or more of the following processes: (1) diffusion, (2) active transport, (3) filtration, and (4) osmosis.
- The kidneys are the primary regulators of fluid balance in the body, and the nephrons conduct the work of the kidneys through the processes of filtration, reabsorption, and secretion.
- Hormones that have a major effect on fluid balance include renin, aldosterone, antidiuretic hormone (ADH), and atrial natriuretic factor (ANF).
- Renin is secreted when blood volume or blood pressure falls. It stimulates release of aldosterone and helps produce angiotensin I, which is converted to angiotensin II—a potent vasoconstrictor.
- Aldosterone is secreted by the adrenal glands and promotes sodium retention. Antidiuretic hormone, produced by the hypothalamus and secreted by the posterior pituitary gland, promotes water retention.
- ANF is secreted when stretch receptors in atria detect an increase in blood volume. It promotes excretion of water and sodium, decreases renin synthesis, inhibits release of aldosterone and ADH, and causes vasodilation.
- The thirst center creates a desire to drink fluids when extracellular fluid becomes concentrated.
- In a healthy adult the 24-hour fluid intake and output are approximately equal.
- The body attempts to compensate for fluid volume deficits by increasing the heart rate and conserving water in the kidneys.
- The body attempts to compensate for fluid volume excess by increasing urine output.
- The kidneys are the primary regulators of electrolytes in the blood.
- Two electrolytes that cause the majority of problems when there is an imbalance are sodium (Na^+) and potassium (K^+).
- Change in body weight is a good indicator of fluid loss or retention.
- Edema reflects sodium retention, which can result from excessive reabsorption or inadequate secretion because of failing kidney function.
- Potassium excess or deficit can lead to life-threatening cardiac dysrhythmias.
- Because older adults often have a reduced thirst sensation and may not conserve water efficiently, they are at risk for fluid volume deficit.
- Acid-base balance is the homeostasis of the hydrogen ion (H^+) concentration in the body fluids.
- Mechanisms that maintain acid-base balance are blood buffers, respiratory control of carbon dioxide, and renal regulation of bicarbonate (HCO_3^-).
- Acid-base imbalances occur when an imbalance in the functioning of the lungs, kidneys, or both exists. The four major acid-base imbalances are (1) respiratory acidosis, (2) respiratory alkalosis, (3) metabolic acidosis, and (4) metabolic alkalosis.

REVIEW QUESTIONS

1. Fluid surrounding the cells is called:

1. intracellular.
2. lymph.
3. intravascular.
4. interstitial.

2. The largest portion of a person's body weight is contributed by:

1. water.
2. fat.
3. bone.
4. muscle.

3. Anions include:
   1. sodium.
   2. calcium.
   3. chloride.
   4. magnesium.

4. The movement of water across a membrane from a less concentrated solution to a more concentrated solution defines:
   1. diffusion.
   2. osmosis.
   3. filtration.
   4. active transport.

5. A hormone with physiologic effects that decrease blood pressure is:
   1. antidiuretic hormone.
   2. renin.
   3. aldosterone.
   4. atrial natriuretic factor.

6. Which of the following statements best describes the risk of fluid and electrolyte imbalances in the older adult?
   1. Most older adults can maintain fluid and electrolyte balance just as well as younger adults.
   2. Older adults have limited reserves to maintain fluid balance when abnormal losses occur.
   3. Body water increases with age, putting the older adult at risk for fluid volume excess.
   4. The amount of extracellular fluid declines, leaving the patient with reduced fluid stores.

7. A patient is receiving diuretics to eliminate excess fluid that has been retained in body tissues. In 2 days the patient lost 4.4 lbs (2 kg) in body weight. This represents how much fluid loss?
   1. 1 liter
   2. 2 liters
   3. 3 liters
   4. 4.4 liters

8. You gently pinch the skin over a patient's sternum. The skin does not flatten right away, leading you to suspect:
   1. recent weight loss.
   2. history of excessive sun exposure.
   3. dehydration.
   4. need for increased diuretics.

9. Fluid volume excess can be classified as intracellular or:
   1. extracellular.
   2. intravascular.
   3. interstitial.
   4. extravascular.

10. When a patient has a potassium imbalance, which of the following nursing assessments is *most* important?
    1. Auscultate bowel sounds.
    2. Evaluate muscle strength.
    3. Monitor heart rate and rhythm.
    4. Assess reflexes.

11. Which answer lists *in correct order* the mechanisms that maintain acid-base balance?
    1. Renal regulation, respiratory regulation, buffers
    2. Buffers, respiratory regulation, renal regulation
    3. Buffers, renal regulation, respiratory regulation
    4. Respiratory regulation, buffers, renal regulation

12. What is the physiologic function of deep, rapid respirations in metabolic acidosis?
    1. Eliminates excess carbon dioxide that is formed in the presence of acidosis
    2. Raises the PaO_2, which reduces the pH of the blood
    3. Supplies additional oxygen needed because of the increased metabolic rate
    4. Reduces $Paco_2$, resulting in a rise in blood pH and correction of acidosis

CHAPTER

14 Pain Management

MARY L. HEYE and KATHLEEN A. REEVES

objectives

1. Define pain.
2. Explain the physiologic basis for pain.
3. Identify situations in which patients are likely to experience pain.
4. Explain the relationships between past pain experiences, anticipation, culture, anxiety, or activity and a patient's response to pain.
5. Identify differences in the duration of pain and patient responses to acute and chronic pain.
6. Explain the special needs of the elderly patient with pain.
7. List the data to be collected in assessing pain.
8. Describe interventions used in the management of pain.
9. Describe the nursing care of patients receiving opioid and nonopioid analgesics for pain.
10. List the factors that should be considered when pain is not relieved with analgesic medications.

key terms

Acute pain (p. 171)
Addiction (p. 182)
Analgesia (ăn-ăl-JĒ-zē-ă, p. 170)
Analgesic (ăn-ăl-JĒ-zĭk, p. 168)
Anesthesia (ăn-ĕs-THĒ-zē-ă, p. 170)
Chronic pain (p. 171)
Nociceptor (nō-sē-SĔP-tĕr, p. 168)
Pain (p. 168)
Pain threshold (p. 170)
Pain tolerance (p. 170)
Physical dependence (p. 182)
Tolerance (p. 182)

Pain is one of the most complex experiences to understand and treat. It is also the most common problem that nurses encounter. Research about pain, **analgesics** (drugs that relieve pain), and the mind-body influence is just beginning to filter down to nursing practice. Still, many questions about pain remain unanswered.

Pain is influenced by many variables: the individual experiencing it, the cause of the pain, and the environment. Pain may arise from a new source, from an old injury, or from nerve injury. Sometimes the cause is unknown. Pain relief rests primarily with the nurse, who must assess the patient and implement appropriate interventions.

Nurses have many categories of pain-relieving interventions to choose from, yet they frequently administer only analgesics. Most nurses believe that pain is easily managed with analgesic drugs. Patients, however, often report that pain remains moderate to severe despite these medications. Research indicates that nurses fail to assess pain, tend to undermedicate for pain, and have inadequate knowledge of pain relief measures. Because of these findings, the Joint Commission on Hospital Accreditation of Healthcare Organizations published standards for the management of pain for all patients. Health care facilities are expected to comply with these standards. These include: (1) recognizing the right of patients to appropriate assessment and management of pain, (2) performing pain assessments, (3) recording results of assessment and follow-up, (4) teaching patients about effective pain management, and (5) addressing needs for pain and symptom management at discharge.

The purpose of this chapter is to enable the nurse to understand pain and provide the most effective interventions for pain relief.

DEFINITION OF PAIN

Pain is defined in many ways. The International Association for the Study of Pain defines it as an unpleasant sensory and emotional experience associated with actual or potential tissue damage. McCaffery, a nurse and leader in the pain management field, has a more useful definition for nurses. She says, "Pain is whatever the person experiencing it says it is and exists whenever he says it does."

PHYSIOLOGY OF PAIN

Pain consists of various sensory experiences such as experiences of time and space, emotions, and cognition. The perception of pain involves afferent pathways, the central nervous system, and efferent pathways. Afferent pathways are nerves that carry messages to the brain for interpretation. Efferent (or descending) pathways are nerves that carry messages away from the brain to the rest of the body via the spinal cord.

Afferent pathways are activated by pain receptors called **nociceptors.** These pain receptors are unevenly distributed in muscles, tendons, subcutaneous tissue, and the skin. This may explain why parts of the body are more sensitive to pain than other parts. Pain receptors are sensitive to chemical changes, temperature, mechanical stimuli, and tissue damage. Some receptors are sensitive to more than one type of stimulus. Pain receptors are unable to adapt to repeated stimuli and thus continue to react until the stimuli are removed.

When pain receptors are stimulated, impulses are transmitted to the spinal cord. The impulses then travel up the spinal cord to the brain. In the brain, the cortex interprets the impulses as pain and identifies the location and qualities of the pain. Other structures involved in the interpretation of pain signals produce the unpleasant qualities associated with pain like fear and activate the stress response. Once pain is perceived in the brain, the descending pathway is activated and several substances like endorphins and enkephalins are released.

Endorphins and enkephalins are the body's natural opioid-like substances that block the transmission of painful impulses to the brain. Differences in the amount of endorphins in individuals may explain why some people seem to experience more pain than others. Research suggests that prolonged stress and pain, as well as the prolonged use of morphine and alcohol, decrease endorphin levels. Factors that increase endorphin levels include brief stress and pain, laughter, exercise, acupuncture, transcutaneous electrical nerve stimulation (TENS), massive trauma, and sexual activity.

GATE-CONTROL THEORY

Although many theories have been proposed to explain pain, none fully describe the pain experience. One of the best known theories is Melzack and Wall's gate-control theory. It assumes that the pain experience reflects both physical and psychosocial factors. Painful impulses are transmitted to the spinal cord through small-diameter nerve fibers in the afferent pathway. When these small-diameter fibers are stimulated, the gating mechanism opens in the spinal cord, which permits the transmission of impulses from the spinal cord to the brain. Consequently the patient perceives pain. Factors that cause the gate to open include tissue damage, a monotonous environment, and fear of pain. These small-diameter fibers end in the spinal cord along with large-diameter fibers. The stimulation of large-diameter fibers can close the gate and interfere with impulse transmission between the spinal cord and the brain. This causes diminished pain perception. Large-diameter nerve fibers are stimulated by cutaneous (skin) stimulation through massage, position change, and heat or cold applications. Sensory input such as distraction, guided imagery, and preparatory information also may close the gate. Figure 14-1 shows the structures and mechanisms associated with the gate-control theory.

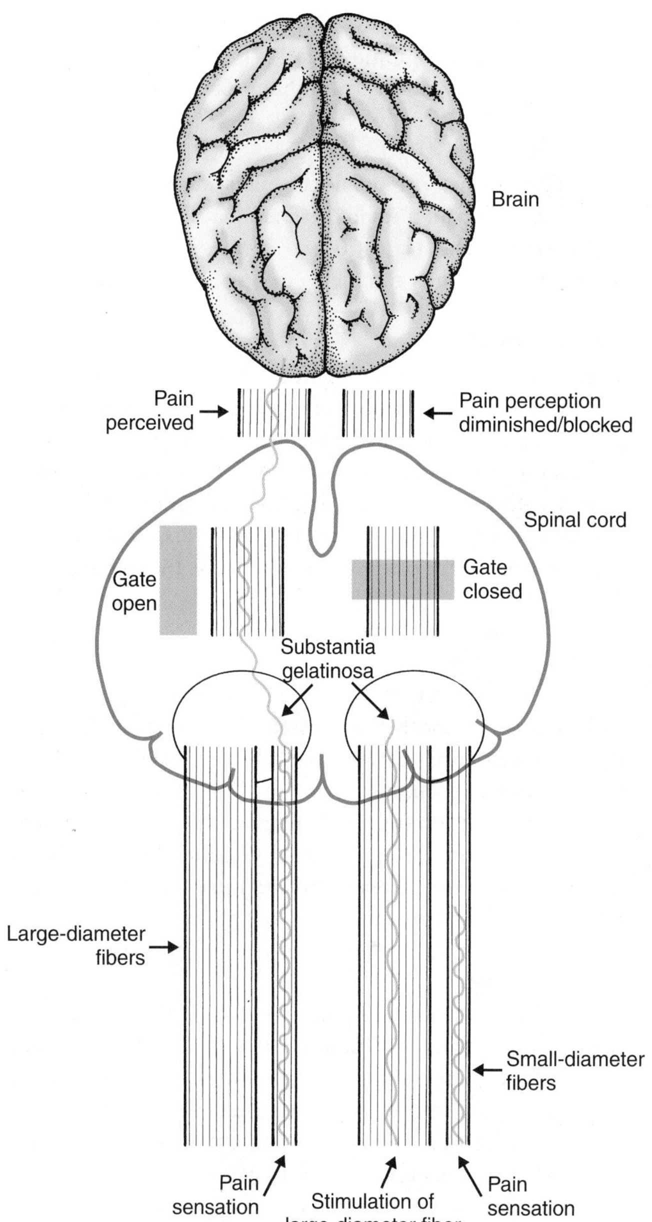

FIGURE **14-1** The gate-control theory of pain.

FACTORS INFLUENCING RESPONSE TO PAIN

Consider the following example: Miss Smith and Mrs. Johnson are roommates in Room 200. Miss Smith, age 19, underwent a cholecystectomy the previous day, as did Mrs. Johnson, age 67. The nurses discussed the difference in behavior of each patient: "Miss Smith constantly wants more pain medication. She moans and groans all the time. She won't even turn, cough, or breathe deeply for more than 10 seconds. She always rates her pain a 9 or a 10 on the pain scale. On the other hand, look at Mrs. Johnson. She's already ambulating. She rarely rates her pain as more than a 5 or a 6 on the pain scale. She usually just complains of aching, and she sure doesn't ask for as much pain medication as Miss Smith. You'd never guess they had undergone the same procedure."

This example illustrates that although people may have the same injury or insult (in this case surgery), they may respond differently. This is because many physical and psychosocial factors affect the response to pain. It is important for health professionals to be nonjudgmental and to avoid comparing one individual in pain with another individual in pain.

PHYSICAL FACTORS

Many physical factors influence the pain experience, including the individual's pain threshold, pain tolerance, age, physical activity, nervous system integrity, and, in cases of surgery, the type of surgery performed and the type of anesthesia used.

Pain Threshold

The pain threshold is the point at which a stimulus causes the sensation of pain. Anger, fatigue, anxiety, insomnia, depression, and uncontrolled pain all lower the pain threshold. With a lower threshold, the person experiences pain more readily with less stimuli. During hospitalization or illness, a patient may experience anxiety, fatigue, or loss of sleep, all of which can lower the pain threshold or cause the patient to experience pain more easily.

Pain Tolerance

Pain tolerance refers to the intensity of pain that a person will endure. It is another factor influencing response to pain. Pain tolerance varies between patients and varies for an individual patient, depending on the situation. Increasing or prolonged pain may lower the pain tolerance because the patient fears the pain will not be relieved. Low pain tolerance or high pain tolerance must be respected and must not interfere with adequate pain management.

Age

Age may also influence response to pain. At times, older patients do not report their pain, or they report that their pain is much less severe than it really is. Some do not report pain because they are stoic or they have been told incorrectly that pain is a normal part of aging. Some older patients may not want to bother the nurse, or they may fear rejection from the care giver. Pain is *not* a normal part of aging, although elderly persons often suffer from chronic conditions such as arthritis, cancer, and bone fractures that are associated with pain.

Physical Activity and Nervous System Integrity

Physical activity and the integrity of the nervous system also can influence the reaction to pain. Physical activity may aggravate or precipitate pain. However, with some patients, physical activity may be used to relieve pain. Because pain is perceived and interpreted within the nervous system, the integrity of the system affects the response to pain. For example, patients with diabetic neuropathy may lose sensation in the extremities and may not feel pain there.

Surgery and Anesthesia

In surgical patients, the type of surgery performed and the type of anesthesia used can influence the response to pain. Surgery on the upper abdominal region of the body is thought to be the most painful type because of the numerous tissues traumatized during the procedure. Within this group are cardiac, pulmonary, gastric, and gallbladder procedures. The type of anesthetic agent used can influence postoperative pain. For example, ketamine has analgesic properties. Some anesthetic agents injected at the operative site may prolong analgesia for 12 to 24 hours after surgery. When these types of agents are used, patients may experience much less pain after surgery than those who do not receive these anesthetic agents.

Surgery or invasive procedures may be performed to relieve pain that is severely debilitating. Rhizotomy and cordotomy are surgical procedures that cut or destroy selected nerve tissue to interrupt the pain pathway. These operations intentionally leave the patient with some neurologic deficit. For example, the patient may be unaware that a body area is painful and may not protect that area from harm. Pain relief from these procedures may not be permanent because nerve tissue regenerates. Nerve blocks are procedures that involve destruction or anesthesia of a nerve root with injection of a chemical to achieve pain relief in a specific body area. For example, intercostal (between the ribs) anesthetic nerve blocks may be performed with cardiac operations to reduce postoperative pain in the thoracic area. Drugs are injected into the nerve to block the pain signal. Acupuncture is another invasive technique that produces anesthesia or analgesia. It is an ancient Chinese practice in which tiny needles are inserted into the skin or subcutaneous tissues at specific points on the body. This technique may be used to relieve acute and chronic pain such as headache, menstrual cramps, and low back pain.

PSYCHOLOGICAL FACTORS

Along with physical factors, several psychological factors can influence the response to pain, including culture, religion, past experiences with pain, anxiety, and situational factors.

Culture and Ethnicity

Although studies have been conducted to determine the effect of culture and ethnicity on people's reaction to pain, it is critical to avoid making judgments based on how you think a person should react or behave. Some persons may deny pain, remain calm and unemotional, or withdraw. Other persons may cry, moan and groan, and involve their families in the painful experience. Be aware of the different ways of expressing pain and respect individual variations in the response to pain.

Religious Beliefs

Religious beliefs also may have an impact on reaction to pain. Some patients may pray and believe that divine intervention will help them to endure the pain. Others may view pain as a punishment for sins. Some individuals believe that suffering is required before pain relief can be obtained.

Past Experiences and Anxiety

Past experiences and anxiety may affect a person's response to current pain. A person may have developed positive coping strategies to deal with previous painful experiences. If, however, previous coping strategies were unsuccessful, the patient may be very anxious and overwhelmed by another painful experience.

Situational Factors

Finally, situational factors may influence response to pain. If the pain is associated with a serious illness such as cancer, the pain may have a greater impact on mood and activity than if the pain were associated with a less serious condition. The pain associated with childbirth is relatively short-lived and usually results in a beautiful outcome, whereas cancer pain may be chronic and increasing and may be associated with progression of the disease and death.

What Does Culture Have to do with Pain?

The way a person behaves in response to pain is, in part, determined by cultural norms. Therefore, people from some cultures quietly endure pain, whereas people from other cultures loudly express their pain. As nurses, we must accept each response and assess and intervene to promote maximum comfort.

RESPONSES TO PAIN

AUTONOMIC NERVOUS SYSTEM

The pain signal is interpreted by the brain as a stressor. The autonomic nervous system activates the fight-or-flight response, and certain physiologic responses are initiated. Table 14-1 indicates some of the responses that occur and the associated effects. The patient in pain may exhibit these physiologic responses, along with behaviors such as grimacing, moaning, and verbalizing pain, or withdrawing. The nervous system responses are measured by an increased heart rate, respiratory rate, and blood pressure. These are predictable responses to acute pain; however, the pain behavior will vary from individual to individual. Acute and chronic pain elicit different kinds of responses. Table 14-2 lists some differences between acute and chronic pain.

table 14-1 *Autonomic Nervous System Responses to Pain*

SYMPATHETIC NERVOUS SYSTEM RESPONSES	PARASYMPATHETIC NERVOUS SYSTEM RESPONSES
↑ Blood pressure	Constipation
↑ Pulse rate	Urinary retention
↑ Respiratory rate	
Dilated pupils	
Perspiration	
Pallor	

ACUTE PAIN

Most pain experienced in the hospital is acute pain. Acute pain follows the normal pathway for pain from nociceptor activation to the brain and may be called nociceptive pain. Examples are postoperative pain from incisions, renal colic pain from kidney stones, bone fractures, and pain in childbirth. Acute pain is temporary, and its cause is known and treatable. It serves as a warning of tissue damage and subsides when healing takes place. Nurses observe behavioral and physiologic signs of acute pain when the patient guards or rubs a body part, wrinkles the brow, bites the lip, and has changes in the heart rate, blood pressure, and respiratory rate. These responses may be absent or lessened in chronic pain.

CHRONIC PAIN

Chronic pain is usually defined as pain that persists or recurs for more than 3 to 6 months; it may last a lifetime. Chronic pain may also be nociceptive; however, most chronic pain is called neuropathic pain because it follows an abnormal pathway for pain. This is a new term that encompasses some puzzling and challenging pain syndromes classified as chronic pain. Neuropathic pain results from nerve damage resulting from a wide variety of anatomic and physiologic conditions and underlying diseases. It includes unusual sensations such as burning, shooting pain, and abnormal sensations that occur when there is no painful stimulus present.

The cause of the pain may be unknown. Treatment may or may not be helpful in relieving the pain. There are several types of chronic pain. Some classes of chronic pain and examples are

table 14-2 *Differences in Acute and Chronic Pain*

CHARACTERISTIC	ACUTE	CHRONIC
Time	Limited, short duration	Lasts 3-6 months, longer duration
Purpose	Sign of tissue injury	No purpose
Verbal	Reports pain, focuses on pain	No report of pain unless questioned
Behavioral	Restless, thrashing, rubbing body part, pacing, grimacing, and other facial expressions of pain	Tired-looking, minimal facial expression, quiet, sleeps, rests, attention on other things
Physiologic	Increased heart rate, blood pressure, respiratory rate	Normal heart rate, blood pressure, respiratory rate
Interventions	Responds to analgesics Standard doses effective Parenteral or oral route used Additional drugs seldom needed to manage pain	Less responsive to analgesics Higher doses needed for pain relief Oral route preferred Additional drugs (adjuvant) often needed to manage pain

table 14-3 ***Chronic Pain***

CLASS	EXAMPLES
Acute pain: recurrent episodes	Neuralgia (herpes zoster) Migraine headaches Sickle cell crisis
Chronic malignant	Cancer pain syndromes
Chronic nonmalignant or benign	Low back pain Rheumatoid arthritis Phantom limb pain

shown in Table 14-3. Chronic pain is associated with a variety of diagnoses, including cancer, arthritis, peripheral vascular diseases, and traumatic injuries.

Chronic nonmalignant or benign pain is pain that cannot be explained or that persists after healing has taken place. It usually occurs daily and is not life-threatening. Treatments may or may not be successful in relieving the pain. Intractable pain is another word used to describe pain that cannot be relieved and has no known effective treatment.

Many conditions common in older adults may be associated with chronic pain. Phantom limb pain, in which the patient still feels sensations and pain in the amputated limb, is an example of chronic benign pain and neuropathic pain. It can be extremely debilitating if it is not recognized and treated early. It may occur in any related body part that has been amputated or traumatized, e.g., amputation of the breast or leg. A number of therapies may be used to reduce this type of pain (e.g., analgesic opioids, antidepressants, nerve block, surgical revision, and physical therapy).

Chronic malignant pain or cancer-related pain may be considered acute and chronic pain. Cancer pain may be chronic pain if it lasts longer than 3 to 6 months. Cancer may also cause the development of new pain when the cancer causes pressure or damage to tissue or nerves. This would be acute pain. Pain related to cancer can be very complex because it may include a variety of pain problems that can be nociceptive and/or neuropathic in nature.

Chronic pain is poorly understood, and new and challenging pain syndromes are currently being identified and classified. Among the new treatments that are being tried for chronic pain are surgically implanted stimulators in the back or brain that can block pain impulses.

COMPARISON OF ACUTE AND CHRONIC PAIN

In contrast to acute pain, which warns of tissue damage and trauma, chronic pain serves no useful purpose. It can have a debilitating and destructive effect on a person's life. Chronic pain can lead to depression, marital difficulties, loss of self-esteem, immobility, and isolation. The patient in chronic pain often does not report pain and shows little facial expression or few physical signs of pain. When pain is chronic, adaptation may occur. The sympathetic nervous system adapts. The heart rate, blood pressure, and respiratory rate may not be elevated, and the patient may rest, sleep, or turn attention to other activities despite severe pain.

The nurse may underestimate the severity of the pain or undermedicate a patient with chronic pain. Nursing assessment of pain is essential to identify (1) the type and amount of pain, (2) whether the pain is chronic or acute, and (3) whether the patient has both acute pain and chronic pain at the same time. When the patient reports pain but shows no physical symptoms, this does not mean there is no pain. It may simply mean that the patient has learned other ways to deal with the pain, or the patient may be taking medications that block the response of the sympathetic nervous system to pain.

NURSING CARE *of the Patient in Pain*

Pain management continues to be a challenge for every nurse. Every individual experiences pain differently and reacts to pain with a variety of physiologic and behavioral responses. Based on an accurate assessment of pain, the physician prescribes treatment and the nurse provides nonpharmacologic and pharmacologic measures together to provide pain relief. The nurse plays a key role by assessing, intervening, and evaluating the patient in pain. Figure 14-2 shows the variety of interventions you can use to relieve pain.

Assessment

Assessment is the first step in pain management. Assessment of pain should be done on admission and on a regular basis. Anticipate pain as a result of procedures, surgery, or progression of a disease. A pain assessment done with vital signs is called the fifth vital sign. Accurately record the data and compare with previous information. This permits evaluation of the pattern of pain or the effectiveness of an intervention.

It can be difficult to assess pain in some patients, especially older adults. Visual, speech, hearing, and motor impairments may limit the ability of older patients to communicate pain or to use scales to rate pain. Patients with cognitive impairment may be unable to report pain or recall pain sensations. Pain can also cause confusion, irritation, and depression in older adults. Consider these aspects when assessing the older adult.

When the patient cannot communicate verbally, he or she may be able to point to or direct your attention to a location on a body chart or pain intensity scale. You may also have to use family observations and patient behaviors to assess pain and pain relief in this type of situation.

The six steps in pain assessment are listed in Table 14-4 and discussed below.

Accept the Patient's Report

The first step in pain assessment is to establish rapport with the patient and accept what the patient says about the pain. When possible, all information about pain should be obtained directly from the patient. The person in pain is the only authority on the pain; no one else can really know what the pain feels like. Accept the report in a nonjudgmental and caring manner. Obtain specific details about the pain, and respond positively that action will be taken to relieve the pain.

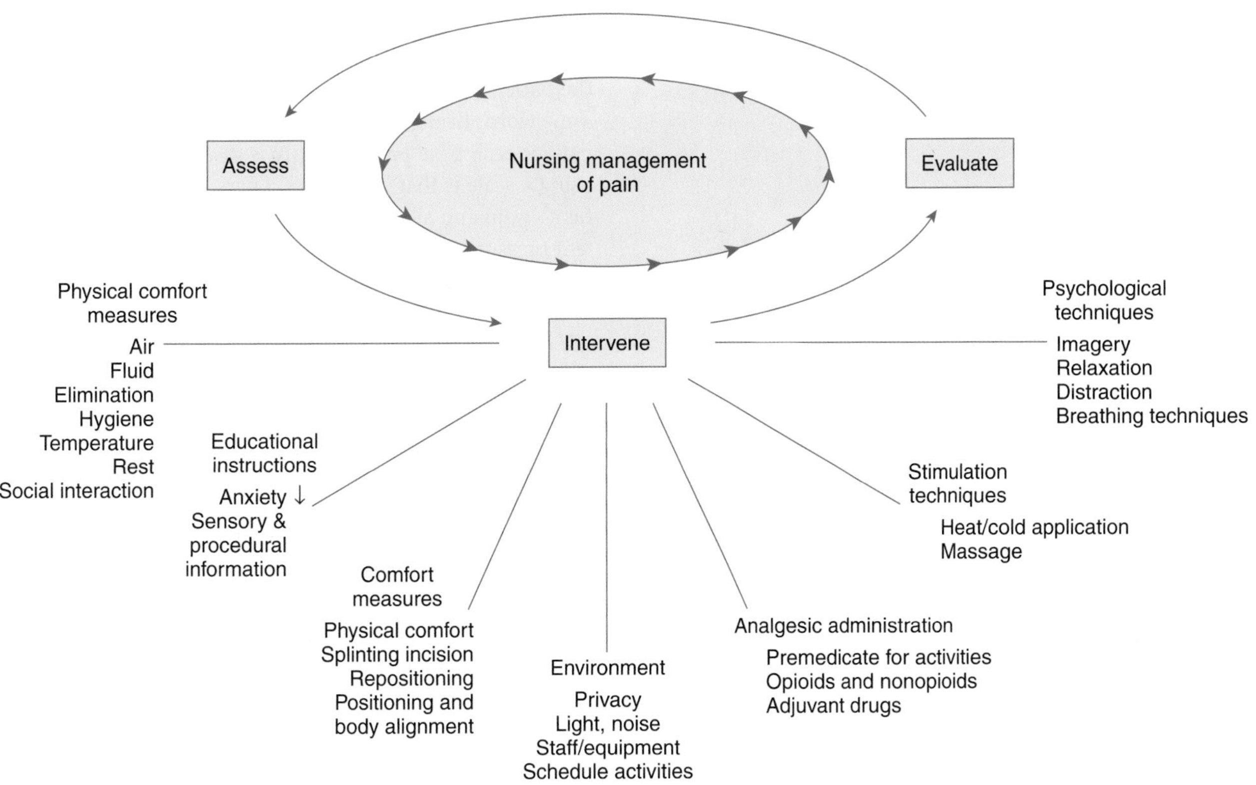

FIGURE **14-2** Nursing management of pain.

table 14-4 ***Six Steps in Pain Assessment***

1. Accept the patient's report
2. Determine the status of the pain
3. Describe the pain
   a. Location
   b. Quality
   c. Intensity
   d. Aggravating and alleviating factors
4. Examine the site
5. Identify coping methods
6. Record assessment, interventions, and evaluation of interventions

The assessment of pain requires excellent therapeutic communication skills. Important attitudes are conveyed through verbal and nonverbal behaviors. Listen patiently without interruption, use eye contact, touch the patient, and repeat and clarify information in an unhurried manner to establish trust and obtain information. Do not compare one patient's report of pain with another's report because pain is an individual experience.

Determine the Status of the Pain

The second step in pain assessment is to determine whether the pain is a new occurrence or has been experienced before. Ask the patient if he or she has had this pain before, and whether it was diagnosed by a physician. On the basis of the patient's responses and history, decide whether the pain is chronic in nature or acute pain that needs immediate treatment. For example, a patient who is recovering from a prostatectomy may suddenly have chest pain. The patient identifies this discomfort as the typical angina pain for which he has taken medication in the past. A similar patient with chest pain and no previous cardiac history should be seen by a physician immediately because this is a new pain that the patient has not had before. Although both patients need to be evaluated by a physician, an accurate nursing assessment is essential to determine the difference between these two types of pain and consequently the action to be taken.

Describe the Pain

The third step in pain assessment is to describe the pain in terms of its location, quality, intensity, and aggravating and alleviating factors.

Location. Have the patient describe where the pain is and point to the exact location with one finger. If there is more than one location of pain, use a body chart, as shown in Figure 14-3. Have the patient shade in or mark an X at the locations of pain. Then number the various locations on the body chart so that you can refer to the number rather than writing the exact location each time. Also determine whether the pain is confined to one area or whether it starts at one place and moves to another.

The location identified as painful does not always correspond with the disease or operative site. For example, patients may experience back and neck spasm after surgical procedures. Another example is referred pain. Referred pain is

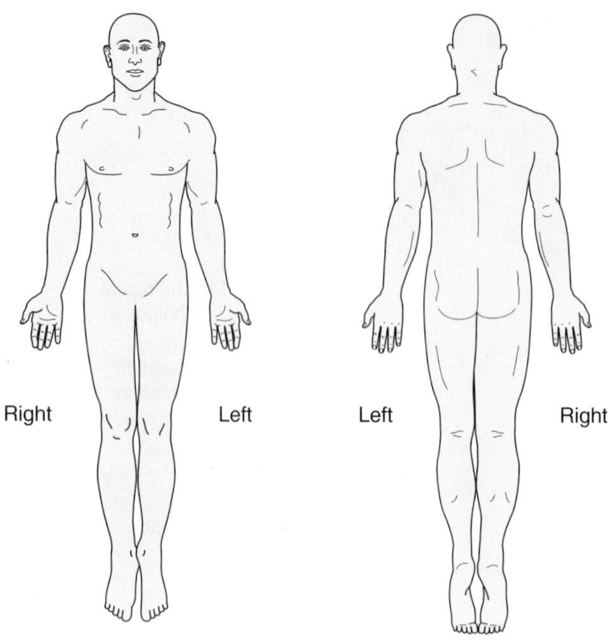

FIGURE **14-3** Body chart.

often experienced in a location different from its source (Fig. 14-4). To illustrate, pain from appendicitis is usually felt around the umbilicus and is of the aching, cramping type. The pain impulses come from an inflamed appendix in the right lower quadrant of the abdomen, where there may also be sharp pain. Anginal pain is another type of referred pain. It is caused by lack of blood flow to the heart muscle and may be experienced as pain in the jaw, arm, and neck as well as in the chest.

Quality. Ask the patient, "What words do you use to describe your pain?" or "What would you do to me to have me feel the pain you have?" If the patient has difficulty describing the pain, suggest words. Commonly used words are sharp, dull, cramping, aching, gnawing, burning, heavy, tender, and throbbing. However, it is best to allow the patient to use his or her own words, and record these in the chart.

Intensity. Because pain is a subjective experience, nurses must have some way to measure the severity of pain. The purpose of asking about intensity is to put the patient's description into an objective term or number. To determine intensity, use one of the several scales shown in Figure 14-5. A simple descriptive scale uses words of varying intensity—for example, mild, moderate, or severe. Some patients have difficulty with these words, and it may be better to use a scale with words such as "a little pain," "a lot of pain," or "too much pain." A numeric scale can be 0 to 10 or 0 to 5, with 0 meaning "no pain" and the highest number meaning "the worst pain experienced." A visual analog scale (or VAS) allows the patient to mark an X anywhere on a line that shows intensity of pain at one end as "no pain" and at the other end as "pain as bad as it could possibly be."

Explain the scale to the patient and ask, "Where would you rate your pain right now?" The scale used should make sense to the patient, be easy to use, and be consistently used with the same words or numbers. Remember to explain the scale to the patient each time pain intensity is assessed. The advantage of using a scale is that it provides a personal measure of the patient's pain and allows evaluation of pain relief using a consistent measure. A scale that is meaningful to the patient and that can be used repeatedly requires less effort for the patient in pain.

For example, a 42-year-old man with multiple fractures in the right arm used the numeric scale from 1 to 10 for rating pain. The patient complained of throbbing in his right arm and a backache. He rated the intensity of both pains at 7 on the scale at 8 PM. The nurse applied heat to the lower back as ordered, massaged his back, and administered 10 mg of morphine intramuscularly. At 9 PM, the patient rated the intensity of both pains at 2 and stated that the pain was slowly going away. The nurse recorded this information and identified that the interventions were effective in relieving the pain because the pain intensity had decreased from 7 to 2 on the 0-to-10 scale. The nurse also noted that she would reassess the patient's pain every 2 hours. Some hospital policies set a number or "comfort goal" that automatically triggers pain intervention. For example, any pain rating 4 or above on the pain scale requires a nursing intervention for pain relief because research has shown that a pain rating of 4 or above interferes with function and recovery.

Aggravating and Alleviating Factors. Ask if any event or activity causes the pain or makes it better or worse. Ask, "What were you doing when the pain occurred?" Aggravating factors are those that make the pain worse. Certain positions, temperatures, or times of day or night may cause the pain to be more severe. Similarly, alleviating factors might include specific positions, application of heat, cold, or menthol, or physical activities that reduce pain in specific areas.

Patients can usually identify factors that aggravate or reduce pain and what specific pain relief methods have worked in the past. For example, four patients having abdominal surgery may have arthritic shoulder pain and have four different methods of reducing the pain. The first patient obtained relief with elevation and rest of the right arm. The second applied an analgesic balm, a menthol ointment. The third patient used a heating pad on the area, and the fourth increased the anti-inflammatory drug dose as prescribed by the physician.

Examine the Site of the Pain

The fourth step in the assessment of pain is to examine the location that the patient states is painful. Assess the area for heat, redness, swelling, tenderness, abnormal position, or other factors that may be causing local irritation.

Patients may identify a location of pain that is not expected as part of their medical problem. This pain location may be due to a complication or an injury that was sustained during a procedure or hospitalization. For example, one patient who had undergone orthopedic surgery on the ankle had also sustained a large burn on his back at some time during the

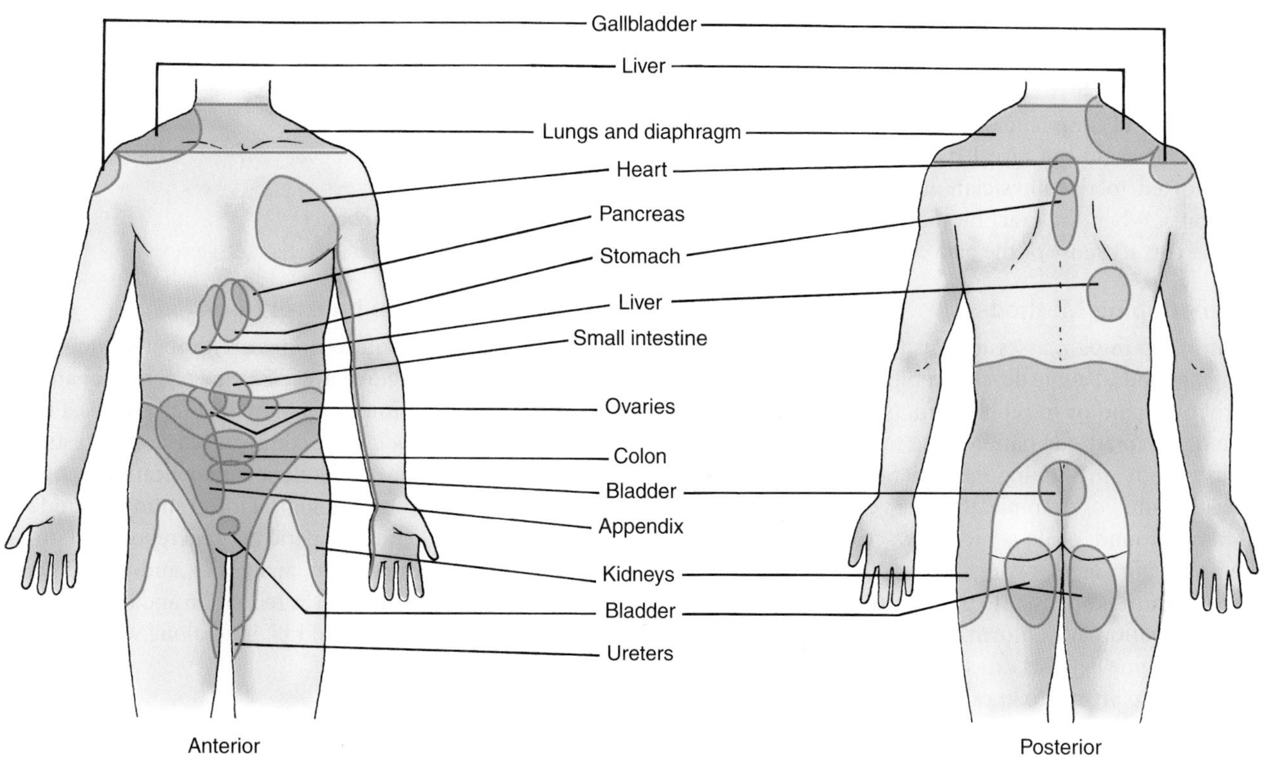

FIGURE 14-4 Anterior and posterior referred pain sites.

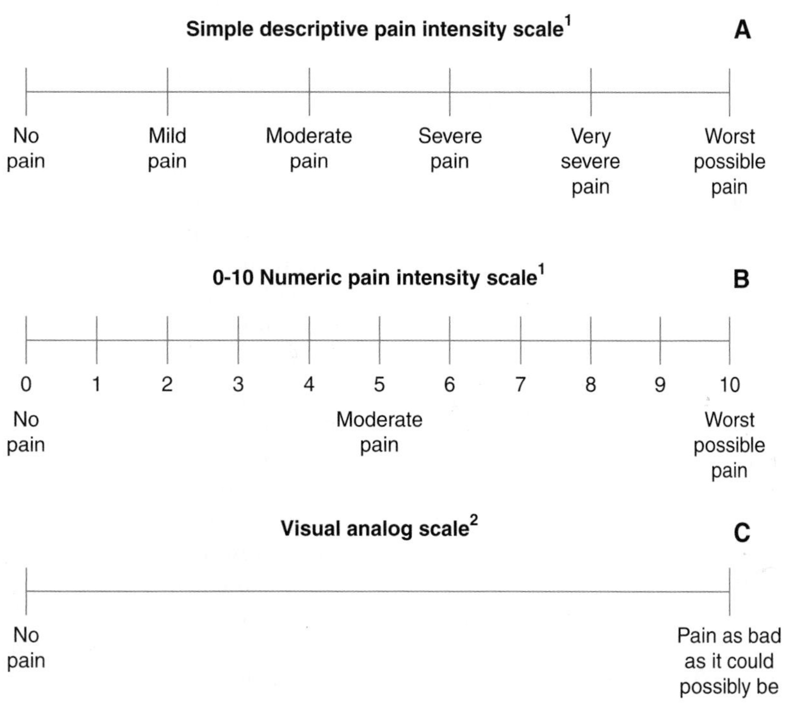

FIGURE 14-5 Examples of pain intensity scales. *A,* Simple descriptive pain intensity scale; *B,* 0-10 numeric pain intensity scale; *C,* visual analog scale (VAS).

procedure. When the nurse examined the pain location, the burn was discovered.

Another example is a patient who had undergone abdominal surgery and complained of pain in the right calf. Examination of the right calf revealed a red, firm, tender area that was reported to the physician and diagnosed as thrombophlebitis. When the exact location of the pain was examined, the correct cause of the pain could be identified.

Identify Coping Methods

The fifth step in pain assessment is to identify the patient's coping methods. People develop coping methods to increase control over pain or to relieve pain. Nurses should become aware of the methods patients use to cope with pain and should support the coping method. Some patients actively deal with pain. For example, they may complain and get up and move around, or do some other activity. Some patients cope by staying quiet, praying, sleeping, or withdrawing.

Nurses must emphasize to patients and their families that their cooperation and information are critical to achieving pain relief. Some patients expect nurses to know that they are experiencing pain and to know what to do about it. Confirm how the patient copes with pain by discussing observations of the patient's behavior with him or her. You can also suggest other coping methods that could be used to relieve pain (e.g., changing positions, imagery, and distraction).

Document Assessment Findings and Evaluate Interventions

The sixth and last step in the pain assessment is to write the information in the patient's chart so that this information can be conveyed to nurses on other shifts and to other health professionals. Identify the location, quality, and intensity of the pain, related factors, and how the patient copes with pain. After interventions, record the intensity of the pain again. Include whether the pain relief intervention was effective or not. If the nursing intervention was not effective, record what was done about the pain.

Put on your THINKING CAP!!

Think of one of your patients who had pain. Discuss with your classmates how you knew that the patient had pain. Compare and contrast how different patients expressed pain, the interventions that were being used for pain control, and the effectiveness of the interventions.

Nursing Diagnoses, Goals, and Outcome Criteria: Patients in Pain

NURSING DIAGNOSES	GOALS AND OUTCOME CRITERIA
Potential or actual **pain** related to surgery	Pain relief: Patient states pain is relieved, has relaxed manner
Chronic pain related to arthritic joint inflammation	Pain reduction or relief: Patient states pain is lessened or relieved, has relaxed manner

You may also use the following diagnoses to identify other problems that often accompany pain:

- **Activity intolerance**
- **Anxiety**
- **Fatigue**
- **Self-care deficit**
- **Sleep pattern disturbance**

Interventions

Nonpharmacologic Interventions

Nonpharmacologic interventions are those that do not employ drugs. They include a wide range of physical and psychological interventions for pain relief (Table 14-5). Physical interventions usually involve comfort measures, adjusting the patient's environment, and cutaneous application techniques such as heat or cold. Psychological interventions include unconditionally accepting the patient's pain report and providing information about pain, analgesics, and procedures or psychological strategies such as relaxation and imagery. These types of interventions should be used along with analgesics to obtain optimal pain relief.

Physical Interventions

Physical comfort measures. These nursing interventions focus on the patient and the environment. Comfort may increase pain tolerance and the patient may experience less pain. Since adequate air, food and fluid, elimination, mobility, hygiene, temperature, and rest and sleep are essential to comfort, monitor these areas for potential problems. For example, patients who are sleep deprived or fatigued may have increased pain. Therefore providing for uninterrupted sleep and periods of rest can enhance pain relief.

For some patients in pain, progressive exercise or immobility may be prescribed as a treatment for pain. The patient with an injury or incision should be moved carefully so that further trauma is avoided. Turning the patient carefully from side to side or supporting an affected extremity during activity can reduce pain. Usually the patient can describe which movements or positions increase or decrease the pain.

Administer analgesic medications prior to painful experiences to reduce the pain intensity and anxiety associated with the event. Aggressively treat pain, nausea, vomiting, appetite suppression, constipation, and other problems. Assist and teach patients how to splint abdominal and thoracic wounds to minimize pain when deep breathing, coughing, and ambulating. A change of bed linen and sheets free of wrinkles can be refreshing and reduce irritation of the skin. Apply ointment to cracked lips and provide ice chips for a dry mouth. Any tubes or equipment attached to the patient should be secure but should not produce tension on the skin. Correct body alignment and frequent changes of position will relieve monotony, increase circulation, and prevent muscle contractures and spasms, which aggravate pain.

PHARMACOLOGY CAPSULE Analgesics should be administered before painful activities to reduce the pain and anxiety associated with these events.

table 14-5 Nonpharmacologic Interventions

INTERVENTION	COMMENTS
PHYSICAL	
Heat, cold, massage, TENS	Increase pain threshold, reduce muscle spasm, and decrease congestion in injured area. Effective in reducing pain and improving physical function. Techniques require skilled personnel and special equipment. May be useful as adjuncts to drug therapy.
PSYCHOLOGICAL	
Relaxation	
Jaw relaxation Progressive muscle relaxation	Effective in reducing mild-to-moderate pain and as an adjunct to analgesic drugs for severe pain.
Simple imagery	Use when patients express an interest in relaxation. Requires 3-5 minutes of staff time for instructions.
Music	Both patient-preferred and "easy listening" music are effective in reducing mild-to-moderate pain.
Imagery	Effective for reduction of mild-to-moderate pain. Requires skilled personnel.
Educational Instruction	Effective for reduction of pain. Should include sensory and procedural information and be aimed at reducing activity-related pain. Requires 5-15 minutes of staff time.

Adapted from Acute Pain Management Guidelines Panel. (1992). *Acute pain management: Operative and medical procedures and trauma. Clinical practice guidelines* (AHCPR Publication No. 92-0032). Rockville, MD: Agency for Health Care Policy and Research, Public Health Service, U.S. Department of Health and Human Services.

Environmental control. Each patient has individual preferences that affect comfort. Some patients prefer an active environment in which they can be distracted from pain. Listening to tapes or music, watching television, working with the hands, walking around, or visiting with others allows a person to focus attention on stimuli other than the pain sensation. On the other hand, lights, noise, and constant activity of the hospital environment often cause sensory overload for the patient in pain. This can increase pain. When this occurs, coordinate with staff to promote a quiet environment with nonglaring lights and scheduled rest and activity periods that meet the patient's needs.

Stimulation techniques. Stimulation of the skin and underlying tissues relieves pain. Various types of skin or cutaneous stimulation can be applied, and each has variable effects. These techniques are not curative; rather, they can decrease the intensity of pain or change the sensation so that it is more acceptable. The exact mechanism for pain relief is unknown, but it is thought that superficial stimulation may block the transmission of pain impulses to the brain. Applications of heat, cold, massage, and TENS are examples of cutaneous stimulation. These interventions tend to be most effective for mild to moderate pain, well-localized pain, and acute and chronic pain. The effects of these therapies last as long as or slightly longer than the application.

The physician may prescribe the application of heat or cold for pain. Heat or cold is used to reduce muscle spasm and decrease congestion or swelling in an injured area. Either therapy may be applied to the painful site, at a location beyond the site, between the site and the brain, or on the opposite side of the body. These therapies should be applied intermittently, not continuously. Heat and cold may be alternated. Both therapies should be applied at a temperature that is comfortable for the patient, and the patient's skin and circulation should be monitored frequently.

Cold may be applied with ice packs or cooling pads to decrease initial tissue injury and swelling (e.g., with musculoskeletal sprains or orthopedic procedures). Cold is contraindicated for patients with peripheral vascular disease or heart disease because it may cause further vasoconstriction of blood vessels and thus decrease circulation. Cold application should be limited to 15 minutes per session to avoid tissue injury or frostbite.

Moist or dry heat can be applied with heating pads, hot-water bottles, towels, gel packs, or warm tub baths or showers. Superficial heat has been shown to be effective for gastrointestinal cramps and muscle and joint pain. Treatment should be limited to 30 minutes to avoid tissue injury. Heat should not be applied to a site of malignancy, to areas of decreased sensation or circulation, or to patients who cannot communicate their discomfort.

Massage involves rubbing, kneading, manipulating, and applying pressure and friction to the body. Rubbing or massaging an area is a natural response when one has an injury or ache. Massage may be used to promote relaxation and relieve muscle cramps. Massage is commonly applied to the back, neck, and large leg muscles; however, massage of the hands and feet is more easily performed and perhaps more effective. Massage should not be applied to areas with injury, phlebitis, or skin lesions or to patients with bleeding problems.

Cold, heat, and massage are easy to apply, inexpensive, effective, and simple for the patient or family to learn. For each therapy, the nurse should evaluate whether the method or location of application is effective, and monitor for any side effects.

Compared with the above therapies, TENS is much more expensive and less widely available. It requires a physician's order, and often the physical therapy department handles the equipment. The therapy involves external electrical stimulation of the skin and underlying tissues through electrodes attached to a small unit that the patient can carry around. The electrodes are placed over, above, or below painful sites and attached to a battery-operated device that delivers low-voltage electrical currents. The electrical current is adjusted through a dial on the unit. The patient should feel a mild tingling or vibrating or prickly sensation over the area of application. Nursing responsibilities with TENS include the following:

1. Apply electrodes in the correct locations and with good contact with the skin.
2. Check that all connections are secure, from skin electrodes to unit.
3. Adjust the current to the prescribed level and/or the patient's level of comfort.
4. Document and evaluate pain relief.

The major disadvantage of TENS is irritation of the skin under the electrodes. The electrodes should be changed daily, the sites rotated, and the skin inspected. Figure 14-6 shows the application of electrodes and a TENS unit.

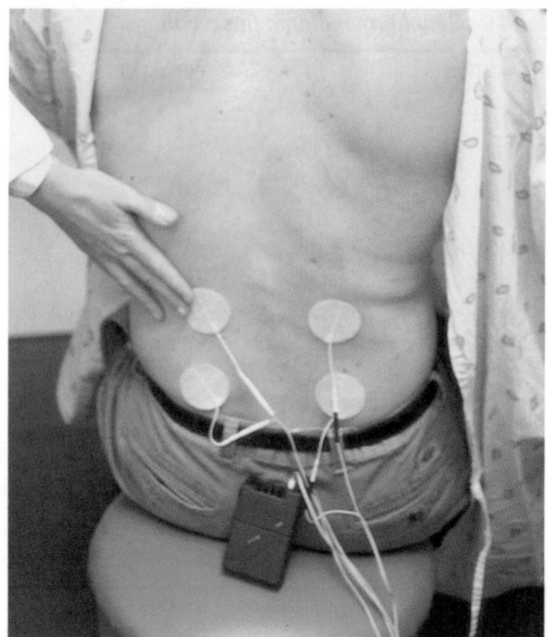

FIGURE **14-6** Application of a TENS unit.

Psychological Interventions

Anxiety reduction. Anxiety, fear of the unknown, and feelings of loss of control may be directly related to the level of pain experienced. The patient who is anxious and uncertain will tend to rate pain high. If the nurse can increase the predictability and control of painful stimuli, pain may be reduced. An important aspect of relieving anxiety associated with pain is the relationship between the nurse and the patient. The nurse can be with the patient, assure the patient that everything possible is being done, and provide timely and appropriate interventions for pain relief.

Several strategies are used to decrease anxiety and increase control. Telling the patient about events and providing descriptions of the sensations or feelings that may accompany the event can reduce anxiety. However, some patients may prefer not to know this information, and their wishes should be respected. Allowing the patient to choose physical comfort measures and the time for treatments or to rearrange items in the room also provides control.

Preoperative teaching should include skills to help patients cope with their pain, such as breathing, relaxation, or imagery techniques. Providing strategies to help the patient cope with pain and anxiety also provides the patient with a sense of control. Table 14-5 describes such psychological interventions used for pain relief.

Distraction. Distraction refers to focusing on stimuli other than pain. Distraction may help the patient gain a sense of control as well as increase pain tolerance, decrease pain intensity, and alter the quality of pain, but it does not eliminate pain. Because the pain is not eliminated, the patient will usually need analgesics and other methods of pain relief. A patient using distraction may not appear or behave as if in pain, which may cause other people to doubt that the pain exists. After a patient has used a distraction technique, he or she may once again focus on the pain and experience a heightened awareness of pain.

Distraction techniques are often most helpful with mild to moderate pain or during brief periods of pain associated with painful procedures such as dressing changes, intramuscular injections, and venipunctures. Examples of distraction methods include rhythmic breathing, listening to music, laughing, counting, watching television, reading, exercising, resting, talking on the phone, and visiting with others. Elderly persons may find reminiscing (relating past experiences) to be an effective distraction technique. It is helpful to include several distraction techniques in the plan of care so that the patient can choose the methods most effective for his or her individual pain relief.

Relaxation. Patients should be aware that relaxation is one of the options for pain relief. Patients may already know this technique or may be taught relaxation techniques. Be aware that the patient is using relaxation, know the rationale for using relaxation, and know the effects of relaxation.

Relaxation is a cognitive approach to pain management. It is a self-hypnotic technique that may, but does not always, produce the relaxation response. The relaxation response counteracts the stress response. It is characterized by decreased muscle tension, a decreased heart rate, decreased respiratory rate, and normal or decreased blood pressure. Relaxation decreases mental stress and physical tension; this is helpful because pain is often accompanied by increased anxiety and muscle tension. Relaxation is more effective for mild to moderate pain than for severe pain.

Rhythmic breathing is a relaxation technique that focuses on just breathing, as described in Table 14-6. Relaxation techniques that focus on total body relaxation require the patient's active participation. Each part of the body is deliberately relaxed, usually in an orderly sequence such as head to toe or vice versa. Relaxation often involves breathing exercises combined with other methods to promote freedom from anxiety and muscle tension. Methods may include yoga, meditation, and music.

table 14-6 ***Sample Relaxation Exercise: Slow Rhythmic Breathing***

1. Breathe in slowly and deeply.
2. As you breathe out slowly, feel yourself beginning to relax; feel the tension leaving your body.
3. Now breathe in and out slowly and regularly at whatever rate is comfortable for you. You may wish to try abdominal breathing. If you do not know how to do abdominal breathing, ask your nurse for help.
4. To help you focus on your breathing and to breathe slowly and rhythmically, do the following:
   a. Breathe in as you say silently to yourself, "in, two, three."
   b. Breathe out as you say silently to yourself, "out, two, three."
   c. Each time you breathe out, say silently to yourself a word such as "peace" or "relax."
5. You may imagine that you are doing this in a position and a place you have found very calming and relaxing, such as lying on a beach in the sun.
6. Do steps 1 through 4 only once, or repeat steps 3 and 4 for up to 20 minutes.
7. End with a slow, deep breath. As you breathe out, say to yourself, "I feel alert and relaxed."

ADDITIONAL POINTS

If you intend to do this for more than a few seconds, try to get into a comfortable position in a quiet environment. You may close your eyes or focus on an object. This technique has the advantage of being very adaptable in that it may be used for only a few seconds or for up to 20 minutes.

Adapted with permission from McCaffery, M., & Beebe, A. (1989). *Pain: Clinical manual for nursing practice.* St. Louis: Mosby.

The patient may be taught relaxation through coaching by the nurse, the use of a script, or an audiotaped relaxation exercise. Emphasize to patients that the use of relaxation does not indicate that the pain is thought to be psychological or that the patient must substitute relaxation for analgesics. Relaxation is a technique to be used in addition to analgesics to enhance pain control and reduce anxiety that contributes to pain.

Imagery. Imagery is another cognitive approach to pain control that encourages physical and mental relaxation. Imagery uses a person's imagination to help control pain. Besides promoting relaxation, imagery may be used for distraction or may help the patient imagine pain relief.

Patients are asked to describe the quality of pain they are experiencing. On the basis of this description, imagery can be used to modify the patient's experience. For example, if the pain is described as "burning," an image of something cool may help reduce pain intensity. As with relaxation, the use of imagery does not mean that medical personnel view the pain as imaginary. In both relaxation and imagery, a script or a prerecorded tape may be used to guide the patient through the experiences. Encourage the patient to practice relaxation or imagery, or both, in order to evaluate their potential effectiveness.

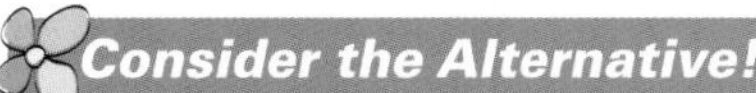

Massage and relaxation with music or imagery are examples of complementary therapies that can be used with analgesics to obtain optimal pain relief.

Pharmacologic Interventions

Drug therapy continues to be the mainstay of pain management. Although the physician orders specific analgesics, it is the nurse's responsibility to assess the pain, to decide which analgesic and how much to administer, and to evaluate the drug's effectiveness.

When administering analgesics, keep in mind that it is critical to use a preventative approach to pain management. When pain is predictable, such as with postoperative pain and cancer pain, analgesics are more effective when given around the clock (ATC) rather than as needed (PRN). An ATC schedule maintains therapeutic blood levels of the analgesics. With a PRN schedule, the patient may have frequent periods of unrelieved pain and may also have more significant and frequent side effects such as sedation. Even when a physician orders analgesics PRN, the analgesics can be given on an ATC schedule. The ATC schedule is usually based on how long the drug lasts; thus, when the order reads every 3 to 4 hours, the analgesic should be administered every 3 to 4 hours to maintain pain relief. Of course, you should assess the patient's pain before the analgesic is administered. The duration of analgesic effect varies among patients.

When pain is unpredictable, it may be appropriate to administer analgesics on a PRN basis. In these situations, instruct the patient to request medication as soon as the pain begins rather than waiting for the pain to become more severe. Patients often report that they wait to call for analgesics, thinking that the pain will decrease with time. Unfortunately, waiting often results in pain reaching an intensity level that is difficult to control.

The three categories of drugs that are used to relieve pain are (1) nonopioid analgesics, (2) opioid analgesics, and (3) adjuvant drugs. Figure 4-7 shows how these categories of drugs are used by themselves or in combination to relieve mild, moderate, and severe pain.

Nonopioid Analgesics

Nonopioid analgesics include aspirin, acetaminophen, and nonsteroidal anti-inflammatory drugs (NSAIDs) such as ibuprofen. The nonopioids are generally the initial treatment choice for mild pain. These analgesics may also be combined with opioids to control moderate-to-severe pain.

Nonopioid analgesics act mostly on the peripheral nervous system and are used for pains such as arthritic pain, backache, headache, dysmenorrhea, postoperative pain, cancer pain, and bone pain. Nonopioids may have antipyretic (fever-reducing), analgesic (pain-reducing), and/or anti-inflammatory (inflammation-reducing) properties. This range of actions makes them especially useful for many conditions.

Most of the nonopioids are oral preparations, but a few are available for rectal administration. A parenteral NSAID,

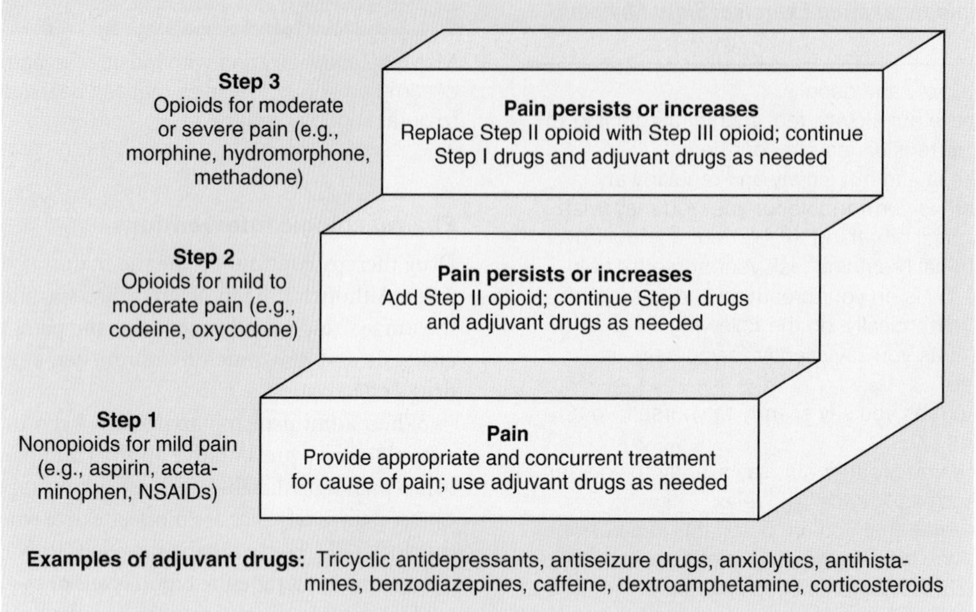
Step 3
Opioids for moderate or severe pain (e.g., morphine, hydromorphone, methadone)
Pain persists or increases
Replace Step II opioid with Step III opioid; continue Step I drugs and adjuvant drugs as needed
Step 2
Opioids for mild to moderate pain (e.g., codeine, oxycodone)
Pain persists or increases
Add Step II opioid; continue Step I drugs and adjuvant drugs as needed
Step 1
Nonopioids for mild pain (e.g., aspirin, acetaminophen, NSAIDs)
Pain
Provide appropriate and concurrent treatment for cause of pain; use adjuvant drugs as needed
Examples of adjuvant drugs: Tricyclic antidepressants, antiseizure drugs, anxiolytics, antihistamines, benzodiazepines, caffeine, dextroamphetamine, corticosteroids

FIGURE **14-7** The World Health Organization three-step analgesic ladder.

ketorolac (Toradol), also is available. It is generally used for the short-term management of postoperative pain. Approximately 30 mg of ketorolac given intramuscularly provides the same amount of pain relief as 12 mg of morphine or 100 mg of meperidine (Demerol) given intramuscularly. Ketorolac has a longer duration of action than many of the opioid analgesics and, like other NSAIDs, can cause nausea and possibly bleeding.

The nonopioids, unlike the opioids, have a ceiling effect on analgesia. This means that, beyond a certain dosage, improved analgesia will not occur. However, these drugs do have side effects, including stomach irritation, fluid retention, and an increased bleeding time. Therefore, they are usually not recommended for patients with liver or kidney disorders, thrombocytopenia, or neutropenia. (Thrombocytopenia is a deficiency of platelets in the blood. Neutropenia is a decreased percentage of neutrophils, the white blood cells that respond to inflammation). Some nonopioids should be used cautiously in patients with congestive heart failure or hypertension because they cause fluid retention, which may aggravate these conditions. Because nonopioids have many side effects, you should assess the patient's history and present condition before administering prescribed analgesics. Some patients have better pain relief with certain types of nonopioids compared to others. It is important to ask which nonopioids work best to relieve their pain.

Table 14-7 identifies commonly used NSAIDs and some considerations to keep in mind when administering these drugs. Older adults may be more sensitive to NSAIDs and may experience more side effects. Carefully monitor each patient's reaction to the analgesic. Older adults especially should be monitored for signs of increased bleeding time, gastrointestinal irritation, and unusual drug reactions such as confusion, constipation, and headaches.

Many nurses forget to administer nonopioids because they fail to recognize the importance of using these drugs for the types of mild to moderate pain mentioned previously. The nonopioids can be administered along with opioids and may be as effective as lower doses of opioids. For instance, 650 mg of aspirin or acetaminophen taken orally provides the same amount of analgesia as 32 mg of codeine or 50 mg of meperidine taken orally. Nonopioids tend to block pain transmission peripherally, whereas opioids block pain transmission in the central nervous system. It is advantageous to administer both for pain relief.

PHARMACOLOGY CAPSULE The adverse effects of nonopioid analgesics include stomach irritation, fluid retention, and increased bleeding time.

Opioid Analgesics

Opioid analgesics are generally used for moderate to severe acute pain, chronic cancer pain, and some other types of pain. The opioids vary in potency and duration of action.

There are currently two types of opioid analgesics:

Opioid agonists. Examples include codeine, methadone (Dolophine), hydromorphone (Dilaudid), meperidine (Demerol), morphine, and fentanyl.

Opioid agonist-antagonists. Examples include buprenorphine (Buprenex), nalbuphine (Nubain), butorphanol (Stadol), and pentazocine (Talwin).

Both types of opioids relieve pain at the level of the central nervous system. Agonist drugs fit into receptor sites on the

table 14-7 ***Nonopioid Analgesics: Commonly Used NSAIDs***

DRUGS	COMMENTS
ORAL NSAIDs	
Acetaminophen	Lacks the peripheral anti-inflammatory activity of other NSAIDs
Aspirin*	The standard against which other NSAIDs are compared. Inhibits platelet aggregation; may cause postoperative bleeding
Choline magnesium (Trilisate)	May have minimal antiplatelet activity; also available as trisalicylate oral liquid
Fenoprofen calcium (Nalfon)	
Ibuprofen (Motrin, others)	Available in several brand-name formulations and as a generic product; also available as oral suspension
Ketoprofen (Orudis)	
Magnesium salicylate	Many brands and generic forms available
Naproxen (Naprosyn)	Also available as oral liquid
Naproxen sodium (Anaprox)	
Salsalate (Disalcid, others)	May have minimal antiplatelet activity
Sodium salicylate	Available in generic form from several distributors
PARENTERAL NSAIDs	
Ketorolac	IM administration not to exceed 5 days

Adapted from Acute Pain Management Guidelines Panel. (1992). *Acute pain management: Operative and medical procedures and trauma. Clinical practice guidelines* (AHCPR Publication No. 92-0032). Rockville, MD: Agency for Health Care Policy and Research, Public Health Service, U.S. Department of Health and Human Services.
*Contraindicated in the presence of fever or other evidence of viral illness.
NSAIDs, Nonsteroidal anti-inflammatory drugs; *IM,* intramuscularly.
Note: Only the NSAIDs listed in the table have been approved by the U.S. Food and Drug Administration for use as simple analgesics, but clinical experience has also been gained with other drugs as well.

cell to "turn on" the site and produce the drug effect. Antagonists are drugs that block drug effects at the receptor sites. Opioid agonists bind to opioid receptors to produce analgesia, but they also bind to other receptors to produce unwanted side effects such as decreased respiration, drowsiness, and nausea. Opioid agonist-antagonists are drugs designed to produce analgesia and also to block certain side effects. The agonist-antagonists block some of the effects of the pure opioid agonists in much the same way that naloxone (Narcan) acts to block or reverse the effects of opioids. Drugs classified as agonist-antagonists (e.g., pentazocine, nalbuphine, buprenorphine) produce analgesia, but they can also block the effects of opioids such as morphine or meperidine if the patient has been receiving these drugs. Thus, a patient receiving pure opioid agonists for pain relief should not be given opioid agonist-antagonists because they may block analgesia, precipitate withdrawal symptoms, and increase pain. For example, if a patient has been receiving morphine intramuscularly for several days, it would not be advisable to administer nalbuphine (Nubain), because it may block some of the analgesic effects of morphine.

Older adults are generally more sensitive to the analgesic effects of opioids because of delayed excretion and slower metabolism. Also, side effects may be more pronounced in older adults. Thus, the recommended adult dose should be reduced 25% to 50% initially, then titrated (adjusted) for optimum pain control with minimal side effects. Some elders are small and thin and weigh less than 100 pounds. In this case, charts with recommended opioid doses for adults and children

table 14-8 ***Opioid Analgesics: Starting Oral Dose Commonly Used for Severe Pain***

NAME	EQUIANALGESIC DOSE (mg) ORAL	PARENTERAL*	STARTING ORAL DOSE ADULTS (mg)
Morphine	30	10	15-30
Hydromorphone (Dilaudid)	7.5	1.5	4-8
Fentanyl	—	0.1	—
Methadone (Dolophine)	20 acute pain 2-4 chronic pain	10 acute pain 2-4 chronic pain	5-10

From The American Pain Society. *Principles of analgesic use in the treatment of acute pain and cancer pain,* 4th ed. Glenview, IL, 1999, The American Pain Society, p. 14.
*These are standard intramuscular doses for acute pain in adults. Equianalgesic doses should be based on the opioid characteristics, and patient characteristics such as age, weight, liver and renal function, and reaction to the drug.

weighing less than 50 kg or less than 110 pounds are available. Table 14-8 provides guidelines for dosing opioids.

It is important to refer to an equianalgesic (approximately equal analgesia) table when changing to a new opioid or a different route. Table 14-8 is such a table showing approximately equianalgesic oral and parenteral doses. The information in the table helps to estimate the new dose, which should then be modified based on the specific patient reaction and drug. An equianalgesic table shows that oral doses are two to six times larger than parenteral doses of the same drug to achieve the same effect. This is because oral opioids must pass through the liver after absorption, which reduces the amount of medication absorbed. Therefore, larger doses of oral opioids must be ordered to provide the same amount of analgesia as parenteral opioids. For example, a patient receives 10 mg of morphine intramuscularly for pain relief, and the order is changed to oral morphine. To receive an equianalgesic dose of morphine, the patient should be given 30 mg of morphine orally.

Meperidine or Demerol continues to be used for moderate-to-severe pain. You should be aware that one of the products of meperidine metabolism is normeperidine, which is a central nervous system stimulant. Clinical practice guidelines state that meperidine may cause central nervous system toxicity. When this metabolite accumulates in the body, the patient may exhibit anxiety, twitching, tremors, muscle jerking and generalized seizures. This opioid is contraindicated for long-term administration, specifically over 48 hours and for diminished renal function. Since many elderly people have decreased renal function, meperidine should be avoided.

PHARMACOLOGY CAPSULE Older adults are more sensitive to opioid analgesics and should be monitored frequently for side effects.

Misconceptions about opioid analgesics. When discussing opioid analgesics, it is critical to review a few terms that are often misunderstood, resulting in undertreatment of pain. Patients, families, nurses, and physicians have misconceptions about addiction; therefore, the term must be defined and differentiated from the terms tolerance and physical dependence. Table 14-9 contains information about these terms.

table 14-9 ***Characteristics of Tolerance, Physical Dependence, and Addiction***

TOLERANCE

Physiologic changes that occur from repeated doses of opioids.

Result: Higher doses are needed to achieve pain relief.

PHYSICAL DEPENDENCE

Physiologic changes that occur from repeated doses of opioids.

Result: Withdrawal symptoms (e.g., irritability, chills, sweating, nausea) may occur if the opioid is stopped abruptly.

ADDICTION

Psychological dependence characterized by continued craving for opioid for other than pain relief.

Result: Compulsive and continued use for psychic effects despite harm.

Note: Risk of addiction is not a concern in treating acute or cancer pain.

When patients take opioids over a period of time for pain, tolerance and physical dependency may occur. The patient who is tolerant requires higher doses of a drug to achieve an analgesic effect. The patient who is physically dependent on an opioid will experience unpleasant withdrawal symptoms when the opioid is stopped. Both tolerance and physical dependence are normal responses to continued opioid administration for pain relief; they do not lead to a craving for the drug for its mind-altering effects. Fear of addiction is greatly exaggerated, and addiction rarely occurs ($<1\%$) in patients taking opioids for pain relief. Remind patients that pain relief is an important goal and they should not worry about addiction. Most patients simply stop taking opioids when the pain stops.

Routes of administration. The opioids can be administered through various routes, depending on the needs of the patient. If tolerated, the oral route is preferred, especially for patients with chronic pain. Oral opioids can control severe pain when given in adequate dosages.

The intramuscular route may be used to administer opioids for breakthrough pain, that is, pain that occurs between regularly scheduled doses of pain medication. Breakthrough pain would require immediate-acting or short-acting analgesic medication such as morphine. Consider the drug being administered when selecting appropriate needle-gauge size and administration site for intramuscular medication. For example, to administer 10 mg of morphine intramuscularly, use at least a 1.5- to 2.5-inch needle to reach the muscle, depending on the patient's size. Some drugs such as Demerol are more irritating to muscle tissue and should be administered deep into the muscle with the *Z*-track method. You can use the ventrogluteal, dorsogluteal, and vastus lateralis muscles. The intramuscular route is impractical for repeated injections. Absorption is often unpredictable with intramuscular injections, particularly in older adults, who have reduced muscle mass. This route is also painful. An accessible and appropriate site for the intramuscular injection of analgesics is the ventral gluteal muscle, especially in older adults.

A limited number of opioids, such as morphine, hydromorphone, and oxymorphone, may be administered rectally. This route is useful when the patient is nauseated or has difficulty swallowing.

Opioids may also be administered sublingually (under the tongue). Intermittent bolus injections, continuous infusions, or patient-controlled analgesia (PCA) are methods of administering medications subcutaneously. These methods may be used in patients in whom the oral and rectal routes cannot be used and who also have poor intravenous access.

The intravenous route is another method of administering opioids. Intravenous PCA is commonly used postoperatively. With PCA, the patient is able to self-administer doses of analgesics in order to control pain. Opioids, when administered intravenously, have a rapid onset but shorter duration of action than when given by any other route. Although the registered nurse is usually responsible for the PCA, the practical nurse may be responsible for monitoring the patient's response and the effectiveness of the medication. Side effects should be reported to the registered nurse.

PATIENT TEACHING PLAN
Patient-Controlled Analgesia (PCA)

- Safety features: The pump has a delay feature and a lockout interval that prevent you from receiving more than the prescribed amount of medication.
- Use: Press the PCA button when pain begins to return, then put it down and wait 10-15 minutes to evaluate pain relief. If pain returns, push the PCA button again and repeat the process until the pain is relieved.
- If pain is not relieved: Notify the RN, who can recommend changes in the opioid, bolus amount, or lockout interval to the physician to achieve satisfactory pain relief.

Opioids can also be administered via the spinal route epidurally (in the epidural space) or intrathecally (in the subarachnoid space). The epidural or intrathecal route may be selected in patients with postoperative pain and chronic cancer pain. The practical nurse may participate in monitoring the patient. Side effects such as itching, hypotension, nausea, urinary retention, sedation, and respiratory depression may occur more frequently in patients receiving opioids epidurally or intrathecally than by other routes of administration. The older adult who has received a spinal opioid infusion is at increased risk for respiratory depression. If anesthetics such as bupivacaine are used with spinal opioids, the nurse must be alert for the side effects of sensory loss and motor weakness. Side effects, as well as any adverse effects, should be reported promptly. A sedation assessment scale should be used with patients receiving spinal opioid infusions. Sedation is usually seen before signs of respiratory depression.

Other routes of administration of opioids also are available. Liquid morphine may be administered sublingually. Duragesic or fentanyl transdermal patches are used to treat cancer and chronic pain by producing constant delivery of the opioids for 72 hours through the skin surface. Intranasal butorphanol is available and may be used preoperatively for sedation and postoperatively for analgesia. Package inserts should be reviewed for doses, precautions, and administration guidelines.

PHARMACOLOGY CAPSULE Oral analgesics are preferred for the treatment of chronic pain.

Side effects. Regardless of the route of administration, opioid analgesics have specific side effects. A common side effect is constipation. Tolerance for this side effect does not develop. Assess the patient for abdominal distention, cramping, and abdominal pain. Stool softeners and laxatives, along with increased fluid, exercise, and bulk-containing foods, may prevent this side effect.

Opioids may also cause nausea, with or without vomiting. Some patients develop a tolerance for nausea but may require antiemetic therapy until tolerance develops. At times, the order may need to be changed to a different opioid to relieve this problem.

Sedation is another side effect that may occur initially with opioids, but it usually subsides in a few days. In patients who have had unrelieved pain for some time and have been sleep deprived, the control of pain may allow the patient to rest, which may be misinterpreted as sedation. When sedation is noted, however, the dose of the opioid may need to be titrated to a level that does not cause sedation but does provide pain relief. Box 14-1 shows a sedation scale. Be aware that drugs such as promethazine (Phenergan), which are sometimes ordered to be given with opioids, may also contribute to sedation. Promethazine does not potentiate or increase the analgesic effects of opioids but does potentiate sedation, respiratory depression, and hypotension. If sedated, the patient may benefit from having separate orders for the opioid and for the promethazine. Work with the physician and ordered drug(s) to reduce sedation to a rating of 1-2 on the scale and achieve the most effective pain relief.

Respiratory depression can occur but does not occur as frequently as commonly thought. If a patient is easily arousable, it is highly unlikely that respiratory depression has occurred. If severe respiratory depression occurs (less than 6-8 respirations a minute) and stimulation does not awaken the patient, this is an emergency. Stay with the patient and call for help. The RN may administer naloxone (Narcan) intravenously to reverse the opioid if prescribed.

Other side effects may be noted with the use of opioid analgesics. These include confusion, hypotension (especially orthostatic), dizziness, itching, and urinary retention. Nonopioid analgesics given with opioids may allow a decrease in the opioid dose to one that maintains pain control with fewer opioid side effects.

Put on your THINKING CAP!!

Ask five people (patients, friends, strangers) what helps when they have pain. Compile a list with your classmates and sort the treatment measures into pharmacologic and nonpharmacologic. Include home remedies and herbal remedies.

Placebos

Placebos are inactive substances (e.g., saline) used in research or clinical practice to determine the effects of a legitimate

box 14-1 *Sedation Scale*

S Sleeping but easy to arouse when called or stimulated
1 Awake and alert
2 Slightly drowsy but easily aroused
3 Frequently drowsy, arousable but drifts off to sleep during conversation—alert the RN
4 Somnolent, minimal or no response to physical stimulation—emergency

table 14-10 ***Adjuvant Analgesics and Medications***

DRUG CLASSIFICATION	TYPE OF PAIN OR PROBLEM ASSOCIATED WITH PAIN
ANTIDEPRESSANTS	Neuropathic pain; dull, aching pain
Amitriptyline (Elavil)	Pain associated with herpes zoster (shingles)
Doxepin (Sinequan)	Sleep disturbances
MUSCLE RELAXANTS	Muscle spasms and anxiety
Methocarbamol (Robaxin)	
Cyclobenzaprine (Flexeril)	
BENZODIAZEPINES	Muscle spasms and anxiety
Alprazolam (Xanax)	
Lorazepam (Ativan)	
ANTIHISTAMINES	Nausea, anxiety
Hydroxyzine (Vistaril, Atarax)	
CORTICOSTEROIDS	Spinal cord or nerve compression
Prednisone (Deltasone)	Bone pain
Dexamethasone (Decadron)	
ANTICONVULSANTS	Neuropathic pain, stabbing pain
Carbamazepine (Tegretol)	Trigeminal neuralgia
Phenytoin (Dilantin)	Pain associated with herpes zoster (shingles)
Gabapentin (Neurontin)	Other nerve pain
LOCAL ANESTHETICS/ANTIDYSRHYTHMICS	Postherpetic neuralgia, diabetic neuropathy, other chronic pain conditions
Lidocaine	
Mexiletine	
MISCELLANEOUS	Pain from spinal cord injury, phantom limb pain, peripheral nerve injuries
Clonidine	
PSYCHOSTIMULANTS	Analgesic effect, postoperative pain
Dextroamphetamines (Dexedrine)	Analgesic effect, cancer pain
Methylphenidate (Ritalin)	

Consider the Alternative!

Patients who have migraines may be taking feverfew, an herbal supplement, for headache prevention. There is no evidence of effectiveness in treating other conditions. Advise patients that feverfew can increase the risk of bleeding in patients taking aspirin, warfarin, or heparin.

drug or treatment. Placebos are appropriately used in studies in which patients consent to participate in the study. Many professional health care organizations take the position that placebos should not be used to assess or manage pain. Nurses have an ethical obligation to ensure that patients are not deceived and that institutional policies related to placebos are followed.

PHARMACOLOGY CAPSULE The adverse effects of opioid analgesics include constipation, nausea, sedation, respiratory depression, confusion, hypotension, dizziness, itching, and urinary retention.

Adjuvant Analgesics and Medications

Drugs that are not usually classified as analgesics may relieve pain in certain situations. For instance, a patient who has undergone back surgery may complain more about muscle spasms than incisional pain. A muscle relaxant may be more effective in relieving pain than an opioid alone. Specific pain syndromes may be controlled with drugs other than the commonly known analgesics. Table 14-10 lists adjuvant drugs and the conditions they effectively treat.

Problem Solving with Pain Medication

Nurses are often faced with patients whose prescribed analgesic drugs do not relieve pain. In these situations, use all of the information presented here. Ask questions about the analgesic drug and the "five rights" (right dose, right patient, right time, right route, right analgesic) to determine why the patient is not getting adequate pain relief. Table 14-11 provides a method for problem solving when analgesic drugs do not provide effective pain relief. Table 14-12 provides a nursing plan of care checklist.

The administration of analgesics is simply one intervention in the nursing care of a patient in pain. Nurses should provide many interventions along with analgesics to relieve

table 14-11 **Problem Solving with Pain Medication**

When the analgesic medication prescribed for pain is not effective in relieving pain, the nurse should take the following steps to solve the problem:

1. Check the analgesic order.
   a. **Right dose:** Is the dose prescribed a recommended starting dose for analgesia, or is the dose prescribed less? If a range of medication is prescribed, has the maximum dose been administered? If the order states morphine, 10-20 mg IM PRN for pain, and 10 mg morphine is ineffective for pain relief, has 20 mg been administered? *Solution:* Adjust the dose up as ordered until pain is relieved without serious side effects or minimal side effects.
   b. **Right patient:** Is the patient experiencing side effects of the analgesic at the present dose? Can the patient tolerate the increase in dose with few side effects?
   c. **Right time:** What is the onset, peak, and duration of the analgesic? Is the analgesic administered around-the-clock based on the duration or properties of the drug? *Solution:* Evaluate pain intensity periodically to see if correct timing of drug is more effective in relieving pain.

If the patient's pain is still not relieved, the following steps should be taken:

2. Consider an alternative prescription.
   a. **Right patient:** What is the diagnosis or source of pain, and what analgesic is most effective for this type of pain? What are patient characteristics to consider (e.g., age, liver or renal problems, NPO status)?
   b. **Right route:** Which route is most appropriate for the patient condition, severity of pain, and medication prescribed (e.g., IV, IM, PO, or topical administration)?
   c. **Right analgesic:** Which analgesic or adjuvant drug is best for this type of pain? Which analgesic has proven effective for the patient in the past or in a similar condition? Can the opioid or nonopioid prescribed be switched to another drug in the class that may provide more effective pain relief? Have both opioids and nonopioids been prescribed to increase pain relief?
   d. **Right dose:** Has the dose of opioid been titrated up or adjusted to a higher dose to reduce the pain? Has the patient been receiving opioids over time and require increased doses of opioids to control pain because of the development of tolerance? If switching opioid drugs, is the correct equianalgesic dose calculated to make sure you have the approximate same level of analgesia?
   e. **Right time:** What is the time interval at which the analgesic should be administered or evaluated given its duration of action and patient?
3. Collaborate with patient, other nurses, pharmacist, and family.
   a. Collect information.
   b. Establish credibility with facts about the patient, analgesics, and written references (articles or drug guides).
   c. Anticipate questions.
   d. Be assertive and keep trying.
   e. Always use other nursing interventions in addition to the analgesic to relieve pain.

IM, Intramuscularly; *PRN*, as needed; *NPO*, nothing by mouth; *IV*, intravenously; *PO*, orally.

pain. Table 14-12 includes the expected patient outcomes and guidelines for nursing care.

key points

- Pain is the most common problem that nurses encounter.
- "Pain is an unpleasant sensory and emotional experience associated with actual or potential tissue damage" (International Association for the Study of Pain).
- When pain receptors are stimulated, impulses are transmitted to the spinal cord and then to the brain, where the cortex interprets the signals as pain.
- Endorphins are natural opioid-like substances that block the transmission of painful impulses to the brain.
- According to the gate-control theory, stimulation of large-diameter fibers in the spinal cord interferes with the transmission of painful impulses to the brain.
- Physical factors that influence the pain experience are pain threshold, pain tolerance, age, physical activity, nervous system integrity, and, in surgical patients, the type of surgery and anesthesia.
- Psychological factors that influence the pain experience include culture, religion, past experiences with pain, anxiety, and situational factors.
- Based on the duration and cause, pain is classified as acute, chronic, chronic benign (nonmalignant), and chronic malignant pain (cancer-related pain).
- Most chronic pain is neuropathic because of nerve damage.
- Assessment is the first step in pain management.
- Pain can be described in terms of location, quality, intensity, and aggravating and alleviating factors.
- It is essential to document assessment findings and the effects of pain interventions.
- Nursing diagnoses for the patient in pain may include pain, chronic pain, activity intolerance, anxiety, fatigue, self-care deficit, and sleep pattern disturbance.
- Examples of nonpharmacologic interventions are comfort measures, control of environmental factors, stimulation techniques, and measures to reduce anxiety.

table 14-12 ***Southwest Texas Methodist Hospital Nursing Plan of Care: Pain***

NURSING DIAGNOSIS/PATIENT PROBLEM	STANDARDS OF PRACTICE/GUIDELINES FOR CARE
Alteration in comfort/pain (acute/chronic) related to: **Date/Initials** ________ Disease processes/illness ________ Surgery ________ Injury/trauma ________ Diagnostic procedures ________ ________ ________ ________ **As evidenced by:** ________ Verbalization of pain/discomfort ________ Verbalization of spasms (specify bladder, back, muscle) ________ ________ Facial grimacing ________ Tense body posture ________ Rubbing/guarding of body parts ________ Inability to concentrate ________ Increased vital signs ________ Restlessness/difficulty sleeping ________ Crying, moaning ________ Withdrawal ________ Change in appetite ________ Decreased activity ________ ________ ________ ________ **STANDARD OF CARE/EXPECTED OUTCOME** Patient will verbalize/demonstrate minimal discomfort or absence of pain AEB: ________ Statements of pain relief and effectiveness of pain medications and/or other interventions ________ Decreased need for pain medication ________ Relaxed facial expression and body part ________ Increase in voluntary movement, ambulation, and ADL ________ Increased ability to concentrate ________ Stable vital signs ________ Statements or demonstrations of coping behaviors and/or factors that reduce or eliminate discomfort or pain ________ Able to sleep/rest ________ Increased appetite ________ ________ ________ ________	________ Accept patient's level/tolerance of pain ________ Assess pain characteristics to include location, intensity, duration, type, precipitating factors ________ Provide the patient with prescribed medication as ordered ________ Provide and teach alternative methods of pain relief based on individual needs and/or physician orders: ________ Positioning ________ Back rub ________ Massage ________ Application of heat ________ Application of cold ________ Diversion/distraction ________ Relaxation/imagery ________ Exercise/ambulation ________ Range of motion ________ Other: ________ Consults: ________ ________ Teach patient and/or significant other pain management strategies: ________ Use of PCA ________ Medications ________ Explain procedures to decrease/relieve anxiety ________ Validate patient's understanding/coping ________ Evaluate effectiveness of interventions and reintervene as necessary

From Southwest Texas Methodist Hospital, San Antonio, TX.
ADL, Activities of daily living; *PCA*, patient-controlled analgesia.

- Predictable pain is best controlled by around-the-clock (ATC) analgesics rather than as-needed (PRN) medication.
- The categories of drugs used to relieve pain are nonopioid analgesics, opioid analgesics, and adjuvant drugs.
- Fear of addiction to opioids is greatly exaggerated. Addiction rarely occurs when opioids are taken for pain relief.
- Placebos are inactive substances such as saline that are used as a control to determine the effects of a legitimate drug or treatment.
- Most professional health care organizations take the position that placebos should not be used to assess or manage pain.
- Opioid side effects to monitor and treat include constipation, nausea, sedation, and respiratory depression.

REVIEW QUESTIONS

1. Pain is best defined by the:
   1. patient.
   2. nurse.
   3. physician.
   4. physiologist.

2. When you cut your finger, which of the following represents the steps involved in your experiencing pain?
   1. Afferent pathways activate nociceptors, which transmit information to the spinal cord for interpretation.
   2. Nociceptors are stimulated, afferent pathways send impulses to the spinal cord, then to the brain.
   3. Efferent pathways stimulate nociceptors, which transmit impulses to the brain.
   4. The brain stimulates nociceptors, which trigger efferent pathways to send impulses to the spinal cord.

3. Mr. A and Mr. B both had back surgery yesterday. Mr. A has used his PCA regularly. He says that he is "pretty comfortable," and he sleeps most of the time. Mr. B has used the maximum analgesic permitted by his PCA and has required additional analgesic twice while continuing to complain of some discomfort. Of the following, which is the most likely explanation for the difference in the pain experience of these two patients?
   1. Mr. B is a complainer who is seeking attention.
   2. Mr. B has higher pain tolerance than Mr. A.
   3. Mr. B has a lower pain threshold than Mr. A.
   4. Mr. B is more anxious, which has raised his pain threshold.

4. Autonomic nervous system responses to pain include:
   1. decreased respiratory rate.
   2. flushing.
   3. urinary frequency.
   4. constipation.

5. A patient says she has pain whenever she bends over. Which aspect of the pain assessment is she describing?
   1. Location
   2. Alleviating factor
   3. Quality
   4. Aggravating factor

6. A frail, elderly patient who is being cared for by her family at home says she finds a heating pad soothing to stiff joints. What patient/family teaching is needed for safe and effective heat therapy?
   1. "It is more effective to use the heating pad continuously rather than intermittently."
   2. "Do not apply heat to any area that lacks normal sensation or circulation."
   3. "Set the heating pad at the highest temperature that the patient can tolerate."
   4. "Heat application is not a safe or effective strategy for pain management."

7. Which statement correctly describes a nonpharmacologic approach to pain control?
   1. Imagery is the use of the patient's imagination to help control pain.
   2. Distraction is most effective in the management of chronic pain.
   3. Relaxation therapy requires that the nurse must be able to hypnotize the patient.
   4. Patient education is usually all that is needed to reduce anxiety.

8. Nonopioid analgesics must be used cautiously in patients with hypertension because they cause:
   1. peripheral vasoconstriction.
   2. potassium loss.
   3. sleep disturbances.
   4. fluid retention.

9. You should question an NSAID order for a patient who is also taking:
   1. antibiotics.
   2. decongestants.
   3. anticoagulants.
   4. hormone replacements.

10. When patients take opioid analgesics, the nurse must assess for:
    1. diarrhea.
    2. deficient fluid volume.
    3. respiratory depression.
    4. urinary incontinence.

UNIT **THREE** ACUTE CARE

CHAPTER 15 First Aid and Emergency Care

objectives

1. List the principles of emergency and first aid care.
2. List the steps of the initial assessment and interventions for the person requiring emergency care.
3. Describe the components of the nursing assessment of the person requiring emergency care.
4. Outline the steps of the nursing process for emergency or first aid treatment of victims of cardiopulmonary arrest, choking, shock, hemorrhage, traumatic injury, burns, heat or cold exposure, poisoning, bites, and stings.
5. Explain the legal implications of administering first aid in emergency situations.

key terms

Avulsion (ă-VŬL-shŭn, p. 196)
Cardiac tamponade (KĂR-dē-ăk tăm-pŏn-ĀD, p. 196)
Cardiopulmonary arrest (kăr-dē-ō-PŬL-mō-nĕr-ē, p. 189)
Epistaxis (ĕp-ĭ-STĂK-sĭs, p. 193)
Evisceration (ĕ-vĭs-ĕr-Ā-shŭn, p. 196)
Flail chest (flāl, p. 196)
Hemorrhage (HĔM-ŏr-ĭj, p. 193)
Hemothorax (hē-mō-THŌ-răks, p. 196)
Hyperthermia (hī-pĕr-THĔR-mē-ă, p. 198)
Hypothermia (hī-pō-THĔR-mē-ă, p. 198)
Pneumothorax (nū-mō-THŌ-răks, p. 196)
Poison (p. 200)
Respiratory arrest (RĔS-pĭ-ră-tō-rē, p. 189)
Shock (p. 192)
Sprain (p. 194)
Strain (p. 194)

In the inpatient setting, the nurse is often the first on the scene when accidents or emergencies occur. Nurses also need to be prepared to act in emergency situations in homes and other community settings. Prompt intervention can make a dramatic difference in patient outcomes. Knowledge of first aid can make the difference between life and death in many situations. This chapter addresses first aid interventions for common emergencies. Some emergency conditions that require further medical attention are covered in greater detail elsewhere in this book.

GENERAL PRINCIPLES OF EMERGENCY CARE

When accidents or emergencies occur, the victim and any observers are often understandably frightened. It can be very reassuring to them to know that a nurse is present, but you must remember a cardinal rule: remain calm! Victims react to emergencies in various ways, from stunned silence to hysteria. Although your priority is to preserve life and minimize effects of injuries, the manner in which you conduct yourself also can soothe and reassure the victim.

The nursing process is used in emergencies just as it is in other nursing situations. The important difference is that assessment and intervention must be done very quickly and very efficiently to identify and treat priority needs immediately.

Assessment begins when approaching the victim. Try to determine the nature of the emergency, that is, was the injury caused by an automobile accident, a fall, a diving accident, or an electrocution? Also, look for any hazards to the victim and the rescuer. For example, is the victim in a burning vehicle or lying in the middle of the highway? Failure to recognize such dangers may result in injuries to the rescuer and additional injuries to the victim.

Initial assessment and immediate intervention proceed in the following sequence:

1. Assess the ABCs: airway, breathing, circulation.
2. Initiate cardiopulmonary resuscitation or rescue breathing as needed.
3. Look for uncontrolled bleeding, identify the source, and apply pressure to the source.
4. Systematically assess for injuries from the head to the feet, and immobilize spine, limbs, or both as indicated.
5. Look for a medical alert tag, usually a necklace or a bracelet.

After the initial assessment, once again go back through the assessment process to detect significant changes and other findings that might have been missed initially.

GUIDELINES FOR FIRST AID TREATMENT

General guidelines for first aid treatment of emergency patients are the following:

1. Splint injured parts in the position they are found.
2. Prevent chilling, but do not add excessive heat.
3. Do not remove penetrating objects.
4. Do not try to give anything by mouth to an unconscious person or to one with potentially serious injuries.

5. Stay with the injured person until medical care or transportation arrives.

NURSING ASSESSMENT IN EMERGENCIES

Patient emergencies can occur in every setting. Sometimes nurses observe the events and know what has happened, but at other times evidence at the scene is needed to determine the circumstances. It is difficult to intervene appropriately in emergencies that cannot be immediately understood. Be prepared to do a quick assessment and then act promptly to provide appropriate care that may save a life. The health history and physical examination are presented separately here but, in fact, may be done almost simultaneously in emergencies.

HEALTH HISTORY

If the victim is able to speak or a witness is available, obtain a brief health history of the victim. Data collection is limited in emergency situations and should include the chief complaint, the treatment given, and the relevant medical history.

Chief Complaint

Determine the nature of the problem, the signs and symptoms, and the circumstances under which the injury or illness occurred. If the victim is or has been unconscious, note the length of time unconscious if possible.

Medical Treatment

Determine whether any treatment has been given and if so, what effect the treatment had. In the event of an injury, note whether the victim has been moved.

Past Medical History

If possible, determine known health problems including diabetes and cardiac or pulmonary disease, which may provide important clues to the immediate problem or influence the care provided. Check for a medical alert tag, which may provide essential information if the patient cannot. If possible, identify current medications and known allergies. Note any evidence of alcohol or other drugs.

PHARMACOLOGY CAPSULE The medical alert tag can provide clues about medical emergencies and alert rescuers to known allergies and chronic conditions.

PHYSICAL EXAMINATION

Begin collecting objective data as soon as the victim is seen and quickly determine whether the patient is responsive. The first assessment priorities must be the ABCs: airway, breathing, and circulation. Watch the victim's chest for rhythmic breathing and listen near the patient's mouth and nose for air movement. Palpate the carotid and peripheral pulses. Once the adequacy of respiration and circulation has been established, assess for uncontrolled bleeding and shock. If there is no evidence of uncontrolled bleeding or shock, the next step is a systematic head-to-toe assessment. At each step, look for obvious injury, bleeding, swelling, bruising, and drainage. Note circulation, mobility, sensation, and alignment of the entire body. Also assess skin color, warmth, and temperature at each step.

The systematic assessment begins with inspection of the head. Speak to the victim and evaluate the response to assess level of consciousness (alert, disoriented, unresponsive). Evaluate comprehension by asking the patient to follow simple commands such as opening and closing the eyes. Inspect the eyes to assess pupil size, equality, and reaction to light. Ask the alert victim about neck pain or stiffness and the ability to swallow. Inspect the chest for symmetry of the chest wall movement. Next assess respiratory effort, dyspnea, and abnormal sounds associated with respirations. Examine the contour of the abdomen to detect distention. Use light palpation to detect areas of pain or tenderness. Inspect the extremities for deformity or injury, and evaluate movement. Then assess peripheral pulses and warmth and sensation in the extremities (Table 15-1).

table 15-1 ASSESSMENT *of the Patient Who Requires First Aid or Emergency Care*

HEALTH HISTORY

Chief Complaint: Nature of illness or injury, signs and symptoms, circumstances of illness or injury, how long unconscious
Treatment: What has been done, effects, whether moved after injury
Past Medical History: Current health problems, current medications, allergies

PHYSICAL EXAMINATION

ABCs: Airway, breathing, circulation
Skin: Color, temperature, obvious injury
Head: Level of consciousness
Eyes: Opening, pupil size, equality, response to light
Neck: Stiffness, pain, ability to swallow
Chest: Symmetry of movement, dyspnea, respiratory rate and effort
Abdomen: Contour, rigidity, distention, pain, tenderness
Extremities: Deformity, movement, sensation, peripheral pulses

SPECIFIC EMERGENCIES

CARDIOPULMONARY ARREST

When the heart stops beating, a person is in cardiac arrest. When respirations cease, the person is in **respiratory,** or pulmonary, **arrest. Cardiopulmonary arrest** is the absence of a heartbeat and respirations. The cardiac and respiratory systems are so dependent on each other that when one fails, the other quickly fails as well.

Nerve tissue is so susceptible to hypoxia (low levels of oxygen) that in most circumstances the brain cells begin to die after 4 minutes without oxygen. Unless circulation and oxygenation are restored very quickly after cardiopulmonary arrest, permanent brain damage results. Prompt recognition and treatment of cardiopulmonary arrest can maintain the oxygen supply to the brain until circulation and respiration are restored.

Cardiopulmonary resuscitation (CPR) can be part of basic life support or advanced life support. Basic life support is the immediate care given to maintain oxygenation of the brain until advanced medical support is available. This chapter focuses on basic life support given outside of the health care setting. Key points only are emphasized here, but literature published by the American Heart Association or the American Red Cross provides additional, more specific information. Advanced life support is discussed in Chapter 33.

Causes

Examples of causes of cardiopulmonary arrest are myocardial infarction, heart failure, electrocution, drowning, drug overdose, anaphylaxis, and asphyxiation.

Signs and Symptoms

Victims of cardiopulmonary arrest collapse and quickly lose consciousness. They have no pulse or respiration.

Nursing Assessment

In cardiopulmonary arrest, assessment and interventions are quickly interwoven. The steps of CPR therefore include assessment and intervention and are presented in sequence below. Only CPR for adults is addressed here.

Nursing Diagnoses, Goals, and Outcome Criteria: Cardiopulmonary Arrest

Cardiopulmonary arrest is a medical diagnosis rather than a nursing diagnosis. Nursing diagnoses that may be appropriate are as follows:

Nursing Diagnoses	Goals and Outcome Criteria
Ineffective Tissue Perfusion related to cessation of heartbeat	Adequate oxygenation until heartbeat and respirations are restored: improving skin color, palpable pulse, spontaneous respirations
Decreased Cardiac Output related to cessation of heartbeat	
Ineffective Breathing Pattern related to inadequate or absent respirations	

Interventions

Refer to the latest American Heart Association guidelines for CPR because the guidelines are revised at intervals.

Open Airway

1. When cardiopulmonary arrest is suspected, tap the victim urgently and ask, "Are you okay?"

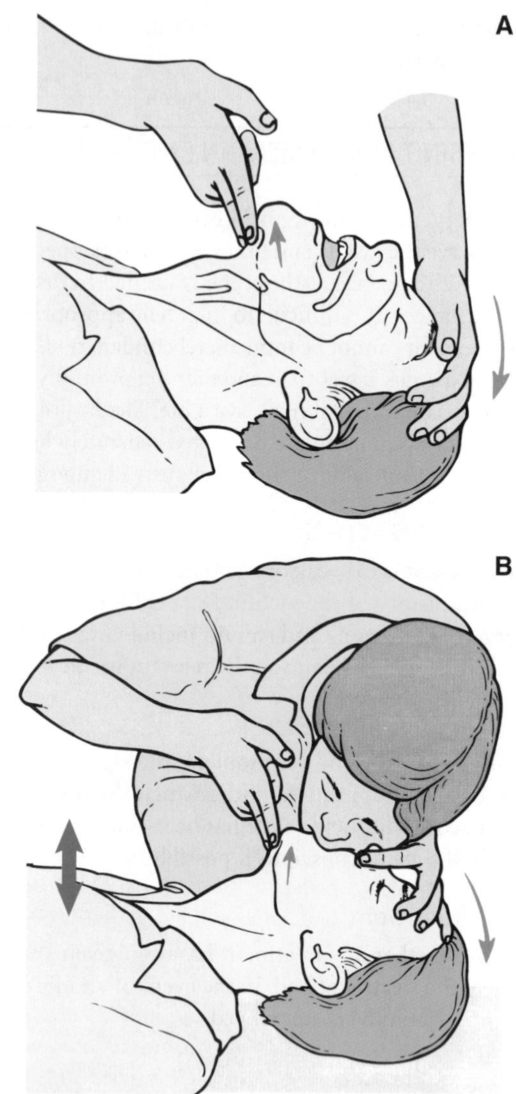

FIGURE **15-1** *A,* To open the airway when no neck injury is suspected, apply pressure to the victim's forehead with one hand and use the other hand to lift the chin forward. *B,* To ventilate the victim, pinch the nostrils shut, take a deep breath, seal your mouth over the victim's, and breathe into the victim's mouth.

2. If there is no response, call for someone to contact the emergency medical service.
3. In the event of near drowning or cardiac arrest associated with trauma or drug overdose, provide CPR for one minute, call EMS, and then resume CPR.
4. Place the victim supine on a firm, flat surface.
5. If no neck injury is suspected, open the airway by applying pressure to the forehead with one hand and using the other hand to lift the chin forward (Fig. 15-1A).
6. If a neck injury is suspected, use the jaw-thrust method of opening the airway. The jaw thrust is done by lifting the lower jaw with both hands (Fig. 15-2).

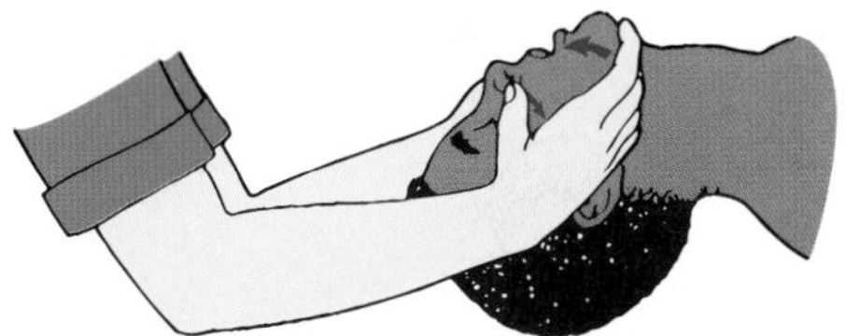

FIGURE **15-2** To open the airway when a neck injury is suspected, lift the lower jaw with both hands.

Check for Breathing (Look, Listen, Feel)

7. Put your ear near the victim's nose and mouth to listen and feel for breathing for 3 to 5 seconds. Watch to see if the chest rises and falls.
8. If the victim is not breathing, give two slow breaths at a rate of 1.5 to 2.0 seconds per breath. To do this, first pinch the victim's nostrils shut (Fig. 15-1B). Take a deep breath, seal your mouth around the victim's, and breathe slowly over 2 full seconds into the victim's mouth. The appropriate volume of air causes a minimal rise of the victim's chest. If the chest does not rise, treat for airway obstruction as described below (see Choking or Airway Obstruction). Allow the patient to exhale between breaths. Various masks and airways are available to avoid direct mouth-to-mouth contact. These should be available in health care facilities but may not be on hand in community settings. For that reason, some health care providers routinely carry disposable masks.

Check Circulation

9. Check for cardiac arrest by palpating the carotid artery on the side of the neck nearest you. Look for normal breathing, coughing, or other movements.
10. If there is no pulse, begin cardiac compressions to restore circulation (Fig. 15-3).
    A. Locate the proper place to compress. Run the middle finger along the lower rib margin to the notch where the rib meets the sternum (the xiphoid process).
    B. Place the index finger next to the middle finger on the lower part of the sternum.
    C. Place the heel of the other hand next to the index finger.
    D. Place the hand used to locate the tip of the sternum over the other hand and keep fingers off the victim's chest.
    E. Lean over the victim so that your shoulders are above your hands and your arms are straight.
    F. Apply pressure to depress the sternum 1.5 to 2 inches, counting "one and two and three and four" for 15 compressions.
    G. Keep your hands in contact with the chest at all times.
    H. At the completion of 15 compressions, ventilate the victim twice.

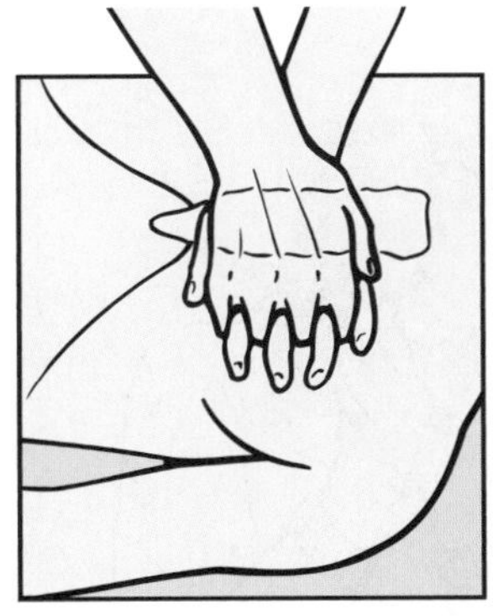
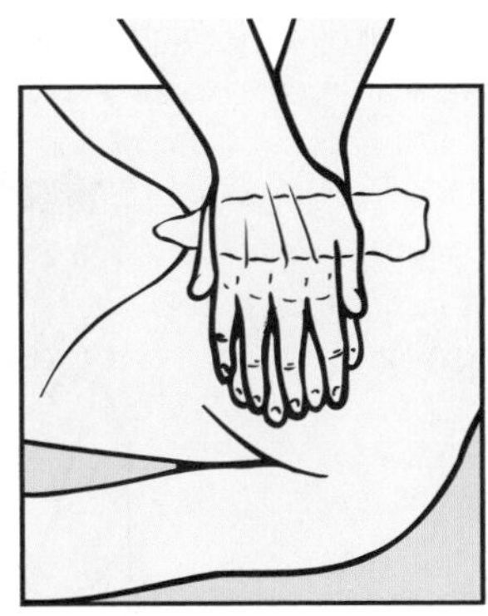
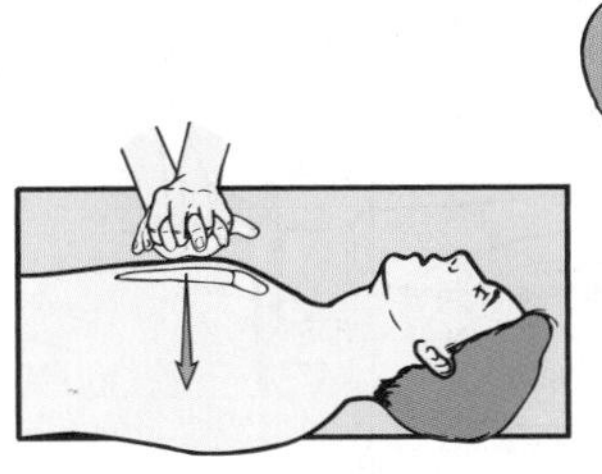
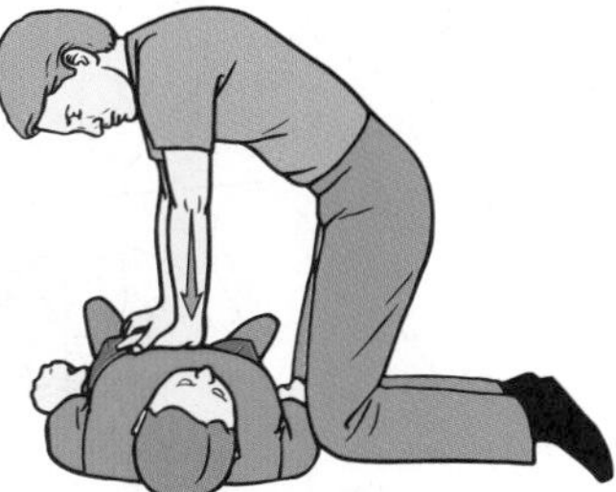

FIGURE **15-3** The proper place for compression is located two finger widths above the tip of the sternum.

11. Perform four cycles of 15 compressions and 2 ventilations and then reassess circulation at the carotid artery for 5 seconds.
12. If there is no carotid pulse, resume CPR with 15 compressions followed by 2 ventilations until help arrives or until you are exhausted.

Two-Rescuer CPR

If two trained people are present to perform CPR, one rescuer compresses the chest fifteen times, then pauses briefly for the second rescuer to ventilate the victim twice. The cycle is repeated until the compressor tires. The compressor calls for a switch and trades places with the ventilator at the end of a cycle.

Recovery Position

The unresponsive victim who is breathing should be log-rolled to one side (the *recovery position*) if no cervical trauma is suspected.

Documentation

When emergency assistance arrives, provide information about the victim and the incident, including time that elapsed, interventions performed, and victim response. Identify yourself and tell how you can be reached if additional information is needed.

CHOKING OR AIRWAY OBSTRUCTION

Choking is airway obstruction caused by a foreign body that enters the airway.

Assessment

The universal sign of choking is grabbing the throat with one or both hands (Fig. 15-4). Fear of suffocation is terrifying,

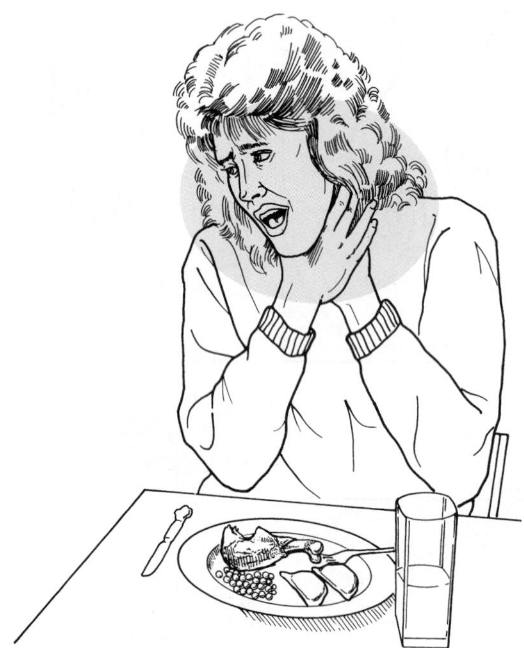

FIGURE **15-4** The universal choking sign.

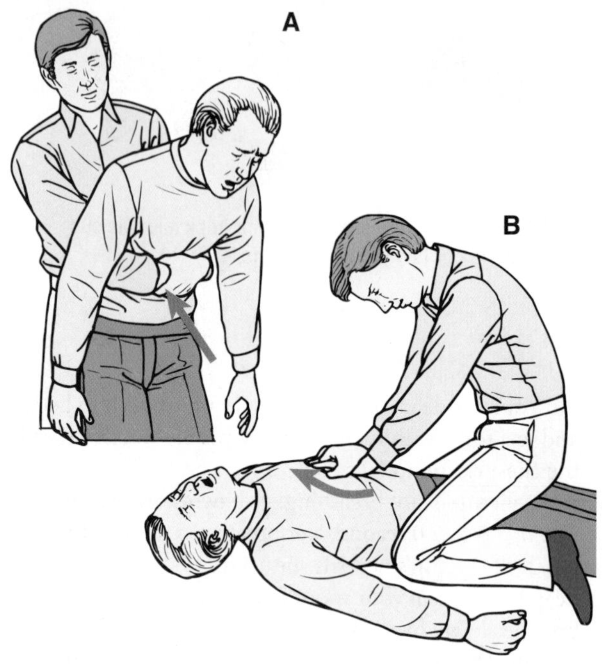

FIGURE **15-5** *A,* The Heimlich maneuver for the conscious choking victim. *B,* The Heimlich maneuver for the unconscious choking victim.

and the victim may look panicky. First determine whether the victim's airway is completely blocked. If the victim is *able* to speak, breathe, or cough with good air exchange, do nothing. If the victim is *unable* to speak, breathe, or cough with good air exchange, quick action is necessary to prevent suffocation.

Nursing Diagnoses, Goals, and Outcome Criteria: Choking

Nursing Diagnoses	Goals and Outcome Criteria
Ineffective Airway Clearance related to inability to expel an aspirated foreign object **Risk for Suffocation** related to aspirated foreign object	Patent airway with normal respirations: expulsion of foreign object, audible respirations, improving skin color, decreased coughing, reduced anxiety, normal pulse

Interventions

If the choking victim is conscious, perform the Heimlich maneuver, a "bear hug" procedure named for the physician who first described it. Stand behind the victim and reach around the victim slightly above the umbilicus and below the xiphoid process (Fig. 15-5A). Make a fist with one hand and use the other to press the fist against the victim. Tighten your arms around the victim and perform quick upward thrusts into the victim's abdomen. This motion exerts pressure upward on the diaphragm, forcing air out of the lungs. If effective, the air expels the foreign body from the airway. If not, repeat the maneuver until the object is expelled or the victim loses consciousness.

If the victim is already unconscious or loses consciousness, position the victim supine and call for an emergency medical service). Then perform three maneuvers:

1. Lift the jaw and sweep a finger through the mouth to try to remove the object.
2. Tilt the head back, lift the chin, pinch the nostrils, and try to ventilate the victim by breathing into the mouth once. If the airway is still obstructed, attempts at ventilation will fail. Reposition the head and attempt once more to ventilate. If unsuccessful, proceed to the next step.
3. Straddle the victim's thighs, place one hand on top of the other, and deliver up to five abdominal thrusts in the same area as that described for the Heimlich maneuver (Fig. 15-5B).

Repeat these three steps until the airway is clear. Once the airway is open, CPR may be necessary to restore cardiac and respiratory function. Even if the obstruction is removed and the victim remains conscious, the victim should see a physician as soon as possible.

Prevention

Most choking deaths could be prevented if people would do the following:

1. Cut food into small pieces, eat slowly, and chew food thoroughly before swallowing
2. Not laugh and talk while chewing and swallowing.
3. Perform the Heimlich maneuver promptly when a person is in distress because of an obstructed airway

SHOCK

Shock results from acute circulatory failure caused by inadequate blood volume, heart failure, overwhelming infection, severe allergic reactions, or extreme pain or fright. Because of the complexity of the topic, shock is covered in detail in Chapter 18.

HEMORRHAGE

Hemorrhage is the loss of a large amount of blood. The loss of more than 1 liter (L) of blood in an adult may lead to hypovolemic shock. Continued uncontrolled bleeding, of course, results in death. Bleeding may be external or internal. Internal bleeding is suspected if a trauma victim shows signs of shock but no external bleeding.

Assessment

Assess for signs and symptoms of hemorrhage, which may include obvious bleeding; cool, sweaty, pale skin; thready pulse; rapid respirations; and decreasing alertness. The victim who is bleeding internally also may have abdominal distention, pain, hematemesis, or dyspnea, depending on the site of the bleeding.

Nursing Diagnoses, Goals, and Outcome Criteria: Hemorrhage

Nursing Diagnoses	Goals and Outcome Criteria
Decreased Cardiac Output related to hypovolemia	Increased cardiac output: pulse and blood pressure within normal range, skin warm and dry, no visible bleeding
Fear related to possible impending death	Decreased fear: patient appears more relaxed, states is less fearful

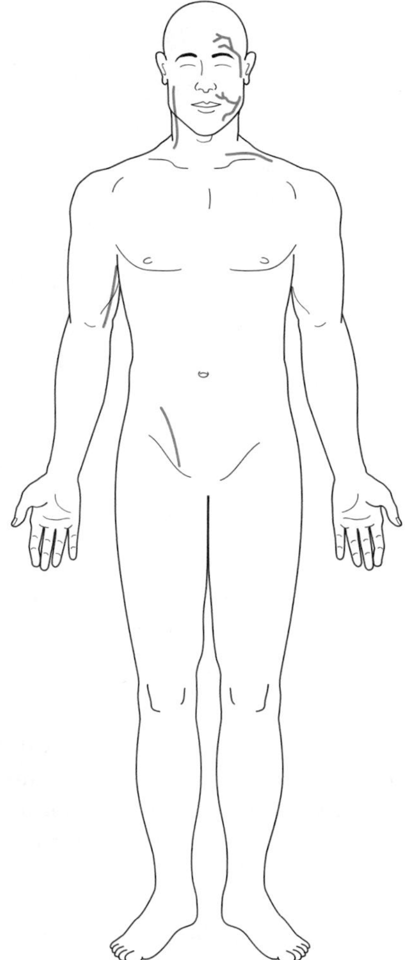

FIGURE 15-6 Major arterial pressure points.

Interventions

The immediate treatment for external bleeding is direct, continuous pressure. Ideally, a sterile dressing is placed over the wound. If sterile supplies are unavailable, use a clean cloth. Elevate and immobilize the injured part (unless fracture is suspected). Elevation decreases blood flow to the area; immobilization prevents dislodging of clots that have formed. After bleeding stops, secure a large dressing, if available, over the wound. Reinforce the dressing but do not change it.

If direct wound pressure and elevation fail to control bleeding, apply indirect pressure, that is, pressure to the main artery that supplies the area (Fig. 15-6).

The use of a tourniquet to control severe bleeding in an extremity is controversial. Tourniquets that are inappropriately placed or left in place too long may result in unnecessary amputations. Therefore they should be applied only by people with advanced training in first aid. Some sources do not recommend it under any circumstances. Others indicate it should be used only as a last resort when a limb is mangled, crushed, or amputated. The least dangerous tourniquet is a pneumatic one, such as a blood pressure cuff, that allows control of pressure. Inflate the cuff above the victim's systolic blood pressure. If the victim's blood pressure cannot be measured, the cuff should be inflated until the bleeding stops. Once the cuff is inflated, only a physician should remove it. When a victim with a tourniquet is transferred, it is critical for the receiving caregiver to know that a tourniquet is in place.

Epistaxis

One type of bleeding that requires special intervention is epistaxis (nosebleed). Blood may come from the anterior or the posterior portion of the nose. Most anterior nosebleeds respond to pressure. Instruct the patient to sit down and lean the head *forward.* Pinch the nostrils of the patient shut for at least 10 minutes (Fig. 15-7). In most cases, this stops the bleeding. Afterward, advise the patient not to blow or pick at the nose for several hours. Continued bleeding or bleeding from the posterior area of the nose requires medical treatment (see Chapter 51).

TRAUMATIC INJURY

Traumatic injuries result from a variety of events. Sports injuries, motor vehicle accidents, falls, and acts of violence often require emergency treatment at the scene of the injury.

Fractures

A fracture is a break in a bone that may be described as simple or compound, open or closed, complete or incomplete. A

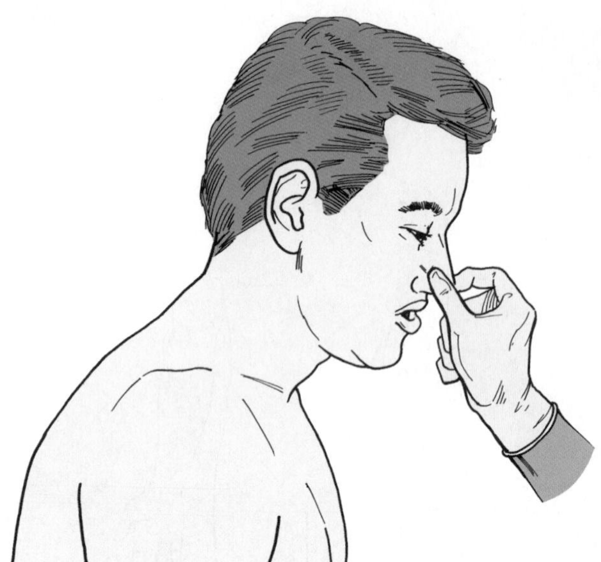

FIGURE **15-7** Epistaxis may be controlled by having the patient sit up and lean forward slightly. Then pinch the patient's nostrils.

simple (closed) fracture does not break the skin. A compound (open) fracture is one in which the ends of the broken bone protrude through the skin. In a complete fracture, the broken ends are separated. The bone ends in an incomplete fracture are not separated. (See Chapter 40 for a discussion of other types of fractures.)

Assessment

Assess the victim of traumatic injury for signs and symptoms of fractures. The primary symptom is pain, although some people, especially the elderly, do not always have severe pain with fractures. Numbness and tingling may be present as a result of injury to nerves and blood vessels. Objective signs of fracture include deformity, swelling, discoloration, decreased function, and bone fragments protruding through the skin. Suspected fractures should be treated as such until they are ruled out by the physician.

Nursing Diagnoses, Goals, and Outcome Criteria: Fractures

The primary nursing diagnosis for the emergency treatment of the person with a suspected fracture is **Risk for Trauma** related to movement of unstable fractures. The goal is reduced risk for trauma and the outcome criterion is stabilization of the fractured bone.

Interventions

The key to emergency management of fractures is immobilization. Immobilize the injured part, including the joints above and below the injury, to avoid further trauma to the bone and surrounding soft tissue. Do not attempt to straighten a broken bone. Instead, splint the bone in the position in which it was found, with as little movement as possible. Boards, sticks, magazines, and strips of cloth can all be used to immobilize an injured limb. A cool pack may be applied to reduce swelling.

Severe bleeding may be present with compound fractures. In such cases, apply direct pressure to the artery above the injury. Give the victim nothing by mouth and seek transportation to a medical care facility as soon as possible.

Strains and Sprains

Strains are injuries to muscles or to the tendons that attach muscles to bones, or to both. Sprains are injuries to ligaments. Ligaments are bands of tissue that hold bones in position in the joints. These injuries are painful, and swelling may be present. Emergency treatment for both of these injuries is immobilization, elevation, and application of a cool pack. The victim should see a physician for further evaluation.

Head Injury

Head injury is not always apparent immediately after an accident. It should be suspected with any type of blow to the head or any unexplained loss of consciousness. A critical complication of head injury is increased intracranial pressure caused by bleeding or swelling associated with trauma. Increased intracranial pressure progressively impairs brain function and may lead to cessation of breathing.

Elderly people are at special risk for head injuries because they are more likely to have sensory deficits, unstable gait, or circulatory disorders. Head injury in an older person may be overlooked if a state of confusion is attributed to age without determining the person's usual level of mental function.

Assessment

When head injury is suspected, assessment includes inspection and palpation of the head and evaluation for signs and symptoms of increased intracranial pressure. Signs of increased intracranial pressure are the following:

- Change in behavior, agitation, confusion
- Decreasing level of consciousness
- Pupil dilation or constriction, inequality, slow response or no response to light
- Impaired sensory or motor function
- Increasing blood pressure with widening pulse pressure
- Decreasing pulse and respiratory rates
- Projectile vomiting

Be alert for the leakage of cerebrospinal fluid that occurs with basilar skull fractures. Cerebrospinal fluid leakage is usually seen as clear, colorless fluid draining from the nose or ear. If the fluid drains onto a white cloth, it appears as a yellowish stain. If there is blood in the fluid, it produces a pink "halo" around the yellow center.

Nursing Diagnoses, Goals, and Outcome Criteria: Head Injury

Nursing Diagnoses	Goals and Outcome Criteria
Ineffective Breathing Patterns related to neurologic trauma	Effective breathing pattern: normal respiratory rate and depth, normal pulse
Risk for Injury related to increasing intracranial pressure, improper movement after spinal fracture	Decreased risk for injury: prompt recognition of rising intracranial pressure (altered mental function, unequal pupils, abnormal response of pupils to light), secure immobilization of spine

Interventions

The victim of a head injury must be assessed by a physician as soon as possible. Because head injuries often accompany spinal injuries, always treat the victim as if there were a spinal injury until it is ruled out. This is especially important when the victim is unconscious or when no history can be obtained. Immobilize the neck and keep the victim flat with proper alignment of the neck and head. A backboard should be used for transporting the victim.

Even if the head injury seems to be minor, the physician may admit the victim to the hospital for observation as a precaution. This is because bleeding and swelling are sometimes so slow that signs and symptoms of increased intracranial pressure may not appear until hours or even weeks after the initial injury. (See Chapter 26 for detailed neurological assessment and care of the hospitalized patient with a head injury.)

Neck and Spinal Injuries

Suspect neck and spinal injuries along with head injuries, especially if the victim has had a diving or motor vehicle accident. Do not move the victim during the initial assessment unless absolutely necessary. Improper movement of the patient with a spinal injury may damage the spinal cord, causing permanent paralysis. After a diving injury, the neck and back should be immobilized while removing the victim from the water.

Assessment

When a victim has a neck or spinal injury, first assess the victim's breathing and circulation and then begin resuscitation if needed. Remember to use the jaw-thrust method to open the airway! Then assess the victim's movement and sensation in all extremities.

Nursing Diagnosis, Goal, and Outcome Criteria: Neck/Spinal Injury

The priority nursing diagnosis for the person with a neck or spinal injury is **Risk for Trauma** related to improper movement of the fractured spine. The goal is decreased risk of additional injury. Outcome criteria include continuous immobilization of the spine and transport for medical care.

Interventions

Immediately summon an expert emergency team when neck or spinal injury is suspected. A professional team has the equipment and the expertise to immobilize and transport the victim properly. In remote or life-threatening settings, the victim may have to be moved. If so, a rolled towel or article of clothing can be used as a collar to support the neck. The victim can then be moved by log-rolling to one side and then rolling back onto a board, keeping the spine as straight as possible. Throughout the movement, one rescuer supports the head while two others support the shoulders, hips, and legs.

Eye Injury

Eye conditions that warrant immediate attention include presence of foreign bodies, chemical contact, perforation of the globe, and eyelid trauma.

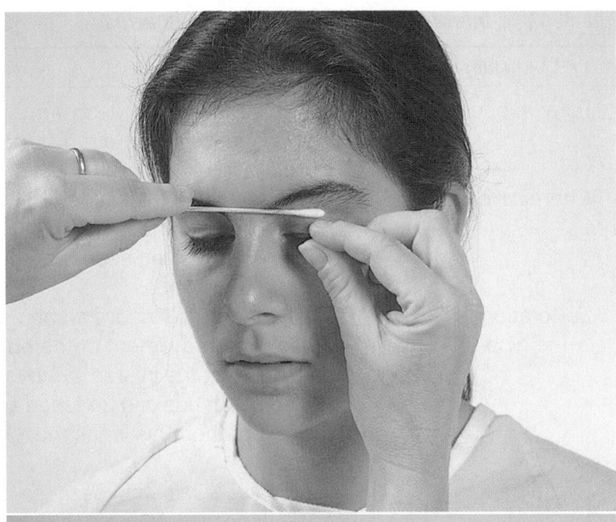
A

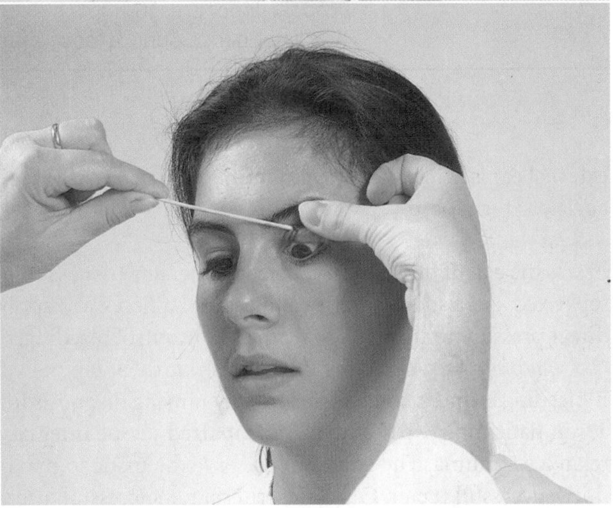
B

FIGURE **15-8** Eversion of the upper eyelid for inspection. *A,* Gently hold a cotton-tipped applicator against the closed lid and lift the lashes up. *B,* Use your thumb to evert the lid over the applicator and hold the lashes against the bony orbit.

Assessment

After an injury of the eye, inspect the patient's eyelid for trauma and the eye itself for redness, foreign bodies, or penetrating objects. To inspect for foreign bodies, evert the eyelids (Fig. 15-8). If the eye has been exposed to an irritant, attempt to determine what the substance is.

Nursing Diagnosis, Goal, and Outcome Criteria: Eye Injury

The primary nursing diagnosis is **Risk for Injury** related to foreign body, direct trauma, or exposure to harmful substances. The goal is to minimize injury to the eye. Outcome criteria, depending on the nature of the injury, may be removal of a foreign body or chemical or protection of the eye from further damage while medical attention is being obtained (Table 15-2).

Ear Trauma

The position and structure of the external ear make it vulnerable to traumatic injury. The most serious injury to the

table 15-2 Interventions for Specific Eye Injuries

TYPE OF INJURY	EMERGENCY INTERVENTION
Foreign bodies	If not embedded: remove by irrigation or by gently touching the object with the corner of a clean cloth or gauze pad or a moistened cotton-tipped applicator. Embedded foreign bodies should be removed only by a physician.
Chemical contact	Immediately flush the eye for 30 minutes. Sterile normal saline or water is ideal, but tap water may be used. Direct the irrigating fluid to flow from the inner canthus to the outer canthus of the eye. Even if the flushing seems to relieve all symptoms, the patient should see a physician to assess the eye for injury.
Perforation of the globe	Do not attempt to remove an object that has perforated the eye! You could cause greater harm. Instead, limit movement of the object and the eye and transport the victim for immediate medical care. Protect the injured eye by covering it with a shield that does not touch the object. An inverted paper cup can be taped over the eye. Patch the unaffected eye as well because the eyes move together. This limits movement in both eyes. Tell the patient why both eyes need to be covered.
Eyelid trauma	Seek medical evaluation because injury of the globe as well as the lid is always possible. Do not apply direct pressure to a bleeding eyelid. If the globe has been injured, pressure could cause greater harm. Apply a loose dressing and transport the victim for medical care.

external ear is avulsion. Avulsion means that all or part of the auricle is torn loose.

Assessment

Assess the extent of the injury; note whether any tissue is fully separated and also the severity of bleeding. If necessary, apply direct pressure to the site of the injury to control bleeding.

Nursing Diagnosis, Goal, and Outcome Criteria: Ear Injury

If bleeding is under control, the priority nursing diagnosis for a traumatic injury to the auricle is **Impaired Tissue Integrity** related to trauma. The goal is to preserve the tissue to maximize successful repair. Outcome criteria for successful interventions are recovery and protection of avulsed tissue.

Interventions

If the injured part is actually separated, reattachment may be possible. Retrieve the tissue, wrap it in plastic, keep it cool, and transport it with the victim.

Chest Injury

Injuries to the chest can result in serious impairment of respiratory function. Chest injuries are described as open or closed. The most critical injuries are open pneumothorax, flail chest, massive hemothorax, and cardiac tamponade. Any injury at or below the nipple line may cause both chest and abdominal injuries.

Assessment

Assessment of respiratory status always takes first priority when the victim has sustained a chest injury. Note the rate and character of the victim's respirations, skin color, pulse rate and rhythm, symmetry of the chest wall movement, and the presence of any apparent injuries to the chest. Signs and symptoms of chest injuries that impair respirations are dyspnea, tachycardia, restlessness, cyanosis, asymmetric or other abnormal chest wall movement, and abnormal sounds associated with breathing. Note the patient's mental state and level of consciousness.

Nursing Diagnosis, Goal, and Outcome Criteria: Chest Injury

For the patient with a chest injury, the priority nursing diagnosis is **Impaired Gas Exchange** related to altered anatomic structure. The goal is adequate oxygenation, and the outcome criteria are absence of dyspnea, normal pulse and respiratory rates, and normal skin color.

Interventions

Interventions for emergency management of specific injuries are briefly described in Table 15-3. (See Care of the Patient with a Chest Wound in Chapter 29 for a more detailed discussion.)

Abdominal Injury

Assessment

Assess the abdomen for evidence of injury. In addition to asking the patient about abdominal symptoms, inspect the abdomen for abnormalities. Suspect internal abdominal injuries when the victim complains of abdominal pain or the abdomen shows evidence of trauma or distention. The protrusion of internal organs through a wound is called *evisceration.* Eviscerated organs are subject to trauma and drying.

Nursing Diagnoses, Goals, and Outcome Criteria: Abdominal Injury

NURSING DIAGNOSES	GOALS AND OUTCOME CRITERIA
Impaired Tissue Integrity related to mechanical destruction	Protection of injured tissue: proper covering of wound to maintain moisture and warmth
Risk for Infection related to break in skin, possible injury to intestinal tract	Decreased risk of infection: wound protected from contamination

Interventions

Possible internal injuries require medical evaluation. Give the patient nothing by mouth while preparing for transport. Do not attempt to replace eviscerated organs in the abdomen, because this may cause additional harm. Cover eviscerated

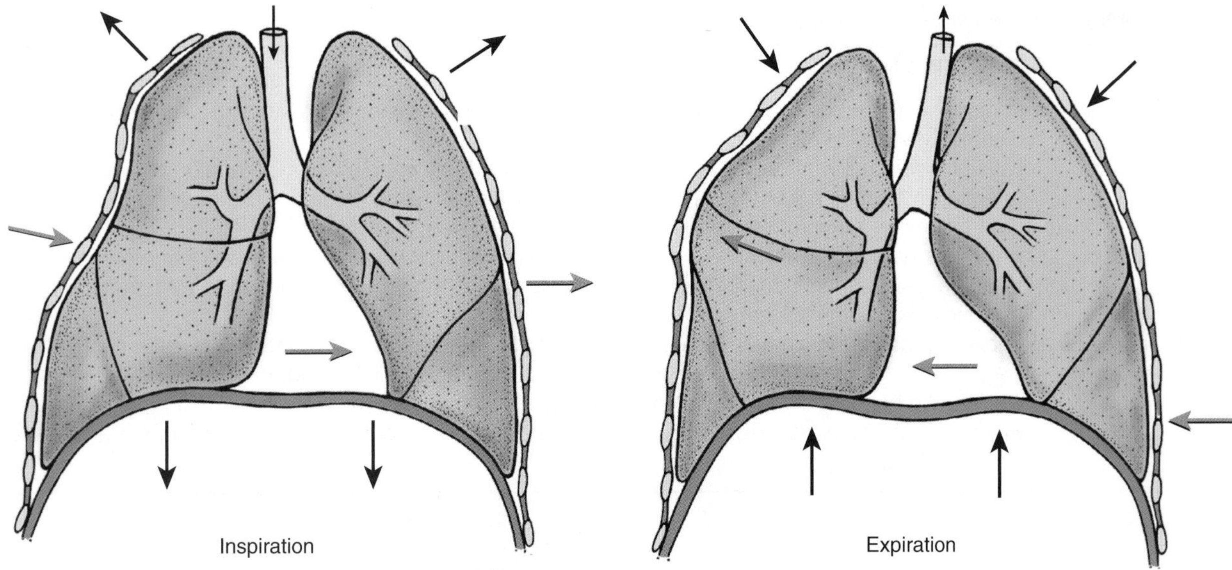

FIGURE 15-9 Paradoxical motion caused by loss of chest wall support.

table 15-3 ***Emergency Interventions for Chest Wounds***

TYPE OF INJURY	EMERGENCY INTERVENTION
Pneumothorax: An open chest wound penetrates the pleural cavity allowing air to enter, which collapses lung on affected side. *Signs and symptoms:* Dyspnea, asymmetric chest wall movement, "sucking" sound as air moves in and out of wound with respirations.	1. Apply vented dressing: sealed on three sides so air can escape, but not enter the wound *OR* 2. Apply airtight dressing. *IF* patient's condition worsens, suspect tension pneumothorax and loosen the dressing.
Flail chest: Several adjacent ribs are broken in more than one place causing a loss of support in the affected section of the chest wall. *Signs and symptoms:* The affected section moves inward on inspiration, and outward on expiration. This abnormal chest wall movement, called *paradoxical motion,* impairs gas exchange (Fig. 15-9).	Provide support for the injured area. Hold or tape a small pad or pillow over the injury to splint the ribs.
Hemothorax: Accumulation of blood in the pleural cavity; causes the lung or lungs to collapse. *Signs and symptoms:* Increasing respiratory or circulatory failure.	Cannot be diagnosed directly or treated by the first aid care provider. The victim requires prompt treatment in a medical facility.
Cardiac tamponade: Presence of blood in the pericardial sac: causes decreased cardiac output. *Signs and symptoms:* Increasing respiratory or circulatory failure.	Cannot be diagnosed directly or treated by the first aid care provider. The victim requires prompt treatment in a medical facility.

organs with some material such as plastic wrap or foil to conserve moisture and warmth. A saline-soaked sterile dressing is ideal but is not likely to be available on the scene of an accident. Cover the wound with a clean cloth and seek transportation to a hospital.

BURNS

Care of the burn patient is discussed in detail in Chapter 48. This chapter addresses only emergency measures for burn care. When a burn accident occurs, the immediate concern is to stop the burning process. A victim whose clothing is burning should be told to drop to the ground and roll to extinguish the flames. Smother the flames with coats or blankets or extinguish the flames with water. Remove burning materials from the victim.

Assessment

First determine the type of burn that has occurred. If the victim has had a flame burn or has been in a closed, smoke-filled area, begin with assessment of respirations. Then determine the extent and depth of the burns. Inspect the skin for color, blisters, and tissue destruction. Superficial burns are typically pink or red and painful. Deeper burns may be red, white, or black and may destroy not only the skin but also the underlying tissues. The deepest burns are not painful because nerves have been destroyed. However, because the depth of a

table 15-4 Emergency Interventions for Burns

TYPE OF BURN	EMERGENCY INTERVENTION
Minor, superficial	Immerse the injured body part in cool water for 2 to 5 minutes. Applying butter to the burn is contraindicated. Medical care not usually required.
Sunburn	Topical preparations with benzocaine may be soothing. Many people believe that aloe vera is very effective in treating minor burns, but this treatment is still being studied. Children and elderly people with extensive sunburn may require hospitalization for dehydration.
Extensive burns	Cover burns with a clean, dry dressing or cloth. Do not apply medications or absorbent materials. Wrap burned fingers and toes separately to prevent sticking together. Have the victim transported for medical care immediately.
Chemical burns	Remove contaminated clothing. Thoroughly dust powdered chemicals from the skin, then flush with water for 30 minutes. If the dry chemical is not removed before flushing, the water may cause the chemical to become caustic, resulting in additional injury. Flush liquid chemicals from the skin with running water for at least 30 minutes. Apply a dressing or covering, and have the victim transported for medical care.

burn often is not uniform, patients with deep burns can still have pain. Determining the extent of the body surface area injured is very important. (See guides for assessing the extent of burn injury in Chapter 48.)

Electrical burns are difficult to assess initially because the full extent of tissue damage may not be apparent for several days. In the event of chemical burns, note and immediately remove any remaining chemical.

Nursing Diagnoses, Goals, and Outcome Criteria: Burns

Depending on the severity and type of the burn, nursing diagnoses and goals for the burn victim immediately after the injury may include the following:

Nursing Diagnoses	Goals and Outcome Criteria
Impaired Gas Exchange related to inhalation or thermal injury, edema of airway tissues	Improved gas exchange: normal pulse and respiratory rates; no dyspnea, confusion, or cyanosis; normal arterial blood gases
Impaired Skin or **Tissue Integrity,** or both, related to thermal destruction, chemical injury	Limited extent of injury: no additional damage after initial burn, skin surfaces protected and free of burning materials
Pain related to thermal injury	Reduced pain: victim calmer, states pain is lessened

Interventions

It is critical to ensure a patent airway and respirations for burn victims. If the burns have been caused by flames, fumes, or chemicals, the victim may have inhaled substances that cause respiratory impairment. Rescue breathing, if needed, is described under cardiopulmonary resuscitation. Other interventions are addressed in Table 15-4 for each of the major types of burns.

HEAT AND COLD EXPOSURE

Extreme heat or cold may have local or systemic effects. A number of mechanisms work to maintain body temperature within a fairly narrow range. If the body temperature rises or falls excessively, vital functions begin to fail. Infants and the elderly are less able to adapt to temperature extremes than other people. This places them at greater risk for excessive alterations in body temperature.

Hyperthermia

Excessive heat exposure may cause hyperthermia, a condition in which body temperature rises above 37.2° C (99° F). Heat edema and heat cramps are mild degrees of hyperthermia. Heat exhaustion and heat stroke are more serious.

Hypothermia

Hypothermia is a decrease in body core temperature below 36° C (95° F). It may be caused by prolonged exposure to cold, extremely cold temperatures, or immersion in cold water. Hypothermia causes depression of vital functions, and if it is not corrected, death results from cardiac dysrhythmias. Elderly people are susceptible to hypothermia because of loss of subcutaneous fat, diminished circulation, and reduced neural control over circulation. They are unable to conserve heat effectively. It has been found that confusion in some older people is the result of hypothermia.

Table 15-5 addresses treatment of systemic responses to heat and cold exposure and local cold injuries. Local thermal injuries were discussed previously under "Burns."

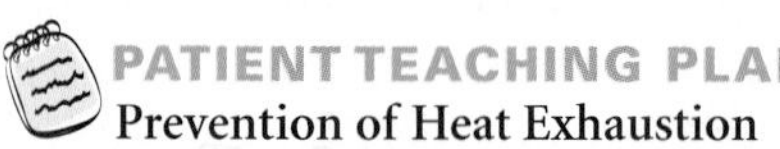

PATIENT TEACHING PLAN
Prevention of Heat Exhaustion

- Avoid strenuous activities outdoors when it is very hot.
- Increase fluid intake to replace excessive fluid loss.
- When working in hot, humid weather, take frequent rest breaks.

table 15-5 ***Emergency Interventions for Heat and Cold Exposure***

TYPE OF EXPOSURE/INJURY	EMERGENCY INTERVENTION
HEAT EXHAUSTION	
Caused by excessive fluid loss when exposed to high environmental temperature and humidity. Rising body temperature and metabolic rate increase oxygen demand. Cardiac output and heart rate first increase, then fall. Loss of fluids causes hypovolemia (low blood volume) and electrolyte imbalances. *Signs and symptoms:* Dizziness, headache, muscle cramps, nausea and vomiting, and collapse. Skin is usually pale and damp. Elevated rectal temperature; may be as high as 41.1° C (106° F).	Move the person to a cooler environment, preferably one that is air-conditioned, and loosen clothing. Splash cool water on the skin. If the victim is alert, offer fluids such as commercially prepared electrolyte drinks, if available.
HEAT STROKE	
Body core temperature of 41.1° C (106° F) or greater. Temperature regulating mechanisms in the brain fail. Heart, kidneys, and central nervous system functions are depressed. The victim is unable to sweat and will die if the temperature is not lowered. Usually associated with strenuous activity in hot, humid weather. *Signs and symptoms:* Similar to heat exhaustion at first: dizziness, weakness, nausea. As the condition worsens, the skin becomes red, hot, and dry. *Perspiration is noticeably absent.* If the condition is not reversed, the victim may collapse and have seizures. The body temperature may reach as high as 43.3° C (110° F).	It is critical to cool the person quickly. Immediate transport for medical care is recommended. Anyone who cannot be transported immediately should be moved into the shade or to an air-conditioned area if possible. Apply wet, cool towels to the trunk and the extremities, and place ice packs on the forehead and axilla. If a tub is available, the victim can be placed in a cool bath. Continue cooling measures until the body temperature falls below 30.3° C (101° F).
FROSTNIP AND FROSTBITE	
Frostnip: mild tissue damage caused by cold Frostbite: more serious cold injury Blood vessels in the skin and the extremities constrict when exposed to extreme cold. Blood clots form, and circulation to the affected areas decreases. Cells die because of lack of oxygen and nutrients and formation of crystals that cause them to swell and rupture. Nose, cheeks, fingers, and toes most often affected. *Signs and symptoms:* pain at first; then tingling followed by numbness.	Immediate treatment of mild cold injury: rapid rewarming. For example, have the patient place cold hands in his axillae or between his thighs. More serious cold injuries: patients should be transported for medical treatment as soon as possible. If transport is delayed, seek a setting where warm water is available. *Do not attempt to thaw the tissue unless warmth can be maintained.* Frostbitten extremities are best rewarmed by immersion in a warm water bath of 37.7° to 40.5° C (100° to 105° F). Handle affected areas very gently to avoid additional tissue trauma. Do not rub, massage, or apply cold to the tissue. As tissue warms, the skin turns bright pink and blisters. Rewarming is very painful. If the procedure is done in a medical facility, analgesics will be ordered before rewarming. After warming the extremities, pat dry and wrap in sterile dressings. Wrap each finger or toe separately to prevent injured tissues from sticking together. Immobilize and elevate affected parts. With severe or deep frostbite, thawed tissue dies and eventually has to be surgically debrided (removed).
HYPOTHERMIA	
Rectal temperature lower than 36° C (95° F). *Signs and symptoms:* Mild hypothermia: shivering and impaired performance. Progressive chilling: decreasing heart and respiratory rates and blood pressure. Irregular heart and breathing patterns; cardiopulmonary arrest if not treated.	Mild hypothermia: Wrap victim in warm, dry clothing and blankets. Severe hypothermia: Transport immediately for treatment. Must be rewarmed aggressively, but gradually, because too rapid rewarming sends lactic acid and cold blood from the extremities to the heart, possibly triggering cardiac dysrhythmias. Warm the torso first. It may be wrapped in blankets or immersed in tepid water. Once the body temperature reaches 36° C (95° F), turn attention to warming the extremities also. Internal rewarming (warmed oxygen and intravenous fluids, peritoneal lavage, and extracorporeal blood warming) may be ordered in a medical facility.

PHARMACOLOGY CAPSULE Diuretics and anticholinergics increase the risk of heat stroke by affecting the body's heat-reducing defenses.

POISONING

A **poison** is any substance that, in small quantities, is capable of causing illness or harm after ingestion, inhalation, injection, or contact with the skin. Large quantities of most chemicals, including all medications, can act as poisons. Even common drugs such as aspirin, acetaminophen, and vitamins can be poisonous if taken in excessive amounts.

PHARMACOLOGY CAPSULE Common drugs such as aspirin, acetaminophen, and vitamins can be poisonous if taken in excessive amounts.

Carbon Monoxide Poisoning

Carbon monoxide is an odorless, invisible gas emitted by automobile engines, gas stoves and furnaces, and burning charcoal and other combustible materials. When carbon monoxide is inhaled, it enters the bloodstream and promptly binds with hemoglobin. Carbon monoxide binds to hemoglobin much more readily than oxygen. Therefore it soon occupies many of the sites on the hemoglobin needed to transport oxygen to the cells. The patient becomes hypoxemic and can die.

Assessment

Assess for early signs and symptoms of carbon monoxide poisoning, which include headache and shortness of breath with mild exertion. Dizziness, nausea, vomiting, and mental changes appear next. As the amount of carbon monoxide in the bloodstream rises, the victim loses consciousness and develops cardiac and respiratory irregularities. A victim usually dies when the carbon monoxide bound with hemoglobin exceeds 70%. A clear indicator of carbon monoxide poisoning is a cherry-red skin color; however, skin color often is found to be pale or bluish with reddish mucous membranes.

Nursing Diagnosis, Goal, and Outcome Criteria: Carbon Monoxide Poisoning

The primary nursing diagnosis for the victim of carbon monoxide poisoning is **Impaired Gas Exchange** related to carbon monoxide poisoning. The goal of nursing care for the emergency treatment of the victim of carbon monoxide poisoning is normal oxygenation. Criteria for evaluating the effects of nursing interventions are regular pulse with a rate of 60 to 100 beats per minute, regular respirations with a rate of 12 to 20 per minute, and mental alertness.

Interventions

Immediately move the victim of carbon monoxide poisoning to fresh air. If the person is not breathing, start rescue breathing. Seek emergency medical assistance immediately. Give the victim oxygen as soon as it is available. At the hospital the patient may be placed in a hyperbaric oxygen chamber. A hyperbaric chamber uses pressure to force oxygen into the blood and tissues.

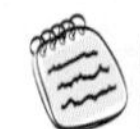

PATIENT TEACHING PLAN
Prevention of Carbon Monoxide Poisoning

- Keep gas furnaces and stoves in proper repair.
- Burners that use gas must be vented to the outside.
- Do not use charcoal or wood-burning devices in a closed area without ventilation.
- Never let an automobile engine run in a closed garage.
- Use a carbon monoxide alarm device.

Drug or Chemical Poisoning

Poisoning by drugs or chemicals can result from accumulation, excessive dosage, drug interactions, or ingestion of inappropriate substances.

Assessment

In situations that suggest poisoning, collect data about relevant signs and symptoms. The signs and symptoms vary with the type of poison. The history is an important part of the assessment of a poisoning victim and should include the following:

1. Name of the drug or chemical involved. If the victim cannot provide the information, look for clues and save the container.
2. Amount of substance consumed.
3. Length of time since the substance was taken.
4. Last food consumed: amount, time.
5. Signs and symptoms that may be caused by poisons.
6. Victim's age and approximate weight.
7. Other medications, drugs, or alcohol ingested.

Nursing Diagnosis, Goal, and Outcome Criterion: Drug or Chemical Poisoning

The primary nursing diagnosis for the victim of drug or chemical poisoning is **Risk for Injury** related to poison. The general goal of nursing intervention for a poisoning victim is decreased or minimized risk for injury caused by the poisoning agent. The criterion for evaluating successful intervention for drug or chemical poisoning is the absence of ill effects from the substance.

Interventions

Specific interventions depend on knowing the exact poison. The product label often provides guidelines for appropriate treatment measures. Some general guidelines for treatment are as follows:

1. Give water to dilute ingested poisons.
2. Contact the local poison control center for information about proper treatment. (Locate the number in your telephone directory, and keep it by your telephone.)
3. Induce vomiting *except:*
   A. With caustic substances or petroleum products
   B. If the victim is already vomiting
   C. If the victim is unconscious
   D. If the victim is having seizures

Syrup of ipecac can be used to induce vomiting. The usual adult dose of syrup of ipecac is 15 to 30 ml taken with a large amount of water. If vomiting has not occurred after 20 minutes, a second dose of 15 to 30 ml may be given.

4. Save urine and emesis (vomited material) for analysis.
5. Seek medical attention promptly.
6. If the victim is unconscious, position on the side and maintain an open airway. Do not try to give oral fluids or drugs.

Once the patient reaches an emergency facility, additional measures may be ordered. Gastric lavage and cathartics may be used to remove the remaining poison from the digestive tract. Activated charcoal may be ordered because it binds to many poisons, thus preventing their absorption.

PHARMACOLOGY CAPSULE Many drugs and chemicals have antidotes. Antidotes are substances that block or reverse the effects of other substances. If the poisonous substance is known, an antidote may be ordered.

Food Poisoning

Food poisoning is caused by ingesting contaminated food. Contaminants can be bacteria, chemicals, or natural toxins. Bacteria most often associated with food poisoning are *Clostridium botulinum, Staphylococcus aureus, Clostridium perfringens,* and *Salmonella* (Table 15-6).

Assessment

Victims of food poisoning often recognize the relationship between their symptoms and the ingestion of food. The most common symptoms of food poisoning are nausea, vomiting, abdominal cramps, and diarrhea. Botulism caused by *C. botulinum* has neurotoxic effects, including difficulty breathing, seeing, and swallowing. An important clue that food poisoning is causing the victim's symptoms is that all who consumed a certain food become ill. To assist in identifying poisons, the nurse should collect samples of stool or vomited materials for possible laboratory analysis.

Nursing Diagnosis, Goal, and Outcome Criterion: Food Poisoning

The primary nursing diagnosis for the victim of food poisoning is **Risk for Injury** related to poisoning. The specific type of injury depends on the action of the contaminant. In general the treatment of food poisoning aims to identify the poison and decrease the symptoms. The goal of nursing care for the victim of food poisoning is the absence or reduction of ill effects from the poison. The criterion for evaluating the effects of intervention for food poisoning is diminished symptoms (e.g., decreased pain, respiratory rate of 12 to 20, depending on the poison).

Interventions

Medical care is necessary if symptoms are severe or persist, especially in children and the elderly. The physician may order antiemetics and antidiarrheals, but sometimes vomiting and diarrhea are allowed to continue within limits to eliminate the offending substances. Intravenous fluids may be

table 15-6 *Food Poisoning*

ORGANISM	SOURCE	SIGNS AND SYMPTOMS	TREATMENT	PREVENTION
Clostridium botulinum	Improper home canning	Onset 18-36 hr after ingestion: nausea and vomiting, headache, dry throat and mouth, dysphagia, diplopia 4-5 days after ingestion: descending paralysis affecting speech, breathing, and swallowing Can be fatal	Gastric lavage, IV fluids, trivalent botulism antitoxin (ABE), mechanical ventilation if needed	Discard food containers that are swollen or have broken seals Spores are not destroyed by boiling Do not depend on taste or odor to detect *C. botulinum*
Staphylococcus aureus	Poor hygiene of food handlers; inadequate refrigeration of food, especially milk products and mayonnaise	Onset within 6 hr: weakness, nausea and vomiting, diarrhea, abdominal cramps Rarely fatal	IV fluids, antiemetics, sedation	Proper refrigeration of food Good hygiene
Clostridium perfringens	Improper canning; inadequately cooked meat or poultry	Onset 6-12 hr after ingestion: abdominal cramps, diarrhea	Antidiarrheals	Thorough cooking
Salmonella	Contaminated food; undercooked meat, eggs	Abdominal cramps, diarrhea, nausea and vomiting	Antidiarrheals, antiemetics, IV fluids	Thorough washing and cooking

IV, Intravenous.

prescribed with severe vomiting and diarrhea. Patients with botulism may require ventilatory support.

Prevention

Most cases of food poisoning can be attributed to improper storage or preparation of perishable foods. People need to be taught the importance of cleanliness when handling and cooking food and the correct way to prepare food for storage.

BITES AND STINGS

Snakes, ticks, bees, wasps, household pets, and even humans are capable of causing serious harm by their bites or stings. The most serious effects of bites are anaphylactic shock, infection, and tissue destruction.

Assessment

In the assessment, the nurse should try to determine the type of bite the patient has received. Inspect the bite wound to identify the characteristics of the actual bite site and any changes in surrounding tissue. Ask the patient about any symptoms that developed after the bite, such as pain, edema, numbness, tingling, nausea, fever, dizziness, and dyspnea.

Nursing Diagnoses, Goals, and Outcome Criteria: Bites and Stings

NURSING DIAGNOSES	GOALS AND OUTCOME CRITERIA
Risk for Infection related to break in skin by bite of human, animal, or insect	Reduced risk for infection: clean wound
Risk for Injury related to exposure to allergens or toxins	Reduced risk for injury: absence of dyspnea, absence of specific toxic effects

Interventions

See Table 15-7 for interventions related to bites.

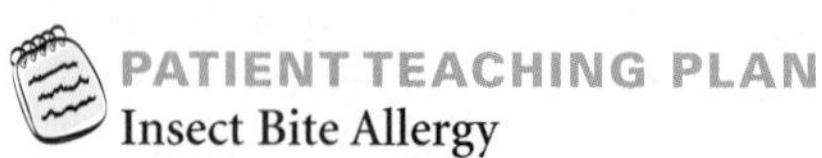

PATIENT TEACHING PLAN
Insect Bite Allergy

People who are very sensitive to venom should be taught how to avoid and treat bites. The teaching plan should include the following:

- Always wear a medical alert tag stating "Allergic to insect bites."
- Obtain an emergency allergy treatment kit. Learn to use it. Teach a family member to use it. Carry it with you at all times.
- Avoid perfumes, hair spray, and bright colors when working outside. Insects are drawn to strong scents and bright colors.
- Wear long pants and sleeves, shoes and socks, and gloves when gardening.
- Keep the car windows closed when driving.
- Consider desensitizing injections if recommended by a physician. These injections gradually reduce sensitivity to venom.
- Use an insect repellant containing DEET.

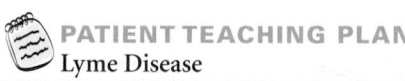

PATIENT TEACHING PLAN
Lyme Disease

Untreated Lyme disease, transmitted by the deer tick, can have serious chronic effects on the brain, eyes, joints, muscles, heart, blood vessels, lungs, skin, liver, spleen, stomach, and intestines. Adherence to the following guidelines can reduce the risk of contracting Lyme disease:

- After engaging in outdoor activities, inspect body folds and hairy areas for ticks. If ticks are removed within 36 hours, the odds of getting Lyme disease are greatly reduced.
- If you have a tick bite and develop flulike symptoms within 7 to 10 days, seek medical care. Antibiotic therapy can arrest Lyme disease at this early stage.
- The vaccine, LYMErix, which has been recommended for people who are at high risk, has been linked with activating an incurable form of autoimmune arthritis. Discuss risks and benefits with your physician.

Put on your THINKING CAP!!

You are traveling with your spouse when a van in front of you swerves, runs off the road, and rolls over. You summon help on your mobile phone, then stop to help. You find the following: Mr. A in the driver's seat complains of severe chest pain from striking the steering wheel; Mrs. B lying on the ground with an open compound fracture that is bleeding heavily; Teenager C in the back seat complains of severe neck pain; Teenager D beside the van with blood streaming from her nose and a cut on her forehead; and Grandmother E wandering around in a dazed state with her hands to her head. Fill in the table below to show the type of injury you think each may have sustained, assessment and interventions for each injury, and the sequence of your interventions. Compare your completed table with your classmates' and reach agreement on the best answers.

VICTIM	TYPE OF INJURY	PRIORITY	ASSESSMENT	INTERVENTIONS
Mr. A	______	______	______	______
Mrs. B	______	______	______	______
Teen C	______	______	______	______
Teen D	______	______	______	______
Grandmother E	______	______	______	______

table 15-7 ***Interventions for Specific Bites***

TYPE OF BITE	EFFECTS	INTERVENTIONS
Snake	Venom that is injected through the fangs into the victim may affect the nervous system or the blood and blood vessels. Venom that affects the nervous system is *neurotoxic* and can cause nausea, vomiting, dizziness, tachycardia, muscle twitching, respiratory distress. *Local effects:* Discoloration, pain, mild to severe edema. Bites of poisonous snakes usually leave two distinct fang marks, although a finger or a toe may be pierced by only one fang.	Seek medical care immediately. A description of the snake (shape of head, color) assists in identification, which may affect treatment. To limit absorption of venom, immobilize the part where the bite is located and keep it at or below the level of the heart. Try to keep the patient still. Wipe the wound. If available, a suction cup can be applied to aspirate the wound. Antivenom may be given to counteract the effects of the venom. Some tissue around the bite often becomes necrotic and must be removed surgically. *No longer recommended* (risks outweigh benefits): Tourniquet, ice, incision and suction.
Insect bite or sting	*Common reactions:* Local itching, edema, and erythema. People who have serious allergies react with systemic symptoms of urticaria (hives), edema, and possibly fatal anaphylaxis. Characteristics of anaphylaxis are difficulty breathing and a drop in blood volume and blood pressure. If the process is not reversed, the victim quickly loses consciousness and dies (see Chapter 32).	Especially anticipate anaphylaxis in victims who develop systemic symptoms rapidly. *Mild reactions:* Calamine lotion or a paste of baking soda or meat tenderizer is soothing. *Severe allergic responses:* The patient with severe allergies should be taken to a medical facility. Epinephrine (subcutaneous), diphenhydramine chloride (Benadryl), aminophylline, and hydrocortisone may be administered after a bite or sting to prevent anaphylaxis. *Prevention:* People who are severely allergic to insect venom should carry emergency epinephrine that can be given subcutaneously after a bite or sting to prevent anaphylaxis. Only the honeybee leaves its stinger, which continues to inject venom into the victim. Immediately remove the stinger with a scraping motion rather than by grasping and pulling on it. Pinching the stinger to grasp it injects more venom.
Animal	All animal bites should be taken seriously because of the risk of wound infections and rabies. Rabies is an infection of the central nervous system that is almost always fatal.	Clean the wound thoroughly; apply a bulky dressing. Advise the patient to have a tetanus booster if immunizations are not current. Patient should see a physician for antibiotic therapy. Follow local protocol to assess whether animal has rabies. If the animal shows signs of rabies or cannot be located, the victim will be given a prophylactic (preventive) rabies vaccine in five doses over a 1-month period. If the victim was bitten on the face or head, the virus may reach the central nervous system more quickly. Therefore treatment may be started before the disease is confirmed in the animal.
Human	Human bites are potentially very dangerous because of the risk of infection. The most common site is the hand or fingers, caused by hitting a person in the mouth.	Clean thoroughly and apply a dressing. Advise the victim to seek medical attention for antibiotic therapy.

Continued

table 15-7 ***Interventions for Specific Bites—cont'd***

TYPE OF BITE	EFFECTS	INTERVENTIONS
Tick	Tick bites require attention because ticks carry organisms that cause Lyme disease and Rocky Mountain spotted fever.	When a tick is discovered, remove it promptly. *CDC recommendation:* Grasp the tick near the skin with tweezers and use a firm, steady motion to remove the tick. After tick removal, inspect to see if it is intact (no part remaining in the victim's skin). Wash the site with soap and water; apply antiseptic.
	Lyme disease: *Early localized stage:* Flulike symptoms with or without a ring-shaped reddened area around the bite ("bull's-eye lesion"). *Early disseminated stage:* Fatigue, anorexia, vomiting, neurological symptoms. *Late disseminated stage:* Joint (Lyme "arthritis") and muscle involvement, progressive neurological symptoms ("arthritis").	*Lyme disease:* Tell patient to notify the physician if flulike symptoms or a "bull's-eye lesion" develop in next 7 to 10 days. *Diagnosis:* Skin biopsy to detect the causative organism, *Borrelia burgdorferi.* A blood test can detect antibodies about 2 months after onset of the infection. *Treatment:* Early localized or disseminated stages: doxycycline or amoxicillin. *Lyme "arthritis" and neurological symptoms:* Penicillin, cephalosporin, or chloramphenicol.
	Rocky Mountain spotted fever: *Symptoms:* Appear 3 to 10 days after the bite: chills, fever, headache, pain behind the eyes, joint and muscle pain, and a rash that begins on the wrists and ankles and spreads to the extremities, the trunk, and sometimes the face. Can be fatal if not treated.	*Rocky Mountain spotted fever treatment:* Tetracycline and chloramphenicol.
Spider bites	Most spider bites cause only local irritation.	For any bite, wash the site and apply a cool compress. Transport the victim for medical care if bite was by black widow or brown recluse.
Black widow	Venom is neurotoxic; causes pain, nausea and vomiting, fever, weakness, muscle cramps, headache. *More serious effects:* Respiratory distress, hypertension, seizures, and shock. Been found to reduce the effects of the venom.	*Black widow* is shiny black with red hourglass on abdomen. Antivenin is available for black widow spider bites. *Not* recommended: Constricting bands.
Brown recluse	Bite not especially painful, area usually swells within a few hours. Initially, a bluish ring appears around the bite. Later it is surrounded by a white ring with a red "halo." Some people experience nausea and vomiting, fever, and joint pain. Severe cardiac, renal, and neurological reactions are uncommon. In 3 to 4 days after a bite, the affected tissue becomes necrotic.	*Brown recluse* is light brown with a fiddle-shaped mark on the thorax. Medical attention should be sought for these bites. There is no specific antivenin to counteract the venom of the brown recluse. Eventually the tissue sloughs off or needs to be debrided. The injury can be so extensive that reconstructive surgery is needed.

LEGAL ASPECTS OF EMERGENCY CARE

Although we do not ordinarily treat people without their permission, in emergencies they may be unable to consent to care. In such cases treatment can be provided under the assumption (called the *emergency doctrine*) that the patient would have consented if able.

In the first aid treatment of emergencies outside the hospital, the nurse is expected to demonstrate the same skill, knowledge, and care that would be provided by other nurses in the same community with the same credentials. Good Samaritan laws in most states limit liability and provide protection against malpractice claims when health care providers render first aid at the scene of an emergency. Although many Samaritan laws cover nurses, not all do. Importantly, these laws do not protect the nurse in the event of gross negligence or willful misconduct.

Be aware that situations involving legal matters may depend on evidence at the scene of the injury. Remember that clothing and other materials may provide important information and should not be discarded. Victims requiring first aid have the same rights to privacy and confidentiality as those treated in health care facilities. Do not disclose to the public any information about the victim's condition or treatment. In cases involving possible criminal activity, preserving all evidence such as soiled or damaged clothing and body fluids may be critical.

key points

- Knowledge of first aid can make the difference between life and death in many situations.
- The cardinal rule in emergency situations is: Remain calm!
- The initial assessment includes evaluation of airway, breathing, and circulation; CPR or rescue breathing if needed; application of pressure to control bleeding; head-to-toe inspection; immobilization of spine/limbs; and location of medical alert tags.
- Because brain cells begin to die after 4 minutes without oxygen, treatment of cardiopulmonary arrest must begin immediately.
- The universal sign of choking is grabbing the throat with one or both hands.
- The Heimlich maneuver uses pressure on the diaphragm to force air and obstructions out of the airway.
- Shock results from acute circulatory failure as a result of inadequate blood volume, heart failure, overwhelming infection, severe allergic reactions, and extreme pain or fright.
- The immediate treatment for external bleeding is direct, continuous pressure.
- Tourniquets should be used to control bleeding only as a last resort.
- For epistaxis, the patient should be told to sit down and lean forward; then pinch the victim's nostrils shut for at least 10 minutes.
- The key to emergency management of fractures is immobilization.
- Sprains and strains are treated initially with immobilization, elevation, and cool packs.
- Assess for increased intracranial pressure with any head injury.
- Improper movement of the patient with a spinal injury may damage the spinal cord, causing permanent paralysis.
- Only a physician removes foreign bodies embedded in the eye.
- When tissue is actually torn from the body, it should be retrieved, wrapped in plastic, kept cool, and transported with the patient for possible reattachment.
- When there is a chest injury, assessment of respiratory status always takes first priority.
- Open chest wounds that penetrate the pleural cavity allow air to enter (pneumothorax), causing the lung on the affected side to collapse.
- Cover eviscerated organs with some material such as plastic or foil to conserve moisture and warmth; do not attempt to replace the organs in the abdomen.
- The first concern with burns is to stop the burning process and then to ensure a patent airway and respirations.
- Cover large burns with clean, dry dressings, and transport the victim to a care facility immediately.
- Extreme heat or cold can have serious local or potentially fatal systemic effects.
- People with heat stroke will die if the body temperature is not lowered quickly.
- Perspiration is noticeably absent with heat stroke.
- Victims of severe hypothermia must be rewarmed gradually to prevent triggering cardiac dysrhythmias.
- A hyperbaric oxygen chamber may be used to treat carbon monoxide poisoning.
- Instructions about treatment of poisoning can be obtained from the Poison Control Center; instructions also may be found on product labels.
- Syrup of ipecac can be used to stimulate vomiting in poisoning victims unless contraindicated.
- The most serious effects of bites and stings are anaphylactic shock, infection, and tissue destruction.
- Lyme disease, transmitted by tick bites, can lead to chronic cardiac, neuromuscular, and musculoskeletal disorders.
- The emergency doctrine assumes that people would give consent for treatment of life-threatening conditions if they were able.
- Good Samaritan laws do not protect nurses against gross negligence or willful misconduct.

REVIEW QUESTIONS

1. After determining that an accident victim is breathing and has a pulse, you should next assess for:
   1. bleeding.
   2. spinal injury.
   3. fractures.
   4. chest injury.

2. Circulation must be restored within 4 minutes of cardiopulmonary arrest because:
   1. irreversible kidney failure develops.
   2. the blood begins to coagulate.
   3. the lungs fill with fluid.
   4. brain cells begin to die.

3. When one person is performing CPR, the correct ratio of compressions to ventilations is 15 to _____.
   1. 1
   2. 2
   3. 3
   4. 4

4. The Heimlich maneuver is used to:
   1. close an open chest wound.
   2. dislodge a foreign body from the airway.
   3. correctly align the ends of a fractured bone.
   4. restore circulation after cardiopulmonary arrest.

5. What first aid treatment is most appropriate for a fractured leg?
   1. Immobilize the leg in the position in which you found it.
   2. Gently straighten the leg and immobilize it.
   3. Apply a tourniquet above the fracture if bleeding is present.
   4. Elevate the injured part above the level of the victim's heart.

6. Your assessment of a person who has sustained a head injury reveals the following: headache, decreasing blood pressure, increasing respiratory rate, unequal pupils. Which finding would cause you to suspect increased intracranial pressure?
   1. Headache
   2. Decreasing blood pressure
   3. Increasing respiratory rate
   4. Unequal pupils

7. While at a picnic on the lake, a person catches his clothing on fire while trying to start a charcoal fire. You should first:
   1. tell him to run and jump in the lake.
   2. try to extinguish the flames with your hands.
   3. tell him to drop to the ground and roll.
   4. run to a telephone to call for help.

8. A high school football player collapses during practice on a hot, humid day. He is breathing but not responding verbally. His skin is hot, red, and dry. You should:
   1. have him go take a cool shower.
   2. call for EMS and apply cool, wet towels.
   3. notify his parents to take him to the hospital.
   4. encourage him to take sips of ice cold liquids.

9. The patient with hypothermia must be *gradually* rewarmed to prevent:
   1. pain in the extremities.
   2. formation of blood clots.
   3. fingers from sticking together.
   4. cardiac dysrhythmias.

10. You notice a peculiar ring-shaped reddened area on the leg of a child in the immunization clinic. When asked about it, the mother stated that she had removed a tick from that area last week. What should you do?
    1. Suspect early Lyme disease and refer the child for medical treatment.
    2. Advise the mother to apply antibiotic ointment to the lesion daily.
    3. Recognize the bite of a black widow spider and apply a constrictive band.
    4. Contact the physician for an order for brown recluse spider antivenin.

CHAPTER 16 Surgical Care

objectives

1. State the purpose of each type of surgery: diagnostic, exploratory, curative, palliative, and cosmetic.
2. List data to be included in the nursing assessment of the preoperative patient.
3. Assist in identifying the nursing diagnoses, goals and outcome criteria, and interventions during the preoperative phase of the surgical experience.
4. Outline a preoperative teaching plan.
5. List the responsibilities of each member of the surgical team.
6. Explain the nursing implications of each type of anesthesia.
7. Explain how the nurse can help prevent postoperative complications.
8. List data to be included in the nursing assessment of the postoperative patient.
9. Identify nursing diagnoses, goals and outcome criteria, and interventions for the postoperative patient.
10. Explain patient needs to be considered in discharge planning.

key terms

Anesthesiologist (ăn-ĕs-thē-zē-ŎL-ō-jĭst, p. 217)
Anesthetic (ăn-ĕs-THĔT-ĭk, p. 217)
Dehiscence (dē-HĬS-ĕns, p. 223)
Evisceration (ĕ-vĭs-ĕr-Ā-shŭn, p. 223)
Hypothermia (hī-pō-THĔR-mē-ă, p. 221)
Nurse anesthetist (p. 217)
Palliative (PĂL-ē-ă-tĭv, p. 207)
Sanguineous (săng-GWĬN-ē-ŭs, p. 229)
Serosanguineous (sĕ-rō-săng-GWĬN-ē-ŭs, p. 229)
Serous (SĒ-rŭs, p. 229)

Surgical treatments have been attempted since early times, but until fairly recently surgery was considered the last resort, to be used only when more conservative measures had failed. However, twentieth century advances brought antibiotics, safe anesthesia, refined surgical techniques, and improved diagnosis and treatment of illness and injury. Through these advances surgery became safer, and now is almost commonplace (Fig. 16-1).

Surgical procedures are performed in physicians' offices, clinics, ambulatory surgery centers, and full-service hospitals. In the past decade, cost control measures resulted in a tremendous shift toward ambulatory surgery centers for many procedures. In all of these settings, nurses play important roles. Nurses who care for patients before, during, and after surgery are called *perioperative* nurses. They admit surgical patients, do initial assessments and prepare them for surgery, assist in the procedures, and provide postoperative care. Since hospital stays for surgical procedures have shortened dramatically and many procedures are done in ambulatory settings, nurses now provide (or teach patients and families to provide) much postoperative care in the home. The importance of good patient and family education cannot be overemphasized.

PURPOSES OF SURGERY

Surgery may be done for a variety of reasons. Surgical procedures classified by purpose include diagnostic, exploratory, curative, palliative, and cosmetic.

Diagnostic surgery involves the removal and study of tissue to make an accurate diagnosis. An example is a biopsy of a skin lesion or a lump in breast tissue.

Exploratory surgery is a more extensive procedure than a biopsy. It usually requires opening a body cavity to diagnose and to find out the extent of a disease process. A common example is an exploratory laparotomy, in which the abdomen is opened to find the cause of unexplained pain. Some exploratory surgery can be done using specialized scopes inserted into the body through small incisions.

Curative surgery is done to remove diseased tissue or to correct defects. The term *ablation* refers to removal of tissue. Removal of an inflamed appendix, for example, is curative for appendicitis. Defects that can be corrected include cleft lip, arthritic joints, and hernias. The repair of damaged tissue is a reconstructive procedure, whereas a constructive procedure repairs congenitally malformed structures.

Palliative surgery relieves symptoms or improves function without correcting the basic problem. For example, palliative surgery may be done just to remove a malignant tumor obstructing the intestine even though the cancer is widespread elsewhere in the body.

Cosmetic surgery can be done to correct serious defects that affect appearance but is often done simply because the patient wants to change a physical feature. Common

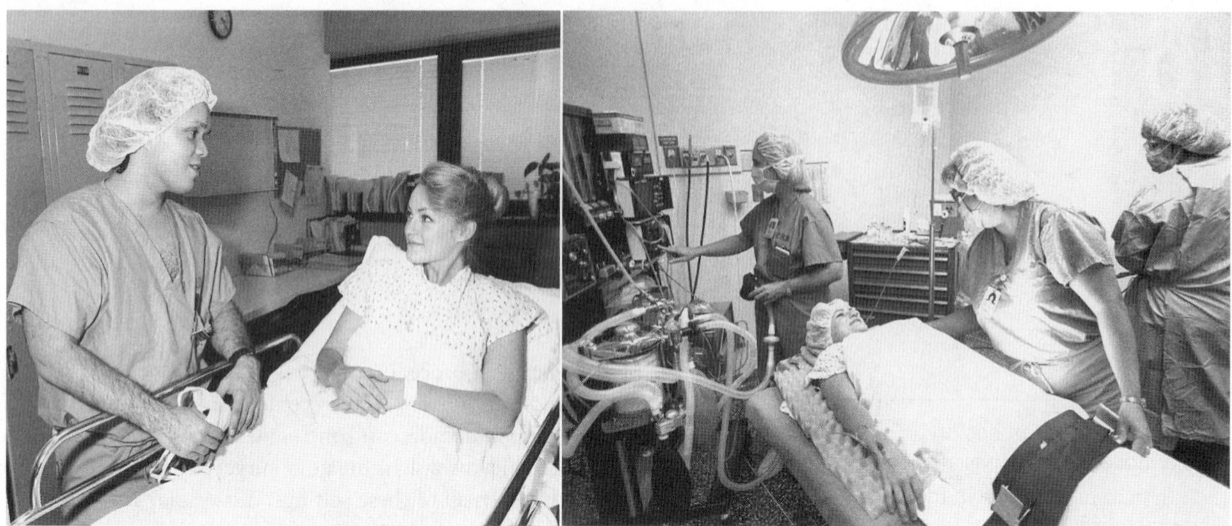

FIGURE **16-1** The nurse provides continuity of care for the surgical patient.

cosmetic procedures are performed to change the shape of facial features, remove wrinkles, flatten the abdomen, and change the size or shape of the breasts.

VARIABLES AFFECTING SURGICAL OUTCOMES

Among the variables that must be considered when caring for surgical patients are age, nutritional status, fluid and electrolyte balance, medical diagnoses, drugs, and habits.

AGE

Health care providers and the elderly themselves often believe that surgery is dangerous for older people. This is unfortunate, because modern surgical techniques can restore many lost functions and often greatly improve the patient's quality of life. It is true that people over age 70 who are frail or have cardiovascular disease or diabetes are at greater risk for surgical complications. Hospitalization and surgery may disrupt control of chronic conditions, leading to impaired healing and recovery. However, elders who are in good health are likely to do just as well in surgery as younger people.

As a general rule, inactivity is not good for anyone. It is especially bad for the older person, who takes longer to regain strength. One other important consideration is that older people may respond differently to drugs because of age-related changes in liver and kidney function and drug interactions.

Surgical risks for the elderly person can be greatly reduced if chronic conditions are well controlled, drug therapy is carefully evaluated, and the patient is well hydrated and nourished before surgery. For that reason, emergency procedures carry greater risks for older patients than scheduled procedures.

NUTRITIONAL STATUS

Patients who are overweight or underweight present special problems. The patient who is malnourished is at risk for poor wound healing and infection. Obese patients are generally in surgery longer and are more likely to have postoperative respiratory and wound complications. Effective deep breathing exercises are limited by the excess weight. Because adipose tissue has poor blood supply, the healing process is slower. The obese patient also takes longer to recover from anesthesia because the drug tends to remain longer in adipose tissue.

FLUID BALANCE

Fluid and electrolyte status can have a significant bearing on the outcome of surgery. Adequate fluids are necessary to maintain blood volume and urine output. Excess body fluid can overload the heart, aggravating the stress of surgery. Electrolyte imbalances may predispose the patient to dangerous cardiac arrhythmias. Physicians usually order laboratory tests to measure serum electrolytes before surgery. Fluid and electrolyte imbalances can then be corrected preoperatively.

MEDICAL DIAGNOSES

A number of medical conditions increase surgical risks or require special attention in the perioperative period. Patients with bleeding disorders are at risk for excessive bleeding and must be closely monitored. People with heart disease are at risk for cardiac complications related to anesthesia and the stress of surgery. Chronic respiratory disease increases the risk of pulmonary complications as a result of anesthesia or hypoventilation. A patient who has liver disease may have impaired wound healing and may experience drug toxicity arising from the inability to metabolize drugs effectively. Patients with diabetes mellitus also heal more slowly and are at greater risk for infection. In addition, the control of chronic conditions may be disrupted by surgery, which may mandate adjustments in therapy. Also, patients who undergo surgery in life-threatening situations are at greater risk of complications.

DRUGS

Many drugs have the potential to interact with anesthetic agents (Table 16-1). Serious adverse effects may result. In

table 16-1 **DRUG THERAPY | *Drug Interactions with General Anesthetic Agents***

DRUGS	EFFECTS OF INTERACTION	NURSING IMPLICATIONS
DRUGS THAT INCREASE EFFECTS OF GENERAL ANESTHETICS		
Some antibiotics: bacitracin, aminoglycosides, polymixin B	Excessive muscle relaxation	Assess motor function Monitor respirations
Antihypertensives	Hypotension	Monitor blood pressure
Catecholamines: dopamine, epinephrine	Cardiac dysrhythmias	Monitor heart rate and rhythm
CNS depressants: alcohol, antianxiety agents, anticonvulsants, antihistamines, antidepressants, antipsychotics, barbiturates, opioid analgesics, sedative-hypnotics	Excessive CNS depression	Monitor blood pressure, level of consciousness, respirations, and blood pressure
Corticosteroids	Hypotension	Monitor blood pressure
MAO inhibitors; isoniazid, procarbazine	CNS depression	Monitor respirations and blood pressure
Muscle relaxants: succinylcholine, tubocurarine	Excessive skeletal muscle relaxation	Assess motor activity
DRUGS THAT DECREASE EFFECTS OF GENERAL ANESTHESIA		
Alcohol	Patients with history of chronic alcohol intake develop tolerance to alcohol and require more general anesthesia	Monitor vital signs and alertness
Atropine	Given to reduce risk of reflex bradycardia with some anesthetics	Monitor pulse
DRUGS THAT INCREASE EFFECTS OF LOCAL ANESTHETIC AGENTS		
Cardiac depressants: general anesthetic agents, propranolol (Inderal)	Hypotension and dysrhythmias	Monitor blood pressure and pulse
CNS depressants	Excessive CNS depression	Monitor respirations and blood pressure
Epinephrine	Prolongs effects of local anesthetic agents	Protect anesthetized tissue
Succinylcholine (Anectine)	Risk of apnea	Monitor respirations
DRUGS THAT INCREASE EFFECTS OF NEUROMUSCULAR BLOCKING AGENTS		
Aminoglycoside antibiotics Potassium-wasting diuretics General anesthetics Local anesthetics MAO inhibitors Opioid analgesics Antidysrhythmics: procainamide and quinidine	For all drugs in this category: Additive respiratory depression, prolonged muscle relaxation	For all drugs in this category: Monitor respirations and assess muscle activity
DRUGS THAT DECREASE EFFECTS OF SUCCINYLCHOLINE		
Anticholinesterase drugs (e.g., neostigmine)	Respiratory depression	Monitor respirations

Data from Abrams, A. C. (2001). *Clinical drug therapy* (6th ed). Philadelphia: Lippincott.

addition, drugs taken long term may require dosage adjustments because of the effects of surgery or additional drugs.

PHARMACOLOGY CAPSULE Drugs that should be held or modified before surgery include anticoagulants, NSAIDs, aspirin, and herbal products including ginkgo and ginseng.

HABITS

Habits that alert the nurse to the possibility of specific perioperative complications are smoking and alcohol use. Smoking increases the risk of pulmonary complications because secretions are more copious and tenacious and ciliary activity is less effective. Alcohol interacts with many drugs. In addition, patients who use alcohol excessively may need a higher dose of anesthetic agent because of increased drug tolerance. If liver damage has occurred, the metabolism of drugs, including anesthetic agents, can be impaired. In addition, patients with liver disease are at increased risk for bleeding.

THE PREOPERATIVE PHASE

PREOPERATIVE NURSING CARE

The preoperative phase begins when a decision is made to perform a surgical procedure. It ends when the patient enters the operating room. During the preoperative phase the goals of nursing care are to inform the patient of what to expect, reduce patient anxiety, and decrease the risk of complications during and after surgery.

Assessment

When nonemergency surgery is scheduled, a thorough assessment is made that starts with the patient's health history and physical examination. This is usually done before admission to the nursing care unit. Laboratory studies of blood and urine, blood grouping and crossmatching, chest radiography, and electrocardiography (ECG) may be done. Often these and other procedures are done on an outpatient basis before admission.

Most surgical facilities have standardized forms for assessing the newly admitted patient. The nursing assessment should obtain important data needed to plan preoperative, intraoperative, and postoperative care. It also provides baseline data for monitoring the patient's status (Table 16-2). For outpatient surgery, it is especially important to obtain some assessment data in advance because the time available for a comprehensive assessment will be limited.

table 16-2 ASSESSMENT *of the Preoperative Patient*

HEALTH HISTORY
Identifying Data: Age, marital status
History of Present Illness: Problem being treated surgically
Past Medical History: Acute and chronic conditions, previous hospitalizations and surgeries, allergies, recent and current medications
Review of Systems: Disabilities and limitations: hearing or vision loss, paralysis, stiffness, weakness, cognitive impairment; any current health deviations
Functional Assessment: Occupation, roles, responsibilities, diet and fluid intake, exercise, tobacco and alcohol use, sources of stress and support, coping strategies, expectations of surgery
PHYSICAL EXAMINATION
General Survey: Emotional state, ability to communicate, response to directions
Height and Weight
Vital Signs
Skin: Color, lesions, bruises, warmth, turgor, moisture
Thorax: Respiratory pattern and effort, breath sounds, apical pulse
Abdomen: Distention, scars, bowel sounds
Extremities: Color, hair distribution, lesions, deformities, range of motion, crepitus, pain, weakness
Prostheses: Hearing aids, eyeglasses, contact lenses, dentures, artificial limbs, other devices

Health History

Identifying Data. Record identifying data, including the patient's age.

History of Present Illness. Describe the problem that is being treated surgically.

Past Medical History. Include acute and chronic conditions, hospitalizations, surgeries, allergies, and drug history. Record all chronic health problems such as diabetes, heart failure, pulmonary disease, or kidney disease.

Document any known allergies (food, drug, tape, chemical) according to agency policy. An allergy alert bracelet is placed on the patient's wrist if there are any allergies. A number of drugs are routinely given to surgical patients. During and immediately after surgery, the patient is unable to report allergies, so if an emergency should arise, any allergies can be determined promptly by checking the patient's alert bracelet.

Compile a complete list of medications the patient is taking or has recently taken. Knowledge of the patient's drug history enables you to anticipate possible effects of drug interactions.

PHARMACOLOGY CAPSULE Long-term drug therapy with agents such as anticoagulants and hypoglycemics may require dosage adjustments before and after surgery.

Review of Systems

Assess each body system, noting any abnormalities. Record any disabilities or limitations. Include the presence of acute problems, for example, a cold or a bout of diarrhea that could necessitate delay of a surgical procedure. In addition to the conditions identified in the past medical history, document problems that may be significant during the surgical experience, such as vision or hearing loss, partial paralysis or joint stiffness, weakness, or cognitive impairment.

Functional Assessment

Describe the patient's usual activity pattern, including occupation, roles, and responsibilities. Determine the usual diet and fluid intake as well as the use of tobacco and alcohol. Note exercise and rest patterns. Ask about sources of stress and support, usual coping mechanisms, and specific fears or concerns about this surgery. Although some anxiety is normal, be alert for indications of excessive anxiety (for example, tearfulness, trembling, tachycardia).

Physical Examination

Throughout the physical examination, assess the patient's emotional state, ability to communicate, and ability to understand directions.

Height and Weight. Measure height and weight. Unless the patient is very ill or malnourished, the admission weight provides a goal weight to be maintained after surgery.

Vital Signs. Vital signs measured shortly after admission provide a baseline for evaluating readings following surgery. If the patient's pulse and blood pressure are slightly higher than expected on admission, it may be due to anxiety. After allowing the patient to rest, retake the vital signs. If they remain abnormal, notify the physician.

Skin. Inspect the skin for color, lesions, and bruises. Palpate to assess texture, warmth, turgor, and moisture.

Thorax. Observe the patient's respiratory rate, pattern, and effort. Auscultate lungs to assess breath sounds. Assess the apical heartbeat for rate and rhythm.

Abdomen. Inspect the abdomen for distention and scars, and auscultate bowel sounds.

Extremities. Inspect the extremities for skin color, hair distribution, lesions, and deformities. Assess range of motion while listening for crepitus and noting pain or weakness.

Prostheses. Note the presence of any prosthetic devices, including hearing aids, contact lenses, eyeglasses, dentures, artificial limbs, or other devices used to maintain appearance or function.

Nursing Diagnoses, Goals, and Outcome Criteria

Some of the nursing diagnoses and goals that might be made during the preoperative phase are:

Nursing Diagnoses	Goals and Outcome Criteria
Anxiety related to uncertain outcome of surgery, anticipated pain, potential disfigurement, or loss of function	Patient's anxiety is reduced: patient calm, states anxiety is reduced
Deficient Knowledge related to the surgical experience	Patient understands the surgical experience: patient describes preoperative and postoperative routines, what to expect

More specific diagnoses and goals are made based on individual patient data and specific surgical procedures.

Interventions

Anxiety

Most patients are somewhat anxious about surgery. Determine the presence and the level of anxiety, the contributing factors, and the need for intervention. It is especially important to find out the patient's previous experiences, if any, with hospitalization and surgery. If a patient admitted for heart surgery had an acquaintance who died after similar surgery, the patient might understandably be frightened. However, a person whose previous experiences have been positive is more likely to expect this procedure to go well. If it seems that the patient is excessively nervous or fearful about the surgery, report this to the surgeon or to the anesthesia personnel. Extreme fear is associated with surgical complications, so it should be controlled with preoperative medication and other therapeutic interventions. Sometimes surgery is postponed until anxiety is reduced.

Deficient Knowledge

Patient teaching may be done in the physician's office, the clinic, during the preadmission workup, or after admission to the hospital. Ideally, it is not left until shortly before surgery, when many activities are scheduled and the patient may be distracted. A cost-saving trend is to admit patients very early in the morning on the day of surgery. In this case, the burden of preoperative teaching rests heavily on the physician, the office nurse, the admission nurse, or the clinic nurse.

Preoperative teaching should include the patient and those who will be with the patient during the recovery period. An attentive family member or companion can reinforce instructions and help reassure the patient. Telling the patient and family or friends what to expect in the immediate postoperative phase can prevent unnecessary stress. An appropriate teaching plan is based on an assessment of what the patient already knows, wants to know, and needs to know (Fig. 16-2). Verbal instructions should be supplemented with written material.

Teaching Methods

The teaching methods selected depend on the situation. Direct patient teaching by the nurse is probably used most often. This has advantages in that the teaching plan can be individualized and the patient can ask questions freely. The main disadvantage of one-to-one instruction is that it is time-consuming.

Some hospitals have group classes for all preoperative patients. The main advantage of group classes is economy of time. Also, some people like talking to others who are having similar procedures. Group classes have several disadvantages. It may be difficult to schedule times that are accessible to multiple patients before admission. Some patients are less

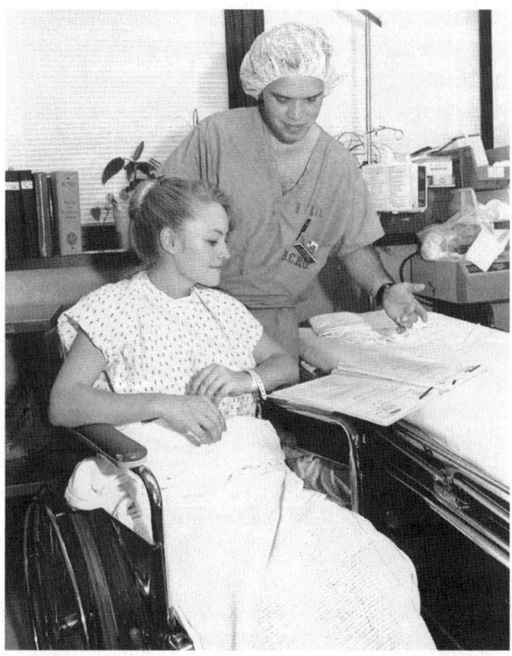

FIGURE **16-2** Preoperative teaching prepares the patient for the surgical experience.

likely to ask questions or express fears in a group setting. Also, information presented to mixed groups of patients is necessarily rather general.

Books, pamphlets, audiotapes, and videotapes are available for patient use. Whatever approach is used for patient teaching, it may be supplemented with these audiovisual materials. Ideally, they are used along with other teaching strategies. Provide the materials for the patient's use and return later to answer questions and assess understanding of the material.

Unfortunately, many patient teaching materials are appropriate only for a limited audience. The reading level may be above the patient's ability, or too many technical terms may be used. We sometimes forget how we felt the first time we encountered medical terminology. In the United States many people do not speak or read English well enough to learn from these materials. So, although audiovisual materials can be very helpful, do not depend on them completely for patient teaching.

PATIENT TEACHING PLAN
Preoperative Patient

The nurse determines how much detail is appropriate for each patient. Most people need basic information and simple explanations without technical details. The family will probably want to know the expected time of surgery, where to wait for the patient, and how they will be informed when the procedure is over. The teaching plan should include an orientation to the unit and the following:

- In preparation for surgery, you will have specific treatments based on the specific surgical procedure, agency protocols, and physician's orders.
- In the postanesthesia care unit (commonly called the PACU or recovery room):
  - You may have tubes, dressings, or equipment in place.
  - Nurses will take your pulse and blood pressure often and perform other procedures specific to your surgery.
  - You will be asked to deep breathe, cough, turn, and exercise your legs to help you eliminate your anesthesia and to prevent complications.
  - You may be asked to respond to various commands, depending on your surgery.
  - You need to report pain so that measures can be taken to provide pain relief.

Preparation for Surgery

Preparation of the patient for surgery starts before or shortly after admission. Patients admitted for emergency surgery may not have the benefit of preoperative teaching.

Informed Consent

Before surgery a patient must sign a legal document called a *consent form* (Fig. 16-3). It states that the patient has been informed about the procedure to be done, the alternative treatments, and the risks involved, and that the patient agrees to the procedure. Written consent is intended to protect the patient from unwanted procedures. It also protects the health care facility and care givers. It is the physician's responsibility to explain the procedure and risks to the patient, but the nurse may obtain and witness the patient's signature on the form if agency policy allows. If the patient has questions or seems to be in doubt, contact the physician.

Because the consent form is a legal document, the patient must be fully alert and aware of what it contains when signing it. If the patient is a minor, a parent or guardian must sign the form. The age at which a person is considered an adult varies from state to state. Know the law in the state in which you practice.

A patient who is confused, mentally incompetent, or under the influence of drugs cannot give informed consent. For that reason, the consent form is always signed before the patient is given preoperative medications.

The patient should sign the consent form in the presence of a witness who also signs the form. The witness's signature confirms that the patient was observed signing the form. The consent form becomes part of the patient's record.

Preparation of the Digestive Tract

The extent of bowel preparation, if any, depends on the type of anesthesia and the type of surgery planned. For surgery on the abdomen or the digestive tract, laxatives and enemas are generally given to empty the bowel. Sometimes patients are instructed to do this at home before being admitted to the hospital.

Bowel cleansing serves three purposes. First, it reduces the risk of contamination from fecal matter during the operation. Second, it helps prevent postoperative distention until normal bowel function returns. Third, it avoids constipation and straining in the postoperative period. Straining can create pressure on the surgical wound. Surgery may be canceled if bowel preparation is inadequate.

Food and Fluid Restriction

Even if bowel cleansing is not ordered, ingestion by mouth of fluids and foods is restricted for a specific period of time. The evening meal before the day of surgery may be restricted to fluids. Typically, adult patients are given nothing by mouth (nil per os, NPO) from midnight before the scheduled surgery. This reduces the risk of vomiting and aspiration during or after anesthesia. Occasionally the physician makes an exception and orders a shorter NPO period, especially for pediatric and geriatric patients. If a patient routinely takes an oral medication that is considered essential, it may be ordered early on the morning of surgery with a few sips of water or given parenterally.

Skin Preparation

When an incision is made in the skin, microorganisms can enter the wound. Skin preparation is intended to reduce the number of organisms near the incision site. It usually includes scrubbing and removing hair from a wide margin around the planned surgical site (Fig. 16-4). The exact skin preparation is ordered by the physician or outlined in a procedure manual.

NORTHWEST HOSPITAL CENTER

REQUEST AND AUTHORIZATION FOR MEDICAL AND/OR SURGICAL TREATMENT

1. I HEREBY REQUEST AND AUTHORIZE DR.____________________ AND/OR HIS ASSOCIATES AND WHOMEVER THEY MAY DESIGNATE AS THEIR ASSISTANTS, TO ADMINISTER SUCH TREATMENT AS IS NECESSARY, AND TO PERFORM THE FOLLOWING OPERATION____AND SUCH ADDITIONAL OPERATIONS OR PROCEDURES AS ARE CONSIDERED NECESSARY ON THE BASIS OF CONDITIONS THAT MAY BE REVEALED DURING THE COURSE OF SAID OPERATION OR TREATMENT.

2. I REQUEST AND AUTHORIZE THE ADMINISTRATION OF SUCH ANESTHETICS AND/OR OTHER MEDICATIONS AS ARE NECESSARY.

3. FINAL DISPOSITION OF ANY TISSUES OR PARTS SURGICALLY REMOVED IS TO BE HANDLED IN ACCORDANCE WITH THE CUSTOMARY PRACTICES OF THE HOSPITAL.

4. REASONS WHY THE ABOVE NAMED SURGERY AND/OR TREATMENT IS CONSIDERED NECESSARY, ITS ADVANTAGES, PROBABILITY OF SUCCESS, POSSIBLE COMPLICATIONS, AND RISKS, AS WELL AS POSSIBLE ALTERNATIVE MODES OF TREATMENT WERE EXPLAINED TO ME BY DR.____________________.

5. I AM AWARE THAT THE PRACTICE OF MEDICINE AND SURGERY IS NOT AN EXACT SCIENCE AND I ACKNOWLEDGE THAT NO GUARANTEES HAVE BEEN MADE TO ME CONCERNING THE RESULTS OF THE OPERATION OR PROCEDURE.

6. I HEREBY ACKNOWLEDGE THAT I HAVE READ AND FULLY UNDERSTAND THE ABOVE REQUEST AND AUTHORIZATION FOR MEDICAL AND/OR SURGICAL TREATMENT.

DATE:____________________ TIME: ____________________

SIGNED: ____________________
Patient

OR: ____________________
Legal representative

____
WITNESS

____
Relationship (if any)

/PL/2736N
702/1019-E-R-5/90 40-1331

FIGURE **16-3** Surgical consent form.

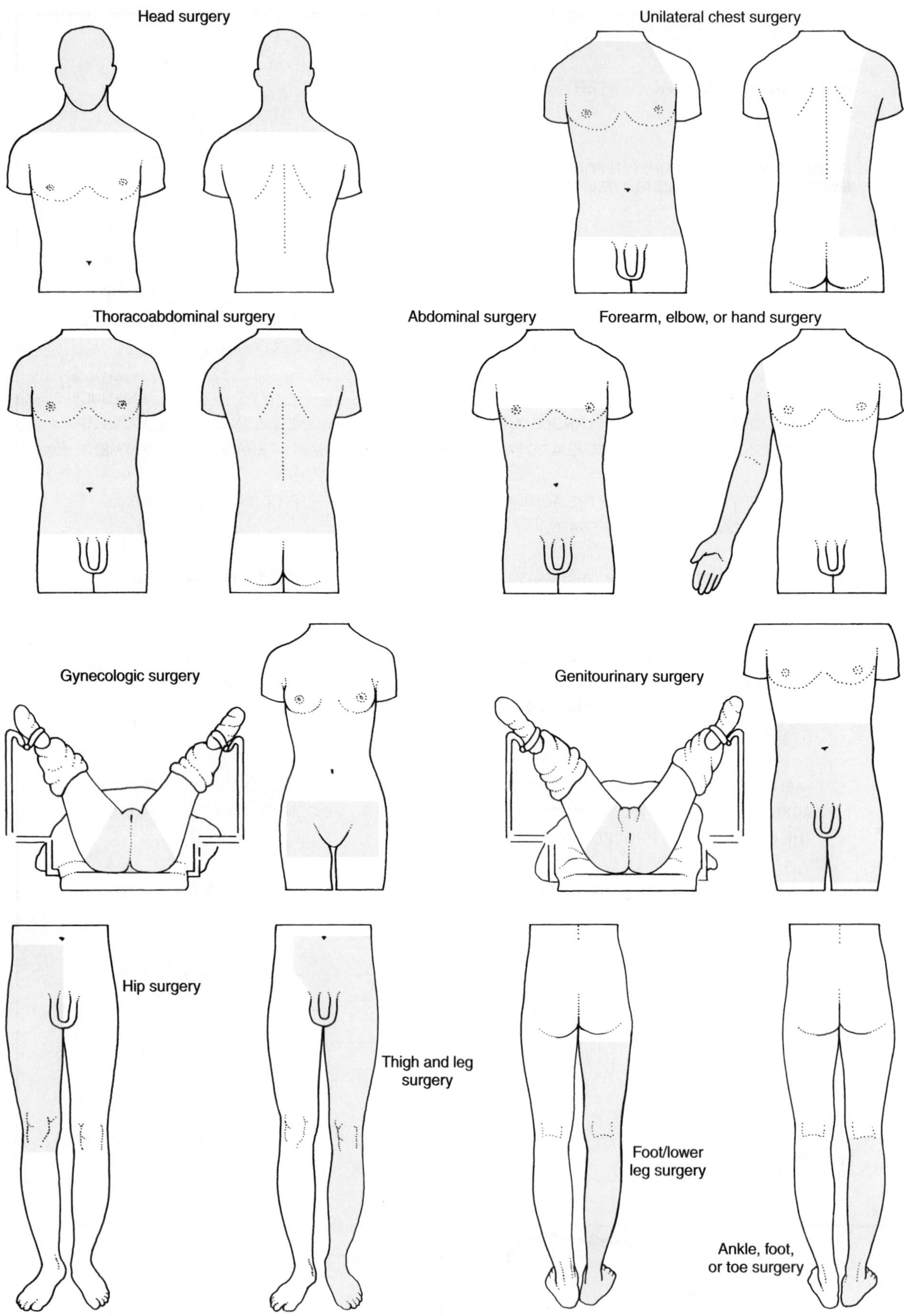

FIGURE **16-4** Skin preparation of common surgical sites.

A typical procedure requires the patient (if able) to shower and wash with an antiseptic soap the evening before the surgery and again the next morning. The perioperative nurse or operating room technician scrubs the operative site and gently removes hair in the operative area shortly before surgery.

Hair can be removed by clipping with electrical surgical clippers, using a depilatory cream, or shaving. Shaving was once routine, but current thinking is that shaving causes tiny nicks in the skin that shelter organisms. Therefore, shaving, if done, is often delayed until shortly before surgery to allow less time for organisms to multiply. Test for allergy before using depilatory cream on a patient.

Dress and Grooming

On the morning of surgery, provide a clean gown and instruct the patient to remove all undergarments. Jewelry should be removed. If a ring cannot be removed or the patient refuses to remove it, it can be secured in accordance with agency policy. Because jewelry often has considerable sentimental as well as monetary value, handle it carefully. The patient may leave jewelry with a relative or friend. It should not be left at the bedside or accepted by the nurse for safekeeping. Most hospitals have a process for valuables to be collected, signed for, and stored in a safe until the patient asks for them to be returned. Document the disposition of jewelry and dentures in the patient's chart.

Braid or secure long hair with a rubber band. Remove hair pins or clips. Provide a cap to cover the hair. Traditionally, dentures have been removed and placed in a denture cup and stored in a safe place. Many anesthesiologists and nurse anesthetists today prefer that dentures be left in. Institutional policies should be specific about this.

Remove nail polish to permit assessment of nail beds for circulation. If the patient has acrylic nails, consult with the anesthesiologist or perioperative nurse about the need to remove them. At least one acrylic nail is usually removed so the pulse oximeter can be used. Makeup, including mascara, is also removed.

A patient identification band must be in place on the patient's wrist on admission. Other wristbands are placed to indicate allergies and blood type. Before surgery, check to be sure all bands are in place. Allergies must be clearly identified on a wristband and in the patient's chart because the anesthetized patient cannot report them to the surgical staff.

Prostheses

Prostheses are usually removed, marked, and secured before surgery to prevent them being lost or damaged and to prevent them from causing injury during anesthesia. Be sure that the devices are returned to the patient when needed. A hearing-impaired patient without a hearing aid may seem uncooperative with postoperative instructions. If the patient is very stressed at having to go to surgery without the prosthesis, consult with the perioperative nurses about making an exception to the rule.

Preoperative Medications

Physicians' orders for the surgical patient often include a preoperative medication to be given shortly before the patient is transported to surgery or when the patient is in a holding area. If the drug is ordered "on call," operating room personnel will notify you concerning when it should be given. If the exact time of surgery is known, the order may specify that the drug be given at a certain time.

Preoperative medication may include an opioid to decrease anxiety and promote sedation, an antiemetic to control nausea and vomiting, and an anticholinergic drug to decrease secretions. Examples are listed in Table 16-3.

table 16-3 DRUG THERAPY | *Preoperative Medications*

DRUG	USE/ACTION	SIDE EFFECTS	NURSING INTERVENTIONS
TRANQUILIZERS			
Chlorpromazine (Thorazine)	Anticholinergic Sedative Antiemetic	Hypotension, dizziness and fainting with parenteral administration Dry mouth, blurred vision, urinary retention, constipation Extrapyramidal symptoms: akathesia, parkinsonism, dystonias	Keep patient in bed after parenteral administration Intramuscular (IM) dose: inject slowly, deeply; massage site Contraindicated with severe central nervous (CNS) depression Monitor blood pressure Take safety measures for drowsiness
Diazepam (Valium)	CNS depressant Skeletal muscle relaxation	Intravenous (IV) route: respiratory depression, dysrhythmias, thrombophlebitis Drowsiness, ataxia, orthostatic hypotension, headache, blurred vision, confusion	Do not mix parenteral form with other drugs IM injection in deep deltoid site; IV route should use large vein Monitor pulse and respirations Contraindicated with acute narrow angle glaucoma or acute alcohol intoxication Keep in bed after parenteral administration

Continued

table 16-3 DRUG THERAPY | *Preoperative Medications—cont'd*

DRUG	USE/ACTION	SIDE EFFECTS	NURSING INTERVENTIONS
TRANQUILIZERS—cont'd			
Hydroxyzine hydrochloride (Vistaril, Atarax)	CNS depressant Anticholinergic	Tissue damage with IM route Drowsiness, dry mouth, pain at injection site, dizziness, ataxia	IM dose should be given deep in large muscle mass using Z technique Maintain oral hygiene Take safety measures for drowsiness
Promethazine hydrochloride (Phenergan)	Sedative Antihistamine Anticholinergic Anti-emetic	Drowsiness, disorientation, hypotension, confusion Fainting in elderly Dry mouth, urinary retention, thickening of bronchial secretions Paradoxical reaction: excitation	IM dose must be deep IV dose given through IV infusion tube Contraindicated with CNS depression, acute asthma attack Monitor pulse and blood pressure Maintain oral hygiene Take safety precautions for drowsiness
OPIOID ANALGESICS			
Meperidine hydrochloride (Demerol)	Analgesic Decreases response to CO_2 Decreases gastrointestinal (GI) secretions	Sedation, nausea, vomiting, lightheadedness, dizziness, sweating, constipation Respiratory depression with overdose Tolerance and physical dependence with repeated use	Slow parenteral injection Monitor pulse, blood pressure, and respirations Withhold if respiratory rate less than 12/min Take safety precautions for drowsiness Contraindicated with monoamine oxidase (MAO) inhibitors
Morphine sulfate (MS Contin, Duramorph)	Analgesic Decreases response to increased CO_2 Decreases GI secretions	Circulatory collapse, cardiac arrest with rapid IV administration Dizziness, hypotension, nausea and vomiting Respiratory depression Occasional: sedation, vomiting, flushing, urinary retention	Administer parenteral forms slowly; rotate sites Dose should be reduced in elderly Monitor respirations and blood pressure Take safety precautions if drowsy Contraindicated with surgical anastomosis, after biliary tract surgery
ANTICHOLINERGICS			
Atropine sulfate Glycopyrrolate (Robinul)	Decreases secretions Decreases GI and urinary motility Mydriatic Reduces salivation, respiratory and GI secretions	Dry mouth, decreased sweating, constipation, blurred vision, drowsiness, urinary retention Tachycardia, palpitations, tachypnea with overdose	Oral hygiene Monitor vital signs; record bowel movements and urine output Take safety precautions if drowsy Numerous contraindications
SEDATIVES AND HYPNOTICS			
Pentobarbital sodium (Nembutal sodium) and Secobarbital sodium (Seconal Sodium)	Produces sedation	Drowsiness, sedation, lethargy, irritability, nausea, anorexia, muscle aches and pain, gastric distress Severe CNS depression with overdose Tolerance/dependence with prolonged use	Deep IM injection in large muscle Monitor vital signs before and after IV administration Administer IV at prescribed rate Take safety precautions if drowsy Dosage should be reduced for elderly Monitor pulse, blood pressure, and respirations
Chloral hydrate (Noctec)	CNS depression	Occasional nausea, vomiting, flatulence, diarrhea, disorientation Somnolence, confusion, respiratory depression, coma with overdose	Monitor pulse, blood pressure, and respirations

PHARMACOLOGY CAPSULE Preoperative medications usually consist of a combination of an antianxiety agent, sedative-hypnotic, opioid analgesic, antiemetic, and anticholinergic drug.

Preoperative medications must be given at the time they are ordered because they interact with the anesthesia. For safety reasons, ask the patient to void immediately before the preoperative medication is given. Tell the patient that the medications will cause drowsiness and dry mouth. Raise side rails, place the call bell within reach, and instruct the patient to remain in bed.

Preoperative Checklist

Most agencies have a preoperative checklist that must be completed and signed before the patient leaves the unit. Check to be sure that all laboratory and radiology reports are with the chart; that jewelry, prostheses, and nail polish have been removed; that the patient has voided; that premedication has been given; that vital signs have been recorded; and that the consent form has been signed (Fig. 16-5).

PHARMACOLOGY CAPSULE Because preoperative medications have a sedative effect, the surgical consent form must be signed before medications are given. After the medications are given, instruct the patient to remain in bed to prevent falls.

Put on your THINKING CAP!!

What observations would lead you to think a patient is excessively anxious before surgery? What are some things you could do that might reduce the patient's anxiety?

THE INTRAOPERATIVE PHASE

Operating room personnel transfer the patient from the nursing unit to the surgical suite. They assist the patient onto a gurney (wheeled stretcher) and take the patient and the chart to the surgical area.

The patient may be taken directly to an operating room or may go to a holding room first. In the holding room, skin preparation may be done and intravenous fluids started, if these procedures were not done earlier. In some settings, preoperative medications are not given until the patient is received in the holding area. The patient who has been told earlier what to expect will feel more secure in the surgical area.

When moved into the operating room, the patient can expect to see many pieces of equipment, bright lights, and various people. The patient is helped to move to the operating room table and positioned in a specific way for the type of surgery being done. Safety straps are applied carefully because there is a risk of impaired circulation or nerve damage caused by pressure. Comfort and alignment are confirmed while the patient is awake (Fig. 16-6). Anesthesia is then administered and is maintained throughout the procedure.

THE SURGICAL TEAM

On arrival in the surgical suite, the patient is greeted by the nurse, the physician, the anesthesiologist, or the nurse anesthetist. A number of people participate in the intraoperative period. They include the following:

- The surgeon who actually performs the procedure.
- An assistant surgeon, a nurse first assistant, or a physician assistant, who assists the surgeon in the procedure.
- The registered nurse, who circulates. This nurse is responsible for assessing the patient, planning intraoperative nursing care, and maintaining patient safety. This person is in charge of the operating room. Responsibilities include setting up the room, monitoring aseptic technique, assisting in positioning and monitoring the patient, preparing the skin, and providing needed supplies and equipment (Fig. 16-7).
- A registered nurse or technician, who scrubs and handles instruments within the sterile field during the procedure.
- The nurse anesthetist or anesthesiologist, who administers anesthetics and monitors the patient's status throughout the procedure. A **nurse anesthetist** is a registered nurse with special training in anesthesia. An **anesthesiologist** is a physician who specializes in anesthesia.
- Other technical personnel with specialized jobs. For example, a perfusionist operates the heart bypass machine during open heart surgery.

ANESTHESIA

Although surgery has been done since prehistoric times, anesthesia has been used only for approximately 150 years. **Anesthetic** agents are used to alter sensation so that surgical procedures can be done painlessly and safely. Agents used for anesthesia include local and general anesthetics.

Regional Anesthesia

Regional anesthesia is achieved by using local anesthetics that block the conduction of nerve impulses in a specific area. These anesthetics do not cause the patient to lose consciousness. For some procedures, intravenous sedatives are given in addition to the local anesthetic.

Examples of local anesthetics are lidocaine hydrochloride (Xylocaine), bupivacaine hydrochloride (Marcaine HCl), tetracaine (Pontocaine), and ropivacaine (Naropin). They are commonly used for dental procedures, eye surgery, cosmetic surgery on the face, repair of lacerations, childbirth, and other procedures in which general anesthesia is not needed or desired by the patient. Local anesthetics are often the agents of choice for elderly patients because of other medical conditions.

Local anesthetics may be administered topically, by local infiltration, and by nerve-blocking techniques. Topical anesthetics are applied directly to the area to be anesthetized. For

Preoperative checklist

Allergies: **Date of surgery:**____________ **Addressograph plate**

CLINICAL DATA:	Yes	No	Comments
Authorization for surgical treatment completed			
Height and weight charted			
History and physical			
Chest x-ray			
ECG report			
Urine report			
Blood glucose within acceptable range (50-300 mg/dL)			
Hematocrit within acceptable range (30-50 mL/dL)			
Potassium within acceptable range (3.5-5.0 mEq/L)			
Unacceptable test results reported to physician	Time	By	
CLIENT PREPARATION	**Yes**	**No**	**Comments**
Jewelry removed			
Hairpiece, wig, hairpins, barrettes, beads, rubber bands removed			
Loose teeth or caps noted			
Dentures removed			
CLINICAL DATA:	**Yes**	**No**	**Comments**
Artificial eye, contact lenses, glasses removed			
Any prosthetic appliance removed			
Voided or catheterized–I&O sheet on chart			
Identification bracelet in place			
Parenteral fluids patent and infusing at ______ mL/h			
B/P, T.P.R. charted			
Premedication given as ordered			
Side rails up–care data and care plan on chart			
CLIENT PREPARATION	**Normal**	**Abnormal**	**Comments**
Vision			
Hearing			
Mental			
Speech			
Other			
Patient's preferred name:			
NURSE TO NURSE REFERRAL			
Limb for burial ______ **Yes** ______ **No at** ____________ **Funeral home**			

FIGURE **16-5** The preoperative checklist must be completed before the patient goes to surgery.

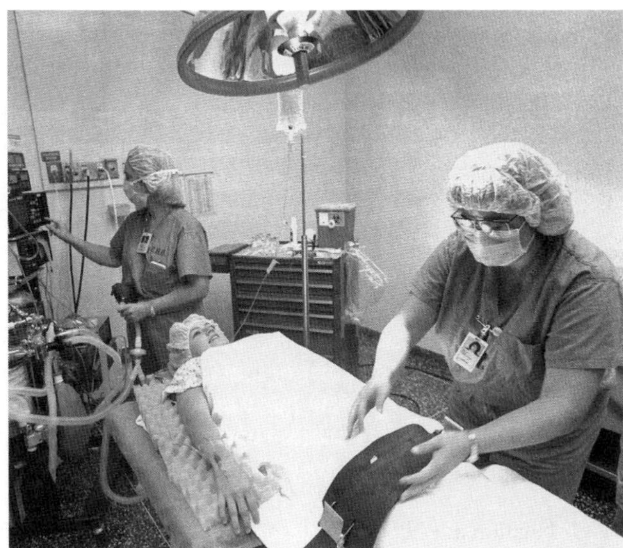

FIGURE 16-6 The nurse ensures the patient's safety on the operating table.

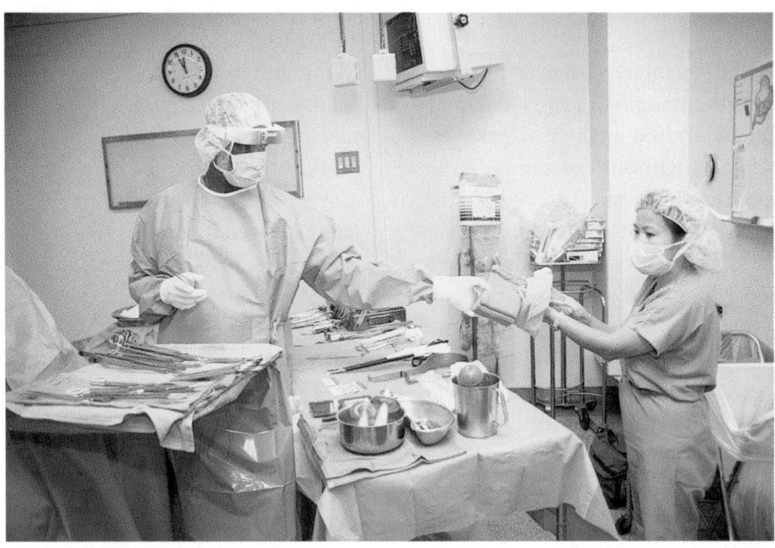

FIGURE 16-7 The nurse sets up the operating room.

local infiltration, the anesthetic agent is injected into and under the skin around the area of treatment. A nerve block is done by injecting an anesthetic agent around a nerve to block the transmission of impulses. Epidural anesthesia and subarachnoid anesthesia are examples of regional nerve blocks. Both are achieved by injecting the anesthetic agent into the area around the spinal nerves. Motor and sensory functions are blocked below the level of the anesthetic administration. This anesthesia is especially useful for surgical procedures on the lower abdomen and legs. The level of anesthesia is controlled by the amount of the drug injected and the position of the patient on the operating table.

As a rule, spinal and epidural anesthesia pose less risk for respiratory, cardiac, and gastrointestinal complications than general anesthesia. If the level of spinal or epidural anesthesia rises higher than intended, there is a risk of respiratory and cardiovascular depression.

One complication of spinal anesthesia is postspinal headache. It is caused by the leaking of cerebrospinal fluid at the puncture site. Postspinal headache can be severe and may last for several weeks. It is relieved by lying flat. It is more common in women, especially postpartum women. Keeping the patient flat for a specified period of time after spinal anesthesia may reduce the risk of headache. The nurse should always check the postoperative orders, however, for any positioning or activity restrictions. Forcing fluids in the postoperative period, if allowed, may help.

Severe spinal headache is sometimes treated by injecting a small amount of the patient's blood into the epidural space at the site of the previous subarachnoid puncture. The blood clots, forming a "blood patch" that prevents further leaking. The procedure can be repeated if it is unsuccessful the first time. A successful patch relieves the headache immediately. Postanesthesia headache should not occur with epidural anesthesia.

As the effect of a regional anesthetic wears off, the patient often reports that the affected limbs feel numb and heavy. You should reassure the patient that this is normal and that movement and sensation gradually return to normal. It is vital to do passive range-of-motion exercises until motility returns, to prevent thrombus (clot) formation. Typically, motor function returns before sensory function. At that time, the patient is susceptible to injury resulting from trauma or pressure because movement is possible but pain is not perceived.

Complications of local anesthesia include toxic effects caused by overdose, local tissue damage, and allergic responses. Initial signs and symptoms of toxic effects are excitement and central nervous system stimulation, followed by depression of the central nervous system and the cardiovascular system. Local tissue effects may be inflammation and edema. Abscesses and necrosis sometimes develop at the injection site. This is thought to be caused by poor technique rather than by the anesthetic agent.

Preanesthetic Agents

Prior to receiving anesthesia, the patient may be given preanesthetic agents, which can include antianxiety agents, sedative-hypnotics, anticholinergics, and opioid analgesics. Preanesthetic medications reduce anxiety without causing excessive drowsiness, induce perioperative amnesia, and reduce the amount of anesthesia required. In addition, they reduce the risk of some adverse effects of anesthetic agents, effects such as salivation, bradycardia, coughing, and vomiting.

General Anesthesia

General anesthesia acts on the central nervous system (CNS), causing loss of consciousness, sensation, reflexes, pain perception, and memory. Combinations of drugs are used to achieve these effects without excessive CNS depression. This use of multiple drugs, referred to as *balanced anesthesia,* allows lower dosages of each drug, which reduces the risks of adverse effects. General anesthetic agents are most often given by inhalation or intravenous infusion. Although the intramuscular and rectal routes can be used to administer anesthetic agents, the use of those routes is uncommon.

Near the end of procedures done under general anesthesia, the anesthetist or anesthesiologist administers drugs to reverse the effects of the anesthetic. When the procedure is completed, a member of the surgical team escorts the patient to the postanesthesia care unit, where careful monitoring can be done until the patient recovers from the anesthesia.

Inhalation Agents

Inhalation agents include isoflurane (Forane), sevoflurane (Ultane), enflurane (Ethrane), desflurane (Suprane), methoxyflurane (Penthrane), and nitrous oxide. For most procedures using inhalation agents, the patient is first induced with a short-acting intravenous agent that causes rapid loss of consciousness. Then an endotracheal tube is inserted into the patient's trachea to permit administration of the maintenance inhalation anesthesia and to control mechanical ventilation. A cuff on the endotracheal tube is inflated to prevent leakage during mechanical ventilation and aspiration of gastric contents while the patient is unconscious (Fig. 16-8).

Intravenous Agents

Intravenous agents include thiopental sodium (Pentothal), methohexital sodium (Brevital Sodium), propofol (Diprivan), midazolam (Versed), etomidate (Amidate), sufentanil (Sufenta), alfentanil (Alfenta), fentanyl (Duragesic), droperidol (Inapsine), and ketamine hydrochloride (Ketalar).

Other Agents

Muscle relaxants and opioids are often given with the anesthetic agents. Muscle relaxants such as succinylcholine, vecuronium (Norcuron), rocuronium (Zemuron), and cisatracurium (Nimbex) prevent movement of muscles during the surgical procedure. Opioids supplement anesthetic agents and support postoperative pain management.

Complications

Inhalation anesthetic agents and the endotracheal tube itself can cause irritation of the respiratory tract and the larynx. Individual agents may have the potential to cause serious adverse effects such as cardiac dysrhythmias, seizures, liver damage, nausea and vomiting, and death.

Malignant hyperthermia

Malignant hyperthermia is a rare but life-threatening complication that occurs in response to certain drugs. Susceptibility to this response is inherited. It may occur when succinylcholine is used with some general anesthetic agents. It is characterized by increasing body temperature and metabolic rate, tachycardia, hypotension, cyanosis, and muscle rigidity. When malignant hyperthermia occurs, the surgery is interrupted and measures are taken to cool the patient (for example, with iced intravenous solutions and/or ice packs). One

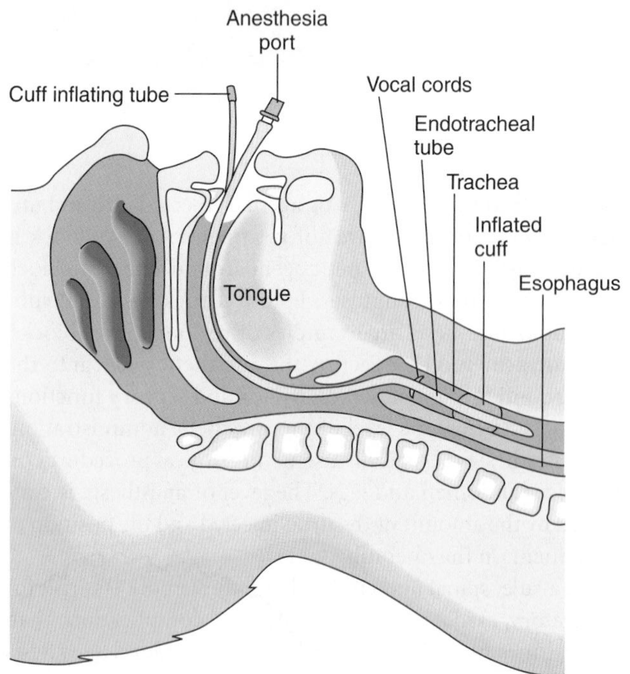

FIGURE 16-8 Inhalation anesthesia is given through an endotracheal tube.

hundred percent oxygen is administered, and the patient is given furosemide (Lasix), mannitol, sodium bicarbonate, diuretics, and dantrolene sodium.

Hypothermia

Hypothermia refers to a condition in which the body temperature is lower than normal. For some surgical procedures, the body temperature is deliberately lowered to reduce the metabolic rate and the need for oxygen. Cooling or freezing of a local area to block pain impulses is called *cryoanesthesia.*

Conscious Sedation

Conscious sedation employs intravenous drugs to reduce pain intensity or awareness without loss of reflexes. It is used with some diagnostic and therapeutic procedures, including cardiac catheterization and endoscopy. Only patients who meet specific psychological and physiologic criteria are candidates for conscious sedation. Registered nurses with specialized training may administer the drugs used for conscious sedation. During the procedure, the patient's vital signs, oxygen saturation, airway, level of consciousness, and electrocardiogram must be closely monitored. Documentation must include assessment data, interventions such as oxygen therapy, and the time, dosage, route, and effects of all drugs administered. Complications include respiratory depression and apnea, hypotension, excessive sedation approaching that of general anesthesia, and agitation and combativeness.

After procedures using conscious sedation, the patient may be discharged home with a responsible person when the following conditions are met: stable vital signs, patent airway, intact motor function and reflexes, satisfactory surgical site, no nausea or vomiting, patient is alert and able to void.

INTRAOPERATIVE NURSING CARE

Intraoperative nursing care is a specialty and is beyond the scope of this chapter. Only potential nursing diagnoses and goals are listed here.

Nursing Diagnoses, Goals, and Outcome Criteria

Nursing Diagnoses	Goals and Outcome Criteria
Risk for Injury related to the effects of anesthesia, positioning, use of restraints	Absence of physical injury: complete recovery from anesthesia, no pressure or traumatic tissue damage associated with positioning or restraints
Impaired Gas Exchange related to the effect of anesthesia and immobility	Adequate gas exchange: normal arterial blood gases
Decreased Cardiac Output related to drug effects or blood loss	Adequate cardiac output: heart rate and blood pressure consistent with patient norms
Risk for Deficient Fluid Volume related to blood loss, insensible loss of water, NPO status	Normal fluid volume: balanced intake and output, pulse and blood pressure consistent with patient norms

THE POSTOPERATIVE PHASE

When the surgical procedure is completed, the patient is usually transferred to the postanesthesia care unit (PACU or recovery room) or the critical care unit before returning to the nursing unit. Exceptions are patients who have undergone minor procedures with only local anesthesia.

SURGICAL COMPLICATIONS

The postoperative patient is at risk for a number of complications. These complications may be related to the surgical procedure itself, to the drugs used before and during the procedure, or to immobility during and after the procedure. The types of postoperative complications vary depending on the length of time elapsed since the surgical procedure. For example, shock and hypoxia are most likely to occur in the immediate recovery period. Wound infection, however, does not appear until several days after surgery. Complications in the immediate and later postoperative periods are described in Table 16-4. Prevention, recognition, and nursing implications are discussed in the section on nursing care.

Shock

Shock is most likely to occur as an effect of anesthesia or loss of blood. If opioid analgesics are given before the anesthesia wears off, they may contribute to a drop in blood pressure.

PHARMACOLOGY CAPSULE Opioid analgesics given before the effects of general anesthesia wear off may cause a drop in blood pressure and slow respirations.

Shock may also result from low blood volume (hypovolemic shock). Bleeding is an obvious cause of low blood volume, but other factors may contribute as well. Dehydration without adequate fluid replacement or fluid losses through wounds and suction can explain low blood volume.

There is growing interest in "bloodless" surgical procedures. These procedures employ a variety of strategies to reduce the need for blood replacement necessitated by excessive blood loss. Such strategies include drug therapy to stimulate production of red blood cells; the use of gamma-knife radiosurgery, electrocautery, and laser beam coagulation; and the collection and reinfusion of the patient's own blood during the procedure.

Hypoxia

Hypoxia refers to inadequate oxygenation of body tissues. The patient is at risk for hypoxia in the immediate postoperative phase for several reasons. First, general anesthetics depress respirations, so that the patient's breathing efforts may be inadequate initially. Second, when the patient is unconscious, the tongue may fall back and block the airway. Third, anesthesia depresses the cough and swallowing reflexes. Until these reflexes return, vomitus and saliva can enter the airway. A fourth reason that hypoxia may occur in the immediate postoperative period is the risk of laryngospasm or

table 16-4 ***Surgical Complications***

COMPLICATIONS	PREVENTION	TREATMENT
Shock	Assess wound dressing Report excessive drainage or bleeding Monitor vital signs every 15 min until stable Note early changes in vital signs Report tachycardia, tachypnea, hypotension Monitor input and output Keep intravenous fluid rate on schedule Assess respirations before giving opioids	Fluid or blood replacement Vasopressors (drugs to raise blood pressure) as ordered Additional surgery may be needed to control bleeding
Hypoxia	Keep airway in place until patient awakens Position unconscious patient on side, if not contraindicated Suction as necessary Monitor vital signs every 15 min until stable Encourage deep breathing	Position to promote effective ventilation Suction as necessary Administer oxygen Encourage deep breathing and coughing
Impaired wound healing Dehiscence Evisceration Infection	Adequate fluids and nutrition Splint incision during activity, coughing and deep breathing Good hand washing; sterile or clean technique for wound care as appropriate	Cover open wound with sterile dressing If organs protrude, saturate the dressing with normal saline and cover wet dressing with dry, sterile dressing; notify physician Keep patient still and quiet with knees flexed Anticipate return to surgery; withhold opioids until consent form signed
Inadequate oxygenation Pneumonia Atelectasis	Change position at least every 2 hr Assist to cough and deep breathe hourly Incentive spirometry	Rest Oxygen and antibiotics as ordered
Digestive disturbances		
Nausea and vomiting	Withhold oral fluids until nausea subsides Give antiemetics to prevent vomiting as soon as nausea is reported	Antiemetic drugs as ordered
Altered elimination Urine retention	Provide privacy; offer warm bedpan; position comfortably; take to bathroom or bedside commode chair if allowed; pour warm water over the perineum; let tap water run	Catheterization as ordered
Kidney failure	Promptly report urine output of less 30 ml/hr	
Abdominal distention	Nothing by mouth until bowel sounds return	Use rectal tube, heat to abdomen, bisacodyl suppositories as ordered Position on right side Nasogastric intubation with suction as ordered
"Gas" pains	Encourage ambulation as allowed	Ambulate frequently when permitted
Constipation	Encourage fluids, food, and ambulation as ordered; use stool softeners as ordered	Laxatives or enemas, or both, as ordered
Thrombophlebitis	Avoid pressure on blood vessels Leg exercises q 1-2 hr Early, frequent ambulation as ordered Elastic or automatic compression stockings	Bedrest Anticoagulant therapy as ordered
Fluid and electrolyte imbalances	Monitor intravenous fluid rate Provide a variety of oral fluids when permitted Treat vomiting Recognize signs of imbalances (see Chapter 13)	Give intravenous fluids as ordered Encourage oral intake when allowed

bronchospasm. Spasm of the larynx or bronchi narrows the airway and obstructs air flow.

Injury

Immediately after surgery, the patient is at risk for injury because of the decreased level of consciousness associated with general anesthesia or other sedatives. If regional anesthesia was used, the affected body part may be injured because it lacks sensation and movement.

PHARMACOLOGY CAPSULE Regional anesthesia blocks sensation and movement, so the affected body part is at risk for injury.

Pneumonia and Atelectasis

Drug effects and immobility place the surgical patient at risk for pneumonia and atelectasis. Patients who are most prone to these complications are the elderly, the obese, those with chronic pulmonary disease, and those who have undergone chest or abdominal surgery. General anesthetics and opioid analgesics depress respiratory function. Anticholinergics cause pulmonary secretions to be drier and thicker.

PHARMACOLOGY CAPSULE General anesthetics and opioid analgesics depress respirations.

Immobility limits lung expansion and allows fluids to pool in the lungs. Fluid provides a medium for infectious organisms to grow. An infection of the lungs associated with immobility is called *hypostatic pneumonia.*

As secretions accumulate, they begin to block off branches of the respiratory tree. When gases can no longer enter or leave the affected alveoli, they collapse. *Atelectasis* is the term used to describe collapse of a portion or all of a lung. Because atelectasis impairs the exchange of gases, it can be very serious.

Wound Complications

Complications in wound healing include dehiscence, evisceration, and infection. All are, to some extent, preventable.

Dehiscence and Evisceration. *Dehiscence* is the reopening of the surgical wound. It involves one or more layers of tissue. Dehiscence is most likely to happen when strain on the suture line is excessive. Factors that increase the risk of dehiscence include wound infection, malnutrition, obesity, dehydration, and extensive abdominal wounds or injuries. Dehiscence is most likely to occur between the 5th and 12th postoperative days. *Evisceration* is the term used when body organs protrude through the open wound. Dehiscence and evisceration are illustrated in Figure 16-9.

Infection. The risk of wound infection is greatest in cases of traumatic injuries, wounds that were not treated promptly, and wounds that were infected before surgery.

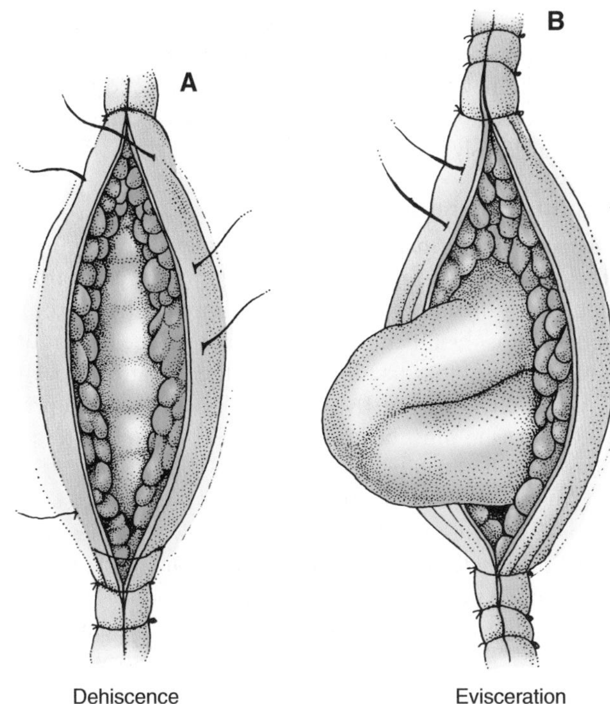

FIGURE 16-9 Complications of wound healing. *A,* Dehiscence. *B,* Evisceration.

Gastrointestinal Disturbances

The primary gastrointestinal problems that follow surgery are nausea, vomiting, impaired peristalsis, and constipation. Nausea and vomiting are most common in the early postoperative period. Causative factors include anesthesia, pain, opioids, decreased peristalsis, and resuming oral intake too soon.

Factors that cause peristalsis to be impaired after surgery include anesthesia, immobility, opioid analgesics, and handling of the bowel during surgery. Patients who develop metabolic imbalances, respiratory problems, or shock are also at risk for gastrointestinal disturbances.

The effects of slowed peristalsis can be mild or severe. Gas normally forms in the digestive tract. When peristalsis is slow, the gas builds up and causes cramping pain and distention. Mild effects are generally seen as gas pains that typically occur on the second or third postoperative day. Constipation is also related to slow peristalsis.

If peristalsis stops completely, the patient is said to have a paralytic ileus. The patient with a paralytic ileus has abdominal distention that may be severe enough to impair lung expansion and decrease blood return from the legs, causing cardiac output to fall. Distention also causes strain on an abdominal incision.

Urinary Retention and Renal Failure

With urinary retention, the kidneys produce urine, but the patient is unable to empty the bladder. Urinary retention can be caused by the effects of anesthesia or opioids, trauma to the urinary tract, or anxiety about voiding. Urine output may also be decreased because of dehydration or blood loss.

With kidney failure, the kidneys are unable to produce enough urine to remove wastes from the body. Urine output falls dangerously low.

Thrombophlebitis

The risk of hemorrhage and shock decreases after the immediate postoperative period. A more common circulatory problem in the later period is thrombophlebitis. Thrombophlebitis is the inflammation of veins with the formation of blood clots. It occurs most often in the legs after a period of immobility. Patients who have very lengthy surgical procedures or who must be immobilized are most likely to develop thrombophlebitis.

Clots that cling to the walls of blood vessels are called *thrombi*. Thrombi that break loose and flow with the blood are called *emboli*. Emboli formed in the legs are most likely to pass through the heart and lodge in the pulmonary circulation. If they are large enough to seriously impair pulmonary blood flow, the patient develops severe respiratory distress and may even die.

IMMEDIATE POSTOPERATIVE NURSING CARE *in the PACU*

Assessment

When the patient is admitted to the postanesthesia care unit (PACU), determine the medical diagnosis and the surgical procedure. Promptly assess the patient's status (level of consciousness, vital signs) and inspect the wound or dressing. Check and set up equipment, such as suction devices, oxygen, urinary drainage, and intravenous lines, as needed. When the patient returns to the nursing unit, a more complete assessment will be done.

Nursing Diagnoses, Goals, and Outcome Criteria

Depending on the severity and type of the burn, nursing diagnoses and goals for the burn victim immediately after the injury may include the following:

Nursing Diagnoses	Goals and Outcome Criteria
Decreased Cardiac Output related to excessive loss of blood and other body fluids or the effects of drugs	Normal cardiac output: pulse and blood pressure consistent with patient norms, normal skin color
Ineffective Breathing Patterns and/or **Ineffective Airway Clearance** related to effects of anesthetic agents or pain	Adequate oxygenation: respiratory rate, effort, and pattern consistent with patient norms; normal arterial blood gases; breath sounds clear
Acute Pain related to tissue trauma or to positioning during surgical procedures	Decreased pain: relaxed expression, patient statement of pain relief
Disturbed Thought Processes related to the effects of anesthetic agents	Normal thought processes: absence of confusion; orientation to person and place
Risk for Injury related to decreased level of consciousness or loss of sensation and movement as effect of anesthesia	Patient remains safe during recovery period: no falls, bruises, trauma when under effects of anesthesia

Interventions

Decreased Cardiac Output

Be alert to the possibility of shock. To detect impending shock, the patient's vital signs are monitored every 5 to 15 minutes in the PACU. Signs and symptoms of impending shock include a rapid, thready pulse, restlessness, decreasing blood pressure, and decreasing urine output. Use the patient's preoperative vital signs to evaluate whether postoperative vital signs are normal. An increasing pulse usually precedes a fall in blood pressure. Monitor intravenous fluid intake and urinary output. When blood volume is low (hypovolemia), the kidneys reduce urine production. Continuous cardiac monitoring is often done to identify early signs of hypovolemia or potentially dangerous changes in cardiac rhythm.

Measures to reduce the risk of shock include prompt recognition and treatment of bleeding, replacement of lost fluids, and the cautious use of opioid analgesics. Frequently inspect wound dressings and drains for the color and amount of drainage. The amount of bleeding expected varies with different surgical procedures.

An open intravenous route must be maintained during the early postoperative period. This permits the infusion of fluids, blood, and emergency medications if needed. Therefore, check the venipuncture site to be sure the fluid is infusing properly. The intravenous fluid infusion rate is ordered by the physician, but the nurse regulates the rate. If the rate falls behind, the patient may not receive adequate fluids to replace losses during surgery. If given too rapidly, intravenous fluids can overload the circulatory system, causing heart failure.

Ineffective Breathing Patterns

To detect early signs of hypoxia in the PACU, monitor the patient's respiratory status. Assess respiratory depth, rate, and effort. Listen for abnormal breath sounds that suggest breathing difficulty. Also be alert for changes in the pulse rate because an increasing pulse rate is often an early indicator of poor oxygenation. An oximeter is used to monitor the oxygenation of the blood. The oximeter is a device with a wire that clips to a finger or an earlobe.

The patient's color, especially in the nail beds and lips, provides a clue to oxygenation. Because cyanosis is a late sign of hypoxia, however, you should detect problems long before color changes develop.

Take measures to reduce the risk of hypoxia during the immediate postoperative period. An airway is inserted to keep the air passages open until the patient begins to awaken. Position the unconscious patient (if permitted) on one side to reduce the risk of aspiration of fluids. Suction if necessary to remove secretions or vomitus. When the gag reflex returns, the airway can be removed.

Acute Pain

Decisions to medicate for pain in the early postoperative phase are based on physician's orders and nursing judgment. If opioid analgesics are given too early, their effects, when combined with the effects of the anesthesia, may lead to shock. However, severe pain also may cause shock.

Disturbed Thought Processes

As patients begin to regain consciousness, they may move around and touch dressings and drains. Tell them where they are, that the surgery is over, and what is happening. Simple explanations and gentle reminders are often sufficient to calm and reassure them. The amnesic effects of anesthetics may cause the patient to forget what was said, making it necessary to repeat information.

Risk for Injury

Patients who have had local anesthesia may be sent to the PACU postoperatively, or they may be returned directly to the nursing unit or the ambulatory surgery unit. In the immediate postoperative period they are usually drowsy because preoperative and intraoperative sedatives typically have been given.

When regional block anesthesia is used, remember that sensation in that area is impaired. Take care, therefore, to prevent injury to the anesthetized body region.

Following spinal anesthesia the patient regains the ability to move the legs before sensation returns. Chart the times that the patient regains both movement and sensation. Assess the bladder for distention because the patient is unable to feel pressure. Patients may be kept flat for a specific period of time in the belief that it may help prevent spinal headache.

The Patient's Family

The time between the patient's leaving the nursing unit and returning can be 3 or 4 hours, even for relatively simple procedures. This may seem like a very long time for family and friends who are waiting. Most hospitals have some system for communicating the patient's status to those who wait. These visitors are usually relieved to know when the patient is in the recovery room. Many surgeons take time to speak with the visitors shortly after the surgery is completed. When problems arise, it is thoughtful to offer visitors privacy and the services of a patient representative or a spiritual counselor.

Discharge from the Postanesthesia Care Unit

The patient's progress in the PACU is carefully monitored. Several systems of scoring have been used to determine when recovery is adequate and the patient can be transferred. In general, the patient can be moved from the recovery room when the following conditions are met:

1. Vital signs are stable.
2. Respiratory and circulatory functions are adequate.
3. The patient has minimal pain.
4. The patient is awake or can be wakened easily.
5. Complications are absent or are under control.
6. The gag reflex is present.

Most patients remain in the PACU for 1 to 2 hours, although the time varies considerably. Patients who are unstable or who need very close observation may be transferred to a critical care unit.

Put on your THINKING CAP!!

Use the "Stress Response" discussed in Chapter 7 to explain the signs and symptoms of deficient fluid volume during the immediate postoperative period.

POSTOPERATIVE NURSING CARE *on the Nursing Unit*

When the patient is transferred to the nursing unit, the PACU nurse reports on the patient to the nurse who will be caring for that patient. Several people are usually necessary to move the patient safely from the gurney to the bed. Be careful to prevent pulling or dislodging tubes and to prevent a shearing force on the skin. Hang intravenous fluids and set at the ordered rate. Connect nasogastric suction tubes to suction equipment. Identify and arrange drains to avoid obstruction. Safety precautions include raising the side rails, lowering the bed, placing the call button within reach, and instructing the patient not to get up without assistance (see Nursing Care Plan: The Postoperative Patient).

NURSING CARE PLAN

The Postoperative Patient

ASSESSMENT

Health History: 27-year-old Susan Matthews was admitted for a hysterectomy and surgical excision of endometriosis implants. She is a secretary, married, and the mother of a 3-year-old child. Is 1 day post-surgery. Complains of moderate abdominal and incisional pain. Has been out of bed three times since surgery. Ambulated well with assistance. Foley catheter removed 3 hours ago. Has not voided since. Intravenous fluids infusing at 100 ml/hr. No nausea, but nothing by mouth (NPO) until noon, when 550 ml of clear liquids was taken and retained.

Physical Examination: Alert and oriented. Vital signs: temperature 99.4° F orally; pulse 90, respirations 16, blood pressure 130/86. (Admission vital signs were temperature 99° F orally; pulse 94, respiration 20, blood pressure 126/82.) Breath sounds diminished in lower lobes. Abdomen soft. No bladder distention. Wound covered with dry dressing. Bowel sounds present but hypoactive.

Continued

NURSING CARE PLAN—cont'd

Nursing Diagnosis	*Goals and Outcome Criteria*	*Interventions*
Acute pain related to tissue trauma.	Patient will report pain relief and appear more relaxed.	Assess nature, location, and severity of pain. Evaluate effectiveness of patient-controlled analgesia. Assure patient that opioids can be taken safely for acute pain for a limited time. Assist to change positions at least every 2 hours. Give back rub. Coach in relaxation exercises and mental imagery. Assess anxiety and explore causes. Be available. Reassure.
Impaired tissue integrity related to surgical incision.	Patient's wound edges will remain clean and closed until discharge.	Check dressing hourly for bleeding first 24 hours, then twice each shift. Report bleeding to physician. Protect wound by supporting during respiratory exercises. Treat nausea promptly.
Risk for infection related to break in skin, invasive devices, and procedures.	Patient will remain free of infection, as evidenced by oral temperature less than 100° F, decreasing redness of incision, no purulent drainage, clear breath sounds, no dysuria, no phlebitis.	Monitor vital signs every 4 hours. Report increasing temperature. Assess wound for increasing redness, edema, or drainage each shift. Inspect for purulent drainage. Exercise good hand washing. Aseptic technique for wound care. Monitor and encourage fluid intake. Collect specimens for culture if ordered. Teach patient how to care for wound after discharge.
Impaired gas exchange related to stasis of pulmonary secretions.	Patient's breath sounds will remain clear and respiratory rate will be between 12 and 20 without dyspnea.	Help patient support incision and turn, cough, and deep breathe or use incentive spirometry at least q 2 hr. Teach to take 10 deep breaths each hour. Auscultate breath sounds for crackles or atelectasis q 2 hr. Encourage fluid intake.
Urinary retention related to effects of anesthesia.	Patient's urine output will be approximately equal to fluid intake; no bladder distention.	Measure all fluid intake and output. Palpate for distended bladder q 2 hr. Provide privacy and try to stimulate voiding. Catheterize using sterile technique as ordered if patient is unable to void.
Constipation related to effects of drugs, immobility, bowel manipulation during surgery.	Patient will have bowel sounds and pass flatus prior to discharge.	Assess bowel sounds and ask patient to report passage of flatus ("gas"). Count and document gurgles per minute. Encourage frequent ambulation as allowed. Position the patient on the right side. Report distention.
Risk for deficient fluid volume related to wound drainage, NPO status.	Patient's fluid intake and output will be approximately equal; serum electrolytes will remain within normal limits.	Measure fluid intake and output. Assess fluid status: tissue turgor, mucous membranes, pulse quality. Administer antiemetics promptly for nausea or vomiting. Offer fluids as prescribed.
Impaired physical mobility related to weakness, tissue trauma.	Patient will gradually increase activity and assume more self-care.	Assist out of bed until patient can do so alone. Teach patient importance of ambulation to promote healing and prevent complications.
Disturbed body image related to abdominal wound.	Patient will state any concerns about appearance of wound.	Observe patient's reaction to the incision. Ask if there are any questions or concerns. Answer questions honestly or refer to surgeon. Tell the patient the incision will fade and the edema will diminish.
Deficient knowledge related to postoperative routines	Patient will correctly describe postoperative routines and self-care during hospitalization and after discharge. Patient will identify complications that should be reported to the physician.	Reinforce physician's instructions for wound care and activity limitations. Encourage consideration of adaptations needed in work or home roles and responsibilities. Stress need for good nutrition. Explain any drugs being prescribed: dosage, schedule, side effects, and adverse effects that should be reported to the physician. Include husband in teaching.

Assessment

Health History

Review the patient's preoperative assessment (outlined in Table 16-2), noting long-term conditions, disabilities, prostheses, drugs, and allergies. When the patient is able to respond, ask about significant symptoms, including pain, nausea, and altered sensations (Table 16-5).

Physical Examination

Vital Signs. Take vital signs and compare the results with the preoperative readings. Assess the respiratory rate, depth, and effort. Take the pulse, noting rate, rhythm, and quality. Record the blood pressure. Measurements are usually repeated every 15 minutes until the vital signs stabilize.

Neurological Status. The assessment of neurologic status includes level of consciousness and pupil size, equality, and reaction to light. Evaluate sensation in affected body areas. Note spontaneous movements and the patient's ability to move affected parts on command. For example, when a cast has been applied to a fractured arm, test the patient's ability to move the fingers.

Integument. Inspect the skin color and palpate for temperature. Inspect the surgical area. If the wound is visible, assess the incision for intactness of the wound margins, drainage, and excessive redness or swelling. If a dressing covers the incision, inspect the dressing for bleeding or other drainage. If closed drains are in place, observe the amount and appearance of the drainage.

Thorax. Observe chest expansion with respirations. Chest movement should be symmetric. Auscultate for breath sounds to detect atelectasis, crackles, and wheezes.

Heart. Take the apical pulse if the peripheral pulse is weak or irregular or if the patient has heart disease.

Abdomen. Inspect the abdomen for distention and auscultate for bowel sounds. Light palpation also may be done to assess bowel and bladder distention and tenderness. Check the patency of gastrointestinal tubes.

Extremities. Assess the color and capillary refill of nail beds and the presence and quality of peripheral pulses in affected extremities. Note the presence of edema or excessive warmth or redness. Simultaneously assess the color and temperature of both arms or legs to detect differences. Dorsiflex the foot to assess for pain in the calf, a finding called a *positive Homans's sign.* This finding is suggestive of thrombophlebitis.

table 16-5 ASSESSMENT *of the Postoperative Patient*

HEALTH HISTORY

Reason for surgery, name of procedure, medical diagnosis, disabilities, prostheses, drugs, allergies
Presence of pain, nausea, altered sensations

PHYSICAL EXAMINATION

Vital Signs
Neurological Status: Level of consciousness; pupil size, equality, response to light; sensation; spontaneous movement, response to commands
Integument: Color, temperature, incision or dressing appearance, amount and appearance of drainage
Thorax: Chest expansion, symmetry, breath sounds
Heart: Apical pulse
Abdomen: Contour, bowel sounds, bladder distention, tenderness
Extremities: Color, capillary refill, pulses, edema, warmth, redness, Homans's sign

Nursing Diagnoses, Goals, and Outcome Criteria

Once the immediate postoperative phase has passed, the type of potential complications changes somewhat. The risks of shock and hypoxia lessen. The nurse's attention turns toward other nursing diagnoses and goals, which are detailed in this chart.

Nursing Diagnoses	Goals and Outcome Criteria
Acute Pain related to tissue trauma	Reduced pain: relaxed expression, patient statement of pain reduction or relief
Impaired Tissue Integrity related to poor wound healing	Normal wound healing: intact wound margins
Risk for Infection related to break in skin or invasive devices and procedures	Absence of infection: minimal redness, clear drainage, no purulence; no fever
Impaired Gas Exchange related to stasis of pulmonary secretions, thrombosis, or emboli	Adequate oxygenation: respiratory rate and effort consistent with patient norms; normal arterial blood gases Absence of thrombophlebitis: no redness or swelling in legs; negative Homans's sign
Urinary Retention related to the effects of anesthesia or restricted position	Normal bladder emptying: urine output equal to fluid intake; no bladder distention
Constipation related to the effects of drugs, immobility, or bowel manipulation during surgery	Normal bowel function: bowel sounds present, passage of flatus
Risk for Deficient Fluid Volume related to wound drainage, inadequate intake, vomiting, or gastrointestinal decompression	Normal hydration: approximately equal fluid intake and output, normal serum electrolytes, pulse and blood pressure consistent with patient norms
Imbalanced Nutrition: Less than Body Requirements related to nausea and vomiting or medical restriction of intake	Adequate nutrition for metabolic demands: retention of oral food and fluids, stable body weight
Impaired Physical Mobility related to weakness, tissue trauma, or medical activity restrictions	Improved physical mobility: gradual increase in mobility to maximal level
Disturbed Body Image related to change in body appearance and function	Adaptation to changes in body image: patient looks at and touches affected area, patient verbalizes acceptance of physical changes

Interventions

Acute Pain

Pain is expected in the early postoperative phase. Pain receptors are stimulated because tissues are cut and stretched during surgery. Muscle spasms in the area around the incision add to the patient's discomfort. The pain is usually most severe during the first 48 hours after surgery. During that time opioid analgesics such as meperidine or morphine are most appropriate. The physician may order doses to be given at 3- to 4-hour intervals when needed, or patient-controlled analgesia may be used. Patient-controlled analgesia is discussed in Chapter 14. By the third postoperative day most patients need less medication for pain relief. The dosage or frequency may be reduced, or the order may be changed to an oral analgesic such as acetaminophen with codeine.

When postoperative patients complain of pain, determine the exact nature of the complaint. Where is the pain located? It is easy to assume that the pain is incisional when in fact the patient may have a headache or a backache. Chest pain, leg pain, or gas pain requires additional assessment and interventions. How severe is the pain? Ask the patient to rate the severity of the pain on a scale of 1 to 10, with 1 being mild pain and 10 being the worst pain imaginable. This provides a system for evaluating response to comfort measures.

During the first few days after surgery, promptly medicate the patient for pain. Pain is controlled better if it is treated before it becomes severe. Some physicians will order routine (rather than PRN) analgesics for the first 24 to 36 hours. This maintains consistent therapeutic blood levels of the analgesic and reduces episodes of acute pain. Pain medication can also be given before activities that normally cause pain. Some patients are afraid that they will become addicted to opioids. Assure them that the short-term use of opioids for acute pain relief generally has not been associated with addiction.

A patient whose pain is controlled adequately is better able to participate in the exercises necessary to prevent postoperative complications. Schedule turning, coughing, deep breathing, and even walking to take advantage of periods when the patient is most comfortable. Of course, a medicated patient must be closely supervised when out of bed.

Although drugs are the mainstay of pain management in the early postoperative phase, other nursing measures can be used to help reduce pain. Position changes and backrubs can be very soothing. Relaxation exercises and mental imagery are often very effective alone or in combination with other nursing measures.

One source of discomfort in the postoperative patient is singultus, commonly known as hiccups. Hiccups are caused by intermittent spasms of the diaphragm. They are uncomfortable and may put stress on the incision, disrupt rest, and interfere with the intake of food and fluids. If hiccups persist, notify the physician.

Anxiety seems to intensify discomfort. Measures to decrease anxiety may therefore enhance the effects of pain relief measures. Recognize when the patient is tense and try to discover the source of the anxiety. Patients need to feel safe and need reassurance about what is happening to them.

Pain management in the elderly can pose special challenges. The older patient may be stoic, reluctant to request analgesics, and fearful of addiction and overdose. Nurses, fearing greater risk of adverse effects or believing that the older person experiences less pain, may fail to treat the older person adequately. Good management of postoperative pain in the older person can often be attained with nonsteroidal anti-inflammatory drugs or acetaminophen in combination with opioids at somewhat reduced dosages. The rule of thumb with opioids is to start with a low dose and gradually increase it. Drugs that are more likely to have adverse effects in the older person are meperidine (Demerol) and long-acting benzodiazepines like diazepam (Valium). Well-prepared patients, regardless of age, can participate in pain management by describing and rating their pain, informing the nurse of the effects of treatment, and using patient-controlled analgesia when appropriate.

The management of pain in cognitively impaired elders is especially difficult. You may have to rely on your observations of patient behavior or family perceptions to recognize pain. Inappropriate behaviors such as pulling at tubes, striking out, and yelling may be manifestations of pain. Some impaired elders can use pediatric pain rating scales, which provide you with some measure of pain intensity. After procedures that are known to be painful, pain should be assumed and analgesics given in combination with other comfort measures.

Impaired Tissue Integrity

Various techniques are used to close the wound after surgery. The patient's incision may be closed with sutures, staples, or tape as shown in Figure 16-10. When the patient returns to the nursing unit, a dressing probably covers the wound. After some procedures such as rectal, vaginal, nasal, or ear surgery, the operative site may be packed with gauze. In some situations wounds are left open and covered with a dressing.

In healthy people surgical wounds begin to heal immediately. By the third or fourth day, the healing is stronger. Although the wound appears to be healed after about 10 days, complete healing may take as long as a year.

Clean sutured incisions heal by first *(primary)* intention. Because the wound edges are closed, tissue bonds with little scarring. An infected wound is left open to heal from the bottom up. This is called *healing by secondary intention.* Some sources refer to healing by *tertiary intention.* This term may be used when the wound is initially left open and later closed. Figure 16-11 illustrates these three types of healing.

The physician usually does the first dressing change, inspects the wound, and orders specific wound care. For the first 24 hours, check the dressing hourly for bleeding or drainage. If dressings become saturated, reinforce them using aseptic technique. Depending on physician preference and agency policy, reinforcement may be done several ways. One method is simply to place dry dressings over the wet ones. Another method is to remove bulky outer layers of the wet dressing and replace them with dry dressings. After the first 24 hours, check the dressing once or twice each shift. Bleeding should be minimal and should stop within a few

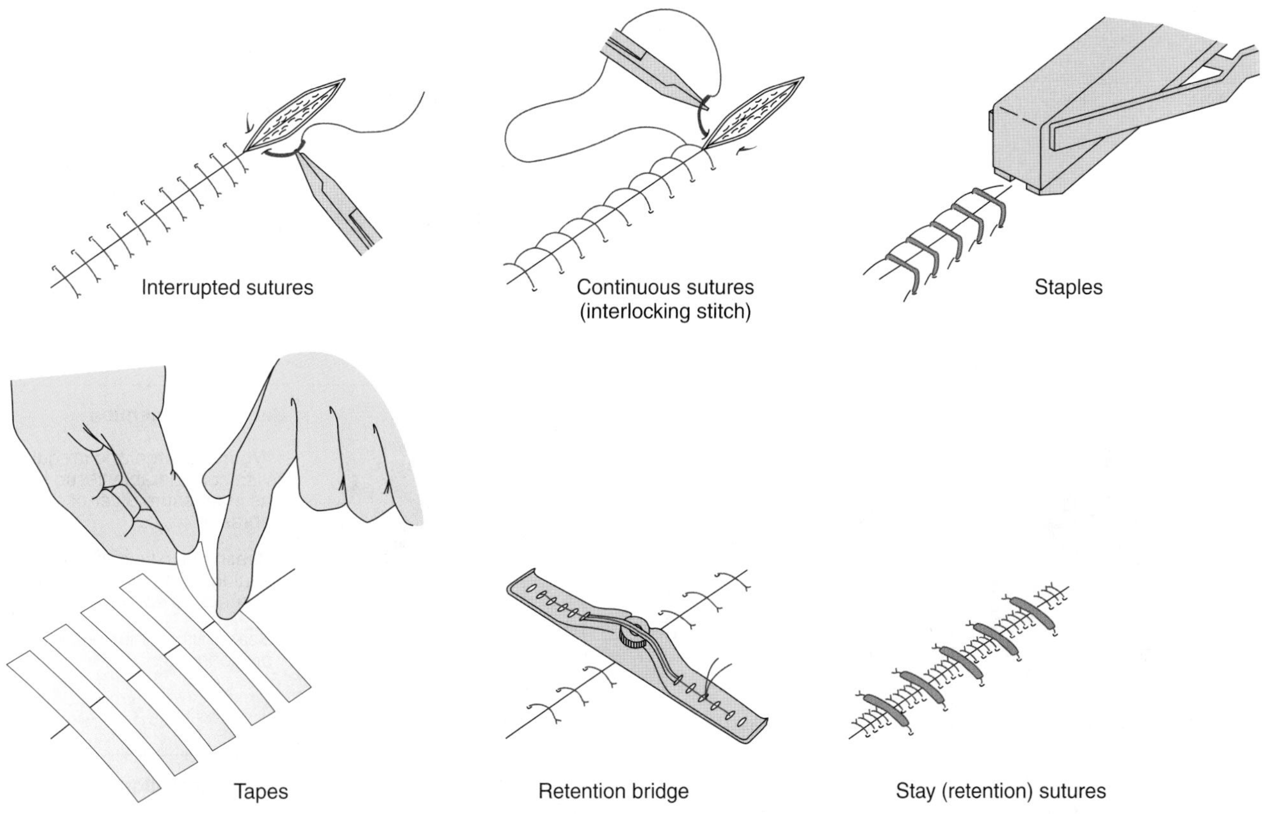

FIGURE **16-10** Methods of wound closure.

hours after the wound is closed. Report continued or excessive bleeding to the physician.

Some wounds have drains in a "stab" wound close to the incision (Fig. 16-12). Drains remove fluids from the operative site. Fluid accumulation in a wound interferes with healing. A Penrose drain is a soft tube that permits passive movement of fluids from the wound. The drainage is absorbed by the wound dressing.

Other types of drains are attached to collection devices that create suction to draw fluid from the wound. This type of drain is called an *active drain.* Examples of low-suction active drains are the Hemovac and the Jackson-Pratt drain. Both create negative pressure when they are compressed. As they fill with fluid, the collection devices expand. They must be emptied and recompressed ("recharged") to maintain their effectiveness. The frequency of emptying depends on the amount of drainage and the physician's orders. Wound drains may also be connected to sump drains. Record drainage as output. Vacuum-assisted closure devices are used to apply negative pressure to certain open wounds.

In the immediate postoperative phase, wound drainage is often bright red (sanguineous). As the amount of blood in the drainage decreases, the fluid becomes pinkish (serosanguineous). It should become progressively lighter in color and thinner until it is straw-colored and clear (serous). At the same time that the color is changing, the amount of drainage should steadily decrease.

Take care to reduce the risk of wound complications: dehiscence, evisceration, and infection. Although dehiscence is not expected in a clean wound, always avoid strain on the suture line. Teach the patient to support the incision during coughing and when getting in and out of bed (Fig. 16-13). Patients who have had abdominal surgery should not use trapeze bars to move themselves. Promptly treat nausea to avoid the stress of retching and vomiting. Because many surgical patients go home in less than a week, they need verbal and written instructions about safe activities. The exact type of surgery that was performed determines the restrictions. Consult with the physician about correct instructions.

Wounds that are healing normally are unlikely to undergo dehiscence. If infection develops under surgical sutures, the sutures dissolve too soon. Fluid accumulates in the wound, and the wound dehisces. A sudden increase in wound drainage may precede wound dehiscence. When the suture line ruptures, the patient may feel like the wound is "pulling apart."

If dehiscence occurs, keep the patient in bed and in a position to decrease strain on the wound and decrease the risk of evisceration. For example, the patient with an abdominal wound should be in semi-Fowler's position with the knees flexed. If dehiscence or evisceration occurs, the usual practice is to cover the wound with sterile dressings saturated with normal saline and to notify the physician. The saline is thought to prevent damage from drying of the exposed organs. Some are concerned, however, that moisture increases the risk of wound contamination by promoting bacterial movement through the dressings. Covering the saline-soaked gauze with a dry dressing may prevent this complication. After inspecting the wound, the physician may order an

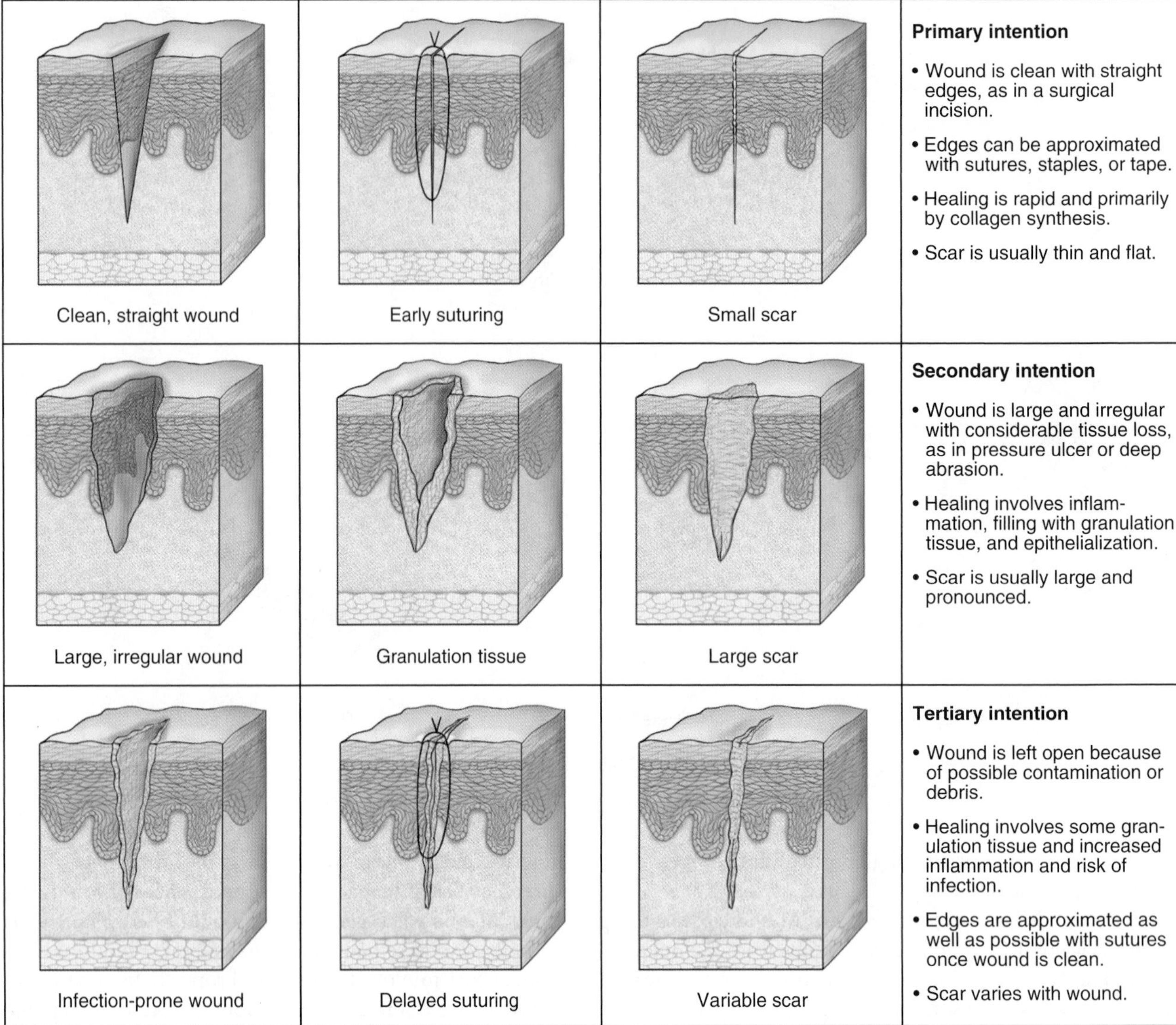

Clean, straight wound
Early suturing
Small scar
Primary intention
• Wound is clean with straight edges, as in a surgical incision.
• Edges can be approximated with sutures, staples, or tape.
• Healing is rapid and primarily by collagen synthesis.
• Scar is usually thin and flat.
Large, irregular wound
Granulation tissue
Large scar
Secondary intention
• Wound is large and irregular with considerable tissue loss, as in pressure ulcer or deep abrasion.
• Healing involves inflammation, filling with granulation tissue, and epithelialization.
• Scar is usually large and pronounced.
Infection-prone wound
Delayed suturing
Variable scar
Tertiary intention
• Wound is left open because of possible contamination or debris.
• Healing involves some granulation tissue and increased inflammation and risk of infection.
• Edges are approximated as well as possible with sutures once wound is clean.
• Scar varies with wound.

FIGURE **16-11** Wound healing.

abdominal binder. Anticipate a possible return to surgery, and do not administer opioid analgesics until surgical consent is obtained. Infected wounds may be allowed to heal by secondary intention.

Risk for Infection

Continuously assess the patient for indications of infection. Signs and symptoms of wound infection usually do not develop until the third to fifth day after the operation. They may appear as late as a week after surgery. The classic signs and symptoms of wound infection include pain, fever, redness, swelling, and purulent drainage. Surgical pain should decrease as the days go by. Continued or increasing pain suggests the possibility of infection. A low-grade fever is common during the first 2 postoperative days because of the normal inflammation stage of healing. If the temperature is higher than 38° C (100.4° F) or lasts more than 2 days, however, it may be due to infection. Early signs of infection are sometimes hard to detect in elderly surgical patients because they typically do not develop high fevers even with serious infections. Some redness is expected at the wound suture line and around the sutures or staples. Increasing redness or redness that spreads to surrounding tissue is not normal.

Prevention of wound infection requires decreasing the exposure to microorganisms and maintaining the patient's resistance to infection. Good hand washing, the use of sterile or clean gloves (as appropriate), aseptic dressing changes, and diligent wound care prevent the introduction of infectious organisms. Good hydration and nutrition support the patient's healing and resistance to infection.

If infection is suspected, a culture of any drainage may identify the infectious organism or organisms. The antibiotics that are most likely to be effective can then be prescribed. Collect the culture specimen before antibiotic therapy is be-

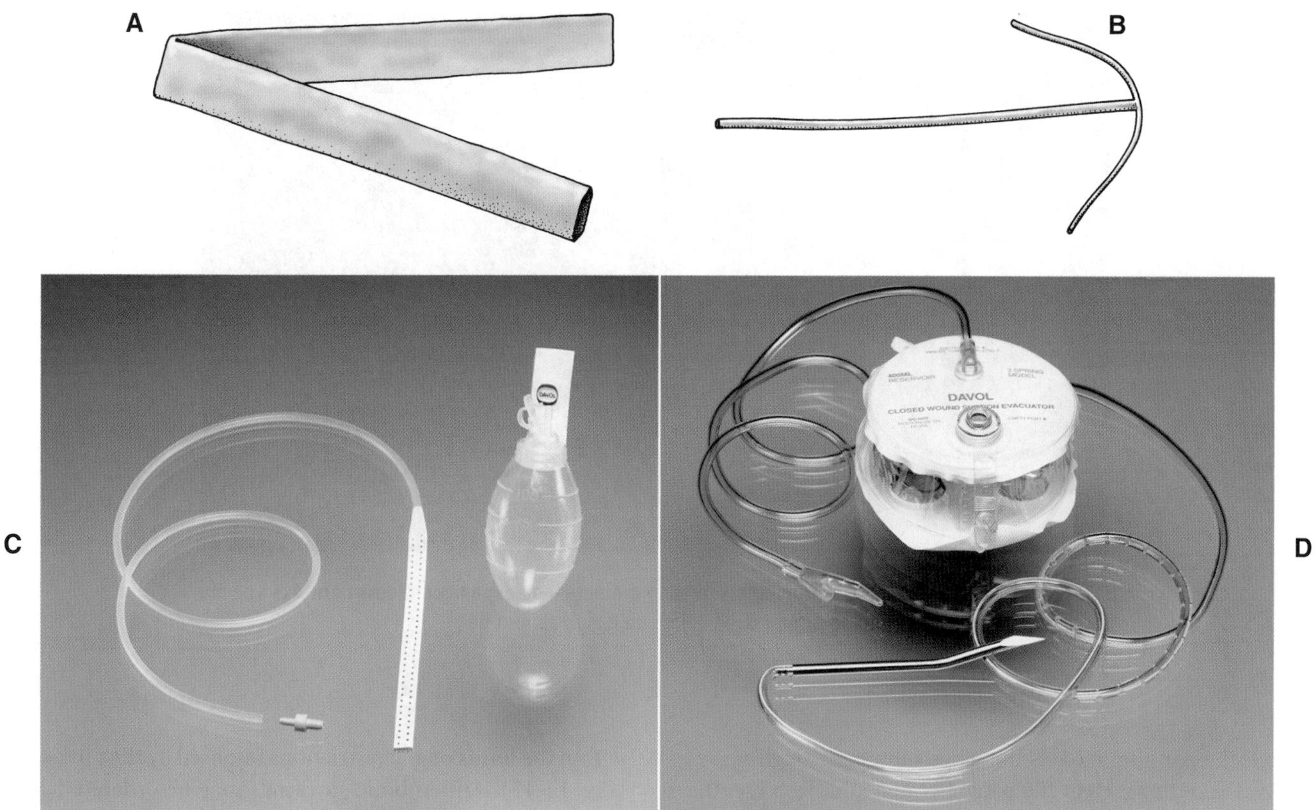

FIGURE **16-12** Types of surgical drains used to remove fluid from wounds. Passive or gravity drains include the Penrose drain *(A)* and the T-tube *(B)*. Drains that work by creating negative pressure when the receptacle is compressed are the Jackson-Pratt drain *(C)* and the Hemovac *(D)*.

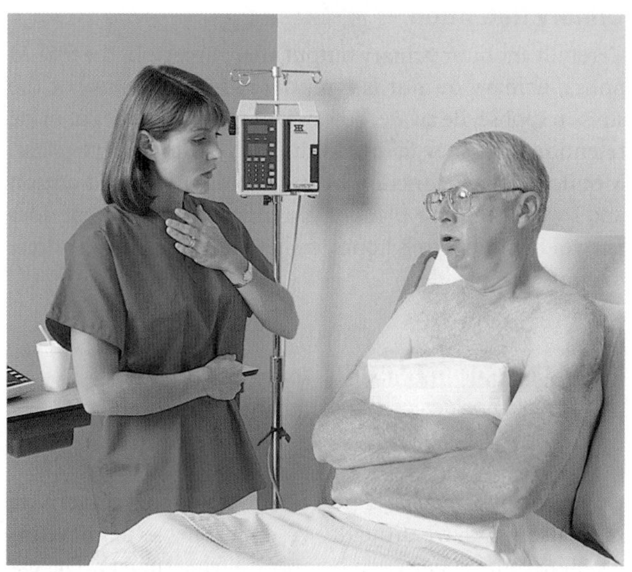

FIGURE **16-13** Splinting supports the incision during coughing.

gun. While awaiting results of the culture and sensitivity tests, the physician often orders a broad-spectrum antibiotic. Various cleansing procedures may also be ordered. The patient may need to be isolated from other patients to prevent transfer of the organisms. The presence of highly contagious organisms such as methicillin-resistant *Staphylococcus aureus* requires patient isolation.

Because infection may develop after the patient is discharged, patient teaching should include signs and symptoms of infection that should be reported to the physician. The patient also should know whether the wound requires any special treatment. If wound care is needed at home, make sure the patient or a family member is able to do it before the patient leaves the hospital.

Impaired Gas Exchange

Assess the patient's respiratory status every hour for the first 24 hours and once or twice a shift after that. Signs and symptoms of pneumonia include dyspnea, fatigue, fever, cough, purulent or bloody sputum, and "wet" breath sounds. When gas exchange is impaired, as with pneumonia or atelectasis, the pulse rate generally increases. Breath sounds are absent in areas of atelectasis.

The most important nursing measures to prevent pneumonia and atelectasis are frequent position changes and coughing and deep breathing exercises. Initially, assist the patient to turn at least every 2 hours. Patients are often assisted out of bed on the day of surgery. They are usually ambulated several times daily, beginning on the second day. Early ambulation has been found to reduce the respiratory complications of surgery greatly.

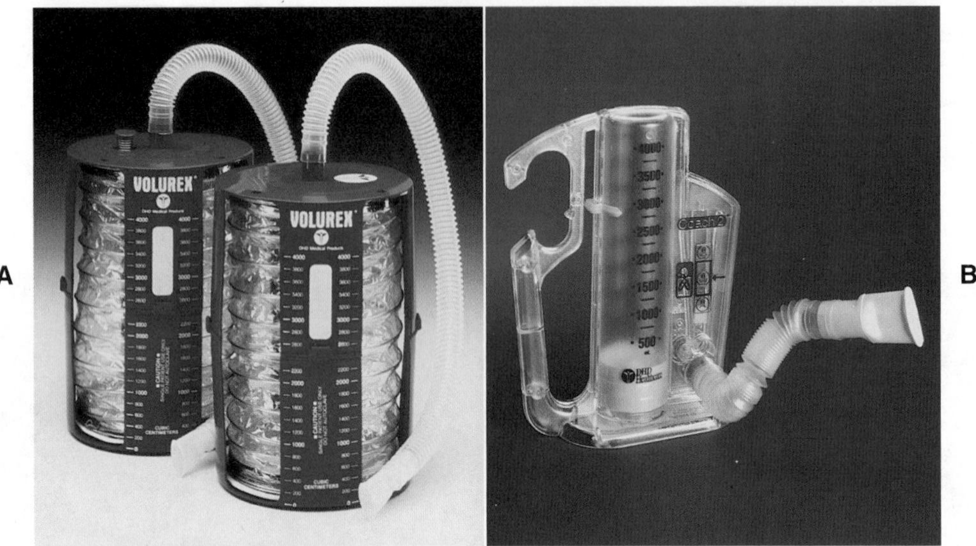

FIGURE **16-14** The incentive spirometer is used to promote lung expansion. Shown are *A,* a volume displacement incentive spirometer and *B,* a volume incentive spirometer.

Deep breathing inflates the lungs fully, and coughing removes secretions. Help the patient cough and deep breathe every hour. Instruct the patient to take in a deep breath through the nose and gradually blow out through the mouth. After taking several deep breaths, a cough should be attempted to bring up secretions.

The incentive spirometer is a device used to promote lung expansion (Fig. 16-14). It consists of a tube through which air is inhaled and a cylinder containing a ball. The ball rises in the cylinder as the patient inhales through the tube. The more air taken in, the higher the ball moves. Markings on the cylinder indicate the volume of air taken in. This gives the patient a measurable goal to work for while using the spirometer.

Deep breathing and coughing are painful for the patient who has had abdominal or chest surgery. To reduce discomfort, coordinate the exercises with analgesics and splint the incision. The patient can splint by holding a pillow firmly over the surgical area while coughing.

It is best to teach turning, deep breathing, coughing, and use of the incentive spirometer before surgery. A patient in pain or drowsy from anesthesia is not in the best condition for learning. There are a few instances in which coughing is contraindicated. They include surgeries for hernias and cataracts, as well as brain surgery.

If the patient develops pneumonia, it is treated with rest, oxygen, and antibiotics. Care of the patient with pneumonia is discussed in Chapter 29.

Another factor that may cause severe, sometimes fatal, respiratory complications is pulmonary embolism. Pulmonary emboli usually arise from thrombi that develop in veins, especially the veins of the legs and pelvis. Measures to prevent thrombophlebitis and related pulmonary emboli include leg exercises, early ambulation, and frequent position changes within the limits of any restrictions imposed by the physician (Fig. 16-15). Antiembolic stockings may be ordered. Signs and symptoms that alert the nurse to possible pulmonary embolism are dyspnea, tachypnea, chest pain, and hemoptysis. If the embolus is very large, the patient may become cyanotic and go into shock. Emboli may be treated with heparin, thrombolytic agents, or both.

Urinary Retention

Carefully monitor urinary output after surgery. In the first 24 hours, urinary output is typically reduced because of the stress response. Be aware, however, of the possibilities of urine retention or kidney failure in the early postoperative phase. Monitor urinary function by measuring intake and output and by checking for bladder distention. If the patient does not void within 6 to 8 hours, catheterization is usually done to empty the bladder.

PHARMACOLOGY CAPSULE Anesthesia, anticholinergics, and opioid analgesics can contribute to urinary retention.

Patients who have had perineal or abdominal surgery are most likely to have difficulty voiding. They often have indwelling catheters inserted before or during surgery. The patient with a urine retention problem usually reports feelings of fullness and pressure over the lower abdomen. Some patients are unable to void at all. When a patient passes small amounts of urine frequently without feeling relief of the fullness, suspect retention with overflow. The bladder releases just enough urine to reduce the pressure but without complete emptying. Gentle palpation of the lower abdomen usually reveals the smooth, rounded, full bladder.

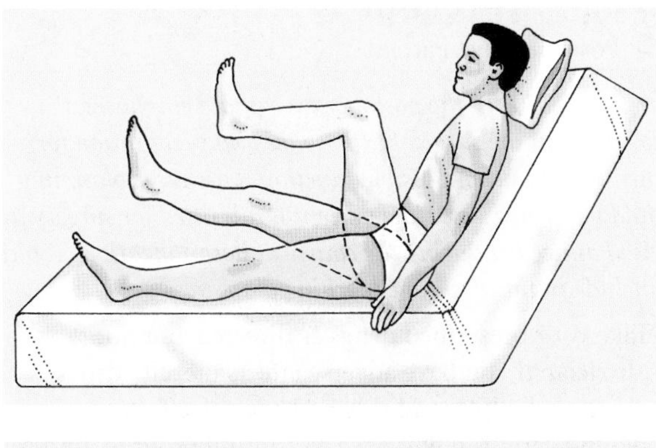

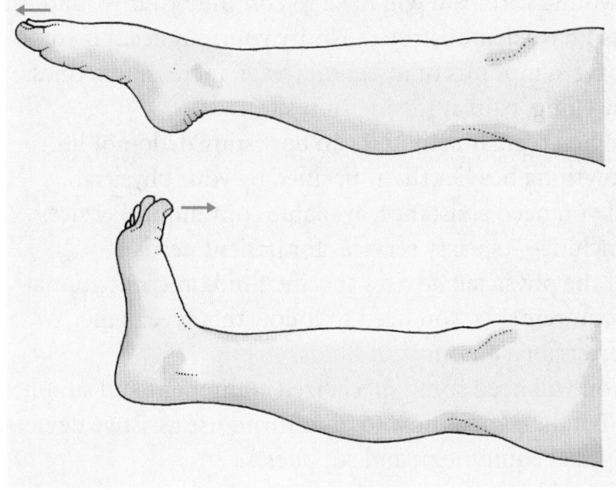

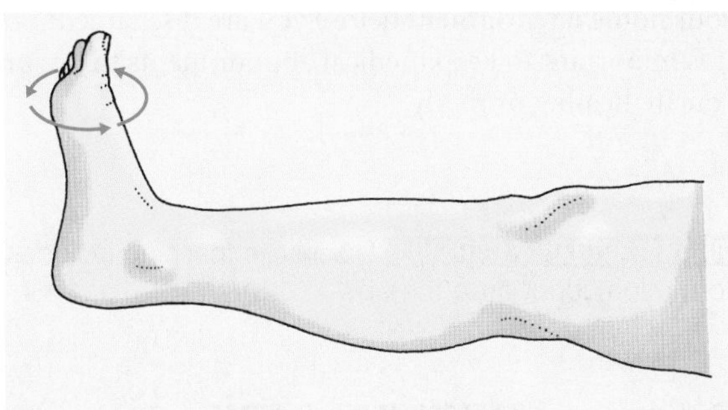

FIGURE 16-15 Postoperative leg exercises promote venous return.

If the patient is unable to void, catheterization is necessary. Because catheterization can cause urinary infection, it should be done only if other interventions fail. Interventions must take the physician's activity orders into consideration. The patient should be provided privacy while attempting to void. The toilet is preferred if the patient can go to the bathroom. If a bedpan has to be used, raise the head of the bed, if permitted, to create a normal position for voiding. Men who need to stand to void should be assisted to do so if not contraindicated.

Sensory stimuli help some people overcome difficulty voiding. The sound of running water or the sensation of warm water poured over the perineum or hands may encourage voiding. Use a measured amount of the water so it can be subtracted from the urine output.

If all independent measures fail, a physician's order is required for catheterization. There is usually an "as necessary" order to empty the bladder with a catheter if the patient does not void within 6 to 8 hours after surgery.

Some agencies have policies that limit the amount of urine that can be drained from a full bladder at one time. These limits are usually 750 to 1,000 ml. After the removal of the allowed amount of urine, the catheter may be clamped for a specified period of time before the bladder is drained again. This procedure is referred to as *bladder decompression.* Research in this area has raised some question as to whether draining the bladder completely is, in fact, dangerous.

If the patient has to be catheterized several times, the physician may order the insertion of an indwelling catheter. Catheterization and the care of the patient with a catheter are discussed in Chapter 38.

If there are no signs of bladder distention but little or no urine output, the patient may be in kidney failure. The minimal urine output is considered to be 30 ml/hr. Failure to produce at least 30 ml/hr should be reported promptly to the physician. The diagnosis and treatment of kidney failure are discussed in Chapter 38.

Constipation

Gastrointestinal function is disrupted by surgery. Postoperatively, inspect and palpate for abdominal distention and auscultate for bowel sounds. Document the passage of flatus and the first bowel movement. The patient may not realize the significance of passing flatus and may wonder why it should be reported. Explain that passing flatus means the digestive tract is beginning to function again. Most patients pass flatus about 48 hours postoperatively.

Early, frequent ambulation is the best way to prevent gastrointestinal discomfort. The intake of oral fluids and ingestion of a normal diet also help to stimulate peristalsis. Oral intake is usually withheld, however, until bowel sounds return (normally 24 to 48 hours after surgery).

Measures to promote the passage of flatus may be ordered, including early ambulation, insertion of a rectal tube for 20 minutes every 2 to 3 hours, application of heat to the abdomen, positioning the patient prone or on the right side, and insertion of bisacodyl suppositories.

If gastrointestinal function does not resume, the patient has a paralytic ileus, manifested by abdominal pain, distention, tenderness, and absence of bowel sounds. Other signs and symptoms of paralytic ileus are nausea, vomiting, and not passing flatus or feces.

Severe abdominal distention develops if normal bowel activity does not resume within a few days. In that case, a nasogastric tube may be ordered to permit decompression of the intestines. If the surgical procedure is one that often causes gastrointestinal problems, the nasogastric tube may be inserted during surgery to prevent problems.

The patient should have a bowel movement within a few days after resuming the intake of solid foods. Sometimes a suppository or an enema is necessary to stimulate emptying of the bowel.

Deficient Fluid Volume and Imbalanced Nutrition: Less Than Body Requirements

Depending on the type of surgery done, fluid and nutrition needs are met in a variety of ways. Some patients are given regular diets the evening of surgery. Others receive nothing by mouth for several days. Most patients return from the PACU with intravenous infusions. Patients are traditionally given clear liquids at first, then full liquids. If liquids are retained, the diet is advanced to include soft foods, then regular foods. Physiologically, there is no reason to delay the introduction of solids once gastrointestinal function has returned and a few oral liquids are retained, but this practice persists.

When the patient is able to tolerate liquids well, the intravenous infusion is usually discontinued unless it is needed for the administration of medication. Monitor the flow rate and the patient response. Nursing care of the patient receiving intravenous fluids is discussed in Chapter 17.

To promote healing, the patient's diet must provide adequate carbohydrates, protein, zinc, iron, folate, and vitamins C, B_6, and B_{12}. Alternative methods of feeding may be ordered if the patient is unable to resume oral intake for a long time. These methods are discussed in Chapter 36.

Fluid intake and output are usually measured for several days after surgery. In addition, laboratory studies of serum electrolytes are often ordered.

Nausea and vomiting interfere with the intake of food and fluids and can cause considerable fluid loss. Antiemetics (drugs used to control nausea and vomiting) are usually ordered as necessary. General nursing measures for the patient with nausea and vomiting are discussed in Chapter 36.

PHARMACOLOGY CAPSULE Antiemetic drugs control postoperative nausea and vomiting.

Impaired Physical Mobility

After general anesthesia and invasive surgical procedures, patients are usually weak and tire quickly. The physician prescribes measures to increase the patient's activity level–progressive ambulation in most cases. Assist the patient out of bed the first few times until it is evident the patient can safely get up alone. Help the patient sit on the bedside, press the feet on the floor, stand, and then walk increasingly greater distances. Monitor for weakness and dizziness associated with orthostatic hypotension. Emphasize the physical benefits of early ambulation to the patient.

Disturbed Body Image

The effects of surgery (scars, loss of body organs, altered physical functions) can be very traumatic. A sense of loss can be demonstrated by anger, depression, or even denial. The nurse should understand and accept these responses. Nursing care of the grieving patient is discussed in detail in Chapter 23. Surgery can also produce positive changes in body image when it improves appearance or function, or relieves symptoms.

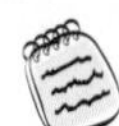

PATIENT TEACHING PLAN
Postoperative Patient

Patient teaching in the postoperative phase emphasizes recovery from the surgical experience and preparation for return to maximum possible function. Discharge planning should be started when the patient is admitted for surgery and revised as needed during the course of hospitalization. Topics to include in the discharge teaching plan are:

- Take your prescribed drugs as directed, but notify the physician if you have adverse effects (specify drug, dosage, schedule, and side and adverse effects).
- Wound care: You will need to continue your wound care as I have demonstrated. Notify your physician if you have symptoms of infection (fever, increasing redness, swelling, pain at the incision site).
- When regular activities can be resumed, do not lift anything heavier than specified by your physician.
- If you need assistance, available community services include—(specify services for patient needs).
- If the physician advises specific fluids and nutritional requirements, you need to follow this special diet, or take prescribed amounts of fluids.
- You will need some specialized equipment and supplies. (Tell the patient how to obtain and use assistive devices, special equipment, and supplies.)
- Can you identify any adaptations that will be needed in your home environment before you are discharged?
- It is important to keep medical appointments to be sure you are healing properly.

PHARMACOLOGY CAPSULE Discharge teaching includes information about drug therapy.

Put on your THINKING CAP!!

Observe the room of a recent postoperative patient and identify four ways the environment can be modified to promote safety.

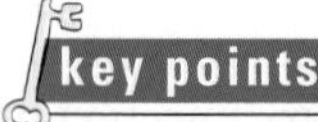

- Surgical procedures classified by purpose are diagnostic, exploratory, curative, palliative, and cosmetic.
- Variables that affect surgical outcomes are age, nutritional status, fluid and electrolyte balance, medical diagnoses, drugs, and habits such as use of tobacco and alcohol.
- The phases of the surgical experience are preoperative, intraoperative, and postoperative.
- Nursing measures to reduce patient anxiety and increase knowledge about the surgical experience may actually decrease complications.
- Preoperative teaching should include surgical preparation; what to expect in the surgical suite and postanesthesia care unit (PACU); what tubes, dressings, or equipment

may be in place after surgery; and how patient participation can promote recovery.

- Before surgery, the patient or legal guardian must sign a legal consent form. Consent from the patient must be obtained *before* premedications are given.
- Preparation for surgery may involve bowel cleansing, food and fluid restriction, skin scrubbing and shaving, securing and covering hair, and administering preoperative medications as ordered. Clothing, jewelry, nail polish, and prostheses are usually removed.
- After preoperative medications are given, the patient should remain in bed.
- The surgical team consists of nurses who circulate, nurses who scrub, one or more surgeons, an anesthesiologist or a nurse anesthetist, and other technical personnel.
- Anesthetic agents are used to induce unconsciousness, alter sensation, and prevent movement so that surgical procedures can be done painlessly and safely.
- The nursing diagnoses in the intraoperative phase may include Risk for Injury, Impaired Gas Exchange, Decreased Cardiac Output, and Risk for Deficient Fluid Volume.
- Postoperative surgical complications may include shock, hypoxia, wound infection, wound dehiscence and evisceration, injury, pneumonia, atelectasis, nausea and vomiting, impaired peristalsis, urinary retention, renal failure, and thrombophlebitis.
- Nursing diagnoses in the immediate postoperative period are Decreased Cardiac Output, Ineffective Breathing Patterns, Acute Pain, Disturbed Thought Processes, and Risk for Injury.
- Advise visitors on where to wait and how they will be informed of the patient's status.
- Nursing diagnoses after recovery from anesthesia may include Acute Pain, Impaired Tissue Integrity, Risk for Infection, Impaired Gas Exchange, Urinary Retention, Constipation, Risk for Deficient Fluid Volume , Imbalanced Nutrition, Impaired Physical Mobility, and Disturbed Body Image.
- Patient teaching for discharge emphasizes drug therapy, wound care, activity limitations, fluid and nutrition needs, equipment and supplies needed, adaptation of the home environment, and the importance of follow-up care.

REVIEW QUESTIONS

1. An elderly relative who is scheduled for a surgical procedure expresses fear that he is too old for surgery and asks what you think. Your response should be based on knowledge that:
   1. older adults are twice as likely to have surgical complications as younger people.
   2. an older adult in good health is likely to do just as well in surgery as a younger person.
   3. for most older adults, the risks of surgery are too great to justify any possible benefits.
   4. older adults who have chronic health problems are poor candidates for surgery.

2. If you obtain a patient's signature on a surgical consent form, your responsibility includes:
   1. explaining the surgical procedure to the patient.
   2. obtaining the signature before the patient is given sedatives.
   3. informing the patient of possible risks associated with the procedure.
   4. assessing the patient's understanding of the surgical procedure.

3. Why is it especially important to assess the affected extremities of a patient who is recovering from regional anesthesia?
   1. Regional anesthesia can impair blood flow to the extremities, causing gangrene.
   2. The patient cannot move the extremities despite feelings of pain or pressure.
   3. The extremities are susceptible to injury because movement returns before sensation.
   4. The effects of regional anesthesia may persist for several weeks.

4. One complication that is most likely to occur during the immediate postoperative period is:
   1. wound infection.
   2. pneumonia.
   3. shock.
   4. thrombophlebitis.

5. In a PACU, a patient's vital signs are as follows: 98° F, pulse 66 regular, respirations 14, BP 100/56. What other information do you need to evaluate these vital signs?
   1. Medications given during surgery
   2. Length of time under general anesthesia
   3. Whether the patient is having pain
   4. Patient's preoperative vital signs

6. A patient with an abdominal incision reports that his dressing is soaked with drainage and that he felt a pulling sensation when getting out of bed. On inspection, you find that the wound margins have separated. You should:
   1. lower the head of the bed and have the patient lie flat.
   2. gently reapply the surgical dressing and call the physician.
   3. administer a dose of prescribed opioid analgesic for pain.
   4. apply saline-soaked gauze and cover with a sterile dry dressing.

7. Following surgery, a patient voids 20 to 30 ml of urine at frequent intervals. You should suspect:
   1. urinary retention with overflow.
   2. damage to the bladder during surgery.
   3. fluid volume excess.
   4. kidney failure.

8. During report, you learn that your postoperative patient has a paralytic ileus. You would expect:
   1. the patient will not be able to walk.
   2. a nasogastric tube and suction may be in place.
   3. to monitor breath sounds every 2 hours.
   4. the patient will be limited to a liquid diet.

CHAPTER

17 Intravenous Therapy

objectives

1. List the indications for intravenous fluid therapy.
2. Describe the types of fluids used for intravenous fluid therapy.
3. Describe the types of venous access devices and other equipment used for intravenous therapy.
4. Given the prescribed hourly flow rate, calculate the correct drop rate for an intravenous fluid.
5. Explain the causes, signs and symptoms, and nursing implications of the complications of intravenous fluid or drug therapy.
6. Explain the nursing responsibilities when a patient is receiving intravenous therapy.

key terms

Cannula (KĂN-ū-lă, p. 238)
Embolism (ĔM-bō-lĭz-ŭm, p. 247)
Embolus (*pl.* Emboli) (ĔM-bō-lŭs, ĔM-bō-lī, p. 247)
Extravasation (ěks-trăv-ă-SĀ-shŭn, p. 246)
Hypertonic (hī-pěr-TŎN-ĭk, p. 237)
Hypotonic (hī-pō-TŎN-ĭk, p. 237)
Infiltration (ĭn-fĭl-TRĀ-shŭn, p. 246)
Isotonic (ī-sō-TŎN-ĭk, p. 237)
Phlebitis (flě-BĪ-tĭs, p. 246)
Solution (p. 237)
Thrombus (*pl.* Thrombi) (THRŎM-bŭs, THRŎM-bī, p. 247)
Tonicity (tō-NĬS-ĭ-tē, p. 237)

Intravenous therapy is the administration of fluids directly into a vein. Most hospitalized patients receive some form of intravenous therapy. Home infusion of intravenous products is becoming increasingly common.

INDICATIONS FOR INTRAVENOUS THERAPY

Intravenous therapy is used to administer drugs, fluids (including nutrients), and blood or blood components. Intravenous administration of drugs may be ordered when a rapid drug effect is needed, when the drug is not available in an oral form, or when the patient is unable to take drugs by mouth. The intravenous route is also recommended when a drug must be maintained at a certain level in the blood.

In addition to drugs, intravenous fluids can provide water, electrolytes, amino acids, lipids, vitamins, and glucose. Intravenous lines may also be used to provide continuous venous access for intermittent drug administration and emergency drug administration.

Whole blood and blood components are also given intravenously. Blood components include packed red blood cells, frozen red blood cells, platelets, and plasma proteins. Blood transfusions are discussed in Chapter 31.

TYPES OF INTRAVENOUS FLUIDS

By definition, a fluid is any liquid or gas. A **solution** is a liquid containing one or more dissolved substances. The terms *fluid* and *solution* are often used interchangeably in relation to intravenous therapy.

TONICITY

Fluids can be classified by **tonicity**, a measure of the concentration of electrolytes in the fluid. The normal concentration of electrolytes in body fluids is about 285 milliequivalents per liter (mEq/L). Solutions that have the same concentration as body fluids are called **isotonic.** When the concentration of a solution is greater than 300 mEq/L, the solution is said to be ***hypertonic. Hypotonic*** solutions have a concentration of less than 280 mEq/L. The tonicity of fluids is important because it affects blood volume. Fluid that is hypertonic draws and retains water in the circulation, increasing the blood volume. Hypotonic fluid allows water to shift out of the capillaries into body tissues, resulting in decreased blood volume.

COMPONENTS

Many types of fluids are available for intravenous use. The physician selects the appropriate fluid to meet the patient's needs. The most commonly used intravenous solutions are specific combinations of water, sugar (in the form of dextrose), sodium chloride, and other electrolytes.

In most intravenous solutions, dextrose is the only source of calories. The patient receives 34 calories for each 1% of dextrose in a liter of fluid; thus, 1 liter of 5% dextrose provides 170 calories ($34 \times 5 = 170$). Dextrose fluids given in a peripheral vein are 2.5%, 5.0%, or 10.0% dextrose. Fluids infused into a larger (central) vein may have a much higher percentage of dextrose.

Sodium chloride solutions also are commonly used. An isotonic solution is 0.9% sodium chloride and is called *normal saline.* It is used to supply balanced amounts of water and sodium chloride. A hypotonic solution of 0.45% sodium chloride may be ordered if the patient's body fluids are concentrated owing to excessive water loss. More concentrated hypertonic solutions are needed when the patient has had excessive losses of both sodium and chloride.

Dextrose, sodium chloride, and other electrolytes are available in numerous combinations. Some commonly used electrolyte solutions are Plasma-Lyte and lactated Ringer's solution. Dextrose 5% in Ringer's is a combined dextrose and electrolyte solution.

When a patient needs long-term or aggressive intravenous therapy for nutrition, total parenteral nutrition may be indicated. A catheter is placed in a large vein, usually the subclavian, for administering total parenteral nutrition fluids. These fluids provide dextrose, water, amino acids, electrolytes, vitamins, and minerals. Fat emulsions can also be given intravenously. Total parenteral nutrition is discussed in greater detail in Chapter 8.

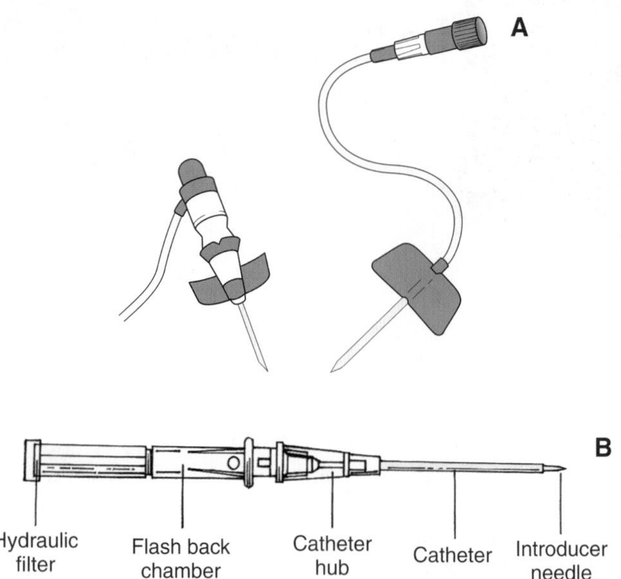

FIGURE **17-1** Venous access devices. *A,* Winged infusion needles. *B,* Catheter.

VENOUS ACCESS DEVICES

Intravenous fluid is delivered by various types of venous access devices (Fig. 17-1). These include needles, over-the-needle catheters, inside-needle catheters, subcutaneous infusion ports, and subcutaneously implanted pumps. The term *cannula* can be used to describe both a needle and a catheter. Cannula size is based on the inside diameter and is expressed as a *gauge.* The smaller the gauge, the larger is the inside diameter of the cannula. Therefore, a 14-gauge cannula is larger than a 22-gauge cannula.

The intravenous administration of fluids requires placement of the venous access device into a peripheral or central vein. Peripheral veins are those located in the extremities (and in the scalp of an infant). They are used for short-term therapy, when a patient has healthy veins, and when relatively nonirritating fluids are given. Figure 17-2 shows common peripheral infusion sites for intravenous fluids.

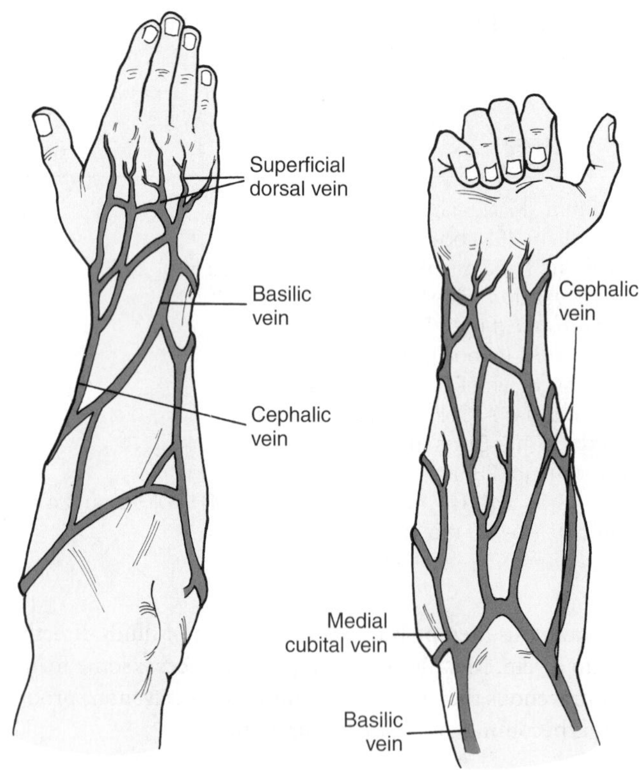

FIGURE **17-2** Common peripheral intravenous infusion sites.

Central veins, large vessels located nearer the heart, are used when long-term therapy is required, when the patient has poor peripheral veins, and when irritating fluids are to be administered. Central lines are inserted into the subclavian or jugular vein or into the superior vena cava. The line may be placed in the subclavian vein through a surgical incision, inserted into a peripheral vein and advanced to the desired location, or inserted through a skin incision and tunneled under the skin and into the large vessel. Devices placed through a cutdown incision are referred to as percutaneous catheters. The central line threaded through a peripheral vein is called a peripherally inserted central catheter (PICC). Examples of central venous tunneled catheters are the Hickman, Broviac, Groshong, Hickman-Broviac, Raaf, and the implanted venous access ports.

A port is a device with a central catheter that is surgically implanted in the subcutaneous tissue. It consists of a venous catheter and a port through which fluids can be injected, but it has no external parts (Fig. 17-1B).The catheter is inserted into a central vein, and the port, which has a rubber septum, can be felt under the skin. A specialized needle that does not damage the septum is used to puncture the skin and deliver fluid and medications through the port and into the catheter (Fig. 17-3). A port requires less care and is less restrictive than other access devices, but does require a needle puncture for each infusion.

A

Subclavian vein
Collar bone
Silicone catheter
Superior vena cava
Port
Right atrium

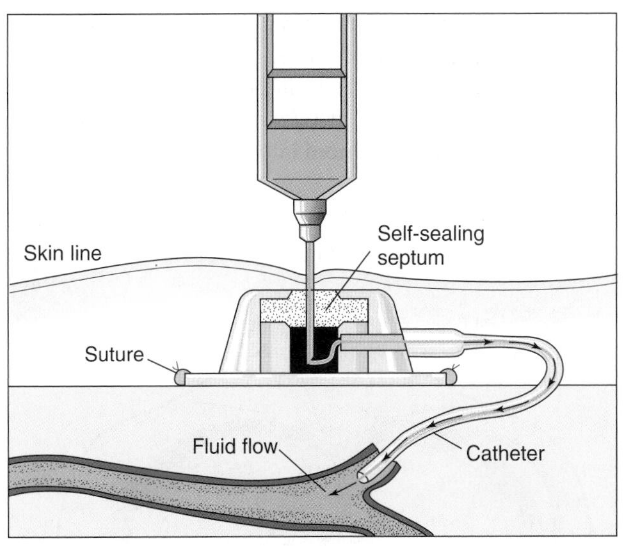

FIGURE **17-3** *A,* An implantable port in place. The entire unit is under the skin. *B,* Injection of medication into the port.

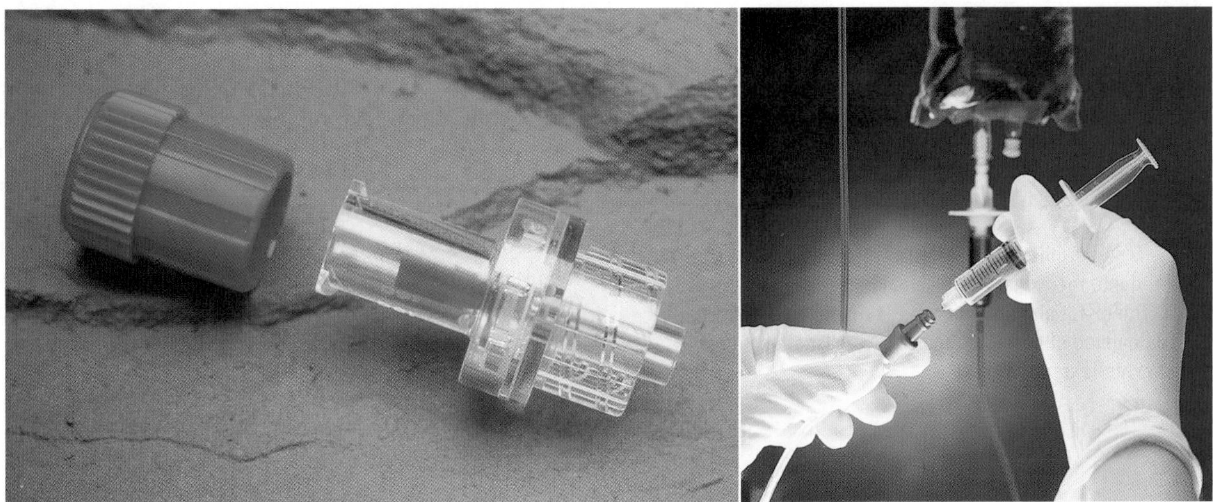

FIGURE **17-4** Needleless system.

For therapy over a period of days to weeks, the percutaneous catheter or midline catheter is preferred. Tunneled catheters and implanted ports are more appropriate for long-term use.

NEEDLES

One type of needle used is a winged ("butterfly") infusion needle, a short needle with two plastic wings that are held during insertion. A winged infusion needle is useful in infants when a scalp vein is used for intravenous therapy. It is also used at times in adults who have very poor or small veins, for one-time therapy, to draw blood samples, and for therapy of short duration (less than 24 hours).

To reduce the risk of blood-borne injuries acquired through needlesticks, various devices have been developed. One style has a self-sheathing stylet that retracts into a rigid chamber at the catheter hub after insertion. Others use Luer-Lok connections rather than diaphragms that must be punctured with a needle (Fig. 17-4).

CATHETERS

A catheter is a small plastic tube that fits over or inside a needle. After insertion into the vein, the needle is withdrawn, leaving the catheter in the vein. The tubing that will deliver the fluid is then connected to the plastic catheter, which remains in the vein. Catheters are less likely than needles to puncture the vein once they are in place. They come in a variety of lengths. Short catheters are only ¾ to 2 inches in length. Midlength catheters are designed for therapy of 2 to 4 weeks. Midlength catheters are inserted near the antecubital region of the arm and advanced 3 to 10 inches. Nurses generally insert only short (¾ to 2 inch) catheters unless they receive special training.

A central catheter that can be inserted by trained nurses is the PICC (Fig. 17-5). The PICC is inserted into a vein in the antecubital space and advanced into the axillary, subclavian, or brachiocephalic vein or the superior vena cava. Advantages of the PICC over other central catheters include easier insertion, cost savings, and less risk of pneumothorax, hemothorax, infection, or air embolism. Compared with peripheral cannulas, PICCs can be left in place longer, do not restrict arm movement, and are less traumatic to the vein.

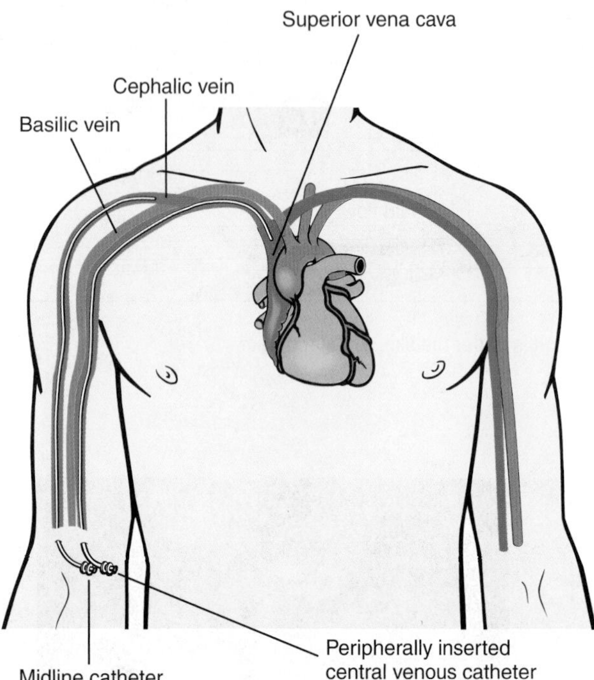

FIGURE **17-5** A peripherally inserted central catheter. The catheter is inserted into the axillary vein, subclavian vein, or superior vena cava. The exact placement depends on the type of fluid to be infused. The midline catheter extends only 3-10 inches into a larger vessel of the upper arm.

Tunneled catheters are inserted only by the physician. An incision is made at the entrance site, a tunnel created in the subcutaneous tissues, and the catheter threaded through the tunnel and into the subclavian vein. Scar formation of a small section of the tunneled catheter holds it in place after a week or two. However, some surgeons leave sutures in place as long as they do not create inflammation. Some special catheters may be inserted at the patient's bedside, whereas others require a surgical procedure. Placement of any central catheter must be confirmed by radiograph before use.

Subclavian catheters can have from one to four lumens. Figure 17-6 depicts a triple-lumen catheter, which is essentially one catheter with three separate channels or tubes. Each catheter has a port through which blood can be drawn. One port can be used to measure central venous pressure. The other ports can be used to give drugs, fluids, or blood.

IMPLANTED DEVICES

Some devices can be implanted to allow immediate access to a vein without repeated, painful venipunctures. They include infusion ports, described earlier, pumps that are implanted under the skin, and external infusion pumps. Infusion ports consist of a catheter and a chamber into which fluids can be injected directly into a vein or an artery. They are also used for intraspinal infusions. The chamber is easily felt directly under the skin. Infusion pumps are filled using a special needle that is inserted through the skin into the port. They dispense the fluid into the vein at a very slow rate. The rate of in-

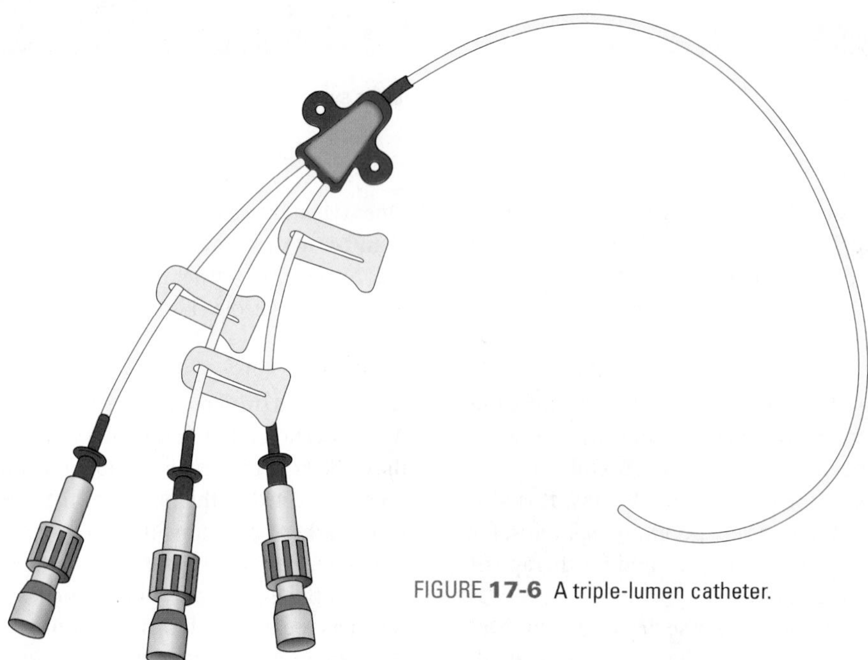

FIGURE **17-6** A triple-lumen catheter.

fusion is sometimes affected by body temperature, with fever increasing the delivery rate. The infusion rate of some infusion pumps can be set electronically by passing a wand over the pump. Infusion pumps are often used to administer chemotherapy drugs for cancer.

INTERMITTENT INFUSION DEVICES

Many patients need intravenous medications at specific intervals, such as every 4 or every 6 hours. Such drugs are often "piggybacked," that is, the drug is given through an injection port in the tubing of a continuous infusion. An option for the patient who does not need continuous intravenous therapy is a latex resealable lock, sometimes called a heparin lock.

PHARMACOLOGY CAPSULE A drug given "piggyback" is administered through the tubing of a continuous infusion using the injection port that is closest to the fluid bag. The injection port closer to the patient is used for IV push medications. If the patient does not need continuous fluids, a resealable latex lock can be used to give the medication.

A resealable lock is a short cannula with an attached injection port. It is taped in place, and medications are injected when needed through the port. It may be called a heparin lock because it may be flushed with a dilute heparin solution after each use to keep clots from forming and blocking the catheter. Although research suggests that flushing with normal saline may be just as effective as, and less expensive than, using heparin, the use of heparin persists in some settings. One concern about the use of heparin is that it prolongs the time required for blood to clot, whereas saline does not. You must know the agency's procedure for flushing these devices and exactly what the licensed practical nurse is permitted to do. Any intravenous cannula (needle or catheter) can be converted to intermittent administration by attaching a resealable cap or an extension with a cap.

INITIATION OF INTRAVENOUS THERAPY

Nurse practice acts and agency policies determine which nurses can perform venipunctures, administer intravenous fluids, and give intravenous medications by various routes.

EQUIPMENT

To start intravenous fluids, gather the equipment needed to start the infusion: cannula (needle or catheter), tourniquet, alcohol swabs, skin cleansing solution, tape, dressing supplies, gloves, tubing, solution container, a pole to suspend the container, and possibly an infusion pump. The size of the cannula depends on the patient's condition and the type of fluid to be administered. For patients with multiple trauma or those facing transplantation or heart surgery, a 14- or 16-gauge cannula is appropriate. Other surgical patients and those receiving blood require an 18- or 20-gauge cannula. Smaller-gauge cannulas can be used in children, in adults with small veins, and for administration of most other nonirritating fluids. Read the product literature to identify any special requirements such as a filter or special tubing. Obtain the prescribed solution or drug using the "five rights": right solution or drug, right dose or strength, right patient, right route, and right time. Attach tubing to the solution container, fill the drip chamber halfway, and allow some fluid to run through the tubing until the tubing is completely filled with fluid and there are no air bubbles in the tubing.

PHARMACOLOGY CAPSULE The intravenous administration of nitroglycerin, blood, or fat emulsions requires special administration sets.

SITE SELECTION

Select the venipuncture site for the infusion. The site chosen should be the least restrictive (i.e., not over a joint or on the hand). It should have a large vein that is in good condition. A soft, straight vein is best. Avoid veins that are hard and bumpy, bruised, swollen, near previously infected areas, or close to a recently discontinued site. A device called a Vein Light may facilitate locating a vein. The preferred site is usually the patient's nondominant arm. Begin with the most distal veins, and then move proximally as needed. Venipuncture should not be done in an arm that has impaired circulation or poor lymphatic drainage, as in a patient who has had a radical mastectomy. Also, do not use an arm that has been affected by a stroke. Although veins on the legs are accessible, they are not normally used in adults.

Put on your THINKING CAP!!

Why should you use the most distal site to start an intravenous infusion?

PROCEDURE

Wash your hands thoroughly, and explain the procedure to the patient. Apply a tourniquet above the venipuncture site to distend the vein. The tourniquet should be flat, at least one-half inch wide, should not obstruct arterial blood flow, and should be used on only one patient. Vigorously cleanse the venipuncture site in a circular pattern first with alcohol and then with a recommended solution. Recommended cleansing solutions include 1% to 2% tincture of iodine, iodophor (povidone-iodine), 70% isopropyl alcohol, and chlorhexidine. Allow the site to air dry after each cleansing step. Do not blow on the site or fan it.

Perform the venipuncture using standard precautions. Carefully insert the cannula through the skin and guide it into the vein in the direction of blood flow. If the first attempt is unsuccessful, select another site, change cannulas, and try again. After two unsuccessful attempts, call a more experienced nurse to start the infusion. When using the most common cannula, the catheter over needle, the needle is threaded only ¼ inch into the vein. Then the catheter is threaded into the vein as the needle is removed. This technique reduces the risk of trauma to the vein. After threading the cannula into the vein, tape it securely but without restricting circulation. Do not apply tape to the site where the cannula enters the skin.

In accordance with your agency procedures, dress the site with a sterile gauze pad or with a clear occlusive dressing that allows inspection of the insertion site. On peripheral sites, gauze dressings are changed every 48 hours and occlusive dressings every 3 to7 days. Dressings on central lines are changed every 48 hours. Some agencies may use antimicrobial barrier patches that fit around the cannula and under the dressing. The application of antibiotic ointment to the insertion site is controversial. Antibiotic ointments without antifungals have been associated with *Candida* infections.

Put on your THINKING CAP!!

What's wrong with this picture? A nurse preparing to start an IV tears strips of tape and sticks them on the edge of the overbed table. The nurse cleanses the site with alcohol and iodophor and blows on the site to hasten drying.

Pain

Venipuncture and cannula placement are painful. Clinicians are seeking measures to reduce the discomfort without making the procedure more difficult. Drugs that have been used to decrease the pain of venipuncture include intradermal lidocaine (Xylocaine), transdermal lidocaine, and prilocaine (EMLA cream). There are some disadvantages to each of these. Intradermal lidocaine may cause vasospasm, allergic reactions, and anaphylaxis. Both lidocaine and EMLA cream must be applied and covered with an occlusive dressing for 60 minutes to be effective. Another option is iontophoresis of lidocaine, a noninvasive system that uses an electrical current to deliver lidocaine to the skin and takes effect in about 10 minutes. Again, there is a risk of reaction to the lidocaine. Intradermal injection of normal saline alongside the vein also produces anesthesia. The Intravenous Nurses Society does not recommend lidocaine or normal saline for this purpose.

DOCUMENTATION

Place a piece of tape on the site dressing with the date and time that the cannula was inserted as well as the length and gauge of the cannula and your initials. Label every bag of fluid and tubing with the date and time that it was hung and the fluid's expiration date.

MAINTENANCE OF INTRAVENOUS THERAPY

The physician orders the type of fluid and the rate at which it is to be given. The nurse is responsible for maintaining the correct rate of flow and for monitoring the patient's response to the infusion. Intravenous fluids can be allowed to flow by gravity or can be regulated by an electronic infusion control device. When gravity flow is used, the rate must be adjusted with the roller clamp or screw clamp on the tubing. The clamp should be positioned on the upper third of the tubing. The slide clamp should *not* be used to set the rate; it is not reliable!

Check the infusion rate hourly even if an infusion control device is used. If the fluid is running too slowly, adjust the flow rate. Do not attempt to "catch up" by administering extra fluid rapidly. If the fluid is running too quickly, slow the rate and assess the patient for signs of fluid volume excess.

If the patient is ambulatory, attach the fluid container to a pole with wheels. Tell the patient to protect the infusion by keeping the solution container above the infusion site and to avoid pulling on the tubing or applying pressure to the infusion site.

FACTORS AFFECTING INFUSION RATE

Even after the infusion rate is set, many factors can alter that rate. The main determinants of the infusion rate are the following:

- The height of the fluid container over the patient's heart. When the container is raised, the fluid flows faster. Lowering the container causes the fluid to run more slowly. The optimal height is 30-36 inches above the patient.
- The volume of fluid in the container. A full container causes the fluid to run faster. As the container empties, the rate slows down.
- Viscosity of the fluid. Thin fluids such as normal saline flow more quickly than thick fluids such as blood.
- Cannula diameter. Fluid flows more quickly through a large cannula than through a small cannula.
- Venting of the fluid container. Soft plastic bags collapse as they empty, but glass containers and rigid plastic containers cannot do that. Therefore, rigid containers must be vented to allow air to enter as fluid leaves. Without proper venting, the fluid does not flow.
- Position of the extremity. With peripheral lines, certain movements or positions may interfere with the flow of fluid. If that happens, the extremity may need to be splinted with an arm board to limit movement, or the patient may be advised to avoid certain movements or positions.

CALCULATING THE INFUSION RATE

You should know how to calculate infusion rates even if infusion control devices are used routinely. To calculate the infusion rate, first determine (1) how much fluid to give each hour and (2) how many drops equal 1 ml in the delivery set used (called the drop factor).

The physician's order specifies the amount of fluid to be administered in a specific period of time. The instructions on the delivery set package state how many drops equal 1 ml using that set. Standard delivery sets (sometimes called macrodrop sets) deliver 10, 12, 15, or 20 drops per milliliter. Microdrop sets deliver 50 or 60 drops per milliliter. They are used in children and when small volumes of fluid are being given.

Once the infusion rate per minute is known, use the roller clamp or screw clamp on a gravity infusion to adjust the flow rate until the correct number of drops per minute is infusing. Recheck the rate hourly. Common practice is to put a timed tape on the fluid container that shows where the fluid level should be each hour. This allows a quick assessment of whether the fluid is running on schedule.

Put on your THINKING CAP!!

A patient is to receive an antibiotic intravenously in 100 ml of IV fluid. Directions are to administer the drug over 30 to 60 minutes. Drop factor: 10 drops/ml. Calculate the minimum and maximum allowable flow rates.

INFUSION CONTROL DEVICES

Electronic infusion control devices maintain an infusion rate set by the nurse. The most commonly used types also have alarms that sound when the fluid bag is empty, when there is air in the line, or when there is resistance to infusion. A variety of infusion control devices are available (Fig. 17-7). Ambulatory pumps are available that allow the patient to

Example

PHYSICIAN'S ORDER: 1,000 ml 5% dextrose in 0.45% normal saline every 8 hours. Delivery set: 20 drops = 1 ml.

Step 1 Calculate how many milliliters should be given in 1 hour. Divide the total number of milliliters to be given by the prescribed number of hours.

1,000 ml ÷ 8 hr = 125 ml/hr

Step 2 Calculate how many drops should be given in 1 hour. Multiply the number of milliliters to be given each hour times the number of drops in 1 ml using the specific delivery set.

125 ml × 20 = 2,500 drops/hr

Step 3 Calculate how many drops should be given in 1 minute. Divide the number of drops per hour by 60 to find out how many drops should be given in 1 minute.

2,500 drops ÷ 60 min = 41.6, or 42 drops/min

Some people prefer to use a formula to calculate the drop rate. The formula is:

(Fluid volume to be infused) × (Number of drops per ml with selected infusion set) ÷ Time (min) = drops per minute.

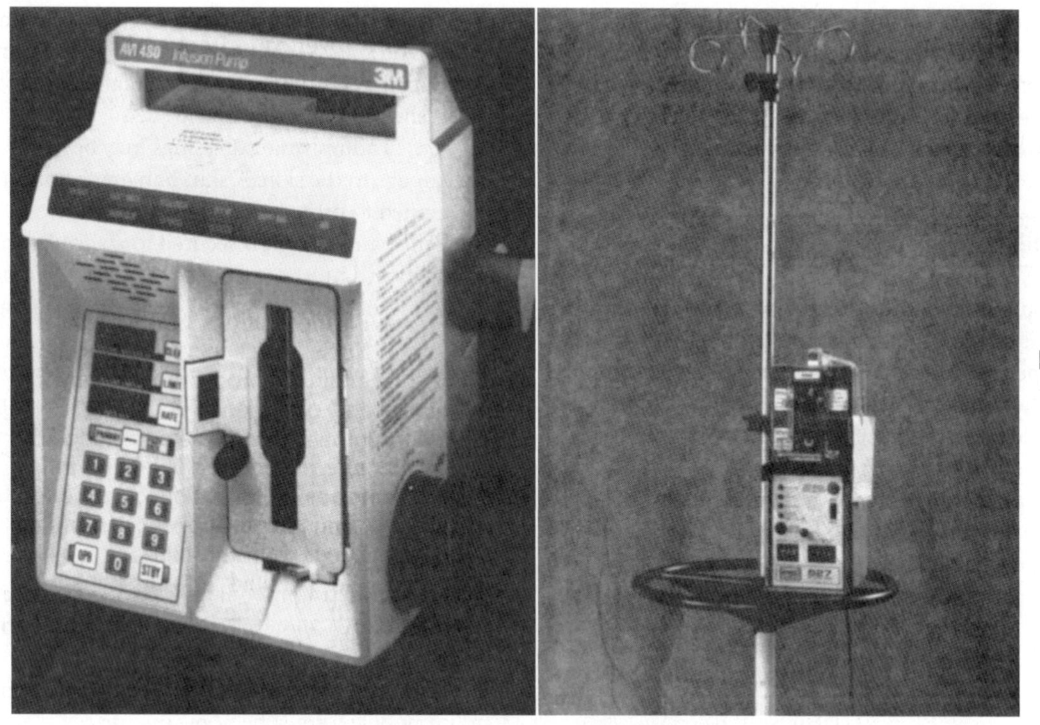

FIGURE **17-7** Electronic infusion pumps. *A,* The AVI 480 infusion pump. *B,* The IMED 927 infusion pump attached to an intravenous line pole.

resume normal activities. You must become familiar with the type used in your work setting. Infusion control devices save time and should prevent accidental delivery of large amounts of fluid. They do not excuse you, however, from monitoring the flow rate at intervals and assessing the catheter or needle insertion site.

INTRAVENOUS INFUSION OF MEDICATIONS

Agency policies usually dictate what medications the nurse may give by piggyback or by direct injection through a cannula into the vein (intravenous push). Many states do not permit licensed practical nurses to give medications by intravenous push. When giving such medications, you must know how to dilute the medication and the correct rate of infusion. Improper administration of intravenous medications can be extremely dangerous. You also must be aware that some medications and intravenous solutions are incompatible, that is, they cannot be given together.

CHANGING VENOUS ACCESS DEVICES AND ADMINISTRATION SETS

Short peripheral cannulas and the tubing are usually changed every 48 to 72 hours in accordance with standards of the Intravenous Nurses Society. If complications occur with 72-hour intervals, the interval should be limited to 48 hours.

Administration sets for continuous peripheral and central infusions are usually changed every 72 hours. PICC lines should be changed every 6 weeks. Tunneled catheters and ports can be left in place for years. Tubing that is used to administer blood, total parenteral nutrition, or lipids must be changed every 24 hours. An intravenous fluid container should not be used for more than 24 hours. Agency policies are generally quite specific about the schedule.

TERMINATION OF INTRAVENOUS THERAPY

To discontinue intravenous therapy with needles or short catheters, put on gloves, stop the flow of fluid, loosen or remove the tape and dressing, and gently remove the cannula. Dispose of the needle or catheter according to standard precautions guidelines. Apply pressure to the puncture site with a sterile gauze pad for 1 or 2 minutes to prevent bleeding. Once bleeding has stopped, apply a sterile dry dressing to the puncture site. Record the appearance of the site, the condition of the catheter, and how the patient tolerated the procedure. Removal of midlength and long catheters requires special training.

PRECAUTIONS

When performing a venipuncture or handling used needles or catheters, always be aware of the risk of exposure to blood-borne pathogens. The most serious pathogens that can be transmitted by this route are the human immunodeficiency virus and hepatitis B virus.

A number of products for venipuncture and intravenous therapy that reduce the risk of needle punctures or other exposure to blood are available. Every nurse should be familiar with the agency needle puncture and body fluid exposure guidelines. In the event of an accidental needlestick, most policies require blood specimens to be drawn from the nurse and the patient to test for blood-borne infections. Drug therapy may be advised if the patient has an infectious disease. Documentation of the incident and the health status of the nurse at the time of the exposure may be very important if the nurse becomes ill as a result of the exposure.

COMPLICATIONS OF INTRAVENOUS THERAPY

Intravenous therapy is so widely used that it is easy to take its safety for granted. Several potential complications of intravenous therapy can be very serious, however. Complications include tissue trauma, infiltration, inflammation, infection, fluid volume excess, bleeding, and embolism. Each of these is discussed in detail under Nursing Care During Intravenous Therapy.

THE OLDER PATIENT AND INTRAVENOUS THERAPY

The elderly patient requires special consideration during intravenous therapy. Key points include:

- When performing the venipuncture, you may be able to distend the vessel by simply pressing the vein. If a tourniquet is needed, protect fragile skin by wrapping a washcloth under the tourniquet.
- Special adhesives or dressings may be needed to prevent damage to the skin. A skin polymer solution can be applied to protect the skin from adhesives.
- If the hand or arm is secured to an armboard, the armboard must be padded; pre-back the tape with gauze or another strip of tape to avoid direct contact of the adhesive with the skin.
- Because older people have less subcutaneous tissue, infiltrated fluid may drain away from the cannula insertion site. For example, if the hand is elevated, fluid may collect in the elbow area.
- If the patient is confused or restless, protect the infusion site and tubing with a commercial securement device or conceal the site under long sleeves.
- If a soft wrist immobilizer is justified, secure the immobilizer to the armboard, then secure the arm with the infusion to the armboard.
- Never apply an immobilizer *over* an infusion site; the immobilizer must be *below* the site.
- Confusion during acute illness is common. Reassure the confused patient, use a calm and gentle approach, and frequently reinforce instructions.

- With dementia patients, distraction may take their attention away from the IV. Keeping the infusion equipment out of sight may reduce attempts to handle it.
- Monitoring for fluid volume excess is especially important, as older people often have less efficient cardiac and renal function.

NURSING CARE *during Intravenous Therapy*

Assessment

When a patient is receiving intravenous therapy, frequent assessment is needed to ensure that the correct fluid is infusing at the correct rate and that the patient is not suffering any complications from this therapy (see Nursing Care Plan: The Patient Receiving Intravenous Therapy).

NURSING CARE PLAN

The Patient Receiving Intravenous Therapy

ASSESSMENT

Health History: Gary Edwin, age 67, was admitted for nausea and vomiting of 3 days' duration. He reported fluid intake of only water and cola for the previous 2 days and complained of dizziness and fatigue. Intravenous fluids were begun at 150 ml/hr via a 21-gauge cannula.

Physical Examination: Lethargic but oriented. Vital signs: blood pressure, 96/58; pulse, 102; respirations, 22; temperature, 101.6° F orally. Mucous membranes dry and sticky. Urine dark yellow. Intravenous infusion site: no swelling or redness.

Nursing Diagnosis	*Goals and Outcome Criteria*	*Interventions*
Risk for injury related to the trauma, infiltration.	The patient will experience minimal trauma, as evidenced by absence of bruising, bleeding, swelling.	Use gentle technique to start the infusion. Inspect the infusion site for swelling and bleeding. Palpate for warmth or coolness. Anchor the tubing securely. Exercise caution to prevent movement of the cannula. Stop the infusion if there are signs of infiltration (swelling near infusion site, pain, slow infusion rate), and restart it.
Risk for infection related to disruption of skin integrity, presence of cannula in vein.	The patient will remain free of infection at infusion site, as evidenced by absence of redness, swelling, edema, or drainage.	Use strict aseptic technique when starting the infusion and handling the site. Assess for signs of inflammation and infection: redness, swelling, warmth, purulent drainage, fever. Report signs to physician. Administer antibiotics and apply warm compress to inflamed site as ordered.
Fluid volume excess related to rapid fluid infusion.	The patient's fluid status will be normal, as evidenced by normal vital signs and fluid intake approximately equal to output.	Monitor rate of fluid infusion and maintain correct rate of flow. Measure all fluid intake and output. Assess for signs and symptoms of fluid volume excess (hypervolemia): increasing blood pressure, bounding pulse, dyspnea. If patient is hypervolemic, slow infusion rate, elevate patient's head, and notify physician.
Decreased cardiac output related to blood loss.	The patient will have no bleeding at infusion or tubing connections	Check connections to be sure they are secure. Tape tubing to prevent accidental disconnection.
Altered tissue perfusion related to obstruction of blood flow by embolus.	The patient will maintain normal circulation, as evidenced by usual skin color and absence of respiratory distress.	Do not irrigate obstructed cannula. Aspirate gently or administer thrombolytic if permitted per agency protocol. Assess and report any signs of respiratory distress.
Self-care deficit (feeding, dressing, hygiene, toileting) related to restricted movement of infusion site and connection to fluid delivery system	The patient will accomplish self-care activities without disruption of intravenous therapy.	Provide assistance with meals, hygiene, dressing, and toileting as needed. Provide gown that unfastens at the shoulder. Assure the patient that he can move with the infusion.
Deficient knowledge of management of intravenous therapy	The patient will demonstrate ability to protect and manage the infusion.	Tell the patient the purpose of the infusion and what symptoms should be reported: pain, bleeding, swelling. Assure the patient that movement is possible with the infusion as long as it is protected and the tubing is not disconnected.

Check the physician's order to be sure the correct intravenous solution is infusing. Determine the prescribed rate of flow, and assess the actual flow rate. Inspect the infusion site for edema, pallor or redness, bleeding, and drainage. Palpate the infusion site for edema and warmth or coolness. Ask the patient if the infusion site is painful.

Many people believe that the infusion is not infiltrating if blood flows into the tubing when the fluid container is lowered. This is not an accurate sign, as blood may return even when fluid is escaping into the tissue. Interestingly, the lack of blood return does not necessarily mean the needle is out of the vein either. Therefore, this time-honored test for needle placement is not reliable. Inspection and palpation of the infusion site remain the best means of evaluating for infiltration.

Take the patient's vital signs and compare the readings with previous findings to detect increased pulse and blood pressure. Measure and record the fluid intake and output, and auscultate the patient's lungs for crackles.

Nursing Diagnoses, Goals, and Outcome Criteria

When a patient is receiving intravenous therapy, nursing diagnoses address the risk for complications, the need for assistance with activities of daily living, and the need for patient teaching. Specific nursing diagnoses and related goals are the following:

Nursing Diagnoses	Goals and Outcome Criteria
Risk for Injury related to trauma, infiltration, inflammation	Absence of trauma, inflammation, infiltration: no bruising, bleeding, edema, pallor, redness, or drainage at infusion site
Risk for Infection related to disruption of skin integrity or presence of a cannula in a vein	Absence of infection: normal body temperature, no purulent drainage or redness at venipuncture site
Fluid Volume Excess related to rapid fluid infusion	Normal fluid volume: fluid output equal to intake, no dyspnea or edema
Decreased Cardiac Output related to blood loss through disrupted intravenous line	Normal cardiac output: pulse and blood pressure within normal limits, skin warm and dry, tubing connection intact
Altered Tissue Perfusion related to obstruction of blood flow by an embolus	Unobstructed blood flow: normal skin color and warmth in extremities
Self-Care Deficit (feeding, grooming, hygiene, dressing, toileting) related to restricted movement of infusion site and connection to fluid delivery system	Patient's performance of self-care activities: activities completed without disruption of intravenous therapy

Interventions

Risk for Injury

Trauma. The insertion of a cannula is traumatic to the skin and underlying tissues. Tape may irritate or tear the skin. Use gentle technique when performing the venipuncture, and anchor the cannula to reduce tissue trauma. Apply a commercial site protector, if available, to shield the intravenous site.

Infiltration. Infiltration is the collection of infused fluid in tissue surrounding the cannula. The term *extravasation* is often used interchangeably with *infiltration,* but extravasation specifically refers to leakage of fluid from a blood vessel. Infiltration can be caused by leakage at the point where the cannula enters the vein or by puncture of a second site in the vein by the cannula. Drugs that are especially toxic to subcutaneous tissues are called *vesicants.* Common vesicants are vasopressors, potassium chloride, and antineoplastic agents.

Frequently assess for signs and symptoms of infiltration. When the infusion is infiltrated, the patient may report pain or a burning sensation in the area. On inspection, the site may be pale and puffy. If a lot of fluid is in the tissue, it may feel hard and cool. When there is evidence of infiltration, stop the infusion and restart it in a different vein; otherwise the patient may not be receiving the drug or fluid as intended. Tissue that is edematous with infiltrated fluid is fragile, so handle it gently. Elevate the affected arm on a pillow to promote reabsorption of excess fluid.

Because many medications harm subcutaneous tissue, the physician should be notified if solutions containing toxic drugs infiltrate. When administering vesicants, it is especially important to select a large, soft vein. Use the smallest appropriate cannula, ensure cannula placement before giving the vesicant, and flush the cannula after the vesicant is given.

Put on your THINKING CAP!!

A patient complains of pain at an IV insertion site. The site feels cool and is slightly swollen. When the IV fluid container is lowered, blood flows back into the tubing. Do you think the infusion is infiltrated? What should you do?

Risk for Infection

Inflammation of the vein is called *phlebitis.* With intravenous fluid therapy, phlebitis may be due to irritation by the cannula or by medications. Redness, swelling, warmth, and tenderness near the insertion site suggest phlebitis. In addition, an infected site may have purulent drainage, and the patient might have a fever. The inflammation may be mild or severe and carries the possibility of the formation of blood clots in the vein (thrombophlebitis).

Infection of a venipuncture site can be caused by contamination of the site itself, by the intravenous fluid, or by the tubing used to deliver the fluid. The infected site is red and warm and may have purulent drainage.

To reduce the risk of inflammation and infection, use strict aseptic technique when starting and handling intravenous infusions. Agency policy describes specific site care, including the frequency of dressing changes.

If the infusion site appears to be inflamed or infected, stop the infusion and restart it in another site. If agency policy permits, a warm compress can be applied to the inflamed site. If there is evidence of infection, notify the physician. Antibiotic therapy may be ordered.

PHARMACOLOGY CAPSULE Drugs that are toxic to body tissues are called vesicants. They can cause phlebitis or tissue necrosis.

Fluid Volume Excess

The patient's blood volume may increase excessively when fluid is delivered directly into the bloodstream. This is most likely to happen when large volumes of fluid are infused, especially in patients who have impaired renal or cardiac function.

Signs and symptoms of fluid volume excess include rising blood pressure, bounding pulse, and edema. Severe fluid volume excess produces congestive heart failure and pulmonary edema (discussed in Chapter 33).

The risk of fluid volume excess is reduced by controlling the rate of fluid infusion. If the infusion falls behind schedule, correct the rate as noted previously, but do not increase it to make up for the slow infusion. Normally, fluid intake and output are approximately equal. When the heart or kidneys are unable to handle excess blood volume, heart failure may develop. Young children and elderly adults must be monitored closely for fluid volume excess because they do not adapt to fluid changes as readily as a young adult. If indications of fluid volume excess (increasing blood pressure, bounding pulse, dyspnea) appear, slow the infusion rate, elevate the patient's head, and notify the physician.

PHARMACOLOGY CAPSULE Rapid intravenous administration of drugs or fluids may cause fluid volume excess, leading to heart failure.

Decreased Cardiac Output

Bleeding may occur if the cannula is moved excessively after insertion. Even more serious bleeding is possible if the tubing becomes disconnected from the cannula, allowing blood to flow freely from the vein.

To prevent bleeding, make sure all connections in the infusion set are secure. Tape tubing so that it is not pulled loose easily. Protect the infusion site and tubing when the patient moves. If a large amount of blood is lost, take the patient's vital signs and notify the physician. Institute emergency measures if the patient is in shock.

Altered Tissue Perfusion

An **embolus** (*pl.* **emboli**) is an unattached blood clot or other substance in the circulatory system. An embolus can have serious, even life-threatening effects if it lodges and obstructs blood flow in a critical blood vessel. The obstruction created by a trapped embolus is called an ***embolism.***

With intravenous therapy, there are risks of emboli from blood clots, air, and broken catheters. A blood clot or **thrombus** (*pl.* **thrombi**) can develop in intravenous needles or catheters. Air can enter the bloodstream if the infusion system is opened. As little as 10 cc of air can cause serious complications. The risk of air embolism with peripheral lines has been greatly reduced by the use of plastic rather than glass fluid containers. The danger is greatest with central venous lines such as the subclavian, Hickman-Broviac, and triple-lumen catheters. If a port is disconnected, air may be drawn into the bloodstream. The patient experiences shortness of breath, hypotension, and possibly shock and cardiac arrest.

A rare occurrence is a catheter embolus. This occurs when a piece of the catheter breaks off in the vein. Broken catheters may be due to defects in the catheter, reintroduction of the needle into the catheter, accidental cutting with scissors, and pulling catheters through needles.

Chest discomfort may be due to a catheter embolism and should be reported to the physician immediately. If a catheter breaks in a peripheral vein, keep the patient quiet with the head elevated. Notify the physician. A radiograph will be ordered to locate the broken catheter, usually in the right ventricle or pulmonary artery. The fragment may be removed with a snare that is passed through the femoral vein.

When the cannula seems to be obstructed, blood clots may have formed in it. Irrigation of the cannula is not recommended, as it may force clots into the bloodstream. Depending on agency policy, gentle aspiration may be attempted to remove the obstruction. Alteplase (tPA) may be ordered to dissolve clots that are obstructing the cannula.

Exercise extra caution to prevent an air embolism when a patient has a central line. The infusion set must remain closed. When hanging new bags of fluid, clamp the catheter port to prevent air entering the bloodstream. When a central catheter is inserted or removed, instruct the patient to take a deep breath and bear down. This helps prevent air entering the bloodstream. If air accidentally enters the line, close the leak immediately. Turn the patient on the left side with the head lowered. This position traps the air in the right atrium, where it can be absorbed gradually. Air in the bloodstream is an emergency situation in which cardiac arrest is possible, so close monitoring is vital. Immediately notify the physician, and keep the emergency supply cart close at hand. One hundred percent oxygen with a nonrebreather mask may be ordered.

Self-Care Deficit

Provide assistance as needed with eating, dressing, toileting, and hygiene. Dressing may be easier if the patient is provided with a gown or shirt that unfastens at the shoulder. These garments are simpler to remove than garments that must be removed over the arm. Some patients are fearful of moving with an intravenous infusion. Explain what restrictions, if any, are needed to protect the infusion. If a commercial intravenous shield is available, consider using one to reduce the risk of trauma at the insertion site.

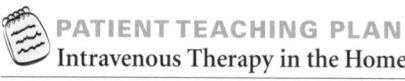

PATIENT TEACHING PLAN
Intravenous Therapy in the Home

When intravenous therapy is ordered outside the acute care setting, explain what will be done and why. Teaching should begin well before discharge so that the patient's ability to do the care can be assessed. With long-term therapy, it is

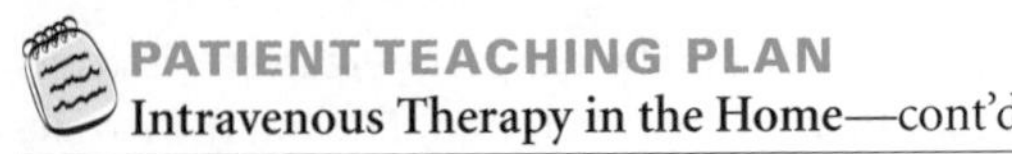

PATIENT TEACHING PLAN
Intravenous Therapy in the Home—cont'd

especially important to teach the patient (and family, if appropriate) the following:

- Infusion site care
- Proper administration of fluids or drugs
- Signs that should be reported to the physician or home health nurse
- How to flush infusion ports if appropriate
- Care of central lines or implanted infusion ports

Details depend on the situation.

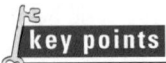

key points

- Intravenous therapy is used to administer drugs, fluids including nutrients, and blood or blood products.
- The terms *fluid* and *solution* are used interchangeably in relation to intravenous therapy.
- Tonicity is a measure of the concentration of electrolytes in a fluid.
- Hypertonic intravenous solutions tend to increase blood volume, whereas hypotonic intravenous solutions tend to decrease blood volume.
- A patient receives 34 calories for each 1% of dextrose in a liter of fluid.
- Devices used to deliver intravenous fluids include needles, over-the-needle catheters, inside-needle catheters, subcutaneous infusion ports, and subcutaneously implanted pumps.
- Central veins are large veins located nearer the heart that are used for long-term therapy, when the patient has poor peripheral veins, and when irritating fluids are administered.
- Peripheral veins in the extremities and scalp are used for short-term therapy, when a patient has healthy veins, and when relatively nonirritating fluids are given.
- Nurse practice acts and agency policies govern who can perform venipuncture, administer intravenous fluids, and give intravenous medications.
- Cannula size is selected based on the patient's condition and the type of fluid to be administered.
- Use the "five rights" when administering intravenous fluids as well as drugs.
- Cannulas and tubing are usually changed every 48 hours in accordance with standards of the Intravenous Nurses Society.
- On the site dressing, record the date and time that the cannula was inserted, the length and gauge of the cannula, and your initials.
- When an infusion flows by gravity, the rate is influenced by the height of the fluid container, fluid volume in the container, fluid viscosity, cannula diameter, venting of the fluid container, and position of the extremity.
- If your state permits you to give drugs per IV push, you must know how to dilute the medication, the correct rate of infusion, and whether the drug is compatible with the infusing fluid!
- Use standard precautions when starting infusions, providing site care, and discontinuing infusions.
- Complications of intravenous therapy are tissue trauma, infiltration, inflammation, infection, fluid volume excess, bleeding, and embolism.
- Monitor for fluid volume excess in the older person who is receiving intravenous fluids.
- When a cannula appears to be obstructed, irrigation is not recommended, as you may force blood clots into the bloodstream.
- With central lines, take precautions to prevent air entering the line, which can cause an air embolism—a potentially fatal complication.

REVIEW QUESTIONS

1. Which intravenous cannula is largest?
   1. 12-gauge
   2. 14-gauge
   3. 18-gauge
   4. 22-gauge
2. The tonicity of an IV solution of 0.45% sodium chloride is:
   1. isotonic.
   2. hypotonic.
   3. hypertonic.
   4. concentrated.
3. A patient is to receive 1000 ml of IV fluid every 8 hours at a rate of 34 drops/min. If the infusion has slowed so that he has received only 700 ml near the end of one 8 hour shift, the correct course of action is to:
   1. quickly infuse an additional 300 ml before the end of your shift.
   2. increase the infusion rate to deliver an additional 300 ml over the next shift.
   3. notify the physician to determine what action should be taken.
   4. reset the infusion rate at 34 drops/min to continue the infusion.
4. An elderly patient is receiving intravenous fluids to treat dehydration. When she complains of shortness of breath, your assessment reveals a 20 point increase in her systolic blood pressure, and a heart rate of 100. You should suspect:
   1. shock caused by deficient fluid volume.
   2. anxiety associated with hospitalization.
   3. fluid volume excess related to fluid overload.
   4. renal failure caused by circulatory collapse.
5. The greatest danger of irrigating an obstructed intravenous line is:
   1. embolism.
   2. trauma to the blood vessel.
   3. rupture of the cannula.
   4. infusion site irritation.

CHAPTER 18 Shock

18 Shock

objectives

1. List the types of shock.
2. Describe the pathophysiology of each type of shock.
3. List the signs and symptoms of each stage of shock.
4. Explain the first aid emergency treatment of shock outside the medical facility.
5. Identify general medical and nursing interventions for shock.
6. Explain the rationale for medical/surgical treatment of shock
7. Assist in developing care plans for patients in each type of shock.

key terms

Ischemia (ĭs-KĒ-mē-ă, p. 251)
Metabolic acidosis (mĕt-ă-BŎL-ĭk ăs-ĭ-DŌ-sĭs, p. 251)
Multiple organ dysfunction syndrome (MODS) (p. 257)
Sepsis (SĔP-sĭs, p. 257)
Shock (p. 249)
Systemic inflammatory response syndrome (SIRS) (p. 257)

DEFINITION OF SHOCK

Shock is a state of acute circulatory failure and impaired tissue perfusion. Inadequate tissue perfusion deprives cells of essential oxygen, forcing cells to rely on anaerobic (without oxygen) metabolism and permitting waste products to accumulate in the cells. If untreated, **shock** progresses first to systemic inflammatory response syndrome (SIRS), and then to multiple organ dysfunction syndrome (MODS) or death. There are a number of types of shock, each with a different cause. Regardless of the cause, the physiologic responses and most of the signs and symptoms of shock remain the same. Some aspects of treatment are appropriate for treating the effects of all types of shock. However, correction of the underlying causes often has additional specific interventions. Continual and astute nursing assessments and prompt interventions are critical to the patient's survival.

TYPES OF SHOCK

Shock is classified as hypovolemic, cardiogenic, or distributive, depending on the cause.

HYPOVOLEMIC SHOCK

Hypovolemic shock occurs when the circulating blood volume is inadequate to maintain the supply of oxygen and nutrients to body tissues. Blood volume falls when there is excessive blood or fluid loss, inadequate fluid intake, or a shift of plasma from the blood vessels into body tissues or organs. Some causes of blood or fluid loss are hemorrhage, severe diarrhea or vomiting, and excessive perspiration. Excessive shift of plasma can occur with pathologic states, including burns, peritonitis, and intestinal obstruction.

CARDIOGENIC SHOCK

Cardiogenic shock occurs when the heart fails as a pump. It can be associated with congestive heart failure, acute myocardial infarction, disturbances in cardiac rhythm, and structural abnormalities in the heart. Some classification systems include the term *obstructive shock* to refer to the type of shock associated with pulmonary embolism, fluid accumulation in the pericardial sac, and tension pneumothorax. All of these conditions can be factors in cardiogenic shock.

DISTRIBUTIVE SHOCK

In distributive shock, the problem is not loss of blood, but excessive dilation of blood vessels causing the blood to be improperly distributed. To demonstrate this point, imagine pouring 5 ml of water into a test tube and another 5 ml into a mixing bowl. The water would nearly fill the test tube, exerting even pressure against the walls of the tube. The water in the mixing bowl, however, might just barely cover the bottom of the bowl. The diameter of the mixing bowl is so large that the water exerts pressure primarily against the container bottom. This is similar to what happens in the vascular system when the diameter enlarges. Fluid pools in the dependent areas of the body and is not returned to the arterial circulation to supply critical cellular metabolic needs. Distributive shock can be complicated by increased capillary permeability, which permits plasma to leak into the interstitial compartment, thereby decreasing intravascular blood volume. The three types of distributive shock are anaphylactic, septic, and neurogenic.

Anaphylactic Shock

Anaphylactic shock occurs when a person has a severe allergic reaction that results in the release of chemicals that dilate blood vessels and increase capillary permeability. Fluid leaks out of the capillaries into the tissues. Pooling of blood in peripheral tissues and the shift of fluid out of the capillaries cause venous return and cardiac output to fall. In addition, the allergic reaction causes constriction of the bronchi and airway obstruction. People can be allergic to many substances including drugs, vaccines, contrast media, insect bites and stings, foods and food additives, pet dander, molds, and pollens. The onset of anaphylaxis is typically sudden and dramatic following exposure to a substance to which the patient has developed antibodies.

Septic Shock

Septic shock is hypotension that develops when pathogenic organisms (e.g., bacteria, fungi, viruses, rickettsiae) release toxic substances that cause blood vessels to dilate and increase capillary permeability. Vasodilation causes the skin to remain warm and dry initially. Especially in older adults, the clinical manifestations are often subtle. Chemicals released in response to tissue ischemia depress the myocardium. Myocardial depression, along with poor venous return, causes cardiac output to fall.

Neurogenic Shock

Neurogenic shock may occur after injury to the head or spinal cord, in response to drugs that depress the vasomotor center, including anesthetic agents, or with severe pain. Blood vessels dilate so that blood pools in the peripheral tissues, and preload (venous return) and cardiac output fall. The body is unable to compensate with vasoconstriction because the vasomotor center is incapacitated. The patient usually has hypotension and bradycardia.

EFFECTS OF SHOCK ON BODY SYSTEMS AND FUNCTIONS

- **Respiratory system:** tissue hypoxia and anoxia, respiratory failure, acute respiratory distress syndrome (ARDS)
- **Acid–base balance:** metabolic acidosis
- **Cardiovascular system:** myocardial depression, disseminated intravascular coagulation (widespread clotting caused by sluggish flow of acidic blood combined with bacterial endotoxins or clotting factors released by destruction of red blood cells [RBCs])
- **Neuroendocrine system:** release of catecholamines (epinephrine and norepinephrine), mineralocorticoids (aldosterone and desoxycorticosterone), glucocorticoids (hydrocortisone), and antidiuretic hormone; decreased level of consciousness when cerebral blood flow falls
- **Immune system:** depressed immune response
- **Gastrointestinal system:** decreased peristalsis, ischemia of intestinal submucosa, impaired liver function
- **Renal system:** reduced glomerular filtration, inadequate renal perfusion, tubular necrosis, renal ischemia

STAGES OF SHOCK

The three stages of shock are compensatory, progressive, and irreversible.

COMPENSATORY STAGE

The compensatory stage of shock begins when a fall in blood volume triggers sympathetic nervous system and hormonal responses. In response to falling blood pressure, the following events occur:

1. Activation of baroreceptors in the carotid arteries and the aorta stimulate the sympathetic nervous system.
2. Sympathetic stimulation causes increased heart rate, constriction of peripheral blood vessels, and reduced blood flow to the kidneys, lungs, muscles, skin, and gastrointestinal (GI) tract.
3. Decreasing renal blood flow triggers the release of renin and a sequence of events that produces angiotensin II, a potent vasoconstrictor.
4. The adrenal cortex secretes aldosterone, which promotes sodium retention by the kidneys.
5. Antidiuretic hormone is released by the posterior pituitary, resulting in additional retention of water by the kidneys.
6. Falling blood pH and increasing arterial carbon dioxide are detected by chemoreceptors in the carotid arteries, which stimulate the respiratory center. Increased respiratory rate and depth help to eliminate excess carbon dioxide and normalize the blood pH.

Assessment findings in the compensatory stage are likely to include:

- **Mental status:** irritability, restlessness
- **Blood pressure:** normal or slightly decreased, decreasing pulse pressure, orthostatic hypotension
- **Pulse:** increased rate; may be thready (as a result of vasoconstriction) or bounding (caused by vasodilation)
- **Respirations:** increased rate and depth
- **Urine output:** decreased
- **Skin:** cool and pale. *Exception:* warm and dry with septic shock.
- **Abdomen:** decreased bowel sounds
- **Blood glucose:** increased
- **Other:** thirst

If the compensatory mechanisms are effective, the patient's blood pressure will remain normal. If the compensatory mechanisms fail, the patient enters the progressive stage. Table 18-1 summarizes the compensatory mechanisms activated in the first stage of shock.

PROGRESSIVE STAGE

In the progressive stage of shock, despite increased sympathetic activity, cardiac output and arterial blood pressure fall. Deprived of adequate oxygen, cells must resort to anaerobic

table 18-1 ***Compensatory Mechanisms in Shock***

MECHANISM	RESPONSE	BENEFITS
Baroreceptors activate SNS.	Increased heart rate	Speeds up delivery of oxygen and nutrients to tissues
	Peripheral vasoconstriction	Shunts blood to vital organs, helps maintain BP
	Constriction of renal arteries	Activates renin-angiotensin-aldosterone system
	Renin-angiotensin-aldosterone system activated	Vasoconstriction shunts blood to vital organs and helps maintain BP.
	Angiotensin is a potent vasoconstrictor.	
	Aldosterone causes the kidneys to retain sodium, which induces ADH secretion and water retention.	Fluid retention increases blood volume by decreasing urine output.
Chemoreceptors in the carotid arteries respond to acidic blood pH and increased arterial carbon dioxide by stimulating the respiratory center.	Increased respiratory rate and depth	This helps eliminate the excess carbon dioxide and normalize the blood pH. Takes in additional oxygen.

SNS, Sympathetic nervous system; *BP,* blood pressure; *ADH,* antidiuretic hormone.

metabolism, which produces lactic acid. Metabolic acidosis has a depressant effect on myocardial cells. Typical assessment findings are:

- **Mental status:** listlessness, confusion
- **Blood pressure:** decreased; narrow pulse pressure
- **Pulse:** tachycardia, weak and thready
- **Respirations:** increased
- **Temperature:** subnormal, except with septic shock
- **Urine output:** decreased; possible renal failure
- **Skin:** cold, pale, clammy, slow capillary refill, cyanosis
- **Other:** dry mouth, thirst, sluggish pupillary response, and muscle weakness

It is still possible to reverse the patient's condition during this stage. However, the liver, lungs, heart, and kidneys begin to deteriorate as areas of ischemia, then necrosis, develop.

IRREVERSIBLE (REFRACTORY) STAGE

The final stage of shock is marked by irreversible changes in vital organs as compensatory mechanisms fail. Cardiac function is depressed, fluid shifts out of the capillaries into the tissues, and cells are unable to maintain metabolic processes. Death is imminent. Even patients who are resuscitated during this stage often die within a week or two from MODS. Assessment findings in the irreversible stage include:

- **Mental status:** loss of consciousness
- **Blood pressure:** systolic continues to fall; diastolic approaches zero
- **Pulse:** progressive slowing, irregular
- **Respirations:** slow, shallow, irregular
- **Urine** output: minimal
- **Skin:** cold, clammy, cyanosis

DIAGNOSIS

A diagnosis of shock is based on the history and physical examination. Tests and procedures that help to establish the type of shock, the stage, and the cause include blood and urine studies, measurement of hemodynamic pressures, chest radiograph, ECG and continuous cardiac monitoring, pulse oximetry and arterial blood gases, and urine output.

FIRST AID FOR SHOCK OUTSIDE THE MEDICAL FACILITY

Treatment that is provided to patients in shock before medical care is available can have a significant impact on the chances of survival. Table 18-2 describes emergency first aid care.

GENERAL MEDICAL TREATMENT

General medical interventions for the patient in shock are directed toward maintaining perfusion of vital organs until the cause is corrected. A priority in shock treatment is to improve blood flow and oxygen supply to the vital organs. Remember that brain cells begin to die after 4 minutes without oxygen. Treatment measures include positioning, oxygen therapy, fluid replacement, correction of acid-base imbalances, management of complications such as cardiac dysrhythmias, and correction of the underlying cause. Tables 18-3 and 18-4 summarize commonly used antishock drugs. Details related to specific drugs and nursing interventions are included in Table 33-8.

table 18-2 ASSESSMENT *and First Aid for the Patient in Shock*

PHYSICAL EXAMINATION

Pulse: Rapid and weak, "thready"
Respirations: Air hunger initially, then increased rate; shallow
Blood Pressure: Stable initially, then decreased
Skin: Cool and moist at first; diaphoresis; later, cyanosis of lips and nail beds
Mental Status: Restless, then listless; confused; unconscious
Thirst: Increased

INTERVENTIONS

- Summon medical assistance.
- Maintain blood flow to the brain.
- Keep still and quiet.
- Position flat; legs may be elevated unless the shock is caused by heart failure, the head or neck is bleeding, spinal injury is possible, intracranial pressure is increased, or the patient has dyspnea.
- Protect the patient from cold but do not overheat (victim should not shiver or perspire).
- Even if the patient complains of thirst, withhold oral fluids in case surgical intervention is needed.
- Tell victim what is being done, that someone will stay with him, and that help is coming.

POSITIONING

To maintain blood flow to vital organs, use the supine position with the legs elevated 45 degrees, trunk horizontal, head and chest at same level, and knees straight (Fig. 18-1). Trendelenburg's (head down) position is *not recommended* because it can impair cerebral blood flow, interfere with respirations and filling of coronary arteries, and increase intracranial pressure.

OXYGENATION

To promote delivery of oxygen to the cells, the patient is given drug therapy and fluids to improve cardiac output, blood products to increase hemoglobin, and supplementary oxygen to increase oxygen saturation. Mechanical ventilation may be necessary. Sedatives and analgesics may be ordered to decrease oxygen requirements.

FLUID REPLACEMENT

Except for cardiogenic shock, all types of shock require significant fluid volume replacement. Normal saline is usually administered initially. Subsequent fluids may include various crystalloids and colloids depending on the situation. Crystalloids provide replacement water and electrolytes for all fluid compartments. Colloids, on the other hand, remain in the vascular system and draw fluid into the bloodstream. Colloids are especially important when large amounts of plasma proteins have been lost. The hemorrhaging patient will require

table 18-3 DRUG THERAPY | *Drugs Used to Treat Shock*

DRUG CLASSIFICATION	DRUG ACTION	SPECIFIC EXAMPLES
Alpha-adrenergic agonists	Vasoconstriction increases peripheral resistance and raises blood pressure	Norepinephrine (Levophed) Phenylephrine (Neo-Synephrine)
Beta-adrenergic agonists	Increase myocardial contractility and heart rate Raises blood pressure	Dobutamine (Dobutrex) Isoproterenol (Isuprel)
Alpha- and beta-adrenergic agonists	Raises blood pressure by constricting blood vessels and increasing myocardial contractility	Dopamine (Intropin) Epinephrine (Adrenalin)
Inotropic/cardiotonic agents	Improve myocardial contractility without increasing heart rate	Digoxin (Lanoxin) Amrinone (Inocor) Milrinone (Primacor)

table 18-4 DRUG THERAPY | *Drugs Used to Increase Cardiac Output*

DRUG	EFFECTS ON HEART RATE	EFFECTS ON PRELOAD (VENOUS RETURN)	EFFECTS ON AFTERLOAD (PERIPHERAL RESISTANCE)	EFFECTS ON CONTRACTILITY
Dobutamine (Dobutrex)	No effect	Decreased	Decreased	Increased
Dopamine (Intropin)	Increased	Decreased at low doses	Decreased at low doses	Increased
Amrinone (Inocor)	No effect	Decreased	Decreased	Increased
Epinephrine (Adrenalin)	Increased	Decreased at low doses	Decreased at low doses	Increased
Norepinephrine (Levophed)	No significant effect	Increased	Increased	Increased

Adapted from F. D. Monahan & M. A. Neighbors (1998). *Medical-surgical nursing: Foundations for clinical practice* (2nd ed, p. 405). Philadelphia: Saunders.

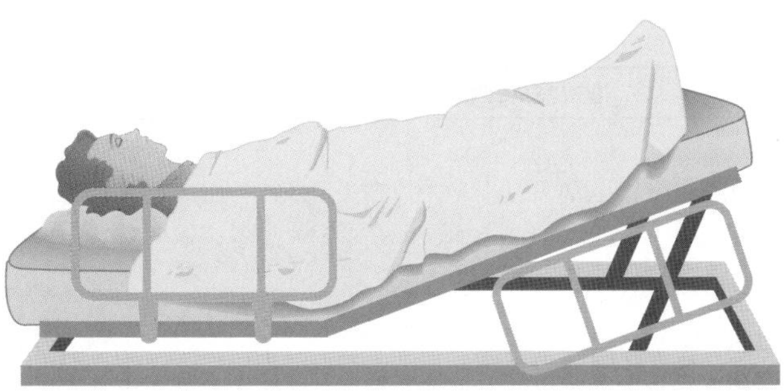

FIGURE **18-1** Positioning of the person in shock. The trunk should be horizontal, the head and chest on the same level, and the legs elevated up to 45 degrees.

blood to replace deficient hemoglobin. Fluid needs of the patient in cardiogenic shock are determined based on individual patient assessments.

Patient response must be closely monitored during fluid replacement to assure adequate, but not excessive, replacement. Fluid replacement is best determined by monitoring pulmonary artery wedge pressure, cardiac output, and urine output. Once adequate fluids have been administered, an inotropic agent may be ordered to increase myocardial contractility.

ACID-BASE IMBALANCE

Specific fluids and mechanical ventilation are used to correct acid-base imbalances. With profound acidosis (pH below 7.2), sodium bicarbonate may be ordered.

SPECIFIC MEDICAL TREATMENT FOR EACH TYPE OF SHOCK

In addition to the general medical treatment for shock, specific interventions are necessary for each type of shock. These are summarized in Table 18-5. Mechanical devices used in the treatment of shock are described in Table 18-6.

Put on your THINKING CAP!!

Three patients are in the emergency department. All are in the compensatory stage of shock. Patient A is in hypovolemic shock. Patient B is in cardiogenic shock. Patient C is in septic shock.

1. What assessment finding would you expect in Patient C, but not Patient A or B?
2. For which patient(s) would colloid intravenous fluids be contraindicated? Why?
3. Which patient would you expect to have a history of:
   a. Coronary artery disease
   b. Severe vomiting and diarrhea
   c. Urinary tract infection

NURSING CARE *of the Patient in Shock*

Assessment

Assessment of the patient who is at risk for shock should include continuous monitoring of cardiac rate and rhythm; blood pressure; body temperature; hemodynamic values; respiratory rate, rhythm, and depth; and arterial blood gases. In the routine nursing assessment, observe the color of the skin and palpate skin warmth and moisture. Note pupil size, equality, and response to light. Describe the patient's level of consciousness and response to commands, and assess reflexes. Auscultate heart, lung, and bowel sounds. Observe the movement of the chest wall with respirations. Inspect and palpate the abdomen for distention. Palpate for bladder distention and note the appearance of urine and the hourly output. Inspect the extremities for color and palpate for peripheral pulses and edema. Inspect intravenous infusion sites for pallor, swelling, or coolness that suggests extravasation.

Nursing Diagnoses, Goals, and Outcome Criteria: Shock (General)

Nursing Diagnoses	Goals and Outcome Criteria
Infeffective Tissue Perfusion related to failing cardiac pump, hypovolemia, or inadequate venous return	Normal tissue perfusion: urine output at least 1.0 ml/kg/hr, patient alert and oriented, normal heart rate and rhythm, normal blood pressure, active bowel sounds, extremities warm with palpable pulses
Decreased Cardiac Output related to hypovolemia, peripheral vasodilation, myocardial disorders	Normal cardiac output: normal hemodynamic values, vital signs consistent with patient norms, mental alertness
Disturbed Thought Processes related to inadequate cerebral perfusion, metabolic acidosis	Normal thought processes: patient alert and oriented, responds to commands appropriately, behaves appropriately
Deficient Fluid Volume related to hemorrhage, inadequate fluid intake, excessive fluid loss	Normal fluid balance: vital signs consistent with patient norms, capillary refill in 3 to 5 seconds
Anxiety related to hypoxia, life-threatening situation	Reduced anxiety: patient calm, states is less anxious
Risk for Injury related to confusion, adverse effects of drugs, invasive treatments	Absence of injury: no trauma
Risk for Infection related to trauma, invasive therapeutic procedures	Absence of infection: body temperature within normal range, normal WBC count
Ineffective Family Coping related to anxiety, uncertainty of patient's outcome	Effective coping: family members are supportive of the patient and each other and indicate that they have adequate resources to cope with present situation

table 18-5 ***Interventions for Each Type of Shock***

TYPE OF SHOCK AND ETIOLOGY	INTERVENTIONS	DRUGS/ACTIONS
HYPOVOLEMIC		
Blood loss: trauma, gastrointestinal bleeding, ruptured blood vessel, DIC	Direct pressure. Surgical repair. Replacement of whole blood, blood components, plasma expanders. Crystalloid fluid replacement. Autotransfusion (patient's own blood is collected and administered) in some circumstances. Pneumatic antishock (MAST) garment is controversial.	N/A
Plasma loss	Intravenous fluids. Albumin, fresh frozen plasma, hetastarch, dextran.	Low-dose inotropics
Crystalloid loss	Intravenous fluids and electrolytes as indicated.	N/A
CARDIOGENIC		
Myocardial and valvular disease or injury	Hemodynamic monitoring. Intravenous fluids. Intra-aortic balloon pump. Surgery for valve disorders. External counterpulsation. Cardiac transplantation.	Inotropics/cardiotonics to improve myocardial contractility. Vasodilators to improve myocardial blood flow. Diuretics to decrease blood volume and reduce workload of the heart.
External pressure on the heart:		
Pericardial tamponade	Pericardiocentesis, surgical repair.	N/A
Ascites	Paracentesis	N/A
Massive pulmonary embolism		Thrombolytics to dissolve blood clots or anticoagulants to prevent clot formation.
Tension pneumothorax	Air removed with needle or chest tube.	N/A
Cardiac dysrhythmias	Cardiac pacing, cardiopulmonary resuscitation.	Antidysrhythmics to restore normal cardiac rhythm.
ANAPHYLACTIC		
Allergy to food, drugs, chemicals, insect bites or stings	Maintain airway. Endotracheal intubation or tracheostomy if needed. Ice pack to injection or sting site. Gastric lavage for ingested antigens. Isotonic intravenous fluids.	Epinephrine and theophylline for bronchospasm. Epinephrine also increases the cardiac rate and strength of contraction. H_1 receptor blockers (antihistamines) to block antigen–antibody response. Corticosteroids to reduce inflammatory antigen–antibody response. Vasopressors to constrict peripheral blood vessels and raise blood pressure.
SEPTIC		
Infection, usually gram negative	Culture and sensitivity tests to identify site of infection, causative agent, and effective antimicrobials. Intravenous fluids: normal saline. Maintain body temperature in normal range.	Antimicrobials: (e.g., vancomycin) if suspected gram positive. Penicillin or cephalosporin and aminoglycoside if suspected gram negative. Cardiotonics/inotropics to improve cardiac output. Vasopressors to raise blood pressure. Monoclonal antibodies to inhibit endotoxins. Heparin, clotting factors, blood product to treat DIC.
NEUROGENIC		
Spinal cord injury, spinal anesthesia	Flat with legs elevated 45 degrees. Intravenous normal saline.	Atropine for bradycardia. Vasopressors to raise blood pressure and improve cardiac output.
Pain, emotional distress (vasovagal response)	Recumbent position.	Analgesics for pain. Atropine for bradycardia.

Adapted from Black, J.M., Hawks, J.H., & Keene, A.M. (2001). *Medical-surgical nursing: Clinical management for positive outcomes* (6th ed., pp. 2249-2250). Philadelphia: Saunders.

DIC, Disseminated intravascular coagulation.

table 18-6 ***Mechanical Devices Used in the Treatment of Shock***

DEVICE	DESCRIPTION	PURPOSE
Medical antishock trousers (MAST garment) (Fig. 18-2)	Trousers with inflatable chambers for each leg and the abdomen. Most often used outside hospital for massive blood or fluid loss. *Use is controversial because of possible restriction of lung expansion and accumulation of lactic acid in extremities.*	When chambers are inflated, blood vessels are compressed. Impedes blood flow to raise blood pressure and improve perfusion of vital organs. May reduce leakage of fluid into tissues of legs.
Intra-aortic balloon pump (IABP) (Fig. 18-3)	A balloon-tipped catheter is inserted into the descending thoracic aorta. The balloon inflates during diastole and deflates just before systole.	Reduces preload with cardiogenic shock. Heart pumps more efficiently; increases cardiac output.
External counter-pulsation device	Air- or water-filled devices are applied to the legs. A pump applies pressure during diastole and relieves pressure during systole.	Reduces preload with cardiogenic shock. Heart pumps more efficiently; increases cardiac output.
Ventricular assist devices (VAD)	Various devices include pulsatile and nonpulsatile pumps, external and implantable devices.	Decreases myocardial workload and oxygen demand. Supports circulation until the heart recovers or is replaced.
Extracorporeal membrane oxygenation (ECMO)	Blood is removed from the inferior vena cava, oxygenated, and returned via the femoral artery.	Used for short-term stabilization.

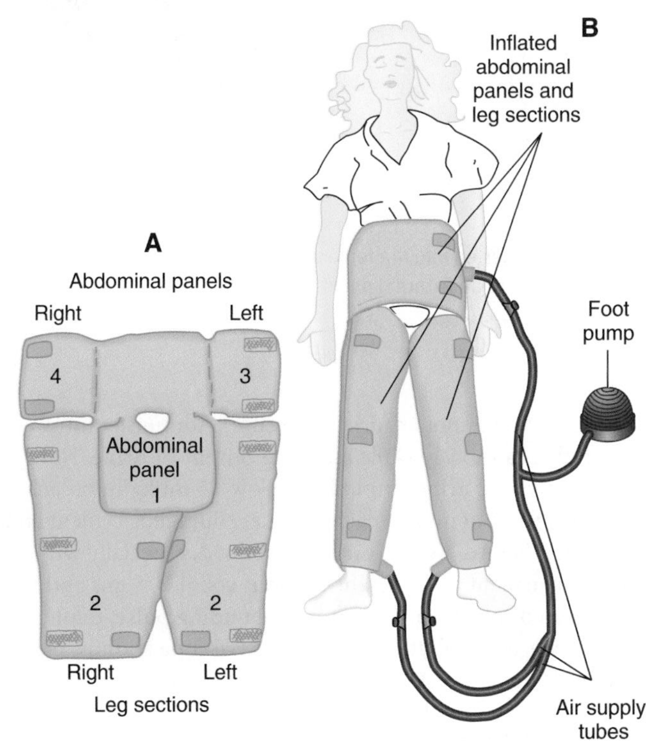

FIGURE **18-2** MAST garment. *A,* Compartments allow compression of the legs and the abdomen. *B,* Garment in place. Compartments are inflated with a foot pump.

Interventions

Ineffective Tissue Perfusion

Your continuous assessment must include all body systems because shock, if not corrected, eventually results in failure of all major organs. Specific organ failures are addressed here under other nursing diagnoses.

Decreased Cardiac Output

Administer intravenous fluids as ordered, and assess for both fluid volume deficit and excess. With cardiogenic shock, it is especially important to monitor hemodynamic parameters. Administer inotropic and antidysrhythmic agents as ordered. Continuous cardiac monitoring enables you to assess the effectiveness of these drugs. You can reduce oxygen requirements by handling the patient gently and coordinating care to allow for rest. Maintain adequate body heat to prevent shivering, which also increases metabolic (and circulatory) demands. Fever may be treated with acetaminophen or nonsteroidal anti-inflammatory drugs. In some situations, a tepid sponge bath or a cooling blanket is ordered.

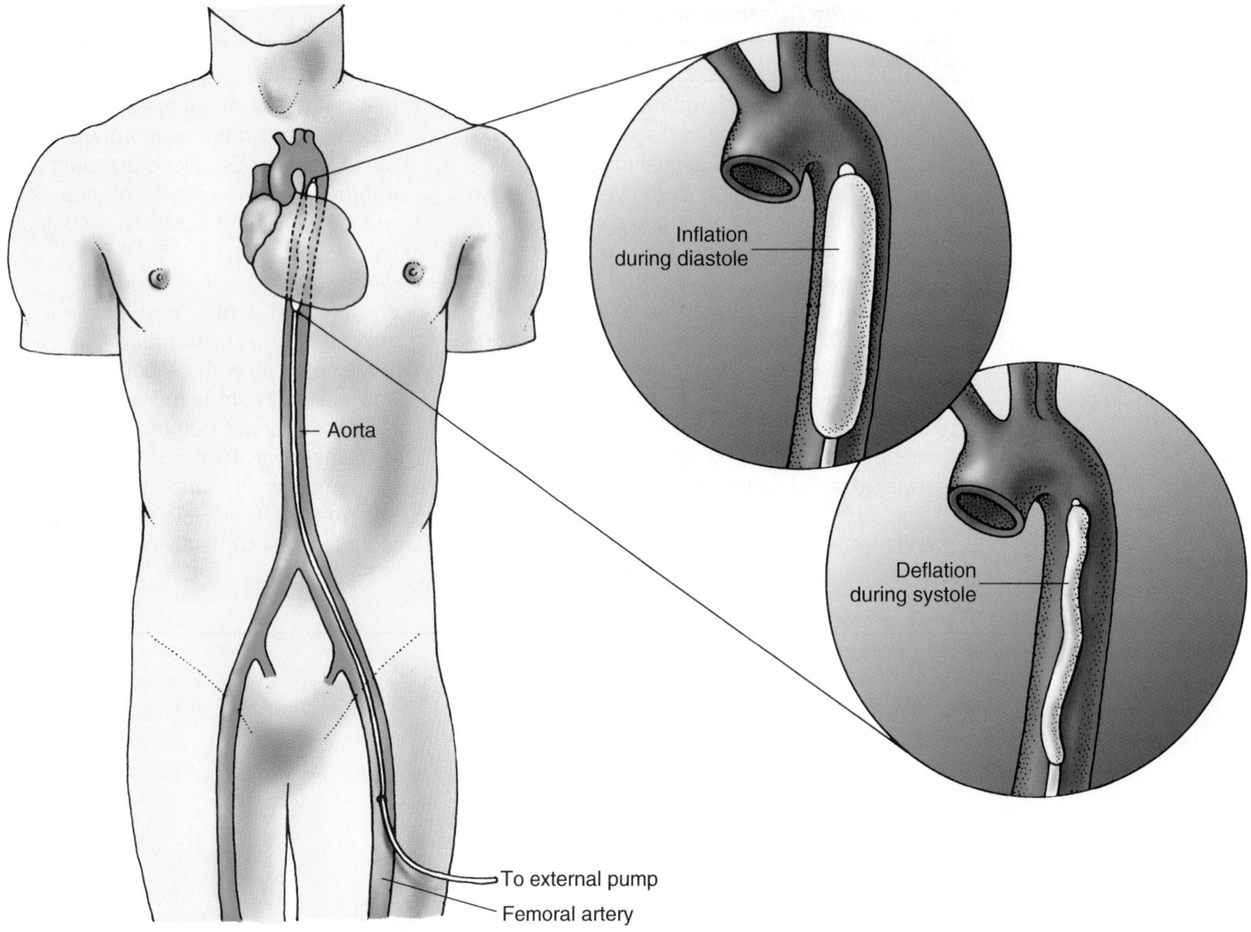

FIGURE **18-3** Intra-aortic balloon pump (IABP). An IABP is inserted into the femoral artery and advanced into the ascending aorta. The catheter is connected to an external pump that inflates the balloon during diastole and deflates it during systole.

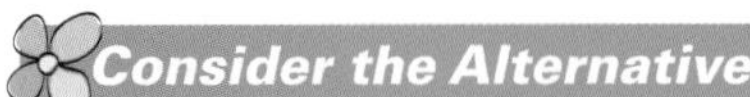

Prayer and religious objects are comforting to many patients.

Disturbed Thought Processes and Anxiety

As patients progress through the stages of shock, they may be anxious, then confused and disoriented, and finally unconscious. For the anxious patient, you must remain calm and give simple explanations of what is being done. Remember that the intensive care environment is foreign and frightening to most people. As much as possible, protect the patient from constant, excessive noise and light.

Protect confused patients from harm. Repeat orientation, instructions, and reassurance often. In the presence of unconscious patients, remember that they may hear even when they cannot respond. Continue to speak to the patient and beware of negative comments in the patient's presence.

Deficient Fluid Volume

Monitor for hypovolemia (tachycardia, hypotension, tachypnea, decreased urine output, decreased central venous pressure and pulmonary artery pressure). Administer intravenous fluids cautiously while assessing output of urine. Notify the physician if urine output falls below 0.5 ml/kg/hr because low urine output may signal inadequate fluid replacement and/or renal failure. Assess for fluid overload, especially with renal impairment and with intravenous colloids. Signs and symptoms of overload include full, bounding pulse; dilute urine, increased respiratory rate; abnormal lung sounds; dyspnea; and edema.

Risk for Injury

In addition to the risk for injury related to changes in consciousness, the patient in shock can be harmed by the therapeutic measures being used. For example, antidysrhythmics can depress cardiac activity, anticoagulants can permit excessive bleeding, and extravasation of vasopressors (drugs that raise blood pressure by vasoconstriction) can cause local tissue necrosis. Therefore, you must closely monitor the patient for both therapeutic and adverse effects of drugs used to treat the patient in shock.

Because of poor peripheral tissue perfusion and the need to minimize activity, the patient in shock is at high risk for complications of immobility. Institute measures to prevent prolonged pressure on susceptible sites. Pressure ulcers can develop very rapidly. Also, personal hygiene may be limited by the patient's tolerance of such activity. A partial bath and gentle range of motion may be done if the patient is stable enough. Mouth care provides some comfort and helps prevent cracking of the lips and dryness of the oral mucosa. Apply water-soluble lubricant to the lips and moisten the mouth with normal saline.

Put on your THINKING CAP!!

Why would a vasopressor be harmful to surrounding tissues if it leaked out of the vein?

Risk for Infection

Intravenous lines, indwelling urinary catheters, chest tubes, airways, ventricular assist devices, and other equipment all provide avenues for infection in the patient in shock. The risk of infection is greatest in very young, very old, and immunocompromised patients. To reduce the risk of infection, wash your hands thoroughly between patients. Follow agency guidelines for care of intravenous and urinary catheters. Use aseptic technique when inserting these devices, caring for insertion sites, and providing wound care. Monitor for signs of infection (elevated body temperature and white blood cell [WBC] count; redness, swelling, and warmth of wounds and tube insertion sites; purulent drainage; abnormal breath sounds; and yellow or green sputum). When antibiotics are ordered, administer them on schedule to maintain a therapeutic blood level.

Ineffective Family Coping

The patient in shock often has one or more family members present. Members of the health care team should be sensitive to the needs of the family for information and support. You can explain the nursing care and encourage them to ask questions. Offer the services of a counselor or patient representative.

What Does Culture Have to do with Shock?

A Japanese or Vietnamese family would expect to participate in patient care or to remain at the bedside. Extended families may gather to be near the patient and to support one another. In Mexico, important decisions may be deferred to male relatives in traditional families. In Italy, a fatal prognosis would not be discussed by patients and families before death. In many cultures, rituals related to illness and death are very important to the patient and the family.

SYSTEMIC INFLAMMATORY RESPONSE SYNDROME (SIRS)

Inflammation is a normal response to tissue injury. However, in certain clinical situations, generalized inflammation occurs that threatens vital organs. This state is called systemic inflammatory response syndrome, or SIRS. In addition to shock, some of the conditions that can lead to SIRS are multiple transfusions, massive tissue injury, burns, and pancreatitis.

The effects of SIRS are damage to the endothelium of blood vessels and a hypermetabolic state. Damaged endothelium increases capillary permeability, allowing fluid to leak into body tissues. Hypotension, microemboli, and shunting of blood flow compromise organ perfusion. The hypermetabolic state is characterized by increased serum glucose, which eventually depletes carbohydrate, fat, and protein stores.

A diagnosis of SIRS is made when a patient manifests two or more of the following:

- Temperature less than 97° F (36° C) or more than 100.4° F (38° C)
- Heart rate more than 90 bpm
- Respiratory rate more than 20/min, or $Pa{CO_2}$ less than 32 mm Hg.
- WBC count less than 4,000 cells/μl or more than 12,000 cells/μl, or more than 10% immature (band) neutrophils.

The term *sepsis* is used when a patient has SIRS with a confirmed infection. Manifestations of SIRS range from mild to severe. With advanced SIRS and MODS, deterioration of the cardiac, pulmonary, renal, and central nervous systems, liver, pancreas, and GI tract occurs. Thrombocytopenia may develop and progress to disseminated intravascular coagulation. If three or more organs fail, the prognosis is very poor.

If more than one organ begins to fail as a result of SIRS, the patient is said to have multiple organ dysfunction syndrome (MODS). As various organs are affected, the patient shows signs of failure specific to the organs affected.

MEDICAL TREATMENT AND NURSING INTERVENTIONS

Detailed care of the patient with SIRS and MODS is beyond the scope of this text. The patient is critically ill and requires critical care nursing. The goals of medical and nursing care for SIRS and MODS are to prevent and treat infection, maintain tissue oxygenation, provide nutritional and metabolic support, and support individual failing organs.

Prevent and Treat Infection

Monitor potential infection sites and assess for signs and symptoms of infection. Maintain strict asepsis with invasive procedures and equipment. Exercise scrupulous handwashing. Administer antimicrobials as ordered. Administer enteral feedings as ordered to enhance perfusion of the GI tract.

Maintain Tissue Oxygenation

Administer sedatives and analgesics as ordered to reduce oxygen requirements. Monitor the patient on mechanical ventilation. Administer drugs to improve cardiac output and tissue perfusion as ordered. Plan care to minimize physical demands on patient.

Nutrition Concepts

1. Hypermetabolism in shock causes protein-calorie malnutrition.
2. Early enteral feedings are thought to improve perfusion of the GI tract and reduce the movement of bacteria through the intestinal walls into the bloodstream.
3. Nutritional status of the patient in shock is assessed by monitoring serum protein, nitrogen balance, and blood urea nitrogen (BUN), serum glucose, and serum electrolytes.

Provide Nutritional and Metabolic Support

Provide enteral or parenteral nutrition as ordered. Monitor blood glucose and weight.

Support Failing Organs

Examples of measures to support failing organs could include mechanical ventilation for respiratory distress syndrome and replacement therapy for renal failure.

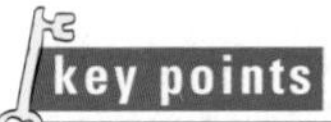

key points

- Shock is a state of acute circulatory failure and impaired tissue perfusion.
- Untreated shock progresses to systemic inflammatory response syndrome and then to multiple organ dysfunction syndrome or death.
- The types of shock are hypovolemic, cardiogenic, and distributive.
- Hypovolemic shock results from inadequate circulating blood volume.
- Cardiogenic shock occurs when the heart fails as a pump.
- Distributive shock results from the excessive dilation of blood vessels that causes blood to be improperly distributed.
- The three types of distributive shock are anaphylactic, septic, and neurogenic.
- Compensatory responses to shock represent stimulation of the endocrine and sympathetic nervous systems.
- In the progressive stage of shock, cardiac output and blood pressure continue to fall, and cells must resort to anaerobic metabolism that leads to acidosis.
- The final stage of shock is marked by irreversible changes in vital organs; death is imminent.
- Because brain cells begin to die after 4 minutes without oxygen, a priority in shock treatment is to improve blood flow and oxygen supply to vital organs.
- The patient in shock should be positioned supine with the legs elevated 45 degrees, the trunk horizontal, the head and chest at the same level, and the knees straight.
- During fluid replacement, a minimum urine output of 1 ml/kg/hr is consistent with adequate fluid volume. Notify the physician if output falls below 0.5 ml/kg/hr.
- Assessment of the patient in shock includes monitoring of vital signs, hemodynamic values, and arterial blood gases.
- General nursing diagnoses for the patient in shock include ineffective tissue perfusion, decreased cardiac output, disturbed thought processes, deficient fluid volume, anxiety, risk for injury, risk for infection, and ineffective family coping.
- Systemic inflammatory response syndrome (SIRS) is generalized inflammation that damages the lining of blood vessels and creates a hypermetabolic state.
- Failure of more than one organ is called multiple organ dysfunction syndrome (MODS); failure of three or more organs presents a very poor prognosis.
- The goals of care with SIRS and MODS are to prevent and treat infection, maintain tissue oxygenation, provide nutritional and metabolic support, and support individual failing organs.

REVIEW QUESTIONS

1. A patient with peritonitis is at greatest risk for which type of shock?
   1. Cardiogenic
   2. Anaphylactic
   3. Neurogenic
   4. Hypovolemic
2. The basic cause of distributive shock is:
   1. blood or fluid loss.
   2. dilation of blood vessels.
   3. an antigen–antibody reaction.
   4. failure of the heart as a pump.
3. A patient in anaphylactic shock has massive edema. What would explain this?
   1. Increased capillary permeability
   2. Pooling of blood in dependent parts of the body
   3. Retention of excess water by the kidneys
   4. Overproduction of antidiuretic hormone
4. What do anaphylactic shock, septic shock, and neurogenic shock all have in common?
   1. Infection
   2. Allergic reactions
   3. Vasodilation
   4. Heart failure
5. Which acid-base disturbance would you anticipate with shock?
   1. Metabolic alkalosis
   2. Respiratory alkalosis
   3. Metabolic acidosis
   4. Respiratory acidosis
6. The best indicator of cerebral perfusion is:
   1. presence of reflexes.
   2. level of consciousness.
   3. emotional state.
   4. mean arterial pressure.

7. The most appropriate position for the patient in hypovolemic shock is:
   1. Trendelenburg's.
   2. flat with legs elevated.
   3. semi-Fowler's.
   4. side-lying with head elevated.

8. When patients have lost large amounts of plasma proteins, which fluid is most appropriate for restoring blood volume?
   1. Packed red blood cells
   2. Crystalloid fluids
   3. Normal saline
   4. Colloids

9. With adequate tissue perfusion, you would expect a minimum hourly urinary output of:
   1. 0.1 ml/kg.
   2. 0.5 ml/kg.
   3. 5 ml/kg.
   4. 30 ml/kg.

10. A patient in shock has been given blood, crystalloids, and osmotic fluids. Your assessment reveals: P = 80, bounding, regular; R = 30; BP = 140/86. Dyspnea. Crackles throughout lung fields. You should suspect:
    1. sepsis.
    2. multiple organ failure.
    3. pneumonia.
    4. circulatory overload.

CHAPTER 19 Falls

objectives

1. Define falls.
2. Give the incidence of falls.
3. Describe factors that increase the risk of falls.
4. Discuss the relationship between restraint use and falls, types of restraints, and regulations for restraint use.
5. Describe fall prevention techniques.
6. Describe nursing interventions to use when a fall occurs.

key terms

Chemical restraint (p. 261)
Extrinsic factors (ĕks-TRĬN-sĭk, p. 260)
Fall (p. 260)
Intrinsic factors (ĭn-TRĬN-sĭk, p. 260)
Omnibus Reconciliation Act (OBRA) (p. 262)
Physical restraint (p. 261)

If you were to ask several people whether or not they had fallen in the past 6 months, the chances are that many would say yes. The chances are even better that those who had fallen, particularly the young and healthy ones, had not sustained a significant injury. Although falls do not necessarily result in serious physical injuries or death, many older people who have fallen become less confident in their ability to function independently. Those who fear falling tend to restrict their physical and social activities, become more dependent, and have an increased need for long-term care. In addition, care givers tend to restrict older persons' activity out of concern that ill or frail people who have been weakened from sickness, hospitalization, or aging may fall and injure themselves.

DEFINITION OF FALLS

Definitions of falls vary from "unexpected displacement" to "an unintentional change in position" to "inadvertent events in which the subject comes to rest unintentionally on the ground." A useful definition that seems more descriptive of an actual **fall** is "a circumstance in which one unintentionally falls to the ground or hits an object such as a chair or stair."

INCIDENCE AND RISK FACTORS

Although falls and fall-related injuries occur at every age, the greater severity of injuries in old age, combined with longer recovery periods, makes a fall a particularly serious threat to the health and functioning of older people. One in three persons aged 65 or older falls in a given year. There appears to be a steady increase in the number of falls among those aged 75 and older. Older women residing in community and long-term care facilities appear to be at higher risk of falling than older men. However, older men are more likely to fall in a hospital setting.

The risk of injury from falls is highest in people over age 65, and falls are the most frequent cause of accidental injury and death among the elderly. The elderly constitute only 12%-13% of the total U.S. population; however, they account for 72% of total deaths due to falls. The rate of death from falls increases from 5 in 100,000 for persons between ages 45 and 64 to 200 in 100,000 for those older than 85.

The U.S. Public Health Service has estimated that two thirds of the deaths due to falls are preventable. Potentially avoidable environmental factors cause 40% to 50% of fatal falls. Adequate medical evaluation and treatment for underlying medical conditions could probably prevent most of the remaining 50% to 60% of fatal falls, according to the Public Health Service.

The elderly are at particular risk for accidents because of changes brought about by aging, a greater potential for injury, and poorer clinical outcomes. Falls occur because of two major factors: (1) ***intrinsic factors,*** or factors related to the functioning of the individual, such as the aging process or physical illness, and (2) ***extrinsic factors,*** or environmental factors. Intrinsic factors enhance the possibility of falling, whereas extrinsic factors enhance the opportunity to fall.

Intrinsic factors related to falls include age-related sensory changes such as reduced vision and hearing; age-related changes in posture and gait; confusion or depression; lack of exercise, leading to weakness and decline in physical vigor; multiple medications related to the increased incidence of chronic illness in the elderly; psychotropic medications; diseases affecting the central nervous system that may affect balance by causing dizziness and gait disorders; and overestimation of abilities.

Extrinsic factors may differ according to setting. For example, potential hazards in the home environment include

NURSING CARE PLAN

The Patient with a History of Falls

ASSESSMENT

Health History: A 75-year-old woman has been placed in a long-term care facility because of chronic health problems, including emphysema, dementia, and a history of several falls at home. She has sustained several fractures as a result of these falls in the past. The nursing staff has used several methods to prevent her from falling, such as restraints, sedation, and sitters, but she continues to have problems. When she is restrained she becomes very agitated, and the staff is unable to calm her without administering sedatives.

Physical Examination: Vital signs: blood pressure, 144/76; pulse, 92; respiration, 22; temperature, 97° F. Height, 5'1"; weight, 98 lb. Her skin is warm and dry. Wheezing is noted on expiration. The patient is not oriented to time and place; she is oriented to person.

Nursing Diagnosis	*Goals and Outcome Criteria*	*Interventions*
Risk for injury related to confusion.	Patient will remain free from fall-related injury.	Approach patient in a calm manner. Assess patient and environment for possible hazards and remove. Orient patient frequently to person, place, and time. Keep bed at lowest level; keep wheelchair brakes on. Have patient wear glasses or hearing aid when appropriate. Have someone familiar stay with patient to monitor as frequently as possible. Provide restraints only as a last resort to maintain safety; use type that is least restrictive; monitor frequently while restraint is on patient; remove at least every 2 hours for 10 minutes for range of motion exercises, toileting, nourishment, and restorative activities. Get patient up and out of room as tolerated.

low-lying and poorly visible tables, trailing electrical wires, pets, steep and unlit stairs, loose carpeting, unsafe walking aids, and inconvenient bathroom or kitchen arrangements. Falls occurring in the institutional setting as a result of various environmental factors are often related to changes in position, such as transferring to and from a bed or chair, toileting procedures, and unstable and defective equipment (nonfunctioning brake locks on wheelchairs, wet or excessively waxed floors, and improper placement of food trays in the hallway). Falls often occur during periods of high activity when staff persons are busy. In addition, falls may result from imposed immobility. Patients may be confined to a bed or chair or be physically restrained, resulting in weakness or problems with balance.

Injury-causing falls are more likely to occur in long-term care facilities than in the community. However, in about 65% to 75% of all reported falls, no injuries occur. Contusions, cuts, or lacerations occur in about 25% to 30% of all reported falls, and deep tissue damage or concussion occurs in about 5%. Fractures result in about 1% to 4% of all reported falls.

People who are at greatest risk for injury are those with:

- A history of previous falls (see Nursing Care Plan: The Patient with a History of Falls)
- Osteoporosis (especially white women over age 75)
- A prior stroke that has left the individual with hemiparesis (weakness or paralysis of one side of the body) or sensory impairment (vision or hearing deficits)
- Anticoagulation therapy
- Parkinson's disease
- Diabetes with peripheral neuropathies (decreased circulation and feeling in the lower extremities) and poor healing
- Falls associated with loss of consciousness or on a hard surface

Put on your THINKING CAP!!

Assess one of your patients in the clinical setting to identify intrinsic and extrinsic risk factors for falling. Develop nursing interventions to prevent falls in this specific situation.

RESTRAINTS

Restraints are frequently used to prevent falls. Restraints restrict individuals' movement and are classified as either physical or chemical. Physical restraints consist of vest, waist, wrist, or ankle ties. Wrist and ankle restraints may be made of soft material or leather. Anything that restricts movement, such as geriatric chairs or side rails, is considered a **physical restraint.** If patients are able to apply or release a safety device themselves, it is not considered a restraint. A **chemical restraint** is usually a psychotropic medication that is given to subdue agitated or confused patients.

PHYSICAL RESTRAINTS

Older patients are more likely to be physically restrained than younger patients, probably because of their greater likelihood of falling and confusion. The most common reasons given for using "protective" restraints with elderly patients in hospitals or long-term care facilities are (1) to protect the patient, equipment, or others from harm, (2) to prevent falls from the bed or chair, and (3) to prevent wandering. The most common incidents precipitating the use of restraints involve attempts to get out of bed or resistance to treatment while confused or disoriented.

Restraints seldom eliminate the risk of injury, however, and may actually cause or worsen problems. Patients are often able to untie their restraints and wriggle out of them, resulting in falls from wheelchairs and beds. In addition, accidental strangulation can occur when some forms of physical restraint, particularly a restraint vest, are used. The Food and Drug Administration has reported at least 100 restraint-related deaths each year. Nurses have long been taught to raise side rails so that vulnerable patients will either stay in bed or call for help. The wisdom of using side rails is now in question. Patients have been injured, sometimes fatally, after crawling over side rails or becoming trapped between side rail bars or between side rails and the mattress. A study of patients who had fallen out of bed revealed that 41% had raised side rails.

Restraints may have damaging psychological effects on older patients. Patients may experience anger, discomfort, resistance, and fear in response to physical restraint. Other behaviors noted include loss of self-image, growing dependency, increased confusion and disorientation, regressive behavior, and withdrawal.

Because the use of physical restraints can have so many negative effects, policies for use and alternatives have been developed. The Omnibus Reconciliation Act (OBRA) of 1987 was enacted to protect patients from unnecessary restraint in long-term care facilities. The law specifies that residents of such facilities have the right to be free from any physical restraints imposed and any psychoactive drug administered for the purposes of discipline or convenience and not required to treat residents' medical symptoms. Additionally, a physician's order is required for restraint use, and the order must specify the duration and the circumstances under which the restraint may be used. When OBRA regulations were enacted, health care providers predicted a surge of fall-related injuries. Although the number of falls did rise, most of those incidents did not result in serious injury. In fact, the most serious injuries occurred among patients who were restrained.

According to OBRA regulations, the only people who are considered restrainable are those who:

- Have a history of severe falls or are at extremely high risk of taking a fall that is *life-threatening*
- Are neurologically, orthopedically, or muscularly impaired and need postural support for safety or comfort, or both
- Experience any of a number of mental dysfunctions that may cause patients to be a *serious hazard* to themselves, objects, or others
- Have medical symptoms that are life-threatening, and a restraint is used *temporarily* to provide necessary treatment

If a physical restraint is used, the least restrictive device is best. For example, use a mitt rather than a wrist restraint that limits movement. Check the patient frequently, at least every 15 to 30 minutes. A patient who is agitated or combative must be monitored continuously. Make sure that the patient's condition is good and that the restraint is used properly and is providing adequate protection and comfort without impeding circulation or breathing. Remove and release physical restraints *every 2 hours* for 10 minutes to provide for range of motion, toileting, nourishment, and restorative activities such as physical therapy, ambulation, and mental stimulation.

Identify patients at risk for restraint so that you can try alternatives. Several alternatives to physical restraint include physical therapy, sitting and talking with patients for short periods of time, and asking staff to be responsible for wanderers in small blocks of time (Table 19-1). In addition, patients, family members, or both, should be involved in the decision to use or not to use physical restraint.

CHEMICAL RESTRAINTS

The same guidelines that apply to the use of physical restraints apply to chemical restraints. Never use psychoactive drugs for the purposes of discipline or convenience. Use them only when there is a danger of self-injury or injury to others. The administration of a psychoactive drug requires a physician's written order that specifies the duration and circumstance under which the medication is to be used.

table 19-1 ***Alternatives to Physical Restraint***

1. Provide general comfort measures.
2. Position with pillows, recliners, etc.
3. Change forms of treatment contributing to restraint use; e.g., substitute oral feedings for intravenous or nasogastric tubes and remove catheters or external urinary drains.
4. Provide companionship and supervision by involving staff, family, friends, or volunteers, especially at night.
5. Use therapeutic touch when appropriate.
6. Distract attention with television, radio, tape player, or other activities.
7. Use a circular or semicircular room arrangement around nursing station for maximal visibility.
8. Redesign furniture; e.g., lower beds or put mattress on floor, or remove wheels from furniture.
9. Manipulate environment to provide easy access to nurse and equipment; e.g., call bell accessible, bedside commode accessible, bed rails in down position, adequate lighting.
10. Provide a policy for a restraint-free environment that is supported by administration and staff.

Data from Strumpf, N. E., Evans, L. K., & Schwartz, D. (1991). Physical restraint of the elderly. In W. C. Chenitz, J. T. Stone, & S. A. Salisbury (Eds.), *Clinical gerontological nursing* (pp. 329-344). Philadelphia: Saunders.

Many psychoactive drugs are used, but the most commonly prescribed are lorazepam (Ativan), haloperidol (Haldol), and thioridazine (Mellaril). All have the potential for causing serious adverse effects, such as greater confusion, agitation, and an increased number of falls.

Psychotropic drugs, especially neuroleptics, antidepressants, and sedatives, commonly cause orthostatic hypotension, which may result in falls. Also, some antihypertensives and diuretics may produce orthostatic hypotension, leading to lightheadedness and falls.

Avoid the use of psychoactive drugs if at all possible. The same alternatives to physical restraints apply to chemical restraints (see Table 19-1).

NURSING ASSESSMENT AND INTERVENTION

FALL PREVENTION

The most important intervention for falls is prevention. The best prevention is education of patients and care givers about ways to prevent falls. Prevention is aimed toward minimizing both the intrinsic and the extrinsic factors causing falls and the potential for injury.

The first step in preventing falls and injury is to determine who is at greatest risk. People who are at greatest risk for falls and injury are those who have fallen before and those who have multiple intrinsic risk factors. Table 19-2 lists intrinsic risk factors for falling and possible interventions.

Fall prevention strategies are carried out in the home and institutional environments. Fall prevention guidelines for the home are listed in Table 19-3, and those for use in institutional settings are listed in Table 19-4.

In summary, basic strategies for reducing all types of falls include:

- Increase physical activities that enhance and maintain muscular strength, endurance, and flexibility.
- Increase regular, moderate physical exercise.
- Reduce visual impairments.
- Increase provider review of prescribed and over-the-counter medications.
- Increase provider screening and referral for alcohol and drug problems.
- Modify the environment to reduce or eliminate environmental factors that can cause falls, or to minimize injury if a fall occurs.

WHEN A FALL OCCURS

Some falls will occur no matter what precautions are taken. In some societies, such as in Great Britain, falls are viewed as indicators of greater activity and independence. Health care

table 19-2 ***Intrinsic Risk Factors for Falling and Possible Interventions***

RISK FACTORS	INTERVENTIONS
IMPAIRED VISION	
Reduced visual acuity	Be sure individual wears glasses, if appropriate. Keep glasses clean. Encourage regular eye examinations.
Impaired dark adaptation	Maintain adequate lighting; reduce glare from shiny floors and allow time to adjust to light levels (e.g., as patient moves from a dark room to outside). Use a night light in bedroom and bathroom.
IMPAIRED HEARING	
Impacted cerumen (ear wax)	Remove ear wax.
Presbycusis	Speak slowly; use low voice; decrease background noise. Encourage use of hearing aid.
BALANCE AND GAIT PROBLEMS	
Musculoskeletal disorders	Encourage balance and gait training and muscle-strengthening exercises.
Balance disorders	Encourage balance exercises.
Peripheral neuropathy	Encourage patient to use correctly sized footwear with firm soles.
FOOT DISORDERS	Trim toenails. Encourage patient to wear appropriate footwear.
CARDIOVASCULAR DISEASE	
Postural hypotension	Encourage dorsiflexion exercises. Use pressure-graded stockings. Elevate head of bed. Teach individual to get up from chair or bed slowly. Individual should avoid tipping head backward.
NEUROLOGIC DISEASE	
Stroke	Place call bell in visual field and within reach of arm that has use. Anticipate needs for toileting, dressing, eating, and bathing. Assist with transfer. Provide passive range-of-motion exercises to improve functional ability.

Data from Chenitz, W. C., Kussman, H. L., & Stone, J. T. (1991). Preventing falls. In W. C. Chenitz, J. T. Stone, & S. A. Salisbury (Eds.), *Clinical gerontological nursing* (p. 316). Philadelphia: Saunders.

table 19-3 ***Fall Prevention Guidelines for the Home: Instructions for the Client***

LIGHTS AND LIGHTING

1. Eyes tire quickly in improper lighting. Illuminate reading material or the object worked on. Illuminate steps, entranceways, and rooms before entering. Use 70- or 100-watt bulbs, not 60-watt bulbs.
2. Avoid glaring light caused by highly polished floors or large expanses of uncovered glass. Use sunglasses to avoid the glare of highway driving, but use light tints or photoray lenses.
3. Allow more time to adjust to changes in light levels. When going from a dark to a light room or vice versa, allow a minute or two for the eyes to accommodate to the change in light before proceeding.
4. Dirty glasses or outgrown prescription lenses inhibit vision. Keep glasses clean. Have regular eye examinations to identify changes and get new glasses when needed. If possible, do not use bifocals when walking because you cannot see the ground clearly.
5. Ability to see up, down, and sideways decreases with age. Observe the "lay of the land"; learn to look ahead at the ground to spot and avoid hazards such as cracks in the sidewalks. Use canes, walking sticks, and walkers that are prescribed.
6. At night, keep a night light on in your bedroom and bathroom. When getting out of bed at night, put the light on and wait a minute or two for the eyes to adjust before getting up. Have a telephone in the bedroom so you don't have to get out of bed to answer the phone. Before you go out in the evening or late afternoon, turn a light on for your return.

ACTIVITY

1. Get up from a chair slowly.
2. When getting out of bed, sit up, then wait a minute or two. Move to the side of the bed and wait another minute. Rest after sitting for a few minutes.
3. If you are dizzy, sit down immediately. Sit on a step or a chair, or ease yourself to the sidewalk if you are outdoors.

ACTIVITY—cont'd

4. Avoid tipping the head backward (extending the neck). Activities to avoid (because they extend the neck) are washing windows, hanging clothes, and getting things from high shelves.
5. Use shelves at eye level. Avoid rapid turning of the head.
6. If weather is rainy and windy, avoid going out.
7. Use alcohol and tranquilizers with caution.
8. Exercise programs keep bodies limber. Consult your physician and then enroll in a senior exercise program.
9. Shoes and slippers should be flat and rubber-soled. Avoid clothing such as long robes and loose-fitting garments that may catch on furniture or doorknobs.

AROUND THE HOUSE

1. Avoid scatter rugs and small bathroom mats that can slide. Repair loose, torn, wrinkled, or worn carpet.
2. Avoid slick, high polish on floors.
3. Put things in easy reach, and avoid reaching to high shelves.
4. Use nonskid treads on stairs and nonskid mats in tub.
5. You may wish to install a grab rail in the bath, in the shower, and also by the toilet.
6. Install handrails on both sides of the stairs. Paint stair edge in bright contrasting color.
7. Remove door thresholds.
8. Remove low-lying objects, such as coffee tables and extension cords.
9. Wipe up spills immediately.
10. Watch for pets underfoot and scattered pet food.
11. Check for even, nonglare lighting in every room, with easily accessible light switches.
12. Avoid floor coverings with complex patterns.
13. Avoid clutter in living areas.
14. Select furniture that provides stability and support, such as chairs with arms.
15. Check walking aids routinely, such as rubber tips on canes and screws on walkers.

From Chenitz, W. C., Stone, J. T., & Salisbury, S. A. (Eds.). (1991). *Clinical gerontological nursing* (p. 310). Philadelphia: Saunders.

providers accept a high number of falls as an inevitable risk that is outweighed by the benefits of physical activity and rehabilitation.

When a fall occurs in a hospital or long-term care facility, assess the circumstances of the fall and any injuries sustained. Document the fall according to the agency protocol. Note what the patient was doing at the time of the fall, the patient's mental and emotional status, and environmental factors that may have contributed to the fall. When the cause of the fall is determined, take steps to remove or correct the cause. Have the patient begin ambulating as soon after the fall as possible and at least several times a day in order to prevent the hazards of bedrest and to restore confidence. It is tempting to apply restraints after a fall, but avoid the use of restraints at all costs.

Dealing with falls in the home requires the cooperation of the person who is at risk, the family, and possibly neighbors. A plan of action for when a fall occurs should include information about getting up and seeking help.

There are several ways to get up after a fall in the home (Table 19-5). These techniques should be practiced by the potential faller to ensure confidence in managing the problem. If none of the methods is possible, a person who is at risk for falling would be wise to have a call system to obtain help from others. Devices worn around the neck that can send signals to a control center are very effective and provide a feeling of well-being for the potential faller. Additionally, having a person or agency call every day can provide reassurance.

table 19-4 ***Fall Prevention Techniques Used in Hospitals and Long-Term Care Facilities***

PATIENT ORIENTED

1. Encourage exercise to strengthen muscles and prevent weakness.
2. Use electronic alarm devices, such as Bed-Check Ambularm.

MEDICATIONS

1. Note hypnotic or sedative drugs given at night, especially to elderly or postoperative patients.
2. Note diuretics and laxatives given at night.

ACTIVITIES OF DAILY LIVING

1. Assist patient to void every 4 hours.
2. Check for proper slippers and footwear (nonskid footwear).
3. Keep patient's belongings close to bed.
4. Provide rehabilitation training to improve functional ability.

ENVIRONMENT ORIENTED

1. Relocate patients with high fall risk to rooms close to nurses' station or in hallway.
2. Place nurse call light system within reach (e.g., pinned to pillow).
3. Teach patient and family about use of call light system, bed controls, bathroom facility, and movable furniture.
4. Use bed rails judiciously; half rails best.
5. Keep bed in low position (ideally 14-20" above the floor, including the mattress)
6. Keep room light on, illumination bright and even.
7. Place TV controls within reach.
8. Keep rooms and hallways free of clutter.

ENVIRONMENT ORIENTED—cont'd

9. Carpet all hard surfaces. Use nonskid wax.
10. Clean up spills, including urine.
11. Lock all equipment with wheels.
12. Keep equipment on one side of hallway.
13. Maintain equipment in good repair.
14. Place night lights in rooms.
15. Place safety (grab) bars in bathroom and hall.
16. Install higher-seated lounge chairs and toilets, or use bedside commodes. Remove wheels from bedside commodes. Place safety posters in room to encourage patients to ask for help.

PATIENT EDUCATION

1. Hand out safety brochure to patient and family on admission.
2. Teach patient about safety and equipment; proper use of assistive devices.
3. Encourage patient to request help.
4. Encourage use of bathroom and corridor handrails.
5. Teach transfer from bed to chair.

NURSING ASSESSMENT

1. Perform assessment at admission and throughout hospital stay.
2. Assign safety risk.
3. Make frequent rounds/checks/observations.

OTHER

1. Monitor falls, watch for trends, and conduct in-service training when trend emerges.
2. Have staff move slowly around ambulatory, unsteady patients.

Adapted from Chenitz, W. C., Kussman, H. L., & Stone, J. T. (1991). Preventing falls. In W. C. Chenitz, J. T. Stone, & S. A. Salisbury (Eds.), *Clinical gerontological nursing* (pp. 309-328). Philadelphia: Saunders.

table 19-5 ***Methods for Getting Up After a Fall: Instructions for the Client***

THE ROLL

1. Roll onto your right side.
2. Bend the right knee.
3. Lever upward to the kneeling position by pressing down on the right forearm.
4. Reach out with the left arm to a nearby chair or bed.
5. With a twist of the trunk, pull yourself into a sitting position.
6. Sit on the chair or bed to recover.

THE CRAWL

1. Roll to a prone position.
2. Get up on all fours.
3. Crawl to a sturdy couch, chair, or bed and place your hands on it.
4. Bring one foot forward, putting the foot flat on the floor.

THE CRAWL—cont'd

5. Pull yourself up to a standing position.
6. Sit on chair or bed to recover.

THE SHUFFLE

1. Pull yourself to a sitting position on the floor.
2. Shuffle on the buttocks to a nearby piece of furniture.
3. Pull yourself up onto your knees directly in front of the item of furniture.
4. Stand up.

THE STAIR SHUFFLE

1. Pull yourself to a sitting position on the floor.
2. Shuffle on the buttocks to the stairs.
3. Gradually move up and backward to a stair height suitable for standing.
4. Grab onto the handrail and pull up.

Data from Chenitz, W. C., Kussman, H. L., & Stone, J. T. (1991). Preventing falls. In W. C. Chenitz, J. T. Stone, & S. A. Salisbury (Eds.), *Clinical gerontological nursing* (pp. 321-322). Philadelphia: Saunders.

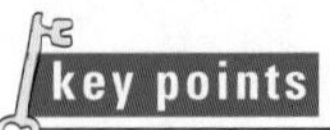

- The risk of injury from falls is highest in people over age 65, and falls are the most frequent cause of accidental injury and death among the elderly.
- The U.S. Public Health Service estimates that two thirds of the deaths due to falls are preventable.
- Falls occur in the elderly because of intrinsic factors, or factors related to the functioning of the individual, such as the aging process or physical illness, and extrinsic factors, or environmental factors.
- In an institutional setting, falls often occur during periods of high activity when the staff are busy.
- In about 65% to 75% of all reported falls, no injuries occur; fractures occur in about 1% to 4% of all reported falls.
- People who are at greatest risk for falls and injury are those who have fallen before and those who have multiple intrinsic risk factors.
- Older patients are more likely to be physically restrained than younger patients, probably because of their greater likelihood of falling and confusion.
- Restraints seldom eliminate the risk of injury and may actually cause or worsen problems.
- The Omnibus Reconciliation Act (OBRA) of 1987 was enacted to protect patients from unnecessary restraint in long-term care facilities.
- A physician's order is required for restraint use, and the order must specify the duration of use and the circumstances under which the restraint may be used.
- Alternatives to using physical restraint include physical therapy, sitting and talking with patients for short periods of time, and asking staff to be responsible for wanderers in small blocks of time.
- The most important intervention for falls is prevention, and the first step in preventing falls and injury is to determine who is at greatest risk.
- When a fall occurs in a hospital or long-term care facility, nurses should assess the circumstances of the fall and any injuries sustained and report the fall according to the protocol of the institution.
- When the cause of a fall is determined, steps should be taken to remove or correct the cause.
- Remove restraints for 10 minutes every 2 hours.

REVIEW QUESTIONS

1. **Of all falls among older adults, what percentage results in serious injury such as concussions or fractures?**
   1. Less than 10%
   2. 25%
   3. 40%
   4. 65%

2. **Of the following residents of an assisted living facility, which is at greatest risk for falling?**
   1. 72 year old male who has had 2 heart attacks and takes digitalis.
   2. 90 year old female with arthritis in her hips and hands.
   3. 85 year old male with early stage Alzheimer's disease.
   4. 80 year old female with osteoporosis and Parkinson's disease.

3. **Which statement is true regarding the use of restraints?**
   1. Anything that restricts movement and cannot be released by the patient is a restraint.
   2. Restraints greatly reduce the risk of injury.
   3. Side rails have been found to be very effective means of preventing falls.
   4. Restraints must be removed once each shift for exercise and to assess skin and circulation.

4. **Psychotropic drugs used to control agitation may contribute to falls because they often cause:**
   1. hallucinations and delusions.
   2. constipation.
   3. orthostatic hypotension.
   4. insomnia.

CHAPTER

20 Immobility

objectives

1. Describe common problems associated with immobility.
2. Discuss the impact of exercise and positioning on preventing complications related to immobility.
3. Identify the risk factors for pressure ulcers.
4. Describe the stages of pressure ulcers.
5. Describe methods of preventing and treating pressure ulcers.
6. Discuss the effects of immobility on respiratory status, nutrition, and elimination.

key terms

Active exercise (p. 269)
Contracture (kŏn-TRĂK-chŭr, p. 269)
Erythema (ĕr-ĭ-THĒ-mă, p. 270)
Immobility (p. 267)
Isometric exercise (ī-sō-MĔT-rĭk, p. 269)
Passive exercise (p. 269)
Pressure ulcer (ŬL-sĕr, p. 270)
Range-of-motion exercise (p. 269)
Shearing forces (p. 270)

Immobility (the inability to move) is a restriction imposed on all or part of the body. People become immobilized for various reasons, including chronic illness, pain, and age-related changes. Therapeutic reasons for **immobility** include (1) to obtain relief from pain and prevent further injury of a part, as in a fractured bone; (2) to reduce the workload of the heart in a cardiac or renal condition; (3) to promote healing and repair; and (4) to reverse the effects of gravity, as in abdominal hernias and prolapsed organs.

Immobility can have a profound impact on both the mind and the body. Psychosocial effects may include depression, fear, anxiety, social withdrawal, apathy, loss of financial and personal independence, and a feeling that one's life has no meaning. Almost every body system can be affected by immobility, depending on the extent and time of immobilization. The physiologic effects of immobility are described in Table 20-1.

Common aging changes, combined with common medical conditions, place the elderly at risk for immobility and its consequences. Examples of physical changes with age are decreased flexibility and strength and changes in posture and gait. In addition, the elderly typically have one or more chronic illnesses that increase the likelihood of immobilization. Examples of such medical conditions are arthritis, stroke, Parkinson's disease, cardiovascular disease, anemia, pulmonary disease, and foot deformities. Pain associated with chronic disease such as arthritis also may be a factor leading to immobility in the elderly. Drugs that cause drowsiness, hypotension, vertigo, or loss of sensory function can affect mobility as well.

PHARMACOLOGY CAPSULE Drugs that cause drowsiness, hypotension, vertigo, or loss of sensory function can impair mobility.

Psychosocial changes that can impair mobility include depression, dementia, bereavement, lack of motivation, fear of falling, isolation, and loss of friends. The older person's environment also can promote or hinder mobility. An unsafe home setting, hospitalization, or institutionalization, for example, may be associated with reduced activity. The older person who is hospitalized may quickly become debilitated and dependent as a result of the combined effects of inactivity, pain, drugs, various therapies such as bedrest or traction, and an unfamiliar environment.

The impact of immobilization on an individual depends on the duration, degree, and type of mobility limitation. Immobility begins a vicious cycle that can lead to an ever-increasing loss of independence for patients. As they become less able to move, they become more dependent. As they become more dependent, they are less able to care for themselves, which in turn leads to an increasing number of adverse effects from immobility.

Whatever the reason for resting a part or all of the body, some effort must be made to prevent the adverse effects of immobility. You can prevent the vicious cycle of events from the beginning by helping patients maintain normal functioning as much as possible and for as long as possible (see Nursing Care Plan: Preventing Hazards of Immobility). Once patients begin to suffer the ill effects of immobility, therapeutic interventions must be implemented immediately. The health care team must work together to develop a plan of care that includes preventive and therapeutic measures that address individual patients' needs. Remember that the patient and family are central members of the health care team. If able, they should participate in care planning.

table 20-1 ***Consequences of Immobility on Body Systems***

BODY SYSTEM	CONSEQUENCES
Musculoskeletal	Thickening of joint capsule; loss of smoothness of cartilage surface; decreased flexibility of connective tissues; changes similar to osteoarthritis—joint contractures, demineralization of bone, bone loss; atrophy and shortening of muscle; decrease in muscle strength; decreased muscle oxidative capacity; decline in aerobic capacity
Pulmonary	Arterial oxygen desaturation; increased hypostatic pooling; increased risk of atelectasis and infection
Cardiovascular	Decreased cardiac output and stroke volume; increased peripheral resistance; net loss of total body water and total blood volume
Integumentary	Pressure ulcers
Gastrointestinal	General weakening of muscles, causing altered colonic motility, constipation
Urinary	Increased nitrogen, phosphorus, total sulfur, sodium, potassium, and calcium excretion; renal insufficiency; decreased glomerular filtration rate; loss of ability to concentrate urine; lower creatinine tolerance
Metabolic	Decreased basal metabolic rate; increased storage of fat or carbohydrate; negative nitrogen and calcium metabolic balance due to decreased absorption of protein and calcium intake; decreased glucose tolerance; metabolic alkalosis
Sensory	Decreased sensory stimulation (kinesthetic, visual, auditory, tactile); decreased social interaction; changes in affect, cognition, and perception

Modified from Chenitz, W. C., Stone, J. T., & Salisbury, S. A. (1991). *Clinical gerontological nursing* (p. 234). Philadelphia: Saunders.

NURSING CARE PLAN

Preventing Hazards of Immobility

ASSESSMENT

Health History: An 84-year-old woman has been living in a long-term care facility for the past 2 years after falling and breaking a wrist, which interfered with her ability to shop, cook, and dress herself. While in the facility, she continues to fall many times and prefers to keep to herself in her room. She stays in her bed or in a chair most of the time and has become so weak that she has to use a wheelchair to move about. She is incontinent of urine and mildly confused.

Physical Examination: Blood pressure, 130/78; pulse, 96; respiration, 26; temperature, 96.7° F. Height, 5'3"; weight, 126 lb. Unable to hold urine long enough to void in the bathroom. Skin intact. Appears quiet, sad, and depressed. Does not interact with others. Daughter visits two to three times a week.

Nursing Diagnosis	*Goals and Outcome Criteria*	*Interventions*
Risk for injury related to weakness	The patient will remain free of injury due to weakness.	Walk with patient three times daily, gradually increasing distance as tolerated. Teach isometric exercises that can be done while lying and sitting to increase strength. Teach and assist in active range-of-motion exercises. Carry out exercises while assisting with daily care.
Functional urinary incontinence related to immobility	The patient will maintain continence as evidenced by lack of soiling of underwear and clothes.	Place on a schedule for toileting. Remind patient q 2 hr to go to the bathroom to urinate.
Risk for impaired skin integrity related to pressure	The patient's skin will remain intact.	Change position at least every 2 hr. Maintain adequate nutrition.
Social isolation related to declining health	The patient will demonstrate social interaction, as evidenced by attendance at functions and visits and phone calls with significant others.	Encourage patient to attend activities that are offered. Have the patient go to the bathroom immediately before activity to decrease the possibility of accidents. Encourage family members and friendly visitors to make short, periodic visits. Visit with patient at least once per shift for at least 10 minutes. Encourage patient to listen to favorite radio and television shows.

NURSING ASSESSMENT AND INTERVENTION

A thorough assessment of the patients' needs and limitations is essential to planning interventions. Physicians may write specific orders related to immobility, or it may be up to the nurse to carry out independent measures to prevent the side effects of immobility. Nursing interventions include promoting exercise, adequate respiratory status, adequate food and fluid intake, proper elimination, and maintaining proper positioning and skin integrity (see Case Study).

CASE STUDY

Mrs. Smith is an 84-year-old woman who has resided in an intermediate care facility for 2 years. She was admitted to the facility because she had been living at home alone and had become unable to shop and cook for herself or to dress herself after sustaining a broken wrist as a result of a fall. She was incontinent of urine and was mildly confused.

Mrs. Smith had previously been quite active in the community, but in the residential home she remained confined to her room and was not interested in interacting with other people. Her daughter visited her two or three times a week.

Because Mrs. Smith preferred to stay in bed or in a chair most of the time, the nurses and other members of the interdisciplinary team were concerned about the consequences of her immobility. She had fallen many times, usually on the way to the dining room to eat. It had reached the point where she stayed in a wheelchair most of the time because she had become too weak to walk.

The team held a case conference and identified problems associated with her immobility: (1) continued falling, (2) incontinence, and (3) isolation and perhaps depression. They formulated a plan to get her up and moving while at the same time avoiding falls. Every day the nurse walked with Mrs. Smith three times a day. The first week they walked around the bed. The second week they walked to the door and back. The third week they walked a few feet outside the door to her room. As the weeks progressed, Mrs. Smith was able to walk to the dining room at the end of the hall without falling. The nurses encouraged the in-bed and in-chair exercises to further build up her strength.

Eventually, Mrs. Smith was able to walk to the bathroom independently. The nurses worked with her to develop a regular schedule of toileting so that the number of "accidents" decreased. Because she was a little bit confused and disoriented, the nurses provided gentle reminders for her to go to the bathroom. After a meal, they would guide her back to her room to use the bathroom. At other times they would stop by her room, look in, and suggest that she go to the bathroom.

With all of the increased activity, Mrs. Smith became more outgoing and involved in activities. She sat with the same group at meals and developed friendships with others around her. The nurses found that taking small steps with a walking program can have many benefits for a person of any age in any condition.

EXERCISE

Exercise is the best medicine for immobility. Exercise can be done anywhere. A well individual of any age can walk, participate in aerobic exercises, swim, engage in sports activities, garden, or do housework. Those who are ill or disabled can perform modified exercise regardless of the acuity of their disease. For example, patients with fractures can tighten and relax muscles in an immobilized extremity; debilitated patients can gradually increase their range of movement, number of movements, or resistance against movement; and patients in pain can move slowly and smoothly while breathing deeply to ease pain and anxiety.

Exercises may be *active* (performed by the patients themselves), or *passive* (movement of the patient's body performed by the therapist or nurse without assistance from the patient). Active and passive exercises may be done with the patient lying down in bed, sitting in a chair, or standing upright. The exercises do not have to be done as a separate part of care. They can easily be carried out while giving other care, such as during a bed bath or other activities. Examples of bed and chair exercises are listed in Table 20-2.

Range-of-Motion Exercises

Range-of-motion exercises are effective in preventing disabilities of the musculoskeletal system as well as other systems. Each of the joints of the body has a range of motion—that is, the limits to which the joint may be moved. Muscular activity maintains range of motion by allowing the joint to remain flexible and functional. When there is little or no movement of a joint, its structures change. Normal muscle tissue is replaced by fibrous tissue. Muscles shorten and lose their elasticity. Shortening of muscles and tendons is called a *contracture.* A contracture can severely and permanently limit joint movement.

The purpose of range-of-motion exercises is to put each joint that is at risk for loss of motion through its full range of motion to the highest degree possible. The major motions are rotation, flexion, extension, abduction, and adduction. The exercises may be active or passive. Range-of-motion exercises should be initiated very early in immobile patients to prevent contractures.

Isometric Exercises

Isometric exercises maintain muscle tone without moving the joint. In these exercises, the muscle is contracted and held in that position for several seconds. The muscle is then relaxed for a few seconds and contracted again. This type of exercise is especially helpful in maintaining muscle strength after a fracture.

POSITIONING

Proper positioning in a bed or chair is extremely important for preventing many of the side effects of immobility. Change the position of the patient *at least every 2 hours* to prevent undue pressure on the skin. Maintain joints in their functional positions so that they are not abnormally flexed or extended.

Use foot boards, splints, and bed boards to maintain proper positioning for patients lying in bed. Foot boards keep the feet at right angles to the legs so that foot drop is avoided. Splinting the limbs keeps them straight. Using a bed board

table 20-2 ***Sample Exercises***

IN-BED EXERCISES	IN-CHAIR EXERCISES
Deep breathing (slow inhalation and full exhalation)	Deep breathing
Neck rolls (neck forward flex, backward extend, lateral flex, rotate)	Head rolls (neck forward flex, backward extend, lateral flex, rotate)
Knee to chest (on back or side, bring one knee to chest, wrap arms around, hold and breathe, straighten leg slowly)	Knee to chest
Pelvic tilts (on back, knees bent, feet flat, tuck in tummy, relax)	Head to knees
Bridging (on back, feet flat on bed, raise hips, lower slowly)	Shoulder rolls (forward and back)
Head raising in prone and supine positions	Weight shifts (hip to hip)
Unilateral leg lifts	Hands on head, elbows out and in, lateral trunk flex-extension, trunk rotation
Foot dorsiflexion	Leg lifts
Rolling	Ankle rotation and dorsiflexion
Prone lying	Ankle on knee (external hip rotation, put ankle on opposite knee and lower the bent leg)
Arms straight over head of bed in supine position	Push down on legs as if to stand, lean forward, bear weight
Arms out to sides, palms up, in supine position	
Hands behind head, elbow bent	
Hands at lower back	

From Giduz, B. H., Snow, T. L., Wildman, D. L., & McConnell, E. S. (1986). *Geriatric first aid kit* (p. 5). Chapel Hill, NC: Program on Aging, University of North Carolina.

prevents curvature of the spine. In addition, placing a firm splint in the hands keeps the fingers from drawing up into a tight fist. Avoid positioning the patient with the knees and hips flexed. Picture how people look while standing and try to achieve that position while they are lying down.

SKIN INTEGRITY

To reduce the risk of pressure ulcers, position patients so that they are not resting on pressure points of the skin. *Pressure ulcers* are localized areas of tissue necrosis (tissue death) that tend to develop when soft tissue is compressed between a bony prominence and an external surface for a prolonged period. Pressure points are areas over bony prominences such as the elbows, hips, shoulders, and sacrum (Fig. 20-1). The most frequent sites of skin breakdown are the sacrum (35%), ischial tuberosities (16%), heels (11%), trochanters (7%), ankles (3%), and scapulae (2%). The National Pressure Ulcer Advisory Panel prefers the term *pressure ulcers* for what are commonly called "bed sores," "decubitus ulcers," or "decubiti." The word *decubitus* means "lying down," and an ulcer is a lesion produced by the sloughing of necrotic, inflammatory tissue (Fig. 20-2). Thus a decubitus ulcer is an open wound that is associated with lying in bed. However, skin breakdown can just as easily develop in patients who are sitting for a long period of time, as a result of pressure against blood vessels.

Development of Pressure Ulcers

An area of *erythema* (redness) is the beginning of a pressure ulcer and a sign that capillaries in the area have become congested because of impaired blood flow. Erythema can occur within an hour or two in a person with healthy skin and adequate circulation. It is even more likely to develop and to progress rapidly to an ulcerated stage in persons who are malnourished, obese, aged, or suffering from circulatory disease.

Factors in addition to immobility that contribute to the development of pressure ulcers are shearing forces, chemical irritants such as urine, sedation, and poor nutrition. *Shearing forces* exert a downward and forward pressure on tissues underlying the skin. Shearing action occurs when a patient slumps down while sitting in bed or in a chair; it also can occur when boosting a patient up in bed.

Pressure ulcers are expensive to treat, result in longer hospital stays, increase the likelihood of placement in a long-term care facility, and increase mortality. Therefore, it is important to prevent their development whenever possible. *Nursing care is a major factor in pressure ulcer prevention.*

Preventing Pressure Ulcers

The first step in prevention of pressure ulcers is to identify patients who are at risk for developing them. The Norton scale is a useful instrument for identifying those at risk (Fig. 20-3). The scores for all five categories are added. If the total score is greater than 14, there is little risk of pressure ulcer development. If the score is less than 14, there is significant risk for pressure ulcer development. Any patient with a score of less than 14 needs a formal pressure ulcer prevention program started as soon as the risk is recognized. The skin of "at risk" patients should be assessed and documented every day.

A pressure ulcer prevention protocol consists of the following:

1. In accordance with a *written* schedule, reposition the bed patient *at least* every 2 hours (more often if redness persists).
2. Teach wheelchair patients to shift their weight every 15 minutes if able. Patients who cannot do this should be repositioned at least hourly.
3. Keep bed linens dry, smooth, and free of wrinkles.
4. Gently cleanse the skin when soiled and at regular intervals, using warm water and a mild cleansing agent.

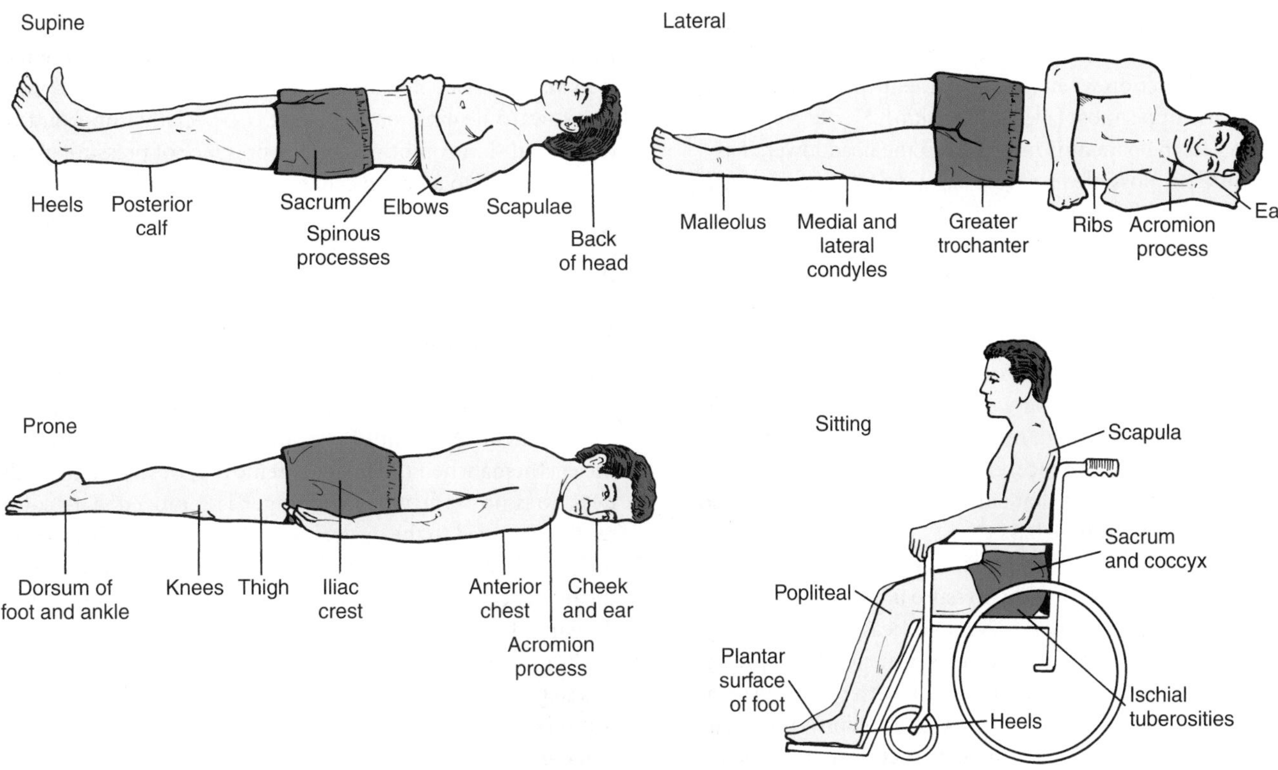

FIGURE **20-1** Possible locations of pressure ulcers.

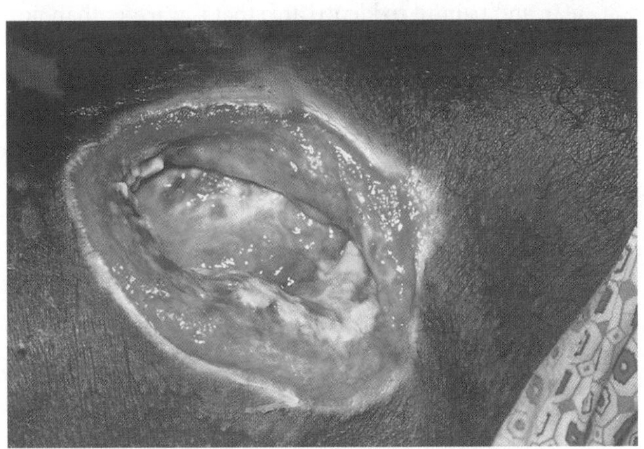

FIGURE **20-2** Stage IV pressure ulcer, with full-thickness involvement of all soft tissue.

NORTON SCALE

		PHYSICAL CONDITION	MENTAL CONDITION	ACTIVITY	MOBILITY	INCONTINENT	
		Good 4 Fair 3 Poor 2 Very bad 1	Alert 4 Apathetic 3 Confused 2 Stupor 1	Ambulant 4 Walk/help 3 Chairbound 2 Bedrest 1	Full 4 Slightly limited 3 Very limited 2 Immobile 1	Not 4 Occasional 3 Usually/urine 2 Doubly 1	TOTAL SCORE
Name	Date						

FIGURE **20-3** Norton scale for identification of those at risk for the development of pressure ulcers.

5. Use moisturizers, lubricants, protective films, barriers, and dressings to reduce friction and shearing.
6. Avoid friction when moving patients to prevent damage to the uppermost layers of the skin.
7. When the patient is in bed, keep the head lowered as much as possible to reduce shearing force caused by sliding down in bed.
8. Use a special mattress or bed designed to reduce pressure, such as an egg crate foam (minimum 2 inches thick), static air, alternating air, gel, fluidized air, or water mattress (Fig. 20-4).
9. Apply sheepskin boots to prevent shearing forces to the feet and use pillows or wedges to prevent heel pressure.
10. Protect the skin from moisture (absorbent pads or briefs for incontinence, etc).
11. Institute measures that enhance patient mobility, such as installing trapeze bars.
12. Instruct the patient and family about risk factors and strategies for preventing pressure ulcers.

Remember that the best preventive measure is frequent position change. Massage is *not* recommended for pressure points. Any kind of massage around or on a reddened area of skin can damage fragile capillaries. In addition, rubber rings should *not* be used to elevate heels or sacral areas. Rings cause a concentrated area of pressure that puts patients at higher risk for developing pressure ulcers. *Remember: No massage on reddened skin, and no rings!* One other important factor that must be considered is the patient's nutritional status. Adequate nutrients are essential to maintain or restore skin integrity.

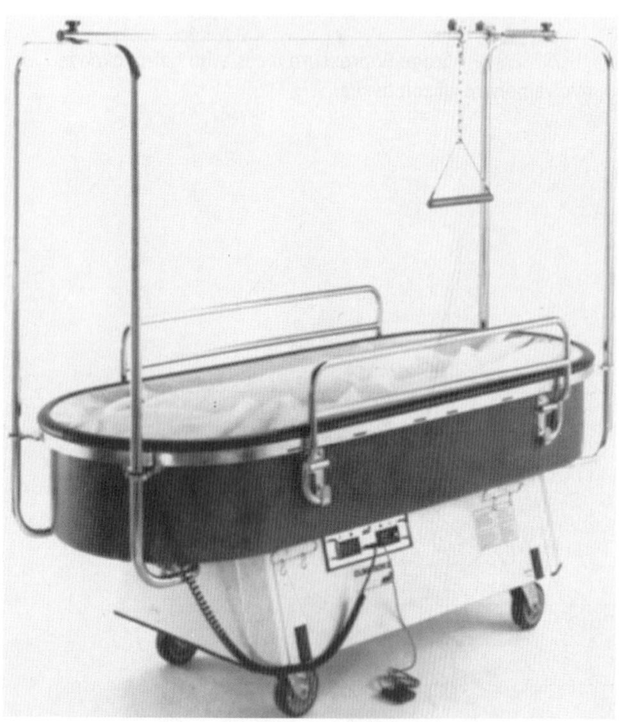

FIGURE **20-4** CLINITRON Air Fluidized Therapy Unit.

If pressure ulcers develop despite all preventive measures, assess the stage and describe it precisely. Proper documentation helps to evaluate the effectiveness of treatment and progress toward healing and repair. It is especially important to document skin condition and the presence of pressure ulcers on admission to a health care facility.

Stages of Pressure Ulcers

Pressure ulcers are classified into four stages (Fig. 20-5).

Stage I

The major characteristic of stage I is erythema (redness) that does not blanch when pressed. Before stage I begins, a finger pressed on a reddened area causes temporary blanching (whiteness at the point of pressure), followed by a return of the erythema when the finger is removed. In stage I, the redness does not fade when the finger is removed. The color ranges from red to the dusky blue called *cyanosis*. The area of pressure is irregular and ill-defined and reflects the shape of the object creating the pressure or the bony prominence underlying the skin. Pain and tenderness may be present, with swelling and hardening of the tissue and associated heat. At this stage there is little destruction of tissue, and the condition is reversible.

Stage II

In stage II, there is some skin loss in the epidermis and dermis. A shallow ulcer develops and appears blistered, cracked, or abraded (scraped). The ulcer is surrounded by a broad, irregular, and painful reddened area that is warmer than normal.

Stage III

Stage III is characterized by full-thickness skin loss involving damage or necrosis of the dermis and subcutaneous tissue. There is a crater-like sore with a distinct outer margin formed as the epidermis thickens and rolls over the edge toward the ulcer base. The wound may be infected, and it is usually open and draining, with a loss of fluid and protein. The patient may have fever, dehydration, anemia, and leukocytosis (increased white blood cells in the blood).

Stage IV

There is full-thickness skin loss with extensive destruction of the deeper underlying muscle and possibly of the bone tissue. The ulcer is usually extensively infected and may appear black, with exudation, foul odor, and purulent drainage.

Treatment

The first step in treating pressure ulcers is to continue all preventive measures. A pressure ulcer cannot heal unless measures are taken to relieve the pressure that initially caused it. Numerous treatments are used to promote wound healing. These treatments vary from institution to institution because research has not yet shown one method of treatment to be the best.

In general, stages I and II pressure ulcers should be cleaned with mild soap and water or normal saline. Avoid using pastes, creams, ointments, and powder because they may promote infection in the ulcer. Also avoid using alcohol, antiseptics, disinfectants, topical and oral antibiotics, and massage because their effectiveness has not been proved, and they may actually

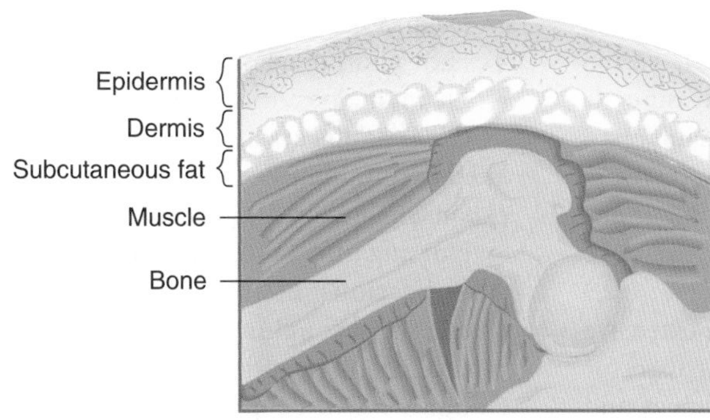
Stage I
Epidermis
Dermis
Subcutaneous fat
Muscle
Bone
Non-blanching erythema of intact skin; the heralding lesion of skin ulceration

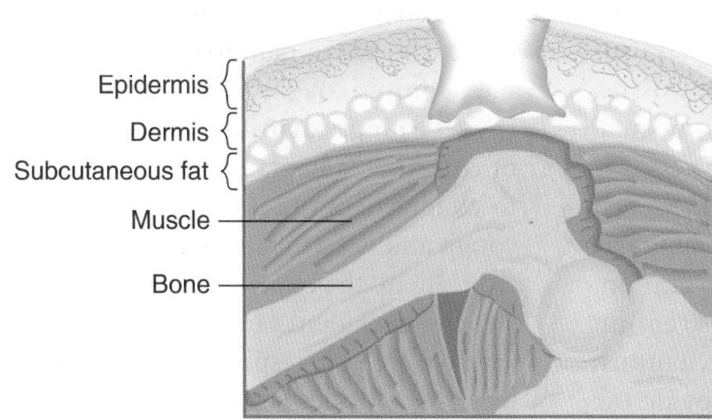
Stage II
Epidermis
Dermis
Subcutaneous fat
Muscle
Bone
Partial-thickness skin loss involving epidermis and/or dermis. The ulcer is superficial and presents clinically as an abrasion, blister, or shallow crater.

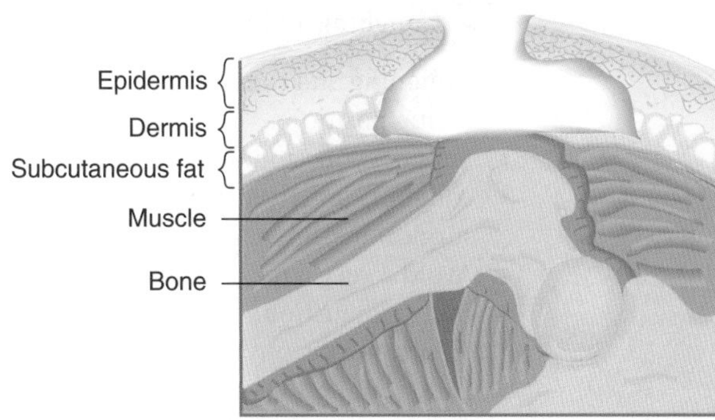
Stage III
Epidermis
Dermis
Subcutaneous fat
Muscle
Bone
Full-thickness skin loss involving damage or necrosis of subcutaneous tissue, which may extend down to, but not through, the underlying fascia. The ulcer presents clinically as a deep crater with or without undermining of adjacent tissue.

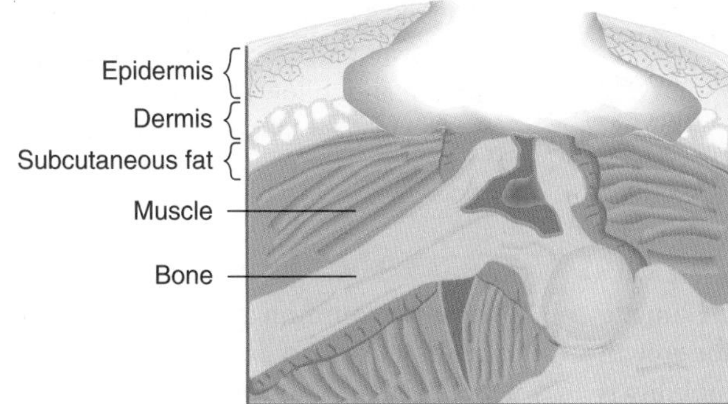
Stage IV
Epidermis
Dermis
Subcutaneous fat
Muscle
Bone
Full-thickness skin loss with extensive destruction, tissue necrosis, or damage to muscle, bone, or supporting structures (e.g., tendon, joint capsule, etc.)

FIGURE **20-5** Classification of pressure ulcers.

cause harm. The use of a heat lamp is not recommended because a rise in temperature increases the metabolic demands of the tissue and places additional stress on the affected area.

The most effective dressing for a stage I or II pressure ulcer is one that provides a moist environment and maintains a temperature close to body temperature. All wound covers should allow oxygen to pass through. Wound healing is enhanced when the ulcer and surrounding tissues can freely take up oxygen and eliminate carbon dioxide.

Stages III and IV pressure ulcers require more extensive treatment and supportive care. Mechanical devices used for irrigation include spray bottles, bulb and piston syringes, and other specialized irrigating devices including a Water Pik. Note that excess pressure can cause trauma and may force bacteria into the wound. The Water Pik should be used only on the lowest setting. Debridement of necrotic tissue is usually necessary to promote granulation of new, healthy tissue. Wet-to-dry dressings and whirlpool baths are used for small amounts of debridement. Surgery is preferred for very advanced cases. Debridement is sufficient when the ulcer bed appears pink, indicating healthy granulation tissue. Supportive care consists of measures to treat anemia, dehydration, protein depletion, and infection. Nutritional intervention consists of oral supplements high in protein and vitamins, nasogastric feedings, or parenteral nutrition to provide the additional nutrients necessary for healing.

Stages II, III, and IV are normally colonized with bacteria. Good wound care usually prevents the bacteria from causing a clinical infection. Topical broad-spectrum antibiotics may be ordered if the wound fails to heal despite good care. If there is evidence of widespread infection, systemic antibiotics are indicated.

In addition to preventive measures, three major principles of wound management should be followed in the treatment of pressure ulcers:

1. Keep the area clean.
2. Promote the formation of granulation tissue by removing debris and dead tissue.
3. Ensure adequate nutritional intake for wound healing.

RESPIRATORY STATUS

Oxygen and carbon dioxide exchanges occur in the thin, moist mucous membrane that lines the airway passages and the alveoli. Most healthy people take about six to eight deep, sighing breaths every hour. Sighs help keep the lungs expanded and move secretions upward along the air passages. When a person remains immobile or does not take deep breaths, thick secretions can accumulate and pool in the lower respiratory structures. These secretions interfere with the normal exchange of gases, can cause areas of the lung to collapse (atelectasis), and provide an environment for growth of pathogens. A lung infection associated with immobility is called hypostatic pneumonia.

Individuals who are at risk for impaired gas exchange related to immobility include those who:

- Are given drugs that depress respirations, such as general anesthetic agents, narcotics, or sedatives
- Have tight binders or bandages that limit chest expansion
- Have abdominal distention from gas, fluid, or feces
- Lie in one position for extended periods of time

Older adults are also at risk for respiratory problems related to immobility because age-related changes reduce lung expansion and breathing capacity.

Nursing interventions for patients at risk for respiratory complications include frequent turning and position changes and coughing and deep breathing exercises. These interventions must be done every 2 hours to be effective. Coughing and deep breathing exercises are done at the same time to allow for periods of rest and to obtain the best results.

Effective coughing may be difficult for patients, especially those who are in pain from a surgical incision or those who have chronic coughs and are worried that the coughing may trigger a long, exhaustive coughing experience. The objective of coughing is to gradually move the secretions upward and to cough them out a little at a time. Teach patients how to cough and deep breathe effectively.

Evaluate the effectiveness of nursing interventions by assessing the patient's respiratory status. Count the respiratory rate, observe the respiratory effort and chest movement, and listen for crackles in the lung fields.

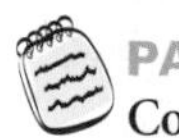

PATIENT TEACHING PLAN
Coughing and Deep Breathing

- Coughing and deep breathing are most effective in a sitting position.
- Support your abdomen to minimize discomfort while coughing and deep breathing (especially if you have a surgical incision and sutures).
- Avoid a very large, explosive cough that can be painful or cause exhaustion.
- To breathe deeply, expand the lower chest and use the abdominal muscles and diaphragm.
- Concentrate on exhaling slowly while pursing your lips.
- Focus on how much air you can exhale rather than the force with which you exhale it.
- The most effective technique for clearing secretions from the lower parts of the air passages is to take a single deep breath and follow it with three consecutive coughs, trying to clear all the air from the lungs with each cough.

FOOD AND FLUID INTAKE

The most common problem associated with immobility in relation to food and fluid intake is *anorexia* (loss of appetite). Factors that contribute to anorexia are worry, depression, anxiety about dependence on others, and decreased metabolic needs resulting from inactivity. *Hypoproteinemia* (protein deficiency) can develop in immobilized patients.

Immobilized patients also may have inadequate fluid intake. Getting up for a drink of water may be too difficult and time-consuming for inactive individuals, or they may not think to drink liquids regularly. Older people are particularly prone to becoming dehydrated from an inadequate fluid intake, resulting in complications such as confusion, constipation, or urinary tract infection.

Keep accurate records of patients' dietary and fluid intakes. Small, frequent meals are usually more effective than three large meals for anorectic patients. Dietary supplements with high protein content also may be encouraged. Offer fluids, even small sips of water, juice, or other liquids, at least every hour. Fluids need to be within reach so that patients may have easy access to them if they are able to drink without help. Encourage family members to offer fluids while they are visiting.

ELIMINATION

Constipation

One of the most common disorders associated with inactivity and immobility is constipation. Factors that contribute to constipation in the immobile patient include changes in the usual routine and environment, inability to defecate on a bedpan because of embarrassment or discomfort, and weakened muscle tone. Also, many medications cause constipation by slowing intestinal motility. Constipated individuals may strain to defecate, causing an increase in intra-abdominal pressure. This is called the *Valsalva maneuver* or vasovagal reflex, and it can lead to cardiovascular alterations and, ultimately, to lightheadedness and fainting. The vasovagal reflex can be especially problematic in older persons, whose circulation may be somewhat impaired.

Confused patients may ignore the normal urge to have a bowel movement. If the impulse is ignored for a considerable time, the natural urge to defecate can diminish and eventually disappear.

Long-standing constipation can result in a fecal impaction. *Fecal impaction* is the presence of hardened or puttylike feces in the rectum and sigmoid colon. If the condition is not relieved, intestinal obstruction can occur. Symptoms of a fecal impaction include painful defecation, a feeling of fullness in the rectum, abdominal distention, and sometimes cramps and watery stool. The presence of diarrhea does not mean that a fecal impaction has been removed because the liquid fecal material may flow around the hardened mass.

When an impaction develops, the mass of feces must be broken up with a gloved finger (a doctor's order usually is needed). Before digital removal of the mass, it may be helpful to give an oil retention enema to soften the mass. In addition, an analgesic may be given 1 hour before digital removal of an impaction.

Inactivity, medications, decreased fluid intake, and lack of adequate fiber in the diet can combine to cause constipation. The vicious cycle of immobility promotes inactivity, decreased fluid intake, and poor appetite. Patients become weaker, more immobile, and less likely to eat and drink adequately. Encouraging proper foods with adequate roughage, fluids, and as much activity as possible can help prevent or relieve constipation. Whenever possible, patients should use a bedside commode or be taken to the bathroom to defecate to avoid the difficulties of using a bedpan. Laxatives should be used sparingly; however, stool softeners may be helpful if the stools are hard and difficult to pass. Patients with long-established laxative dependence may require continued laxative therapy during the period of immobility.

Urinary Incontinence

The urinary system functions best when the body is upright. Urine flows from the kidney downward, drawn by the pull of gravity. When the body is in a reclining position, the kidney must force urine into the ureters against the pull of gravity. Urine is continually being formed in the kidney, but the peristaltic action of the ureters is not strong enough to maintain a constant flow of urine. If the body remains in a supine (lying down) position for even a few days, the flow becomes sluggish and the urine pools. This sets the stage for the development of a urinary tract infection.

Lying in bed also can cause loss of control of the urinary sphincter muscles and result in incontinence. Without the downward pressure of the full bladder against the sphincter muscles, there is less awareness of the need to void. The result can be bladder distention and an overflow or a dribbling of urine that the patient cannot control.

Elderly individuals who have problems with mobility may have functional incontinence because they are unable to respond to the urge to void in time. The bladder is usually more full when the urge to void occurs, so there is less time to get to the bathroom. In addition, their bodies may not be able to move quickly enough because of the slowed reflexes and responses associated with older age or infirmities associated with chronic illness.

The most effective way to prevent urinary incontinence associated with immobility is to set up a toileting program. Patients should have scheduled toiletings with adjustments in schedule based on the patient's voiding patterns. If voiding patterns cannot be assessed, patients should at the very least be taken to the bathroom or commode or offered a bedpan every 2 hours during the waking hours. Some individuals restrict fluids at certain times of the day, especially after dinner and through the night to avoid nighttime incontinence. However, studies have been inconclusive regarding the effectiveness of limiting fluids. Incontinence is covered in greater detail in Chapter 22.

Put on your ***THINKING CAP!!***

1. With pencil and paper in hand, note the time. Now, sit perfectly still for 10 minutes. At the end of that time, note what sensations and thoughts you experienced. When the time was up, what was the first thing you did? Discuss what a nurse could have done to make you more comfortable. Compare your experience with that of a patient who is immobilized.
2. Observe a person during class, church, a movie, or other situation where people are expected to stay seated. Note the number of movements by that person in a 5-minute period. Identify the therapeutic value of those motions.

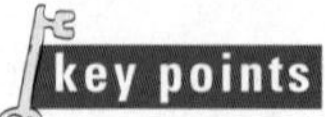

- The psychological effects of immobility may include depression, fear, anxiety, social withdrawal, apathy, loss of financial and personal independence, and lack of meaningful existence.
- Some of the most problematic physiologic side effects of immobility are pressure ulcers, respiratory problems, impaired nutrition, constipation, and urinary tract infection and incontinence.
- Exercise is the best medicine for immobility.
- Exercises may be active (performed by the patient) or passive (movement of the patient's body performed by the therapist or nurse without assistance from the patient).
- Pressure ulcers are expensive to treat, result in longer hospital stays, increase the likelihood of placement in a residential care facility, and increase mortality.
- Good nursing care is a major factor in pressure ulcer prevention.
- The best preventive measure for pressure ulcers is frequent position changes.
- The major principles of pressure ulcer wound management are the following: (1) clean the area, (2) promote the formation of granulation tissue, and (3) ensure adequate nutritional intake for wound healing.
- Especially in older adults, immobility can contribute to respiratory problems, including impaired gas exchange, atelectasis, and hypostatic pneumonia.
- Factors that contribute to respiratory complications of immobility include drugs that depress respirations; tight binders or bandages that limit chest expansion; abdominal distention from gas, fluid, or feces; and lying in one position for extended periods of time.
- Nursing interventions for patients at risk for respiratory complications include frequent turning and position changes, and encouraging coughing and deep breathing exercises.
- The most common problem associated with immobility in relation to nutrition is anorexia (loss of appetite).
- Immobility causes constipation by causing a change in the usual routine and environment, an inability to defecate on a bedpan because of embarrassment or discomfort, and a weakening of muscle tone.
- Immobility can promote a loss of control of the urinary sphincter muscles, resulting in incontinence.
- The most effective way to prevent urinary incontinence associated with immobility is to set up a toileting program.
- Urinary stasis increases the risk of urinary tract infections.

REVIEW QUESTIONS

1. A patient who sustained a head injury has not regained consciousness. The nurse moves the patient's joints through their normal movements twice a day. This intervention is called:

1. isometric exercise.
2. active exercise.
3. passive exercise.
4. isotonic exercise.

2. The home health nurse is teaching family members how to move a patient up in bed by using a draw sheet to prevent:

1. tissue trauma from shearing force.
2. strain on the care giver.
3. disturbing the bed linens.
4. extension contractures of the spine.

3. The nursing care plan for an immobilized patient includes the following interventions. Which one is specifically intended to maintain skin integrity?

1. Keep joints in functional positions.
2. Reposition patient at least every 2 hours.
3. Perform range-of-motion exercises twice daily.
4. Give at least eight 8-ounce glasses of fluids each day.

4. During a bed bath, you observe a reddened area over the sacrum. You should:

1. document erythema and instruct nursing assistants to keep the patient off his back.
2. gently massage the reddened area with skin lotion to provide protective moisture.
3. place a round inflatable cushion under the patient's buttocks to relieve pressure on the sacrum.
4. position the patient on one side and use a heat lamp to stimulate circulation to the area.

5. Instructions in effective coughing for the postoperative patient should include:

1. Try not to use the abdominal muscles during coughing and deep breathing exercises.
2. Assume a comfortable side-lying position to reduce strain on the incision.
3. Exhale as forcefully and as long as you can.
4. Take one deep breath and then cough three times, trying to clear all air from the lungs.

6. A postoperative patient reports that she was straining to have a bowel movement when she became lightheaded. You should suspect:
   1. the Valsalva maneuver.
   2. internal hemorrhage.
   3. dehydration.
   4. wound dehiscence.

7. What is the effect of immobility on the urinary tract?
   1. Decreased urine production by the kidneys
   2. Pooling of urine in the urinary system
   3. Increased blood flow to kidneys
   4. Increased bladder sensitivity to fullness

CHAPTER

21 Confusion

objectives

1. Define delirium and dementia.
2. Identify the causes of acute confusion.
3. Explain the differences between delirium and dementia.
4. Discuss nursing assessment and interventions related to delirium and dementia.

key terms

Delirium (dĕ-LĬR-ē-ŭm, p. 278)
Dementia (dē-MĔN-shē-ă, p. 278)

Confusion is a symptom experienced by various patients under varying circumstances. Older people often experience confusion as a first symptom of disease. People of all ages may experience confusion in the intensive care unit or in the post anesthesia care unit after surgery. Confusion may be acute, transient, or permanent. It has many causes and names and can be very difficult to manage.

The collection of symptoms associated with confusion falls into two categories: (1) acute confusional states, or delirium, and (2) chronic confusion, or dementia. ***Delirium*** is a short-term confusional state that has a sudden onset and is typically reversible. It is more prevalent in children and the elderly. ***Dementia*** is a syndrome that is chronic and irreversible. It is characterized by impairment in memory and accompanied by many other cognitive deficits. Dementia is most prevalent in the elderly. Delirium and dementia have been called *organic brain syndrome, acute brain syndrome, chronic brain syndrome, senile dementia,* and *senility.*

DELIRIUM

Delirium is characterized by disturbances in consciousness that impair a person's awareness of the environment. People with delirium may have difficulty focusing or paying attention, so that they are easily distracted. It may be difficult to engage people with delirium in a conversation, and questions often must be repeated several times. Impaired recent memory is common, along with disorientation and language problems. Speech may be slurred and disjointed, with aimless repetitions. Individuals may misinterpret what is going on in the environment and may develop delusional thinking and experience hallucinations. For example, they may think that the banging of a door is a gunshot, and may develop the delusion that someone is trying to shoot them. There can be a disturbance in the sleep-wake cycle. A delirious person may alternate between hyperactivity and hypoactivity. The level of consciousness may fluctuate from drowsiness to stupor or coma. At the other extreme, the individual may be hyperalert and agitated. Other symptoms include anxiety, depression, irritability, anger, apathy, or euphoria. Acute confusion begins abruptly and usually lasts a short period of time, perhaps as long as a week, but rarely more than a month. However, if the underlying cause is not identified and treated, delirium can become a permanent condition, especially in older adults. The symptoms tend to fluctuate and often become worse at night.

Examples of factors that can contribute to delirium are listed in Table 21-1.

DEMENTIA

Dementia is characterized by impaired intellectual function, problem-solving ability, judgment, memory, and orientation, and inappropriate behavior (Table 21-2). There are several types of dementia with various causes and symptoms. Some examples are Alzheimer's disease, vascular dementia, Pick's disease, Huntington's disease, and Creutzfeldt-Jakob disease. It should also be noted that some patients who have Parkinson's disease develop dementia as well. Other conditions that are associated with dementia include normal pressure hydrocephalus, subdural hematoma, brain tumors, neurosyphilis, and acquired immunodeficiency syndrome (AIDS). Dementia is not a disease itself but a clinical syndrome, a collection of symptoms that can occur with many types of diseases. The two most prevalent types of dementia are Alzheimer's disease (AD) and vascular dementia. The cause of AD is unknown, but the disease is characterized by the presence of amyloid (a protein) deposits in brain tissue, neurofibrillary tangles (tangled microtubules in neurons), and a deficiency of acetylcholine (a chemical that transmits signals in the brain). These changes affect the structure and function of the neurons in the brain. Vascular dementia results from damage to brain cells caused by inadequate blood supply. Patients with vascular dementia often have had a series of small strokes that cause progressive damage.

table 21-1 ***Systemic and Central Nervous System Causes of Delirium***

SYSTEMIC CAUSES		CENTRAL NERVOUS SYSTEM CAUSES	
Cardiovascular Disease Congestive heart failure Arrhythmias Cardiac infarction Hypovolemia Aortic stenosis Infections Pneumonia Urinary tract infections Bacteremia Septicemia Medications Alcohol Amphetamines Analgesics Anticholinergics Antidepressants Antihistamines Antiparkinsonian agents Cimetidine Digitalis glycosides Diuretics Neuroleptics Sedative/hypnotics	Metabolic Electrolyte and fluid imbalance Hepatic, renal, or pulmonary failure Diabetes, hyperthyroidism, hypothyroidism, or other endocrine disorder Nutritional deficiencies Hypothermia and heat stroke Neoplasm Postoperative state Poisons Heavy metals Solvents Pesticides Carbon monoxide Trauma Head injury Burns Hip fracture	Infections Meningitis Encephalitis Septic emboli Neurosyphilis Brain abscess Neoplasm Primary intracranial Metastatic Trauma Subdural hematoma Extradural hematoma Contusion	Vascular Transient ischemic attack Stroke Chronic subdural hematoma Vasculitis Arteriosclerosis Hypertensive encephalopathy Subarachnoid hemorrhage Seizure Ictal and postictal states

From Zisook, S., & Braff, D. L. (1986). Delirium: Recognition and management in the older patient. *Geriatrics, 41*(6), 67-78.

table 21-2 **Diagnostic and Statistical Manual of Mental Disorders, Fourth Edition *(DSM-IV-TR)* Criteria for Dementia**

A. The development of multiple cognitive deficits manifested by both
   1. memory impairment (impaired ability to learn new information or to recall previously learned information)
   2. one (or more) of the following cognitive disturbances:
      a. aphasia (language disturbance)
      b. apraxia (impaired ability to carry out motor activities despite intact motor function)
      c. agnosia (failure to recognize or identify objects despite intact sensory function)
      d. disturbance in executive functioning (i.e., planning, organizing, sequencing, abstracting)

B. The cognitive deficits in criteria A1 and A2 each cause significant impairment in social or occupational functioning and represent a significant decline from a previous level of functioning.

C. The deficits do not occur exclusively during the course of delirium.

FEATURES OF SPECIFIC DEMENTIAS

Dementia of the Alzheimer's Type

The course is characterized by gradual onset and continuing cognitive decline.

The cognitive deficits in criteria A1 and A2 are not due to any of the following:

1. other central nervous system conditions that cause progressive deficits in memory and cognition (e.g., cerebrovascular disease, Parkinson's disease, Huntington's disease, subdural hematoma, normal-pressure hydrocephalus, brain tumor)
2. systemic conditions that are known to cause dementia (e.g., hypothyroidism, vitamin B_{12} or folic acid deficiency, niacin deficiency, hypercalcemia, neurosyphilis, human immunodeficiency virus [HIV] infection)
3. substance-induced conditions

Dementia Due to Other General Medical Conditions

There is evidence from the history, physical examination, or laboratory findings that the disturbance is the direct physiologic consequence of one of the following medical conditions: dementia due to HIV disease, dementia due to head trauma, dementia due to Parkinson's disease, dementia due to Huntington's disease, dementia due to Pick's disease, dementia due to Creutzfeldt-Jakob disease, dementia due to normal-pressure hydrocephalus, etc.

Vascular Dementia

Focal neurologic signs and symptoms (e.g., exaggeration of deep tendon reflexes, extensor plantar response, pseudobulbar palsy, gait abnormalities, weakness of an extremity) or laboratory evidence indicative of cerebrovascular disease (e.g., multiple infarctions involving cortex and underlying white matter) that is judged to be etiologically related to the disturbance.

Substance-Induced Persisting Dementia

There is evidence from the history, physical examination, or laboratory findings that the deficits are etiologically related to the persisting effects of substance use (e.g., a drug of abuse, a medication).

Modified with permission from American Psychiatric Association (2000). *Diagnostic and statistical manual of mental disorders* (4th ed., Text Revision). Washington, DC: American Psychiatric Association.

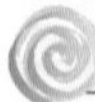

What Does Culture Have to do with Dementia?

Caregivers from lower socioeconomic families are more likely to be caring for elderly parents at an earlier age when the caregiver is employed or still has children at home.

NURSING CARE *and Intervention*

Assessment

The first step in assessing a confusional state is to observe the patient's behavior and to collect data about orientation, memory, and sleep habits. Family members may be able to provide helpful information if the patient cannot. Ask when the symptoms of confusion started and whether the confusion is constant or intermittent. List any known acute or chronic illnesses, and all medications the patient has been taking (including home remedies and over-the-counter drugs). Drugs that most often cause confusion include anticholinergics, digoxin, H_2-receptor blockers, benzodiazepines, nonsteroidal anti-inflammatory drugs, and many antiarrhythmics and antihypertensives.

These assessment data help the physician to determine whether the patient is suffering from delirium or dementia. Some major differences between the clinical features of delirium and dementia are described in Table 21-3. Nursing care of delirium and dementia are addressed separately even though they have some common interventions.

Nursing Diagnoses, Goals, and Outcome Criteria: Delirium

Nursing Diagnoses	Goals and Outcome Criteria
Disturbed Thought Processes related to drugs, infection, dehydration, unfamiliar setting, sensory overload or deprivation, etc.	Improved thought processes: orientation to person, place, and time; calm, no combative behavior
Disturbed Sleep Pattern related to agitation, mood alterations, drug effects	Restoration of patient's usual sleep pattern: fewer nighttime awakenings, patient reports feeling rested.
Risk for Injury related to agitation, disorientation, unfamiliar setting	Safety maintained: absence of injury

Interventions: Delirium

When managing delirium, the physician focuses on identifying and treating the cause of the problem. During an episode of confusion, you should focus your attention on supporting the patient to provide safety and comfort and to reduce anxiety (see Nursing Care Plan: The Patient with Delirium). Nursing care can be more effective than drugs in managing confusion.

Disturbed Thought Processes

Patients with delirium often need hospitalization. If possible the patient should be in a private room with continuous supervision. Keep the room quiet and uncluttered to avoid agitation caused by extraneous stimuli. Lighting should be soft and diffuse to avoid shadows that may be misinterpreted and add to the patient's fears. Familiar objects such as pictures, a clock, and a large calendar placed in the room can help orient the patient to place and person (Fig. 21-1). Patients who normally wear hearing aids and glasses should be allowed to use them.

Communication with a confused patient should be simple and direct. Anyone dealing with a delirious patient should be calm, warm, and reassuring. It is helpful if the same personnel are assigned to care for the patient. Avoid sudden movements and handle the patient gently during procedures or turning.

Patients with delirium may have frightening hallucinations that cause them to lash out, cry, or scream. The best response is to orient the patient to the reality of being sick and hospitalized and to explain that the hallucinations are not real even though they seem to be. You might say, "You are sick in the hospital, and what you are seeing is part of the illness." Hallucinating patients in a delirious state need one-to-one nursing observation and repeated verbal reorientation. They need to be assured that the medical and nursing staff are helping them and keeping them safe.

table 21-3 ***Clinical Features in Delirium and Dementia***

FEATURE	DELIRIUM	DEMENTIA
Duration	Few weeks to 3 months	In progress at least 1-2 years
Paranoid states	Prominent while cognitive impairment is mild or variable	More consistent with degree of impairment; less prominent paranoia
Fluctuations	Marked contrasts in levels of awareness	Not seen in such contrast; progressive decline
Persecutory delusions	Ordered and cohesive	Vague, random, contradictory
General intellectual powers	Preserved during lucid intervals	Consistent loss and decline
Affect	Intermittent fear, perplexity, or bewilderment	Flat or indifferent affect
Perceptual disturbances	Hallucinations often disturbing and very clearly defined	Hallucinations vague, fleeting, ill-defined; in many cases difficult to make a clear judgment that they exist

From Chenitz, W. C., Stone, J. T., & Salisbury, S. A. (Eds.). (1991). *Clinical gerontological nursing* (p. 485). Philadelphia: Saunders.

NURSING CARE PLAN

The Patient with Delirium

ASSESSMENT

Health History: An 81-year-old man was admitted for hip replacement surgery 2 days ago. Before his surgery he lived alone and cared for himself. He was active, alert, and independent. However, since his surgery he has been confused and at times combative with the nurses. His physician believes that he is suffering from delirium related to the anesthesia from surgery and that it should resolve within a few days.

Physical Examination: Blood pressure, 165/95; pulse, 98 with slight irregularity; respiration, 20; temperature, 97.4° F measured orally. Height, 5'7"; weight, 178 lb. Alert, disoriented to time, place, and sometimes person; combative. Awakens during the night. Dark circles around eyes. Refuses food or fluids.

Nursing Diagnosis	*Goals and Outcome Criteria*	*Interventions*
Disturbed thought processes related to anesthesia during surgery.	The patient will have improved thought processes, as evidenced by orientation to time, place, and person and absence of combative behavior.	Place in a private room with minimal stimuli, soft lighting. Request a family member to stay with patient. Maintain consistency with the nursing staff caring for the patient. Approach and communicate with the patient in a calm, reassuring manner. Have patient use hearing aid or glasses if used previously. Reorient patient frequently and consistently. Place familiar objects in the room: pictures, clock, calendar.
Disturbed sleep pattern related to agitation and mood alterations.	The patient will have adequate sleep and rest, as evidenced by fewer awakenings during the night, absence of dark circles around the eyes, and no complaints of fatigue.	Provide a back rub or offer milk at bedtime. Engage in soothing conversation to relax the patient. Plan activities for long periods (at least 2-4 hours) of uninterrupted sleep.
Imbalanced nutrition: less than body requirements related to confused state and inability to feed self.	The patient will have adequate fluid and food intake, as evidenced by eating meals as offered and maintenance of normal body weight.	Assist the patient with feeding. Offer small light meals more frequently. Stay with the patient during meals to monitor and provide safety.

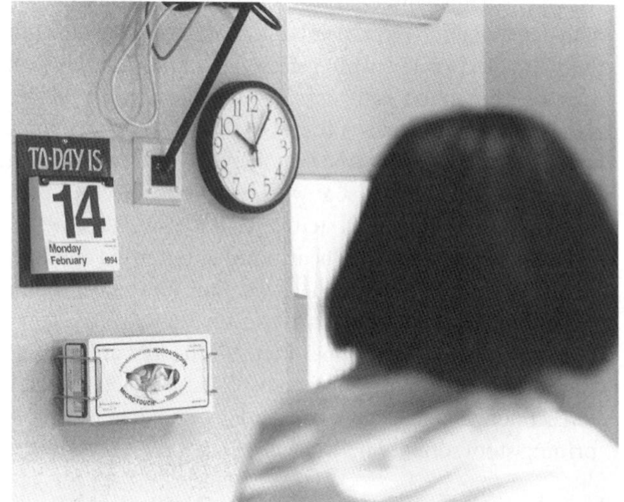

FIGURE **21-1** A clock and calendar may help orient a patient with delirium; however, they must be in a place where they can be seen easily. In addition, patients with visual impairments should wear their glasses, if possible.

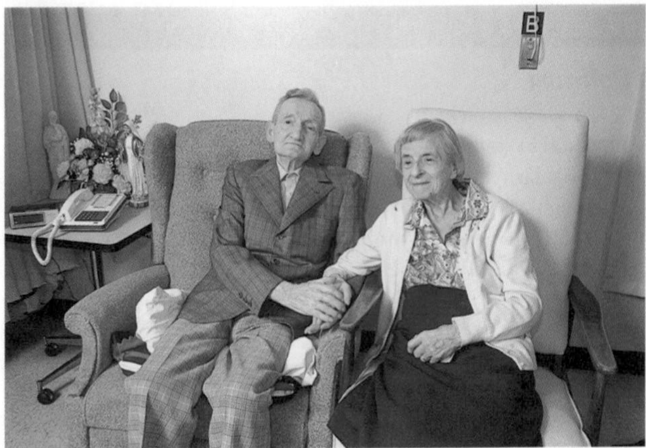
FIGURE 21-2 The presence of a family member may help calm a confused patient.

Frequent orientation to the surroundings and the situation is important for patients with delirium. Orienting phrases such as "here in the hospital" or "now that it is evening" can be woven into the conversation. Keep choices to a minimum. Simple, direct statements ("Now it is time to take your bath") are better than questions ("When would you like to take a bath?"). All communication and nursing care should be carried out in a way that conveys respect and preserves the patient's dignity.

Disturbed Sleep Pattern

Adequate sleep is important to avoid further disorientation and the confusion that can result from sleep deprivation. Nursing measures such as giving a back rub, providing a glass of warm milk, and having a soothing conversation may help the patient relax and fall asleep. Schedule medications or treatments at times that do not interrupt nighttime sleep. The presence of a family member may help calm an agitated and confused patient (Fig. 21-2).

Risk for Injury

The patient with delirium may pull on tubes, try to get out of bed unassisted, or attempt to leave the setting. It can be challenging to protect the patient from harm without imposing excessive restrictions. Avoid using physical restraints, which tend to increase anxiety and agitation in confused patients and often result in injuries. Rather, ask a family member to remain with the patient or assign a staff member to do so. Use common sense. Position tubes out of sight. Put the bed in low position. Postpone activities that are flexible. If there is no reason that confused patients have to stay in bed, try sitting them in chairs, or even "visiting" the nurses' station in a wheelchair. Avoid arguing with delirious patients. Gently explain what you are doing and why. Try to elicit their cooperation.

These nursing diagnoses are only a few that might apply to the patient with delirium. Depending on the situation, there will be different priorities.

Nursing Diagnoses, Goals, and Outcome Criteria: Dementia

Nursing Diagnoses	Goals and Outcome Criteria
Self-Care Deficit related to impaired thinking, sensory and motor dysfunction	Maximum possible independence in ADLs: patient participation in bathing, grooming, feeding, toileting with assistance as needed.
Imbalanced Nutrition: Less than Body Requirements related to difficulty with self-feeding, inattention	Adequate nutrition: stable weight (within 5 lb. of ideal)
Disturbed Sleep Pattern related to neurologic changes, altered perceptions	Adequate sleep: patient rests at night and remains physically active and awake during the day.
Risk for Injury related to poor judgment, physical decline, sensorimotor changes	Absence of injuries: patient has no falls, suffers no bruises, cuts, fractures.
Disturbed Thought Processes/Impaired Verbal Communication related to memory loss, altered perception, impaired judgment, anxiety, etc.	Cooperative behavior: patient calm, no combative behavior, no dangerous behavior. Effective communication: patient needs are recognized by caregiver.

Interventions: Dementia

Most people with dementia suffer from chronic, debilitating illnesses with little hope for recovery. The goal for patients with dementia is to maintain the highest level of functioning possible as their abilities gradually diminish (see Nursing Care Plan: The Patient with Dementia).

Self-Care Deficit

As with patients with delirium, the first priority for patients with dementia is to meet their basic needs. Adequate nutrition, fluid and electrolyte balance, sleep, elimination, and hygiene must be maintained. Patients with dementia have varying levels of competence when it comes to carrying out these functions. Assess the patient to determine the level of functioning that exists, and then assist at whatever level is needed. Break down tasks into individual steps to be done one at a time.

Dementia patients may be incontinent of urine and feces. Frequent, routine toileting helps prevent unwanted voiding and soiling. Observe for signs of constipation. Avoid laxatives if possible; instead, high-fiber foods in the diet are more effective for promoting regular bowel movements. If constipation cannot be managed with diet, fluids, and exercise, a bulk-forming stool softener may be needed.

Imbalanced Nutrition: Less than Body Requirements

People with dementia may eventually need help with eating. Assistance with meals may mean cutting food or total feeding. Finger foods high in protein and carbohydrates allow patients to feed themselves more easily. Small, frequent meals

NURSING CARE PLAN

The Patient with Dementia

ASSESSMENT

Health History: A 75-year-old woman is admitted to a long-term care facility by her daughter because she has been unsafe living alone at home. Her daughter reports that the patient has been in good health, but during the past 5 years she has gradually had more and more problems with her memory, and during the past year, she has refused to take a bath or change her clothes. Lately she has had times that she has not even known her daughter. At times she has been unable to find the bathroom and has been incontinent of urine. She often forgets to eat, and when she does eat, prefers only junk foods. Recently she has begun "wandering." She was found at a local park not knowing who she was or where she lived. Her physician has diagnosed Alzheimer's disease.

Physical Examination: Blood pressure, 170/95; pulse, 88; respiration, 22; temperature, 98.2° F. Height, 5'3"; weight, 126 lb. Inability to bathe and dress self. Disoriented to time, place, and person.

Nursing Diagnosis	*Goals and Outcome Criteria*	*Interventions*
Self-care deficit related to impaired thinking, sensory and motor dysfunction.	The patient will perform activities of daily living (ADL) as independently as possible, as evidenced by participation in bathing and dressing with the assistance of the nurse as needed.	Assess the patient's ability to perform own ADL. Allow the patient to perform as many of own ADL as possible. Remain with the patient while she performs ADL to maintain safety. Work out a routine toileting schedule and encourage patient to go to bathroom at regular intervals.
Imbalanced nutrition: less than body requirements related to difficulty with self-feeding, inattention.	The patient will maintain adequate nutrition, as evidenced by keeping within 5 lb. of ideal weight.	Cut the food into small portions. Offer finger foods. Offer foods high in protein and carbohydrates. Offer small, frequent meals and snacks. Offer fluids frequently. Stay with the patient while eating.
Disturbed sleep pattern related to neurologic changes, altered perceptions.	Patient will have adequate sleep as evidenced by quiet restfulness at night and remain physically active and awake during the day.	Try to keep her awake during the day and encourage sleep only at night. Minimize activities late in the day to allow her to "wind down" by bedtime. Have a quiet hour in the evening with soft music. If she awakens during the night and becomes confused or agitated, reassure in a soft, soothing manner to avoid precipitating extreme agitation and loss of control. Try gently stroking and singing to her. Provide a comfort object if she has one (blanket, doll, etc.).
Risk for injury related to poor judgment, physical decline, sensorimotor changes.	Absence of injuries: patient has no falls, suffers no bruises, cuts, fractures.	Provide a safe environment: no clutter, no medications or dangerous chemicals in reach. Avoid use of restraints. Provide opportunities for safe, supervised walking. Monitor exits to prevent wandering from the premises.
Disturbed thought processes/ impaired verbal communication related to memory loss, altered perception, impaired judgment, anxiety.	The patient will remain calm, free of combative behavior, as evidenced by a calm, cooperative manner during times when nursing care is performed.	Speak to patient in a calm, reassuring manner. Avoid confrontations with patient. Break tasks down into individual steps to be done one at a time. Provide consistency in nursing care. Attempt to understand what patient is communicating verbally and nonverbally.

are less confusing to the patients. Remove distractions from the eating area. Group meals may be helpful because patients often imitate behaviors of others. Offer fluids frequently during the day.

Disturbed Sleep Pattern

Sleep and awakening are often reversed in dementia patients. It is helpful to try to keep them awake during the day and get them to sleep at night. Tests and treatments can be scheduled during the morning and early afternoon to allow the patients time to wind down by bedtime. Some caregivers have found that a quiet hour in the afternoon with soft music playing promotes sleep at night. Patients who awaken during the night and become confused and agitated should be reassured in a soft, soothing manner to avoid precipitating extreme agitation and loss of control.

Risk for Injury

A safe, structured environment is essential for a person with dementia. Nothing should be left around that could harm the patient. Falls and injuries may be prevented with careful observation, muscle strengthening, and a fall prevention program.

Disturbed Thought Processes/Impaired Verbal Communication

Communication usually becomes increasingly difficult. Patients with dementia are disoriented and their thinking ability is impaired. They are confused by what is going on around them. Communication should be simple and direct. Patients must be approached gently, calmly, and quietly. They tend to copy the behavior of people around them, so a caregiver who is anxious or upset can easily convey these feelings to a patient. Nonverbal communication is extremely important. Look for cues from patients' actions and facial expressions because they frequently are not able to express their needs verbally. When patients resist activities such as bathing or dressing, avoid confrontations. Confrontations only provoke agitation and possible violence; it is better to come back at another time. A consistent schedule of care given by the same caregivers provides security for a dementia patient.

Whereas constant reality orientation is helpful for the patient with delirium, such orientation is not effective for the patient with dementia. Clocks, calendars, constant mention of the date and time, and other such orientation reminders used to be a staple of care for demented patients. However, it is now thought that reality orientation tends to agitate people with dementia by pointing out to them their forgetfulness and confusion. It is better to assist them in a nonconfrontational manner and redirect activities without constantly reminding them of their deficits.

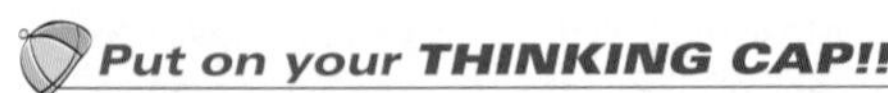

A patient's daughter is distressed because her mother does not seem to recognize her at times. What could you say to help the daughter? What suggestions could you give her to promote communication with her mother?

GUIDELINES FOR WORKING WITH DEMENTIA PATIENTS

It is helpful to keep in mind two important concepts when taking care of patients with dementia: (1) they usually forget things relatively quickly, and (2) they are usually unable to learn new things. For example, if persons with dementia start to become very restless, anxious, or agitated and are becoming more so by the minute, it is best to divert their attention somewhere else. They may be gently guided to another activity, and usually within a relatively short period of time they will forget what was bothering them in the first place and focus on the new activity (Fig. 21-3). Take advantage of the fact that patients with dementia are usually slow or unable to learn new things. For example, putting new locks on the doors in new places may prevent wandering patients from opening exit doors. You can be very creative in the care of dementia patients by using these two concepts as a basis for their care.

One approach that can also guide care for dementia patients is the Cognitive Developmental Approach (CDA). The CDA adapts interventions based on the patient's cognitive

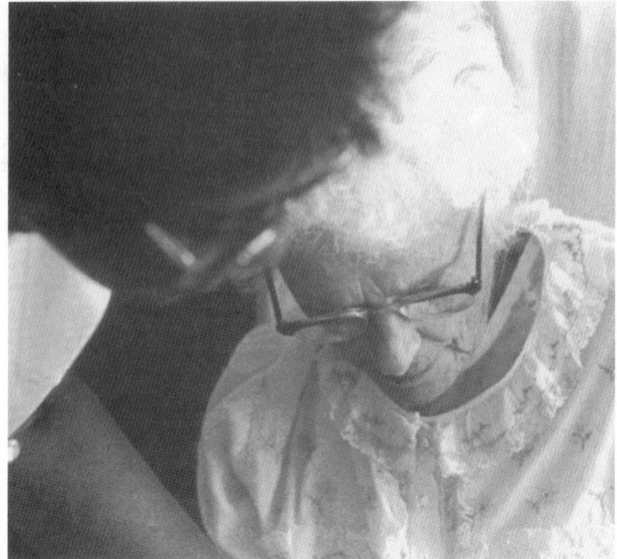

FIGURE **21-3** It is best to calmly divert the attention of confused, agitated patients somewhere else by gently guiding them to another activity.

abilities. It is thought to reduce patient stress and frustration by eliminating unrealistic expectations and allowing the patient to do as much as he or she is able. Some principles derived from the CDA that you can apply include:

- Accept that the patient with dementia may no longer be able to make adult decisions and behave as a healthy adult would. Offer limited choices to simplify decision-making.
- Adapt the environment to the patient rather than trying to adapt the patient to the environment. For example, create a safe environment for wandering instead of trying to keep the patient from wandering.
- Encourage self-care at whatever level the patient can function. If the patient can eat independently with his hands, but not with utensils, provide finger foods.
- Recognize irrational fears such as fear of the bathtub and arrange alternative ways to give personal care.
- Accept that, in advanced dementia, patient behaviors and thinking are not typical of a healthy adult. Some strategies that work with children often work with dementia patients also.
- Recognize that the patient deserves to be treated with dignity regardless of abilities or behaviors. Even the most impaired patient can probably perceive compassion in a caregiver.

key points

- The two major types of confusion are (1) acute confusional states, or delirium, and (2) chronic confusion, or dementia.
- Elderly individuals are the most susceptible to confusion associated with delirium or dementia.

- Delirium is a short-term confusional state that usually develops over a short period of time and is often reversible.
- Delirium is characterized by disturbances in attention, thinking, perception, orientation, short-term memory, and sleep.
- Delirium is usually caused by some underlying illness such as neurologic, pulmonary, or cardiovascular disease or conditions such as infection, dehydration, and overmedication.
- Dementia is chronic and irreversible.
- Dementia is characterized by inappropriate behavior and impairment of intellectual function, problem-solving ability, judgment, memory, and orientation.
- Dementia is not a disease entity itself but a clinical syndrome, a collection of symptoms that may be part of the profile of many diseases, including Alzheimer's disease, vascular dementia, Huntington's disease, and Parkinson's disease.
- The first step in assessing a confusional state is to observe the patient's behavior, and to evaluate orientation, memory, and sleep habits.
- Try to determine how long the symptoms of confusion have been present and how and when they started.
- In caring for a patient with delirium, provide safety and comfort and provide frequent orientation to the surroundings and the situation.
- The goal for patients with dementia is to maintain the highest level of functioning possible as their abilities gradually diminish.
- A safe, structured environment is essential for patients with dementia, and tasks should be broken down into individual steps that can be performed one at a time.
- When patients with dementia resist activities such as bathing or dressing, it is best to avoid confrontations and divert their attention elsewhere.
- The Cognitive Developmental Approach adapts interventions to the patient's cognitive level.

REVIEW QUESTIONS

1. What is the primary difference between delirium and dementia?
   1. Delirium is typically reversible; dementia is irreversible.
   2. Agitation is constant with delirium, but intermittent with dementia.
   3. The onset of delirium is gradual; the onset of dementia is typically rapid.
   4. Delirium usually lasts only a few minutes; dementia lasts weeks to months.
2. A confused patient repeatedly cries out for her daughter in the middle of the night. What is the best intervention?
   1. Check to see if she has an order for a sedative.
   2. Call her daughter and ask her to come see her mother.
   3. Calmly tell her where she is and that her daughter is not here.
   4. Tell her she needs to be quiet because she is disturbing other patients.
3. A patient with Alzheimer's disease wanders away from the table during meals, leaving most of his food uneaten. What should you do?
   1. Consult with the dietitian about providing finger foods.
   2. Restrain the patient in his seat during meals.
   3. Tell him he must sit down and finish his meal.
   4. Ask another patient to try to keep him at the table.
4. Which message is most appropriate for the patient with dementia?
   1. "You need to be dressed for church in 30 minutes."
   2. "Put your arm in the sleeve of your shirt."
   3. "Put your shirt on."
   4. "What would you like to wear today?"
5. A new nurse on the Alzheimer's special care unit repeatedly asks patients what time it is and if they know where they are. What information should you share with her?
   1. If a patient cannot answer the questions correctly, wait 5 minutes and ask again.
   2. Consistently tell patients the time, date, and place to keep them oriented.
   3. Frequent attempts at orientation tend to agitate Alzheimer's patients.
   4. Have the patient repeat the date, time, and place after you say them.
6. If you applied principles of the Cognitive Developmental Approach, you would:
   1. consistently follow very specific interventions for dementia patients.
   2. have the patient confront irrational fears so they can be overcome.
   3. insist that the patient behave as a mature adult at all times.
   4. adapt your expectations and interventions to the patient's abilities.

CHAPTER

22 Incontinence

objectives

1. Identify the types of urinary and fecal incontinence.
2. Explain the pathophysiology and treatment of specific types of incontinence.
3. Identify common therapeutic measures used for the incontinent patient.
4. List nursing assessment data needed to assist in the evaluation and treatment of incontinence.
5. Assist in developing a nursing care plan for the patient with incontinence.

key terms

Anorectal incontinence (ā-nō-RĔK-tăl ĭn-KŎN-tĭ-nĕns, p. 300)
Crede's technique (kră-DĀZ, p. 293)
Fecal incontinence (p. 286)
Functional incontinence (p. 293)
Micturition (mĭk-tū-RĬSH-ŭn, p. 286)
Neurogenic bladder (nū-rō-JĔN-ĭk, p. 293)
Neurogenic incontinence (p. 300)
Overactive bladder (p. 291)
Overflow incontinence (fecal) (p. 299)
Overflow incontinence (urine) (p. 292)
Reflex incontinence (p. 291)
Stress incontinence (p. 293)
Symptomatic incontinence (p. 300)
Transient incontinence (TRĂN-zē-ĕnt, p. 291)
Urge incontinence (p. 291)
Urinary incontinence (p. 286)
Void (p. 286)

Incontinence is the term used to describe the inability to control the passage of urine (**urinary incontinence**) or feces (**fecal incontinence**). Many conditions and situations can cause either temporary or permanent incontinence. Incontinence deserves special attention because of the toll it takes on the individual. The person who is troubled by incontinence faces physical, psychosocial, and financial burdens. The management of incontinence also requires many hours of nursing care.

The goals of treatment for the incontinent person include restoration or improvement of control for treatable incontinence, management of irreversible incontinence, and prevention of complications.

URINARY INCONTINENCE: PREVALENCE AND COSTS

The U.S. Department of Health and Human Services estimates that more than 13 million Americans suffer from urinary incontinence. Exact figures are difficult to obtain because people often do not report the problem to health care providers. However, among elderly people in institutions and those who are homebound, approximately 50% are reportedly incontinent. Among people ages 60 and over who live outside of institutions, the prevalence rate is estimated as 15% to 35%. The problem is twice as common among women as it is among men. Even though it is more common in older people, urinary incontinence should not be considered a normal age-related change. It often can be improved or cured, no matter how old the patient is.

The cost of managing the incontinence of institutionalized elderly people in the United States is estimated to be more than $15 billion each year. Health care providers need to recognize the economic and personal value of treating incontinence aggressively. Nurses play an important role in educating people about the need for evaluation and treatment.

PHYSIOLOGY OF URINATION

The passage of urine is called *urination* or ***micturition.*** Nurses and physicians more commonly refer to the process of urinating as voiding. For that reason, the terms ***void*** and *voiding* are used in this chapter.

Normal controlled voiding requires healthy bladder muscle (detrusor muscle), a patent (open) urethra, normal transmission of nerve impulses, and mental alertness. Alterations in any of these factors may result in incontinence.

The urinary bladder receives urine continuously from the kidneys. The function of the bladder is to store urine until it can be eliminated. The walls of the bladder are muscular and capable of stretching. When 200 to 250 ml of urine collects in the bladder, stretch and tension receptors are stimulated. The bladder contracts, and the internal sphincter relaxes. A message is sent to the brain, making the person aware of the need to void. Because the act of voiding is normally voluntary, it can be delayed until an appropriate time. Then the external sphincter can be relaxed, permitting urine to flow out through the urethra (Fig. 22-1).

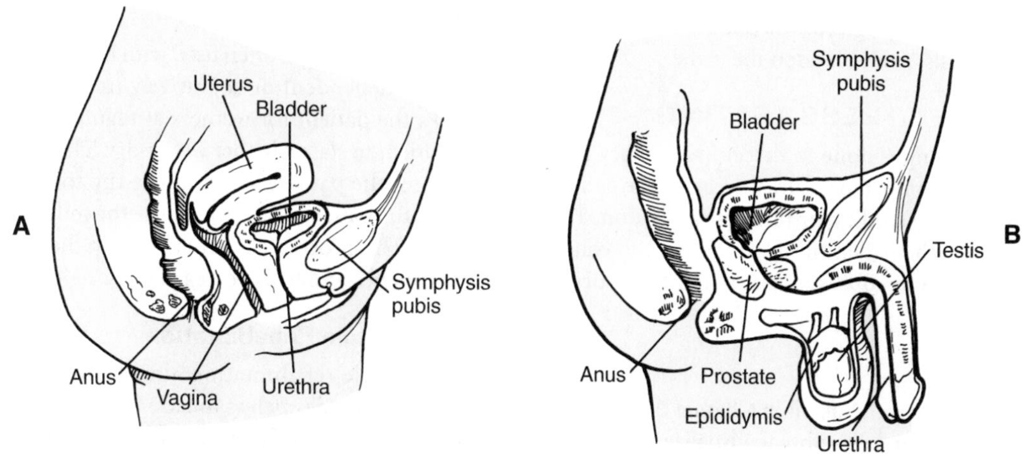

FIGURE 22-1 The bladder, urethra, and adjacent structures. *A*, Female. *B*, Male.

There is, of course, a limit to the amount of urine the bladder can hold. When the limit is exceeded, pressure causes the bladder to contract and force urine out involuntarily. If the bladder cannot be emptied, urine backs up into the kidneys (a condition called hydronephrosis) and can cause kidney damage.

DIAGNOSTIC TESTS AND PROCEDURES

The presence and specific type of urinary incontinence are diagnosed on the basis of the patient's history, physical examination, and various diagnostic tests and procedures. Diagnostic studies may include laboratory tests, measurement of urine volumes, imaging procedures, endoscopy, stress tests, and urodynamic studies. Other helpful tools are voiding diaries and wet pad counts. The results help to define the type of incontinence, which in turn guides treatment decisions.

LABORATORY TESTS

A clean-catch urinalysis with culture and sensitivity testing is usually ordered to assess for infection. The specimen is studied for bacteria, red blood cells, white blood cells, and glucose. If the patient cannot cooperate with the clean-catch procedure, catheterization may be necessary. A blood sample may be collected to measure blood urea nitrogen, creatinine, glucose, and calcium.

POSTVOID RESIDUAL

It is useful to know whether the patient is emptying the bladder completely. The amount of urine remaining in the bladder after voiding is called the *postvoid residual* (PVR). Several methods are used to determine the PVR. One method is to catheterize the patient immediately after voiding and measure the amount of urine obtained by catheterization. A second method is to use an ultrasound device to estimate the amount of urine remaining in the bladder after voiding. Some physicians estimate PVR by abdominal palpation and percussion. Normally less than 50 ml of urine remains after voiding. An amount greater than 199 ml reflects inadequate emptying.

Imaging Procedures

Imaging procedures such as computed tomography or magnetic resonance imaging may be ordered to create images of the urinary structures. Imaging procedures for the urinary tract are discussed in Chapter 38.

Urodynamic Testing

Urodynamic procedures assess the neuromuscular function of the lower urinary tract. These tests are indicated when the cause of incontinence cannot be determined by simpler means.

UROFLOWMETRY

Uroflowmetry measures voiding duration and the amount and rate of urine voided. The patient voids into the funnel of the flowmeter. Sometimes serial measurements are made over 2 to 3 days. The patient is advised to void before defecating and not to allow stool or bathroom tissue to enter the funnel. The patient's position for each voiding is recorded. Fluid intake is measured during the testing period. Additional urodynamic tests are discussed in Chapter 38.

CYSTOMETRY

Cystometry is used to evaluate the neuromuscular function of the bladder. Signed consent is obtained before beginning the procedure. The patient voids into a flowmeter, after which a catheter is inserted and the postvoid residual is measured. Fluid or air, or both, is instilled into the bladder, and the patient's sensations and bladder response are determined. The bladder is filled until the patient feels uncomfortable or it is apparent that the patient is unable to sense the pressure. The bladder is then drained, or the patient is permitted to void. The physician may administer a drug that stimulates bladder tone and repeat the test. After the test, the patient should force fluids if not contraindicated. The nurse advises the patient to report difficulty voiding or signs of infection (fever, burning during urination, chills, pain, blood in the urine).

PROVOCATIVE STRESS TESTING

Provocative stress testing is done to detect involuntary passage of urine when abdominal pressure increases. The patient may be positioned in a standing or lithotomy position. The physician encourages the patient to relax and then to cough vigorously. The examiner observes for urine loss during coughing.

CYSTOSCOPY

Cystoscopy is covered in more detail in Chapter 38. In brief, a scope is inserted through the urethra to visualize the urethra and bladder. Signed consent is required, and the procedure may be done under local or general anesthesia. Postprocedure care includes monitoring urine output and encouraging fluid ingestion (if not contraindicated). The patient is advised to report difficulty voiding, continued blood in the urine (it is normally pink-tinged at first), and fever, chills, or pain, which may indicate infection.

COMMON THERAPEUTIC MEASURES

Depending on the type of urinary incontinence, a number of therapeutic measures may be prescribed. These are generally classified as behavioral, pharmacologic, or surgical treatments.

BEHAVIORAL INTERVENTIONS

Behavioral interventions include bladder training or retraining, habit training, prompted voiding, and pelvic muscle exercises. These techniques are low risk and are often effective in decreasing the frequency of incontinent episodes.

Bladder Training

Bladder training uses patient education, scheduled toileting, and positive reinforcement. The teaching plan includes information about normal urinary anatomy and physiology and the bladder training program. With scheduled voiding, the patient is encouraged to delay voiding and void only at scheduled times. Initially, voiding is usually scheduled every 2 to 3 hours while the patient is awake. The length of time between voidings is gradually increased. If the patient voids ahead of schedule, the next voiding may be rescheduled at the prescribed interval. Another approach is to ignore the unscheduled voiding and have the patient void again at the previously scheduled time. The patient's efforts and improvement are positively reinforced throughout the treatment period, which usually lasts several months.

Habit Training

Habit training is also called timed voiding. It is similar to bladder training in that the patient is encouraged to void at scheduled intervals. The difference is that the patient is not advised to resist the urge and delay voiding. The voiding schedule is based on the patient's usual pattern.

Prompted Voiding

Prompted voiding is often used with habit training for people who are dependent or cognitively impaired. The caregiver checks the patient for wetness at regular intervals and asks the patient to state whether wet or dry. The caregiver then encourages the patient to try to use the toilet. The caregiver praises the patient for trying to use the toilet and for remaining dry. This process is intended to help the patient recognize incontinence and to ask caregivers for help with toileting.

Pelvic Muscle Rehabilitation

Pelvic muscle rehabilitation aims to strengthen the pelvic floor and includes pelvic muscle exercises, with or without biofeedback, pelvic floor electrical stimulation, and vaginal weight training. Pelvic muscle exercises, commonly called Kegel exercises, are described in the Patient Teaching Plan. They actively exercise the pubococcygeus muscle, which helps close the urethra and strengthen muscles of the pelvic floor.

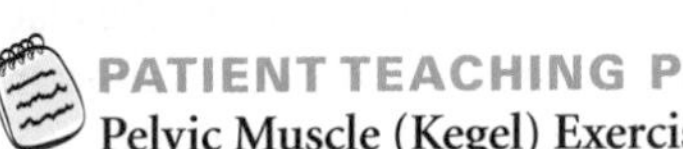

PATIENT TEACHING PLAN
Pelvic Muscle (Kegel) Exercises

- Uncontrolled loss of urine is commonly caused by weakness in the perineal muscles that normally control urination.
- Strengthening perineal muscles, which are located around the vagina and the rectum, can improve urinary control.
- To identify the correct muscles that you need to exercise, practice tightening the perineal muscles as if you were trying to control the passage of intestinal gas. Try to hold the contraction up to 10 seconds, and then relax for 10 seconds.
- Your goal is to work up to 10 repetitions in a set, done three to four times each day for a total of 30 to 40 contractions or as recommended by your physician.
- It may take 6 to 8 weeks before you notice improvement in urinary control.
- Continue the exercises indefinitely to maintain control.
- You can do these exercises anywhere: at your desk, while driving, standing in line at the grocery store. No one can tell!

Biofeedback may be used in conjunction with other pelvic muscle exercises. Electronic or mechanical sensors are used to help the patient isolate the appropriate pelvic muscles to contract while keeping the abdominal muscles relaxed. Electrical stimulation of the muscles of the pelvic floor can also be employed to cause muscle contraction along with Kegel exercises.

Sometimes vaginal weights ("cones") are used with pelvic muscle training in women. The cones are ceramic devices of various weights that are inserted into the vagina. The patient begins with the lightest cone, inserts it, and tries to retain it for up to 15 minutes twice daily. When the lightest cone is successfully retained, the heavier cones are then used in succession.

REFLEX TRAINING

Reflex training is sometimes employed by people with spinal cord injury. This technique uses the Valsalva maneuver with rectal stretching to force urine from the bladder. The Valsalva maneuver is performed by taking a deep breath, holding it, and bearing down. At the same time the rectum is stretched by inserting a gloved finger into the rectum and pulling toward the back. This creates pressure on the urinary sphincter and relaxes the pelvic floor, allowing urine to flow. Patients who use this method of emptying the bladder should be checked for residual volume at times. Ideally, the residual volume will be less than 100 ml. Patients who learn to use this method successfully may no longer need catheterization.

DRUG THERAPY

Drug therapy may be used to treat stress and urge incontinence. Classifications of drugs that are being used include anticholinergics, smooth muscle relaxants, calcium channel blockers, tricyclic antidepressant agents, nonsteroidal anti-inflammatory drugs, alpha-adrenergic agonists, and estrogen. Examples of these drugs, their side effects, and nursing considerations are presented in Table 22-1. Fat or glutaraldehyde cross-linked collagen (Contigen) may be injected into the tissues around the urethra. The substance adds bulk to the bladder neck, thereby increasing resistance to urine outflow. This procedure, called periurethral bulking, is helpful in certain situations for both men and women. The long-term effects of Contigen injection are still being studied.

In addition to drugs used to control incontinence, a variety of creams and sprays are available to coat and protect the skin of the perineum and buttocks of the incontinent patient. A light dusting powder can be used to absorb moisture. Cornstarch is not recommended because it promotes the development of yeast infections. Do not use talc and lotion together on the same area because the combination creates an abrasive paste.

URINE COLLECTION DEVICES

External Devices

External urine collection devices are useful for males. These latex sheaths, sometimes called condom catheters or Texas catheters, drain urine into a bag that is usually secured to the leg. These are quite effective in maintaining dryness, but the adhesive may cause skin irritation on the penis. The directions for applying a condom catheter must be followed carefully. *Make sure the patient and all caregivers know not to encircle the penis with tape.* To do so can restrict circulation. Elastic tape should be used and wrapped in a spiral pattern. There is no external device for women in common use at this time, although several are being tested.

Indwelling Catheters

An indwelling catheter may be ordered to control urinary incontinence. This is usually done when all other measures have failed and skin integrity is endangered. A catheter may also be needed temporarily if urine is coming in contact with a wound. Care of the patient with an indwelling catheter is covered in Chapter 38.

Intermittent Self-Catheterization

Some patients are quite successful at using intermittent self-catheterization. Of course, this requires dexterity, adequate vision, and ability and motivation to learn. Clean technique rather than sterile is usually taught for use in the home setting. Initially the bladder is drained every 4 hours. If more than 500 ml of urine is obtained, the time interval is shortened. If less than 200 ml is obtained, the time is extended. Most people produce more urine at certain times of day. Individual schedules can be adjusted to accommodate this variation.

GARMENTS AND PADS FOR INCONTINENCE

A variety of incontinence products are available that help maintain dryness. Disposable briefs and pads are found in most pharmacies and grocery stores. Some elderly women wear perineal pads to absorb urine. "Geri pads" are used in some nursing homes. These are washable waterproof briefs with absorbent cotton liners. Another style has a stretchy brief with a perineal pouch through which absorbent pads can be changed. The best product is one that draws urine away from the skin through a liner that remains dry. These products do not, however, protect the skin against feces.

Those who discourage the use of incontinence briefs and pads say it encourages patients to void in their clothing. This may be true at times, but there is a place for these items. It may give a person the confidence to be socially active without the risk of having an embarrassing accident. When trying to restore control, it is best to use briefs that can be removed easily for toileting. For patients who will never be continent, these products may be an acceptable management tool.

For the immobile patient, an absorbent pad with a waterproof backing may be used instead of briefs. These pads can also be placed under the buttocks of a bedridden patient wearing briefs in case leakage occurs. One factor to remember is that multiple layers of padding interfere with special beds or mattresses designed to prevent decubitus ulcers. Some paper pads stick to the skin and become lumpy when wet. The patient should never be placed directly on a plastic surface because this keeps the skin wet from perspiration as well as urine.

PENILE CLAMP

The penile clamp is a device that is applied to the penis. It compresses the urethra, preventing the passage of urine. To prevent circulatory impairment and pressure sores, the clamp must be removed and repositioned frequently. Use of the penile clamp is controversial (Fig. 22-2).

PELVIC ORGAN SUPPORT DEVICES

A *pessary* is a device that is inserted into the vagina to hold the pelvic organs in place. It is sometimes used as a tool to treat incontinence in women with relaxation of pelvic structures. A doughnut-shaped pessary exerts pressure on the vaginal wall, lifting the uterus and holding it in the pelvis. When incontinence occurs because the bladder prolapses into the vagina, other types of pessaries may be used to support the

table 22-1 **DRUG THERAPY** | ***Drugs Used to Treat Urinary Incontinence***

DRUG	USE	ACTION	NURSING INTERVENTIONS
CHOLINERGICS			
Bethanechol chloride (Urecholine)	Atonic bladder (overflow incontinence)	Bladder contraction	Common side effects: sweating, flushing, GI distress, headache, visual disturbances Toxicity: nausea, dyspnea, irregular pulse, headache Antidote: atropine Contraindications: bladder or intestinal obstruction, asthma, hyperthyroidism, ulcer, cardiac disease, parkinsonism Works quickly: 15-30 min after SC route, 1 hr after PO route; be sure bedpan or toilet is accessible *Warning:* dosages are very different for SC and PO administration
ANTICHOLINERGICS			
Propantheline bromide (Pro-Banthine)	Urge incontinence	Bladder relaxation and sphincter contraction Delayed desire to void	Common side effects: constipation, dry mouth, blurred vision (pupil dilation), fatigue, tachycardia Contraindications: glaucoma, severe coronary artery disease, some GI disorders Use cautiously in the elderly
ANTISPASMODICS			
Oxybutynin chloride (Ditropan) Tolterodine (Detrol)	Urge incontinence	Bladder relaxation Increased bladder capacity Delayed urge to void	Side effects: (less with tolterodine) dry mouth, constipation, tachycardia, drowsiness, urinary retention, insomnia, blurred vision. Give 1 hour AC. Provide oral care. Potentiates other CNS depressants.
ALPHA-ADRENERGICS			
Ephedrine	Stress incontinence Enuresis (with atropine)	Sphincter contraction	Common side effects: cardiac dysrhythmias, nervousness, palpitations Contraindications: Severe hypotension, narrow-angle glaucoma Elderly people are more likely to have hallucinations, convulsions, CNS depression, insomnia, and urinary retention
ALPHA-ADRENERGIC BLOCKERS			
Prazosin hydrochloride (Minipress) Phenoxybenzamine hydrochloride (Dibenzyline)	Overflow incontinence	Relaxation of internal sphincter	Side effects: postural hypotension (especially in the elderly), tachycardia, headache, dizziness, nasal congestion After the first dose, the patient should lie down for 2 hr to prevent fainting; elastic stockings may help During dosage adjustments, monitor blood pressure; most side effects decrease over time
BETA-ADRENERGIC BLOCKERS			
Propranolol hydrochloride (Inderal)	Stress incontinence	Improved sphincter tone	Side effects: cardiac depression Contraindications: asthma
COLLAGEN			
Glutaraldehyde cross-linked collagen (Contigen)	Stress incontinence	Adds bulk to sphincter to increase resistance to urine	Injected around urethra by physician Monitor voiding and assess bladder for distention

GI, Gastrointestinal; *SC*, subcutaneous; *PO*, by mouth; *CNS*, central nervous system.

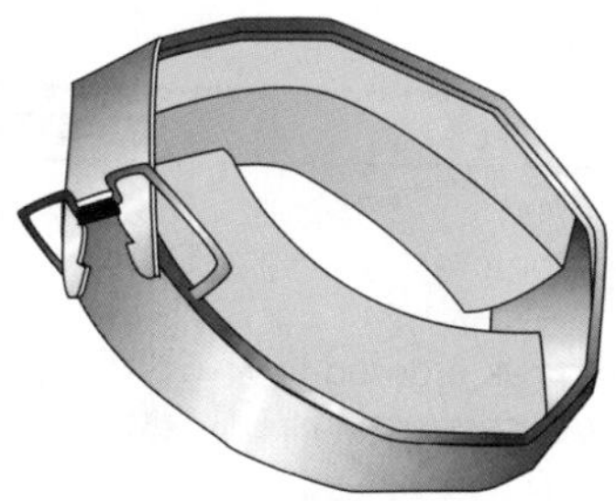

FIGURE 22-2 A penile clamp used for urinary incontinence.

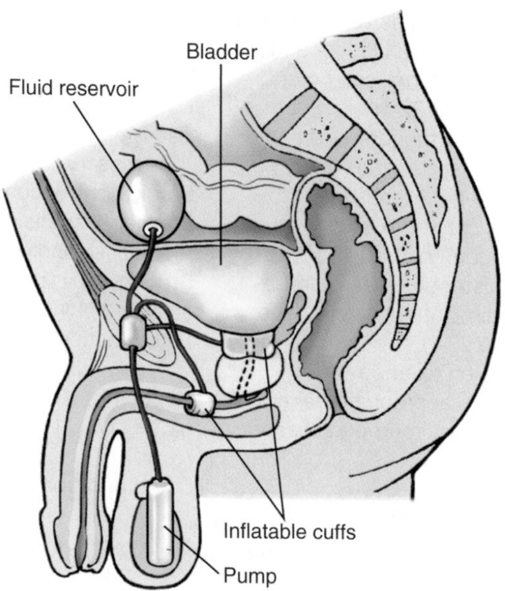

FIGURE 22-3 An artificial urinary sphincter in place.

urethra as well. Pessaries are generally recommended for patients who are awaiting surgical treatment or those for whom surgery is contraindicated. Within 24 hours after pessary placement, the patient must be re-examined to assure proper placement and to rule out urinary obstruction. The device must then be removed periodically for cleansing and replacement as needed. *Be sure to document that the patient has a pessary, so it will not be forgotten.*

For women with stress incontinence, a bladder neck support prosthesis may be helpful. When the Silastic device is fitted into the vagina, it supports the area where the urethra connects to the bladder thereby reducing the incidence of involuntary urine loss.

SURGICAL TREATMENT

Surgical intervention may be recommended for some conditions that cause urinary incontinence. Specific surgical procedures may be done to remove obstructions, treat severe bladder instability, implant an artificial sphincter, reposition the sphincter unit, implant electrodes that inhibit the micturition reflex, improve perineal support, and inject substances that increase urethral compression. Nursing care of the patient undergoing surgery on the urinary tract is described in Chapter 38.

The artificial sphincter illustrated in Figure 22-3 consists of an inflatable cuff, a reservoir of fluid that fills the cuff, and a pump. The cuff is positioned around the urethra or bladder neck. The reservoir is placed in the abdomen and the pump in the scrotum or labia. Fluid fills the cuff, applying pressure to the urethra to prevent urine passage. To void, the patient compresses the pump, which deflates the cuff by transferring fluid from the cuff to the reservoir and allowing urine to pass through the urethra.

TYPES OF URINARY INCONTINENCE

There are six basic types of urinary incontinence. They are urge, overflow, reflex, stress, functional, and total incontinence (Table 22-2). It is possible for a patient to have more than one type at the same time (mixed incontinence). Urinary incontinence may be transient or persistent. **Transient incontinence** is caused by reversible conditions and is often corrected by treatment of the underlying problem. A related condition is **overactive bladder.** Symptoms of overactive bladder are urinary frequency, urgency, and urge incontinence, alone or in combination, in the absence of pathology. Note that patients with overactive bladder may or may not be incontinent.

URGE INCONTINENCE

Description

Urge incontinence is the involuntary loss of urine shortly after a strong, abrupt urge to urinate. It most often results from involuntary detrusor contractions described as detrusor overactivity or hyperreflexia. It may be associated with neurologic disorders such as stroke, multiple sclerosis, and spinal cord lesions. Inability to control the passage of urine because of injury to the spinal cord above the 12th thoracic vertebra is called **reflex incontinence.** Detrusor overactivity is the most common cause of incontinence in older adults.

If no neurologic disorder is found, the patient is said to have an unstable bladder or detrusor instability. Some patients with urge incontinence have involuntary urethral relaxation in addition to abnormal detrusor activity. Urinary tract infection and fecal impaction sometimes cause temporary urge incontinence.

Management

Treatment of urge incontinence is aimed at correcting the cause, if possible: antibiotics for infection, removal of impaction. When the problem is not related to reversible conditions, behavioral techniques, drug therapy, or surgical intervention may be employed. Bladder training with scheduled voiding and positive reinforcement may be effective. Pelvic muscle exercises may be prescribed to supplement bladder

table 22-2 ***Types of Urinary Incontinence***

TYPE	DESCRIPTION	CAUSES	NURSING CARE	TREATMENT
Urge	Loss of urine that usually follows a strong desire to void	Nervous system disorders Urinary tract infection Bladder obstruction	Scheduled toileting Limit fluids 2 hr before bedtime Administer drugs as ordered to control bladder contractions (see Table 22-1) Keep incontinence record	Behavior modification Drug therapy: anticholinergics Surgical procedures to increase bladder capacity or decrease bladder contractions
Overflow	Loss of urine associated with a full bladder Frequent voiding Volume usually small	Urethral obstruction Disorders of bladder, nerves, or muscles Spinal cord injury Postanesthesia	Catheterize as ordered; teach self-catheterization as appropriate Administer drugs as ordered to stimulate the bladder and relax the internal sphincter (see Table 22-1)	Surgery to relieve obstruction Drug therapy to stimulate the bladder and relax the sphincters Catheterization
Reflex	Loss of urine due to reflexive contraction	Spinal cord injury Radiation cystitis	Cutaneous triggers; teach stimulation techniques	Catheterize as necessary
Stress	Loss of urine during physical exertion	Relaxation of pelvic floor muscles Urethral trauma Sphincter injury	Teach Kegel exercises Advise patient to void frequently Administer drugs as ordered to stimulate sphincter (see Table 22-1)	Surgical correction Bladder suspension Artificial sphincter Drug therapy to improve sphincter contraction
Functional	Bladder functions normally but subject voids inappropriately	Dementia Head injury Cardiovascular accident (stroke)	Scheduled toileting Reinforce appropriate behavior Remove environmental barriers	
Total	Loss of urine when other types of incontinence have been ruled out	May be unclear; possibly neurologic, or bladder sphincter injury	Timed voiding Incontinence briefs	Catheterization

training. Anticholinergics and antispasmodics are the drugs most commonly used for urge incontinence. Be aware that anticholinergics may cause confusion and agitation that could be mistaken for dementia in the elderly. Tolterodine (Detrol) is an antispasmodic that is effective in many people, particularly those with overactive bladder. It generally has fewer side effects than the anticholinergics. If behavioral techniques, drugs, or both do not work, some surgical procedures may be recommended. These include stretching the bladder, cutting some of the bladder nerves, and enlarging the bladder surgically.

REFLEX INCONTINENCE

Description

Reflex incontinence is caused by neurologic dysfunction associated with radical pelvic surgery, spinal cord injury, or radiation cystitis. Urine may flow out of the bladder back into the ureters and kidneys, and cause hydronephrosis—a condition that can damage the kidneys.

Management

'or patients who have reflex incontinence, bladder drainage 't be maintained! Overdistention of the bladder may trigger a very serious reaction called *autonomic dysreflexia*, in which the blood pressure rises to life-threatening levels. This can be prevented by emptying the bladder often enough to prevent overdistention. Among the techniques that may be used to stimulate bladder emptying in patients with reflex incontinence are cutaneous triggering methods and include tapping the suprapubic area and stroking the inner thigh. These techniques and others are more fully described in texts on rehabilitation. Crede's method is *not* used for patients with reflex incontinence. Chapter 28 discusses care of the patient with spinal cord injury in detail.

OVERFLOW INCONTINENCE

Description

Overflow incontinence is the involuntary loss of urine associated with an overdistended bladder. Small amounts of urine are lost either continuously or at frequent intervals. Patients who have normal sensation usually feel uncomfortable because of bladder distention.

Factors that contribute to overflow incontinence are obstruction to urine flow, an underactive detrusor muscle, or impaired transmission of nerve impulses. In addition, some females have overflow incontinence after anti-incontinence surgery. Patients with certain types of spinal cord injuries have neurogenic bladders. These patients are not aware of bladder fullness, and the bladder becomes overdistended. Urinary retention with overflow is also fairly common after general anesthesia or childbirth or following removal of an indwelling catheter. Drugs that may cause retention include antihistamines, epinephrine, anticholinergics, and theophylline (Table 22-3).

Management

The medical treatment of overflow incontinence depends on the cause. The physician may prescribe drugs to stimulate the bladder (bethanechol chloride) and relax the internal sphincter (prazosin). A common reason for obstruction in males is prostate enlargement. Surgical removal of all or part of the gland often restores normal bladder emptying.

In some cases intermittent or indwelling catheterization is necessary. Postoperative and postpartum patients usually need intermittent catheterization only once or twice before normal bladder function returns. The indwelling catheter is considered the measure of last resort in the management of overflow incontinence. Self-catheterization using clean technique may be taught to patients who are able to do it in the home setting. This technique works very well for many patients.

Other techniques that may be used to empty the bladder are Crede's method, the Valsalva maneuver, and the anal stretch maneuver. Crede's technique involves using the open hand to gently press the abdomen over the bladder and promote urine passage. Ask the physician about the safety of this procedure for individual patients. These techniques and others are described more fully in rehabilitation texts.

table 22-3 *Drugs that Cause Urinary Retention or Incontinence*

CLASSES AND EXAMPLES OF DRUGS THAT CAN CAUSE URINARY RETENTION
Anticholinergics: atropine sulfate
Antihistamines: diphenhydramine hydrochloride (Benadryl)
Sympathomimetics: epinephrine hydrochloride (Adrenalin chloride)
Xanthine: theophylline (Theo-Dur)
CLASSES AND EXAMPLES OF DRUGS THAT MAY CONTRIBUTE TO INCONTINENCE
Alpha-adrenergic blockers: prazosin hydrochloride (Minipress)
Anticholinergics: atropine sulfate
Antihistamines: diphenhydramine hydrochloride (Benadryl)
Antiparkinson agents: levodopa (Dopar), trihexyphenidyl hydrochloride (Artane)
Antipsychotics: chlorpromazine (Thorazine)
High-ceiling diuretics: furosemide (Lasix)
Opiate agonists: morphine sulfate (Epimorph)
Sedatives or hypnotics: phenobarbital sodium (Luminal sodium), diazepam (Valium)
Sympathomimetics: phenylephrine hydrochloride (Neo-Synephrine), isoproterenol hydrochloride (Isuprel)

STRESS INCONTINENCE

Description

Stress incontinence is the involuntary loss of small amounts of urine during physical activity that increases abdominal pressure. Coughing, laughing, sneezing, and lifting are examples of activities that often result in urine loss. In women it is usually caused by relaxation of the pelvic floor muscles and the urethrovesical juncture as a result of pregnancy, childbirth, obesity, and aging. Urethral trauma, sphincter injury, congenital sphincter weakness, urinary infection, neurologic disorders, and stress can cause stress incontinence in men and women. It may occur after prostatectomy or radiation therapy.

Management

Sometimes stress incontinence is successfully treated with behavioral methods such as scheduled voiding and pelvic muscle exercises (see Nursing Care Plan: The Patient with Stress Incontinence). In addition, the patient is advised to maintain a fluid intake of at least 2,000 ml/day. Fluids that have a diuretic effect (tea, coffee, cola) should be avoided. Alpha-adrenergic drugs such as pseudoephedrine HCl (Sudafed) may be prescribed to increase bladder outlet resistance. Oral or topical estrogen may be given to strengthen the bladder outlet in postmenopausal women. The most common surgical intervention is bladder suspension.

FUNCTIONAL INCONTINENCE

Description

Functional incontinence is the term used when a person voids inappropriately because of inability to get to the toilet or to manage the mechanics of toileting. The problem can be caused by confusion, immobility, or barriers in the environment.

Management

The treatment of functional incontinence depends on the cause. The environment should be arranged to permit independent toileting. Assistive devices that enable the immobile patient to void appropriately are provided. The confused patient may respond well to scheduled or timed voiding and efforts to improve orientation to toilet facilities. In long-term care facilities, it is important to promote the attitude that incontinence can usually be improved even in physically and cognitively impaired patients.

TOTAL INCONTINENCE

Description

Some sources use the term *total incontinence* to describe urine loss when all other types of incontinence have been ruled out. Total incontinence may be demonstrated by constant dribbling or just occasional events of urine loss. Causes may include injury to bladder sphincters and some neurologic disorders.

NURSING CARE PLAN

The Patient with Stress Incontinence

ASSESSMENT

Health History: Mrs. Seigel is an 80-year-old resident in a long-term care facility. She complains of having trouble "holding my urine." She is unable to control urination if she strains, coughs, or laughs. She is the mother of five children, all born at home. She reports no other physical complaints except for arthritis in her hips and knees and hypertension. Her medications are acetaminophen, 325 mg q.i.d., and hydrochlorothiazide, 25 mg/day. Fear of losing control of her urine has caused her to avoid leaving her room except for meals. She is wearing perineal pads to keep her clothing dry.

Physical Examination: Vital signs: temperature, 98° F orally; pulse, 72; respiration, 20; blood pressure, 130/86. Height, 5'3"; weight, 179 lb. Heart and breath sounds normal. Abdomen obese and soft. No bladder distention. Faint urine odor present. Rises with some difficulty. Walks slowly with walker. Limited range of motion in knees and hips.

Nursing Diagnosis	*Goals and Outcome Criteria*	*Interventions*
Stress incontinence related to weak pelvic muscles and high intra-abdominal pressure.	Improved urinary control: patient will report fewer incidents of stress incontinence.	Explain to the patient how weak perineal muscles cause stress incontinence. Instruct her on how to do Kegel perineal exercises: contract the perineal muscles and hold the contraction for 10 sec; repeat the contraction three more times; repeat the set of four contractions four times a day. Advise the patient to empty her bladder every 2 hr while awake. Encourage intake of normal amounts of fluid but discourage liquids with diuretic effects: coffee, tea, and alcohol. Explain that obesity increases intra-abdominal pressure and contributes to stress incontinence. Explore interest in weight loss and refer to dietitian.
Risk for impaired skin integrity related to prolonged contact of urine with skin.	The patient's skin will remain intact and free of excessive redness.	Inspect the perineal area and buttocks and report signs of irritation: redness, breaks in the skin. Apply skin protectants as ordered or per agency protocol. Teach the patient the importance of good perineal care to remove urine from the skin. Encourage her to cleanse the area with mild soap, rinse, and gently dry twice daily. Perineal pads or other incontinence pads should be changed promptly if they are wet.
Social isolation related to fear of embarrassment due to incontinence.	The patient will report resumption of previous activities and participation in social activities.	Identify activities that patient would like to resume. Discuss strategies to decrease embarrassment about incontinent episodes: (1) Empty bladder before leaving room. (2) Wear perineal pads or special incontinence pads to absorb urine and protect clothing and furniture. Avoid any comments that could humiliate the patient, such as references to "diapers," and avoid discussing her problem in front of others.

Management

Timed voiding may help these patients empty the bladder often enough to avoid incontinence. For some, the use of a catheter or incontinence briefs is necessary.

NURSING CARE *of the Patient with Urinary Incontinence*

Assessment

Health History

Your assessment helps in the identification of the type of incontinence, the possible causes, and the patient's response to treatment.

Chief Complaint

A thorough description of the chief complaint is essential. Assessment includes awareness of the need to void and ability to hold the urine once aware of the need to void. Determine the pattern of incontinent voiding, urine volume, and related symptoms.

Pattern. Ask the patient to describe the frequency of incontinent episodes and whether they occur during any particular activities, such as sneezing or laughing. A voiding diary is a helpful tool in identifying the pattern of urinary incontinence. Many patients are able to keep their own diaries. If the patient is unable to maintain an accurate record, you or another caregiver must do it.

Volume. If a patient is incontinent, measurements of urine can only be estimated, but the patient can probably describe the amount voided as being large, moderate, or small. If pads or briefs are used, record the number used and the degree of saturation. When assessing the patient in the long-term care facility or a hospital, measure and record the amount of urine passed with continent voiding as well.

Related symptoms. Assess the presence of dysuria (painful voiding), pain in the suprapubic area (the lower abdomen where the bladder is located), and polyuria (large urine volume).

Past Medical History

Past problems that might be related to incontinence include urologic, gynecologic, neurologic, and endocrine conditions. Specifically ask if the patient has diabetes mellitus. People who have diabetes may develop neurologic problems that affect the bladder. Also, if their diabetes is poorly controlled, they may produce large volumes of urine that quickly fill the bladder.

Document all abdominal disorders, surgeries, and trauma. Record the number of pregnancies and types of deliveries. Inquire about current and recent medications because many drugs can affect kidney or bladder function in some way. Drugs that might contribute to urinary incontinence are high-ceiling (loop) diuretics, major tranquilizers, anticholinergics, antihistamines, decongestants, some sedatives or hypnotics, and antiparkinsonian drugs. Other drugs that can disrupt normal voiding are epinephrine, theophylline, isoproterenol, and prazosin.

PHARMACOLOGY CAPSULE When urinary incontinence develops suddenly, check the patient's drug profile for drugs known to contribute to incontinence.

Review of Systems

The review of systems may detect clues to conditions that contribute to incontinence. For example, the patient with severe arthritis in the hands or severely impaired vision may have difficulty managing toileting independently. Constipation is a common problem that can contribute to incontinence.

Functional Assessment

For the functional assessment, document the patient's usual activities and habits. Of special interest when assessing incontinence are usual fluid intake and consumption of alcohol.

Physical Examination

The physical examination begins with the measurement of vital signs and height and weight. Be alert for fever, tachycardia, and weight gain. Assess the patient's level of awareness and appropriateness of responses. Inspect the skin for edema.

Sometimes incontinence is first recognized when you detect an odor of urine during the assessment or when providing care. When assessing the incontinent patient, palpate the abdomen for masses, tenderness, fullness, or distention. A distended bladder or abdominal distention associated with constipation are important findings. Examination of the male genitalia includes inspection for abnormalities and for skin irritation. Inspect the female perineum for redness or irritation. The physician or nurse practitioner performs a pelvic examination on the female patient to inspect for prolapse of abdominal organs and to evaluate perineal muscle tone. A rectal examination is done to determine sensation, sphincter tone, and presence of fecal impaction. In males, the prostate is palpated for contour and consistency.

Assessment of the patient with urinary incontinence is outlined in Table 22-4. In addition, the environment must be assessed, including toilet accessibility, grab bars, lighting, and availability of toileting options (urinals, commode chairs).

table 22-4 ASSESSMENT *of Patients with Urinary Incontinence*

HEALTH HISTORY

Chief Complaint: Pattern of continent and incontinent voiding, behaviors or activities associated with incontinent voiding, amount of urine passed with continent and incontinent voiding, awareness of need to void, ability to hold urine once aware of need to void, dysuria

Past Medical History: Urologic, gynecologic, neurologic, and endocrine problems; abdominal operations, trauma, disorders; mental confusion; current and recent medications

Review of Systems: Disorders that might contribute to incontinence: diabetes mellitus, CVA, paralysis

Functional Assessment: Usual activities, fluid intake, alcohol consumption

PHYSICAL EXAMINATION

Vital Signs: Fever, tachycardia

Height and Weight: Weight gain

Level of Consciousness: Orientation

Odor of Urine

Abdomen: Masses, tenderness, fullness, or distention

Male Genitalia: Abnormalities of foreskin, glans penis, perineal skin

Female Genitalia: Redness, irritation

Rectal Examination: Sensation, sphincter tone, fecal impaction

Nursing Diagnoses, Goals, and Outcome Criteria: Urinary Incontinence

Nursing diagnoses and goals for the patient with urinary incontinence may include the following:

Nursing Diagnoses	Goals and Outcome Criteria
Deficient Knowledge of causes of incontinence and corrective measures	Patient understands condition and management: accurately describes and participates in treatment plan
Functional Urinary Incontinence related to physical, cognitive, or environmental barriers	Continent voiding with appropriate support: decreased episodes of incontinent voiding
Reflex Urinary Incontinence related to neurologic impairment	Adequate management of irreversible incontinence: bladder emptying accomplished with minimal involuntary leakage

Nursing Diagnoses, Goals, and Outcome Criteria: Urinary Incontinence—cont'd

Nursing Diagnoses	Goals and Outcome Criteria
Stress Urinary Incontinence related to weak pelvic structures, increased intra-abdominal pressure	Improved control of urine flow: decreased episodes of involuntary voiding when under stress
Total Urinary Incontinence related to neurologic dysfunction	Adequate management of irreversible incontinence to prevent spillage: bladder emptying accomplished with minimal involuntary leakage
Urge Urinary Incontinence related to decreased bladder capacity or bladder spasms	Ability to hold increasing volume of urine: time between voiding increases without leakage
Social Isolation related to fear of embarrassment	Decreased social isolation: patient participates in usual social activities
Situational Low Self-Esteem related to loss of control over voiding	Improved self-esteem: patient demonstrates positive self-image (confidence, pride in appearance)
Risk for Impaired Skin Integrity related to the presence of urine on the skin	Reduced risk of skin breakdown: skin kept clean, dry, and free of urine or feces
Risk for Infection related to chronic bladder distention or catheterization	Absence of urinary tract infection: normal body temperature and white blood cell count

Interventions

Deficient Knowledge

Patient and caregiver education are key elements in the management of urinary incontinence. Often you must overcome the assumption that the condition is not treatable, especially in frail, elderly people. Emphasize that improvement or correction is possible for most people. Sometimes the incontinent patient is very discouraged and reluctant to try retraining techniques. Be positive, encouraging, and praise attempts and successes. Many people believe that patients will be more motivated if they are dressed in street clothes and are not wearing incontinence garments.

In the teaching plan include an overview of normal urination, an explanation of the type of incontinence the patient is experiencing, and detailed explanations of the prescribed treatment. Supplement verbal information with written material. Tell the patient that improvement takes time and not to expect immediate results. Praise the patient's interest in working toward continence, participation in the treatment plan, and successful voiding. Specific methods for improving continence were discussed earlier. The appropriate methods for managing various types of incontinence are emphasized in the next section.

Incontinence

Nursing interventions for various types of incontinence overlap. Therefore, interventions are discussed in general terms here. Table 22-2 summarizes the treatments for each type of incontinence.

Bladder Training or Retraining

Bladder training or retraining may be recommended for stress and urge incontinence. Teach the patient (and caregiver, if appropriate) the basic principles of bladder training. Establish a schedule for voiding every 2 to 3 hours. The patient is not usually asked to get up during the night, so pads or an external collection device may be needed during sleep. Emphasize the importance of the patient trying to delay voiding until the scheduled time. Praise the patient's efforts and encourage the caregiver to do so as well.

Habit Training

If habit training is prescribed, you may initiate an incontinence record to help establish the schedule for timed voiding (Fig. 22-4). You or other caregivers must then remind the patient to try to void at the scheduled times. It might be argued that the caregiver, rather than the patient, is being trained. This is true to some extent, but in many cases the patient is able to take responsibility for toileting on the prescribed schedule and remain continent.

If the patient has difficulty voiding at the scheduled time, try to stimulate voiding. Measures to promote voiding include establishing a comfortable position for the patient, ensuring privacy, and using specific stimuli. Stimuli that may encourage voiding include stroking the inner thigh, pouring warm water over the perineum, running water in the lavatory or tub, and drinking water while on the toilet.

Fluid intake may be spaced at 2-hour intervals to provide regular filling of the bladder. Nighttime wetness can be reduced by limiting fluids after 7 P.M. Patients or their caregivers sometimes decrease fluid intake excessively to reduce urinary incontinence. This makes it harder to schedule toileting and can lead to other problems (urinary tract infection, urinary calculi). Most references recommend 2,000 to 3,000 ml of fluid daily unless contraindicated. If a patient has cardiovascular or renal disease, consult the physician about the ideal fluid intake. Gradually increase the fluid intake for older patients, because they often do not adapt well to rapid changes in blood volume.

Social Isolation

The person with urinary incontinence may curtail social activities out of fear of having embarrassing accidents. Also, access to toilets in public places is often limited, so patients who cannot delay voiding may be afraid to venture far from home. If continence is unlikely or not yet established, a variety of incontinence products are available that may permit the patient to venture out without fear of wetness or odor. Specially designed pads and undergarments as well as some external urine collection devices may be used. As was mentioned earlier, external collection devices are more readily available and more satisfactory for men than for women. The patient also can be encouraged to maintain the voiding schedule during the social outing. If the patient has an incontinent episode, be careful not to show disapproval.

Situational Low Self-Esteem

The ability to control elimination is an important childhood accomplishment. Adults who are incontinent may be so

INCONTINENCE MONITORING RECORD

INSTRUCTIONS: EACH TIME THE PATIENT IS CHECKED:
1) Mark *one* of the circles in the BLADDER section at the hour closest to the time the patient is checked.
2) Make an X in the BOWEL section if the patient has had an incontinent or normal bowel movement.

● = Incontinent, small amount ○ = Dry X = Incontinent BOWEL
● = Incontinent, large amount △ = Voided correctly X = Normal BOWEL

PATIENT NAME ______ ROOM # ______ DATE ______

	BLADDER				BOWEL			
	INCONTINENT OF URINE		DRY	VOIDED CORRECTLY	INCONTINENT X	NORMAL X	INITIALS	COMMENTS
12 am	●	●	○	△ cc ___				
1	●	●	○	△ cc ___				
2	●	●	○	△ cc ___				
3	●	●	○	△ cc ___				
4	●	●	○	△ cc ___				
5	●	●	○	△ cc ___				
6	●	●	○	△ cc ___				
7	●	●	○	△ cc ___				
8	●	●	○	△ cc ___				
9	●	●	○	△ cc ___				
10	●	●	○	△ cc ___				
11	●	●	○	△ cc ___				
12 pm	●	●	○	△ cc ___				
1	●	●	○	△ cc ___				
2	●	●	○	△ cc ___				
3	●	●	○	△ cc ___				
4	●	●	○	△ cc ___				
5	●	●	○	△ cc ___				
6	●	●	○	△ cc ___				
7	●	●	○	△ cc ___				
8	●	●	○	△ cc ___				
9	●	●	○	△ cc ___				
10	●	●	○	△ cc ___				
11	●	●	○	△ cc ___				
TOTALS:								

C 1984

FIGURE 22-4 An incontinence record.

embarrassed that they are reluctant to tell anyone about it. Nurses often discover that a newly admitted patient has concealed incontinence from family and physicians. Some older people do not seek help for incontinence because they think it is caused by old age and cannot be corrected.

You can help patients learn to manage incontinence and see that it is not a barrier to achieving a full life. Your attitude toward the patient and toward incontinence influences how the patient deals with the change in body function. Caregivers must be committed to efforts to help patients avoid incontinence. The situation described below should not be allowed to happen:

> A stroke patient in a long-term care facility calls out, "I need to go to the bathroom!" A busy nursing staff member rushes by, pats her on the hand, and says, "That's all right. You have a diaper on. Go ahead and pee."

Encourage the patient to attend to dress and grooming to promote a more positive self-image. The patient who takes an active role in carrying out the treatment plan may feel less helpless and better able to cope with incontinence. Advise caregivers not to refer to incontinence pads and undergarments as "diapers" because of that term's association with infants.

Impaired Skin Integrity

A major problem for the incontinent patient is the risk of skin breakdown. Urine and feces, if left in contact with the skin, cause a rash. Continuous moisture causes the skin to lose its oily protective barrier. Skin breakdown may follow. The key to preventing breakdown is to keep the skin clean, dry, and free of urine or feces. If a patient is incontinent and unable to report voiding, check hourly for wetness. Immediately remove wet garments and linens. Wash the skin with mild soap and warm water, rinse, and gently pat dry. Inspect the genitals, perineum, thighs, and buttocks for redness and skin breakdown. Apply protective creams as ordered or according to agency policy. If breakdown does occur, notify the registered nurse or physician and provide treatment as ordered or according to agency policy.

Risk For Infection

The patient who is incontinent of urine is at risk for urinary tract infection and urinary calculi (stones). These complications are most likely to occur in patients who retain urine and in those who restrict their fluids. Retained urine is a good medium for bacterial growth, and the overstretched bladder wall is susceptible to infection. Patients may restrict fluid intake to try to reduce the frequency of incontinence. Concentrated urine is a risk factor for infections and calculi. Patients with indwelling catheters are at even greater risk for urinary tract infections.

The risk of urinary tract infection can be reduced by having the patient empty the bladder as scheduled, providing adequate fluids, and using strict aseptic technique during catheterization. Also, keep the perineal area clean. Encourage the intake of 2,000 to 3,000 ml of fluid daily unless contraindicated. Details of catheter care are covered in Chapter 38.

FECAL INCONTINENCE

Fecal incontinence is less common than urinary incontinence, but it can be very distressing for patients who are affected by it. Fecal incontinence is usually related to anal sphincter dysfunction caused by anal surgery, trauma during childbirth, Crohn's disease affecting the anus, and diabetic neuropathy. Some patients experience temporary incontinence with severe diarrhea because they do not have time to reach the toilet. Incontinent diarrhea may also be present with fecal impaction. Diminished muscle strength associated with aging also may be a factor.

PHYSIOLOGY OF DEFECATION

The structures that maintain bowel control are the internal and external sphincters and the puborectal muscle. The muscles of the pelvic floor and the external sphincter are under voluntary control (Fig. 22-5). The bowel has its own nerve network that stimulates peristalsis when it is distended. Therefore, disorders of the central nervous system and spinal cord do not impair bowel control as much as they do bladder control.

The fecal mass enters the rectum by mass movement. The presence of feces in the rectum creates a desire to defecate. Defecation occurs when the anal sphincter relaxes and the rectum contracts. Tightening of the diaphragm and abdominal muscles promotes defecation by increasing pressure in the abdomen. If defecation does not occur soon after this pressure is felt, the sensation of needing to defecate soon fades. People who often ignore or delay defecation tend to become constipated.

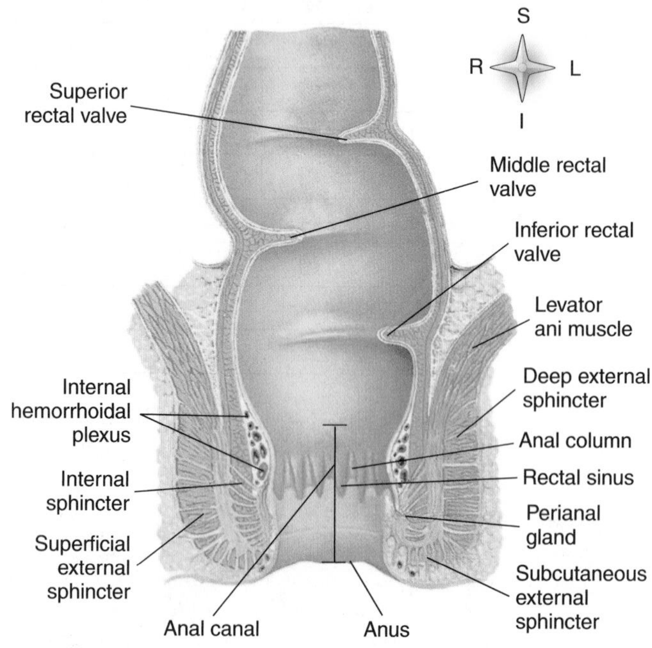

FIGURE 22-5 The anal sphincters and musculature.

DIAGNOSTIC TESTS AND PROCEDURES

Evaluation of fecal incontinence may include assessment of rectal sphincter tone, laboratory examination of a stool specimen for blood or pathogens, and endoscopic or radiologic procedures to detect underlying problems. Diagnostic tests and procedures for the gastrointestinal system are presented in detail in Chapter 36.

COMMON THERAPEUTIC MEASURES

ENEMAS

Enemas may be necessary to stimulate emptying of the bowel in the patient who is prone to impaction. Various types of enemas and nursing considerations are discussed in Chapter 36. In general, frequent use of large-volume enemas is not advised because it overstretches the bowel and contributes to loss of muscle tone. Sometimes, however, enemas are necessary. The patient with poor rectal sphincter tone may have difficulty retaining enema solutions. An adapter can be placed on the enema tubing and inserted into the anus. The nipple-like adapter helps the patient retain the solution.

POUCHES

Plastic pouches, much like ostomy bags, may be applied to the perianal area and held in place with adhesive. They are helpful for patients who have frequent stools. Because they are bulky and uncomfortable, they are not usually used on ambulatory patients. Another disadvantage is the skin irritation caused by the adhesive. When the pouch is changed, always provide meticulous skin care. An alternative to the pouch is an adult incontinent brief or (for bed patients) linen protectors.

DRUG THERAPY

Types of drugs employed to treat fecal incontinence include laxatives, stool softeners, and antidiarrheal drugs, depending on the underlying problem. These drugs are discussed in Chapter 36.

Put on your THINKING CAP!!

When would a patient with fecal incontinence need laxatives?

BIOFEEDBACK

Patients who are motivated and able to follow directions and whose external anal sphincter is capable of responding to rectal distention may achieve bowel control with biofeedback. A balloon is inserted into the rectum and inflated. A manometer creates a tracing of the normal response of the sphincter to rectal pressure. The patient tries to consciously reproduce the pattern by contracting the muscles that delay defecation. The size of the balloon is progressively decreased to help the patient recognize and respond to the amount of rectal distention expected with normal stool volume. Biofeedback has been effective for many patients but has not proved useful for patients with fecal incontinence associated with diabetes, spinal cord injury, rectal trauma, or radiation injury. Pelvic muscle strengthening exercise as described with urinary incontinence may be helpful.

DIETARY CHANGES

Some foods can contribute to fecal incontinence. For example, chocolate, coffee, tea, and other caffeinated beverages all stimulate the anal sphincters to relax. Raw fruits, fruit juices (especially prune and grape juice), raw vegetables, cabbage, sweets, alcohol, and highly spicy foods stimulate stool production. The patient can be advised to avoid these foods and to consume more foods that thicken the stool. These include bananas, rice, bread, potatoes, cheese, yogurt, oatmeal, oat bran, boiled milk, and pasta. Until fecal incontinence is corrected, the patient may also wish to avoid foods that cause odor and gas. Odor-causing foods include cabbage family vegetables, beans, garlic, eggs, fish, and turnips. Gas-producing foods include beans, beer, carbonated beverages, cucumbers, cabbage, broccoli, dairy products, and corn.

TYPES OF FECAL INCONTINENCE

There are four types of fecal incontinence: overflow, anorectal, neurogenic, and symptomatic. Table 22-5 summarizes the features of each type.

OVERFLOW INCONTINENCE

Description

Fecal overflow incontinence is caused by constipation in which the rectum is constantly distended. The fecal mass backs up until the entire colon is full. There may or may not be a fecal impaction. The patient passes semisolid stools frequently. This condition may be related to a long-standing dependence on laxatives or enemas.

Medical Treatment

Medical management of fecal overflow incontinence is concerned with immediate relief of the constipation and long-term control of the problem. The first step is to cleanse the colon. Phosphate enemas and suppositories may be ordered to empty the rectum. Daily enemas for 7 to 10 days are then needed to empty the entire colon. Instead of the enemas, the physician may order oral laxatives such as bisacodyl or mannitol. If hard masses of stool are present, they can be softened with oil retention enemas and then removed digitally.

Once the colon has been cleansed, regular evacuation is essential. Increased fluids and fiber may be helpful, but some patients need regular aids to elimination. The physician may order enemas or suppositories twice a week or daily laxatives. For elderly patients, senna or lactulose is preferred by many geriatric specialists. Mineral oil should be avoided because it interferes with absorption of fat-soluble vitamins and because it may be aspirated, causing lipid pneumonia.

table 22-5 ***Types of Fecal Incontinence***

TYPE	DESCRIPTION	CAUSES	NURSING CARE
Overflow	Uncontrolled, frequent passage of small, semisoft stools Fecal impaction may be present	Constipation in which entire colon is full of fecal matter	Administer laxatives and enemas as ordered Increase fluids and fiber as appropriate
Anorectal	Uncontrolled passage of stool several times a day	Weak pelvic muscles Loss of anal reflexes Poor rectal sphincter tone Rectal prolapse	Teach Kegel exercises Prepare for surgery, if planned
Neurogenic	Formed stools are passed after meals Usually seen in dementia patients	Gastrocolic reflex stimulates defecation Patient does not delay until appropriate time	Scheduled toileting
Symptomatic	Incontinent stools, usually diarrhea Not related to other types of fecal incontinence	Colon or rectal disease	Comfort measures; skin care Prepare for diagnostic tests and procedures

NEUROGENIC INCONTINENCE

Description

Many people report having a bowel movement shortly after the first meal of the day. This is caused by the gastrocolic reflex. When food enters the stomach, it stimulates activity throughout the digestive tract and causes the movement of the fecal mass into the rectum. Patients who do not voluntarily delay defecation are said to have neurogenic incontinence. This occurs most often in patients with dementia. These patients usually have one or two formed stools daily after meals.

Medical Treatment

Neurogenic incontinence is usually treated with scheduled toileting based on the patient's usual time of defecation. If this is not successful, some physicians order a constipating drug (such as codeine) each morning and a laxative (senna or milk of magnesia) each night. This routine results in a controlled bowel movement each morning and avoids later accidents. It does not, however, correct the underlying problem.

SYMPTOMATIC INCONTINENCE

Description

Symptomatic incontinence is the result of colorectal disease. These patients usually have incontinence with diarrhea. Blood or mucus may be seen in the stool.

Medical Treatment

When a patient has symptomatic incontinence, medical care should be sought to identify and treat the cause.

ANORECTAL INCONTINENCE

Description

Anorectal incontinence is associated with nerve damage that causes the muscles of the pelvic floor to be weak. There may be rectal abnormalities, including loss of anal reflex and loss of anal sphincter tone. Patients typically have several incontinent stools a day.

Medical Treatment

Anorectal incontinence is treated with pelvic muscle exercises and sometimes biofeedback. If these techniques are ineffective, surgical repair of the anal sphincter may be advised.

NURSING CARE *of the Patient with Fecal Incontinence*

Assessment

A thorough nursing assessment can help diagnose the type and cause of fecal incontinence and guide the selection of treatment.

Health History

Chief Complaint

When a patient has fecal incontinence, assess the usual bowel pattern, changes, stool characteristics, and related symptoms such as pain or cramping.

Bowel Pattern

Bowel patterns are usually well established in the adult. The frequency of bowel movements may range from several times daily to several times a week. Document the patient's usual frequency of bowel movements. In relation to incontinent episodes, ask if the patient is aware of the need to defecate. For dementia patients, a caregiver may be able to detect clues that the patient is about to have a bowel movement. If the patient is confused, initiate a record of times and circumstances when defecation occurs.

Characteristics of Stools

Assess the consistency, color, and constituents of the patient's stools. Terms used to describe consistency include liquid, watery, pasty, tarry, semiformed, formed, and hard. Most of these terms are self-explanatory. Tarry is used to describe stools that are shiny, sticky, and black. Stool is normally brown in color. Abnormal colors are black, red, green, and white. Abnormal stool constituents might include blood, mucus, or undigested food.

Past Medical History

Document chronic illnesses, past acute illnesses, and surgeries or trauma to the abdomen or rectum. Neurologic conditions, including stroke, spinal cord injury, and dementia, are significant. List recent and current medications and all allergies. It is especially important to determine the use of laxatives, enemas, or suppositories. Because these are often purchased without a prescription, the patient may not mention them when reporting medications. Record the obstetric history, including the number of pregnancies, types of deliveries, and complications of childbirth.

Review of Systems

The review of systems identifies problems that may be related to fecal incontinence such as motor, sensory, or cognitive impairments.

Functional Assessment

The functional assessment focuses on habits that may be related to bowel function, including diet, fluid intake, and exercise or activity pattern. Determine whether the patient has the mobility and dexterity to manage toileting independently. Recent travel to other countries may be significant, because travelers sometimes acquire uncommon intestinal infections.

Physical Examination

Inspect and palpate the abdomen for distention and auscultate for bowel sounds. Inspect the perianal area for irritation or breakdown. The physician or nurse practitioner may perform a rectal examination and test the strength of the rectal sphincter.

Assessment of the patient with fecal incontinence is outlined in Table 22-6.

table 22-6 ASSESSMENT *of Patients with Fecal Incontinence*

HEALTH HISTORY

Chief Complaint: Bowel pattern changes, stool characteristics (consistency, color, constituents), awareness of need to defecate, symptoms associated with passage of incontinent stool

Past Medical History: Chronic illnesses, past acute illnesses, abdominal or rectal trauma or surgery, abdominal radiotherapy, recent and current medications, dementia, allergies

Review of Systems: Motor, sensory, or cognitive dysfunction that could affect continence

Functional Assessment: Diet, fluid intake, exercise or activity pattern, foreign travel

PHYSICAL EXAMINATION

Abdomen: Distention, bowel sounds

Perianal Area: Irritation, breakdown

Nursing Diagnoses, Goals, and Outcome Criteria: Fecal Incontinence

Nursing diagnoses and goals for the patient with fecal incontinence may include the following:

Nursing Diagnoses	Goals and Outcome Criteria
Bowel Incontinence related to impaction, cognitive impairment, neurologic impairment, environmental barriers, or impaired mobility	Controlled bowel elimination: regular voluntary bowel evacuation of soft, formed stool
Impaired Skin Integrity related to contact of feces with skin	Normal skin integrity: no redness or skin breakdown
Situational Low Self-Esteem related to loss of control over elimination	Improved self-esteem: patient's comments and behavior reflect a positive view of self (confidence, takes pride in appearance)

Interventions

Bowel Incontinence

Continued assessment is an essential part of the nurse's role in caring for the patient with incontinence. Documentation of the patient's usual bowel pattern provides a guideline for scheduled elimination and for setting realistic goals. To establish a bowel program, take the patient to the toilet at the usual time of defecation, usually 30 minutes after eating. If suppositories or enemas are ordered, administer them and document the results.

When enemas or laxatives are prescribed on a routine basis for overflow incontinence, caregivers often fear creating laxative or enema dependency. For these patients, however, normal bowel function may not be a realistic goal. They may do better with a program that promotes regular bowel evacuation. It is far better than the miserable process of emptying a full colon every few weeks.

Explain normal bowel physiology and interventions for incontinence to the patient. Advise the patient to consume adequate fluids and fiber to prevent constipation and impaction. A fluid intake of 2,000 ml/day is recommended if not contraindicated. Increase fluids gradually in the elderly patient because fluid overload can lead to heart failure. Work with the dietitian to teach the patient that fresh fruits and vegetables provide bulk and fiber that keep the stool moist and soft. Encourage ambulation if the patient is able to walk. If perineal exercises are prescribed, advise the patient to practice contracting the muscles that control defecation. The contraction should be held up to 10 seconds and repeated several times each day.

Impaired Skin Integrity

After each incontinent stool, cleanse the patient's perianal area thoroughly. Apply protective creams or ointments as ordered or per agency policy. Incontinence undergarments may be needed to prevent soiling and embarrassment, but they must be checked frequently so that stool does not remain in contact with the skin. Fecal pouches may be used, but the adhesive and plastic can irritate the skin, so good skin care is still a priority.

Situational Low Self-Esteem

Loss of bowel control can be devastating for the patient. Express understanding of the patient's distress and encourage the patient to strive for as much improvement as possible. Praise the patient for participation in the treatment program and for decreased frequency of incontinent stools. Encourage the patient to practice good grooming and to resume social activities. Help patients coordinate their social schedule with their bowel programs.

Put on your THINKING CAP!!

Three of the patients you have cared for in the past week have had diagnoses of "urinary incontinence." Mrs. A., age 55, was admitted for treatment of her asthma. She has five adult children and often babysits for two toddlers. She says she loses a small amount of urine when she coughs or picks up a toddler.

Mr. B., age 72, had a prostatectomy 2 weeks ago. His catheter has been removed, but he was readmitted with a severe urinary tract infection. He complains of constant dribbling of urine that requires wearing incontinence pads. His bladder is not palpable.

Mrs. C., age 25, had an appendectomy. The afternoon of the procedure, she voided 25 to 60 ml of urine at frequent intervals. Her bladder was distended and she complained of a constant urge to void.

Mr. D., age 85, was admitted with pneumonia. He has a diagnosis of moderate dementia. On two occasions he was found out of bed, and there was urine on the floor. On another occasion, he urinated in the wastebasket.

Decide which type of incontinence each patient probably had, and fill in the chart with the probable cause(s) for the specific patient, the recommended treatment, and the appropriate nursing interventions for each patient in relation to incontinence.

PATIENT	TYPE OF INCONTINENCE	PROBABLE CAUSE(S)	TREATMENT	NURSING CARE
Mrs. A	______	______	______	______
Mr. B	______	______	______	______
Mrs. C	______	______	______	______
Mr. D	______	______	______	______

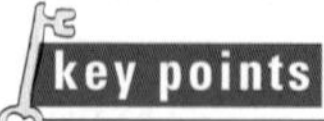

- Incontinence is the inability to control the passage of urine or feces.
- Normal controlled voiding requires healthy bladder muscle, a patent urethra, normal transmission of nerve impulses, and mental alertness.
- Assessment of urinary incontinence includes recording the voiding pattern, urine volume, associated signs and symptoms, medications, past medical history, and physical findings.
- The types of urinary incontinence are transient, urge, stress, overflow, reflex, functional, and total.
- Transient incontinence is caused by reversible conditions and is often corrected by treatment of the underlying problem.
- Urge incontinence, involuntary loss of urine after a strong urge to void, may be corrected by treating the cause with behavior modification and drug therapy.
- Overflow incontinence, involuntary loss of urine associated with a full bladder, may be corrected by treating the cause (enlarged prostate) or by using drugs that stimulate the bladder and relax the internal sphincter.
- Stress incontinence, the involuntary loss of urine during physical exertion, may be improved by strengthening the perineal muscles, by surgical intervention, or by placement of an artificial sphincter.
- Functional incontinence is inappropriate voiding despite normal urinary function.
- Assessment of fecal incontinence includes recording the usual bowel pattern, stool characteristics, related symptoms, activity, diet, fluid intake, medications, and use of aids to help elimination as well as performing an abdominal assessment.
- Types of fecal incontinence include overflow, anorectal, neurogenic, and symptomatic.
- Fecal overflow incontinence is caused by constipation in which the rectum is constantly distended and is treated by relieving the constipation and preventing future episodes.
- Anorectal incontinence is caused by abnormalities in the pelvic muscle, anus, or rectum and may require pelvic floor muscle exercises or surgery.
- Neurogenic incontinence is automatic defecation seen in people (such as patients with dementia) who do not voluntarily delay defecation; it may be corrected by scheduled toileting.
- Symptomatic incontinence results from colorectal disease and requires correction of the basic problem.
- Nursing care of the patient who is incontinent may address measures to correct the specific type of incontinence, to maintain skin integrity, to improve situational low self-esteem, and to improve knowledge of management.
- Techniques to restore bladder control include bladder retraining using scheduled toileting, Crede's technique for emptying the bladder, Kegel exercises to strengthen pelvic floor muscles, and reflex training.
- Bowel training may be accomplished by scheduled toileting, stimulation techniques, or both.

REVIEW QUESTIONS

1. Which of the following diagnostic tests/procedures is done under anesthesia and requires signed consent?
   1. Cystometry
   2. Postvoid residual
   3. Uroflowmetry
   4. Cystoscopy
2. Habit training is being used to treat a patient with urinary incontinence. What will you instruct the nursing assistant to do?
   1. Check the patient for wetness every 2 hours and ask the patient to state whether wet or dry.
   2. Encourage the patient to void every 2 hours on a schedule based on the patient's usual pattern.
   3. Encourage the patient to delay voiding and to void only at scheduled times.
   4. Have the patient practice interrupting urine flow by contracting perineal muscle.
3. Patient teaching for performing pelvic muscle exercises includes:
   1. Contract perineal muscles for 30 seconds, then relax for 30 seconds.
   2. Anticipate improvement within 1 week after starting exercises.
   3. To do these exercises correctly, you must be in a sitting position.
   4. You will need to continue the exercises indefinitely to maintain control.
4. How does intermittent self-catheterization in the home setting differ from that in an institution?
   1. Clean technique may be used at home, but not in a hospital.
   2. Sterile technique must be used regardless of the setting.
   3. Clean technique may be used anywhere as long as the patient performs the procedure.
   4. Clean technique can be used in long-term care facilities because patients live there.
5. Care of the patient with a pessary includes:
   1. evaluation of placement position within 1 week after insertion.
   2. documentation of pessary placement so it will not be forgotten.
   3. monitoring for signs of bowel obstruction.
   4. removal for cleansing each time perineal care is done.
6. Which of the following is true of urge incontinence?
   1. A strong, abrupt urge to urinate occurs shortly before involuntary urine loss.
   2. Urge incontinence is often caused by anticholinergic drugs.
   3. It commonly occurs in patients who have fecal impactions.
   4. The bladder overfills so that small amounts of urine are passed to relieve pressure.
7. The most serious complication of reflex incontinence is:
   1. urinary tract infection.
   2. skin breakdown.
   3. autonomic dysreflexia.
   4. bladder rupture.
8. Which type of urinary incontinence is sometimes associated with antihistamines or anticholinergic drugs?
   1. Urge
   2. Reflex
   3. Overflow
   4. Stress
9. Patient teaching related to stress incontinence should include:
   1. It is usually caused by relaxation of the pelvic floor muscles.
   2. Limit fluid intake to 1,500 ml a day.
   3. Fluids containing caffeine stimulate contraction of perineal muscles.
   4. The only effective treatment for stress incontinence is surgical repair.
10. Patients with fecal incontinence should be advised to avoid:
    1. bananas.
    2. alcohol.
    3. pasta.
    4. cheese.
11. A bedridden patient with no history of fecal incontinence has been involuntarily passing semisolid stools for 2 days. You should suspect:
    1. the gastrocolic reflex is being stimulated.
    2. the patient is too confused to control defecation.
    3. the patient may have a fecal impaction.
    4. the pelvic muscle floor has been injured.

CHAPTER

23 Loss, Death, and End-of-Life Care

CHERYL ROSS STAATS

objectives

1. Describe beliefs and practices related to death and dying.
2. Describe responses of patients and their families to terminal illness and death.
3. Identify nursing diagnoses that are appropriate for the terminally ill.
4. Identify nursing goals that are appropriate for the terminally ill.
5. Identify nursing interventions to meet the needs of terminally ill and dying patients.
6. Discuss the needs of the terminally ill patient's significant others.
7. Discuss the ways nurses can intervene to meet the needs of the terminally ill patient's significant others.
8. Explore the responses of the nurse who works with the terminally ill.
9. Explore the needs of the nurse who works with terminally ill patients.
10. Identify issues related to caring for the dying patient, including advance directives, do-not-resuscitate decisions, brain death, organ donations, and pronouncement of death.

key terms

Advance directive (p. 314)
Algor mortis (ĂL-gŏr MŎR-tĭs, p. 311)
Autopsy (ĂW-tŏp-sē, p. 312)
Cerebral death (sĕ-RĒ-brăl, p. 310)
Denial (p. 306)
Grief (p. 305)
Livor mortis (LĪ-vŏr MŎR-tĭs, p. 311)
Loss (p. 304)
Palliative care (PĂL-ē-ă-tĭv, p. 304)
Rigor mortis (RĬG-ŏr MŎR-tĭs, p. 311)
Shroud (p. 313)

A time to be born and a time to die . . .
Ecclesiastes 3:2

Throughout history life and death have intrigued humankind. Artists, writers, philosophers, scientists, religious leaders, and ordinary people have pondered the meaning of life and death. Yet human mortality and the death experience have not been a priority in American society. The culture of the United States tends to be youth and beauty oriented, generally approaching the life cycle in an unrealistic way. Death is a real part of life, just as birth and aging are.

The concepts of death and dying were rarely studied before the 1960s. Many times patients who were not expected to survive were placed in isolated hospital areas and given less than quality care. Many patients who were dying went without appropriate care and technically could have been termed abandoned by the medical profession. Family members, church associates, or both were usually the care providers.

Today, with the reality of the "graying of America" and the increasing number of persons with acquired immunodeficiency syndrome (AIDS), the aging process, terminal illness, and dying are not viewed as the taboo topics they once were. The specialized needs of the dying and the terminally ill are no longer ignored, nor are they denied. The processes associated with dying and death are researched by scientists, health care professionals, theologians, and lay persons. Information concerning death and dying can be found in popular as well as professional literature and is openly discussed.

A **palliative care** movement is aimed toward providing care rather than toward curing treatments. The trend toward palliative care is refocusing health care toward allowing natural death in a pain- and symptom-controlled environment with psychosocial support. Palliative care can take place outside the traditional hospital setting. The environment may be in an institutional setting, in a community setting, or in the home.

This chapter presents information concerning the death process in persons for whom death is imminent. The grieving process for the dying person and the person's friends and family is presented, with a special emphasis on nursing care.

CONCEPT OF LOSS

Death, like birth, is a natural part of the life cycle. Death favors no age, social, religious, economic, or racial groups. It is inevitable for everyone. People in general experience similar feelings and thoughts related to loss, whether the loss is real or potential.

Loss may be defined as a real or potential absence of someone or something that is valued. Real losses occur when something actually happens so that valued people or possessions are no longer available. Potential losses relate to an individual's perceptions of what *might* occur if a valued person or object were lost permanently. Anxiety, fear, and grief are common with both real and potential losses. An example of a potential loss is a 45-year-old woman, pregnant for the first time, who is concerned that her infant may be born with congenital disabilities.

TYPES OF LOSSES

Loss is experienced in many ways. Changes in self-image, developmental changes, loss of possessions, and loss of significant others are common types of loss.

Change in Self-Image

In addition to a perception of self, within each individual's life ideas about personal worth, usefulness, roles, and beliefs are created. Each aspect of the person may be subject to change. Some change is planned. Some change is beyond the individual's control. Situations that lead to a perceived change in body image, such as pregnancy, hair loss, disability, or radical surgery, can alter a person's self-concept. New parenthood and forced retirement often lead to lifestyle changes. These changes include uncertainty about roles, functions, and usual patterns of productivity. The uncertainties and insecurities in role changes result in perceived loss in terms of former roles.

Developmental Changes

Within the life cycle, changes or milestones take place. Insecurities, fears, and feelings of loss result. During infancy and childhood, parents experience a loss of control over their children as children gain independence and self-control. Examples of increasingly independent function are weaning, toileting, walking, talking, and attending school.

As maturation progresses, additional changes take place. As they grow into adulthood, individuals may relate loss to changes in routines that were previously secure and dependable. These changes include moving away from parents, getting a job, and a general loss of dependence and innocence.

Multiple losses can occur throughout the life span. Frequently the losses associated with old age happen rapidly. Age-related physical and body function changes as well as a return to dependence lead many individuals to a loss of self-concept in addition to the developmental loss. Dying and death at any age challenge the individual with multiple, successive losses.

Loss of Possessions

Loss of valued possessions may affect the individual. Generally, a possession has a perceived value to the owner, and its value may not be readily apparent to others. An object may be irreplaceable because of the memories associated with it, or it may be valuable from a monetary standpoint. Loss of an appointment calendar may be as tragic as the loss of a family heirloom. The loss of a pet can affect the owner as significantly as the loss of a family member. For aged persons, the loss of a lifetime's accumulation of possessions through placement into housing for the elderly can be devastating. When a significant object is lost or left behind, the individual loses a part of his or her identity.

Loss of Significant Others

Loss of significant others occurs through death but may also occur through separation, growth of children, change of residence, divorce, or lack of communication.

Separation from significant others may be related to actual distance, or it may be emotional in nature. Children leaving their parents to go to school or to start their own families can produce feelings of loss for all concerned. Placement of a family member in an institution for long-term care or acute care can lead to prolonged separation and feelings of loss.

Emotional aspects of loss of significant others may be related to a lack of fulfillment of expected roles. Feelings of disappointment for persons who have remained unmarried or who have not had children can lead to perceptions of loss. Communication breakdowns or barriers can divide significant others as completely as changing their place of residence.

The loss of a loved one through death is a permanent loss. In nonindustrialized societies death is looked on as a natural, normal event. In American society death is frequently seen as a negative and unacceptable event. This society values preserving and prolonging life. Americans expect to live into old age, even if old age is not considered as attractive as youth.

A death by accident or by unexpected illness is related to a specific situation. Loss that occurs during normal development, such as children leaving home or the retirement and death of aging friends and family members, can be anticipated and possibly prepared for.

No matter who or what is lost, those left behind react to the event. Not all people react in the same fashion to similar situations.

GRIEF

Grief is a normal, natural response to a loss. It is an emotional reaction that is necessary to maintain quality in both emotional and physical well-being. The grieving process involves a total individual experience associated with thoughts, feelings, and behaviors. The grief process is usually most profound when the loss experienced is death. In particular, grieving during a death loss is a complex and intense emotional experience.

In conjunction with grief, significant others who survive respond to the loss of the loved one through bereavement. Bereavement is the individualized response to the loss of a significant person.

Working through the grief process helps the dying person and the significant others adapt to the loss. Grief that is helpful or that assists the person in accepting the reality of death is called adaptive grief. Grief that is prolonged, unresolved, or disruptive to the experiencing person may be termed maladaptive or dysfunctional grief.

Adaptive grief is a healthy response. It may be associated with grieving before a death actually occurs or when the reality that death is inevitable is known. This adaptive response is termed anticipatory grief. Anticipatory grief is usually related to a loss or death. It may be a healthy or an unhealthy response to the grief process. Both the patient and the family members can experience anticipatory grieving. After an actual loss or a death occurs, the grief is considered to be reactive. That is, with reactive grief the loss has already happened.

Grief that is delayed or exaggerated may be identified as dysfunctional. Dysfunctional grieving may relate to a real loss or a perceived loss. It may occur in the absence of anticipatory grief, when grief is not resolved from a prior experience, or when the expression of grief is blocked in some way. Within dysfunctional grief, feelings and behaviors may become exaggerated and disruptive to a person's typical lifestyle.

Specific behaviors are associated with dysfunctional grief. Many times there are expressions of distress at the loss. Unresolved issues may be identified and past experiences reviewed. Emotions such as anger, sadness, guilt, and denial may be present in all types of grief. Some people have difficulty expressing these feelings. The person experiencing grief may show signs of changes in eating, sleeping, and other activities of daily living.

THE GRIEVING PROCESS

People experiencing the inevitability of death, the final loss, are in need of caregivers who are knowledgeable about personal attitudes that affect the experience. The attitudes of the dying person, those of the significant others, and the nurse's own attitudes affect the death experience.

You must be able to understand various aspects of the dying person's life to provide appropriate care. An adequate understanding of cultural, religious, familial, and developmental influences is beneficial in focusing on the dying person's needs, wants, and fears. Although there may be influences from culture, religion, family, and stages of development, the uniqueness of each person causes responses to vary.

Culture, religious beliefs, and age affect a person's understanding of and reaction to death or loss. Frequently, beliefs and attitudes are interrelated between culture and religion. The American work ethic is closely related to the Protestant ethic, which emphasizes independence, self-reliance, hard work, and rugged individualism. With these attitudes, many people believe that privacy is imperative. Death and dying tend to be private matters shared only with significant others. Often feelings are repressed or internalized. People who believe in "toughing it out" or "being strong" may not express themselves when they have experienced a tragic loss.

Some cultural groups, such as African Americans and Latinos, may express their feelings more easily. In some predominantly African American churches, expressing emotions plays an important role. Kinship tends to be very strong within the Latino culture. Family members, both immediate and extended, provide support for one another. Expressing feelings of loss is encouraged and accepted easily.

Religious beliefs influence a person's reaction to loss and death. Most religious groups have common practices related to dying and death. Practices and beliefs vary from group to group regarding dying and the care of the body after death. Specific information should be obtained from the family concerning religious preferences.

Family beliefs and practices and family members' stages of development are responsible for attitudes surrounding death and dying. Past experience with facing the death of a loved one provides a frame of reference for members of the family. The past abilities of persons to adapt and accept losses can help them adapt to the death of a loved one.

The age or stage of development affects a person's reactions to death and dying. Through experience with other losses, a generalized acceptance of dying can take place. Maturity contributes toward understanding and accepting death. Table 23-1 identifies some common age-related attitudes associated with death.

Children have a different understanding of loss and death from adults. Some adults believe that children should be protected from the pain associated with the death of a loved one. Often, however, children who are "protected" may feel abandoned, frightened, and alone with their feelings. A child who loses a loved one to death may regress or be delayed in emotional development until the grief can be resolved.

Adults generally become experienced in accepting the inevitability of death. During adulthood, people must come to terms with the death of their parents and other older family members. Coping with the death of one's parents is often identified as a developmental crisis. During adulthood people have to confront their own mortality.

For elderly adults, the impact from the death of a spouse is profound. Elderly adults may also outlive their children. Loss of one's child at any age is an especially traumatic event. With the increase in the elderly population, it stands to reason that the majority of deaths are among the elderly. What seems to be an increase in health problems for widowed persons during the first year of widowhood has been reported. Elderly adults comprise the largest group of people needing health care services, so it is imperative that nurses be sensitive to their individual needs concerning loss.

STAGES OF GRIEVING

Many researchers have identified stages of grief. Among them are Kübler-Ross, Martocchio, and Rando.

Kübler-Ross

One of the most prominent and popular authors is Kübler-Ross, who in 1969 identified five stages of grieving. The five stages are denial, anger, bargaining, depression, and acceptance. The stages represent a series of responses to an anticipated or actual loss. Kübler-Ross identified specific behaviors for each stage.

Denial. The person refuses to acknowledge the loss and may put forth a cheerful appearance to prolong the denial of the loss. Denial serves to protect the patient, family, or both from the reality of the loss.

Anger. The patient or family members may become angry or outraged with situations. The anger and resentment may

table 23-1 ***Age-Related Beliefs About Death***

AGE RANGE	BELIEFS
Infancy to 5 years (preschool)	Little or no understanding of death Death is temporary and reversible, like sleep
6 to 9 years (school age)	Death is final Own death can be avoided Death is related to violence Wishing or hoping for death can make it happen
10 to 12 years (preadolescent)	Death is an inevitable end to life Grasps own mortality by discussing fear of death or life after death Expresses feelings of death based on adult attitudes
13 to 18 years (adolescent)	Afraid of prolonged death May act out defiance for death through dangerous or self-destructive acts Has a philosophical or religious approach to death Seldom thinks about death
19 to 45 years (young adulthood)	Cultural and religious beliefs influence attitudes Death is seen as a future event
45 to 65 years (middle adulthood)	Accepts own mortality as inevitable Faces death of parents and peers May experience death anxiety
65 years and older (older adulthood)	Afraid of prolonged health problems Faces death of family members and peers Sees death as inevitable Examines death as it relates to various meanings, such as freedom from discomfort

be a result of a comparison between their sadness and the happiness of others. The anger may be directed toward the nurse, the staff, or the institution, as well as toward significant others.

Bargaining. In the bargaining stage, the person wishes for more time to avoid the loss. The individual may express feelings that the loss is occurring as a punishment for past actions and may try to bargain with a higher power to gain time.

Depression. The patient may speak openly or may withdraw from feelings concerning past losses. The patient needs to review his or her life. In this stage, the person realizes that the loss is final and that the situation cannot be altered.

Acceptance. The patient identifies the loss as inevitable and may want to make plans. Acceptance can involve peaceful acknowledgment of the loss. There is a sense of inner resolution of the loss.

The stages may alternate with the individual and the situation. Not all people experience all stages, and there is no predictable timetable for the stages to occur.

Martocchio

In 1985, Martocchio presented five clusters of grief. These five clusters are shock and disbelief; yearning and protest; anguish, disorganization, and despair; identification in bereavement; and reorganization and restitution.

Shock and Disbelief. Persons may feel numb. Feelings of anger, sadness, or guilt may be expressed. Denial may be present.

Yearning and Protest. Anger may be directed toward God, health care providers, survivors, and even toward the deceased for dying. Surviving loved ones may withdraw into themselves, not wishing to share their feelings.

Anguish, Disorganization, and Despair. There may be a decreased interest in the future. Decision making is difficult. Survivors may express a general lack of purpose for living. Crying at this stage is common.

Identification in Bereavement. Behaviors unique to the deceased such as habits, traits, or goals may be imitated by the survivors.

Reorganization and Restitution. Grieving does not simply stop all at once. Typical patterns of life gradually return. No timetable can be set for the process of grieving. Some people seem to recover from grief quickly, whereas others may experience recurrent grief throughout their lives.

Rando

Phases of the grief response were refined in 1993 by T. A. Rando. The three phases of responses that were identified include avoidance, confrontation, and accommodation.

Avoidance. Individuals respond to grief with denial, shock, and disbelief regarding the loss.

Confrontation. Feelings are intense and charged with great emotion. Individuals face the loss, and experience emotional upheaval.

Accommodation. There is a beginning of emotional healing. The intensity of grief gradually subsides. Individuals learn to deal with the loss.

A comparison of Kübler-Ross's stages of grief, Martocchio's clusters of grief, and Rando's phases of grieving is found in Table 23-2.

table 23-2 **Comparison of Stages of Grieving**

KÜBLER-ROSS (1969)	MARTOCCHIO (1985)	RANDO (1993)
Denial	Shock and disbelief	Avoidance
Anger	Yearning and protest	
Bargaining	Anguish, disorganization, and despair	Confrontation
Depression	Identification of bereavement	
Acceptance	Reorganization and restoration	Accommodation

COMMON SIGNS AND SYMPTOMS OF GRIEF

Common signs and symptoms of grief are shared by the terminally ill person and those who lose a significant other. Knowledge of the signs and symptoms allows you to better communicate with everyone involved.

Physical symptoms are experienced during the grief process. The physical symptoms are a reaction to stress. Some symptoms include tightness in the chest, sensations of shortness of breath, suffocation, generalized weakness, intense tightening in the abdomen, and emptiness or churning in the stomach. These symptoms may fluctuate throughout the grief process. Generally, they may occur with the initial acknowledgment of death as the outcome. The patient and the family members may experience the symptoms of a stress reaction.

You should be aware that the stress reaction is a very real experience. Nursing intervention may be needed to assist a person in regaining a sense of physical function.

Awareness of Terminal Illness

Awareness of terminal illness and impending death affects the dying person and the family emotionally and physiologically. Strauss and Glaser have identified three states of awareness: closed awareness, mutual pretense, and open awareness.

Closed Awareness. When closed awareness occurs, the family and the patient recognize that the patient is ill. They may not understand the severity of the illness. There is a lack of awareness related to impending death.

Mutual Pretense. With mutual pretense, the patient, the loved ones, and the care providers know of the terminal prognosis. No one discusses the issue openly, and people may make every effort to avoid the subject. Frequently the patient avoids the subject to protect the family and the caregivers from discomfort.

Open Awareness. Most health care providers prefer open awareness in most situations. With open awareness, the patient and others involved freely discuss the impending death. The discussions may be difficult, but they allow the patient and the family to become comfortable with the topic. The patient can participate in making final arrangements for personal business. Open awareness is not necessarily appropriate for all people. Some people are unable to cope emotionally with an open, honest discussion of death.

Generally, honesty is the best choice in dealing with death. Many times ethical dilemmas occur over whether to "tell" the patient about the terminal illness and impending death. At times the physician may decide not to tell the patient about the expected outcome of the illness or disease, frequently opting to discuss the patient's condition with family members. The decision may be the physician's alone or it may be based on family wishes. More often than not, the patient knows the prognosis even if he or she is not told directly. If such is the case, the patient may feel distrustful and suspicious of the care providers and the family based on a breach in confidentiality. This suspicion can be a source of great discomfort for the patient.

Honesty in most cases provides patients with the opportunity to accept their fate. Through understanding of the illness and participation in their own care, patients can work through and take control of their grief.

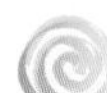

What Does Culture Have to do with Grief?

Culture strongly influences the way people handle grief. For example, traditional Vietnamese value stoicism, traditional Mexicans express grief openly, and traditional Swedes accept quiet or open grief. Traditional widows in Greece wear black for the rest of their lives.

FEARS ASSOCIATED WITH TERMINAL ILLNESS AND DEATH

Fear is a typical feeling associated with dying. The nurse is frequently called on to deal with the dying person's fears. Williams identified three specific fears associated with dying. They are fear of pain, fear of loneliness, and fear of meaninglessness.

Fear of Pain

There is a tendency to associate death with pain. Common sayings such as "on pain of death" or "a violent death" have colored the way we perceive death. A dying person who has lost a loved one to a painful death may expect the same type of experience. Subsequently many people assume that pain always accompanies death.

Physiologically, there is no absolute indication that death is always painful. Psychologically, pain may occur based on the anxieties and separations related to the loss through dying.

Terminally ill patients who do experience physical pain should have medication available. The patient and family need assurance that medication will be given promptly when it is needed. Patients can participate in their own pain relief by discussing pain relief measures and their effects. Most patients want their pain relieved without the side effects of grogginess or sleepiness. Pain relief measures such as medication need not deprive the patient of the ability to interact with others.

Prevention of pain and relief from discomfort should be handled with compassion. Pain control must be consistent. It is necessary to provide constant relief rather than to wait until the pain is unbearable and then try to relieve it. Addiction to narcotics is of little concern when dealing with the terminally ill patient. When death is inevitable, nursing interventions are aimed at maintaining comfort rather than promoting wellness. Pain management is discussed in Chapter 14.

PHARMACOLOGY CAPSULE The terminally ill patient should not be denied pain relief measures. Pain relief is best achieved by scheduled administration of analgesics rather than administration as necessary.

What Does Culture Have to do with Pain?

Culture influences how patients respond to pain. Some readily report pain, whereas others try to be stoic. Assess all patients for pain and explain how it can be reduced or relieved to improve quality of life.

Fear of Loneliness

Most terminally ill and dying people do not want to be alone. Many are afraid that they will be abandoned by loved ones who cannot cope with imminent death. Dying patients typically want someone whom they know and trust to stay with them. It may be a loved one or a caregiver. The simple presence of someone provides support and comfort. Neither words nor actions are necessary unless the patient requires something. Holding hands, touching, and listening are quality nursing responses. Simply providing companionship allows the dying person a sense of security.

Fear of Meaninglessness

During the dying process most people review their lives. They review their intentions during life, examining actions and expressing regrets about what might have been. Patients need to look at positive aspects of their lives. Relatives can help patients review their lives. The worth of the dying person needs to be expressed.

You can assist patients and their families by pointing out the positive qualities of the patient's life. Prayers, thoughts, and feelings may provide comfort for the patient. While remaining nonjudgmental during interventions, you can respect and accept the practices and rituals associated with the patient's life review.

CLINICAL SIGNS OF IMPENDING DEATH

Death occurs when all vital organs and systems cease to function. During the death process, systems and organs slow and lose their ability to maintain life. There is a general loss of muscle tone, a decrease in the cardiovascular system, a decrease in respiratory function, and a decrease in sensory abilities. All systems are involved. Table 23-3 lists the systems and the associated clinical signs of impending death.

LOSS OF MUSCLE TONE

The muscular system weakens gradually. Body movements are slowed. Facial muscles lose tone, and the jaw may sag. Speech may be difficult because of decreased muscle coordination. Swallowing becomes increasingly difficult, and the gag reflex is eventually lost. The functions of the gastrointestinal and the genitourinary systems slow down. Peristalsis diminishes, which can lead to constipation, gas accumulation, distention, and nausea. Pain medications may enhance the gastrointestinal slowing. Loss of sphincter control may produce fecal and urinary incontinence.

CIRCULATORY AND RESPIRATORY CHANGES

Vital signs provide valuable information related to cardiovascular and respiratory changes that precede death. The pulse slows and weakens. Blood pressure drops. Temperature may be elevated. Respirations may be rapid, shallow, and irregular, or they may be very slow. Breathing may sound wet and noisy. The noisy, wet-sounding respirations, termed the death rattle, are a response based on mouth breathing and accumulation of mucus in the upper airways. Cheyne-Stokes respirations are irregular with periods of apnea and develop as a person nears death.

Decreased circulation causes the skin to become fragile. The extremities become mottled and cyanotic. The skin feels cool to the touch, first in the feet and legs, then progressing to the hands and arms. It is important to remember that the patient may feel warm because of an elevated temperature.

SENSORY CHANGES

Sensation decreases. Sensory changes include decreasing pain and touch perception, blurred vision, and decreasing sense of taste and smell. The blink reflex is lost eventually, and the patient appears to stare. Lubrication of the eyes with liquid tears may be ordered by the physician.

The sense of touch decreases first in the lower extremities in response to circulatory changes. Hearing is commonly believed to be the last sense to remain intact during the death process. You should assume that the patient can hear and understand. Speaking slowly and clearly may increase the patient's understanding. You must explain to the patient's family and visitors that the patient may still be able to hear. Family members should be encouraged to talk to the patient.

During the death process, the body gradually relaxes until all function ends. Generally, the respirations cease first. The heart stops beating within a few minutes. The physician is responsible for ordering discontinuation of life support if it is in use. The physician is also responsible for pronouncement of death in most situations.

In 1968, a committee of the Harvard Medical School faculty developed the Harvard Criteria for determining a permanently nonfunctioning brain. The criteria deal with specific functions that must be evaluated before a physician can determine death. According to the Harvard Criteria the following must occur:

1. Unresponsiveness to external stimulation that would normally be painful
2. A complete absence of spontaneous movement and breathing

table 23-3 ***Physical Manifestations of Approaching Death***

	MANIFESTATION
Hearing	Is usually last sense to disappear *Remember that comatose patients may still be able to hear.*
Touch	Decrease of sensation Decrease of pain and touch perception
Taste	Decreases as illness progresses
Smell	Decreases with disease progression Related to loss of taste
Sight	Blurring of vision Sinking and glazing of eyes Blinking stops and eyelids remain half-opened
Skin	Mottling on hands and feet Cold, clammy skin High fever due to improper functioning of thermo-regulator in the brain or dehydration "Wax-like" skin appearance very near death
Respiration	Breathing becomes rapid and deep with periods of apnea (Cheyne-Stokes breathing) Becomes irregular, gradually slowing down to terminal gasps (may be described as "guppy breathing") Grunting and noisy tachypnea (death rattle) is common *Families need to be reassured that those symptoms do not signal emotional/physical distress.*
Urinary Tract	Becomes incontinent of urine or unable to excrete/pass urine
Bowel	Slowing of digestive tract and possible cessation of function (may be enhanced by pain medications) Accumulation of gas, distention, and nausea due to diminished peristalsis Loss of sphincter control may produce incontinence Experiences a very large bowel prior to their imminent death
Muscle tone	Sagging of jaw due to loss to tone of the facial muscles Speaking may be difficult due to decreased muscle coordination Swallowing can become more difficult; therefore taking food, fluids, and medications by mouth becomes harder and harder Loss of gag reflex Jerking seen in patients on large amounts of opioids (myoclonic jerking)
Circulation changes	Slowing and weakening of pulse Blood pressure drops

3. A total lack of reflexes that are normally found on a neurologic examination, particularly the reaction of the pupils to light
4. A flat electroencephalogram (EEG) for 24 hours, which indicates that there is no electrical activity in the brain
5. The lack of circulation to the brain for 24 hours as identified by technology

Usually the first three criteria are enough for a pronouncement of death. The EEG and other technology are generally used when life support equipment is in use. The Harvard Committee recommended that if the final two criteria are used, the tests be repeated 24 hours later.

Another definition associated with the diagnosis of death is cerebral or brain death. Cerebral death occurs when the cerebral cortex stops functioning or is irreversibly destroyed. The cerebral cortex or the higher brain is responsible for voluntary movement and actions as well as for thought. Many people believe that cerebral cortex function *is* the individual.

Since technology has been developed that assists in supporting life, many controversies have arisen. Questions and discussions have developed around whether cerebral or brain death occurs when the whole brain (cortex and brain stem) ceases activity or when cortical function alone stops. In 1995, the Quality Standards Subcommittee of the American Academy of Neurology recommended diagnostic criteria guidelines for clinical diagnosis of brain death in adults. The criteria include coma or unresponsiveness, absence of brain stem reflexes, and apnea as three findings in brain death: Specific assessments by a physician are required to validate each of the criteria.

Currently, legal and medical standards require that all brain function must cease for brain death to be pronounced and life support to be disconnected by the physician. Diagnosis of brain death is of particular importance when organ donation is an option.

In some states under specific circumstances Registered Nurses are legally permitted to pronounce death. Policies and procedures may vary from state to state, among Boards of Nurse Examiners for Registered Nurses in each state, and among institutions, as well.

PHYSICAL CHANGES AFTER DEATH

After death, many changes take place in the body rapidly. After body functions cease, decomposition takes place. Three specific changes are rigor mortis, algor mortis, and livor mortis.

Immediately following death, some involuntary jerking movements may take place. Within 2 to 4 hours the body stiffens, a condition referred to as rigor mortis. Rigor mortis is caused by chemical changes within the body's cells that prevent muscle relaxation. It is usually fully developed in 6-12 hours and will disappear with the decomposition process within 36 hours.

After death the body begins to cool. This is known as algor mortis. Body temperature falls until it reaches the environmental temperature in approximately 24 hours. As the body cools, the skin tends to lose elasticity and can be broken easily.

The breakdown of red blood cells after death causes a discoloration in the skin, which is called livor mortis. The skin may appear bruised with reddish purple discoloration. Generally, the blood settles in the dependent parts of the body. Livor mortis usually occurs within 30 minutes to 2 hours.

Decomposition of the body happens faster in warmer temperatures or environments because of bacterial growth. To slow decomposition, the body must be kept cool. Embalming reverses the process of decomposition by replacing the body's fluids with chemicals that prevent further growth of the bacteria that cause decomposition.

NURSING CARE *of Terminally Ill and Dying Patients*

Nursing care of terminally ill and dying patients deals with the psychological and physical aspects of care. Nursing care focuses on the grieving process as well as the physical changes that are associated with dying. The patient and the family need to be the focus of nursing care. Respect, dignity, and comfort are important for the patient and for the family. In addition, nurses and other care providers must recognize their own needs when dealing with grief and dying.

Assessment

Assessment of the terminally ill or dying patient varies with the patient's condition. In general, the assessment is limited to essential data.

The nurse documents the specific event or change that brought the patient into the health care facility. The patient's medical diagnoses, medication profile, and allergies are recorded. If the patient is alert, briefly review the body systems to detect important signs and symptoms. Document discomfort such as pain or nausea for prompt intervention.

The functional assessment of activities of daily living elicits information about the patient's abilities, food and fluid intake, patterns of sleep and rest, and response to the stress of terminal illness. Determine how the patient (if able to communicate) and family are coping. You can draw inferences about the stage of grief and the coping mechanisms based on statements reflecting sorrow, anger, guilt, or denial.

The physical assessment is abbreviated and detects changes that accompany terminal illness. The frequency of assessment depends on the patient's stability but is done at least every 8 hours. As changes occur, documentation is done more frequently.

Neurologic assessment is especially important and includes level of consciousness, reflexes, and pupil responses. Evaluation of vital signs, skin color, and temperature indicates changes in circulation. Monitor the respiratory status and describe the character and pattern of respirations and the characteristics of breath sounds. Renal and gastrointestinal functions are assessed by monitoring nutritional and fluid intake, urinary output, and bowel function. Skin condition must also be monitored, as skin becomes very fragile and may break down. Detailed assessment of the immobile patient is covered in Chapter 20.

To reemphasize, it is important to be sensitive and not to impose repeated, unnecessary assessments on the dying patient. If health history data are available in the chart, you can use that resource rather than tiring the patient with an interview. However, it is important to check on the patient frequently so the patient does not feel abandoned.

Nursing Diagnoses, Goals, and Outcome Criteria

The nursing care plan for the grieving patient must be individualized depending on individual patient data. Below is an example of nursing diagnoses, goals, and outcome criteria frequently used during the process of grieving. Discussion of other diagnoses follows.

Nursing Diagnoses	Goals and Outcome Criteria
Grieving related to an actual or perceived loss	Resolution of grief: patient expresses feelings related to grief, progresses through stages of grief resolution
Anticipatory Grieving related to terminal illness	Resolution of grief: patient acknowledges impending loss, demonstrates behaviors that reflect progress in grief resolution
Dysfunctional Grieving related to the inability to adapt to the loss	Resolution of grief: patient verbalizes feelings related to grief process, begins to move toward resolution of grief

Additional diagnoses for the dying patient and family may be pain, fear, impaired skin integrity, imbalanced nutrition: less than body requirements, ineffective airway clearance, spiritual distress, hopelessness, powerlessness, and ineffective individual or family coping. Refer to Chapter 20 for specific nursing diagnoses and interventions for the immobile patient and to Chapter 14 for pain management.

The general nursing diagnosis of grieving deals with the normal grieving that a person experiences following a loss. It involves psychosocial and physiologic reactions to a loss. Outcome criteria, nursing interventions, and the evaluation of goals center on the patient's abilities to express and share feelings of grief with others.

Resolution of grief is the primary goal for diagnoses of anticipatory and dysfunctional grieving. Goals and interventions are similar to these two types of grieving, and therefore they are addressed together. Specific goals are formulated for the stage of the grief process or the specific feelings expressed by the patient. Examples of goals for anticipatory and dysfunctional grief are patient expression of feelings related to grief, acknowledgment of the impending loss, and demonstration of behaviors that reflect progress in grief resolution.

Evaluation of patient-centered goals focuses on specific coping skills learned and expressed by the patient or the significant others. Outcome criteria for goal achievement include verbalization of specific feelings related to the grief process, expression that the loss is real, and identification of specific progress in the resolution of grief. The criteria are evaluated based on specific behaviors and verbalizations exhibited by the patient or the significant others.

Interventions

Nurses need to be aware of how grief affects them personally. The nurse who is responsible for the care of terminally ill or dying patients is not immune to feelings of loss. It is common for nurses to feel helpless and powerless when dealing with death. Your feelings of sorrow, guilt, and frustration need to be expressed. Also, remember there are many interventions that help to ease physical and emotional suffering. It is necessary to recognize and acknowledge what you can and cannot control. The basic recognition of your own feelings allows an openness with the patient and family in exchanging feelings. You must realize that it is okay to cry with the patient or family during the grief process. It is okay to be human.

Priority interventions for anticipatory and dysfunctional grief must focus on providing an environment that allows the patient to express feelings. Open discussion of feelings helps the patient and family work toward resolution of the grief process. The patient should be free to express feelings of anger, fear, or guilt without judgment on the part of the nurse. The patient and family need to know that the grief reaction is normal. Respect for the patient's privacy and need or desire to talk (or not to talk) is important. Honesty in answering questions and giving information is essential.

Families and patients need encouragement to continue their usual activities as much as possible. They need to discuss their activities and maintain some control over their lives. At times, it helps to discuss what can and cannot change.

Grieving relatives, friends, and significant others can provide emotional support for one another. Health care providers need to be sensitive to the importance of significant others who are not necessarily relatives. Resources such as community counseling and local support may assist some people in working through their grief. Generally, simply allowing the involved people to express their feelings helps to resolve the grief.

It is useful to identify the stage of grief (denial, anger, bargaining, depression, acceptance) that the person is experiencing. Awareness of the stage permits the nurse to react according to individual needs. Respect for the person's right to privacy, right to have emotions, and right to talk when he or she chooses is necessary for developing the nurse–patient relationship. Assistance with planning for the future or for the funeral may be needed based on the patient's or family's coping abilities.

Anger is a common and normal response to grief. It is important to understand that the grieving person cannot be forced to accept the loss. You need to acknowledge and encourage the expression of feelings but at the same time realize how difficult it is to come to terms with grief. Nurses are sometimes the target of the anger, and must understand what is happening and not react on a personal level.

Feelings of hopelessness and powerlessness are common in terminal illness and during grief. Encourage realistic hope within the limits of the situation. The patient and the family should be allowed to identify and to deal with what is within their control and to recognize what is beyond their control. Patient-identified goals can be encouraged to restore some sense of power.

During terminal illness and after death, physical care is important. Nursing care during the last stages of life involves comfort measures and physical maintenance care.

Meeting the patient's physiologic needs and needs for safety are the priorities. Physical requirements for oxygen, nutrition, pain relief, mobility, elimination, and skin care remain throughout the life cycle. Physical care should be maintained and monitored. People who are dying deserve and require the same physical care as people who are expected to recover.

CARE OF THE BODY AFTER DEATH

Following death, the body must be prepared for transfer to the morgue or the funeral home. Nurses are responsible for the care and preparation of the body. Dignity and privacy for the deceased and the family must be maintained. Table 23-4 identifies nursing management in preparation of the body for family viewing after death.

Legal and moral issues may affect the care required for the disposition of the body. In certain instances an autopsy may be required. An **autopsy** is a postmortem examination of the deceased. An autopsy may be requested by the next of kin, suggested by the physician, or required by law. Consent for an autopsy must be signed before the procedure can be performed unless the law requires that the procedure be performed.

Each state has its own laws regarding autopsy. Under the law in most states, an autopsy is required if a person expires by suicide, homicide, within 24 hours of admission to a health care facility, or from unknown causes. In such cases the coroner or the medical examiner must be notified.

During an autopsy, organ specimens and samples may be removed for examination. Body parts that are removed are either disposed of or preserved for burial, depending on the situation and the family's wishes. Signs of an autopsy are not apparent following embalming.

Typically, the family wants to view the body before it is transported to the mortuary or the morgue. It is important to make the environment as comfortable for the family as possible. It is your responsibility to prepare the body for viewing before the transfer.

Normally, following death you will place the body in the supine position with the arms at the sides or with the hands across the abdomen. Identification bands should remain in place. A single pillow is placed under the head and shoulders

table 23-4 Preparation of the Body for Family Viewing after Death

TOPIC	NURSING MANAGEMENT
Autopsy	Identification band remains on the body. Contact Medical Examiner/Coroner if required. Consent form signed by next of kin if autopsy is requested. Follow legal requirements and agency policy.
Positioning	Place body in supine position with arms at sides or hands folded across the abdomen. Place small pillow under the head/shoulders. Close eyelids gently, hold for a few minutes, or apply moist cotton balls as needed. Close mouth. Place a rolled towel under the chin, as needed. Follow agency policy.
Hygiene	Wash soiled areas of the body. Apply a clean gown. Place linen savers under the buttocks. Comb hair. Apply clean top linens and cover body to shoulder level. Follow agency policy.
Personal Effects	Insert dentures gently. Do not force. If dentures cannot be inserted, place in denture container marked with appropriate identification. Secure with tape jewelry that cannot be removed easily. Inventory all valuables and possessions with the family, the funeral director, or the Medical Examiner/Coroner staff. Clearly document the disposition of possessions. Follow agency policy.

to prevent discoloration of the face from pooling of the blood. Large overstuffed pillows should be avoided.

Gently holding the eyelids closed for a few seconds helps them to remain closed. If the eyelids do not remain closed after a few seconds, the application of moist cotton balls for a few minutes may help.

Dentures may be inserted gently to maintain the normal facial appearance. If the dentures cannot be inserted easily, do not force them. Dentures that are not in place should be stored in a denture container, marked with identification, and sent with the body to the mortuary. The mouth should be closed. A rolled towel placed under the chin helps hold the mouth closed.

Areas of the body that are soiled should be washed. Linen savers are placed under the buttocks to absorb urine or feces that may be released as the sphincters relax. A clean gown is applied, and the hair is combed.

Tubes that are present in the body may be removed unless an autopsy is required. Some agencies require that tubes remain in place or that they be trimmed to approximately 1 inch and taped in place. It is important to review state and agency requirements.

Jewelry is generally removed except for the wedding band, which may be taped to the finger. If rings cannot be removed easily, they should be taped in place. An inventory of the deceased's possessions and valuables is done with the family. Each valuable is listed and signed for by the family. If no family is available, the inventory of valuables is listed and signed for by the funeral home director. The disposition of possessions is documented in the medical record.

Following the positioning and preparation of the body, straighten the top linens and pull them up to the shoulder level. The family may view the body after preparation is complete.

Many times the family needs the nurse's emotional support while viewing the body. If only one family member is present, it is wise to accompany the person who is viewing the body. The door may be closed to allow for privacy. The family should be allowed as much time as desired.

When the family leaves, apply additional identification tags to the wrist and ankle or toe of the deceased. The gown is removed, and the body may be wrapped in a **shroud.** The shroud may be a large square or rectangle of cloth or plastic material. An identification tag is placed on the outside of the shroud. Additional identification markings may be required if the deceased had a communicable disease. The body is then transported to the morgue or removed by the mortician. Agency policy regarding the transport of a body from the room may vary. Some agencies require that all patient doors be closed before transport and that service elevators be used. Table 23-5 lists the nursing management for preparation of the body for transfer.

What Does Culture Have to do with Care after Death?

Cultural practices related to care of the body after death must be respected. Examples of traditional practices include:

Greece: Body is washed by a relative or elderly woman.

Roman Catholics: Body should not be shrouded until sacraments have been performed.

table 23-5 ***Preparation of the Body for Transfer***

TOPIC	NURSING MANAGEMENT
Body Identification	Identification band remains on the body. Apply additional identification tags to the wrist, ankle, or toe per agency policy. Place additional identification on the outside of the shroud. Communicable disease identification should be listed both on the body and outside of the shroud. Follow agency policy.
Autopsy	Tubes and medical appliances frequently are left as originally placed in accordance with agency policy and legal requirements. Follow agency policy.
Positioning	Place body in supine position with arms at sides or hands folded across the abdomen. Wrists and ankles may be bound following agency policy. Remove gown. Apply shroud. Follow agency policy.
Personal Effects	Inventory all valuables and possessions with the family, the funeral director, or the Medical Examiner/Coroner staff. Clearly package and document the disposition of possessions. Follow agency policy.
Transport	Transport via stretcher to the morgue following agency policy. Assist with transfer of the body to the mortician's stretcher for transport.

What Does Culture Have to do with Care after Death?—cont'd

Orthodox Jews: Dying person is not left. Body is not left alone between death and burial, which must occur within 24 hours. Body is not be touched for up to 30 minutes after death. Only designated Orthodox persons or Jewish Burial Service care for the body.

ISSUES RELATED TO TERMINAL ILLNESS AND DEATH

Patients and families struggle with many emotional decisions during the terminal illness and dying experience. The decisions often focus on physical and emotional comfort. Many people decide that the outcomes should be based on their own wishes. The decisions may involve the choice for an advance directive, medical power of attorney, living wills, organ donations, and resuscitation (Figs. 23-1 and 23-2).

ORGAN DONATION

Organ donation may be made by any person who is legally competent. Any body part or the entire body may be donated. The decision to donate organs or to provide anatomic gifts may be made by a person before death. The decision to donate organs may be made by immediate family members following death.

Some people carry donor cards. Some states allow for organ donation to be marked on drivers' licenses. The names of agencies that handle organ donation will vary by locale. Some common names for such an agency might be the organ bank, organ-sharing network, and organ-sharing alliance. Organ donation follows specific legal guidelines. Legal requirements and facility policy for organ donation must be followed. The physician should be notified immediately when organ donation is intended because some tissues must be used within hours after death.

CARDIOPULMONARY RESUSCITATION

In the past 30 years, cardiopulmonary resuscitation (CPR) has become common practice in health care. Patients who suffered respiratory or cardiac arrest have been given CPR unless a do-not-resuscitate (DNR) order was given by the physician. Many times patients and families have had no choice as to whether CPR was used.

In recent years, much has been written concerning the right to die and the right to choose. Many people believe that the patient or the patient's family has the right to decide whether CPR will be used. It is no longer the sole decision of the physician.

In 1991, the Omnibus Reconciliation Act of 1990 became effective. It is frequently known as the Patient Self-Determination Act. This act requires that all institutions that participate with Medicare must provide written information to patients concerning their rights to accept or refuse treatment. The information must explain the patient's right to initiate advance directives. **Advance directives** are written statements of a person's wishes regarding medical care. The first advance directive was developed by the Euthanasia Education Council in 1974. It was called the Living Will.

Most states have replaced the idea of living wills with natural death acts. Within many of these acts are specific aspects related to the individual's wishes and durable powers of attorney for health care. Directives to physicians may be included. Under the natural death acts an individual can tell the physician exactly what is desired. Each state will have its own unique requirements.

FLORIDA LIVING WILL

Declaration made this ______ day of ________________, ________________,
(day) *(month)* *(year)*

I, ____________________________, willfully and voluntarily make known my desire that my dying not be artificially prolonged under the circumstances set forth below, and I do hereby declare that:

If at any time I am incapacitated and
__ I have a terminal condition, or
__ I have an end-stage condition, or
__ I am in a persistent vegetative state

and if my attending or treating physician and another consulting physician have determined that there is no reasonable medical probability of my recovery from such condition, I direct that life-prolonging procedures be withheld or withdrawn when the application of such procedures would serve only to prolong artificially the process of dying, and that I be permitted to die naturally with only the administration of medication or the performance of any medical procedure deemed necessary to provide me with comfort care or to alleviate pain.

It is my intention that this declaration be honored by my family and physician as the final expression of my legal right to refuse medical or surgical treatment and to accept the consequences for such refusal.

In the event that I have been determined to be unable to provide express and informed consent regarding the withholding, withdrawal, or continuation of life-prolonging procedures, I wish to designate, as my surrogate to carry out the provisions of this declaration:

Name: ____
Address: ______________________________________
________________________________ Zip code: ____________
Phone: ____

I wish to designate the following person as my alternate surrogate, to carry out the provisions of this declaration should my surrogate be unwilling or unable to act on my behalf:

Name: ____
Address: ______________________________________
________________________________ Zip code: ____________
Phone: ____

Additional instructions (optional):

I understand the full import of this declaration, and I am emotionally and mentally competent to make this declaration.

Signed: ____

Witness 1:
Signed: ____
Address: ______________________________________

Witness 2:
Signed: ____
Address: ______________________________________

FIGURE **23-1** Sample advance directive: Florida Living Will. (Reprinted by permission of Partnership for Caring, 1620 Eye St. NW, Suite 202, Washington, DC, 20006, 800-989-9455.)

Continued

FLORIDA DESIGNATION OF HEALTH CARE SURROGATE

Name: ____
(Last) (First) (Middle initial)

In the event that I have been determined to be incapacitated to provide informed consent for medical treatment and surgical and diagnostic procedures, I wish to designate as my surrogate for health care decisions:

Name: ____
Address: ____
______________________________ Zip code: ____________
Phone: ____

If my surrogate is unwilling or unable to perform his or her duties, I wish to designate as my alternate surrogate:

Name: ____
Address: ____
______________________________ Zip code: ____________
Phone: ____

I fully understand that this designation will permit my designee to make health care decisions and to provide, withhold, or withdraw consent on my behalf; to apply for public benefits to defray the cost of health care; and to authorize my admission to or transfer from a health care facility.

Additional instructions (optional):

I further affirm that this designation is not being made as a condition of treatment or admission to a health care facility. I will notify and send a copy of this document to the following persons other than my surrogate, so they may know who my surrogate is:

Name: ____
Address: ____
Name: ____
Address: ____

Signed: ____
Date: ____

Witness 1:
Signed: ____
Address: ____

Witness 2:
Signed: ____
Address: ____

FIGURE **23-1, cont'd** For legend see p. 315.

Special forms for durable power of attorney, medical power of attorney, and directives for physicians, family members, or surrogates can be obtained from local medical associations and the Internet. Specific details as to withholding or withdrawing treatments must be included. What is to be done and what is not to be done must be included in very clear terms.

A person may write a durable power of attorney or directive to physicians without special forms. Verbal directives may be given to physicians with specific instructions in the presence of two witnesses. Attorneys and notaries are not necessarily required.

In the event that the person is not capable of communicating his or her wishes, the family and the physician can agree on what measures will or will not be taken. The physician should document the family's decision.

Several different types of CPR decisions can be made. Complete and total heroic measures, which may include CPR, medications, and mechanical ventilation, can be referred to as a full code. Some people choose variations of the full code. A chemical code involves the use of medications for resuscitation without the use of CPR. A "no code" or a DNR order allows the person to die without the interference of technology.

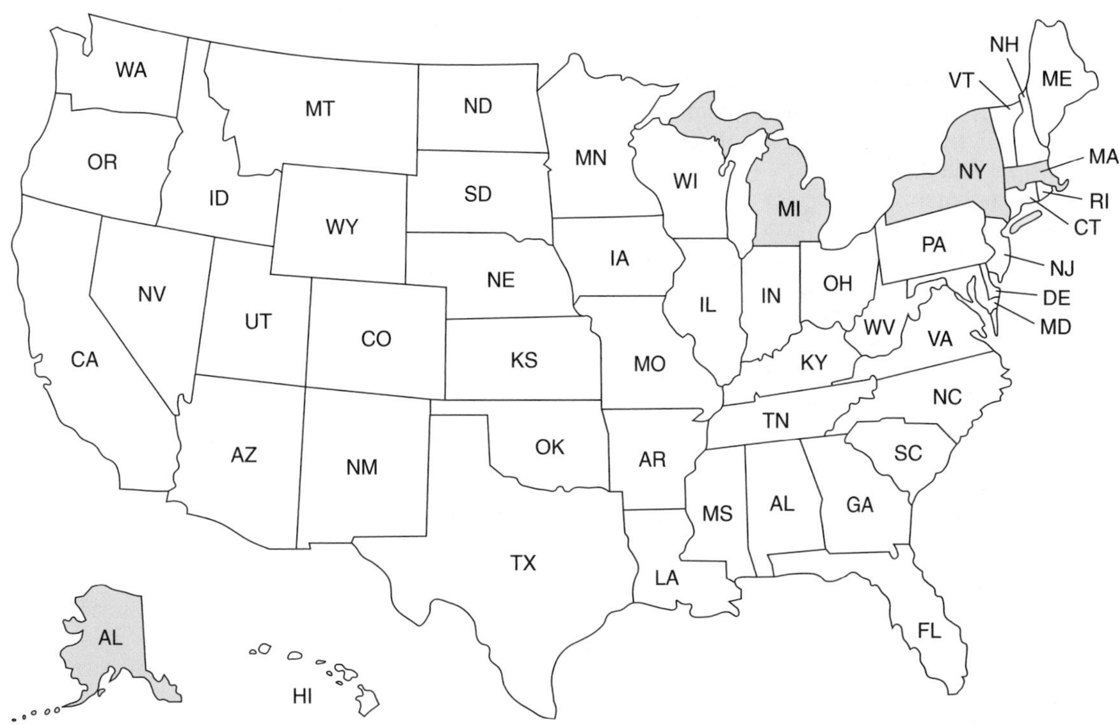

Jurisdictions with legislation that authorizes both living wills and the appointment of a health care agent **(the District of Columbia and 46 states: Alabama, Arizona, Arkansas, California, Colorado, Connecticut, Delaware, Florida, Georgia, Hawaii, Idaho, Illinois, Indiana, Iowa, Kansas, Kentucky, Louisiana, Maine, Maryland, Minnesota, Mississippi, Missouri, Montana, Nebraska, Nevada, New Hampshire, New Jersey, New Mexico, North Carolina, North Dakota, Ohio, Oklahoma, Oregon, Pennsylvania, Rhode Island, South Carolina, South Dakota, Tennessee, Texas, Utah, Vermont, Virginia, Washington, West Virginia, Wisconsin, and Wyoming)**.

Alaska's Power of Attorney Act precludes health care agent authority to terminate life-sustaining medical procedures. The Act does provide that the health care agent may enforce a Declaration.

States with legislation that authorizes only the appointment of a health care agent **(three states: Massachusetts, Michigan, and New York)**.

Note: The specifics of living will and health care agent legislation vary greatly from state to state. In addition, many states also have court-made law that affects residents' rights. For information about specific state laws, please contact Partnership for Caring.

FIGURE **23-2** State Statutes Governing Living Wills and Appointment of Health Care Agents. (Reprinted by permission of Partnership for Caring, 1620 Eye St. NW, Suite 202, Washington, DC, 20006, 800-989-9455.)

Another option is the durable power of attorney for health care or medical power of attorney. This document allows individuals to select someone to make health care decisions for them if they are unable to do so for themselves. This power of attorney can be used only if the physician certifies in writing that the person is incapable of making decisions. Until the physician does this, the individual remains in control of his or her own decisions.

You need to be aware of legal issues and the wishes of the patient. Advance directives and organ donor information should be located in the medical record and identified on the Kardex or the nursing care plan. All caregivers responsible for the patient need to know the patient's wishes.

Terminal illness and dying are very personal events that affect the patient, the family, and the caregivers. Grief is experienced by everyone differently but with similar patterns of behavior. The dying process and death require specific physical, emotional, spiritual, and legal nursing interventions. Caring for the terminally ill and dying is a challenging and rewarding experience.

Put on your ***THINKING CAP!!***

1. Write down the customs and rituals that are followed in your family in relation to deaths: care of the body, viewing, wake, spiritual counselors, services, burial or cremation, types of memorials, support for survivors.
2. Discuss your answers with others in your clinical group.
3. Consider how you reacted to others' customs and rituals. Recognize the importance of your customs and rituals to you, and appreciate the need to be accepting of different practices. Do not assume that your patients will handle death the same way you do.

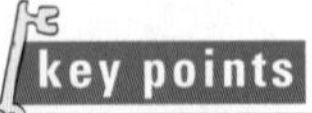

- Terminal illness and dying are no longer viewed as the taboo topics they once were, and health care providers are more sensitive to the special needs of people who are terminally ill and dying.
- Loss is the real or potential absence of someone or something that is valued.
- People experience loss when faced with changes in self-image, developmental changes, loss of possessions, and loss of significant others through death or other means.
- The response to loss, called grief, is similar regardless of the nature of the loss but is usually most profound when the loss experienced is death.
- Adaptive grief is a healthy response to loss; dysfunctional grief is a delayed or an exaggerated response.
- Anticipatory grieving is the response to a loss before it happens.
- Culture, religion, and age affect a person's understanding and reaction to death or loss.
- Kübler-Ross's stages of grieving are denial, anger, bargaining, depression, and acceptance.
- Martocchio's five clusters of grief are shock and disbelief; yearning and protest; anguish, disorganization, and despair; identification in bereavement; and reorganization and restitution.
- Rando's three phases of grieving are avoidance, confrontation, and accommodation.
- The stages of awareness of terminal illness are closed awareness, mutual pretense, and open awareness.
- Common fears associated with terminal illness and dying are fear of pain, fear of loneliness, and fear of meaninglessness.
- Clinical signs of impending death are loss of muscle tone, bradycardia, hypotension, abnormal respiratory pattern, abnormal breath sounds, cyanosis, cool skin, blurred vision, and sensory changes.
- Current legal and medical standards require that all brain function must cease for brain death to be pronounced.
- Changes in the body after death are rigor mortis, algor mortis, and livor mortis.
- Assessment of the terminally ill or dying person varies with the person's condition but is often limited to essential data.
- Nursing diagnoses for the patient who is terminally ill or dying may include grieving, anticipatory grieving, dysfunctional grieving, pain, fear, impaired skin integrity, altered nutrition, ineffective airway clearance, spiritual distress, hopelessness, powerlessness, and ineffective coping.
- The nurse is responsible for the care and preparation of the body after death.
- An autopsy is a postmortem examination of the body that requires family consent unless the procedure is required by law.
- Decisions that terminally ill patients and their families may record in advance directives include desired medical interventions and organ donations.
- Cultural and religious beliefs strongly influence the grief experience and rituals related to death.

REVIEW QUESTIONS

1. The focus of palliative care is:
   1. finding alternative methods of treatment of disease.
   2. providing supportive care while allowing natural death.
   3. delaying death as long as possible by any means.
   4. hastening death when there is no hope for a cure.

2. An example of a loss related to a change in self image is:
   1. The first child in a family begins school.
   2. Love letters are destroyed in a house fire.
   3. An adult child accepts a job in another country.
   4. A patient's hair falls out due to chemotherapy.

3. When a patient was diagnosed with a terminal illness, his wife began to grieve. Her grief is an example of:
   1. dysfunctional grief.
   2. anticipatory grief.
   3. reactive grief.
   4. exaggerated grief.

4. Ms. A has been diagnosed with terminal lung cancer. She tells the nurse, "If God will just let me live to see my children finish school, I will never smoke another cigarette." This illustrates which stage of grief according to Kübler-Ross?
   1. Denial
   2. Anger
   3. Bargaining
   4. Depression

5. Martocchio defines the last cluster of grief as:
   1. yearning and protest.
   2. anguish, disorganization, and despair.
   3. confrontation and avoidance.
   4. reorganization and restitution.

6. Rando describes emotional healing as:
   1. acceptance.
   2. avoidance.
   3. confrontation.
   4. accommodation.

7. Which principle should guide health care providers when a terminally ill person has pain?
   1. Relief of pain must be a priority.
   2. Use caution to prevent addiction.
   3. Keep the patient heavily sedated.
   4. Only medicate when pain is severe.

8. During the last few days of Ms. B's life, family members visited her and talked about shared happy memories and how much Ms. B. meant to them. How might this be helpful to Ms. B?
   1. This would probably benefit the visitors more than Ms. B.
   2. Reviewing her life can help Ms. B. find meaning in her life.
   3. Visitors will keep Ms. B from focusing on her impending death.
   4. Ms. B will pretend to feel better in the presence of her visitors.

9. The assessment of a dying patient reveals irregular respirations with periods of apnea. This observation should be documented as:
   1. intermittent breathing.
   2. decreasing respirations.
   3. Cheyne-Stokes respirations.
   4. ineffective airway clearance.

10. As Mr. C. nears death, his wife says, "I wish I could do something for him." What could the nurse tell her?
    1. It may be comforting if you will talk to him slowly and clearly.
    2. Unfortunately, there is nothing that you can do at this point.
    3. He probably cannot hear you, but may be able to feel your touch.
    4. It is just a matter of time now. Why don't you take a break?

11. A new nursing assistant leaves the room in tears the first time one of her patients dies. What should the nurse say to her?
    1. Get back in there and take care of your patient.
    2. It hurts to lose a patient, but you will get used to it.
    3. You really can't get so emotionally involved with patients.
    4. It is normal for you to feel sad. How can I help you?

UNIT **FIVE** CANCER

CHAPTER 24 The Patient with Cancer

objectives

1. Explain the differences between benign and malignant tumors.
2. List the most common sites of cancer in men and women.
3. Describe measures to reduce the risk of cancer.
4. Define terms used to name and classify cancer.
5. List nursing responsibilities in the care of patients having diagnostic tests to detect possible cancer.
6. Explain the nursing care of patients undergoing each type of cancer therapy: surgery, radiation, chemotherapy, and biotherapy.
7. Assist in developing a nursing care plan for the terminally ill patient with cancer and the patient's family.

key terms

Alopecia (ăl-ō-PĒ-shē-ă, p. 330)
Antineoplastic (ăn-tĭ-nē-ō-PLĂS-tĭk, p. 331)
Benign (bĕ-NĪN, p. 320)
Biotherapy (p. 331)
Carcinogen (kăr-SĬN-ō-jĕn, p. 321)
Chemotherapy (kē-mō-THĔR-ă-pē, p. 330)
Malignant (mă-LĬG-nănt, p. 321)
Metastasis (mĕ-TĂS-tă-sĭs, p. 321)
Neoplasm (NĒ-ō-plăzm, p. 320)
Oncofetal antigen (ŏn-kō-FĒ-tăl ĂN-tĭ-jĕn, p. 327)
Radiotherapy (p. 328)

WHY STUDY CANCER?

Specific cancers are discussed with every body system in this book. Why, then, is a separate chapter devoted to the subject? The American Cancer Society defines cancer as a large group of diseases characterized by uncontrolled growth and spread of abnormal cells. More than 200 diseases are classified as cancer. They share some common characteristics, progress in similar ways, and respond to similar types of treatments. To reduce repetition throughout the text, this chapter addresses the common features of those diseases known as cancer.

Health statistics often group all types of cancer together. Not surprisingly, cancer is listed as the second most common cause of death in the United States. Almost everyone has been touched by cancer. It is estimated that one in four Americans will have cancer at some time. The most common sites of cancer in men and in women are shown in Figure 24-1. Because so many die of cancer, many people assume that a diagnosis of cancer is a death sentence. In reality, more than 8 million Americans who have a history of cancer are alive today.

Some cancers can be prevented by avoidance of causative agents. Early diagnosis has been found to make a significant difference in survival with many types of cancer, and advances in treatment have prolonged the lives of many cancer patients.

Nurses use their teaching and assessment skills in the prevention and detection of cancer. They also care for patients undergoing diagnostic procedures and treatments for cancer. In almost any specialty, nurses work with patients who are being treated for cancer.

WHAT IS CANCER?

NORMAL BODY CELLS

A normal cell has the following characteristics:

- A distinct, recognizable appearance typical of all cells from a particular tissue ("tissue of origin"); has a single small nucleus
- The ability to perform a specific function when mature
- The production of substances that hold cells from the same type of tissue closely together
- Ability to recognize other cells and identify the cells' tissue of origin
- Reproduce in a controlled manner to produce additional identical cells only as needed for growth and replacement
- Cell division inhibited by inadequate space or insufficient nutrients
- Remain in their tissue of origin (except for white and red blood cells, which migrate)

Cells that reproduce abnormally and in an uncontrolled manner form **neoplasms** or tumors. Such cells may be benign or malignant.

BENIGN TUMORS

Benign tumors are relatively harmless, primarily because they do not spread to other parts of the body. Benign tumors present problems, however, if they create pressure on or obstruct body organs. Because of this, surgical removal of benign tumors is often recommended.

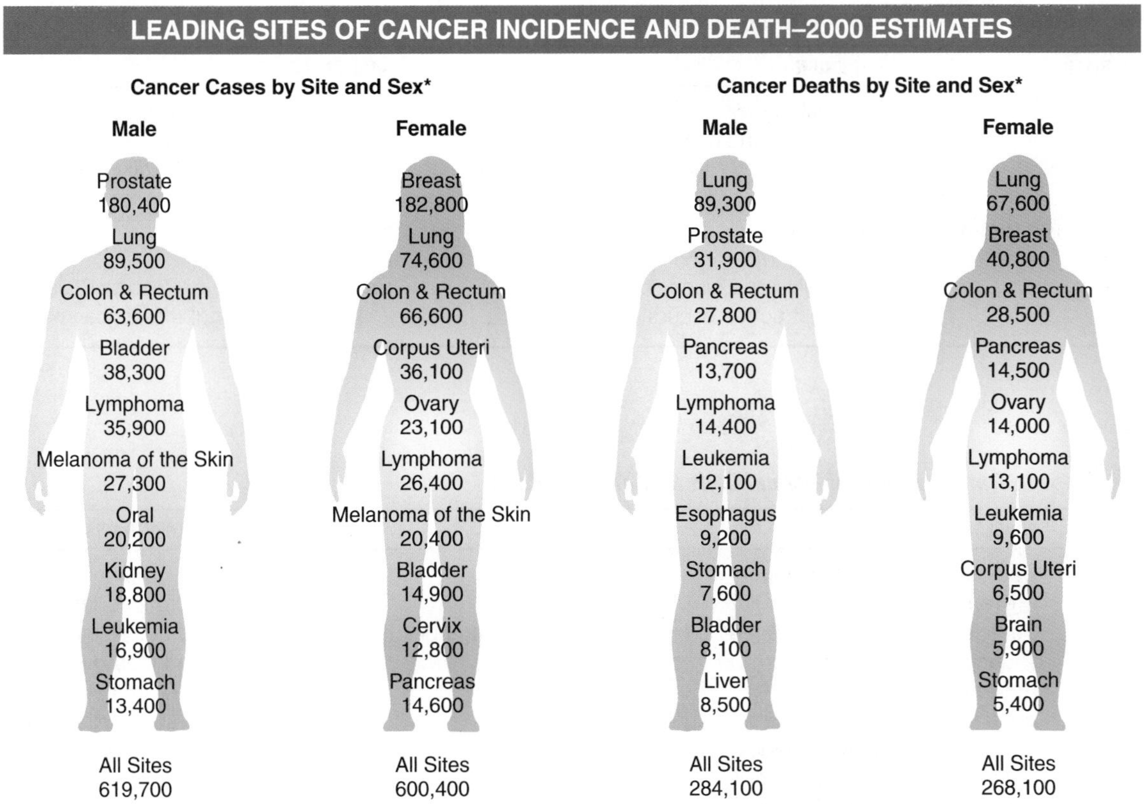

LEADING SITES OF CANCER INCIDENCE AND DEATH–2000 ESTIMATES

Cancer Cases by Site and Sex*		Cancer Deaths by Site and Sex*	
Male	**Female**	**Male**	**Female**
Prostate 180,400	Breast 182,800	Lung 89,300	Lung 67,600
Lung 89,500	Lung 74,600	Prostate 31,900	Breast 40,800
Colon & Rectum 63,600	Colon & Rectum 66,600	Colon & Rectum 27,800	Colon & Rectum 28,500
Bladder 38,300	Corpus Uteri 36,100	Pancreas 13,700	Pancreas 14,500
Lymphoma 35,900	Ovary 23,100	Lymphoma 14,400	Ovary 14,000
Melanoma of the Skin 27,300	Lymphoma 26,400	Leukemia 12,100	Lymphoma 13,100
Oral 20,200	Melanoma of the Skin 20,400	Esophagus 9,200	Leukemia 9,600
Kidney 18,800	Bladder 14,900	Stomach 7,600	Corpus Uteri 6,500
Leukemia 16,900	Cervix 12,800	Bladder 8,100	Brain 5,900
Stomach 13,400	Pancreas 14,600	Liver 8,500	Stomach 5,400
All Sites 619,700	All Sites 600,400	All Sites 284,100	All Sites 268,100

*Excluding basal and squamous cell skin cancer and carcinoma in situ.
Source: American Cancer Society, *Estimated new cancer cases and deaths by sex for all sites*, United States, 2000. Retrieved from http://www3.cancer.org, June 10, 2001.

FIGURE **24-1** Leading sites of cancer incidence and deaths—2000 estimates.

MALIGNANT TUMORS

The presence of malignant cells is the basis for a diagnosis of cancer. Characteristics of cancer cells are:

- Change in appearance from normal cells of tissue or origin (said to be *undifferentiated* if tissue of origin cannot be determined); large nucleus or multiple nuclei
- Inability to properly perform function of tissue of origin; may assume functions of other cells
- Cells not readily recognized by other cells
- May have abnormal proteins (called *tumor markers*) on cell surface
- Random, disorganized, uncontrolled growth pattern
- Continue dividing even when there is no need for additional cells, inadequate space, or inadequate nutrients
- Ability to migrate from one tissue or organ to another

As they grow, malignant tumors cause some of the same problems as benign tumors. They press on normal tissues and compete with normal cells for nutrients. Malignant growths are more threatening, however, because they can invade nearby tissues or disperse cells to colonize distant parts of the body. *Regional invasion* is the term used to describe the movement of cancer cells into adjoining tissue. The process by which cancer spreads to distant sites is called *metastasis.* Tumors found away from the original site of malignant cells are called metastatic growths. The most common sites of metastasis are liver, brain, bone, and lungs. Once metastasis has occurred, cancer treatment is more difficult and less likely to be curative.

A comparison of the features of benign and malignant cells is presented in Table 24-1.

MALIGNANT TRANSFORMATION

Malignant transformation occurs when normal cells are exposed to substances (called *carcinogens*) that damage cell DNA. The transformation occurs in four steps as depicted in Table 24-2. It seems that carcinogens stimulate the initial change of normal cells, making them susceptible to malignant changes. Examples of factors that then promote the transformation of normal cells to malignant cells are increasing age, diet, hormones, and chronic irritation. A person's general emotional and physical health also may be factors in promoting or slowing the growth of cancer cells.

CLASSIFICATION OF TUMORS

Tumors are classified by anatomic site, stage, and cell appearance and differentiation. The term *differentiation* refers to how different cells are from their parent cells ("tissue of origin"). It is difficult to identify the original type of tissue from which poorly differentiated cells developed. The tissue of origin is recognizable in well-differentiated cells.

table 24-1 A Comparison of Benign and Malignant Tumors

CHARACTERISTIC	BENIGN	MALIGNANT
Growth rate	Usually slow	Usually rapid, but may be slow
Growth mode	Enlarges and expands	Invades surrounding tissue
Cell structure and differentiation	Cells closely resemble those of tissue of origin	Tissue of origin not readily identifiable
Recurrence after removal	Unlikely	Common
Metastasis	No	Yes
Tissue destruction	Usually none unless compression or obstruction occurs	Can cause necrosis, ulceration, perforation, tissue sloughing; effects can be fatal

table 24-2 Steps in Transformation of Normal Cells to Malignant Cells

STEP	PROCESS	EFFECTS ON CELLS AND TISSUE
Initiation	DNA exposed to a carcinogen Irreversible changes occur in DNA	Cell appears somewhat abnormal Continues to function normally
Promotion	Sufficient exposure to an agent (a *promoter*) to encourage or enhance cell growth	Latent period before increased growth forms tumors
Progression	Accelerated growth rate Enhanced invasiveness Altered appearance and biochemical activity	Tumor development Cells mutate so that they are not all identical and have differing sensitivities to treatment
Metastasis	Tumor develops internal blood vessels Tumor cells extend into normal tissue by producing enzymes that dissolve substances that hold normal cells together Tumor penetrates capillaries, other body structures, and cavities Tumor cells are transported throughout the body; most destroyed by body's defenses Tumor cells are trapped in capillary bed and form a fibrin meshwork that prevents detection by immune system Enzymes dissolve lining of blood vessels; cell invades surrounding tissue Cells attempt to establish blood supply to support development of metastatic colony	Transformed cells relocate by direct extension, invasion, establishment of remote sites

Anatomic Site

The suffix *-oma* means "tumor." Technically, a tumor is a swelling. The word is most commonly used, however, to refer to a malignant or benign neoplasm. Tumors are named according to the type of tissue from which they developed originally. These names are summarized in Table 24-3.

Additional prefixes may be used to designate the exact type of malignant tissue. For example, a sarcoma could be an osteosarcoma or a chondrosarcoma. An osteosarcoma is a tumor of the bone, whereas a chondrosarcoma is a cartilage tumor. Many other combinations of terms are used to describe tumors precisely by origin and location.

Staging System for Cancer

Because cancers tend to grow and spread in predictable ways, their progress can be described in stages. There are specific stages for all types of cancer. Staging is done at the time of diagnosis and at intervals during and after treatment. Such staging is helpful in planning treatments and in predicting long-term survival.

One method of describing the extent of cancer is shown in Table 24-4. A second, more specific system is the TNM staging system (Table 24-5), which specifies the status of the primary tumor, regional lymph nodes, and distant metastases. In the TNM system, *T* refers to the tumor, *N* to regional lymph nodes, and *M* to distant metastases. To illustrate, a patient whose primary tumor has grown and spread to regional lymph nodes but not to distant sites would be staged *T2, N1, M0.*

Put on your THINKING CAP!!

You are assigned to care for a patient who has cancer. The cancer has been staged T4, N3, M1. How would you interpret this information?

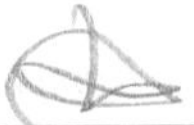

table 24-3 Tumor Names by Anatomic Site

TYPE OF TUMOR BY ANATOMIC SITE	TISSUE OF ORIGIN
BENIGN TUMOR	
Fibroma	Fibrous connective tissue
Lipoma	Fat tissue
Leiomyomas	Smooth muscle tissue
MALIGNANT TUMOR	
Carcinoma	Skin; glands; linings of digestive, urinary, and respiratory tracts
Sarcomas	Bone, muscle, other connective tissue
Melanomas	Pigment cells in the skin
Leukemias and lymphomas	Blood-forming tissues: lymphoid tissue, plasma cells, and bone marrow

table 24-4 Staging Classification for Cancer

STAGE	DESCRIPTION
Stage I	The malignant cells are confined to the tissue of origin. There is no invasion of other tissues.
Stage II	There is limited spread of the cancer in the local area, usually to nearby lymph nodes.
Stage III	The tumor is larger or has spread from the site of origin into nearby tissues, or both. Regional lymph nodes are likely to be involved.
Stage IV	The cancer has metastasized to distant parts of the body.

table 24-5 The TNM Staging System for Cancer

T = PRIMARY TUMOR	N = REGIONAL LYMPH NODES	M = DISTANT METASTASIS
T0 - no sign of tumor after treatment	N0 - no regional lymph nodes involved	M0 - no distant metastasis
Tis - malignancy in epithelial tissue but not basement membrane	N1 - minimal regional lymph node involvement	M1 - distant metastasis present
T1 - minimal size and extension	N2 - increased involvement of regional lymph nodes	
T2, T3 - progressively increasing size and extension	N3 - extensive involvement of regional lymph nodes	
T4 - large size and extension		

RISK FACTORS

A single, specific cause of cancer has not been identified. Both genetic and environmental factors appear to increase the risk for development of cancer. Changes in genetic information of a normal cell can cause alterations that lead to malignancies. Cancer-causing agents, called *carcinogens,* include a variety of chemicals, radiation, and viruses. Table 24-6 is a partial list of carcinogens. Carcinogens such as cigarette smoke, asbestos, and nitrites are commonly found in the environment. Drugs that may act as carcinogens include diethylstilbestrol, androgenic steroids, and high-dose unopposed synthetic estrogens.

Other factors thought to be associated with cancer development are heredity and hormones. Cancers that appear at a higher rate than expected in one family are called *familial cancers.* In these situations, no single genes have been identified to explain the frequency. Hereditary cancers, on the other hand, have clearly predictable patterns of inheritance based on a single gene. For people with family histories of familial or hereditary cancers, genetic counseling can direct the person to appropriate screening and lifestyle changes, and serve as a basis for making decisions about reproductive options.

PHARMACOLOGY CAPSULE Some drugs are carcinogenic, meaning they can cause cancer. Examples are diethylstilbestrol, androgenic steroids, and high-dose unopposed synthetic estrogens.

SEVEN WARNING SIGNS

The signs and symptoms of cancer vary with the location and severity of the disease. The American Cancer Society has

table 24-6 Common Carcinogens

VIRUSES	**HORMONES**
CHEMICALS	Synthetic estrogens
Tar	Androgenic anabolic steroids
Soot	**IMMUNOSUPPRESSANTS**
Asphalt	Antimetabolites
Aniline dyes	Corticosteroids
Hydrocarbons	Alkylating agents
Crude paraffin oils	Antilymphocyte serum
Nickel	**CYTOTOXIC DRUGS**
Arsenic	Phenylalanine mustard
Benzene	Cyclophosphamide
Cadmium	
PHYSICAL AGENTS	
Radiation	
Asbestos	
Tobacco smoke	

box 24-1 Warning Signs of Cancer

Change in bowel or bladder habits
A sore that does not heal
Unusual bleeding or discharge
Thickening or lump in a breast or elsewhere
Indigestion or difficulty swallowing
Obvious change in a wart or a mole
Nagging cough or hoarseness

identified seven warning signs that are associated with many common types of cancer. They can serve to guide the nurse and the public in identifying signs and symptoms that require medical evaluation. The first letters of the warning signs spell out CAUTION, making it easier to remember them (Box 24-1).

PREVENTION AND EARLY DETECTION

A number of things can be done to reduce the risk of development of cancer or to detect it in the early stages. They include (1) general measures to promote health, (2) avoidance of known carcinogens, (3) identification of high-risk people, and (4) cancer screening.

Health Promotion

Many behaviors associated with good health may reduce the risk of some cancers. The recommended diet is low in fat, calories, and preservatives, and high in fiber with at least five servings of various fruits and vegetables daily. Alcoholic beverages and foods that are salt-cured, smoked, or nitrite-preserved should be taken in limited quantities. Appropriate calorie intake to maintain or attain normal body weight is also important because obesity is a risk factor for some cancers. A balanced program of activity and rest with stress management may enable the body to resist diseases, including cancer.

Avoidance of Carcinogens

Some specific carcinogens were mentioned earlier. They include cigarette smoke, alcohol, a variety of chemicals and drugs, and even excessive sun exposure. Public education has focused attention on carcinogens, and people are becoming more aware of the need to avoid them.

For example, smoking tobacco has long been known as a risk factor for cancers of the lung, bladder, head and neck, mouth, and stomach. Only in the past few years, however, have anti-smoking programs had a real impact on tobacco use. The fact that 1 million people quit smoking each year demonstrates that public education is making a difference. On a broader scale, legal restrictions on public smoking are reducing the exposure of nonsmokers to so-called "second-hand smoke."

A harmful effect associated with use of smokeless tobacco is the increased risk of oral cancers. Alcohol consumption also increases the risk of cancers of the mouth, head and neck, and stomach. Many industrial products are recognized as carcinogens as well. Their use is regulated by the Occupational Safety and Health Administration's guidelines for the safety of workers and consumers. Unprotected sun exposure is a risk factor for skin cancers including the most deadly type—melanoma. Increased awareness of the dangers of excessive sun exposure has boosted the use of sunscreens.

Identification of High-Risk People

Identifying people at risk for development of specific cancers serves several purposes. It helps researchers recognize factors that may contribute to the development of various cancers. Also, people who are known to fall into high-risk categories can be monitored closely to detect cancer early. Examples of people at risk for specific cancers are those with familial rectal polyposis, those with family histories of breast cancer, and those with Down's syndrome, who are at increased risk for leukemia. In addition, certain racial and ethnic groups have increased risk of specific cancers.

What Does Culture Have to do with Cancer?

Of all racial and ethnic groups, African-American men have the highest rates of prostate, colon and rectum, and lung and bronchus cancers and are most likely to die of those cancers. Although white women have the highest rates of breast cancer, African-American women are more likely to die from breast cancer. Nurses should encourage African-Americans to participate in screenings and to seek early treatment for warning signs of cancer.

Screening for Cancer

When cancer does occur, early diagnosis and treatment often increase the chance of cure. Public education should emphasize the following:

The value of early detection and treatment
The seven warning signs of cancer
How to do self-examinations (breast, skin, testicular)

table 24-7 ***American Cancer Society Recommendations for Early Cancer Detection in Asymptomatic People***

SITE	GENDER	AGE	RECOMMENDATION
Breast	F	20-39	Clinical breast exam by health professional every 3 yr Monthly self breast examination
		40 and older	Annual mammogram Annual clinical breast exam by health professional Monthly self breast exam
Colon and rectum	M & F	50 and older	Fecal occult blood test every year and flexible sigmoidoscopy every 5 yr *or* colonoscopy every 10 yr *or* double-contrast barium enema every 5-10 yr NOTE: People at moderate or high risk should discuss appropriate testing schedule with physician.
Prostate	M	50 and older with life expectancy of at least 10 yr High-risk younger men (start at age 45 for African-Americans)	Annual prostate-specific antigen and digital rectal exam
Uterus (cervix)	F	18 and older who are sexually active	Annual pelvic exam and Pap test (frequency may be decreased after normal findings for 3 or more years)
Uterus (endometrium)	F	Women at high risk	Endometrial biopsy at onset of menopause
Cancer-related checkup	M & F	20-40	Checkup every 3 yr: thyroid, oral cavity, lymph nodes, testes, ovaries
		40 and older	Checkup every 3 yr: thyroid, oral cavity, lymph nodes, testes, ovaries

From American Cancer Society. (2000). *Summary of American Cancer Society Recommendations for the Early Detection of Cancer in Asymptomatic People.* Retrieved from http://www3.cancer.org/ on June 10, 2001.

The importance of periodic examinations for common cancers

The American Cancer Society recommends specific examinations or procedures to detect cancers of the colon, prostate, cervix, endometrium, and breast. The recommendations are summarized in Table 24-7.

Put on your THINKING CAP!!

1. What are possible reasons that minorities in the United States have higher rates of several types of cancer and are more likely to die from cancer?
2. How can you use your knowledge of culture to intervene?

DIAGNOSIS OF CANCER

The health history and physical examination often provide the first clues to the presence of cancer. Diagnostic procedures may be used when cancer is suspected, when high-risk people are screened, or when determining the extent of known disease. Diagnostic procedures rely on tissue examinations, imaging studies, endoscopic procedures, and laboratory tests. Combinations of procedures may be indicated for cancers that are difficult to locate or to determine whether there is more than one site. It is important to note that many laboratory tests are nonspecific for cancer. Abnormal laboratory results can have many causes, but combined with other data, they assist in the diagnostic process. Also, the same diagnostic tests and procedures may be used during and after cancer treatment to assess treatment effectiveness. Table 24-8 presents examples of tests and procedures that might be employed in the diagnostic process.

MEDICAL TREATMENT OF CANCER

Methods of treating cancer include surgery, radiotherapy, chemotherapy, biotherapy, transplantation of bone marrow and hematopoietic stem cells, and hormone therapy. Various complementary therapies may be employed as well. One treatment or a combination may be recommended, depending on the type and location of the cancer.

SURGERY

Surgery may be done to diagnose cancer, relieve symptoms, maintain function, effect a cure, or reconstruct affected structures. Although not common, surgery is sometimes done prophylactically in people who are at very high risk for development of specific cancers. For example, those with familial polyposis may have a portion of the colon removed to prevent colon cancer. Surgery is commonly used in the treatment of cancers. Increasingly, surgery is employed in combination with other therapies. Surgery for cancer may be extensive or simple. A thorough preoperative diagnostic

table 24-8 **DIAGNOSTIC TESTS AND PROCEDURES | *for Cancer***

TEST/PROCEDURE	EXAMPLES OF USES
TISSUE EXAMINATION	
Specimens of body fluids, secretions, or tissues are obtained and examined microscopically to detect the presence of malignant cells. Fluids and secretions can be obtained by swabs or smears, by venipuncture, or by withdrawal of fluids from body structures.	Papanicolaou test detects cancer cells in cervical smear. Examination of body fluids from digestive and respiratory tracts for presence of cancer cells. Blood cells examined to diagnose leukemias and lymphomas.
Tissue samples are obtained by biopsy (the removal of cells from living tissue). Specimen may be entire growth, sample cut from the growth, or cells drawn from the growth with a needle.	Biopsy: samples can be taken from any accessible growth. Tissue is examined for cancer cells.
IMAGING STUDIES	
Plain Radiographs	Chest radiographs detect changes in lung tissue and bones. Can reveal organ size, position, abnormal structures/shapes. Mammography detects potentially malignant breast calcifications before they can be felt.
Contrast Radiographs Use contrast media given orally or intravenously to outline hollow organs. Shadows of abnormal structures can be visualized.	Used primarily to detect cancers of the digestive and urinary tracts.
Computed Tomography (CT Scan) Provides cross-sectional, three-dimensional views of body tissue (Fig. 24-2). Details much clearer than radiographs. Can be done plain or with contrast media.	Used to detect cancers of the head and trunk, spine, joints, and soft tissue. Also useful in staging bronchogenic and gastrointestinal tumors.
Positron Emission Tomography A nuclear scan that reveals patterns of tissue metabolism. Two intravenous lines are started: one to deliver an isotope, another to draw blood samples.	Used to detect solid tumors in the brain and breast and to assess the effects of cancer treatment.
Magnetic Resonance Imaging Uses radiofrequency waves in the presence of a strong magnetic field. Energy changes are measured and converted to computer images. Does not expose patient to radiation.	Used to detect cancers of the central nervous system, spinal column, neck, bones, joints, lung, kidney, and others.
Radionuclide Scans Radionuclides are radioactive substances that are taken up by specific body tissues. The patient is given a radionuclide, usually intravenously, and is then scanned to study the pattern of uptake of the radionuclide in target tissues. The radionuclide accumulates in target tissue, with greater uptake in abnormal tissue.	Used to detect tissue abnormalities. For example, technetium tagged with phosphorus is used for bone scans because technetium is absorbed in increased amounts in bone tissue where abnormal activity or increased metabolism is evident. Other radionuclides are used to detect cancers of the thyroid, liver, lung, and breast as well as lymphoma and melanoma.
ENDOSCOPIC PROCEDURES	
Lighted tubes are inserted into hollow organs or body cavities to visualize and take specimens of suspicious tissue for examination.	Examples: Bronchoscopy: bronchi Colonoscopy: colon Cystoscopy: urinary bladder Laparoscopy: abdominal cavity

table 24-8 DIAGNOSTIC TESTS AND PROCEDURES | *for Cancer—cont'd*

TEST/PROCEDURE	EXAMPLES OF USES
LABORATORY TESTS	
Oncofetal Antigens Oncofetal antigens are substances found on fetal cells and the surface of cancer cells. They are called tumor markers because elevations are associated with certain cancers. Can be elevated by nonmalignant conditions also. Often used to monitor response to cancer treatments. If treatment is successfully destroying the cancer, the antigen level goes down. Note that elevated oncofetal antigens can have causes other than cancer. For example, oncofetal antigens may be elevated with cirrhosis of the liver and ulcerative colitis.	The following are examples of oncofetal antigens and the types of cancers they are associated with: Carcinoembryonic antigen: digestive tract, breast; also elevated in heavy smokers Alpha-fetoprotein: liver, testicle CA-50: gastrointestinal tract, biliary tract, pancreas, transitional cell carcinoma, non–small cell lung cancer CA-125: ovary, breast, cervix, colon, endometrium, fallopian tube, gastrointestinal tract, liver, lung, lymphoma, non-Hodgkin's lymphoma, pancreas Prostate-specific antigen: prostate CA-19-9: pancreas, liver, lung, colon, rectum Pancreatic oncofetal antigen: pancreas and lung CA 15-3: breast, liver, lung, prostate BTA: urinary bladder
Other Other laboratory studies of body fluids do not specifically diagnose cancer, but may suggest possible malignancies.	Examples of other useful laboratory tests are: Serum alkaline phosphatase: elevated with metastatic bone cancer or hyperparathyroidism Serum acid phosphatase: elevated with metastatic bone cancer, hairy cell leukemia, prostate cancer Serum and urine calcium: elevated with bladder, breast, kidney, lung, endocrine, leukemia, lymphoma Thyroid antithyroglobulin antibody: elevated with thyroid cancer NOTE: Elevations can be caused by numerous other, nonmalignant conditions.

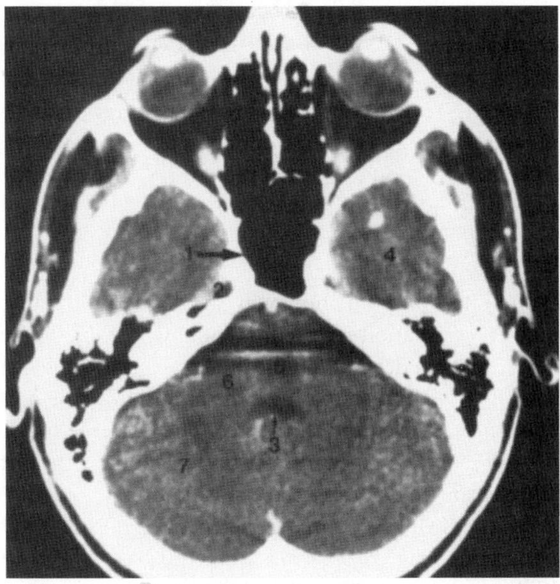

FIGURE 24-2 Computed tomography provides cross-sectional, three-dimensional views of body tissue. 1, sphenoid sinus; 2, trigeminal ganglion; 3, fourth ventricle; 4, temporal lobe; 5, pons (partially obscured by streak artifact); 6, middle cerebellar peduncle; 7, cerebellar hemisphere.

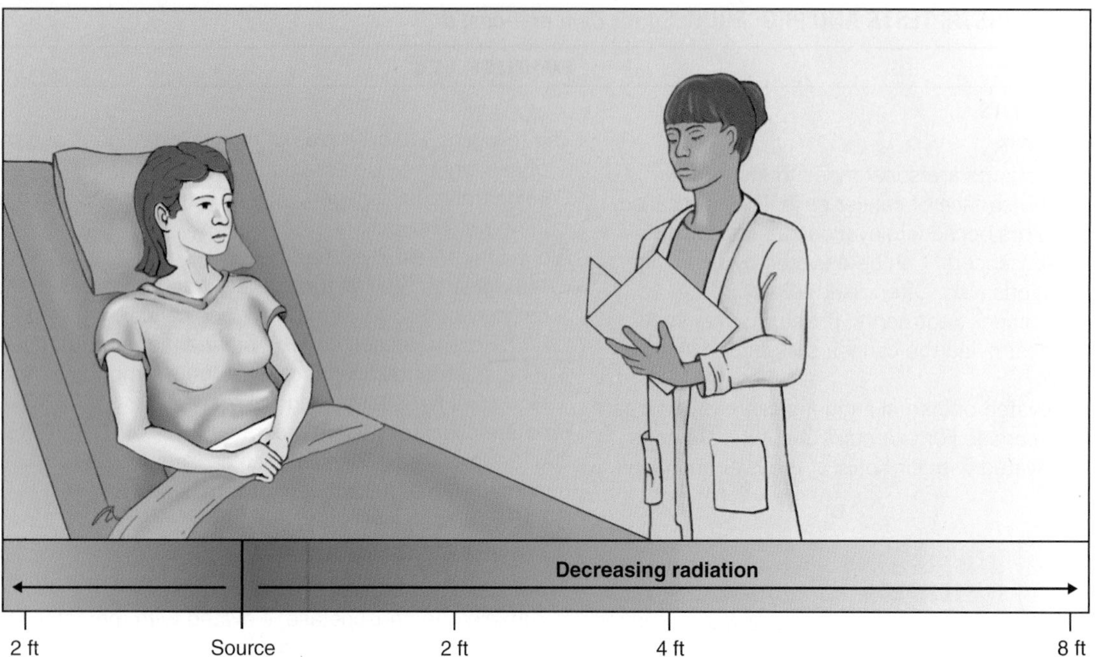

FIGURE **24-3** Radiation exposure decreases as distance from the source increases.

evaluation enables the surgeon to plan the most appropriate procedure.

Surgery is most likely to be curative when tumors are slow growing, confined to one area, and do not invade vital body structures. Surrounding tissues, including lymph glands, are often removed to eliminate malignant cells that have escaped the tumor mass. When surgery is extensive, it is often referred to as a *radical procedure.*

The preoperative and postoperative care of the surgical cancer patient varies with the specific surgery. General care of the surgical patient is detailed in Chapter 16. Specific surgeries are discussed in individual chapters. After surgery, other therapies may be recommended. The recommended treatment is based on the type of cancer, its location, and the extent of metastasis. The surgeon often consults with a radiologist and an oncologist (a physician who specializes in treating patients who have cancer) to determine the best therapy.

Adjuvant and neoadjuvant therapies are relatively recent approaches to cancer treatment. Adjuvant therapy may be used when a patient has had surgery or radiotherapy and is free of signs of disease but has a high likelihood of recurrence. Such patients may be given chemotherapy to eradicate any remaining undetected cells. Adjuvant therapy is often used in the treatment of breast cancer. Neoadjuvant therapy uses chemotherapy to reduce the extent of the tumor before surgery or radiotherapy.

RADIOTHERAPY

Radiotherapy is the use of ionizing radiation in the treatment of disease. The unit of measure for radiation doses is now the *Gray.* Formerly, the *rad* was the unit of measure. One Gray (Gy) equals one hundred rads. Radiation is used to treat cancer because malignant cells are more sensitive than are normal cells to radiation. Radiation has immediate and delayed effects on cells. The immediate effect is cell death due to damage to the cell membrane. The delayed effect is alteration of DNA, which impairs the cell's ability to reproduce. Types of cancer cells vary in their sensitivity to radiation. A tumor is considered *radiosensitive* if it can be destroyed by radiation at a dose that is tolerated by surrounding normal tissue.

Radiotherapy may be given internally or externally. Internal radiation requires the introduction of the radioactive substance into the body. External radiation is given by way of a beam directed at the tumor.

Caregiver Safety

If you understand radiation, you can work with it safely. The amount of radiation received by those who come in contact with the patient depends on the time of exposure, the distance from the radiation source, and the amount of shielding between the caregiver and the source. The less time spent near the source, the less exposure is incurred. Doubling the distance from the source decreases the exposure to one fourth. When the distance from the source is tripled, the exposure is reduced to one ninth (Fig. 24-3). Unless direct care is being given, remain at least 6 feet away from the source. Effective shielding depends on the type of rays being emitted. In general, the denser the material composing the shield, the better protection it provides. Therefore, lead is more protective than concrete or wood. Because shielding is awkward and cannot provide complete protection during patient care, many agencies rely more on time and distance to limit exposure.

External Radiation

Procedure

With external radiation therapy, the source of the radioactivity is located outside the body. A special type of x-ray machine is used to deliver a beam of radiation to the area being treated. Beams may be directed from several different angles to provide the greatest dose to the tumor and minimal exposure of other tissues. The number of treatments given is based on the radiologist's recommendation. It is not unusual for a patient to be treated five times a week for 2 to 8 weeks. A variation of this therapy is intraoperative radiation therapy (IORT), a technique in which the tumor or tumor bed is radiated directly during surgery.

Patient Preparation

Before the first radiation treatment, the patient goes through a treatment simulation to determine the exact dosage needed, the site to be treated, and the treatment schedule. The patient is positioned in various ways while radiographs are taken. The radiologist then marks the skin over the area to be treated. The markings are usually made with waterproof ink; however, tiny permanent marking are sometimes made. The markings must remain visible throughout the course of radiation. Instruct the patient not to remove the markings until given permission by the radiologist. For the actual treatments, various devices are used to shield healthy tissue.

Internal Radiation

Internal radiation involves the introduction of a radiation source into the body. Sources of radiation used for therapy include radioactive forms of iodine, phosphorus, radium, iridium, radon, and cesium. The source may be either sealed or unsealed. In general, patients being treated with internal radiation emit radiation and *do* pose a threat to others until the source is removed or excreted. An exception is the patient who has small radioactive beads permanently implanted to treat localized prostate cancer or inoperable lung cancer.

Sealed-Source Radiation. Sealed-source radiation is inserted into the body in a sealed container. One example of sealed-source radiation is cesium, which is contained in a sealed applicator that is inserted into body cavities to treat cancer of the mouth, tongue, vagina, and cervix. Sealed-source radiation also may be placed in threads, beads, needles, or seeds and implanted into body tissues, or enclosed in a mold and applied externally. The radiologist determines how long the source is left in place. The patient's body fluids are not radioactive and neither are objects touched by the patient radioactive because the radiation source is closed. Because radiation is emitted from the source while it is in the patient, however, the following safety measures are necessary in most cases to protect all visitors and nurses from excessive exposure to radiation:

1. The patient is placed in a private room, preferably one that is lined with lead.
2. A sign is placed on the door to the patient's room indicating that the room is a radiation area. A standard sign is usually available for this purpose (Fig. 24-4).

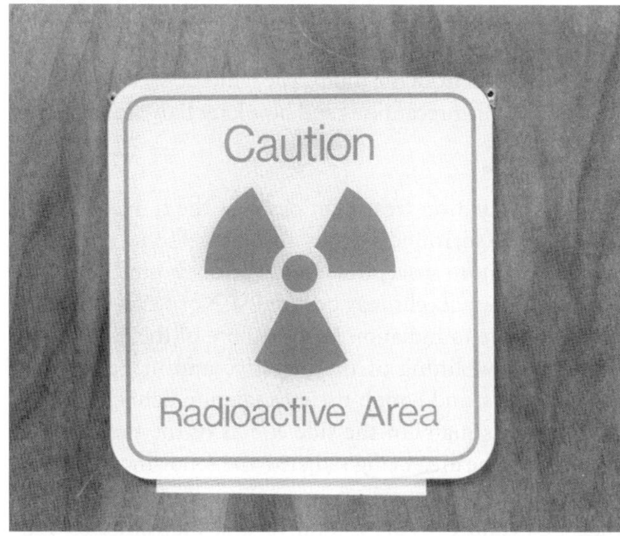

FIGURE **24-4** The radiation sign alerts others to the dangers of radiation.

3. Anyone who might enter the room for any reason is informed of the proper precautions to be taken. People younger than 18 years of age and any pregnant woman should not enter the room. This restriction applies to staff as well as others. Exposure to radiation is potentially harmful to a fetus.
4. The amount of radiation exposure is reduced by limiting time spent in the room and by working as far as possible from the radiation source. Institutional policies prescribe the time restrictions with implants. Nursing personnel who spend the most time with the patient should wear film badges to monitor their radiation exposure.
5. Work must be organized efficiently. For most patients, care can be provided in a total of 30 minutes each shift. Portable lead shields can be used to provide some protection. Lead aprons do not provide adequate protection in this situation.
6. Recognize that sealed sources can be dislodged accidentally. The placement of the source is selected to exert the direct effects of radiation on the area being treated. Specific positions may be ordered for the patient to decrease the risk of displacing the source. Check bedpans and linens for any dislodged source before disposal. If the source moves out of position, immediately notify the physician and the radiation safety personnel. If the source comes out of the patient's body, *do not touch it with bare hands.* Forceps and a lead container (called a *pig*) that are routinely placed in the room are used to retrieve and contain the source.

Unsealed-Source Radiation. When unsealed sources are used, there are some additional considerations. Because body fluids may be contaminated, you must wear gloves when working with the patient. Contaminated fluids, dressings, and the like may require special care, as outlined in the agency policy. Disposable utensils are recommended. Equipment used in the room may need to be checked for radioactivity before it can be removed from the room. The radiologist can advise the staff on specific precautions and how long they are necessary.

Side Effects

The ideal radiation treatment destroys the tumor with the least harm to surrounding cells. Because cells that regenerate rapidly are more susceptible to radiation, both cancer cells and some normal cells may be harmed. Normal cells that are most sensitive to radiation include those of the hair follicle, bone marrow, lining of the digestive and urinary tracts, ovaries, testes, and lymph tissue. Radiation damage to these cells explains many of the side effects of the therapy. Depending on the area being radiated, the following additional side effects may occur: bone marrow suppression, alopecia (hair loss), anorexia, dry mouth, nausea and vomiting, diarrhea, and inflammation of the esophagus (esophagitis), lungs (pneumonitis), and bladder (cystitis). Regardless of the site treated, radiation therapy commonly causes skin toxicity, fatigue, and anorexia. Side effects are usually not evident until at least a week after treatments are started. Some people tolerate therapy well, whereas others become very ill. Factors that influence the severity of side effects include total and daily radiation doses, volume of tissue treated, method of treatment, and individual factors.

Bone Marrow Suppression

In healthy people, the bone marrow produces red blood cells, white blood cells, and platelets. Radiation suppresses the production of these cells. Anemia results from a deficiency of red blood cells. Without adequate white blood cells, the patient's ability to resist infection is reduced. Without adequate platelets, the patient is at risk for bruising and bleeding. Bone marrow suppression is most common among patients being treated for prostate or uterine cancer or for metastatic disease of the long bones.

Blood counts are usually ordered every week during radiation therapy to detect excessive bone marrow suppression. If blood counts are too low, transfusions may be required. The radiation treatments may have to be temporarily stopped until the bone marrow recovers. White blood cell and platelet counts usually recover in 2 to 6 weeks.

Alopecia

Because the cells in the hair follicles are very sensitive to radiation, radiation of the head often produces partial or complete alopecia (loss of hair). Whether the hair grows back depends on the radiation dosage. If the hair does grow back, it may be different in color or texture than it was before treatment.

Anorexia

Anorexia is a loss of appetite. Factors that may cause the patient undergoing radiation therapy to have anorexia include inflammation of the mouth and tongue, altered taste perception, and nausea. Anorexia is a significant problem because it can lead to inadequate nutrition and weight loss. It is especially problematic for patients being treated for cancer of the esophagus, stomach, neck, or head. Depression may contribute to anorexia in the patient undergoing radiation therapy.

Dry Mouth

Dry mouth, called *xerostomia,* is a special problem with radiation of the head and neck. The production of saliva decreases, putting the patient at risk for infections of the teeth and gums. Diseased teeth are often extracted before radiation of the head or neck because the risk of osteoradionecrosis is so great. Osteoradionecrosis is destruction of bone caused by radiation. It is a debilitating complication of head and neck radiation.

Effects on Reproduction

Radiation is potentially harmful to reproductive cells as well as to the developing fetus and embryo. Therefore, radiotherapy is not recommended during pregnancy, and patients are advised to avoid becoming pregnant during the therapy.

The major side effects of radiation are summarized in Table 24-9.

CHEMOTHERAPY

Chemotherapy is the use of chemical agents in the treatment of disease. Chemical agents specifically used to treat cancer are called *antineoplastic* or *anticancer drugs.* The terms *chemotherapy, anticancer,* and *antineoplastic drugs* are used interchangeably in this chapter, just as they are in common practice. These drugs act by destroying rapidly dividing cells and may be used alone or in combination with other forms of treatment. In some cases, chemotherapy is curative. In other circumstances, it may reduce the number of cancer cells, causing symptoms to decrease and often prolonging life.

Types of Antineoplastic Drugs

Types of antineoplastic drugs now commonly used in chemotherapy include cytotoxic agents, hormones and hormone antagonists, and biologic response modifiers. Various types of cancer are sensitive to different drugs or drug combinations. Combinations are sometimes used to attack cells at different stages of development. Drugs that are effective only during a particular phase of cell development are said to be *cell-cycle phase-specific.* Drugs that are effective during any phase of cell development are said to be *cell-cycle phase-nonspecific.* Table 24-10 gives examples of drugs used in chemotherapy and the cancers for which they are used. A new class of drugs that is being studied for cancer treatment is called *angiogenesis inhibitors.* These agents prevent the development of new blood vessels in tumors so that they cannot grow. Angiogenesis inhibitors will not eliminate tumors but are expected to be safe enough for continuous use because they are less toxic than current drugs.

Chemotherapy is administered by a physician or a nurse who has had specialized education. The drugs may be given in an inpatient or outpatient setting. The route may be oral, intramuscular, intravenous, intracavity, or intrathecal. *Intracavity* means the drug is instilled into a body cavity such as the bladder. Intrathecal chemotherapy is given in the subarachnoid space.

Perfusion is a technique in which the drug is injected directly into an artery supplying the tumor. Perfusion has been

table 24-9 ***Side Effects of Radiation Therapy and Nursing Implications***

SITE	SIDE EFFECTS	NURSING IMPLICATIONS
Skin	Erythema (redness), desquamation (peeling), permanent darkening	Skin is easily injured. Avoid exposure to sun, trauma, harsh chemicals, or soaps. Until therapy is completed, no lotions or topical medications should be applied. Do not remove markings.
Scalp	Partial or complete alopecia (hair loss); may be permanent	New hair may be different color and texture. Cover scalp with wig, cap, or scarf if patient desires. Refer to American Cancer Society for free hairpieces and help with styling and care.
Digestive tract	Anorexia, inflammation and dryness of the mouth, decreased or altered sense of taste	Small, frequent feedings. Respect patient preferences. Frequent oral hygiene. Suggest artificial saliva. Monitor weight to assess nutritional state.
	Dental caries	Encourage dental care. Mouth care per protocol.
	Painful swallowing	Antacids and viscous lidocaine as ordered.
	Nausea, vomiting	Antiemetics as ordered. Monitor intake.
	Diarrhea	Antidiarrheals as ordered. Perianal care.
Urinary tract	Cystitis	Increase fluid intake.
	Contracted bladder	Have patient empty bladder often.
	Crystalluria	Keep intake and output records.
Bone marrow	Suppressed production of red blood cells, white blood cells, and platelets	Schedule activities to prevent overtiring. Protect from infection. Protect from injury. Watch for excessive bruising or bleeding. Check results of blood tests. Report fever. Use soft toothbrush, electric razor.
Lungs	Pneumonitis	Encourage coughing and deep breathing to prevent pneumonia. Use humidifier if ordered. Protect from respiratory infections.
Reproductive organs	Harm to embryo or fetus; sterility, impotence	Patient advised not to become pregnant during therapy or for specified time afterward. Physician may counsel male patient about banking sperm.

used experimentally in the treatment of metastatic liver cancer and melanoma. The advantages of this approach, if any, are yet to be determined.

Side Effects

Like radiotherapy, antineoplastic drugs act on both normal cells and malignant cells. The major systemic side effects of antineoplastic drugs are the same as those of radiation: bone marrow suppression, nausea and vomiting, and alopecia. Depending on the specific antineoplastic agent, the patient is also at risk for toxic effects to the heart, lungs, nerve tissue, kidneys, and bladder. These problems and related nursing interventions are discussed in the section on nursing care and are summarized in Table 24-11.

PHARMACOLOGY CAPSULE The most dangerous adverse effect of antineoplastic drugs used in chemotherapy is bone marrow suppression.

Although bone marrow suppression is the most *dangerous* side effect, nausea and vomiting are likely to be the most distressing. Antineoplastic drugs simultaneously irritate the lining of the digestive tract and stimulate the vomiting center in the brain. Some agents, especially doxorubicin (Adriamycin), have toxic effects on the heart that may lead to heart failure. Bleomycin (Blenoxane) causes pulmonary inflammation and fibrosis that usually reverses after the therapy is completed. Vinblastine (Velban) and vincristine (Oncovin) are neurotoxic, with effects manifested most often by numbness and tingling of extremities and loss of deep tendon reflexes. Hypersensitivity reactions can occur with paclitaxel (Taxol) and most other chemotherapeutic agents. Like radiation, antineoplastic drugs are hazardous to reproductive cells, and some cause erectile dysfunction and sterility.

Antineoplastic agents also can cause very serious tissue injury to the vein during administration. If the agent leaks out of the vein, surrounding tissue destruction may occur. When extravasation is suspected, immediately stop the infusion. Various interventions may be used by the physician or clinical nurse specialist in an effort to limit the harm caused by the agent.

PHARMACOLOGY CAPSULE Tissue destruction can result from leakage of intravenous antineoplastic agents into surrounding tissues.

BIOTHERAPY

Agents that work by affecting biologic processes (referred to as biotherapy) include hematopoietic growth factors,

table 24-10 ***Examples of Drugs Used to Treat Cancer***

CYTOTOXIC DRUGS

Mitotic Inhibitors (Plant Alkaloids)

Docetaxel (Taxotere)
Paclitaxel (Taxol)
Vinblastine (Velban)
Vincristine (Oncovin)
Vinorelbine (Navelbine)

Alkylating Agents

Busulfan (Myleran)
Carboplatin (Paraplatin)
Carmustine (BCNU)
Chlorambucil (Leukeran)
Cisplatin (Platinol)
Cyclophosphamide (Cytoxan)
Ifosfamide (Ifex)
Lomustine (CCNU)
Mechlorethamine hydrochloride (Mustargen)
Melphalan (Alkeran)
Streptozocin (Zanosar)
Temozolomide (Temodar)

Antitumor Antibiotics

Bleomycin (Blemoxane)
Dactinomycin (Cosmegen)
Daunorubicin (Cerubidine, and others)
Doxorubicin (Adriamycin)
Epirubicin (Ellence)
Idarubicin hydrochloride (Idamycin)
Mitomycin (Mutamycin)
Mitoxantrone (Novantrone)
Plicamycin (Mithramycin)
Valrubicin (Valstar)

Antimetabolites

Folic Acid Analog
- Methotrexate (Folex)

Pyrimidine Analogs
- Capecitabine (Cytosar-U, and others)
- Cytarabine (Cytosar-U)
- Fluorouracil (Adrucil)
- Floxuridine (FUDR)
- Gemcitabine (Gemzar)

Purine Analogs
- Fludarabine (Fludara)
- Mercaptopurine (Purinethol)
- Pentostatin (Nipent)
- Thioguanine (Thioguanine)

Topoisomerase Inhibitors

Etoposide (Etopophos, VePesid, and others)
Irinotecan (Camptosar)
Teniposide (Vumon)
Topotecan (Hycamtin)

Miscellaneous

Altretamine (Hexalen)
Asparaginase (Elspar)
Dacarbazine (DTIC-Dome)
Hydroxyurea (Hydrea)
Pegaspargase (Oncaspar)
Mitotane (Lysodren)
Procarbazine (Matulane)

HORMONES AND HORMONE ANTAGONISTS

Androgens

Fluoxymesterone (Halotestin)
Testosterone (generic only)
Testolactone (Teslac)

Gonadotropic-Releasing Hormone Analogs

Leuprolide (Lupron)
Goserelin (Zoladex)

Androgen Receptor Blockers

Flutamide (Eulexin)
Bicalutamide (Casodex)
Nilutamide (Nilandron)

Estrogens

Diethylstilbestrol diphosphate (Stilphostrol)
Ethinyl estradiol (Estinyl)

Estrogen Mustard

Estraumustine (Emcyt)

Antiestrogens

Tamoxifen (Nolvadex)
Raloxifene (Evista)
Toremifene (Fareston)

Progestins

Medroxyprogesterone acetate (Depo-Provera)
Megestrol acetate (Megace)

Aromatase Inhibitors

Anastrozole (Arimidex)
Letrozole (Femara)
Exemestane (Aromasin)

Glucocorticoid

Prednisone (Deltasone, et al)

BIOLOGIC RESPONSE MODIFIERS (IMMUNOSTIMULANTS)

Interferons

Interferon alfa-2a (Roferon-A)
Interferon alfa-2b (Intron A)
Interferon alfa-n3 (Alferon N)
Interferon beta-1a (Avonex)
Interferon beta-1b (Betaseron)
Interferon gamma-1b (Actimmune)

Interleukins

Aldesleukin/Interleukin-2 (Proleukin)
Oprelvekin/Interleukin 11 (Neumega)

Vaccines

BCG vaccine (TheraCys, and others)

Colony-Stimulating Factors

Erythropoietin (EPO, Epogen, Procrit)
Filgrastim/Granulocyte CSF (G-CSF, Neupogen)
Sargramostim/Granulocyte-macrophage CSF (GM-CSF, Leukine)
Interleukin-3
Macrophage CSF

Other

Levamisole (Ergamisol)

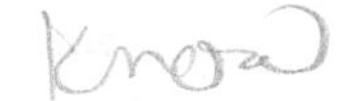

table 24-11 ***Side Effects of Antineoplastic Therapy and Nursing Implications***

SITE	SIDE EFFECTS	IMPLICATIONS
Bone marrow	Suppressed production of red blood cells, white blood cells, and platelets	Monitor blood test results. Allow rest. Prevent overtiring. Protect from infection. Report fever. Watch for excessive bruising or bleeding. Apply pressure to injection sites. Avoid rectal temperatures if white blood cell count is low. Use soft toothbrush and electric razor.
Digestive tract	Nausea and vomiting	Give antiemetics as ordered. Assess for dehydration. No fluids with meals. Pleasant environment. Respect food preferences.
	Anorexia	Small, frequent feedings. Frequent oral hygiene. Monitor weight. Give supplements as ordered.
	Xerostomia	Increase fluid intake. Recommend artificial saliva, sugarless gum or hard candy, ice chips. Moisten dry food.
	Stomatitis	Encourage dental care. Mouth care as ordered or per protocol. Assess for lesions.
	Diarrhea	Antidiarrheals as ordered. Perianal care.
	Constipation	Encourage fluids and high-fiber foods and exercise as tolerated. Give laxatives, stool softeners, enemas as ordered.
Heart	Cardiomyopathy Heart failure	Monitor for dyspnea, edema, increasing pulse pressure. Request electrocardiograms as ordered.
Lungs	Inflammation, fibrosis	Encourage turning, coughing, and deep breathing to prevent pneumonia. Use humidifier as ordered. Elevate head if dyspneic. Protect from respiratory infections. Monitor activity tolerance.
Nerve tissue	Numbness, tingling, loss	Assess sensation. Protect affected areas from injury of deep tendon reflexes.
Scalp	Alopecia	Cover scalp with hairpiece, scarf, turban if patient wishes. Refer to American Cancer Society for free hairpieces and help with grooming.
Veins	Phlebitis at infusion site	Possible necrosis of surrounding tissue with extravasation. Monitor infusion carefully. Protect infusion site. Report signs of extravasation immediately.
Reproductive cells	Harm to developing embryo or fetus. Sterility, impotence with some agents.	Pregnancy discouraged while on therapy and for specified period thereafter. Physician may discuss banking sperm with male patients.

biologic response modifiers (BRMs), and monoclonal antibodies. Hematopoietic growth factors include erythropoietin, oprelvekin (Neumega), and colony-stimulating factors (CSFs). Erythropoietin is specifically used to stimulate production of red blood cells, and oprelvekin is used to stimulate production of platelets. Because antineoplastic agents suppress the bone marrow, colony-stimulating factors may be used to stimulate the bone marrow to produce white blood cells in patients on chemotherapy. This reduces the risk of infection by shortening the period of neutropenia associated with chemotherapy. Chapters 31 and 32 provide additional information about CSFs. With CSFs, higher doses of chemotherapy can be given for longer periods of time.

Surgery, radiotherapy, and chemotherapy work by destroying malignant cells and thereby reduce the size of the tumor. It is hoped that the body's natural defenses will then destroy the remaining malignant cells. Therapy using BRMs is intended to boost the body's existing defenses. BRMs act directly on malignant cells or stimulate the immune system to act against them. Such therapy is most effective if the immune system is functioning adequately. A skin test may be performed to evaluate the immune response before therapy is started. Examples of BRMs are interferons and interleukins.

PHARMACOLOGY CAPSULE Biologic response modifiers boost the body's natural defenses to combat malignant cells.

Because the effectiveness of BRM therapy for cancer is still being studied, it is not usually the first line of treatment. The most common side effects are extreme fatigue, headache, muscle aches, chills, and fever. Side effects are more common in older people and in people who are dehydrated, anemic, and malnourished. Previous cardiac, neurologic, gastrointestinal, hepatic, or renal disease also increases the risk of side effects. Table 24-12 outlines side effects of BRM therapy. The patient should be told to report a rash, blister, or pain at the injection site or a fever.

Monoclonal antibodies (MoAbs) are specific for proteins on the surface of certain cancer cells. The use of MoAbs in both the diagnosis and treatment of cancer is the subject of numerous studies.

table 24-12 **Common Side Effects of Biologic Response Modifiers and Nursing Implications**

SITE	SIDE EFFECTS	NURSING IMPLICATIONS
Generalized	Flulike symptoms: fever, chills, muscle aches, severe fatigue, malaise, headaches, tachycardia	Side effects may mask signs and symptoms of infection, so assess carefully. Give acetaminophen as ordered (meperidine is sometimes ordered for severe chills). Help patient plan for adequate rest.
Heart	Serious dysrhythmias, myocardial infarction	Monitor heart rate and rhythm. Report abnormal findings.
Capillaries	Increased permeability, pulmonary and dependent edema, hypotension	Assess for edema. Monitor blood pressure. Have patient change positions slowly; avoid prolonged standing, hot baths, and showers. For hypotension, give colloids or vasopressors as ordered.
Bronchi and lungs	Anaphylaxis with bronchial constriction	Note signs of allergy: rash, wheezing, itching. For anaphylaxis, give epinephrine or diphenhydramine as ordered. Maintain airway.
	Pulmonary edema	Assess lungs for crackles. Position for comfort (head elevated).

NOTE: Many other side effects occur with individual biologic response modifiers. They include nausea, diarrhea, anorexia, weight loss, skin redness or rash, pruritus, desquamation, bone pain, renal toxicity, anemia, thrombocytopenia, leukopenia, leukocytosis, altered mental status, and liver toxicity. The nurse should identify the specific effects and implications for the specific agents the patient is receiving.

table 24-13 **DRUG THERAPY | *Antiemetics Used with Cancer Therapy***

CLASSIFICATION	SPECIFIC DRUGS	SIDE EFFECTS
Phenothiazines	Prochlorperazine maleate (Compazine)	Sedation, hypotension, extrapyramidal symptoms
	Chlorpromazine hydrochloride (Thorazine)	
	Thiethylperazine maleate (Torecan)	
	Promethazine hydrochloride (Phenergan)	
	Perphenazine hydrochloride (Trilafon)	
	Fluphenazine hydrochloride (Prolixin)	
Antihistamines	Diphenhydramine (Benadryl)	Sedation, dry mouth, constipation
	Hydroxyzine hydrochloride (Vistaril)	
	Cyclizine hydrochloride (Marezine)	
	Meclizine hydrochloride (Bonine, Antivert)	
	Dimenhydrinate (Dramamine)	
Butyrophenones	Droperidol (Inapsine)	Extrapyramidal symptoms, sedation, hypotension
	Haloperidol lactate (Haldol)	
Corticosteroid	Dexamethasone (Decadron)	Fluid retention
Hypnotics or sedatives	Diazepam (Valium)	Sedation, ataxia
	Lorazepam (Ativan)	Amnesia, sedation, dizziness
Cannabinoids	Dronabinol (Marinol)	Visual hallucinations, somnolence, ataxia, hypotension
5-HT_3 Blockers	Ondansetron hydrochloride (Zofran)	Constipation, diarrhea, headache
	Granisetron (Kytril)	Headache, constipation, somnolence, diarrhea, asthenia, fever, taste disorders
Miscellaneous	Metoclopramide hydrochloride (Reglan)	Sedation, diarrhea, dizziness, extrapyramidal symptoms

BONE MARROW AND STEM CELL TRANSPLANTATION

Bone marrow transplantation is most often used after treatment of leukemias and lymphomas with chemotherapy or radiation that destroys the patient's bone marrow. Stem cell transplantation can be used to treat bone marrow depression caused by chemotherapy or radiotherapy. Transplantation of bone marrow or peripheral blood stem cells is done to restore the blood manufacturing cells. See Chapter 32 for additional discussion of CSFs and bone marrow and stem cell transplants.

HORMONE THERAPY

Because some tumors are affected by hormones, various treatments may be used to suppress natural hormone secretion, block hormone actions, or provide supplemental hor-

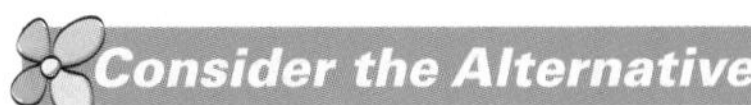
Consider the Alternative!

The American Cancer Society identifies some complementary therapies that can help to relieve symptoms or side effects, ease pain, and increase enjoyment of life. These include:

Aromatherapy	Music therapy
Art therapy	Prayer, spiritual practices
Biofeedback	T'ai chi
Massage therapy	Yoga

mones. For example, hormones may be used to block the male sex hormones in the treatment of prostate cancer.

COMPLEMENTARY AND ALTERNATIVE THERAPIES

Some patients choose to use nontraditional treatments such as relaxation techniques, guided imagery, music, meditation, herbal remedies, and acupuncture. If a nontraditional therapy is used with conventional treatment, it is called *complementary* therapy. The term *alternative* is used if the patient uses nontraditional therapy in place of traditional treatment. Research is being conducted by the National Center for Complementary and Alternative Medicine in the National Institutes of Health to determine the therapeutic value of nontraditional therapies.

UNPROVEN METHODS OF CANCER TREATMENT

Studies have found that 6% to 9% of patients with cancer admit to using some questionable method of cancer treatment. The American Cancer Society discourages the use of treatments that have not been studied and found to be safe and effective. Alternative therapies can be harmful in themselves and may delay treatment with potentially effective conventional therapies. A partial list of treatments considered unproven with regard to safety and effectiveness is presented in Table 24-13. You can direct patients to the American Cancer Society for further information about questionable therapies. The website for the American Cancer Society also provides information on this topic (http://www.cancer.org/alt_therapy/index.htm).

NURSING CARE *of the Patient Who Has Cancer*

When working with people who have cancer, it is easy to focus on the cancer and forget the person. There are many things we can do to help the person who has cancer (see Nursing Care Plan: The Patient with Cancer) that can significantly affect the person's quality of life. Assessment of the patient who has cancer is discussed along with nursing care for each phase of illness: diagnostic phase, treatment phase, rehabilitation, and recurrence of terminal illness.

THE DIAGNOSTIC PHASE

People who develop one of the common signs of cancer are often aware of how serious the condition might be. Out of fear, some ignore the signs until the disease is advanced. When people seek evaluation of the signs, they are likely to be very worried. Patients often say that just "not knowing" is the hardest part. They go through tests and procedures, some uncomfortable, and then wait for the final word. Cancer is often what they fear most.

Assessment

When a patient is having diagnostic procedures related to an actual or a potential diagnosis of cancer, collect data needed in the planning and provision of care.

Health History

Chief Complaint. Begin the assessment with the chief complaint. The patient may complain of pain, lesions, lumps, or changes in some body function. Elicit a complete description of the problem and the related signs and symptoms.

Past Medical History. Document chronic illnesses, serious injuries, surgeries, and hospitalizations.

Family History. Inquire about the incidence of cancer and other serious diseases in the patient's immediate family.

Review of Systems. In the review of systems, record any of the following signs and symptoms, if present: pain, lumps, fatigue, activity intolerance, lesions of the skin or mucous membranes, easy bruising or bleeding, headache, vision or hearing disturbances, hoarseness, cough, dyspnea, hemoptysis, loss of appetite, difficulty swallowing, digestive disturbances, blood in the urine or stool, and change in bowel pattern.

Functional Assessment. Describe the patient's diet, use of alcohol and tobacco, activity, and sleep routines. Document the occupation and describe a usual day. Assess health practices, including frequency of breast self-examination, testicular examination, and medical checkups. Identify the patient's concerns. Ask about sources of stress and of support and usual coping strategies.

Physical Examination

The physical examination begins with measurement of vital signs, height, and weight. Note whether there has been a change in weight. Inspect the face, scalp, and oral mucosa for lesions. Palpate the neck for enlarged lymph nodes. Throughout the examination, inspect the skin for color, lesions, edema, and bruising. Auscultate breath sounds and observe respiratory effort. Inspect the breasts for symmetry, dimpling, and abnormal skin color, and palpate for lumps or thickened areas. Inspect the abdomen for distention, auscultate for bowel sounds, and palpate for masses. Inspect the genitalia for lesions. Palpate the scrotum for descended testicles and, if present, for testicular lumps.

Nursing Diagnoses, Goals, and Outcome Criteria: Diagnostic Phase

Nursing Diagnoses	Goals and Outcome Criteria
Ineffective Denial related to fear of diagnosis of cancer	Acceptance of need for medical evaluation and treatment: patient seeks medical evaluation and treatment

NURSING CARE PLAN

The Patient with Cancer

ASSESSMENT

Health History: Mr. Silas Wilson is a 63-year-old African-American man who was recently diagnosed with lung cancer that is being treated with radiotherapy and chemotherapy. He reports a chronic nonproductive cough but denies dyspnea or hemoptysis. He states that he has been fatigued and weak since starting his therapy. He has had mild nausea, anorexia, and occasional diarrhea. He complains of dry mouth and is having some dysphagia. The skin over the area being radiated is tender. He is married, the father of three grown children, and is an insurance salesman. He has smoked one pack of cigarettes a day for 30 years, having quit smoking in 1996. He continues to work part time and expresses concern about his financial situation. He states he has excellent insurance coverage.

Physical Examination: Height, 5'9", weight, 175 lb; Vital signs: pulse, 72; respirations, 18; blood pressure, 176/92; temperature, 98° F (oral). Alert and oriented but does not initiate conversation. Dry mucous membranes and cracked lips. Skin on upper chest and neck is more darkly pigmented. Central venous catheter in place; insertion site free of swelling or drainage. Respirations are not labored, and breath sounds are clear throughout lung fields. Abdomen is soft and bowel sounds present. Extremities are warm with strong peripheral pulses. No edema. Unable to distinguish warm and cold or sharp and dull sensations in lower legs.

Nursing Diagnosis	*Goals and Outcome Criteria*	*Interventions*
Anxiety related to effects of treatment of uncertain outcomes.	Patient will experience reduced anxiety as evidenced by patient statements and by more relaxed behavior.	Encourage patient to talk about his illness and his feelings about it. Listen attentively and use touch to convey concern. Help patient identify sources of anxiety and strategies to deal with it, such as teaching, counseling, spiritual guidance, and support groups.
Ineffective coping related to multiple stressors.	Patient will identify stressors and strategies to deal with them to improve coping.	Help patient set priorities during therapy. Provide information about management of therapy side effects. Encourage self-care as much as possible. Emphasize his strengths. Teach relaxation techniques. Refer to American Cancer Society for information about support services in the community.
Deficient knowledge of the prescribed therapy, effects, and precautions.	Patient will correctly describe his disease, treatment, the effects of therapy, and the precautions needed.	Determine what the patient already knows and what additional information he wants. Reinforce pretreatment teaching. Remind him not to wash off skin markings until radiologist gives permission. Do not apply lotion to irritated skin. Recommend cotton clothing over irritated skin. Provide information about specific drugs used in his chemotherapy. Refer to Cancer Information Service (1-800-4CANCER) if interested.
Risk for injury related to side effects of therapy.	Patient will have no injuries related to therapy as evidenced by absence of bleeding, dyspnea, skin lesions, or bruises.	Monitor for excessive bruising or prolonged bleeding, edema, dyspnea, impaired sensation. Report blood in stool, urine, or sputum. Handle gently. Apply pressure for 5 minutes after venipunctures or injections. Instruct to use a soft toothbrush and an electric razor. Protect feet and legs from trauma. Inspect daily for injury. Advise to wear shoes whenever out of bed.
Risk for infection related to decreased white blood cells, venous access devices.	Patient will remain free of infection as evidenced by normal body temperature and absence of swelling or warmth at central line insertion site.	Advise patient to avoid crowds and people with infection. Report fever, foul wound drainage, or confusion to physician promptly. Teach patient proper care of central venous catheter and have him return demonstration.
Imbalanced nutrition: less than body requirements related to anorexia and nausea.	Patient will maintain adequate nutrition as evidenced by body weight within 10 lb of usual (180 lb).	Emphasize the importance of good nutrition. Request a dietary consult. Consider frequent feedings. Respect preferences and aversions. Suggest soft diet eaten slowly for dysphagia. Tell the patient not to drink alcohol while receiving chemotherapy. Advise not to drink fluids with meals and to decrease intake of sweets and fatty foods. Create a pleasant environment without offensive odors. Suggest mild exercise before meals and rest afterward. Give ordered antiemetics as necessary.

NURSING CARE PLAN—cont'd

Nursing Diagnosis	*Goals and Outcome Criteria*	*Interventions*
Impaired oral mucous membranes related to decreased salivation, inflammation.	Patient will report successful management of dry mouth, and oral mucous membranes will be intact.	Tell patient to do frequent, gentle mouth care. Recommend artificial saliva for dryness. Encourage increased fluids, sugarless gum or candies, and ice chips. Suggest moistening food before eating. When the mouth is inflamed, avoid acidic, salty, or spicy foods.
Fatigue related to anemia, effects of cancer.	Patient will report adaptations in lifestyle that reduce fatigue.	Assess patient's need for assistance and schedule activities to conserve energy.
Interrupted family processes related to illness and therapy.	Patient and family will discuss need to alter roles and relationships during treatment.	Include the family in patient teaching. Encourage them to plan with the patient for accomplishment of family tasks and responsibilities. Acknowledge family stress and fears. Refer to sources of help as needed. Ask the social worker to assist with financial arrangements.

Nursing Diagnoses, Goals, and Outcome Criteria: Diagnostic Phase—cont'd

Nursing Diagnoses	Goals and Outcome Criteria
Anxiety related to threat of or change in health status	Reduced anxiety: patient states anxiety reduced, demonstrates calm manner
Deficient Knowledge of diagnostic tests and procedures	Knowledge of tests and procedures: patient correctly describes tests and follows directions in relation to tests

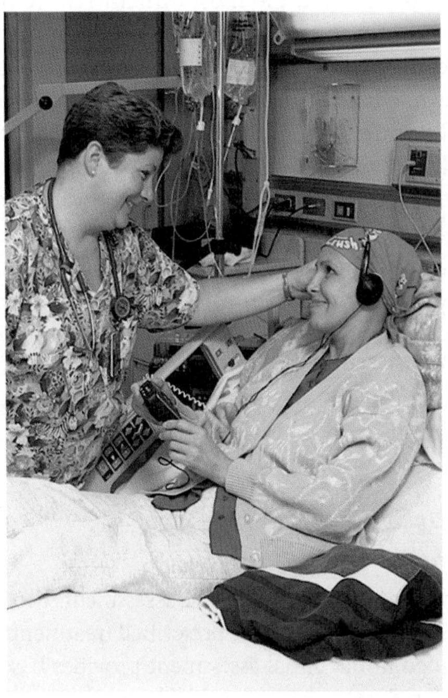

FIGURE **24-5** Listening and touching convey acceptance and caring.

Interventions

Ineffective Denial

When people detect possible signs or symptoms of cancer, they may be so anxious that they cannot deal with their fears. Instead, they deny the seriousness of the situation and do not seek medical care. Such delays may allow the disease to progress, making treatment more difficult and less likely to be successful. Encourage people to learn the warning signs of cancer and to report them promptly. Emphasize that these signs may be caused by conditions other than cancer, but medical evaluation is needed for a correct diagnosis. Stress the fact that many cancers are curable, especially in the early stages.

Anxiety

During the diagnostic phase, the patient needs encouragement, support, and honest information. Be careful to remain hopeful yet not give false reassurance ("I'm sure it will not be cancer."). Clichés are not helpful either ("Everything has a purpose."). It *is* helpful to recognize what the patient seems to be feeling ("You seem to be very worried."). Information about tests and procedures allows the patient to prepare mentally.

Remember that patients who are being evaluated for cancer are under stress. They may show this stress through anger, irritability, fear, or depression. All of these reactions are normal under the circumstances and should be accepted with understanding (Fig. 24-5).

The physician reports findings to the patient and informs the patient of the diagnosis. In the past, it was not uncommon for the diagnosis of cancer to be kept from the patient. Now most patients are told of their diagnoses. This change has come about because patients are better informed, cancer treatment has improved the odds of survival, and the patient's right to know is recognized. Nevertheless, you should know what the patient has been told to avoid giving the patient conflicting messages. At times, you may need to help patients communicate their needs and questions to the physician.

Once a diagnosis of cancer has been made, the patient needs support to adapt to the situation. Even at this phase of the illness, the patient may show various responses related to grief. Responses could include denial, shock and disbelief, anger, depression, bargaining, and acceptance. It is useful to understand and recognize how to help the grieving patient. Chapter 23 discusses nursing care of the grieving patient.

Patients struggle to adjust to the knowledge that they have cancer. For many, this is the first time they have seriously considered the possibility of their own deaths. They are typically preoccupied with what will happen to them.

People have different ways of coping with a diagnosis of cancer. Poor coping is sometimes related to lack of information about the disease and its treatment. In that case, the oncology clinical nurse specialist may be consulted to provide patient education. Some coping styles are more effective than others. Weisman's research, cited in Dodd et al. (1993), found that patients who had the most difficulty were those who tended to try not to think about the situation, passively accepted treatment, lacked personal support, and tended to expect the worst. Patients who handled the stress of cancer better usually confronted problems directly, wanted to be well informed, had personal support, and were optimistic.

In the diagnostic phase of cancer care, patients typically use their usual methods of dealing with stress. When coping is not effective, a referral to a psychiatric clinical nurse specialist or a mental health counselor may be in order.

Deficient Knowledge

Tell the patient about diagnostic procedures, including preparation, what the procedure is like, and any specific postprocedure care.

THE TREATMENT PHASE

Assessment

During the treatment phase, specific assessments depend on the type and site of cancer and the prescribed treatment. Information obtained in the initial assessment provides baseline data. Frequently and systematically assess the patient for changes related to the disease process and for effects and side effects of therapy. Areas of ongoing assessment are presented here.

Health History

Note the patient's diagnosis and treatment plan. Take the past medical history to reveal other acute and chronic conditions that require attention during cancer therapy. Obtain a complete drug profile, and record allergies prominently. Review the systems to detect significant symptoms related to cancer or the treatment, including fatigue, weakness, headache, sore or dry mouth, dyspnea, palpitations, altered taste sensations, nausea, diarrhea, constipation, blood in stools, change in urinary frequency, hematuria or dysuria, sexual dysfunction, numbness, and tingling sensations. In the functional assessment, determine the effects of the illness and therapy on the patient's daily functioning. Assess the patient's knowledge, fears, concerns, and coping strategies. Also explore adaptations made by the patient and family during this phase.

table 24-14 ASSESSMENT *of the Patient with Cancer in the Treatment Phase*

HEALTH HISTORY

Chief Complaint: Diagnosis, prominent symptoms related to disease or treatment
Past Medical History: Acute and chronic conditions, previous surgeries and hospitalizations, drug profile, allergies
Review of Systems: Fatigue, weakness, headache, sore mouth, dyspnea, palpitations, altered taste sensation, nausea and vomiting, diarrhea, constipation, blood in stools or urine, urinary frequency, dysuria, numbness or tingling sensations, sexual dysfunction
Functional Assessment: Effects of illness and treatment on functioning, patient knowledge and concerns, stresses and coping strategies, family adaptation

PHYSICAL EXAMINATION

General Survey: Level of consciousness, posture and gait, eye contact, mannerisms, tone of voice
Height and Weight: Present and previous weight
Vital Signs: Present and previous readings, fever, tachypnea, tachycardia, hypotension, hypertension
Skin: Lesions, bruises, darkened or irritated areas
Scalp: Hair loss
Mouth: Condition of mucous membranes, dryness
Thorax: Respiratory effort, breath sounds
Abdomen: Distention, bowel sounds
Extremities: Color, edema, peripheral pulses, reflexes, sensation

Physical Examination

Note the patient's general appearance, level of consciousness, posture, and gait. Be alert for clues to the patient's mental and emotional state (e.g., eye contact, mannerisms, tone of voice). Measure weight and vital signs and compare with previous measurements. Assess the skin for lesions and bruises. Inspect the scalp for hair loss. Inspect the oral mucous membranes for lesions and inflammation. Observe the patient's respiratory effort and auscultate the lung fields for atelectasis or abnormal breath sounds. Inspect the abdomen for distention, and auscultate bowel sounds. Inspect and palpate the extremities for color, edema, and peripheral pulses. Test reflexes and sensation in the extremities.

Assessment of the patient with cancer during the treatment phase is summarized in Table 24-14.

Nursing Diagnoses, Goals, and Outcome Criteria: Treatment Phase

NURSING DIAGNOSES	GOALS AND OUTCOME CRITERIA
Anxiety related to effects and outcomes of treatment	Reduced anxiety: patient states anxiety is reduced, demonstrates relaxed manner

Ineffective Coping related to multiple stressors or overwhelming threat to self	Effective coping: patient identifies and uses strategies that decrease distress
Risk for Injury related to side effects of therapy	Absence of injury/serious adverse effects: patient has no signs/symptoms of injuries (e.g., bleeding, dyspnea, edema, diarrhea, dysuria) associated with therapy
Risk for Infection related to decreased white blood cells or venous access devices	Absence of infection: body temperature normal, no purulent drainage
Imbalanced Nutrition: Less than Body Requirements related to anorexia, nausea, and vomiting	Adequate nutrition: stable body weight
Impaired Oral Mucous Membranes related to decreased salivation or inflammation (stomatitis, mucositis)	Decreased oral discomfort: moist mucous membranes, patient states is more comfortable
Risk for Constipation related to decreased activity or drug side effects	Normal bowel elimination: bowel movement at least every 3 days
Fatigue related to anemia or effects of cancer	Adaptation to decreased energy level: patient completes essential activities without dyspnea, tachycardia, exhaustion
Disturbed Body Image related to alopecia, surgical scars, loss of function, stoma	Adaptation to change in body image: patient demonstrates acceptance of hair loss and scars or conceals them; adapts to functional changes; adjusts to stoma, learns to care for stoma
Dysfunctional Grieving related to loss of body part or altered appearance or function	Patient recognizes losses and moves toward resolving grief: patient discusses feelings of loss, touches affected body parts
Interrupted Family Processes related to illness and therapy	Adjustment of family roles and relationships: reassignment of roles and responsibilities within family
Ineffective Therapeutic Regimen Management related to lack of knowledge, inadequate resources, denial, hopelessness	Effective management of treatment program: patient describes treatment plan, self-care measures; patient carries out plan of care

Interventions

Anxiety

The thought of having surgery or of receiving cancer therapy may be very frightening to the patient. Suspect anxiety when a patient seems tense, apprehensive, or helpless. The patient may have poor eye contact, increased pulse and respirations, perspiration, and trembling. Tactfully share your observations and offer the patient an opportunity to talk. Encourage the patient to express feelings and identify the source of the anxiety. Listening and touch can be very effective in reducing anxiety. Recognize the need for patient teaching or for referrals.

Ineffective Coping

The patient may need help in setting priorities and in coping with the side effects of therapy. Strategies to promote coping include teaching, encouraging self-care within the patient's limitations, treating physical signs and symptoms, emphasizing abilities, coaching in relaxation strategies, and encouraging the use of coping strategies that have been effective in the past.

Support groups may be most effective at this phase. People who have been through the same treatments as the patient can be especially informative and supportive. The local chapter of the American Cancer Society can provide information about services in the patient's community. Some agencies can arrange transportation for therapy and medical care. The Reach for Recovery program trains women who have had mastectomies to counsel others in adapting to their losses. Groups are also available to help patients with ostomies resulting from cancer of the colon, bladder, or larynx.

When a patient must be isolated physically (as when receiving internal radiotherapy), it is difficult to provide emotional support. Remember to check on the patient frequently. Intercom conversations let the patient know he or she has not been forgotten.

Risk for Injury

The patient may exhibit various signs and symptoms of tissue injury associated with cancer therapy. Specific nursing measures are described below for some of the injurious effects of cancer therapy.

Pneumonitis and Pulmonary Fibrosis. Encourage patients with pneumonitis to do coughing and deep-breathing exercises to reduce the risk of pneumonia. Protect the patient from exposure to people who have upper respiratory infections. If the patient has dyspnea, elevate the head and schedule care to allow adequate rest and avoid exhaustion.

Cardiac Toxicity. Patients receiving doxorubicin (Adriamycin) may show signs of heart failure, so monitor for dyspnea, increasing pulse pressure, and edema. Notify the registered nurse promptly if these signs occur. Care of the patient with heart failure is covered in Chapter 33.

Neurotoxicity. The patient who has neurotoxic effects of chemotherapy has special needs as well. Extremities that lack normal sensation are prone to injury and must be protected.

Cystitis and Diarrhea. If the abdomen or lower back is irradiated, encourage the patient to increase fluid intake and empty the bladder often because of the risk of cystitis. Assessments of tissue turgor and mucous membrane moisture help detect dehydration. Diarrhea may require the administration of antidiarrheal drugs and special perianal care.

Thrombocytopenia. Both radiation and chemotherapy can suppress the production of platelets. When a patient has a low platelet count (thrombocytopenia), the blood does not clot promptly. Gentle handling is necessary to avoid trauma and bruising. Invasive procedures, including rectal temperatures, should be minimized. After venipunctures or injections, apply pressure for 5 minutes to control oozing. Instruct the patient to use a soft toothbrush and an electric razor to prevent trauma to the oral tissues or the skin.

Immediately report any blood in the stool, urine, or sputum to the physician. Signs and symptoms of internal bleeding include increased pulse and respirations, restlessness, pallor, decreased urine output, and falling blood pressure (a late sign).

Anemia. Anemia is less common than thrombocytopenia but should be anticipated approximately 3 months after therapy with cisplatin. Therefore, those patients should have hemoglobin and hematocrits done after treatment. Anemia is treated with packed red blood cells and erythropoietin (Epoetin Alfa). A diet high in iron is recommended. Tell the patient to report palpitations, pallor, and excessive fatigue to the physician.

Reproductive Cells. Because of the potential for harm to the developing embryo or fetus, women are usually advised not to become pregnant within 2 years of chemotherapy or while receiving radiotherapy. Female patients of childbearing age should discuss specific guidelines with their physicians. Because sperm production is reduced, male patients are counseled about the advisability of banking sperm before beginning therapy with certain drugs.

Risk for Infection

Patients with low white blood cell counts due to radiation or chemotherapy must be protected from infection. They should avoid crowds and close contact with others who have infectious diseases. Promptly report any signs of infection (elevated temperature, foul wound drainage, confusion).

If the white blood cell count is very low, compromised host precautions (or neutropenic precautions) may be needed to protect the patient. Such precautions include a private room and strict hand washing by all who enter the room. Fresh flowers, fruits, and vegetables are not allowed in the room because they harbor organisms. Additional details on compromised host precautions are presented in Chapters 12 and 32.

Patients who receive chemotherapy may have a venous access device implanted to permit frequent intravenous access without repeated venipunctures. An access device also delivers the antineoplastic agent into a large vein with turbulent blood flow. This decreases the local tissue injury caused by the drug. The venous access device presents a potential portal for infection. Most agencies have standard procedures for care of the device. Because the device usually remains in place for the entire treatment period, the patient or a helper must know how to care for it at home. Care of venous access devices is discussed in Chapter 17.

Imbalanced Nutrition: Less Than Body Requirements

Anorexia is common with cancer therapy, but maintaining good nutrition is essential. The patient is advised to eat a high-protein, high-calorie diet. Small, frequent feedings are sometimes easier to take than three large meals a day. Light exercise before meals may stimulate the appetite. If patients have specific food preferences and aversions, they should be respected. Many patients find that red meat and some other foods taste bitter when on chemotherapy. Use of plastic utensils may decrease the bitter taste. Nutritional supplements (such as Carnation Instant Breakfast, Ensure, or Sustacal), enteral feedings, or both may be ordered if the patient has excessive weight loss.

Be familiar with the specific antineoplastic agents so that the patient can be advised of any specific food restrictions. For example, patients taking procarbazine (Matulane) may have severe hypertensive reactions if they consume foods containing tyramine while on this drug. Foods rich in tyramine include aged cheeses, bananas, beer, beverages containing caffeine, yogurt, and liver. Alcohol should not be consumed if the patient is taking procarbazine.

Persistent nausea and vomiting can lead to dehydration and malnutrition. Various combinations of antiemetics and sedatives can be tried as ordered to obtain relief (Table 24-15). Newer antiemetics such as ondansetron (Zofran) and granisetron (Kytril) sedatives have greatly improved the management of nausea and vomiting associated with chemotherapy and have fewer side effects.

Contrary to common belief, not all patients with cancer have problems with weight loss. Patients with breast cancer and with Hodgkin's disease often are nauseated but actually gain weight during therapy possibly because they eat often to settle their stomachs. The important point for the nurse is to assess and treat each patient individually.

While antineoplastic drugs are being administered, sedatives are sometimes ordered so the patient can sleep. Nursing

table 24-15 ***Unproven Methods of Cancer Management***

Antineoplastons
Brych, Vlastimil (Milan)
Contreras methods
Dimethylsulfoxide (DMSO)
Electronic devices
Fresh cell therapy
Gerson method
Greek cancer cure
Hoxsey method/Bio-Medical Center
Hydrogen peroxide and other "hyperoxygenation" therapies
Immunoaugmentative therapy
Iscador
Kelley malignancy index and ecology therapy
Laetrile
Livingston-Wheeler therapy
Macrobiotic diets
Metabolic therapy of Harold W. Manner, Ph.D.
"Psychic surgery"
Questionable cancer practices in Tijuana and other Mexican border clinics
Questionable "nutritional" therapies
Revici method

From American Cancer Society. (1993). *Questionable methods of cancer treatment* (p. 15). Atlanta, GA: Author.

measures to manage nausea and vomiting are detailed in Chapter 36. Additional suggestions from the National Cancer Institute (1987) are the following:

1. Don't drink fluids with meals.
2. Decrease intake of sweets and fatty foods.
3. Eat food at room temperature.
4. Eat slowly and chew well.
5. Drink clear, cool, unsweetened liquids.
6. Avoid offensive odors.
7. Rest after eating.

Impaired Oral Mucous Membranes

A number of measures are helpful when the patient has xerostomia (dry mouth). Try frequent, gentle mouth care and offer artificial saliva to increase comfort. Several commercial products on the market moisten the mouth. Various protocols for mouth care can be used. For example, the patient can rinse the mouth with normal saline, a solution of 1 tablespoon of hydrogen peroxide in a glass of water, or a solution of ½ teaspoon of bicarbonate of soda in a glass of water. Encourage the patient to increase fluid intake, chew sugarless gum or candies, suck on ice chips, and moisten dry food before eating. Lemon and glycerin swabs are no longer recommended because lemon juice dehydrates oral tissues and glycerin provides a medium for bacterial growth.

Mucositis is inflammation of the mucosa and may extend from the mouth throughout the intestinal tract. It is a painful condition that can interfere with adequate food intake. The patient who has stomatitis should continue mouth care as prescribed, eat soft foods, and avoid foods that are acidic, salty, or spicy. A soft-bristled or foam toothbrush should be used. Normal saline alone or with sodium bicarbonate makes a soothing mouthwash and should be used at least four times a day.

Constipation

Some patients are constipated while on cancer therapy because of reduced activity, opioid analgesics, and the effects of some antineoplastic agents. Monitor the patient's bowel movements to detect constipation. The physician may prescribe a high-fiber diet, stool softeners, laxatives, and phosphate or biphosphate enemas to prevent or treat constipation.

Fatigue

Fatigue is a common symptom in the patient with cancer. In addition, side effects of therapy may cause the patient to tire easily. Assess the patient's need for assistance and schedule activities to conserve energy. Encourage the patient to prioritize activities and ask others to assume less important ones. Daily naps and mild exercise may be helpful.

Disturbed Body Image

The effects of cancer and cancer treatments can alter physical appearance and function. For example, patients receiving chemotherapy may have hair loss. Surgical interventions may result in visible scars, altered functioning, loss of body structures, and ostomies.

Be sensitive to the patient's concern about hair loss. At first, the patient may just note extra hair in the brush or comb. Later, the hair often comes out in clumps. Hair loss may be partial or complete. Typically, hair begins to grow back soon after the completion of chemotherapy and 4 to 6 months after the completion of radiotherapy. It is not unusual for the new hair to be a different color or texture. After large doses of radiation to the head, hair in the treated area may not return. Although some patients take this in stride, others may wish to use wigs, scarves, or hats to cover the head. Some insurance companies cover the price of wigs; others do not. The American Cancer Society loans wigs to patients free of charge. The society also sponsors the "Look Good-Feel Better" program to assist patients in looking their best during therapy.

Whereas hair usually grows back, other effects of cancer treatment are often permanent. Patients need time and support to incorporate those changes into their body images and to regain a healthy self-concept.

Dysfunctional Grieving

Treatment of cancer often results in temporary or permanent changes in body appearance or function. Changes or losses often trigger a grief response. The patient may be sad, tearful, or verbalize feelings about the loss. Listen in an accepting way that lets the patient know the feelings are understood. Behaviors that suggest that the patient is beginning to accept the loss or change include talking about the loss and looking at or touching the affected part. Support the patient as needed and provide practical information about adapting to the loss. Participation in a support group may help the patient learn new coping strategies and begin to resolve the grief process.

Impaired Family Processes

While undergoing treatment for cancer, the patient may be concerned with meeting responsibilities at home and at work. Some treatments extend over many months and make it difficult to maintain one's usual activities. Side effects of the treatment may make the patient feel tired and discouraged. Family and friends need to understand what the patient is going through and what they can do to help. Encourage them to remain involved with the patient. Family members may need some help themselves to handle their responses to the patient's illness.

Financial concerns may be very serious for the patient and family. Obtain a social work consultation if necessary to assist them with insurance and disability claims and financial assistance referrals.

Ineffective Therapeutic Regimen Management

A pretreatment teaching plan informs the patient of what the prescribed therapy involves and what the experience will be like. Know what the physician has told the patient and reinforce that teaching. One source of information is the National Cancer Institute's Cancer Information Service (CIS). Booklets on cancer, cancer therapy, and coping can be obtained by calling CIS at 1-800-4CANCER. A variety of materials are available from the American Cancer Society that can be accessed by calling 1-800-227-2345, or at the internet address http://www.cancer.org.

PATIENT TEACHING PLAN
External Radiation Therapy

- Having the treatment is much like having a radiograph (x-ray). You are positioned on a table, and the machine is adjusted to direct the beam appropriately. During the treatment, you are alone in the room, but closed-circuit television permits the staff to see you.
- The treatment is not painful. In fact, there are no sensations at all related to the radiation. The machine that houses the radiation is controlled by a radiologist or technician. You will hear whirring or clicking sounds as the machine operates.
- These treatments do not cause you to be radioactive. The radioactive material remains in the machine. Only the rays emitted by the material come in contact with you. When the machine is turned off, there is no radiation exposure.
- The skin markings made by the radiologist are used to direct the radiation to the treatment site. Do not wash the marks off until the radiologist gives permission.
- Skin over the area being treated may become irritated. Irritated skin should be kept clean and dry, but do not apply lotions. Cotton clothing may feel more comfortable over irritated skin. Antiperspirants should not be applied to a treatment site, but cornstarch can be used to absorb moisture.

PATIENT TEACHING PLAN
Internal Radiation Therapy

- The radioactive material is given orally, injected into a vein, or implanted by a physician.
- You are placed in a private room for a specified period of time for the treatment.
- Visitors and staff are restricted in the amount of time they can spend in your room to limit their exposure to radiation. They also will maintain some distance from you when they are in the room.
- If a sealed source is to be placed in a body cavity, you may be required to maintain a certain position to keep the source positioned correctly.

Chemotherapy. If chemotherapy is prescribed, the teaching plan includes a description of the drugs to be administered, the potential side effects, and related precautions. Provide written information to supplement the verbal teaching. Explore what the patient has heard about chemotherapy and correct any misconceptions. Many patients have heard horror stories about drug side effects, especially nausea and vomiting. Inform the patient of measures that can be taken that usually make the side effects more tolerable.

Put on your ***THINKING CAP!!***

You are assigned to two patients who are being treated for cancer. One is receiving external radiation, the other is receiving chemotherapy.

1. Identify nursing diagnoses that might appear in the care plans of *both* of these patients.
2. Identify one adverse effect that occurs with radiation but not with chemotherapy.
3. Identify one adverse effect that occurs with chemotherapy but not with radiation.

RECOVERY AND REHABILITATION

If the outcome of treatment appears to be a cure, the patient and family are usually overjoyed. Some patients, however, become excessively concerned with their bodies, constantly monitoring for new evidence of cancer. Periodic checkups are essential but may be dreaded because the patient realizes that complete or permanent recovery cannot be guaranteed. If any signs of a possible recurrence appear, patients are understandably concerned.

As patients recover from the effects of cancer and cancer therapy, rehabilitation may be needed to restore them to the highest possible level of functioning.

TERMINAL ILLNESS

Although increasing numbers of people are surviving cancer, it is still the second leading cause of death. If treatment is unsuccessful, the patient eventually begins to decline. Patients need to know what resources are available to them and their families. The oncology clinical nurse specialist is an excellent resource person for the patient. Provide information about home health care, hospice, and voluntary and charitable organizations whose services might be needed. For patients who wish to die at home, hospice provides the support and teaching needed for this to be honored. The focus of hospice is to keep the patient's symptoms, especially pain, under control during the final period of the illness. In addition, hospice staff provide bereavement care after the patient's death.

To work effectively with these patients, you must be aware of your own feelings about dying. You can help the terminal patient in many ways. Continue to be attentive and accepting. New nurses often fear that patients will ask them questions they cannot answer. It's alright to admit you don't know, but acknowledge the patient's concerns. Listening carefully is more important than talking. Guide patients to claim their accomplishments and find peace with their failures. Terminally ill patients should remember that although they are going to die eventually, they are living now and can still have some pleasure. Chapter 23 discusses care of the dying patient in more detail.

People with terminal cancer often express fear of having great pain as the disease progresses. Although cancer is usu-

Nutrition Concepts

1. Thirty-five percent of all cancers are believed to be related to diet.
   a. Diets high in salt-cured, smoked, and nitrate-cured foods are associated with esophageal and stomach cancers.
   b. Obesity is associated with cancers of the colon, breast, prostate, gallbladder, ovary, and uterus.
   c. Cancers of the breast, colon, and prostate may be associated with high-fat diets.
   d. High alcohol intake is associated with cancers of the oral cavity, larynx, esophagus, liver, colon, and breast.
2. To *reduce the risk* of cancer, the American Cancer Society recommends:
   a. Fruits and vegetables: five or more servings each day
   b. Grains, rice, pasta, beans: several servings each day
   c. Fats: limit consumption
   d. Physical activity: at least moderate activity 30 min or more on most days; maintain healthy weight
   e. Alcohol: none or limited
3. Impaired nutrition in patients with cancer can result from the disease itself or from the various treatment modalities, such as chemotherapy and radiation.
4. Cancer cachexia is a complex metabolic problem characterized by weight loss, anemia, and abnormalities in fat, protein, and carbohydrate metabolism.
5. The goals of nutritional care for patients with cancer are to prevent or correct nutritional deficiencies and to minimize weight loss.
6. Interventions for common problems associated with cancer therapy (nausea and vomiting, food aversions, anorexia, dry mouth, diarrhea, and constipation) should be geared toward individual needs.
7. Immunotherapy indirectly affects nutrition by causing fatigue, chills, fever, and flulike symptoms, which may affect appetite.
8. Diets for cancer patients must be individualized depending on their baseline nutritional status, symptoms, and therapy side effects.
9. If oral intake is inadequate, enteral tube feedings or parenteral nutrition are considered.

ally painless in the early stages, advanced disease often causes pain. Cancer pain can be caused by pressure on nerves, interference with circulation, obstruction of hollow structures (e.g., ureter, bowel, bronchi), and local tissue destruction.

General medical and nursing measures for the management of pain are discussed in Chapter 14. An especially good resource is the Agency for Healthcare Research and Quality (AHRQ—formerly AHCPR) publication on management of cancer pain. A variety of approaches should be tried to keep the patient as comfortable as possible. With severe, chronic pain, it is appropriate to medicate the patient at fixed intervals rather than on request. The patient may have pain at specific times or during certain activities despite the routine analgesic. This is referred to as *breakthrough pain.* If that happens, there may be an order for the additional prn use of a short-acting drug with a rapid onset of action. Do not withhold ordered opioids out of concern about causing addiction. Analgesics that may be ordered include long-acting opioids (morphine sulfate [MS Contin, Roxanol], fentanyl patches) that may be supplemented with short-acting opioids for breakthrough pain. Combinations of drugs, including opioids, a stimulant, and an antiemetic, may be effective for the patient with cancer. These "cocktails," although not used as much as they once were, often control pain when given regularly without causing excessive sedation. Advise the physician if pain control is not achieved.

ONCOLOGIC EMERGENCIES

In the patient with cancer, conditions sometimes develop that require emergency intervention as a result of the disease process or the therapy. Some of the conditions requiring prompt recognition and action are hypercalcemia, syndrome of inappropriate antidiuretic hormone, disseminated intravascular coagulation, superior vena cava syndrome, and spinal cord compression. Characteristics of these conditions and related interventions are outlined in Table 24-16.

Put on your THINKING CAP!!

A patient who is receiving outpatient chemotherapy for cancer tells you he is using natural vitamins and herbal products to help combat his cancer. He says, "They are all natural products, so they can't be harmful, right?"

1. How should you answer him?
2. What should you advise him to do?

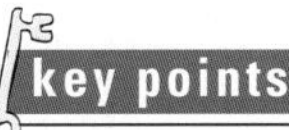

key points

- Cancer is the second most common cause of death in the United States.
- Early diagnosis and treatment increase the chances of survival with many types of cancer.
- The risk of developing certain types of cancers, and dying from some cancers, varies with race and ethnicity.
- Cells that reproduce abnormally and in an uncontrolled manner form neoplasms that can be benign or malignant.
- Benign neoplasms do not spread to other parts of the body, whereas malignant neoplasms invade nearby tissues and can form metastases in distant parts of the body.
- Tumors are classified by anatomic site, cell appearance and differentiation, and staging.
- Carcinogens are factors that appear to increase the risk for development of cancer.
- The seven warning signs of cancer are change in bowel or bladder habits, a sore that does not heal, unusual bleeding or discharge, thickening or a lump, indigestion or difficulty swallowing, obvious change in a mole or wart, and a nagging cough or hoarseness.

table 24-16 ***Oncologic Emergencies***

EMERGENCY	RISK FACTORS	SIGNS AND SYMPTOMS	TREATMENT	NURSING CARE
Hypercalcemia	Multiple myeloma, metastatic bone cancer; cancer of lung, breast, or kidney; prolonged immobility	Fatigue, confusion, weakness, constipation, polyuria, hypertension, tachycardia, poor muscle tone If untreated, renal failure, coma, cardiac dysrhythmias, or death can occur.	IV normal saline and furosemide (Lasix). Drugs to promote excretion of calcium: plicamycin, calcitonin, etidronate disodium.	Monitor fluid status. Give IV fluids and drugs as ordered. Record intake and output.
Syndrome of inappropriate antidiuretic hormone	Thoracic or mediastinal tumors, thymoma, lymphomas, pancreatic cancer, cyclophosphamide (Cytoxan) or vincristine (Oncovin) therapy	Water intoxication and dilutional hyponatremia due to water retention: nausea and vomiting, anorexia, weakness. Lethargy at first, followed by confusion, psychosis, loss of deep tendon reflexes, seizures, coma, and death.	Fluids restricted to 500 ml/day. Demeclocycline (Declomycin). IV fluids and diuretics administered only in late stage.	Explain and enforce fluid restriction. Monitor vital signs. Keep intake and output records. Do not give demeclocycline with food or dairy products.
Disseminated intravascular coagulation	Septicemia, transfusion reaction. Some drugs: vincristine, methotrexate, mercaptopurine, prednisone, asparaginase	Normal clotting process is exaggerated, which depletes clotting factors. Early signs: petechiae, ecchymoses, prolonged bleeding from venipuncture. Late signs: signs of vascular obstruction, tachycardia, dyspnea, gastrointestinal bleeding, heart failure, and shock.	Platelets, fresh frozen plasma, other blood components. Heparin may be prescribed.	Avoid trauma. Handle gently. Give blood products and heparin as ordered. Monitor vital signs. Look for bleeding.
Superior vena cava syndrome	Breast or lung cancer, lymphoma, Kaposi's sarcoma, or metastatic testicular cancer that puts pressure on the superior vena cava	Redness and edema of face, conjunctiva; distended neck and thoracic veins; dyspnea, cough, tachypnea, tachycardia, cyanosis progressing to increased intracranial pressure.	Radiation therapy, diuretics, steroids.	Give medications as ordered. Elevate head and arms but not legs. Tell patient not to bend forward. Reassure patient that symptoms usually subside in 2-3 days.
Spinal cord compression	Lung and breast cancers, lymphomas	Tumor in epidural space presses on spinal cord, causing intense pain, weakness, altered sensation in arms or legs, impaired bowel and bladder function.	High-dose radiation, corticosteroids, surgery to relieve pressure.	Give analgesics as ordered. Assess for full bladder, constipation. Do neurologic checks on affected extremities.

From Gribben, M. E. (1990). Could you detect these oncological crises? *RN, 53*(6), 36-42. Copyright(c) 1990 by Medical Economics Publishing, Montvale, N.J. Reprinted by permission.
IV, Intravenous.

- A diagnosis of cancer is based on tissue studies, laboratory tests, endoscopic examinations, and radiologic and imaging procedures.
- Surgery is a common treatment for malignant tumors.
- Internal or external radiotherapy is used to treat cancer because malignant cells are more sensitive than are normal cells to radiation.
- Chemotherapy is the use of chemical agents in the treatment of disease.
- Radiotherapy and chemotherapy have serious side and adverse effects, including bone marrow suppression, anorexia, alopecia, nausea and vomiting, and local inflammation.
- Patients who receive internal radiation emit rays that can be harmful to others.
- Biologic response modifiers act directly on malignant cells and promote the body's natural defenses against cancer.
- Patients who have suspected or confirmed cancer are under great stress and may respond with anger, irritability, fear, denial, or depression.
- In addition to helping with specific physical problems, nursing care of the patient with cancer addresses Ineffective Coping, Grief Response, Imbalanced Nutrition, Risk for Infection, and Ineffective Management of Therapeutic Regimen.

REVIEW QUESTIONS

1. Benign and malignant tumors are alike in that *both:*
   1. press on normal tissues and compete with normal cells for nutrients.
   2. usually grow very rapidly.
   3. invade nearby tissues or disperse cells to colonize distant parts of the body.
   4. contain cells that closely resemble the tissue of origin

2. A carcinogen is a:
   1. drug that is used in the chemotherapeutic treatment of cancer.
   2. cell or group of cells that is undergoing abnormal reproduction.
   3. chemical, viral, or radioactive substance that can cause cancer.
   4. substance that helps the body resist the development of cancer cells.

3. Dietary recommendations to reduce the risk of some cancers include:
   1. No dairy products or red meat; green, leafy vegetables; low calories.
   2. High fiber; variety of fruits and vegetables; low fat and calories.
   3. Fish and poultry as primary protein source; high fiber; no alcohol.
   4. Limited smoked and nitrate-preserved foods; low fiber and calories.

4. A patient's blood level of the oncofetal antigen CA-125 has continued to rise during 6 months of chemotherapy for ovarian cancer. What is the most likely explanation?
   1. The chemotherapy is effectively destroying the cancer cells.
   2. The patient is having an adverse response to the chemotherapy.
   3. The cancer is continuing to grow despite chemotherapy.
   4. The patient's immune system has been strengthened.

5. When working with a patient who has an internal radiation source, safety precautions include:
   1. Always wear a lead apron when providing direct care to the patient with internal radiation.
   2. If the radiation source comes out of the patient's body, wear gloves to pick it up.
   3. When not providing direct care, stay at least 3 feet away from the source.
   4. No pregnant visitors or staff should enter the patient's room.

6. Adverse effects of radiation therapy commonly affect the bone marrow, hair follicles, and gastrointestinal tract. What makes these tissues especially sensitive to the effects of radiation?
   1. They have inadequate defenses against harmful substances.
   2. These tissues attract radioactive substances.
   3. These tissues have very poor circulation.
   4. They regenerate rapidly.

7. What is the rationale for giving colony-stimulating factors (CSFs) to patients on chemotherapy?
   1. CSFs stimulate the production of white blood cells by the bone marrow.
   2. With CSFs, the dosage of chemotherapy drugs can be reduced.
   3. CSFs reduce the risk of anemia that commonly occurs with chemotherapy.
   4. CSFs eliminate the need for bone marrow or stem cell transplantation.

8. The most dangerous adverse effect of antineoplastic drugs used in chemotherapy is:
   1. gastrointestinal bleeding.
   2. increased intracranial pressure.
   3. bone marrow suppression.
   4. nausea and vomiting.

9. The action of biologic response modifiers (BRMs) is to:
   1. treat mental depression that is common during cancer treatment.
   2. promote the body's natural defenses against cancer cells.
   3. immunize patients against some types of cancer.
   4. prevent the spread of cancer cells before metastasis occurs.

10. Three patients at a urology clinic received diagnoses of prostate cancer. All were in an early stage and had similar expectations of cure. Mr. A. asked many questions and started planning his work schedule around his treatments. Mr. B. stalked out of the office and slammed the door saying he would rather die than give up sex. Mr. C. was stunned and seemed unable to take in any more information at that time. Which of these patients' responses would be considered "normal" in this situation?
    1. Mr. A's
    2. Mr. B's
    3. Mr. C's
    4. They are all normal reactions to grief.

CHAPTER

25 The Ostomy Patient

objectives

1. List the indications for ostomy surgery to divert urine or feces.
2. Describe nursing interventions to prepare the patient for ostomy surgery.
3. Explain the types of procedures used for fecal diversion.
4. Assist in developing a nursing process to plan care for the patient with each of the following types of fecal diversion: ileostomy, continent ileostomy, ileoanal reservoir, and colostomy.
5. Explain the types of procedures done for urinary diversion.
6. Assist in developing a nursing care plan for the patient with each of the following types of urinary diversion: ureterostomy, ileal conduit, and continent internal reservoir.
7. Discuss content to be included in teaching patients to learn to live with ostomies.

key terms

Anastomosis (ă-năs-tŏ-MŌ-sĭs, p. 349)
Colostomy (kŏ-LŎS-tō-mē, p. 354)
Continent (p. 352)
Ileostomy (ĭl-ē-ŎS-tō-mē, p. 348)
Nephrostomy (nĕ-FRŎS-tō-mē, p. 363)
Ostomy (ŎS-tō-mē, p. 347)
Prolapse (PRŌ-lăps, p. 355)
Stoma (STŌ-mă, p. 347)
Ureterostomy (ŭ-rē-tĕr-ŎS-tō-mē, p. 358)
Vesicostomy (vĕs-Ī-KŎS-tō-mē, p. 363)

Ostomy is the term used to describe the surgical creation of an artificial opening into a body cavity. The site of the opening on the skin is called a *stoma.* An ostomy in the digestive tract may be a gastrostomy, jejunostomy, duodenostomy, ileostomy, or colostomy. The gastrostomy is used for long-term feedings and is discussed in Chapter 8. Jejunostomies, duodenostomies, ileostomies, and colostomies are created to drain fecal matter from the intestines. Examples of stomas in the urinary tract are the ureterostomy, ileal or colonic conduit, cystostomy, vesicostomy, and continent internal reservoir. Ostomies of the urinary tract drain urine from the kidney, ureters, or bladder. Ostomies are sometimes described as means of urinary or fecal diversion. The term *ostomate* refers to a person who has an ostomy. Many people, however, prefer to be thought of as individuals with ostomies rather than as ostomates. This chapter describes the care of patients with ostomies created to pass urine or feces.

INDICATIONS AND PREPARATION FOR OSTOMY SURGERY

Ostomy surgery is done for a number of reasons. A temporary ostomy may be indicated after surgery or trauma or when there is severe inflammation or infection. The ostomy bypasses the affected portion of the bowel or urinary tract, giving it time to heal. Permanent ostomies are usually necessitated by cancer of the bladder or colon or severe inflammatory bowel disease. Pouches are external appliances that are used with most ostomies to collect drainage. Whether ostomies are temporary or permanent, patients require considerable assistance and support to learn to manage them.

Ideally, the patient is prepared for the ostomy before surgery. The physician informs the patient of the need for the ostomy, what it is, and whether it will be temporary or permanent. Sometimes the procedure is done in emergency situations, as when treating acute bowel obstruction or trauma. In these situations, the ostomy may come as a great shock to the patient.

An important resource for both the nurse and the patient is the enterostomal therapist (ET). The ET is a registered nurse who has passed a certification examination following completion of specialized training in stoma care. The ET is often an appropriate person to assess and teach the ostomy patient. This does not, however, relieve the staff nurse of all teaching responsibility. The staff follows up and reinforces the instructions of the ET. In settings in which specialists are not available, the responsibility for teaching may fall primarily on the staff nurse.

The exact placement of the stoma is very important. The ET often consults with the surgeon regarding the ideal site. Two factors must be considered: secure pouch placement and ease of self-care. To provide a good seal, the site must not be too close to the umbilicus, bony prominences, scars, folds, or creases. If the pouch does not fit smoothly around the stoma, liquid stool or urine may leak around it. The stoma is placed below the waistline if possible. If it can be placed within the margins of the rectus muscle, the muscle will help prevent peristomal hernias. The stoma must also be placed where it can be seen and touched by the patient. A patient cannot learn to care for a stoma that is located where it cannot be seen.

What Does Culture Have to do with Colon Cancer?

In the United States, African-Americans have the highest rates of colon and rectal cancers, which commonly are treated with ostomies. Therefore nurses should counsel African-American patients about the importance of periodic screening. Emphasize that early detection and treatment improve chances of cure.

NURSING CARE *of the Patient Having Ostomy Surgery*

General preoperative nursing care is discussed in detail in Chapter 16. This section emphasizes only those aspects that are unique to the patient with an ostomy.

Assessment

Before ostomy surgery, you should be especially concerned with assessing the patient's expectations, understanding of the procedure, information desired, and fears. The health history reveals the reason for the procedure. The medical history documents other acute and chronic conditions that will require management before and after surgery. Note drug therapy and allergies. During the physical examination, expect to see a mark on the abdominal skin where the stoma will be created. See Chapter 16 for other details of the preoperative assessment.

Nursing Diagnoses, Goals, and Outcome Criteria: Ostomy Surgery

The nursing diagnoses and goals that require particular attention are:

Nursing Diagnoses	Goals and Outcome Criteria
Anxiety related to perceived threat to self-image, anticipated changes in body appearance and function	Reduced anxiety: patient states anxiety is reduced; relaxed manner
Deficient Knowledge of what to expect after surgery in relation to the stoma	Patient understanding of postoperative routines and procedures in relation to ostomy care: patient describes routines correctly and participates in postoperative care

Interventions

Anxiety

Be accepting of the patient's anxiety and try to help the patient identify exactly what his or her concerns are. Some patients may be concerned about appearance, and others about how their jobs or family lives might be disrupted. Encourage patients to talk and to use coping strategies that have been effective in the past. Be aware that moderate or severe anxiety interferes with learning and, therefore, attempt to reduce anxiety before teaching.

Deficient Knowledge

Basic aspects of ostomy care should be taught before surgery. Let the patient's responses and questions guide you as to how much detail is appropriate. Remember, however, that preoperative teaching usually requires repetition and reinforcement after surgery.

In addition to the ET, an important resource is a volunteer from an organization like the American Cancer Society or the United Ostomy Association. Volunteers are people with ostomies who have been trained to counsel other patients about adjustment to their ostomies. Their personal experiences in everyday ostomy management can make them very effective role models. Another good reason for using these volunteers is that the patient has a chance to see a well-groomed, active person who is living fully with an ostomy. When a patient is referred to an ostomy group (with the patient's permission, of course), the organization tries to send a volunteer who is similar in age, sex, and occupation.

FECAL DIVERSION

Intestinal ostomies divert fecal matter through a surgically created opening. Although the various types of ostomies have much in common, there are also differences that should be noted. The characteristics of the fecal material vary with the location of the ostomy and influence the type of care needed. Fecal matter in the ileum is liquid. Normally, the colon absorbs water from the fecal mass as it moves toward the rectum so that it becomes progressively more solid. When the mass is diverted from the colon, it may be liquid, semisolid, or formed depending on the section of the colon where the ostomy is created. The closer the ostomy is to the rectum, the more formed the fecal matter will be.

Before fecal diversion, a low-fiber diet may be prescribed for several days. Antibiotics may be given to reduce the bacterial flora in the intestines. Cathartics and laxatives are usually ordered to empty the digestive tract.

ILEOSTOMY

An ileostomy is an opening in the ileum. The ileum is the distal portion of the small intestine that empties into the large intestine. An ileostomy is necessary when the entire colon must be bypassed or removed. Conditions that require colon bypass include congenital defects, cancer, inflammatory bowel disease, bowel trauma, and familial conditions such as multiple polyposis. Multiple polyposis is characterized by the presence of many polyps in the colon. Because these polyps often become malignant, removal of the colon may be recommended.

Procedure

A surgical incision is made in the abdomen, and a loop or the end of the ileum is brought out through a second abdominal incision. The edges of the loop or the end of the ileal segment are everted and sutured to the abdominal skin to create a stoma. Loops may be supported with a device such as a rod or bridge instead of being sutured to the skin. Even though the patient is allowed nothing by mouth before surgery, digestive secretions quickly begin to drain from the stoma. The physician applies a temporary plastic pouch or a fluffy dressing in the operating room. The pouch collects fecal drainage to keep it from contaminating the surgical incision and to protect surrounding skin. The plain ileostomy frequently or intermittently drains liquid to pasty stool, so the patient will always have to wear a pouch. A newer procedure, the Kock pouch, creates a reservoir for the liquid stool so that it can be drained at intervals. The ileal J pouch–anal anastomosis essentially creates a new rectum from the terminal ileum. This procedure allows for nearly normal bowel evacuation. The patient may have a temporary ileostomy while the pouch heals.

PHARMACOLOGY CAPSULE Ileostomy patients are usually not given timed-release capsules or enteric-coated tablets because they are likely to be eliminated before they can dissolve and be absorbed.

POSTOPERATIVE NURSING CARE *of the Patient with an Ileostomy*

The immediate postoperative care of the patient with an ileostomy is like that of most other patients having abdominal surgery. The patient has a nasogastric tube attached to low intermittent suction. Intravenous fluids are ordered for several days, after which oral intake is gradually increased.

General care of the surgical patient is covered in Chapter 16. This section emphasizes only the special needs of the ileostomy patient beyond the immediate recovery period.

Assessment

Health History

After surgery, document significant symptoms such as pain, anorexia, nausea, vomiting, weakness, thirst, and muscle cramps in the review of systems. The functional assessment reveals how the patient is reacting to the surgery and how he or she thinks it will affect usual functioning. Also determine what stressors the patient perceives, usual coping strategies, and sources of support. Assess the patient's understanding of ileostomy care.

Physical Examination

Begin the physical examination with observation of the patient's general status: level of consciousness, orientation, posture, and expression. Take vital signs and weight and compare with preoperative findings. Assess the skin for color, warmth, and turgor. Inspect the oral tissues for moisture. Observe respiratory effort, and auscultate breath sounds. Assess the abdomen for distention and bowel sounds.

Inspect the stoma for color and bleeding. A new intestinal stoma should be beefy red. When healed, it should be rose red, somewhat darker than the color of the oral mucosa. A very pale, bluish, or black stoma has impaired circulation and MUST be reported to the registered nurse or the physician immediately.

Swelling of the stoma is expected initially, after which it shrinks over a period of 6 to 8 weeks. Inspect the base of the stoma for redness, skin breakdown, and purulent drainage. A small amount of bleeding around the base of a new stoma is not unusual. In fact, it may be a positive sign indicating an adequate blood supply. If edema occurs later, it is probably due to pressure created by an improperly fitting collection device. Ileostomy drainage begins 24 to 48 hours after surgery. Note the characteristics of draining fluid or fecal matter. The presence of some blood and mucus in the drainage is normal at first.

Assess urine appearance and volume. Palpate the extremities for warmth and peripheral pulses. Observe for neuromuscular symptoms such as trembling, twitching, or cramping.

General postoperative assessment of the patient with an ostomy is summarized in Table 25-1.

Nursing Diagnoses, Goals, and Outcome Criteria: Ileostomy

Nursing diagnoses and goals common to most postoperative patients (acute pain, ineffective airway clearance, risk for infection, impaired tissue perfusion, and urinary retention) are covered in Chapter 16. Additional diagnoses specific to the ileostomy patient in the immediate postoperative phase are the following:

Nursing Diagnoses	Goals and Outcome Criteria
Risk for Deficient Fluid Volume related to nothing by mouth status, nasogastric suction, passage of liquid stool	Normal fluid balance: pulse and blood pressure consistent with patient norms, moist mucous membranes, urine output equal to fluid intake
Impaired Skin Integrity related to adhesive, fecal drainage	Normal skin integrity: skin intact with minimal redness around stoma
Disturbed Body Image related to presence of stoma, altered body function	Adjustment to change in body image: patient makes positive statements about ability to adapt; learns, and takes over ostomy care
Sexual Dysfunction and/or **Ineffective Sexuality Patterns** related to altered body structure and function or reactions to those changes	Fulfilling sexual expression: patient reports satisfying sexual expression, makes adaptations as necessary
Ineffective Therapeutic Regimen Management related to lack of understanding of self-care with ostomy, failure to accept ostomy, lack of resources for proper care	Patient effectively manages ostomy: patient accepts responsibility for self-care, demonstrates proper care of ostomy, obtains necessary supplies

Interventions

Risk for Deficient Fluid Volume

The loss of fluids and electrolytes through nasogastric suction and the passage of liquid stool can lead to deficient fluid volume and electrolyte imbalances. Administer intravenous

table 25-1 POSTOPERATIVE ASSESSMENT *of the Patient with an Ostomy*

HEALTH HISTORY

Chief Complaint and History of Present Illness: Type of ostomy procedure done and reason
Past Medical History: Acute and chronic conditions, prescribed drugs, allergies
Review of Systems: Pain, anorexia, nausea, vomiting, abdominal cramping or pain, weakness, thirst, muscle cramps
Functional Assessment: Response to surgery, anticipated effects on lifestyle, sources of stress and support, usual coping strategies

PHYSICAL EXAMINATION

General Survey: Level of consciousness, orientation, posture, expression
Skin: Color, warmth, turgor
Mouth: Moisture
Thorax: Respiratory effort, breath sounds
Abdomen: Distention, bowel sounds
Stoma: Color, bleeding, edema; condition of skin at base of stoma
Characteristics of Drainage: Amount, color, odor, blood, mucus
Extremities: Warmth, peripheral pulses
Neuromuscular: Trembling, twitching, cramping

fluids as ordered, with careful monitoring of hydration status. Keep accurate intake and output records. Measure output from all sources, including urine, gastric contents, and fecal drainage. Closely monitor serum electrolytes, and be alert for signs and symptoms of imbalances: changes in mental status (confusion, anxiety), changes in neuromuscular status (twitching, trembling, weakness), poor tissue turgor, edema, and dry mucous membranes.

When the patient resumes oral intake, advise a daily fluid intake of 2 to 3 liters. During hot weather or illness, additional fluids may be required. It is best to consume a variety of fluids, rather than plain water, to obtain electrolytes. The loss of bicarbonate in ileostomy drainage can result in metabolic acidosis. To prevent this, the physician may order bicarbonate replacement.

Impaired Skin Integrity

Check the pouch hourly at first to detect leakage. When the pouch is emptied or changed, try to keep fecal matter from contaminating the primary incision. Clean the skin around the stoma gently but thoroughly. Maintaining skin integrity is an ongoing problem for the patient with an intestinal ostomy. The presence of fecal matter on the skin provides a medium for bacterial, fungal, and yeast infections. In addition, the materials used to hold the pouch securely can cause traumatic injuries and allergic responses.

A protective barrier must be maintained to prevent skin breakdown. A plastic pouch is used to collect fecal drainage. A good pouch is one that protects the skin, contains wastes and gas, is odor proof, permits freedom of movement, provides security for the patient, and is not noticeable. Many kinds of pouches are available, as seen in Figure 25-1, but the features are basically the same. Some type of adhesive is needed to secure the pouch around the stoma. The pouch has an opening at the bottom that allows for emptying and rinsing. Some have gas filters that allow gas to escape while minimizing odor. There are reusable and disposable pouches, including one that is even flushable for easy disposal. The ET is a good resource person to help the patient find the right appliance.

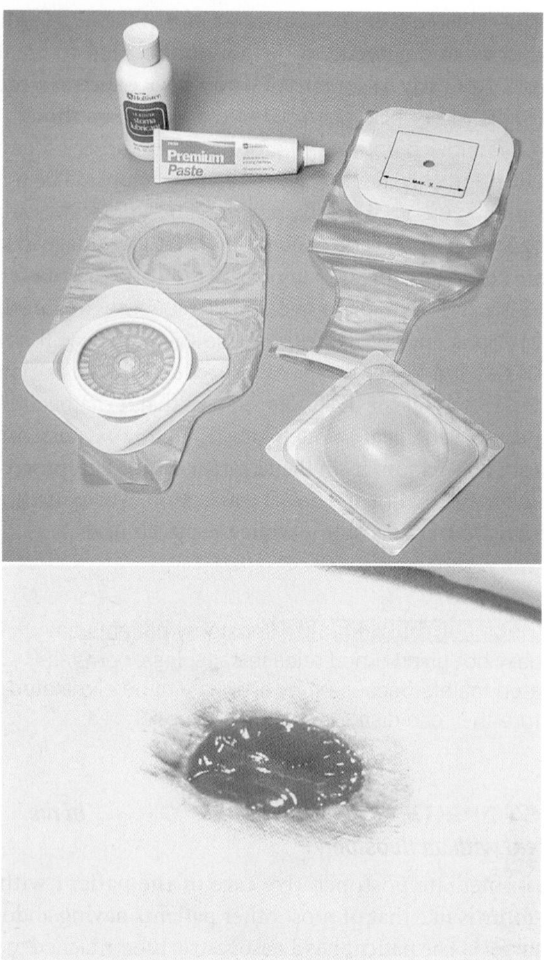

FIGURE 25-1 Supplies needed to pouch an ostomy may include a pouch with an attached or separate skin barrier, a pouch closure device, skin barrier, stomahesive paste, and adhesive remover.

Periodically (usually every 3 to 5 days) remove the appliance for thorough cleansing of the skin surrounding the stoma. Very gently peel the adhesive off the skin. Rough handling and frequent changes contribute to skin breakdown. Commercial adhesive removers are available if needed. After removing the adhesive, wash the stoma and the area around it with water. If soap is used, it should be nonoily and must be rinsed off thoroughly. Then pat the skin dry. The patient may be surprised to find that the stoma itself has no sensation, but the surrounding skin may be tender.

A protective barrier must be applied before the pouch can be replaced. Skin sealants that come in the form of gels, wipes, sprays, liquids, and roll-ons may be applied to the skin. Sealants protect the skin; they do not hold the pouch in place. Next, apply a skin barrier. Commonly used skin barriers include powders, pastes, wafers, and washers. If the skin around the stoma is irritated, powder may be applied. Dust away excess powder before the wafer is applied. Wafers and washers may be precut or may have to be cut to fit around the stoma. The opening should be no more than ⅛ inch (some experts favor 1/16 inch) larger than the stoma because a larger opening permits more fecal matter to come in contact with the skin. If a paste is used, apply it around the stoma or on the cut edge of the wafer. Place the wafer over the stoma and press down. Some pouching systems have the pouch attached to the wafer. Other systems consist of a wafer that is placed around the stoma and a pouch that then adheres to the wafer. After the pouch is securely placed, clamp it. Initially, the pouch opening will probably need to be custom cut. As the stoma heals and shrinks, precut appliances may work well. Custom cut pouches can be ordered for stomas of unusual size or shape. Patients whose barriers quickly erode and those with very convex stomas can obtain special barriers to maintain good fit. Once the stoma heals, some patients will prefer to cleanse the peristomal skin in the shower.

Disturbed Body Image

Establishment of bowel control is an important developmental task of childhood. The patient who has an ileostomy is no longer able to control the passage of fecal matter and must learn to manage bowel elimination in a new way. This can be very distressing to the adult who fears spillage and exposure.

Inability to control odor associated with passage of gas through the stoma is another concern for the patient with an intestinal ostomy. The characteristic odor of stool is generally considered unpleasant. Because the ostomy patient may have fecal matter draining intermittently, the source of odor is almost always present.

Assure the patient that odor is normal when the pouch is being changed or emptied, but that it can be controlled at other times. Causes of odor include certain foods and poor hygiene. Foods that produce gas or stimulate bowel activity are most likely to contribute to odor problems. These generally include spicy foods, onions, garlic, some vegetables like cabbage and beans, and high-fiber foods like whole grains and fresh fruits and vegetables. Reactions to specific foods depend on the individual. Therefore, advise the patient to delete and reintroduce various foods to find those that are most troublesome. Because flatus is usually evident several hours after eating gas-forming foods, the patient can eat those foods selectively at times when flatus would not be embarrassing.

Good hygiene also helps control odor. Reusable collection pouches should be washed with soap and water. Rinsing with a vinegar solution neutralizes odors that cling to the pouch. Odor-proof pouches and commercial pouch deodorizers are available as well.

Sexual Dysfunction and/or Ineffective Sexuality Patterns

One area that often worries patients with ostomies is sexuality. Encourage patients to ask questions about how the ostomy might affect sexual function or behavior. Patients may feel unattractive or fear rejection by their partners. Some men have erectile dysfunction or disruption of emission, especially if they have had nerve damage associated with perineal surgery. The surgeon and the ET counsel these men about options, which may include penile implants. Other patients have problems because of psychological factors, which may improve with counseling.

Some practical suggestions may help the patient resume sexual activity. The pouch should be emptied and taped down before sexual intercourse. Pouch covers are available to conceal the appliance and its contents. The partner wearing the pouch should experiment with positions that are most comfortable. Female patients should know that ostomy surgery does not interfere with pregnancy or delivery.

Ineffective Therapeutic Regimen Management

After surgery, some teaching should be included every time stoma care is done. At first, you may simply tell the patient what is being done and why. Then, encourage the patient to take over more and more of the procedure. Have the patient demonstrate and practice as much as possible before discharge.

Some patients adjust more easily than others to an ostomy. A first step in accepting the stoma is looking at it. Note when the patient begins to watch stoma care. Encourage, but do not force, patients to participate in the care. If a patient does not begin to show some interest in learning self-care after a few days, consider supportive resources such as the ET or an ostomy club volunteer. You may feel frustrated if patients seem unwilling to learn self-care. Be sensitive to the patient's feelings. An ostomy requires adjustments in body image and self-concept. Patients also have a grief response to this type of surgery. Chapter 23 explores nursing interventions to help the patient cope with feelings of loss.

PATIENT TEACHING PLAN
Ostomy Surgery

The nurse or ET, or both, must help the patient plan for discharge. General topics to include in the teaching plan after ostomy surgery are outlined here. Specifics must be individualized to the patient and the surgical procedure.

- Stoma and skin care: recommended procedure and supplies
- Appliances: list of supplies needed, where to purchase
- Irrigation (if appropriate) or drainage: frequency, procedure, supplies
- Other helpful points include:
- You can bathe or shower with your appliance in place because the pouch and the seal are waterproof.
- You can wear regular clothing, but avoid direct pressure over stoma.

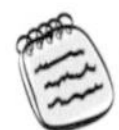

PATIENT TEACHING PLAN
Ostomy Surgery—cont'd

- You will learn to recognize foods that cause excess gas or odor, so these can be avoided.
- Maintain a fluid intake of at least 2,000 ml daily.
- Avoid heavy lifting and strenuous activities at first; there are usually no restrictions after approximately 3 months; ask your physician about specific activities and contact sports.
- Adaptations for sexual activity can include concealing the pouch and experimenting with positions.
- Contact your physician or the ET if you observe skin breakdown, prolapse (bulging out) of the stoma, or obstruction (output absent or markedly decreased).
- Resources for information about living with an ostomy include the American Cancer Society, United Ostomy Association, Crohn's and Colitis Foundations of America, and home health agencies.
- If you enjoy traveling, you can continue doing that. Tips on traveling include the following:
- Take adequate supplies.
- If flying, keep the supplies in a hand-carried bag. This could avoid problems if luggage is lost or delayed.
- Include sealable plastic bags to dispose of used supplies.
- Exercise caution with new foods that may cause diarrhea or gas.
- If visiting a country where drinking the water is not advised, do not irrigate a colostomy with the water.
- Provide written care instructions, and some temporary supplies when the patient is discharged.

Put on your ***THINKING CAP!!***

Locate a resource in the area where you live that provides information for people with ostomies. Share these with classmates.

CONTINENT (POUCH) ILEOSTOMY

The continent ileostomy has an internal pouch created from a loop of ileum for storing fecal matter. The advantage of this type of ileostomy is that the patient does not have continuous drainage and so does not have to wear a pouch.

Not all patients are candidates for the continent ileostomy. It cannot be done for people who cannot drain the pouch or for those who do not have enough ileum for the valve to be constructed. People with ulcerative colitis are candidates for the continent ileostomy, but patients with Crohn's disease are usually not eligible.

Procedure

To create a continent ileostomy, a loop of the ileum is sutured together and then opened. A portion of the distal end of the ileum is inverted within itself to create a nipple valve. The valve prevents the leakage of fluid from the pouch. The looped section of the ileum is then closed, leaving a pouch capable of expanding and storing fecal matter. The distal end of the ileum is brought through the abdominal wall and sutured into place to create a stoma (Fig. 25-2). During surgery, a catheter is placed through the stoma into the pouch and sutured in place. The catheter is connected to low intermittent suction to keep the pouch empty. This prevents stress on the suture lines while the pouch heals.

POSTOPERATIVE NURSING CARE *of the Patient with a Continent Ileostomy*

In general, postoperative nursing care is like that described for the patient with an ileostomy. This section provides information on additional nursing measures that are specific to the patient with a continent ileostomy.

Assessment

Postoperative assessment of the patient who has a continent ileostomy is essentially the same as that of the patient with an ileostomy. When the patient has a continent ileostomy, it is especially important to assess for continuous drainage because obstruction of the catheter may occur. Absence of drainage or patient complaints of a feeling of fullness in the pouch suggest obstruction. The drainage from the catheter is bloody at first, then brownish.

Nursing Diagnoses, Goals, and Outcome Criteria: Continent Ileostomy

Nursing diagnoses and goals in addition to those previously listed are the following:

Nursing Diagnoses	Goals and Outcome Criteria
Risk for Injury related to obstruction of the pouch drainage	Absence of injury: patient's pouch drains readily
Deficient Knowledge of technique for draining pouch and caring for stoma pouch	Patient understands pouch and stoma care: patient demonstrates proper pouch drainage and stoma care

Interventions

Risk for Injury

In the initial postoperative period, the patient is given only intravenous fluids. This allows the bowel to heal and peristalsis to resume. The catheter is removed after several days, and the pouch is drained at intervals. At first, the pouch can hold only 70 to 100 ml of fluid. Later, it can hold as much as 600 ml. For the first 2 weeks, the pouch is drained every 3 to 4 hours. Over the next 2 weeks, the interval is lengthened to every 5 hours. Eventually, the patient will need to drain the pouch only two to four times a day. As the patient's body adapts to the ileostomy, the drainage gradually becomes thicker and the color of normal stool.

Deficient Knowledge

Key points in draining the continent ileostomy are as follows:

1. Have the patient sit or lie down for the procedure.
2. Gather supplies: lubricant, No. 28 catheter, drape, basin, irrigating syringe, irrigating solution, gauze dressing.

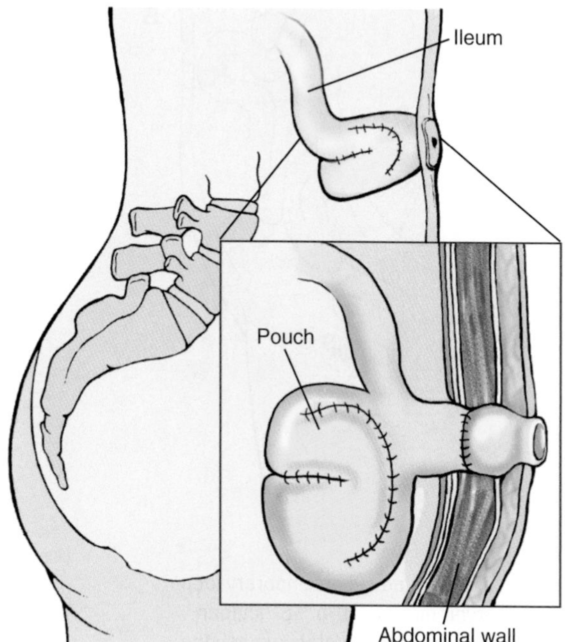

FIGURE **25-2** Continent ileostomy (Kock pouch). The pouch to hold fecal matter is created from a loop of ileum folded back on itself.

3. Lubricate the catheter and insert it gently into the stoma.
4. Resistance will be felt when the catheter reaches the nipple valve (approximately 2 inches past the stoma). Instruct the patient to bear down, then roll the catheter between your fingers and advance it into the pouch.
5. As soon as the catheter is in the pouch, gas and fecal matter begin to drain. Drainage usually continues for approximately 10 minutes and produces a total volume of 50 to 200 ml.
6. If the drainage is too thick, instill 30 ml of normal saline as ordered. Gently aspirate. Do not do this unless necessary because it may cause dislocation of the nipple.
7. When drainage stops, quickly remove the catheter.
8. Place a gauze dressing over the stoma to absorb any secretions.
9. Measure, describe, and discard the drainage.
10. Instruct the patient in how to perform this procedure as soon as possible.
11. Advise the patient to wear a medical alert bracelet at all times that states he or she has a continent diversion that must be drained.

Request a postoperative dietary consult because the patient with a continent ileostomy will have some dietary restrictions. The diet is intended to avoid excess gas, maintain a soft stool, and avoid obstruction of the catheter. The following are foods to avoid:

Coffee, alcohol, and gas-forming foods (initially)
Skins, seeds, or nuts (including corn, olives, peas)
Pineapple, berries, fresh fruit (initially)
Milk products if they cause excessive gas

ILEOANAL RESERVOIR

An ileoanal reservoir is somewhat like the pouch ileostomy except that fecal matter is stored and then eliminated through the rectum. It is an alternative to an ostomy and is included in this chapter because the patient has a temporary ileostomy and the nursing care is similar to that of the ostomy patient.

Procedure

The ileoanal reservoir requires a complex set of surgical procedures that are done in two stages. In the first stage, the colon is removed and an internal pouch that is created from the ileum is attached to the anorectal canal. A temporary ileostomy commonly is made to allow the reservoir to heal. Approximately 2 months later, barium radiographs are taken to be sure that the reservoir is intact. If the reservoir does not leak, the ileostomy is closed (Fig. 25-3). The procedure is not recommended for patients with Crohn's disease or poor rectal sphincter control.

Complications

The major complications of the ileoanal reservoir are small bowel obstruction, leaking of suture lines leading to peritonitis, and inflammation of the reservoir.

Obstruction. Scar tissue or strictures may cause obstruction. Signs and symptoms of small bowel obstruction are abdominal distention, nausea and vomiting, decreased bowel sounds, and a change in bowel pattern.

Peritonitis. If fecal matter leaks through the suture lines of the reservoir into the abdominal cavity, abscesses or peritonitis can develop. Signs and symptoms are increased pulse, respirations, and temperature; rigid abdomen and abdominal pain; and elevated white blood cell count.

Inflammation. Inflammation of the reservoir may be manifested by bloody diarrhea, anorexia, and pain.

POSTOPERATIVE NURSING CARE *of the Patient with an Ileoanal Reservoir*

Assessment

The nursing assessment after surgery to create an ileoanal reservoir is the same as for the patient with an ileostomy. In addition, assess for rectal drainage and condition of the perianal skin.

Nursing Diagnoses, Goals, and Outcome Criteria: Ileoanal Reservoir

In addition to the nursing diagnoses and goals for the patient with an ileostomy, the following diagnoses may be appropriate for the patient with an ileoanal reservoir:

Nursing Diagnoses	Goals and Outcome Criteria
Risk for Impaired Skin Integrity related to frequent passage of liquid stool through the rectum	Healthy skin: intact skin without excessive redness around the rectum and the perianal area
Bowel Incontinence related to inability to control passage of frequent liquid stools	Control of bowel elimination: decreasing number of incontinent episodes

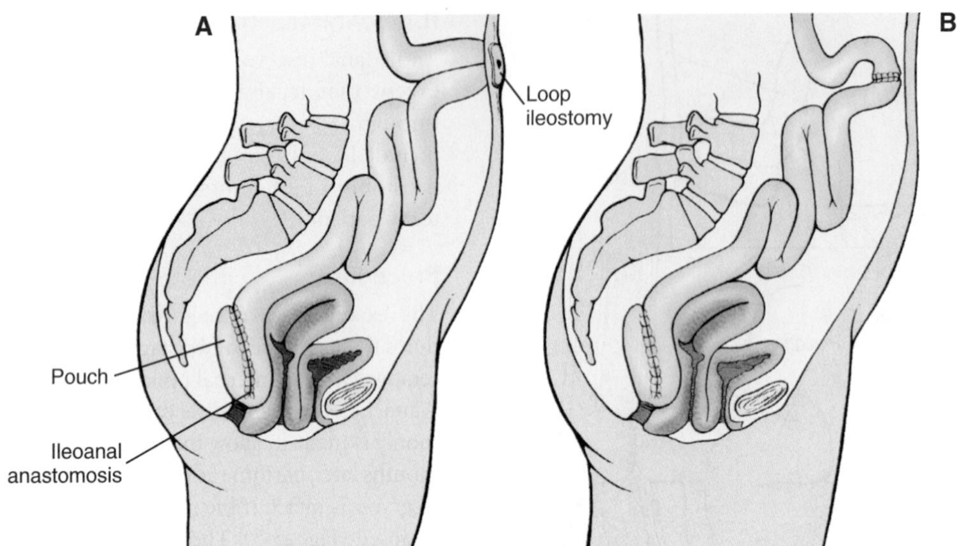

FIGURE 25-3 Creation of an ileoanal reservoir. Stage 1 *A,* The colon is removed, a temporary loop ileostomy is created, and an ileoanal reservoir is formed. The reservoir may be "J" or "S" shaped depending on the technique used. Stage 2 *B,* After the reservoir heals (usually several months), the temporary loop ileostomy is reversed and stool drains into the reservoir for storage until it is eliminated through the rectum.

Nursing Diagnoses, Goals, and Outcome Criteria: Ileoanal Reservoir—cont'd

Nursing Diagnoses	Goals and Outcome Criteria
Risk for Injury related to possible small bowel obstruction, leaking of reservoir suture line, inflammation of reservoir	Absence of signs and symptoms of obstruction, suture leakage, or reservoir inflammation: no fever, abdominal pain or distention, bloody stools

Interventions

Risk for Impaired Skin Integrity

After the first surgical procedure, the patient's skin around the ileostomy stoma and in the perianal area needs special care. Ileostomy care is covered earlier in this chapter. Until the reservoir is well healed, liquid discharge may be expelled without warning. Thorough, gentle cleansing and protective creams help prevent skin breakdown.

Bowel Incontinence

Initially, the patient may have as many as 20 stools a day. After a week, the number decreases to 8 to 10 daily. By 6 months, the frequency is usually only approximately four to six a day. Nighttime control may continue to be a problem. Perineal pads may be needed to prevent soiling of clothing.

The patient must learn to strengthen perineal muscles to restore control of fecal elimination. A recommended exercise is to tighten the anus, count to 10, and relax. This should be repeated five to six times, four times daily. Also, drugs can be prescribed to decrease the frequency of stools and to make them less watery.

Advise patients to avoid fatty foods at first. There are no absolute restrictions. The patient learns through trial and error how his or her body handles specific foods. Caffeine and fresh fruits and vegetables tend to cause loose, frequent stools. Pasta, boiled rice, and low-fat cheese tend to produce thicker stools.

Risk for Injury

Be alert for signs and symptoms of bowel obstruction (abdominal distention, pain, no stool passage), peritonitis (pain, fever), and inflammation (pain, bloody stools) that should be reported to the physician. If obstruction occurs, the patient is given intravenous fluids and nothing by mouth. A nasogastric tube is inserted to decompress the bowel. If the obstruction is caused by adhesions (scar tissue), surgery may be necessary to release the restriction.

Sometimes a stricture or narrowing develops at the site where the ileum is joined to the rectum. This is most likely to happen in the fourth week after surgery. The physician may be able to stretch the tissue manually and relieve the obstruction. If an abscess or peritonitis develops, the infection is treated with antibiotics. Intravenous fluids are ordered, and a nasogastric tube is inserted for decompression of the bowel. Surgery may be necessary to drain abscesses and repair the leaking suture line.

If the inner lining of the reservoir becomes inflamed or infected, the physician may do a proctoscopic examination to identify the cause. The condition may be treated with metronidazole (Flagyl) and steroids given orally.

COLOSTOMY

A colostomy is an opening in the colon through which fecal matter is eliminated. The location of the colostomy affects

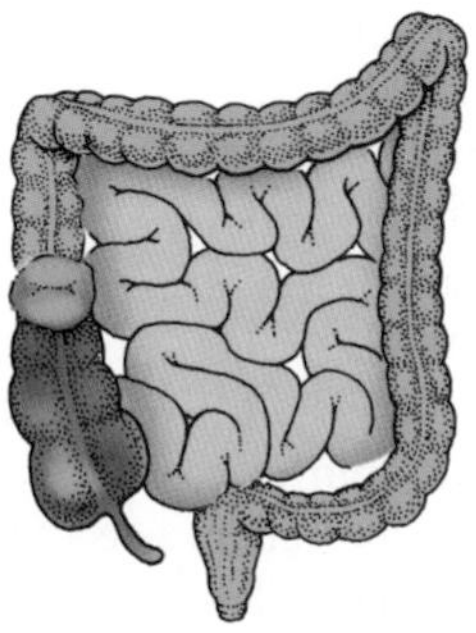

The **ascending colostomy** is done for right-sided tumors.

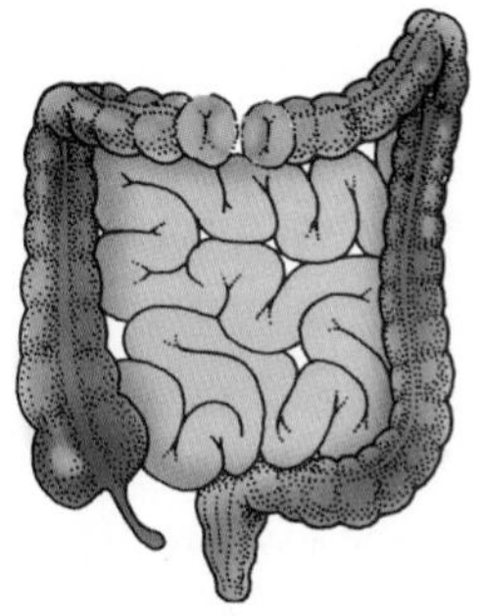

The **transverse (double-barreled) colostomy** is often used in such emergencies as intestinal obstruction or perforation because it can be created quickly. There are two stomas. The proximal one, closest to the small intestine, drains feces. The distal stoma drains mucus.

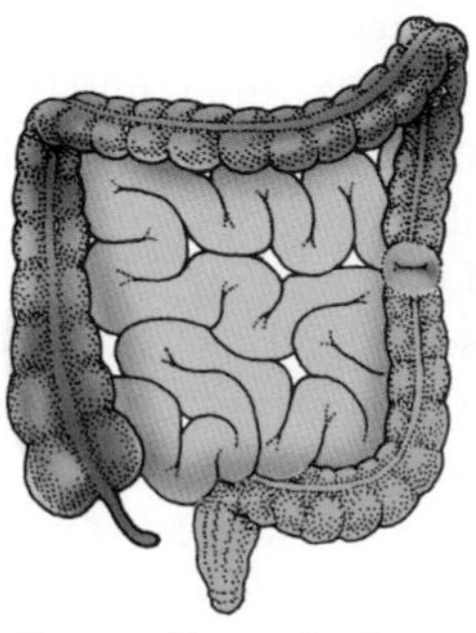

Descending colostomy

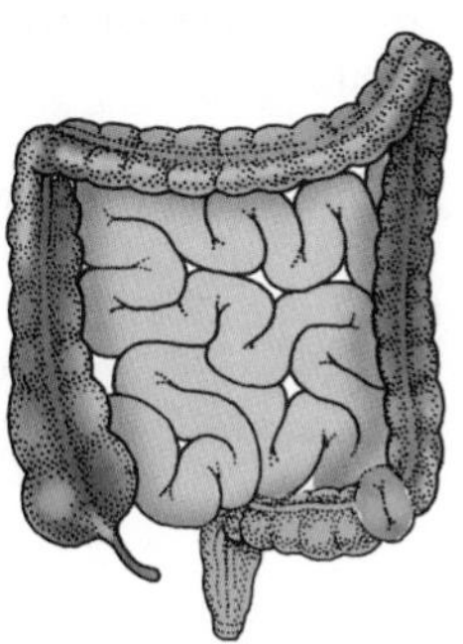

Sigmoid colostomy

FIGURE **25-4** Colostomy location depends on the reason for the surgery and, in the case of cancer, the location of tissue that must be removed.

the characteristics of the fecal drainage: the closer to the rectum, the more formed the stool.

Procedure

A colostomy is performed by bringing a loop or an end of the intestine through the abdominal wall and creating a stoma for the passage of fecal matter. The location of the stoma depends on the portion of the intestine removed. Colostomies are classified by location in the colon. Therefore, there are ascending, transverse, descending, and sigmoid colostomies (Fig. 25-4). An ascending colostomy passes relatively liquid material. The drainage from a transverse colostomy is liquid to semisolid. A descending or sigmoid colostomy passes softly formed stool. The colostomy begins to function on the third to fifth postoperative day.

A colostomy may be temporary or permanent. A temporary colostomy is done to allow healing of the intestine after surgery or in certain disease states. Because the intestine below the colostomy is intact, the temporary colostomy may have two stomas. The stoma that drains fecal matter from the intestine is the proximal stoma. The distal stoma opens into the portion of the colon connected to the rectum. This is called a *double-barreled colostomy.* Sometimes the opening of the distal portion is brought through another location on the abdominal wall, creating a fistula through which mucus drains. An end colostomy with a Hartmann pouch for the distal segment is now more common than the double-barreled colostomy. A Hartmann pouch is created by closing the distal bowel and leaving it in place. The patient with a Hartmann pouch passes mucus through the rectum.

When it is necessary to remove a large part of the colon or the rectum, a permanent colostomy is made. Sometimes the colostomy is created in two stages. The patient returns from the first procedure with a loop of intestine protruding from an abdominal wound. The loop is held in place by a rod or a bridge. Later, the surgeon cuts the loop to create the stoma.

The main long-term complications of colostomy are prolapse and stenosis. A prolapsed stoma protrudes farther out than usual. It is caused by increased abdominal pressure, as can occur with coughing or sneezing. Other contributing factors might include an abdominal opening that is too large or a poorly attached stoma. Stenosis is the narrowing of the abdominal opening around the base of the stoma. If severe, stenosis blocks the passage of feces. Additional complications are associated with poor blood supply to the stoma, leading to necrosis and peristomal hernia. Peristomal hernia can limit bowel function, causing constipation, strangulation of the bowel, and poor results from colostomy irrigation.

POSTOPERATIVE NURSING CARE *of the Patient with a Colostomy*

Assessment

The postoperative care of the patient with a colostomy is essentially the same as that for the patient with an ileostomy.

Nursing Diagnoses, Goals, and Outcome Criteria: Colostomy

In addition to the nursing diagnoses and goals already identified, the following may also apply to the patient with a colostomy:

Nursing Diagnoses	Goals and Outcome Criteria
Ineffective Therapeutic Regimen Management related to lack of knowledge of irrigation procedure (if ordered), lack of confidence, failure to accept colostomy, lack of resources	Patient manages colostomy effectively: patient demonstrates irrigation (if ordered), and other ostomy care correctly; uses resources as needed
Risk for Injury related to prolapse or stenosis	Absence of signs of prolapse: no protrusion of stoma Patent stoma with lumen of adequate diameter: regular elimination of feces through stoma

Interventions

Most aspects of care are the same as those discussed in relation to the patient with an ileostomy. A few points specific to the patient with a colostomy are presented here (see also Nursing Care Plan: The Patient with a Colostomy).

Ineffective Therapeutic Regimen Management

In the past, people with sigmoid colostomies were taught to irrigate them daily to maintain regular, controlled elimination. This procedure is no longer routinely recommended. Many patients have regular bowel movements without irrigation. Others are unlikely to establish controlled elimination and may find the procedure not worth the trouble. Patients who have liquid stools do not benefit from irrigation because they drain fecal matter continuously. Irrigation is unlikely to establish control if the patient has diarrhea when under stress, has had radiotherapy, has a poor prognosis, or has a history of inflammatory bowel disease.

Irrigation can cause complications. The tube used to introduce irrigating fluid can perforate the bowel. A perforated bowel permits fecal matter to flow into the abdominal cavity, causing peritonitis, a very serious infection. The risk of perforation can be reduced greatly by using a cone-tipped catheter. Other complications are caused by the type, amount, or temperature of the solution used. Plain tap water may cause fluid and electrolyte imbalances if used repeatedly or in large amounts. If too much solution is used or if it is too cold, the patient may experience cramping, nausea, and dizziness. The physician should be advised if weakness occurs after irrigation even after the amount and temperature of the solution are adjusted.

If irrigations are indicated, you or the ET may perform them initially. The goal, however, is for the patient or significant other to learn to do the procedure, so an explanation of the process must be provided.

The following are key points to remember when irrigating a colostomy:

1. Have the patient select the time of day that is most convenient. The procedure should be done at approximately the same time every day. The entire process takes 45 minutes to 1 hour.
2. Have the patient sit on or in front of the toilet if possible. If the patient cannot get out of bed, the procedure can be done while the patient is in bed.
3. Remove the old pouch and apply an irrigating sleeve. This device opens at the top so that the tubing can be inserted into the stoma, and at the bottom so that fecal matter can drain into the toilet.
4. Pour 500 to 1,000 ml of lukewarm irrigating solution into an enema fluid container and hold it at the level of the patient's shoulder. Five hundred milliliters is used initially, but adults eventually increase the fluid to 1,000 ml.
5. Clear the air from the tubing, lubricate the tubing, and insert it gently 2 to 4 inches into the stoma. The direction to insert the tubing can be assessed by first inserting a gloved, lubricated finger into the stoma. Do not use force! If a cone-tipped catheter is used, the catheter can be inserted only approximately 1 inch. This reduces the risk of perforation.
6. Allow the solution to flow slowly into the stoma. If the patient has cramping, slow down or stop the flow for a few minutes. Remove the catheter after the solution has been administered.
7. If the solution does not drain promptly, close the bottom of the sleeve so that the patient can carry out other activities. Complete emptying may take 20 to 30 minutes.
8. When elimination is complete, remove, wash, and dry the sleeve.
9. Apply a clean pouch if additional drainage usually occurs during the day. Some patients need only a small dressing or a stoma cap.
10. Rectal suppositories can be inserted into a colostomy stoma to stimulate evacuation.
11. Patients who have double-barreled colostomies can be given rectal medications through the distal stoma.

Risk for Injury

Be alert for indications of colostomy complications. Although a prolapsed stoma may look frightening, it is not usually serious. There is no reason for immediate action if it continues to drain feces. It can usually be gently put back in place by the surgeon or ET. If the prolapse is severe or causes fecal obstruction, surgical repair is indicated.

NURSING CARE PLAN

The Patient with a Colostomy

ASSESSMENT

Health History: Mr. Chin is a 47-year-old Asian American who had a bowel resection and permanent colostomy in the descending colon to remove a malignant tumor. He is 3 days postsurgery. He has been receiving intravenous morphine by patient-controlled analgesia and reports adequate pain control. He has had no nausea or vomiting but has a nasogastric tube attached to low suction. He is allowed nothing by mouth (NPO) and is receiving intravenous fluids at 150 ml per hour. He participates in turning, coughing, deep breathing, and using incentive spirometry every 2 hours. He has discussed his fear of cancer with the nurse, stating that his mother died of stomach cancer.

Physical Examination: Vital signs: temperature, 100° F orally; pulse, 92; respiration, 20; blood pressure, 118/64. The patient is alert and oriented. His skin is warm and dry with good turgor. Oral mucous membranes are moist. Breath sounds are clear to auscultation. The abdomen is soft, and bowel sounds are present in all four quadrants. The stoma is beefy red and edematous. A temporary drainage device is in place, and the collection pouch has approximately 100 ml of greenish brown liquid stool. Extremities are warm with palpable peripheral pulses. No muscle twitching or cramps are noted.

Nursing Diagnosis	*Goals and Outcome Criteria*	*Interventions*
Risk for deficit fluid volume related to NPO status, nasogastric suction, passage of liquid stool.	Patient will maintain normal fluid balance as evidenced by pulse and blood pressure consistent with patient's baseline, moist mucous membranes, and approximately equal fluid intake and output.	Monitor for signs of hypovolemia: tachycardia, hypotension, decreasing urine output, dry mucous membranes. Keep accurate intake and output (urine, liquid stool, gastric fluid) records. Monitor for signs of electrolyte imbalances: confusion, anxiety, twitching, trembling, muscle weakness, cardiac dysrhythmias. Give intravenous fluids as ordered, monitoring rate of flow carefully.
Impaired skin integrity related to stoma adhesive, fecal drainage.	Skin at the base of the stoma will be healed by time of discharge.	Check pouch hourly to detect leakage. When pouch is removed for emptying, prevent fecal matter from contaminating incision. When changing appliance, gently remove adhesive. Cleanse skin around stoma with soap and water, rinse, and pat dry. Apply a protective skin barrier before replacing pouch. If washers or wafers are used, make the opening not more than ⅛ inch larger than the stoma. Report rash or skin breakdown.
Disturbed body image related to presence of stoma, altered body function.	Patient will adapt to colostomy as evidenced by self-care and ability to resume normal activities.	Provide an opportunity for patient to share his thoughts about colostomy. Identify specific concerns such as activity limitations, stoma care, odor control, and impact on sexuality. Provide information. Be accepting of patient's feelings. Encourage him to attend to grooming and appearance. Offer to have a volunteer from American Cancer Society or United Ostomy Association visit him. Advise of services of enterostomal therapist, mental health counselor, and spiritual counselor if patient desires.
Ineffective therapeutic regimen management related to lack of understanding of self-care with ostomy, lack of resources, failure to accept ostomy.	Patient will manage therapeutic regimen effectively: patient demonstrates proper ostomy care, uses available resources, resumes valued activities with adaptations as needed.	During stoma care in early postoperative period, tell patient what is being done and why. When patient begins to watch procedure, gradually encourage him to participate and then to take over care. Recognize patient's need to grieve and that patient may use denial as a coping mechanism. Develop a teaching plan that includes skin care, pouches, diet, fluids, irrigation if appropriate, activity, sexuality, complications, tips on traveling, and resources.

Inform the physician if the ostomy is not draining properly. The surgeon may be able to dilate the stoma and enlarge the opening. If dilatation is not successful, surgery may be needed.

What Does Culture Have to do with Ostomies?

Consider how culturally based individual variables can affect how a person adapts to an ostomy. Culture shapes values related to body image, self-esteem, independence, sexuality, and hygiene.

URINARY DIVERSION

The most common types of urinary diversion are ileal conduits and continent internal reservoirs. Other diversions include cutaneous ureterostomy, colonic (sigmoid) conduit, cystostomy, vesicostomy, and nephrostomy (Fig. 25-5). Ureterosigmoidostomy and ureteroileosigmoidostomy are not performed as commonly now as in the past; however, you may encounter patients who have had them.

Urinary diversion may be temporary or permanent. Permanent urinary diversion is necessary when the bladder is congenitally absent or removed because of malignancy or trauma or when extensive pelvic malignancy obstructs urine flow. Temporary diversion may be used when there is obstruction to urine flow, as might be caused by a urinary calculus, or to permit healing of the ureters or bladder.

Preparation of the patient for ostomy surgery is discussed at the beginning of this chapter. Postoperative care after each type of diversion is discussed separately.

CUTANEOUS URETEROSTOMY

A cutaneous ureterostomy is created when one or both ureters are brought out through an opening in the abdomen or flank. Often the two ureters are joined surgically so that

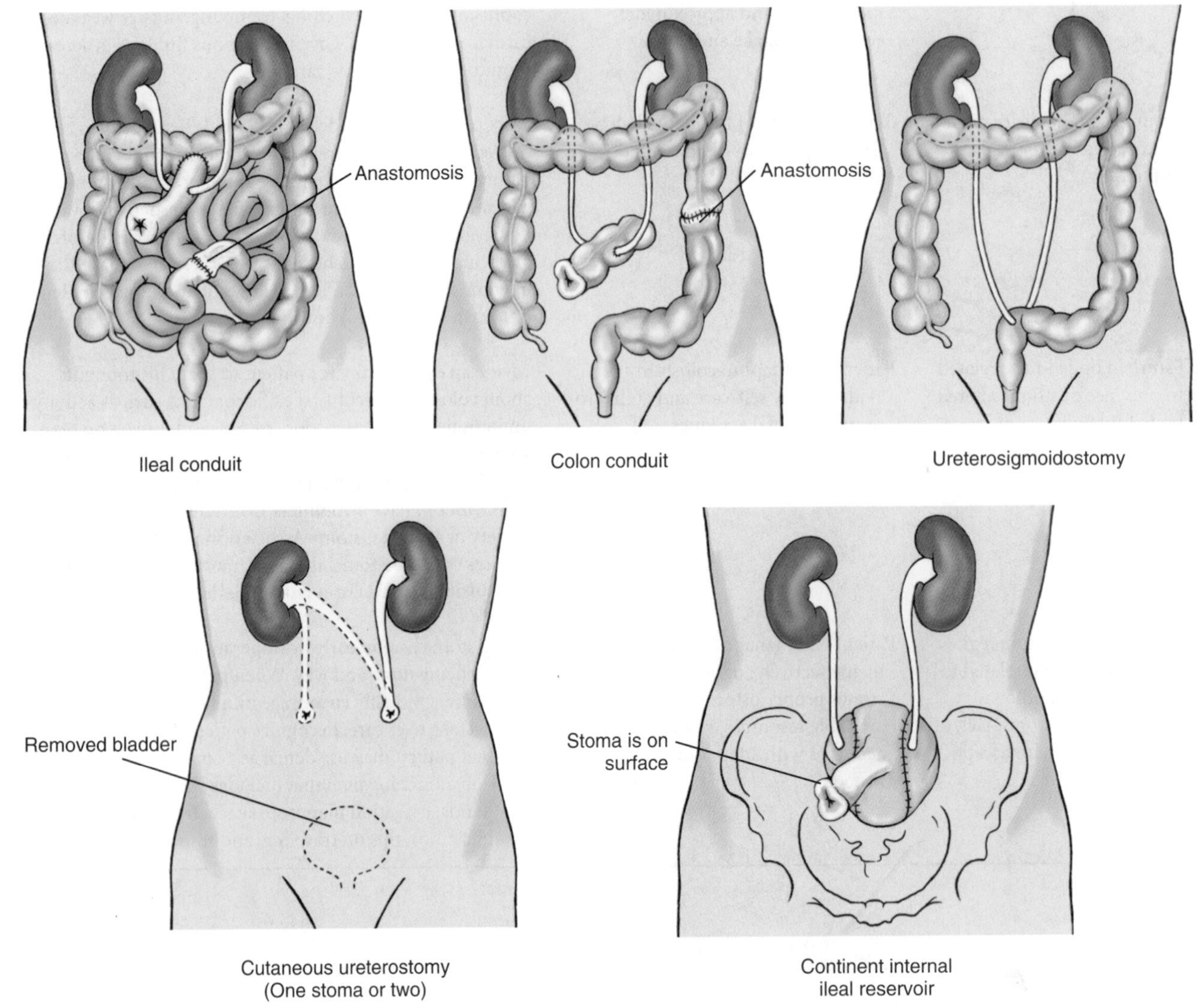

Anastomosis
Ileal conduit

Anastomosis
Colon conduit

Ureterosigmoidostomy

Removed bladder
Cutaneous ureterostomy (One stoma or two)

Stoma is on surface
Continent internal ileal reservoir

FIGURE **25-5** Types of urinary diversion.

only one stoma is needed. In some situations, a stoma is created from each ureter.

A ureterostomy stoma is much smaller than an intestinal stoma. Immediately after surgery, the urinary stoma is pink, but it quickly fades to a lighter color. Because there is no reservoir to hold it, urine drains from the stoma continuously. A pouch is needed to collect the urine and protect the skin.

Complications

Complications experienced by patients with cutaneous ureterostomies include stenosis and urinary tract infections. Stenosis is a narrowing of the opening that interferes with the flow of urine. If the obstruction is not relieved, urine backs up in the kidney. The kidney may become swollen with urine, a condition called *hydronephrosis,* which leads to serious kidney damage. The kidneys can also be damaged by urinary tract infections.

POSTOPERATIVE NURSING CARE *of the Patient with a Cutaneous Ureterostomy*

Assessment

Health History

The preoperative health history may be used to determine the reason for ureterostomy as well as pertinent past medical history, drug profile, and allergies. In the postoperative period, the review of systems should include assessment of the presence of flank or abdominal pain, fatigue, malaise, and chills. Also assess the patient's response to the ostomy, knowledge about it, and readiness to learn.

Physical Examination

Begin the physical examination with a survey of the patient's general state. Take vital signs and compare with preoperative readings. Observe respiratory effort and auscultate breath sounds. Assess the abdomen for distention and bowel sounds. Inspect the stoma. It is usually much smaller than an intestinal stoma and lighter in color. Document the amount, appearance, and odor of the urine. Some blood in the urine is normal at first, but it should gradually clear. Ureterostomy drainage should not contain mucus.

Nursing Diagnoses, Goals, and Outcome Criteria: Cutaneous Ureterostomy

In addition to the common diagnoses and goals for postoperative patients (see Chapter 16), the following diagnoses may apply to the patient who has a cutaneous ureterostomy:

Nursing Diagnoses	Goals and Outcome Criteria
Impaired Skin Integrity related to contact of urine with skin	Normal skin around stoma: healed stoma base without redness or edema
Risk for Infection related to contamination of stoma	Absence of infection: no fever or foul urine odor
Risk for Injury related to obstruction of urine flow	Unobstructed urine flow: urine output equal to fluid intake
Disturbed Body Image related to presence of stoma, altered body function	Adjustment in body image: patient acknowledges stoma, shows increasing interest in self-care, resumes previous sexual activity
Self-Care Deficit related to management of ostomy	Patient understands self-care with an ostomy: patient demonstrates proper techniques of ostomy care and describes self-care with an ostomy

Interventions

Impaired Skin Integrity

After a ureterostomy, the patient has a ureteral catheter for a week or two. The catheter is attached to a collection device. Once the catheter is removed, an appliance is needed to collect urine drainage. A variety of pouches are available (see Fig. 25-1). Some have antireflux valves to prevent the flow of urine back into the stoma. A skin barrier product can be used around the stoma for protection. Karaya products are used for intestinal ostomies but not for urinary drainage because urine breaks down the product. Belts can be worn with some appliances to hold them in place. Some pouches can be connected to a leg bag for urine collection.

The pouch is usually cleaned once or twice daily. It is changed every 4 to 6 days or when it leaks because frequent changes are irritating to the surrounding skin. When it is changed, gently remove any adhesive. A gauze pad, tampon, or tissue may be placed at the opening of the stoma to absorb urine. Pouch changes are usually done in the morning when urine production is lowest. Steps in the application of a urinary pouch are illustrated in Figure 25-6. Wash the peristomal area with water and pat dry. If soap is used, it should be nonoily and rinsed off thoroughly. If there are crystals present, a gauze pad saturated in a dilute vinegar solution can be used to dissolve them. Urinary stoma problems are summarized in Table 25-2.

Risk for Infection

The stoma serves as a portal for pathogens to enter the urinary tract, causing infection. Urinary tract infections can have serious consequences, including kidney damage and septicemia. Pouch care is treated as a clean rather than sterile procedure because the stoma is not sterile. Still, you should take care to avoid introducing organisms to the area.

Yeast infections that sometimes develop around the stoma are characterized by a skin rash surrounding the stoma. These are usually treated with nystatin powder applied under the skin barrier.

Risk for Injury

If urine does not flow readily, suspect obstruction and notify the registered nurse or the surgeon immediately.

Disturbed Body Image

Adjustment to a stoma can be very difficult. The patient may be afraid of leakage and odor and may feel disfigured.

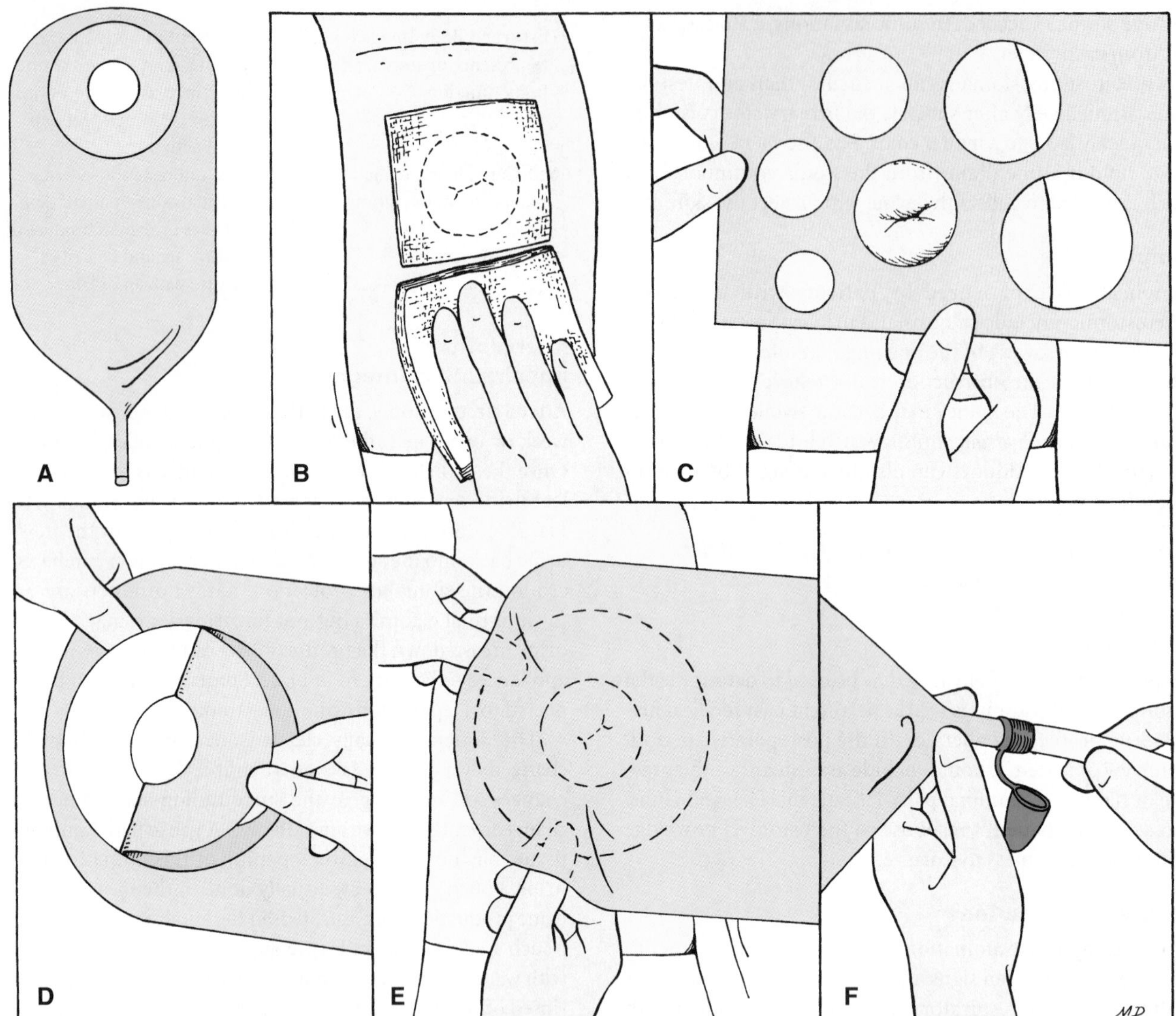

FIGURE **25-6** Procedure for applying pouch. *A,* Gather supplies: pouch, ostomy belt, skin barrier, stoma template, gauze pads, pouch clamp or rubber band, safety pin, and clean gloves. Wash hands and put on gloves. *B,* After removing the old pouch and cleaning the area around the stoma, place a gauze square over the stoma to absorb the drainage. *C,* Use a stoma template to measure the size of the stoma, and then cut an opening the same size as the stoma into the skin barrier and adhesive. *D,* Remove the backing from the adhesive of the new pouch. *E,* Place the opening in the new pouch over the stoma and gently press into place with the pouch drain pointed toward the floor. *F,* Connect the drain to the tubing or close the drain if appropriate. Secure the tubing to sheets or according to agency policy.

Demonstrate acceptance of the patient and care for the stoma in a matter-of-fact manner. Also express understanding of the patient's feelings. Encourage the patient to groom and dress normally. If odor is a problem, the pouch can be soaked in vinegar water for 20 to 30 minutes. Odor-proof pouches also should be recommended. Learning to care for the ureterostomy boosts the patient's self-confidence and may help to restore a more positive body image.

Patients with ostomies commonly experience grief in response to the loss of normal function and perceived disfigurement. This may be exhibited as denial, shock, anger, bargaining, or depression. Chapter 23 offers guidance for dealing with the patient who is grieving.

The change in body image may affect the patient's sexuality. Provide opportunities for patients with an ostomy to ask questions or discuss how the ostomy might affect sexual function or behavior. Patients may feel unattractive or fear rejection by their partners. People who have had radical perineal surgeries may have physical barriers to sexual performance; other patients have problems because of psychological factors.

The same practical suggestions identified for the patient with an intestinal ostomy may be useful to the patient with a urinary ostomy. The pouch should be emptied before sexual intercourse. Pouch covers are available to conceal the appliance and its contents. The partner wearing the pouch should experiment with positions that are most comfortable. Female

table 25-2 ***Problems Associated with Urinary Stomas***

PROBLEM	CAUSE	ASSESSMENT/INTERVENTION
Stomal laceration	Pouch opening too small Pouch not positioned correctly	Enlarge pouch opening Reposition pouch Monitor healing
Peristomal laceration	Improperly fitting pouch Improper pouch removal technique	Evaluate pouch fit with patient in sitting, lying, and standing positions. Check fit of belt. Consider need for adhesive removers, and/or specialized pouching systems
Bleeding	Trauma	Apply cool cloth Cleanse gently
	Urinary tract infection	Treat infection, acidify urine
Stenosis	Scar formation	Dilatation by or under physician's direction
Crystal formation		Apply vinegar compress to stoma during dressing change Put 1-2 oz of vinegar solution in pouch 20 min bid, then rinse Use vinyl or plastic pouch rather than rubber
Skin irritation	Skin barrier or wafer too small Leaking appliance	Adjust size of skin barrier or wafer to cover skin around stoma Check belt; if too tight, can break seal Replace appliance PRN
	Hair follicle inflammation	Use topical antimicrobial powder and skin barrier powder Cover lesions with non-stick dressing and cover with barrier before applying pouching system Use adhesive remover; remove sealants gently After skin returns to normal, shave or cut hair around stoma
	Perspiration under pouch	Dry skin well Apply protective barrier Apply powder to skin under pouch Use a soft pouch cover
	Allergy to pouching products	Spot test other brands to find one that does not cause irritation
	Candida ("yeast") infection	Dry well Apply nystatin powder as ordered Cover with sealant
Hernia/prolapse	Muscle weakness Increased intraabdominal pressure	Surgical repair
Wart-like lesions	Excessive peristomal wetness	Reduce pouch opening size or acquire custom cut system to reduce moisture on skin. May require debridement by physician.
Odor	Urinary tract infection Appliance soiled or leaking	Treat infection Check seal; change appliance Deodorant tablets PRN, as needed.

patients should know that ostomy surgery does not interfere with pregnancy or delivery.

Self-Care Deficit

Many aspects of teaching the patient with a ureterostomy are the same as those identified for the patient with an ileostomy. The topics to include in the teaching plan are ostomy care, pouches, diet, fluids, activity, sexuality, complications, and resources. See the teaching plan in the section on Ileostomy.

From the early postoperative period, try to help the patient learn independent ostomy care. At first, patient teaching may take place each time stoma care is done by simply telling the patient what is being done and why. Encourage the patient to participate and gradually assume more responsibility for the care. Practice builds confidence and provides the patient with the opportunity to identify problems while you are available to help.

Some people adapt more readily to the stoma than others, but you must be sensitive to their feelings and encourage them in a kind way. A volunteer from the American Cancer Society or the United Ostomy Association can be especially helpful as a role model to the patient with a new ostomy. With the patient's and the physician's approval, the agency can be contacted about sending a volunteer to visit the patient.

The nurse or ET, or both, must help the patient plan for discharge. Provide written care instructions. The patient needs a list of supplies and places where they can be purchased. In addition, send some temporary supplies home with the patient. Also provide information and make referrals as needed for resources such as home health care and community organizations.

In general, normal activities can be resumed within 3 months, but specific directions should be obtained from the physician or ET. Because the pouch and seal are waterproof, the patient can bathe or shower with the appliance in place. Regular clothing can be worn but should not apply pressure to the stoma.

Patients with an ostomy who enjoy traveling are encouraged to continue to do so. When traveling, patients are advised to take adequate supplies, including sealable plastic bags to dispose of used materials. If the patient is flying, his or her supplies should be kept in a hand-carried bag to avoid problems if luggage is lost or delayed. On a long flight, a leg bag attached to the pouch may be beneficial in case the patient must remain seated owing to turbulence.

ILEAL CONDUIT

The ileal conduit is the most common type of urinary diversion. Other names for the ileal conduit are ureteroileostomy, ureteroileocutaneous anastomosis, ileal loop, and Bricker procedure.

Procedure

The ileal conduit is a urinary drainage system made out of a portion of small intestine. A 6- to 8-inch segment of ileum is first removed. The remaining ends of the ileum are then anastomosed (joined) to restore bowel function. The ureters are cut from the bladder and attached to the ileal segment at an angle to prevent reflux. One end of the ileal segment is sutured closed. The other end of the ileal segment is brought through an abdominal incision and sutured to create a stoma for urine drainage. A similar procedure that uses a segment of large intestine is called a colonic or sigmoid conduit. The stoma of an ileal or colonic conduit is bright red because it is intestinal mucosa.

Complications

During the postoperative period, the patient is at risk for a number of complications. Complications related to the surgical procedure include leakage of the anastomosed ureters and intestinal segments, ureteral obstruction, and separation of the stoma from surrounding skin.

Other problems include wound infection, necrosis of the stoma, and paralytic ileus. The stoma may become necrotic if the blood supply in the resected segment is inadequate. If the stoma turns gray or black, circulation is impaired; the physician should be notified at once.

Complications that may occur in the later postoperative period are infection, crystal formation, and calculi (stones). The patient may also have problems with the stoma, including retraction, prolapse, or hernia.

POSTOPERATIVE NURSING CARE *of the Patient with an Ileal Conduit*

Nursing care of the patient who has an ileal conduit is essentially the same as that for the patient with an ileostomy. There are a few special points to make about the ileal conduit. This patient will have a nasogastric tube attached to suction to prevent abdominal distention and stress of the resected portion of the ileum while it heals. The patient is allowed nothing by mouth and is given intravenous fluids until bowel sounds return. A temporary ileus (absence of bowel activity) is expected after bowel resection. A ureteral catheter or stent may be in place to drain urine. If one is present, output is monitored because obstruction can occur. Mucus is normally present in drainage from a conduit because it is produced by the lining of the bowel segment. All patients with ileal conduits are advised to attach the pouch to a collection device during the night.

CONTINENT INTERNAL RESERVOIRS

All of the methods of urinary diversion already discussed permit urine to flow steadily through a stoma. Newer procedures have been developed that allow for the storage and controlled drainage of urine. An example of these, called continent internal reservoirs, is the Kock pouch. An even more recent development is the ileum neobladder, which eliminates the need for any stoma. The neobladder is an internal urinary reservoir constructed using a resected segment of the colon that is attached to the urethra. Urine drains into the reservoir and is eliminated through the urethra instead of a stoma. The neobladder is used more in men than in women. Continence varies with the neobladder, so an artificial urinary sphincter is sometimes implanted. Another option for patients who cannot achieve continence with the neobladder is intermittent self-catheterization. Even though the procedure is well received by patients, some surgeons are reluctant to spare the urethra with bladder cancer, fearing the urethra could be a site for recurrent cancer.

The Kock pouch is constructed with a segment of ileum. The ureters are implanted in one side of the ileum segment. A nipple valve is constructed from the other side and attached to the skin, where a stoma is created. The valve prevents urine from flowing from the reservoir. A catheter is used to drain the reservoir at 4- to 6-hour intervals.

The Indiana pouch is similar to the Kock pouch except that it is made of a portion of the terminal ileum and the ascending colon. This reservoir is larger than that of the Kock pouch. The Indiana pouch is also drained with a catheter every 4 to 6 hours.

Complications

Complications of the continent pouches are incontinence, difficult catheterization, and urinary reflux leading to pyelonephritis, obstruction, and bacteriuria.

POSTOPERATIVE NURSING CARE *of the Patient with a Kock or Indiana Pouch*

Immediately after surgery, the patient may have a Penrose drain to remove fluid from the operative site and a clear tube in place for continuous urine drainage. Irrigations may be ordered to remove clots and mucus. When the tube is removed, the pouch may be drained every 2 to 3 hours at first. Later, the patient may need to drain the pouch only every 4 to 6 hours during the day and once during the night. If the pouch functions properly, the patient does not have to wear an external appliance. A small gauze dressing may be placed over the stoma to absorb mucus drainage. Advise the patient to wear a medical alert bracelet that identifies the presence of a continent device that needs intubation to drain.

URETEROSIGMOIDOSTOMY AND URETEROILEOSIGMOIDOSTOMY

Ureterosigmoidostomy and ureteroileosigmoidostomy are not done as often now as in the past. You may care for patients, however, who have had these diversions for some time and have adapted well to them. In a ureterosigmoidostomy, the ureters are implanted into the sigmoid colon. Urine drains into the colon and is eliminated through the rectum. For a ureteroileosigmoidostomy, a segment of the ileum is anastomosed to the sigmoid and the ureters implanted into that part of the ileum. Neither procedure provides continence, and both present problems with kidney infections and urinary calculi (stones). Additional complications are caused by the colon's absorption of electrolytes from the urine. Patients are at risk for deficits in potassium and bicarbonate and for excesses in sodium, chloride, and hydrogen. These imbalances may lead to metabolic acidosis.

VESICOSTOMY

Vesicostomy or cystostomy is an opening into the urinary bladder. There are several types. Some are drained continuously through a catheter, others have a nipple valve and are drained at intervals.

NEPHROSTOMY

A nephrostomy tube diverts urine directly from the kidney through a tube that exits through the skin. This device may be used as a temporary or permanent method of urinary diversion. Conditions that may be treated with these tubes are discussed in Chapter 38.

Put on your THINKING CAP!!

1. Use a procedure manual or fundamentals text to identify supplies Mr. Chin will need for ostomy care.
2. Locate a source of ostomy supplies. Determine the cost of supplies for 1 month.

Nutrition Concepts

1. The patient with an ileostomy or colostomy may eat a normal diet and simply omit foods that seem to cause problems.
2. The main concern of the patient with an ileostomy or colostomy is odor, which is caused by flatulence.
3. Patients should be encouraged to avoid foods tending to cause bad odor, especially corn, dried beans, onions, cabbage, spicy foods, and fish.
4. Fibrous vegetables should be avoided, and all food should be chewed well.

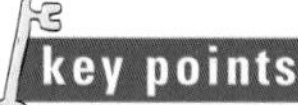

key points

- An ostomy is an artificial opening into a body cavity; a stoma is the site of the opening on the skin.
- Ostomy surgery may be done to bypass a section of the digestive or urinary tract either temporarily or permanently.
- An important resource for nurses and ostomy patients is the enterostomal therapist, a nurse with specialized training in ostomy management.
- Before ostomy surgery, assess the patient's expectations, understanding of the procedure, information desired, and fears.
- Intestinal ostomies include the ileostomy, the continent ileostomy, the ileoanal reservoir, and the colostomy.
- The characteristics of fecal material depend on the location of the ostomy, with liquid stool draining from the ileum and softly formed stool from the descending colon.
- The new intestinal stoma should be beefy red, and a small amount of bleeding around the base is not unusual.
- Postoperative nursing care after intestinal ostomy surgery addresses deficient fluid volume, impaired skin integrity, disturbed body image, sexual dysfunction, and ineffective management of therapeutic regimen.
- Protective barriers are applied around the stoma to fill creases and create a seal, and a pouch is secured over the stoma with adhesive to collect fecal drainage.
- Elimination of gas-forming foods and good hygiene can help control odor associated with an intestinal ostomy.
- The continent pouch ileostomy and the ileoanal reservoir both store fecal matter, but the continent ileostomy is drained periodically with a catheter whereas the ileoanal reservoir allows fecal elimination through the rectum.
- Routine colostomy irrigations are no longer recommended.
- The most common types of urinary diversion are cutaneous ureterostomy, ileal conduit, colonic conduit, and continent internal reservoirs.
- A urinary stoma is pink immediately after surgery but quickly fades to a light color.
- Ureterostomies and ileal conduits drain urine continuously, so collection pouches are needed and meticulous skin care must be provided.
- A continent internal reservoir allows for storage and controlled drainage of urine.
- Complications of urinary stomas include urinary infections, obstruction of urine flow, and skin breakdown.

REVIEW QUESTIONS

1. An example of a surgically created opening that drains fecal matter from the intestines is a/an:
   1. gastrostomy.
   2. ileostomy.
   3. ileal conduit.
   4. vesicostomy.
2. Which of the intestinal ostomy sites will produce the most formed stool?
   1. Jejunostomy
   2. Duodenostomy
   3. Ileostomy
   4. Colostomy
3. The nurse is assessing a new intestinal stoma on the first postoperative day. The stoma should be:
   1. beefy red.
   2. rose red.
   3. pale pink.
   4. white.
4. What is the main reason that a patient with an ileostomy is at risk for fluid and electrolyte imbalances?
   1. There is a significant loss of blood during the surgical procedure.
   2. Patients with ileostomies often have anorexia, nausea, and vomiting.
   3. Fluid normally reabsorbed in the colon is lost through the ileostomy.
   4. Fluid intake will be restricted until the stoma heals completely.
5. Aspects of stoma care include:
   1. Remove the drainage appliance daily to cleanse skin around the stoma.
   2. Wash the stoma and surrounding skin with a moisturizing soap.
   3. Vigorously rub the skin surrounding the stoma to stimulate circulation and healing.
   4. Cut the opening on the wafer no more than ⅛ inch larger than the stoma.
6. When teaching a new colostomy patient how to control odor, the nurse provides list of foods that commonly cause gas. The patient says, "You mean I can't eat any of these foods?" The most appropriate reply is:
   1. Gradually try one at a time to see how you tolerate them.
   2. That is correct. You can never eat any of these foods again.
   3. Since flatus production is unpredictable, you never know what will happen if you eat these foods.
   4. It would be better if you took vitamins instead of eating fresh fruits and vegetables.
7. A good strategy for helping patients adjust to a stoma and learn how to do self-care is to:
   1. shield the stoma from the patient's sight until he/she asks to see it.
   2. tell the patient "If you don't do your stoma care, no one will do it for you."
   3. encourage patients to participate in care once they start looking at the stoma.
   4. teach a family member how to do the care in the presence of the patient.
8. In a patient with a new continent ileostomy, which assessment finding most suggests an obstruction?
   1. Bloody drainage from the catheter in the stoma
   2. Patient complaint of pain in the incision area
   3. Absence of drainage from the stoma catheter
   4. Abdominal distention and hypoactive bowel sounds
9. Which type of urinary diversion does not require the patient to wear a pouch?
   1. Cutaneous ureterostomy
   2. Ileal conduit
   3. Kock pouch
   4. Ureteroileostomy
10. The main advantage of the ileum neobladder is that:
    1. the patient does not have a stoma for urine drainage.
    2. urinary continence is always maintained.
    3. urine is eliminated through the rectum.
    4. the neobladder only has to be drained once a day.

UNIT SIX NEUROLOGIC DISORDERS

CHAPTER 26 Neurologic Disorders

LESLIE GODDARD

objectives

1. Identify common neurologic changes in the older person and the implication of these for nursing care.
2. Describe the diagnostic tests and procedures used to evaluate neurologic dysfunction and the nursing responsibilities associated with each.
3. Identify the uses, side effects, and nursing interventions associated with common drug therapies employed in patients with neurologic disorders.
4. Describe the signs and symptoms associated with increased intracranial pressure and the medical therapies used in treatment.
5. List the components of the nursing assessment of the patient with a neurologic disorder.
6. Describe the pathophysiology, signs and symptoms, complications, and medical or surgical treatment for patients with selected neurologic disorders.
7. Assist in developing a nursing care plan for the patient with a neurologic disorder.

key terms

Aura (ĂW-ră, p. 387)
Automation (ăw-TŎM-ăh-shŭn, p. 386)
Contralateral (kŏn-tră-LĂT-ĕr-ăl, p. 376)
Decerebrate (dē-SĔR-ĕ-brāt, p. 383)
Decorticate (dē-KŎR-tĭ-kāt, p. 383)
Encephalitis (ĕn-sĕf-ă-LĪ-tĭs, p. 393)
Hemiparesis (hĕm-ē-pă-RĒ-sĭs, p. 382)
Hemiplegia (hĕm-ē-PLĒ-jă, p. 382)
Intracranial (ĭn-trăh-KRĀ-nē-ăl, p. 371)
Ipsilateral (ĭp-sĭ-LĂT-ĕr-ăl, p. 376)
Neuralgia (nū-RĂL-jă, p. 404)
Neurotransmitter (nū-rō-trăns-MĬ-tĕr, p. 365)
Paresthesia (păr-ĕs-THĒ-zē-ă, p. 394)
Postictal (PŌST-ĭk-tĕl, p. 386)
Seizure (SĒ-zhŭr, p. 385)

Neurologic disease and injury present some of the greatest challenges in health care today. Nurses face the challenge of caring for neurologic patients during the acute and rehabilitation phases of recovery from injuries and diseases. The long-term effects of many neurologic disorders are frequently devastating to both the patient and the family. An important aspect of care is assisting the patient and family to adjust physically and emotionally to the alterations that often result from neurologic dysfunction.

ANATOMY AND PHYSIOLOGY OF THE NERVOUS SYSTEM

In this age of computers, it may be helpful to think of the nervous system as an elaborate control system. The system coordinates and regulates all bodily functions. It receives and interprets information from the external environment and initiates responses to the received information.

The functional unit of the nervous system is the neuron (nerve cell), which conducts electrical impulses from one area of the brain to another. The main cell body has branches called axons and dendrites (Fig. 26-1). Axons conduct impulses away from the cell body and dendrites convey impulses toward the cell body. Many axons and dendrites are covered with a material called myelin, which enhances conduction along nerve fibers. Myelin gives the axons a white appearance (white matter), whereas cell bodies without myelin are gray (gray matter).

Neurons are classified according to their particular functions. Those that transmit information from distal parts of the body or environment toward the central nervous system (CNS) are sensory neurons, also known as afferent ("bearing toward") neurons. Motor information is carried from the CNS to the periphery by motor neurons, also known as efferent ("bearing away from") neurons. There are interneurons, which are like relay stations between sensory and motor neurons.

Coordinated, organized function is a result of a well-integrated system of impulse transmission. When the end of a dendrite is stimulated, a series of electrochemical events is initiated. At the point of stimulation, sodium and potassium ions are exchanged, resulting in a process called depolarization. This process continues down the dendrite to the axon, until the ions return to their resting state. This return to the resting state is known as repolarization.

Impulses must be able to pass from one neuron to another across the neural synapse—the space between the axons of one neuron and the dendrites of the next neuron. When an impulse reaches the end of its axon, a biochemical messenger called a **neurotransmitter** is released. Common neurotransmitters are

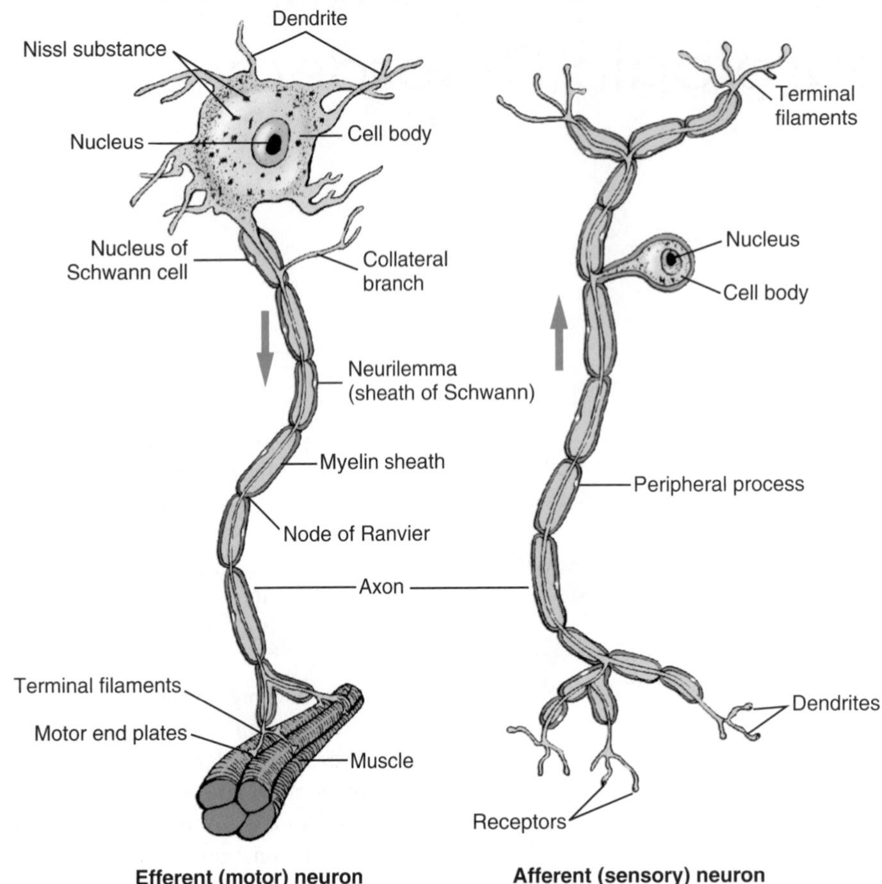

FIGURE **26-1** A neuron (nerve cell). The dendrites receive incoming messages. The axons convey outgoing signals. Diagram of a motor neuron and a sensory neuron. *Arrows* indicate the direction of impulse conduction.

table 26-1 ***Functions of the Major Parts of the Brain***

BRAIN STEM AND DIENCEPHALON

Controls awareness or alertness through reticular activating system, composed of fibers scattered throughout the midbrain, pons, and medulla.

MEDULLA

Links higher brain centers to other parts of the body through spinal cord. Controls muscles of respiration through respiratory reflex center. Controls heartbeat (to some extent) through cardiac reflex center. Constricts blood vessels to raise blood pressure through vasomotor reflex center. Is point of origin for some cranial nerves.

PONS

Relays messages from medulla to higher centers in brain. Is reflex center for some cranial nerves.

CEREBELLUM

Coordinates movement, balance, posture, and spatial orientation.

HYPOTHALAMUS

Controls pituitary. Controls appetite, sleep, and some emotions. Controls much activity of autonomic nervous system.

FOREBRAIN (CEREBRUM)

Controls higher functions and activities: conscious mental processes, sensations, emotions, and voluntary movements.

FRONTAL LOBE

Controls voluntary muscle movements, verbal and written speech.

PARIETAL LOBE

Contains sensory reception areas to interpret pain, touch, temperature, distances, sizes, and shapes.

TEMPORAL LOBE

Contains auditory center for hearing and understanding spoken language. Contains olfactory center for smell.

OCCIPITAL LOBE

Contains visual center for seeing and reading.

Data from Jacob, S. W., & Francone, C. A. (1989). *Elements of anatomy and physiology* (2nd ed.). Philadelphia: Saunders.

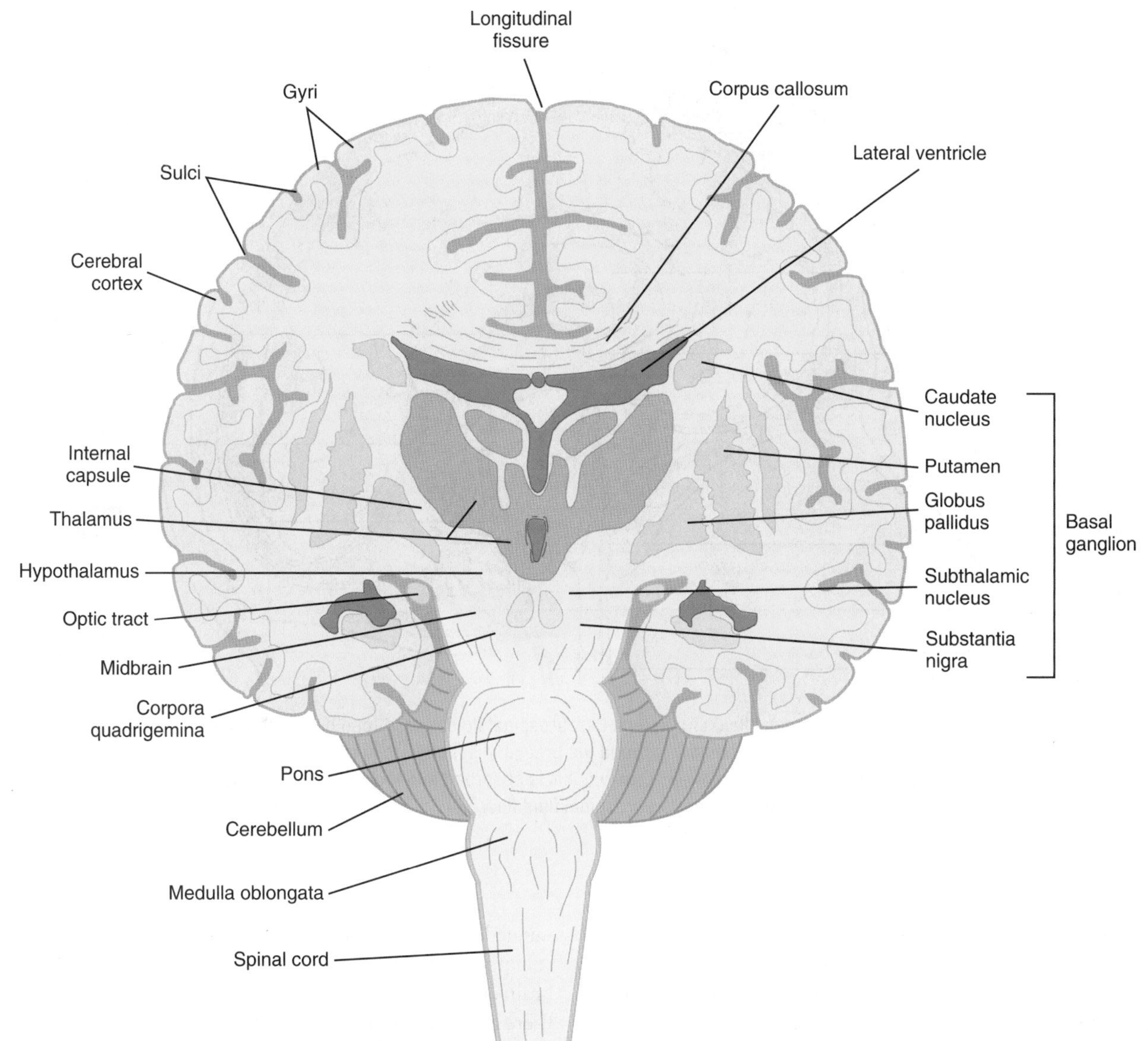

FIGURE **26-2** Structures of the brain (coronal section).

acetylcholine, norepinephrine, epinephrine, and dopamine. The neurotransmitter crosses the synapse to the neighboring dendrite, where it stimulates an electrical impulse. The process of depolarization then continues down the length of the nerve cells.

Structurally, the nervous system is divided into two main parts: (1) the central nervous system (CNS), made up of the brain and spinal cord, and (2) the peripheral nervous system, which comprises all the nerves of the peripheral parts of the body. The brain is divided into the cerebrum, cerebellum, and brain stem (Fig. 26-2). The cerebrum is composed of left and right hemispheres, which are subdivided into specific lobes. The thalamus, hypothalamus, and basal ganglia are other important structures identified in the cerebrum. Table 26-1 lists the functions of the major parts of the brain.

Cerebrospinal fluid (CSF) is composed primarily of water, glucose, sodium chloride, and protein. It is produced in the ventricles of the brain in the arachnoid granulations. CSF circulates within the subarachnoid space, the ventricles, and the central canal of the spinal cord (Fig. 26-3). The fluid is reabsorbed in the arachnoid villi. The CSF acts as a shock absorber for the brain and spinal cord. If excess fluid forms or if fluid is not normally reabsorbed, pressure within the ventricular system increases.

The spinal cord extends from the border of the first cervical vertebra (C1) to the level of the second lumbar vertebra (L2). Thirty-one pairs of spinal nerve roots exit from the spinal cord, each consisting of a posterior sensory (afferent) root and anterior motor (efferent) root (Fig. 26-4). These nerve roots, along with the 12 cranial nerves, make up the peripheral nervous system.

Part of the peripheral nervous system, known as the autonomic nervous system, helps to maintain homeostasis for the body. The autonomic nervous system controls the involuntary

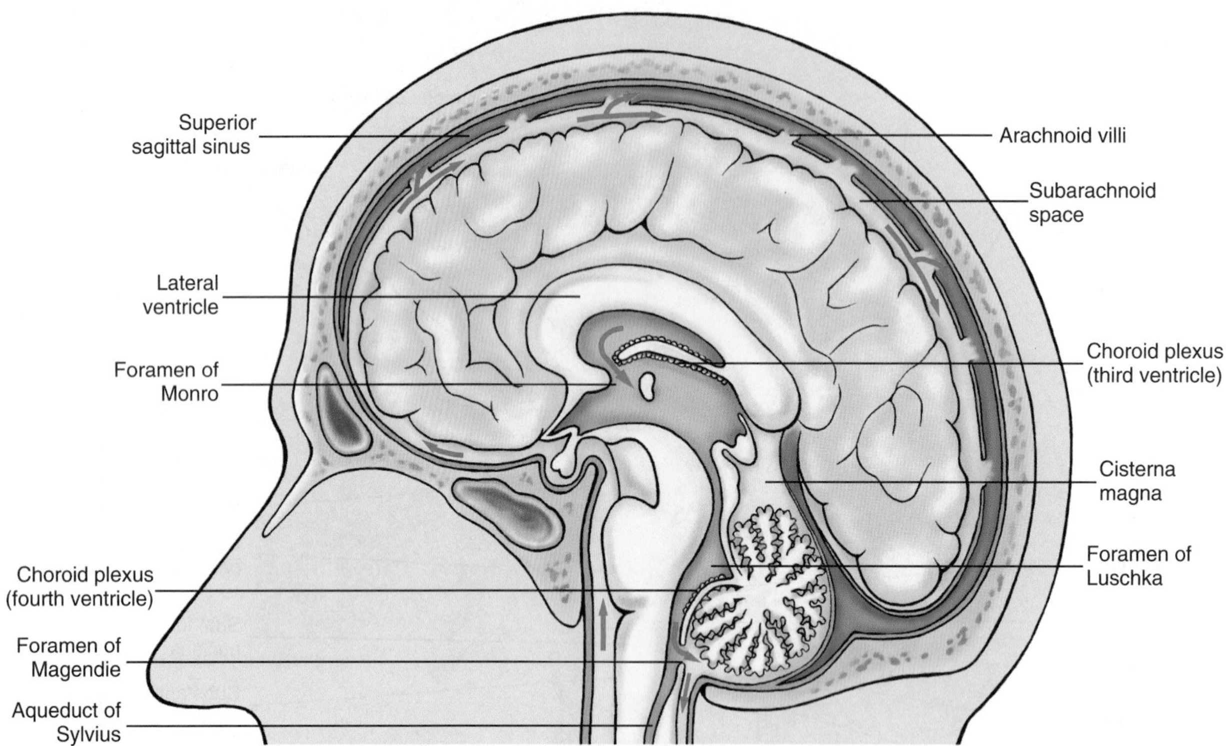

FIGURE **26-3** Cerebro spinal fluid circulation. Cerebrospinal fluid is produced by the choroid plexus in the lateral ventricles and flows around the brain and spinal cord in the subarachnoid space until it reaches the arachnoid villi, from which it is absorbed into the venous circulation. *Arrows* indicate the major pathway of cerebrospinal fluid flow.

activities of the viscera, including smooth muscles, cardiac muscle, and glands. The two major subdivisions of the autonomic nervous system are the sympathetic nervous system and the parasympathetic nervous system.

The sympathetic nervous system is activated by stress to increase the secretion of epinephrine and norepinephrine. These neurotransmitters increase the heart rate and constrict peripheral blood vessels, causing the blood pressure to rise. This reaction to stress is called the "fight or flight" response. The sympathetic nervous system is also referred to as the thoracolumbar system.

Conversely, the parasympathetic nervous system mediates a rest response. Stimulation of this system results in decreased heart rate and blood pressure. The parasympathetic nervous system is also known as the craniosacral system. Specific effects of the stimulation of the sympathetic and parasympathetic nervous systems are outlined in Table 26-2.

AGE-RELATED CHANGES

With normal aging, the number of nerve cells decreases. Brain weight is reduced, and the ventricles increase in size. An aging pigment called *lipofuscin* is deposited in nerve cells along with amyloid, a type of protein. Increased plaques and tangled fibers are found in nerve tissue. These changes are associated with Alzheimer's disease but are also seen in the brains of people without evidence of dementia. Fortunately, there are many more nerve cells present than are needed for normal function. Therefore, most older people retain normal cognition and behavior despite the decreasing number of nerve cells.

The physical examination reveals some neurologic changes typical of aging. The pupil of the eye is often smaller and may respond to light more slowly. When asked to track (follow with the eyes) a moving object, the older person's eye movements may be jerky rather than smooth. Reflexes are usually intact except for the Achilles tendon jerk, which is often absent.

Older people often demonstrate some changes in functional abilities as well. Reaction time increases with aging, especially for complex reactions. Tremors in the head, face, and hands are common. Some older people develop dizziness and problems with balance, but these are not considered normal age-related changes.

Put on your THINKING CAP!!

Identify three implications for nursing care related to normal neurologic changes that occur with age.

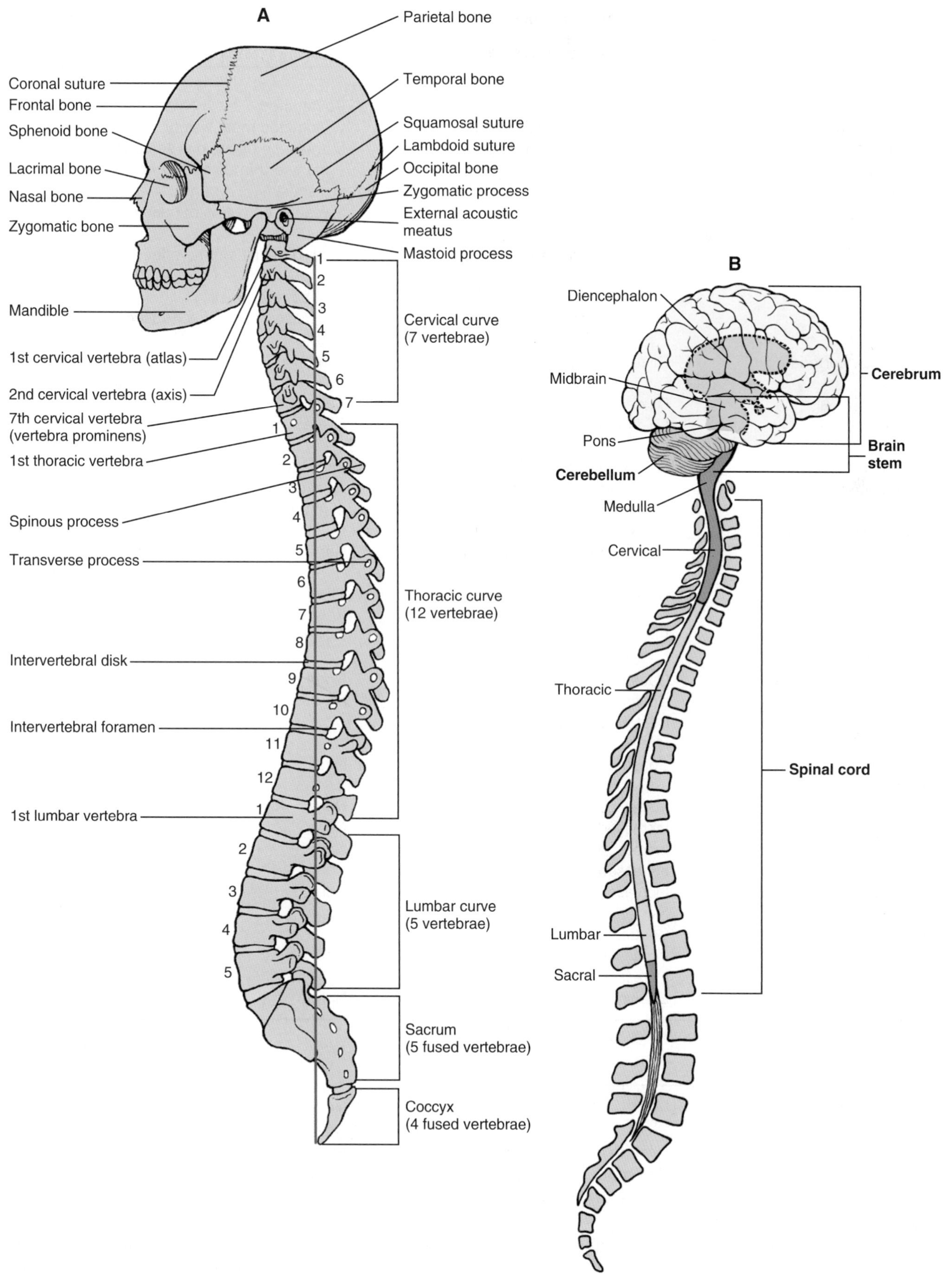

FIGURE 26-4 *A,* Bony structure of the skull and vertebral column. *B,* Lateral view of the central nervous system, showing its main divisions.

table 26-2 ***Effects of Sympathetic and Parasympathetic Stimulation***

ORGAN	EFFECT OF SYMPATHETIC STIMULATION	EFFECT OF PARASYMPATHETIC STIMULATION
Eye		
Pupil	Dilated	Constricted
Ciliary muscle	Slight relaxation (far vision)	Constricted (near vision)
Glands: nasal, lacrimal, parotid secretion, submandibular, gastric, pancreatic	Vasoconstriction and slight secretion	Stimulation of copious secretion (containing many enzymes for enzyme-secreting glands)
Sweat glands	Copious sweating (cholinergic)	Sweating on palms of hands
Apocrine glands	Thick, odoriferous secretion	None
Blood vessels	Mostly constricted	Most often little or no effect
Heart		
Muscle	Increased rate Increased force of contraction	Slowed rate Decreased force of contractions (especially atria)
Coronary arteries	Dilated ($beta_2$), constricted (alpha)	Dilated
Lungs		
Bronchi	Dilated	Constricted
Blood vessels	Mildly constricted	Dilated
Gut		
Lumen	Decreased peristalsis and tone	Increased peristalsis and tone
Sphincter	Increased tone (most times)	Relaxed (most times)
Liver	Glucose released	Slight glycogen synthesis
Gallbladder and bile ducts	Relaxed	Contracted
Kidney	Decreased output and renin secretion	None
Bladder		
Detrusor	Relaxed (slight)	Contracted
Trigone	Contracted	Relaxed
Penis	Ejaculation	Erection
Systemic arterioles		
Abdominal viscera	Constricted	None
Muscle	Constricted (alpha adrenergic) Dilated ($beta_2$ adrenergic) Dilated (cholinergic)	None
Skin	Constricted	None
Blood		
Coagulation	Increased	None
Glucose	Increased	None
Lipids	Increased	None
Basal metabolism	Increased up to 100%	None
Adrenal medullary secretions	Increased	None
Mental activity	Increased	None
Piloerector muscles	Contracted	None
Skeletal muscle	Increased glycogenolysis Increased strength	None
Fat cells	Lipolysis	None

From Guyton, A. C., and Hall, J. E. (1996). *Textbook of medical physiology* (9th ed., p. 775). Philadelphia: Saunders.

PATHOPHYSIOLOGY OF NEUROLOGIC DISEASES

Potential causes of neurologic disorders include developmental and genetic disorders, trauma, infections and inflammation, neoplasms, degenerative processes, vascular disorders, and metabolic and endocrine disorders.

Developmental and genetic disorders. Developmental disorders include structural problems such as hydrocephalus. An example of a genetic disorder is Huntington's disease.

Trauma. Central nervous system injuries resulting from trauma can be life-threatening or severely disabling. Physical trauma to the nervous system may follow accidental injury, violent crime, or chemical injury caused by drugs, alcohol, or other harmful substances.

Infections and inflammation. Meningitis and encephalitis are examples of disease states that cause inflammation of meningeal and brain tissue, respectively. Causative agents may be viruses or bacteria and may be transmitted by a variety of vectors and routes.

Neoplasms. Central nervous system tumors may be primary or metastatic in origin. Although considerable progress has been made in treating these tumors, definitive therapy is often difficult to achieve, depending on the cell type involved in the tumor and the degree of invasion of surrounding tissue.

Degenerative processes. The primary degenerative disease of the brain is Alzheimer's disease, a progressive condition that begins with memory loss and eventually results in severe mental and physical deterioration. Alzheimer's disease is discussed in Chapter 21. Other degenerative disorders are multiple sclerosis, Parkinson's syndrome, amyotrophic lateral sclerosis, and Huntington's disease.

Vascular disorders. Any factor that interferes with blood flow to nervous tissue can lead to cell death, with resulting loss of function. Nerve tissue is so sensitive to hypoxia that cells begin to die after being deprived of oxygen for 4 minutes. Neurologic disorders associated with impaired blood flow include cerebrovascular accident (see Chapter 27) and multi-infarct dementia. Vascular abnormalities, including aneurysms and arteriovenous malformations, can rupture or they can prevent the delivery of adequate oxygen to affected tissue.

Metabolic and endocrine disorders. The brain is dependent on constant supplies of glucose and other nutrients. Disturbances in glucose metabolism and electrolyte imbalances can lead to deterioration in thought processes and level of consciousness. Neurologic dysfunction can also result from accumulation of toxins, as in poisoning, renal failure, and liver failure.

NURSING ASSESSMENT OF NEUROLOGIC FUNCTION

A number of diagnostic tests may be done to evaluate and diagnose neurologic problems. However, any evaluation begins with an accurate assessment, which may be initiated by the nurse. Much of the assessment requires simply observing the patient and then recording the findings.

Health History

The general nursing assessment of the patient with a neurologic disorder is described here. Throughout the assessment, note the patient's speech, behavior, coordination, alertness, and comprehension. More sophisticated assessments are discussed in the section on diagnostic tests and procedures.

Chief Complaint and History of Present Illness

An initial portion of the neurologic assessment includes an investigation of the health history of the patient, particularly as it relates to the chief complaint. Document the event that prompted the patient to seek medical attention. Describe any injuries. If the patient has pain, note the onset, severity, location, and duration.

Past Medical History

Past neurologic disorders and pertinent signs and symptoms are vital pieces of information. Ask about a history of head injury, seizures, diabetes mellitus, hypertension, heart disease, and cancer. Record dates and types of immunizations, including influenza. List current medications. Record current drugs and highlight allergies according to agency policy.

> **PHARMACOLOGY CAPSULE** Many drugs stimulate or depress the CNS.

Family History

Questions about the presence of neurologic disease or other diseases in the immediate family may elicit valuable information about risk factors, such as those for stroke or neuromuscular diseases. Therefore, ask whether any immediate family members have had heart disease, stroke, diabetes mellitus, cancer, seizure disorders, muscular dystrophy, or Huntington's disease.

Review of Systems

Important signs and symptoms to be collected in reviewing the system are fatigue or weakness, headache, dizziness, vertigo, changes in vision or hearing, tinnitus, drainage from the ears or nose, dysphagia, neck pain or stiffness, vomiting, problems with bladder or bowel function, sexual dysfunction, fainting, blackouts, tremors, paralysis, uncoordination, numbness or tingling, memory problems, and mood changes.

Functional Assessment

Document whether present symptoms interfere with the patient's usual activities and occupation. Explore sources of stress, usual coping strategies, and sources of support.

Physical Examination

A complete physical examination, including the neurologic examination, should be done when the patient is stable. A neurologic assessment provides baseline data to compare with ongoing assessments and serves as the basis for developing the nursing care plan. Four major components of a routine neurologic examination that provide valuable information regarding the overall integrity of the CNS are level of consciousness, pupillary evaluation, neuromuscular response, and vital signs. You must look at the trends in the patient's neurologic status. A single finding considered in isolation may not provide a true picture of the patient's status. For example, one elevated blood pressure reading may not be significant, but continuing increases may be associated with increased intracranial pressure (ICP).

Basic Neurologic Examination

Level of consciousness. The most accurate and reliable indicator of neurologic status is level of consciousness. Evaluate patients for orientation to person, place, and time by asking them to state their names, where they are, and what time it is. It is important to consider the degree of stimulation required to evoke a response from the patient. If the patient responds only to vigorous physical stimulation, then consciousness is more impaired than if the patient immediately responds to a verbal greeting. Consider patient behavior in response to stimulation. Does the patient respond pleasantly, or is he or she combative, agitated, or lethargic? All these observations provide additional information regarding mental status.

Some of the common terms used to describe altered levels of consciousness are somnolence, lethargy, stupor, semicoma, and coma. Somnolence is unnatural drowsiness or sleepiness. Lethargy also is used to describe excessive drowsiness. Stupor suggests decreased responsiveness accompanied by lack of spontaneous motor activity. If a patient is in a stupor (stuporous) but can be aroused, the term *semicomatose* is used. A patient who cannot be aroused even by powerful stimuli is said to be in a coma, or comatose.

Because the above terms related to altered levels of consciousness are open to interpretation, it is clearer to describe the patient's response to specific stimuli. Always begin with the mildest stimuli and stop when a response is elicited. The mildest stimulus is simply approaching the patient. This can be followed in order with verbal stimuli, tactile stimuli (shaking the shoulder gently), and finally with painful stimuli. Appropriate methods of applying painful stimuli include applying pressure on the nail bed using an object such as a pen or pinching the trapezius muscle firmly between the thumb and forefinger and twisting.

Pupillary evaluation. The second major component of the neurologic assessment is the pupillary evaluation. To evaluate the pupils, assess and compare their size, shape, and reactivity. Pupils are normally about 3 mm in size, round, and react briskly to light. Changes in equality or reactivity from one assessment to the next may indicate neurologic deterioration.

Neuromuscular response. Assessment of neuromuscular response provides a means of evaluating cerebral and spinal cord function. All electrical impulses responsible for eliciting motor responses are initiated in the frontal lobe of the cerebral cortex. The impulses travel down the brain stem into the spinal cord. Motor spinal nerve roots then stimulate muscle movement. Additional techniques for assessing specific neuromuscular responses can be found in Table 28-6.

Vital signs. Monitoring pulse, respirations, and blood pressure provides highly reliable information regarding neurologic well-being. However, changes in vital signs are late indicators of deterioration. The significance of these values is discussed in detail in the section on increased ICP. Elevated temperature may be associated with infection or with impaired thermoregulation.

General Physical Examination

Once the neurologic assessment is done, complete the remaining physical examination. If possible, measure height and weight. Throughout the examination, inspect the skin for lesions and color change, and palpate for temperature. Assess hydration status by evaluating tissue turgor and moisture of mucous membranes. Inspect the head for lesions and palpate for masses or swelling. Observe respiratory effort, and auscultate breath sounds. Inspect the abdomen, auscultate bowel sounds, and palpate for bowel and bladder distention. Inspect the extremities for injuries or abnormal positions. Assessment of motor and sensory function is detailed in Chapter 28.

Assessment of the patient with a neurologic disorder is summarized in Table 26-3.

table 26-3 ASSESSMENT *of the Patient with a Neurologic Disorder*

HEALTH HISTORY

Chief Complaint and History of Present Illness: Event requiring medical attention
Past Medical History: Head injury, seizures, other neurologic disorders, other diseases (diabetes mellitus, hypertension, heart disease, cancer), dates of immunizations, current medications, allergies
Family History: Stroke, neuromuscular diseases, heart disease, diabetes mellitus, cancer, seizures
Review of Systems: Fatigue, weakness, headache, dizziness, vertigo, changes in vision or hearing, tinnitus, drainage from nose or ears, dysphagia, neck pain or stiffness, vomiting, bladder or bowel dysfunction, fainting, blackouts, tremors, paralysis, uncoordination, numbness or tingling, memory problems, mood changes
Functional Assessment: Usual occupation and activities, impact on life, changes in sexuality, changes in activities of daily living, sources of stress, usual coping strategies, sources of support

PHYSICAL EXAMINATION

Level of Consciousness: Response to stimulation
Pupils: Size, shape, response to light, equality
Neuromuscular Status: Voluntary movement, reflexes
Vital Signs: Blood pressure, pulse, respirations, temperature
When stable:
Height and Weight
Skin: Lesions, injuries, turgor
Head: Lesions, injuries, masses, swelling
Oral Cavity: Moisture
Thorax: Respiratory effort, breath sounds
Abdomen: Distention, bowel sounds
Extremities: Injuries, abnormal positions

DIAGNOSTIC TESTS AND PROCEDURES

Once an initial evaluation and history have been obtained, more detailed diagnostic tests and procedures are often indicated. Table 26-4 summarizes the information that may be obtained from diagnostic tests and procedures.

Advanced Neurologic Examination

Baseline and serial examinations are critical in the evaluation of the patient with a neurologic disorder. Cranial nerve function, coordination and balance, neuromuscular function, and reflexes are those components that can assist the practitioner in localizing the area of injury or disease and in developing a plan of care relevant to the individual patient. Figure 26-5 shows a flow sheet used to record the findings on periodic neurologic assessments.

Cranial Nerves

Various motor and sensory functions are mediated by the cranial nerves. The cranial nerves enter and exit the brain

table 26-4 **DIAGNOSTIC TESTS AND PROCEDURES | *Neurologic Disorders***

TEST/PURPOSE	PATIENT PREPARATION	POSTPROCEDURE NURSING CARE
LUMBAR PUNCTURE		
Used to diagnose infections and other CNS disorders. CSF pressure is measured. A CSF sample is taken for analysis	Informed consent is required. Tell the patient a fluid sample will be taken from the spinal column. Have the patient void to reduce the discomfort of a full bladder. Support the patient on one side in a knee-to-chest position during the procedure (Fig. 26-8).	The risk of headache may be reduced by lying flat for a specific period after the procedure. Encourage oral fluids. Assess for numbness, tingling, or pain in the extremities, CSF or bleeding from the puncture site, and changes in vital signs. Promptly deliver labeled specimens to the lab. The puncture site is covered with a small bandage
ELECTROENCEPHALOGRAPHY (EEG)		
Used to detect seizure activity by monitoring electrical activity in the brain.	Explain that electrodes will be applied to the scalp; patient will not feel any electrical shocks. Shampoo hair before EEG. Withhold medications (anticonvulsants, sedatives, stimulants, tranquilizers) and caffeine, for up to 48 hr before EEG as ordered.	Help patient shampoo hair to remove electrode paste.
ELECTROMYOGRAPHY (EMG)		
Useful in diagnosing neuromuscular abnormalities such as ALS, peripheral neuropathy, myasthenia gravis, and carpal tunnel syndrome.	Signed consent is required. Tell patient procedure takes 1-2 hrs. No caffeine or smoking for 3 hrs before EMG.	Inspect the sites of needle electrode placement. Patient may be instructed to return within 5 days to have blood drawn for enzyme tests (AST, CK, LD).
IMAGING STUDIES		
Brain Scan		
Depicts pattern of distribution of a radioactive isotope that has been injected IV. Used to diagnose brain abscesses, tumors, contusions, vascular occlusions or hemorrhage, and hematomas.	Informed consent required. Contraindicated during pregnancy. KCl is given several hrs before the procedure. Tell patient that scan is painless, and that radiation exposure is minimal. An isotope will be injected and the patient will lie on a stretcher while the scanner moves over the head. The scan will be repeated an hour later.	Encourage oral fluids to promote elimination of the isotope.
Cerebral Angiography		
Uses computer-based images taken after injection of contrast media to assess abnormalities in cerebral, carotid, and vertebral blood vessels.	Informed consent required. Inform radiologist if allergic to contrast media, shellfish, or iodine. Remove any metal from head area. Tell patient a "dye" will be injected and radiographs taken as the patient lies on a stretcher. When media is injected, patient may feel flushed, warm, nauseated, and report a salty taste.	Apply pressure to puncture site, and monitor for bleeding. Bedrest may be ordered for specified period. Extremity used to inject contrast media; may be immobilized for a specified period of time; assess circulation and neurologic function. Allergic response to contrast medium causes hives, nausea, swollen salivary glands. Treat with antihistamines as ordered.

CNS, Central nervous system; *CSF,* cerebrospinal fluid; *ALS,* amyotrophic lateral sclerosis; *AST,* aspartate aminotransferase; *CK,* creatine kinase; *LD,* lactic dehydrogenase; *KCl,* potassium chloride; *IV,* intravenously; *NPO,* nothing by mouth.

Continued

table 26-4 **DIAGNOSTIC TESTS AND PROCEDURES | *Neurologic Disorders—cont'd***

TEST/PURPOSE	PATIENT PREPARATION	POSTPROCEDURE NURSING CARE
IMAGING STUDIES—cont'd		
Computed Tomography (CT)		
Shows intracranial structures. Used to diagnose tumors, inflammation, edema, hematomas, and infarctions. Distinguishes normal from clotted blood. May be done along with angiography.	Patient may be NPO 4-8 hrs before scan if contrast medium is planned; can take prescribed meds and diabetic diet. Patient must lie still on a stretcher that fits into a donut-shaped frame that moves around the head. A mechanical sound can be heard. Procedure is painless and takes 15-20 minutes. Give sedatives as ordered for patients who cannot stay still.	No special aftercare needed. Observe patient who receives contrast for a delayed allergic reaction.
MAGNETIC RESONANCE IMAGING (MRI)		
Magnetic Resonance Angiogram (MRA)		
Creates images of intracranial structures without radiation.	Tell patient he or she will lie on a stretcher that passes into a tubular structure. Loud drumming noises will be heard while imager is in use. No special preparation is required. Sedation may be ordered for confused patients or those who are claustrophobic. Open MRI may be available for claustrophobic patients. Patients with some metal implants cannot be exposed to MRI because magnet can cause metal to move in the body. Special oxygen equipment, ventilators, and infusion pumps must be used.	No special aftercare needed.
Pneumoencephalography		
Uses injected gas by lumbar puncture and radiography to provide outline of the cerebral ventricles and cisterns. Used to diagnose masses, congenital abnormalities, cysts, and atrophy of cerebral and cerebellar cortex.	Informed consent required. Remove metal objects from head area. Support patient during lumbar puncture.	Perform neurologic checks per agency protocol. Keep patient flat and log-roll for up to 48 hrs as ordered. Inspect puncture site for CSF leakage or bleeding. Encourage oral fluids if permitted.
BLOOD FLOW STUDIES		
Doppler Flow		
Uses ultrasound to assess carotid blood flow. Can be used with a duplex scanner to detect plaques in blood vessels.	Signed consent required. Inform patient that test is painless and not to smoke for 30 minutes before test. Patient will need to lie supine while instrument is moved over the neck area.	No special aftercare needed unless activity restrictions are ordered.

CNS, Central nervous system; *CSF*, cerebrospinal fluid; *ALS*, amyotrophic lateral sclerosis; *AST*, aspartate aminotransferase; *CK*, creatine kinase; *LD*, lactic dehydrogenase; *KCl*, potassium chloride; *IV*, intravenously; *NPO*, nothing by mouth.

MISSION HOSPITAL
REGIONAL MEDICAL CENTER

ADULT NEURO FLOW SHEET

		TIME	0700	0800	0900	1000	1100	1200	1300	1400	1500	1600	1700	1800	1900	2000	2100	2200	2300	2400	0100	0200	0300	0400	0500	0600
GLASGOW COMA SCALE		Eyes open																								
		Best motor																								
		Best verbal																								
		TOTAL																								
VOLUNTARY MOTOR	Right	Upper extremity																								
		Lower extremity																								
	Left	Upper extremity																								
		Lower extremity																								
CRANIAL NERVES	PUPILS Right	Size																								
		Reaction																								
	PUPILS Left	Size																								
		Reaction																								
	EOMS	Conjugate																								
		Disconjugate																								
		Tracking Right																								
		Left																								
	Blink reflex																									
	Gag reflex																									
	Facial symmetry																									
		TIME	0700	0800	0900	1000	1100	1200	1300	1400	1500	1600	1700	1800	1900	2000	2100	2200	2300	2400	0100	0200	0300	0400	0500	0600

KEY

MOTOR
5+ Normal power
4+ Weakness
3+ Anti-gravity
2+ Not anti-gravity
1+ Trace
0 No movement

Pupil Size
B = Brisk
S = Sluggish
A = Absent

2 mm 3 mm 4 mm 5 mm

6 mm 7 mm 8 mm

✓ = Present
O = Absent
S = Symmetrical
A = Asymmetrical

Date

Speech patterns: ____________________

Comments: ____________________

GLASGOW COMA SCALE		
Eyes Open	4	Spontaneously
	3	To verbal command
	2	To pain
	1	No response
Best Motor Response	6	Obeys command
	5	Localize pain
	4	Flexion to pain withdraw
	3	Flexion decorticate
	2	Extension to pain (decerebrate)
	1	No response to pain
Best Verbal Response	5	Oriented
	4	Confused
	3	Inappropriate words
	2	Incomprehensive sounds
	1	No response

Unit ____________________

R.N. signature ____________________ Shift: __________

R.N. signature ____________________ Shift: __________

R.N. signature ____________________ Shift: __________

Form: 408 5/92 **Adult Neuro Flow Sheet**

ADDRESSOGRAPH

FIGURE **26-5** A neuro flow sheet is used to record the assessment of neurologic function.

rather than the spinal cord. The primary function of the cranial nerve is to control sensory and motor activities of the head and neck, but the vagus nerve also affects cardiac, respiratory, gastric, and gallbladder function. Each nerve may be assessed individually by the examiner with advanced assessment skills.

Coordination and Balance

Both the cerebellum and the cerebral cortex influence coordination and balance. Cerebellar dysfunction creates loss of steady, balanced posture and gait on the ipsilateral side (same side) as the brain lesion. Lesions of the cortex, however, cause motor dysfunction on the contralateral side (opposite side) of the lesion.

Observation of routine activity, such as ambulation, feeding, or performing activities of daily living, can provide valuable information regarding coordination and balance. In the assessment of balance, ask the patient to walk 10 to 20 feet away from you, turn, and walk back toward you. Observe gait and arm swing. Then ask the patient to walk a straight line in a heel-to-toe fashion.

To perform Romberg's test, have the patient stand, with feet together and arms at sides. Instruct the patient to close the eyes and maintain that position. Stay close by in case the patient starts to fall. Normally, there will be only slight swaying.

To evaluate coordination of movements:

1. Ask the patient to pat his or her knees with the palms of the hands and then with the backs of the hands in a rapid, alternating pattern.
2. Hold up one of your fingers and instruct the patient to touch it with his or her index finger.
3. Ask the patient to touch his or her nose with the index finger, first with the eyes open and then with the eyes closed.
4. Ask the patient to run the heel of one foot down the shin of the other leg then repeat with the opposite heel.
5. Alternate tapping with the heel and then the toes of one foot and then the other foot.

Normally these responses are done smoothly and rapidly.

Neuromuscular Function

Evaluate individual muscle groups by assessing their size, tone, and strength. Upper arm strength is evaluated by having the patient squeeze your fingers. Put one finger on top of another so that a firm squeeze will not painfully press your knuckles together. You can also instruct the patient to lift each hand or to raise a finger on each hand. Another means of assessing upper arm strength is to have the patient extend both arms forward with the palms up. Ask the patient to close his or her eyes and maintain the position for 10 to 20 seconds. With normal strength, the arms remain steady. In the presence of a slight weakness, the weak arm will internally rotate and drift slightly downward. This is referred to as ulnar or motor drift.

To evaluate strength of the legs, position the patient supine and ask him or her to raise one leg at a time. The patient with normal strength can lift the leg 90 degrees. Test the strength of other muscles as indicated.

Sensory Function

There are many tests of sensory function, including evaluation of the patient's perception of pain, touch, temperature, vibration, position, and tactile discrimination. All sensory testing is done with the eyes closed. Apply various stimuli to the skin and ask the patient to identify the type of stimulus perceived.

Pain. Pain can be evaluated by using a wooden applicator that is broken to create a sharp point. This broken applicator is used as the "sharp" stimulus, whereas the cotton end is used as a "dull" control stimulus. Ask the patient to state whether sharp or dull sensations are felt. Recognition of sharp pricks indicates ability to perceive painful stimuli.

Temperature. Temperature perception can be tested by touching test tubes containing hot or cold water to the patient's skin and asking the patient to distinguish hot from cold.

Light touch. A wisp of cotton brushed against the skin is used to assess perception of light touch. Ask the patient to state when the sensation is felt.

Vibration. Strike a tuning fork and touch the base to a joint in the great toe or a finger. Ask the patient to report when the vibration is felt and when it stops. The examiner actually stops the tuning fork from vibrating. If the sensation is not perceived, repeat the test on a more proximal joint until the patient perceives it.

Position. Lightly hold the patient's great toe or a finger on the sides and move it up and down. Ask the patient to identify the direction of the movement.

Tactile discrimination. Tests for fine tactile discrimination include stereognosis, graphesthesia, and point location. In testing stereognosis, place a familiar object (paper clip, cotton ball) in the patient's hand and request identification. Graphesthesia tests the patient's ability to recognize a number or letter "written" on the palm with a dull object. To test point location, briefly touch the skin and ask the patient to touch the place where the sensation was felt.

Reflexes

A reflex is an unconscious, involuntary response that is entirely mediated at the level of the spinal cord, without input from higher brain centers. The knee jerk represents a simple reflex. When a stimulus is applied to the patella, the sensory root of the spinal nerve transmits the impulse to the spinal cord. At the cord, the impulse is relayed to the motor nerve root, which then elicits the knee jerk (Fig. 26-6). Other commonly tested reflexes are listed in Table 26-5.

Although these common reflexes are normal, others appear only with pathologic states. Babinski's reflex accompanies abnormalities in the motor pathways originating in the cerebral cortex. Assess for it by stroking the lateral side of the bottom of the foot and across the ball of the foot with a blunt object and observing the resulting movement of the toes. Normally, the toes curl downward. However, in the presence of cortical dysfunction, the big toe bends upward, and the other toes fan out. Figure 26-7 illustrates the response.

Lumbar Puncture

A lumbar puncture is an invasive procedure that is most often used to detect infections and other disorders of the CNS, tumors, and hydrocephalus. A local anesthetic agent is used to anesthetize the puncture site. Then a cannula is inserted into the subarachnoid space at the level of the third lumbar verte-

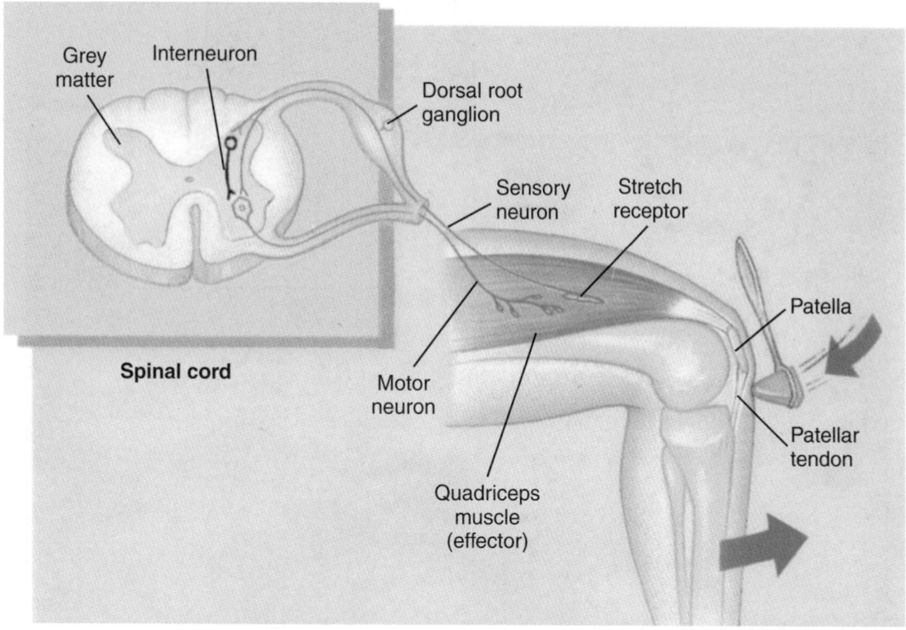

FIGURE **26-6** Reflexes are elicited by stimulating a sensory nerve, which conveys an impulse to the spinal cord. An impulse is then conveyed by a motor nerve to cause the muscle to contract.

table 26-5 ***Commonly Tested Reflexes***

REFLEX	EXPECTED RESPONSE
Biceps	Flexion of forearm
Triceps	Extension of forearm
Brachioradialis	Flexion and supination of forearm
Quadriceps	Extension of lower leg
Achilles (ankle jerk)	Plantar flexion of foot
Clonus	Repetitive movement after brisk dorsiflexion of foot

bra (Fig. 26-8). Entering at this level allows the physician to avoid traumatizing the spinal cord, which ends at the level of the second lumbar vertebra. Once the needle is in place, a sample of CSF is collected for laboratory analysis. CSF specimens are placed in test tubes and labeled, with the first specimen usually being discarded because it may contain blood from the puncture. Normal CSF has the following characteristics: pressure, 50 to 175 mm H_2O; pH, 7.30 to 7.40; clear, colorless appearance; fasting glucose, 40 to 80 mg/dL; WBC, 0 to 5 small lymphocytes/mm^3.

Injuries resulting from lumbar puncture are rare. However, some patients experience severe headaches resulting from a CSF leak. Leaks are sometimes treated with a blood patch, which is created by injecting a small amount of the patient's blood into the lumbar puncture site. The blood clots, sealing the puncture site and preventing further loss of CSF.

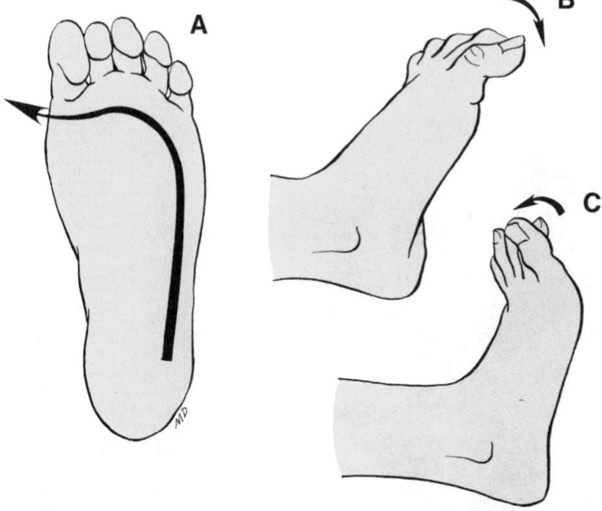

FIGURE **26-7** Babinski's reflex. *A,* The examiner scrapes the foot as shown using a blunt point. *B,* The normal response (absence of Babinski's response) is plantar flexion of the toes. *C,* An abnormal response (presence of Babinski's response) is characterized by dorsiflexion of the big toe and often fanning of the other toes.

Electroencephalography

The electroencephalogram (EEG) is a graphic representation of electrical activity in brain cells. Small electrodes are placed at various positions on the head to detect electrical signals generated from neurons located near the surface of the cerebral cortex. It is an excellent tool in the diagnosis of seizure activity (Fig. 26-9).

Some people have misconceptions about EEG. Assure the patient that no electrical shock will be experienced, that the examiner is not able to "read the patient's mind," and that the test is not done to detect mental illness. Fatigue stresses the brain and may evoke abnormal activity not usually seen on the EEG. Therefore, patients may be evaluated with a

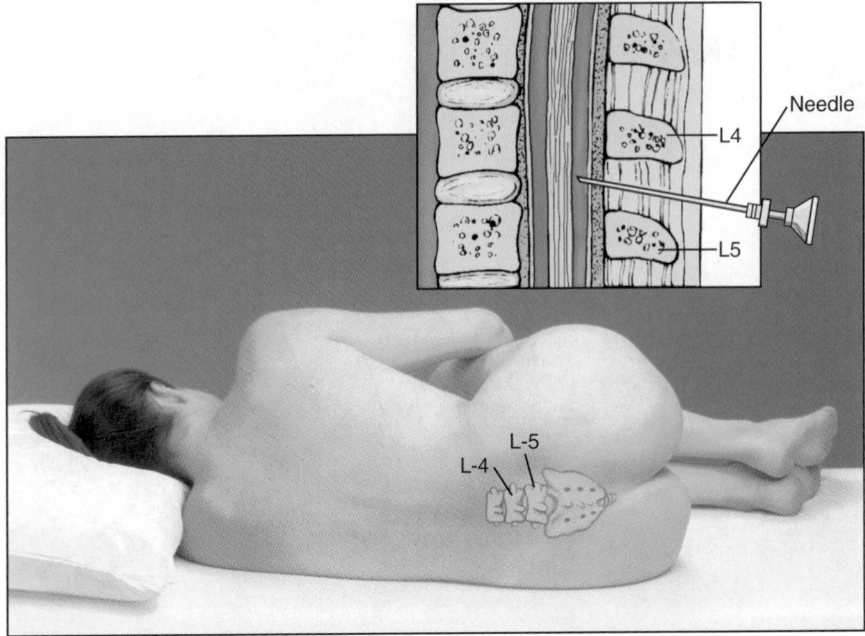

FIGURE 26-8 Lumbar puncture. With the patient in a flexed position to maximize the space between vertebrae, the lumbar puncture needle is inserted between L-4 and L-5 to gain entry to the subarachnoid space. During the actual procedure, the patient would be gowned and draped to protect privacy.

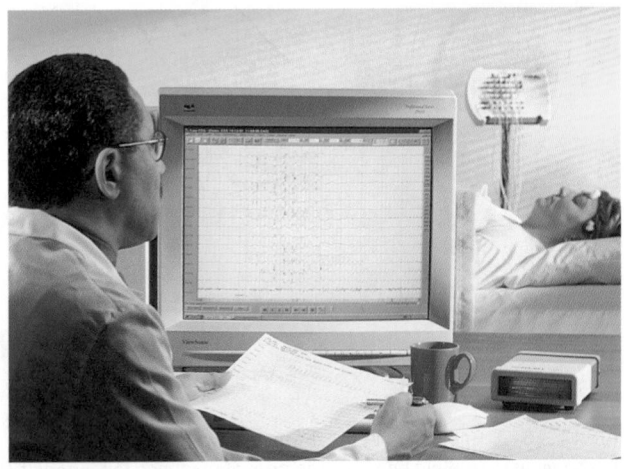

FIGURE 26-9 Client undergoing an electroencephalogram.

sleep-deprived EEG, in which they are awakened after a short sleep period in an effort to elicit such activity during the test.

Electromyography

Electromyography studies the response of peripheral motor and sensory nerves to electrical stimuli. Needle electrodes are placed on several points over a nerve and over the muscles supplied by the nerve. Stimuli are administered, and the effects are recorded on an oscilloscope.

Radiologic Studies

Brain Scan

The brain scan shows the pattern of distribution of a radioactive isotope injected intravenously. It is useful in detecting brain abscesses, tumors, contusions, vascular occlusion or hemorrhage, and hematomas. The patient is given potassium chloride 2 hours before the isotope is injected to prevent excessive isotope uptake. The isotope is given immediately before the scan is done. While the patient lies still on a stretcher, the scanner, which is somewhat like an x-ray machine, moves back and forth over the head. There is no sensation associated with the scanning process. The scan is repeated 1 hour later.

Cerebral Angiography and Digital Subtraction Angiography

Cerebral angiography provides images of the cerebral, carotid, and vertebral blood vessels. A catheter is inserted into an artery (usually femoral) and advanced to the carotid or vertebral arteries. A contrast dye is injected, and a series of radiographs is taken. Angiography is the most definitive diagnostic test in the diagnosis of cerebral aneurysm or congenital vascular disorders, such as arteriovenous malformation. Risks include severe allergy to contrast media, embolus, hematoma, hemorrhage, renal toxicity, transient ischemic attack, infection, and loss of consciousness. Digital subtraction angiography (DSA) is a complementary, computer-assisted radiographic procedure for visualization of cerebral vessels.

Computed Tomography

The evolution of computed tomography (CT) represents one of the most significant developments in neurologic diagnostic procedures. CT is an excellent tool in the evaluation of

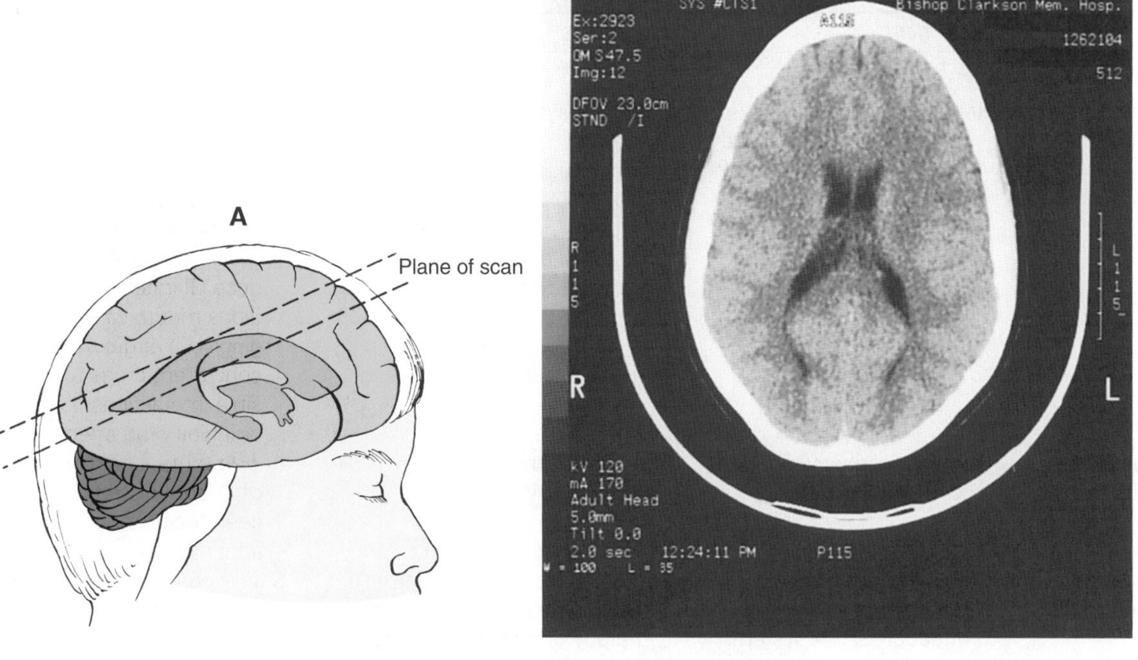

FIGURE **26-10** Computed tomography scans are taken at various cross-sections of the brain. The image in *A* illustrates the cross-section used for the scan shown in *B.*

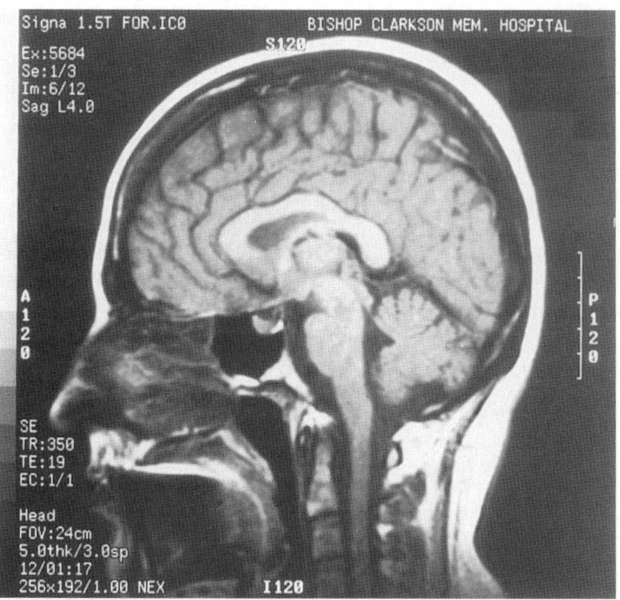

FIGURE **26-11** Magnetic resonance imaging uses magnetic fields to create cross-sectional views of the brain. This sagittal section shows the cerebrum, ventricles, cerebellum, and medulla.

trauma, tumors, and hemorrhage (Fig. 26-10). Enhancement of an area may be achieved by injecting contrast medium; therefore, any allergy to such media must be reported to the radiologist in advance. The entire scanning procedure lasts 15 to 20 minutes and generally requires no advance preparation or postprocedure care.

Magnetic Resonance Imaging

One of the latest tools in neuroradiology is magnetic resonance imaging (MRI). Unlike CT, MRI does not expose the patient to radiation. It is a noninvasive examination that involves placing the patient in a strong magnetic field and then applying bursts of radiofrequency waves. Sophisticated technology converts information about the movement of molecules in the tissue into precise, clear images (Fig. 26-11). Magnetic resonance angiography (MRA) is a special technique that allows the measurement of flow through blood vessels. Depending on the type of equipment available, metal prostheses, pacemakers, and various implants may contraindicate MRI. This noninvasive diagnostic procedure is painless, has no known risks, and requires no preparation.

COMMON THERAPEUTIC MEASURES

DRUG THERAPY

A number of drugs are used to treat neurologic disorders. They include antimicrobials, analgesics, anti-inflammatories, corticosteroids, anticonvulsants, diuretics, chemotherapeutic agents, dopaminergics, anticholinergics, cholinergics, and antihistamines. Examples of specific drugs are presented in Table 26-6.

SURGERY

A craniotomy (surgical opening of the skull) may be done to treat tumors, correct defects, evacuate hematomas, and relieve pressure associated with trauma. A craniectomy is the

table 26-6 **DRUG THERAPY | *Neurologic Disorders***

DRUG	USE/ACTION	SIDE EFFECTS	NURSING INTERVENTIONS
ANTICONVULSANTS			
Phenytoin (Dilantin)	Reduces neuron hyperexcitability; inhibits seizure activity. Reduces pain of trigeminal neuralgia.	Sluggishness, ataxia, slurred speech, nystagmus, constipation, nausea, vomiting, overgrowth of gingiva, skin rashes. Hypotension with IV route. Unusual: aplastic anemia, agranulocytosis.	With IV doses, monitor BP pulse and report bradycardia. Do not exceed recommended rate of IV administra-tion per minute. Safety precautions if ataxic, drowsy. Give with food to reduce GI irritation. Provide meticulous mouth care to prevent gingival overgrowth. Identify concurrent drugs to detect possible interactions that enhance or inhibit drug effect.
Fosphenytoin (Cerebrex)	Precursor of phenytoin. Used for acute seizures.	Side effects the same as phenytoin.	IV or/n route. Less irritation at site of IV administration. Do not exceed recommended rate of IV administration.
Gabapentin (Neurontin)	Unique gabapentin-specific binding site in brain; no effect on GABA system.	Somnolence, dizziness, ataxia particularly after initiation of therapy or dosage increase. Weight gain, edema. Dyspepsia, nausea, vomiting, constipation. Rhinitis, pharyngitis.	Safety precautions if drowsy. Give with food to prevent GI distress. Notify physician of side effects. Encourage periodic rest periods to help with fatigue.
Lamotrigine (Lamictal)	Inhibits release of excitatory amino acid glutamate. Blocks Na channel.	Dizziness, headache, insomnia, somnolence, ataxia, diplopia. Nausea, vomiting. Potentially life threatening rash.	Safety precautions if drowsy. Notify physician of rash. Identify current drugs to detect possible interactions that enhance or inhibit drug effect. Monitor renal and hepatic function. Take drug with food or milk. Medicate for headache.
Topiramate (Topamax)	Blocks voltage-dependent sodium and calcium channels; enhances GABA activity at some GABA receptors; blocks excitatory receptors (kainite/glutamate).	Somnolence, abnormal thinking, dizziness, agitation, confusion, ataxia, nystagmus, nephrolithiasis, nausea, dyspepsia, anorexia, weight loss, dysmenorrhea, upper respiratory tract infection.	Safety precautions if drowsy. Inform physician of agitation, confusion, abnormal thinking. Administer with food if GI upset occurs. Caution not to chew or break tablet because of bitter taste. Maintain adequate hydration to prevent renal stones. Suggest use of barrier contraceptives due to decreased effectiveness of oral contraceptives. Encourage avoidance of alcohol due to increased CNS depression.
Vigabatrin (Sabril)	Inhibits GABA metabolism.	Drowsiness, dizziness, fatigue.	Safety precautions if drowsy. Monitor for possible drug interactions. Encourage rest periods for fatigue.
Tiagabine (Gabitril)	Increases level of GABA by inhibiting reuptake systems.	Tiredness, dizziness, headache, nervousness, asthenia, somnolence, nervousness, difficulty concentrating. GI upset, pain, Serious skin rash.	Safety precautions if drowsy. Note other drugs for possible drug interactions. Give with food. Monitor weight, liver function studies, neurologic status. Avoid alcohol and sleep-inducing drugs.

BP, Blood pressure; *IV,* intravenous; *GI,* gastrointestinal; *GABA,* inhibitory amino acid that increases seizure threshold; *CNS,* central nervous system.

table 26-6 **DRUG THERAPY | *Neurologic Disorders—cont'd***

DRUG	USE/ACTION	SIDE EFFECTS	NURSING INTERVENTIONS
ANTICONVULSANTS—cont'd			
Zonisaminde (Zonegran)	Sulfonamide; mechanism of action is unclear. Decreases seizure activity by inhibiting sodium and calcium channels	Skin rash; somnolence, anorexia, dizziness, headache, nausea, agitation/irritability. Renal calculi, bone marrow depression. Nausea, vomiting, dry mouth, unusual taste.	Safety precautions if drowsy. Adequate hydration to prevent renal calculi. Monitor hepatic, renal, and cardiac function. Monitor closely at beginning of therapy and with dosage changes.
Oxcarbazepine (Trileptal)	Inhibits seizure activity by preventing sodium shift that causes neuron hyperexcitability.	Dizziness, drowsiness, double vision, fatigue, ataxia, nausea, vomiting, abdominal pain, tremor, dyspepsia, gait abnormalities.	May be taken with or without food. Implement safety precautions if CNS effects occur. Encourage rest periods for fatigue.
Levetiracetam (Keppra)	Unknown mechanism of action.	Somnolence, dizziness, impaired coordination, abnormal behavior, fatigue, infection.	Safety precautions if drowsy. Give with food to prevent GI side effects. Be aware of interactions with other drugs. Advise to use barrier contraceptives. Implement safety precautions if CNS side effects occur.
BARBITURATES			
Phenobarital (Luminal) Primidone (Myidone)	Depresses CNS and raises seizure threshold.	Drowsiness, respiratory depression, nausea, vomiting, diarrhea, constipation, rash, photosensitivity, muscle aches. With IV route: laryngospasm, bronchospasm, hypotension.	Safety precautions if drowsy. Monitor respiratory rate and BP, especially with IV route. Note other drugs for possible drug interactions. Tell patient not to stop drug without consulting physician and to avoid alcohol and excessive sunlight.
Carbamazepine (Tegretol)	Slows transmission of impulses in CNS; prevents seizures. Reduces pain of trigeminal neuralgia.	Drowsiness, ataxia, blurred vision, BP increase or decrease, heart failure, urinary retention, rash, hepatitis, aplastic anemia, agranulocytosis.	Safety precautions if drowsy. Monitor BP. Teach patient: avoid alcohol and excessive sunlight, do not change dosage or stop drug without physician's guidance, immediately report fever, sore throat, excessive bruising or bleeding, jaundice.
Diazepam (Valium)	Depresses CNS; inhibits impulse conduction.	Drowsiness, rash, nausea, vomiting, diarrhea, constipation, respiratory depression, psychological and physical dependence. IV route: hypotension, phlebitis.	Safety precautions if drowsy. Monitor infusion site for extravasation. Monitor BP. Give with food to decrease GI distress. Tell patient not to stop or change drug dose without physician's guidance.
Clonazepam (Klonopin)	Raises seizure threshold.	Drowsiness, ataxia, agitation, rash, edema, nocturia, blurred vision, dry mouth, excitement in elderly. Toxicity causes lethargy, confusion, coma.	Safety measures if drowsy. Advise patient that abrupt withdrawal may cause restlessness, insomnia, status epilepticus.

excision of a segment of the skull, and a cranioplasty is any procedure done to repair a skull defect. General care of the surgical patient is covered in Chapter 16, but interventions specific to neurologic surgery are emphasized here.

Preoperative Nursing Care

Preoperatively, assess and document neurologic status to provide a baseline for evaluating postoperative progress. Encourage the patient to ask questions and to express fears. If the patient has cerebral edema, parenteral corticosteroids may be ordered to help reduce cerebral swelling. All or part of the scalp is usually shaved, and the shaved hair is saved for the patient. Recognize that shaving the head can be very stressful for patients, and assure them that it will grow back. Sometimes shaving is done after the patient is anesthetized to reduce the trauma. Advise the family that a craniotomy can take as long as 12 hours and that they will get progress reports during the procedure.

Postoperative Nursing Care

Postoperative craniotomy assessment includes evaluation of level of consciousness, vital signs, movement and strength, pupil size and response to light, and speech. Signs and symptoms that may be related to complications are headache, visual disturbances, vomiting, seizures, and respiratory depression. Vital signs are recorded and neurologic checks are done hourly until the patient is stable. Maintain intake and output records. Inspect the dressing for bleeding or CSF drainage. Note drainage from the ears or nose. A dressing may be placed loosely to absorb the drainage. Replace it when it becomes wet because the moisture can harbor bacteria. On dressings, CSF appears as a pink stain surrounded by a lighter ring described as a "halo." It is no longer recommended to check CSF with a dipstick for glucose because dipsticks are calibrated only for the specific fluids they were designed to test. Report signs of deteriorating neurologic status to the physician immediately. The physician prescribes the patient's position. It usually specifies that the head of the bed be elevated about 30 degrees.

If the patient has an external ventricular drainage system, use strict aseptic technique when changing the insertion-site dressing and the drainage bag. Keep the zero reference point of the drip chamber of the drainage bag at the level of the external auditory canal or at the level prescribed by the physician to prevent drainage of excessive CSF. When the patient is being repositioned, clamp and then restore the drainage tube to the correct level and unclamp.

In addition to the usual surgical complications, the patient having a craniotomy is at risk for increased ICP, CSF leak, meningitis, and seizures. Other complications depend on the area of the brain affected and could include paralysis, memory loss, confusion, and impaired speech, vision, or hearing. Because increased ICP is a concern with cranial surgery as well as with many neurologic disorders, it is described here.

Increased Intracranial Pressure

Increased intracranial pressure (ICP) poses an extremely serious threat to the neurologic patient. Understanding the physiology as well as the signs and symptoms can enable you to recognize the problem and respond appropriately to prevent life-threatening consequences.

Pathophysiology. Anatomically, the skull is an empty cavity with rigid sides and an opening at the bottom. This cavity contains the brain, blood, and CSF, which are the components that exert pressure in the cranium. This pressure, or ICP, is normally 0 to 15 mm Hg.

In the course of a day, ICP fluctuates minimally because alterations are usually corrected rapidly. The Monro-Kellie hypothesis describes the adaptations that must occur in the three components (brain, blood, or CSF) for ICP to remain normal. If the volume of one component increases, ICP will rise unless there is a subsequent decrease in the other two components. For example, if a brain tumor increases the volume of brain tissue, ICP will rise unless the volume of both blood and CSF decreases.

As ICP increases, the perfusion (delivery of blood and oxygen) to brain tissue decreases. This can be measured by calculating cerebral perfusion pressure (CPP):

$$\text{CPP} = \text{MAP} - \text{ICP}$$

A minimum perfusion pressure of 70 mm Hg is necessary to ensure adequate cerebral functioning. If perfusion pressure falls to 40 mm Hg, ischemia occurs. A perfusion pressure of 30 mm Hg or less is incompatible with life. Perfusion pressure can be increased by decreasing ICP.

Signs and Symptoms. You can detect increases in ICP and assess the adequacy of perfusion based on the presence of specific signs and symptoms. Assess level of consciousness, pupillary characteristics, motor function, sensory function, and vital signs to detect signs of increasing ICP so that treatment can be initiated promptly.

Level of consciousness is the most reliable indicator of mental status because of its extreme sensitivity to oxygen levels in the cerebral blood. As ICP increases and perfusion is reduced, oxygen delivery to cerebral tissue also is reduced. Changes in level of consciousness are the earliest changes seen in ICP. These changes may be very subtle, with minimal agitation or drowsiness, or may be quite extreme, with profound unresponsiveness.

Classic pupillary changes are seen with increasing ICP. As pressure rises, the pupil progresses from its normal size to a dilated state described as a "blown pupil." The pupil becomes dilated and fixed, and no longer reacts to light. These changes occur because of pressure on the oculomotor nerve (third cranial nerve). This is a late sign of increased ICP.

Another major indicator of increased ICP is altered motor function. As the motor areas of the frontal lobe are compressed by rising pressure, deficits develop on the side opposite the expanding mass. When deficits are on the opposite side from brain injury, they are said to be contralateral to the injury. For example, if there is a tumor in the right side of the brain, motor deficits will appear in the left side of the body. The deficits may involve a single extremity or an entire side. **Hemiparesis** (weakness on one side) or **hemiplegia** (paralysis on one side) may be seen.

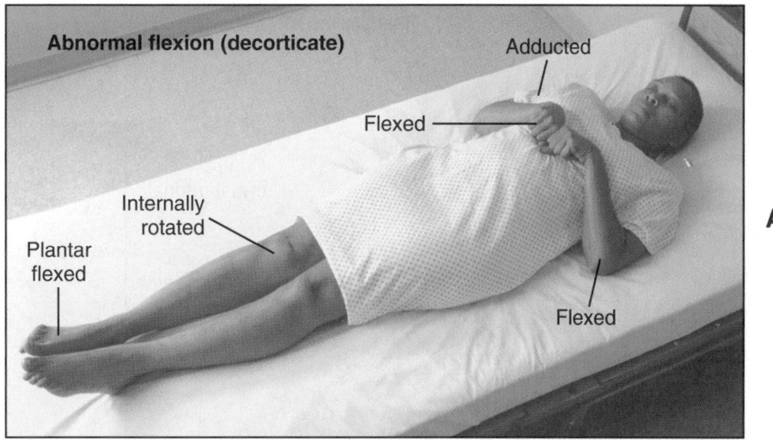

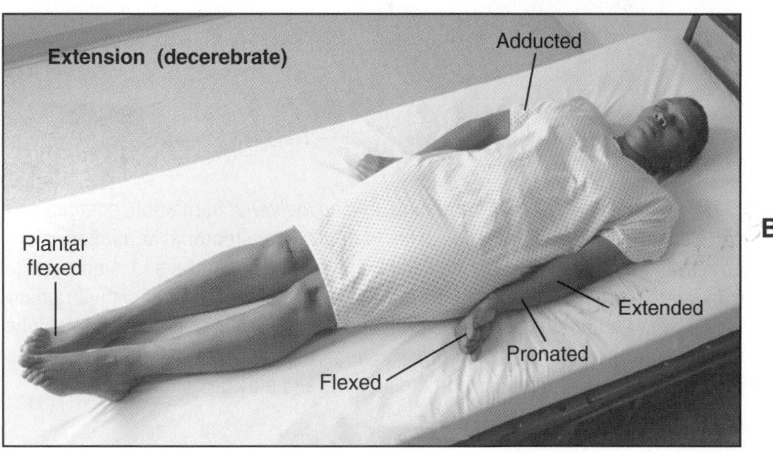

FIGURE **26-12** Abnormal postures may be seen in the patient with neurologic impairment. *A,* Abnormal flexion posturing (decorticate rigidity). *B,* Abnormal extension posturing (decerebrate rigidity).

As increased pressure becomes more extensive, abnormal posturing may be evident. As increasing pressure is exerted on the cerebral tissue above the midbrain, a pattern known as abnormal flexion (decorticate) posturing can be observed. The patient exhibits abnormal flexion in the upper extremities, with extension of the lower extremities. Increasing pressure affecting the midbrain or upper pons causes extension (decerebrate) posturing. The lower extremities remain extended, and the upper extremities are abnormally extended as well. These motor changes may occur spontaneously or may be seen only with painful stimuli (Fig. 26-12).

Hypothalamic impairment results in the loss of temperature control. As ICP compresses the tissue around the hypothalamus, it becomes ischemic and unable to regulate body temperature.

ICP elevations evoke an increase in systolic blood pressure with little or no associated increase in diastolic pressure. This results in a widening pulse pressure, defined as an increasing difference between systolic and diastolic blood pressure values. Initially, the heart rate may be slightly accelerated. However, as ICP compresses the center for cardiac control in the brain stem, the heart rate becomes slow and irregular. Alterations in respiratory pattern are directly related to the extent of tissue compression. Figure 26-13 illustrates areas of tissue compression (types of "herniation" syndromes).

Although it is extremely important to monitor vital signs in the neurologic patient, remember that changes in pulse, respiratory pattern, and blood pressure are late signs of increasing ICP. The combination of hypertension, bradycardia, and a widening pulse pressure is known as Cushing's triad. Cushing's triad is generally associated with increased ICP, but it is unreliable in determining the severity of neurologic compromise.

Medical Treatment. Prompt treatment of increased ICP is vital for survival. Measures to lower ICP include positioning, hyperventilation, fluid management, mechanical drainage, and drug therapy.

The jugular vein is the primary route for venous outflow from the brain. It has long been thought that raising the head of the bed 30 to 45 degrees improves the flow of venous blood from the brain, thereby decreasing cerebral blood volume and ICP. However, recent research indicates that perfusion

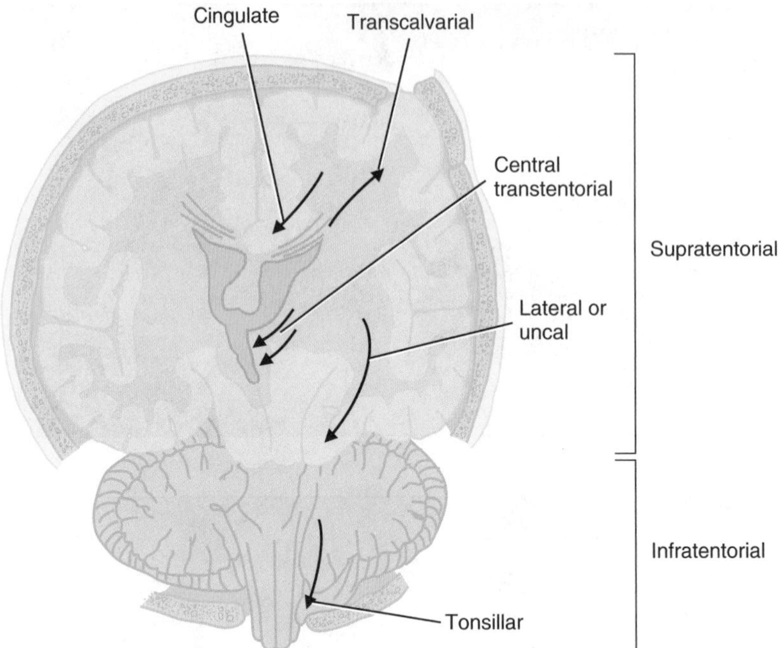

FIGURE **26-13** Types of intracranial herniation. In *transcalvarial* herniation, edematous brain tissue is extruded through a fracture in the skull. In *central* transtentorial herniation, the lesion is located centrally or superior in the cranium, and compression of central and midbrain structures may result. In *lateral,* or *uncal,* herniation the lesion is located laterally within the cranium and can cause pressure on the midbrain. *Cingulate* herniation occurs between the two frontal lobes; the brain is pressed under the falx cerebri. In *tonsillar* herniation, the cerebellar tonsils are driven between the posterior arch of the atlas and the medulla and may be compressed.

pressure may be better preserved if the head of the bed is elevated no more than 30 degrees. Further investigations may lead to some changes in current practice.

As oxygen delivery to cerebral tissue becomes more impaired, the level of carbon dioxide in the tissue increases. Increased carbon dioxide leads to dilation of cerebral blood vessels, thereby increasing the cerebral blood volume and ICP. With controlled hyperventilation, the excess carbon dioxide is eliminated, causing blood vessels to constrict and ICP to fall. Controlled hyperventilation is best achieved by mechanical ventilation. It effectively decreases ICP within 1 to 2 minutes, but its effectiveness is diminished after 36 to 48 hours. Hyperventilation does have risks. Excessive vasoconstriction reduces cerebral oxygenation and worsens ischemia. Hyperventilation may be reserved for situations in which other treatments fail to reduce ICP.

The patient must have adequate fluids to maintain CPP. Fluid volumes are often increased in an effort to boost perfusion. Patients with questionable cardiac function must be monitored closely for fluid volume excess. A specialized catheter, called a ventriculostomy catheter, can be placed in the brain to drain excess CSF. After placement, the catheter is connected to tubing and a collection bag for gravity drainage. Drainage of CSF lowers ICP. Absolute sterility must be maintained in managing this system, because it presents an open avenue for contamination.

Intravenous mannitol administration is one of the mainstays in the treatment of increased ICP. Mannitol is a hyperosmolar diuretic that draws edema fluid from the tissue spaces into the bloodstream. The mannitol and excess fluid are then eliminated through the kidneys. Other diuretic agents, such as furosemide, also may be used in an effort to reduce edema.

Corticosteroids, although controversial, may be used to help decrease cerebral edema and ICP. They decrease the edema, thereby lowering the elevated ICP associated with CNS tumors. Dexamethasone (Decadron) is a major agent used for patients with neurologic disorders. Additional information about drugs is presented in Table 26-6.

PHARMACOLOGY CAPSULE Diuretics used to treat increased intracranial pressure can cause fluid and electrolyte imbalances.

DISORDERS OF THE NERVOUS SYSTEM

HEADACHE

Headache is the most common type of pain. It is a symptom, rather than a disease, that has many causes. Four common types of headaches are migraine headache, cluster headache,

Consider the Alternative!

Complementary and alternative therapies are excellent adjuncts in the management of headache. Progressive muscle relaxation techniques, imagery, acupuncture, and electromyography (EMG) biofeedback can be used to reduce the frequency and intensity.

tension headache, and headache related to disorders of the eyes, teeth, or sinuses. For headaches associated with these and other conditions, treatment depends on the underlying cause.

Migraine Headache

Migraine headache is thought to be due to intracranial vasoconstriction followed by vasodilation. Although no single cause is known, it may be triggered by menstruation, ovulation, alcohol, some foods, and stress.

Patients may experience depression, irritability, vision disturbances, nausea, and paresthesias before the onset of pain. The pain is usually unilateral, often begins in the temple or eye area, and is often very intense. Tearing and nausea and vomiting may occur. The patient is hypersensitive to light and sound and prefers a dark, quiet environment.

Mild migraines may be treated with acetaminophen or aspirin, but more severe ones may be treated with ergotamine (Cafergot) or sumatriptan (Imitrex) administered as a tablet or by autoinjector for self-injection. Prevention, however, should be emphasized. Medications such as beta-blockers or calcium channel blockers may help control the vascular influences. Identification and avoidance of triggering agents, such as particular foods (chocolate, yogurt, aged meats, and cheeses), beverages (alcohol and red wine), or emotional stress, may also prove helpful.

Cluster Headache

Cluster headaches occur in a series of episodes followed by a long period with no symptoms. They are intensely painful and seem to be related to stress or anxiety. Unlike migraines, cluster headaches usually have no warning symptoms. They are also shorter in duration than migraines. Treatment may include cold application, indomethacin (Indocin), and tricyclic antidepressants.

Tension Headache

Tension headaches result from prolonged muscle contraction associated with anxiety, stress, or stimuli from other sources such as a brain tumor or an abscessed tooth. The location of the pain may vary, and the patient may have nausea and vomiting, dizziness, tinnitus, or tearing. Tension headaches may persist for days or even years. Treatment measures include correction of known causes, psychotherapy, massage, heat application, and relaxation techniques. Analgesics, usually nonopioid, may be prescribed along with other drugs to reduce anxiety.

SEIZURE DISORDER

The electrical impulses generated in the brain normally spread in a very organized fashion. However, in the patient with a seizure disorder, electrical impulses are conducted in a highly chaotic pattern that yields abnormal activity and behavior. Seizure activity involves a large number of hyperactive neurons that use excessive oxygen and glucose. Therefore, oxygen and glucose stores may be depleted, leading to permanent neurologic damage.

Seizure activity may be related to trauma, reduced cerebral perfusion, infection, electrolyte disturbances, poisoning, or tumors. There may also be a genetic tendency for such activity.

Medical Diagnosis

Diagnostic testing for seizure activity is often directed toward ruling out specific problems. An accurate history of the seizure disorder can provide clues to the type of seizure disorder, possible triggering events, and the origin of activity. Because unexpected seizure activity is often very frightening to the family, the nurse or other health care provider may be the first reliable eyewitness. If you observe a seizure, note the patient's behavior before, during, and after the seizure as well as the duration of the seizure.

The patient's electroencephalogram (EEG) tracing, which records the electrical activity of the brain, is used to detect abnormal brain activity.

Seizure Classification

The two broad classifications of seizures, based on the patterns of activity, are partial seizures and generalized seizures. Abnormal electrical activity may be generated in a specific area of the brain, remain localized, and stop; or the activity may spread to adjacent neurons but remain fairly localized. These patterns of activity are termed *partial* (or focal) *seizures* because they involve only a part of the brain. The observed activity corresponds to the area of the brain affected.

Additionally, partial seizures may recruit a sufficient number of adjacent cells and the activity can spread throughout the cerebral hemispheres. This is known as a partial seizure with secondary generalization. *Generalized seizures* involve the entire brain from the onset and are associated with loss of consciousness.

Some sources use the term *unclassified seizures* for those that are not readily classified as partial or generalized.

Partial Seizures

Partial seizures are described as simple or complex. Simple seizures affect part of one cerebral hemisphere and consciousness is not impaired. A simple partial seizure may include motor, somatosensory, autonomic, or psychic symptoms. Focal motor seizures are a subtype of simple seizures in which the abnormal brain activity remains localized to a specific motor area. This may occur with or without *Jacksonian march,* the term used when the abnormal activity begins in one area, then "marches" (spreads) to adjacent motor areas. For example, the simple focal motor seizure may begin with the eyelid, then spread to the same side of the face and continue on to involve the arm and leg on that side.

In a complex partial seizure (previously called a psychomotor or temporal lobe seizure), the patient's consciousness is impaired and the patient may exhibit bizarre, repetitive behavior. Simple partial and complex partial seizures can progress to involve the entire brain.

Generalized Seizures

Generalized seizures involve the entire brain from the onset. Consciousness is lost during the *ictal* (seizure) period. One type of generalized seizure is the tonic-clonic seizure, previously referred to as a grand mal seizure. The tonic phase of the seizure is characterized by stiffening of the muscles or extremities with loss of consciousness. After the tonic phase, there is a rhythmic movement of the extremities called the clonic phase of the seizure. These phases are illustrated in Figure 26-14. The patient may be incontinent of urine during a generalized seizure.

Other types of generalized seizures are absence, myoclonic, and atonic seizures. Absence seizures (previously called petit mal) are brief periods of loss of consciousness in which the person may appear to be daydreaming. Absence seizures may be associated with automations such as eye blinking and lip smacking. These seizures are generally identified during childhood. During a myoclonic seizure, the person has only brief jerking or stiffening of the extremities. Atonic seizures were formerly called "drop attacks" because a sudden loss of muscle tone causes the patient to collapse.

Status epilepticus. Status epilepticus is a medical emergency in which the patient has continuous seizures or repeated seizures in rapid succession for 30 minutes or more. The prolonged seizure activity depletes the brain of oxygen and glucose, which can lead to permanent brain damage.

Aura. Some people experience an aura preceding a seizure. The aura is a sensation such as dizziness, numbness, visual or hearing disturbance, perception of an offensive odor, or pain.

A

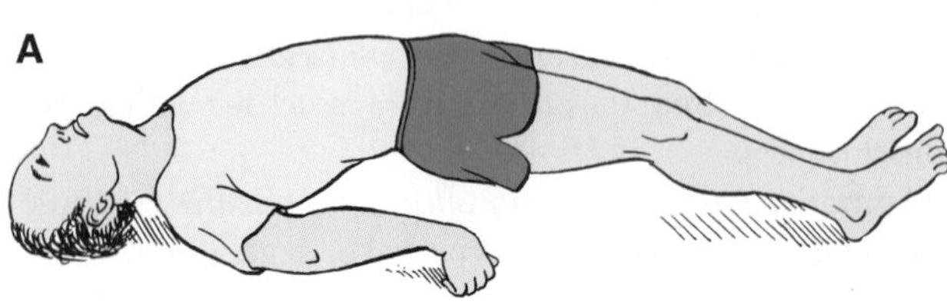

Tonic phase

B

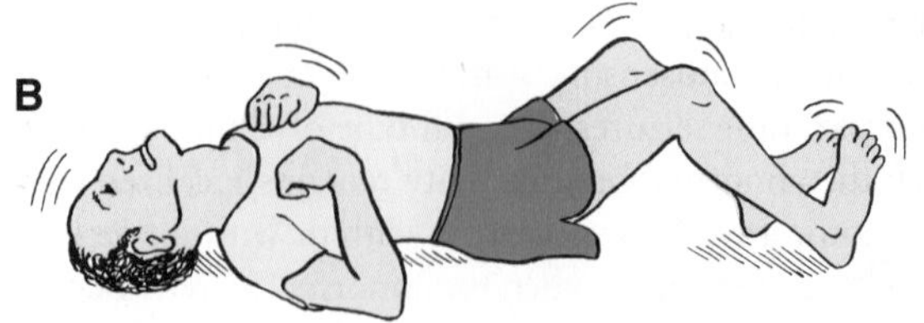

Clonic phase

FIGURE 26-14 Phases of a grand mal seizure. *A,* Tonic phase is marked by loss of consciousness, falling, crying, and generalized stiffness. There may be incontinence. *B,* During the clonic phase, there is jerking of the limbs and salivary frothing.

Medical Treatment

The most desirable treatment of a seizure disorder is the resolution of the underlying condition. For example, if a tumor is causing seizure activity, surgical excision of the tumor would be the most desirable therapy. However, if a cause is not readily identifiable or correctable, medical management is implemented.

Anticonvulsant drug therapy provides satisfactory chemical control of seizure activity in about 75% of patients. A variety of drugs are available, some being more effective in particular seizure disorders than others. The selected drug is introduced and the dosage is gradually increased until a therapeutic level is achieved. If good seizure control is not accomplished with one drug, combinations of drugs may be prescribed. Table 26-6 summarizes the major drugs used in the medical management of seizure disorders.

Status epilepticus is treated with intravenous anticonvulsant drugs. If the patient does not respond to anticonvulsants, general anesthetic agents and neuromuscular blocking agents may be used.

PHARMACOLOGY CAPSULE Sudden discontinuance of anticonvulsant drugs can trigger seizure activity.

Surgical Treatment

Patients whose seizures are poorly controlled with medication may be candidates for surgical procedures to decrease or control seizures. Procedures include removal of seizure foci in the temporal lobe and pallidotomy or vagal nerve stimulator.

NURSING CARE *of the Patient with a Seizure Disorder*

Assessment

Assessment of the neurologic patient is summarized in Table 26-3. With a seizure disorder, it is especially important to describe the seizure episode including the postictal period (following the seizure), and to document drug therapy.

Nursing Diagnoses, Goals, and Outcome Criteria: Seizure Disorder

Nursing Diagnoses	Goals and Outcome Criteria
Risk for Injury related to seizure activity	Absence of injury: no bruises, breaks in skin, or fractures
Ineffective Coping related to social stigma of seizure disorder or chronicity	Effective coping: patient makes positive statements about life with a seizure disorder, patient adheres to prescribed therapy
Deficient Knowledge of seizure disorders, treatment, and self-care	Patient understands self-care: patient and family accurately describe condition, drug therapy, and care, demonstrate appropriate care

Interventions

Risk for Injury

You must protect the patient from injury during and after a seizure. Most agencies require that the side rails of the bed be up and padded, a suction machine be readily available, and the bed be maintained in the low position. Some experts believe that padding the side rails is unnecessary, is cumbersome, and may have a negative emotional impact on the patient and visitors. It is, however, a common practice used in an effort to protect the patient in case the patient strikes the rails during a seizure.

If the patient has a seizure, quickly move objects away from the patient. If the patient falls to the floor, the head may be cradled in your lap to prevent injury. Do not attempt to restrain the patient. In the past it was common practice to attempt to insert a tongue blade or oral airway between the teeth to prevent biting the tongue. This is no longer recommended. Attempts to force an object between clenched teeth may result in injury to the mouth and do not help if the tongue has already been bitten. The patient will not "swallow his tongue," but it may fall back and occlude the airway. Turning the patient to one side can help maintain a patent airway.

When seizure activity ceases, the patient is typically drowsy and needs to rest. Provide for quiet and privacy. Measures to prevent injury are described in Table 26-7. Afterward, document the conditions and any unusual behaviors that preceded the seizure, the length of the seizure, associated patient activity, deviation of the eyes, and any incontinence. Also, document any lingering effects and the time before recovery.

Ineffective Coping and Deficient Knowledge

Ineffective coping can be related to lack of information or misconceptions and may be reflected in noncompliance with prescribed therapy, in anxiety, or in social isolation. Important aspects of nursing management include not only the care of the patient during hospitalization but also teaching the family and patient about the seizure disorder and the therapy. The teaching plan should include the following:

PATIENT TEACHING PLAN
Seizures

- A sensation that warns of an impending seizure is called an aura; common sensations include dizziness, numbness, visual or hearing disturbance, pain, and perception of an offensive odor.
- Factors that may trigger a seizure are fatigue, stress, fever, visual disturbances, alcohol, failure to take medication, and large caffeine intake.
- When you perceive an impending seizure, immediately seek a safe place.
- Know your prescribed drug names, dosages, schedules, and side effects to be reported to the physician.
- Consult your physician regarding the use of generic substitutions for your drugs.
- Never stop taking your seizure medication without direction from your physician.
- Psychological counseling may help you deal with stress associated with this disorder.
- Always wear a medical alert tag, which states that you have a seizure disorder, and carry a card that specifies drug therapy, physician, and individuals to be contacted in an emergency.
- The local chapter of the Epilepsy Foundation is an excellent resource. The telephone number is 1-800-332-1000. The Internet address is www.EFA.org.

Because a seizure disorder is often a lifelong problem, patient teaching must be directed toward helping the patient and family adjust to a chronic condition. Patients must adjust physically, psychologically, and vocationally to the changes brought on by the disorder itself as well as to the side effects of the medications. Encourage the patient to ask questions and to express concerns.

HEAD INJURY

Traumatic brain injury is a leading cause of death due to trauma in the United States. The most common causes of head injury are motor vehicle accidents, assaults, and falls, with drug and alcohol abuse being major contributing factors. Several different types of injuries can be identified.

Types of Head Injuries

Scalp Injuries

Scalp injuries include lacerations, contusions, abrasions, and hematomas. They may bleed profusely and may or may not be associated with skull or brain injuries.

Concussion

A concussion is head trauma in which there is no visible injury to the skull or brain. The patient has a loss of consciousness

table 26-7 ***Management of Seizures***

"DO'S"	"DON'T'S"
DO remove any objects that could cause harm. DO turn the person to one side if possible. DO note the time the seizure began and how it progressed. DO assess and document postictal (postseizure) status. DO allow person to rest quietly. DO call a medical emergency if a generalized tonic-clonic seizure lasts more than 4 min or if seizures occur in rapid succession.	DO NOT restrain unless in grave danger of severe injury. DO NOT attempt to force anything between teeth.

lasting less than 5 minutes and may have a headache, amnesia about the event, nausea, and vomiting.

Contusion

A contusion is more serious than a concussion because there is actual bruising and bleeding in the brain tissue. Contusions can be very serious, especially if the brain stem is affected.

Hematomas

A hematoma is a collection of blood, usually clotted, that may be classified as subdural or epidural.

Subdural Hematoma

A subdural hematoma is usually the result of tearing of the veins that drain the brain, allowing blood to accumulate in the space beneath the dura (Fig. 26-15A). The three types of subdural hematomas are acute, subacute, and chronic. Acute subdural hematomas develop within 24 hours of the injury. Subacute subdural hematomas are seen more than 24 hours and less than 1 week after the initial injury. Chronic subdural hematomas occur within weeks or even months of the original injury and are associated with low-impact injuries that cause very slow, diffuse bleeding. Because the bleeding associated with any hematoma can cause potentially serious consequences, astute assessment is needed to determine patient status. Surgical intervention is usually indicated for these types of injuries.

Epidural hematoma. An epidural hematoma forms in the space between the inner surface of the skull and the outermost meningeal covering of the brain, known as the dura (Fig. 26-15B). Generally, epidural hematomas result from arterial bleeding secondary to a laceration and tearing of the middle meningeal artery. The patient typically has a momentary lapse of consciousness, then a period of alertness followed by rapid deterioration. Therefore, you must be alert for any indication of increasing ICP, especially drowsiness progressing to coma. Surgical intervention may be necessary to relieve pressure, remove the clot, and stop the bleeding.

Intracerebral Hemorrhage

Intracerebral hemorrhages result from lesions within the tissue of the brain itself (Fig. 26-15C). These injuries may be small or large and may be accompanied by massive neurologic deficits.

Penetrating Injuries

Penetrating injuries result from sharp objects that penetrate the skull and brain tissue. In addition to the obvious brain injury, there is also a scalp laceration along with the skull fracture. All penetrating injuries require prompt surgical intervention and pose an extremely high risk of infection for the patient because of the wound contamination that occurs.

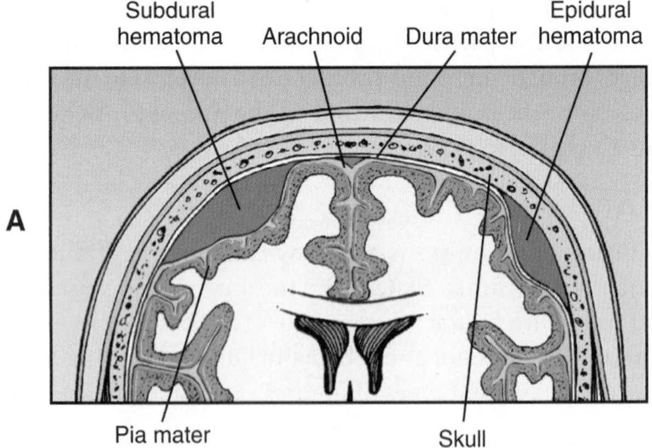

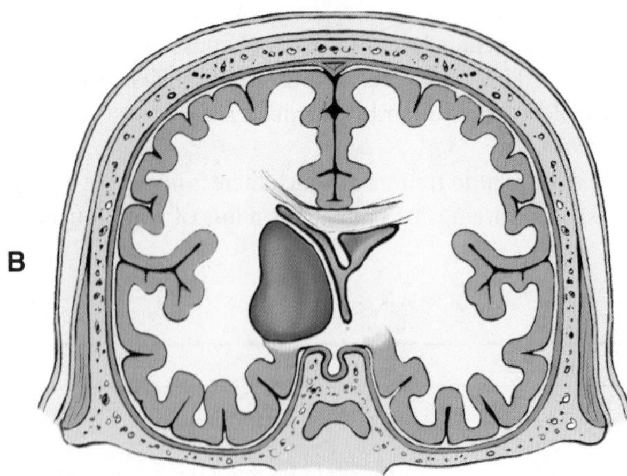

FIGURE 26-15 Epidural hematoma, subdural hematoma, and intracerebral hematoma.

Surgical Treatment

Surgical intervention for each of these types of trauma is directed at evacuating (removing) hematomas and débriding damaged tissue.

NURSING CARE *of the Patient with a Head Injury*

Assessment

Nursing assessment of the patient with a neurologic disorder is outlined in Table 26-3 (see also Nursing Care Plan: The Patient with a Head Injury).

Nursing Diagnoses, Goals, and Outcome Criteria: Head Injury

Nursing Diagnoses	Goals and Outcome Criteria
Ineffective Tissue Perfusion related to increased ICP	Adequate cerebral tissue perfusion: patient alert and oriented
Ineffective Breathing Patterns related to increased ICP	Normal oxygenation: respiratory rate of 12 to 20 per minute with normal arterial blood gas values
Risk for Injury related to seizures, decreased level of consciousness, disorientation, vision disturbances	Absence of injury: no abrasions, fractures, or severe bruising incurred during seizures or falls

NURSING CARE PLAN

The Patient with a Head Injury

ASSESSMENT

Health History: Austin Mandrel is a 17-year-old boy who was injured in a motorcycle accident 2 weeks ago. He reportedly struck his head on the pavement and was unconscious on admission. He is now alert and oriented to person and place but not to time. He is reluctant to discuss his injuries and refers to himself as a "gimp." He had a seizure the evening of admission but is now being given anticonvulsants and has had no seizures since. His mother reports that he has had no serious illnesses, hospitalizations, or operations and that he has no known allergies. He is a high school junior and football player. He has two close friends who visit frequently.

Physical Examination: Vital signs: temperature, 98° F orally; pulse, 62; respiration, 12; blood pressure, 150/84 mm Hg. Laceration on the forehead, well healed; healing abrasions on the forehead and right cheek without edema or drainage. Pupils equal and react to light. No drainage from the ears. No stiffness of the neck. Reflexes normal in right extremities but decreased in left extremities. Patient moves left extremities on command, but they are weaker (4/5) than the right. Ambulates with a walker.

Nursing Diagnosis	*Goals and Outcome Criteria*	*Interventions*
Ineffective tissue perfusion related to increased intracranial pressure (ICP).	Patient will have adequate cerebral tissue perfusion as evidenced by alertness and orientation to person, place, and time.	Monitor for signs of increased ICP: decreasing level of consciousness, pupil inequality or dilation without response to light, increasing motor deficits, abnormal posture, fever, increasing blood pressure, bradycardia, respiratory depression. If increased ICP is suspected, notify physician, elevate head of bed as ordered. Monitor rate of fluid administration to ensure adequate cerebral perfusion. Administer diuretics and anti-inflammatory drugs as ordered.
Ineffective breathing patterns related to increased ICP.	Patient will have adequate oxygenation, as evidenced by respiratory rate of 12-20 min with normal arterial blood gas values.	Monitor for changes in LOC; decreasing respiratory rate and depth; and tachycardia. Check results of arterial blood gas studies.
Risk for injury related to lethargy, possible seizures.	Patient will remain free of injury during hospitalization.	Employ seizure precautions per agency policy. Place bed in low position. Have call light available and within reach of patient's right hand. Provide assistance with transferring.
Risk for infection related to traumatic wounds.	Patient will remain free of infection, as evidenced by normal temperature and white blood cell count.	Assess temperature for elevation. Assess wounds for increasing redness, edema, and foul drainage. Use standard precautions for wound care and when handling invasive equipment. Administer antibiotics as ordered.
Impaired physical mobility related to neuromuscular impairment, lethargy.	Patient will retain normal range of motion in all extremities and will participate in activities to restore strength to left extremities.	Explain importance of frequent position changes (at least every 2 hours) and assist patient to do so. Position affected extremities in functional alignment. Assist in active range-of-motion exercises at least three times a day. Apply antiembolism stockings as ordered. Assess skin, especially bony prominences, for signs of pressure or breakdown. Monitor elimination to detect urinary retention or constipation. Encourage fluids and high-fiber diet as needed.
Disturbed body image related to loss of function.	Patient will adapt to altered body function, as reflected in positive statements about self.	Encourage patient to ask questions and to express thoughts and feelings about injuries. Include him in planning sessions. Show acceptance through touch and genuine interest. Encourage friends to continue visits. Explain healing process and how rehabilitation measures can help. Emphasize abilities rather than disabilities. Promote independence in light of abilities. Refer to support group.
Ineffective role performance related to neurologic impairment.	Patient will participate in rehabilitation efforts and explore potential new roles and activities.	Explain healing process and how rehabilitation measures can help. Help patient learn to perform activities of daily living with limitations.

Nursing Diagnoses, Goals, and Outcome Criteria: Head Injury—cont'd

Nursing Diagnoses	Goals and Outcome Criteria
Risk for Infection related to traumatic wounds or invasive procedures	Absence of infection: normal body temperature without signs of wound infection (redness, edema, purulent drainage) or urinary infection (cloudiness, foul odor), or phlebitis (redness, tenderness)
Impaired Physical Mobility related to neuromuscular impairment, decreased mental alertness	Absence of complications of immobility, (contractures, pressure ulcers, pneumonia, atelectasis, constipation, urinary retention): intact skin, mobile joints, regular bowel movements, no bladder distention, breath sounds clear on auscultation
Disturbed Body Image related to loss of function	Adaptation to altered body function: patient verbalizes way to compensate for changes in body function
Ineffective Role Performance related to neurologic impairment	Adjustment of roles and responsibilities consistent with abilities: patient assumes new roles within abilities

Interventions

Ineffective Tissue Perfusion

Monitor the patient closely for signs of increased ICP and impaired cerebral blood flow: decreasing level of consciousness, pupillary dilation with no response to light, motor deficits, abnormal posture, fever, increased blood pressure, bradycardia, and respiratory depression. Particularly note early signs of deterioration including restlessness, agitation, or lethargy. Promptly report changes to the physician or the registered nurse. Nursing care that can decrease ICP includes positioning to prevent neck and hip flexion, limiting suctioning, spacing nursing care, and preventing isometric muscle contraction. Elevate the head of the bed as ordered. Carefully regulate the rate of administration of intravenous fluids to prevent fluid volume excess. Monitor urine output to assess fluid balance. If a ventriculostomy catheter is in place, inspect and measure the drainage fluid as ordered using strict aseptic technique. Administer diuretics and anti-inflammatory drugs as ordered.

Ineffective Breathing Patterns

Closely monitor the patient's respiratory status using pulse oximetry or measurement of arterial blood gases. Immediately advise the physician of signs of respiratory depression or changes in the respiratory pattern.

Risk for Injury

Nursing measures to prevent injuries associated with seizures and decreased level of consciousness were discussed earlier in this chapter and are summarized in Table 26-7.

Risk for Infection

The patient who has suffered a head injury may have serious lacerations or abrasions that can admit pathogenic organisms. Intravenous lines and urinary catheters also place the patient at risk for infection. Use standard precautions when handling all invasive lines or when dressing wounds. Monitor the patient's temperature and inspect wounds for increasing redness, swelling, or foul drainage. Administer antibiotics as ordered.

Impaired Physical Mobility

After a head injury, the patient may have temporary or permanent motor impairment. While confined to bed, the patient should be turned and positioned and encouraged to deep breathe at least every 2 hours. Routinely inspect the skin for signs of pressure or breakdown. Use antiembolism stockings if ordered. Perform range-of-motion exercises, and position joints in functional alignment. Frequently assess urine and bowel elimination to detect retention or constipation. As soon as permitted, assist the patient out of bed and encourage as much activity as possible. Unfortunately, some head-injured patients have permanent impairments that necessitate lifelong care. Care of the immobile patient is covered in detail in Chapter 20.

Disturbed Body Image and Ineffective Role Performance

The losses associated with a serious head injury can render the patient unable to resume usual activities. The injury also may leave disfiguring scars or distorted features. Demonstrate acceptance of the patient through touch and genuine interest. Encourage the patient to ask questions, express concerns, and anticipate problems and solutions. Be realistic about the patient's disabilities while emphasizing abilities.

Patients with serious deficits are usually treated by a team that includes rehabilitation specialists. These experts help the patient regain physical mobility, learn to carry out activities of daily living, learn new job skills, and deal with the emotional trauma of the injury and its effects.

Include the family in the rehabilitation process. In many cases, family members serve as the caregivers after head injury. Carson (1993) described behaviors of family members of patients who had sustained head injuries. Behaviors included providing personal care, obtaining rehabilitation services, providing a safe environment, seeking reminders of the preinjury person, exploring what abilities might be regained, encouraging return to preinjury activities, encouraging active decision making, becoming active members of the rehabilitation team, and staying open to potential gains.

Put on your THINKING CAP!!

You are caring for a patient with a head injury. The patient has been lethargic most of the day, but now seems more difficult to arouse. His vital signs and pupils are the same as they have been. What do you think is your best course of action in this situation?

BRAIN TUMORS

Brain tumors account for a relatively small percentage of cancer deaths annually. Brain tumors develop in some cancer patients as a result of metastasis from other primary sites. Tumor cells can spread to the CNS through the blood and CSF.

Not all brain tumors are malignant. Some tumor types, such as the meningioma, a tumorous growth of the meningeal tissue, are often benign. One might assume that benign tumor cells would suggest an excellent chance of complete recovery. However, the invasion of any kind of tumor into normal brain tissue is never insignificant. This invasion can cause significant damage that may prove fatal because of increasing ICP or surgical inaccessibility of the tumor.

Etiology and Risk Factors

The causes of brain tumors are generally unknown, but some appear to be congenital in origin, whereas others may be related to heredity. In addition, drug influences and environmental factors may play a role in the development of some brain tumors.

Signs and Symptoms

The signs and symptoms of brain tumors are directly related to the area of the brain that is invaded by the tumor. Motor and sensory symptoms, visual disturbances, and headache all may be early manifestations of tumor growth. New-onset seizure activity in an adult patient often indicates the presence of a tumor. Cerebellar tumors may cause difficulties with balance and coordination. Other tumors, depending on their location, may involve cranial nerves.

Medical Treatment

Management of the patient with a brain tumor depends on the type of cells present in the tumor. Surgery can be done to remove as much of the tumor tissue as possible. If the tumor is malignant, surgery is often followed by radiation therapy with or without chemotherapy.

NURSING CARE *of the Patient with a Brain Tumor*

Nursing care of the patient with a brain tumor depends on the specific deficits, treatment, and prognosis and may be similar to the care of the patient with a head injury. Care of the patient with cancer is discussed in Chapter 24.

Assessment

The complete neurologic assessment is summarized in Table 26-3. The assessment is especially important before brain surgery to provide a baseline for comparing postoperative findings.

Nursing Diagnoses, Goals, and Outcome Criteria: Brain Tumor

Nursing diagnoses vary with the patient's specific symptoms and disabilities and the type of treatment employed. Common nursing diagnoses and goals include the following:

Nursing Diagnoses	Goals and Outcome Criteria
Acute Pain related to pressure of expanding tumor mass	Pain relief: patient states pain relieved, has relaxed manner
Disturbed Thought Processes related to effects of tumor on brain tissue	Adaptation to altered thinking: improved mental orientation
Disturbed Sensory Perception related to impaired conduction of sensory information	Recognition of disturbed perceptions: absence of injury associated with sensory or perceptual impairment
Impaired Physical Mobility and **Self-Care Deficits** related to motor disturbances, impaired cognition	Accomplishment of activities of daily living: maximum possible patient mobility level and absence of complications of immobility (contractures, pneumonia, constipation, urinary retention)
Ineffective Coping related to life-threatening disease, changes in behavior function	Effective coping: patient and family make positive statements about ability to deal with the illness

Interventions

Acute Pain

Document pain and administer analgesics as ordered. Codeine or acetaminophen is often used. Small doses of morphine also may be used for pain relief. If pain relief is not achieved, inform the physician and assess for signs of increased ICP.

Disturbed Thought Processes

Monitor for changes in cognitive function by assessing orientation and response to instructions. Patients may demonstrate cognitive dysfunction, including impaired short-term memory, poor judgment, poor decision making, and impaired problem solving. Investigate *sudden* changes in mental status that may be caused by the tumor or by correctable factors such as drugs, hypoxia, and fluid and electrolyte imbalances. Listen carefully to the patient and present reality in a straightforward manner. Devices to help the patient maintain orientation include clocks, calendars, and seasonal decorations.

Disturbed Sensory Perception

Explain that the effects of the brain tumor may cause unusual sensations and perceptual disturbances. Implement safety measures as needed to prevent injury due to impaired vision, spatial perceptual problems, or sensation.

Impaired Physical Mobility and Self-Care Deficits

Patients with brain tumors may have varying degrees of physical impairment. Assess the patient's ability to perform activities of daily living and provide assistance as needed. Encourage the patient to remain as active as possible. If the patient's mobility is severely impaired, there is a high risk for disuse syndrome and the associated complications. Care of the immobilized patient is described in Chapter 20.

Ineffective Coping

You must assist the patient and family in dealing with a difficult diagnosis in addition to the obvious residual physical effects. A diagnosis of a malignant brain tumor is devastating for the family, and emotional support is vital to help them understand the nature of the disease and the anticipated problems and outcomes. Nursing care depends on the specific deficits, treatment, and prognosis and may be similar to the care of the patient with a head injury. Care of the patient with cancer is discussed in Chapter 24.

INFECTIOUS AND INFLAMMATORY CONDITIONS

Meningitis

Meningitis is inflammation of the meningeal coverings of the brain and spinal cord caused by either viruses or bacteria. Organisms may reach the meninges through the blood, through head wounds, or from other cranial structures such as the sinuses or inner ear. A number of organisms may be responsible for bacterial infection, including *Neisseria meningitidis, Streptococcus pneumoniae,* and *Haemophilus influenzae.*

Complications of meningitis include seizures, septicemia, vasomotor collapse, and increased ICP. *Neisseria meningitidis* is particularly problematic because septicemia develops in approximately 10% of patients.

Signs and Symptoms

The common signs and symptoms of meningitis are generally related to meningeal irritation. These include headache, nuchal rigidity (stiffness of the back of the neck), irritability, diminished level of consciousness, photophobia (sensitivity to light), hypersensitivity, and seizure activity. The presence of Kernig's sign and Brudzinski's sign also is indicative of meningeal irritation. To assess for Kernig's sign (Fig. 26-16A), flex the patient's hip to a 90-degree angle and then extend the knee. In the presence of a meningeal infection, this movement produces pain in the hamstring area. Brudzinski's sign (Fig. 26-16B) is flexion of both hips when the examiner flexes the patient's neck.

Medical Diagnosis

A lumbar puncture is done to obtain a CSF sample for laboratory analysis. The sample is examined to detect the presence of microorganisms in the CSF and to identify the infecting organism. With bacterial meningitis, the CSF appears milky and purulent because of white blood cells suspended in the fluid.

Medical Treatment

Management of bacterial meningitis requires prompt recognition and treatment with antimicrobials. In severe infections, broad-spectrum antimicrobials such as penicillin G are initiated immediately. Changes in therapy may be made when the results of culture and sensitivity tests are reported. Bacterial infections usually respond to antimicrobial therapy, but there are no specific drugs effective against most viral infections of the CNS. Anticonvulsants are used to control seizure activity if necessary.

If needed, isolation precautions should be initiated. Organisms responsible for meningococcal meningitis are spread by the respiratory route, and appropriate safeguards must be employed to protect other patients, family, and staff. (See Chapter 12.)

NURSING CARE *of the Patient with Meningitis*

Assessment

The routine neurologic assessment is summarized in Table 26-3. When a patient has meningitis, assess vital signs and neurologic status frequently to determine further deterioration or the onset of complications.

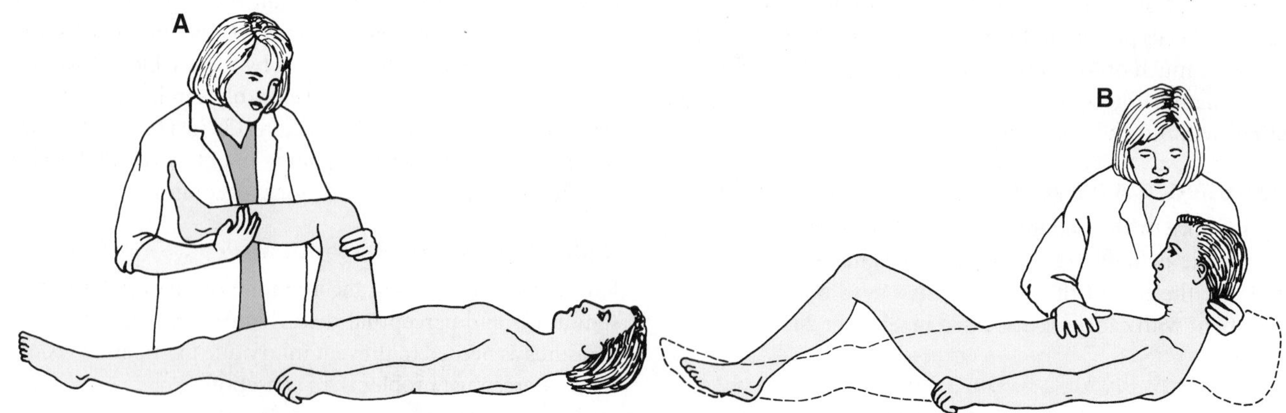

FIGURE 26-16 *A,* Positive Kernig's sign: When the patient's leg is flexed as shown, the patient is unable to completely extend the leg. *B,* Brudzinski's sign: When the nurse flexes the patient's neck, hip flexion occurs.

Nursing Diagnoses, Goals, and Outcome Criteria: Meningitis

Nursing Diagnoses	Goals and Outcome Criteria
Altered Tissue Perfusion related to increased ICP	Adequate cerebral tissue perfusion: vital signs and level of consciousness consistent with patient norms
Ineffective Breathing Patterns related to depression of the respiratory center	Adequate oxygenation: respiratory rate of 12 to 20 per minute
Acute Pain related to irritation of meninges and increased ICP	Pain relief: patient states pain has been relieved, relaxed manner
Risk for Injury related to confusion, seizures, restlessness	Absence of injury: no falls or other trauma
Deficient Fluid Volume related to vomiting and fever	Normal fluid balance without vomiting or fever: fluid intake and output equal, moist mucous membranes, blood pressure within patient norms
Risk for Disuse Syndrome related to bedrest	Absence of complications of immobility: clear breath sounds, intact skin, normal muscle strength and joint mobility, regular bowel movements without straining

Interventions

Ineffective Tissue Perfusion

Elevate the head of the patient's bed as ordered. Instruct the patient to avoid coughing and not to hold his or her breath during turning, because these behaviors increase ICP. Do not use restraints unless they are absolutely necessary. Monitor for signs of increasing ICP: decreased level of consciousness, headache, nausea, vomiting, abnormal pupillary responses, and respiratory depression. If ICP does increase, administer prescribed treatments (e.g., diuretics, barbiturates, opioids). Measures to lower the body temperature may be ordered to reduce the metabolic rate.

Ineffective Breathing Patterns

Monitor the respiratory status and gag and swallowing reflexes. Position the patient to maintain a patent airway and suction if necessary. Arterial blood samples are drawn and analyzed for gas values as ordered. Report a decreasing respiratory rate to the physician.

Acute Pain

Assess the location and severity of any discomfort. Nursing measures to decrease pain include position changes, massage, and a quiet environment. Give analgesics as ordered, and document their effect. Chapter 14 provides additional information about the nursing management of pain.

Risk for Injury

Because of the prevailing risk of seizures, take appropriate precautions to ensure patient safety. A subdued environment should be maintained to reduce irritability and contribute to patient comfort. Keep the bed in a low position, with the side rails padded and raised. Reorient the patient to the setting as needed, and keep the call button within easy reach. Remind patients who are dizzy not to get up without assistance.

Deficient Fluid Volume

Monitor the patient's vital signs, tissue turgor and moisture, and fluid intake and output. Weight may be measured daily to assess fluid status. Encourage oral fluid intake if it is permitted and if the patient is alert. Provide intravenous fluid therapy as ordered and monitor to ensure the correct flow rate. Antipyretics may be ordered for fever and antiemetics for vomiting.

Risk for Disuse Syndrome

The patient who is confined to bed is at risk for all the complications of immobility, especially stasis of pulmonary secretions, pressure sores, muscle weakness, joint stiffness, and constipation. Measures to prevent these complications are discussed in detail in Chapter 20.

Encephalitis

Encephalitis is inflammation of brain tissue that is usually caused by one of several viruses. These viruses may be prevalent during certain times of the year or in a specific geographic area. For example, certain types of mosquitoes found in the United States are carriers of a virus commonly associated with encephalitis. In addition, toxic substances or other types of viral infections, such as herpes simplex, may precipitate encephalitis.

Signs and Symptoms

The patient with encephalitis presents with symptoms directly related to the area of the brain that is involved. Fever, nuchal rigidity (stiff neck), headache, confusion, delirium, agitation, and restlessness are commonly seen. However, the patient also may become comatose or exhibit aphasia, hemiparesis, facial weakness, and other alterations in motor activity.

Medical Treatment

Care for the patient with encephalitis is focused on enhancing patient comfort and increasing strength. Because seizure activity is a potential problem, you must take appropriate safety precautions.

NURSING CARE *of the Patient with Encephalitis*

The nursing plan of care parallels that of the patient with meningitis.

GUILLAIN-BARRÉ SYNDROME

Although its specific cause is unknown, Guillain-Barré syndrome is believed to be an autoimmune response to a viral infection. It is a rapidly progressing disease that affects the motor component of the peripheral nervous system. Although the spinal nerves are usually affected, the cranial nerves also may be involved.

Patients with Guillain-Barré syndrome often report some recent viral infection or vaccination. This apparently triggers an autoimmune response that destroys the myelin sheath around the peripheral nerves, slowing the conduction of impulses across the involved nerves.

Signs and Symptoms

Guillain-Barré syndrome has three phases: initial, plateau, and recovery, as described in Table 26-8. The initial phase is characterized by symmetric muscle weakness that typically begins in the lower extremities and ascends to the trunk and upper extremities. The disease process may affect cranial nerves, resulting in visual and hearing disturbances, difficulty chewing, and lack of facial expression. The muscles of respiration also may be affected, resulting in the need for mechanical ventilation.

Mild paresthesias (abnormal sensations) or anesthesia (numbness) in the feet and hands may be present in a glove or stocking distribution pattern. In addition, some patients experience pain associated with the sensory changes. Despite all the motor and sensory changes, level of consciousness and intellectual functioning remain unchanged.

Effects on the autonomic nervous system may include hypertension, orthostatic hypotension, cardiac dysrhythmias, profuse sweating, paralytic ileus, and urinary retention. Dysautonomia, characterized by the above effects, occurs most frequently in patients with respiratory involvement and is potentially life threatening.

In the plateau phase, the patient with Guillain-Barré syndrome remains essentially unchanged. There is no further neurologic deterioration, but there is no improvement either.

As recovery begins and progresses, remyelinization occurs and muscle strength returns in a proximal to distal pattern (head to toes). Because the underlying axon generally remains undamaged, approximately 95% of patients with Guillain-Barré syndrome have a nearly complete recovery. Others have residual numbness, stiffness, or paresis.

Medical Diagnosis

The characteristic onset and pattern of ascending motor involvement provide the basis for the diagnosis of Guillain-Barré syndrome. An elevated protein level in the CSF obtained by lumbar puncture provides additional evidence for the diagnosis. Nerve conduction velocity studies reveal slowed conduction speed in the involved nerves.

Medical Treatment

Management during the acute phase of the illness is directed at preserving vital function, particularly respiration. Respiratory status is closely monitored and mechanical ventilation initiated if the vital capacity falls to 15 ml/kg of body weight. Massive doses of corticosteroids may be prescribed to suppress the inflammatory process.

Because Guillain-Barré syndrome is believed to be an autoimmune disease, plasmapheresis has emerged as a major treatment intervention. Plasmapheresis is a process in which blood is removed, centrifuged, and returned to the patient. In the process, antibodies that trigger the autoimmune disease are removed from the blood by a machine equipped with a special filtration system. The patient with Guillain-Barré syndrome generally undergoes a series of treatments, ideally delivered within 7 to 14 days after the onset of the disease. Those patients benefiting from plasmapheresis often recover faster.

NURSING CARE *of the Patient with Guillain-Barré Syndrome*

Assessment

Assessment of the patient with a neurologic disorder is summarized in Table 26-3. When Guillain-Barré syndrome is suspected, the health history describes the progression of symptoms. Note the patient's fears, coping strategies, and sources of support. Record information about important social data such as occupation and family roles and responsibilities. The physical examination focuses on cranial nerve, motor, respiratory, and cardiovascular function.

Nursing Diagnoses, Goals, and Outcome Criteria: Guillain-Barré Syndrome

Nursing Diagnoses	Goals and Outcome Criteria
Ineffective Breathing Patterns related to neurologic impairment	Adequate oxygenation: normal arterial blood gases and skin color
Decreased Cardiac Output related to labile blood pressure, cardiac dysrhythmias	Normal cardiac output: regular pulse with rate of 60 to 100 beats per minute and blood pressure consistent with patient norms
Risk for Disuse Syndrome related to motor impairment	Absence of complications of immobility: intact skin, no contractures, clear breath sounds, regular bowel movements

table 26-8 *Phases of Guillain-Barré Syndrome*

PHASE	CHARACTERISTICS	DURATION
Initial	Begins with onset of symptoms Ends when disease ceases to progress	Usually 1-3 wk
Plateau	No further changes; neither deterioration nor improvement	Several days to 2 wk
Recovery	Gradual improvement	May be as long as 2 yr; some residual effects may be permanent

Imbalanced Nutrition: Less than Body Requirements related to dysphagia, endotracheal tube	Adequate nutrition: stable body weight
Risk for Injury related to loss of sensation in hands and feet, motor impairment, inability to speak	Absence of injury in affected body areas: no falls, bruises, corneal damage, or other injuries
Anxiety related to paralysis, doubts about recovery, loss of verbal communication	Decreased anxiety: patient states anxiety is reduced, calm manner
Deficient Knowledge of Guillain-Barré syndrome and its treatment	Knowledge of Guillain-Barré syndrome and its treatment: patient confirms understanding and (if possible) demonstrates self-care

Interventions

Ineffective Breathing Patterns

About 25% of patients with Guillain-Barré syndrome need mechanical ventilation because of neuromuscular failure. Assess the patient's oxygenation status frequently. A respiratory rate greater than 30, abnormal chest and abdominal movements, and decreasing vital capacity signal increasingly ineffective breathing. Turn the patient at least every 2 hours and suction when indicated by increased pulse or adventitious breath sounds.

Decreased Cardiac Output

Be alert to rapid or slow cardiac dysrhythmias and administer antidysrhythmic drugs as ordered.

Risk for Disuse Syndrome

Immobility is a major issue to address in the patient with Guillain-Barré syndrome. If mobility is severely impaired, the patient is at high risk for disuse syndrome. These patients generally benefit from the use of rotational bed therapy to help promote pulmonary hygiene, peristalsis, and urinary bladder emptying. Careful positioning is crucial, with emphasis on maintaining joint function, muscle tone, and range of motion. Active and passive exercises, splints, and continuous passive motion machines may be used to prevent contractures.

Risk for Injury

Progressive weakness makes the patient susceptible to falls. When the patient is in bed, raise the side rails, place the call bell within reach, and put the bed in low position. If the eyes do not close completely, apply ophthalmic drops or ointments as ordered. A moisture chamber for the eye is used to prevent eye injury from excessive drying. Carefully inspect the skin, especially areas without sensation, to detect pressure or injury.

Imbalanced Nutrition: Less than Body Requirements

Impaired swallowing or the presence of an endotracheal tube mandates an alternative means of feeding. Enteral feedings are usually provided by way of a gastrostomy or nasoduodenal tube. Feedings may be given continuously or intermittently. Elevate the head of the bed 30 degrees during feedings to reduce the risk of aspiration. Aspirate and measure the residual (amount of feeding remaining in the stomach) at intervals to assess emptying of the stomach and prevent overfilling. In some cases, total parenteral nutrition may be employed.

Anxiety

Anxiety is understandable with progressive paralysis and increasing dependence on others for basic needs. You must work to develop trust and establish a therapeutic relationship with the patient. If the patient is able to speak, encourage discussion of thoughts, fears, and feelings. Explore previously used coping strategies. To promote some sense of control, give the patient some choices about aspects of care. Explain equipment and procedures to the patient. Other strategies to reduce anxiety include the use of imagery, music, deep breathing (if possible), and controlling anxiety-producing thoughts. Boredom is a problem that must be considered for the patient with Guillain-Barré syndrome. Orienting devices such as clocks, calendars, and daily schedules are helpful. The patient may enjoy television, radio, tapes, and visits from friends and family.

One source of anxiety for many patients is impaired communication. While the patient is able to speak, establish a system of communication such as blinking (one blink means yes, two blinks mean no) or a communication board. Then, if the condition does affect speech or if mechanical ventilation is required, the patient will have a simple means of expression.

Deficient Knowledge

From admission through rehabilitation, the patient with Guillain-Barré syndrome needs education about the condition and its usual course. Patients can deal with the condition better if they know how the symptoms progress, and that reversal and improvement are expected.

Rehabilitation

As function is restored, emphasis is placed on both respiratory and physical rehabilitation. Total recovery of respiratory function determines how quickly physical rehabilitation can begin. Once rehabilitation is initiated, attention must be devoted to maximizing motor function through exercises and occupational therapy. Because complete recovery may take several years, a prolonged rehabilitation period is sometimes necessary. Before the patient is discharged from the hospital, referrals may be made to rehabilitation or home health agencies as appropriate. The patient and family may benefit from a support group for people with long-term or chronic illnesses. The Guillain-Barré Foundation is a source of information

Consider the Alternative!

Strategies to reduce anxiety include music therapy and massage. The herb valerian is used by some people to reduce anxiety and promote rest.

(telephone number: 1-610-667-0131; website http://www.guillain-barre.com).

PARKINSON'S SYNDROME

Parkinson's syndrome is a progressive degenerative disorder of the basal ganglia that results in an eventual loss of coordination and control over involuntary motor movement. It is generally recognized as a disease of the elderly, first appearing in individuals in their fifties, with men affected more often than women. Idiopathic Parkinson's syndrome has no known cause but is related to decreased levels of dopamine in the basal ganglia. A deficiency of dopamine, a neurotransmitter, contributes to the loss of motor function. Other types of parkinsonism are caused by atherosclerosis, the long-term use of phenothiazines, and some toxins.

Signs and Symptoms

Several symptoms are characteristic of Parkinson's syndrome. The major triad of symptoms is tremor, rigidity, and bradykinesia. Tremor is a trembling or shaking type of movement most often seen in the upper extremities of the patient with Parkinson's syndrome. Tremors are more pronounced during resting postures and often relieved by movement. Typically they disappear during sleep. A movement associated with the tremor is pill rolling, in which the tremor repetitively moves the individual's thumb against the fingertips as if rolling a small object. Rigidity is stiffness, and bradykinesia refers to extremely slow movements. Other signs and symptoms are loss of dexterity and power in affected limbs, aching, monotone voice, handwriting changes, drooling, lack of facial expression, rhythmic head nodding, reduced blinking, and slumped posture. Those with advanced disease demonstrate cogwheel rigidity (jerky movements with passive muscle stretching) and gait disturbances. The individual may appear to freeze and may have difficulty initiating the action of walking. Depression is common, and dementia develops in some patients. Figure 26-17 illustrates the typical facial appearance, posture, and gait of individuals with Parkinson's syndrome.

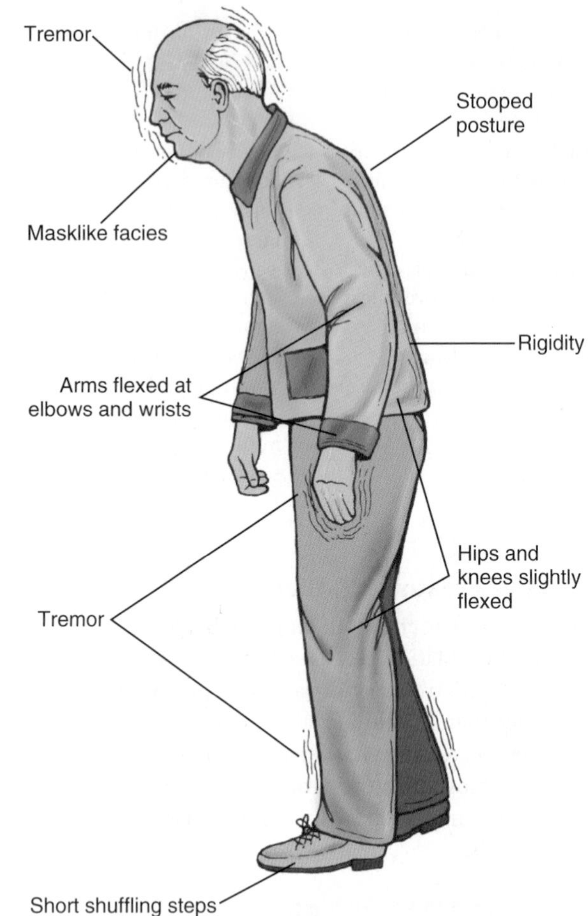

FIGURE **26-17** Clinical manifestations of Parkinson's syndrome.

Medical Diagnosis

Parkinson's syndrome is diagnosed from the health history and the physical examination results. MRI may be done to rule out other causes of the symptoms.

Medical Treatment

Management of the patient with Parkinson's syndrome is directed toward controlling the symptoms with physical therapy and drug therapy. The most beneficial physical therapy programs incorporate massage, heat, exercise, and gait retraining. Speech therapy has been tried, but results have generally not been encouraging.

Drug therapy relieves many of the symptoms of the disease. The cornerstone of therapy is the use of L-dopa (l-dihydroxyphenylalanine). L-dopa can cross the blood-brain barrier and is converted to dopamine in the basal ganglia, thereby supplementing levels of the neurotransmitter and reducing the symptoms of the disease. The conversion of L-dopa to dopamine must occur in the basal ganglia and not in the peripheral tissue. To ensure this, inhibitors are administered to prevent the breakdown of L-dopa by decarboxylase enzymes. The decarboxylase inhibitor most commonly used is carbidopa (Sinemet). When the two drugs are used in combination, therapeutic levels may be achieved with lower dosages. Because the benefits of L-dopa tend to decline after about 2 years, various other drug combinations may be used in an effort to control symptoms. A newer agent that is being used in combination with L-dopa is selegiline hydrochloride (Eldepryl). Selegeline extends the duration of action of L-dopa and may actually slow the progression of the disease.

Anticholinergic drugs such as trihexyphenidyl (Artane) may be used in patients who have less severe symptoms or who are unresponsive to L-dopa. These are useful in managing tremors, rigidity, or cramping. Although the exact mechanism of action is unclear, amantadine (Symmetrel), an antiviral compound, also is used in the management of Parkinson's syndrome. Amantadine is thought to release dopamine from storage sites in the neurons. It is often used in combination with L-dopa.

Treatment for depression may include antidepressant drug therapy, psychotherapy, and electroconvulsive therapy.

Additional information about drug therapy is presented in Table 26-6.

Several surgical procedures, among them thalamotomy, thalamic stimulation, and pallidotomy, may be used to treat parkinsonism, although the benefits are variable. Surgical implantation of fetal dopamine-producing cells continues to be done experimentally. Adrenal medullary transplant entails implantation of the patient's own adrenal cells into the brain. It has produced limited improvement in some patients and is not widely accepted. All of these surgical procedures are considered palliative rather than curative.

Put on your THINKING CAP!!

Write a short teaching plan for a home health patient who has started taking selegiline (Eldepryl) for Parkinson's syndrome.

NURSING CARE *of the Patient with Parkinson's Syndrome*

Nursing management for the patient with Parkinson's syndrome is primarily related to maintaining mobility and preventing injury.

Assessment

The complete neurologic assessment is summarized in Table 26-3. The health history of a patient with Parkinson's syndrome should specifically include assessment for weakness, fatigue, muscle cramps, sweating, dysphagia, constipation, difficulty voiding, and unusual movements. Describe the effects of the disease on the patient's life. During the physical examination, be alert for lack of facial expression, eyes fixed in one direction, drooling, slurred speech, tearing, tremors, muscle stiffness, and poor balance and coordination.

Nursing Diagnoses, Goals, and Outcome Criteria: Parkinson's Syndrome

Nursing Diagnoses	Goals and Outcome Criteria
Impaired Physical Mobility and **Self-Care Deficit** related to neuromuscular disease	Maximum possible self-care: patient participates in prescribed exercise program and performs self-care within abilities
Risk for Injury related to poor balance and coordination	Absence of injury: no bruises, lacerations, or fractures due to trauma
Impaired Nutrition: Less than Body Requirements related to dysphagia, difficulty with self-feeding	Adequate nutritional intake: stable body weight
Ineffective Coping related to physical changes and effects of disease on lifestyle	Effective coping with disease effects: patient makes statements confirming ability to deal with condition, adheres to plan of care
Noncompliance related to lack of understanding of disease, management, and self-care	Compliance with the prescribed plan of care: patient correctly describes and adheres to drug therapy, demonstrates exercise routine, uses resources, adapts to continue self-care

As the disease progresses, the patient becomes more immobilized, requiring additional nursing diagnoses, as addressed in Chapter 20.

Interventions

Impaired Physical Mobility

Assess the patient's mobility and ability to perform self-care. Provide assistance as needed, but encourage the patient to remain as independent in self-care as possible. Assistive devices, including walkers and wheelchairs, may enable the patient to be mobile despite some deterioration in coordination and balance. Stress the value of exercise in maintaining strength and mobility. Active and passive range-of-motion exercises may be done. Both the physical therapist and the occupational therapist may participate in designing programs to maintain or improve function.

Suggestions to improve mobility with Parkinson's syndrome include:

- Scoot to the edge of a chair before trying to stand.
- Use satin sheets to make it easier to move in and out of bed.
- March in place before starting to walk.
- Practice lifting the foot as if to step over an object on the floor to initiate walking.

Risk for Injury

The patient with Parkinson's syndrome is at special risk for injury related to falls. Place the call button within easy reach and instruct the patient to call for assistance when getting up. If the patient is ambulatory, remove obstacles on the floor. Recommend firm shoes, which provide better support than soft slippers. Provide assistive devices (canes, walkers, wheelchairs) as needed. Allow the patient to move at his or her own speed to decrease the risk of injury. Because this is a chronic condition, the patient's home setting should be evaluated and adapted for safe ambulation.

Imbalanced Nutrition: Less than Body Requirements

To promote ease of swallowing, position the patient comfortably for meals, with the head elevated and food conveniently arranged. Provide assistance as needed. It may involve only cutting meat and opening containers or may entail actually feeding the patient. Do not rush patients while they are eating. If the patient chokes on liquids, consult the dietitian about the need for semisolids and thick liquids, which are often easier to swallow. Thickening agents can be added to thin fluids to facilitate swallowing. Small, frequent meals may be

Consider the Alternative!

St. John's wort is used widely as an antidepressant. It is an MAO inhibitor and can interact with prescribed drugs. Ask the patient to report use of herbal remedies to the physician. Other measures to treat depression are physical exercise, massage, and light therapy.

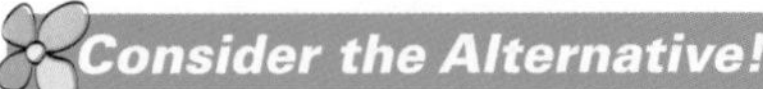

Consider the Alternative!

Caution patients with Parkinsons not to use herbal supplements without physician approval. Kava can worsen symptoms of Parkinson's syndrome. Chaste tree fruit interferes with the drug selegiline. Indian snakeroot interferes with the actions of levodopa and carbidopa.

better tolerated than three large ones. Monitor the patient's weight to assess the adequacy of nutritional intake. Some researchers believe that Parkinson's patients benefit from a low-protein diet during the day and an evening meal high in protein, but this is still experimental.

Ineffective Coping

Patients with Parkinson's syndrome must deal with loss of mobility that may affect their jobs, home and family responsibilities, social relationships, and leisure activities. Voice changes may severely impair verbal communication. Explore how the patient is dealing with these changes. Nurses and other members of the health care team help the patient identify strategies to adapt to changing abilities. Be alert to expressions of depression and inform the physician of such findings. A referral may be made to a mental health counselor, clinical nurse specialist, or support group. Administer antidepressant drugs as ordered and monitor their effects.

Deficient Knowledge

Management of this progressive condition requires the patient or a caregiver to be knowledgeable about Parkinson's syndrome and how it is treated. Supplement information with written material.

PATIENT TEACHING PLAN
Parkinson's Syndrome

- Drugs relieve symptoms but do not cure Parkinson's. You must continue therapy as prescribed to control symptoms.
- Know your drug names, dosages, schedule, and adverse effects that should be reported to your physician.
- Exercise is essential to maintain mobility.
- Resources: American Parkinson Disease Association (1-800-223-2732); Parkinson's Disease Foundation (1-222-923-4700, website: http://www.parkinsons-foundation.org); National Parkinson Foundation, Inc. (1-800-327-4545), website: http://www.parkinson.org)

MULTIPLE SCLEROSIS

A chronic, progressive degenerative disease, multiple sclerosis (MS) attacks the protective myelin sheath around axons and disrupts the conduction of impulses through the CNS (Fig. 26-18). It may affect motor, sensory, cerebellar, and other pathways. The course of the disease is variable. It may follow one of four patterns. The disease may progress steadily (chronic, progressive MS); may be characterized by exacerbations and remissions (exacerbating-remitting MS); may have less stable periods than exacerbating-remitting (relapsing-progressive MS); or may become stable with no active disease for at least a year (stable MS). MS is the second most common neurologic cause of disability. The incidence is highest in persons between 20 and 40 years of age, and affects women more often than men.

Etiology

Although the exact cause of MS is unknown, viral infections and autoimmune processes have been implicated. Some studies have implicated a retrovirus in the disease process, but more research is needed to determine whether this is indeed the cause of MS. The myelin sheath surrounding the axons is destroyed, eventually leaving areas of sclerotic tissues (Fig. 26-18). As the sclerotic tissue develops, the patient may have a period of remission. The involved fibers eventually degenerate, resulting in permanent damage. Nerve impulses, then, are no longer able to travel down the affected axon.

Signs and Symptoms

Because the exact pattern of damage varies from patient to patient, the signs and symptoms are varied as well. The most common symptoms of MS are fatigue, weakness and tingling in one or more extremities, visual disturbances, problems with coordination, bowel and bladder dysfunction, spasticity, and depression.

For patients who have exacerbating-remitting MS, the progression is variable. As the disease progresses, the periods of remission become shorter and the neurologic deficits present during exacerbations become more severe and permanent.

Medical Diagnosis

The diagnosis of MS is based primarily on the physical examination and history of cyclic remission-exacerbation periods. A familial history of the disease is significant, as is worsening of symptoms when the patient is exposed to warm weather. Magnetic resonance imaging of the brain and spinal cord may reveal plaques characteristic of MS.

Medical Treatment

Because of its chronic, progressive nature, the treatment of MS is symptomatic and supportive. Drug therapy during pe-

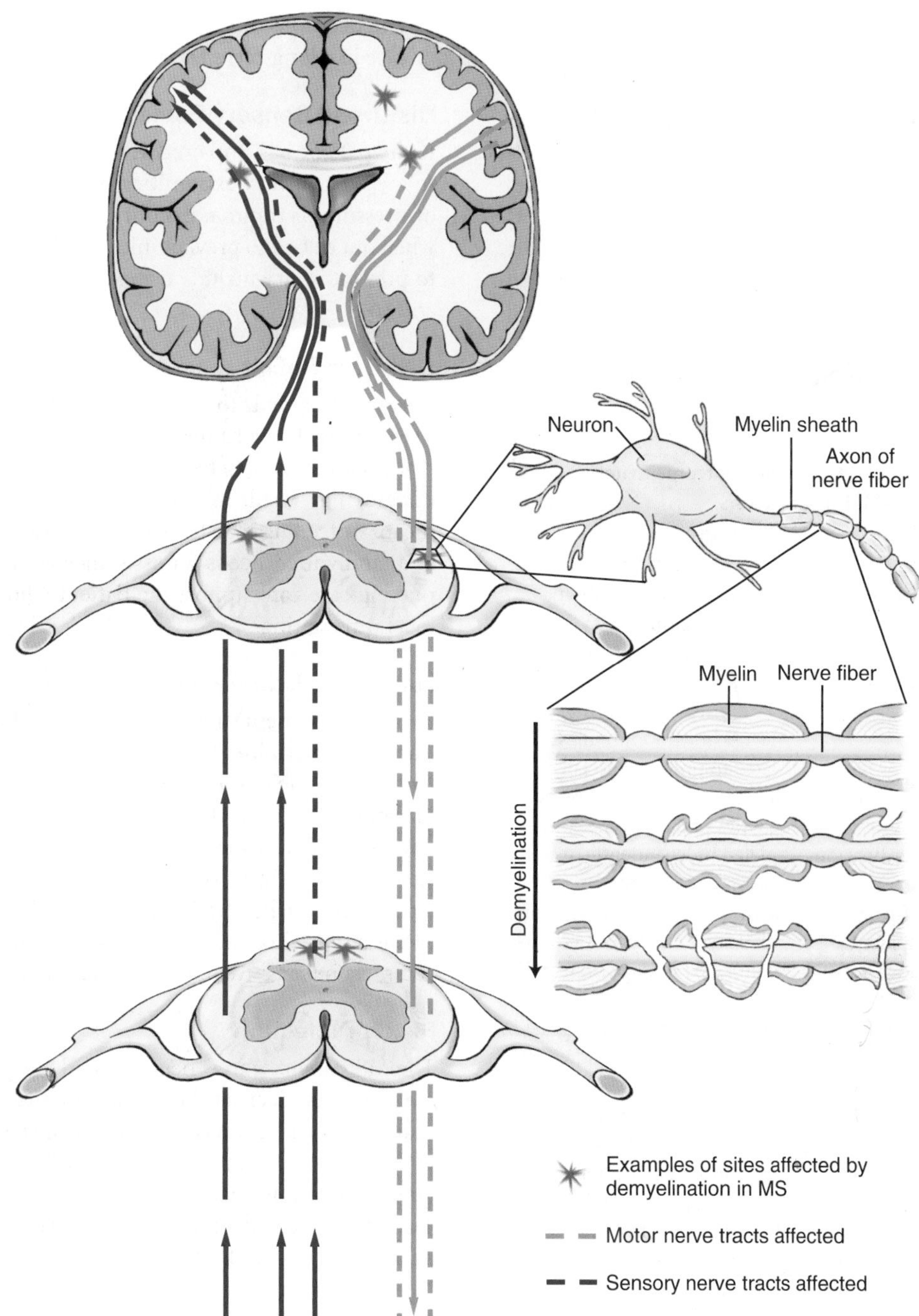

FIGURE **26-18** The lesions in multiple sclerosis: location and effects.

riods of exacerbation may involve administration of adrenocorticotropic hormone. Prednisone may be used to control exacerbations, but it does not slow the progression of the disease. Treatment often includes drugs that modulate the immune response. The specific drug will depend on the type of MS. Drugs in this category include interferon 1B (Betaseron) and interferon 1A (Avonex); glutiamer acetate (Copaxone); and mitoxantrone (Novantrone). The spasticity experienced by MS patients may respond to treatment with baclofen (Lioresal) or tizanidine (Zanaflex). Carbamazepine (Tegretol) and gabapentin (Neurontin) are used to relieve neuropathic pain. Amantadine (Symmetrel) is used to relieve fatigue associated with the disease. Immunosuppressive agents may be used, but these carry the risk of bone marrow suppression and must be carefully monitored. Electrical neuromuscular stimulation is being used to decrease spasticity and improve active movement and function, but studies of its effectiveness have not found consistent evidence of improvement.

NURSING CARE *of the Patient with Multiple Sclerosis*

Assessment

Complete assessment of the patient with a neurologic disorder is summarized in Table 26-3. When a patient has MS, the health history specifically includes the onset and progression of symptoms, especially those that affect mobility, vision, eating, and elimination. Explore the effects of the disease on the person's lifestyle. Identify the patient's usual coping strategies. Important aspects of the physical examination are evaluation of range of motion and strength and observation for gait abnormalities, tremors, and muscle spasms.

Nursing Diagnoses, Goals, and Outcome Criteria: Multiple Sclerosis

Nursing Diagnoses	Goals and Outcome Criteria
Impaired Physical Mobility related to weakness or spasticity	Maximal possible mobility: patient continues physical activity within capabilities
Disturbed Sensory Perceptions related to neurologic impairment	Absence of injury associated with impaired sensation: intact skin without redness related to pressure, no falls
Self-Care Deficit related to impaired voluntary movements and poor coordination	Achievement of self-care: activities of daily living completed independently or with assistance as needed
Functional Urinary Incontinence related to impaired conduction of bladder nerve impulses	Absence of bladder distention: bladder not palpable, no uncontrolled passage of urine
Risk for Infection related to inadequate resistance	Absence of infection: normal body temperature and white blood cell count
Ineffective Coping related to chronic illness, uncertain course of disease	Adaptation to changes in physical functioning: behavior and statements reflect intent to maximize abilities
Deficient Knowledge of disease, treatment, and self-care	Patient understands disease, treatment, and self-care: patient accurately describes MS, its treatment, and self-care measures to reduce risk of complications

Interventions

Impaired Physical Mobility

Encourage the patient to be as independent as possible. Provide assistance with ambulation as needed. A cane or walker may enable the patient to walk safely. If the patient has muscle spasms, administer muscle relaxants as ordered. Perform range-of-motion exercises to prevent contractures, and teach a caregiver to do the exercises. Physical therapy may be ordered. The patient who is not able to move independently is at risk for disuse syndrome. Care of the immobile patient is covered in Chapter 20. If the patient becomes disabled to this extent, decisions must be made about home nursing services or care in a long-term facility.

Disturbed Sensory Perceptions

If the patient has impaired sensation, give special attention to the skin. Inspect extremities and pressure points for signs of pressure or trauma. Encourage the patient to wear shoes when out of bed to prevent injury. Other measures instituted to prevent injury include using caution with sources of heat and cold.

Self-Care Deficit

Encourage patients to do as much as they can for themselves. Provide assistance as needed to carry out activities of daily living. Difficulty with feedings, especially if the patient is dysphagic, may result in inadequate food intake. Alternative means of feeding may be necessary. Discuss with the patient and family their needs for assistance with caregiving. Home nursing care can support the patient who wishes to remain in a home setting.

Functional Urinary Incontinence

Palpate the patient's lower abdomen for bladder distention. Carry out intermittent catheterization as ordered. If urine retention is a problem, assess the patient for signs and symptoms of urinary tract infection: fever, burning on urination, foul odor, sediment. If the patient has urinary incontinence, take steps to reduce the incontinent episodes as described in Chapter 22. Incontinence briefs may be needed, and meticulous skin care is a must. Loss of bladder control is very distressing, and you must be sensitive in helping the patient deal with it.

Risk for Infection

The MS patient who is being treated with immunosuppressive drugs has decreased resistance to infection. Take steps to reduce the risk of infection. Protect the patient from people with infections. Encourage intake of fluids to maintain adequate hydration, and emphasize good hygiene practices. Teach the patient and family the signs of infection that should be reported promptly to the physician.

Ineffective Coping

Multiple sclerosis is a chronic, progressive disease. Patients have increasing disability, requiring considerable adaptation. Because the initial symptoms typically occur in young adults, patients must often learn to balance work, home, and family responsibilities. Provide the patient opportunities to talk about the illness and its effects. Be accepting of the patient's concerns and guide the patient to identify strengths, abilities, and usual coping strategies. With the patient's permission, a referral may be made to the clinical nurse specialist, mental health counselor, or spiritual counselor. Support groups can be helpful to many patients and their families.

Deficient Knowledge

Assess what the patient knows about MS and what he or she would like to know. The teaching plan is individualized to the

Consider the Alternative!

Imagery, breathing exercises, and progressive relaxation can help the MS patient reduce stress. Various specials diets and nutritional supplements (commonly fatty acids, niacin, zinc, magnesium, selenium, beta carotene, and vitamins C, B_6, and B_{12}) have been proposed, but research has not consistently shown benefits to the MS patient.

patient's needs and may include problems associated with immobility and measures to prevent complications.

AMYOTROPHIC LATERAL SCLEROSIS

Etiology

Amyotrophic lateral sclerosis (ALS), also known as Lou Gehrig's disease, is a degenerative neurologic disease. It affects males two to four times as often as females and strikes most often in the populace in those between 40 and 70 years of age. The disease generally progresses rapidly, and death ensues approximately 3 years after the onset of symptoms. Although a viral cause has been suspected, the exact cause is unknown.

Pathophysiology

In ALS, there is degeneration of the anterior horn cells and the corticospinal tracts, so the patient exhibits both upper and lower motor neuron symptoms. Evidence of upper motor neuron disease includes spasticity and hyperreflexia. Lower motor neuron disease is demonstrated by weakness, atrophy, cramps, and muscle twitching. Some patients have difficulty swallowing and slurred speech. Despite involvement of the motor nuclei of the brain stem, intellectual ability, sensory perception, vision, and hearing are all unaffected.

Signs and Symptoms

Initially, the patient exhibits weakness of voluntary muscles of the upper extremities, particularly the hands. In addition, some patients may experience difficulty swallowing and speaking, because of progressive weakness of the oropharyngeal muscles. Spasticity of the involved muscle groups may be evident. The disease progresses steadily until the patient is completely incapacitated. Eventually, respirations become shallow and the patient has difficulty clearing the airway of pulmonary secretions. Death results from aspiration, respiratory infection, or respiratory failure.

Medical Diagnosis

The patient's history and physical examination findings lead to the diagnosis of ALS. Electromyography provides supporting evidence of impaired impulse conduction in the muscles. More sophisticated tests are used to rule out other degenerative motor diseases such as MS or myasthenia gravis.

Medical Treatment

Because there is no known cure or treatment for ALS, therapy is supportive, focusing on the prevention of complications and the maintenance of maximum function.

NURSING CARE *of the Patient with Amyotrophic Lateral Sclerosis*

Assessment

The complete neurologic assessment is outlined in Table 26-3. When a patient has ALS, the nurse's history assessment of the patient determines the presence of dyspnea, dysphagia, muscle cramps, weakness, twitching, and joint stiffness. Describe the effects of the disease on the patient's lifestyle. During the physical examination, anticipate finding weakness, muscle atrophy, abnormal reflexes and gait, and paralysis.

Nursing Diagnoses, Goals, and Outcome Criteria: ALS

Nursing Diagnoses	Goals and Outcome Criteria
Ineffective Airway Clearance related to paralysis of respiratory muscles	Patent airway: respiratory rate of 12 to 20 without crackles or wheezes
Impaired Physical Mobility related to progressive weakness and atrophy	Maximal possible mobility: patient participates in activities to maintain joint mobility
Imbalanced Nutrition: Less than Body Requirements related to dysphagia	Adequate nutritional intake: stable body weight
Impaired Verbal Communications related to oropharyngeal muscle weakness	Effective communication: patient conveys needs without excessive frustration
Impaired Skin Integrity related to immobility	Normal skin integrity: intact skin without signs of pressure (redness, blanching)
Anticipatory Grieving related to progressive, fatal disease	Adaptation to losses: patient verbalizes losses, their importance, and acceptance of losses; makes realistic plans
Situational Low Self-Esteem related to loss of independence	Stable or improved self-esteem: patient makes positive statements about self
Interrupted Family Processes related to progressive illness of patient	Family adapts to patient condition: positive family communication and interactions, patient's role shifted

Interventions

Ineffective Airway Clearance

Monitor the patient's respiratory rate and effort, breath sounds, and pulse rate to detect inadequate oxygenation. Instruct or assist the immobile patient in turning, coughing, and deep breathing at least every 2 hours. Chest physiotherapy may be ordered to mobilize secretions to prevent atelectasis and pneumonia. If the patient has difficulty removing secretions, gentle suction may be needed. Oxygen therapy is indicated if there is evidence of hypoxia (restlessness, tachycardia).

Impaired Physical Mobility

Progressive muscle wasting, spasticity, and paralysis cause increasing immobility. Perform active or passive range-of-motion exercises to prevent contractures. Give antispasmodic drugs as ordered. Maintain extremities in functional positions. Encourage use of assistive devices (cane, walker, wheelchair) as needed to maintain mobility as long as possible. Monitor the patient's ability to perform activities of daily living and provide assistance as needed. The patient who is immobile is at high risk for complications of immobility. Nursing care of the immobile patient is covered in Chapter 20.

Imbalanced Nutrition: Less than Body Requirements

Muscle weakness and cranial nerve involvement eventually make it difficult for the patient to consume adequate food for good nutrition. Monitor the patient's weight to assess adequacy of the diet. Meals may be supplemented with high-protein snacks. Recommend high-fiber foods if the patient can eat them because constipation is a common problem. Adequate fluids are needed but may be difficult to swallow. The patient may be able to increase fluid intake by eating semisolids such as ice cream, milk shakes, or gelatin desserts.

The patient with ALS is at risk for aspiration because of impaired swallowing. While the patient is eating, the head of the bed must be elevated or the patient must be seated in a chair. Consult the dietitian about providing a diet of the appropriate texture for the patient. Arrange dietary instruction for any caregivers who might be involved in preparing foods for the patient. A speech therapist can recommend techniques to facilitate swallowing. Eventually, oral intake becomes inadequate. The decision to insert a feeding tube should be based on the desires of the patient and family. If a feeding tube is in place, administer feedings and monitor for tube placement and residual. Teach the family or other caregivers how to do the feedings.

Impaired Verbal Communication

Speech becomes impaired by muscle weakness and dyspnea. You need to establish alternatives to verbal communication. These might include the use of blinks or gestures, or the use of boards with pictures, words, or letters that the patient can select. Use questions that can be answered with "yes" or "no," and allow the patient time to respond.

Impaired Skin Integrity

Muscle wasting, incontinence, and immobility put these patients at risk for skin breakdown. Reposition them at least every 2 hours, and inspect bony prominences for redness. Special beds that alternate or distribute pressure may be used. Promptly change wet or soiled clothing to avoid skin irritation. Meticulous skin care is essential. Once again, if the patient will be cared for at home, be sure caregivers are able to care for the skin.

Anticipatory Grieving

Once the implications of a diagnosis of ALS are understood, patients and their families may begin the grieving process. Encourage patients to talk, listen compassionately, and help them make realistic plans. Remember the stages of grief and be understanding when patients and families show anger, denial, and depression. Referrals to visiting nurse agencies and hospice services can provide needed emotional and physical support at various times in the progress of the disease.

Situational Low Self-Esteem

Explore the patient's thoughts, feelings, and concerns about living with this progressive, terminal disease. Although it is difficult not to offer false reassurance, let the patient ventilate, cry, or express anger. Stress the patient's strengths, abilities, and contributions. Identify and enlist sources of support (family, friends, support groups, spiritual counselors, therapists). Stress-reducing techniques include imagery, breathing exercises, and progressive relaxation. Preserve the patient's dignity by providing privacy during personal care and by helping the patient attend to grooming and appearance.

Interrupted Family Processes

The disease is painful for both the patient and the family as it steadily takes its toll. Patients with ALS are often middle-aged, with family responsibilities, jobs, and places in the community. The family must plan for transfer of responsibilities and care of the patient when he or she becomes disabled. Issues that need to be discussed are patient feelings about advance directives, insurance, and wills. These topics may be difficult for them to address but are best handled while the patient can participate. Care of the dying patient is covered in Chapter 23.

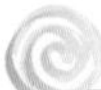

What Does Culture Have to do with Incurable Illness?

Patients facing progressive, incurable illness may find comfort in religious symbols, charms, incense, candles, and native healers.

HUNTINGTON'S DISEASE

Huntington's disease is an inherited degenerative neurologic disorder. It usually begins in middle adulthood with abnormal movements, emotional disturbance, and intellectual decline. Symptoms progress steadily, with increasing disability and death in 15 to 20 years. Medical and nursing care are supportive only; there is no cure.

MYASTHENIA GRAVIS

Myasthenia gravis is a chronic, progressive disease in which there is a defect at the neuromuscular junction, where electrical impulses are transmitted to muscle tissue.

Etiology

There is evidence that myasthenia gravis may have an autoimmune basis. Some patients present with an increase in the titer of acetylcholine receptor antibody. The presence of these antibodies interferes with the normal activity at the acetylcholine receptor sites and reduces muscle strength.

Pathophysiology

Normally, as a nerve impulse travels down a peripheral nerve, the neurotransmitter acetylcholine is released at the presynaptic membrane (Fig. 26-19). The impulse is then transmitted

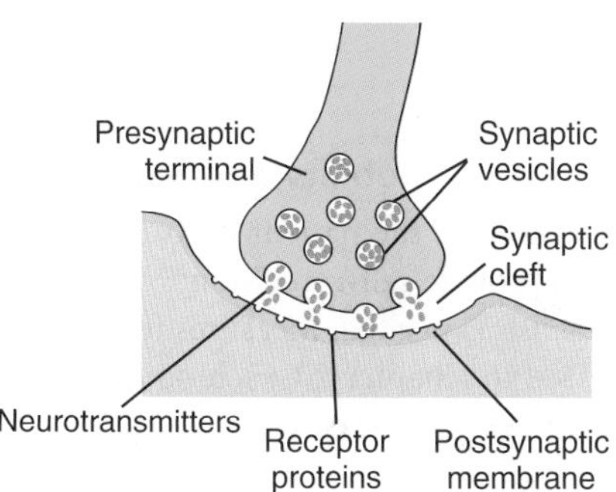

FIGURE **26-19** Neurotransmitters (norepinephrine, acetylcholine, dopamine) are released from the axon, travel across the synaptic cleft, and produce some response in the receptors of target cells.

across the synaptic junction to postsynaptic receptor sites on the effector muscle. This causes contraction of the involved muscle.

In myasthenia gravis, there are insufficient receptor sites at the junction of the motor nerve with the muscle. With repeated stimulation, the muscle becomes exhausted and is eventually unable to contract at all. If respiratory muscles become involved, death from respiratory insufficiency or arrest is a possibility.

Signs and Symptoms

Myasthenia gravis is characterized by the following features: weakness of voluntary muscles, particularly those of chewing, swallowing, and speaking; partial improvements of strength with rest; and dramatic improvement with the use of anticholinesterase drugs.

The onset of symptoms is gradual, and early weakness may be so subtle that it goes unnoticed. Muscles responsible for fine movements, such as eye, facial, or hand muscles, are often affected early in the disease process. Ptosis and diplopia are commonly seen. The patient becomes unable to perform any activity that demands sustained muscular contractions, such as brushing the hair, walking upstairs, or holding the hands over the head. The fatigue may abate with rest but rapidly returns when the activity is tried again. If the diaphragm or intercostal muscles are involved, breathing is compromised.

Medical Diagnosis

The diagnosis is made by administering edrophonium (Tensilon). This is an anticholinesterase agent that increases the relative amount of acetylcholine in the neuromuscular junction by destroying acetylcholinesterase. In the patient with myasthenia gravis, muscle tone is markedly improved within 1 minute of injection, and this improvement persists for 4 to 5 minutes. The serum is tested for antiacetylcholine receptor antibodies. CT and MRI are performed to screen for thymoma.

Medical Treatment

Anticholinesterase Drugs

Therapy is primarily directed toward pharmacologic management with anticholinesterase agents and corticosteroids. Neostigmine and pyridostigmine (Mestinon) are anticholinesterase drugs that increase the availability of acetylcholine at the neuromuscular junction. Both drugs inhibit the action of cholinesterase, the enzyme that destroys acetylcholine. The availability of acetylcholine is improved, thereby enhancing muscle strength. Dosages are individualized for each patient, based on response and needs. Stress or sustained levels of activity can alter the need for these agents.

Neuromuscular blocking agents must be used very cautiously in the patient with myasthenia gravis.

Corticosteroids

Corticosteroids may be useful in those patients who do not respond well to the anticholinesterase agents. Adrenocorticotropic hormone or prednisone is administered concurrently with the anticholinesterase agent in an effort to induce remission. During the first 7 to 10 days of therapy, symptoms may worsen, requiring hospitalization to monitor for respiratory depression. With improvement, corticosteroids may be tapered and maintained at the lowest effective dose.

Cytotoxic Therapies

Cytotoxic therapies are useful in patients who are unable to significantly taper corticosteroids. Azathioprine and cyclosporine have been used in these cases.

Thymectomy

Because a large number of patients with myasthenia gravis have hyperplasia of the thymus gland, thymectomy is performed early after the initial diagnosis. Close monitoring is essential postoperatively because there is a risk of respiratory compromise because of possible pneumothorax. About 40% of patients enjoy some degree of remission after thymectomy.

Plasmapheresis

Plasmapheresis is an adjunctive therapy based on the autoimmune theory of myasthenia. It is a process of plasma exchange in which the acetylcholine receptor antibodies are washed from the plasma. A temporary catheter, similar to a renal dialysis access catheter, is used for venous access. Blood is then routed through a pheresis field, where the antibodies are separated from the plasma. The washed blood is then returned to the patient. The procedure takes 3 to 4 hours and is repeated over several days to ensure adequate treatment. Improvement in muscle strength may be noted within 24 to 48 hours after treatment. As progress is made with plasmapheresis, drug dosages may be decreased.

Myasthenic and Cholinergic Crises

Emergency respiratory support requiring mechanical ventilation may be necessary in the event of myasthenic or cholinergic crises. Myasthenic crisis is marked by a sudden exacerbation of myasthenic symptoms, including difficulty swallowing and breathing, with possible respiratory arrest. Infection often precipitates the event, and symptoms do not decrease even with higher doses of medications.

Cholinergic crisis presents with sudden, extreme weakness and respiratory impairment. It is precipitated by overmedication with anticholinesterase drugs, which literally bombard the receptor sites with excess amounts of acetylcholine. Intubation and mechanical ventilation are required to manage the respiratory compromise.

Because the two crises present similarly, differentiation is critical. Once again, edrophonium is used to distinguish the two entities. Rapid improvement in muscle strength after administration of edrophonium indicates an underlying myasthenic crisis. If no improvement is observed, the patient is experiencing a cholinergic crisis.

Because myasthenia gravis is a chronic neurologic disease, the patient is generally managed at home. However, hospitalization is likely on the initial diagnosis and during periods of crisis and respiratory compromise.

PHARMACOLOGY CAPSULE Edrophonium rapidly reverses a myasthenic crisis but has no effect on a cholinergic crisis.

NURSING CARE *of the Patient with Myasthenia Gravis*

Assessment

The complete neurologic assessment is outlined in Table 26-3. When the patient has myasthenia gravis, the health history describes the onset of symptoms, particularly muscle weakness, diplopia, dysphagia, slurred speech, breathing difficulties, and loss of balance. Record the effects of the condition on the patient's lifestyle. In the physical examination, evaluate muscle strength, balance, respiratory effort, and oxygenation status.

Nursing Diagnoses, Goals, and Outcome Criteria: Myasthenia Gravis

Nursing Diagnoses	Goals and Outcome Criteria
Ineffective Breathing Patterns related to impaired conduction of nerve impulses	Adequate oxygenation: respiratory rate of 12 to 20 per minute without dyspnea
Impaired Physical Mobility and Self-Care Deficit related to muscle weakness, fatigue	Improved mobility and self-care: performance of activities of daily living without excessive fatigue
Impaired Verbal Communication related to weakness of the muscles involved in speech	Effective communication: patient makes needs known
Impaired Swallowing related to muscle weakness	Adequate intake of fluids and food: stable body weight and absence of respiratory distress associated with aspiration
Deficient Knowledge of disease and treatment	Patient understands disease and treatment: patient accurately describes condition and treatment, follows plan of care

Interventions

Ineffective Breathing Patterns

You must monitor the patient for early signs and symptoms of ineffective breathing and hypoxia (tachycardia, restlessness). Progressive symptoms that do not respond to prescribed drug therapy may require mechanical ventilation. Management of the patient on a ventilator is discussed in Chapter 29.

Impaired Physical Mobility and Self-Care Deficit

Because of weakness, the patient may be relatively inactive and unable to provide self-care. Monitor the patient's capabilities and assist as needed. Measures to prevent complications, discussed in Chapter 20, include turning and repositioning at least every 2 hours.

Impaired Swallowing

Patients may have difficulty chewing and swallowing. Anticholinesterase drugs may be ordered 30 minutes before meals to improve muscle strength. Seat the patient upright for meals and allow or assist the patient to eat in an unhurried manner. Teach patients to rest their chins on the chest area when swallowing to help prevent aspiration. Small, frequent meals may be tolerated better than three large ones. A soft diet is usually ordered so that minimal chewing is required. If swallowing is severely impaired, a feeding tube may be inserted and liquid feedings given as ordered. Adequate fluid intake is important to maintain hydration and prevent constipation.

Deficient Knowledge

Patient teaching with myasthenia gravis is essential because this chronic condition requires lifelong treatment.

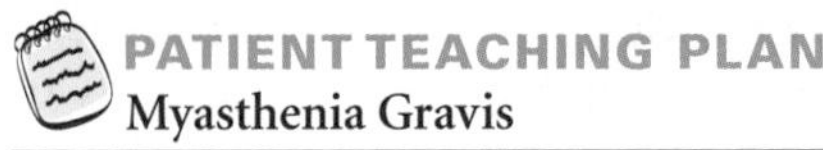

PATIENT TEACHING PLAN
Myasthenia Gravis

- Myasthenia gravis is a chronic disease that can be treated but not cured.
- You must know your drug names, dosages, schedule, side effects, and adverse effects that should be reported to the physician. It is very important to take the prescribed drugs on time.
- Myasthenic crisis indicates too little acetylcholine.
- Cholinergic crisis occurs when there is too much acetylcholine.
- Difficulty swallowing and breathing are symptoms of both types of crises, and each requires immediate medical treatment.
- You will need to adjust your routine based on your symptoms.
- A good source of information is the Myasthenia Gravis Foundation (1-800-541-5454; website: http://www.myasthenia.org), which may have a local chapter where you live.

TRIGEMINAL NEURALGIA (TIC DOULOUREUX)

Trigeminal **neuralgia** is characterized by intense pain along the distribution of one of the three branches of the trigeminal nerve (fifth cranial nerve): ophthalmic, mandibular, or maxillary (Fig. 26-20). The pain has an abrupt onset and is usually unilateral in nature, lasting from seconds to a few minutes. Despite the intense pain, there is no associated mo-

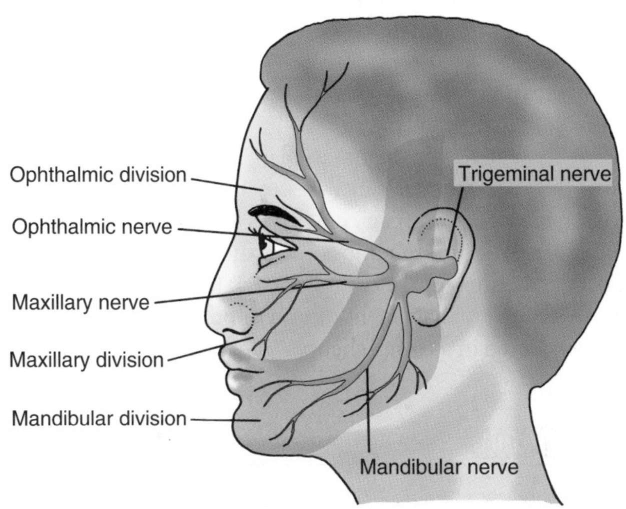

FIGURE **26-20** Distribution of the trigeminal nerve and its three divisions: ophthalmic, maxillary, and mandibular.

tor or sensory deficit. The pain may be crippling, restricting the patient's daily routine. Attacks may be triggered by ingestion of hot or cold liquids, chewing, shaving, or washing the face. Between episodes the patient may experience a dull ache or be pain free.

Etiology

Although the exact cause of trigeminal neuralgia is undetermined, various contributing factors can be identified. Trauma or infection may precipitate the characteristic pain, as may compression on the nerve by an aneurysm, artery, or tumor.

Medical Diagnosis

Because there is no specific test, the diagnosis is based on the history. Stimulation of certain trigger points may precipitate the pain.

Medical Treatment

Pharmacologic management is the preferable course of therapy. Phenytoin (Dilantin) and carbamazepine (Tegretol) are most commonly used to suppress the pain episodes. During the acute attack, alcohol or phenol may be injected into the affected branch of the trigeminal nerve, with pain relief lasting from 8 to 16 months.

Patients with the most severe, debilitating pain may undergo surgical intervention. Electrocoagulation, a procedure in which heated electrodes are used to destroy the sensory fibers of the nerve, is effective in providing lasting pain relief without compromising motor or tactile function.

NURSING CARE *of the Patient with Trigeminal Neuralgia*

Assessment

Assessment of the patient with trigeminal neuralgia focuses on describing the pain, factors that trigger it, and treatments found to be effective or ineffective. The effects of the condition on the patient's life are recorded.

Nursing Diagnoses, Goals, and Outcome Criteria: Trigeminal Neuralgia

Nursing Diagnoses	Goals and Outcome Criteria
Chronic Pain related to disease process	Reduced frequency and severity of attacks: patient reports attacks are less frequent and pain is lessened
Self-Care Deficit related to debilitating pain	Self-care activities accomplished: activities of daily living completed independently
Imbalanced Nutrition: Less than Body Requirements related to pain associated with chewing	Adequate nutrition: stable body weight
Fear related to anticipated painful episodes	Lessened fear: patient expresses less fear and greater confidence in ability to manage condition
Deficient Knowledge of trigeminal neuralgia and its treatment	Patient understands condition and treatment: patient accurately describes condition, prevention of episodes, and treatment

Interventions

The focus of nursing care for the patient with trigeminal neuralgia is pain assessment and management. It may be beneficial to assist the patient in developing alternative strategies for pain relief, such as guided imagery or relaxation therapy. Because of the debilitating nature of the pain, the patient may need assistance in performing self-care activities. Nutrition may be affected because chewing may trigger pain. Psychological effects are also a consideration in management because the fear of engaging in some activity that may trigger pain can lead to social isolation. Chapter 14 provides additional information about care of the patient in pain. Patient teaching emphasizes the nature of the condition and avoidance of factors that trigger episodes.

NEUROFIBROMATOSIS

Neurofibromatosis, also known as von Recklinghausen's disease, is characterized by multiple tumors of the peripheral, spinal, and cranial nerves. The tumors are benign but may be removed to relieve compression on the nerves or for cosmetic reasons. The patient also may have bone, muscle, and skin involvement.

BELL'S PALSY

Bell's palsy is acute paralysis of the seventh cranial nerve, which serves the face. The condition usually begins with pain behind the ear or on the face. The patient then has a drawing sensation followed by paralysis of the muscles on the affected side. The affected eyelids do not close, taste is impaired, and eating may be difficult. Most patients recover over a period of weeks or months, but some have residual weakness.

Bell's palsy is treated on an outpatient basis with prednisone and analgesics. Artificial tears are needed if the eyelids do not close, and the affected eye should be closed and an eye shield should be used on the affected eye at night to prevent drying of the cornea. When function begins to return, the patient can do simple exercises to improve muscle tone: grimacing, opening and closing the eye, whistling, and puffing out the cheeks. Be sensitive to the patient's concerns about the condition and his or her appearance.

CEREBRAL PALSY

Cerebral palsy is a paralysis associated with a loss in motor coordination caused by cerebral damage. Although the etiology is uncertain, the damage is generally believed to occur at birth and to be related to hypoxia, premature birth, or birth trauma.

Individuals with cerebral palsy are often frustrated by people who equate the disorder with mental retardation. Although the staggering gait and unclear speech may resemble a partial picture of a person with mental retardation, the individual with cerebral palsy is fully capable of comprehending his or her situation and is willing to strive for as much independence as possible.

Types of Cerebral Palsy

Three general types of cerebral palsy can be identified, based on symptoms: spastic paralysis, athetoid, and ataxic. Spastic paralysis is characterized by overall exaggerated reflexes and muscle spasms. Random, purposeless movement with extreme muscle tone is indicative of the athetoid type, whereas the ataxic variety is characterized by poor balance, an uncoordinated, staggering gait, and speech or vision defects.

Medical Treatment

Although there is no cure for cerebral palsy, early muscle training and exercises can be beneficial in an effort to prevent complications and promote optimal function. Orthopedic surgery, braces, and casts may be useful in limiting deformities and disabilities.

NURSING CARE *of the Patient with Cerebral Palsy*

Nursing care of the patient with cerebral palsy is covered in depth in pediatric nursing texts because it is typically a lifelong condition diagnosed in infancy. Therefore although many adults have cerebral palsy, it is not discussed in detail here.

POSTPOLIO SYNDROME

Before the advent of the polio vaccine, many people suffered varying degrees of motor impairment caused by the polio virus. Many years after having had the initial infection, some patients once again experience progressive muscle weakness, fatigue, pain, and respiratory problems typical of polio infections. The reason for the recurrence of symptoms is not known. Medical and nursing care are primarily supportive, aimed at helping the patient adapt to the symptoms and maintain maximum possible function.

SUMMARY

Management of the patient with a neurologic disorder can be demanding and challenging. Astute observation and assessment are vital to any treatment plan, and other therapies are often based on the nursing assessment. As is apparent from this chapter, many nursing diagnoses and modes of management are common to almost any patient with a neurologic disorder. Because of the complicated nature of many of these disorders, the management of other body systems also must be considered in a comprehensive care plan.

key points

- The functional unit of the nervous system is the neuron (nerve cell), which conducts electrical impulses from one area of the brain to another.
- The brain and the spinal cord compose the central nervous system, whereas the nerves in the peripheral parts of the body compose the peripheral nervous system.
- Cerebrospinal fluid circulates through the central nervous system.
- The neurologic assessment includes evaluation of the level of consciousness, pupillary size and response, coordination and balance, sensory function, reflexes, and vital signs.
- Increased intracranial pressure may impair cerebral tissue perfusion, resulting in ischemia and possibly respiratory arrest.
- Signs and symptoms of increased intracranial pressure and impaired cerebral blood flow are decreasing level of consciousness, pupil dilation with no response to light, motor deficits, abnormal posture, fever, increased blood pressure, bradycardia, and respiratory depression.
- Measures to decrease intracranial pressure include positioning, hyperventilation, fluid restriction, mechanical drainage, and drug therapy.
- Seizures are abnormal activity and behavior caused by abnormal electrical impulses in the brain that may be treated with anticonvulsant therapy and, when possible, measures to correct the cause.
- Nursing care of the patient with a seizure disorder addresses Risk for Injury, Ineffective Coping, and Deficient Knowledge.
- Nursing care of the patient with a head injury may focus on Altered Tissue Perfusion, Ineffective Breathing Pattern, Risk for Injury, Risk for Infection, Impaired Physical Mobility, Disturbed Body Image, and Altered Role Performance.
- Meningitis and encephalitis are infections of the nervous system.
- Guillain-Barré syndrome, thought to be an autoimmune response to a viral infection, is characterized by progressive ascending neurologic deficits that, in most cases, eventually resolve.
- Nursing care of the patient with Guillain-Barré syndrome addresses Ineffective Breathing Patterns, Decreased Cardiac Output, Risk for Disuse Syndrome, Imbalanced

Nutrition, Risk for Injury, Anxiety, and Deficient Knowledge.

- Parkinson's syndrome, a progressive disorder that results in loss of coordination and control over involuntary movement, is treated with physical therapy and drugs that increase dopamine levels in the brain.
- The focus of nursing care for the patient with Parkinson's syndrome is Impaired Physical Mobility, Risk for Injury, Imbalanced Nutrition, Ineffective Coping, and Deficient Knowledge.
- Multiple sclerosis is a progressive degenerative disease that disrupts the motor pathways of the central nervous system that may lead to severe neurologic disabilities.
- Amyotrophic lateral sclerosis is a rapidly progressive degenerative disease that usually results in death from respiratory complications within 3 years.
- The patient with amyotrophic lateral sclerosis has increasing needs for nursing care, eventually becoming completely dependent for all aspects of care.
- Myasthenia gravis is caused by a defect in impulse conduction that is manifested as weakness of voluntary muscles and is treated with anticholinesterase drugs and corticosteroids.
- Trigeminal neuralgia is intense pain along a branch of the trigeminal nerve that may be treated with drug therapy or surgical intervention.
- Cerebral palsy is associated with a loss in motor coordination caused by cerebral damage.

REVIEW QUESTIONS

1. The known neurotransmitters include acetylcholine, norepinephrine, epinephrine, and:
   1. dopamine.
   2. acetylcholinesterase.
   3. dendrites.
   4. interneurons.
2. Which statement best describes normal aging of the neurologic system?
   1. The size of neurons increases to make up for the loss in number of neurons.
   2. Decreasing lipofuscin and amyloid slow the transmission of impulses.
   3. Despite loss of neurons, most older people retain normal cognition.
   4. By age 80, only the Achilles tendon jerk reflex remains intact.
3. A patient who is being treated for a closed head injury is lying still and appears to be sleeping even in the noisy emergency room. When you shake his shoulder and call his name, he opens his eyes and says, "huh?" Then he closes his eyes again. A term to describe his level of consciousness is:
   1. somnolent.
   2. lethargic.
   3. stuporous.
   4. semicomatose.
4. To evaluate neuromuscular function, the patient is instructed to raise one leg at a time while lying supine. A patient with normal strength would be able to lift each leg at least:
   1. 25 degrees.
   2. 45 degrees.
   3. 60 degrees.
   4. 90 degrees.
5. A postoperative craniotomy patient has an external ventricular drainage system. Proper management of the system includes:
   1. do not clamp the drainage tube under any circumstances.
   2. use clean technique to cleanse the insertion site every shift.
   3. keep the zero point of the drip chamber at the level of the external auditory canal.
   4. irrigate the tube with sterile normal saline at least every 8 hours.
6. A patient with a head injury is being monitored for increased intracranial pressure. The earliest sign of increased intracranial pressure is a change in:
   1. pupil response to light.
   2. level of consciousness.
   3. blood pressure.
   4. motor and sensory function.
7. Factors that may trigger migraine headaches include:
   1. alcohol.
   2. sleep disturbances.
   3. exposure to bright light.
   4. changes in environmental temperature.
8. Nursing measures when a patient has a generalized seizure include:
   1. apply soft arm restraints to prevent injury
   2. insert a tongue blade between the teeth to prevent biting the tongue.
   3. turn the patient to one side to prevent swallowing the tongue.
   4. move objects away from the patient to prevent injury.
9. One nursing measure used to decrease intracranial pressure is to:
   1. suction the patient frequently.
   2. encourage isometric exercises.
   3. avoid flexing the neck and hips.
   4. provide continuous stimulation.

CHAPTER 27 Cerebrovascular Accident

JANEAN JENKINS

objectives

1. Discuss the risk factors for cerebrovascular accident (CVA).
2. Identify the four types of CVA.
3. Describe the pathophysiology, signs and symptoms, and medical treatment for each type of CVA.
4. Describe the neurologic deficits that may result from CVA.
5. Explain the tests and procedures used to diagnose a CVA, and nursing responsibilities for patients undergoing those tests and procedures.
6. List data to be included in the nursing assessment of the CVA patient.
7. Assist in developing a nursing care plan for a CVA patient during the acute and rehabilitation phases.
8. Specify criteria used to evaluate the outcomes of nursing care for the CVA patient.
9. Identify resources for the CVA patient and family.

key terms

Aphasia (ă-FĀ-zhă, p. 414)
Diplopia (dĭp-LŌ-pē-ă, p. 422)
Dysarthria (dĭs-ĂR-thrē-ă, p. 415)
Dysphagia (dĭs-FĀ-jē-ă, p. 415)
Dyspraxia (dĭs-PRĂK-sē-ă, p. 415)
Expressive aphasia (p. 414)
Hemiplegia (hĕm-ē-PLĒ-jă, p. 415)
Homonymous hemianopsia (hō-MŎN-ĭ-mŭs hĕ-mē-ă-NŎP-sē-ă, p. 416)
Intracerebral (ĭn-trăh-sĕ-RĒ-brăl, p. 412)
Nonfluent aphasia (p. 415)
Ptosis (TŌ-sĭs, p. 411)
Receptive aphasia (p. 414)
Subarachnoid (sŭb-ăh-RĂK-noid, p. 412)
Transient ischemic attack (TIA) (TRĂN-zē-ĕnt ĭs-KĒ-mĭk ă-TĂK, p. 410)

The brain is the body's center of thinking, feeling, and physical function. A continuous blood supply is essential to maintain function in the brain. A cerebrovascular accident (CVA) is an interruption of blood flow to part of the brain. Without normal blood flow, the affected area is deprived of oxygen, and cell death begins to occur in as little as 4 minutes. The effects of oxygen deprivation vary depending on the area of the brain involved and the length of time the brain is deprived of oxygen.

ANATOMY AND PHYSIOLOGY OF THE BRAIN

The central nervous system structures of the brain include the cerebrum, the brain stem, and the cerebellum. A brief review of the anatomy and physiology of the brain is presented here. Refer to Chapter 26 for a more detailed review.

CEREBRUM

The cerebrum has many complex functions, including initiation of movements, recognition of sensory input, higher-order thinking, regulation of emotional behavior, and regulation of endocrine and autonomic functions.

The cerebrum is divided into two halves, called hemispheres. Each hemisphere controls the opposite side of the body; that is, the right hemisphere controls the left side of the body and the left hemisphere controls the right side of the body. For most people the left hemisphere is dominant. This hemisphere controls the more analytic mental processes such as language acquisition and use, mathematics, and reasoning powers. The right hemisphere encompasses emotional and artistic tendencies.

A folded layer of nerve cells, the cortex, covers each hemisphere. The cortex of each hemisphere is divided into the parietal, frontal, temporal, and occipital lobes. Each lobe has a different area of function (Fig. 27-1).

BRAIN STEM

The brain stem includes the midbrain, pons, medulla, and part of the reticular activating system. The brain stem controls vital, basic functions, including respiration, heart rate, and consciousness.

CEREBELLUM

The cerebellum uses information received from the cerebrum, muscles, joints, and inner ear to coordinate movement, balance, and posture. Unlike the cerebrum, the right side of the cerebellum controls the right side of the body and the left side of the cerebellum controls the left side of the body.

CIRCULATION

The brain is rich with arterial circulation to satisfy its high need for oxygen. Figure 27-2 shows the major cerebral arter-

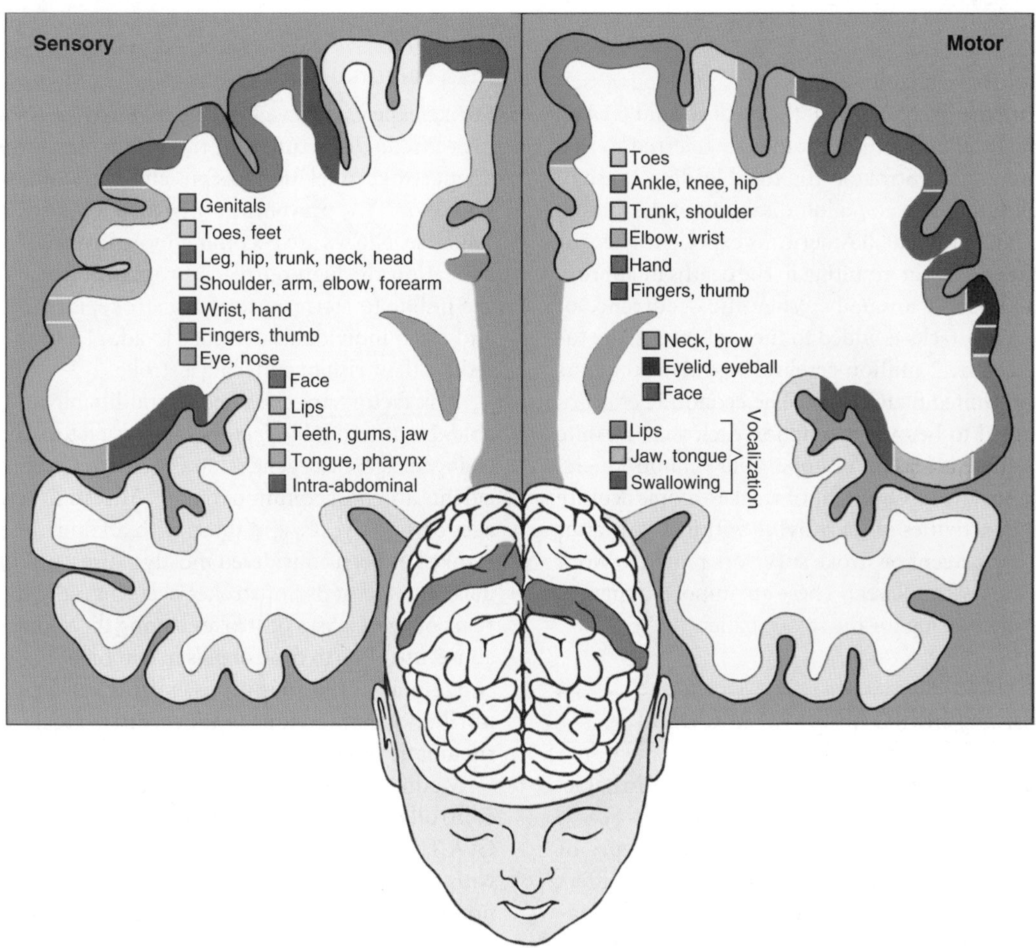

FIGURE **27-1** Control zones of the brain. This drawing represents a slice of each side of the brain. The diagram on the left shows the areas of the cerebral cortex that receive sensory information for specific body areas. The diagram on the right shows where motor activity is initiated for various areas of the body.

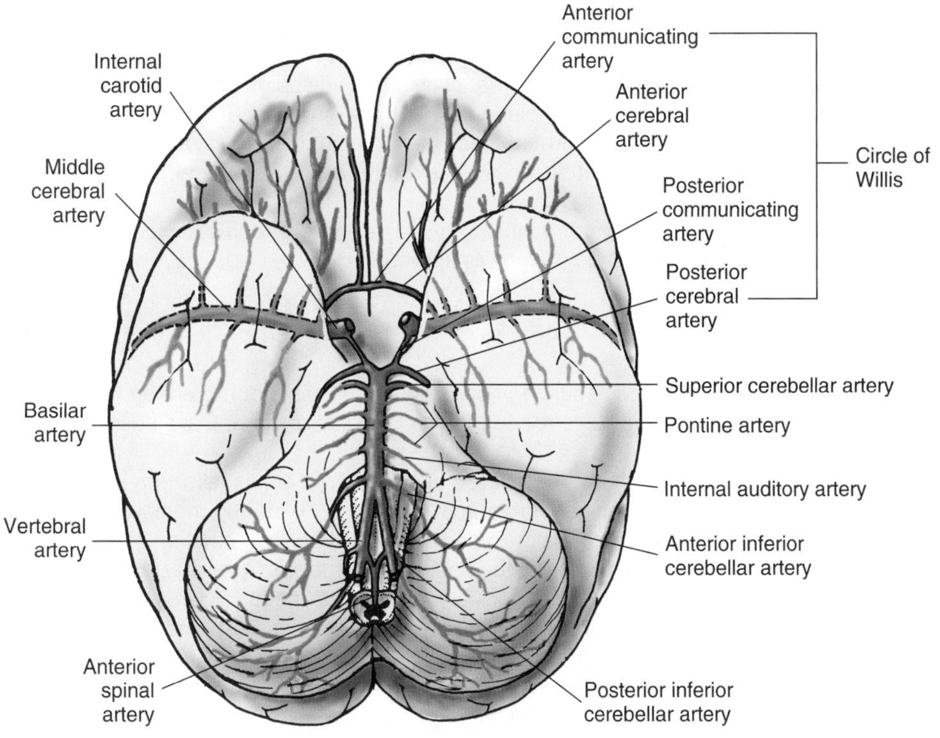

FIGURE **27-2** Cerebral circulation.

ies. Some people have anatomic differences in blood vessels that can increase the likelihood that they will sustain CVAs.

A cerebrovascular accident is commonly referred to as a stroke or "brain attack." Stroke is the third leading cause of death and the leading cause of adult disability in the United States. Approximately 750,000 Americans experience new or recurrent strokes each year, resulting in the deaths of approximately 160,000 people annually. When the occurrence of transient ischemic attacks is added to these numbers, the total is estimated to be 2 million cerebral vascular accidents each year in the United States alone. The economic effect of stroke is estimated to be over $45 billion each year. Despite these statistics, there is reason for hope. Four million Americans are stroke survivors. Over half of stroke victims acquire independence in activities of daily living within 1 year after the stroke. Thirty percent of stroke survivors return to work or productive lives within 1 year. These are important figures to remember when caring for the stroke patient.

TYPES OF CEREBROVASCULAR ACCIDENTS

There are two types of strokes, ischemic and hemorrhagic. They are further classified as transient ischemic attack (TIA), stroke in evolution, and completed stroke. Many types of CVAs share common signs and symptoms. There are differences, however, among the types of CVAs in relation to duration and progression of symptoms.

Risk Factors

Stroke experts believe that the majority of strokes could be prevented. Unfortunately, the public has little knowledge about stroke in relation to signs and symptoms of impending stroke or TIA, prevention of stroke, or medical treatment available. Nurses are becoming more involved in community education through outreach programs directed at assisting the public to learn more about stroke, identify risk factors, and teach individuals methods to adopt a healthy lifestyle to reduce their risk of suffering a stroke.

Risk factors are classified as modifiable and nonmodifiable. Nonmodifiable factors are risk factors that cannot be changed: age, race, gender, and heredity. Cerebrovascular accidents are most common in men, African Americans, people ages 51 to 74 years, and those with a family history of CVA. Stroke has been considered mostly a disease of older individuals but at least 5% of strokes occur in individuals under 45 years of age. Causes of strokes among the young include drug abuse, use of birth control pills in combination with smoking, congenital heart conditions, mitral valve prolapse, atrial fibrillation, infectious endocarditis, sickle-cell anemia, rheumatic fever, and leukemia.

Modifiable risk factors are those that can be eliminated or controlled, thereby dramatically reducing the risk for CVA. The modifiable risk factors are listed in Table 27-1 along with the interventions used for each factor. A common denominator of many of the risk factors (hypertension, cardiac disease, diabetes mellitus) is atherosclerosis. Therefore, many

table 27-1 ***Modifiable CVA Risk Factors and Related Interventions***

MODIFIABLE RISK FACTOR	INTERVENTIONS TO MODIFY EFFECTS OF RISK FACTOR
PATHOLOGIC DISORDERS	
Hypertension	Antihypertensive drugs. Weight control. Stress management. Smoking cessation. Limited alcohol consumption. Low-fat diet. Reduced sodium intake.
Cardiac disease	Drug therapy to improve blood flow and prevent clots. Treatment of atrial fibrillation.
Diabetes mellitus	Balanced program of drug therapy, diet, weight control, exercise. Blood glucose monitoring.
Hypotension	Maintain good hydration, especially in the elderly. Monitor effects of diuretic and antihypertensive therapy.
Migraine headaches	Drug therapy to abort impending migraines or for prophylaxis.
Conditions that increase risk of blood clotting (e.g., sickle-cell anemia)	Good hydration. Drug therapy as appropriate.
LIFESTYLE FACTORS	
Excessive alcohol consumption	Limit alcohol to one ounce of pure alcohol or less (not more than 1 ounce of pure alcohol per day: 2 cans beer, 2 small glasses of wine, 2 average cocktails). Avoid binge drinking.
Cigarette smoking	Advise patient of risks of tobacco use. Explain that risk falls with smoking cessation. Recommend self-help programs. Refer to MD for drug therapy.
Obesity	Encourage patient to maintain normal body weight. Instruction in proper diet. Weight control programs that help patients modify eating behaviors and establish healthy nutritional practices. Exercise programs as specified by the physician.
High-fat diet	Instruction in meal planning and preparation. Reduce saturated fats in diet.
Drug abuse	Drug abuse treatment programs

interventions include measures to slow the progression of atherosclerosis (see Chapter 33 for more complete coverage).

TRANSIENT ISCHEMIC ATTACK

A TIA is a temporary neurologic deficit caused by impairment of cerebral blood flow. Blood vessels may be occluded by spasms, fragments of plaque, or blood clots. It is believed that at least 85% of blood flow to an area must be blocked before signs and symptoms of a TIA appear.

It is difficult to say how common TIAs are because the temporary signs and symptoms may be overlooked, not reported, or attributed to old age and dismissed. This is unfortunate because a TIA is an important warning sign of a possible future stroke.

Signs and Symptoms

With a TIA, neurologic signs and symptoms last from a few minutes to 24 hours, with no permanent effects. Some common signs and symptoms are dizziness, momentary confusion, loss of speech, loss of balance, tinnitus, visual disturbances, ptosis, dysarthria, dysphagia, drooping mouth, weakness, and tingling or numbness on one side of the body. The nature and severity of the symptoms depend on the area of the brain involved and the extent of tissue deprived of oxygen.

Medical Diagnosis

A TIA is generally diagnosed from the health history, physical examination findings, and results of brain imaging studies. In addition, laboratory studies, electrocardiography (ECG), duplex ultrasonography, and cerebral angiography may be ordered to detect risk factors for TIA and stroke. Angiography and radiologic studies can show narrowing of cerebral blood vessels. Doppler studies may also be done to assess cerebral blood flow. Ultrasonic duplex scanning is useful in detecting carotid artery disease. Computed tomography and electroencephalography (EEG) may be employed to rule out intracranial lesions such as tumors, aneurysms, and abscesses. Key features of diagnostic tests are presented in Table 26-1 (previous chapter).

On auscultation, a swooshing noise may be heard over a carotid artery. Its sound is similar to that of a rush of water through a narrow or dammed-up area. This sound, called a *bruit,* reveals that the artery is partially obstructed.

Medical Treatment

Treatment of a TIA depends on the location of the narrowed vessel and the degree of narrowing. Medical treatment may include drug therapy with aspirin, ticlopidine hydrochloride (Ticlid), Aggrenox, or clopidogrel (Plavix) to decrease platelet clumping. Warfarin (Coumadin) and heparin are anticoagulants that may be given alone or in combination in patients exhibiting a cardioembolic TIA. The dosage for warfarin therapy is based on the prothrombin time and the international normalized ratio (INR). For therapeutic anticoagulation, the prothrombin time is usually kept in a therapeutic range of 1.5 to 2.0 times normal and the INR at 2.0 to 3.0. The effect of heparin therapy is monitored with the activated partial thromboplastin time (aPTT). Additional information about drug therapy is provided in Table 27-2.

PHARMACOLOGY CAPSULE When patients are taking antiplatelet or anticoagulant medications, take care to prevent injuries and bleeding.

Because of the operative risks and controversy about the value of surgical intervention in terms of stroke prevention, surgery is often reserved for the most serious stenosis. The most common surgical procedures are carotid endarterectomy (Fig. 27-3) and transluminal angioplasty. Carotid endarterectomy is the surgical removal of plaques in the artery to permit improved blood flow. A stent may be placed in the artery to keep it open. Transluminal angioplasty improves blood flow by dilating the narrowed artery with a balloon that is inserted into the artery. Extracranial-intracranial (EC-IC) bypass is intended to improve blood flow by connecting a branch of an artery outside the cranium to one inside the cranium that is beyond the obstruction. The benefit of EC-IC is in doubt, and it is rarely used now.

STROKE

Stroke is the third leading cause of death and the leading cause of adult disability in the United States. Approximately 750,000 Americans experience new or recurrent strokes each year, resulting in the deaths of approximately 160,000 people annually. When the occurrence of transient ischemic attacks is added to these numbers, the total is estimated to be 2 million cerebral vascular accidents each year in the United States alone. The economic impact of stroke is estimated to be over $45 billion each year. Despite these statistics, there is reason for hope. Four million Americans are stroke survivors. Over half of stroke victims acquire independence in activities of daily living within 1 year after the stroke. Thirty percent of stroke survivors return to work or productive lives within 1 year. These are important figures to remember when caring for the stroke patient.

A stroke is an abrupt impairment of brain function resulting in a set of neurologic signs and symptoms that are caused by impaired blood flow to the brain and that last more than 24 hours. When symptoms progress over hours or days, the condition is described as stroke in evolution. When the neurologic deficits do not change for 2 to 3 days, the stroke is said to be completed. Unlike TIA, a completed stroke causes lingering motor, sensory, or cognitive damage with varying disabilities.

Pathophysiology

The two main classifications of stroke are hemorrhagic and ischemic.

Hemorrhagic Stroke

Hemorrhagic stroke accounts for only about 20% of all strokes. In hemorrhagic stroke, a blood vessel in the brain

table 27-2 **DRUG THERAPY | *Cerebrovascular Accident***

DRUGS	USE/ACTION	SIDE EFFECTS	NURSING INTERVENTIONS
CORTICOSTEROIDS			
Dexamethasone (Decadron)	Reduces ICP by reducing inflammation in brain after stroke.	Fluid retention, hypertension, hypokalemia, hyperglycemia, suppressed response to infection, fat deposits in cheeks and upper back, gastric ulcers, insomnia, easy bruising, mood swings. Dose usually tapered over 7-10 days to prevent acute withdrawal and adrenal insufficiency.	Monitor I & O, BP, blood glucose in people with diabetes. Protect from infection. Report even minor signs of infection. Protect from bumps and other minor injuries.
HYPEROSMOTIC AGENTS			
Mannitol (Osmitrol) Urea (Ureaphil) Glycerin (Osmoglyn)	Induces diuresis, which reduces ICP. Mannitol is first choice drug.	Circulatory overload. Heart failure. Hypertension. Renal failure.	15%-25% mannitol solutions should be filtered. Monitor infusion site; stop flow and have restarted if infiltrated to avoid tissue damage. Monitor for signs of fluid volume excess: hypertension, bounding pulse, edema, urine output less than fluid intake.
ANTICOAGULANTS			
Heparin sodium (Liquaemin sodium)	Prevents formation of new blood clots; does not dissolve existing clots.	Bleeding or hemorrhage due to excessive anticoagulation; hyperkalemia; alopecia (hair loss); allergy. Contraindicated with active bleeding.	Effect is monitored by partial thromboplastin time (PTT) or by activated partial thromboplastin time (aPPT). Therapeutic goal is 1.5-2.0 times the control of 30-40 sec. If patient's aPPT is greater, withhold drug and contact physician. Assess for bruises, bleeding from gastrointestinal and urinary tracts, mouth, or nose. Heparin antidote is protamine sulfate. Caution with venipuncture—apply pressure to site.
Warfarin sodium (Coumadin, Panwarfin)	Prevents formation of new blood clots; does not dissolve existing clots.	Bleeding or hemorrhage due to excessive anticoagulation. Contraindicated with severe cardiac, renal, or liver disease. Interacts with many other drugs	Effect is monitored by prothrombin time (PT) and international normalized ratio (INR). Therapeutic goal is a PT of 1.5-2.0 times control and INR of 2.0-3.0. Check PT/ INR before initiating medication and daily until maintenance dose is reached. Assess for bruising, bleeding from gastrointestinal and urinary tracts, mouth, or nose. Apply pressure after venipuncture. Antidote for warfarin overdose is vitamin K_1 (AquaMEPHYTON).

ruptures and bleeding into the brain occurs. As a result, intracranial pressure may increase, disrupting normal cerebral function. Hemorrhagic strokes are further classified by location. An intracerebral (within the cerebrum) hemorrhage is associated with trauma, uncontrolled hypertension, and aneurysms. When a hemorrhage occurs within the spaces of the brain, the terms subdural, subarachnoid, or ventricular will be used to describe the location. Hemorrhagic strokes are often sudden in onset and require emergent, life-sustaining treatment.

A subarachnoid hemorrhage occurs between the arachnoid and pia mater layers of the brain covering. The pia mater is the thin membrane covering the brain. The arachnoid covers the pia mater. Subarachnoid hemorrhage may be caused by congenital malformations of blood vessels in the brain or by rupture of an aneurysm.

table 27-2 **DRUG THERAPY | *Cerebrovascular Accident—cont'd***

DRUGS	USE/ACTION	SIDE EFFECTS	NURSING INTERVENTIONS
THROMBOLYTICS			
Streptokinase	Dissolve fibrin clots and clot components to destroy thrombi	Increased risk of minor and major bleeding, especially at injection sites. Mild fever, mild allergic reaction. Extensive list of contraindications to be reviewed carefully before administration.	Avoid unnecessary injections; watch puncture sites closely. After arterial puncture, apply pressure at least 30 minutes. For major bleeding, streptokinase infusion must be stopped; whole blood, packed cells, or plasma may be ordered. Antidote for excessive bleeding: aminocaproic acid (Amicar).
Tissue plasminogen activator (tPA) Recombinant tPA (rt-PA)	Initiates dissolution of clots by breaking down fibrin.	Hemorrhage, especially within the first 24 hr after administration.	Minimize venipunctures; protect arterial line sites; assess for bleeding; monitor coagulation sites.
PLATELET AGGREGATION INHIBITORS			
Aspirin	Reduces risk of stroke in male patients with recurrent ischemic attacks.	Excessive bruising, bleeding; bronchoconstriction; nausea, vomiting, gastric bleeding, urticaria, confusion, drowsiness, tinnitus. May be given in combination with other antiplatelet agents.	Tinnitus and confusion suggest overdosage. Teach patients that aspirin can be harmful if not taken properly.
Dipyridamole (Persantine)	Prevents thromboembolism with heart valve prostheses. Used with coumarin anticoagulants.	Hypotension, dizziness. Caution with hypotensive patients. MI, dysrhythmias with IV use. Constipation, dry mouth.	Teach patient to manage orthostatic hypotension. Monitor P and BP.
Aggrenox (Aspirin/extended-release dipyridamole)	Prolongs bleeding time, decreasing the risk of stroke.	Rash, diarrhea, itching, bruising. Not associated with neutropenic purpura as with Ticlid.	May be given with or without food; assess for bruising.
Ticlopidine (Ticlid)	Prolongs bleeding time, decreasing the risk of stroke.	Diarrhea, nausea, dyspepsia, rash; occasionally neutropenia, purpura. Overdose: hypotension.	Give with food or after meals; assess for bruising, signs of infection.
Clopidogrel (Plavix)	Reduces risk of stroke by inhibition of clotting.	GI bleeding, epistaxis, neutropenia, intracranial hemorrhage, hypertension, dyspnea.	Give with food. Advise patient of need for periodic lab studies, including liver function tests with long-term therapy.
CALCIUM CHANNEL BLOCKERS			
Nimodipine (Nimotop)	Prevents spasms in cerebral blood vessels after a hemorrhagic stroke.	Headache, fatigue, depression, confusion, dysrhythmias, hypotension, myocardial infarction, renal failure.	Monitor pulse and blood pressure. Assess for edema. Monitor urine output. Count pulse before each dose; withhold if less than 60 beats per min.

Ischemic Stroke

An ischemic stroke is caused by the obstruction of a blood vessel by an atherosclerotic plaque, a blood clot, or a combination of the two, or by other debris released into the vessel that impedes blood flow to an area of the brain. Brain cells deprived of blood flow become ischemic and die. Ischemic strokes account for 80% of all strokes including embolic and thrombotic strokes. In an embolic stroke, the clot or plaque fragment is "traveling" through a blood vessel from an area outside of the brain until it lodges in a cerebral artery. Mitral valve stenosis, atrial fibrillation, and myocardial infarction are cardiovascular conditions that may lead to the development of clots that become emboli.

A thrombotic stroke develops when an obstruction forms in a blood vessel of the brain. The atherosclerotic process, which often affects large cerebral arteries, produces most of

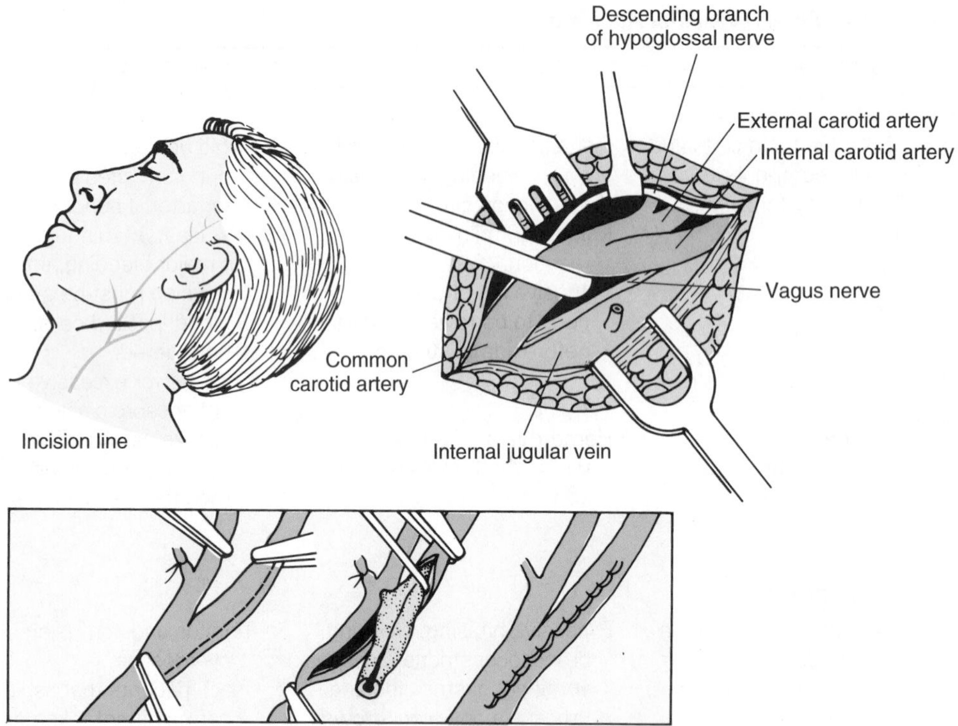

FIGURE **27-3** Carotid endarterectomy. Plaques are removed from the artery to improve blood flow.

the thrombotic strokes. Patients may experience stroke in evolution, in which symptoms worsen over approximately 48 hours. As the obstruction progresses, neurologic impairment increases. Figure 27-4 illustrates each type of stroke. Patients who have thrombotic strokes may have a history of TIAs.

A lacunar stroke results from occlusion of the small penetrating arteries deep within the brain. The occlusive process in these small arteries is different from that of the larger arteries. The clinical features associated with lacunar strokes are usually less severe and produce less pronounced neurologic changes.

***Put on your* THINKING CAP!!**

Why would patients with atrial fibrillation be treated with anticoagulants?

Signs and Symptoms

A stroke may produce different signs and symptoms, depending on the type, location, and extent of brain injury. Symptoms of a hemorrhagic stroke generally occur suddenly and may include severe headache that the patient describes as "the worst headache of my life." Other symptoms are stiff neck, loss of consciousness, vomiting, and seizures.

Symptoms of an embolic stroke also often appear without warning. The specific symptoms depend on the area of the brain affected by the lack of blood supply. One or more of the following signs and symptoms may be present: one-sided (unilateral) weakness, numbness, visual problems, confusion and memory lapses, headache, dysphagia (difficulty swallowing), and language problems. Language problems may be in the form of difficulty understanding, speaking, or both. Reading and writing may also be affected.

The signs and symptoms of a thrombotic stroke may be the same as those of an embolic stroke. Because the obstruction forms gradually through the atherosclerotic process, however, the symptoms may develop more gradually. Sudden onset of symptoms may occur with either embolic or thrombotic stroke.

Regardless of the type of stroke, symptoms can be devastating. Whereas some symptoms improve with time and therapy, others may be permanent. Many signs and symptoms are related to the location of the damage and whether the right or the left side of the brain is affected. Figure 27-5 compares right-sided and left-sided stroke. Long-term effects that merit more discussion are: aphasia, dysarthria, dysphagia, dyspraxia, hemiplegia, homonymous hemianopsia, personality change, emotional lability, impaired cognition, and bladder dysfunction.

Aphasia

The speech center is located in the left hemisphere in more than 90% of all people. In left-handed persons, the speech center is sometimes located in the right hemisphere. If the speech center is damaged, communication is affected. Aphasia is a defect in the use of language; speech, reading, writing, or word comprehension. Aphasia is classified as receptive or expressive. The patient with receptive aphasia has difficulty understanding spoken or written words. Receptive aphasia is characterized as *fluent,* meaning the speech sounds normal but the patient makes little sense. The patient with expressive aphasia has difficulty speaking and writing. Expressive apha-

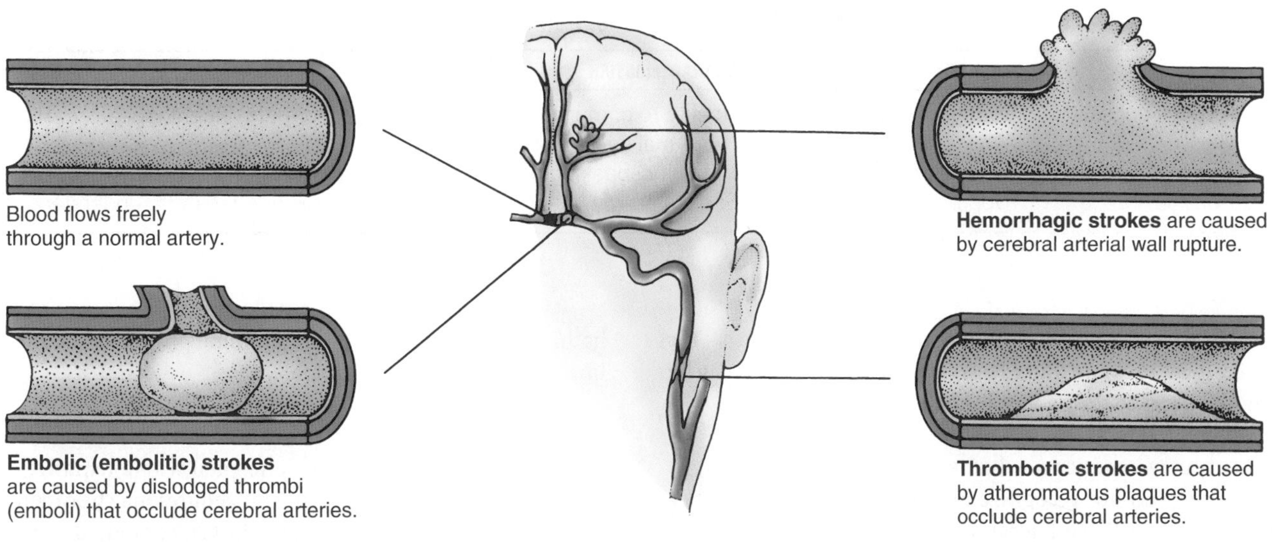

Blood flows freely
through a normal artery.
Embolic (embolitic) strokes
are caused by dislodged thrombi
(emboli) that occlude cerebral arteries.
Hemorrhagic strokes are caused
by cerebral arterial wall rupture.
Thrombotic strokes are caused
by atheromatous plaques that
occlude cerebral arteries.

FIGURE **27-4** Types of stroke.

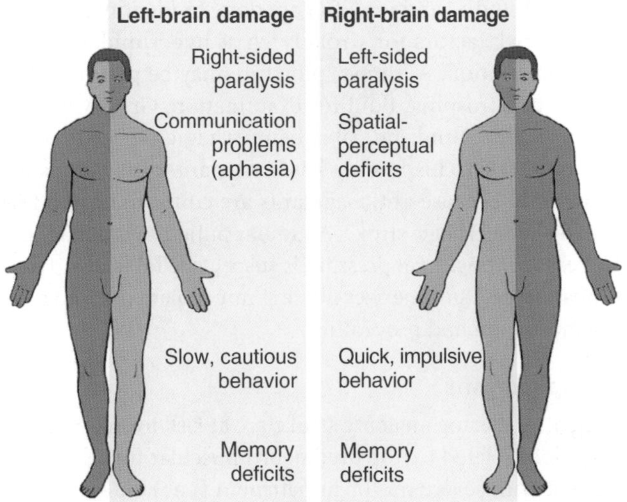

FIGURE **27-5** Comparison of right-sided and left-sided stroke.

sia is described as ***nonfluent aphasia,*** meaning the person has difficulty initiating speech. Although these types of aphasia are distinctly defined, some patients have components of both types. The term *global aphasia* is sometimes used when speech is impaired to the point that the person has almost no ability to communicate. Terms describing communication problems of the stroke patient are defined in Table 27-3.

Dysarthria

Dysarthria is the inability to speak clearly. It is caused by neurologic damage that prevents normal control of muscles used in speech. Dysarthric patients are difficult to understand, but they understand what is said and have no difficulty putting together their thoughts.

Dysphagia

Patients with dysarthria are also likely to have dysphagia (swallowing difficulty), which may require extensive rehabilitation. This is a very serious problem because of the risk of aspiration and because it can interfere with adequate nutrition. Dysphagia can be especially discouraging for the patient when attempts to eat result in choking, frustration, and fear. A gastrostomy tube may be inserted for long-term feeding purposes. Speech therapists are trained to help patients with dysphagia.

Dyspraxia

Dyspraxia is the partial inability to initiate coordinated voluntary motor acts. Any part of the body with motor function may be affected. For instance, the patient may not be able to walk or transfer to a chair without assistance even though the patient is not paralyzed. Dyspraxic patients may be able to spontaneously perform a motor act, yet be unable to initiate such an act willfully. This contradictory behavior can lead uninformed family, friends, or caretakers to assume the person is being "difficult." The difficulty initiating motor actions seen in dyspraxia is quite different from the inability to perform motor acts due to hemiplegia. The person who has apraxia can move the affected parts but cannot perform specific purposeful actions such as walking or dressing.

Hemiplegia

Hemiplegia is defined as paralysis of one side of the body. The affected side is opposite from the side of the brain in which the stroke occurred because nerve fibers in the brain cross over as they pass into the spinal cord (see Fig. 25-5). Hemiplegia is characterized at first by flaccidity (decreased muscle tone), then by spasticity (increased muscle tone). Recovery from hemiplegia is a gradual process, and the extent of improvement varies widely.

Sensory Impairment

Impaired sensory function is common after a stroke. The patient may be unable to feel touch, pain, or temperature in affected body parts. Conversely, some hemiplegic individuals with sensory impairment perceive every sensation to the affected area as painful. Patients may feel as if their body were

table 27-3 Types of Communication Disorders After Cerebrovascular Accident

TYPE	LOCATION OF BRAIN LESION	CHARACTERISTICS
Receptive aphasia	Wernicke's area	Unable to comprehend spoken or written words. Fluent: speaks easily but makes little sense.
Expressive aphasia	Broca's area	Difficulty speaking or writing. Nonfluent: much effort to initiate speech.
Dysarthria	Upper motor neurons	Speaks slowly with great effort. Words prolonged, hard to understand.

limp or flaccid. Altered sensations put the patient at risk for injury from pressure and excess heat or cold. Injuries may be ignored because the patient is not aware of them.

Unilateral Neglect

Patients may experience what is called *unilateral neglect,* in which they do not recognize one side of their body as belonging to them. Unilateral neglect is most common with right hemisphere damage and results in failure to attend to the left side of the body. The condition often resolves after about 3 months.

Homonymous Hemianopsia

Homonymous hemianopsia is a perceptual problem that involves loss of one side of the field of vision. Homonymous hemianopsia translates to a half-blinded field of vision that occurs on the same side in both eyes. At mealtime, the patient may leave half the plate untouched, the half on the affected side. Or the patient may shave his face completely on one side and leave the whiskers untouched on his affected side.

Intellectual and Emotional Effects

Many patients experience emotional changes after a stroke, sometimes to the point of personality change. Emotional lability is a frequent problem after a stroke. The patient may seem quite happy, then suddenly burst into tears for no apparent reason. Angry outbursts, childlike behavior, and inappropriate sexual behavior may occur. Emotional changes such as these are thought to be caused by neurochemical imbalances in the brain or by loss of the brain's ability to inhibit inappropriate behavior. It has also been found that cognitive processes may be slowed after a stroke even without obvious deficits in thinking and responding.

Elimination Disturbances

In the acute phase of stroke, and sometimes into the rehabilitation phase, the patient may experience a neurogenic bladder. A neurogenic bladder is further classified depending on the type of symptoms identified. A flaccid bladder (one without muscle tone) cannot empty completely. In some cases, the coordination to be able to store urine in the bladder or wait once the urge to void is felt is lost (dyssynergia), which also leads to incontinence.

Bowel incontinence may also be a physiologic consequence of stroke. However, confusion, disorientation, and immobility may contribute to incontinent episodes and to chronic constipation.

With both bladder and bowel incontinence, it is important to determine if the cause is physiologic or related to other factors such as infection from a urinary catheter or the inability of the patient to communicate the need to go to the bathroom. Bladder and bowel retraining programs should be implemented as soon as possible.

Medical Diagnosis

When a patient is admitted to a hospital with a tentative diagnosis of a stroke, the following procedures may be ordered: blood studies, electrocardiogram (ECG), computed tomography, magnetic resonance imaging, carotid ultrasound studies, cerebral and carotid angiography, electrocardiography, positron emission tomography, and single-photon emission computed tomography.

Blood studies and the ECG are done to identify the presence of risk factors for stroke such as hyperlipidemia and atrial fibrillation. A lumbar puncture may be performed to obtain cerebrospinal fluid for examination. Grossly bloody cerebrospinal fluid indicates hemorrhagic rather than ischemic stroke. This finding has important implications for treatment, because anticoagulants are contraindicated following hemorrhagic stroke. A lumbar puncture is *not* done if increased intracranial pressure is suspected. Table 26-1 (previous chapter) summarizes nursing care of patients who have diagnostic test and procedures.

Complications

Patients suffering an acute stroke are at risk for many complications related to impaired neuromuscular function. The patient with severe motor impairment is at risk for constipation, dehydration, contractures, urinary tract infections, thrombophlebitis, decubitus ulcers, and pneumonia. Sensory losses put the patient at risk for traumatic and thermal injuries.

Prognosis

The prognosis for stroke patients is becoming increasingly hopeful. The critical variables that affect recovery are the patient's condition before the stroke, the length of time between the occurrence of stroke and the diagnosis, the support for the patient in the acute phase (usually the first 48 hours), the severity of the patient's symptoms, and access to rehabilitative therapy. A stroke patient who is comatose for more than 36 hours has a poor chance of recovery. In addition, the recovery prospects for hemorrhagic stroke victims are significantly poorer than for ischemic stroke victims. Most recovery from stroke takes place in the first 3 months but progress may continue long after that.

The long-term recovery of the stroke patient may well depend on the care received immediately after the stroke. Therefore, the nurse's role in providing care to stroke patients is a vital one.

Medical Treatment in the Acute Phase

The acute phase of a stroke begins with the onset of signs and symptoms and continues until the patient's vital signs, particularly blood pressure and neurologic condition, stabilize. This phase usually lasts 24 to 48 hours. The patients are often placed in a monitored setting for close observation and treatment during the acute phase.

The majority of patients admitted with an acute stroke have high blood pressure during and immediately after a stroke. It is important to be cautious in treating high blood pressure during this phase, as sudden reductions in blood pressure have been associated with decreased cerebral perfusion and may lead to worsening of brain tissue damage. Blood pressure naturally decreases within 48 hours, even without treatment. A small group of patients may present or develop low blood pressure after a stroke. This is often related to dehydration and should be identified and treated right away to avoid a decrease in blood flow to the brain.

Medical treatment usually includes oxygen therapy, drugs, and measures to maintain essential functions. Surgical intervention is indicated in some situations. A challenge for the physician is to provide immediate care for acute problems while considering preexisting conditions as well. Management of chronic conditions such as diabetes mellitus, heart disease, arthritis, and gastrointestinal disturbances must be continued during the acute phase of stroke.

Many medical management interventions are directed at minimizing complications and deterioration of the patient's condition after a stroke. Recent studies support keeping the patient's temperature as close to normal as possible. Hyperthermia of any degree has now been shown to extend the area of damage and worsen the outcome after stroke. In addition, hyperglycemia during the acute phase of a stroke has also been shown to worsen the outcome of a patient. It is very important to monitor patients and report any changes in vital signs or glucose levels.

Oxygen

Oxygenation is a priority immediately after a stroke, especially if the patient is unconscious, because hypoxemia can extend the area affected and therefore worsen the stroke. Oxygen therapy and monitoring of oxygen saturation may be ordered. For patients who are comatose, intubation and mechanical ventilation may be required to provide adequate ventilation. Respiratory exercises, including incentive spirometry, may be ordered for the alert patient.

Drug Therapy

Tissue plasminogen activator (tPA, Alteplase, Activase) may be given to dissolve clots in patients with acute ischemic strokes. This is the only FDA-approved medication to reverse the effects of an ischemic stroke. This medication must be initiated intravenously within 3 hours from the onset of stroke symptoms. This narrow window of time has limited the use of rt-PA with acute ischemic stroke. Patient selection criteria are also very strict, as this medication is associated with a higher risk of cerebral hemorrhage in patients who have received it. Although thrombolytic agents such as rt-PA and streptokinase are being tested for intra-arterial treatment of acute ischemic stroke, none have FDA approval at this time.

The trauma of a CVA causes edema in the affected tissues and surrounding tissues. Cerebral edema is sometimes treated with osmotic diuretics such as mannitol. Corticosteroids may be prescribed to reduce intracranial pressure by reducing cerebral inflammation. Nimodipine (Nimotop), a calcium channel blocker, may be ordered to prevent spasms in cerebral blood vessels after subarachnoid hemorrhage. Phenytoin (Dilantin) and phenobarbital are anticonvulsants that may be ordered if the patient has seizures. The efficacy and safety of heparin and heperanoids have been challenged in recent years and are no longer routinely used as a first line treatment with a TIA or an acute ischemic stroke unless a cardioembolic stroke is suspected. Small doses of these medications given subcutaneously are recommended in the prevention of deep vein thrombosis associated with acute stroke. When appropriate, heparin is given intravenously followed by oral warfarin. Later the regimen may be changed to aspirin, which decreases the risk of thrombus by preventing platelets from clumping.

Medical management is often directed at preventing a subsequent or future stroke. Examples of drugs given in an effort to prevent strokes caused by thrombi include acetylsalicylic acid (aspirin), ticlopidine hydrochloride (Ticlid), Aggrenox, and clopidogrel (Plavix). Drugs used to prevent or treat CVA are included in Table 27-1.

PHARMACOLOGY CAPSULE Tissue plasminogen activator, which is used to dissolve clots, must be given within 3 hours of the onset of stroke symptoms.

Surgical Intervention

Surgical intervention is an option for some patients with hemorrhagic strokes. Decisions about surgery are based on the patient's age, the intracranial pressure, and the location of the hemorrhage.

Fluids and Nutrition

An order for intravenous fluids will probably be given for the stroke patient in the acute phase. This route provides fluids, electrolytes, and an access for the intravenous administration of drugs. The dietary order is based on the patient's nutritional requirements and ability to eat. Food may be regular, soft, or pureed, depending on how well the patient can chew and swallow. Vitamins and electrolyte supplementation may also be ordered.

Total parenteral nutrition may be ordered for the malnourished patient. Sometimes a nasogastric tube is inserted for feeding purposes. If long-term enteral feedings are indicated, a gastrostomy tube may be placed.

Urine Elimination

Sometimes an indwelling catheter is ordered to manage urinary incontinence. Intermittent catheterization is a method of controlling incontinence caused by a flaccid bladder that is less likely to lead to infection. Intermittent catheterization is done every 4 to 6 hours as ordered. The frequency of catheterization is based on the amount of urine obtained each time.

NURSING CARE *in the Acute Phase of Stroke*

The most important aspects of care during the acute phase of a stroke are assessment and support. Management in this phase focuses on maintenance or improvement of vital physiologic functions (see Nursing Care Plan: The Stroke Patient).

Assesment

The nursing assessment reveals risk factors for CVA and identifies nursing care needs. It also provides a record of baseline data for comparison. Details of the neurologic assessment are covered in Chapter 26 and summarized in Table 26-3. Data specific to the stroke patient are outlined in Table 27-4.

Health History

The health history may be obtained from the patient or from a family member if the patient is too ill or unable to communicate. On introduction to the stroke patient, begin to assess the patient's ability to understand language and to respond verbally and nonverbally. Responses to simple yes-or-no commands provide a good basis for initial assessment. Evaluate verbal responses, facial expressions, and physical reactions for appropriateness. If responses are not appropriate, try to identify the source of difficulty. Does the patient have trouble finding words? Do clues help the patient respond? Does the patient speak fluently? If the patient cannot provide the data needed, attempt to obtain them from a family member or friend. Note the informant (person who provides the history). Assess the patient's orientation to person, place, and time.

Chief Complaint and History of Present Illness. In the history of the present illness, assess the events that led the patient to seek medical care. A complete description of the illness includes the initial symptoms and how the symptoms progressed.

Medical History. Record past serious illnesses or conditions, including hypertension, heart disease, diabetes mellitus, liver disease, gout, head trauma, and previous strokes or transient ischemic attacks. Record previous hospitalizations, operations, and injuries.

Family History. The health history includes a family history of neurologic or cardiovascular disease as well as strokes.

Review of Systems. Ask the patient about significant problems in the review of systems. Important items to assess include

NURSING CARE PLAN

The Stroke Patient

ASSESSMENT

Health History: Mr. Gonzales is an obese 82-year-old Latino who was admitted with weakness on the right side and slurred speech. His daughter assisted with the health history since the patient had some difficulty responding verbally. He has had type 2 diabetes mellitus for 10 years, which he treats with an oral hypoglycemic agent, and had a myocardial infarction at age 75. He has no changes in vision but does wear reading glasses. He has good hearing and no headaches. He is right-handed. He was unable to stand when he awoke this morning. He tried to drink some water but had difficulty swallowing. He has had no loss of bowel or bladder control. Mr. Gonzales is divorced. An adult daughter and her two teenagers live with him. He is a retired construction worker; his hobbies are carpentry and watching television.

Physical Examination: Vital Signs: Temperature, 97° F orally; pulse, 96; respirations, 22; blood pressure, 210/104. Patient is alert. Acknowledges he is in the hospital but is uncertain about day or date and time. Uses gestures to respond to some questions when he seems unable to find the right word. Pupils are equal and react to light. Ptosis of right eyelid is noted. Hand grips, voluntary movements, and reflexes of leg, arm, and hand are normal on left side but diminished on right side. Leans toward right side when not supported.

Nursing Diagnosis	*Goals and Outcome Criteria*	*Interventions*
Deficient fluid volume related to inadequate intake, dysphagia.	The patient will maintain adequate hydration, as evidenced by moist mucous membranes, dilute urine, pulse and blood pressure within usual range.	Record fluid intake and output. Administer intravenous fluids as ordered. Monitor oral fluid intake and assess swallowing. Assist patient to sit up while eating and drinking. If thin fluids are difficult to swallow, try semisolids such as ice cream, puddings, and popsicles. Have oral suction device available in case of choking or aspiration. Detect and report signs and symptoms of fluid volume deficit: tachycardia, concentrated urine, dry mucous membranes.
Imbalanced nutrition: less than body requirements related to dysphagia, inability to feed self.	The patient will maintain adequate nutrition, evidenced by stable weight.	Assess food intake. Assist with meals as needed. Seat upright for meals. Do not make him feel rushed. Provide alternative means of feeding (nasogastric or gastrostomy tube, total nutrition) as ordered. Weigh weekly to assess adequacy of food intake.

NURSING CARE PLAN—cont'd

Nursing Diagnosis	*Goals and Outcome Criteria*	*Interventions*
Impaired verbal communication related to aphasia.	The patient will use nonverbal means to supplement verbal communication and will participate in speech therapy exercises.	Establish a code system of blinks or nods for nonverbal communication, use pictures or cards that patient can select to express his needs. Encourage verbalization but recognize frustration and provide words if patient cannot retrieve them. Discuss referral for speech therapy with physician. Tell the patient that improvement is usually possible with therapy.
Impaired physical activity related to weakness, paralysis, poor balance.	The patient will maintain intact skin, joint mobility, regular bowel and bladder elimination, good peripheral circulation, and normal breath sounds.	While on bedrest, assist him to change positions at least every 2 hours. He should not lie on his right side for more than 30 minutes at a time. Use positioning techniques and devices to reduce pressure points. Inspect skin for redness and edema associated with pressure. Position limbs in functional alignment and perform range of motion exercises three times a day. Do not pull on the affected side. Monitor bowel and bladder function. Administer stool softeners and laxatives as ordered. Encourage fluids and fiber when able to take orally. Palpate lower abdomen for bladder distention and catheterize as ordered as necessary. Assess for Homans's sign. Report tenderness, pain, or swelling in calves. Exercise legs with each position change. Apply elastic stockings or alternating pressure wraps as ordered. Ambulate when able. Encourage coughing and deep breathing with each position change. Assess lung fields for atelectasis, wheezes, or rales. Report temperature elevation.
Risk for injury related to paralysis.	The patient will have no falls or injuries associated with motor impairment or altered sensory perception.	Keep the bed in low position with the side rails raised according to hospital policy. Put the call button in reach and instruct patient to call for help to get up. A bed check device may be implemented when patients have difficulty understanding directions or are in a confused state. Check on him frequently. Monitor position of affected extremities to prevent trauma that might not be detected because of poor sensation. Use sling or brace if ordered to support affected limbs. Assess effects of ptosis on vision. If vision is impaired, approach patient from unaffected side and arrange personal articles on that side. When patient is out of bed, be sure he is seated safely. Use pillows to prevent excessive leaning to one side. When ambulatory, use gait belt if needed and assist as appropriate.
Anxiety related to loss of function or fear of disability. Provide information about what is happening, what you are doing, and what he can expect. Check on him often. Encourage family to visit.	The patient will have a reduction in anxiety, as evidenced by calm manner and patient statement.	Acknowledge signs of anxiety and attempt to identify sources.
Altered family processes related to anticipated need of patient for assistance after discharge.	The patient and family will plan for altered roles and responsibilities to support the patient during and after discharge.	Give family members an opportunity to ask questions and share their concerns. Provide information and facilitate communication with physician as needed. Refer to sources of support and resources, including social worker and community agencies. Start planning for discharge. Assess family strengths and resources, willingness to help care for patient after discharge. Identify new responsibilities they might need to assume and discuss how these can be carried out.

table 27-4 ASSESSMENT *of the Cerebrovascular Accident Patient*

HEALTH HISTORY

Source of Data: Reliability and ability of patient to provide information
Present Illness: Description of onset and progression
Past Medical History: Cardiovascular conditions, liver disorder, diabetes mellitus, gout, previous cerebrovascular accidents, head injury, current medications
Family History: Neurologic or vascular conditions
Review of Systems: Visual disturbances, motor or sensory impairments, pain, dysphagia, incontinence, mental-emotional changes
Functional Assessment: Usual activities, diet, occupation, use of alcohol and tobacco, interpersonal relationships, stressors

PHYSICAL ASSESSMENT

General Appearance: Level of consciousness, behavior, gait, posture
Height and Weight
Vital Signs: Blood pressure, temperature, pulse, respiration
Face: Symmetry
Eyes: Pupil size, equality, alignment, reaction to light; gross visual acuity, eyelid closure, ptosis
Skin: Moisture, turgor, color
Abdomen: Bowel or bladder distention
Genitalia and Anus: Presence or odor of urine or stool
Extremities: Muscle tone, strength, voluntary movement, sensation

weakness, impaired movement, pain (especially headache), dysphagia, bowel or bladder incontinence, visual disturbances, mental or emotional changes, and altered sensation.

Functional Assessment. The last component of the health history, the functional assessment, addresses the patient's usual activities and health practices. Inquire about activity level, dietary pattern, occupation, use of alcohol and tobacco, drug use, interpersonal relationships, and current stressors.

Physical Examination

During the physical examination, observe the patient's general appearance, responsiveness, and behavior. Record restlessness or agitation. The level of consciousness is important because subtle changes in level of consciousness such as confusion, irritability, or a decrease in level of consciousness may suggest a stroke in evolution or increasing intracranial pressure. Measure vital signs. The breathing pattern and effort are especially important. Obtain the patient's weight and height if possible.

Inspect the face for symmetry. Assess the mouth for moisture and drooling. Evaluate the alert patient's ability to swallow. Inspect the pupils for size, equality, and reaction to light. Conduct a gross vision assessment by asking the patient to read something. Inspect the skin for color and palpate for moisture and turgor. Assess extremities for muscle tone and strength, sensation, and voluntary movement. Instruct the patient to move each extremity individually and observe responses. Impaired movement or inappropriate response may be due to aphasia or dyspraxia as well as to neuromuscular damage. The patient who has aphasia has difficulty interpreting the messages and may not perform the requested movement for that reason. The patient with dyspraxia may comprehend the instruction but be unable to direct the body part to move. Also record any evidence of incontinence or bladder distention.

Frequently repeat neurologic checks consisting of evaluating level of consciousness, pupil appearance and response to light, the patient's ability to follow commands, and the movement and sensation of extremities. For additional neurologic assessment, see Chapter 26.

The National Institute of Health (NIH) Stroke Assessment Scale is a tool sometimes used to assess patients who have experienced a stroke. This tool provides a method to guide systematic assessment of neurologic deficits often associated with an acute stroke. It was designed by a research neurologist to standardize and document neurologic assessments of stroke patients. Most facilities that use this assessment tool require those administering the examination to go through a certification process to ensure accuracy and consistency among examiners.

Nursing assessment of the stroke patient is summarized in Table 27-4.

Nursing Diagnoses, Goals, and Outcome Criteria: Acute Phase of Stroke

Depending on location and extent of brain damage, appropriate diagnoses and goals may include the following:

NURSING DIAGNOSES	GOALS AND OUTCOME CRITERIA
Ineffective Airway Clearance related to impaired cough reflex, altered consciousness, impaired swallowing	Patent airway: breath sounds clear to auscultation
Ineffective Breathing Patterns related to impaired cerebral circulation, increased intracranial pressure	Effective breathing pattern: normal respiratory rate and depth, arterial blood gases within normal limits
Risk for Injury related to seizure activity, confusion, motor impairment	Absence of injury: no bruising, skin breaks, falls, or fractures
Risk for Deficient Fluid Volume related to inadequate intake or excessive diuresis	Adequate hydration: balanced fluid intake and output
Risk for Fluid Volume Excess related to overhydration	Normal extracellular fluid volume: pulse and blood pressure consistent with patient norms, no edema, breath sounds clear
Imbalanced Nutrition: Less than Body Requirements related to dysphagia, inability to feed self, inability to chew	Adequate intake of nutrients: maintenance of body weight

Disturbed Sensory Perception related to neurologic impairment	Adaptation to sensory perceptual alterations
Ineffective Thermoregulation related to effects of neurologic impairment and/or metabolic processes	Effective thermoregulation: temperature within patient's normal range
Disturbed Thought Processes related to impaired cerebral circulation	Improved mental function: patient is oriented to self and environment
Impaired Verbal Communication related to aphasia	Effective communication: patient successfully communicates needs
Impaired Physical Mobility related to weakness, paralysis, spasticity, impaired balance	Absence of complications of immobility: joints have full range of motion, skin intact
Total or Functional Incontinence related to impaired control, inability to manage toileting process	Improved control of urine elimination: episodes of uncontrolled voiding decrease; patient voids voluntarily
Constipation related to immobility, dehydration, drug side effects	Normal bowel elimination: regular passage of soft, formed stool without straining
Bowel Incontinence related to impaired conduction of impulses	Controlled bowel elimination: no involuntary bowel evacuation
Ineffective Coping related to adapting to neurologic deficits	Effective coping strategies: patient verbalizes acceptance of stroke and strives for maximum recovery
Interrupted Family Processes related to disruption of family roles and functions	Adaptation of the family to the patient's condition: family demonstrates willingness and ability to adapt to patient's condition

Interventions

Ineffective Airway Clearance and Ineffective Breathing Patterns

Closely monitor the patient's respiratory status. Maintaining a patent airway is a priority for patients who have suffered strokes. Neurologic deficits may cause altered breathing patterns and impaired swallowing, gag, and cough reflexes. Increasing intracranial pressure may affect the respiratory center in the brain, causing respiratory depression. If the patient exhibits signs of increased intracranial pressure (rising blood pressure, bradycardia, abnormal pupil response, decreasing level of consciousness), elevate the head of the bed 30 degrees and notify the physician.

The stroke patient is at risk for airway obstruction, for a number of reasons. If the patient is unconscious, the tongue may fall back and block the airway. A side-lying position helps prevent such obstruction. An oral or nasal airway is sometimes employed to keep the airway open.

Immobility and dehydration cause thick secretions to be retained in the respiratory tract, possibly leading to pneumonia and atelectasis. Good hydration helps to thin respiratory secretions for easier expectoration. Dysphagia may cause the patient to aspirate fluids or food, causing airway obstruction and contributing to the development of pneumonia. Pneumonia is, in fact, the most frequent cause of death after stroke. Feeding the patient with dysphagia is discussed in Chapter 36.

Suctioning and frequent position changes can help prevent aspiration and promote removal of secretions. Respiratory treatments for the patient, with regular reminders to do deep breathing exercises, can be helpful. Forceful coughing may be discouraged in the acute phase after a hemorrhagic stroke as it tends to increase intracranial pressure. Ask the physician if and when coughing is permitted. Administer oxygen therapy as ordered.

Risk for Injury

Many factors place the stroke patient at risk for injury. Seizures may occur, causing the patient to lose consciousness and to have abnormal motor activity. Raise side rails and pad them according to agency protocol to reduce the trauma should the patient strike the rails. During a seizure, turn the patient to one side and move hard objects away from the patient. Never force anything between clenched teeth. To do so may injure the teeth and gums. Additional information about seizures is presented in Chapter 26.

Safety precautions are also essential for confused patients and patients with motor impairments. Orient patients to their surroundings and explain why they should not get up unassisted. The staff must respond promptly to the patient's calls for help. Although restraints are needed at times, they should be used as a last resort because they often agitate the patient and can actually cause injuries. A bed check system may be of more benefit when the patient is having difficulty understanding directions. Get sufficient help or use mechanical devices to assist the patient in and out of the bed.

Deficient Fluid Volume or Fluid Volume Excess

Close monitoring of fluid status is especially important in the acute phase of stroke. Accurate intake and output records are essential. Take vital signs and compare for trends suggesting fluid volume excess or deficit. Assess the mouth for moisture. In a well-hydrated person the mucous membranes of the mouth are moist. Evaluate tissue turgor, but remember it is not a very reliable indicator of fluid status in the older person. Age-related changes in the skin and subcutaneous structures cause a loss of tissue elasticity that may be mistaken for dehydration. Laboratory studies, including urine specific gravity, serum electrolytes, and hematocrit, are also useful indicators of fluid balance.

The patient is at risk for fluid volume excess if excessive intravenous fluids are administered or if the patient's kidneys are unable to eliminate excess fluid rapidly enough. Fluid volume excess may lead to edema and heart failure. Signs of fluid volume excess are fluid intake greater than output, bounding pulse, venous distention, increased blood pressure, crackles in the lungs, and edema. Report evidence of excess fluid to the registered nurse or the physician. The rate of intravenous fluid may be decreased and diuretics given as ordered. Explain to the patient and family the need to temporarily restrict fluids. If the patient is thirsty, frequently provide small amounts of fluids in small containers and record all intake.

Factors that place the stroke patient at risk for fluid volume deficit include age, dysphagia, drug therapy with diuretics, and immobility. The stroke patient is likely to be older, and older people are less able to conserve water through the kidneys. The patient with dysphagia may be unable to take adequate oral fluids. If diuretics are given for fluid volume excess or increased intracranial pressure, they can precipitate excess loss of water and electrolytes. The patient with motor deficits may not be able to obtain fluids independently.

Fluid volume deficit contributes to constipation, skin dryness, urinary tract infections, and renal calculi (stones). Signs of fluid volume deficit are a thready pulse, tachycardia, low blood pressure, low urine output, concentrated urine, dry mucous membranes, and sometimes confusion. Report evidence of fluid volume deficit to the registered nurse or the physician. If intravenous fluids are being administered, the physician may order an increase in the hourly flow rate. Fluids may also be given through enteral feeding tubes.

To reduce the risk of fluid volume deficit, monitor the fluid intake record to be sure the patient is getting at least eight 8-ounce glasses of fluids each day (unless contraindicated). Be sure all staff and family members know to offer fluids and record the amounts taken. Place fluids within sight and easy reach of the patient and explain the need for adequate hydration. If the patient has hemiplegia, be sure the fluids are placed on the nonparalyzed side. Spillproof containers that are easily held with one hand can facilitate independent drinking. If the patient is able to take oral fluids but has difficulty swallowing, proceed slowly. Have suction equipment on hand in case of aspiration. Thin liquids are more readily aspirated. Jello, ice cream, popsicles, and frozen juice may be substituted to provide adequate fluids. There are also thickening agents that can be added to other liquids as needed.

Imbalanced Nutrition

The patient's nutritional status is of concern throughout stroke treatment. Factors that may lead to inadequate nutrition include dsyphagia, paralysis, difficulty chewing, and depression. The patient who is malnourished is at risk for skin breakdown and infection. Obesity hampers mobility and can interfere with rehabilitation.

The patient who has dysphagia may not be able to consume adequate nutrients orally. Sometimes a nasogastric tube is inserted for feeding purposes. The physician may order total parenteral nutrition for the malnourished patient. Aggressive treatment of dysphagia is delayed until the rehabilitative phase. Dysphagia often resolves spontaneously during the first few months of recovery. Feeding the dysphagic patient is discussed in Chapter 36.

If the patient has a nasogastric or nasointestinal feeding tube in place, check its placement and residual according to agency policy. Provide the correct formula and ensure that it flows at the prescribed rate. Bolus feedings may be ordered at intervals, or pumps may be used to dispense continuous feedings. Monitor the rate of administration. Slightly elevate the head of the bed to reduce the risk of fluid flowing back into the esophagus and being aspirated. The nasogastric tube irritates the naris and the nasal passages. Gently cleanse the naris several times a day. Assess tube placement according to agency policy. Concentrated formulas may cause diarrhea. If that happens, the physician should be consulted about diluting the formula or changing to another type of formula.

Total parenteral nutrition is given through an intravenous line inserted into a large vein (a central line). Unlike enteral feedings, the flow of total parenteral nutrition fluids is always controlled with a mechanical infusion pump. The nurse hangs new bottles of prescribed fluids. Take special care to prevent air from entering the tubing. The insertion site also requires special care to prevent infection. Do dressing changes according to agency protocol, using strict aseptic technique. Patients on total parenteral nutrition may develop hyperglycemia; therefore, monitor blood glucose levels at regular intervals. Care of the patient receiving total parenteral nutrition is discussed in detail in Chapter 8.

Disturbed Sensory Perception

Sensory perceptual problems in the stroke patient may include visual disturbances, sensory deprivation or overload, and impaired tactile sensation. Among the visual disturbances are **diplopia** (double vision), loss of the corneal (blink) reflex, ptosis (drooping of the upper eyelid), homonymous hemianopsia, and inability to close the eyelids on the affected side. All of these pose threats to safety and to self-care. They may also contribute to confusion. The cornea is susceptible to injury when not protected and kept moist by the closed eyelid and the blink reflex. Artificial tears may be used to provide moisture.

Patients who have homonymous hemianopsia see only half the field of vision. Some patients have unilateral neglect, a condition in which visual fields are intact but the patient does not attend to certain parts of the fields. Unilateral neglect is most common in patients with right brain damage. These patients may not attend to one side of the body and may overlook objects on one side of the visual field.

It is helpful to encourage patients to scan the affected side. Differences in the nursing approaches during the acute and rehabilitative phases are well contrasted here. In the acute phase, position patients with homonymous hemianopsia so that their unimpaired side is approached by the staff, to reduce stress to the patient. In rehabilitation, position the patient so that deliberate scanning and use of the affected side are required. This is designed to stimulate return of function. Balanced sensory input is essential to reduce the risk of sensory deprivation or overload. The environment should be pleasant but not overly stimulating.

Another type of sensory disturbance after stroke is diminished sensation in affected body parts. The patient who does not feel pressure or pain is susceptible to injury. A paralyzed foot can easily slip down in-between the bed frame and side rails. Catheter tubing under the leg may create pressure that the patient cannot feel. Protect susceptible areas and remind the patient of the need for extra caution. Check positioning of affected extremities to ensure that they are free of pressure and reposition as needed.

Ineffective Thermoregulation

After a stroke, the body's temperature-regulating mechanism may be impaired, causing the temperature to rise. There are also metabolic processes in play that may increase the body temperature. It is important to monitor the patient's temperature and treat elevations promptly. Fever is treated aggressively with antipyretics and, if necessary, cooling blankets. Some studies even suggest a decrease in infarction size in those patients aggressively treated for hyperthermia. Always assess the patient for an underlying infection as a potential cause for any temperature elevation.

Disturbed Thought Processes

After a stroke, patients may suffer functional losses, alterations in sensation and perception, and impaired communication. In addition, they find themselves in the hospital, where they are poked, monitored, and prodded by strangers and where days and nights all seem the same. All these factors combined can cause the patient to become disoriented or confused. Neglect associated with right brain strokes may also be manifested as denial. In extreme cases, patients deny that they have even had a stroke.

To orient patients, introduce yourself, remind patients where they are, and tell them what is being done and why. Be sure that eyeglasses and hearing aids are worn if the patient normally uses them. Place clocks and marked calendars in view. Tell the patient what time it is and what to expect next. Confused patients require frequent reassurance and reinforcement. Instructions and information should be concise and repeated as needed. Sometimes a familiar person is helpful with a confused patient. If the visitor is disturbed by the patient's behavior, provide guidance in how to deal with the patient.

Impaired Verbal Communication

The alert patient who has aphasia is understandably anxious about the inability to speak, to understand words, or both. Use brief, clear statements accompanied by gestures, pictures, and facial expressions. Questions that can be answered yes or no may allow the patient to respond more easily. Pause attentively when the patient struggles to respond. Excessive chatter can be distressing to the aphasic patient. Explain the communication problem and approaches to the family. Speech therapy may be initiated once the medical condition of the patient is stable. Speech rehabilitation is discussed further in the section Nursing Care in the Rehabilitation Phase.

Impaired Physical Mobility

Impaired motor function is common after stroke and places the patient at risk for complications of immobility. Care of the immobilized patient is discussed in detail in Chapter 20 and is summarized here.

Skin Integrity. The potential for skin breakdown in this patient population is great because of motor impairment, altered consciousness or ser
incontinence. Measures t
cleanliness, pressure relief,
When skin is dry, as it c
bathing frequency, use so
retain skin moisture.

It is essential to turn an
tient at least every 2 hours. S
nerable pressure points after j
dened pressure areas remain
patient, shorten the intervals be
the patient to lie on the affected s... more than 30 minutes. Because of impaired sensation, the risk of excessive pressure and trauma is much greater on the affected side. Pressure must be alternated on main pressure points such as hips, knees, heels, and lower back. An air flotation mattress or fluidized bed may be used for the high-risk patient. Some of the newer therapeutic beds automatically turn patients. These beds do not stress the usual pressure points of the patient, but regular skin assessments and breathing exercises are still required. As soon as possible, position the patient comfortably in a chair for brief periods. Remember to monitor for a drop in blood pressure when getting the patient out of bed.

Good nursing care is time-consuming, so take advantage of this time to stimulate the patient with conversation and explanations of care. This is important even if the patient is unresponsive.

Joint Mobility. The immobilized patient is at risk for muscle atrophy and joint contractures. In the stroke patient, the affected side is especially vulnerable when there is loss of voluntary movement. During the acute phase, be concerned with maintaining joint mobility. This can be done with frequent gentle range-of-motion exercises and proper positioning. Determine whether the patient had any preexisting limitations of joint mobility. Older patients may have arthritic changes that reduce the range of motion. *Never* force resistant joints. Once the acute phase has passed, the patient is usually referred for vigorous physical therapy.

Support affected extremities. It is important never to grab or pull the extremities on the patient's affected side. Dislocation or further injury can easily occur, as the patient may not be able to accurately perceive the pressure or pain that is normally felt.

Circulation. Deep vein thrombosis (DVT) is a major complication of immobility, especially in this patient population. Regular passive and active range-of-motion exercises encourage venous blood return, thereby reducing the risk of thrombus formation. The physician may order elastic stockings or alternating pressure wraps to promote venous return. Low-dose anticoagulation therapy should be initiated to help prevent thrombus formation. Ambulation is generally encouraged (if the patient is able) as soon as possible after the medical condition stabilizes.

Total or Functional Urinary Incontinence

It is not unusual for urinary incontinence to occur after stroke. This may due to a temporarily flaccid bladder or an

to coordinate information to be able to bladder or wait once the urge to void is felt. ent hourly for wetness. Promptly remove wet d linens. Wash the skin, rinse, and pat dry. A vari- ncontinence products are available to minimize the act of urine with the skin (see Chapter 22). Sometimes n indwelling catheter is ordered to prevent incontinence. The catheter protects the skin and allows for more accurate measurement of output. The disadvantage is that an indwelling catheter is frequently the cause of urinary tract infections. A regular toileting schedule with intermittent catheterization is a better alternative to indwelling catheterization. External condom catheters are options for male patients. Bladder retraining, discussed in Chapter 22, is actively pursued in the rehabilitative phase.

Many older men have prostatic hypertrophy, which can cause dribbling of urine or urine retention. Scheduled toileting may be helpful, but catheterization may be required. The enlarged prostate makes catheterization more difficult. If the catheter cannot be inserted easily, *never* force it. Notify the registered nurse or physician. Sometimes a special type of catheter is needed for the patient with prostate enlargement.

Constipation and/or Bowel Incontinence

As with urinary incontinence, the ability of the brain to coordinate the information to wait once the urge to move their bowels is felt may be damaged. During the acute phase of stroke, it is especially important to monitor bowel elimination, because the patient may develop constipation or incontinence. It is helpful to know the patient's usual patterns of elimination, although they cannot always be determined.

Constipation may develop as a result of immobility, dehydration, and drug therapy. A bowel program, consisting of a mild laxative or stool softener and a high-fiber diet, can help prompt regular fecal elimination. Explain to patients and family members the importance of sufficient fluids to prevent dry stools. Some older people are laxative dependent. It is unrealistic to try to reverse the effects of years of laxative use during the acute phase of stroke. Inform the registered nurse or physician of the pattern and document bowel movements. Laxatives and enemas may be needed to maintain bowel elimination in these patients.

Bowel incontinence may be related to the inability to toilet independently or to confusion, and can often be prevented in the alert patient by taking the patient to the toilet at the usual time of defecation. A raised toilet seat with arm rests is easier and safer for the patient with hemiplegia. If incontinence occurs, take special care to clean the skin thoroughly. Be careful not to make comments that embarrass the patient. Remember that incontinence, especially with liquid stools, may indicate a fecal impaction. Removal of an impaction usually requires repeated enemas and manual removal of hard stool. Restoration of bowel control receives more attention in the rehabilitative phase and is detailed in Chapter 22.

Ineffective Coping

The effects of stroke may be temporary or permanent. It is difficult to predict how much function will be lost permanently or returned during recovery. Patients typically exhibit responses that reflect the grief process: shock, denial, depression, withdrawal, and bargaining. Determine how the patient is coping and whether the coping strategies are constructive and/or effective.

An example of unhealthy coping is the patient who denies having problems with vision or balance and refuses to call for help when getting out of bed. Another example is the depressed and withdrawn patient who resists doing therapeutic exercises that would minimize complications. You can point out the behavior to the patient, explain its consequences, and encourage the patient to take an active role in rehabilitation activities. Depression is a major problem associated with stroke and can occur in up to 70% of stroke patients. The depression seen post stroke may be the result of a loss of brain chemicals that are damaged by the injury or a reaction to the loss of one's functional abilities. Antidepressant medications may be ordered for patients experiencing depression after a stroke and have been associated with improved outcomes in those patients treated. Sometimes a mental health counselor or support group is beneficial to help the patient learn to deal with the effects of stroke more constructively.

Interrupted Family Processes

In the acute phase of stroke, family members are often frightened and confused. They may fear the patient's death or severe disability. They may also experience emotional and financial strain during the long rehabilitation process. Family members have to assume roles and responsibilities normally carried by the patient. Recognize that the family, as well as the patient, experiences a sense of loss when a loved one has a stroke. Provide support by telling family members what is happening, what is being done, and how they can help the patient. If necessary, a referral may be made to a social worker, mental health specialist, or spiritual counselor.

NURSING CARE *in the Rehabilitation Phase*

A patient's transition from the acute phase to the rehabilitation phase of stroke is an important one. Early and attentive care for the stroke patient shortens the recovery time and hastens the return of function. The general goals of treatment in the rehabilitation phase are to maximize functional abilities and to teach new ways to compensate for losses. Stabilization of vital signs, with no further neurologic deficits, indicates that the patient has entered the rehabilitation phase of stroke. At this time the patient's functional and cognitive problems can vary widely, depending on the location and extent of brain damage. The patient may regain complete independent functioning, partially recover previous abilities, or lose functional abilities completely.

The rehabilitation phase is usually managed by an interdisciplinary team that includes nurses, physicians, physical therapists, occupational therapists, speech therapists, social workers, psychologists, recreational therapists, vocational rehabilitation counselors, and dietitians.

During the rehabilitation phase of a stroke, vast changes can occur in the brain. The extent to which collateral blood circulation and alternative neuronal pathways develop affects the ultimate outcome for the patient. The goals of rehabilitation to enhance the ultimate recovery of functional abilities are reached through a program of stimulation and practice. It has been said that rehabilitation is the respectful challenging of the patient facing a chronic health problem. With this in mind, the next section describes nursing care in the management of long-term problems that can follow a stroke.

Assessment

Nursing assessment of the stroke patient was described earlier in this chapter and is summarized in Table 27-4. In the rehabilitation phase, reassess the patient's abilities as well as his or her expectations, knowledge, motivation, and resources.

Nursing Diagnoses, Goals, and Outcome Criteria: Rehabilitation Phase of Stroke

Nursing Diagnoses	Goals and Outcome Criteria
Self-Care Deficits related to sensory and motor impairments	Self-care needs met: care accomplished with assistance as needed
Risk for Injury related to sensory and motor impairments	Absence of injury: no falls, bruises, skin tears, pressure sores
Ineffective Coping related to cognitive impairments	Effective coping: patient uses adaptive strategies to cope with disability
Impaired Verbal Communication related to aphasia, dysarthria	Effective communication: meaningful verbalizations or effective use of nonverbal communication to make needs known
Imbalanced Nutrition: Less than Body Requirements related to dysphagia, anorexia	Adequate nutrition: achievement and maintenance of ideal body weight
Impaired Physical Mobility related to residual motor impairment	Improved physical mobility: increasing independent physical activity
Constipation related to inactivity	Normal bowel elimination: regular, formed stools without straining
Total and Functional Incontinence related to neurologic and motor impairment	Normal urine elimination

Interventions

Self-Care Deficits

The main focus of the rehabilitation phase is to return the stroke patient to the highest level of functioning possible. One of the most frustrating problems following a stroke for many patients and caregivers is the patient's inability to complete activities of daily living. To improve, patients need to use affected parts as much as they are able. It is important for the nurse to demonstrate patience and a supportive attitude. Allow time for patients to try to do things for themselves. Discouragement is a major factor in unsuccessful rehabilitation and demands prompt attention by the rehabilitation team.

A variety of personal devices and environmental adaptations can foster a return to independence. Prosthetic devices that assist patients with dressing, bathing, and eating are available. Simple measures such as replacing buttons with Velcro fasteners and replacing complicated trousers with elastic-waist pants can make a big difference.

A referral for follow-up at home should be initiated so that the safety and accessibility of the home environment can be assessed before discharge. The trend toward shorter hospital stays means this must be addressed very early. Many patients are discharged to rehabilitation or skilled nursing facilities until they are ready to return home. A home visit by the patient, home health nurse, and occupational therapist can be made to identify problems and make plans for adaptations. Adaptations should promote access in and out of the home and enable patients to be as independent as possible. The addition of a raised commode seat, bathtub handrails, shower seats, or other devices can facilitate toileting and bathing. Cooking may be assisted by adjusting the height of counters, creating shelves that roll out, and rearranging cabinet contents to improve access. Patients need to practice daily tasks under conditions similar to those at home. Rehabilitation centers usually have activity centers that allow patients to practice self-care skills with their disabilities (Fig. 27-6).

Risk for Injury

Alterations in motor function, sensation, and vision are distressing changes that affect the patient's ability to carry out self-care and pose a threat to safety.

Motor. Alterations in motor functioning may leave the patient at risk for injury. Safety precautions are a vital part of

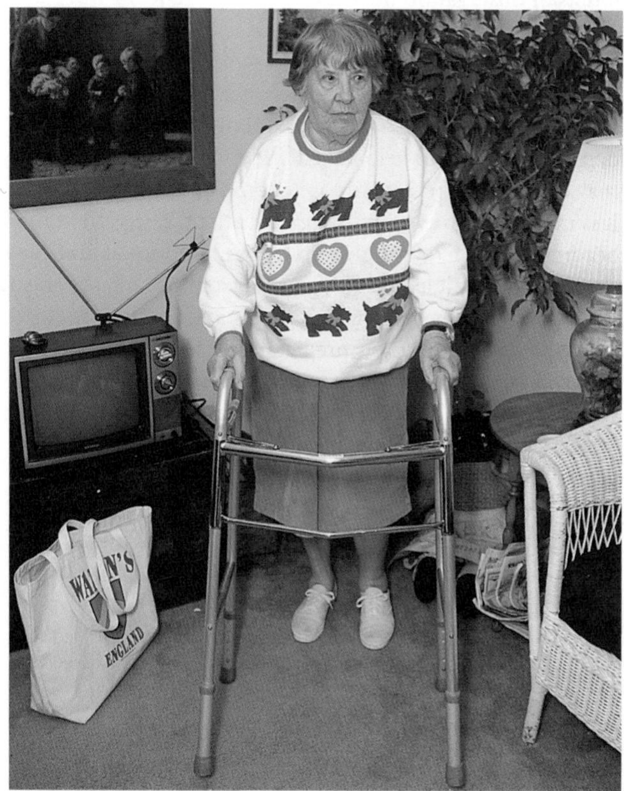

FIGURE **27-6** Assistive devices enable the patient to be active at home.

nursing care of the patient. Teaching should include calling for assistance as needed, use of assistive devices for mobilization, and adaptation of the environment to promote safety. Physical and occupational therapists are invaluable in assisting with providing a safe environment.

Sensation. As noted previously, patients may have altered sensation in the affected body parts after a stroke. This may appear as loss of sensation or as exaggerated response in which every sensation is perceived as painful. The patient may be injured without even knowing it because of impaired sensation. Teach the patient and family to assess the affected area frequently for signs of pressure and to protect it from injury. In addition to teaching the patient how to avoid pressure, advise the patient not to apply heat or cold to that area because of the risk of injury. Remind the patient and family not to pull on the affected side or use that side to move or support the patient in ambulation.

Patients with abnormal pain perception may benefit from regular physical therapy, using a kind of desensitization. During therapy, the patient is reminded and encouraged that the pain is not real and is only misinterpreted by the brain.

Vision. Homonymous hemianopsia, in which half of the field of vision is lost, also presents problems with self-care and safety. In the acute phase, the patient's environment is arranged so that people approach and important items are available on the unaffected side. In rehabilitation, the patient is challenged more to promote adaptation to the disability. Place objects in the field of the visual deficit. Remind and encourage the patient to scan the affected visual field, especially when walking, wheeling, and eating. The patient forms new habits of observation through constant practice.

Ineffective Coping

Intellectual and emotional changes after stroke are distressing to patients and their families. Explain these changes and demonstrate how to help patients adapt. Cognitive processes may continue to be slow for quite some time after the stroke. It is important to avoid rushing the patient. The patient may become frustrated and give up trying. Emotional ability is manifested as sudden laughing, crying, or outbursts of anger without apparent reason. Caregivers and families may attribute this emotional unpredictability to depression. It is generally believed that depression is frequently associated with brain trauma of any kind. The patient can often be easily distracted from crying or from anger with simple redirection to the task at hand. This is an indication that the depression, if it exists, may be of a different type than the usual emotional state and require specific interventions. Treatment of depression, whatever the cause, is an important part of the rehabilitation process. Research clearly demonstrates a positive relationship to outcomes when patients are identified and treated aggressively for depression after a stroke.

Impaired Verbal Communication

Helping the patient improve or regain effective communication is an extremely important goal of the rehabilitation phase. Aphasia may affect the ability to understand spoken words or to use words to express oneself. Types of aphasia were explained with signs and symptoms of stroke (see Table 27-3).

Patients with aphasia need encouragement as they struggle to communicate. Be patient, as the aphasic person requires more time to plan and deliver a response. Take time to allow this to happen, but provide verbal cues or picture boards before patients become overly frustrated trying to respond. The physician often refers patients with severe communication impairments to speech therapists.

Imbalanced Nutrition

The patient with dysphagia must be reevaluated at intervals for ability to swallow. If the patient is able to swallow saliva, the physician may allow liquids to be introduced. Initially, ¼ teaspoon of ice chips might be given with a spoon. The amount is increased and water may be added until the patient is able to swallow a teaspoon of water. If problems with this simple assessment occur, a video fluoroscopic test of swallowing may be ordered. This test traces the route of swallowed fluid to detect swallowing abnormalities. Because water is thin, some patients find it difficult to swallow. It may be helpful to add a thicker substance to liquids to facilitate swallowing.

The patient who has some difficulty swallowing may be placed on a supervised feeding program. Speech therapists are trained to help patients relearn swallowing, but everyday feeding falls to the nursing staff. The best position for eating is sitting with the head tilted forward and toward the unaffected side. Fluid intake must still be encouraged for the dysphagic person, despite the increased work for patient and staff. Special utensils can greatly facilitate self-feeding (Fig 27-7). Acknowledge even small improvements as the patient struggles in rehabilitation.

Impaired Physical Mobility

Mobility can continue to be a problem for patients in the rehabilitation phase. Hemiplegia, dyspraxia, and visual field disturbances all create unique problems. Hemiplegia is rarely a motor problem alone. It is often accompanied by disturbances in balance and spatial perception (Fig. 27-8).

Regular physical therapy and occupational therapy promote optimal return of motor function. Regular exercise can facilitate a dramatic return of function for some patients. Therefore, affected arms and legs need to be used to maintain muscular function and circulation if and until neurologic ability is recovered. In the meantime, assistance is needed with motor activities. When the patient is moving, assess gait (if applicable), strength in arms and legs, and balance. Correct body mechanics and transfer techniques are essential when working with the patient. A gait belt helps the patient in transfers and in ambulation and may protect staff members from injury. This is a fabric belt with a toothed buckle that is applied between the nipple line and the waist and is used to support and assist the patient. Assistive devices such as the quad cane and walkers may improve safety with ambulation (Fig. 27-9).

Patients who have dyspraxia are unable to initiate voluntary motor acts. Interestingly, they sometimes exhibit those

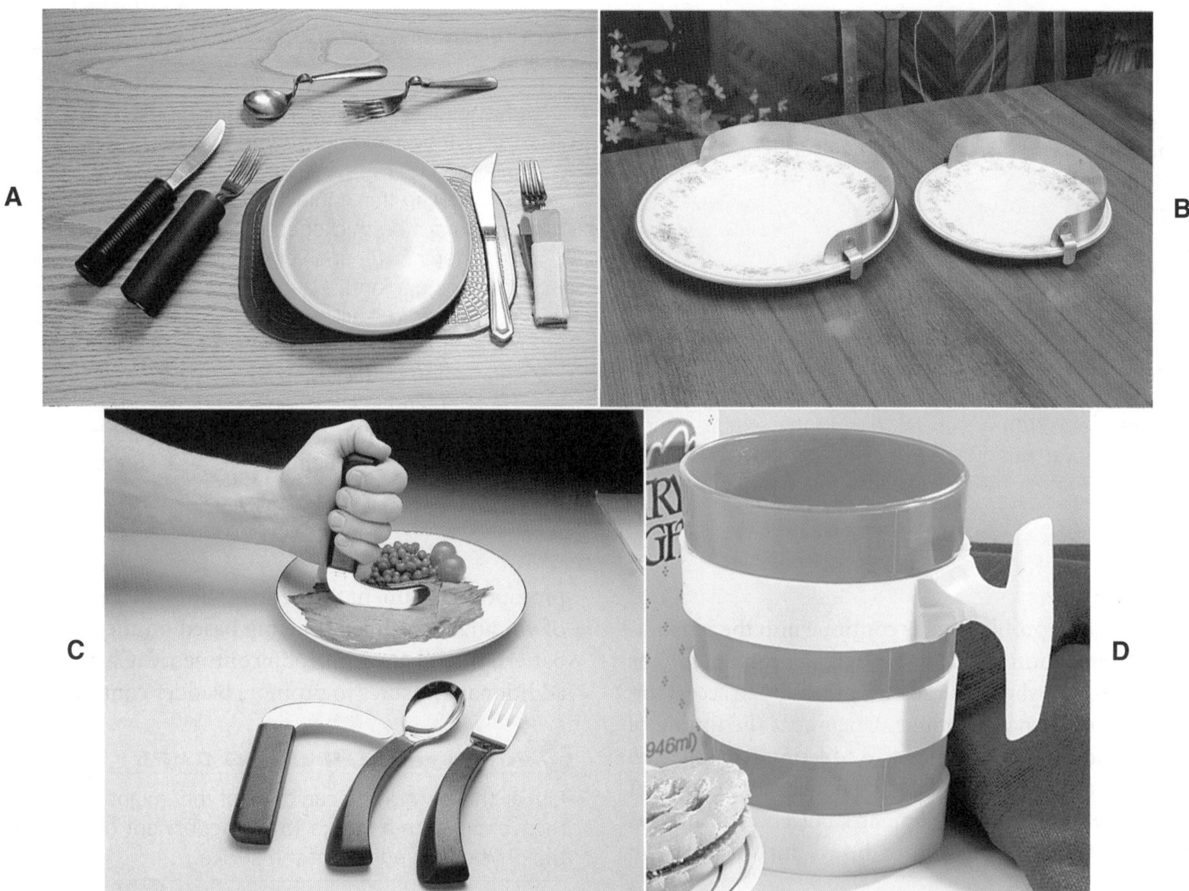

FIGURE 27-7 Assistive devices for eating. *A,* Utensils adapted to special needs. A plate that keeps food from being pushed off. *B,* Plate guards keep food on the plate. *C,* The round-blade knife allows a person to cut with only one hand. *D,* Special handle is easier to grasp and hold.

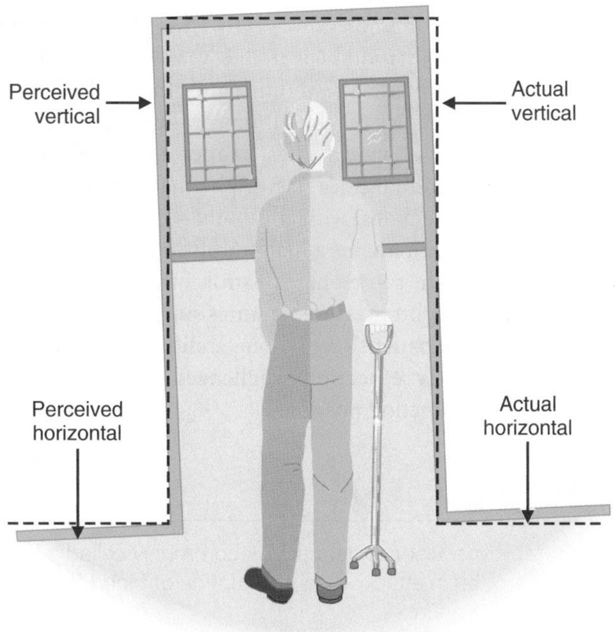

FIGURE 27-8 Perceptual disturbances in hemiplegia may affect the patient's ability to maneuver safely in the environment.

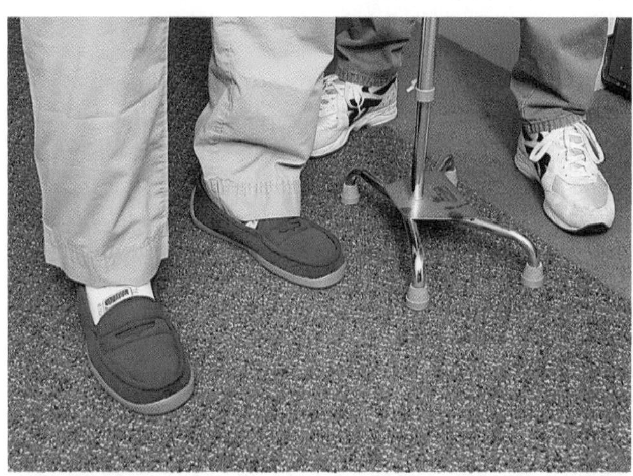

FIGURE 27-9 A quad cane provides good support for a patient with hemiplegia.

actions spontaneously. To help the patient remember to initiate voluntary responses, provide verbal cues. Teach family members about dyspraxia and advise them to be patient and employ cues to induce the desired motor performance. Remind the patient who has unilateral neglect to use and support the affected side.

Put on your THINKING CAP!!

Use a towel or other material to make an arm sling. Place your dominant arm in the sling while you prepare a meal, eat, and clean up. Immediately after this exercise, write down: 1) what adaptations you had to make, 2) what things you were unable to do unassisted, 3) how you felt during the exercise, and 4) how you behaved during the exercise. Compare responses with your classmates. Discuss implications for patient care.

Nutrition Concepts

1. A major nutritional concern for the stroke patient is dysphagia (difficulty swallowing), which may lead to malnutrition and dehydration because of inadequate intake.
2. Swallowing thin liquids is frequently a problem. Thin liquids can be thickened with dry milk powder, cornstarch, fruit and vegetable flakes, or commercial thickening agents.
3. Very warm or chilled foods stimulate the swallowing reflex better than bland, lukewarm foods.
4. In addition to thickened liquids, foods that are better for chewing and swallowing are soft bread, cooked cereal, ice cream, yogurt, cooked eggs, moist ground beef, canned fruits and vegetables, thick soups, and puddings.

Constipation

Bowel elimination problems may continue into the rehabilitation phase. Incontinence is not usually a problem for the alert patient except when it is caused by inability to access toileting devices or manage clothing. Document the timing of incidents of bowel incontinence so a toileting schedule can be developed. Often simply taking the patient to the toilet at the usual time of defecation eliminates bowel incontinence. There is additional discussion of bowel incontinence in Chapter 22.

Constipation is a more common challenge in the rehabilitation phase. A regular bowel program with toileting, orientation, and reminders is needed. Provide sufficient fluids to promote bowel regularity. Many stroke patients do not receive adequate fluid intake because of dysphagia or fear of incontinence. Also, caregivers may not take the extra time needed to provide fluids for the patient who responds slowly. Stool softeners, laxatives, and suppositories may be used to reestablish regular bowel elimination and then gradually discontinued. Some patients continue to need stool softeners. As noted earlier, some patients with long-standing laxative dependency may not respond to more conservative measures to promote bowel elimination.

Total and Functional Urinary Incontinence

If an indwelling catheter was inserted in the acute phase of stroke treatment, it will probably be removed and efforts made to restore bladder control. Immediately after the catheter is removed, the patient may have poor sphincter control or may retain urine. Therefore, monitor urine output and check for bladder distention until normal voiding is established. Perineal muscle exercises (see Chapter 22) may be prescribed to improve sphincter control.

Intermittent catheterization may continue to be necessary in the rehabilitation phase. The urine volume obtained is measured, and intermittent catheterization is done every 4 to 6 hours, depending on the volume obtained.

Incontinence of urine is more difficult to correct than bowel incontinence. A bladder program should be initiated promptly. Document the patient's fluid intake and frequency of voiding. Scheduled toileting based on the patient's usual pattern often helps control incontinence. Chapter 22 details additional measures to promote bladder control.

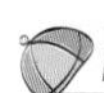

Put on your THINKING CAP!!

List all the factors you can think of that might cause a patient recovering from a stroke to be incontinent of urine *besides* the physiologic effects of the stroke.

Discharge

Patients may be discharged to their homes or may go to specialized rehabilitation centers for continued therapy. Outpatient therapy is an option for some patients. The rehabilitation phase is defined in various ways. When no improvements in function are noted in a 1- to 2-week period, some consider the rehabilitation phase to be over. Medicare defines the rehabilitation phase as 3 months after the stroke. Rehabilitation specialists say rehabilitation continues indefinitely, but progress slows down. During and after the rehabilitation phase, patients and families need to be made aware of resources to help them deal with continuing disabilities.

Although stroke remains a major health problem, the risk can be reduced. The acute phase of stroke, from diagnosis to stabilization of blood pressure, requires support and careful evaluation of the patient's remaining abilities. In rehabilitation, the patient is respectfully challenged to return to the highest level of function possible.

key points

- A cerebrovascular accident (CVA), commonly called a stroke or brain attack, is an interruption of blood flow to part of the brain.
- The risk factors for CVA are atherosclerosis, atrial fibrillation, hypertension, diabetes mellitus, cardiac disease, excessive alcohol consumption, and, for women, smoking while taking oral contraceptives.

- A cerebrovascular accident can be classified as a transient ischemic attack, a stroke in evolution, or a completed stroke.
- A transient ischemic attack is a temporary neurologic deficit caused by impaired cerebral blood flow.
- A transient ischemic attack, sometimes considered a warning sign of impending stroke, is treated with diet modification, exercise, drug therapy to prevent clot formation, surgery to clear or bypass obstructed blood vessels, or a combination of these.
- A stroke is a set of neurologic signs and symptoms caused by impaired blood flow to the brain that persists for more than 24 hours.
- When neurologic symptoms continue to progress over hours or days, the condition is described as stroke in evolution; with a completed stroke, the symptoms do not change for several days.
- A hemorrhagic stroke is caused by rupture of a blood vessel in the brain, and an ischemic stroke is caused by obstruction of a blood vessel by an embolus or a thrombus.
- Signs and symptoms of stroke depend on the type, location, and extent of brain injury but may include one-sided weakness, numbness, visual problems, confusion and memory lapses, headache, dysphagia, and speech problems.
- Some symptoms of stroke improve, but patients may be left with impairments in speech, language comprehension, motor function, vision, cognition, and bladder control, as well as with personality changes and emotional liability.
- Aphasia is the inability to understand words or respond with appropriate messages.
- Dysarthria is the inability to speak clearly because of neurologic damage that affects the muscles of speech.
- Dysphagia is difficulty swallowing.
- Dyspraxia is the partial inability to initiate coordinated voluntary motor acts in an unparalyzed extremity.
- Paralysis of one side of the body (the side opposite the brain injury) is called hemiplegia.
- Medical treatment of CVA may employ oxygen therapy, diuretics, corticosteroids, anticoagulants, thrombolytics, intravenous fluids, dietary modifications, and catheterization, as well as treatment of risk factors.
- The focus of nursing care after stroke is on ineffective airway clearance, ineffective breathing patterns, risk for injury, deficient fluid volume, fluid volume excess, imbalanced nutrition: less than body requirements, sensory perceptual alterations, ineffective thermoregulation, disturbed thought processes, impaired verbal communication, impaired physical mobility, total or functional urinary incontinence, constipation, bowel incontinence, ineffective coping, and altered family processes.
- After experiencing a stroke, the patient may regain complete independent functioning, partially recover previous abilities, or lose functional abilities completely.
- The goal of rehabilitation after stroke is to enhance the recovery of functional abilities through a program of stimulation and practice.

REVIEW QUESTIONS

1. The structures of the brain that control respirations and heart rate are located in the:
   1. cerebrum.
   2. brain stem.
   3. cerebellum.
   4. cortex.

2. Recognition of a transient ischemic attack (TIA) is important because a TIA:
   1. is a symptom of a brain tumor.
   2. can cause permanent disability.
   3. is a warning sign of future stroke.
   4. occurs shortly before a hemorrhage.

3. How are TIAs and strokes different?
   1. Weakness and loss of balance are symptoms of TIA, but not stroke.
   2. Imaging studies show circulatory changes with stroke, but not with TIA.
   3. Anticoagulants are used with some strokes, but not with TIA.
   4. TIA symptoms resolve within 24 hours; stroke symptoms persist longer.

4. When anticoagulants are used to reduce the risk of stroke, the INR should not exceed:
   1. 1.5.
   2. 2.0.
   3. 2.5.
   4. 3.0.

5. The most common type of stroke is:
   1. ischemic.
   2. incomplete.
   3. hemorrhagic.
   4. subarachnoid.

6. Mr. X was admitted to the hospital with signs and symptoms of a stroke. After 24 hours, his symptoms are more severe than on admission. This sequence of events is called:
   1. completed stroke.
   2. stroke in evolution.
   3. progressive stroke.
   4. terminal stroke.

7. Ms. Y is recovering from a stroke. She is able to follow directions and communicate nonverbally. However, she struggles to speak and the words are slurred. When you can understand her, her message is appropriately expressed. This pattern describes:
   1. amnesia.
   2. dysarthria.
   3. dysphagia.
   4. dyspraxia.

8. Modifiable risk factors for stroke include:
   1. age.
   2. race.
   3. gender.
   4. hypertension.

9. Successful use of tissue plasminogen activator in the stroke patient requires:
   1. Deep intramuscular administration into a large muscle mass.
   2. Administration only to patients who have had hemorrhagic strokes.
   3. Intravenous administration within 3 hours of the onset of symptoms.
   4. Concurrent use with heparin to prevent additional clots from forming.

10. Nursing interventions for patients with aphasia include:
    1. Insist that patients try to express needs verbally.
    2. Help them find the right word if they become frustrated.
    3. Give praise only when patients verbalize successfully.
    4. Encourage families to speak for patients rather than forcing patients to speak.

CHAPTER

28 Spinal Cord Injury

LESLIE GODDARD

objectives

1. Explain the impact of spinal cord injury.
2. Describe the diagnostic tests used to evaluate spinal cord injuries and related nursing responsibilities.
3. Explain the physical effects of spinal cord injury.
4. Describe the medical and surgical treatment during the acute phase of spinal cord injury.
5. List the data to be included in the nursing assessment of the patient with a spinal cord injury.
6. Identify nursing diagnoses, goals, interventions, and outcome criteria for the patient with a spinal cord injury.
7. Describe the nursing care for the patient undergoing a laminectomy.
8. State the goals of rehabilitation for the patient with spinal cord injury.

key terms

Autonomic dysreflexia (aw-tō-NŌM-ĭk dĭs-rē-FLĔKS-ē-ă, p. 439)
Dermatome (DĔR-mă-tōm, p. 444)
Flaccid (FLĂS-ĭd, p.439)
Myelinated (MĪ-ĕ-lĭ-nāt-ĕd, p. 433)
Paraplegia (păr-ă-PLĒ-jă, p. 436)
Quadriplegia (kwŏd-rĭ-PLĒ-jă, p. 436)
Spasticity (spăs-TĬS-ĭ-tē, p. 440)

Few injuries are as physically and emotionally devastating to a person as a permanent spinal cord injury. The latest National Head and Spinal Cord Injury survey estimates that 10,000 people sustain permanent injuries each year. One third of victims die before reaching a hospital. The remaining injured have varying degrees of disabilities, requiring care that costs more than $10 billion annually.

The incidence of spinal cord injury peaks in individuals in their early twenties, with a small increase seen in the elderly as a result of falls and degenerative disease. The leading cause of spinal cord injury is trauma sustained in vehicular accidents, falls, assaults, and sports-related mishaps. The cord also can be damaged by degenerative conditions and tumors.

Medical advances and more rapid transport of accident victims to trauma centers have made it possible for an individual with spinal cord injury to achieve a normal life expectancy. The effects of the injury, however, may lead to other health problems that require long-term care and impair quality of life. Quality nursing care during the acute and rehabilitative phases of injury can minimize the impact of lifelong problems that plague the spinal cord–injured person. Consequently, the potential for rehabilitation and full quality of life can be enhanced.

ANATOMY AND PHYSIOLOGY OF THE SPINAL CORD

To understand the effects of spinal cord injury fully, it is important to know the anatomy and physiology of the spinal cord. Normal spinal cord function requires an intact cord with a good blood supply and bony support. Disruption of any one of these components can result in neurologic dysfunction.

VERTEBRAL COLUMN

The bony vertebral column consists of 33 vertebrae: 7 cervical (C1 through C7), 12 thoracic (T1 through T12), 5 lumbar (L1 through L5), 5 sacral (S1 through S5), and 4 coccygeal, which are fused (Fig. 28-1). The individual vertebra consists of a body and an arch, as shown in Figure 28-2. The body is the round structure that forms the anterior portion of the vertebra. The arch is the posterior portion of the vertebra. The spinal cord passes through an opening in the center of each arch. The structures that form the posterior section of the arch are called laminae. Each arch has articulating surfaces against which adjacent vertebrae smoothly glide with movement. In addition, each arch has locations for the attachment of ribs and muscles. The bony column is supported by muscles and ligaments, which permit mobility and flexibility.

DISKS

Vertebrae are separated by intervertebral disks, which serve as shock absorbers for the vertebral column. Disks are composed of the anulus fibrosus and the nucleus pulposus. The anulus fibrosus is the fibrous ring of tissue that encircles the nucleus pulposus. The nucleus pulposus is the central sac-like structure with a gelatinous filling that has a high water content. As a person ages, the nucleus pulposus loses a great deal of its water, so it becomes less effective as a shock absorber. Therefore, older people are at greater risk for back injuries and herniated disks.

SPINAL CORD

The spinal cord extends from the brain stem to the level of L2 in the pelvic cavity (Fig. 28-3). It has a central canal, which

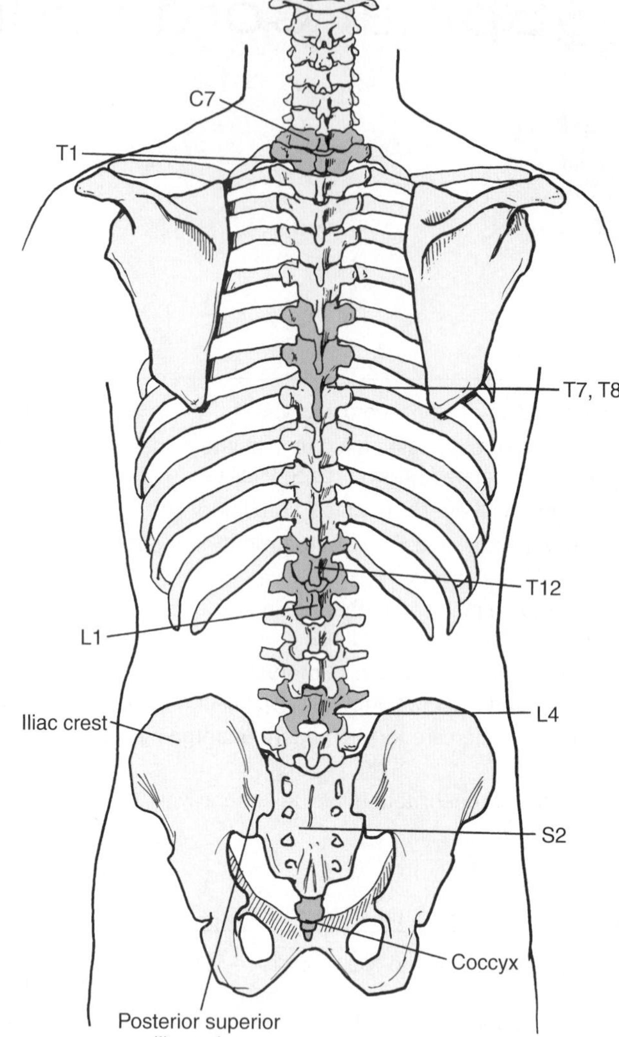

FIGURE **28-1** The bony vertebral column consists of 33 vertebrae.

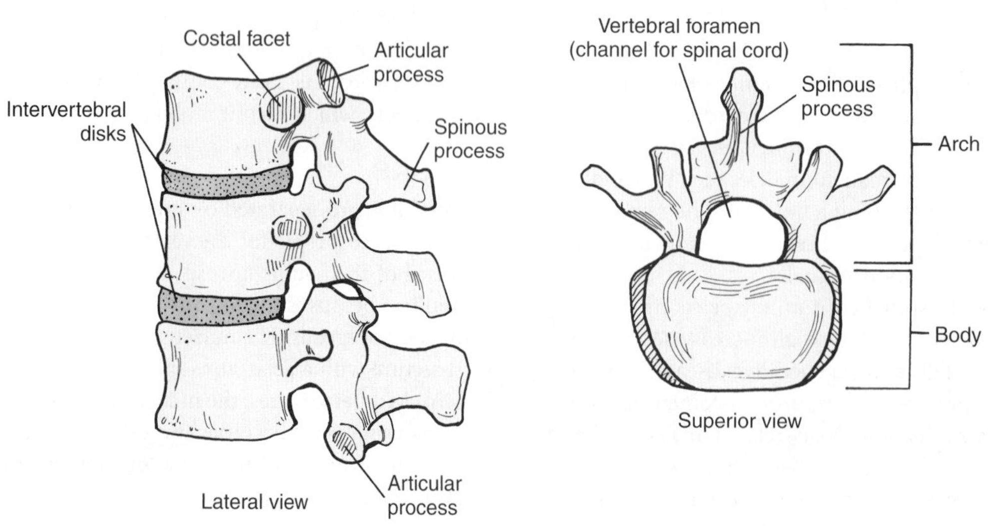

FIGURE **28-2** Intervertebral disks separate the vertebrae, each of which consists of a body and an arch.

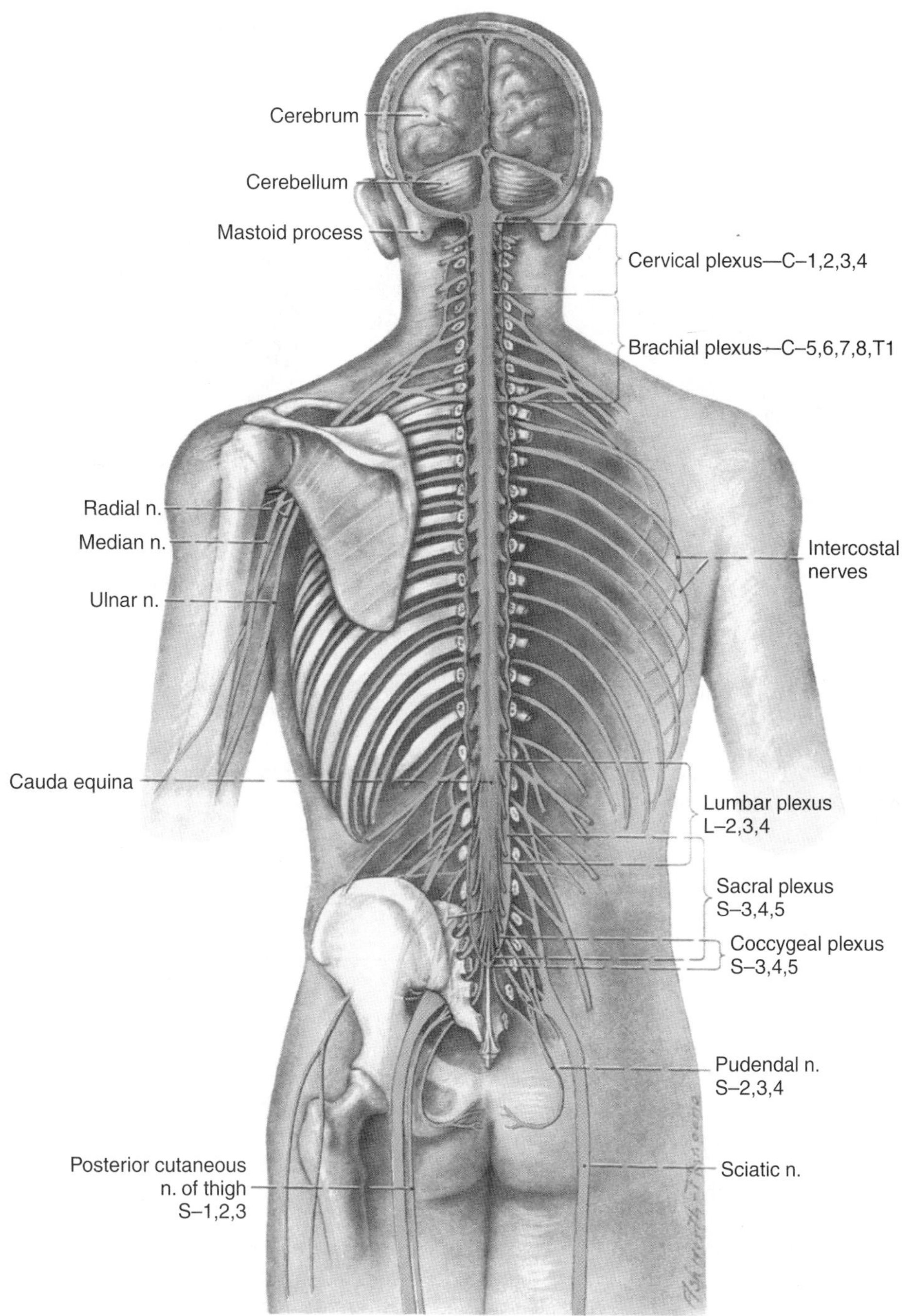

FIGURE 28-3 The spinal cord extends from the brain stem to the level of the second lumbar vertebra.

is continuous with the fourth ventricle of the brain. The cord is surrounded by three protective meningeal layers: the dura mater, the arachnoid, and the pia mater. The dura mater is the outermost layer. The arachnoid, the middle layer, is a network of spaces containing cerebrospinal fluid (CSF). The pia mater is the innermost layer; it directly covers the spinal cord. The cerebrospinal fluid circulates through the brain and spinal column, bathing and protecting the entire central nervous system.

A cross section of the spinal cord reveals an inner area of H-shaped gray matter surrounded by white matter. The gray matter consists of the bodies of nerve cells that control motor and sensory activities. The white matter, which is myelinated (surrounded by a sheath), consists of bundles of fibers. These fibers, known as columns or tracts, convey information between the brain and the spinal cord. The tracts may be either ascending or descending. Ascending tracts carry sensory information from the spinal cord to the brain. Descending tracts

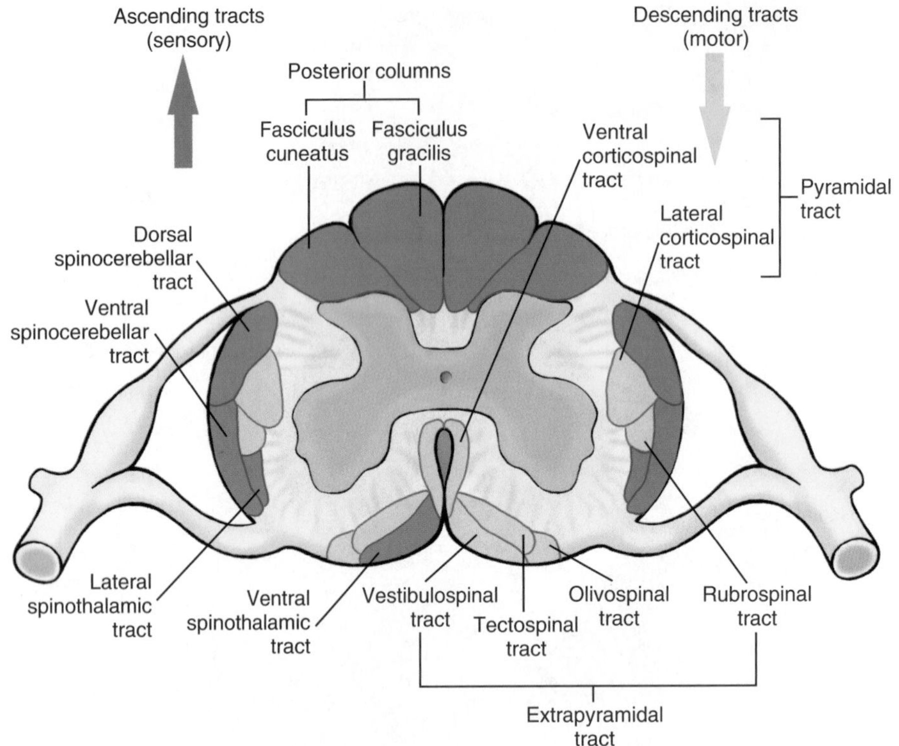

FIGURE **28-4** Cross section of spinal cord. Sensory *(S)* tracts convey sensory information to the brain. Motor *(M)* tracts convey information from the brain.

table 28-1 ***Summary of the Four Major Spinal Cord Tracts***

TRACT	TYPE	FEATURES	FUNCTION
Spinothalamic, lateral	Ascending (sensory: pain and temperature)	Originates in spinal cord and ascends to thalamus in brain. On entering cord, impulses cross over to opposite side (contralateral).	Carries pain and temperature sensation from opposite side.
Corticospinal, lateral	Descending (motor)	Initiates in motor tract of brain, crosses over to opposite side at level of medulla, proceeds down to appropriate spinal cord level.	Controls voluntary motor action.
Spinocerebellar	Ascending (sensory)	Initiates in spinal cord and terminates in cerebellum.	Assists in coordination of muscle contraction.
Posterior columns	Ascending (sensory: touch, vibration, position sense)	Made up of several tracts that relay messages from body to brain. Initiates in sensory fibers of spinal nerves, crosses over in medulla, and terminates in sensory cortex of opposite hemisphere.	Carries touch, deep pressure, vibration, and position sense.

carry motor information from the brain to the spinal cord (Fig. 28-4).

Blood supply to the spinal cord is vital. Any disruption in blood flow can ultimately lead to neurologic damage. The major arterial supply to the spinal cord consists of the vertebral arteries posteriorly and the anterior spinal artery.

Spinal cord function may be classified as either reflexive or relay in nature. With reflexive activity, the sensory stimulus is received and a response is initiated at the level of the spinal cord. The knee jerk is an example of reflexive activity. When the knee is tapped, impulses travel by sensory neurons to the spinal cord, where they are relayed to motor neurons. The impulse travels back to the muscles at the front of the thigh, causing muscle contraction and jerking of the leg. This circuit of impulse transmission is called a reflex arc.

With relay activity, the stimulus enters the spinal cord and travels up the ascending tracts to relay sensory signals from the external environment to the brain. Information is processed in the brain, and responses are initiated by impulses transmitted to the body by way of descending tracts.

The descending white matter tracts also participate in the relay function of the spinal cord. These tracts relay motor information, with messages being sent from the brain, down the cord, to muscles, which effect various kinds of responses. Four of the most important spinal cord tracts are summarized in Table 28-1.

Information is conveyed by the senses to the brain and spinal cord via the peripheral nervous system. This system consists of 31 pairs of spinal nerves, which branch from the cord and pass between the vertebrae to muscles and visceral organs. Each spinal nerve has a dorsal root, which transmits sensory information, and a ventral root, which transmits motor information. The 12 cranial nerves, arising from the brain stem, also are part of the peripheral nervous system.

DIAGNOSTIC TESTS AND PROCEDURES

Emergency care of the patient with a spinal cord injury is discussed in Chapter 15. When the victim of spinal cord injury arrives at the hospital, the extent of injury must be assessed. Specific tests are performed to determine the type of injury and to provide direction for treatment. Throughout the diagnostic process, the spine must be immobilized continuously.

NEUROLOGIC EXAMINATION

The initial neurologic evaluation of the spinal cord–injured patient provides the nurse with a baseline assessment of both function and problems. Ongoing assessment is necessary to monitor the effects of neurologic injury, detect related complications, and determine the patient's need for assistance in activities of daily living.

In the patient with spinal cord injury, neurologic evaluation focuses on the motor and sensory systems. Movement, muscle strength, and reflex activity are evaluated on an ongoing basis as described in the section on assessment. Basic neurologic assessment is covered in Chapter 26. A textbook on physical assessment should be referred to for the detailed steps of the neurologic evaluation.

IMAGING STUDIES

Radiography

Standard radiographs are obtained to detect vertebral compression, fractures, or problems with alignment. The entire spine may be radiographed because patients sometimes have multiple fractures separated by sections of normal spine. The physician also may order special radiographs, called coned-down views, that reveal fractures more clearly. Radiography is repeated at intervals to evaluate the achievement of proper alignment with treatment.

Computed Tomography

Computed tomography (CT) is a truly revolutionary diagnostic tool. This noninvasive procedure is used to examine small sections of tissue within any organ, allowing anatomic structures and pathologic processes to be viewed. The specific levels of the spinal cord can be visualized on the scan, as can the bony vertebrae and the spinal nerves. The physician can readily identify bony fractures, floating bone fragments, dislocations, tumors, hemorrhage, and cord and nerve compressions. In some injuries, soft tissue swelling may obscure some structures and make visualization of the cord and vertebrae difficult.

Although no special physical preparation is needed for a patient undergoing computed tomography, this imaging procedure should be explained to the patient. The patient is told that he or she will be asked to lie very still for a period of time while on a small table that slowly moves through the scanner. Enhanced scanning also may be done, in which a radiopaque dye is infused intravenously into the patient. This testing is contraindicated in the patient who is allergic to this type of dye. The patient receiving the dye must be encouraged to take plenty of fluids after the procedure to promote renal excretion.

Magnetic Resonance Imaging

Magnetic resonance imaging (MRI), unlike computed tomography, does not expose the patient to radiation. The patient is slowly moved through a strong magnetic field and then subjected to short bursts of radio waves. Sophisticated technology translates information about body tissue to produce precise, clear images of internal structures.

This noninvasive diagnostic imaging study is painless, has no known risks, and requires no preparation. The nurse tells the patient to expect to hear a humming sound as the radio waves are turned on and off. The patient must have no metal materials or equipment on (including pacemakers or prostheses) when entering the scanning suite. Because the magnetic field in the scanner is very strong, any metal object may be attracted into the field. A quartz watch would be disrupted because the magnetic field has a detrimental effect on the battery. If an intravenous pump is being used, the site must first be converted to a heparin lock because the pump cannot be placed in the scanning room. If oxygen is required, adequate tubing is needed to allow the oxygen tank to be placed a safe distance outside the suite. Patients with pacemakers cannot undergo magnetic resonance imaging because the magnetic field would inactivate the pacer.

Myelography

A myelogram is obtained to visualize the spinal cord and vertebrae. A puncture is made in the lumbar area between L3 and L4. Radiopaque dye is then injected into the subarachnoid space of the spinal cord. Any obstruction that impedes the flow of the dye can be seen on radiography. Because of the invasive nature of the procedure, informed consent must be obtained. Nursing care before and after myelography is summarized in Table 28-2.

table 28-2 *Nursing Care of the Patient Having Myelography*

PREPARATION	POSTPROCEDURE CARE
Ensure that signed consent has been obtained.	Frequently assess vital signs and neurologic status.
Inquire about allergy to dye, iodine, or shellfish; inform radiologist if the patient is allergic.	Encourage increased fluid intake to promote elimination of dye, if not contraindicated.
Allow nothing by mouth for 4-6 hr before the procedure, according to agency protocol.	Measure and record fluid intake and output.
Administer prescribed premedications.	Position as ordered: flat or head of bed elevated 30-45 degrees, depending on type of contrast medium used.
Have patient empty bladder if able.	Administer analgesics as ordered for headache.
Determine whether any medications should be withheld.	Assess for back pain, increased temperature, difficulty voiding, neck stiffness, and nausea and vomiting.

PATHOPHYSIOLOGY OF SPINAL CORD INJURY

Traumatic injury creates abnormal forces on the neck and structural components of the spinal cord. The cervical vertebrae support the head and neck and permit movement in various directions. The thoracic vertebrae, on the other hand, permit little movement because of the restrictions of the ribs. Because the thoracic spine has limited flexibility, the neck and cervical spine are extremely vulnerable to injury.

TYPES OF INJURIES

Spinal cord injuries may be classified (1) by location, (2) as open or closed, and (3) by extent of damage to the cord. Injuries classified by location are described as cervical, thoracic, or lumbar, depending on the level of the cord affected.

Closed injuries involve trauma in which the skin and meningeal covering that surround the spinal cord remain intact. Keep in mind, however, that stretching or twisting the spinal cord can lead to injury as extensive as partial or complete transection. Common causes of closed injuries include compression, flexion, hyperextension, rotation, and blunt trauma (Fig. 28-5). Degeneration of the vertebrae or intervertebral disks, hematomas, or spinal cord tumors also may compress the cord or one of the spinal nerves. Fractures of the vertebral bodies may cause a subluxation (partial dislocation) of bone fragments, which may further damage the cord. Open injuries with damage to protective skin and meninges are most commonly caused by bullets or stabbing.

The injury may be classified as complete or incomplete, depending on the extent to which the cord is transected (cut across). A complete spinal cord injury occurs when the cord has been completely severed, whereas an incomplete injury results from partial cutting of the cord. Open injuries often result in either complete or partial transection (cutting across) of the cord.

EFFECTS OF SPINAL CORD INJURY

Early recognition of the effects of spinal cord injury is vital to maintain maximum possible function. Factors that determine the effects of spinal cord injury include the extent of the cut and the level of the injury. Sometimes the extent of injury cannot be fully determined because the symptoms of spinal cord edema may mimic partial or complete transection. A complete injury cuts all descending and ascending tracts. The result is disruption of all motor and sensory activity below the level of the injury. However, reflex activity continues below the level of injury because it occurs by completing the reflex arc without the transmission of impulses to and from the brain.

Trauma also may produce a variety of incomplete spinal cord injuries. These are injuries in which some function remains below the level of the injury. Specific tracts may be involved, causing particular patterns of neurologic dysfunction (Fig. 28-6). Table 28-3 describes the major types of incomplete injuries and the resulting neurologic losses.

The higher the level of the injury, the more devastating is the neurologic dysfunction, for increasingly more of the body is affected. High cervical spine injuries may result in the loss of motor and sensory function in all four extremities, known as **quadriplegia**. Injuries at or below T2 may cause **paraplegia**, which is paralysis of the lower part of the body. Table 28-4 describes those activities that are possible with spinal cord injury at various levels.

Respiratory Impairment

The diaphragm is innervated by the phrenic nerve, which is formed by the nerve roots of C1 through C4. Therefore, injuries at or above the level of C5 (called high cervical injuries) may result in instant death because the nerves that control respiration are interrupted. Many patients with high cervical injuries die before reaching the hospital. If these patients are fortunate enough to receive immediate attention and rapid transport to a skilled facility, mechanical ventilation may be possible. However, they remain dependent on ventilators and present great challenges for rehabilitation.

Modern technology affords the ventilator-dependent patient a variety of options for pulmonary rehabilitation. A small portable ventilator can be mounted on the back of a mechanized wheelchair, enabling the patient to be mobile. Phrenic nerve stimulators also may be implanted in the patient to help stimulate diaphragmatic movement and enhance respiratory function. Even with a ventilator or phrenic nerve

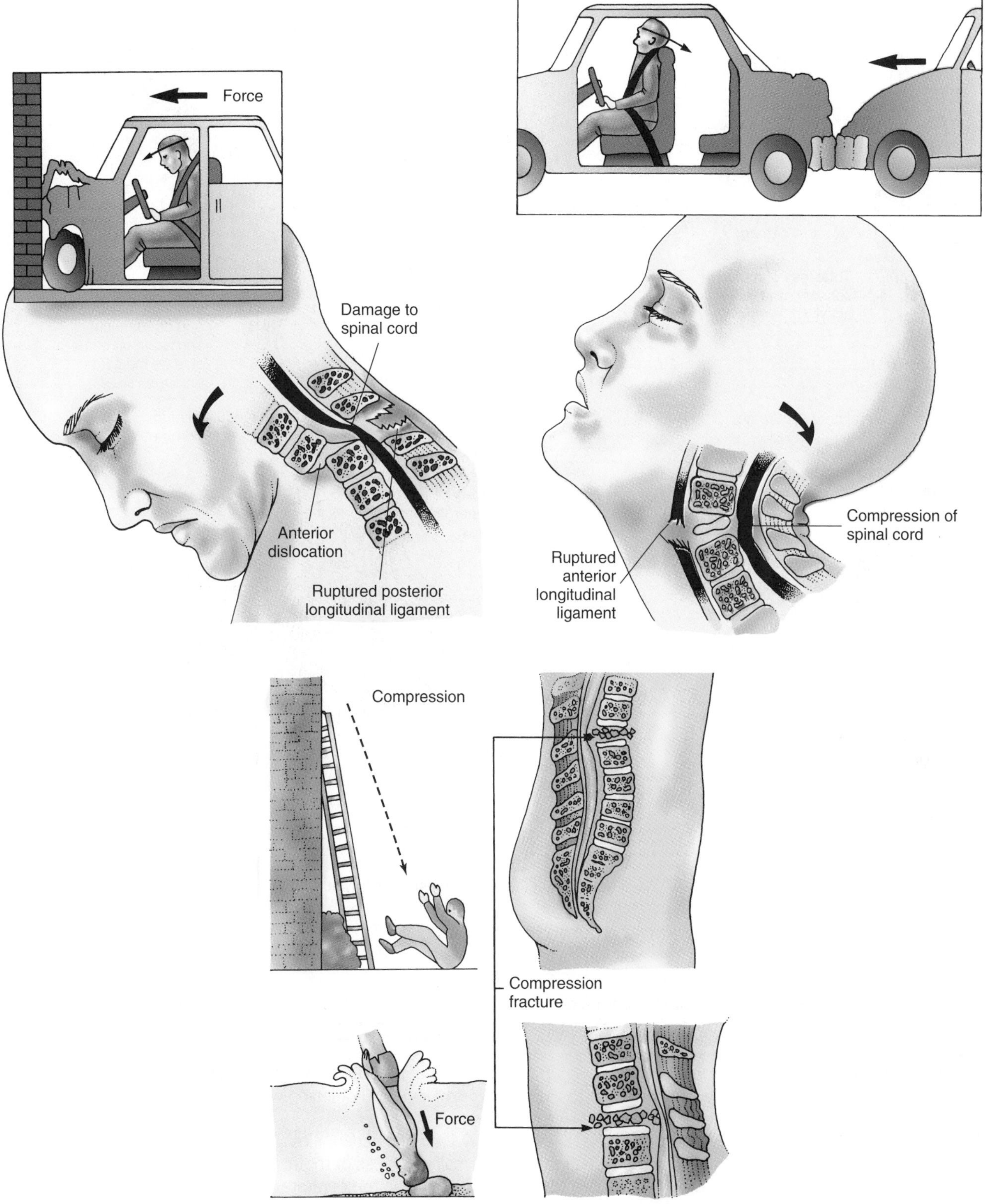

FIGURE 28-5 Mechanisms of spinal cord injury.

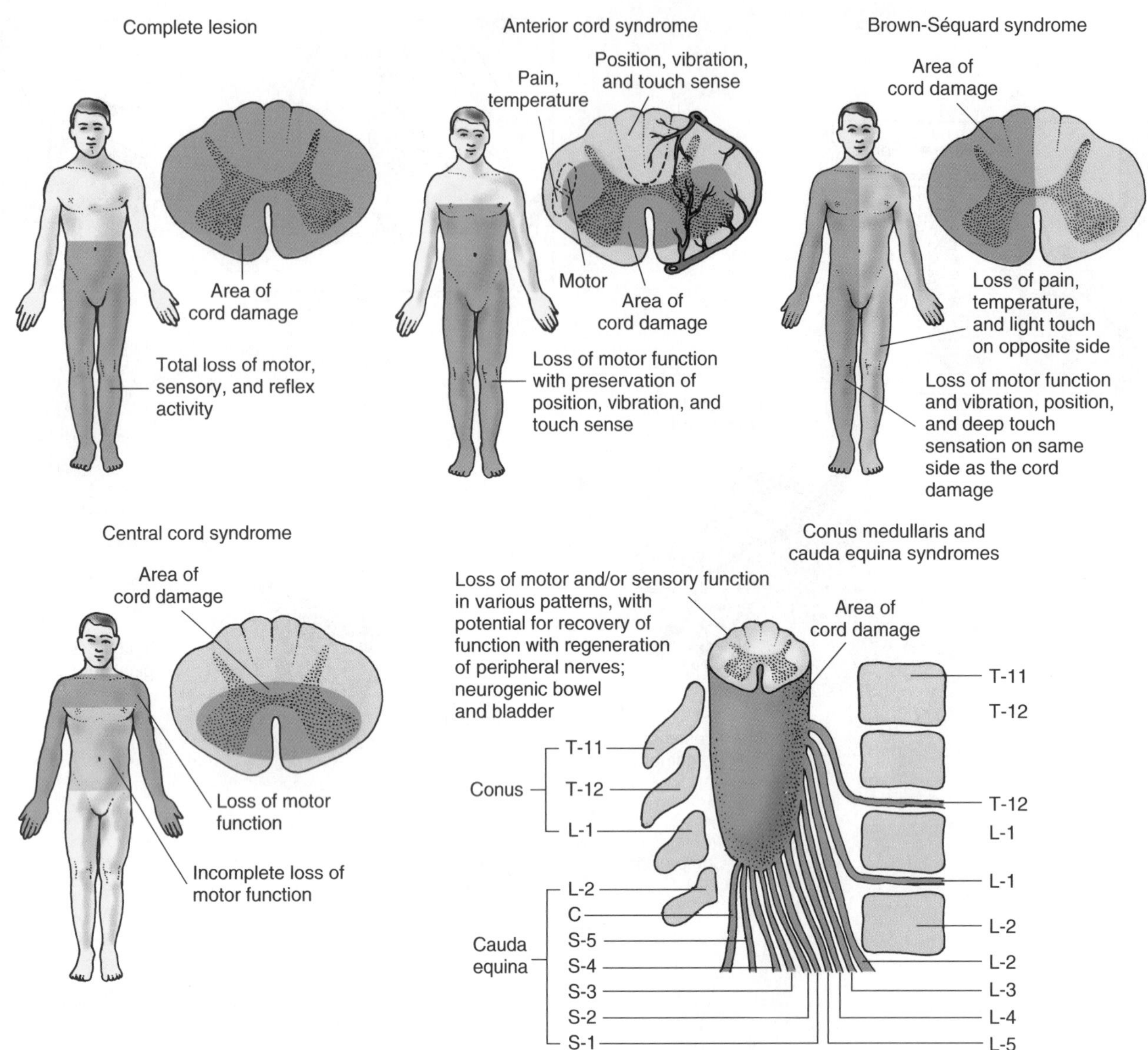

FIGURE **28-6** Patterns of injuries and neurologic dysfunction.

table 28-3 ***Incomplete Injuries and Related Neurologic Deficits***

INJURY	MECHANISM OF INJURY	ACCOMPANYING DEFICIT
Anterior cord syndrome	Herniation of disk occurring with flexion injury or dislocation of vertebrae	Loss of bilateral pain and temperature and motor function below level of lesion without loss of position sense
Central cord syndrome	Hyperextension injury	Motor and sensory loss in upper extremities
Brown-Séquard syndrome	Transverse hemisection of cord	Ipsilateral loss of motor function with contralateral loss of pain and temperature

table 28-4 Degree of Loss and Functional Capability with Injury to Each Level of the Spinal Cord

CORD LEVEL	DEGREE OF LOSS	FUNCTIONAL CAPABILITY
C1 through C4	Motor and sensory function from neck down Respiratory function Bowel and bladder control	Mechanical ventilation with home care
C5	Motor and sensory function below shoulders Intercostal function in ventilation Bowel and bladder control	Has remaining head control, which facilitates use of "joystick" for writing, typing, and control of mechanical wheelchair
C6	Motor and sensory function below shoulders but greater degree of sensation in arm and thumb Intercostal function in ventilation Bowel and bladder control	Requires some assistive devices for upper extremity use but may be able to help feed and dress self Requires mechanical wheelchair but may be capable of utilizing hand control
C7	Motor control of portions of upper extremities Sensation below clavicle Intercostal function Bowel and bladder control	Remaining intact muscles enhance ability to carry out activities of daily living (ADL) Increased ability to manage specially equipped wheelchair and automobile
C8	Motor control of portions of upper extremities Sensation below chest Intercostal function Bowel and bladder control	Improved upper extremity mobility enhances hand grasp, independence in ADL, and use of wheelchair Capable of self-catheterization
T1 through T6	Trunk muscles below midchest Sensation from midchest Some intercostal function Bowel and bladder control	Complete control of upper extremities makes independence in wheelchair and ADL possible Employment possible
T6 through T12	Motor control below waist Sensation below waist Bowel and bladder control	Capable of unassisted respiratory function Good upper back and abdominal strength, making increased wheelchair activities and athletics possible
L1 through L3	Motor and sensory function to lower extremities Sensation to lower abdomen Bowel and bladder function	Full control of upper extremities allows independence in wheelchair and appropriate athletic activity
L3-4	Motor and sensory function to distal portions of lower extremities Bowel and bladder control	Control of hip extensors remains, making ambulation possible with leg braces
L4-S5	Variable motor and sensory function to knee, ankle, and foot Sensation to perineum Variable bowel and bladder control	Ambulation with braces possible Considerable independence in ADL can be expected

stimulator, pulmonary hygiene is an issue because these patients may have difficulty clearing the airway.

Cervical injuries below the level of C4 spare the diaphragm but can involve impairment of intercostal and abdominal muscles. Patients with these injuries can usually breathe independently but often experience some degree of respiratory compromise related to weakened exhalation and cough.

Spinal Shock

Spinal shock is an immediate, transient response to injury in which reflex activity below the level of the injury temporarily ceases. It may appear as early as 30 to 60 minutes after the injury and may persist intermittently for days, weeks, or months. During the period of spinal shock, paralysis is described as **flaccid,** meaning the involved extremity or muscle group has no tone. The involved neurons in the spinal cord gradually regain their excitability. Resolution of spinal shock is marked by the appearance of spastic, involuntary movements of the extremities.

Autonomic Dysreflexia

One of the most serious and potentially dangerous problems for the spinal cord–injured patient is **autonomic dysreflexia,** an exaggerated response of the autonomic nervous system to some noxious (painful) stimuli. It occurs in patients whose injury is at or above the level of T6. As spinal shock begins to subside and reflex activity returns, the risk of autonomic dysreflexia increases. It may even occur in patients with long-standing injuries.

Excessive stimulation of sensory receptors below the level of the injury precipitates autonomic dysreflexia. The sympathetic nervous system is stimulated, but an appropriate response cannot be elicited because of the spinal cord injury. Arterioles constrict, causing severe hypertension, which may lead to seizures or a stroke if not corrected. In an attempt to reduce the excessively increased blood pressure, regulatory mechanisms cause the blood vessels to dilate. The vasodilating response is effective only above the level of the injury, where superficial vasodilation, flushing, and profuse sweating occur.

Increased blood pressure also stimulates the vagus nerve, causing bradycardia. Normally, vagal stimulation also would serve to dilate the constricted vessels. But, because the cord has been severed, these impulses never reach the affected blood vessels.

Autonomic dysreflexia is commonly triggered by a distended bladder, constipation, renal calculi, ejaculation, or uterine contractions, but it also may be caused by pressure sores, a skin rash, enemas, or even sudden position changes. In the event of autonomic dysreflexia, indwelling catheters must be inspected for possible occlusions or kinks. If there is no indwelling catheter and the bladder is distended, intermittent catheterization may be done. If constipation is the triggering event, disimpaction may be necessary.

Spasticity

Most spinal cord–injured patients display some degree of spasticity (increased muscle tone) following their injury. Muscle spasms may prove to be quite incapacitating for these patients, hampering efforts at rehabilitation. Generally, after 1 or 2 years, there is a gradual reduction in spastic episodes.

Muscle tone is evaluated by assessing the amount of resistance to passive movement. The spastic muscle displays a brief period of increased resistance, which is followed by a sudden relaxation. Reflexes also are assessed because hyperactive reflexes accompany spasticity. Spastic activity may be elicited by passive movement, positioning, or even the slight stimulation of a sheet moving over the lower extremities. A number of drugs are available to treat spasticity.

Impaired Sensory and Motor Function

As stated earlier, the higher the level of the lesion, the more extensive is the neurologic dysfunction. Any complete cord injury results in the loss of both motor and sensory function below the level of the lesion. The effects of incomplete lesions on sensation and motor function are variable. Impaired motor function can significantly affect the patient's mobility and self-care and thus result in complications from immobility. Loss of sensation puts the patient at risk for skin breakdown and other injuries because pressure and pain are not perceived.

Put on your THINKING CAP!!

1. Observe a person in a public setting who is seated for at least 10 minutes. You might choose an office worker at a desk, someone on a bus, someone watching television, someone waiting in a doctor's office, or someone in a lecture class. Try not to be obvious so that the person will not realize you are observing. Note the types and frequency of movements.
2. Try sitting perfectly still for 10 minutes. You can move your head. Were you able to do it? Describe your feelings. What bothered you most?
3. Describe any insights this experience provided that could help you take care of a spinal–cord injured person in a wheelchair.

Impaired Bladder Function

During the period of spinal shock, all bladder and bowel function ceases. An indwelling catheter is inserted to empty the bladder and permit close monitoring of urinary output. As soon as the patient's fluid status is stabilized, the indwelling catheter often is removed and the bladder drained by intermittent catheterization. Once spinal shock resolves, reflex activity returns. The bladder becomes spastic and may spontaneously empty. Bladder retraining protocols can be specifically designed for individual patients.

Medications may be used to aid in the prevention of urinary tract infections. Methenamine mandelate (Mandelamine) is a urinary antiseptic that may be used in the regimen. Because the action of methenamine is enhanced in an acidic environment, vitamin C (ascorbic acid) often is prescribed to lower urine pH.

Impaired Bowel Function

Loss of bowel activity in the first day or two after injury may require insertion of a nasogastric tube for decompression. Peristalsis usually returns by the third postinjury day. Most spinal cord–injured patients can maintain bowel function because the large bowel musculature has its own neural center that responds to distention by the fecal mass. To assist in evacuation of the bowel, the patient must take advantage of the abdominal muscles as well as have an appropriate diet. Bowel retraining programs are initiated to aid in the regular evacuation of the bowel.

Impaired Temperature Regulations

Depending on the level of the injury, the patient may have difficulty maintaining body temperature within a normal range. If a person becomes too cold, the body normally responds with vasoconstriction and shivering to increase the temperature. If a person becomes too hot, sweating helps to dissipate heat. The spinal cord–injured patient may lose these regulatory mechanisms and be unable to adapt to temperature extremes. The quadriplegic person is especially vulnerable to environmental temperature changes because such a large part of the body is affected.

Impaired Sexual Function

Spinal levels S2, S3, and S4 control sexual function, so injury at or above these levels results in sexual dysfunction. The ability of the male patient to achieve erection and ejaculation is variable, depending on the level of injury. In females, menses resumes normally after injury. Women with spinal cord injuries can have sexual intercourse but lack vaginal sensation. Some women with spinal cord injuries do experience orgasm, although it is not vaginally triggered. They also can bear children, regardless of the level of the lesion. In the event of pregnancy, vaginal delivery is possible if pelvic proportions are adequate. If the lesion is high, however, the woman will not be aware of labor contractions.

Impaired Skin Integrity

Immobility and loss of sensation put the patient at risk for skin problems. One of the most common complications in the spinal cord–injured patient is pressure ulcers. Because the immobile patient is unable to change positions, skin in the sacral area and across the bony prominences may break down. This presents a portal for infection in the patient. In addition, the presence of a pressure sore in the sacral area impedes early rehabilitation efforts because the patient is unable to begin wheelchair training until the ulcer heals.

The complete spinal cord injury also interrupts the vasomotor tone of the vascular system. This loss of tone results in vasodilation and pooling of blood in the periphery, impeding perfusion of the skin and encouraging the development of pressure sores.

Altered Self-Concept and Body Image

The impact of spinal cord injury on the patient's self-concept and body image is tremendous. Depending on the extent of the injury, every aspect of the patient's life (occupation, family roles and responsibilities, socialization, hobbies) may be affected. French and Phillips (1991) have described the effects of spinal cord injury on body image as occurring in four phases: impact, retreat, acknowledgment, and reconstruction. In the impact phase, the patient becomes aware of the devastating changes that have taken place. He or she is in emotional shock and may express a desire to die. The retreat phase is marked by depression and withdrawal as the patient considers the implications of the injury. In the acknowledgment phase, the patient begins to face the injury and deal with it realistically. The patient moves into the reconstruction phase when he or she is ready to tackle the work of rehabilitation and begins to plan for the future. A new body image has been constructed that incorporates the injury.

MEDICAL TREATMENT IN THE ACUTE PHASE

The goals of medical treatment guide the plans for the spinal cord–injured patient through all phases of the injury. The three major medical goals for the patient with spinal injury are to save the patient's life, to prevent further injury to the cord, and to preserve as much cord function as possible. Each medical goal has specific implications for nursing care and is directed at maximizing the patient's potential for recovery and rehabilitation.

SAVING THE PATIENT'S LIFE

The patient with a spinal cord injury may have additional life-threatening injuries. As mentioned earlier, patients with high cervical cord injuries often die from impaired respiratory function before arriving at the hospital.

The first priority is to establish a patent airway. The conventional head-tilt–chin-lift method of opening the airway is inappropriate in spinal injury patients because of the risk of increasing cord damage. The risk of additional damage is especially high with cervical injury. Flexion of the neck, even that caused by a pillow or other support, must be avoided. The jaw-thrust method of opening the airway is preferred for these patients. Once the airway has been opened, 100% oxygen may be administered by mask and manual resuscitator (e.g., an Ambu bag).

An endotracheal or tracheostomy tube may be placed to allow direct access to the airway and to facilitate optimal oxygenation. Any injury that compromises ventilation must be treated immediately.

PREVENTING FURTHER CORD INJURY

Immobilization is essential to prevent further damage to the spinal cord after the initial injury. At the scene of an accident, emergency personnel will apply a hard cervical collar, also known as a Philadelphia collar, around the patient's neck to immobilize the spinal column. Various types of devices and traction may be utilized once the patient arrives at an acute care facility.

Traction

Immobilization with skeletal traction often is used to manage cervical spinal cord injuries acutely. A variety of skull traction devices may be used, including Gardner-Wells and Crutchfield tongs. Gardner-Wells tongs are secured just above the ears but do not actually penetrate the skull. Crutchfield tongs, which are less commonly used now than in the past, are applied directly to the skull, just behind the hairline. The tongs allow traction to be applied, which separates and aligns the vertebrae to prevent further cord damage and reduces painful muscle spasms (Fig. 28-7). After the tongs are applied, radiographs are ordered to confirm alignment of the spine. Ongoing neurologic assessment is done to monitor for further deficits.

The halo ring is used to immobilize and align the cervical vertebrae and usually is placed at the time of surgery that is

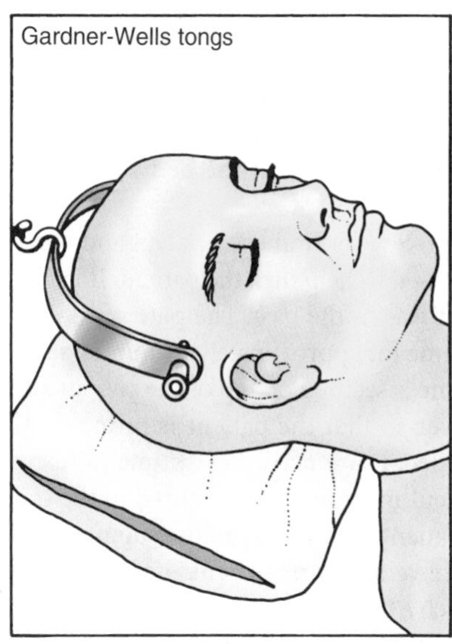

FIGURE 28-7 Gardner-Wells tongs are used to immobilize the cervical spine.

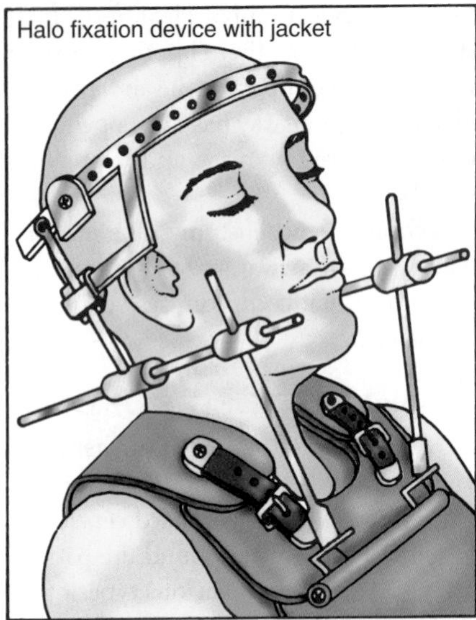

FIGURE 28-8 The halo device immobilizes and aligns the cervical vertebrae.

done to internally stabilize fractures and relieve the compression of nerve roots (Fig. 28-8). It is applied to the skull using four pins and then to a fiberglass jacket by adjustable rods. The jacket allows the paralyzed patient to be moved out of bed and allows the patient who is not paralyzed to be ambulatory. Because such good immobilization is achieved, attention can be turned to other aspects of treatment, and rehabilitation can be initiated.

Special Beds and Cushions

A number of special beds are available to help prevent complications of immobility while maintaining spinal immobilization. A kinetic bed such as the Roto-Rest bed slowly but continually rotates the patient from side to side (Fig. 28-9). This rotation is especially helpful in preventing pulmonary complications by mobilizing secretions. Overlay air mattresses are flotation devices that are placed on standard hospital beds. Air-fluidized and flotation beds may be used *after* the spine has been stabilized, but they are *never* used when a patient is in tongs because of the potential damage that could occur if the bed should unexpectedly deflate.

The Wedge-Stryker frame is a canvas and metal frame bed that may be used to help turn the patient. It is no longer used as often as it was in the past. The patient lies supine on the posterior frame for approximately 2 hours at a time. Then the anterior frame is secured on top of the patient and the device is turned over so that the patient is prone on the anterior frame. Two people are needed each time to turn the patient, and the patient must be tightly secured to the frame. Every 2 hours, the patient is turned from the supine to the prone position or vice versa. Many patients have a difficult time adjusting to such a bed because the prone position leaves the patient feeling as though suspended in midair. Because of this, most patients are managed on a conventional or specialty bed.

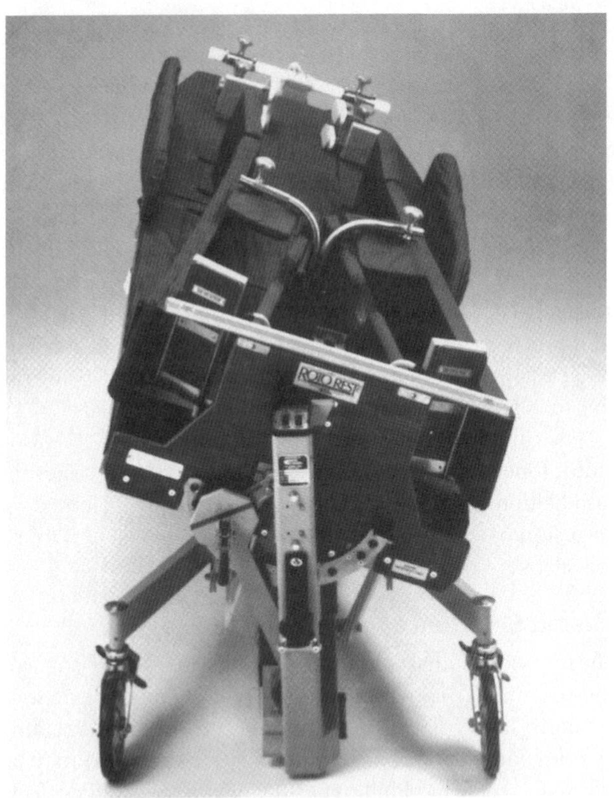

FIGURE 28-9 The Roto-Rest bed slowly turns the patient from side to side.

Once the patient is able to be up in a chair, cushioning is needed to prevent excessive pressure and pressure ulcers. Types of cushions include those inflated with air, flotation devices, and gel pads. Examples of pressure-reducing cushions are the ROHO cushion, BBD-Bye Bye decubiti cushion, Jay cushion, Akro cushion, and Vari-Lite cushion. The cushion that best meets the needs of the individual patient is selected. The physical therapist is a good resource person to consult for this recommendation.

Drug Therapy

Until the early 1990s, management of the spinal cord–injured patient relied almost exclusively on surgical and immobilization techniques. However, the use of methylprednisolone to reduce the damage to the cellular membrane has become standard practice in the acute management of spinal cord injury. The optimal time of administration is within the first 8 hours of injury. Completely paralyzed patients have been found to regain about 20% of function, while those partially paralyzed have regained up to 75% of function.

PHARMACOLOGY CAPSULE The administration of high doses of methylprednisolone sodium succinate during the first 8 hours after spinal cord injury may help limit the neurologic effects of injury.

PRESERVING CORD FUNCTION

Early surgical intervention may be necessary to repair cord damage. Situations in which surgery is required include cord compression by bony fragments, compound vertebral fractures, and gunshot and stab wounds. In these cases, surgery within the first 24 hours is most desirable.

A laminectomy involves removing all or part of the posterior arch of the vertebra. This may be done to alleviate compression on the cord or spinal nerves. If multiple vertebrae are involved, spinal fusion also may be done to stabilize the area. A spinal fusion entails placing a piece of donor bone, commonly taken from the hip, into the area between the involved vertebrae. After healing, the fusion immobilizes the affected section of the spine. Postoperative immobilization of the area is necessary to allow for adequate healing, permanent fusion, and correct alignment. If the cervical area is involved, a halo jacket will be utilized. If the thoracic or lumbar area is involved, other brace-like devices may be fitted to the patient. Neither laminectomy nor spinal fusion can be attempted until the patient has been fully stabilized during the acute phase of the injury.

NURSING CARE *in the Acute Phase*

Assessment

A complete assessment as described here may be delayed until the patient is stabilized. Until then, monitor the patient's level of consciousness, vital signs, respiratory status, motor and sensory function, and intake and output.

Health History

Present Illness

Record the event that brought the patient to the hospital. Note specific injuries incurred in the incident. This may be the initial hospitalization after the injury, or the patient may be admitted at a later time for other reasons. Describe pain and other symptoms in detail.

Past Medical History

It is important not to overlook other medical problems when the patient has a spinal cord injury. Inquire about other accidents or injuries and chronic illnesses such as diabetes, hypertension, heart disease, cancer, or seizure disorder. Record previous hospitalizations and operations. Obtain an obstetric history from the female patient. Identify and record current medications and allergies.

Family History

A routine family history is taken but is not considered specifically relevant to a diagnosis of spinal cord injury resulting from trauma.

Review of Systems

Inquire about signs and symptoms that may be related to neurologic dysfunction or its consequences. Data to be collected include skin condition, headache or dizziness, vision disturbances, hearing impairment or tinnitus, nasal or ear drainage (especially if there was a head injury), dyspnea, nausea and vomiting, constipation or diarrhea, fecal incontinence, bladder dysfunction, sexual dysfunction, and impaired motor and sensory function.

Functional Assessment

Assess the patient's self-care abilities. Explore the patient's roles and responsibilities as a family member. Record occupation, hobbies, usual activity pattern, habits (including use of tobacco and alcohol), and diet. It is important to know who the patient's significant others are and whether those relationships are supportive. In addition, determine the patient's emotional response to the spinal injury. Assess usual coping strategies. Determine spiritual beliefs and other sources of support.

Physical Examination

Record the patient's reported height and weight. An actual weight measurement may have to be deferred until the patient can tolerate the procedure. Assess vital signs. Be alert for hypertension and bradycardia typical of autonomic dysreflexia (discussed earlier in this chapter). Take the temperature to detect alterations that may reflect failure of regulatory mechanisms or infection. In the general survey, observe the patient's level of responsiveness, posture, and spontaneous movements.

Inspect the skin for lesions (lacerations, bruises) that may have occurred at the same time as the spinal cord injury, or for signs of pressure that may have resulted from immobility. Assess tissue turgor. Inspect the head for lesions and palpate for masses and swelling. Ask the patient to read available print to assess visual acuity. Examine the pupils of the eyes for size, equality, and reaction to light.

Observe the patient's respiratory effort and auscultate breath sounds. Inspect the abdomen for distention and auscultate for bowel sounds. Inspect the extremities for open fractures or abnormal positions. Assess range of motion, voluntary and involuntary movement, muscle strength, spasms, and sensory perception in all extremities. If the patient is conscious, ask him or her to move the extremities through the various ranges of motion. This simply indicates whether or not the patient is capable of such movement and gives some early indication as to the involvement of particular spinal cord levels.

Assess muscle strength by using passive range-of-motion exercises and by testing strength against gravity as well as against resistance applied by the examiner. Instruct the patient to try to move the extremity against the examiner's hand. Evaluate both upper and lower extremities, and compare one side with the other. Function is graded on a scale of 0 (complete paralysis) to 5 (normal strength) (Table 28-5). If the patient is unconscious, some noxious stimulus, such as pressure on the nail bed, must be applied to determine whether movement is possible. In the event of cranial involvement, such movement in response to noxious stimuli may be described as decorticate or decerebrate posturing. Both of these are described in Chapter 26.

Involuntary movement also may be observed in the injured patient. This type of movement is evidenced by the appearance of muscle spasms. Record the location and severity of such spasms. Techniques for assessing the movement of the major muscle groups in both the upper and the lower extremities are described in Table 28-6.

table 28-5 ***Grading Scale for Muscle Strength***

SCORE	FINDINGS
0	No movement, total paralysis
1	Weak contraction palpated or observed
2	Muscle moves when supported against gravity
3	Active muscle movement against gravity
4	Full active range of motion against gravity but with some weakness when resistance is tested
5	Full active range of motion against gravity and resistance

table 28-6 ***Assessment Techniques for Major Muscle Groups***

NERVE ROOT	MUSCLE ACTION	ASSESSMENT TECHNIQUE
C4-5	Abduction of shoulder	Shrug shoulder against downward pressure
C5-6	Elbow flexion (biceps)	Arm flexed toward body against resistance
C7	Elbow extension (triceps)	Arm extended away from body against resistance
C8	Hand grasp (finger flexors)	Hands grasped around examiner's fingers with attempts to withdraw fingers from grasp
L2 through L4	Hip flexion	Leg raised against resistance
L2 through L4	Knee extension	Knee extended away from body against resistance
L5	Foot dorsiflexion	Foot pulled upward against resistance
L5-S1	Knee flexion	Knee flexed toward body against resistance
S1	Plantar flexion	Foot and toes pointed downward against resistance

To evaluate sensory function, determine the patient's ability to perceive sharp and dull sensations and touch with the eyes closed. As with the motor evaluation, compare one side of the body with the other to assess equality. Include the hands, forearms, upper arms, trunk, thighs, lower legs, feet, and perineal area in the assessment. Sensory loss is best described with the aid of a dermatome chart (Fig. 28-10). A **dermatome** defines an area of the skin that is innervated by a particular subcutaneous nerve root. In the initial postinjury period, frequently reassess sensation because the injury may ascend (rise) and affect vital functions.

To test proprioception (position sense), have the patient close his or her eyes and identify the position of a toe or finger as you move it up or down.

Nursing assessment of the patient with a spinal cord injury is summarized in Table 28-7.

Nursing Diagnoses, Goals, and Outcome Criteria: Acute Phase of Spinal Cord Injury

NURSING DIAGNOSES	GOALS AND OUTCOME CRITERIA
Ineffective Breathing Patterns related to neurologic impairment	Adequate oxygenation: normal respiratory rate and measures of oxygenation (blood gases, oximeter)
Risk for Injury related to involuntary muscle spasms, lack of motor and sensory function, orthostatic hypotension, and **Disturbed Sensory Perception** (kinesthetic, tactile) related to altered sensory transmission	Reduced risk for injury: protective measures are taken to prevent injury associated with uncontrollable movement or with sensory loss Absence of injury: patient has no bruises, breaks in skin, signs of pressure, or fractures
Risk for Autonomic Dysreflexia related to bladder or bowel distention, renal calculi, pressure sores	No signs of autonomic dysreflexia: pulse and blood pressure consistent with patient norms
Risk for Disuse Syndrome related to pathologic or prescribed immobility, or both	Absence of complications of immobility: no pressure sores, maximal possible range of motion, clear breath sounds
Bowel Incontinence related to impaired conduction of impulses	Controlled bowel elimination: regular bowel movements under controlled circumstances
Impaired Urinary Elimination related to sensory motor impairment	Absence of urinary retention and urinary infection: no bladder distention, urine clear with normal odor
Risk for Infection related to skeletal traction pins	Pin sites free of infection: minimal redness and swelling around pins, no purulent drainage

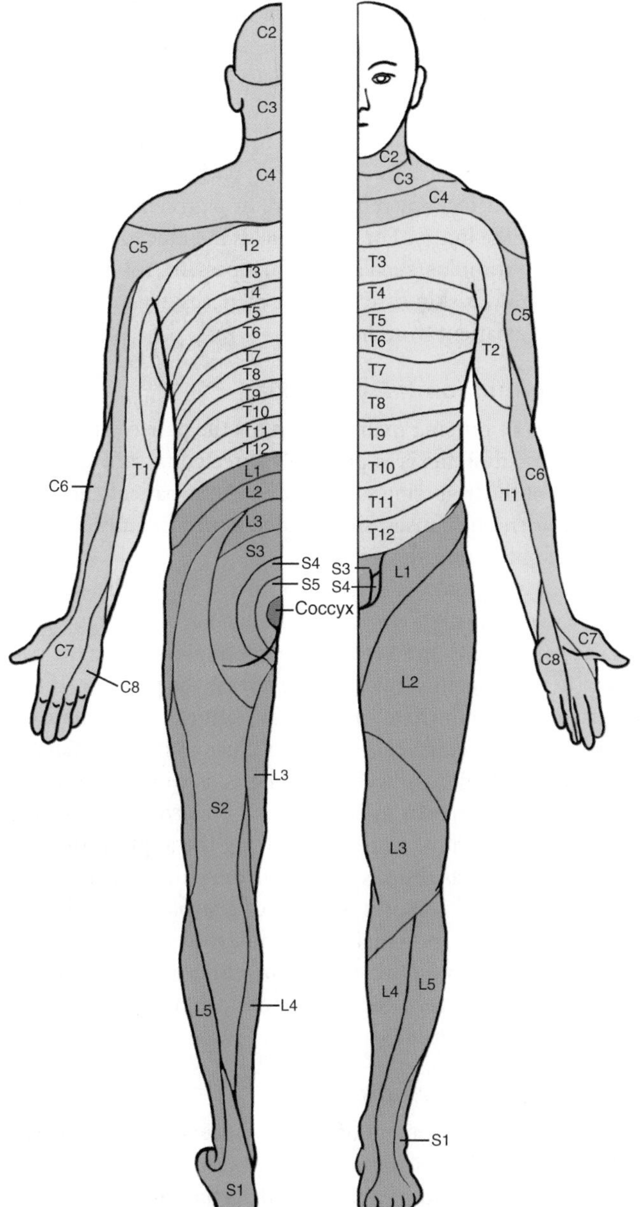

FIGURE 28-10 A dermatome chart. A dermatome is an area of the skin that is innervated by a particular nerve root.

table 28-7 ASSESSMENT *of the Patient with a Spinal Cord Injury*

HEALTH HISTORY

Present Illness: Specific event that caused injury, other apparent injuries, pain location and severity
Past Medical History: Past accidents, injuries, hospitalizations, and operations; history of diabetes mellitus, hypertension, heart disease, cancer, seizure disorder; obstetric history; current medications; allergies
Family History: Routine family history
Review of Systems: Skin condition, headache, dizziness, vision disturbances, hearing impairment, tinnitus, nasal drainage, dyspnea, nausea, vomiting, constipation, diarrhea, fecal incontinence, bladder dysfunction, sexual dysfunction, impaired motor or sensory function
Functional Assessment: Self-care abilities, roles and responsibilities, occupation, hobbies, usual activity pattern, use of tobacco and alcohol, diet, interpersonal relationships, emotional response to injury, usual coping strategies, spiritual beliefs, sources of support

PHYSICAL EXAMINATION

Height and Weight
Vital Signs
Level of Consciousness, Posture, Spontaneous Movements
Skin: Lesions, bruises, redness, tissue turgor
Head: Lesions, masses, swelling
Eyes: Visual acuity, pupil size, equality, reaction to light
Thorax: Respiratory effort, breath sounds
Abdomen: Distention, bowel sounds
Extremities: Range of motion, voluntary and involuntary movements, muscle strength, spasms, sensory perception, abnormal posturing, ability to recognize position of digits without looking

Ineffective Thermoregulation related to spinal cord trauma	Maintenance of normal body temperature: temperature within normal range
Feeding/Dressing/Grooming Self-Care Deficit related to neurologic impairment	Adaptation to self-care deficits: patient participates in self-care as much as possible, accepts help as needed
Sexual Dysfunction related to altered body function	Adaptation to altered sexual function: patient verbalizes sexual capabilities and adaptive techniques
Ineffective Coping related to overwhelming losses and limited potential for recovered function	Effective coping: patient expresses feelings about losses, makes realistic plans for future
Ineffective Therapeutic Regimen Management related to lack of knowledge, denial, depression	Patient effectively manages self-care within capabilities: follows plan of care, plans realistically, uses resources

Interventions

Ineffective Breathing Patterns

Respiratory problems may result from neurologic damage or may be associated with immobility. The patient with an injury at or above C5 has complete loss of spontaneous respirations and requires mechanical ventilation. When a person has an injury to the lower thoracic cord, abdominal and intercostal muscles are affected, resulting in weakened exhalation and cough. Nursing care is individualized for these patients depending on the extent of respiratory impairment. Ventilator-dependent patients may be taught techniques to allow independent breathing for limited periods of time. The ventilator-dependent patient needs special care, as described in Chapter 29.

A variety of techniques may be used to help patients with spontaneous but impaired breathing to clear the airway more effectively. These include breathing exercises, assisted coughing, and vibration and percussion with postural drainage. For assisted coughing, apply firm pressure to the diaphragm just below the rib cage as the patient exhales or coughs. Because timing is important, establish some form of communication with the patient (such as a blink) to identify when inspiration is completed. You should be properly trained in this technique before using it.

Turn and reposition the immobile patient as permitted to decrease pooling of secretions in the lungs. If the patient is breathing independently, coach the patient in deep-breathing exercises and use of the incentive spirometer. Adequate hydration helps to thin secretions so that they can be more readily removed.

Risk for Injury and Disturbed Sensory Perception

Safety is of prime consideration during the period of spastic paralysis. Involuntary muscle spasms can be so violent that the patient may be thrown from the wheelchair or bedside chair. It is imperative that the patient be adequately secured with a protective strap across the chest. Even while in bed, the patient requires protection. Avoid undue stimulation of the spastic extremity or muscle group. When performing range-of-motion exercises or positioning the patient, avoid grasping the muscle itself. Rather, support the joints above and below the affected muscle groups with the palms of the hands.

For the patient maintained in cervical traction on a conventional bed, position changes must be done by "log rolling." A minimum of three nurses is needed to correctly log roll the patient. Some prior planning must be done so that the movement is coordinated. Identify the desired position, and place pillows and equipment in the proper locations before turning the patient. One nurse stands at the head of the bed and stabilizes the traction by placing his or her hands firmly on the patient's head and neck without flexing the neck. The second nurse prepares to move the patient's shoulders while the third prepares to move the patient's hips and legs. After explaining the procedure to the patient, turn the patient as a unit ("log rolled") to the desired position while maintaining proper alignment. Then place pillows to the patient's back and shoulders and between the legs to protect any pressure spots and to promote comfort. The nurse holding the head and neck should not release the patient until all movement has been completed to ensure that traction does not slip out of place.

Pressure stockings are used as ordered to promote venous return, prevent a sudden drop in blood pressure, and reduce the risk of thrombophlebitis.

If injections are necessary, administer them above the level of paralysis. There are two reasons for this. First, circulation is impaired below the level of injury, causing drug absorption to be poor. Second, the patient is at increased risk for infection when the skin integrity is broken in affected parts of the body.

Sensory loss presents definite implications for nursing care. The spinal cord–injured patient with a complete lesion is unable to detect any temperature or pain sensation below the level of the injury. The individual is not able to determine if a painful stimulus, such as a burn, is present. You must provide meticulous skin care and take all necessary measures to protect the patient from harm.

Risk for Autonomic Dysreflexia

The focus of nursing management for the patient at risk for autonomic dysreflexia is primarily directed toward the prevention of the triggering stimulus. Teach the patient and family members the causes, signs and symptoms, and management of autonomic dysreflexia.

When autonomic dysreflexia occurs, it is a medical emergency. Once it is recognized, immediate action is required. Raise the patient's head to a 45-degree angle or place the patient in a sitting position to help decrease the pressure. If the cause can be identified, make every effort to eliminate it. Check the indwelling catheter for occlusion. If the bladder is distended and no indwelling catheter is present, straight catheterization may be indicated. Fecal impactions, if present, need to be digitally removed following the application of a local anesthetic as ordered. Monitor the patient with severe hypertension for seizures or signs of a stroke. Immediately notify the physician so that appropriate medications or other interventions can be initiated. Administer antihypertensive drugs as ordered. Features of autonomic dysreflexia are summarized in Table 28-8.

Risk for Disuse Syndrome

To avoid the development of pressure ulcers, turn the patient at least every 2 hours. Massage of the bony prominences may be harmful and is not recommended. As the patient is turned, inspect the back and sacral area for skin breakdown or signs of pressure. Provide back care using a gentle lotion or other agent designed specifically to prevent skin breakdown. Relieve pressure on any reddened or broken areas. When the patient is resting in the lateral supine position, place a pillow between the legs to keep the heels free of pressure and to prevent pressure between the knees. Keep bed linens clean, dry, and free of wrinkles. Teach the patient and caregiver how to inspect the skin and recognize signs of pressure.

Specialty beds and cushions also may be used to help alleviate pressure and enhance circulation. Even if special padding is used, patients in wheelchairs should still be instructed or assisted to reposition at least every 15 minutes. Some wheelchairs designed for quadriplegic patients can be tilted backward to allow shifting of body weight.

Patients with tongs are maintained on strict bedrest. Therefore, it is imperative that meticulous skin care be provided. With the vertebral column stabilized, the patient may be turned for position changes and skin assessment.

table 28-8 Autonomic Dysreflexia

CAUSES
Distended bladder or plugged catheter
Fecal impaction
Urinary calculi
Pressure ulcer
Ejaculation
Uterine contractions
SIGNS AND SYMPTOMS
Sudden hypertension
Pounding headache
Anxiety
Flushed face
Diaphoresis
Nasal congestion
Bradycardia
Vasoconstriction below lesion with cold skin and "goose flesh"
Vasodilation above lesion with warm, moist skin
POTENTIAL EFFECTS
Seizures
Stroke
MANAGEMENT
Assessment to identify cause
Elevation of head of bed
Irrigation or replacement of urinary catheter
Intermittent catheterization
Application of topical anesthetic and digital disimpaction
Removal of pressure from irritated skin
Administration of antihypertensives as ordered

When the patient has spasticity, nursing management is directed toward preventing contractures and muscle atrophy. Pharmacologic agents, such as diazepam (Valium), baclofen (Lioresal), and dantrolene sodium (Dantrium), may be effective muscle relaxants. Electrical stimulators, used with heat and physiotherapy, also may help relieve spasms. Nursing management of the patient with muscle spasms is summarized in Table 28-9.

During the time of flaccid paralysis, you must diligently perform passive range-of-motion exercises and position and align the patient's extremities to reduce the risk of subluxation or contractures. A more complete discussion of the nursing care of the immobilized person is given in Chapter 20.

PHARMACOLOGY CAPSULE Muscle relaxants may be ordered to control muscle spasticity.

Bowel Incontinence

In the early postinjury period, an ileus may develop, meaning that peristalsis ceases. The abdomen becomes distended, and bowel sounds are absent. If this happens, fluids are administered intravenously and nothing is given by mouth. A nasogastric tube may be inserted and connected to suction for decompression. Peristalsis usually returns by the third day after the injury.

Once peristalsis resumes, the patient is given oral fluids and food. Encourage adequate fluids and high-fiber foods to promote soft stools. Administer bulk laxatives, stool softeners, suppositories, and lubricants as ordered. Document bowel movements, and institute measures to prevent constipation and impaction. Work with the patient to determine the best schedule for bowel elimination and to help the patient carry out the program. A bowel retraining program must be a cooperative effort between the caregiver and the patient. The program can succeed only when the patient is prepared physically and emotionally. Bowel retraining is discussed in detail in Chapter 22.

table 28-9 Management of Spasticity in the Spinal Cord–Injured Patient

Perform passive range-of-motion exercises at least four times a day
Properly position and splint extremities to prevent contractures
Limit tactile stimuli
Avoid incidence of noxious stimuli, such as anxiety, pain, bladder or bowel distention, and pressure ulcers
Turn and reposition at least every 2 hr
Properly administer medications to reduce spasms

Impaired Urinary Elimination

While the patient has an indwelling catheter, meticulous catheter care is essential. Because catheterization increases the risk of urinary tract infections, monitor the patient's temperature and assess the urine for cloudiness and foul odor. Administer prescribed urinary acidifiers, antiseptics, and antimicrobials. Encourage the oral intake of fluids, when permitted, to maintain dilute urine. Discourage the ingestion of dairy products because they contain calcium, which may promote formation of urinary calculi.

In the rehabilitation phase, bladder retraining is addressed. As a bladder retraining program is instituted, work with the patient to carry out the program. To help improve tone and relieve bladder spasms, the catheter may be periodically clamped and then released in an effort to increase bladder capacity. When the bladder can hold 300 to 400 ml of urine, the catheter may be removed for a trial period. Details of bladder retraining are covered in Chapter 22.

Risk for Infection

The risks of pulmonary and urinary infections have already been discussed. If the patient has skeletal traction (Gardner-Wells tongs, halo ring), there is also a risk of infection at the pin insertion sites. Provide specific skin care as ordered or per agency policy. Pin care in some agencies involves the application of polymyxin B (Neosporin) ointment covered with sterile, dry dressings. Report increasing redness or purulent drainage at the pin sites to the physician.

PHARMACOLOGY CAPSULE Topical antimicrobial ointments may be applied to the pin insertion sites to decrease the risk of infection.

Ineffective Thermoregulation

Maintain the environmental temperature at a level that avoids chilling or overheating the patient. A room temperature of 70° F (21° C) will keep the quadriplegic's body temperature stable at 95° F. To prevent hypothermia, provide adequate clothing and blankets. Immediately change wet clothing and linens.

To prevent excessive warming (hyperthermia), the patient should avoid the outdoors during very hot, humid weather. Some patients carry a water spray bottle when outdoors in the heat or during intense activity. The water can be sprayed on the skin, where it evaporates and cools the body. Fans also can help cool the patient. An increase in temperature after exercise is normal.

Feeding/Dressing/Grooming Self-Care Deficit

Continually reassess the patient's abilities and need for assistance with self-care activities. The patient may need total care initially. As soon as the patient is able, begin preparing him or her for self-care consistent with the patient's expected abilities. During rehabilitation, the patient learns to use specialized equipment and strategies in order to be as independent as possible in self-care.

Sexual Dysfunction

Sexuality and sexual function in the spinal cord–injured patient must be addressed when the patient first brings up the subject. Because sexual gratification is an important aspect of emotional and psychological well-being, it is an issue that requires thoughtful discussion and counseling. Patients must be apprised of their physical abilities to achieve erection or to bear children. Provide information about the possibility of pregnancy and about birth control, if the patient expresses a desire to know.

Advise the patient of resources available in the agency and in the community. The expertise of a trained counselor often is needed, and the counselor is usually a member of the rehabilitation team. Honest discussion must occur between the patient and the counselor. Both parties must be willing to explore the physical and emotional aspects of the injury. Additional information on management of impaired sexual function is presented in Chapters 45 and 46.

Ineffective Coping

Ineffective coping may occur at any phase but is particularly evident during rehabilitation as the patient begins to deal with the realities of the situation. Ineffective coping may present as hopelessness. Hopelessness may be manifested by withdrawal, passive behavior, and decreased affect. A person who feels hopeless sees few or no personal choices available and cannot mobilize the energy needed to move forward. Offer opportunities for the patient to discuss feelings about his or her situation and future. Listen actively and accept the patient's feelings. When the patient is withdrawn, encourage, but do not force, participation in self-care. As the patient begins to acknowledge the injury and assess its impact, encourage him or her to identify strengths and coping strategies. Begin rehabilitation efforts in earnest, and give generous praise for effort.

The health care team also works with the patient's significant others to create a supportive atmosphere that conveys hope, acceptance, and confidence. Patients and families often continue to hope for physical improvement that is unlikely. For example, they may interpret the movement associated with spastic paralysis as a return of voluntary motor function. You can avoid this misconception by explaining this phenomenon in advance and emphasizing that it is expected and does not signify improved function.

Ineffective Therapeutic Regimen Management

During the acute phase of spinal cord injury, explain routines and procedures. The physician or clinical nurse specialist usually informs the patient of the extent of the injury and probable effects. The nurse reinforces that information and helps the patient and family obtain any additional information requested. An important resource is the National Spinal Cord Injury Association (website: http://www.spinalcord.org; telephone: 1-800-962-9629), which has a 24-hour service to provide information about rehabilitation, research, organizations, and local contacts. Many communities have local chapters of the Spinal Cord Society, Paralyzed Veterans of America, and National Spinal Cord Injury Association that can provide information and resources.

The following are the essential components of the teaching plan. The details will vary with the level of the injury:

- Effects of spinal cord injury
- Types of treatments and their purposes
- Breathing exercises and adaptive techniques
- Range-of-motion exercises and positioning
- Management of orthostatic hypotension
- Skin care and assessment (Table 28-10)
- Management of bowel and bladder elimination
- Recognition of signs and symptoms of infection
- Changes in sexual function and resources for information about adaptation
- Protection of body areas that lack sensation
- Adaptive techniques and devices to maximize self-care
- Emotional responses to spinal cord injury and coping strategies
- Community resources

Put on your THINKING CAP!!

What is the most important reason for monitoring elimination in the patient with a spinal cord injury at the level of T5?

REHABILITATION

The saying "rehabilitation begins at admission" may sound trite, but for the spinal cord–injured patient its truth is as-

table 28-10 Skin Care: Key Points for the Patient with a Spinal Cord Injury

Avoid excessive pressure, shearing force, and trauma.
Bathe in tepid water with mild soap; dry thoroughly.
Soak feet for 20 min once a week; keep toenails trimmed and smooth.
Keep skin dry and free of contact with urine or stool.
Avoid tight clothing with heavy seams.
Wear cotton undergarments and avoid clothing made of fabrics that do not absorb moisture.
Eat a balanced diet with adequate vitamins A and C and protein.
Drink 2,000 to 3,000 ml of fluid (8 to 12 8-ounce glasses) each day unless directed otherwise.
When in bed, turn at least every 2 hr.
When in a chair, shift weight at least every 15 min.
Inspect skin every morning and every evening for redness, bruising, blisters, and dryness and feel for swelling and hardness.
If redness is present, try to determine cause. Ask yourself if you are turning or shifting weight often enough, if you are transferring correctly, and if your cushions are in good condition.

tounding. The newly paralyzed person is faced with many sobering physical and psychological challenges. Both the acute care staff and the rehabilitation staff strive to see that the patient is fully equipped to face the challenge.

Nursing care during the acute phase of the injury focuses on preventing further disability and avoiding complications that could prolong hospitalization and hamper rehabilitation. Rehabilitation is best described as those activities that assist the individual to achieve the highest possible level of self-care and independence.

The rehabilitation process involves a well-organized interdisciplinary team that can address all aspects of function. Members of the team include the physician, nurse, physical therapist, occupational therapist, speech therapist, dietitian, social worker, psychologist, and counselor. Each plays a vital role in helping the patient achieve the highest level of independence. What was once regarded by the patient as a normal lifestyle or occupation may no longer be possible. Rather, modifications and adjustments must be made. Both the patient and the family must be emotionally and physically prepared to make those adjustments. The team not only helps the patient accomplish activities of daily living and self-care but also addresses successful adjustment to social integration and gainful employment in the workplace. Although this phase of treatment may take more than a year to accomplish, the patient, family, and rehabilitation team can take pride in the realization that a life can once again be productive and happy.

NURSING CARE *of the Laminectomy Patient*

General care of the surgical patient is discussed in Chapter 16. This section focuses on the specific needs of the spinal cord–injured patient undergoing a laminectomy. However, laminectomy may be done for reasons other than traumatic cord injury.

Preoperatively, assess the patient's vital signs and neurologic status to establish baselines. Determine the patient's understanding of surgical routines. Tell the patient what to expect in the immediate postoperative period.

For the patient who has undergone a laminectomy, postoperative care focuses on ongoing assessment of neurologic status and on promoting healing at the operative site. Specific nursing responsibilities are summarized in Table 28-11.

table 28-11 Nursing Care after Laminectomy

NEUROLOGIC ASSESSMENT AND VITAL SIGNS

Frequently assess movement, strength, and range of motion
Assess ability to localize sensory stimulus
Frequently measure vital signs to determine any postoperative complications, such as hemorrhage or infection

CIRCULATION AND RESPIRATION

Maintain elastic stockings on lower extremities to prevent deep vein thrombosis
Encourage range-of-motion exercises four times a day
Encourage deep breathing exercises every 2 hr
Auscultate breath sounds every 2-4 hr
Have patient perform incentive spirometry every 2 hr while awake

PROGRESSIVE AMBULATION

Help patient progress from sitting at edge of bed to ambulating with assistance
Encourage increasing distances and independence while ambulating
Ensure that patient uses back brace or other apparatus as ordered

BED OR POSITIONING

Maintain bed flat or only slightly elevated to reduce strain on operative site
Maintain soft collar for cervical laminectomy
Encourage position changes every 2 hr

BOWEL AND BLADDER FUNCTION

Measure urinary output
Assess for urinary distention and complete emptying of bladder after spontaneous void
Encourage fluid intake
Perform intermittent catheterization (as needed) if patient is unable to void
Auscultate bowel sounds
Initiate bowel program as appropriate

SURGICAL INCISION

Change dressing aseptically
Check dressing for blood or cerebrospinal fluid drainage

PAIN OR DISCOMFORT

Medicate for pain and spasms as needed
Encourage ambulation to reduce spasms

Assessment

After a laminectomy, monitor the patient's vital signs, neurologic status, and breath sounds. Frequently assess movement, strength, range of motion, and ability to localize sensory stimulus. Measure fluid intake and output. Auscultate the abdomen for bowel sounds and palpate for bladder distention. Inspect the surgical dressing for bleeding, clear cerebrospinal fluid drainage, and foul drainage. If the patient has pain, obtain a complete description.

Nursing Diagnoses, Goals, and Outcome Criteria: Post Laminectomy

Nursing Diagnoses	Goals and Outcome Criteria
Risk of Injury related to immobility, neurologic trauma, spinal fluid leakage	Freedom from injury: stable or improving neurologic and vital signs, absence of bleeding or cerebrospinal fluid drainage, absence of fever, normal white blood cell count
Ineffective Tissue Perfusion related to hypovolemia, obstruction to blood flow	Adequate tissue perfusion: normal pulse, blood pressure, respirations, skin color, and tissue turgor
Acute Pain related to tissue trauma, muscle spasms	Pain relief: patient states pain relieved, relaxed expression
Impaired Urinary Elimination related to sensory motor impairment, prescribed position restrictions	Normal urine elimination: spontaneous, controlled voiding; no bladder distention; urine output equal to fluid intake
Constipation related to immobility, neurologic trauma, drug therapy	Normal bowel elimination: regular passage of formed stool without discomfort
Impaired Physical Mobility related to neuromuscular impairment, weakness, prescribed restrictions	Improved physical mobility: daily increase in walking distance without fatigue
Deficient Knowledge of course of recovery, self-care activities, and limitations	Patient understands routines, self-care, and limitations: patient describes and demonstrates appropriate self-care

Interventions

Risk for Injury

Monitor the patient for complications of surgery. Notify the physician of deviations in vital signs, including increased pulse and respirations, hypotension, and fever. Compare neurologic findings with preoperative assessments. Report decreasing sensory or motor responses to the physician. Assist the patient with measures to prevent complications of immobility (breathing and leg exercises) within the limitations of postoperative restrictions. Inform the physician if clear drainage is observed draining from the incision, because this usually indicates a cerebrospinal fluid leak. When the dressing is changed, use aseptic technique to reduce the risk of wound contamination.

Ineffective Tissue Perfusion

Measures are taken to promote oxygenation and circulation. Apply elastic or pneumatic stockings to the lower extremities as ordered to promote venous return and prevent deep vein thrombosis. Instruct or assist the patient to do range-of-motion exercises at least four times daily or as ordered. Auscultate breath sounds every 2 to 4 hours, and support the patient in deep breathing and coughing to remove pulmonary secretions. The incentive spirometer may be used every 2 hours while the patient is awake. Position the patient in good alignment. Teach the patient to keep the back straight and avoid twisting when turning or getting out of bed.

A soft collar may be ordered after cervical laminectomy. Back braces may be prescribed after lumbar or thoracic spinal fusions. Typically, the braces are worn at all times at first. Use of the device is decreased as muscle strength returns. In some situations, corsets and casts are used to support and stabilize the spine. When supportive devices are worn, inspect the skin carefully to make sure they are not creating pressure that could result in skin breakdown.

Acute Pain

Assess and record the patient's level of discomfort. Keep the bed flat or with the head slightly elevated to reduce strain on the operative site. Administer analgesics and muscle relaxants as ordered. Other pain-control measures, such as relaxation techniques, cutaneous stimulation, and imagery, are described in detail in Chapter 14. If the prescribed medications and nursing interventions do not provide pain relief, discuss the problem with the physician to see if other measures can be tried.

Impaired Urinary Elimination

Take measures to promote voiding. Intravenous fluids are usually ordered, but fluids also can be given orally as soon as the patient is able to tolerate them. Document voiding, measure urine output, and assess the bladder for emptying. Promote voiding by providing privacy and positioning the patient as comfortably as allowed. Running water may stimulate voiding. If the patient is unable to void, intermittent catheterization may be ordered.

Constipation

Stool softeners may be ordered to prevent constipation. In addition, ingestion of adequate fluids and fiber is helpful. Ambulation, when permitted, also promotes normal bowel elimination.

Impaired Physical Mobility

Patient activity progresses from sitting on the edge of the bed to ambulating with assistance. Encourage the patient to gradually increase distance and independence in ambulating. If the patient is to wear a back brace or other apparatus, ensure that it is properly applied. Physical therapy may be ordered.

Deficient Knowledge

Postoperative teaching is directed toward promoting recovery from the surgery and preventing future injuries. Determine activity restrictions and discuss these with the patient.

Put on your THINKING CAP!!

You are assigned to a 19-year-old male who sustained a C8 spinal cord injury 2 weeks ago. His condition is stable at this time and he is alert and oriented. When the nursing assistant brings his breakfast tray, he closes his eyes, says he isn't hungry, and asks her to turn off the lights and close the drapes.

1. What phase of adjustment do you think the patient's behavior represents?
2. With adequate support, education, and encouragement, the patient will move into the next phase of adjustment. Describe expected behaviors at that time.

key points

- Spinal cord injury most often results from trauma but also may be caused by degenerative conditions and tumors.
- Spinal cord injuries may be classified by location, as open or closed, and by extent of damage to the cord.
- After spinal cord injury, motor and sensory function is monitored by assessing movement, muscle strength, sensation, and reflex activity.
- Effects of spinal cord injury may include respiratory impairment, spinal shock, autonomic dysreflexia, spasticity, impaired sensory and motor function, impaired bladder function, impaired bowel function, impaired temperature regulation, impaired sexual function, impaired skin integrity, and altered self-concept and body image.
- Injuries at or above the level of the fifth cervical vertebra may result in instant death because of interruption of the nerves that control respirations.
- Autonomic dysreflexia is an exaggerated sympathetic response to stimuli such as bladder distention, constipation, renal calculi, ejaculation, and uterine contractions that produces severe hypertension with the potential for seizures and stroke.
- Muscle tone is usually flaccid immediately after injury, but spasticity develops when spinal shock resolves.
- The goals of medical care after spinal injury are to sustain life, prevent further cord injury, and repair cord damage.
- Immobilization is essential to prevent further damage to the cord after injury.
- Nursing care after spinal cord injury is concerned with Ineffective Breathing Patterns, Risk for Injury and Disturbed Sensory Perception, Risk for Autonomic Dysreflexia, Risk for Disuse Syndrome, Bowel Incontinence, Impaired Urinary Elimination, Risk for Infection, Hyperthermia, Hypothermia, Self-Care Deficits, Sexual Dysfunction, Ineffective Coping, and Ineffective Therapeutic Regimen Management.
- Rehabilitation assists the patient to achieve the highest possible level of self-care and independence.

REVIEW QUESTIONS

1. A patient's chart notes that he has had complete transection of the spinal cord at T2. You would expect the patient to be:
   1. ventilator dependent.
   2. paraplegic.
   3. comatose.
   4. tetraplegic.
2. Which assessment finding would indicate that spinal shock is resolving?
   1. Spastic, involuntary movements of the extremities
   2. Blood pressure returns to normal range
   3. No muscle tone in extremities
   4. Patient responds to light touch and pressure
3. Autonomic dysreflexia in a patient with a spinal cord injury is caused by:
   1. an emotional reaction to pain.
   2. stimulation of the sympathetic nervous system.
   3. dilation of blood vessels below the level of the injury.
   4. constriction of blood vessels above the level of the injury.
4. After spinal shock resolved, a patient's bladder began to empty spontaneously. This could be interpreted to mean:
   1. the spinal cord is beginning to heal.
   2. the patient is regaining normal bladder control.
   3. intact reflex activity is causing bladder emptying.
   4. the patient is not a candidate for bladder retraining.
5. Patient teaching for women with spinal cord injuries should include:
   1. Pregnancy is unlikely.
   2. Sexual intercourse is impossible.
   3. If pregnancy occurs, cesarean section will be necessary.
   4. Although vaginal sensations are lacking, some women have orgasms.
6. Immediate care after a suspected spinal cord injury should include:
   1. Gently lift the patient's chin and tilt the head.
   2. Prop the patient's head to maintain slight flexion.
   3. Administer 100% oxygen by nasal cannula.
   4. Use the jaw-thrust method to open the airway.

7. The purpose of a skeletal traction device after spinal cord injury is to:
   1. align and immobilize the vertebrae to prevent further cord damage.
   2. apply tension to the spinal cord to keep it straight.
   3. maintain the neck in the best position to assure an open airway.
   4. permit healing of the spinal cord injury.

8. A patient admitted with a spinal cord injury may be given methylprednisolone to:
   1. prevent allergic reactions to dyes used in diagnostic procedures.
   2. boost the patient's immune system.
   3. reduce damage to the cellular membrane of the spinal cord.
   4. promote regeneration of neurons.

9. Nursing care during the acute phase of spinal cord injury should include:
   1. Never use restraints of any kind because the pressure tends to stimulate spastic muscle contractions.
   2. Encourage patients in cervical traction to turn themselves every 2 hours to maintain muscle strength.
   3. For the best absorption and to avoid injury, administer injections above the level of paralysis.
   4. Because the patient will require a permanent indwelling catheter, begin teaching catheter care.

10. Postoperative nursing care for the laminectomy patient should include:
   1. Inspect the skin under a back brace for signs of pressure or irritation.
   2. Adjust the bed to keep the patient in a high Fowler's position.
   3. Discourage use of analgesics that sedate the patient.
   4. Observe the bloody drainage, which is usually cerebrospinal fluid.

CHAPTER 29

Acute Respiratory Disorders

VIRGINIA SHAW and ADRIANNE DILL LINTON

objectives

1. Identify data to be collected in the nursing assessment of the patient with a respiratory disorder.
2. Identify the nursing implications of age-related changes in the respiratory system.
3. Describe diagnostic tests or procedures for respiratory disorders and nursing interventions.
4. Explain nursing care of patients receiving therapeutic treatments for respiratory disorders.
5. For selected respiratory disorders, describe the pathophysiology, signs and symptoms, complications, diagnostic measures, and medical treatment.
6. Assist in developing a nursing care plan for the patient who has an acute respiratory disorder.

key terms

Atelectasis (ă-tē-LĔK-tă-sĭs, p. 458)
Crackles (KRĂK-ŭlz, p. 458)
Dyspnea (DĬSP-nē-ă, p. 457)
Hemothorax (hē-mō-THŌ-răks, p. 487)
Hypercapnia (hī-pĕr-KĂP-nē-ă, p. 482)
Hypoxemia (hī-pŏk-SĒ-mē-ă, p. 468)
Hypoxia (hī-PŎK-sē-ă, p. 458)
Orthopnea (ŏr-thŏp-NĒ-ă, p. 457)
Pneumothorax (nū-mō-THŌ-răks, p. 458)
Rhonchus (*pl.* Rhonchi) (RŎNG-kŭs, RŎNG-kī, p. 458)
Tachypnea (tăk-ĭp-NĒ-ă, p. 472)
Tissue perfusion (pĕr-FŪ-zhŭn, p. 489)

Respiration is basic to life. The respiratory system provides fuel for bodily activities and energy to sustain life. Respiration is defined as the exchange of oxygen (O_2) and carbon dioxide (CO_2) through the inspiration of air from the atmosphere and the expiration of air from the lungs. The function of the respiratory system is to supply oxygen for the metabolic needs of the cells and to remove carbon dioxide, one of the waste products of cell metabolism.

ANATOMY AND PHYSIOLOGY OF THE RESPIRATORY SYSTEM

ANATOMY OF THE RESPIRATORY SYSTEM

To reach the lungs, air must travel through several passages, including the nose, mouth, pharynx, larynx, trachea, and bronchi (Fig. 29-1). Each passage has an effect on the quality of the air that reaches the lungs.

Nose

The nose includes the external nose, the part that is seen on the face, and the nasal cavity, which lies over the roof of the mouth. The external nose is made up of bones and cartilage that are covered with skin. The inside lining of the external nose consists of thick mucous membranes and small hairs. The mucous membranes also line the nasal cavity along with the cilia, which are small, hairlike projections.

The mucous membranes warm and moisten the air that enters the nose. If the air is not warmed as it enters the body, the tissue lining the respiratory tract functions poorly. The mucous membranes, the hairs in the external nose, and the cilia filter out dust particles and bacteria from the air. These cilia wave back and forth approximately 12 times per second to help the mucus clean the air. Air that enters via the nose is warmed and filtered, whereas air that enters via the mouth is not.

Pharynx

The pharynx, or throat, is a 5-inch tube extending from the back of the mouth to the esophagus. It is divided into three parts: nasal, oral, and laryngeal. The nasopharynx lies behind the nose, the oropharynx lies behind the mouth, and the laryngopharynx lies behind the larynx. The pharynx serves as a passage for both the respiratory and the digestive systems. It also has an important function in the formation of sounds, especially vowel sounds. The tonsils are located in the pharynx and may interfere with breathing, particularly nasal breathing, if they become enlarged. In addition, speech may have a nasal sound.

Larynx

The larynx, or "voice box," is the air passage between the pharynx and the trachea. It contains vocal cords and several types of cartilage, including the thyroid cartilage and the

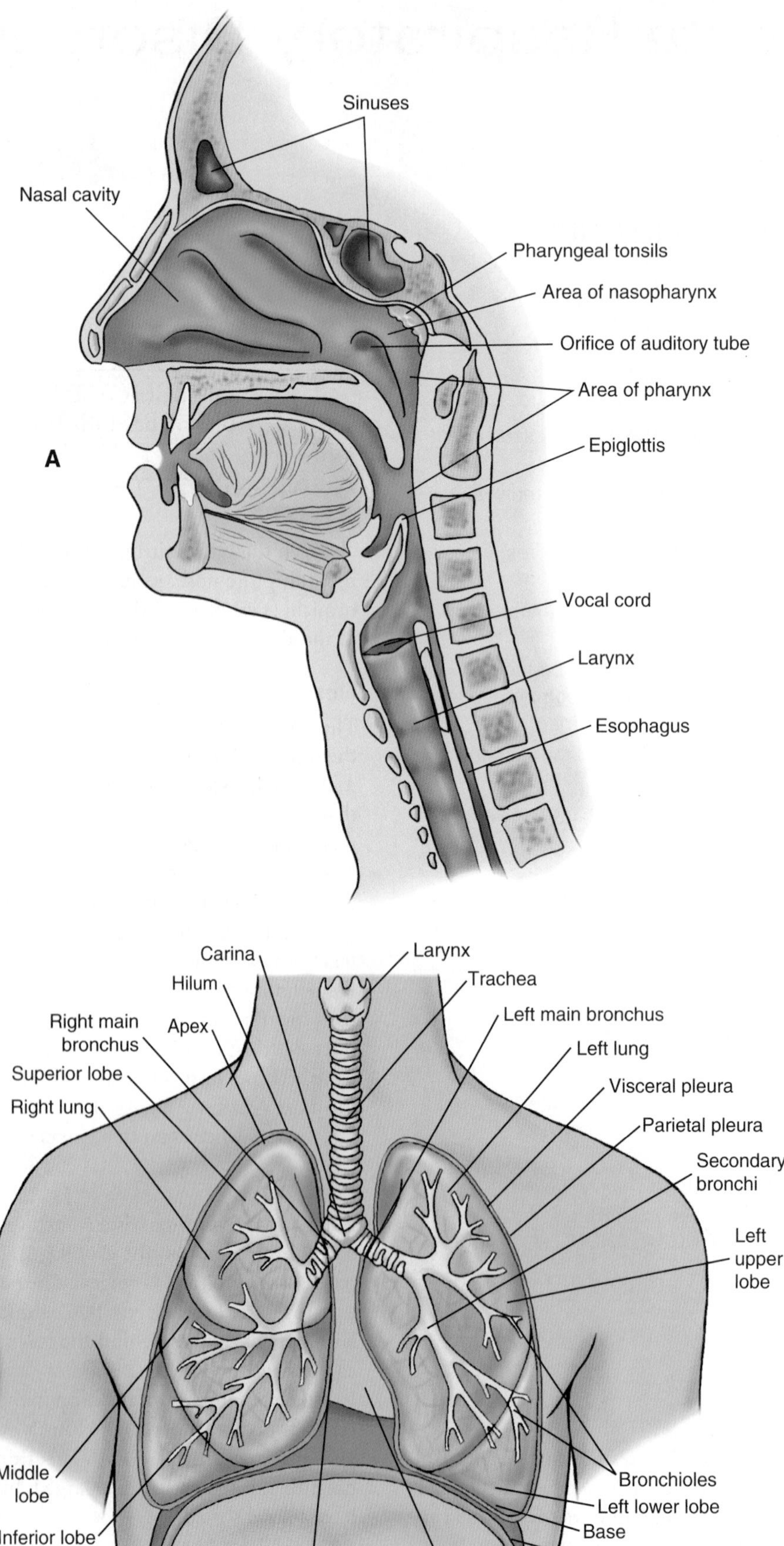

FIGURE **29-1** Structure of the respiratory system. *A,* Upper respiratory tract. *B,* Lower respiratory tract.

epiglottis. The epiglottis has a hinged, door-like action at the entrance to the larynx. During swallowing, it acts like a lid to help prevent aspiration of food into the trachea.

The vocal cords are folds of mucous membranes that are attached to cartilage and extend from the front to the back of the larynx. The space between the folds is known as the *glottis.* Sound is produced when air from the lungs causes a rapid, repeated opening and closing of the glottis. The sounds are transformed into speech through the movements of the lips, jaws, and tongue.

Trachea

The trachea, or windpipe, is a 4- to 5-inch tube descending from the larynx into the bronchi. It is made up of cartilage, smooth muscle, and connective tissue lined by a layer of mucous membrane. The trachea functions as a passageway for air to reach the lungs.

Bronchi

The bronchi provide a passageway for air going to and from the lungs. Two primary bronchi split to the right and left from the trachea. The right bronchus is shorter and wider and runs straighter up and down than the left bronchus. Therefore foreign bodies from the trachea usually enter the right bronchus.

The larger bronchi divide into smaller, or secondary, bronchi, which then divide again into even smaller tertiary bronchi. The tertiary bronchi divide into smaller units called *bronchioles,* which eventually lead into tiny air sacs called *alveoli* located in the lungs. It is through the walls of the alveoli that the exchange of oxygen and carbon dioxide takes place (Fig. 29-2).

Lungs

The lungs are located in the right and left sides of the thoracic cavity within the chest wall. The thoracic cavity is separated from the abdominal cavity by the diaphragm, a large sheet of muscle. The lungs are divided into lobes: three lobes on the right and two on the left. Each lung is covered by a membrane called the *pleura.* The pleura is a sac containing fluid that acts as a lubricant for the lungs when they expand and contract.

RESPIRATORY PHYSIOLOGY

Mechanism of Breathing

The process of air entering into the lungs is called *inspiration,* and the process of air leaving the lungs is called *expiration.* The terms *inhalation* and *exhalation* are used interchangeably with inspiration and expiration. Both of these processes are accomplished by the movement of the diaphragm and the

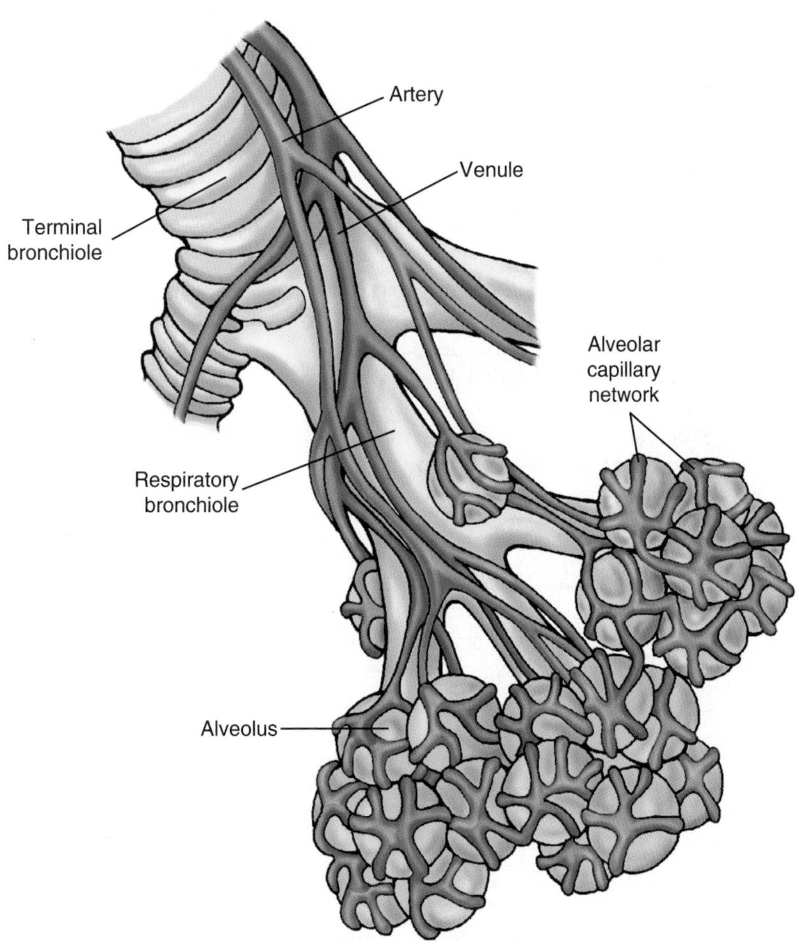

FIGURE **29-2** The terminal bronchioles, alveoli, and capillaries.

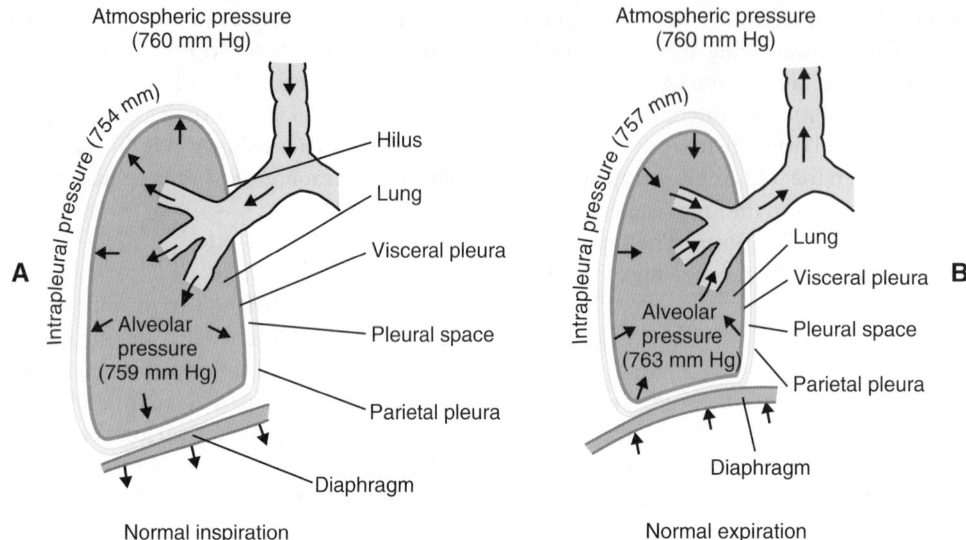

FIGURE **29-3** Normal inspiration *(A)* and expiration *(B)*. Note the visceral pleura, pleural space, and parietal pleura and the changes in pressure in the alveoli and pleural space on inspiration and expiration.

table 29-1 ***Types of Breathing Patterns***

PATTERN	CHARACTERISTICS	CAUSES
Normal	Pattern: regular Depth: even Rate: 12-20 breaths/min	Normal respiratory drive
Tachypnea	Pattern: regular Depth: even Rate: faster than 20 breaths/min	Fever, pain, anxiety
Bradypnea	Pattern: regular Depth: even Rate: slower than 12 breaths/min	Sedatives, narcotics, alcohol; brain, metabolic, and respiratory disorders
Sighing respirations	Pattern: regular Depth: uneven: periodic deep breaths (more than 3 sighs/min) Rate: 12-20 breaths/min	Severe anxiety
Cheyne-Stokes respirations, apnea	Breaths progressively deeper, then becoming more shallow, followed by period of apnea	Severe brain pathology
Kussmaul's respirations (with hyperventilation)	Pattern: regular Depth: deep Rate: faster than 20 breaths/min	Metabolic acidosis Diabetic ketoacidosis, renal failure
Biot's respirations; apnea	Pattern: irregular Depth: varies, sudden periods of apnea	Neurologic disorders
Obstructive breathing, rising end-expiratory level with forced rapid breathing.	Gradual rise in end-expiratory level with each successive breath	Emphysema

Adapted from Kersten, L. D. (1989). *Comprehensive respiratory nursing* (pp. 279-281). Philadelphia: Saunders.

muscles in the chest. Inspiration involves an active contraction of the muscles and diaphragm and can be noted by an enlargement of the chest cavity. Expiration is a passive process during which the muscles relax and the chest returns to its normal size (Fig. 29-3).

During normal, quiet breathing, approximately 500 ml of air is inhaled and exhaled. Most of the air movement occurs because of the contraction and relaxation of the diaphragm. A temporary interruption in the normal breathing pattern in which no air movement occurs is called *apnea*. Difficulty breathing, or shortness of breath, is called *dyspnea*. Difficulty with breathing in a lying position is called *orthopnea*. Different types of breathing patterns are described in Table 29-1.

Respiratory Center

Breathing is controlled by the respiratory center, which is located in the medulla. The medulla is part of the brain stem immediately above the spinal cord. The respiratory center is stimulated by changing levels of carbon dioxide and oxygen in arterial blood. Chemoreceptors in the aorta and carotid artery monitor the pH and the amount of carbon dioxide and oxygen in the bloodstream. Changes in the pH, increased levels of carbon dioxide, or decreased levels of oxygen cause signals to be sent to the phrenic nerves, which in turn send signals to the respiratory muscles to carry out the major work of breathing.

AGE-RELATED CHANGES

Changes that occur with aging in the pharynx and larynx include muscle atrophy, slackening of the vocal cords, and loss of elasticity of the laryngeal muscles and cartilages. These changes may result in a gravelly, softer voice with a rise in pitch. Elders may have a difficult time communicating with one another when they already have impaired hearing and must try to understand speech that is less clear and more muted. Older adults may have a deviation of the trachea if they suffer from scoliosis of the upper spinal column.

Older people may experience difficulty with respiration because they can have loss of lung elasticity, enlargement of the bronchioles, and a decreased number of alveoli. In addition, the respiratory muscles atrophy, the rib cage becomes more rigid, and the diaphragm flattens. The consequences of these changes include reduced chest movement and ability to inhale and exhale, less effective cough, increased work of breathing, and less tolerance for exercise and stress.

NURSING ASSESSMENT OF THE RESPIRATORY SYSTEM

HEALTH HISTORY

The health history encompasses the chief complaint and history of the present illness, the past medical history, the review of systems, and the functional assessment. If the patient is in respiratory distress, the nurse focuses on the immediate problem, any conditions that might affect treatment, and allergies. Detailed assessment may be deferred until the patient's respiratory status improves. The components of a complete assessment of the patient with a respiratory disorder are discussed here.

Chief Complaint and History of Present Illness

Common complaints associated with respiratory disorders are cough, dyspnea, and pain. To describe a cough, include the onset, duration, frequency, type (wet or dry), severity, and related symptoms such as sputum production and pain. Document the frequency of expectoration and the sputum characteristics (color, consistency, odor, amount). Record the patient's effort to treat the cough with measures such as medication, vaporizers, and humidifiers, as well as the response to the treatments.

If the patient complains of dyspnea, determine the onset, duration, severity, and precipitating events. Note whether the dyspnea becomes worse with activity or certain positions and whether it is more frequent during certain seasons. Identify associated symptoms such as fatigue or palpitations. Describe the effectiveness of methods used to manage dyspnea, which might include medications, oxygen, and positioning.

When the patient has chest pain, assess the location, severity, onset, duration, and precipitating events (trauma, coughing, inspiration). Determine whether the pain causes shallow breathing and whether it radiates up to the jaw or down the arms. Record the presence of fever, sweating, or nausea. Document measures that bring relief such as splinting, heat, analgesics, and antitussives.

Past Medical History and Family History

The patient's past medical history determines previous respiratory disorders, allergies, trauma, and surgery. Conditions that are important to document when a patient has a respiratory disorder include allergies, colds, pneumonia, tuberculosis, chronic bronchitis, emphysema, asthma, cancer of the respiratory tract, cystic fibrosis, sinus infections, ear infections, diabetes mellitus, and heart disease. It is especially important to note conditions that suppress the immune response, making the patient more susceptible to infection. Record all recent and current medications, and the dates of the most recent chest radiograph and tuberculosis test. Inquire about immunizations against pneumonia and influenza. Include questions regarding family history. Also describe any major respiratory conditions and the smoking history of members of the household.

Review of Systems

The review of systems assesses signs and symptoms that may be directly or indirectly related to the respiratory disorder. Ask about fatigue, weakness, fever, chills, and night sweats. Other data that may be significant are earaches, nasal obstructions, sinus pain, sore throat, hoarseness, edema, dyspnea, and orthopnea.

Functional Assessment

Describe the patient's occupation, including any exposure to pathogens or to substances that might irritate or harm the respiratory tract. Document exposure to any fumes, toxins, coal dust, silica, or sawdust. Ask the patient to describe a typical day and to give particular attention to any limitations imposed by the respiratory disorder. Assess the usual diet and fluid intake. A smoking history is important and for the cigarette smoker is usually reported in pack years. Pack years are calculated by multiplying the number of years the patient smoked cigarettes times the number of packs smoked each day. To illustrate, a person who smoked two packs a day for 30 years would have a 60-pack-year smoking history. The functional assessment also includes the patient's role in the family, sources of stress, and coping strategies.

What Does Culture Have to do with Smoking?

Among adolescents, smoking is most prevalent among whites followed by Hispanics, then African-Americans. However, programs aimed at smoking prevention and cessation need to target all segments of the population because smoking is a health threat to everyone that typically begins before high school. On a positive note, people who practice Mormonism abstain from using tobacco.

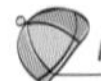
Put on your THINKING CAP!!

A patient has smoked one pack of cigarettes each day for 15 years. Calculate the pack years of his smoking history.

PHYSICAL EXAMINATION

Begin the physical examination with observation of the patient's general appearance. Note facial expression, posture, alertness, speech pattern, and any obvious signs of distress. Take the vital signs, and measure height and weight. Be alert to unusually rapid or slow breathing and to tachycardia, which may be a sign of hypoxia. The normal respiratory rate is 12 to 20 breaths per minute.

Head and Neck

Examine the head and neck. Inspect the nose for symmetry and for deformity and gently palpate for tenderness. Assess the patency of each naris by closing one at a time and asking the patient to breathe in through the nose. Note flaring of the nares because it is a common sign of air hunger. Use a nasal speculum to inspect the nasal cavity for swelling, discharge, bleeding, or foreign bodies. The nasal mucosa is normally light red in color. Tilt back the patient's head to inspect for deviation of the nasal septum, the structure that separates the nares. A deviation may be seen as a hump in the nasal cavity. Palpate the sinuses for tenderness by using the thumbs to apply pressure over the frontal and maxillary sinuses (see Chapter 51).

Inspect the lips, the tip of the nose, the top of the auricles, the gums, and the area under the tongue for cyanosis, a bluish color related to inadequate tissue oxygenation. Document the presence of pursed-lip breathing, a common technique for decreasing dyspnea with chronic respiratory disease. Inspect the pharynx for redness and tonsil exudate or enlargement, which are signs of infection.

Inspect the trachea to see if it is midline; if not midline, it is said to be deviated. A deviated trachea can be indicative of a large atelectasis, pleural effusion, aortic aneurysm, enlargement of part of the thyroid gland, and/or tension pneumothorax. Place the thumbs on either side of the trachea just above the clavicles, and gently move the trachea from side to side. Compare the spaces between the sternocleidomastoid muscles on either shoulder and the trachea. An experienced examiner palpates for enlargement and tenderness of the lymph glands in the neck.

Thorax

Inspect the chest for deformities and lesions and observe the breathing pattern and effort. The rise and fall of the chest should be regular and symmetric. Table 29-1 on p. 456 illustrates the different types of breathing patterns. Palpate the thorax for tenderness and lumps. Additional, more sophisticated aspects of the examination that require special training include palpating for symmetric chest expansion and tactile fremitus. The skilled examiner also may percuss (tap) the thorax in a systematic manner to elicit sounds that give clues about the density of underlying tissues.

Using the diaphragm of the stethoscope, auscultate the lungs bilaterally in a systematic manner (Fig. 29-4), usually the posterior, the sides, then the anterior chest. Listen for the normal movement of air in and out of the lungs and for abnormal breath sounds: wheezes, rhonchi, and crackles. A wheeze is a high-pitched sound caused by air passing through narrowed passageways that may be present with asthma or chronic obstructive pulmonary disease. A rhonchus is a dry rattling sound caused by partial bronchial obstruction. Crackles, also called rales, are abnormal sounds associated with many cardiac and pulmonary disorders. To demonstrate the sound of fine crackles, rub a few strands of hair between the thumb and forefinger next to the ear. Coarse crackles are described as sounding like a Velcro fastener being separated. One other abnormal sound that may be heard on auscultation is a pleural friction rub, which is indicative of pleurisy. A pleural friction rub is a grating, scratchy noise similar to a creaking shoe.

In addition to the examination of the thorax and the auscultation of lung sounds, assess for signs of circulatory disorders that could affect respirations. Inspect the abdomen for distention that might interfere with full expansion of the lungs. Inspect the extremities for color and palpate for edema. Examine the fingers for clubbing, which is associated with chronic respiratory problems (Fig. 29-5). Assess Homans' sign by dorsiflexing the patient's foot. Suspect thrombophlebitis if this maneuver elicits pain behind the knee or in the calf. This is important because the deep veins in the legs and pelvis are the source of most pulmonary emboli.

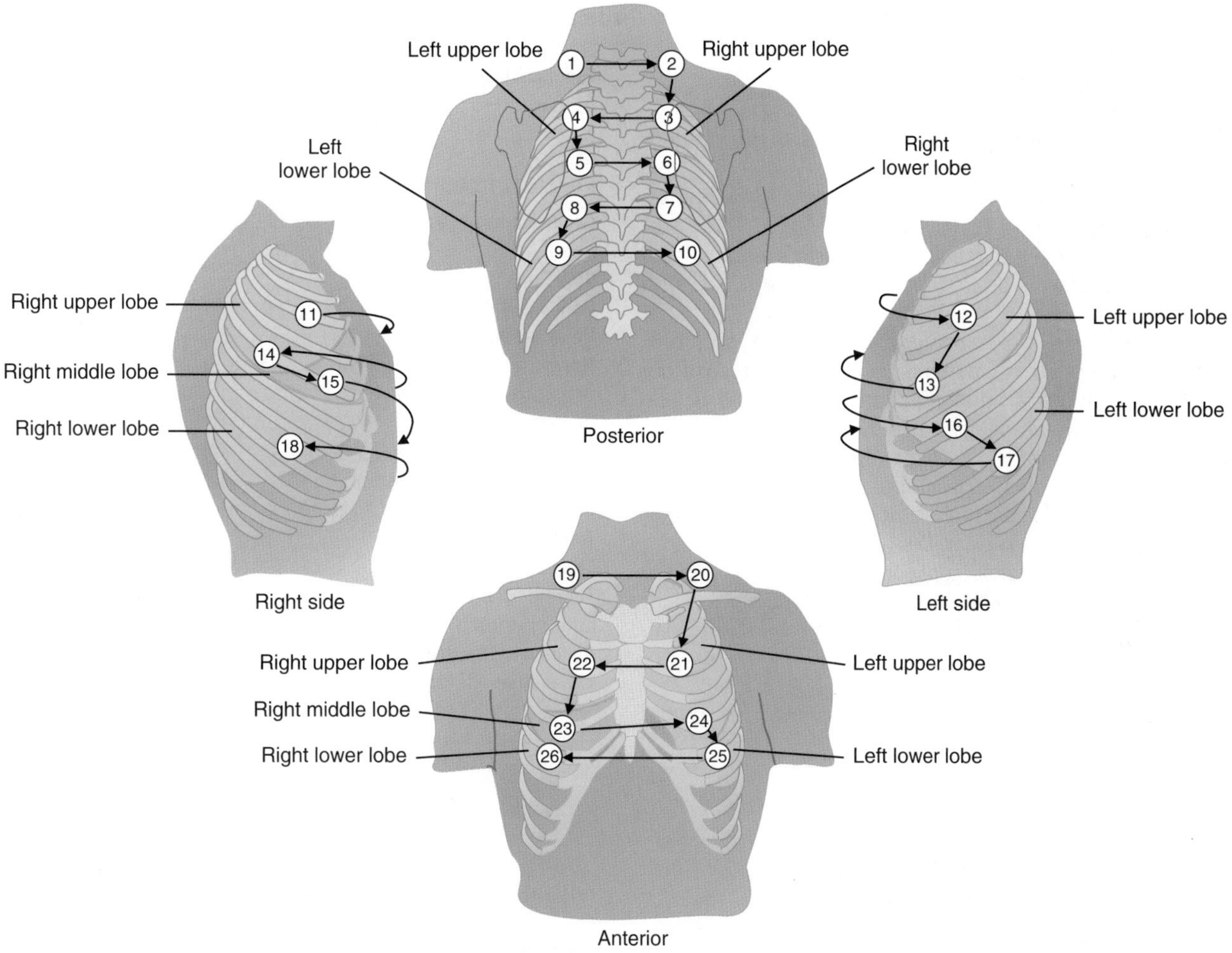

FIGURE 29-4 Sequence for percussion and auscultation of the lungs.

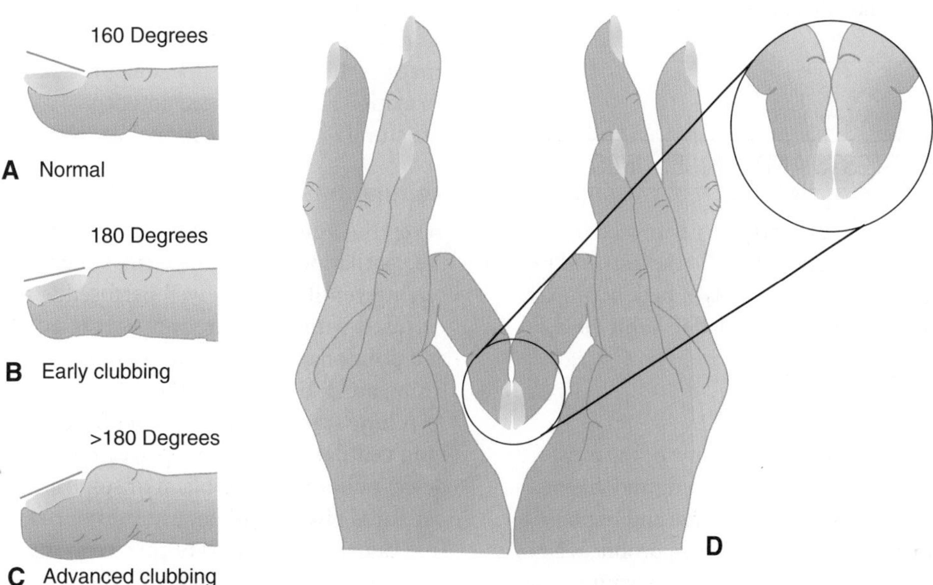

FIGURE 29-5 Clubbing is a flattening of the angle between the nail and the skin. *A,* Normal angle of 160 degrees. *B,* Early clubbing: the angle is flattened to 180 degrees. *C,* Advanced clubbing: the angle is greater than 180 degrees. *D,* The Schamroth technique: The patient puts the nails of the ring fingers of each hand together and holds the other fingers straight up. The examiner looks at the space between the touching nails. If there is no clubbing, the space is diamond shaped.

table 29-2 **ASSESSMENT *of the Patient with a Respiratory Disorder***

HEALTH HISTORY	Functional Assessment
Present Illness: **Cough:** Onset, duration, frequency, type, severity, sputum production and characteristics, pain **Dyspnea:** Onset, duration, severity, precipitating events, associated symptoms **Pain:** Location, onset, duration, precipitating events, effects on breathing, measures that reduce or relieve, associated symptoms **Past Medical History:** Colds, pneumonia, tuberculosis, chronic bronchitis, emphysema, asthma, cancer of the respiratory tract, cystic fibrosis, sinus infections, ear infections, diabetes mellitus, heart disease, allergies, trauma, surgeries, hospitalizations, conditions that suppress the immune response, immunizations against pneumonia and influenza, last chest radiograph, last tuberculosis test, recent and current medications **Family History:** Major respiratory conditions, smoking history **Review of Symptoms:** Fatigue, weakness, fever, chills, night sweats, earaches, nasal obstruction, sinus pain, sore throat, hoarseness, edema, dyspnea, orthopnea	**Functional Assessment:** Occupation, exposure to pathogens or respiratory irritants, typical day, usual diet and fluid intake, smoking history, role in family, stressors, coping strategies **PHYSICAL EXAMINATION** **General Survey:** Appearance, facial expression, posture, alertness, speech pattern, obvious distress **Vital Signs** **Height and Weight** **Head and Neck:** **Nose:** Nasal shape, tenderness, patency, flaring; swelling, discharge, bleeding, foreign bodies in nasal cavity, septal deviation **Sinuses:** Tenderness **Lips:** Pursed-lip breathing, color **Pharynx:** Redness, tonsil exudate or enlargement **Trachea:** Midline **Lymph Nodes:** Enlargement, tenderness **Thorax:** Breathing pattern and effort, accessory muscles, lung sounds **Abdomen:** Distention **Extremities:** Color, clubbing, edema, Homans' sign

The nursing assessment of the patient with a respiratory disorder is summarized in Table 29-2.

Put on your THINKING CAP!!

A patient in respiratory distress usually has tachycardia. Explain why this happens and what purpose the increased heart rate serves.

DIAGNOSTIC TESTS AND PROCEDURES

A variety of tests and procedures may be performed to diagnose disorders of the respiratory system. These tests and procedures are described briefly here. Details of patient preparation and postprocedure care are presented in Table 29-3.

RADIOLOGIC STUDIES

Chest Radiography

Radiographic examination of the chest is one of the most frequently used methods for respiratory screening and diagnosis. It also is used to assess progression of a disease and response to treatment. The radiograph or roentgenogram produces a picture in which the bony structures (e.g., ribs, sternum, clavicle), heart shadow, trachea, bronchi, and blood vessels are visible. Bone appears white on the film because it is very dense and does not absorb much energy. In contrast, the lungs appear black because they are filled with air and absorb the x-ray energy. Chest films usually are taken posteroanterior (back to front), anteroposterior (front to back), and lateral (side) to view the chest cavity from different angles.

Fluoroscopy

Fluoroscopy is a radiograph of the chest taken to observe deep structures in motion. It is possible to observe both lungs at the same time during inspiration and expiration. Instead of producing a single, still image, the screen registers a constant image of the chest. The fluoroscopic examination can give information about the speed and degree of lung expansion and structural defects in the bronchial tree.

Ventilation—Perfusion Scan

When the lungs are working efficiently, there is a balance in the ventilation-**perfusion ratio,** which means that areas receiving ventilation are well perfused with blood, and areas perfused with blood are well ventilated. When the alveolus and pulmonary blood flow are normal, ventilation and perfusion are said to match (Fig. 29-6).

A lung scan or ventilation-perfusion scan is used to assess lung ventilation and lung perfusion. Its chief purpose is to detect pulmonary embolism or some other obstruction. The patient is given a radioactive substance either by inhalation (to evaluate ventilation) or intravenously (to evaluate perfusion). Ventilation images are compared with the pictures taken during the perfusion scan to determine whether there is an equal amount of radioactivity on both the ventilation and the perfusion pictures. Any areas indicating good ventilation but poor perfusion suggest the presence of a pulmonary embolus or obstruction.

table 29-3 **DIAGNOSTIC TESTS AND PROCEDURES | *the Respiratory System***

General nursing implications: Always tell the patient what to expect before, during, and after the procedure. When a venous blood sample is required, tell the patient to expect a venipuncture.

TEST/PURPOSE	PATIENT PREPARATION	POSTPROCEDURE CARE
PULMONARY FUNCTION TESTS (PFTS)		
Evaluate lung function, gas exchanges, pulmonary blood flow, and acid-base balance.	Advise not to smoke or eat a heavy meal 4-6 hr before test. Patient should be dressed comfortably, and should void before the tests. Determine whether any medications or treatments should be withheld.	Resume medications. No special care.
FIBEROPTIC BRONCHOSCOPY		
Used to visualize abnormalities, take biopsy samples of lesions, or remove foreign bodies.	Obtain signed consent. NPO 6-8 hr or as specified. Have patient remove dentures and provide oral hygiene. Document loose teeth. Ask the patient not to smoke. Administer sedatives and anticholinergics as ordered.	NPO until gag reflex returns. Semi-Fowler's position. Monitor vital signs. Monitor for gross hemoptysis, swelling of face and neck, stridor, decreased or asymmetric chest movement, diminished lung sounds, dyspnea. Report abnormal findings to physician.
THORACENTESIS		
Pleural fluid is aspirated and examined for pathogens, other abnormal components. Cells studied for malignancy.	Obtain signed consent. Stress the importance of not moving or coughing during the procedure. Support the patient during the thoracentesis, and monitor skin color, respiratory rate, and general response. Label specimens and send to laboratory.	Monitor vital signs, lung sounds, chest movement. Report dyspnea, asymmetric chest movement. Assess for bleeding. Document amount and color of fluid removed. Check dressing for bleeding..
TUBERCULIN SKIN TEST		
Determine past or present exposure to tuberculosis.	Inform patient the procedure causes pain briefly. Cleanse skin and inject intradermally in lower anterior forearm. Mark and record site. Tell patient skin reaction may persist for a week, do not scratch. Stress need to return in 48-72 hr to read reaction. A reaction (swelling, redness) of 5 mm or more is positive for tuberculosis exposure. A patient who has ever been vaccinated with BCG will test positive regardless of actual exposure.	Follow-up depends on response. If positive, patient will be evaluated for active tuberculosis.
RADIOGRAPHIC AND IMAGING STUDIES		
Chest Radiography		
Used to screen and diagnose some respiratory disorders.	Patient will be asked to remove jewelry on neck and chest and clothing above waist and to put on hospital gown.	No special care.
Fluoroscopy		
Motion radiographs of lungs.	Same as chest radiography.	No special care.
Ventilation-Perfusion Scan (Lung Scan)		
Demonstrates lung ventilation and perfusion. Detects pulmonary embolism and other obstructive conditions.	Assure patient that radiation dose is small and that isotope is quickly eliminated. Procedure is painless except for venipuncture. If sedation is needed for agitated patients or small children, the patient is usually maintained NPO for 4 hr. The procedure takes approximately 2 hr. Monitor patient for 1 hr for anaphylaxis.	Check venipuncture site. Apply small dressing and pressure if needed. Radioactive material is excreted in the urine. Tell patient to wash hands after voiding. Anyone who handles patient's urine should wear rubber gloves. Gloves and hands should be washed after urine is discarded.

NPO, Nothing by mouth.

Continued

table 29-3 **DIAGNOSTIC TESTS AND PROCEDURES | *the Respiratory System—cont'd***

TEST/PURPOSE	PATIENT PREPARATION	POSTPROCEDURE CARE
RADIOGRAPHIC AND IMAGING STUDIES—cont'd		
Computed Tomography (CT, CAT, or CAT Scan)		
Used to visualize lesions and tumors.	Inform the patient that the procedure is painless. Stress the importance of remaining still during the scanning. Assess iodine allergy and report to radiologist in case contrast media is to be used. NPO status may be required.	Assess for side effects of contrast: headache, nausea, vomiting.
Magnetic Resonance Imaging (MRI)		
Produces images of multiple body planes without radiation. Used to detect abnormalities, lesions, and tumors.	Obtain signed consent. Inform patient: will lie on a stretcher that slides into a tubelike device. Mechanical clanging noises are heard as the machine operates. Aneurysm clips, intraocular metal, heart valves made before 1964, and middle ear prostheses generally contraindicate MRI. Metal implants such as cardiac pacemakers and orthopedic implants may be affected by MRI, but are not absolute contraindications. Assess for and report claustrophobia. Patients who are anxious or restless may require sedation. Special equipment must be used for oxygen therapy or mechanical ventilation. Have patient remove metal watch and jewelry.	Safety precautions if sedated; otherwise, no special care is needed.
LABORATORY STUDIES		
Arterial Blood Gas Analysis		
Detects alkalosis or acidosis and alterations in oxygenation status	Tell the patient a blood sample will be drawn from an artery (usually the radial). An Allen's test *must* be done before an arterial puncture to ensure that the arteries to the hand are patent. (Arterial punctures require specialized training.)	Apply pressure to the puncture site for 5-10 min. Note the concentration of any oxygen therapy on the laboratory slip. Transport the blood gas syringe containing the specimen to the laboratory in an ice bath within 15 min.
Sputum Analysis Examination Volume, consistency, odor, color provide clues to clinical disorders. **Culture and Sensitivity (C & S)** Reveals pathogens and effective antimicrobials. **Cytology** Detects malignant cells and inflammatory changes.	Collect the specimen early in the morning before breakfast. Provide a sterile container. Instruct patient to (1) brush teeth and rinse mouth; (2) cough deeply and expectorate directly into the container; (3) immediately cap the container; and (4) inform the nurse that the specimen is ready. *For cytology,* a special container and solution must be used for specimens. Send specimen to the laboratory promptly. Refrigerate if it will be more than an hour before delivery to the laboratory.	No special care.

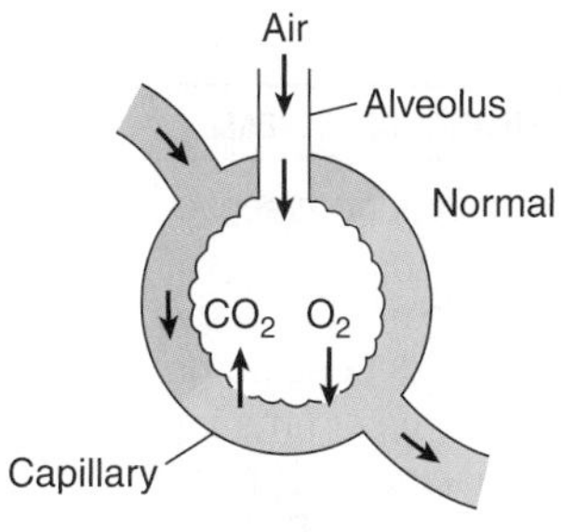

Normal functioning alveolus and pulmonary capillary flow. Ventilation and perfusion match.

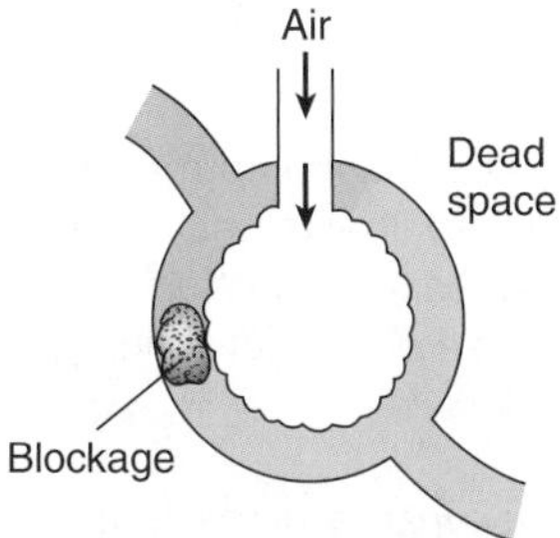

When there is ventilation without perfusion a deadspace unit exists, e.g., pulmonary embolus preventing blood flow through pulmonary capillary.

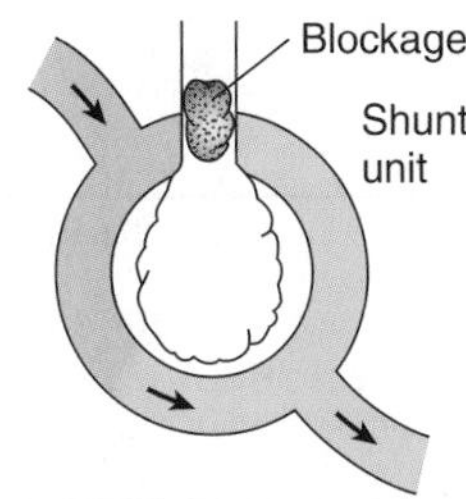

When there is no ventilation to an alveolar unit but perfusion continues, a shunt unit exists and unoxygenated blood continues to circulate, e.g., atelectasis, pneumonia. The alveoli collapse.

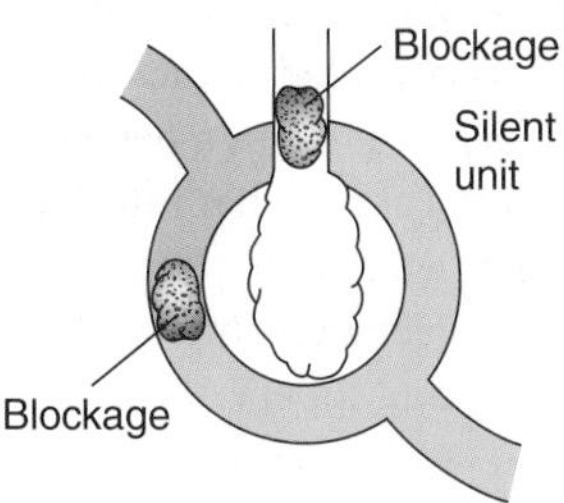

When there is neither ventilation nor perfusion a silent unit develops, e.g., pulmonary embolus combined with ARDS (adult respiratory distress syndrome). The alveoli collapse.

FIGURE **29-6** Normal functioning alveolus and pulmonary capillary blood flow. When both are normal, the ventilation and perfusion match.

IMAGING PROCEDURES

Computed Tomography

Tomography or tomograms allow visualization of slices or layers of the chest. A computed tomography scan is a computerized method of tomography in which a camera rotates in a circular pattern around the body to provide a three-dimensional assessment of the thorax. The test usually is used to look for the presence of lesions or tumors.

Radioactive dye containing iodine may be injected intravenously. Each layer of the chest is photographed before and after the injection of the dye. It is extremely important to find out whether the patient is allergic to iodine before the procedure is carried out. Failure to determine sensitivity to iodine could result in an allergic reaction, anaphylaxis, and death.

PHARMACOLOGY CAPSULE Dyes used in computed tomography contain iodine that can produce fatal reactions in people with iodine allergies.

Magnetic Resonance Imaging

A magnetic resonance imaging (MRI) scan is similar to a computed tomography scan but without the harmful radiation. The MRI scanner encloses the patient in a doughnut-shaped magnet and picks up signals from the body to make electronic images. The patient must remain as quiet and as motionless as possible during the procedure. No preparation is necessary for the procedure, but patients should be warned that no metal may be worn inside the unit (with the exception of dental fillings). Patients with implanted devices such as pacemakers and orthopedic plates, pins, or screws may be ineligible for MRI scanning.

PULMONARY FUNCTION TESTS

Pulmonary function tests are used to diagnose pulmonary disease, monitor disease progression, evaluate the extent of disability, and assess the effects of medication. The tests measure lung volumes and capacities including total lung capacity (TLC), forced respiratory volume (FEV), functional residual capacity (FRC), inspiratory capacity (IC), vital capacity (VC), forced vital capacity (FVC), minute volume (MV), and thoracic gas volume (TGV).

A clip is applied to the nose, and the patient breathes through a mouthpiece as directed while various measurements are taken to assess the mechanics of breathing (flow rates of gas in and out of the lungs), and measure diffusion (the movement of the gas across the alveolar-capillary membrane).

Spirometry

A spirometer is an instrument that measures the ventilatory function of the lung. It measures the volume of air that the lung can hold, the rate of flow of air in and out of the lung, and the compliance (elasticity) of lung tissue. The test enables the physician to detect impaired pulmonary function, classify the pulmonary impairment, estimate the severity of the impairment, monitor the cause of pulmonary disease, evaluate treatment, give information helpful in planning care, and provide preoperative assessment.

The test involves inserting a mouthpiece, taking as deep a breath as possible, and blowing as hard, as fast, and as long as possible. Patients should be encouraged to continue blowing out until exhalation is complete.

Spirometry measures forced vital capacity and forced expiratory volume. These and other lung volumes and capacities are defined in Table 29-4.

table 29-4 *Lung Volumes and Capacities*

VOLUME	DEFINITION	SIGNIFICANCE OF INCREASE	SIGNIFICANCE OF DECREASE
Total lung capacity (TLC)	Total lung volume when fully inflated	Overdistention of lung caused by obstructive lung disease	Restrictive lung disease
Forced expiratory volume (FEV)	Volume of air expired during specified time intervals (0.5, 1, 2, 3 sec)	Not significant	Restrictive or obstructive lung disease depending on measurements at time intervals
Functional residual capacity (FRC)	Volume of air remaining in the lungs after normal exhalation	Chronic obstructive pulmonary disease	Adult respiratory distress syndrome (ARDS)
Inspiratory capacity (IC)	Maximal volume of air that can be inhaled after a normal exhalation	Excessive use of positive end-expiratory pressure	Restrictive lung disease
Vital capacity (VC)	Total volume of air that can be exhaled after maximum inspiration	Not significant Increased or normal VC with normal flow rates: pulmonary edema	Decreased VC with normal or increased flow rates: impaired respiratory effort Obstructive or restrictive lung disease
Forced vital capacity (FVC)	Total volume of air exhaled rapidly and forcefully after maximum inhalation	Not significant	Restrictive parenchymal lung disease; fatigue
Minute volume (MV)	Total amount of air breathed in 1 min	Not significant	Not significant
Thoracic gas volume (TGV)	Total volume of air in the lungs, including ventilated and nonventilated areas	Obstructive lung disease with air trapping	

Data from Chernecky, C. C., & Berger, B. J. (2001). *Laboratory tests and diagnostic procedures.* (3rd ed.) Philadelphia: Saunders; and Jaffe, M. S., & McVan, B. F. (1997). *Davis's laboratory and diagnostic test handbook.* Philadelphia: Saunders.

People who are to undergo spirometry should be taught what to expect during the test and how to prepare. They may be anxious about taking a breathing test if they have respiratory problems because they may fear increased dyspnea or exhaustion. They should be advised not to smoke or use bronchodilator medications for 4 to 6 hours before testing.

PHARMACOLOGY CAPSULE Bronchodilators should not be given before pulmonary function testing because they can alter the results.

Arterial Blood Gas Analysis

Ventilation and diffusion also are measured by testing for concentrations of oxygen and carbon dioxide in the arterial blood to determine whether the exchange is adequate across the alveolar membrane. Blood gas analysis is useful in the care of patients with respiratory disorders, problems of circulation and distribution of blood, body fluid imbalances, and acid-base imbalances. *Drawing an arterial blood sample requires special training.* Samples are often obtained from the radial artery after first performing the Allen's test to ensure adequate circulation to the hand from other arteries (Fig. 29-7). After the arterial puncture, pressure must be applied for 5-10 minutes to assure no bleeding.

The arterial blood sample is analyzed for pH, $PaCO_2$, PaO_2, HCO_3, and O_2 saturation to detect alkalosis or acidosis and alterations in oxygenation status. Normal values for adults are pH: 7.35-7.45; $PaCO_2$: 35-45 mm Hg; PaO_2: 80-100 mm Hg (some references give a lower limit of 75 mm Hg); HCO_3: 22-26 mEq/L; O_2 saturation: 96%-100%.

PULSE OXIMETRY

Pulse oximetry permits the noninvasive measurement of arterial oxygen saturation. A sensor is clipped to an earlobe or fingertip. A beam of light passes through the tissue, and the amount of light absorbed by oxygen-saturated hemoglobin is measured. The oxygen saturation is presented as a percentage and registered on a digital readout. Factors that interfere with accurate measurement of the oximeter are hypotension, hypothermia, vasoconstriction, and finger movement. Normal pulse oximetry is $\geq$95%. Notify your supervisor or the physician of readings $<$90%.

SPUTUM ANALYSIS

Sputum is material that originates in the bronchi. Sputum analysis may be performed when respiratory disease is suspected. The mucous membrane lining of the lower respiratory tract responds to acute inflammation by increasing the production of secretions, which may contain bacterial or malignant cells. These cells may be detected by examination of sputum. Sputum specimens are also examined for volume, consistency, color, and odor. Sputum that is thick, foul smelling, and yellow, green, or rust colored may indicate a bacterial infection. Instruct the patient to expectorate the specimen directly into a sterile container after coughing deeply. If the patient is unable to expectorate a specimen, sputum production may be induced with aerosol therapy or obtained by suctioning.

Culture and Sensitivity

Sputum culture and sensitivity tests are ordered to determine the presence of bacteria, identify the specific organisms, and identify appropriate antimicrobials. Collect specimens before

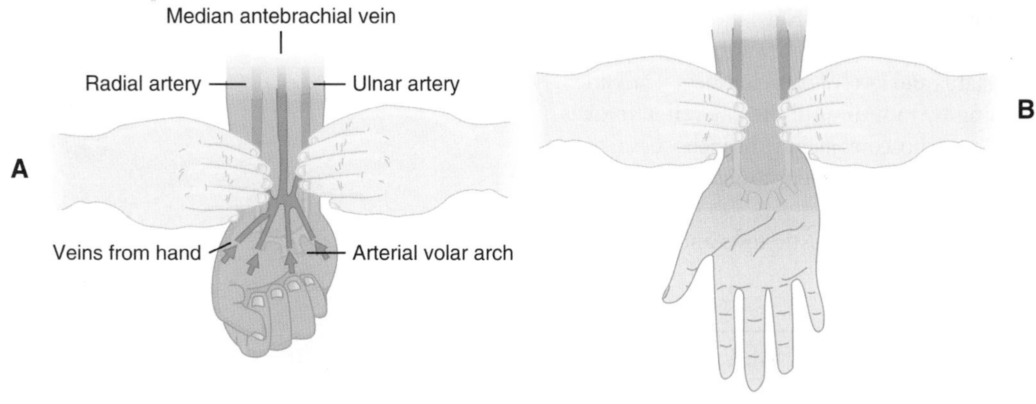

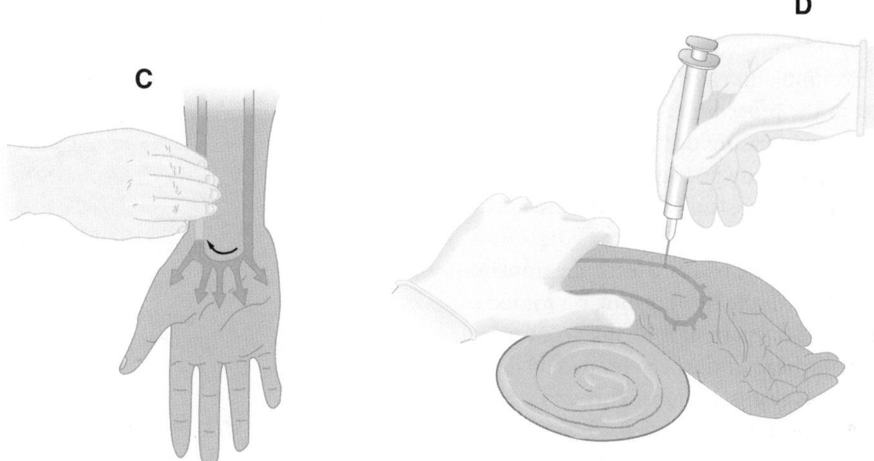

FIGURE **29-7** The Allen test should be done before each radial arterial puncture to ensure adequate collateral circulation. Because an arterial puncture may injure the radial artery, the adequacy of blood supply to the area by other arteries must be determined. A puncture is not done on an artery if the other blood supply is not adequate. To perform the Allen test, occlude the radial and ulnar arteries and have the patient make a fist *(A)*. While maintaining pressure on the arteries, have the patient open the hand. The hand is pale if the arteries are occluded *(B)*. Release the pressure on the ulnar artery. If collateral circulation is adequate, color will return to the hand. This is a positive Allen test result; the puncture can proceed on the radial artery. If color does not return, the Allen test result is negative and the radial artery should not be punctured *(C)*. A blood sample is drawn from the radial artery after a positive Allen test result *(D)*.

antimicrobial therapy is begun to ensure that sufficient bacterial growth is present.

Acid-Fast Test

An acid-fast test on a sputum specimen is performed to determine the presence of acid-fast bacilli, which include the bacteria that cause tuberculosis. Specimens are usually collected on 3 consecutive days. Keep each sputum specimen covered and refrigerated or delivered to the lab within 1 hour. Use a new sterile container for each collection.

Cytologic Specimens

Sputum specimens are obtained for cytologic examination to determine the presence of lung carcinoma or infectious conditions. Because sputum contains cells from the tracheobronchial tree, malignant cells may be detected in the specimen. A special container with fixative solution may be used for this type of specimen collection. Consult the agency laboratory manual for directions.

FIBEROPTIC BRONCHOSCOPY

A bronchoscopic examination is performed by inserting a flexible fiberoptic scope through the nose or mouth into the bronchial tree after local anesthesia of the patient's throat. The scope allows for direct visualization of the bronchial tree structures for assessment, diagnosis, or removal of foreign bodies or mucus plugs. Lesions suggestive of malignancy may be located and a biopsy performed as well. Before the procedure, signed consent should be obtained. Have the patient remove dentures. Give sedatives as ordered. Afterward, monitor the patient's respiratory status and level of consciousness. The patient should take nothing by mouth until the gag reflex returns. Complications of bronchoscopy include bronchospasm, bacteremia, bronchial perforation, pneumonia, laryngospasm, hemorrhage, and pneumothorax.

Additional details about diagnostic tests and procedures are presented in Table 29-3.

COMMON THERAPEUTIC MEASURES

THORACENTESIS

A thoracentesis is the insertion of a large-bore needle through the chest wall into the pleural space. The procedure is usually performed at the bedside by the physician. Thoracentesis is done to remove pleural fluid, blood, or air or to instill medication. Pleural fluid may be removed to reduce respiratory distress caused by fluid accumulation in the pleural space. In addition, fluid obtained in the procedure may be studied to obtain blood cell counts or to measure protein, glucose, lactic dehydrogenase, fibrinogen, or amylase levels. The study of pleural fluids may aid in the diagnosis of infectious diseases and cancer.

The patient sits on the side of the bed and leans the upper torso over the bedside table with the head resting on folded arms or pillows (Fig. 29-8). If the patient is unable to sit up, a side-lying position with the head of the bed elevated 30 degrees may be used. The skin is cleansed thoroughly and a local anesthetic injected. The physician inserts a 20-gauge or larger needle between the ribs and through the parietal membrane. Fluid or air is then aspirated, the thoracentesis needle is removed, and a sterile dressing is applied to the puncture site. The patient is positioned on the unaffected side. A chest radiograph may be ordered after the procedure to detect any pulmonary complications caused by accidental injury to the lung. Complications of thoracentesis include air embolism, hemothorax, pneumothorax, and pulmonary edema. Immediately report uneven chest movements, respiratory distress, or hemorrhage to the supervisor and the physician. Details of nursing responsibilities are included in Table 29-2.

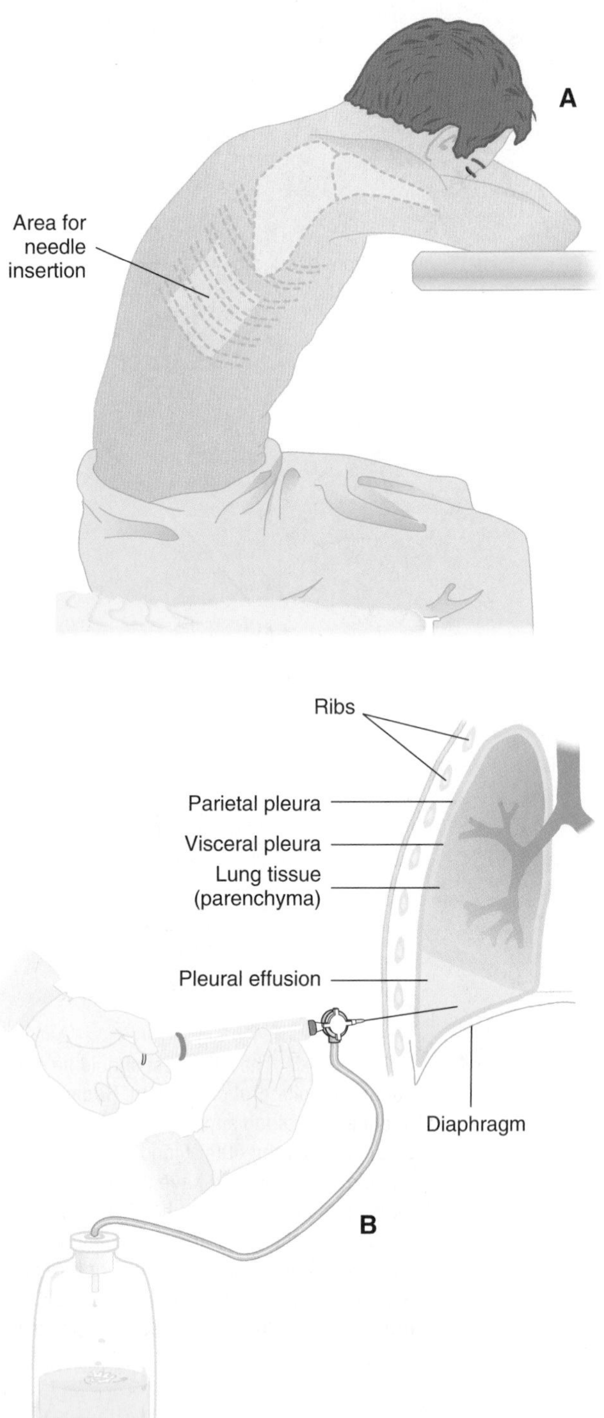

FIGURE **29-8** *A,* The patient is positioned for a thoracentesis. *B,* The needle is inserted into the pleural space, avoiding lung tissue and the diaphragm. The exact location of the puncture varies.

BREATHING EXERCISES

Deep Breathing and Coughing Exercises

Deep breathing and coughing exercises are performed to aid in lung expansion and expectoration of respiratory secretions. They are indicated when patients are immobilized or after general anesthesia. Instructions to the patient include the following:

1. Sit in a semi-Fowler's position for maximal lung expansion.
2. Place one hand on the abdomen to feel it rise and fall with breathing.
3. Inhale deeply through the nose, pause 1 to 3 seconds, and exhale slowly through the mouth.
4. After 4 to 6 deep breaths, cough deeply from the lungs to aid in the expectoration of sputum.
5. After thoracic or abdominal surgery, splint the incision with a pillow to minimize discomfort and support the incision.

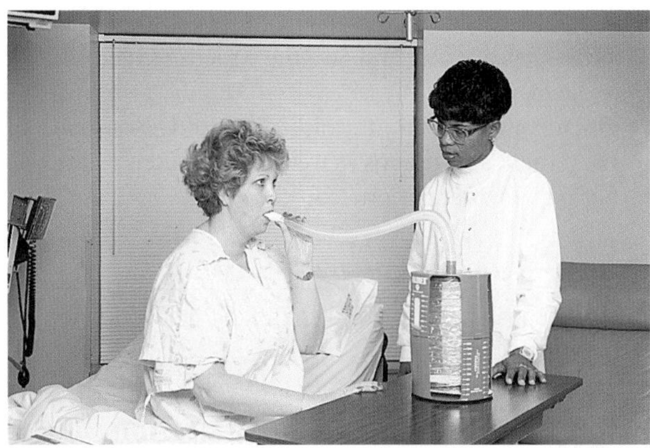

FIGURE 29-9 Incentive spirometry encourages deep breathing by providing a visual cue to the patient about the efficiency of deep breathing.

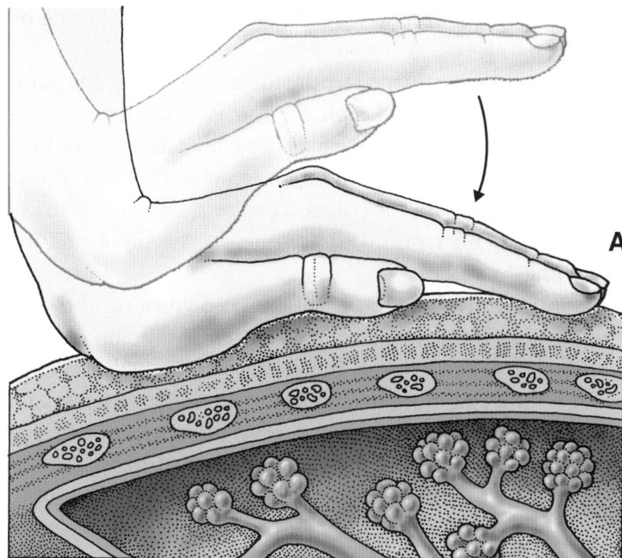

Chest percussion (with cupped hand)

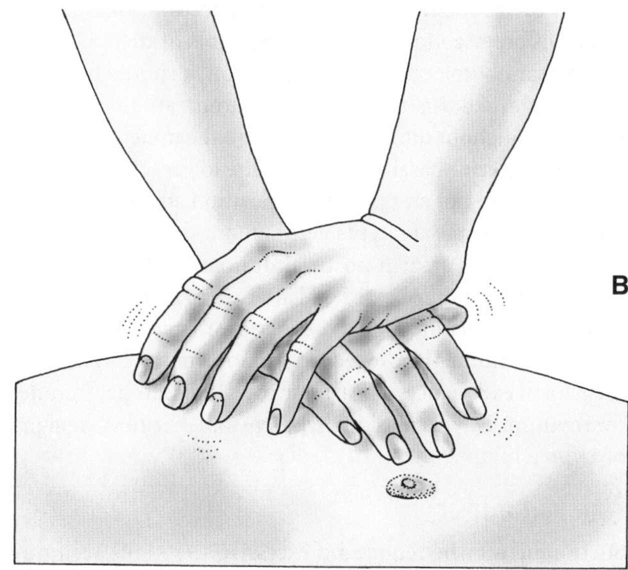

Chest vibration

FIGURE 29-10 Chest physiotherapy. *A,* Percussion. *B,* Vibration.

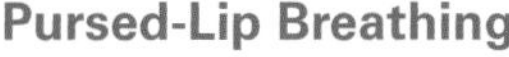

Pursed-Lip Breathing

Another type of breathing exercise is pursed-lip breathing. It is used to inhibit airway collapse and to decrease dyspnea in patients with chronic lung disease. Instruct patients to pucker the lips as if to whistle, blow out a candle, or blow through a straw. They should then inhale through the nose and slowly exhale through pursed lips. Exhalation should last twice as long as inhalation.

Sustained Maximal Inspiration

Sustained maximal inspiration is used to ensure deep inspiration for maximal expansion and aeration of the lungs. An incentive spirometer is an instrument that frequently is used to encourage maximal inspiration. Spirometers basically consist of a cylinder that contains balls or disks and a tube through which the patient inhales. As the patient inhales through the tube, the balls or disks rise (Fig. 29-9). Instruct the patient to inhale deeply to move the balls or disks in the cylinder upward. For maximum effect, the spirometer is kept upright because tilting the device reduces respiratory effort. Some spirometers provide a digital readout of the volume of air displaced. If the patient's maximal inspiration can be measured before surgery, that reading can be used as a target after surgery.

CHEST PHYSIOTHERAPY

Chest physiotherapy consists of percussion, vibration, and postural drainage. These mechanical techniques are used to facilitate the mobilization and expectoration of secretions in patients with large mucus-producing or chronic mucus-retaining respiratory disorders such as chronic bronchitis and cystic fibrosis. Although this therapy is usually performed in the acute care setting by a respiratory therapist, the nurse often does this in long-term and home care settings. Therefore you should be familiar with the procedures and able to evaluate the patient's response. In an outpatient setting, you also may monitor the caregiver's technique in administering the treatment. Chest physiotherapy should be performed before meals to reduce the risk of regurgitation and aspiration of stomach contents.

Chest Percussion and Vibration

Chest percussion and vibration are performed to facilitate the movement of respiratory secretions so sputum can be expectorated. Percussion is clapping of the cupped palms against the chest wall to dislodge and mobilize respiratory secretions (Fig. 29-10A). The procedure is performed with the hands cupped to create a pocket of air when striking the patient's chest, first with one hand, then with the other. Percussion is confined to areas protected by the rib cage and is never done over the sternum, kidney, liver, spleen, stomach, or spine. In general, percussion is done for 20 to 30 seconds, followed by vibration.

Vibration is performed by the therapist placing one hand on the top of the other, keeping the arms straight, and pressing the hands flat against the patient's chest (see Fig. 29-10B). As the patient exhales, the therapist creates a shaking (vibrating) movement with the palms. The therapist pauses during inhalation. The vibration is repeated over three or four breathing cycles.

Contraindications to percussion and vibration include lung cancer, bronchospasm, pain in the area being treated, hemorrhage, hemoptysis, increased intracranial pressure, chest trauma, pulmonary embolism, pulmonary edema, gastric reflux, pneumonectomy with open pericardium, extreme agitation or anxiety, and high risk for rib fractures.

Postural Drainage

Postural drainage is the technique of positioning the patient to facilitate gravitational movement of respiratory secretions toward the bronchi and trachea for expectoration. Various positions are used to drain all 18 segments of the lungs. If a patient cannot tolerate a specific position, it should be omitted or modified. Instruct the patient to breathe slowly and deeply throughout the procedure. Drain the upper lobes first, and the posterior basal segments of the lower lobes last. The patient should not sit up between position changes. Provide tissues and a disposal receptacle. Maintain each position for 5 to 15 minutes. Perform postural drainage before meals or tube feedings. It may be ordered after respiratory treatments with bronchodilators. The frequency is ordered by the physician. Discontinue the procedure and inform the physician if the patient experiences a heart rate over 120 beats per minute, dysrhythmias, hypertension, hypotension, dizziness, or signs of hypoxemia.

SUCTIONING

Suctioning may be required if excessive secretions accumulate in the oral or nasal airway and the patient cannot expectorate. The goal of suctioning is to improve oxygen and carbon dioxide exchange in the lungs by removing excessive mucous secretions with a suction catheter. Consult a procedure manual for details, but key points when suctioning a patient include the following:

1. Use strict aseptic technique.
2. Administer oxygen before inserting the suction catheter because the procedure temporarily interferes with the patient's airflow.
3. Moisten the catheter in sterile water and insert the catheter through the nose or mouth before applying suction.
4. Apply suction as the catheter is withdrawn from the airway.
5. Maintain the pressure gauge between 80 and 100 mm Hg.
6. Limit each suction pass to 10 seconds.
7. Allow the patient to rest briefly, encourage deep breathing, and rinse the catheter with sterile solution between suction attempts.
8. Monitor the patient's response to suctioning.
9. If tachycardia or increased respiratory distress develops, stop the procedure and give the patient oxygen as ordered.
10. Document the amount, color, odor, and consistency of the patient's secretions as well as the patient's status before and after the procedure.

 ***Put on your THINKING CAP!!***

Why is actual suctioning time limited to 10 seconds for each pass of the catheter?

HUMIDIFICATION AND AEROSOL THERAPY

The upper respiratory system is designed to moisturize and warm the air that is inspired through the nose. Humidity is necessary in the respiratory tract to prevent secretions from becoming inspissated (thickened and dried). Inspissated secretions irritate the mucosa, making it more susceptible to bacterial infection.

Humidifiers

A humidifier creates water vapor to raise the relative humidity of inspired gas to 100%. There are several types of humidifying devices available for use. Room humidifiers deliver water vapor directly into the air. Medical oxygen is humidified as it bubbles through a container of water. Humidifiers that require heat to create water vapor pose a risk of heat injury. The fluid reservoir can become contaminated, making it a source of airborne infection. To prevent the spread of bacteria, sterile water should be used to fill the reservoir, and the equipment must be cleaned between each use. Last, the equipment can present an electrical hazard.

Aerosol Therapy

Aerosol therapy is used to liquefy and mobilize respiratory secretions and to deliver medications. Aerosols are suspended liquid particles of bronchodilators or inactive fluids such as water or saline that are delivered by devices called nebulizers. Nebulizers deliver a humidified aerosol through large tubing, which may be connected to an oxygen mask or a handheld device. When hand-held nebulizers are used, the patient should sit upright and slowly inhale the nebulizer aerosol deeply, hold the breath briefly, and exhale slowly. Once secretions are mobilized, the patient may require deep breathing and coughing techniques, postural drainage, suctioning, or a combination of these to clear the secretions. Because aerosols can cause bronchospasm, bronchodilators may be ordered before administering some types of aerosol therapy. There is also a risk of fluid retention, infection, and drug toxicity.

OXYGEN THERAPY

Air in the atmosphere contains approximately 21% oxygen. Usually this is sufficient for oxygenation to maintain the tissue's ability to function appropriately. In the presence of cardiopulmonary disease or injury, it may be necessary to provide a patient with supplemental oxygen, that is, to enrich the atmospheric air with higher concentrations than the patient normally breathes. Oxygen should be treated as a pharmacologic agent in that there may be serious side effects as well as benefits from its use.

PHARMACOLOGY CAPSULE Oxygen should be thought of as a pharmacologic agent with risks of adverse effects.

Oxygen therapy requires a medical order that should be carried out like any drug order. If a patient is observed becoming lethargic or bradypneic (abnormally slow breathing), immediately notify a supervisor or physician because these are symptoms of adverse effects of oxygen therapy.

To administer oxygen to the patient, it is necessary to alter the gas from a compressed form such as a bulk oxygen supply or cylinder to a form with a usable, safe flow rate. Modern hospitals have bulk oxygen systems with wall adapters to which flowmeters can be attached. When patients with oxygen must be transported, a cylinder on wheels is necessary. A regulator with a flowmeter must be used. After a flowmeter has been attached to the oxygen source, it may be necessary to humidify the gas before delivering it to the patient. Humidification is usually unnecessary when using a low-flow cannula at a flow setting of 2 or fewer liters per minute or when using an air entrainment (Venturi) oxygen delivery system.

A tube is needed to connect the flowmeter to the specific oxygen delivery device being used. In some of the devices, the tube is incorporated as an integral component, but in others it is not. It is possible to use extension tubes for some devices, but increasing the length of the tube increases the resistance to gas flow, thus causing pressure to back up in the system, so the patient may not receive the desired oxygen flow.

Oxygen therapy is ordered in liters per minute, or FIO_2. FIO_2 means fraction of inspired oxygen. It is written, for example, as 0.30, which means 30% oxygen concentration. Various devices can deliver different amounts of oxygen (Fig. 29-11).

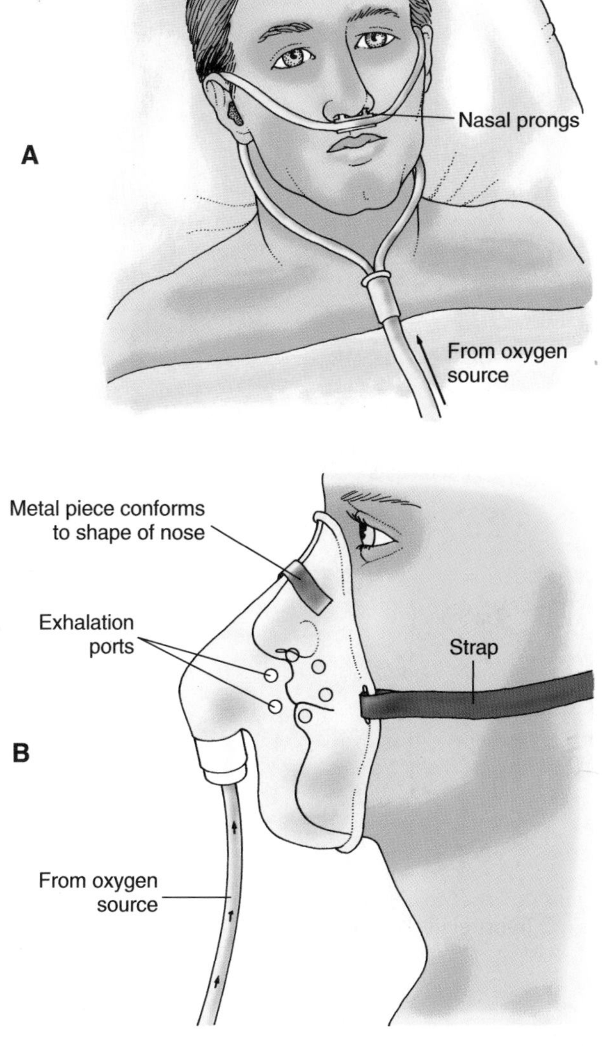

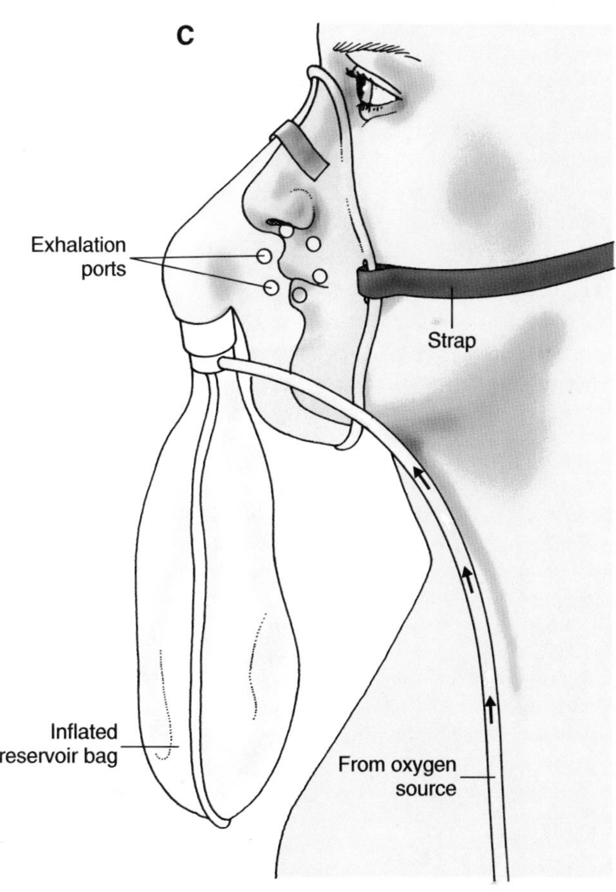

FIGURE **29-11** Oxygen delivery systems. *A*, Nasal cannula. *B*, Standard oxygen mask. *C*, Partial rebreathing oxygen mask.
Continued

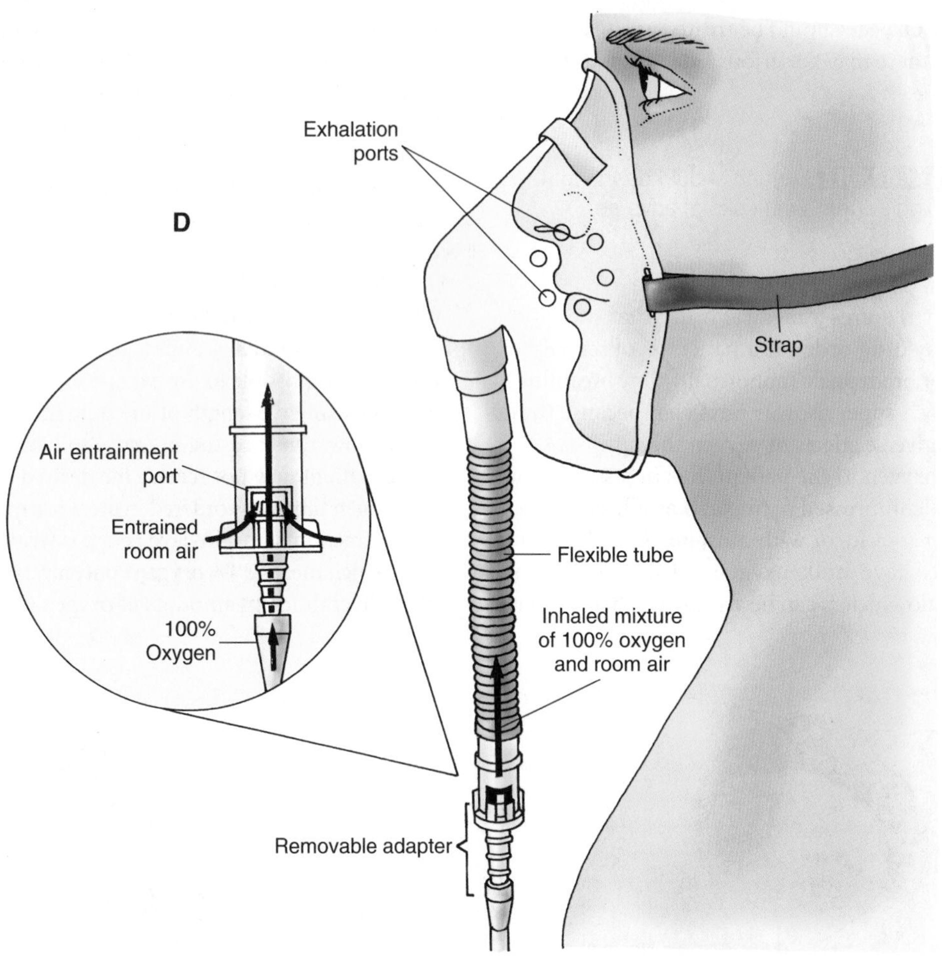

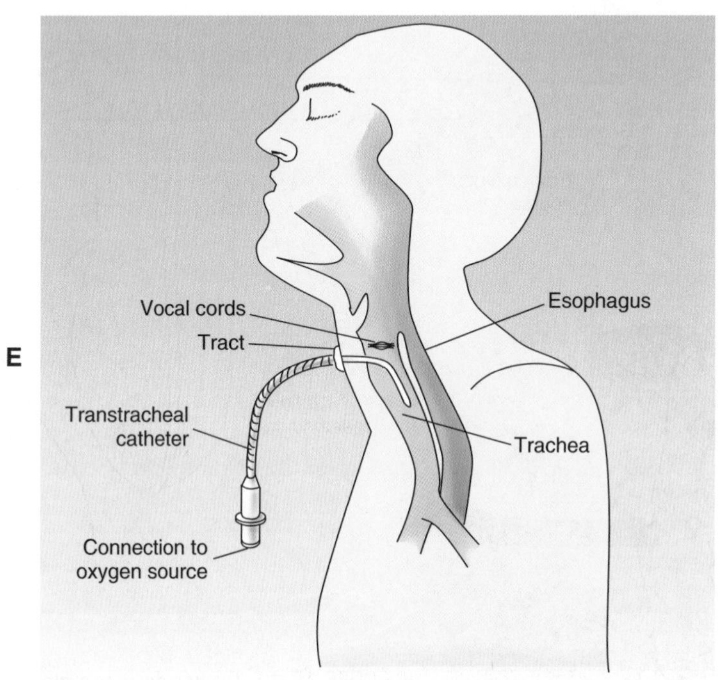

FIGURE **29-11, cont'd** *D,* Venturi oxygen mask. *E,* Transtracheal oxygen delivery.

The most commonly used device is the nasal cannula, which fits around the face and directly into the nares by way of two prongs. It is designed to deliver a low flow of oxygen from 1 to 6 L/min with an approximate FIO_2 of 0.24 to 0.40 (24% to 40% oxygen). The nasal catheter is also a low-flow device that is inserted into one naris and then into the pharyngeal space approximately at the uvula. The FIO_2 and flow rates are the same as those for the cannula. This catheter is rarely used, except during short-term procedures.

Four types of masks are available: the simple oxygen mask, the partial rebreathing mask, the nonrebreathing mask, and the air entrainment (Venturi) mask. The simple oxygen mask is designed to deliver an FIO_2 ranging from 0.35 to 0.55 (35% to 55% oxygen). Flow rates from the flowmeter may be adjusted from 6 to 10 L/min. The minimum flow rate of 6 L/min is necessary to prevent any chance of carbon dioxide buildup from occurring. The partial rebreathing mask includes a reservoir bag to elevate the potential FIO_2. It is unique because the patient actually rebreathes part of the exhaled gas in the system. However, it is designed so that the rebreathed gas contains almost no carbon dioxide from the patient's lungs—only enriched oxygen. The expected FIO_2 range is 0.35 to 0.60 (35% to 60%). The flowmeter setting must be from 6 to 10 L/min. The nonrebreathing mask is so named because none of the patient's exhaled gas is rebreathed. Like the previous mask, it also includes a reservoir bag to enhance the FIO_2, but it has a series of valves to direct the flow of oxygen in such a way that the patient receives a fresh supply of gas with each breath. The expected FIO_2 should be near 1.0 (100%). However, Scanlon and colleagues have shown experimentally that the highest FIO_2 is approximately 0.7 (70%). The air entrainment mask is designed to provide a specific FIO_2. This device has been called a Venti mask or a Venturi mask in the past, and still may be referred to by these names. The manufacturers of these devices list a specific flowmeter setting for the desired FIO_2. It is also necessary either to adjust a setting on the device or to place a specific attachment on the mask to obtain the desired results. Read the literature accompanying the mask, and if there is confusion, consult a respiratory therapist.

Transtracheal oxygen therapy delivers oxygen through a small, flexible catheter that is inserted into the trachea through a small incision or with a special needle. This approach is sometimes used when long-term therapy is indicated.

There may be times when an oxygen mask must be removed, as for oral care or for eating or drinking. Ask the physician to write an order for the temporary use of a cannula during these times.

Advances in outpatient oxygen therapy have the potential to improve greatly the quality of life for patients with chronic pulmonary conditions. Whereas patients used to have to rent large cylinders for home use, they can now rent oxygen concentrators that process room air and deliver air with an increased percentage of oxygen. The concentrator is about the size of a canister vacuum cleaner and has a 50-foot tubing connected to a nasal cannula. This allows the patient considerable freedom of mobility in the home setting.

To leave the home, patients can use small tanks of compressed oxygen. The tanks weigh approximately 3 pounds and can deliver 2 L/min for approximately 3 hours. A device that can be used with the canister delivers oxygen only "on demand," when the patient inhales. This conserves the oxygen, making the canister last longer. Portable liquid oxygen canisters that can deliver a very high flow of oxygen are also available. These canisters can be refilled from a larger tank that can be kept in the patient's home. A weekend version of the tank fits in the back seat of a car and lasts several days. These devices allow considerable freedom for the patient.

The nurse must recognize the complications of oxygen therapy, including hypoventilation, toxicity, atelectasis, and ocular damage. Patients at greatest risk for oxygen-induced hypoventilation are those with chronic respiratory disorders. They may have become insensitive to high carbon dioxide levels in the blood, so that low oxygen levels in the blood serve as the stimulus for respirations ("hypoxic drive"). Oxygen administration raises the level of oxygen in the blood, and the patient who has hypoxic drive may hypoventilate or even have apnea. Oxygen toxicity can result from exposure to a high concentration of oxygen for a prolonged period of time. Toxicity progresses from tracheobronchitis to lung fibrosis and atelectasis, and may be fatal. Atelectasis can result from the replacement of nitrogen normally in the alveoli with oxygen. Oxygen is readily absorbed, predisposing the alveoli to collapse. Exposure to 100% oxygen can cause retinal injury and visual impairment.

Key points when a patient is receiving oxygen therapy are the following:

1. Monitor the liter flow to be sure it is as prescribed.
2. Assess the patient's response to oxygen therapy; monitor reports of blood gas analyses.
3. Inspect the tubing for kinks, obstructions, loose connections; listen for a hissing sound in the oxygen mask; feel for adequate oxygen flow.
4. Maintain sterile water in the humidifier reservoir.
5. Clean and replace oxygen therapy equipment according to agency policy.
6. Post a "No Smoking" sign and advise the patient and visitors that smoking is not allowed because oxygen supports combustion.

INTERMITTENT POSITIVE-PRESSURE BREATHING TREATMENTS

Intermittent positive-pressure breathing (IPPB) treatments are used to achieve maximal lung expansion. The IPPB equipment delivers humidified gas with positive pressure, which forces air into the lungs with inhalation and allows passive exhalation. This facilitates maximal exchange of oxygen and carbon dioxide gases in the alveoli and promotes a productive cough. Aerosol medications, including mucolytics (agents that liquefy secretions) and bronchodilators, can be administered through IPPB treatments with a nebulizer device. Although most IPPB treatments are administered by respiratory therapists, they are done by nurses in some settings.

In the past, IPPB was used for a wide range of conditions. The American Association for Respiratory Care now recommends it only for specific conditions, including atelectasis, decreased lung compliance with kyphoscoliosis, and cardiogenic pulmonary edema. In addition to its limited usefulness, IPPB is losing favor because it may cause a tension pneumothorax in patients with chronic obstructive pulmonary disease. It also may cause respiratory alkalosis because of hyperventilation. The desired effects of IPPB usually can be achieved by other, less expensive measures such as incentive spirometry and hand-held nebulizers.

ARTIFICIAL AIRWAYS

Artificial airways are sometimes required to maintain a patent airway. Artificial airways include the oral airway, nasal airway, endotracheal tube, and tracheostomy tube.

Oral Airway

The oral airway is a curved tube used to maintain an airway temporarily. The oropharyngeal airway is inserted by tilting the head back, opening the mouth, and inserting the airway into the patient's mouth with the tip pointed toward the roof of the mouth. The tube is turned over while being advanced so that the end of the tube rests on the base of the patient's tongue.

Nasal Airway

A nasopharyngeal airway is a soft rubber tube that is inserted through the nose and extended to the base of the tongue. After ruling out a deviated septum, the nasal airway is coated with a water-soluble lubricant and inserted upward into the nose so that the distal end is located in the pharynx at the level of the base of the tongue. A nasal airway should be changed from one naris to the other every 8 hours.

Endotracheal Tube

An endotracheal tube is a long tube inserted through the mouth or nose into the trachea. These tubes have cuffs, inflatable balloons that seal the trachea to prevent aspiration of foreign material and to facilitate mechanical ventilation. Insertion of an endotracheal tube and care of the patient who is intubated require specialized training.

Tracheostomy

A tracheostomy is a surgically created opening through the neck into the trachea. There are a variety of tracheostomy tubes, and they may be used with or without cuffs. Care of the patient with a tracheostomy is covered in Chapter 51.

MECHANICAL VENTILATION

Mechanical ventilation is the process of providing respiratory support by means of a mechanical device called a ventilator. Ventilators are most commonly required for patients with inadequate ventilation and hypoxemia. This may be evidenced by tachypnea or bradypnea with an elevated or a stable arterial carbon dioxide tension ($Pa{CO_2}$), a low arterial oxygen tension ($Pa{O_2}$), or a low pH. To ventilate a patient mechanically, a cuffed endotracheal or tracheostomy tube must be used to deliver the air. Once the tube is in place, the cuff must be inflated to create a closed system in the patient's airway. Otherwise, air being forced into the lungs could simply flow back out of the trachea.

A volume-limited ventilator is most commonly used for patients with acute respiratory failure. It inflates the lungs with a preset volume of oxygenated air that is delivered under pressure during the inspiratory cycle. The expiratory cycle may be conducted passively or with pressure as indicated.

There are three types of positive-pressure ventilators: volume cycled, pressure cycled, and time cycled. A volume-cycled ventilator, which delivers a constant preset amount of oxygenated air to the patient, is the most commonly used type. A pressure-cycled ventilator, which pushes air into the lungs until a preset pressure is reached, is not widely used for continuous mechanical ventilation. Time-cycled ventilators deliver oxygenated air over a preset length of time. This type is used most frequently in infants and children.

Depending on the patient's needs, ventilators may be programmed to control or assist the rate of ventilation. The most frequently used modes are intermittent mandatory ventilation and synchronized intermittent mandatory ventilation. These modes provide assistance with ventilation by allowing the patient to breathe spontaneously between a preset number of ventilator breaths. Ventilators deliver oxygen ranging in concentration from 21% oxygen (atmospheric air) to 100% oxygen. The oxygen concentration, or $F{IO_2}$, is adjusted for individual patient needs.

Tidal volume is the preset amount of oxygenated air delivered during each ventilator breath. This is usually 10 to 15 ml/kg of the patient's body weight.

The respiratory rate setting is the total number of breaths delivered per minute. The rate may be governed by the ventilator alone or by the ventilator and the patient's spontaneous respirations.

Positive end-expiratory pressure may be prescribed to keep the pressure in the lungs above the atmospheric pressure at the end of expiration. This reduces collapse of small airways and alveoli, thereby increasing the functional residual capacity and improving ventilation.

Other mechanical ventilation modalities include options such as pressure support, flow-by, continuous positive airway pressure, and high-frequency ventilation. These are mentioned only for completeness, and not for discussion. If you encounter any of these modalities, specific training is needed that is beyond the scope of this text.

Like much other health care technology, mechanical ventilation can now be managed in the home. With proper training, these devices can be managed by a family member. A device that is used by people with sleep apnea is a continuous positive airway pressure unit. Continuous positive airway pressure (CPAP) maintains positive pressure in the airway during sleep, thereby avoiding periods of apnea. CPAP units are small and have a nose mask that is worn during sleep.

Nursing care of patients on mechanical ventilation requires special training, but key aspects of care include the following:

1. Monitor settings to ensure they are set as prescribed.
2. Be sure high and low pressure alarm settings are turned on.

3. Have a manual resuscitator and oxygen source readily available.
4. Do not allow water to accumulate in the tubing.
5. Monitor the patient's vital signs and breath sounds; suction as necessary.
6. Establish an alternate method of communication because the patient cannot speak while intubated.

CHEST TUBES

Chest tubes are inserted to drain air or fluid from the pleural space of the lungs. This permits reexpansion of a collapsed lung in the patient with a hemothorax, pneumothorax, or pleural effusion. Chest tubes are inserted by the physician under sterile conditions in the operating room or at the bedside. One or two tubes may be inserted. A small incision is made to insert one chest tube in the second to fourth intercostal space to remove air. Another tube may be placed in the eighth or ninth intercostal space to remove fluids. The tubes are sutured in place, and an airtight sterile dressing is applied. The distal ends of the plastic chest tubes are connected to sterile rubber tubing that leads to a pleural drainage device composed of three compartments: the collection chamber, the waterseal chamber, and the suction chamber (Fig. 29-12). Chest fluid and air drain into the collection chamber. Air is diverted to the waterseal chamber, where it can be seen bubbling up through the water. Suction pressure is controlled in the suction control chamber. The tubing in the suction chamber is partially submerged in water; the depth of the tube in the water regulates the amount of suction. After the tubes have been inserted, a chest radiograph is obtained to confirm placement.

Monitor the patient's vital signs and breath sounds frequently. Assess the dressing to be sure a tight seal is maintained. Tape tubing connections, and inspect the connections frequently to detect air leaks. Coil extra tubing on the bed to avoid kinks and keep the drainage system on the floor. Monitor the drainage for blood clots or lung tissue, which may have to be gently kneaded downward to keep the tube patent. Agency and physician preferences dictate whether chest tubes are stripped or milked (Fig. 29-13). Observe the chambers for bubbling. Bubbles are usually seen in the waterseal chamber unless the lung has reexpanded or the tubing is occluded.

The rate of drainage is monitored by marking the drainage level on the drainage receptacle. The middle waterseal chamber is observed for the expected rise in the fluid level with inspiration and the fall with expiration. Continuous bubbling

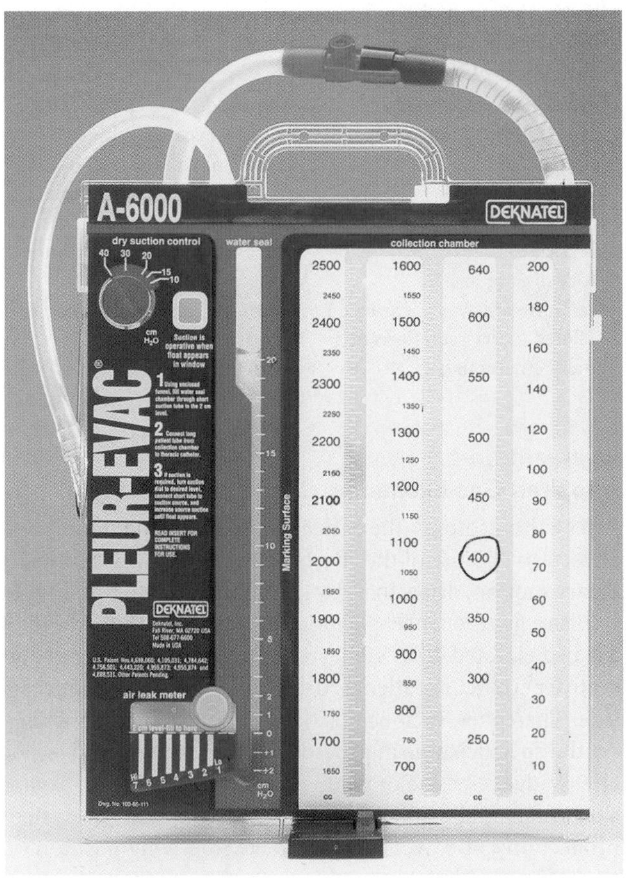

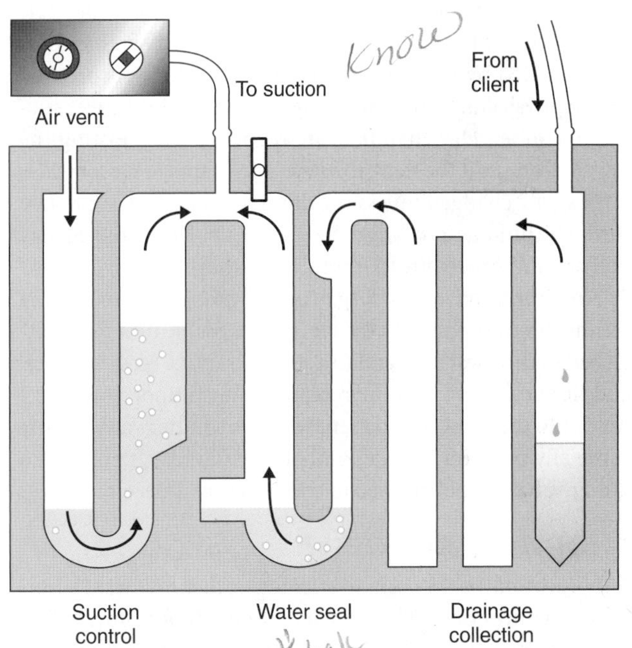

FIGURE 29-12 *A*, A commonly used disposable chest drainage system. *B*, Diagram of chambers of waterseal chest drainage.

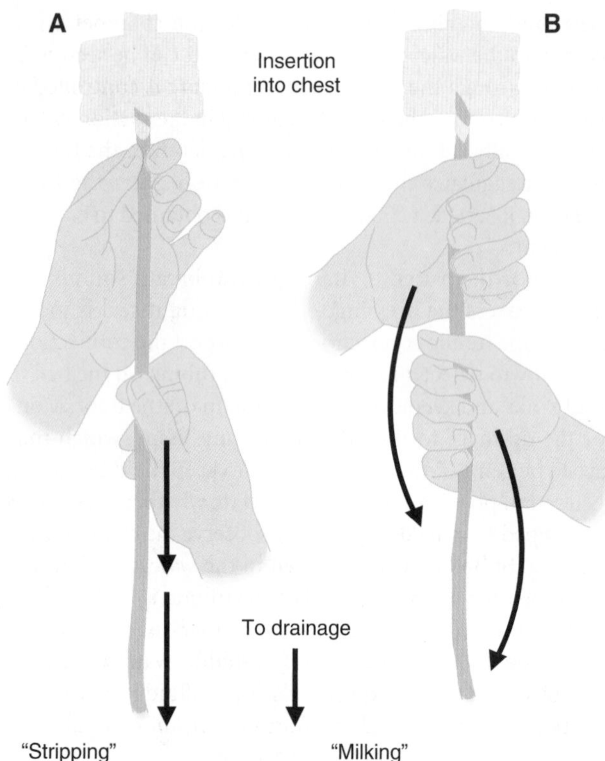

FIGURE 29-13 Two techniques for removing blood clots from chest tubes. *A,* Stripping. *B,* Milking. Both can create excessive negative pressure in the pleural space, but milking is safer than stripping. Follow agency policies and physician orders in relation to these procedures.

in the waterseal chamber suggests an air leak. If an air leak is suspected, agency policy may permit the tubing to be clamped for a maximum of 10 seconds while locating the leak. The suction control chamber may be wet or dry. Wet chambers are regulated by maintaining the water level that is ordered by the physician. Gentle bubbling is expected in the wet suction chamber. Dry chambers are regulated by adjusting the dry suction until the float appears. The drainage receptacle is not usually changed unless the drainage chamber is full. Use sterile technique to change the receptacle. Know the agency policies and procedures for managing chest tubes.

An alternative to the large chest drainage systems is the Heimlich flutter valve. The valve is a disposable unit that is attached to the chest tube and to a sterile drainage receptacle. Air and fluid can flow into the receptacle but cannot flow backward into the chest. The patient who has a flutter valve can assume any position and can ambulate easily. A system with a flutter valve can be attached to chest suction if necessary.

THORACIC SURGERY

A thoracotomy is the surgical opening of the chest wall. Surgical procedures on the lung include pneumonectomy, lobectomy, segmental resection, and wedge resection. Pneumonectomy is the removal of an entire lung, whereas a lobectomy is removal of one lobe of a lung. The extensive dissection and removal of a section of the lung is called a segmental resection. A wedge resection is the removal of a small, triangular section of lung tissue. Other procedures that require a thoracotomy are decortication and thoracoplasty. Decortication is stripping of the membrane that covers the visceral pleura, and thoracoplasty is the removal of ribs. Among the most common purposes for thoracic surgery are evaluation of chest trauma, removal of tumors and cysts, and treatment of empyema.

PREOPERATIVE NURSING CARE *of the Patient with a Thoracotomy*

Preoperative nursing care is described in Chapter 16. Before thoracotomy, emphasize postoperative breathing exercises. If the insertion of a chest tube is anticipated, explain the procedure to the patient.

POSTOPERATIVE NURSING CARE *of the Patient with a Thoracotomy*

Assessment

After surgery, monitor vital signs, lung sounds, mental state, dressings, and chest tube function and drainage.

Nursing Diagnoses, Goals, and Outcome Criteria: Thoracotomy

General postoperative nursing diagnoses are presented in Chapter 16. Diagnoses and goals specific to the patient who has had a thoracotomy may also include the following:

Nursing Diagnoses	Goals and Outcome Criteria
Impaired Gas Exchange related to ventilation-perfusion mismatch	Improved gas exchange: vital signs consistent with patient's norms, arterial blood gases within normal limits
Ineffective Breathing Patterns related to preexisting respiratory disease or pain	Effective breathing patterns: regular respirations without cyanosis or dyspnea
Ineffective Airway Clearance related to dry secretions or ineffective cough	Improved airway clearance: breath sounds clear to auscultation

Interventions

Impaired Gas Exchange

After a thoracotomy, the patient is at risk for pneumonia and atelectasis because of the effects of anesthesia, which impairs ciliary motion, drugs that dry secretions, and immobility. To improve gas exchange, position the patient with the head of the bed elevated 20 to 40 degrees. In the immediate postoperative period, the patient is usually placed on the unaffected side. Thereafter, various positions are permitted depending on the specific surgical procedure. Avoid the operative side after wedge resection or segmentectomy to encourage expansion of remaining lung tissue on the affected side. After pneumonectomy, also avoid the complete side-lying position on the affected side because this may encourage mediastinal shift. Administer oxygen as ordered.

Ineffective Breathing Patterns

Splint the thoracic incision while assisting the patient to breathe deeply and cough. An incentive spirometer may be used to encourage full expansion of the lungs. Adequate pain control enables the patient to breathe more effectively. Chest physiotherapy and bronchodilators are indicated for some patients. When permitted, assist the patient to sit on the edge of the bed with the feet flat on the floor. An overbed table can be placed in front of the patient, who can lean on it with folded arms. This position fosters movement of the diaphragm and chest expansion.

Ineffective Airway Clearance

Good hydration thins secretions; therefore, encourage fluids. If the patient cannot tolerate adequate oral fluids, intravenous fluids may be ordered. For management of chronic respiratory conditions, see Chapter 30.

VIDEO THORACOSCOPY

Many procedures that formerly required thoracic surgery now can be done with video thoracoscopy. Thoracoscopy is performed by inserting an endoscope through a small thoracic incision. Procedures that can be done with this instrument include resection of pulmonary and mediastinal lesions, biopsy, drainage of effusions, sympathectomy, vagotomy, and thymectomy. Potential complications of thoracoscopy include atelectasis, pneumonia, air leaks, and injury to thoracic organs. A chest tube is usually needed to promote full reexpansion of the lung on the operative side. Otherwise, patient care is much less complicated than it is after thoracotomy. Monitor the patient's respiratory status, including lung sounds. Immediately report sudden dyspnea or other signs of respiratory distress to the surgeon. Document the amount and appearance of chest tube drainage. Inspect the closed drainage system for proper functioning. Incentive spirometry may be used to encourage lung expansion. Give analgesics as ordered, although pain is usually not as severe as it is after thoracotomy. Patients are usually permitted out of bed 4 to 6 hours after surgery and can return to work in 1 week. Before discharge, instruct the patient to notify the physician of dyspnea or a temperature higher than 38.3° C (101° F).

DRUG THERAPY

Drugs used to treat respiratory disorders include decongestants, antitussives, antihistamines, expectorants, antimicrobials, bronchodilators, corticosteroids, mast cell stabilizers, leukotriene inhibitors, and thrombolytics (Table 29-5).

Decongestants

Decongestants are sympathomimetic agents. They mimic the action of epinephrine and norepinephrine, causing constriction of nasal blood vessels and reducing the swelling of mucous membranes. Over-the-counter decongestants such as Sudafed are commonly used to treat the common cold. With oral decongestants, constriction of the blood vessels is not limited to the nasal passages, so that systemic vasoconstriction and elevated blood pressure may result. Systemic effects are less severe with topical drops and sprays. Nevertheless, people with hypertension, heart disease, diabetes mellitus, and hyperthyroidism are usually advised to avoid decongestant drugs except under medical supervision.

PHARMACOLOGY CAPSULE People with hypertension, heart disease, and hyperthyroidism should not take over-the-counter cold remedies without consulting a pharmacist or a physician. Many cold remedies stimulate the heart and raise the blood pressure.

Antitussives

Antitussives suppress the cough reflex. Antitussive action is not always desirable because coughing removes secretions from the airways. However, when a cough is nonproductive, creates pain, interferes with sleep, or impairs wound healing, temporary cough suppression may be indicated. Codeine is an effective antitussive, but it is an opioid with many side effects and abuse potential. Therefore, dextromethorphan, which is not an opioid, is more commonly used.

PHARMACOLOGY CAPSULE Use antitussives cautiously. Cough is a protective mechanism that clears the airway.

Antihistamines

Antihistamines are also called histamine 1 blockers because they block the effects of histamine—one of the chemicals that causes allergic symptoms. Antihistamines include a variety of prescription and over-the-counter medications that are frequently used because of their action in drying nasal secretions. First-generation antihistamines such as diphenhydramine (Benadryl) provide short-term relief. However, they also can cause dizziness, dry mouth, constipation, blurred vision, urinary retention, tachycardia, drowsiness, and impaired judgment. Second-generation antihistamines such as loratadine (Claritin) are less likely to cause drowsiness. Antihistamines may worsen a cough by drying up bronchial secretions. These drugs are not usually recommended for people with asthma because dry secretions contribute to difficulty clearing the airway.

Expectorants

Expectorants thin respiratory secretions so they are more readily mobilized and cleared from the airways.

Antimicrobials

Antimicrobials kill or inhibit the growth of bacteria, viruses, or fungi. Antibacterials are used to treat only bacterial infections because they are not effective against viruses or fungi. A limited number of antiviral and antifungal drugs are available. Specific antimicrobials are best selected after culture and sensitivity tests are performed on a specimen of respiratory

table 29-5 DRUG THERAPY | *Drugs Used to Treat Respiratory Disorders*

DRUG	USE/ACTION	SIDE EFFECTS	NURSING INTERVENTION
DECONGESTANTS			
Pseudoephedrine (Sudafed)	Vasoconstriction. Reduces swelling of mucous membranes. Used to treat nasal discharge, common cold.	Occasional mild CNS stimulation, especially in elderly. Toxicity: lightheadedness, tachycardia, palpitations, nausea, vomiting, hallucinations, seizures.	Monitor pulse and blood pressure, mental and emotional state. Contraindicated with severe hypertension, coronary artery disease, lactation. Tell patient to swallow extended-release tablets whole.
ANTITUSSIVES			
Codeine Hydrocodone bitartrate (Hycodan) Dextromethorphan	Suppression of cough reflex. Appropriate uses: control nonproductive cough or cough that interferes with rest or wound healing.	Codeine is an opioid; has abuse potential. Can cause sedation. Dextromethorphan does not have these effects.	Encourage fluids unless contraindicated to facilitate expectoration of secretions. Safety measures with codeine.
ANTIHISTAMINES			
Diphenhydramine (Benadryl)	Block allergic response. Dry respiratory secretions. Also antiemetic and sedative effects.	Drowsiness, dry mouth, blurred vision, photophobia, thickening of mucus secretions, decreased sweating, constipation, urinary retention, increased heart rate.	Safety precautions if drowsy. Monitor respiratory status. Not recommended for patients with asthma. Encourage fluids if not contraindicated. Monitor elimination. Oral hygiene.
EXPECTORANTS			
Guaifenesin (Robitussin)	Thin respiratory secretions for easier expectoration.	Nausea and vomiting with large doses.	Assess cough productivity. Do not crush sustained-release capsules.
ANTIMICROBIALS	Kill or inhibit the growth of bacteria, viruses, or fungi.	Side and adverse effects specific to each antimicrobial classification. Common side effects are nausea, vomiting, and diarrhea. Risk of superinfections such as yeast infections of mouth, genitourinary tract. Risk of severe allergic response.	Assess allergies before administration. Be alert for allergic response: rash, dyspnea, loss of consciousness. Withhold drug if allergy suspected. Instruct patient to complete entire course of therapy. Monitor for improvement and for superinfections. Report continued symptoms.
BRONCHODILATORS	Relax smooth muscle in the bronchial tree to relieve bronchial constriction.		
1. Methylxanthines Theophylline Aminophylline	Methylxanthines also cause increased heart rate and force of cardiac contraction, central nervous system stimulation, and increased gastric acid secretion.	Anxiety, restlessness, tachypnea, tachycardia, dysrhythmias, GI distress. Rapid intravenous administration can cause hypotension, fatal dysrhythmias.	Monitor vital signs, mental state, serum drug levels. Measure intake and output. Give with milk or food to decrease GI distress. Do not administer before bedtime (may keep awake).
2. Sympathomimetics Epinephrine Isoproterenol hydrochloride (Isuprel) Ephedrine	Sympathomimetics also decrease mucus secretion, increase mucociliary clearance, and stabilize mast cells.	Restlessness, anxiety, tachycardia, headache, hypertension, disorientation, nausea, vomiting, diarrhea.	Do not exceed prescribed dosage. Teach patient to use inhaler. Rinse mouth after inhalation to decrease dryness and irritation. Avoid excessive caffeine. Monitor respiratory and cardiovascular status.

Selective $beta_2$ agonists: Albuterol sulfate (Proventil), Terbutaline sulfate (Brethine), Isoetharine hydrochloride (Bronkosol)		Less cardiac stimulation with $beta_2$ agonists.	
3. Inhaled muscarinics: Ipratropium bromide (Atrovent)	Inhaled muscarinics act directly on the respiratory passages to cause bronchodilation. Not effective for acute asthma attacks.	Increased intraocular pressure with narrow-angle glaucoma. Rare: hypotension.	Monitor respiratory status. Evaluate for improvement. Tell patient not to use more than two inhalations at a time. Rinse mouth after inhaling to reduce dry mouth and throat. Avoid excessive caffeine intake.
CORTICOSTERIODS			
Inhalation: beclomethasone (Vanceril, Beclovent) Nasal: beclomethasone (Beconase)	Stabilize mast cells to reduce release of mediators that cause inflammation and edema. Restore bronchodilator response to sympathomimetics in treating acute bronchial constriction. Routes: oral, parenteral, inhalation.	Systemic therapy: water and sodium retention, potassium loss, abnormal fat distribution, hypertension, gastrointestinal distress. Masks signs of infection. Abrupt withdrawal can trigger adrenal insufficiency. Inhaled steroids: hoarseness, oral yeast infections, systemic effects possible with long-term use.	Monitor vital signs, weight, and electrolytes. Assess for subtle signs of infection. Rinse mouth after inhalation.
MAST CELL STABILIZER			
Cromolyn sodium (Intal) Nedocromil (Tilade)	Reduces the production of chemicals by the mast cells that cause bronchial constriction, edema, inflammation. Helps reduce frequency/severity of asthma attacks. Does not *stop* asthma attack. Routes: inhalation, nasal.	Wheezing, sneezing, coughing. Occasional bronchoconstriction. Rare: allergies, headache, nausea, urinary frequency.	Instruct patient in self-medication. Advise that excessive use can actually cause bronchoconstriction. Rinsing mouth after use of inhaler reduces dry mouth effects. Monitor effects.
LEUKOTRIENE INHIBITORS			
Zafirlukast (Accolate)	Inhibit synthesis or receptors of substances that mediate allergic responses.	Zafirlukast: headache, nausea, diarrhea, infection.	Zafirlukast: take on empty stomach.
Zileuton (Zyflo)	Prevent acute asthma attacks.	Zileuton: elevated liver enzymes, pain, nausea, headache.	Zileuton: can take with or without food. Monitor liver function.
Montelukast (Singulair)		Montelukast well tolerated; does *not* seem to cause liver damage	Montelukast: phenytoin can lower blood levels
THROMBOLYTICS			
Streptokinase (Streptase) Urokinase (Abbokinase) Alteplase (Activase)	Dissolve clots; used to treat pulmonary emboli. An IV bolus dose is given, followed by an infusion.	Streptokinase: cerebral hemorrhage, hypotension, allergic reaction, bleeding. Alteplase: bleeding, arrhythmias, rash, itching.	Assess for bleeding. Monitor fibrinogen levels, blood pressure, pulse. Watch for allergic reactions.

secretions. Antimicrobials can cause allergic responses and have many side effects. Instruct the patient in self-medication and stress the importance of completing the prescribed course of therapy to prevent reinfection and the development of resistant strains of pathogens.

Bronchodilators

Bronchodilators relax smooth muscle in the bronchial airways and blood vessels. They are used to treat airway obstruction from respiratory disorders such as asthma and chronic obstructive pulmonary disease. The primary drawback to many bronchodilators is their tendency to cause cardiac and central nervous system stimulation. Some bronchodilators act primarily to prevent bronchial constriction, whereas others relieve it.

Corticosteroids

Corticosteroids are anti-inflammatory drugs that may be administered parenterally, orally, and by inhalation. The drugs may be inhaled orally or nasally. They are important drugs in the treatment of asthma because they reduce inflammation and edema in the respiratory tract. These drugs are less commonly used to treat chronic obstructive pulmonary disease. Among the many systemic effects of steroids are fluid and electrolyte imbalances, hyperglycemia, hypertension, osteoporosis, reduced resistance to infection, and muscle wasting. Oral and parenteral steroids have more side effects than inhaled forms of the drug. Therefore parenteral use is generally confined to short-term, acute situations and oral use is usually limited to 2 weeks. Advise patients not to discontinue steroid therapy abruptly because that may lead to acute adrenal insufficiency.

PHARMACOLOGY CAPSULE Inhaled corticosteroids can have systemic effects if used over a long period of time.

Mast Cell Stabilizers

Cromolyn sodium (Intal) and nedocromil (Tilade) reduce the production of chemicals by the mast cells that cause bronchoconstriction, edema, and inflammation. These drugs, called mast cell stabilizers, are used to prevent acute asthma attacks. They are not useful in stopping an attack after it starts.

Leukotriene Inhibitors

Leukotrienes are substances that mediate allergic responses, including bronchospasm. Drugs that inhibit leukotrienes are useful in the treatment of asthma because they inhibit the allergic response, thereby helping prevent acute asthmatic attacks. Examples are zafirlukast (Accolate) and zileutin (Zyflo).

Thrombolytics

Thrombolytics such as streptokinase (Streptase), urokinase (Abbokinase), and alteplase or tissue plasminogen activator (Activase) may be used to dissolve blood clots in the lungs (pulmonary emboli).

DISORDERS OF THE RESPIRATORY SYSTEM

ACUTE VIRAL RHINITIS (THE COMMON COLD)

Etiology and Risk Factors

Acute viral rhinitis, also called coryza or the common cold, is the most prevalent infectious disease. It is caused by viruses that invade the upper respiratory tract through airborne droplets. The droplets are spread by an infected person through breathing, sneezing, coughing, or by direct hand contact. Touching contaminated surfaces and then carrying the virus to the nasal membranes and eyes is the most important means of spreading a cold. Therefore, careful attention to hand washing is one of the best preventive measures for avoiding a common cold.

Signs and Symptoms

Colds occur most frequently during the winter months when people tend to stay indoors and can more easily contaminate one another. A cold lasts 2 to 14 days, and people are most contagious during the first 3 days. Symptoms include a feeling of nasal dryness and stuffiness, sneezing, runny nose, headache, sore throat, lethargy, and fatigue. In severe cases, chills, fever, and marked prostration may be present.

Complications

Although most people with colds recover without incident, viral or bacterial pneumonitis develops in some patients.

Medical Diagnosis

The common cold is diagnosed on the basis of the patient history and physical examination.

Medical Treatment

The most common treatment for a cold is a combination of rest, fluids, proper diet, antipyretics, and analgesics. Antibiotics and currently available antiviral agents are usually not indicated because they are not effective against cold viruses. Studies have been inconclusive about the value of using large doses of vitamin C for treating and preventing a cold. Other drugs that may be used to relieve the symptoms of the common cold by drying secretions are antihistamines and decongestants.

NURSING CARE *of the Patient with Acute Viral Rhinitis*

Assessment

The complete assessment of the patient with a respiratory disorder is summarized in Table 29-2. The health history may be limited in focus and include a complete description of symptoms, past medical history, and drug history. The physical examination focuses on the nose, throat, ears, neck, and chest.

Nursing Diagnosis, Goal, and Outcome Criteria: Common Cold

The primary diagnosis for the patient with a common cold is ineffective therapeutic regimen management related to lack of understanding of treatment, prevention, and signs and symptoms of complications. The goal of nursing care is effective patient management of the cold with full recovery and no complications. If the patient is at risk for secondary infection, the goal is absence of signs of worsening infection.

Criteria for assessing the effective patient management of the plan of care are the patient's verbalization of content presented and statement of intent to follow plan of care. Absence of infection is evidenced by normal vital signs, clear breath sounds, and clear sputum.

Interventions

The common cold is unlikely to require inpatient care unless a patient is immunosuppressed. Therefore, the primary nursing intervention is usually patient teaching. Advise the patient to rest and to maintain a daily fluid intake of 2 to 3 L, if not contraindicated. Good hydration is essential for keeping secretions thin for easier expectoration. A room humidifier may provide some comfort by keeping mucous membranes moist. Fever can be treated with antipyretics. Identify drugs prescribed or recommended by the physician and inform the patient of the drug names, dosages, and side effects. Many drugs used to treat symptoms of the common cold cause drowsiness, so advise the patient to avoid activities requiring mental alertness.

PHARMACOLOGY CAPSULE Explain to patients that antibacterials are not usually prescribed for the common cold because it is caused by a virus, and antibacterials are effective only against bacteria.

Infection control measures are needed to prevent spread of the cold and to protect the patient who has a cold from secondary bacterial infections. During the first 3 days the patient is most contagious. The patient should avoid contact with others, especially those who are at increased risk for infection (young children, the elderly, people who are immunosuppressed), to prevent the spread of the cold.

PATIENT TEACHING PLAN
Common Cold

To reduce the risk of spreading the cold or of acquiring secondary bacterial infection:

- Avoid close contact with other people who have bacterial infections.
- Avoid crowded places.
- Avoid sharing drinking glasses or eating utensils.
- Practice good hand washing with antibacterial soap.
- Cover the mouth when coughing or sneezing.
- Use disposable tissues for expectorated secretions; dispose of them promptly.
- If you develop purulent (greenish) sputum; chest pain; a temperature higher than 37.8° C (100° F); a red, sore throat; or lung congestion, contact the physician because these signs and symptoms suggest a more severe respiratory condition that may require additional treatment.

ACUTE BRONCHITIS

Etiology and Risk Factors

Acute bronchitis is a common condition that may follow a viral infection such as a cold or influenza. Bronchitis is usually viral in origin, but bacterial causes (*Streptococcus pneumoniae* or *Haemophilus influenzae*) also are common. Irritation and inflammation may occur throughout the upper respiratory tract, resulting in an increased production of mucus. Excess production of mucus leads to coughing and sputum production.

Signs and Symptoms

Symptoms of acute bronchitis include fever, cough, yellow or green sputum, rapid breathing, and occasionally chest pain.

Medical Diagnosis

Acute bronchitis is usually diagnosed on the basis of the health history and the physical findings.

Medical Treatment

Treatment consists of a broad-spectrum antibiotic (ampicillin, tetracycline, or erythromycin) for 7 to 10 days; hospitalization is usually unnecessary.

NURSING CARE *of the Patient with Acute Bronchitis*

Nursing care with acute bronchitis is similar to that for the common cold. In addition, encourage patients who are taking antibiotics to take the full course of the medication.

INFLUENZA

The term *flu* is commonly used to describe a number of ailments involving various body systems. However, influenza is actually an acute viral respiratory infection that is accompanied by a fever. There are several strains of the influenza virus (A, B, C). A strain is further subtyped according to the place and year it was isolated. Influenza usually occurs in epidemics during the winter months. Those most susceptible to the influenza virus are very young children, elderly people, people living in institutional situations, people with chronic diseases, and health care personnel.

Complications

The most common complications of influenza are bronchitis and viral or bacterial pneumonia. Other, less common complications are myocarditis, pericarditis, Reye's syndrome, confusion, seizures, Guillain-Barré syndrome, toxic shock syndrome, myositis, and renal failure.

Signs and Symptoms

Influenza is similar to the common cold in the way that it is spread, that is, through droplet infection; however, its symptoms differ from those of the common cold. People with colds experience nasal symptoms and malaise and usually are afebrile (without fever), whereas those with influenza typically have chills, fever, muscular pain, headache, and dry, hacking cough.

Medical Diagnosis

A diagnosis of influenza is usually based on the patient's history and physical findings. Laboratory tests for confirming infections caused by the influenza virus are improving dramatically and can provide results in less than 48 hours. However, viral tests in general are expensive and may not be available in all facilities.

Medical Treatment

Treatment of influenza is similar to the treatment of the common cold: rest, fluids, proper diet, antipyretics, and analgesics. First-generation antiviral agents like amantadine hydrochloride (Symmetrel) or rimantadine (Flumadine) can be used to treat type A influenza. Second-generation antivirals such as oseltamivir (Tamiflu) and zanamivir (Relenza) treat influenza types A and B. With either generation, therapy must be started within 24 to 48 hours after the onset of symptoms and continued for 10 days.

PHARMACOLOGY CAPSULE Antiviral drugs must be administered soon after the onset of influenza symptoms to be effective.

The best treatment is prevention through immunization, especially for elderly people, people with chronic illnesses, health care personnel, and people living in crowded environments. The Immunization Practices Advisory Committee recommends an annual vaccination using inactivated influenza vaccine. The immunizations are usually given in the fall of the year. The protection rate for influenza vaccines is approximately 70% in the general population, but may be lower among the elderly. Although the incidence of adverse reactions to influenza immunizations is small, some people report sore arm, headache, fever, muscle aches, nausea, and diarrhea. Acetaminophen 325 mg taken every 4 hours for the first 12 hours may reduce these symptoms. Other measures to reduce the risk of influenza are good nutrition and hygiene. An antiviral agent also may be prescribed for people who are at increased risk of acquiring viral infections.

NURSING CARE *of the Patient with Influenza*

Nursing care of the patient with influenza is similar to care of the patient with the common cold. Ongoing assessment is particularly important with influenza because of the risk of serious complications, especially in the elderly. In addition, encourage immunization against influenza for people at high risk: those with serious chronic cardiopulmonary disorders, residents of long-term care facilities, health care providers who have contact with high-risk patients, people older than 65 years of age, and those who have chronic metabolic disorders such as diabetes mellitus.

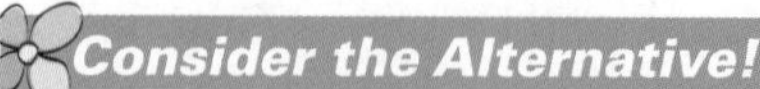
Consider the Alternative!

Echinacea is an herb taken orally to stimulate immune function, suppress inflammation, and treat viral infections such as the common cold and influenza. There is little evidence that it prevents colds, but it may decrease the duration and severity of a cold.

PNEUMONIA

Etiology and Risk Factors

The term *pneumonia* describes inflammation of certain parts of the lung such as the alveoli and bronchioles. Pneumonia may be caused by either infectious or noninfectious agents. Examples of infectious agents are bacteria, fungi, and nonspecific viruses. Noninfectious agents may include irritating fumes, dust, or chemicals that are inhaled or foreign matter that is aspirated. Nosocomial pneumonia is a hospital-acquired infection that may be attributed to inadequate hand washing, poor sterile technique with suctioning, contaminated equipment, and exposure to others who have infectious respiratory conditions.

People who are most likely to contract pneumonia are smokers; those with altered consciousness from alcohol, seizures, anesthesia, or drug overdose; those who are immunosuppressed; chronically ill people who are malnourished or debilitated; and people on bedrest with prolonged immobility.

Patients at increased risk for aspiration pneumonia are those with impaired swallowing or cough reflexes, decreased gastrointestinal motility, esophageal abnormalities, tube feedings, tracheostomies, and endotracheal tubes.

Pathophysiology

Pneumonia may be classified according to the causative organism, usually bacteria or viruses. Gram-positive bacteria cause pneumococcal, staphylococcal, and streptococcal pneumonias, and gram-negative bacteria cause pseudomonal and influenza pneumonias and legionnaires' disease. Pneumococcal pneumonia *(S. pneumoniae)* is the most common cause of bacterial pneumonia. Viral pneumonias are caused by several different viruses, including the influenza virus.

The pathophysiology of pneumonia follows a predictable course. When pathogens invade the lungs, the inflammatory process causes fluid to accumulate in the affected alveoli. In a process called *hepatization,* capillaries dilate and neutrophils, red blood cells, and fibrin fill the alveoli, causing the lung to appear red and granular. Next, blood flow decreases, and leukocytes (white blood cells) and fibrin infiltrate the area and consolidate (solidify). As the infection resolves, the consolidated material dissolves and is ingested and removed by macrophages.

Complications

Although most people recover from pneumonia, it remains among the most common causes of death. Relatively common pulmonary complications of pneumonia include pleurisy, pleural effusion, and atelectasis. Pleurisy is inflammation of the pleura that causes pain with breathing. Pleural effusion is the accumulation of fluid between the pleura that encases the lungs and the pleura that lines the thoracic cavity. A large amount of fluid can lead to collapse of the lung. Atelectasis refers to collapsed alveoli. Other, less common pulmonary complications of pneumonia are lung abscesses, delayed resolution, and empyema. Empyema is the presence of purulent exudate in the pleural cavity. Potential systemic complications include pericarditis, arthritis, meningitis, and endocarditis.

Signs and Symptoms

Usual symptoms of pneumonia are fever, chills, sweats, chest pain, cough, sputum production, hemoptysis (coughing up blood), dyspnea (difficulty breathing), headache, and fatigue. Elderly people, however, may present with confusion, anorexia, and weakness, but no fever or cough. People with bacterial pneumonia may experience an abrupt, almost explosive onset: severe shaking chills; sharp, stabbing lateral chest pain, especially with coughing and breathing; and intermittent cough with rusty sputum. Viral pneumonia is characterized by burning or searing chest pain in the sternal area; a continuous, hacking, barking cough producing small amounts of sputum; and headache.

Medical Diagnosis

Diagnosis of pneumonia is based on the findings of the history and physical examination, sputum culture and Gram stain, chest radiograph, complete blood count, and blood culture.

Medical Treatment

Treatment usually consists of increased fluid intake (at least 3 L every 24 hours), limited activity or bedrest, antipyretics, analgesics, and, in some cases, oxygen and aerosol intermittent positive-pressure breathing therapy. Bacterial pneumonias are treated with appropriate antibacterials; however, antibacterials are not used with viral pneumonias because they do not kill viruses.

Vaccination with the Pneumococcal Conjugate Vaccine is recommended for all children under 24 months of age; children ages 24 to 59 months who have sickle cell disease, HIV infection, chronic disease, or immunosuppression; and children ages 24 to 59 months who are African American, Alaskan native, or Native American.

Vaccination with an unconjugated pneumococcal vaccine (e.g., Pneumovax 23) may be recommended for adults with chronic illnesses, particularly cardiovascular and respiratory diseases and diabetes mellitus; people recovering from a severe illness; people aged 65 years and older; and older adults living in nursing homes or other long-term care facilities. Vaccination with the unconjugated vaccine is not recommended for children younger than 2 years of age. A booster may be given to selected patients after 6 years.

NURSING CARE *of the Patient with Pneumonia*

Assessment

Assessment of the patient with a respiratory disorder is summarized in Table 29-2 (see also Nursing Care Plan: The Patient with Pneumonia).

Nursing Diagnoses, Goals, and Outcome Criteria: Pneumonia

Nursing Diagnoses	Goals and Outcome Criteria
Ineffective Airway Clearance related to increased sputum production, thick secretions, ineffective cough	Effective airway clearance: clear breath sounds without wheezes or crackles
Impaired Gas Exchange related to obstruction of airways by edema and secretions or atelectasis	Adequate oxygenation: normal arterial blood gases, heart rate, and respiratory rate
Activity Intolerance related to obstruction of airways by edema and secretions or atelectasis	Improved activity tolerance: performance of daily activities without fatigue or dyspnea
Imbalanced Nutrition: Less than Body Requirements related to anorexia, dyspnea, fatigue	Optimal nutritional status: stable body weight
Risk for Deficient Fluid Volume related to inadequate fluid intake, fever, mouth breathing	Normal hydration: fluid intake equal to fluid output, moist mucous membranes, blood pressure consistent with patient norms
Acute Pain related to inflammation, cough, muscle aches	Pain relief: patient statement of pain relief, relaxed appearance

Interventions

Ineffective Airway Clearance

Accumulated secretions in the respiratory tract impair gas exchange and may result in alveolar collapse. Therapeutic measures are taken to decrease the production and promote the expectoration of secretions. Administer antimicrobials, decongestants, and expectorants as ordered. A good cough is essential for removal of secretions, but antitussives may be given as ordered if the patient becomes exhausted because of constant coughing. Encourage or assist the patient to change positions at least every 2 hours to help mobilize secretions. Other measures used to mobilize secretions are deep breathing and coughing exercises, chest physiotherapy, and aerosol therapy. The patient who has a very weak cough may require suctioning. Provide tissues and a receptacle for disposal of secretions. Note the amount, color, and consistency of secretions. Auscultate lung sounds frequently to assess the effects of interventions to clear the airways.

Impaired Gas Exchange

The edema and secretions present with pneumonia interfere with the exchange of gases in the lungs. The patient may have hypoxemia, meaning that the level of oxygen in

NURSING CARE PLAN

The Patient with Pneumonia

ASSESSMENT

Health History: Alice Guthrie, 77 years old, is a retired schoolteacher who complains of chills and fever, cough, sore throat, and chest pain. The physician diagnosed viral pneumonia and recommended hospitalization. Ms. Guthrie states she had a cold for about a week and seemed to get progressively worse. She states she has "a little" shortness of breath and tires very easily. Her chest pain is aggravated by coughing. She has been taking over-the-counter cold remedies. She has a history of hypertension and congestive heart failure for which she takes verapamil hydrochloride (Calan SR), 240 mg daily, and digoxin, 0.25 mg daily. Ms. Guthrie lives alone in a one-story apartment. She has a close friend next door who visits frequently.

Physical Examination: Vital signs: temperature, 100.6° F orally; pulse, 92; respiration, 24; blood pressure, 160/94. Alert, slightly dyspneic. Skin color pale. Nail beds slightly dusky. Lung sounds clear to auscultation over right lung fields. Wheezes and crackles auscultated in left lung. Frequent cough producing greenish sputum. No retractions or use of accessory muscles of respiration. Abdomen soft.

Nursing Diagnosis	*Goals and Outcome Criteria*	*Interventions*
Ineffective airway clearance related to increased sputum production and thick secretions.	The patient will have a patent airway as evidenced by clear breath sounds without wheezes or crackles.	Administer decongestants and expectorants as ordered. Administer antitussives as ordered if cough interferes with rest. Suction only if necessary. Turn, deep breathe, and cough at least every 2 hours. Perform chest physiotherapy and provide aerosol therapy as ordered. Assess response. Monitor lung sounds, respiratory rate, and characteristics of secretions. Dispose of tissues in a sanitary manner.
Impaired gas exchange related to obstruction of airways by edema and secretions or atelectasis.	The patient will have adequate oxygenation as evidenced by normal arterial blood gases and vital signs.	Monitor vital signs, lung sounds, skin color, blood gas reports, and level of consciousness. Be alert for signs of hypoxemia: restlessness, tachycardia, tachypnea. Report abnormal findings to physician. Elevate head of bed. Administer oxygen therapy as ordered.
Activity intolerance related to fatigue or hypoxia.	The patient will perform activities of daily living as ordered without excessive fatigue or dyspnea.	Instruct in activity restrictions. Plan care to allow periods of uninterrupted rest. Assist with activities of daily living as needed. Gradually encourage increased activity while monitoring for dyspnea and fatigue. Keep interactions short, and limit visitors.
Imbalanced nutrition: less than body requirements related to anorexia, dyspnea, or fatigue.	The patient will maintain optimal nutritional status as evidenced by stable body weight.	Monitor food intake and weight. If intake is poor, consult with dietitian about patient preferences. Suggest small, frequent meals. Provide pleasant environment for meals. Position for comfort. Use oxygen cannula during meals if permitted. Weigh daily.
Risk for deficient fluid volume related to inadequate fluid intake, fever, or mouth breathing.	The patient's hydration will remain normal as evidenced by fluid intake equal to output, moist mucous membranes, and blood pressure consistent with patient's norms.	Monitor fluid status for signs of fluid volume deficit: decreased skin turgor, concentrated urine, decreased urine output, dry mucous membranes, elevated hemoglobin and hematocrit levels. Administer intravenous fluids as ordered. Encourage fluids by mouth up to 3 L/day as permitted. Record intake and output. Monitor temperature and treat fever as ordered. Keep dry and lightly covered. Administer tepid sponge baths as ordered for fever, but do not induce shivering. Use hypothermia blanket as ordered.
Acute pain related to inflammation, cough, or muscle aches.	The patient will report pain relief, as measured with a pain scale	Use a pain scale to assess pain. Administer analgesics as ordered. Reposition for comfort. Splint painful areas during coughing and deep breathing. Use massage and relaxation techniques. Document effects of interventions.

the blood is low. At the same time, excess carbon dioxide may accumulate in the blood, a condition called *hypercapnia.* Because normal oxygenation is essential for all body tissues, efforts must be made to improve the patient's gas exchange.

To assess gas exchange, monitor vital signs, lung sounds, and skin color. Be alert for signs of hypoxemia: restlessness, tachycardia, and tachypnea. If arterial blood gases are being measured, report abnormal results to the physician. Hemoglobin may also be measured. A low hemoglobin is significant because it indicates the reduced oxygen-carrying capacity of red blood cells.

Measures that mobilize secretions, discussed earlier, are important in improving gas exchange. In addition, elevate the head of the bed. Some patients are more comfortable in a reclining chair that permits alterations in position. A semi-Fowler's position decreases the pressure of the abdominal organs on the diaphragm so the patient breathes more easily. Maintain oxygen therapy as ordered.

Activity Intolerance

Activity is usually restricted for the patient with pneumonia and may range from complete bedrest to limited activities. Schedule nursing care to prevent overtiring and to allow for periods of uninterrupted rest. Provide assistance as needed until the patient is able to resume self-care. Keep conversations short, and encourage visitors not to tire the patient with long visits. When the patient begins to resume activities of daily living, evaluate the ability to tolerate daily activities.

Imbalanced Nutrition: Less than Body Requirements

Good nutrition is essential to combat the infection and to promote healing. Assess the patient's usual dietary habits to provide baseline information so that the diet may be individualized. Monitor weight to determine the adequacy of nutrition. Weigh the patient before breakfast using the same scale each time. Monitor albumin and lymphocyte blood counts to detect low levels that are common with inadequate protein.

A typical diet for the patient with pneumonia is a high-protein, soft diet. Unfortunately, fatigue, dyspnea, and anorexia may interfere with adequate food intake. Provide the diet as ordered, assist the patient with the meal if needed, and document intake. To enhance the appetite, provide oral care before meals, elevate the head of the bed, and arrange the tray in an attractive and convenient manner. The diet should conform to the patient's preferences as much as possible. If oxygen is needed, a nasal cannula is recommended during meals. If the patient tires quickly, more frequent meals with smaller servings may be better received.

Risk for Deficient Fluid Volume

The patient with pneumonia may lose excess fluid because of fever and mouth breathing, and fluid intake may be inadequate because of fatigue and dyspnea. Dehydration causes respiratory secretions to be thicker and more difficult to mobilize. Signs and symptoms of deficient fluid volume include decreased skin turgor, concentrated urine, dry mucous membranes, and elevated hemoglobin and hematocrit levels. Therefore, the patient should consume 3 L of fluid a day unless contraindicated. If the patient's oral intake is low, intravenous fluids may be ordered. Hard candy, if permitted, stimulates thirst and fluid intake. Intake and output records may be kept.

Monitor the patient's temperature every 2 to 4 hours to detect fever. Administer antipyretics as ordered. Keep the patient dry and lightly covered. Keep the room at a comfortable temperature that avoids chilling. Tepid sponge baths may be given for high fevers as ordered, but do not induce shivering. A hypothermia blanket may be needed to reduce body temperature.

Pain

Treat pain with ordered analgesics. Also use positioning, splinting painful areas during deep breathing and coughing, and massage to promote comfort. Other measures to manage pain are detailed in Chapter 14. Document the effects of comfort measures, and notify the physician if pain is unrelieved or worsens.

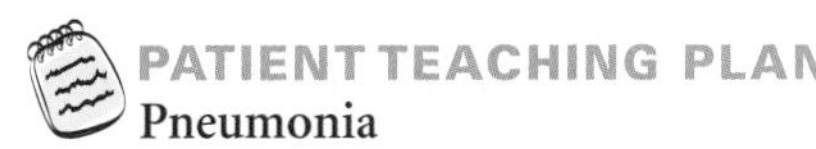

Pneumonia

The teaching plan for the patient with pneumonia should include the following points.

- Gradually increase your activities as you recover because fatigue may persist for several weeks
- Avoid people with colds or other infections
- You need plenty of rest, good nutrition, and 3 L of fluids each day (unless contraindicated!)
- Complete any prescribed drugs after discharge

Prevention of Aspiration Pneumonia

Aspiration pneumonia may be prevented by measures to avoid aspiration or to treat it promptly. If a patient is at risk for aspiration, keep suction equipment on hand. Position patients with dysphagia (difficulty swallowing) upright with the neck in a neutral position or slightly bent forward during meals. Because semisolids are swallowed more easily than thin liquids, thickening agents may be added to liquids.

If a patient is receiving enteral feedings, elevate the head of the bed while the feeding is being delivered and for 30 minutes afterward. Check tube position per agency policy before each bolus feeding or at specified intervals. The aspirated fluid can be tested for acidity to ensure tube placement. Measure residual before each bolus feeding. If it is greater than 100 ml, withhold the feeding and notify the physician.

Stop continuous feedings for 20 to 30 minutes before lowering the patient's head. If a patient must be kept flat, the best position is on the right side. Check residual every 4 hours. If the residual is 20% more than the hourly rate, consult the physician about reducing the rate of feeding.

To reduce the risk of aspiration, position the unconscious patient on alternating sides with the head of the bed elevated unless contraindicated. Do not put fluids in the patient's mouth until the presence of a gag reflex has been established.

If aspiration is suspected, use suction to try to remove the foreign material. A side-lying or slight Trendelenburg position, if not contraindicated, may promote drainage from the airway. Stop the enteral feeding until it is ruled out as the source of the aspirated material. Monitor the patient closely and notify the physician. Administer oxygen as ordered.

PLEURISY (PLEURITIS)

Pleurisy is inflammation of the pleura. The most common causes are pneumonia, tuberculosis, injury to the chest wall, pulmonary infarction, and tumors. The most characteristic symptom of pleurisy is abrupt and severe pain. The pain almost always occurs on one side of the chest, and patients can usually point to the exact spot where the pain is occurring. Breathing and coughing aggravate the pain.

Treatment of pleurisy is aimed at the underlying disease and at pain relief. Analgesics, anti-inflammatory drugs, antitussives, antimicrobials, and local heat therapy may be ordered.

NURSING CARE *of the Patient with Pleurisy*

Assessment

Assessment of the patient with a respiratory disorder is summarized in Table 29-2.

Nursing Diagnoses, Goals, and Outcome Criteria: Pleurisy

The primary nursing diagnoses when a patient has pleurisy are listed here. There may be other diagnoses related to the underlying cause of pleurisy.

Nursing Diagnoses	Goals and Outcome Criteria
Acute Pain related to inflammation	Pain relief: patient statement of pain relief, relaxed expression
Ineffective Breathing Pattern related to splinting, pleural effusion	Effective breathing pattern: vital signs within patient norms, normal breath sounds

Interventions

Acute Pain

When the patient reports pain, obtain a complete description including location, severity, precipitating factors, and alleviating factors. Use analgesics and splinting of the affected side to relieve pain. It also is helpful to splint the rib cage when coughing. If ordered, apply heat to the painful area and give antitussives to decrease painful coughing. If bedrest is prescribed, assist the patient with regular position changes. Administer nonsteroidal anti-inflammatory drugs (NSAIDs) as ordered to reduce pain and inflammation. Monitor patients on NSAIDs for gastrointestinal distress and bleeding.

Ineffective Breathing Pattern

Monitor the patient's breathing pattern with attention to the symmetry of chest movement. Encourage the patient to turn, take deep breaths and cough, and ambulate if permitted to mobilize secretions and maximize ventilation. Elevate the head of the bed to improve lung expansion. If pleural effusion develops, the patient experiences progressive dyspnea, decreased or absent breath sounds in the affected area, and decreased chest wall movement on the affected side. A thoracentesis may be done to remove the accumulated fluid. If the procedure is done at the bedside, the nurse assists as described in the section on Common Therapeutic Measures.

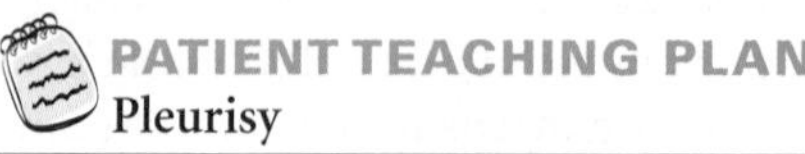

PATIENT TEACHING PLAN
Pleurisy

- Take deep breaths every 1 to 2 hours while awake.
- Sitting upright will make breathing more comfortable.
- If being discharged on NSAIDs:
  Avoid aspirin because it increases the risk of bleeding.
  Take NSAIDs with food, milk, or antacids if gastrointestinal distress occurs.

CHEST TRAUMA

Traumatic chest injuries fall into two major categories: (1) nonpenetrating injuries and (2) penetrating injuries. Nonpenetrating or blunt injuries most commonly result from automobile accidents, falls, or blast injuries. In automobile accidents, 40% of the people killed have sustained blunt injuries from the steering wheel. The extent of the injury depends on the force and impact of the trauma. Common nonpenetrating injuries include rib fractures, pneumothorax, pulmonary contusion, and cardiac contusion. Penetrating injuries most commonly result from gunshot or stab wounds to the chest. Common penetrating injuries include pneumothorax and life-threatening tears of the aorta, vena cava, or other major vessels.

Chest trauma can result in changes in normal pressure relationships between air inside and outside the body, interference with normal breathing patterns and protective mechanisms such as cough, disturbances in blood flow to the lungs, swelling, and pain. Patients are therefore at risk for air entering the pleural space, infection and increased secretions in the tracheobronchial tree, hemorrhage, and abnormal fluid collection in the lung.

Signs and Symptoms

Signs and symptoms of chest injury may include obvious trauma to the chest wall (e.g., bruising); chest pain; dyspnea; cough; asymmetric movement of the chest wall; marked cyanosis of the mouth, face, nail beds, and mucous membranes; rapid, weak pulse; decreased blood pressure; deviation of the trachea; distended neck veins; and bloodshot or bulging eyes.

Medical Treatment

Immediate care of a person with a chest injury is directed at stabilization and prevention of further injury. Remove clothing to assess injury sites and to observe for other injuries such as bleeding. Immediately treat bleeding. Cover any open chest wound with an airtight dressing taped on three sides. This is called a vented dressing; it permits air to escape through the chest wound but prevents additional air from entering the chest through the wound. If you were to completely seal an open chest wound, air could continue to leak from the lung into the pleural space. With no exit, the leaking air could accumulate in the pleural space and create a tension pneumothorax (discussed in the next section).

If an airtight dressing has been applied, be alert for worsening respiratory status (increasing dyspnea, cyanosis, distended neck veins, trachea deviated from midline, decreased breath sounds on the affected side), which requires removal of the airtight dressing. Do not remove impaled objects but stabilize them with bulky dressings. Monitor vital signs and level of consciousness, keeping in mind the potential for shock. Oxygen may be administered by nasal cannula. To facilitate breathing, put the client in a semi-Fowler's position or on the injured side.

PNEUMOTHORAX

Chest injuries often cause pneumothorax, which is an accumulation of air in the pleural cavity that results in complete or partial collapse of a lung. Pneumothorax occurs in nearly half of the people who have chest injuries. Air enters the space between the chest wall and the lung either through a hole in the chest wall or through a tear in the bronchus, bronchioles, or alveoli (Fig. 29-14).

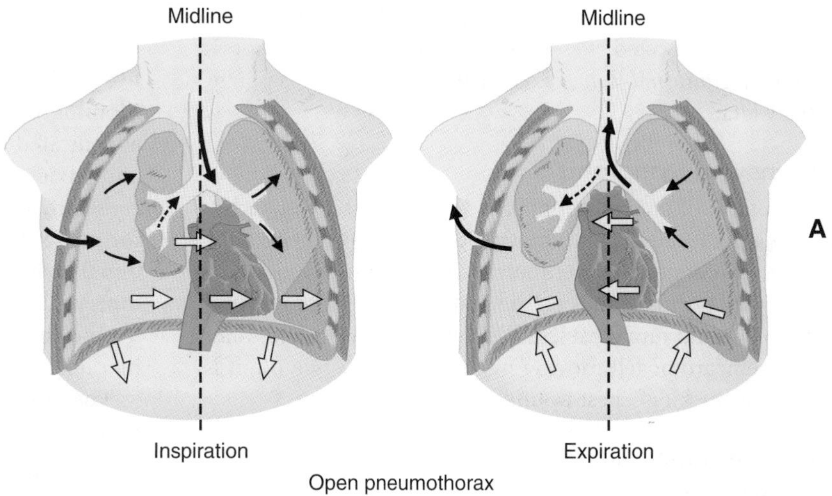

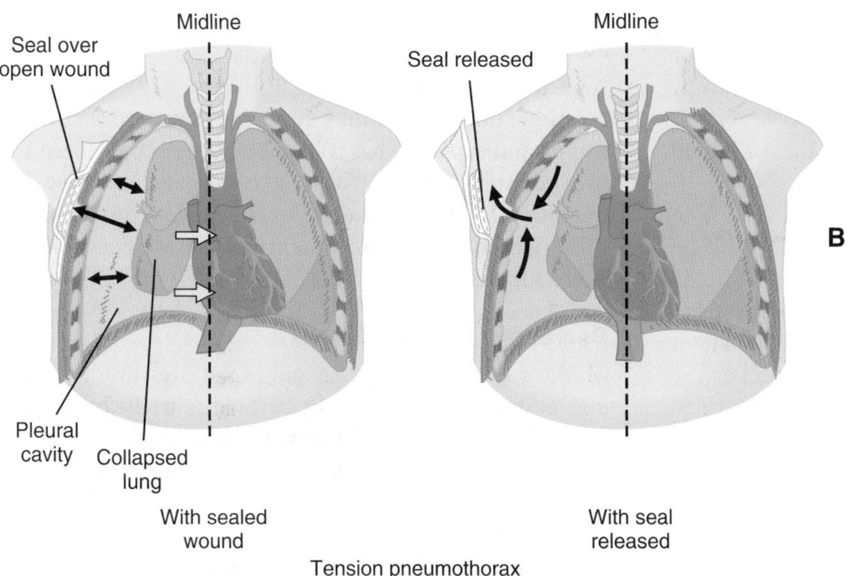

FIGURE **29-14** *A,* Open pneumothorax. *Solid and dashed arrows* = air movement; *open arrows* = structural movement. On inspiration, air is sucked into the pleural space through the open chest wound and the lung on the affected side collapses. The mediastinal contents shift toward the unaffected side. On expiration, air exits through the open wound and the mediastinal contents swing back toward the affected side (mediastinal flutter). *B,* An airtight dressing can cause a tension pneumothorax when air accumulates in the pleural space through a tear in the lung tissue. The air cannot exit if there is no open chest wound, and pressure builds, shifting the contents of the mediastinum toward the unaffected side and impairing circulatory and respiratory function (mediastinal shift).

There are two types of pneumothorax: tension and open. With a tension pneumothorax, air repeatedly enters the pleural space with inspiration, causing the pressure to rise. Because air is not escaping from the wound, the accumulating pressure causes the affected lung to collapse. The heart, trachea, esophagus, and great blood vessels shift toward the unaffected side. This is called a *mediastinal shift,* a condition that interferes with blood return to the heart. If not corrected, cardiac output falls, and the patient dies.

An open pneumothorax results from a chest wound that allows air to move in and out freely with inspiration and expiration. The lung on the affected side collapses. The heart, trachea, esophagus, and great blood vessels may shift back and forth toward the unaffected side with inspiration, then toward the affected side with expiration. This condition is called *mediastinal flutter.* Like mediastinal shift, it is potentially fatal.

Signs and Symptoms

Symptoms of pneumothorax are dyspnea, tachypnea, tachycardia, restlessness, pain, anxiety, decreased movement of the involved chest wall, asymmetric chest wall movement, diminished breath sounds on the injured side, and progressive cyanosis. In trauma cases, there may be a chest wound. If air can be heard or felt moving in and out of the wound, it is called a "sucking" chest wound.

Medical Treatment

The physician may insert an 18-gauge needle through the chest wall into the pleural space and aspirate accumulated air or fluid, and then insert a chest tube. An alternative is to omit the needle aspiration and immediately insert the chest tube. If air is entering the pleural space from a tear in the lung or bronchus, surgery may be needed to repair the tear. A variety of materials are being studied for use in sealing persistent air leaks, including intrapleural tetracycline, autologous "blood patches," and fibrin glue.

NURSING CARE *of the Patient with Pneumothorax*

Assessment

The complete assessment of the patient with a respiratory disorder is outlined in Table 29-2. In addition, if the patient has a chest tube, monitor the insertion site as well as the amount and characteristics of any drainage from the tube. Care of patients with chest tubes is covered earlier in this chapter.

Nursing Diagnoses, Goals, and Outcome Criteria: Pneumothorax

Nursing Diagnoses	Goals and Outcome Criteria
Ineffective Breathing Patterns related to decreased lung expansion	Effective breathing patterns: regular respirations, rate of 12 to 20, normal arterial blood gases, no dyspnea, normal skin color
Fear related to difficulty breathing	Decreased fear: calm demeanor, patient statement that fear is reduced
Decreased Cardiac Output related to mediastinal shift	Adequate cardiac output: pulse and blood pressure consistent with patient norms
Acute Pain related to trauma, altered pressure in chest cavity, chest tube	Pain relief: patient statement that pain is reduced/relieved, relaxed manner
Risk for Infection related to traumatic injury, chest tube insertion	Absence of infection: normal body temperature, normal white blood cell count

Interventions

Ineffective Breathing Patterns

Monitor the patient closely for increasing respiratory distress as indicated by tachycardia, dyspnea, cyanosis, restlessness, and anxiety. Inspect the trachea for deviation that may be caused by mediastinal shift. Check arterial blood gas results for hypoxemia (low blood oxygen) and hypercapnia (high blood carbon dioxide). Immediately report signs and symptoms of deteriorating respiratory status to the physician. After the chest tube has been inserted, protect the tube and monitor its function as described earlier in this chapter.

Position the patient for comfort in a Fowler's or semi-Fowler's position. Avoid the side-lying position until the affected lung has reexpanded because this position could foster mediastinal shift. Support and encourage the patient to do deep breathing and coughing exercises at least every 2 hours while awake. Administer oxygen as ordered.

Fear

A pneumothorax is frightening. Patients feel like they are suffocating and may fear they are dying. Speak to the patient calmly and explain what is happening. Tell the patient that the chest tube will allow the lung to reexpand and relieve the dyspnea. Also, tell the patient how to prevent dislodging the tube. Give the patient the opportunity to ask questions and express fears.

Decreased Cardiac Output

Monitor the patient's pulse and blood pressure. If cardiac output decreases owing to mediastinal shift, the blood pressure falls and the pulse rate increases. Immediately notify the physician of signs of this potentially life-threatening change.

Acute Pain

Be alert for signs of pain and document the characteristics of the patient's pain. Administer analgesics as ordered, and document the effects. In addition to drug therapy, use positioning, massage, distraction, and other measures described in Chapter 14. Notify the physician if pain is not relieved.

Risk for Infection

Monitor the patient for signs and symptoms of infection: fever, increased pulse and respirations, foul drainage from the tube insertion site, and elevated white blood cell count. Various possible sites of infection must be considered: traumatic wounds, chest tube insertion site, intravenous infusion sites, indwelling catheter, and lungs. Use sterile technique for invasive procedures and dressing changes and administer prescribed antimicrobials. Encourage increased activity when permitted. Monitor hydration status and promote fluid intake of 2 to 3 L/day unless contraindicated. Before discharge, instruct the patient to keep the chest tube insertion site clean and dry, and to notify the physician of signs of infection: fever or increasing redness, swelling, or drainage from the insertion site.

HEMOTHORAX

Hemothorax is an accumulation of blood between the chest wall and the lung that is often associated with pneumothorax. Hemothorax results from lacerated or torn blood vessels or lung tissues, lung malignancy, or pulmonary embolus. It may also be a complication of anticoagulant therapy. When air or blood collects in the pleural space, pressure around the lung increases, causing partial or complete collapse. Hemothorax is essentially treated like a pneumothorax, and the nursing care is similar. Surgical intervention may be needed to control the source of bleeding. In addition, the patient is at risk for decreased cardiac output due to hemorrhage.

RIB FRACTURES

Rib fractures are the most common chest injuries. The most common cause is a blunt injury, especially the impact of the steering wheel against the chest in an automobile accident. Ribs 4 to 9 are most frequently fractured because they are least protected by chest muscles. It takes approximately 6 weeks for rib fractures to heal.

Signs and Symptoms

Signs and symptoms of fractured ribs include pain at the site of injury (especially on inspiration), occasional bruising or surface markings, swelling, visible bone fragments at the site of the injury, and shallow breathing or holding the chest protectively to minimize painful chest movements.

Medical Treatment

Treatment is aimed at relief of pain so that the patient can have good chest expansion for adequate breathing. Intercostal nerve blocks with local anesthesia are most frequently used. Analgesics along with mild sedatives also may be given for pain relief. Strapping the chest with tape or binders was once common but is now avoided because this procedure constricts the expansion of the chest and restricts deep breathing, leading to complications such as pneumonia or atelectasis.

NURSING CARE *of the Patient with Rib Fractures*

Assessment

The nursing assessment of the patient with a respiratory disorder is outlined in Table 29-2. After rib fractures, the nurse is especially alert for signs of increasing respiratory distress that may indicate a pneumothorax caused by a bone fragment.

Nursing Diagnosis, Goal, and Outcome Criteria: Rib Fractures

The primary nursing diagnosis for the patient who has fractured ribs is ineffective breathing pattern related to pain that occurs with ventilation. The goal of nursing care when a patient has fractured ribs is for the patient to have an effective breathing pattern. Outcome criteria include vital signs within normal range, absence of dyspnea, and breath sounds clear to auscultation.

Interventions

Breathing exercises are necessary to prevent pulmonary complications after rib fractures. Instruct the patient in supporting the fractured ribs while deep breathing and coughing. The patient will perform these exercises better with adequate pain control. Assess the patient's pain every 2 hours, asking the patient to rank the pain from 0 (no pain) to 10 (worst pain imaginable). Encourage the patient to report pain and offer reassurance that measures will be taken to provide relief. Because pain typically persists for 5 to 7 days, administer prescribed analgesics. After medications are given, provide a calm environment and encourage the patient to rest. Other nursing measures described in Chapter 14 (guided imagery, distraction, rhythmic breathing) may be used to manage pain as well. Evaluate the effects of pain management measures, and inform the physician if the patient's pain cannot be controlled.

FLAIL CHEST

The term *flail chest* refers to an injury in which two adjacent ribs on the same side of the chest are each broken into two or more segments. The affected section of the rib cage is, in a sense, detached from the rest of the rib cage. This permits it to move independently, so that the segment moves in with inspiration, and moves out with expiration. The pattern of movement is exactly the opposite of the movement of an intact chest wall. Therefore, it is called *paradoxical movement.* Ventilation is impaired, and the patient becomes hypoxemic. Also, contusion (bruising) of underlying lung tissue may cause fluid to accumulate in the alveoli. Fractured ribs may tear the pleura or the lung itself, resulting in a pneumothorax or a hemothorax. The loss of chest wall stability and collapse of a lung may permit the mediastinum to flutter, swinging back and forth with respirations. Progressive hypoxemia and hypercapnia may be fatal.

Signs and Symptoms

Signs and symptoms of flail chest include severe dyspnea, cyanosis, tachypnea, tachycardia, and paradoxical movement of the chest.

Medical Diagnosis

Diagnosis is based on the history, physical examination, and chest radiographs. Arterial blood gases may be measured to assess the adequacy of ventilation.

Medical Treatment

The treatment of flail chest varies depending on the severity of the condition. If the patient is able to maintain adequate oxygenation, treatment may consist of deep breathing and coughing, IPPB treatment, and pain management. The patient in respiratory distress usually requires intubation and mechanical ventilation. Radiographs and arterial blood gas tests are often repeated at intervals to monitor oxygenation and detect additional pulmonary complications such as pneumonia.

NURSING CARE *of the Patient with Flail Chest*

Assessment

The nursing assessment of the patient with a respiratory disorder is outlined in Table 29-2. When the patient has flail chest, defer the complete assessment until the patient's condition stabilizes. The initial assessment focuses on respiratory status, vital signs, other medical diagnoses, and a drug history.

Nursing Diagnoses, Goals, and Outcome Criteria: Flail Chest

Nursing Diagnoses	Goals and Outcome Criteria
Ineffective Breathing Patterns related to loss of rib cage integrity	Effective breathing patterns: normal pulse and respiratory rates, normal arterial blood gases, no dyspnea
Acute Pain related to fractures	Pain relief: patient statement of pain relief, relaxed manner
Anxiety related to lack of understanding of injury and treatment	Reduced anxiety: patient statement of reduced anxiety, calm manner

Interventions

Nursing interventions for patients with flail chest are similar to those for the patient with fractured ribs. Because flail chest is more serious and the patient may be acutely ill, anxiety may be very high. To reduce anxiety, respond promptly to the patient's needs, provide simple explanations, and acknowledge the patient's concerns. Anxiety may be especially high if mechanical ventilation is needed. The detailed care of patients who require mechanical ventilation is beyond the scope of this book. A general discussion of mechanical ventilation is included in the section on Common Therapeutic Measures in this chapter.

PULMONARY EMBOLUS

An *embolus* is a foreign substance that is carried through the bloodstream. Emboli are usually blood clots but may be fat, air, tumors, bone marrow, amniotic fluid, or clumps of bacteria.

Etiology and Risk Factors

Risk factors for development of emboli include surgery of the pelvis or lower legs, immobility, obesity, estrogen therapy, and clotting abnormalities. Most pulmonary emboli originate in the deep veins of the thigh or pelvis. A thrombus that develops in the veins can break away and become an embolus. The embolus flows with the blood until it reaches a vessel too narrow to pass through. The embolus lodges and obstructs blood flow so that perfusion to the area is diminished. When a portion of a pulmonary blood vessel is occluded by an embolus, the patient is said to have a *pulmonary embolism* (PE). The effects depend on the extent of the lung tissue that is deprived of blood. Small emboli usually do not cause dramatic symptoms but disrupt perfusion nevertheless. The alveoli in the affected area are ventilated, but without blood flow, gas exchange cannot occur. The result is a ventilation-perfusion mismatch that results in hypoxemia. If a large pulmonary vessel is obstructed, alveoli collapse, cardiac output falls, there is constriction of the bronchi and the pulmonary artery, and sudden death may ensue.

Signs and Symptoms

Classic signs and symptoms of PE include sudden chest pain that worsens with breathing, tachypnea, and dyspnea. The patient may be apprehensive and diaphoretic with a cough and hemoptysis. Crackles may be heard on auscultation of the lungs, and the patient may have fever and tachycardia.

Medical Diagnosis

A diagnosis of PE is suggested by the history and physical findings and is confirmed by arterial blood gas analysis, electrocardiogram, lung scan, and pulmonary angiogram.

Medical and Surgical Treatment

Anticoagulation therapy is the cornerstone of treatment for PE. Intravenous heparin is usually given to establish and maintain a partial thromboplastin time of 2.0 to 2.5 times the normal rate. Heparin prevents the development of new thrombi; it also prevents the extension of existing thrombi but does not dissolve them. The heparin is eventually discontinued, and the patient is maintained on an oral anticoagulant (warfarin sodium) for up to 6 months. Tissue plasminogen activator, a fibrinolytic, may be given intravenously to dissolve the clots.

Hypoxemia may be managed with oxygen therapy, endotracheal intubation, and mechanical ventilation. Intravenous fluids and drugs to improve cardiac function are indicated to treat hypotension. Intravenous morphine sulfate is commonly used to relieve chest pain and apprehension.

A number of surgical interventions have been used for PE, including embolectomy, vena cava interruption, and venous thrombectomy. Embolectomy, surgical removal of the embolus from the obstructed pulmonary arteries, is a risky procedure. Vena cava interruption is most often done by placing a filter in the inferior vena cava to strain clots before they reach the pulmonary circulation (Fig. 29-15). Venous thrombectomy, removal of thrombi from veins, is not often done.

NURSING CARE *of the Patient with a Pulmonary Embolus*

Assessment

Assessment of the patient with a respiratory disorder is outlined in Table 29-2. When a patient has a PE, the nurse must monitor cardiopulmonary function but also must assess risk factors that may have led to the embolism. Homans' sign should be assessed

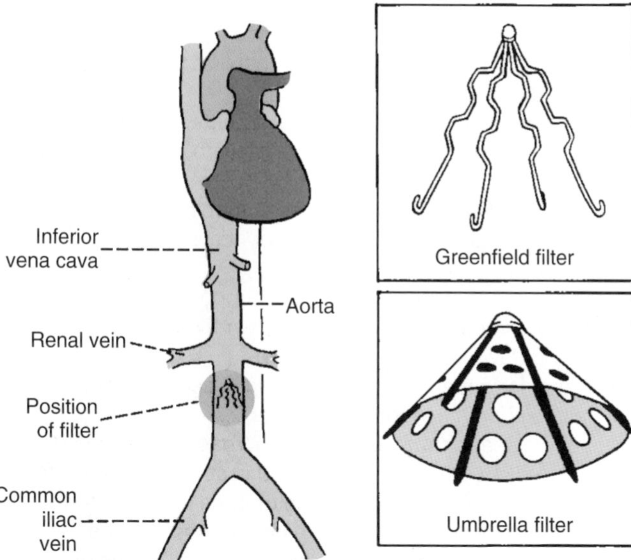

FIGURE 29-15 Greenfield and umbrella filters are examples of filters that may be placed in the inferior vena cava to prevent emboli traveling to the lung.

in each leg. If this causes pain behind the knee or in the calf, the patient is said to have a positive Homans' sign, which is often associated with thrombophlebitis.

Nursing Diagnoses, Goals, and Outcome Criteria: Pulmonary Embolism

Nursing Diagnoses	Goals and Outcome Criteria
Ineffective Tissue Perfusion related to interruption of blood flow to the alveoli	Normal tissue perfusion: vital signs consistent with patient norms, no dyspnea, normal arterial blood gases
Anxiety related to dyspnea, fear of dying	Reduced anxiety: patient statement of less or no anxiety, calm manner
Risk for Injury related to anticoagulant therapy	Decreased risk of excessive bleeding: prothrombin time within therapeutic range, absence of excessive bruising or bleeding

Interventions

Ineffective Tissue Perfusion

Monitor the patient's respiratory rate and effort, breath sounds, skin color, pulse, and blood pressure. Note arterial blood gas results as a measure of tissue perfusion and notify the physician if they are abnormal. Elevate the head of the patient's bed. Administer oxygen as ordered, usually by nasal cannula. Enforce strict bedrest or other prescribed activity limitations to decrease oxygen demands. Administer prescribed intravenous fluids and inotropic drugs. Measure and record fluid intake and output.

Interventions to decrease the risk of further emboli include active and passive range-of-motion exercises for immobilized patients, early ambulation after surgery, and antiembolism and pneumatic compression stockings. Do not place cushions and pillows under the legs where circulation might be impaired.

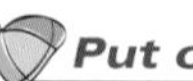

Put on your THINKING CAP!!

To prevent emboli, we recommend compression stockings and avoidance of pressure under the legs. This sounds like a contradiction! How can you explain the value of each intervention?

Anxiety

The patient in respiratory distress and pain is understandably anxious. Remain calm and tell the patient what is being done. Explain equipment and procedures in terms the patient can understand. Encourage the patient to express concerns and ask questions. Permit a reassuring family member to remain with the patient.

Risk for Injury

Anticoagulant therapy poses a risk of uncontrolled bleeding. While the patient is hospitalized, assess for excessive bruising or bleeding. Symptoms that may be caused by internal bleeding include severe headache and abdominal or back pain. Inspect the urine for hematuria. Apply pressure to venipuncture sites to control bleeding.

To reduce the risk of bleeding, the patient's activated partial thromboplastin time is monitored every 1 to 2 days until stabilized at 1.5 to 2.5 times the normal rate. Patients with a PE are usually changed to warfarin sodium (Coumadin), an oral anticoagulant, after receiving heparin for a week or so. The effect of warfarin sodium is monitored by assessing the prothrombin time (PT), which should be 1.5 to 2.0 times the normal (control) rate, and the INR, which should be 2.0 to 3.0. The dosage is adjusted daily based on PT and INR.

PHARMACOLOGY CAPSULE Monitor the patient's activated partial thromboplastin time when on heparin and the prothrombin time and INR when on warfarin sodium to determine the extent of anticoagulation. Watch for bleeding.

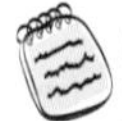

PATIENT TEACHING PLAN
Pulmonary Embolism

Patients who have had a PE must be taught how to manage their anticoagulant therapy because they usually remain on these drugs for at least several months. Important points are:

- Use soft toothbrush and electric razors to avoid trauma and bleeding.
- Report red or dark urine, which suggests urinary bleeding.

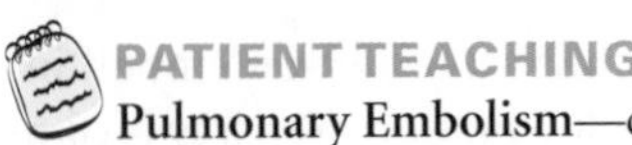

PATIENT TEACHING PLAN
Pulmonary Embolism—cont'd

- Report vomited blood, nosebleed, and red or black stools, which suggest intestinal bleeding.
- Do not take any over-the-counter medications without consulting with the physician or pharmacist. Some drugs, especially aspirin, prolong the bleeding time, which could cause excessive bleeding.
- To reduce the risk of a future PE, avoid constricting clothing such as garters or tight girdles and avoid prolonged pressure on the back of the knee.

RESPIRATORY ARREST

Respiratory arrest, the cessation of breathing, is addressed in Chapter 15.

ACUTE RESPIRATORY DISTRESS SYNDROME

Etiology and Risk Factors

Acute respiratory distress syndrome (ARDS) is a progressive pulmonary disorder that follows some trauma to the lung. From 1 to 96 hours after the trauma, pulmonary infiltrates develop and lung compliance decreases. Fluid shifts into the interstitial spaces in the lungs and into the alveoli, causing pulmonary edema. Production of pulmonary surfactant decreases, leading to atelectasis. Lung compliance decreases, and the patient rapidly becomes hypoxemic.

Some patients recover and heal completely, whereas lung fibrosis develops in others. The fibrosis may be mild or severe and sometimes occurs after the patient appears to be recovering. Progressive fibrosis may lead to death. Systemic complications of ARDS include cardiac dysrhythmias, renal failure, stress ulcers, thrombocytopenia, and disseminated intravascular coagulation. In addition, these patients are at risk for oxygen toxicity and sepsis.

Signs and Symptoms

The first sign of ARDS is usually increased respiratory rate. Auscultation of the lungs may reveal fine crackles. The patient may be restless, agitated, and confused. The pulse rate increases, and a cough may be present. These early signs are followed by progressively worsening dyspnea with retractions, cyanosis, and diaphoresis. Diffuse crackles and rhonchi may be heard on auscultation.

Medical Diagnosis

Acute respiratory distress syndrome is suspected on the basis of the patient's history and physical findings. Diagnostic studies include arterial blood gas analysis and chest radiographs. The blood pH rises and the $PaCO_2$ falls at first because of hyperventilation. The PaO_2 falls below 70 mm Hg despite oxygen concentrations greater than 40% (FIO_2 0.4). This hypoxemia causes respiratory acidosis, as evidenced by pH below 7.35.

Nutrition Concepts

1. Adequate fluids are needed to mobilize pulmonary secretions for expectoration.
2. Approximately 40% of patients admitted to intensive care units with acute respiratory failure are malnourished.
3. Nutritional support for patients with respiratory failure should begin within the first 3 to 4 days of hospitalization.
4. Patients who receive nutritional support are more easily weaned from ventilators than those who receive only intravenous glucose support.
5. A diet for patients who have been in acute respiratory failure should be high in nutrients.
6. Lung disease can substantially increase energy needs.
7. The patient who is malnourished is at increased risk for respiratory infections because of impaired immunity and possible impairment of defense mechanisms.
8. When a patient has a fever, each degree Celsius of elevation increases the metabolic rate 10% to 13%. For each degree Fahrenheit, the metabolic rate rises 7.2%.
9. Excessive intake of vitamin K–rich foods (cabbage, broccoli, cauliflower, asparagus, onions, spinach, fish, liver) can interfere with anticoagulation therapy.

Medical Treatment

Early detection and treatment are critical factors in treating ARDS successfully. The patient is usually intubated and placed on a mechanical ventilator with positive end-expiratory pressure. Patient anxiety and restlessness may require sedation or even pharmacologic paralysis. Specific drug therapy depends on the underlying cause of ARDS. For example, the patient with sepsis is treated with antimicrobials. Corticosteroids are commonly used to reduce inflammation with ARDS, but there is some question about the value of this treatment.

NURSING CARE *of the Patient with Acute Respiratory Distress Syndrome*

The patient with ARDS is critically ill and should be treated in an intensive care setting. Critical care nursing is beyond the scope of this text. However, all nurses must be aware of the risk of ARDS and respond promptly when a patient exhibits progressive respiratory distress. The rapid progression of the condition is frightening to the patient and the family. Recognize their anxiety and fear and offer emotional support and simple explanations.

key points

- The function of the respiratory system is to supply oxygen for the metabolic needs of the cells and to eliminate carbon dioxide, one of the waste materials of cell metabolism.
- Age-related changes in the respiratory system include loss of lung elasticity, enlargement of bronchioles,

decreased number of alveoli, thoracic rigidity, atrophy of chest muscles, and flattening of the diaphragm.

- A thoracentesis is the insertion of a needle through the chest wall into the pleural space to remove fluid, blood, or air or to instill medication.
- Chest physiotherapy, which consists of percussion, vibration, and postural drainage, mobilizes respiratory secretions for expectoration.
- Oxygen therapy is widely used and generally safe but must be used cautiously in chronic respiratory patients to avoid respiratory depression.
- Chest tubes drain fluid and air from the pleural space, permitting a collapsed lung to reexpand.
- Nursing diagnoses after thoracotomy may include impaired gas exchange, ineffective breathing pattern, and ineffective airway clearance.
- Drugs commonly used for treatment of respiratory disorders include decongestants, antitussives, antihistamines, expectorants, antimicrobials, bronchodilators, corticosteroids, mast cell stabilizers, and leukotriene inhibitors.
- Acute viral rhinitis (the common cold), the most prevalent infectious disease, is treated symptomatically because available antimicrobials are not effective against the cold virus.
- Influenza is an acute viral respiratory infection that can lead to pneumonia, especially in debilitated people.
- Influenza immunizations do not protect everyone from influenza but do reduce the incidence of the infection, and are recommended for people who have poor resistance to infection.
- Pneumonia may be caused by pathogenic organisms or by noninfectious agents such as inhaled irritants, including aspirated gastric contents.
- Nursing diagnoses for the patient with pneumonia may include ineffective airway clearance, impaired gas exchange, activity intolerance, imbalanced nutrition: less than body requirements, risk for deficient fluid volume, and acute pain.
- Pleurisy (pleuritis) is inflammation of the pleura that is treated with analgesics, anti-inflammatory drugs, antitussives, antimicrobials, and local heat therapy.
- Nursing diagnoses for the patient with pleurisy may include acute pain and ineffective breathing pattern.
- Pneumothorax is the accumulation of air in the pleural space, which may cause the lung to collapse.
- The immediate treatment of an open chest wound is coverage with a vented dressing followed by careful monitoring to detect signs of a tension pneumothorax.
- With a tension pneumothorax, air accumulates in the affected side, collapsing the affected lung and causing the heart, trachea, esophagus, and great blood vessels to shift toward the unaffected side (mediastinal shift, a life-threatening condition).
- Nursing diagnoses when a patient has chest trauma may include ineffective breathing pattern, fear, decreased cardiac output, acute pain, and risk for infection.
- Flail chest is the loss of thoracic integrity caused by fractures of two adjacent ribs into two or more segments on the same side of the chest.
- A pulmonary embolus is a foreign substance carried through the bloodstream into the lung, where it lodges and blocks blood flow.
- Nursing diagnoses for the patient who has a pulmonary embolism may include ineffective tissue perfusion, anxiety, and risk for injury.
- Adult respiratory distress syndrome, a progressive pulmonary disorder that may lead to fibrosis of lung tissue and death, is treated with mechanical ventilation and treatment of the underlying cause.

REVIEW QUESTIONS

1. Where is the respiratory center located?

1. Lungs
2. Alveoli
3. Brain
4. Aorta

2. Age-related changes in the respiratory system include:

1. elevated diaphragm.
2. atrophy of bronchioles.
3. respiratory muscle hypertrophy.
4. rib cage rigidity.

3. Which of the following is the best example of documentation of the respiratory assessment?

1. Expectorated moderate amount of tenacious, green sputum.
2. Patient reports coughing up lots of mucus this shift.
3. Physical activity seems to cause patient to have severe coughing spells.
4. Patient is coughing up less sputum today than yesterday.

4. Your patient has a pulse oximeter. The current oxygen saturation is 96%. You should:

1. notify the registered nurse or physician immediately.
2. document the reading and continue routine monitoring.
3. increase the patient's oxygen to at least 5 L per minute.
4. request arterial blood gases to confirm the oximetry reading.

5. Several days after thoracic surgery, your patient's respiratory status is normal. When checking the chest tube drainage system, you observe that there is no bubbling in the waterseal chamber. This could mean that:

1. there is a leak in the drainage system.
2. the patient's affected lung has reexpanded.
3. it is time to change the drainage receptacle.
4. the patient's affected lung has collapsed.

6. A community education project is designed to encourage older adults to have influenza immunizations. A participant asks about the difference between influenza and the common cold. What is the most appropriate reply?
   1. Influenza is actually just a very severe cold.
   2. Colds are caused by bacteria; influenza is caused by a virus.
   3. Influenza is more likely to cause fever and chills.
   4. They are equally likely to have serious complications.

7. A patient who has pneumonia has become restless; vital signs are: T = 100° F, P = 110, R = 28, BP 130/72. You should suspect:
   1. fluid volume excess.
   2. dehydration.
   3. excess potassium.
   4. hypoxemia.

8. In the emergency care of a patient who has a sucking chest wound, why is a vented dressing preferred over a dressing that completely seals the wound?
   1. The vented dressing permits the drainage of blood from the pleural sac.
   2. Sealing the wound increases the risk of bacterial contamination.
   3. The vented dressing prevents air from escaping from the injured lung.
   4. Sealing the wound could lead to a tension pneumothorax.

9. A patient who comes into the ER after a traffic accident is in respiratory distress. You observe that a part of the rib cage moves inward with inspiration, and outward with expiration. This pattern is described as:
   1. paradoxical movement.
   2. tension pneumothorax.
   3. compensatory breathing.
   4. Cheyne-Stokes respirations.

10. Measures to prevent pulmonary embolism in postoperative patients include:
    1. splinting extremities to limit movement.
    2. assisting with range-of-motion exercises.
    3. enforcing bedrest until wound healing is complete.
    4. supporting the legs with pillows to promote circulation.

CHAPTER

30 Chronic Respiratory Disorders

ADRIANNE DILL LINTON and LOUIS K. LINTON

objectives

1. Identify examples of chronic inflammatory, obstructive, and restrictive pulmonary diseases.
2. Explain the relationship between cigarette smoking and chronic respiratory disorders.
3. For selected chronic respiratory disorders, describe the pathophysiology, signs and symptoms, complications, diagnostic measures, and medical treatment.
4. Assist in developing a nursing care plan for the patient who has a chronic respiratory disorder.

key terms

Asbestosis (ăs-bĕs-TŌ-sĭs, p. 507)
Asthma (ĂZ-mă, p. 493)
Brachytherapy (brăk-ē-THĔR-ă-pē, p. 509)
Bronchiectasis (brŏng-kē-ĔK-tă-sĭs, p. 503)
Bronchitis (brŏng-KĪ-tĭs, p. 496)
Cor pulmonale (kŏr pŭl-mō-NĂ-lē, p. 496)
Emphysema (ĕm-fĭ-SĒ-mă, p. 496)
Granuloma (grăn-ū-LŌ-mă, p. 507)
Pneumoconiosis (nū-mō-kē-nē-Ō-sĭs, p. 507)
Pneumonitis (nū-mō-NĪ-tĭs, p. 507)

CHRONIC OBSTRUCTIVE PULMONARY DISORDERS

Chronic obstructive pulmonary disease (COPD) is the fifth leading cause of death in the United States. It is characterized as varying combinations of asthma, chronic bronchitis, and emphysema. There are people who have only one or two of these conditions, but the three are usually found together. Other terms used to describe COPD are chronic obstructive lung disease (COLD) and chronic airflow limitation (CAL).

A common diagnostic procedure for COPD is the pulmonary function test. Pulmonary function tests provide information about airway dynamics, lung volumes, and diffusing capacity. *Airway dynamics* refers to the patient's ability to inhale or exhale by force. Some of the lung volumes measured include vital capacity, inspiratory capacity, expiratory reserve volume, residual volume, and total lung capacity. The diffusing capacity is a measurement of the ability of gases to diffuse across the alveolar capillary membrane. "Norms" are based on average measurements for healthy people who are the same age, gender, and weight as the patient. Pulmonary function tests should be performed under laboratory conditions by trained personnel to ensure a maximum degree of accuracy. These tests are effort dependent, meaning that the patient must be mentally alert, cooperative, and able to follow directions. Additional information about pulmonary function tests is presented in Chapter 29.

ASTHMA

Asthma, also called *reactive airway disease,* is a potentially reversible obstructive airway disorder that occurs across the life span, from the very young to the very old. It is a highly complex condition that can be a mild nuisance or a very serious, life-threatening condition. It traditionally has been classified as an obstructive disorder because of the narrowing of the airways and presence of mucus plugs. Now it is often defined as an inflammatory disorder because inflammation appears to be the basic pathological process that leads to obstruction.

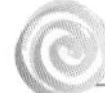

What Does Culture Have to do with Asthma?

African-Americans have a higher incidence of asthma than white Americans.

Pathophysiology

Asthma was once thought to be simply a condition in which allergies induced episodes of bronchoconstriction. We now know that it is much more complicated than that and that it has long-term consequences. Patients with asthma periodically have acute episodes, or attacks, of varying intensity. Attacks have two distinct phases. The early phase of an acute episode begins when "triggers" (allergens, irritants, infections, exercise) activate the inflammatory process. The airways constrict (*bronchoconstriction* or *bronchospasm*) and become edematous. Mucus secretion increases, forming plugs in the airways, and tenacious sputum is produced. Obstruction causes air to be trapped in the alveoli, creating a ventilation-perfusion mismatch. That is, the alveoli are perfused with blood but not ventilated with fresh air. The effect is hypoxemia with compensatory hyperventilation. Acute episodes usually occur within 30 to 60 minutes after exposure to the trigger and resolve some 30 to 90 minutes later. These events characterize the early phase response to the triggers (Fig. 30-1).

The late phase begins 5 to 6 hours after the early phase response when airway inflammation is pronounced. Red and white blood cells infiltrate the swollen tissues of the airways.

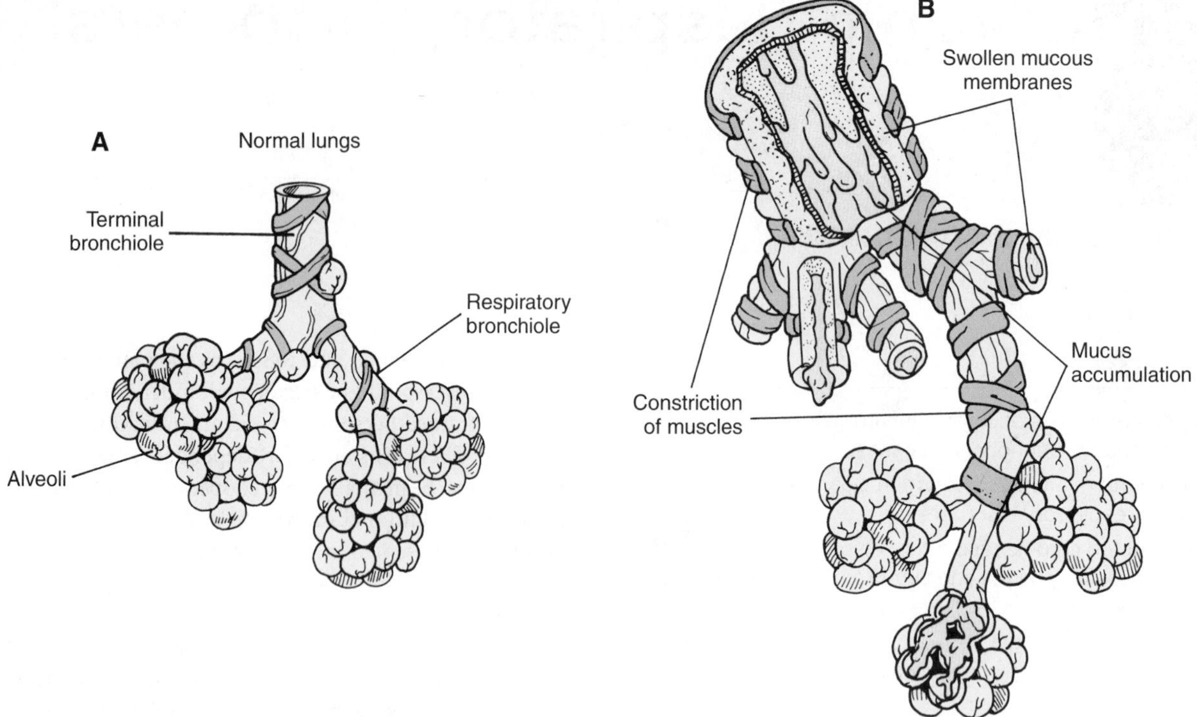

FIGURE **30-1** Comparison of terminal bronchioles, respiratory bronchioles, and alveoli in a normal lung *(A)* and in the lung of a person with bronchial asthma *(B)*.

During this phase, which lasts several hours or days, the airways are hyperreactive (very sensitive). The patient is at risk for another acute episode until the phase subsides.

It is important to note that asthma is not an emotional disorder! Stress does not cause asthma, though there is an understandable emotional response to episodes of difficult breathing. It is possible that the patient's emotional state plays some role in acute episodes, but this is not fully understood.

Complications

Severe, persistent bronchospasm is called *status asthmaticus.* If not corrected, status asthmaticus can lead to right-sided heart failure, pneumothorax, worsening hypoxemia, acidosis, and respiratory or cardiac arrest. Over time, repeated episodes can cause hypertrophy of bronchial smooth muscle, thickening of the tissues in the airways, hypertrophy of mucus glands, air trapping in the alveoli, and hyperinflation of the lungs.

Signs and Symptoms

During an asthma attack, the patient may exhibit dyspnea, productive cough, use of accessory muscles of respiration (scalenes and sternocleidomastoids), audible expiratory wheezing, tachycardia, and tachypnea. The wheezing is caused by air moving through the narrowed airways. Findings that suggest that respiratory arrest is imminent include drowsiness, confusion, absence of wheezing, bradycardia, and retractions above the sternum.

Medical Diagnosis

A diagnosis of bronchial asthma is based on the health history, the physical examination, and the pulmonary function test results. The pulmonary function tests typically reveal that the airflow coming from the patient's lungs is significantly less than expected.

Medical Treatment

The primary goal of medical therapy is to prevent acute asthma attacks by using bronchodilators and anti-inflammatory drugs. Bronchodilators include beta$_2$-receptor agonists, methylxanthines, and anticholinergics. Glucocorticoids, mast cell stabilizers, and leukotriene inhibitors are types of anti-inflammatory drugs. The exact drug therapy varies with the severity of the condition. People with mild asthma may have to use inhaled bronchodilators only when necessary, whereas those with moderate asthma may be advised to use the inhalers daily. Patients with severe asthma may require daily use of inhalers along with other agents, such as aerosol glucocorticoids (Fig. 30-2). Some combination preparations are available that contain both an inflammatory agent and a bronchodilator.

Drugs used to treat asthma can be classified as those that relieve acute symptoms ("relievers") and those that provide long-term control ("controllers"). Beta$_2$-receptor agonists are the most often used relievers; however, some anticholinergics are effective for this purpose. Controllers include inhaled glucocorticoids, leukotriene inhibitors, long-acting beta$_2$-receptor

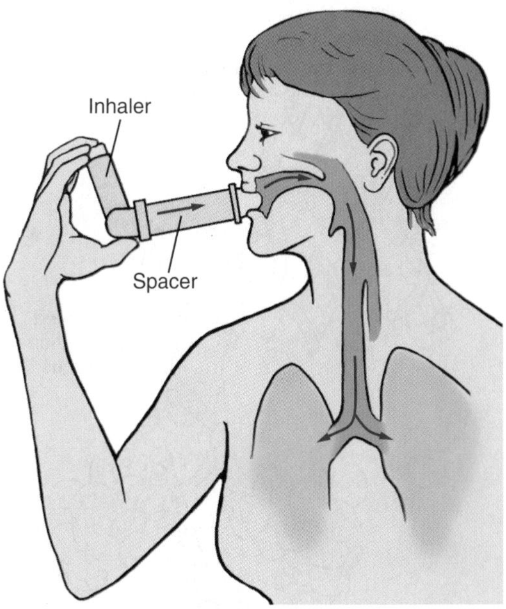

FIGURE **30-2** Use of metered-dose inhaler for administration of inhalant medication.

agonists, mast cell stabilizers, and xanthines (theophylline, aminophylline). Systemic glucocorticoids may be used for asthma that does not respond to other controllers. The course of systemic therapy is usually limited to 2 weeks, although especially severe cases may require them for a longer time.

Status asthmaticus is treated with inhaled and intravenous bronchodilators and oxygen therapy. Endotracheal intubation and mechanical ventilation are sometimes necessary. Drugs used to treat respiratory disorders are presented in Table 29-5.

Put on your THINKING CAP!!

Write a teaching plan (including at least three facts) for an asthma patient who is prescribed zafirlukast (Accolate).

NURSING CARE *of the Patient with Asthma*

Assessment

Complete assessment of the patient with a respiratory disorder is summarized in Table 29-2. When the patient has asthma, obtain essential information (medications, allergies, known cardiac disease, sleep disruption) and immediately take steps to relieve symptoms. Then perform a complete assessment.

Health History

Determine the frequency and severity of attacks, the factors known to trigger attacks, the impact of the condition on the patient's life, the strategies used to manage the condition, the sources of stress and support, and the patient's knowledge about asthma and its treatment. Explore the patient's ability to afford medical care and drug therapy.

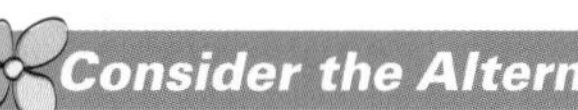

Consider the Alternative!

Ma Huang is an herbal product that has the same effects as ephedrine: relief of bronchospasm and central nervous system (CNS) stimulation. Because Ma Huang is available as an herbal supplement, patients may exceed the therapeutic dose. Educate patients that excessive use of Ma Huang or combining it with other similar drugs could result in toxicity.

Physical Examination

Important aspects of the physical examination include measurement of vital signs and auscultation of lung sounds. In addition, assess the patient's skin color and respiratory effort.

Nursing Diagnoses, Goals, and Outcome Criteria: Asthma

NURSING DIAGNOSES	GOALS AND OUTCOME CRITERIA
Ineffective Breathing Patterns related to air trapping	Effective breathing pattern: regular respirations, 12 to 20/min, without dyspnea or wheezing
Impaired Gas Exchange related to bronchospasm, air trapping, increased secretions	Improved gas exchange: normal skin color, normal pulse and respiratory rates, arterial blood gases within normal limits
Anxiety related to perceived threat of suffocation, hypoxemia	Reduced anxiety: patient statement of lessened anxiety, calm manner

Interventions

Ineffective Breathing Pattern

Monitor the patient's respiratory rate, pattern, and effort. Support the patient in a Fowler's position and give oxygen as ordered. Administer prescribed bronchodilators, and assess for adverse effects of drug therapy. Remain with the patient during an acute attack. If the patient does not respond to these interventions, the condition may be life-threatening and immediate medical care is essential.

Because asthma is a chronic condition, patient teaching is critical. Patients must understand their drugs, how they should be used, and adverse effects that should be reported to the physician. If the patient is unable to afford these drugs, consult a social worker or case manager for assistance. Many patients are now taught to use peak expiratory flow rate (PEFR) meters routinely. The patient uses the meter twice daily to establish a baseline PEFR, then daily to monitor level of control. If the PEFR drops 20% or more below the patient's usual level, the physician should be notified so that adjustments can be made in the treatment plan.

Impaired Gas Exchange

Monitor for signs and symptoms of impending respiratory failure: tachypnea, shallow respirations, diaphoresis, reddening skin, tachycardia, cardiac dysrhythmias, initial hypertension, later hypotension, restlessness, drowsiness, or loss of consciousness. Check arterial blood gas values, and contact the physician if the Pa_{O_2} decreases, the Pa_{CO_2} increases, and the pH falls. Administer oxygen as ordered, usually 4 to 6 L/min unless the patient has chronic bronchitis and emphysema, in which case oxygen therapy is limited to 3 L/min. A nasal cannula is preferred over a face mask because the mask may increase the patient's feeling of suffocation.

If the patient has tenacious secretions that cannot be expectorated, chest physiotherapy and suctioning may be necessary. Because good hydration helps to thin secretions, a daily fluid intake of 2,500 to 3,000 ml is recommended unless contraindicated. Intravenous fluids may be ordered to improve hydration and provide venous access for administration of emergency drugs.

Anxiety

The feeling of not being able to breathe is very frightening. In addition, with moderate to severe asthma, the arterial oxygen decreases, which causes a feeling of restlessness and anxiety. Anxiety may serve to perpetuate the physical symptoms. While taking steps to improve the patient's oxygenation, try to reduce anxiety by remaining calm yourself, responding to the patient's needs promptly, providing quiet reassurance, and explaining what is being done. The family also may need information and reassurance to calm their fears so they can be more supportive to the patient.

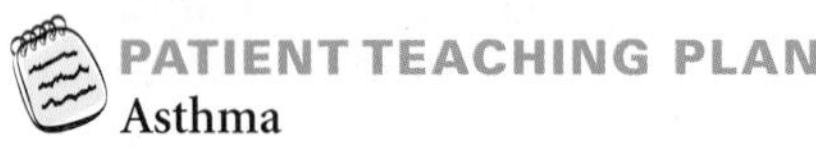

PATIENT TEACHING PLAN
Asthma

Because asthma is a chronic condition, the patient must learn to manage it. After the acute attack has subsided, initiate patient teaching. The teaching plan should include the following:

- Acute asthma attacks can be triggered by allergic reactions to substances in the environment, exercise, or infection, and can be aggravated by stress.
- To reduce the occurrence of attacks, avoid irritating substances, have infections treated promptly, and learn to manage stressful situations.
- If you have symptoms during exercise, use your prescribed inhaler (bronchodilator or mast cell inhibitor) 30 minutes before you exercise.
- Drugs for asthma must be taken as prescribed; report adverse effects to the physician (see Table 29-5).
- Seek emergency medical care if your symptoms worsen and do not respond to your medications.
- Drink 10 to 14 8-ounce glasses of fluids daily if approved by your physician.
- The Asthma and Allergy Foundation of America is a resource for information about treatment and management of asthma.
- To deliver drugs effectively, metered-dose inhalers must be used correctly. (Teach correct use and have patients practice, using the manufacturer's directions).

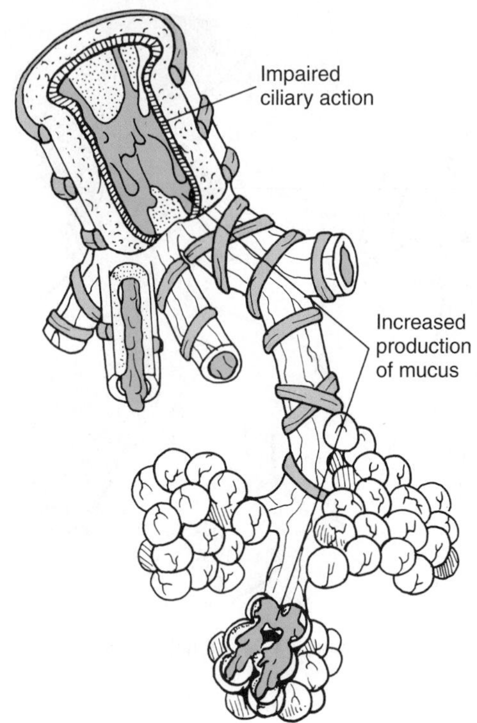

FIGURE **30-3** Chronic bronchitis.

CHRONIC BRONCHITIS AND EMPHYSEMA

Chronic bronchitis and emphysema can occur independently. Because they most often accompany each other, however, the two conditions are discussed together.

Pathophysiology

Chronic Bronchitis

Chronic **bronchitis** is bronchial inflammation characterized by increased production of mucus and chronic cough that persist for at least 3 months of the year for 2 consecutive years and by impaired ciliary action (Fig. 30-3). The inflammation is caused by inhaled irritants, including cigarette smoke. At first, only large airways are affected, but smaller airways are eventually involved. Mucus obstructs the airway, causing air to be trapped in distal portions of the lungs. Alveolar ventilation is impaired, and hypoxemia may develop, leading to heart failure. ***Cor pulmonale*** is the term used to describe right-sided heart failure secondary to pulmonary disease. The patient with chronic bronchitis is susceptible to respiratory infections that aggravate the condition.

Emphysema

Pulmonary **emphysema** is a degenerative, nonreversible disease characterized by the enlargement of the airways beyond the terminal bronchioles. The two types of emphysema are centrilobular and panlobular (Fig. 30-4). Centrilobular emphysema is associated primarily with cigarette smoking, and affects mainly the respiratory bronchioles. The walls of respiratory bronchioles enlarge and break down, whereas the alveoli remain intact. Elastic recoil diminishes, and the airways partially collapse.

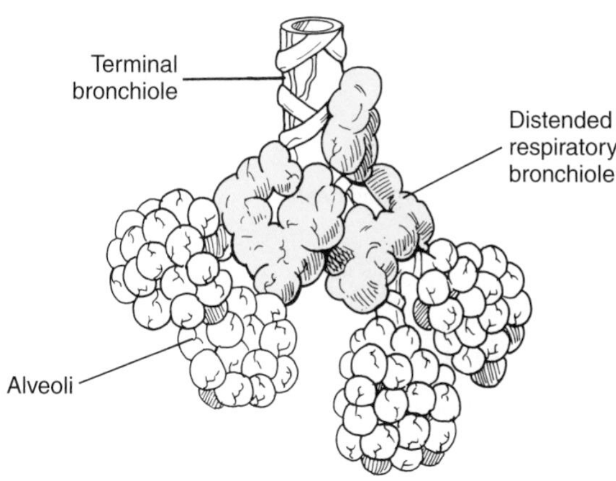

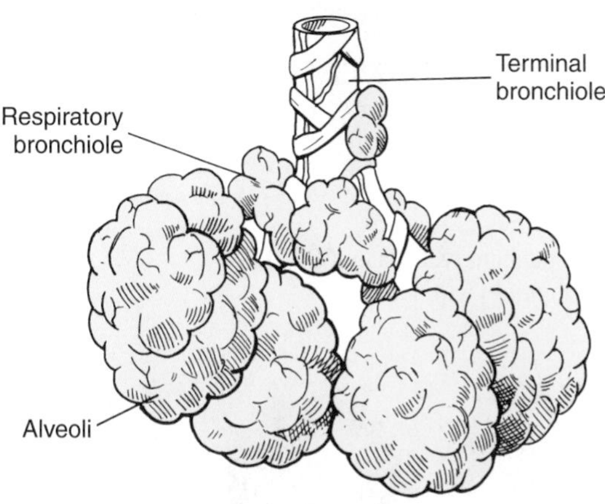

FIGURE **30-4** Types of emphysema.

Pockets of air called bullae and blebs form. Bullae are located between the alveolar spaces, whereas blebs are in the lung parenchyma. Ruptured blebs can cause the lung to collapse. As the functional units of the lung are destroyed, the patient's ability to exchange oxygen and carbon dioxide declines. The lungs become hyperinflated, causing the diaphragm to flatten and increasing the reliance on accessory muscles for breathing. Eventually, as with chronic bronchitis, right-sided heart failure develops. The progression of panlobular emphysema is similar despite differences in the initial pathology. Panlobular emphysema, which affects the respiratory bronchioles *and* the alveoli, is more often caused by a hereditary deficiency of the enzyme inhibitor alpha$_1$-antitrypsin. The walls of both the alveoli and the respiratory bronchioles break down, causing air to be trapped and decreasing the surface area for gas exchange. A patient may have both types of emphysema at the same time.

Put on your THINKING CAP!!

Why is a patient with emphysema likely to develop failure of the right side of the heart before developing left-sided heart failure?

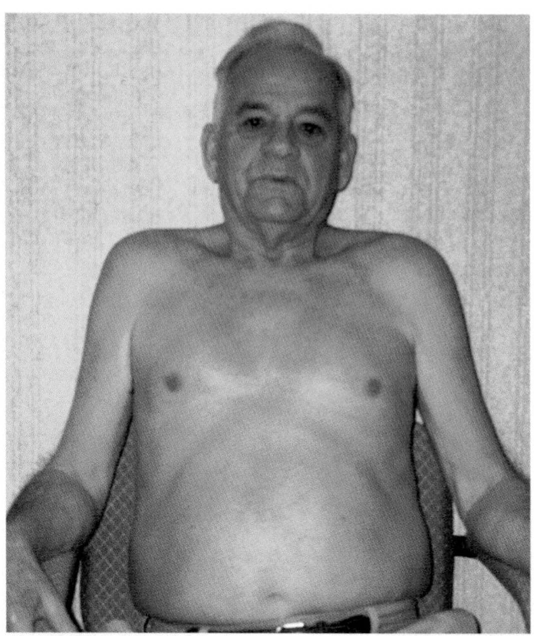

FIGURE **30-5** Patient with chronic bronchitis and all the classic findings of the "blue bloater." Note the elevation of the shoulders and the tense muscles.

Complications

The most serious complications of COPD are respiratory failure and heart failure. Respiratory failure is marked by hypoventilation and ventilation-perfusion mismatch with rising arterial carbon dioxide pressure ($Paco_2$), declining arterial oxygen pressure (Pao_2), and respiratory acidosis. Factors that may lead to complications include infection, air pollution, continued smoking, left ventricular failure, myocardial infarction, pulmonary embolism, spontaneous pneumothorax, and adverse effects of drugs.

Put on your THINKING CAP!!

Refer to Chapter 13, Fluid and Electrolytes, to figure out why a patient with COPD might develop respiratory acidosis.

Signs and Symptoms

Chronic bronchitis and emphysema each have specific signs and symptoms because of the differences in pathologic origin. The signs and symptoms of each are presented separately here, but remember that the two conditions are often found together.

Chronic Bronchitis

Signs and symptoms of chronic bronchitis include productive cough, exertional dyspnea, and wheezing. With chronic hypoxemia, the red blood cell count is typically elevated to compensate for the inadequate oxygen in the blood. The patient with cor pulmonale demonstrates signs and symptoms of heart failure, including increasing dyspnea, cyanosis, and peripheral edema. These signs have given rise to the term *blue bloater* to describe the patient with advanced chronic bronchitis (Fig. 30-5).

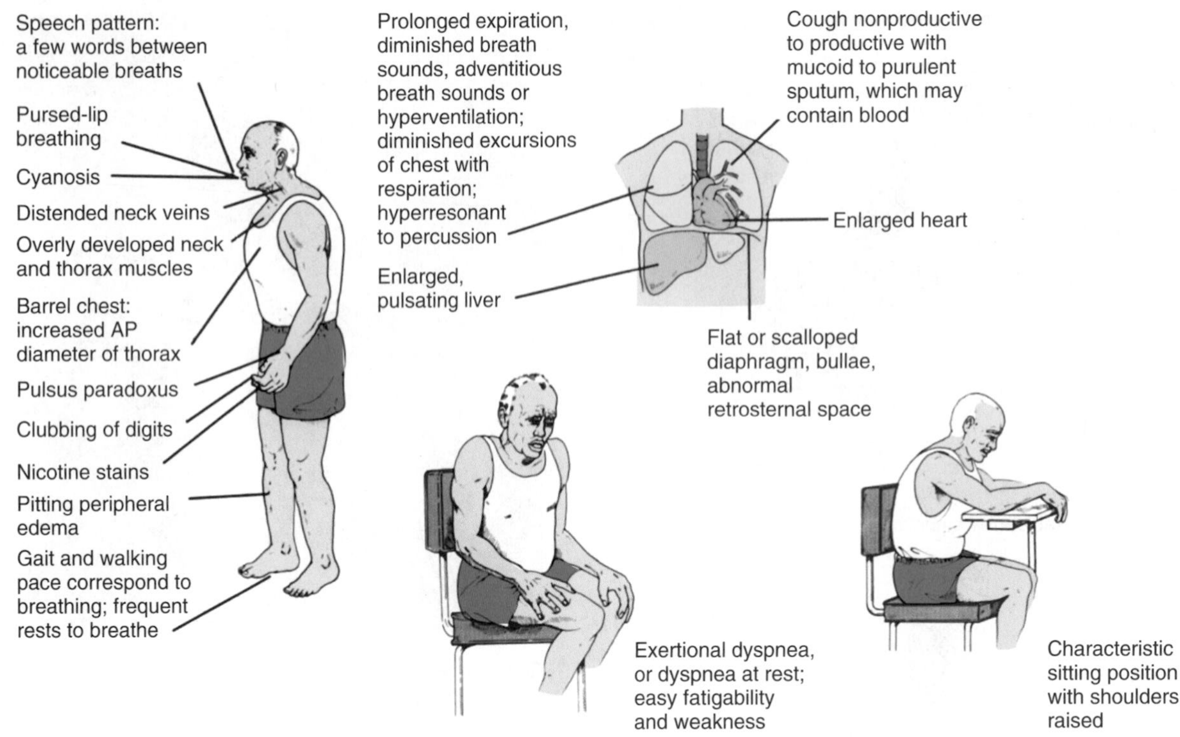

FIGURE **30-6** Signs and symptoms of chronic obstructive pulmonary disease (COPD).

Emphysema

The main symptom of emphysema is dyspnea on exertion (Fig. 30-6). As the disease progresses, the patient also may have dyspnea when at rest. Patients often are thin and may be observed using accessory muscles of respiration. Increased anteroposterior diameter of the chest creates what is called a barrel chest. Despite dyspnea, patients who have emphysema without chronic bronchitis often have normal arterial blood gases until the disease is very advanced. Therefore, skin color may be normal. This explains the term *pink puffer* used to describe the patient with emphysema (Fig. 30-7). Depression and irritability are common in the patient with COPD.

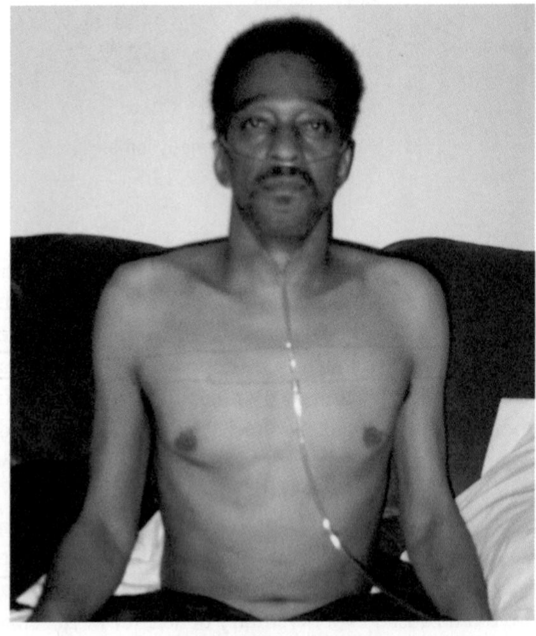

FIGURE **30-7** Patient with emphysema and all the classic findings of the "pink puffer." Note the use of accessory muscles in the neck and chest.

Medical Diagnosis

Chronic obstructive pulmonary disease is suspected on the basis of the patient's health history and physical examination. The most reliable diagnostic tests for COPD are the pulmonary function tests, which reveal a decreased forced expiratory volume and forced vital capacity accompanied by increases in functional residual capacity and residual volume. Total lung capacity can be increased or normal. A computed tomography scan may be done to help differentiate the type of emphysema.

Medical Treatment

Drug Therapy

The goals of medical treatment are improved ventilation and removal of secretions. Drug therapy plays an important part in treating COPD. Bronchodilators, including beta-adrenergics and anticholinergics, are ordered to decrease airway resistance and the work of breathing. The preferred route of administration is by inhalation using a metered-dose inhaler. There is some evidence that anticholinergics such as ipratropium bromide (Atrovent) are more effective than beta-adrenergics for treating COPD.

Oral theophylline is not used as commonly for bronchodilation as it once was because of the risk of drug toxicity. If theophylline is used, the sustained-release form is recommended, and periodic blood levels must be determined. Corticosteroids are useful in the treatment of the inflammatory response in asthma, but whether they are effective with bronchitis and emphysema is controversial. Antidepressants may be indicated and can improve the quality of life.

Theophylline blood levels must be monitored because toxicity can cause fatal cardiac dysrhythmias. The therapeutic blood level is 5 to 15 micrograms per milliliter (μg/ml).

Oxygen Therapy

Oxygen therapy may be prescribed but must be used cautiously. The goal of oxygen therapy is to maintain the PaO_2 between 50 and 60 mm Hg. The initial liter flow is usually 1 to 3 L/min. A pulse oximeter may be used while titrating the liter flow to maintain the SaO_2 (saturation of oxygen in the arterial blood) at 90%. Periodically, the pulse oximeter should be correlated with actual blood gas laboratory values. High levels of oxygen are not administered because patients with COPD may rely on *hypoxic drive* to breathe. A comparison of respiratory stimuli in healthy people and people with COPD helps to explain the concept of hypoxic drive. A healthy person's respirations are stimulated by rising carbon dioxide levels in the blood. The patient with COPD who retains carbon dioxide (as confirmed by blood gas analysis), however, has adapted to high blood carbon dioxide and relies on low blood oxygen to stimulate breathing. A high concentration of oxygen may raise the blood oxygen level so that the patient's stimulus to breathe is lost and respiratory depression may result.

For outpatient use, patients can rent oxygen tanks or cylinders, oxygen concentrators, and portable oxygen therapy equipment. Oxygen concentrators compress and filter room air and deliver oxygen to the patient through a nasal cannula. Using long tubing, the patient can be mobile in the home setting. Suitcase models can be used for travel. Portable equipment includes liquid oxygen reservoirs that are easily carried on a shoulder strap and compressed gas units that deliver oxygen only "on demand," so that a small quantity lasts longer than standard cylinders.

Chest Physiotherapy

Chest physiotherapy, described in Chapter 29, may be ordered to mobilize secretions in the patient with COPD.

Exercise

The patient may be referred to a rehabilitation program that includes exercise reconditioning. Programs are individualized but usually use progressive exercise—either walking or pedaling a stationary cycle. A typical program might have the patient walk 10 to 15 minutes every day or every other day. Every week or two, the exercise time is increased by 5 or 10 minutes. The goal is to enable the patient to exercise comfortably for 45 minutes to 1 hour daily or every other day. Of course, some patients may not improve this much, but improvement in walking performance and general well-being has been found in patients who consistently walked as little as 12 minutes every day for 2 months. Sometimes bronchodilators are prescribed before exercise.

Nutrition

Nutrition is important for the patient with COPD because malnutrition causes decreased energy and decreased resistance to infection and because obesity increases the work of breathing. No special diet is indicated; however, supplementary feedings may be needed for some patients. Good hydration helps thin pulmonary secretions.

Treatment of Respiratory Failure

Respiratory failure is treated with oxygen therapy, aerosol bronchodilators, chest physiotherapy (possibly), and mechanical ventilation (if the patient is becoming exhausted).

Surgical Treatment

If medical interventions fail, a surgical procedure, lung volume reduction surgery (LVRS), may be used in selected patients. Up to 30% of the hyperinflated lung tissue is excised to improve the mechanics of breathing, enabling the patient to breathe more deeply. The short- and long-term benefits of such surgery are still being evaluated. In early studies, about 70% of patients experienced some improvement. However, the recovery period is long, and the mortality rate has been 5% to 10%. One question under study is how to determine which patients are the best candidates for surgical intervention.

NURSING CARE *of the Patient with Chronic Obstructive Pulmonary Disease*

Assessment

Assessment of the patient with a respiratory disorder is summarized in Table 29-2 (see Nursing Care Plan: The Patient with COPD). When a patient has COPD, describe the presenting symptoms—often dyspnea, cough, chest pain, or a combination of these. Obtain a complete medical history unless the patient's symptoms make it difficult to participate in a long interview. Sometimes it is necessary to break the interview into smaller sections so as not to exhaust the patient who is dyspneic. A list of current medications and drug allergies is essential. Obtain a functional assessment to explore the impact of the condition on the patient's activities of daily living. Assess exposure to smoke or other respiratory irritants.

During the physical examination, observe the patient's posture, color, respiratory effort, and use of accessory muscles. Measure vital signs. Observe the patient for signs of hypoxemia, including restlessness, confusion, and lethargy. Note pursed-lip breathing. Inspect the neck for distention of veins. Inspect the shape of the thorax for the classic barrel chest. Auscultate the lung fields for diminished breath sounds. Inspect the nails for clubbing, pallor, or cyanosis. Inspect and palpate the feet and ankles for edema. Note muscle wasting.

Nursing Diagnoses, Goals, and Outcome Criteria: COPD

Nursing Diagnoses	Goals and Outcome Criteria
Impaired Gas Exchange related to damaged alveoli and/or terminal bronchioles, bronchospasm, air trapping	Improved air exchange: vital signs and arterial blood gases consistent with patient norms

NURSING CARE PLAN

The Patient with Chronic Obstructive Pulmonary Disease

ASSESSMENT

Health History: Susan Kellogg is a 73-year-old woman admitted for increasing dyspnea. She has had chronic bronchitis and emphysema for 3 years. Her past medical history includes frequent upper respiratory infections with two hospitalizations for pneumonia in 1999. She had a myocardial infarction in 1995 and is being treated for hypertension, for which she takes verapamil. She also uses an ipratropium (Atrovent) inhaler four times a day. She is allergic to penicillin. The review of systems notes fatigue, increasing dyspnea both with exertion and at rest, orthopnea, and productive cough with yellow sputum. Patient states she is depressed. Ms. Kellogg is a retired nurse who volunteers at a local homeless shelter 1 day a week. She lives alone and has no family in the area. She reports that her appetite is poor and that she has lost "a little" weight over the last few weeks. She has smoked one pack of cigarettes daily for 45 years. She states she knows she should quit and has tried many programs but has never lasted more than a week.

Physical Examination: Vital signs: temperature, 100.6° F orally; pulse, 100; respirations, 28; blood pressure, 140/94. Height, 5'6". Weight, 102 lb. The patient is seated with her hands on her knees to elevate her shoulders. She appears to be in mild distress. Skin color is normal. Pursed-lip breathing noted. Accessory muscles of respiration are tense. The thorax is barrel-shaped. Abdomen soft. Abdominal muscles used in respirations. No peripheral edema.

Nursing Diagnosis	*Goals and Outcome Criteria*	*Interventions*
Impaired gas exchange related to alveolar destruction, bronchospasm, air trapping.	The patient will have improved gas exchange as evidenced by pulse, respirations, and arterial blood gases with normal pH, PaO_2 minimum 60 mm Hg, and $PaCO_2$ at baseline.	Monitor vital signs and arterial blood gases for tachycardia, tachypnea, increasing $PaCO_2$, decreasing pH. Administer oxygen at 1-3 L/min per nasal cannula as ordered. Assist to comfortable position: high Fowler's position in bed or supported at bedside. Reinforce pursed-lip and abdominal breathing techniques. Provide bronchodilator per inhaler as ordered. Assess technique. Assess respiratory status before and after use of bronchodilator. Monitor for adverse drug effects: dry mouth, headache, nausea, blurred vision, palpitations.
Ineffective airway clearance related to increased secretions, weak cough.	The patient will maintain a patent airway as evidenced by absence of crackles on auscultation, expectoration of secretions.	Auscultate breath sounds at least every 4 hours. Support patient during coughing and deep breathing. Document sputum amount and color. Encourage 2,500-3,000 ml of fluid daily. Request chest physiotherapy per order. Have suction equipment available if patient cannot expectorate secretions.
Anxiety related to hypoxemia.	The patient will verbalize decreased anxiety and will appear calm.	Respond to the patient's needs promptly. Provide comfort measures. Be accepting of irritability. Acknowledge anxiety and try to identify stressors in addition to hypoxemia. Include patient in planning care.

Nursing Diagnoses, Goals, and Outcome Criteria: COPD—cont'd

NURSING DIAGNOSES	GOALS AND OUTCOME CRITERIA
Ineffective Airway Clearance related to increased secretions, weak cough	Effective airway clearance: breath sounds clear to auscultation
Anxiety related to hypoxemia	Decreased anxiety: calm manner, patient statement of decreased anxiety
Imbalanced Nutrition: Less than Body Requirements related to anorexia, dyspnea	Adequate nutrition: stable body weight
Risk for Infection related to decreased ciliary action, increased secretions, weak cough	Absence of infection: normal body temperature, white or clear sputum
Activity Intolerance related to inability to meet oxygen demands	Improved activity tolerance: completion of activities of daily living without excess fatigue
Decreased Cardiac Output related to right-sided heart failure	Improved cardiac output: absence of dependent edema and distended neck veins

Interventions

Impaired Gas Exchange

Monitor the patient's vital signs and arterial blood gases for signs of inadequate oxygenation: tachycardia, tachypnea, increasing $PaCO_2$ level, and decreasing pH level. Administer oxygen at 1 to 3 L/min as ordered. Teach the patient and family not to increase the liter flow, because a sudden increase in

NURSING CARE PLAN—cont'd

Nursing Diagnosis	*Goals and Outcome Criteria*	*Interventions*
Imbalanced nutrition: less than body requirements related to anorexia, dyspnea.	The patient will maintain or increase body weight during hospitalization.	Provide pleasant environment for meals. Schedule respiratory treatments at least an hour before meals. Assist with oral hygiene. Offer to arrange smaller, more frequent meals. Consult with dietitian to consider patient preferences.
Activity intolerance related to inability to meet oxygen needs.	The patient will accomplish activities of daily living without dyspnea or excessive fatigue.	Allow periods of uninterrupted rest during the day. Use comfort measures such as backrub and massage to promote rest. Allow patient to do what she can for herself, but assist when needed to avoid excessive tiring. Include occupational therapist and social worker to discuss plans for discharge and ways to reduce effort of activities at home. Discuss pulmonary rehabilitation program with physician. Encourage ambulation as permitted.
Risk for injury related to respiratory infection, effects of continued smoking.	The patient will have a normal body temperature, clear or white sputum, no peripheral edema.	Monitor sputum color and body temperature. Administer antimicrobials as ordered. Encourage fluid intake. Protect from people with respiratory infections. Monitor for signs of heart failure, especially peripheral edema.
	The patient will express intent to attempt smoking cessation.	Explore smoking cessation programs that patient has tried. Be nonjudgmental and avoid scolding. Inform her of newer options such as nicotine patches, gum, and nasal spray. Tell her that drug therapy has been helpful for some people and that she may want to ask the physician about this. Provide literature from American Cancer Society and American Lung Association with suggestions to facilitate smoking cessation.
Decreased cardiac output related to right-sided heart failure.	The patient will have improved cardiac output as evidenced by no dependent edema or distended neck veins.	Monitor for signs of right-sided heart failure, especially peripheral edema

oxygen in the blood may actually depress respirations in people with emphysema. Place the patient in a high Fowler's position or seated on the bedside with the arms folded on the overbed table to promote full expansion of the lungs (Fig. 30-8). Teach pursed-lip breathing by instructing the patient to breathe in through the nose and exhale slowly through the mouth with the lips almost closed. Pursed-lip breathing reduces the collapse of airways with exhalation and reduces dyspnea. Administer prescribed bronchodilators, and assess the patient for therapeutic and adverse effects.

Smoking cessation is an important aspect of the management of chronic bronchitis and emphysema as well as of other cardiovascular and respiratory conditions. One fifth of all deaths in the United States are related to smoking. Health care providers should discourage smoking but must be careful not to be judgmental of the patient. Most patients are aware of the relationship between smoking and respiratory disease, but many find they are unable to overcome the addiction to nicotine. Ask patients if they have considered quitting smoking and if they would like information about programs that might be helpful.

The physician may order nicotine patches, gum, or nasal spray for the patient who wants to try to withdraw from smoking. Some studies have found the success rate for these products is only approximately 25%, but other types of smoking cessation programs typically have less success, with rates of approximately 10% to 20%. Success is defined as abstinence from smoking for at least 1 year. The American Cancer Society and the American Lung Association sponsor programs to support people who are trying to quit smoking.

In addition to nicotine, drugs that have been tried to discourage smoking include bupropion (Wellbutrin) cimetidine hydrochloride (Tagamet), clonidine (Catapres), doxepin hydrochloride (Sinequan), fluoxetine hydrochloride (Prozac), and calcium channel blockers. Although 70% of smokers

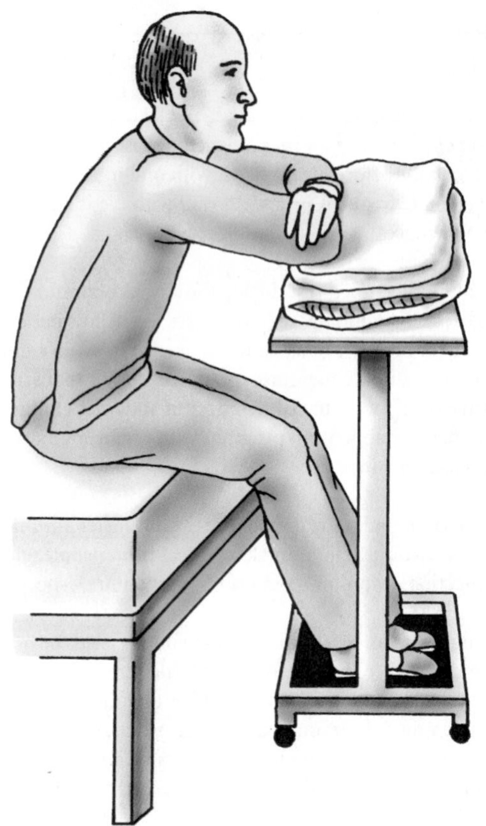

FIGURE **30-8** Sitting on the edge of the bed with the arms folded and elevated allows the accessory muscles of respiration to function more effectively.

indicate they would like to quit, the addictive quality of nicotine makes it very difficult.

PHARMACOLOGY CAPSULE Two drugs that have been approved for smoking cessation are nicotine and bupropion (Wellbutrin).

See Box 30-1 for the facts about smoking.

Strategies to discourage youth smoking include educational activities, reduced accessibility to tobacco, changing social and environmental norms, and deglamorizing smoking (Table 30-1).

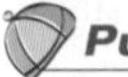

Put on your THINKING CAP!!

Think of some ways to discourage smoking by deglamorizing it. Make a poster to illustrate your strategy.

Ineffective Airway Clearance

Monitor for signs and symptoms of airway obstruction, including tachycardia, increasing dyspnea, and abnormal breath sounds. Demonstrate effective coughing techniques and assess the patient's efforts. Encourage the patient to drink at least 2,500 to 3,000 ml of fluid each day unless contraindicated to help liquefy secretions for easier expectoration. Use a humidifier to decrease the drying of secretions. Perform chest physiotherapy as ordered, and evaluate the effects. If the patient is unable to expectorate, suctioning may be needed to remove secretions.

box 30-1 *Facts About Smoking*

Smoking is *the* major preventable cause of death in the United States, where over 400,000 smoking-related deaths occur each year.

Smoking increases the risk of lung cancer, chronic bronchitis, emphysema, cardiovascular disease, duodenal and gastric ulcers, esophageal reflux, osteoporosis, reproductive complications, premature skin wrinkling, cataracts, and fire-related injuries.

Environmental tobacco smoke is classified as a carcinogen.

Smokeless tobacco is not recommended as an alternative to smoking because it has other adverse effects including oral cancers.

Anxiety

The most important intervention for relieving anxiety is helping the patient breathe more easily. Positioning and oxygen therapy are two simple measures that can be instituted promptly. Also, explain procedures and equipment to the patient. Remain calm and reassuring until the patient is more comfortable and relaxed. It is important to remember that irritability and anxiety are related to hypoxemia and that the patient is not just being difficult. Encourage a family member who has a calming influence on the patient to remain at the bedside. When leaving the patient, place the call button within reach and instruct the patient in its use. Check on the patient often to provide reassurance that help is nearby if needed.

Imbalanced Nutrition: Less than Body Requirements

The work of breathing is increased with COPD, which in turn increases the patient's caloric requirements. Some patients with COPD have difficulty maintaining adequate nutritional intake. Monitor the patient's weight daily or weekly depending on the situation to assess the fluid or nutritional status. A patient with heart failure may gain weight because of fluid retention. Weight loss may indicate elimination of excess fluid or loss of body weight as a result of inadequate nutrition. Inadequate nutrition may be associated with dyspnea, anorexia, depression, or inability to obtain and prepare food.

The patient who is dyspneic may be given a soft diet with frequent small meals rather than three large meals daily. High-calorie, high-protein supplements may be provided as well. Try to plan nursing care so that the patient is not excessively tired or coughing during meals. To combat anorexia, consult with the dietitian to provide foods that are appealing to the patient. Assist the patient with oral hygiene before meals. Create a pleasant environment by removing soiled tissues and emesis basins. If the agency permits, encourage a family mem-

table 30-1 ***Aids to Smoking Cessation***

MEDICATION	PATIENT TEACHING
NICOTINE REPLACEMENT	
Gum	Slowly chew 8-10 pieces a day, each for 20-30 minutes, over a period of at least 3 months.
Transdermal patch	Apply patch in the morning and remove at bedtime or the next morning, depending on product instructions. Use the full dose patch for 1-3 months, then lower dose patches for 2-4 weeks each to taper off.
Nasal spray (Nicotrol NS)	Deliver one spray to each nostril every 30-60 minutes. Initial irritation (nasal burning, sneezing, watery eyes) resolves after 24-48 hours of use.
Inhaler (Nicotrol Inhaler)	The inhaler resembles a plastic cigarette that delivers nicotine flavored with menthol. Most patients use it 6-16 times a day for 3 months, and then taper off over 2-3 months.
Bupropion (Wellbutrin)	Usually prescribed for 7 days before patient attempts to quit smoking and continued for 6-12 weeks. Can be used with nicotine patch.
	Do not exceed prescribed dosage. Overdosage can cause seizures.
	Advise your physician if you have a history of seizures or an eating disorder, both of which are contraindications for bupropion.

ber to eat with the patient to provide a more social atmosphere. If the patient is unable to consume adequate nutrients, tube feeding or total parenteral nutrition may be instituted. If the patient is obese, discuss the benefits of weight loss.

Risk for Infection

Because of pooled secretions and poor nutritional status, the patient with chronic bronchitis and emphysema is at risk for respiratory infections. Monitor for fever and for green or yellow sputum. Promote good hydration and nutrition. Administer prophylactic antimicrobials as ordered. Advise patients to take annual influenza immunizations and to avoid people who are ill with infectious respiratory diseases. The physician may prescribe a Pneumovax vaccine for pneumococcal pneumonia.

Activity Intolerance

During hospitalization, attempt to schedule treatments, meals, and exercise so that the patient has time to rest. If the patient becomes excessively dyspneic or experiences tachycardia during activity, stop that activity until the patient recovers. When preparing for discharge, help the patient plan a daily schedule that spaces more demanding activities and allows scheduled rest periods. Portable oxygen therapy may be ordered to permit greater mobility while receiving supplemental oxygen. At home, environmental adaptations may be needed, such as rearrangement of furniture to permit easy access to bathrooms and ramps to replace steps.

If the patient is participating in a rehabilitation program to improve exercise tolerance, monitor progress and provide encouragement and feedback.

Decreased Cardiac Output

Patients with chronic bronchitis and emphysema are at risk for right-sided heart failure that eventually affects the left side of the heart as well. Therefore, monitor for signs of failure: increasing dyspnea, decreasing urine output, tachycardia, and dependent edema. Management of congestive heart failure is covered in Chapter 33.

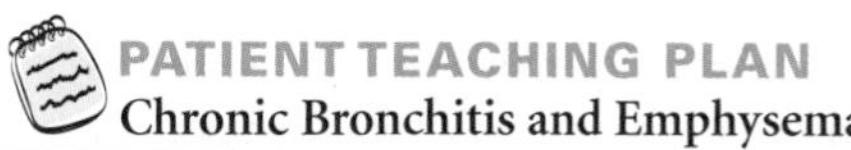

PATIENT TEACHING PLAN
Chronic Bronchitis and Emphysema

Patients with chronic bronchitis and emphysema need to know how they can manage the condition. However, patient instruction is best done in small units to prevent overtiring and overwhelming the patient. Supplement instruction with written material. Include the following:

- Take your prescribed drugs as instructed; report adverse effects to the physician.
- Avoid substances that irritate the airway.
- Cover the nose and mouth when outside in cold weather.
- To reduce risk of infection, avoid infected people.
- Report fever or increased symptoms to your physician promptly.
- Schedule your activities to allow adequate rest.
- If oxygen therapy is ordered, do not exceed the prescribed liter flow; to do so may depress your breathing.
- Smoking cessation can improve your symptoms. Programs and assistance are provided by the local chapter of the American Lung Association and the American Cancer Society.

BRONCHIECTASIS

Bronchiectasis is an abnormal dilation and distortion of the bronchi and bronchioles that is usually confined to one lung lobe or segment. It typically follows recurrent inflammatory conditions, infections, or obstructions but is sometimes congenital. The most prominent signs of bronchiectasis are coughing and the production of large amounts of purulent sputum. The patient also may have fever, hemoptysis, nasal stuffiness, sinus drainage, fatigue, and weakness.

The goals of medical treatment are to control symptoms and to prevent the spread to other areas of the lungs. Treatment consists of antibiotic therapy, bronchodilators, chest physiotherapy, and oxygen therapy. Severe bronchiectasis may be treated with surgical excision of the affected portion of the lung if the condition is confined to a limited area. Nursing care includes administration of prescribed drugs and treatments and documentation of the patient's response.

CYSTIC FIBROSIS

Cystic fibrosis is a hereditary disorder that is characterized by dysfunction of the exocrine glands and the production of thick, tenacious mucus. Cough is the first pulmonary symptom. It eventually becomes productive of thick, purulent sputum that obstructs the airways. Cystic fibrosis also results in obstruction of the pancreatic ducts so that pancreatic enzymes cannot be delivered to the gastrointestinal (GI) tract. Without pancreatic enzymes, patients cannot effectively absorb proteins, fats, and fat-soluble vitamins. Their stools become bulky and foul smelling. Most patients do not develop diabetes because the endocrine function of the pancreas is still adequate. In most males, the vas deferens is absent, rendering them infertile. Women have reduced fertility as well. Patients lose more salt in sweat than normal, putting them at risk for salt depletion, especially in hot environments. Over a period of years, symptoms progress, with increasing dyspnea, decreasing exercise tolerance, and weight loss. Airway obstruction and decreased resistance to infections lead to chronic bacterial infections, emphysema, atelectasis, and respiratory failure.

Treatment

At one time, people with cystic fibrosis were unlikely to survive the early childhood years. Improved treatment, however, has resulted in more people with cystic fibrosis surviving to adulthood, so they are now more commonly seen in adult care settings. Treatment consists of pancreatic enzyme replacement, chest physiotherapy, and aerosol and nebulizer treatments to reduce mucus viscosity. Alternatives to manual chest physiotherapy include the flutter mucus clearance device, a handheld tool that vibrates to loosen secretions and promotes movement of secretions out of the lungs. An inflatable vest is also available that achieves similar results. Infections are treated with antibiotic therapy, usually administered parenterally, although some can be given by inhalation. Treatment of infections is complicated by the emergence of bacterial strains that are resistant to commonly used antibiotics. Other treatments that are used less often or in specific circumstances include bronchodilators, anti-inflammatory agents, inhaled deoxyribonuclease, and lung transplantation. It is hoped that gene therapy eventually will provide effective treatment of cystic fibrosis.

NURSING CARE *of the Patient with Cystic Fibrosus*

The goals of nursing care are effective airway clearance, prevention/treatment of infection, adequate nutrition, and effective therapeutic regimen management by patients and their families. Measures to clear the airway include administering prescribed medications, maintaining hydration, and performing chest physiotherapy. Infection prevention focuses on medical asepsis and protecting the patient from others with infections. To maintain adequate nutrition, administer pancreatic enzymes as ordered, allow for rest around mealtimes, and encourage the patient to consume adequate nutrients. Monitor stools to assess the adequacy of replacement enzymes. Frothy, bulky stools indicate inadequate enzymes. For adult cystic fibrosis patients, the therapeutic regimen has been a way of life. Allow the patient to maintain as much control as possible and try to maintain the patient's usual routines during hospitalization. Nevertheless, identify any teaching needs *with* the patient and family and design a teaching plan as appropriate.

CHRONIC RESTRICTIVE PULMONARY DISORDERS

In general, restrictive pulmonary disorders are those that result in reduced lung volumes with a normal to elevated ratio of forced expiratory volume in 1 second to forced vital capacity. Examples of restrictive disorders presented here are tuberculosis, sarcoidosis, pneumoconiosis, interstitial fibrosis, and lung cancer.

TUBERCULOSIS

Etiology and Risk Factors

Tuberculosis is an infection caused by *Mycobacterium tuberculosis,* an acid-fast aerobic bacterium. It is spread by droplets emitted by infected people during coughing, laughing, sneezing, and singing. Tuberculosis was a leading cause of death in the United States until effective drugs became available in the 1940s and 1950s. The incidence declined dramatically until 1986 when the numbers of reported cases began to rise. The rise was variously attributed to the development of drug-resistant strains (multidrug-resistant TB or MDR-TB), the increasing population of immunosuppressed people with human immunodeficiency virus infection, and the influx of immigrants from developing nations. Even though the national incidence has fallen significantly beginning in 1992, the number of new cases continues to rise in many areas. Anyone may become infected with tuberculosis, but most healthy people are not infected through brief contact. Those at increased risk for tuberculosis include the elderly; the economically disadvantaged and homeless; people who are substance abusers; children younger than the age of 5 years; people who are immunosuppressed; and some racial and ethnic groups.

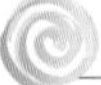

What Does Culture Have to do with Tuberculosis?

In the United States, the incidence of tuberculosis is higher among non-white Americans and immigrants from Asia, Mexico, Africa, the Caribbean, and Latin America. The incidence is greatest in those ages 25 to 44 years among non-whites; among whites, the peak age is 70 years. These populations should be targeted for education and screening.

Pathophysiology

A patient's initial tuberculosis infection is called the *primary infection.* Most people in whom primary infections develop do not acquire active (symptomatic, progressive) tuberculosis. When the tuberculosis bacterium invades the lung, a small area becomes inflamed. The body's immune response attempts to destroy the infecting organisms, but some may escape and be carried into the lymph nodes or throughout the body. The site of the primary infection may undergo necrotic degeneration. Cavities develop that are filled with infectious material, which eventually liquefies. This material can drain into the tracheobronchial tree and be coughed up as sputum. The infected site usually heals, creating scar tissue (the lesion is called a tubercle) and sometimes shelters inactive bacteria. In some patients, however, the infectious process progresses, and active tuberculosis develops. Also, it is possible for inactive bacteria to be reactivated, causing illness at a later time.

Tuberculosis is primarily an infection of the lungs, but the organisms may spread and cause infection in the kidneys, bones, meninges, genitourinary tract, lymph nodes, pleurae, pericardium, abdomen, and endocrine glands. *M. tuberculosis* infection outside the lungs is called *extrapulmonary tuberculosis.*

Signs and Symptoms

Signs and symptoms of pulmonary tuberculosis may include cough, night sweats, chest pain and tightness, fatigue, anorexia, weight loss, and low-grade fever. The cough is often persistent and productive and may produce bloody sputum (hemoptysis). Tuberculosis should be considered in patients who have pneumonia that does not respond to usual therapy.

Medical Diagnosis

The patient's history and physical examination may lead the physician to suspect tuberculosis, especially if there is known exposure to high-risk people. Tests to confirm the diagnosis include sputum cultures, acid-fast smears of potentially infected body fluids, tuberculin skin tests, and chest radiographs. Tuberculin skin tests are commonly used for screening. People who have been infected mount an immune response that causes a local reaction when tuberculin, a protein fraction of the tubercle bacillus, is injected intradermally. The patient is said to have a positive reaction if a hard area (induration) of 5 mm or more develops at the site within 48 to 72 hours. A positive reaction may indicate active or inactive infection (see Table 29-3).

A number of factors including a history of BCG vaccination may cause false-negative reactions, that is, an induration does not develop even though the patient does have the infection. To determine if a person has the ability to respond to any antigen, additional antigens may be used with the tuberculin. If the patient has no response to any of the antigens, additional testing is needed to rule out tuberculosis.

The Tuberculosis Stat Test detects *M. tuberculosis* in respiratory secretions within 48 hours. The test does not distinguish between active and past infections and is very expensive, so it is used less often than the tuberculin skin test. When tuberculosis is suspected, a chest radiograph is useful in detecting the disease.

Medical Treatment

Patients who have positive results for tuberculosis on skin tests and negative results on chest radiographs but are at increased risk for the disease are usually treated prophylactically to prevent development of active tuberculosis. The most common preventive treatment is isoniazid therapy for 9 to 12 months.

For patients with active tuberculosis, drug therapy usually consists of combinations of drugs that may include isoniazid, ethambutol, rifampin, streptomycin, and pyrazinamide. Ciprofloxacin and other fluoroquinolones also are used, but less widely. The course of therapy may range from 6 to 24 months. Most drugs can be given in daily doses or twice-weekly doses. Drug therapy for MDR-TB may use various combinations of the drugs listed above with the addition of others as indicated. The risk of adverse effects with long-term drug therapy is significant, so patient monitoring is essential. Adverse effects are especially common in the elderly. Hospitalization is sometimes indicated when drug therapy is initiated. Because the organism that causes tuberculosis readily develops resistance to drugs, it is extremely important that patients take the correct drug dosages for the prescribed period of time. Incomplete courses of therapy foster resistant organisms and relapses of the infection.

Pyridoxine (vitamin B_6) may be ordered with isoniazid to prevent peripheral neuritis.

PHARMACOLOGY CAPSULE A common treatment plan for tuberculosis begins with a 2-month course of isoniazid, rifampin, pyrazinamide, and ethambutol that is followed by 4 months of isoniazid and rifampin alone.

NURSING CARE *of the Patient with Tuberculosis*

Assessment

Assessment of the patient with a respiratory disorder is outlined in Table 29-2. When tuberculosis is suspected or confirmed, a complete health history and a physical examination are essential because the infection may not be confined to the lung.

Nursing Diagnoses, Goals, and Outcome Criteria: Tuberculosis

Nursing Diagnoses	Goals and Outcome Criteria
Impaired Gas Exchange related to respiratory secretions, effects of the infectious process	Improved gas exchange: no dyspnea
Social Isolation related to medically imposed isolation, fear of contagious disease	Reduced social isolation: less feelings of loneliness or rejection
Risk for Injury related to spread of the infection, reactivation of the infection secondary to lowered resistance	Knowledge of measures to decrease disease progression and reactivation of infection: patient demonstrates precautions
Fatigue related to infection, weight loss, coughing	Improved activity tolerance: patient report of decreased fatigue

Nursing Diagnoses, Goals, and Outcome Criteria: Tuberculosis—cont'd

Nursing Diagnoses	Goals and Outcome Criteria
Imbalanced Nutrition: Less than Body Requirements related to anorexia, fatigue, inadequate financial resources, lack of knowledge	Improved nutritional status: stable body weight; normalization of weight if malnourished
Ineffective Therapeutic Regimen Management related to lack of understanding of treatment and risk of reactivation, lack of financial resources	Effective management of prescribed therapy: patient states intention to comply, obtains and takes drugs as prescribed

Interventions

Impaired Gas Exchange

Routinely monitor the patient's respiratory status. Instruct the patient in effective coughing to expectorate secretions. Encourage ambulation as tolerated and within medically prescribed limits. Assist the patient who has limited mobility to change position at least every 2 hours. Although dyspnea is not common except with pleural effusion, elevate the head of the bed for the patient who is dyspneic.

Social Isolation

The patient who is thought to have active tuberculosis is isolated at first. Practice good hand washing and wear masks (disposable particulate respirators) during contacts. Gowns are unnecessary unless there is gross contamination of clothing. The patient may feel rejected and be fearful that others will avoid contact. Encourage expression of feelings about the diagnosis and the isolation. Instruct visitors in measures to reduce the risk of infection.

Risk for Injury

Once antibiotic therapy has been initiated and the patient's sputum cultures demonstrate low counts of acid-fast bacilli, the patient usually can be discharged. Explain to the patient how the infection is transmitted and how to protect others. The patient should always cover the nose and mouth when sneezing or coughing. Disposable tissues should be used and discarded in a sanitary way. Members of the patient's household are tested for active disease. Those who have positive skin tests but are asymptomatic are usually given prophylactic therapy to prevent development of active tuberculosis. One problem with the homeless population is that it may be impossible to locate contacts. Emphasize the importance of the patient completing the full course of therapy. Otherwise, the infection may be reactivated.

Fatigue

Fatigue is fairly common with tuberculosis. Adjust the patient's schedule to allow for periods of rest. Assure the patient that fatigue diminishes as treatment progresses.

Imbalanced Nutrition: Less than Body Requirements

Anorexia and nausea are common adverse effects of antitubercular drugs. Monitor the patient's weight at regular intervals. Some measures that may reduce the drug's side effects include taking it at bedtime and taking antinausea drugs. Explain the role of nutrition in recovering from an infectious disease and encourage the patient to eat a balanced diet. Five or six small meals may be more acceptable than three large ones to the patient who has a poor appetite. Respect food preferences as much as possible. For patients who are homeless or low income, ask the social worker to locate services that provide food or prepared meals.

Ineffective Therapeutic Regimen Management

A major problem with treating tuberculosis is failure to complete the lengthy prescribed drug therapy. Nurses must realize that there are many reasons that patients do not take drugs as ordered, including denial of the illness, lack of understanding, adverse drug effects, and inadequate money. Intervention should be based on the reason for the patient's noncompliance. Explain the infectious process and its treatment. Reinforce the physician's instructions for the drugs and emphasize that failure to complete the course of therapy results in reactivation of the infection that may be more difficult to treat. Encourage the patient to report adverse drug effects, and seek solutions to make them more tolerable. If the patient cannot afford the drugs, consult a social worker to help the patient obtain financial assistance. Patients who are unable to manage daily self-medication can be given doses twice or three times weekly in a health care setting or the patient's work site or place of residence. This approach is called directly observed therapy.

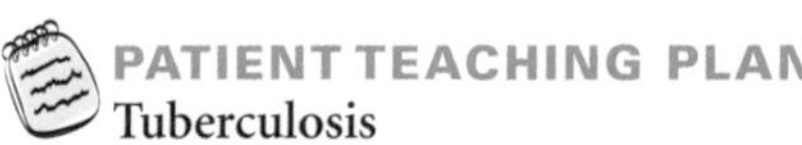

People with tuberculosis are usually hospitalized for just a short time, so you must implement efficient patient teaching. Supplement verbal instructions with written material. Subjects to include in the teaching plan are the following:

- Tuberculosis is spread by airborne droplets. Protect others by covering your mouth when coughing, laughing, or sneezing. Wash your hands often.
- Effective treatment requires taking drugs exactly as prescribed for the full course of therapy to prevent reinfection. Notify your physician of adverse effects of your drugs, but do not stop taking them unless advised by the physician.
- If you are taking isoniazid, you must avoid foods containing tyramine (aged cheeses, smoked fish, for example) and histamine (tuna, sauerkraut). These foods combined with isoniazid can make you very ill.
- Good hygiene, nutrition, and hydration can help you recover.
- Rifampin causes body fluids to become red-orange and may stain soft contact lenses.

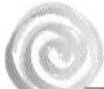

What Does Culture Have to do with Patient Teaching?

To be effective, the teaching plan for the patient with tuberculosis must consider the patient's native language, vocabulary, lifestyle, and financial resources.

SARCOIDOSIS

Pathophysiology

Sarcoidosis is an inflammatory condition that may affect the skin, eyes, lungs, liver, spleen, bones, salivary glands, joints, and heart. An unknown factor triggers a series of immune processes leading to the formation of clusters of cells and debris in affected tissues called *granulomas.* Granulomas in the lungs may resolve or may progress to fibrosis, in which case a restrictive pulmonary condition exists.

What Does Culture Have to do with Sarcoidosis?

In the United States, sarcoidosis more commonly affects African Americans than white Americans and is twice as common in black women as in black men.

Signs and Symptoms

Although many patients with sarcoidosis have no symptoms, others experience dry cough, dyspnea, chest pain, hemoptysis, fatigue, weakness, weight loss, and fever.

Medical Diagnosis

A diagnosis of sarcoidosis is based on results of chest radiography, pulmonary function tests, and flexible bronchoscopy with transbronchial lung biopsy.

Medical Treatment

If the patient is asymptomatic, no treatment is indicated. Symptoms usually respond well to a 6- to 12-month course of systemic corticosteroids. Methotrexate has been used as an alternative to corticosteroids in some situations. Lung transplantation is the only option for patients with end-stage pulmonary disease who do not respond to drug therapy. However, the disease may recur in the transplanted lung.

NURSING CARE *of the Patient with Sarcoidosis*

Nursing care of the patient with sarcoidosis focuses on monitoring the patient for progressive dysfunction and teaching about corticosteroid therapy, if prescribed. Care of the patient with severe pulmonary symptoms is similar to that for patients with COPD.

OCCUPATIONAL LUNG DISEASES

The inhalation of various particles in the work setting can lead to lung conditions classified as occupational lung diseases. Examples of offending substances are dust, ammonia, chlorine, plant and animal proteins, silica, asbestos, and coal dust. The Occupational Safety and Health Administration provides regulations that are intended to protect workers from exposure that could lead to occupational lung diseases.

Categories of occupational lung diseases are described here briefly. The nursing care of patients with occupational lung diseases varies with the severity of symptoms but is similar to that provided to the patient with COPD.

Acute Respiratory Irritation

The inhalation of gases such as ammonia or chlorine causes acute respiratory irritation. The effects are usually temporary, but if the lower airways are affected, the patient may have pulmonary edema or alveolar damage and airway obstruction. The patient may have coughing, wheezing, and dyspnea. Symptoms resolve within a few days to several weeks, and there is usually no permanent lung damage. The treatment focuses on management of the symptoms and avoidance of future exposure.

Occupational Asthma

Inhalation of plant or animal proteins may cause an allergic reaction referred to as *occupational asthma.* Treatment is the same as that for bronchial asthma. Although the initial acute symptoms usually last only a few hours, the patient may continue to have a hyperreactive airway for years. This means that future exposure to irritants may trigger acute asthmatic symptoms. The patient should avoid continued exposure to the offending substance.

Hypersensitivity Pneumonitis

Hypersensitivity pneumonitis is an allergic inflammatory response of the alveoli to inhaled organic particles. The reaction may resolve within a few days, or the patient may contract pulmonary edema or interstitial fibrosis with permanent restrictive or restrictive-obstructive disease. The condition may be treated with corticosteroids and avoidance of the irritants. Respiratory support may be needed if symptoms are severe.

Pneumoconiosis

Lung disease caused by inhalation of various dusts is called *pneumoconiosis.* Pneumoconiosis develops in response to repeated exposure to silica, asbestos, or coal dust and is characterized by diffuse pulmonary fibrosis and restrictive lung disease. The effects are usually aggravated by cigarette smoking, so patients are advised to avoid both the offending dust and the cigarette smoke. Otherwise, treatment is symptomatic.

Asbestosis is a pneumoconiosis caused by occupational exposure to asbestos, an insulating material. Asbestos exposure has been linked to pleural effusions, pleural fibrosis, and malignant mesotheliomas (a specific type of lung cancer). Fear of asbestosis has led to the removal of asbestos insulation from public buildings in many cities, but there is disagreement as to whether the insulation actually poses any public health threat.

DIFFUSE INTERSTITIAL FIBROSIS

Pathophysiology

Diffuse interstitial fibrosis, also known as interstitial lung disease, is an inflammatory condition of the lower respiratory tract. It is characterized by thickening and fibrosis of the alveolar walls, rendering the alveoli nonfunctional. The condition may be caused by inhaled substances or connective tissue disorders, but sometimes no specific cause is identified.

Complications

Severe fibrosis may lead to pulmonary hypertension (increased pressure in the pulmonary artery caused by obstruction to blood flow in pulmonary vessels), cor pulmonale, and ventilatory failure, in which case the patient is said to have end-stage disease.

Signs and Symptoms

The primary symptoms of diffuse interstitial fibrosis are cough and progressive dyspnea. Crackles are heard in the lungs on auscultation. The patient may have clubbing of the fingertips.

Medical Treatment

The condition is treated with corticosteroids to reduce inflammation, bronchodilators, and oxygen therapy. Corticosteroid treatment may prevent additional damage but does not correct existing fibrosis. The patient should avoid additional exposure to the offending substance. Lung transplantation is relatively uncommon but may be recommended for end-stage disease.

NURSING CARE *of the Patient with Diffuse Interstitial Fibrosis*

Assessment

The complete assessment of the patient with a respiratory disorder is summarized in Table 29-2.

Nursing Diagnoses, Goals, and Outcome Criteria: Diffuse Interstitial Fibrosis

NURSING DIAGNOSES	GOALS AND OUTCOME CRITERIA
Impaired Gas Exchange related to alveolar damage	Improved gas exchange: normal pulse and respirations, no cyanosis, normal blood gases
Activity Intolerance related to inadequate oxygenation	Improved activity tolerance: lack of dyspnea on exertion, gradual improvement in tolerance of daily activities
Risk for Infection related to immune suppression by corticosteroids	Reduced risk of infection: patient practices infection control measures
Ineffective Airway Clearance related to increased secretions	Effective airway clearance: clear breath sounds, normal pulse, expectoration of secretions
Anxiety related to dyspnea or possible disabling illness	Decreased anxiety: calm manner, patient statement of lessened anxiety

Interventions

Nursing interventions are similar to those described for the patient with COPD.

LUNG CANCER

Etiology and Risk Factors

Lung cancer is the leading cause of cancer death in the United States. The incidence is decreasing among men but has been rising steadily among women. Since 1987, the death rate from lung cancer has exceeded that from breast cancer in women.

Cigarette smoking is the leading cause of lung cancer. The risk is increased even more for smokers who are exposed to other carcinogenic substances, such as arsenic, asbestos, and radioactive materials. Evidence is increasing that "secondhand" smoke poses a threat to nonsmokers as well. Air pollution may be an additional risk factor.

Pathophysiology

There are two major categories of lung cancer: small cell ("oat cell") lung carcinoma (SCLC), and non–small–cell lung carcinoma (NSCLC), which includes squamous cell carcinomas, adenocarcinomas, large cell carcinomas, and bronchial carcinoids. Small cell and large cell undifferentiated carcinomas grow rapidly: other lung cancers grow slowly. They can all metastasize to other body organs. Enlarging tumors or metastatic lesions may compress the laryngeal and phrenic nerves, the esophagus, and the major blood vessels. SCLCs, which grow rapidly, tend to metastasize early. They can invade the pericardium, causing pericardial effusion (fluid accumulation in the pericardial sac) and possibly triggering dysrhythmias.

Signs and Symptoms

The warning signs of lung cancer are persistent cough, hemoptysis, chest pain, and recurring pneumonia or bronchitis. Patients also may have dyspnea, weight loss, and pain in the shoulder, arm, or hand. There is some variation with the type of cancer as well as the location. Other signs and symptoms may be related to metastatic lesions. For example, invasion of the tumor into the ribs produces bone pain, and invasion of the pericardium may produce cardiac dysrhythmias.

Medical Diagnosis

Diagnostic tests and procedures for lung cancer include radiographic procedures (chest radiography, computed tomography scan, MRI), fiberoptic bronchoscopy, sputum cytology studies, and biopsy of tissue obtained through bronchoscopy, percutaneous transthoracic fine-needle biopsy, thoracotomy, or other methods. Information about specific procedures appears in Table 29-3. Unfortunately, lesions often are not detectable until they are no longer localized. Radionuclide scans of the bones, liver, or brain may be ordered to detect metastatic lesions.

Medical Treatment

Early detection is the key to survival of lung cancer, but this is difficult because metastasis often occurs before the lesion can be seen on radiographs. Treatment decisions are made on the basis of tumor type, lymph node involvement, evidence of metastasis, and the patient's general state of health.

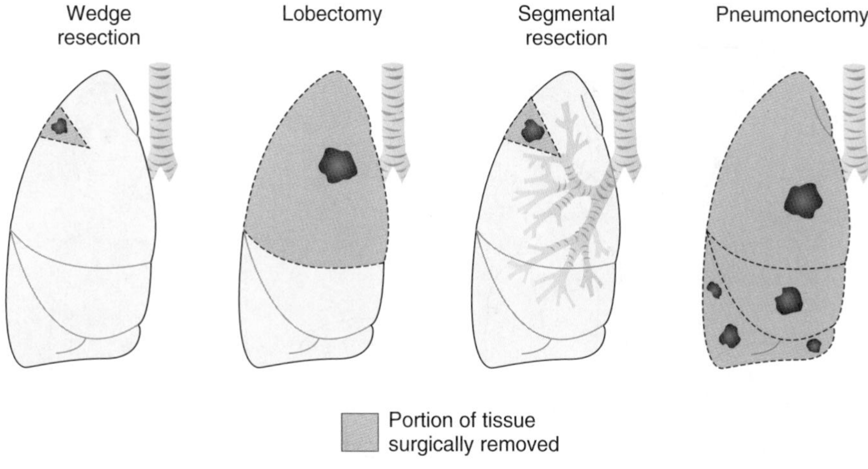

FIGURE **30-9** Pulmonary resections.

Radiotherapy

Radiotherapy may be used alone or in combination with other treatment methods. It may be curative in some situations but also may be used to temporarily relieve symptoms by reducing the size of the lesion. Radiotherapy for lung cancer may include external beam irradiation and brachytherapy. Brachytherapy is direct irradiation by placement of the radiation source at the site of the tumor. Complications of endobronchial irradiation are pulmonary hemorrhage and radiation bronchitis and stenosis. Other general complications of radiotherapy are discussed in Chapter 24.

Chemotherapy

Chemotherapy may be used alone or with radiation and surgery in the treatment of SCLC. There is debate about the value of chemotherapy in other types of lung cancers, but research continues to explore various treatment combinations of agents such as carboplatin, vinblastine, mitomycin C, ifosfamide, and etoposide. Cisplatin and paclitaxel often are used in combination. These and other chemotherapeutic agents are discussed in Chapter 24.

Surgical Treatment

Surgical intervention is the treatment of choice for early NSCLC. The goal of surgery is to remove the entire tumor while removing as little healthy surrounding tissue as possible. Removal of a section of tissue is called a *resection.* With lung surgery, the procedure may be a wedge resection, sleeve lobectomy, segmental resection, lobectomy, or pneumonectomy. These procedures are illustrated in Figure 30-9. Tumors that are accessible with a bronchoscope are sometimes treated with laser therapy. Radiotherapy, chemotherapy, or both may be used before or after surgery.

Despite advances in treatment, the 5-year survival rate for lung cancer remains 14%. Survival improves with early treatment, but American Cancer Society data indicate that only 16% of all lung cancers are detected while still localized. The outlook is best for stages I and II NSCLC treated surgically.

NURSING CARE *of the Patient with Lung Cancer*

Nursing care of the patient with cancer is detailed in Chapter 24. Care of the patient who has a thoracotomy is discussed in Chapter 29. In addition, nurses must continue to educate the public about the dangers of cigarette smoking to help eliminate the primary cause of lung cancer.

EXTRAPULMONARY DISORDERS

This chapter and the previous one describe disorders of the respiratory system. Many other disorders, however, also can result in significant impairment of respiratory function. For example, chest deformities as seen in Figure 30-10 may interfere with lung expansion. Neuromuscular diseases such as myasthenia gravis and amyotrophic lateral sclerosis affect the muscles of respiration. Head or spinal cord injuries can disrupt the breathing center in the brain or the neural control of the diaphragm. Heart failure with pulmonary edema fills the lungs with fluid, interfering with the exchange of gases. The specific interventions are covered with each of these conditions in other chapters.

Nutrition Concepts

1. Malnutrition and pulmonary disease are strongly related.
2. Starvation and malnutrition often cause impaired pulmonary function, and pulmonary disease may result in malnutrition.
3. Pulmonary disease causes an increase in energy expenditure because of increased work of breathing and chronic infection.
4. Reduced dietary intake in lung disease results from fluid restriction, shortness of breath, anorexia, gastrointestinal distress, and vomiting.
5. Approximately 70% of patients with chronic obstructive pulmonary disease exhibit weight loss.
6. Strategies for increasing intake and weight gain include eating high-calorie and high-fat foods; small, frequent meals; and resting before meals.

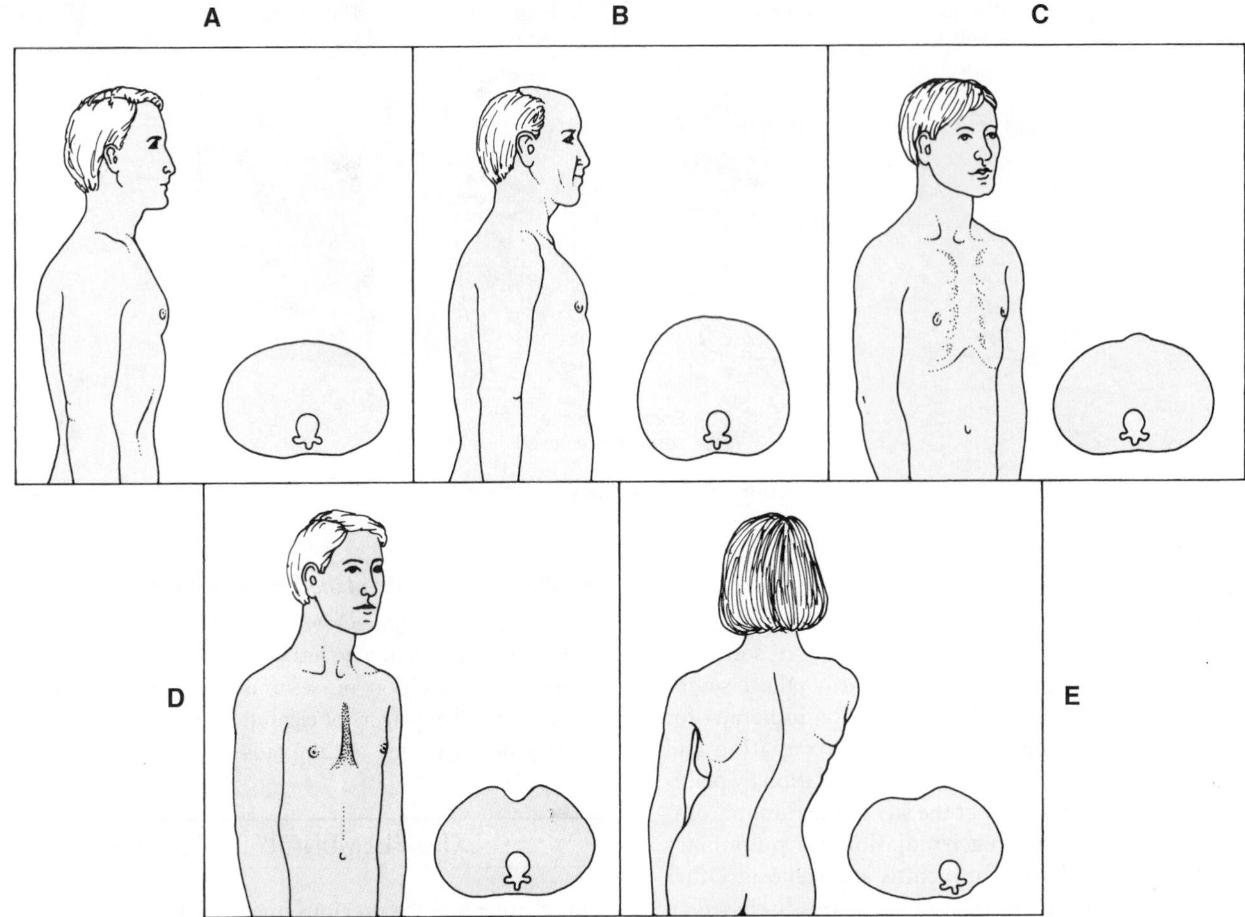

FIGURE **30-10** Normal adult chest *(A)* and chest deformities that may affect respiratory function *(B-E)*. *B,* Increased anteroposterior diameter ("barrel chest"). *C,* Pectus excavatum ("funnel chest"). *D,* Pectus carinatum ("pigeon chest"). *E,* Thoracic kyphoscoliosis.

key points

- Chronic obstructive pulmonary disease (COPD) includes varying combinations of asthma, chronic bronchitis, and emphysema.
- Bronchial asthma is a potentially reversible obstructive airway disorder that is characterized by bronchospasm as a response to a variety of stimuli.
- Status asthmaticus is severe bronchospasm that can be fatal.
- The goal of medical therapy for asthma is to prevent acute asthma attacks using bronchodilators, beta$_2$-receptor agonists, mast cell stabilizers, leukotriene inhibitors, anticholinergics, and corticosteroids.
- Nursing diagnoses for the patient with asthma may include Ineffective Breathing Patterns, Impaired Gas Exchange, and Anxiety.
- Chronic bronchitis is bronchial inflammation characterized by increased production of mucus and chronic cough that persists for at least 3 months of the year for 2 consecutive years.
- Pulmonary emphysema, which often coexists with chronic bronchitis, is a degenerative, nonreversible disease characterized by the breakdown of the alveolar septa distal to the terminal bronchioles.
- Centrilobular pulmonary emphysema is characterized by breakdown of respiratory bronchioles; panlobular pulmonary emphysema by breakdown of alveolar walls and respiratory bronchioles.
- Nursing diagnoses for the patient with chronic bronchitis and emphysema may include Impaired Gas Exchange, Ineffective Airway Clearance, Anxiety, Imbalanced Nutrition: Less than Body Requirements, Risk for Infection, Activity Intolerance, and Decreased Cardiac Output.
- Smoking cessation is an important aspect of management of COPD and other cardiovascular and respiratory conditions, but success rates for stop-smoking programs are low.
- Bronchiectasis is an abnormal dilation and distortion of the bronchi and bronchioles that causes coughing and the production of large amounts of sputum, and is often associated with infection.
- Restrictive pulmonary disorders result in reduced lung volumes.

- Tuberculosis is an infectious disease of the lungs and other body tissues that requires long-term drug therapy.
- Nursing diagnoses for the patient with tuberculosis may include Impaired Gas Exchange, Social Isolation, Risk for Injury, Fatigue, Imbalanced Nutrition, and Ineffective Therapeutic Regimen Management.
- Sarcoidosis is an inflammatory condition that may resolve with corticosteroid treatment or may lead to fibrosis.
- Occupational lung diseases are caused by the inhalation of various substances and include acute respiratory irritation, occupational asthma, hypersensitivity pneumonitis, and pneumoconiosis.
- Diffuse interstitial fibrosis is an inflammatory condition in which there is thickening and fibrosis of the alveolar walls that renders the alveoli nonfunctional.
- Nursing diagnoses for the patient with interstitial fibrosis may include Impaired Gas Exchange, Ineffective Airway Clearance, Activity Intolerance, and Anxiety.
- Lung cancer, the leading cause of cancer death in the United States, is usually caused by cigarette smoking and is most treatable if detected while still localized.
- Extrapulmonary causes of respiratory problems may be skeletal, neuromuscular, neurologic, or cardiac.

REVIEW QUESTIONS

1. The late phase of an acute asthma attack is characterized by:
   1. bronchospasm.
   2. increased mucus secretion.
   3. hypoxemia.
   4. hyperreactive airway.
2. Drugs that are effective in *relieving* acute symptoms of asthma include:
   1. beta$_2$-receptor agonists.
   2. corticosteroids.
   3. mast cell stabilizers.
   4. leukotriene inhibitors.
3. Asthma patients use peak expiratory flow rate meters to:
   1. improve ventilation.
   2. monitor level of control.
   3. prevent hypostatic pneumonia.
   4. measure permanent lung damage.
4. A patient's health history includes "reports persistent productive cough for 3 to 4 months each winter for the past 5 years." You recognize these symptoms as typical of:
   1. centrilobular emphysema.
   2. asthma.
   3. chronic bronchitis.
   4. tuberculosis.
5. What is the nursing implication when a COPD patient has hypoxic drive?
   1. The patient needs deep breathing exercises to improve oxygenation.
   2. The patient's oxygen therapy should not exceed 3 L/min.
   3. The patient is unable to tolerate any activity and should remain in bed.
   4. The patient is in respiratory acidosis and requires emergency care.
6. The home health nurse's assessment of a COPD patient reveals increased dyspnea since last visit, heart rate of 92 bpm, and edematous ankles. The nurse should:
   1. increase the patient's oxygen flow rate to 5 L/min.
   2. encourage the patient to walk more to promote circulation.
   3. document the findings and have the patient return in 1 week for follow up.
   4. contact the physician to report signs of congestive heart failure.
7. The priority nursing diagnosis for the patient with cystic fibrosis is:
   1. Ineffective Airway Clearance.
   2. Risk for Infection.
   3. Imbalanced Nutrition: Less than Body Requirements.
   4. Risk for Deficient Fluid Volume.
8. Patient teaching for the person with active tuberculosis should include:
   1. You can stop taking your medications when your symptoms go away.
   2. Cover your mouth when coughing to prevent spreading the infection.
   3. Antitubercular drugs have no serious side effects.
   4. Tuberculosis only affects people who do not have good hygiene.
9. The primary drug used for the prevention and treatment of tuberculosis is:
   1. rifampin.
   2. streptomycin.
   3. ethambutol.
   4. isoniazid.
10. The leading cause of lung cancer is:
    1. asbestos.
    2. smoking.
    3. coal dust.
    4. silica.

CHAPTER 31 Hematologic Disorders

STACEY YOUNG-MCCAUGHAN

objectives

1. List the components of the hematologic system and describe their role in oxygenation and hemostasis.
2. Identify data to be collected when assessing a patient with a disorder of the hematologic system.
3. Describe tests and procedures used to diagnose disorders of the hematologic system, and nursing considerations for each.
4. Describe nursing care for patients undergoing common therapeutic measures for disorders of the hematologic system.
5. For selected disorders of the hematologic system, describe the pathophysiology, signs and symptoms, medical diagnosis, and medical treatment.
6. Assist in planning nursing care for a patient with a disorder of the hematologic system.

key terms

Anemia (ă-NĒ-mē-ă, p. 522)
Ecchymosis (ĕk-ĭ-MŌ-sĭs, p. 516)
Hemostasis (hē-mŏ-STĀ-sĭs, p. 512)
Orthostatic vital sign changes (ŏr-thō-STĂT-ĭk, p. 514)
Oxygenation (ŏk-sĭ-jĕ-NĀ-shŭn, p. 512)
Petechiae (pĕ-TĒ-kē-ă, p. 516)
Purpura (PŬR-pū-ră, p. 516)
Universal donor (p. 520)
Universal recipient (p. 520)

The primary functions of the hematologic system are oxygenation and hemostasis (control of bleeding). Disorders of the hematologic system can be either a primary disease or a complication of another disease. The diagnosis and treatment of these disorders can be very complex. The nurse plays an important role in helping to assess, plan, and manage the care of these patients.

ANATOMY AND PHYSIOLOGY OF THE HEMATOLOGIC SYSTEM

ANATOMIC STRUCTURES AND COMPONENTS OF THE HEMATOLOGIC SYSTEM

Important structures and components of the hematologic system are the bone marrow, the liver, the spleen, and the blood.

Bone Marrow

The bone marrow is the spongy center of the bones where the red blood cells and platelets are made. The marrow of all bones produces these cells; however, the majority of red blood cells and platelets are produced in the vertebrae, ribs, sternum, skull, pelvis, and long bones of the legs.

Liver

The liver is located in the upper right quadrant of the abdomen, under the rib cage and below the diaphragm. The liver performs many functions for different body systems. As part of the hematologic system, the liver manufactures clotting factors. Additionally, the liver clears old and damaged red blood cells from circulation.

Spleen

The spleen is located in the upper left quadrant of the abdomen. Like the liver, the spleen performs many functions for different body systems. As part of the hematologic system, the spleen removes old red blood cells from circulation.

Blood

Blood is a generic term referring to a mixture of red blood cells, platelets, clotting factors, and plasma as well as white blood cells, proteins, electrolytes, hormones, and enzymes that travel through vessels in the body (Fig. 31-1). Blood serves many functions, but as part of the hematologic system, it transports oxygen from the lungs to tissues and maintains hemostasis. A healthy adult has about 6 liters of blood circulating through the body pumped by the heart.

Red Blood Cells (RBCs or Erythrocytes)

Red blood cells are made in the bone marrow. Once released from the marrow they circulate in the body, transporting oxygen from the lungs to the tissues and carbon dioxide from the

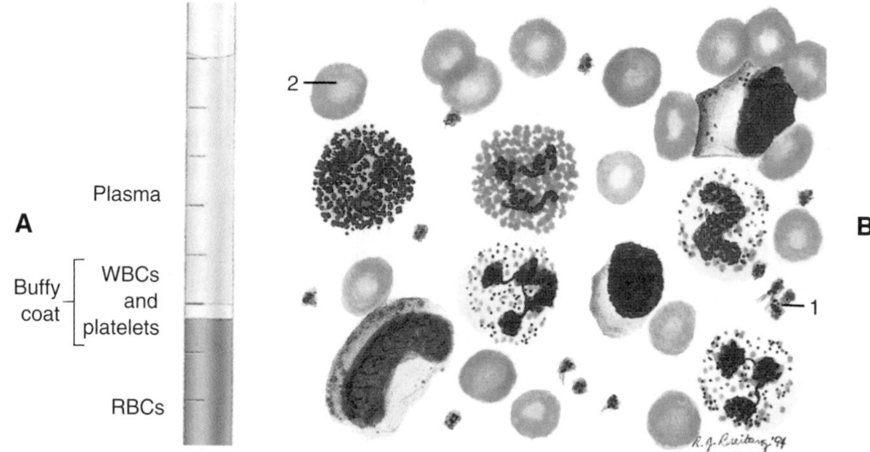

FIGURE **31-1** Blood is composed of plasma (about 55%) and cellular elements *(A)*, including leukocytes *(B)*, thrombocytes (platelets) *(1)*, and erythrocytes (about 45%) *(2)*. There are 600 times as many erythrocytes as leukocytes.

tissues back to the lungs. Hemoglobin in the red blood cells makes the transport of oxygen and carbon dioxide possible. The tough, flexible membrane of the red blood cells allows these disc-shaped cells to maneuver through the smallest capillaries. After about 120 days, the old red blood cells are filtered out of circulation by the liver and spleen. The iron and heme in the old red blood cells are recycled to make new red blood cells.

Red blood cells normally have various proteins, called antigens, as part of their cell membranes. The two major antigens are named A and B. Based on the presence or absence of the A and B antigens, a person's blood type is determined. People with type A blood have the A antigen, those with type B blood have the B antigen, those with type AB blood have both the A and B antigens, and those with type O blood have neither the A nor the B antigen. Rhesus (Rh) is another type of red blood cell antigen that is either present or absent. People with the Rh antigen are designated Rh positive (Rh+), while those without the Rh antigen are designated Rh negative (Rh−).

Platelets (Thrombocytes)

Platelets also are produced in the bone marrow. Platelets activate the blood clotting system by going to a break in a blood vessel and forming a platelet plug. At the same time, other clotting mechanisms are activated, and the body begins repairing itself. Once released into circulation from the bone marrow, the normal life span of a platelet is 10 days.

Clotting Factors

Once platelets activate the blood clotting system, several clotting factors are activated. The clotting factors are numbered I through XIII and include fibrinogen (factor I) and thrombin (factor II). The clotting factors form a stable fibrin matrix over the wounded area, protecting the injured site while the healing process is completed.

Plasma

Plasma is the clear, straw-colored fluid that carries the red blood cells, platelets, and clotting factors through the circulatory system. Plasma is primarily water. The other major components of plasma are the plasma proteins, albumin, and globulins.

PHYSIOLOGIC FUNCTIONS OF THE HEMATOLOGIC SYSTEM

Oxygenation

Red blood cells transport oxygen from the lungs to the tissues and carry carbon dioxide from the tissues back to the lungs for excretion. The hemoglobin in the red blood cells combines easily with both oxygen and carbon dioxide to accomplish oxygenation.

Hemostasis

Hemostasis means control of bleeding. It is how the body maintains the integrity of the circulatory system. If a blood vessel is injured, three things occur: (1) the blood vessel constricts, reducing the amount of bleeding; (2) platelets adhere to the injured blood vessel, forming an unstable platelet plug; and (3) the coagulation cascade is initiated, forming a stable fibrin matrix, which is commonly recognized as a scab. The coagulation cascade is a term used to describe the series of events that occur in the process of blood clotting.

AGE-RELATED CHANGES

With advancing age, the bone marrow becomes less productive. Hematologic function is generally not affected unless a person is unusually stressed with trauma, a chronic illness, or treatment for cancer. Yet even with conditions necessitating a higher production of blood cells, the bone marrow can usually respond to the increased demand, given time.

NURSING ASSESSMENT OF THE HEMATOLOGIC SYSTEM

Many subtle findings on the physical examination can suggest changes in the patient's hematologic system that should be reported to a nurse or physician for evaluation. Table 31-1 outlines the nursing assessment of patients with a disorder of the hematologic system.

HEALTH HISTORY

Chief Complaint and History of Present Illness

Pay special attention to the patient who remarks that he or she bruises easily, bleeds for an unusually long time, or is chronically fatigued. These may be the symptoms of an underlying hematologic disorder.

Past Medical History

A patient could have an underlying hematologic problem if he or she reports any of the following: cancer or prior treatment for cancer, human immunodeficiency virus (HIV) infection, liver disease, kidney disease, malabsorption disease, prolonged bleeding or delayed healing with surgery or dental extractions, a history of blood transfusion, placement of prosthetic heart valves, or placement of an indwelling venous access device, indicating that the patient needed long-term venous access. Note any history of blood transfusions.

Medications the patient is currently using or a recent change in medication may suggest an underlying hematologic problem. It is important to find out what over-the-counter medications the patient uses, as many of these contain aspirin or nonsteroidal anti-inflammatory drugs (NSAIDs) that may prolong bleeding.

Family History

Note any family history of blood disorders such as sickle cell disease or hemophilia. Death of a family member at a young age for reasons other than trauma may indicate a genetic hematologic disorder.

Review of Systems

The review of systems is aimed at finding out what symptoms the patient has been experiencing over the past weeks or months that might provide clues as to what specific medical disorder the patient may now have.

In assessing the integumentary system, ask the patient about changes in skin color, skin dryness, pruritus (itching), and brittle fingernails or toenails. To assess the neurologic system, ask the patient about dizziness, vertigo, confusion, and pain. Patients with low red blood cell counts may have headaches. If the patient has had headaches, record the location, duration, and intensity of the pain as well as what, if anything, relieves the pain. Patients with intracranial bleeding from low platelet counts may report sudden mental status changes or severe headaches. Note changes in vision, which may indicate bleeding behind the eye. While assessing the respiratory and cardiovascular systems, ask the patient about epistaxis (nosebleeds), hemoptysis (coughing up blood), dyspnea (shortness of breath), heart palpitations, or chest pain, which may be symptoms of a low red blood cell count. Heart palpitations accompanied by dizziness may occur with position changes as the heart beats faster in an attempt to move what little blood there is quickly from the lungs to the body tissues to deliver oxygen. In assessing the gastrointestinal sys-

table 31-1 ASSESSMENT *of Patients with Disorders of the Hematologic System*

HEALTH HISTORY

History of Present Illness: Easy bruising, prolonged bleeding, chronic fatigue
Past Medical History: Cancer or prior treatment for cancer, HIV infection, liver disease, kidney disease, malabsorption disorder; prolonged bleeding or delayed healing with surgery or dental extractions; history of having blood transfused; placement of prosthetic heart valves, or placement of an indwelling venous access device, indicating that the patient needed long-term venous access; current medications, including over-the-counter medications and any recent changes in medication
Family History: Blood disorders, death of a family member at a young age for reasons other than trauma
Review of Systems:
Integumentary: Change in skin color, dryness, pruritus, brittle fingernails or toenails
Neurologic: Dizziness, vertigo, confusion, pain, headache, mental status changes, change in vision
Respiratory: Epistaxis, hemoptysis, dyspnea
Cardiovascular: Palpitations, chest pain, dizziness or fainting with position changes
Gastrointestinal: Change in eating habits, nausea, vomiting, bleeding, pain, change in bowel habits, blood in stool
Genitourinary: Blood in urine, heavy menses in women
Musculoskeletal: Numbness or pain in bones or joints
Endocrine: Fatigue, cold intolerance
Functional Assessment: Occupation and hobbies, self-concept, activities and exercise, sleep and rest, nutrition, interpersonal relationships, coping and stress, perception of health

PHYSICAL EXAMINATION

Vital Signs: Tachycardia, tachypnea, hypotension, orthostatic vital sign changes
Height and Weight
General Survey: Responsiveness, mood, expression, posture
Skin: Color, dryness, brittle fingernails and toenails, bruising, petechiae, purpura, ecchymoses
Head and Neck: Bleeding, cracking at the corners of the mouth
Thorax: Respiratory rate, breath sounds, heart rate
Abdomen: Liver enlargement, stool guaiac test, dipstick urine sample for blood

tem, ask the patient to describe any changes in eating habits, including changes in appetite or episodes of nausea or vomiting. Inquire about bleeding or pain in the mouth, gums, or tongue. Describe the patient's normal bowel function and any recent changes in frequency of bowel movements or consistency of the stool. Record any report of blood in the stool. Likewise, note any report of blood in the urine as an abnormality of the genitourinary system. Ask women about unusually heavy menses, which may indicate a bleeding disorder. Describe any musculoskeletal numbness or pain. Joint pain can occur if bleeding has occurred in the joint. Finally, to assess the endocrine system, ask the patient about fatigue or cold intolerance, which may be a symptom of a low red blood cell count.

Functional Assessment

Patients newly diagnosed with blood disorders may not experience dramatic changes in their functional abilities. However, many blood disorders are chronic conditions that the patient has lived with for many years. The functional abilities of these patients may be adversely affected.

Occupation and Hobbies. Knowing a patient's job and hobbies can alert you to unusual chemical exposures. Because the bone marrow and blood can be affected by various chemicals, document any recent chemical exposure. For example, someone who builds models for a hobby may be exposed to unusual glues or paints, which may affect the blood count.

Self-Concept. Assess the patient's self-concept by exploring the patient's feelings about himself or herself. For many people, their self-concept is related to their job. If the patient is unable to work, his or her self-concept can be adversely affected. Additionally, medical insurance is often contingent on employment. Loss of medical insurance and the need to receive state or federal assistance can further erode a patient's self-concept. Another factor that can adversely affect the patient's self-concept is a change in appearance because of the disease.

Activity and Exercise. Assess the patient's current activity level and the effects of the disease and treatment on the patient's usual pattern of activity and exercise. Ask about the layout of the patient's home, specifically the location of bathrooms in relation to living areas and bedrooms. Ask if the patient must climb stairs to enter the home or get to a second floor. Having to climb stairs can quickly tire a patient with a hematologic disorder. Inquire what the patient does for recreation and whether these activities can still be done during times of decreased energy.

Sleep and Rest. Assess the number of continuous hours the patient sleeps every night, whether any sleeping aids are used, what interrupts the patient's sleep, and whether the patient naps during the day.

Nutrition. Ask the patient to describe his or her usual diet and any recent changes in appetite or weight. Identify factors that might be interfering with eating, such as nausea, vomiting, and taste changes. Depression and loneliness can adversely affect a patient's nutritional status. Limited financial resources can also limit a patient's ability to maintain a nutritious diet.

table 31-2 *Assessing for Orthostatic Changes in Vital Signs*

1. Have the patient lie down on a bed or in a reclining chair for at least 1 minute.
2. Record the patient's heart rate and blood pressure.
3. Have the patient sit up.
4. After the patient has been sitting 1 minute, record the heart rate and blood pressure again.
5. Have the patient stand up.
6. After the patient has been standing 1 minute, record the heart rate and blood pressure again.
7. If the blood pressure decreases 15-20 points with change from the lying to the standing position and the heart rate increases 15-20 points from lying to standing, the patient is described as having *orthostatic* or *tilt-positive* changes.

Consider the Alternative!

Be sure to note any herbal products that the patient uses. Herbs that can affect blood clotting include black cohosh, feverfew, garlic, ginkgo, and ginseng.

Interpersonal Relationships. Explore the patient's view of himself or herself as a husband or wife, father or mother, son or daughter, friend, and co-worker. Discuss the effects of the disease on these relationships. Consider the patient's roles in the home. Ask what household chores the patient is responsible for and who does the shopping, cooking, and cleaning. If there are children to care for, ask whether or not the patient is able to perform the usual child care.

Coping and Stress. Ask what worries the patient and how the patient usually deals with stress. Explore sources of support, which might include family, support groups, and spiritual beliefs and practices.

Perception of Health. Discuss the patient's view of his or her own health and health practices. This might include measures taken to prevent complications from the disease, and keeping regular medical appointments.

PHYSICAL EXAMINATION

Begin the physical examination by measuring vital signs, height, and weight. Be alert for tachycardia (pulse greater than 100), tachypnea (respiratory rate greater than 20 per minute), and hypotension (systolic blood pressure less than 90 mm Hg).

Patients with low red blood cell counts may experience orthostatic changes in pulse and blood pressure when they stand up. The body tries to maintain a normal blood pressure when the patient changes position from lying to standing. If the patient's blood volume is inadequate, the heart rate increases and the blood pressure decreases as the patient stands. This can be why patients complain of feeling dizzy or light-headed when they stand up quickly. Table 31-2 describes how to assess for orthostatic changes in vital signs. Patients who have orthostatic changes in their vital signs usually need some type of hydration. Often the patient is simply dehydrated and needs extra fluids. However, a patient with a low red blood cell count needing a blood transfusion can also be orthostatic.

General Survey

Note the patient's responsiveness, mood, expression, and posture. Throughout the examination, carefully inspect and describe any reddened, swollen, or painful areas the patient identifies.

Skin

Note the general color of the skin. A patient with a low red blood cell count may appear pale. In dark-skinned people this may be difficult to assess. Look at the conjunctiva of the eyes, the nail beds, and around the mouth to detect any paleness. Patients also may appear jaundiced, or yellow, if many red blood cells have been destroyed or if the body is having trouble clearing the blood of old red blood cells. Indications of a vitamin deficiency that might cause a blood disorder include dry, itchy skin and scalp, or brittle fingernails and toenails.

Describe any bruising. Petechiae are small (1 to 3 mm), red or reddish purple spots on the skin resulting from blood capillaries breaking and leaking small amounts of blood into the tissues. Petechiae are often confused with a skin rash. Petechiae almost always signal that the patient has a very low platelet count. Severe coughing can cause petechiae on the chest, neck, and face of a patient. A blood pressure cuff pumped up to greater than 250 mm Hg on a patient with a low platelet count can cause petechiae on the arm below the blood pressure cuff as the small capillaries break with the high cuff pressure. This is not dangerous to the patient but can be frightening to both the patient and the nurse if it happens. Red or reddish purple spots denote purpura and are the result of larger blood vessels breaking. Purpura are larger than petechiae, usually 3 mm or more. Purpura can suggest a low platelet count or a problem with clotting factors in the blood. Ecchymoses are larger purplish areas of skin resulting from a larger amount of blood leaking outside the blood vessels. The common name for ecchymosis is a bruise. Ecchymoses do not necessarily indicate a bleeding disorder, but if the patient has a number of these areas or notes that he or she bruises easily, it may be a symptom of a blood disorder.

Head and Neck

When evaluating the eyes, ears, nose, mouth, and throat, note any signs of bleeding. Look for cracking at the corners of the mouth, which may be a symptom of a vitamin deficiency.

Thorax

Lungs

Assess respiratory rate and effort. Auscultate breath sounds, which are usually normal without wheezing, crackles, or rhonchi. Patients with low red blood cell counts often are dyspneic, or short of breath, because they do not have enough red blood cells to carry oxygen to all their tissues. As a result they are tachypneic, with a respiratory rate greater than 20 per minute, in an attempt to oxygenate what little blood they have. Any strenuous activity may exacerbate the shortness of breath.

Heart and Vascular System

Assess heart rate, resting blood pressure, and adaptation of blood pressure to position changes. Patients with low red blood cell counts can be tachycardic, with a heart rate greater than 100 beats per minute. Again, because there are not enough red blood cells to carry oxygen to all the tissues, the heart beats faster in an attempt to move what little blood there is quickly from the lungs to the body tissues to deliver oxygen.

Abdomen

Inspect and palpate the abdomen for distention and tenderness. The examiner with advanced skills may also palpate for organ enlargement. The liver and spleen can become enlarged with blood cell disorders, causing abdominal fullness and tenderness. If a stool specimen is available, a guaiac test may be done to detect microscopic blood. If the patient can provide a urine sample, it also can be tested for blood.

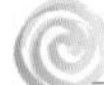

What Does Culture Have to do with Blood Disorders?

Many blood disorders have a genetic basis. Individuals in high-risk groups should be assessed, and genetic counseling made available to those who might be affected. An example is sickle cell disease, which is predominant in African Americans.

DIAGNOSTIC TESTS AND PROCEDURES

Primarily, blood studies determine the function of the patient's hematologic system. Diagnostic tests and procedures done to diagnose disorders of the hematologic system are described in Tables 31-3 and 31-4. Table 31-5 lists normal laboratory values of the various blood tests.

BLOOD TESTS

The red blood cell count, the hemoglobin (Hb or Hgb), and the hematocrit (Hct) are the three main blood tests used to monitor red blood cells. The red blood cell count is the total number of red blood cells found in a cubic millimeter (mm^3) of blood. The hemoglobin indicates the oxygen-carrying capacity in the blood. The hematocrit is the percentage of red blood cells in whole blood. Normally, the hematocrit is approximately three times the hemoglobin value. Iron is an essential part of red blood cells; therefore, serum iron, total iron-binding capacity (TIBC), and ferritin are measured to assess the patient's resources for producing red blood cells.

Normal platelet counts range from 140,000 to 440,000 platelets/mm^3 of blood. Many times the platelet count is abbreviated as a multiple of 1000. For example, a platelet count of 200,000 is abbreviated 200K.

The function of the clotting factors is measured with the prothrombin time (PT), the partial thromboplastin time (PTT), and the bleeding time. If the results of these tests are abnormal,

table 31-3 **DIAGNOSTIC TESTS AND PROCEDURES | *the Hematologic System***

TEST/PURPOSE	PATIENT PREPARATION	POSTPROCEDURE NURSING CARE
Blood tests (CBC, Hb, Hct, serum iron, TIBC, ferritin, platelets, PT, PTT, fibrinogen, TT, FSP, D-dimers, INR, HbS, serum bilirubin, Coombs tests). Blood tests measure various blood components. Blood for different tests is collected in different laboratory tubes containing specific reagents or no reagents at all. Usually the tubes have color-coded tops. Be sure to collect the blood in the blood tube specific for the blood test ordered. Usually each institution's laboratory publishes a manual identifying what colored tube to use for each blood test.	Choose the correct blood tubes to collect the blood. Tell the patient he or she will feel a sharp pain as the needle goes through the skin.	Apply bandage. Have the patient apply pressure to the site for 1 minute. The bandage may be removed in 1 hour.
Bleeding time: measures the time it takes for the platelet plug to form.	Tell the patient a blood pressure cuff is placed above the elbow and inflated to 40 mm Hg. The forearm is cleaned and a puncture is made. A stopwatch is started. The wound is blotted with filter paper every 30 seconds until all the bleeding has stopped. The time is noted.	Apply bandage.

CBC, Complete blood cell count; *Hb,* hemoglobin; *Hct,* hematocrit; *TIBC,* total iron-binding capacity; *PT,* prothrombin time; *PTT,* partial thromboplastin time; *TT,* thrombin time; *FSP,* fibrin split products; *INR,* international normalized ratios; *HbS,* sickle cell hemoglobin.
Data from Fischbach, F. (2000). *A manual of laboratory and diagnostic tests* (6th ed.). Philadelphia: Lippincott.

table 31-4 **DIAGNOSTIC TESTS AND PROCEDURES | *the Hematologic System: Bone Marrow Biopsy***

TEST/PURPOSE	PATIENT PREPARATION	POSTPROCEDURE NURSING CARE
BONE MARROW BIOPSY		
A bone marrow biopsy is used to evaluate how well the bone marrow is making white blood cells, red blood cells, and platelets. The patient is positioned on an examining table according to the location of where the bone marrow biopsy will be collected. The most common site is the posterior iliac crest, although the anterior crest, sternum, and tibia can also be biopsied. The selected site is prepared and draped as for a minor surgical procedure. A local anesthetic is injected. A Jamshidi needle is forced into the bone marrow. Bone marrow fluid is aspirated and a core biopsy is taken through and with the Jamshidi needle. The needle is removed and a pressure dressing applied to the site. A laboratory technician must be present during the procedure to immediately fix and stain the specimens.	Explain the purpose and procedure to the patient. A permit must be signed. No fasting is necessary. Sometimes a short-acting benzodiazepine, such as midazolam (Versed), is ordered to sedate the patient during the procedure. Tell the patient some local discomfort may be experienced as the local anesthesia is injected. The patient usually feels pressure and a momentary sharp pain down the leg. The procedure takes approximately 30 minutes.	If intravenous sedation is used, monitor the patient's pulse, blood pressure, respirations, and pulse oximetry until the patient is fully recovered. The pressure dressing can be removed in 2 hours.

Data from Fischbach, F. (2000). *A manual of laboratory and diagnostic tests* (6th ed.). Philadelphia: Lippincott.

table 31-5 Normal Laboratory Values

Red blood cell (RBC) count
- Men 4.2-5.4 × 10^6 cells/mm^3
- Women 3.6-5.0 × 10^6 cells/mm^3

Hemoglobin (Hb)
- Men 14.0-17.4 g/dL
- Women 12.0-16.0 g/dL

Hematocrit (Hct)
- Men 42%-52%
- Women 36%-48%

Serum iron
- Men 75-175 μg/dL
- Women 65-165 μg/dL

Total iron-binding capacity (TIBC) 240-450 μg/dL

Ferritin
- Men 18-270 μg/L
- Women 18-160 μg/L

Platelets 140,000-440,000 cells/mm^3 (may be annotated 140K-440K)

Prothrombin time (PT) or Activated partial Thromboplastin Time (APTT) 21-35 sec*

Partial thromboplastin time (PTT) 30-45 sec*

Bleeding time 3-10 min*

Fibrinogen (factor I) 200-400 mg/dL

Thrombin time (TT) 7-12 sec*

Fibrin split products (FSPs) Negative at 1:4 dilution

D-dimers <250 ng/mL or <0.25 mg/L

International Normalized Ratios (INR) 0.9-1.1

Hemoglobin S (Sickledex) 0

Serum bilirubin

Total bilirubin 0.2-1.3 mg/dL or 3.4-17.1 μmol/L

Direct 0.0-0.2 mg/dL or 0.0-3.4 μmol/L

Indirect 0.2-1.1 mg/dL or 3.4-13.7 μmol/L

Coombs antiglobulin test

Direct Negative for antibody on RBCs

Indirect Negative for antibody in serum

Note: Normal laboratory values may differ from hospital to hospital. Be sure to check your institution's normal values.
*Normal values depend on the measurement method used.
Data from Fischbach, F. (2000). *A manual of laboratory and diagnostic tests* (6th ed.). Philadelphia: Lippincott.

other blood tests that may be done to determine the specific abnormality include measurements of fibrinogen, thrombin time (TT), fibrin split products (FSP), and D-dimers. If the patient is taking heparin to anticoagulate the blood, the partial prothrombin time is used to monitor therapy. If the patient is taking warfarin (Coumadin) to anticoagulate the blood, the prothrombin time and/or the International Normalized Ratio (INR) is used to monitor therapy.

BONE MARROW BIOPSY

If blood tests show abnormalities, the physician may perform a bone marrow biopsy to see how well the blood cells are being made in the bone marrow. Table 31-4 describes the bone marrow biopsy procedure.

table 31-6 Nursing Actions for the Patient at Risk for Injury from Low Red Blood Cell Counts

1. Administer oxygen as prescribed.
2. Administer blood products as prescribed (see Table 31-8, Commonly Transfused Blood Products; Table 31-9, Administration of a Red Blood Cell Transfusion; and Table 31-11, Blood Transfusion Reactions).
3. Administer the hematopoietic growth factor erythropoietin as prescribed (see Table 31-12, Drugs Used to Treat Disorders of the Hematologic System).
4. Allow for rest between periods of activity, as the anemic patient can tire easily.
5. Elevate the patient's head on pillows for shortness of breath.
6. Provide extra blankets if the patient feels too cool.
7. Teach the patient and family about the underlying pathophysiology and how to manage the symptoms of anemia.

From Young-McCaughan, S., & Jennings, B. M. (1998). Hematologic and immunologic systems. In J. G. Alspach (Ed.). *Core curriculum for critical care nursing* (5th ed., pp. 601-646). Philadelphia: Saunders.

COMMON THERAPEUTIC MEASURES

Treatment of disorders of the hematologic system is aimed at correcting the underlying problem. Blood product transfusions and colony-stimulating factors are used to symptomatically manage the patient.

NURSING ACTIONS FOR THE PATIENT AT RISK FOR INJURY FROM LOW RED BLOOD CELL COUNTS

Table 31-6 outlines typical nursing actions for the patient at risk for injury from low red blood cell counts.

NURSING ACTIONS FOR THE PATIENT AT RISK FOR INJURY FROM BLEEDING

Table 31-7 outlines typical nursing actions for the patient at risk for injury from bleeding.

BLOOD PRODUCT TRANSFUSIONS

Because of the risk of infections, such as with hepatitis or HIV, blood product transfusions are no longer automatically given when the patient's laboratory values fall below a certain value. Instead, the patient is evaluated clinically and a decision is made with the patient whether or not to administer a blood transfusion. Symptoms of a low red blood cell count that would prompt a red blood cell transfusion include shortness of breath, tachycardia, decreased blood pressure, chest pain, lightheadedness, or extreme fatigue. For each unit of packed red blood cells transfused, the patient's hemoglobin should increase approximately 1 gm/dL and the hematocrit approximately 3%. Table 31-8 provides an overview of commonly transfused blood components.

table 31-7 Nursing Actions for the Patient at Risk for Injury from Bleeding

1. Administer blood product transfusions as prescribed. If a platelet transfusion is to be given in preparation for a procedure, it is best to give the transfusion immediately before the procedure so the greatest number of platelets will be available to stop bleeding caused by the procedure (see Table 31-8, Commonly Transfused Blood Products; Table 31-10, Administration of a Platelet Transfusion; and Table 31-11, Blood Transfusion Reactions).
2. Minimize the number of invasive procedures done to the patient that might result in prolonged bleeding.
   a. Draw blood for as much lab work as possible with one venipuncture.
   b. Avoid prolonged tourniquet use.
   c. Apply direct pressure for 5-10 minutes after all invasive procedures such as venipuncture or bone marrow biopsies.
   d. Avoid intramuscular injections.
3. Avoid damage to the rectal mucosa that might cause bleeding by:
   a. Avoiding rectal temperatures
   b. Avoiding suppositories
   c. Avoiding enemas
   d. Preventing constipation by increasing fiber in the diet or administering stool softeners as ordered
4. When measuring blood pressure, inflate the cuff only until the pulse is obliterated to prevent petechiae along the arm. Set automated sphygmomanometers to the lowest appropriate pressure.
5. Instruct the patient to use a soft-bristled toothbrush. If oral bleeding occurs, toothettes or mouth rinses can be used to maintain oral hygiene.
6. Instruct the patient to use an electric razor to shave, not a straight-edged razor.
7. As much as possible, and as prescribed by the physician, avoid the use of drugs that interfere with platelet function such as aspirin, aspirin-containing drugs (e.g., Pepto-Bismol, Percodan), and the nonsteroidal anti-inflammatory drugs (NSAIDs).
8. Teach the patient and family about the underlying pathophysiology that puts the patient at risk for hemorrhage and precautions to minimize the risk of bleeding.

From Young-McCaughan, S., & Jennings, B. M. (1998). Hematologic and immunologic systems. In J. G. Alspach (Ed.). *Core curriculum for critical care nursing* (5th ed., pp. 601-646). Philadelphia: Saunders.

table 31-8 Commonly Transfused Blood Products

BLOOD COMPONENT	INDICATIONS	USUAL AMOUNT IN ONE UNIT	RECOMMENDED INFUSION RATE	SPECIAL CONSIDERATIONS
Packed red blood cells (PRBC)	Symptoms due to a low hematocrit or hemoglobin such as shortness of breath, tachycardia, decreased blood pressure, chest pain, lightheadedness, or fatigue	250-300 ml/unit	2-4 hr/unit	
Platelets	Bleeding from thrombocytopenia	80-60 ml/pack; usually 4-6 packs are pooled for a platelet transfusion	As quickly as the patient can tolerate	
Fresh frozen plasma (FFP)	Clotting deficiencies, hemophilia, rapid reversal of warfarin (Coumadin), massive red blood cell transfusions	180-270 ml/unit	<4 hours	FFP contains all clotting factors except platelets
Cryoprecipitate	Hemophilia A, disseminated intravascular coagulation	10-15 ml/bag; usually 10 bags are pooled for a transfusion	<4 hours	Cryoprecipitate contains factors I (fibrinogen) and VIII

Data from American Association of Blood Banks, America's Blood Centers, & American Red Cross. (2000). *Circular of information for the use of human blood and blood components.* Stock number 00301101L01. Available on the American Association of Blood Banks website, http://www.aabb.org/all_about_blood/coi/aabb-coi.htm and DeVita, Jr. V. T., Hellman, S., & Rosenberg, S. A. (2001). *Cancer: Principles and practice of oncology* (6th ed.). Philadelphia: Lippincott-Raven.

Typing for Transfusions

Prior to a blood transfusion, a sample of the patient's blood is sent to the blood bank for typing and crossmatching. As discussed previously, depending on which antigens are present in the red blood cell membrane, a person has either type A, B, AB, or O blood. Additionally, depending on the presence or absence of the Rh antigen, a person is either Rh+ or Rh−. People with any of these antigens cannot be given blood containing a different antigen. Therefore, persons with type O− blood are considered *universal donors* because their blood does not contain any of the A, B, or Rh antigens and can safely be given to anyone. Those with AB+ blood are considered *universal recipients* because their blood contains the A, B, and Rh antigens. They can safely receive any type of blood. However, usually blood banks exactly match the blood to be transfused with the blood of a patient needing a transfusion.

Transfusions of Packed Red Blood Cells

The patient should be counseled by the physician and a consent signed before any blood transfusion. A blood sample is drawn from the patient and sent to the blood bank for type and crossmatch. One procedure for administering a packed red blood cell transfusion is outlined in Table 31-9. The policies for administering blood products vary from hospital to hospital, so be sure to be familiar with and follow your own institution's policies.

One way to prevent the risks of infection and reactions with blood transfusions is to collect the patient's own blood prior to a planned procedure and then transfuse the patient's own blood back into the patient if needed as an autologous red blood cell transfusion. The patient donates his or her own blood several times before the planned procedure. The blood is stored by the blood bank and reinfused into the patient if needed intraoperatively or postoperatively. Autologous transfusion—using the patient's own blood—is recommended if significant blood loss is expected during the procedure, especially if the patient has a rare blood type or religious beliefs against receiving donated blood.

table 31-9 Administration of a Red Blood Cell Transfusion

1. After the patient has been counseled and has given signed consent for the transfusion, draw a sample of blood and send it to the blood bank with a request for a type and crossmatch. Start an IV of normal saline using an 18- or 20-gauge needle. Blood should not be infused through a cannula smaller than 20 gauge because of the chance of lysing (destroying) the individual blood cells as they go through the cannula.
2. When the blood arrives, it should be checked by two licensed people at the patient's bedside. Be certain to check the expiration date of the blood. Once the blood has arrived from the blood bank, the transfusion should be started within 30 minutes.
3. Take and record the patient's vital signs.
4. To administer blood, use a special blood transfusion tubing that has a filter built in to the system to screen for clots. Piggyback the blood into the normal saline line. Each unit of blood is usually between 250 and 300 ml. Generally blood is infused over 2-4 hours.
5. Stay with the patient for 5-10 minutes after the blood is started to observe for any immediate untoward reactions that might signal a reaction to the transfusion, such as back pain, fever, chills, or a decreased blood pressure.
6. Continue to monitor vital signs during the transfusion per your institution's policy.
7. When the transfusion is complete, document the procedure, the patient's vital signs, and how the patient tolerated the procedure.
8. Subsequent units of blood can be immediately hung as described above. Sometimes the same blood tubing can be used for administering several units of blood.

Platelet Transfusions

Like red blood cell transfusions, platelet transfusions are not automatically administered when the patient's platelet count falls below a certain value. However, the lower a patient's platelet count goes, the greater is the chance of bleeding. Generally, when the platelet count falls below 20,000 cells/mm^3, platelets are administered. If the platelet count is greater than 20,000 cells/mm^3, platelets usually are not given unless the patient is actively bleeding. For each multidonor (from multiple donors) pack of platelets, the patient's platelet count should increase by 5000-10,000 cells/mm^3.

The patient should be counseled by the physician and give signed consent for the platelet transfusion. A blood sample is drawn from the patient and sent to the blood bank for typing. If the patient has been previously typed and crossmatched for either a red blood cell transfusion or a platelet transfusion, the blood bank can usually use this information to provide platelets. Platelets are commonly ordered in four-packs or six-packs. Each pack contains approximately 60 ml. One procedure for administering a platelet transfusion is outlined in Table 31-10. The policies for administering blood products vary from hospital to hospital, so be sure to be familiar with and follow your institution's policies.

If platelets are ordered before an invasive procedure that might cause bleeding, such as a lumbar puncture or endoscopy, the platelets should be administered just before the procedure is started. There is no indication to "get the platelets in early" for a procedure scheduled for later in the day. Instead, plan with the physician doing the procedure to administer the platelets just before the procedure begins.

Fresh Frozen Plasma Transfusions

Plasma is separated from whole blood by centrifugation and quickly frozen. So, when plasma is to be transfused, usually fresh frozen plasma is ordered. Fresh frozen plasma contains all the clotting factors as well as the plasma proteins. Cryoprecipitate, which contains only fibrinogen and factor VIII,

table 31-10 ***Administration of a Platelet Transfusion***

1. After the patient has been counseled and has given signed consent for the transfusion, draw a sample of blood and send it to the blood bank with a request for typing and crossmatch. Start an IV of normal saline using at least a 24-gauge needle. Platelets are smaller than red blood cells, and so a smaller IV needle can be used to administer the platelets without risk of lysing the cells.
2. When the platelets arrive, they should be checked by two licensed people at the patient's bedside. Once the platelets have arrived from the blood bank, the transfusion should be started immediately.
3. Take and record the patient's vital signs.
4. Run the platelets through blood transfusion tubing that has a filter built in to the system. Piggyback the platelets into the normal saline line. Platelets can be infused as fast as the patient can tolerate.
5. Stay with the patient for 5-10 minutes after the platelets are started to observe for any immediate untoward reactions that might signal a reaction to the transfusion, such as back pain, fever, chills, or decreased blood pressure.
6. Continue to monitor the patient's vital signs during the infusion per your institution's policy.
7. When the transfusion is complete, document the procedure, the patient's vital signs, and how the patient tolerated the procedure.

table 31-11 ***Blood Transfusion Reactions***

REACTION	MECHANISM	SYMPTOMS	OCCURRENCE	TREATMENT
Hemolytic	Antigen-antibody reaction to transfusion of ABO-incompatible blood	Fever, chills, nausea, dyspnea, chest pain, back pain, hypotension	Shortly after starting the transfusion	Stop the transfusion. Notify the physician immediately. Be prepared to provide supportive therapy to maintain heart rate and blood pressure.
Anaphylactic	Type I hypersensitivity reaction to plasma proteins	Urticaria, wheezing, dyspnea, hypotension	Within 30 minutes of starting the transfusion	Stop the transfusion. Notify the physician immediately. Be prepared to administer epinephrine and steroids.
Febrile	Recipient's antibodies react to donor leukocytes	Fever, chills	Within 30-90 minutes of starting the transfusion	Stop the transfusion. Notify the physician immediately.
Circulatory overload	Patient's cardiovascular system is unable to manage the additional fluid load	Cough, frothy sputum, cyanosis, decreased blood pressure	Any time during the transfusion and up to several hours afterward	Stop the transfusion. Call for help. Be prepared to administer oxygen and/or furosemide (Lasix).

can be further separated out from plasma and administered alone if indicated.

Reactions to Blood Transfusions

Four main types of transfusion reactions can occur with transfusions of blood or any of the blood components: hemolytic, anaphylactic, febrile, and circulatory overload. If the patient experiences back or chest pain, fever, chills, a decreased blood pressure, urticaria, wheezing, dyspnea, or coughing during the transfusion, stop the transfusion immediately and keep the intravenous line open with normal saline. Immediately notify the physician, nursing supervisor, and blood bank. Be prepared to administer oxygen, epinephrine, Solu-Cortef, furosemide (Lasix), and antipyretics as prescribed by the physician. Save the unused portion of the blood bag for the blood bank. Be prepared to collect blood and urine samples from the patient for evaluation. Documentation of the event is important. Usually each institution has a blood transfusion reaction form that needs to be completed. Table 31-11 outlines the types, symptoms, and treatments for the different blood transfusion reactions.

COLONY-STIMULATING FACTORS

Colony-stimulating factors are naturally occurring hormones that stimulate the bone marrow to produce more blood cells. Certain of the colony-stimulating factors have been isolated and are available for therapeutic use. Erythropoietin (Epogen) stimulates the bone marrow to produce more red blood cells.

table 31-12 **DRUG THERAPY | *Drugs Used to Treat Disorders of the Hematologic System***

DRUGS	USE/ACTION	SIDE EFFECTS	NURSING INTERVENTIONS
Epoetin alfa (Epogen)	Stimulates the bone marrow to produce red blood cells	Hypertension, headache, arthralgias	May be given by intravenous or subcutaneous injection. Patient is usually treated three times per week until the hematocrit is 30-33.
Ferrous sulfate (Feosol, Fer-In-Sol)	Iron replacement	Constipation, black stools, mild nausea	Have the patient take the drug with food but not with milk, eggs, or caffeinated drinks because milk, eggs, and caffeine inhibit drug absorption. If the patient is taking liquid iron, dilute the drug and administer through a straw to prevent the drug from staining the teeth.
Iron dextran	Iron replacement	Hypersensitivity reactions, brown skin discoloration at the injection site	Test dose the patient before starting treatment. Give intramuscular injections only in the upper, outer quadrant of the buttock using the Z-track technique. To give an injection using the Z-track technique, firmly pull the skin over the upper, outer quadrant of the buttock laterally. Insert the needle. Withdraw the plunger to check that no blood enters the syringe. Slowly inject the medication. Remove the needle and let go of the skin. Massage the area.
Vitamin B_{12} (cyanocobalamin)	Vitamin B_{12} replacement		Intramuscular injection. For patients with pernicious anemia, vitamin B_{12} injections must be given every month the rest of the person's life.
Hydroxyurea	Prevention of sickle cell crisis	Nausea, vomiting	Reinforce to the patient that this drug must be taken regularly to prevent sickle cell crises and that it is of no use once a crisis occurs.

Data from Shannon, M. T., Wilson, B. A., & Stang, C. L. (2002). *Health Professional's Drug Guide 2002.* Upper Saddle River, NJ: Prentice Hall.

The effects of erythropoietin on the hematocrit are not apparent for several days; therefore, it is not an option for patients immediately needing to elevate their red blood cell counts. These patients need a red blood cell transfusion. Erythropoietin is predominantly used by hemodialysis patients who are chronically anemic as a result of dialysis, and it has also been used to prevent the complications and relieve the symptoms of anemia in patients with cancer or HIV infection. Table 31-12 describes the nursing care of patients receiving this drug.

DISORDERS OF THE HEMATOLOGIC SYSTEM

RED BLOOD CELL DISORDERS

Patients with red blood cell disorders may have either too many red blood cells (i.e., polycythemia vera) or too few red blood cells (i.e., anemia). Having too few red blood cells is more common. Because the main function of red blood cells is oxygenation, anemia results in tissue hypoxia. Anemia can result from a major blood loss over a short period of time, too few red blood cells being made, or increased red blood cell destruction. Acute blood loss, such as with an arterial rupture, dramatically changes the patient's hemodynamic status, requiring emergency intervention. Chronic blood loss, such as with sickle cell disease, allows the body to compensate. Depending on whether the anemia is acute or chronic, the body compensates in three ways: (1) by increasing heart rate and respiratory rate to circulate the existing red blood cells as quickly as possible with as much oxygen as possible, (2) by redistributing the blood away from the skin, gastrointestinal tract, and kidneys to the brain and heart, and (3) by increasing the production of erythropoietin, the hormone that stimulates the bone marrow to produce more red blood cells. Anemia can be a primary disease or a symptom of another disease. The different types of red blood cell disorders are described below.

Types of Red Blood Cell Disorders

Polycythemia Vera

Polycythemia vera is a condition in which too many red blood cells are produced. The increased number of red blood cells makes the blood more viscous, or thicker, so that it does not circulate freely through the body. Symptoms of polycythemia vera include headache, dizziness, ringing in the ears, and blurred vision. Patients with this disorder may have a ruddy (reddish) complexion.

Treatment for polycythemia vera is to have a unit of blood phlebotomized, or taken off, to keep the patient's hematocrit normal. This procedure is usually done in the blood bank. A large-bore intravenous needle is inserted into the patient's antecubital vein and 1 unit of blood is taken off. This is the same procedure used when a person goes to the blood bank to donate blood; however, the blood taken from the patient with polycythemia vera cannot be used as donor blood.

Aplastic Anemia

Aplastic anemia results from the complete failure of the bone marrow. The term *aplastic anemia* is misleading because patients with this condition have more than an extremely low red blood cell count; they also have extremely low white blood cell counts and low platelet counts because their bone marrow is not making any of these cells. Certain drugs such as streptomycin and chloramphenicol as well as exposure to toxic chemicals or radiation can cause bone marrow failure. Yet in many cases the cause of a patient's bone marrow failure is never identified.

Signs and symptoms of aplastic anemia can include pallor, extreme fatigue, tachycardia, shortness of breath, hypotension, unusually prolonged or spontaneous bleeding, and frequent infections that do not resolve. In addition to abnormally low red blood cell, white blood cell, and platelet counts on blood tests, patients with aplastic anemia have abnormally low numbers of blood-making cells in their bone marrow.

Medical treatment for aplastic anemia focuses on identifying and treating the cause. Transfusions are given to replace red blood cells and platelets. Antibiotics are given to prevent or treat infections. Corticosteroids also may be given. If the patient's bone marrow does not recover on its own, a bone marrow transplant may be considered if a donor can be found. The patient with aplastic anemia is critically ill and requires intensive nursing support similar to the care provided to a patient who is undergoing a bone marrow transplant, as described in Chapter 32.

Autoimmune Hemolytic Anemia

With aplastic anemia, the bone marrow does not make adequate amounts of the blood cells; with autoimmune hemolytic anemia, the bone marrow makes adequate amounts of the blood cells, but they are destroyed once they are released into the circulation. Causes of autoimmune hemolytic anemia can include certain infections, drug reactions, and certain cancers. Hemolytic anemia of the newborn can occur after delivery if the mother has Rh− blood and the baby has Rh+ blood. Blood transfusions can cause a hemolytic anemia if lymphocytes in the transfused blood make antibodies against the person receiving the blood. As with aplastic anemia, many times the cause of the hemolytic anemia is never identified.

Signs and symptoms of hemolytic anemia include pallor, extreme fatigue, tachycardia, shortness of breath, and hypotension. Patients may appear jaundiced. Patients with hemolytic anemia usually have high bilirubin levels in their blood from all the red blood cells being lysed (broken down). Patients with hemolytic anemia have a positive result on a direct Coombs antiglobulin blood test.

Medical treatment of this type of anemia focuses on identifying and treating the cause. Blood transfusions may be needed to replace red blood cells. Corticosteroids may be administered to the patient. The patient usually recovers in a few days to weeks.

Iron-Deficiency Anemia

Iron-deficiency anemia results from a diet too low in iron or from the body not absorbing enough iron from the gastrointestinal tract. As a result, the body does not have enough iron to make adequate amounts of hemoglobin. Older adults with poor eating habits frequently suffer from anemia. Symptoms of this anemia include fatigue and pallor. In severe cases patients may have orthostatic changes in their heart rate and blood pressure. In addition to a low red blood cell count, a low hemoglobin value, and a low hematocrit, patients with iron-deficiency anemia have a low serum iron level, a low ferritin level, and a high total iron-binding capacity.

Physicians treat iron-deficiency anemia by prescribing iron supplements such as ferrous sulfate and iron dextran. Table 31-12 describes the nursing care of the patient taking iron supplements. Nurses caring for patients with iron-deficiency anemia can suggest incorporating foods high in iron into the diet. Foods that are rich in iron include liver, oysters, red meats, fish, dried fruits, legumes (e. g., dried beans and peas), dark green vegetables, and iron-enriched whole grain breads and cereals.

PHARMACOLOGY CAPSULE Large doses of iron can be toxic. Caution patients not to exceed recommended dosage, and to keep the drug out of the reach of children.

Pernicious Anemia (Vitamin B_{12} Anemia)

Pernicious anemia occurs when a person does not absorb vitamin B_{12} from the stomach. The person may lack intrinsic factor, a substance made in the stomach that is essential for B_{12} absorption. The individual may have had a gastrectomy, in which part or all of the stomach was surgically removed, and so cannot make intrinsic factor and therefore cannot absorb vitamin B_{12}. In addition to the fatigue and pallor commonly seen with all anemias, symptoms of pernicious anemia characteristically include weakness, a sore tongue, and numbness of the hands or feet. Physicians treat pernicious anemia by prescribing a monthly intramuscular injection of vitamin B_{12} (cyanocobalamin). Table 31-12 describes the nursing care of patients receiving vitamin B_{12}.

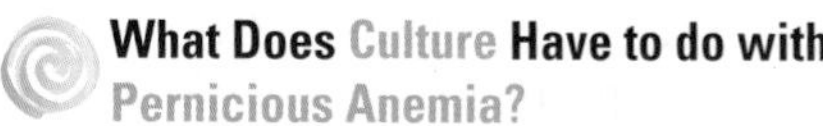

What Does Culture Have to do with Pernicious Anemia?

The incidence of pernicious anemia is high among Scandinavians and African Americans.

Sickle Cell Anemia

Sickle cell anemia is a disease in which the normally disc-shaped red blood cells become sickle-shaped (Fig. 31-2). These misshapen blood cells are much more fragile than normal red blood cells, and as a result, the sickled cells easily rupture as they pass through small capillaries, resulting in a chronic anemia. Additionally, these abnormally shaped, sickled cells become stuck in the small capillaries of the body, obstructing blood flow.

Sickle cell anemia is a genetic disease occurring almost exclusively in African Americans. Eight percent of blacks carry the genetic trait for sickle cell anemia. Because sickle cell anemia is carried on a recessive gene, a person must inherit the gene from both the mother and the father to actually have the disease. Newborn screening for hemoglobin S can be done to identify infants with sickle cell disease and to educate parents about the disease and prevention of crises. Unfortunately, this screening is not required in every state.

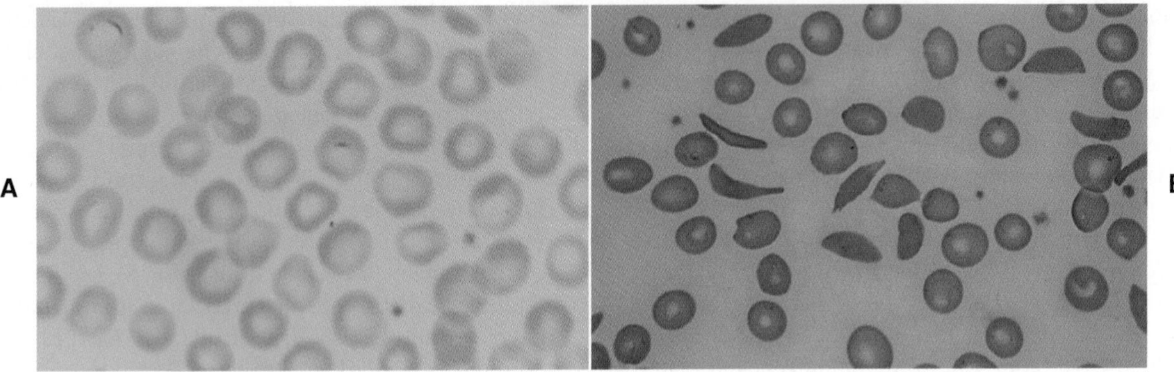

FIGURE **31-2** Comparison of normal red blood cells *(A)* and sickled cells *(B)* (magnification ×875).

Symptoms of sickle cell anemia include persistently low red blood cell counts, fatigue, and jaundice. The chronically low red blood cell counts can cause the heart to enlarge (cardiomegaly) and beat faster in an attempt to oxygenate the body's tissues. A sickle cell crisis occurs when the sickled cells become stuck in larger blood vessels of the body, obstructing blood flow and causing severe pain.

Signs and symptoms of sickle cell crisis. Various stressors can trigger a sickle cell crisis. They include dehydration, infection, overexertion, cold weather changes, excessive alcohol consumption, and smoking. Symptoms vary depending upon where circulation is blocked by the sickled red blood cells. Commonly during a sickle cell crisis, circulation to the chest, abdomen, bones, joints, bone marrow, brain, or penis may be compromised. With circulation obstructed, tissue hypoxia occurs, causing severe pain. Patients in a sickle cell crisis often have a fever, either because infection precipitated the crisis or as part of the inflammatory response to tissue hypoxia.

Medical diagnosis of sickle cell disease. Patients with known sickle cell disease complaining of severe pain are suspected of being in crisis. There is no test to determine that a patient is in sickle cell crisis. Rather, physicians use clinical judgment to make the diagnosis. Crises can last anywhere from 1 to 10 days. Some patients experience crises every few weeks, whereas other patients can go months without experiencing painful episodes. Radiographs and scans of the painful area are usually taken to evaluate for bleeding.

Medical treatment of the patient in sickle cell crisis. There is no cure for sickle cell disease. Medical treatment for patients experiencing a sickle cell crisis is symptomatic. The physician usually prescribes intravenous fluids and pain medication. Aggressive intravenous hydration helps the kidneys clear the metabolic wastes from ruptured red blood cells. The pain can be very severe, and the patient needs adequate pain relief during these episodes even if they last for several days. Intravenous morphine commonly is prescribed for pain relief. Patients with sickle cell disease can become addicted to opioids. Therefore, physicians try to quickly transition the patient from intravenous opioids to oral opioids to nonopioid pain relievers as the crisis resolves. Red blood cell transfusions may be prescribed to correct the anemia and help the body oxygenate tissues. While oxygen therapy is often prescribed, it is of little benefit in reversing the crisis.

For patients who experience frequent crises, the drug hydroxyurea can be prescribed. Hydroxyurea has been used for many years as a treatment for leukemia. The drug also stimulates the production of a certain type of hemoglobin that is resistant to sickling. Patients with sickle cell disease who regularly take hydroxyurea experience fewer crises. However, once a patient is in crisis, hydroxyurea does not work quickly enough to reduce either the severity or the duration of the crisis. Table 31-12 describes the nursing care of patients receiving hydroxyurea.

NURSING CARE *of the Patient in Sickle Cell Crisis*

Patients in sickle cell crisis have specialized needs beyond treatment of the simple anemia. (See Nursing Care Plan: The Patient in Sickle Cell Crisis.)

Assessment

Obtain a complete description of the pain that the patient in sickle cell crisis is experiencing. Document the location, intensity, duration, and precipitating events. Measure vital signs every 4 hours. Be especially alert for a fever, which may indicate an infection that precipitated the crisis. Investigate any symptoms of an infection, such as sore throat, cough, abnormal breath sounds, dysuria, or diarrhea. Also assess the patient for signs and symptoms of dehydration, such as concentrated urine, low blood pressure, or poor skin turgor, which may have precipitated the crisis.

Nursing Diagnoses, Goals, and Outcome Criteria: Sickle Cell Crisis

Nursing Diagnoses	Goals and Outcome Criteria
Acute Pain related to sickle cell crisis	Pain relief: patient states pain has been relieved, relaxed manner
Anxiety related to pain and hospitalization	Reduced anxiety: patient states anxiety is reduced, calm manner

NURSING CARE PLAN

The Patient in Sickle Cell Crisis

ASSESSMENT

Health History: Tabitha Simmons is a 19-year-old African-American woman who was diagnosed with sickle cell anemia at age 12. She has been in stable health until 3 days ago, when she complained of nausea and began to have diarrhea and vomiting. She has taken only soup and cola beverages since that time. When she began to complain of severe pain in her abdomen, she was brought to the emergency room by her mother, who suspected sickle cell crisis.

Physical Examination: T, 102° F; P, 106, regular; R, 24; BP, 110/56. Oral mucosa dry. Skin dry and warm to touch. Breath sounds clear to auscultation. Abdomen soft, but tender to light palpation. Bowel sounds hyperactive in all 4 quadrants. No bladder distention. Mild joint enlargement noted in both knees.

Nursing Diagnosis	*Goals and Outcome Criteria*	*Interventions*
Acute pain related to sickle cell crisis.	Pain relief: patient states pain has been relieved, appears relaxed.	Administer analgesics as prescribed. Assess effects and notify physician if pain is not relieved. Have Tabitha rate pain (1 = least, 10 = most) before and after medication. Use distraction technique. Respond to calls quickly. Reassure.
Anxiety related to pain and hospitalization.	Reduced anxiety: patient states anxiety is reduced, appears calm.	Respond quickly to her needs. Check on her often. Assign consistent caregiver. Listen. Use attention and touch to convey concern.
Risk for injury related to orthostatic hypotension.	Absence of injury: no falls caused by dizziness.	Assist out of bed when permitted. Have her sit on bedside and exercise legs before rising. Check BP in lying, sitting, and standing positions to detect orthostatic hypotension. Advise her to sit and lower her head if dizzy.
Risk for deficient fluid volume related to inadequate intake and excess loss of fluids.	Adequate hydration: consistent intake of 4-6 liters of fluid daily, moist oral tissues, normal urine specific gravity.	Administer intravenous fluids as ordered. Teach importance of fluid intake. Weigh daily to assess change in fluid status. Monitor fluid intake and output. Note urine characteristics.
Ineffective therapeutic regimen management related to lack of knowledge of disease process and self-care.	Effective management of condition: patient accurately describes disease process and implications of self-care measures.	Assess what she knows about sickle cell disease. Initiate teaching when crisis has resolved. She should know to avoid smoking, alcohol, and high altitudes. Emphasize need to maintain good hydration (4-6 liters fluids each day) and to keep regular medical appointments.

Risk for Injury related to orthostatic hypotension	Absence of injury: no falls caused by dizziness
Risk for Deficient Fluid Volume related to inadequate intake or excess loss of fluids	Adequate hydration: consistent intake of 4 to 6 liters of fluid daily
Ineffective Therapeutic Regimen Management related to lack of knowledge of the disease process and self-care	Effective management of condition: patient accurately describes disease process and implications for self-care measures

Interventions

Acute Pain

Give pain medications as prescribed. Usually intravenous morphine is prescribed. Initially it is not unusual for patients to need large amounts of medication to control the pain. One option for medication delivery is patient-controlled analgesia. Closely monitor the patient's pain level and medication usage. Good documentation can contribute to effective pain management. Keeping a flow sheet of patient reports of pain on a 10-point scale can be helpful, especially as different nurses care for the patient throughout the day. A 0 represents no pain, while a 10 represents the worst pain a patient ever experienced. The patient report of pain, coupled with the amount of pain medication he or she is receiving, can guide you and the physician as to the appropriate type and amount of pain medication. A detailed discussion of pain management strategies is presented in Chapter 14.

Anxiety

Sickle cell crises can be extremely frightening to a patient, especially because of the severe pain that accompanies these crises. Patients fear not obtaining adequate pain relief. The unpredictability of both the timing and the severity of the crises can be especially frustrating to patients. Provide consistent care to the patient in sickle cell crisis to establish a trusting relationship. Listening closely to the patient helps establish this trust, thereby reducing patient anxiety. Once the patient is discharged from the hospital, he or she can contact one of the many support groups available for patients with sickle cell disease and their families. Patients should be encouraged to attend meetings of these groups so that they can better cope with this chronic disease.

Risk for Injury

The primary treatment for anemia is red blood cell transfusions. Nursing considerations in administering blood transfusions were outlined earlier in this chapter. Nursing actions that should be taken when patients are anemic are outlined in Table 31-6. Procedures for administering a red blood cell transfusion are outlined in Table 31-9.

Deficient Fluid Volume

Administer intravenous fluids as prescribed and keep records of fluid intake and output. Measure daily weights to assess gross fluid status. Encourage the patient to drink 4 to 6 liters of fluids each day to maintain adequate hydration.

Ineffective Therapeutic Regimen Management

When patients are not in crisis, they should be taught about their disease. Help patients identify stressors that bring on a crisis, and help them take actions to avoid these stressors. Encourage these patients not to smoke or drink large amounts of alcoholic beverages, as these are two common stressors that can bring on a crisis. Traveling to high altitudes where there is less oxygen can bring on an attack, so patients should be warned about vacationing at high altitudes. Drinking 4 to 6 liters of nonalcoholic fluids a day helps to maintain adequate hydration. Regular medical follow-up is extremely important in keeping the patient with sickle cell disease out of a crisis.

Genetic counseling can be done with people who have the sickle cell gene to inform them of the risk of passing on the trait or disease to their children. With this information, some people choose not to have their own children and risk passing on this painful, life-threatening disease. There are several resources available for patients, families, and health care providers including the Sickle Cell Disease Association of America (200 Corporate Point, Suite 495, Culver City, CA 90231-8727; website: http://www.sicklecelldisease.org; telephone: 1-800-421-8453) and the Sickle Cell Information Center sponsored by the Georgia Comprehensive Sickle Cell Center and Grady Health System, Emory University School of Medicine Department of Pediatrics, the Sickle Cell Foundation of Georgia, and Morehouse School of Medicine (PO Box 109, Grady Memorial Hospital, 80 Butler Street SE, Atlanta, GA 30303; website: http://www.emory.edu/PEDS/SICKLE; telephone: 1-404-616-3572). These organizations provide excellent free literature on sickle cell disease and can help locate groups in specific regions of the country.

PATIENT TEACHING PLAN
Sickle Cell Anemia

- To prevent crises, maintain good hydration and avoid smoking, alcoholic beverages, and high altitudes.
- Drink 4 to 6 liters of fluid each day to maintain adequate hydration.
- Genetic counseling can help you with decisions about having children by exploring the risk of passing on sickle cell trait or disease.
- You can get additional information from the Sickle Cell Disease Association of America or the Sickle Cell Information Center.

Put on your THINKING CAP!!

How would a high fluid intake decrease the risk of sickle cell crisis?

COAGULATION DISORDERS

Coagulation disorders can result from a platelet abnormality or from a clotting factor deficiency.

Types of Coagulation Disorders

Thrombocytopenia

Thrombocytopenia is a condition in which a person has too few platelets circulating in the blood. This may be because not enough platelets are being made in the bone marrow or because too many platelets are being destroyed in circulation.

The major cause of thrombocytopenia related to inadequate production of platelets is treatment of cancer with chemotherapy or radiation therapy. Both chemotherapy and radiation therapy kill rapidly dividing cells. Unfortunately, the therapy cannot tell the difference between rapidly dividing cancer cells and rapidly dividing normal cells like those that produce platelets. In patients treated with chemotherapy or radiation therapy, thrombocytopenia can be expected 10 to 14 days following treatment and lasts until the bone marrow is able to make more platelets, which is usually a week.

Two examples of thrombocytopenia resulting from too many platelets being either destroyed or consumed are idiopathic thrombocytopenic purpura (ITP) and thrombotic thrombocytopenic purpura (TTP). Both of these disorders are abnormal immunologic processes that result in thrombocytopenia. ITP and TTP are discussed in more detail in Chapter 32.

Symptoms of thrombocytopenia include petechiae and purpura, gingival bleeding, epistaxis (nose bleeds), or any other unusual or prolonged bleeding. The diagnosis is made with blood tests and a bone marrow biopsy. Treatment for thrombocytopenia is to treat or stop the causative factor. If the cause is cancer chemotherapy or radiation therapy, platelet transfusions may be prescribed. Nursing actions for the patient who is at risk for injury from bleeding are outlined in Table 31-7. Procedures for administration of a platelet transfusion are outlined in Table 31-10.

Disseminated Intravascular Coagulation

Disseminated intravascular coagulation (DIC) is a hypercoagulable state, meaning that blood clotting is abnormally increased. DIC occurs when overstimulation of the normal coagulation cascade results in simultaneous thrombosis and hemorrhage. DIC is always secondary to another pathologic process, such as overwhelming sepsis, shock, major trauma, crush injuries, burns, cancer, acute tumor lysis syndrome, or obstetric complications such as abruptio placentae or fetal demise (death). Coagulation occurs at so many sites in the body that eventually all available platelets and clotting factors are depleted and uncontrolled hemorrhage results.

Blood tests that help diagnose DIC include the prothrombin time, partial thromboplastin time, fibrinogen level, thrombin time, fibrin split products level, and D-dimers.

Blood component replacement therapy may be prescribed. However, some physicians believe additional platelets and clotting factors perpetuate the abnormal DIC feedback loop and so do not prescribe blood component replacement. Heparin may be prescribed to interrupt the DIC cycle and allow the body to replenish platelets and clotting factors. However, heparin therapy is also controversial, as some physicians believe it only makes the bleeding worse. Nursing actions for the patient who is at risk for injury from bleeding are outlined in Table 31-7.

Put on your THINKING CAP!!

Explain how heparin could be helpful for a patient with DIC.

Hemophilia

Hemophilia is a genetic disease in which the affected person lacks some of the blood clotting factors normally found in plasma. The incidence of hemophilia is one to two cases per 20,000 persons. In hemophilia A, factor VIII is missing, whereas in hemophilia B, factor IX is missing. Hemophilia A has a much higher incidence than hemophilia B. Because the trait is carried on the X chromosome, women carry the trait and can pass it on to their sons, who manifest the disease. Because this recessive trait is carried only on the X chromosome, it is rare for women to have the disease.

Signs and symptoms. Uncontrollable bleeding is the hallmark of hemophilia. Bleeding generally occurs after some sort of trauma; however, bleeding can also occur spontaneously for no clear reason. Most commonly, bleeding occurs into the joints, causing swelling and severe pain. Bleeding also can occur into the skin; from the mouth, gums, and lips; and from the gastrointestinal tract. Because any surgical procedure puts the patient at great risk for bleeding, a complete preoperative evaluation must be done. Also, the availability of replacement factors for transfusion must be confirmed.

Medical diagnosis. The diagnosis of hemophilia is made by measuring factors VIII and IX in the blood. Also, the partial thromboplastin time is prolonged in people with hemophilia.

Medical treatment. There is no cure for hemophilia. Medical treatment for patients experiencing a bleeding episode is symptomatic. The physician usually prescribes transfusions of fresh frozen plasma or cryoprecipitate, or both. Patients with hemophilia A need factor VIII, which is found in both fresh frozen plasma and cryoprecipitate. Patients with hemophilia B need factor IX, which is found in fresh frozen plasma. Red blood cell transfusions are frequently used to replace blood lost from the profuse bleeding to which hemophiliacs are prone. The pain can be very severe. The patient needs adequate pain relief during these episodes even if they last several days. Intravenous morphine is commonly prescribed for pain relief. Because patients with hemophilia can become addicted to opioids, pain must be carefully assessed. Usually physicians try quickly to transition the patient from intravenous opioids to oral opioids to nonopioid pain relievers as the crisis resolves.

NURSING CARE *of the Patient with Hemophilia*

Assessment

Assess the patient for bleeding and pain, noting what measures have stopped the bleeding and relieved the pain in the past. Monitor vital signs and urine output.

Nursing Diagnoses, Goals, and Outcome Criteria: Hemophilia

Nursing Diagnoses	Goals and Outcome Criteria
Risk for Injury related to bleeding	Cessation of bleeding: no visible bleeding, stable vital signs
Acute Pain related to bleeding into closed spaces, creating pressure on nerves	Pain relief: patient states pain is relieved, relaxed manner
Ineffective Therapeutic Regimen Management related to lack of knowledge about the disease process and self-care	Effective management of condition: patient accurately describes condition and demonstrates self-care measures

Interventions

Risk for Injury

The primary treatment to control bleeding in hemophilia is to transfuse fresh frozen plasma, cryoprecipitate, or both. Nursing considerations in administering these products are outlined in Table 31-8. Bleeding precautions that should be taken when patients have hemophilia are similar to bleeding precautions taken when patients are thrombocytopenic. Refer to Table 31-7 for these bleeding precautions.

Acute Pain

Give pain medications as prescribed. If the patient is experiencing a great deal of pain, patient-controlled analgesia may be appropriate. Closely monitor the patient's pain level on a scale of 0 to 10. Keeping a flow sheet of patient reports of pain on a 10-point scale can be helpful, especially as different nurses care for the patient throughout the day. The patient's report of pain, coupled with the amount of pain medication he or she is receiving, can guide the nurse and physician as to the appropriate type and amount of pain medication. A detailed discussion of pain management is presented in Chapter 14.

Nutrition Concepts

1. Iron-deficiency anemia is caused by inadequate dietary intake of iron or inadequate absorption of dietary iron.
2. The lack of intrinsic factor, which is normally manufactured in the stomach, prevents the absorption of vitamin B_{12}, and leads to pernicious anemia.

Ineffective Therapeutic Regimen Management

Hemophiliacs bleed with even the smallest bruise or abrasion. Patients and their families should be taught to prevent injury and to safeguard their environment against accidents as much as possible. Some patients and families are taught to administer the replacement concentrate at home so that if an injury does occur, prompt treatment can be initiated and blood loss minimized. Genetic counseling can be done with people with the hemophilia gene to inform them of the risk of passing on the disease to their children. With this information, some people choose not to have their own children and risk passing on this painful, life-threatening disease. The National Hemophilia Foundation (116 West 32nd Street, 11th Floor, New York, NY 10001; website: http://www.hemophilia.org; telephone: 1-212-328-3700 or 1-800-424-2634) provides information and support to patients with hemophilia and their families.

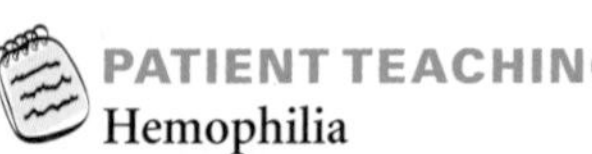

Hemophilia

- Protect yourself from injuries by avoiding activities that could result in trauma.
- Know the emergency treatment of bleeding episodes: first aid measures (apply pressure, immobilize and elevate affected part if possible), seek medical attention, administer replacement concentrate (if prescribed).
- A resource for additional information is the National Hemophilia Foundation.

The views of this author are her own and do not purport to reflect the position of the Army Medical Department, Department of the Army, or the Department of Defense.

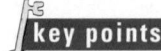

- The hematologic system includes the bone marrow, liver, spleen, and blood.
- A healthy adult has about 6 liters of blood circulating through the body.
- Components of the blood are red blood cells, platelets, clotting factors, and plasma, as well as white blood cells, proteins, electrolytes, hormones, and enzymes.
- Signs of hematologic abnormalities can include petechiae, purpura, and ecchymoses.
- The four major blood groups are A, B, AB, and O; each group may be Rh negative or Rh positive.
- People with type O-negative blood are universal blood donors, and people with type AB-positive blood are universal blood recipients.
- Types of reaction that can occur when blood or blood components are transfused include hemolytic, anaphylactic, febrile, and circulatory overload.
- Anemia is a deficiency of red blood cells or hemoglobin that may be due to blood loss, an iron-deficient diet, vitamin B_{12} deficiency, bone marrow failure, or genetic abnormalities.
- Sickle cell anemia is an incurable genetic condition in which red blood cells can become abnormally sickle-shaped so that they rupture easily and can obstruct capillaries.
- Sickle cell crisis, characterized by severe pain, occurs when blood flow is obstructed.
- Nursing diagnoses during sickle cell crisis focus on the patient's acute pain, anxiety, risk for injury, risk for deficient fluid volume, and ineffective therapeutic regimen management.
- Thrombocytopenia is a deficiency of platelets that can lead to excessive or prolonged bleeding.
- Hemophilia, an incurable genetic disease in which some of the factors needed for blood clotting are absent, is treated with replacement clotting factors.
- Nursing diagnoses for the patient with hemophilia include the patient's risk for injury, acute pain, and ineffective therapeutic regimen management.

REVIEW QUESTIONS

1. If a person has no A or B antigens, what is his blood type?
   1. AB
   2. A
   3. B
   4. O

2. When assessing a patient, you notice multiple ecchymoses and petechiae. This should lead you to suspect a deficiency of:
   1. red blood cells.
   2. white blood cells.
   3. platelets.
   4. protein.

3. A patient says he is a universal donor. This means his blood type is:
   1. AB positive.
   2. O positive.
   3. O negative.
   4. AB negative.

4. While receiving a blood transfusion, a patient complains of chest and back pain and chills. Your initial action should be to:
   1. notify the blood bank.
   2. take vital signs.
   3. administer acetaminophen.
   4. stop the transfusion.

5. Which nursing intervention is appropriate for a patient with a low red blood cell count?
   1. Avoid rectal temperatures and suppositories.
   2. Allow for rest between periods of activity.
   3. Encourage increased fluids and dietary fiber.
   4. Do not allow fresh flowers in the room.

6. A deficiency of red blood cells, white blood cells, and platelets is characteristic of:
   1. aplastic anemia.
   2. hemolytic anemia.
   3. sickle cell anemia.
   4. iron-deficiency anemia.

7. Sickle cell crisis occurs when:
   1. cell lack sufficient hemoglobin to transport oxygen.
   2. sickled cells are unable to transport adequate oxygen.
   3. sickled cells form clumps that obstruct blood flow.
   4. the bone marrow stops producing red blood cells.

8. Factors that can trigger a sickle cell crisis include:
   1. dehydration.
   2. inactivity.
   3. low iron intake.
   4. caffeine consumption.

9. Overstimulation of the normal blood clotting process can result in:
   1. disseminated intravascular coagulation.
   2. idiopathic thrombocytopenic purpura.
   3. thrombotic thrombocytopenic purpura.
   4. hemophilia.

10. Hemophilia A is treated with:
    1. factor VI.
    2. factor VII.
    3. factor VIII.
    4. factor IX.

CHAPTER

32 Immunologic Disorders

STACEY YOUNG-MCCAUGHAN

objectives

1. List the components of the immune system and describe their role in innate immunity, acquired immunity, and tolerance.
2. List the data to be collected when assessing a patient with a disorder of the immune system.
3. Describe the tests and procedures used to diagnose disorders of the immune system and nursing considerations for each.
4. Describe the nursing care for patients undergoing common therapeutic measures for disorders of the immune system.
5. For selected disorders of the immune system, describe the pathophysiology, signs and symptoms, medical diagnosis, and medical treatment.
6. Assist in developing a nursing care plan for a patient with a disorder of the immune system.

key terms

Acquired immunity (p. 533)
Antibody (ĂN-tĭ-bŏ-dē, p. 533)
Antibody-mediated immunity (p. 533)
Antigen (ĂN-tĭ-jĕn, p. 532)
Cell-mediated immunity (p. 534)
Compromised host precautions (p. 544)
Eicosanoid (ĭ-KŌ-săh-noid, p. 533)
Immunity (ĭ-MŪ-nĭ-tē, p. 533)
Immunoglobulin (ĭm-ū-nō-GLŎB-ū-lĭn, p. 532)
Innate immunity (p. 533)
Leukemia (lū-KĒ-mē-ă, p. 535)
Pathogen (PĂTH-ō-jĕn, p. 530)
Phagocytes (FĂG-ō-sīts, p. 533)

The immune system is the body's defense network against infection. It is an inherently complex system that recognizes, isolates, and destroys pathogens as quickly as possible. Disorders of the immune system leave the patient susceptible to overwhelming, life-threatening infections. The nurse plays an important role in helping to assess, plan, and manage the care of patients with these disorders.

ANATOMY AND PHYSIOLOGY OF THE IMMUNE SYSTEM

ANATOMIC STRUCTURES AND COMPONENTS OF THE IMMUNE SYSTEM

Bone Marrow

The bone marrow is the spongy center of the bones where the white blood cells are made. The marrow of all bones produces these cells; however, in adults the majority of white blood cells are produced in the vertebrae, ribs, sternum, skull, pelvis, and long bones of the legs.

Lymph, Lymphatics, and Lymph Nodes

When blood flows through the capillary beds to deliver oxygen and pick up carbon dioxide, not all the plasma returns to the veins to be recirculated. The lymphatic system is a network of open-ended tubes—separate from the blood circulation system—that collects the plasma left behind in the tissues and returns it to the venous system. Additionally, various white blood cells that travel through tissues and organs monitoring for infection reenter the blood circulation via the lymphatic system. This mixture of plasma and cells is known as lymph fluid. Lymph fluid is propelled along the lymphatic system by the normal contraction of skeletal muscles. One-way valves located in the lymphatic vessels prevent the lymph fluid from pooling in the periphery. The lymphatic vessels empty into the venous system through the right lymphatic duct of the right subclavian vein and the thoracic duct of the left subclavian vein. Figure 32-1 shows the flow of lymph fluid and where it empties into these ducts.

Lymph nodes are small patches of lymphatic tissue located along the lymphatic system that filter microorganisms from the lymph fluid before it is returned to the bloodstream. Lymph nodes are located throughout the body, as shown in Figure 32-1. The lymph nodes can become swollen with infection and also with some cancers. The nodes closer to the surface of the body in the neck, under the arm, and in the groin can be palpated when they are swollen. Usually lymph nodes deeper in the body cannot be palpated but can be visualized on computed tomography if they are larger than 2 cm. During surgery for cancer, the surgeon will usually biopsy nearby lymph nodes and have the pathologist check the specimens to see if the cancer might have spread.

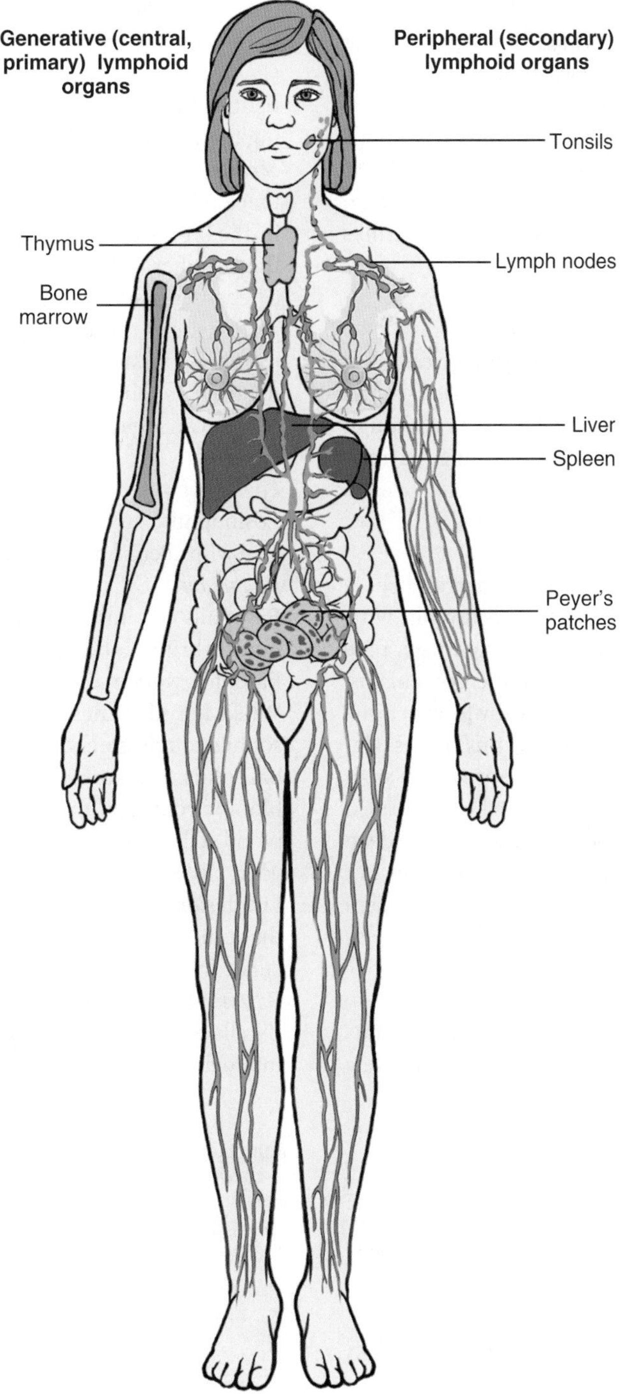

FIGURE **32-1** Diagram of the lymphatic system.

Spleen

The spleen is located in the upper left quadrant of the abdomen. Like the lymph nodes, the spleen filters microorganisms from the blood. Once trapped in the spleen, microorganisms are destroyed by the white blood cells that reside in the spleen.

Under some circumstances the spleen is surgically removed. Trauma from a motor vehicle accident can rupture the victim's spleen, necessitating removal. Patients newly diagnosed with Hodgkin's disease, a form of cancer of the lymph nodes, may have their spleens removed and pathologically examined to help determine the best treatment. Anyone without a spleen is at greater risk for certain kinds of infections such as pneumococcal infections. If possible, patients should receive a Pneumovax vaccine before undergoing splenectomy so that the body can form its own antibodies against pneumococcal bacteria. Vaccinations are not always possible for the individual undergoing an emergency splenectomy.

Thymus

The thymus is a lymphoid organ located in the upper chest below the thyroid. Early in life certain white blood cells, called lymphocytes, migrate from the bone marrow where they are produced to the thymus where they mature into T lymphocytes, or T cells. Mature T lymphocytes are then released into circulation. After puberty, the T cell population has been maximized. The thymus stops growing and eventually shrinks because it is no longer needed to mature T cells.

Stem Cells

Stem cells are called progenitor cells, or precursor cells, because they are capable of developing into the various white blood cells, red blood cells, or platelets (Fig. 32-2). Although the majority of stem cells are located in the bone marrow, some stem cells circulate in the blood.

White Blood Cells (Leukocytes)

White blood cells are produced by the bone marrow. There are five major types of white blood cells: neutrophils, lymphocytes, eosinophils, basophils, and monocytes. Each type of white blood cell combats certain types of microorganisms. Normally, white blood cells identify and destroy foreign antigens or proteins by ingesting them. Because this process destroys the white blood cells themselves, the normal life span for a white blood cell is only about 12 hours. Other cells called macrophages clean up the white blood cell debris. If the dead white blood cells build up faster than the macrophages can clean them up, pus is formed. This is why pus is a classic sign of infection and should immediately be reported to a nurse or a physician and carefully monitored.

Neutrophils

Neutrophils fight bacterial infections. They are the most numerous of the white blood cells, comprising approximately 60% of all the white blood cells. These cells are known by many names, including polymorphonuclear neutrophils (PMNs, polys), neuts, granulocytes (grans), or segmented neutrophils (segs). The bone marrow is capable of producing huge numbers of neutrophils to fight infection.

Monocytes and Macrophages

Once released from the bone marrow, monocytes circulate in the bloodstream for approximately 1 day before leaving the peripheral circulation and entering tissue. When monocytes enter tissue, they are called macrophages. Some macrophages move throughout the body, while others stay in one particular tissue monitoring for microorganisms. Unlike neutrophils, which are destroyed during phagocytosis, macrophages can ingest many foreign antigens and survive months to years.

Eosinophils

Eosinophils combat parasitic infections. They are also associated with allergic reactions and other inflammatory processes.

Basophils

Basophils can initiate a massive inflammatory response that quickly brings other white blood cells to the site of infection. Basophils work in conjunction with immunoglobulin E (IgE). When IgE identifies a foreign antigen, the IgE triggers basophils to release histamine from cell vesicles located in the basophils. Histamine is a potent vasodilator that increases blood circulation to the site, quickly bringing other white blood cells to the site of infection.

Mast Cells

Like basophils, mast cells also store histamine in cell vesicles that can be released by IgE. Whereas basophils normally circulate in the blood, mast cells are located in the tissue.

B Lymphocytes (B Cells)

B cells manufacture antigen-binding proteins, called immunoglobulins, on their cell membrane. When the B cell im-

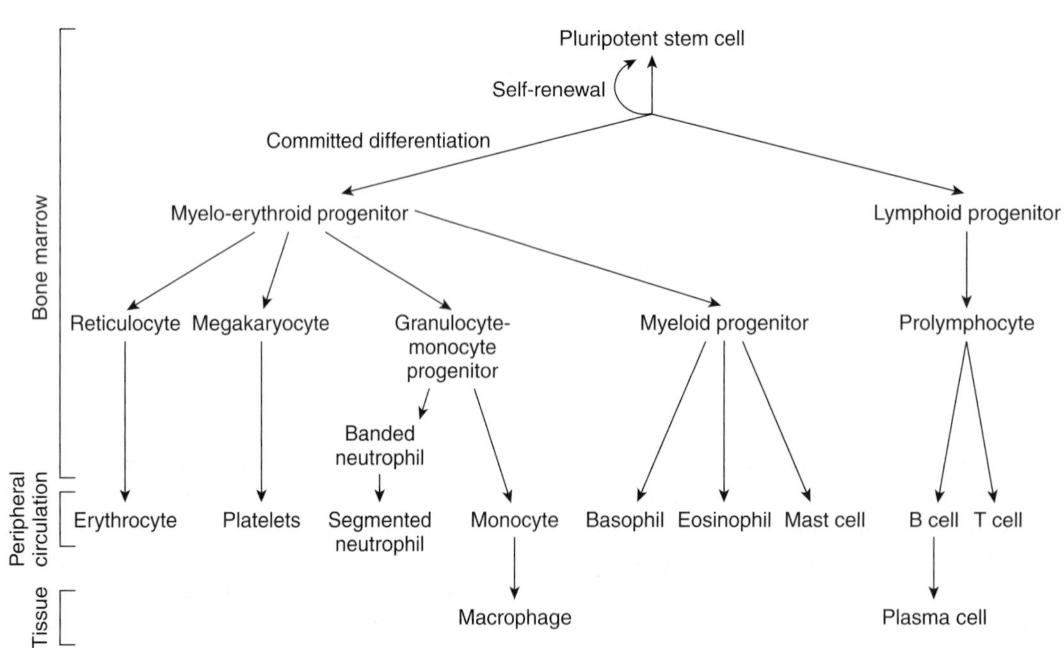

FIGURE 32-2 Maturation of cells constituting the hematologic and immune systems.

munoglobulin binds with a particular antigen, the B cell is stimulated to produce plasma cells and memory B cells. Plasma cells are antibody factories that immediately produce large amounts of immunoglobulin. Memory B cells go into a resting state but can be quickly reactivated to produce plasma cells and antibodies if exposed to the same antigen in the future.

Once the immunoglobulin is released from the membrane of either the B cell or the plasma cell, it is called an antibody. There are four major types of antibodies. IgM is the first immunoglobulin to be secreted during the primary immune response to an antigen.

IgG is secreted during the secondary immune response and is more specific to a particular antigen.

IgA is present in secretions such as mucus and mother's milk. IgE attaches to the cell membranes of basophils and mast cells, where it triggers the cell to release histamine.

T Lymphocytes (T Cells)

There are two major types of T lymphocytes: T helper (T_H) cells and T cytotoxic (T_C) cells. T_H cells are also called CD4 cells because of the protein complex CD4 found on their cell membranes. When T_H cells come in contact with foreign antigens, they secrete cytokines that activate other components of the immune system to facilitate the body's immune response. These are the cells that can become infected with the human immunodeficiency virus (HIV). T_C cells are also called CD8 cells because of the protein complex CD8 found on their cell membrane. When T_C cells come in contact with foreign antigens, they can directly destroy the invader.

Cytokines

Cytokines are hormones secreted by cells to signal other cells. Examples of cytokines include interferon, interleukin, tumor necrosis factor (TNF), granulocyte-macrophage colony-stimulating factor (GM-CSF), granulocyte colony-stimulating factor (G-CSF), and erythropoietin (EPO).

Eicosanoids

Eicosanoids are a class of fatty acids that regulate blood vessel vasodilation, temperature elevation, white blood cell activation, and other physiologic processes involved in immunity. Many commonly prescribed drugs, such as nonsteroidal anti-inflammatory drugs (NSAIDs), disrupt eicosanoid production, thereby affecting a person's ability to mount an immunologic response.

PHYSIOLOGIC FUNCTIONS OF THE IMMUNE SYSTEM

Innate Immunity

Innate immunity is operational at all times, whether a pathogen is present or not. At birth, innate immunologic defense systems are immediately functional. Innate immunologic systems include anatomic and physiologic barriers, inflammatory response, and the ability of certain cells to phagocytose foreign invaders.

Anatomic and Physiologic Barriers

The skin and mucous membranes are the body's first line of defense, acting as a protective covering and secreting substances that inhibit the growth of pathogens. Sweat glands secrete a lysozyme, an antimicrobial enzyme. The skin and the mucosa of the gastrointestinal and genitourinary systems are acidic, which inhibits the growth of many pathogenic organisms. Secretions from the respiratory and gastrointestinal tracts contain the antibody IgA, as well as phagocytes. Skin and mucous membrane surfaces are colonized by normal bacterial flora, which prevents pathogens from attaching and gaining access to the body. Also, coughing and sneezing, peristalsis in the gastrointestinal tract, emptying the bladder, and sloughing of dead skin cells all serve to remove microorganisms from the body, thus preventing their invasion and overgrowth.

Inflammation

The body initially responds to an injury or infection by dilating the capillary bed and increasing the capillary permeability of the affected area. This brings white blood cells to the site and allows them to enter the tissue to attack microorganisms. This multistep process is called inflammation and is recognized by rubor (redness), tumor (swelling), calor (heat), and dolor (pain) at the site of injury or infection.

Phagocytosis

Phagocytosis is the process of ingesting and digesting invading pathogens, dead cells, and cellular debris. Neutrophils, monocytes, and macrophages are capable of phagocytosis and are sometimes called phagocytes.

Acquired Immunity

Whereas innate immunity fights any type of invader and is operational at all times, acquired immunity is specific to a particular pathogen and is activated only when needed. The two types of acquired immunity are antibody-mediated and cell-mediated.

Antibody-Mediated Immunity

An antibody-mediated immune response is initiated when the IgM immunoglobulins on the surface of B lymphocytes detect a foreign antigen. With the help of T_H cells, the B lymphocytes secrete additional IgM and differentiate to produce antibody-secreting plasma cells and memory B cells. The newly made plasma cells can produce and secrete large amounts of IgM antibody. When antibodies bind to an antigen, they do not actually destroy the pathogen, but they make the antigen readily recognizable to neutrophils, monocytes, and macrophages, which can phagocytose the pathogen. If in the future this same pathogen tries to reenter the body, the memory B cells are triggered to immediately produce large amounts of IgG antibody. IgG is like IgM except that it is more specific to one particular pathogen, based on the previous experience with that same pathogen.

Acquired antibody immunity can be active or passive. Active acquired immunity occurs when a person synthesizes his or her own antibodies in response to a pathogen. A person is exhibiting active acquired immunity when he or she manufactures antibodies in response to an infection or a vaccination. Active acquired immunity is permanent. Passive acquired immunity occurs when an antibody produced by one person or an animal is transferred to another person. For example, IgA antibodies in mother's milk confer passive immunity to breast-fed babies. Another example of passive acquired immunity is the gamma globulin that may be given to a person exposed to hepatitis. Gamma globulin contains IgG antibodies that help destroy the hepatitis virus. Passive acquired immunity lasts only 1 to 2 months after the antibodies have been received.

Cell-Mediated Immunity

Antibody-mediated immune responses are aimed primarily at invading microorganisms such as bacteria. In contrast, cell-mediated immunity is aimed primarily at intracellular defects caused by viruses and cancer. Cell-mediated immunity is also responsible for delayed hypersensitivity reactions and rejection of transplanted tissue. T_C cells are the primary component of cell-mediated immunity. When T_C cells recognize foreign antigens in cells, they secrete cytotoxic substances that destroy the defective cells. Unfortunately, a transplanted tissue graft, such as a kidney transplant or a heart transplant, may be recognized by the organ recipient's immune system as foreign and is attacked by T_C cells in this same way.

Tolerance

As part of initiating an immunologic response, the immune system must be able to recognize its own proteins and not mount an immune response against itself. This process of self-recognition occurs as part of normal neonatal growth and development. Autoimmune diseases occur when there is a breakdown of tolerance. The immune system inappropriately identifies its own proteins as foreign and mounts a response to destroy these self-proteins. Examples of autoimmune diseases include idiopathic thrombocytopenic purpura (ITP), thrombotic thrombocytopenic purpura (TTP), acute rheumatic fever, type 1 diabetes mellitus, systemic lupus erythematosus, rheumatoid arthritis, Graves' disease, and Hashimoto's thyroiditis.

AGE-RELATED CHANGES

With advancing age, the bone marrow becomes less productive. Immunologic function is generally not affected unless a person is unusually stressed by trauma, a chronic infection, or treatment for cancer. Yet even with conditions necessitating a higher production of blood cells, the bone marrow usually can respond to the increased demand, given more time. The lymphatic tissue grows very quickly between the ages of 6 and 20 years. With advancing age, lymphatic tissue shrinks, resulting in fewer and smaller lymph nodes. However, as with the bone marrow, this does not generally affect the overall health of an individual.

NURSING ASSESSMENT OF THE IMMUNE SYSTEM

Many subtle findings in the assessment can inform the nurse that changes in the patient's immune system may be occurring and to notify a nurse or physician to evaluate the patient. Table 32-1 outlines the nursing assessment of patients with disorders of the immunologic system.

table 32-1 ASSESSMENT *of a Patient with Disorders of the Immune System*

HEALTH HISTORY

History of Present Illness: Frequent or persistent infections, prolonged bleeding, easy bruising, chronic fatigue
Past Medical History: Cancer or prior treatment for cancer, HIV infection, history of splenectomy, placement of an indwelling venous access device indicating that the patient needed long-term venous access, recent infections, current medications (including over-the-counter medications, recent changes in medication, herbal products), recent immunizations
Family History: Cancer, death of a family member at a young age for reasons other than trauma

REVIEW OF SYSTEMS

Integumentary: Rash, breaks in the skin, ulcers, lesions, or enlarged lymph nodes; red, swollen, or painful areas
Neurologic: Weakness, lethargy, malaise, restlessness, apprehension, headache
Respiratory: Sinus pain, dyspnea, cough
Gastrointestinal: Sore throat, pain with swallowing, pain with defecation, unplanned weight loss or weight gain, diarrhea
Genitourinary: Pain or burning with urination
Musculoskeletal: Pain in bones or joints
Endocrine: Fatigue

FUNCTIONAL ASSESSMENT

Occupation and hobbies, changes in ability to do activities of daily living, roles at home and work, self-concept, activities and exercise, sleep and rest, nutrition, interpersonal relationships, stressors, coping style

PHYSICAL EXAMINATION

Vital Signs: Fever, tachycardia, tachypnea, hypotension
Height and Weight
General Survey: Responsiveness, mood, expression, posture
Skin: Color
Head and Neck: Enlarged, swollen, or draining areas; enlarged lymph nodes
Thorax: Enlarged lymph nodes, respiratory rate, breath sounds, heart rate
Abdomen: Organ enlargement, enlarged lymph nodes

HEALTH HISTORY

Chief Complaint and History of Present Illness

Pay special attention to the patient who remarks that he or she has frequent or persistent infections, bleeds for a long time when cut, bruises easily, or has chronic fatigue, as these symptoms may reflect an underlying immunologic disorder.

Past Medical History

A patient could have an underlying immunologic problem if he or she reports any of the following: cancer or prior treatment for cancer, HIV infection, history of splenectomy, or placement of an indwelling venous access device, indicating that the patient needed long-term venous access. Medications the patient is currently using or a recent change in medication may suggest an underlying immunologic problem. It is important to find out what over-the-counter medications (including herbal products) the patient uses, as many of these products contain aspirin or NSAIDs, which may disrupt immunologic function. Ask the patient about any recent changes in medications and any recent immunizations.

Family History

Note any family history of immunologic disorders such as cancer. Death of a family member at a young age for reasons other than trauma may indicate a genetic immunologic disorder.

Review of Systems

The review of systems is aimed at finding out what symptoms the patient has been experiencing over the past weeks or months. These symptoms might provide clues as to what specific medical disorder the patient may now have. The primary symptom of an immunologic disorder is infection. The patient should be carefully questioned about any reddened, swollen, painful, or unusually warm areas that might indicate an infectious process. Ask the patient about fever, chills, or night sweats. Night sweats can occur when the patient's temperature rises at night but the patient does not awaken until the temperature falls, causing sweating. Night sweats can occur normally in women undergoing menopause. However, night sweats can also be a symptom of infection (such as tuberculosis or malaria), leukemia (cancer of the white blood cells), or lymphoma (cancer of the lymph nodes).

Begin the review of systems with the integument. Ask about any red, swollen, or painful areas, which could be sites of infection. Document any breaks in the skin, ulcers, lesions, or enlarged lymph nodes, which could indicate a cancer or a site of infection. When assessing the neurologic system, ask about weakness, lethargy, malaise, restlessness, apprehension, or headache, which could indicate a central nervous system infection or tumor. When assessing the respiratory system, ask about sinus pain, dyspnea, or cough, which could indicate an infection. If the cough is productive, ask the patient to describe the sputum. When assessing the gastrointestinal system, ask about sore throat, any pain with swallowing, and any pain with defecation, which could indicate an infection. Ask if the patient has had any unplanned weight loss or weight gain. When reviewing the genitourinary system, ask about any pain or burning with urination, which could indicate an infection. Describe any musculoskeletal pain. Bone pain can occur with leukemia as a result of cancerous white blood cells crowding the normal cells in the bone marrow. Finally, when assessing the endocrine system, ask about any unusual fatigue.

Functional Assessment

Patients newly diagnosed with an immunologic disorder may not experience dramatic changes in their functional abilities. However, many immunologic disorders are chronic conditions that the patient has lived with—and been treated for—for many years. The functional abilities of these patients may be adversely affected.

Occupation and Hobbies. Knowing a patient's job and hobbies can alert the nurse to unusual chemical exposures. Because the bone marrow and blood can be affected by various chemicals, any recent chemical exposure should be noted. For example, someone who builds models for a hobby may be exposed to unusual glues or paints that may affect the blood count.

Self-Concept. Assess the patient's self-concept by exploring the patient's feeling about himself or herself. For many people, one's self-concept depends on one's job. If the patient is unable to work because of an immunologic disorder, his or her self-concept can be adversely affected. Additionally, medical insurance is often contingent on employment. Loss of medical insurance and the need to go on state or federal assistance can further erode a patient's self-concept. Another factor that can adversely affect the patient's self-concept is a change in appearance because of the disease or the treatment.

Activity and Exercise. Assess the patient's current activity level and the effects of the disease and treatment on the patient's usual pattern of activity and exercise. Ask about the layout of the patient's home, specifically the location of bathrooms in relation to living areas and bedrooms. Ask whether the patient must climb stairs to enter the home or get to a second floor. Stair climbing can quickly tire a patient with an immunologic disorder. Inquire what the patient does for recreation and whether these activities can still be done during times of decreased energy.

Sleep and Rest. Assess the number of continuous hours the patient sleeps every night, whether any sleeping aids are used, what interrupts the patient's sleep, and whether the patient naps during the day.

Nutrition. Ask the patient to describe his or her usual diet and any recent changes in appetite or weight. Identify factors that might be interfering with eating, such as nausea, vomiting, and taste changes. Depression and loneliness can adversely affect a patient's nutritional status. Limited financial resources can also limit a patient's ability to maintain a nutritious diet.

Interpersonal Relationships. Explore the patient's view of himself or herself as a husband or wife, father or mother, son or daughter, friend, and co-worker. Discuss the effects of the disease on these relationships. The patient's roles in the home must be considered. Ask for what household chores the patient is responsible and who does the shopping, cooking, and cleaning. If there are children for whom to care, ask whether or not the patient is able to perform the usual child care.

Coping and Stress. Ask what worries the patient and how the patient usually deals with stress. Explore sources of support, which might include family, support groups, and spiritual beliefs and practices.

Perception of Health. Discuss the patient's view of his or her own health and health practices. This might include measures taken to prevent complications from disease, and keeping regular medical appointments.

PHYSICAL EXAMINATION

The physical examination begins with measurement of vital signs and height and weight. The nurse is alert for fever, tachycardia, tachypnea, and hypotension.

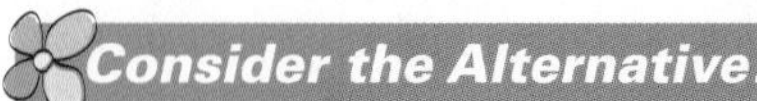

Herbs that are used to boost the immune system include echinacea, ginseng, and goldenseal. Patients should consult with their physicians about taking them, because they have adverse effects and can interact with some medications.

General Survey

Note the patient's responsiveness, mood, expression, and posture. Throughout the examination, carefully inspect and describe any reddened, swollen, or painful areas the patient identifies.

Skin

Inspect the skin from head to toe. Note the general color, texture, turgor, temperature, and integrity of the skin. Assess the skin for any red, swollen, or painful areas.

Head and Neck

When evaluating the eyes, ears, nose, mouth, and throat, note any enlarged, swollen, or draining areas that might indicate an infection. Examples might be swollen, draining sinuses; a canker sore in the mouth; or enlarged tonsils with exudate. The examiner with advanced skills may palpate the neck for enlarged lymph nodes.

Thorax

The examiner with advanced skills may palpate the axilla for enlarged lymph nodes.

Lungs

Assess respiratory rate and effort. Auscultate for wheezing, crackles, or rhonchi. Patients with a respiratory tract infection may have abnormal breath sounds or a cough.

Heart and Vascular System

Assess heart rate and blood pressure. Patients with a severe infection may be tachycardic or hypotensive.

Abdomen

The examiner with advanced skills may palpate the abdomen for tenderness. The liver and spleen can become enlarged with blood cell disorders, causing abdominal fullness and tenderness. Palpate the groin for enlarged lymph nodes.

DIAGNOSTIC TESTS AND PROCEDURES

Various blood studies are used to screen the function of the patient's immunologic system. Blood studies as well as other tests and procedures done to diagnose disorders of the immune system are described in Tables 32-2 and 32-3. Table 32-4 lists normal laboratory values for the various blood tests.

BLOOD TESTS

The complete blood cell (CBC) count is a common blood test done in most laboratories that reports the total number of white blood cells as well as what percentage of the total number of white blood cells are neutrophils, monocytes, eosinophils, basophils, and lymphocytes. Both the total number of white blood cells in the body as well as the differential, or percentage of each of the specific types of white blood cells in the body, are evaluated. Normal white blood cell counts range between 5,000 and 10,000 white blood cells per cubic millimeter (mm^3) of blood. The majority of the white blood cells, 60%, are neutrophils. Physicians and nurses are primarily interested in the number of neutrophils because these are the cells that fight bacterial infections.

A *shift to the left* on a CBC indicates that the percentage of the white blood cells that are neutrophils is greater than 60%. This usually indicates that the bone marrow has been stimulated to produce more neutrophils to fight a severe infection. In contrast, a *shift to the right* on a CBC indicates that only a small percentage of the white blood cells are neutrophils. This can occur either when the body has been completely overwhelmed with an infection, exhausting the supply of neutrophils, or when the bone marrow is not producing neutrophils. To calculate the absolute neutrophil count, multiply the percent neutrophils indicated on the differential of the CBC by the total number of white blood cells. See Figure 32-3 for a sample calculation.

Other blood tests are specific to the diagnosis of a particular disease. Serum protein electrophoresis measures the amount of immunoglobulin proteins present in the blood. This test is used to evaluate the patient suspected of having multiple myeloma, a cancer of the plasma cells. The antinuclear antibody test detects antibodies in the blood that may be indicative of systemic lupus erythematosus or other autoimmune disorders. An enzyme-linked immunosorbent assay and Western blot tests are used to diagnose HIV infection. T cell counts and viral load are tests used to determine the severity of the infection. Table 32-2 describes the procedures for collecting blood specimens for these tests.

URINE TESTS

Urine protein electrophoresis measures the amount of immunoglobulin proteins present in the urine. This test is used to evaluate the patient suspected of having multiple myeloma, a cancer of the plasma cells. Table 32-2 describes the procedures for collecting urine specimens.

CULTURES OF BLOOD, URINE, SPUTUM, AND STOOL

Cultures are done to detect infections in the blood, sputum, urine, or stool. When a patient has a fever without an obvious source of infection, all of these specimens are obtained to look for the source of the infection. Table 32-2 describes the procedures for collecting these specimens for culture.

BONE MARROW BIOPSY

If the CBC is abnormal, the physician may perform a bone marrow biopsy to evaluate the bone marrow. This procedure is also done to diagnose leukemia, cancer of the white blood cells, and multiple myeloma, cancer of the plasma cells. Table 31-4 describes the procedure for a bone marrow biopsy.

table 32-2 Nursing Care: Diagnostic Tests for Evaluating the Immune System

TEST/PURPOSE	PATIENT PREPARATION	POSTPROCEDURE NURSING CARE
Blood tests (CBC, SPEP, ANA, HIV ELISA, HIV Western blot, T cell counts, viral load) Blood tests measure various blood components. Blood for different tests is collected in different laboratory tubes containing specific reagents or no reagents at all. Usually the tubes have color-coded tops. Be sure to collect the blood in the blood tube specific for the blood test ordered. Usually each institution's laboratory publishes a manual identifying what colored tube to use for each blood test.	Choose the correct blood tube to collect the blood in. Tell the patient he or she will feel a sharp pain as the needle goes through the skin.	Apply bandage. Have the patient apply pressure to the site for 1 minute. The bandage may be removed in 1 hour.
Urine tests (UPEP) Electrophoresis of urine is performed to detect abnormal amounts of protein.	Have the patient void into the toilet. Mark the time. Have the patient collect all urine for the next 24 hours. The container should be kept on ice. Exactly 24 hours after the starting time, have the patient void for the last time and submit the entire 24-hour collection to the laboratory.	No special care after this test is required.
Blood culture: detects and identifies microorganisms in the blood	Choose the correct blood culture bottles according to whether aerobic or anaerobic species are to be cultured. The vein is prepared with Betadine and allowed to dry. The tops of the blood culture bottles are prepared with Betadine and allowed to dry. Do not touch the draw site except with sterile gloves. Tell the patient he or she will feel a needle prick as the needle goes through the skin. Draw enough blood so that 5 ml of blood can be placed in each culture bottle. Send the specimens to the laboratory immediately. Blood culture results are evaluated at 48 and 72 hours. Tell the patient not to expect any final results for 3 to 4 days.	Apply bandage. Have the patient apply pressure to the site for 1 minute. The bandage may be removed in 1 hour.
Sputum cultures: detect and identify microorganisms in the sputum.	Give the patient a sterile cup. Have the patient collect sputum the next time he or she coughs. Caution the patient not to collect saliva. Sputum comes from the lungs with coughing. Send the specimen to the laboratory immediately.	No special care after the procedure is required.
Urine culture: detects and identifies microorganisms in the urine	Give the patient wipes and a sterile container. Have the patient clean around the meatus of the urethra. Tell the patient to urinate a small amount into the toilet and stop. Then tell the patient to collect a urine specimen. If the patient is unable to collect the specimen, the physician may request a straight catheterization to collect the specimen. Follow the procedures for catheterizing a patient, as described in Chapter 38. If the patient has an indwelling catheter, clamp the catheter. In approximately 15 minutes, prepare the withdrawal port on the catheter with Betadine and allow the Betadine to dry. Withdraw a sample of urine through the port with a sterile needle and syringe and transfer the specimen into a collection cup. Send the specimen to the laboratory immediately.	No special care after the procedure is required.
Stool culture: detects and identifies microorganisms in the stool.	Have the patient defecate into a clean bedpan or other container. Using a sterile tongue blade, collect a specimen in a sterile container. Send the specimen to the laboratory immediately. Some tests must be done while the specimen is still warm.	No special care after the procedure is required.

CBC, Complete blood count; *SPEP*, serum protein electrophoresis; *ANA*, antinuclear antibody assay; *HIV*, human immunodeficiency virus; *ELISA*, enzyme-linked immunosorbent assay; *UPEP*, urine protein electrophoresis.
Data from Fischbach, F. (2000). *A manual of laboratory and diagnostic tests* (6th ed.). Philadelphia: Lippincott.

table 32-3 **DIAGNOSTIC TESTS AND PROCEDURES | *the Immune System***

TEST/STUDY	PURPOSE/PROCEDURE	PATIENT PREPARATION	POSTPROCEDURE NURSING CARE
Lymphangiography (LAG)	Lymphangiography demonstrates the anatomy of the lymphatic vessels and nodes. The patient is taken to diagnostic radiology, where a 1- to 2-inch incision is made on the dorsum of each foot or hand. The lymphatic vessels are cannulated and dye is injected. Several radiographs are taken as the dye moves up the extremity. The patient returns to diagnostic radiology 12 to 24 hours later for more radiographs of the lymph nodes and higher lymphatic channels.	Explain the purpose and procedure to the patient and obtain signed consent. Ask the patient about any allergies to contrast media. No fasting is necessary. Some local discomfort may be experienced as the local anesthetic agent is injected to numb the top of the foot or hand. Incisions may stain blue from the dye. The procedure takes approximately 3 hours. The patient returns to diagnostic radiology 12 to 24 hours later for more radiographs.	Check the patient's vital signs every 4 hours for 48 hours. Keep the incisions clean and dry after the procedure. The doctor may order the legs or arms to be elevated. Stitches may be in place that should be removed in 5 to 7 days.
Liver-spleen scan	A spleen scan is used to evaluate the size and function of the spleen. In the nuclear medicine department, a radioactive dye is injected into a vein. The amount of dye taken up by the spleen is measured by a machine 20 to 60 minutes after the dye is injected.	Explain the purpose and procedure to the patient. Ask the patient about any allergies to contrast media. No fasting is necessary. An intravenous line must be in place to inject the dye but may be discontinued after the injection. The procedure takes approximately 60 minutes.	No special care after the procedure is required.
Gallium scan	A gallium scan is used to detect the presence, location, and size of chronic infections, abscesses, and malignant tumors primarily of lymphoid origin. In the nuclear medicine department, a radioactive dye is injected into a vein. The amount of dye taken up by malignant lymphoid tissue is measured by a machine 24 to 72 hours after the dye is injected.	Explain the purpose and procedure to the patient. Ask the patient about any allergies to contrast media. An intravenous line must be in place to inject the dye but may be discontinued after the injection. Scanning is usually done 24 to 72 hours following dye injection. If the abdomen is to be scanned, a laxative is usually given the evening before the scanning. However, the patient may eat breakfast the morning of the scan. During imaging the patient must lie quietly for 45 to 90 minutes while scanning is done.	No special care after the procedure is required.
Skin tests	Skin testing is done for several reasons—to detect sensitivity to allergens such as pollen, to determine sensitivity to microorganisms that cause disease (such as tuberculin), and to determine whether cell-mediated immune functions are normal. As part of the evaluation of a patient with HIV infection, skin testing is done to determine whether the cell-mediated immune system is functioning. The inner side of the patient's forearm is cleaned. Generally 0.1 ml of the test material is injected intradermally using a 26- or 27-gauge needle and tuberculin syringe. A common battery of five skin tests used to test immune function in patients with HIV infection includes mumps, *Candida, Trichophyton,* tetanus, and purified protein derivative of tuberculin bacillus.	Explain the purpose and procedure to the patient. Tell the patient he or she will feel a needle prick as the needle goes through the skin.	No special care after the procedure is required. Tell the patient that he or she must be reexamined in 2 to 3 days to determine the results of the testing. Swelling at the site of injection indicates that the body's cell-mediated immune system is functioning.

Adapted from Fischbach F. (2000). *A manual of laboratory and diagnostic tests* (6th ed.). Philadelphia: Lippincott.

table 32-4 ***Normal Laboratory Values***

White blood cell (WBC) count	5,000-10,000 cells/mm³
White blood cell differential	
Neutrophils	50%-62% of total WBC
Bands	3%-6% of total WBC
Monocytes	3%-7% of total WBC
Basophils	0%-1% of total WBC
Eosinophils	0%-3% of total WBC
Lymphocytes	25%-40% of total WBC
Serum protein electrophoresis (SPEP)	
Total protein	6.0-8.0 gm/dl
Albumin	3.8-5.0 gm/dl
Urine protein electrophoresis (UPEP)	Interpreted based on SPEP results
Antinuclear antibody (ANA) assay	Negative
HIV ELISA	Negative
HIV Western blot	Negative
T cell counts	
Total T cells	812-2,318 cells/mm³
T_H cells (CD4 cells)	589-1,505 cells/mm³
T_S cells	325-997 cells/mm³
T_H/T_S ratio	>1.0

Note: Normal laboratory values may differ from hospital to hospital. Be sure to check your institution's normal values.
Data from Fischbach F. (2000). *A manual of laboratory and diagnostic tests* (6th ed.). Philadelphia: Lippincott.

CBC report

6.5	WBC × 10^3
4.51	RBC × 10^6
14.0	HGB g/dl
40.8	HCT %
90.5	MCV fl
30.9	MCH pg
34.2	MCHC g/dl
333	PLT × 10^3

Automated differential

35.0	LYMPH %
10.3	MONO %
46.3	NEUT %
7.3	EOS %
1.0	BASO %

Manual differential

Segmented Neutrophils %	49
Banded Neutrophils %	1
Lymphocytes %	32
Monocytes %	8
Eosinophils %	9
Basophils %	1

HCT, Hematocrit; *HGB*, hemoglobin; *MCH*, mean corpuscular hemoglobin; *MCHC*, mean corpuscular hemoglobin concentration; *MCV*, mean corpuscular volume; *PLT*, platelets; *RBC*, red blood cell; *WBC*, white blood cell.

FIGURE **32-3** Calculating the absolute neutrophil count (ANC) from the complete blood count.

To calculate the ANC, use the *manual differential* because it is more accurate. Multiply the percent of segmented neutrophils (49% in this example) and the percent of banded neutrophils (1% in this example) by the total number of white blood cells (WBCs) (6,500 in this example). Banded neutrophils are included in the calculations of the ANC because they are developmentally nearly mature neutrophils and can function as mature neutrophils (see Fig. 32-2). If a manual differential has not been done, the automated differential can be used; if the total WBC count is >10,000 μl or <3,000/μl, a manual differential should be requested.

Generic Calculation:
(% neutrophils + % bands) (WBC) = ANC
Calculations for this example:
(.49 + .01) (6,500) = 3,250

LYMPHANGIOGRAPHY

Lymphangiography is done to evaluate the anatomy of the lymphatic vessels and the lymph nodes. Dye is injected into the lymph vessels of the foot or hand and radiographs are taken as the dye moves up the lymph channels. Lymphangiography is often done as part of the staging work-up for Hodgkin's disease, a cancer of the lymph nodes. However, with improved diagnostic radiologic techniques, computed tomography may reveal enlarged abdominal lymph nodes and eliminate the need for lymphangiography. Table 32-3 describes the procedure for a lymphangiography.

LIVER-SPLEEN SCAN

A liver-spleen scan is used to evaluate the size and function of the liver and spleen. A radioactive colloid is injected into the patient. A single-photon emission computed tomography machine measures how much of the radioactive colloid is taken up by the liver and spleen. This scan is sometimes used in the staging work-up for Hodgkin's disease, a cancer of the lymph nodes. Table 32-3 describes the procedure for a liver-spleen scan.

GALLIUM SCAN

A gallium scan uses a radioactive tracer to detect the presence of malignant tissue, particularly malignant lymph tissue. Table 32-3 describes the procedure for a gallium scan.

SKIN TESTS

Skin tests can serve as a barometer of immune system functioning, pointing out either hyposensitivities or hypersensitivities to a particular antigen. Examples of allergens used in skin testing include dust, pollen, animal dander, purified protein derivative, tuberculin bacillus, and *Candida albicans.* Table 32-3 describes the procedure for skin tests.

COMMON THERAPEUTIC MEASURES

NURSING ACTIONS FOR THE PATIENT AT RISK FOR INJURY FROM INFECTION

The lower a patient's white blood cell count, in particular the lower the neutrophil count, the greater is the patient's risk of infection. Table 32-5 outlines typical nursing actions for the patient at risk for injury from infection.

table 32-5 Nursing Actions for the Patient at Risk for Injury from Infection: Compromised Host Precautions

1. The patient should have a private room. It does not have to be an isolation room. The door may be left open. A "Compromised Host Precaution" sign should be posted on the door.
2. All persons entering the patient's room must wash hands before touching the patient for any reason. This is the most important way to prevent infection. The patient and family should be encouraged to remind all staff and visitors to wash their hands before touching the patient.
3. Administer hematopoietic growth factors as prescribed. Hematopoietic growth factors, also called colony-stimulating factors (CSFs), are cytokines that stimulate production of various blood cell components. Because hematopoietic growth factors take several days to increase white blood cell counts, they are best used in anticipation of neutropenia (e.g., immediately after cytotoxic chemotherapy).
4. Monitor vital signs every 2-4 hours. Notify physician immediately of temperature >101° F to consider the need for an infectious fever workup and initiating or changing antibiotics. An infectious fever workup usually includes two sets of blood cultures, a chest radiograph, sputum culture, urine culture, wound culture, and cultures of other sites suggestive of infection. Patients with a central line or permanent, indwelling venous access device usually have one set of specimens for culture drawn from the line and one set drawn from a peripheral site. Mark the culture bottles clearly regarding where the specimen was obtained to assist with localization of the infection. Blood cultures are more likely to yield the offending organism if the blood is drawn as the patient's temperature is rising instead of after the patient's temperature has peaked.
5. Invasive procedures should be kept to a minimum. Invasive devices such as catheters and tubes should be removed as soon as the patient's medical condition permits.
6. Careful attention to aseptic technique must be observed, especially when performing phlebotomy, handling intravenous lines, or performing other invasive procedures.
7. Designate a particular stethoscope and thermometer to be used exclusively in caring for the patient.
8. Masks are not required; they are actually discouraged. Staff with upper respiratory tract or other infections should not care for the patient.
9. Clean table tops, equipment, and the floor frequently with hospital-approved disinfectant, clean cloths, and clean mops.
10. The patient should be taught to wash his or her hands before and after eating, using the toilet, and doing any self-care procedure. If possible, the patient should shower every day. Liquid soap instead of bar soap should be used.
11. Encourage the patient to cough and deep breathe every 4 hours. Mobility should be encouraged. Smoking should be discouraged.
12. Only canned or cooked foods should be served. Raw fruits, raw vegetables, and milk products are not served because of the risk of *Escherichia coli, Pseudomonas aeruginosa,* and *Klebsiella* species bacteria on or in these food items. The patient should be encouraged to choose appropriate foods from the menu. The diet roster should be annotated "Compromised Host Precautions" so that the nutrition care staff can verify that appropriate choices are being made.
13. Tests, scans, and appointments away from the patient's room should be coordinated in advance to eliminate or minimize waiting time in common waiting areas.
14. The patient should wear a clean mask when outside the room, especially in heavily traveled public areas such as corridors, elevators, and waiting rooms. The mask may be removed when the patient is in less public areas. A new mask should be used for each trip out of the room.
15. Some hospitals allow flowers and plants in the patient's room; however, they should not be handled by the patient because of the possibility of *Escherichia coli* contamination of the water and dirt.
16. No humidifiers with standing water should be used in the patient's room. If a wall humidifier is needed, the water should be changed every day.
17. Teach the patient and family about the underlying pathophysiology that puts the patient at risk for infection and about precautions to minimize the risk of infection.

From Young-McCaughan, S., & Jennings, B. M. (1998). Hematologic and immunologic systems. In J. G. Alspach (Ed.), *Core curriculum for critical care nursing* (5th ed., pp. 601-646). Philadelphia: Saunders.

COLONY-STIMULATING FACTORS

Colony-stimulating factors (CSFs) are naturally occurring hormones that stimulate the bone marrow to produce more blood cells. Certain of the colony-stimulating factors have been isolated and are available for therapeutic use. Two drugs, granulocyte-macrophage colony-stimulating factor (GM-CSF), or sargramostim (Leukine), and granulocyte colony-stimulating factor (G-CSF), or filgrastim (Neupogen), stimulate the bone marrow to produce more white blood cells. These drugs have revolutionized the treatment of patients with cancer receiving chemotherapy by shortening the duration of neutropenia and thereby reducing the patient's risk of infection. When colony-stimulating factors are used to support the white blood cell count, patients can be treated with higher doses of chemotherapy for longer periods of time. Studies are now under way to determine if these aggressive treatment regimens will improve the long-term survival of patients with cancer. Colony-stimulating factors are administered subcutaneously. The patient or a family member is taught how to administer the drug at home. Table 32-6 describes the nursing care of patients receiving these drugs.

BONE MARROW TRANSPLANT AND PERIPHERAL BLOOD STEM CELL TRANSPLANT

Bone marrow transplantation and peripheral blood stem cell transplantation are done to restore the hematologic and immunologic systems in patients with malignancies who have received extremely high doses of chemotherapy and radiation therapy. Bone marrow transplantation is also used in patients with genetic bone marrow defects and aplastic anemia in an attempt to repopulate the bone marrow with blood-producing cells. The donated bone marrow is administered to the patient just like a blood transfusion through an intravenous line. The infused bone marrow finds its way to the patient's bone marrow, where it starts growing and producing healthy white blood cells, red blood cells, and platelets.

There are three main types of transplants: allogeneic bone marrow transplant, autologous bone marrow transplant, and peripheral blood stem cell transplant. Allogeneic bone marrow transplants have been done the longest. They originally were used to treat people with leukemia, or cancer of the white blood cells. High doses of chemotherapy and radiation therapy are given to destroy all of the cancerous bone marrow. Then bone marrow from a human leukocyte antigen (HLA)–matched donor is reinfused into the patient to restore bone marrow function. HLA typing is similar to blood typing but is much more specific. Because these HLAs are genetically determined, brothers and sisters of the patient are initially tested to determine whether they can be bone marrow donors for their sibling. There is a 25% chance that a sibling will be an HLA match to a patient needing a bone marrow transplant. There is a possibility that someone in the general population might be HLA matched to the patient, but the chances of finding a matched, unrelated donor are very small. For many patients an allogeneic bone marrow transplant is not possible because a matched donor cannot be found.

Another type of bone marrow transplant harvests the patient's own bone marrow before chemotherapy and radiation therapy. Following therapy, the patient's own bone marrow is returned to the patient. This type of bone marrow transplant, called an autologous bone marrow transplant, is the best option for patients with a solid tumor that has not metastasized to the bone marrow, for example patients with breast cancer or lymphoma. An autologous bone marrow transplant is generally not an option for patients with leukemia or who have a cancer that has metastasized to the bone marrow because healthy bone marrow must be reinfused into the patient after chemotherapy and radiation therapy to prevent cancer recurrence.

A third type of bone marrow transplant is a peripheral blood stem cell transplant. For this type of transplant, colony-stimulating factors are administered to the patient to stimulate the bone marrow to produce large numbers of white blood cells. Then apheresis is performed to collect the patient's peripheral stem cells. Apheresis is a procedure similar to hemodialysis. A large-bore apheresis catheter is placed into the subclavian vein that allows simultaneous blood withdrawal and blood reinfusion. The patient's blood is first drawn off into the apheresis machine. The apheresis machine centrifuges, or spins, the blood, separating it into white cells, red cells, and plasma. The stem cells in the white blood cell layer are removed and stored while the rest of the white blood cells, red blood cells, and plasma are returned to the patient. When enough of these peripheral blood stem cells are harvested and stored, the patient is treated with chemotherapy and radiation therapy. After treatment, the peripheral blood stem cells are returned to the patient. Stem cells re-engraft more quickly than bone marrow, reducing the duration of neutropenia and therefore the risk of infection. Often peripheral blood stem cell transplants are administered concurrently with autologous bone marrow transplants. Peripheral blood stem cell transplants have been so successful that they are quickly becoming the most common type of transplant.

Major complications of bone marrow transplantation and peripheral blood stem cell transplantation include infection, thrombocytopenia, renal insufficiency, hepatic veno-occlusive disease, and graft-versus-host disease. Infection is a constant concern in the care of patients undergoing bone marrow transplantation. For approximately 2 weeks after transplantation, when the new bone marrow is engrafting, patients are severely neutropenic and at very high risk for infection. Even when white blood cells and neutrophil counts approach normal levels, the patient's cell-mediated immune function can be compromised for more than a year.

Thrombocytopenia can be profound and prolonged in the patient undergoing bone marrow transplantation or peripheral blood stem cell transplantation because of the high doses of chemotherapy and radiation therapy.

Renal insufficiency can occur if the kidneys are damaged with high doses of nephrotoxic drugs such as cisplatin chemotherapy or the antibiotic gentamicin. Kidney function can be further compromised if blood flow to and through the kidneys is not maintained.

Hepatic veno-occlusive disease can occur if the liver is damaged with high doses of chemotherapy and radiation therapy. Blood flow into and out of the liver can be obstructed, resulting in ischemia, ascites, and increasing serum bilirubin.

Graft-versus-host disease is a complication of allogeneic bone marrow transplants in which T lymphocytes in the transplanted bone marrow identify the patient's tissue as foreign and try to destroy the patient's tissues. The transplanted T lymphocytes primarily attack epithelial cells of the skin, gastrointestinal tract, biliary ducts, and lymphoid system, resulting in a skin rash, large amounts of green watery heme-negative diarrhea, and elevated liver enzyme levels.

Patients undergoing bone marrow transplantation or peripheral blood stem cell transplantation as treatment for a hematologic or immune system disorder need intensive nursing

table 32-6 **DRUG THERAPY** | ***Drugs Used to Treat Disorders of the Immunologic System***

DRUGS	USE/ACTION	SIDE EFFECTS	NURSING INTERVENTIONS
DRUGS USED IN THE TREATMENT OF PATIENTS WITH NEUTROPENIA			
Colony-stimulating factors (e.g., G-CSF or filgrastim [Neupogen], GM-CSF or sargramostim [Leukine])	Used in neutropenic patients to stimulate the bone marrow to produce white blood cells	Bone pain	Teach the patient how to give subcutaneous injections. Generally the patient is treated until the absolute neutrophil count is >10,000 cells/mm^3.
DRUGS USED IN THE TREATMENT OF PATIENTS WITH A TRANSPLANTED ORGAN TO PREVENT REJECTION			
Steroids (e.g., dexamethasone [Decadron], methylprednisolone [Solu-Medrol], prednisone, prednisolone, hydrocortisone [Solu-Cortef])	Used to prevent rejection of a transplanted organ, because glucocorticoids interfere with eicosanoid production; also used to treat acute hypersensitivity reaction type I (anaphylaxis)	Glucose intolerance, muscle wasting, obesity, hyperlipidemia, redistribution of body fat, growth inhibition in children, increased capillary fragility, osteoporosis, stomach irritation and peptic ulcer disease, hypertension, sodium and water retention, mood changes	Give these drugs with meals. An H_2-receptor antagonist such as ranitidine (Zantac) may be prescribed to decrease gastric acid production. If the patient takes these drugs for an extended period of time, the drug should not be stopped abruptly. Instead, the drug dosage should be gradually decreased over time under a physician's direction.
Immunosuppressants (e.g., cyclosporine)	Used to prevent rejection of a transplanted organ by inhibiting T lymphocytes	Tremor, hypertension, vomiting, electrolyte imbalance, nephrotoxicity, hirsutism	Blood levels should be monitored at regular intervals.
Purine and pyrimidine analogues (e.g., azathioprine, mycophenolic acid, brequinar)	Used to prevent rejection of a transplanted organ by interfering with DNA synthesis in rapidly dividing cells such as T cells	Bone marrow suppression, increased susceptibility to infection, stomach irritation, diarrhea, hepatotoxicity	Closely monitor the patient's CBC and liver function studies.

DRUGS USED IN THE TREATMENT OF PATIENTS WITH HIV INFECTION

Nucleoside reverse transcriptase inhibitors (e.g., zidovudine [AZT, Retrovir], 3TCEpivir [Lamivudine], stavudine [d4T, Zerit], didanosine [ddI, Videx], zalcitabine [ddC, Hivid])	Used in patients with HIV infection to slow the replication and progression of HIV by interfering with HIV replication inside the T_H CD4 cell	Headache, nausea, vomiting, fatigue, muscle aches, neutropenia, anemia, peripheral neuropathy, skin rash, elevated liver enzymes, pancreatitis, diarrhea	Some of these drugs should be taken on an empty stomach, while others can be taken with or without food. Administration recommendations for specific drugs should be reviewed with the patient. The CBC is checked periodically to monitor for the patient's WBC/RBC counts. Liver function tests are also monitored. There are multiple drug interactions between these and other drugs. The patient's complete medication record needs to be reviewed before beginning these drugs or adding another drug to the patient's regimen in the future.
Protease inhibitors (e.g., invirase [Saquinivir mesylate], indinavir sulfate [crixivan], nelfinavir [Viracept], norvir [Ritonavir])	Used in patients with HIV infection to slow the replication and progression of HIV by blocking the enzyme protease so that the infected cell cannot produce any more HIV proteins	Diarrhea, nausea, vomiting, kidney stones, jaundice, abdominal pain, headache, skin rash, numbness and tingling around mouth, drooling, dizziness, sleepiness, sore throat, sweating, altered taste	Some of these drugs should be taken on an empty stomach, while others should be taken with food. Administration recommendations for specific drugs should be reviewed with the patient. There are multiple drug interactions between these and other drugs. The patient's complete medication record needs to be reviewed before beginning these drugs or adding another drug to the patient's regimen in the future.
Non-nucleoside reverse transcriptase inhibitors (e.g., viramune [Nevirapine], delavirdine)	Used in patients with HIV infection to slow the replication and progression of HIV by interfering with HIV replication inside the T_H CD4 cell	Skin rash, headache, nausea, diarrhea, fatigue	Can be taken with or without food. There are multiple drug interactions between these and other drugs. The patient's complete medication record needs to be reviewed before beginning these drugs or adding another drug to the patient's regimen in the future.

Data from Shannon, M. T., Wilson, B. A., & Stang, C. L. (2002). *Health Professional's Drug Guide 2002.* Upper Saddle River, NJ: Prentice Hall.

care and long-term follow-up to be sure their new immune system is functioning and that the underlying disease does not recur.

Put on your THINKING CAP!!

Compare and contrast the three types of bone marrow transplants in relation to: patient preparation, source of cells, advantages, disadvantages, and complications.

DISORDERS OF THE IMMUNE SYSTEM

WHITE BLOOD CELL DISORDERS

The main function of the white blood cells is to protect the body against pathogens. Patients are at great risk for infection when the white blood cells are not functioning properly.

Neutropenia

Neutropenia occurs when the total number of neutrophils is abnormally low, putting the patient at increased risk of infection. Neutropenia can be caused by decreased bone marrow production (e.g., because of infiltration with malignant cells), chemotherapy, radiation therapy, certain drugs (e.g., zidovudine, clozapine), or an autoimmune reaction (e.g., systemic lupus erythematosus, rheumatoid arthritis). Neutropenia also can be caused by increased neutrophil utilization because of overwhelming infection. The longer the patient is neutropenic, the greater is the chance of infection. Because these patients do not have adequate numbers of white blood cells to mount an immunologic response, classic signs of infection (redness, swelling, and pain) may be absent. Fever may be the only sign of infection.

The most common sites of infection in neutropenic patients are the lung (pneumonia), blood (septicemia), skin, urinary tract, and gastrointestinal tract (mucositis, esophagitis, perirectal lesions). Usually bacteria cause infections in neutropenic patients; however, fungi and viruses can also infect these patients. The goal of antibiotic therapy is to support the patient until the patient's own white blood cells are available to fight the infection. In addition to administering prescribed antibiotics, it is important to minimize the patient's exposure to infectious agents by instituting compromised host precautions, described in Table 32-5.

Leukemia

Leukemia is a cancer of the white blood cells in which the bone marrow produces too many immature white blood cells. These nonfunctioning, immature white blood cells leave the patient unprotected against microorganisms and at a great risk for life-threatening infections. The American Cancer Society statistics estimated that 30,800 cases of leukemia would be diagnosed in 2002, accounting for 2% of all new cases of cancer diagnosed in that year. Although for most cases no cause is identified, factors that may be associated with the development of leukemia are exposure to large doses of ionizing radiation or exposure to certain chemicals such as benzene, a compound found in gasoline. Persons with Down's syndrome and certain other genetic abnormalities are at increased risk for developing leukemia.

There are two main types of leukemia—myelogenous and lymphocytic. Each type of leukemia can be either chronic or acute. The chronic leukemias—chronic myelogenous leukemia and chronic lymphocytic leukemia—occur most often in adults. In both types of chronic leukemias, the white blood cell count slowly increases over months or years. The disease usually can be controlled with oral chemotherapy agents for many years. Patients being treated for chronic leukemia generally feel healthy. They do not lose their hair and usually do not experience nausea. Most of these patients can continue to work. A new drug now available for patients with chronic myelogenous leukemia, Gleevec (imatinib mesylate), has revolutionized the treatment of this particular leukemia. Gleevec is a protein tyrosine kinase inhibitor that targets the leukemic cells while sparing normal cells. It is an oral medication taken once a day. Only minimal side effects have been reported. Research continues to determine the optimal length of treatment and follow-up needed for these patients. The average life expectancy after diagnosis for a patient with chronic myelogenous leukemia ranges from 3 to 8 years, depending on the stage of the disease. It is anticipated that life expectancy will increase with Gleevec treatment but by how much is currently unknown. The average life expectancy for a patient with chronic lymphocytic leukemia ranges from 2 to 10 years, again depending on the stage of the disease when diagnosed. After this time, the chronic leukemias often transform into an acute leukemia that is very difficult to treat. Patients generally die shortly after they enter this accelerated phase.

Each of the chronic forms of leukemia—lymphocytic and myelogenous—also has an acute form. Acute lymphocytic leukemia occurs most often in children between the ages of 2 and 6 years. Acute nonlymphocytic leukemia, also called acute myelogenous leukemia, occurs more often in adults. The acute leukemias appear very suddenly. The patient's white blood cell count can skyrocket in days, crowding out the normal red blood cells and platelets and leaving the patient at severe risk for infection and bleeding. Treatment with chemotherapy must be started as soon as possible. Between 70% and 80% of children diagnosed with acute lymphocytic leukemia will be alive in 5 years. Only 20% of patients diagnosed with acute nonlymphocytic leukemia will be alive in 5 years.

Signs and Symptoms of Acute Leukemia

Patients with leukemia commonly have infections because their bone marrow is producing huge numbers of immature white blood cells that cannot effectively fight infection. Usually patients with acute leukemia have fevers and night sweats in response to the infection. Because the leukemic white blood cells crowd out the normal cells in the bone marrow, patients may have symptoms related to low red blood cell counts, such as fatigue, paleness, tachycardia, and tachypnea. Concurrently, patients may have symptoms related to low platelet counts, such as petechiae or purpura, epistaxis (nose bleeds), gingival bleeding (from the gums), melena (blood in the stool), or menorrhagia (heavy menstrual bleeding). Some patients may have bone pain because of the crowding created by rapidly dividing leukemic cells in the bone marrow. Patients may report weight loss and swollen lymph nodes.

Medical Diagnosis of Acute Leukemia

A CBC with an extremely high white blood cell count indicates that leukemia might be present. A bone marrow biopsy enables diagnosis of the specific type of leukemia. Tables 32-2 and 32-3 describe the procedure for drawing specimens for a CBC as well as for a bone marrow biopsy.

Medical Treatment of the Patient with Acute Leukemia

The acute leukemias are initially treated using high doses of chemotherapy to destroy the diseased bone marrow and allow the body to regrow healthy bone marrow. Patients are at great risk for infection and bleeding while their healthy bone marrow is growing back, but this is the only way the acute leukemias can be treated. Patients stay in the hospital during the chemotherapy treatments and afterward to receive antibiotics and blood transfusions until their own bone marrow grows back. After the initial high doses of chemotherapy, called *induction therapy,* patients with acute lymphocytic leukemia take lower doses of chemotherapy, called *maintenance therapy,* for 1 to 3 years. Patients with acute nonlymphocytic leukemia immediately receive the same high doses of chemotherapy two to four more times over the next 2 to 4 months but are then finished with treatment. Subsequent chemotherapy for acute nonlymphocytic leukemia is called *intensification* and *consolidation therapy.* Bone marrow transplantation is one form of intensification therapy.

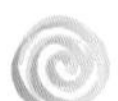

What Does Culture Have to do with Blood Transfusions?

Members of some religious groups do not accept blood transfusions from other people. Autotransfusion may be an acceptable alternative.

NURSING CARE *of the Patient with Acute Leukemia*

Patients with acute leukemia require intensive nursing care. Patients are normally hospitalized only 2 to 3 weeks and are critically ill most of that time. Once a patient's vital signs stabilize and the patient has no signs or symptoms of infection, he or she can be discharged from the hospital and followed as an outpatient until normal bone marrow function returns and adequate numbers of white blood cells, red blood cells, and platelets are being made. The physical and psychological nursing care of these patients is intensive.

Assessment

Infection is the leading cause of death in patients with leukemia. Therefore patients are frequently assessed for any signs or symptoms of infection. The most common sites of infection are the lungs, blood, skin, urinary tract, and gastrointestinal tract. Take complete vital signs every 4 hours. Fever is the hallmark of infection. Other vital sign changes due to sepsis or to widespread infection include tachycardia, tachypnea, and hypotension. Assess breath sounds every shift and note changes. A cough, especially a productive cough, may indicate an early pulmonary infection. If sputum is produced, note the amount and color. The physician may want the sputum cultured. Each day carefully inspect the skin for any reddened, swollen, painful, or draining areas. This is most easily done when helping the patient bathe. Because patients with leukemia do not have normal white blood cells, pus may not be seen even though an infection may be present. Redness, swelling, pain, or a combination of these may be the only symptoms of a serious infection. Inspect the mouth and pharynx, looking for any reddened, swollen, painful, or draining areas. Ask the patient about any pain or burning on urination, indicating a possible bladder infection.

While assessing for infection, also assess for any evidence of bleeding. The lower the platelet count, the greater is the patient's risk for bleeding. A platelet count below 50,000 cells/mm^3 is cause for concern. Note any petechiae, purpura, or ecchymoses. Patients may have or report epistaxis, gingival bleeding, melena, or menorrhagia. Perform a guaiac test to assess for blood on all bowel movements as directed.

Also note any side effects from the chemotherapy itself, such as nausea and vomiting or stomatitis, so the appropriate interventions can be taken. Most patients lose their hair from chemotherapy for acute leukemia beginning 1 to 2 weeks after treatment. This is to be expected.

While doing a physical assessment, also assess how much the patient knows about the disease and treatment as well as how the patient is coping with this life-threatening disease.

Nursing Diagnoses, Goals, and Outcome Criteria: Acute Leukemia

Nursing Diagnoses	Goals and Outcome Criteria
Risk for Injury related to infection, thrombocytopenia, and anemia	Absence of injury from infection, bleeding, and inadequate oxygenation: normal body temperature, no bruising or frank bleeding, pulse and respiratory rates within patient's norms
Fatigue related to the disease process and treatment	Reduction in fatigue: patient reports tolerance of activity has improved
Impaired Oral Mucous Membranes related to stomatitis	Intact mucous membranes: oral tissues normal in color without lesions
Imbalanced Nutrition: Less than Body Requirements related to nausea and vomiting	Adequate intake of nutrients: stable body weight
Anxiety related to the disease, treatment, and uncertain outcome	Reduced anxiety: patient reports anxiety is reduced, calm manner
Ineffective Therapeutic Regimen Management related to lack of knowledge about the disease process and treatment	Patient manages side effects of treatment effectively: patient resumes self-care; verbalizes disease process, treatment, and implications

Interventions

Risk for Injury

Infection. Infection presents the greatest risk to patients with leukemia. Most hospitals institute compromised host precautions when a patient's absolute neutrophil count falls below 1,000 cells/mm^3. Thorough hand washing is of extreme importance in caring for these patients. Microorganisms are transmitted by hospital personnel who do not diligently wash their hands. Encourage patients to shower every day to remove bacteria from the skin and perianal area. Because patients with low white blood cell counts often become infected with their own microorganisms through their gastrointestinal tract, discourage patients from eating fresh fruits or vegetables and from drinking milk products. Any uncooked foods naturally contain the bacteria *Escherichia coli, Pseudomonas aeruginosa,* and *Klebsiella* species. A normal immune system can destroy the bacteria in uncooked foods. However, patients undergoing treatment for leukemia are at high risk of infection after being exposed to even small amounts of these bacteria. Table 32-5 outlines typical compromised host precautions for patients with low white blood cell counts. Once the patient's absolute neutrophil count climbs above 1,000 cells/mm^3, compromised host precautions can be discontinued and a regular diet resumed without restrictions.

Thrombocytopenia. In addition to infection, patients with leukemia are at great risk for bleeding related to thrombocytopenia (a low platelet count). The primary treatment for thrombocytopenia is a platelet transfusion. However, physicians try not to prescribe platelet transfusions for patients unless they are actively bleeding or their platelet count is below 20,000 cells/mm^3 because of the risks associated with blood product administration. Nursing considerations in administering platelet transfusions are outlined in Table 31-10. When patients are thrombocytopenic, take bleeding precautions as outlined in Table 31-7.

Anemia. Anemia, or a hematocrit below 30 and a hemoglobin below 10 gm/dl, is a common finding in patients with leukemia. Expect anemia along with neutropenia and thrombocytopenia. As with neutropenia and thrombocytopenia, anemia may be caused by the leukemic cells crowding out the healthy red cells in the bone marrow, or it may be the result of chemotherapy. The primary treatment for anemia is a red blood cell transfusion. Nursing considerations in administering blood transfusions are outlined in Table 31-9. Other precautions for patients with anemia are outlined in Table 31-6.

Fatigue

Almost all patients with acute leukemia experience fatigue, which has been described as an overwhelming tiredness or exhaustion. Causes of fatigue in these patients can include a low red blood cell count from both the disease and treatment, the buildup of metabolic wastes as the leukemic cells are being destroyed and cleared from the body, disrupted sleep, and the psychological stress of the disease and treatment. A detailed discussion of the nursing management of fatigue is presented in Chapter 24.

Impaired Oral Mucous Membranes

Stomatitis, or an inflammation of the mucous membranes, is also a common side effect of chemotherapy. A detailed discussion of the nursing management of stomatitis is presented in Chapter 24.

Imbalanced Nutrition: Less than Body Requirements

Nausea, with or without vomiting, is a common side effect of chemotherapy. Persistent nausea and vomiting can adversely affect a patient's nutritional status and psychological state. You can play an important role in managing this most distressing side effect. A detailed discussion of the nursing management of nausea and vomiting related to chemotherapy is presented in Chapter 24.

Anxiety

A diagnosis of leukemia is always a shock to patients and their families. Patients must deal not only with the disease and treatment but also with the feelings and emotions of facing a life-threatening illness. Encourage patients to ask questions and talk about their feelings. Often a patient's fears are due to a lack of knowledge about the disease and treatment. The oncology clinical nurse specialist or other specially trained oncology nurse can answer many of the patient's and family's questions. Many times information is what the patient and family need to deal with their anxieties. However, a referral to a social worker, chaplain, or mental health counselor may be indicated if the patient and family are having continued anxiety and difficulty in coping. It is important for you to know what the patient understands about the disease, the treatment, and the prognosis so that correct information can be reinforced.

Ineffective Therapeutic Regimen Management

It is very important that the patient receive accurate, consistent information from all members of the health care team. An oncology clinical nurse specialist or other specially trained oncology nurse can usually provide comprehensive information about the disease and its treatment to the patient and family and answer questions as they arise during hospitalization. All nurses reinforce this teaching. The Leukemia and Lymphoma Society (1311 Mamaroneck Avenue; White Plains, NY 10605; website: http://www.leukemia-lymphoma.org; telephone: 1-800-955-4LSA or 1-914-949-5213) provides excellent, free literature on the different types of leukemia. The National Cancer Institute, through the Cancer Information Service, provides excellent, free literature on chemotherapy for people receiving treatment. They can be reached by calling 1-800-4CANCER or on the Internet at http://www.nci.nih.gov. The American Cancer Society (1599 Clifton Road; Atlanta, GA 30320; website: http://www.cancer.org; telephone: 1-800-ACS-2345) has many support services available for people with all forms of cancer, including leukemia.

OTHER IMMUNE SYSTEM DISORDERS

Hypersensitivity Reactions

Hypersensitivity reactions, or allergies, are exaggerated immune responses that can be uncomfortable and potentially harmful to the patient. There are four types of hypersensitivity reactions, classified according to the time between exposure and reaction, immune mechanism involved, and site of reaction.

Type I immediate hypersensitivity reactions are mediated by IgE reacting to common allergens such as dust, pollen, animal dander, insect stings, or various drugs. Type I reactions can be either local, resulting in local swelling and discomfort, or systemic, resulting in anaphylaxis and possible death if not recognized and treated promptly. Type I anaphylactic hypersensitivity reactions occur in the following way. After a first, sensitizing exposure to a specific allergen, subsequent exposures to the same allergen trigger an exaggerated antibody reaction. For example, in a person with a hypersensitivity reaction to insect stings, one insect sting results in the production of abnormally large amounts of IgE antibodies. When this person is stung again by the same type of insect, the circulating IgE immediately triggers the release of histamine and other cytokines from mast cells, causing bronchiole constriction, peripheral vasodilation, and increased capillary permeability. These individuals can experience airway obstruction, pulmonary congestion, peripheral edema, hypotension, shock, and circulatory collapse. Prompt diagnosis and treatment of anaphylaxis with epinephrine, antihistamines, steroids, and hemodynamic support is of paramount importance.

Type II immediate hypersensitivity reactions are mediated by antibody reactions. Type II hypersensitivity reactions can occur with a mismatched blood transfusion or as a response to various drugs.

Type III immediate hypersensitivity reactions result in tissue damage resulting from precipitation of antigen-antibody immune complexes. Type III hypersensitivity reactions can occur with autoimmune reactions, some occupational diseases, or as a response to various drugs.

Type IV delayed hypersensitivity reactions result from immune cells migrating to the site of exposure days after the exposure to the antigen. Type IV hypersensitivity reactions can occur with contact dermatitis, measles rash, tuberculin skin testing, or various drugs. Transplanted graft rejection occurs because of a type IV hypersensitivity reaction. Hypersensitivity reactions to drugs, or drug allergies, are one of many possible adverse drug reactions. Drug-induced hypersensitivity reactions can be any of the four types of hypersensitivity.

Idiopathic Thrombocytopenic Purpura (ITP)

ITP is an antibody-mediated autoimmune disorder in which IgG mistakenly helps destroy the patient's own platelets. Drugs known to induce ITP include sulfonamides, thiazide diuretics, chlorpropamide, quinidine, and gold. Patients with HIV infection are at increased risk for developing ITP.

Treatment for ITP can include steroids and intravenous immune globulin (IVIG). Approximately 75% of adult patients with ITP will sequester (store) platelets in the spleen, and so splenectomy is done in some patients to remove this storehouse, thereby increasing the circulating blood levels of platelets. Immunosuppressive therapy with cytotoxic drugs (e.g., vincristine or cyclophosphamide) can be used in patients who do not respond to splenectomy. Platelet transfusions are *not* indicated because the underlying problem is platelet consumption, not platelet production. If platelets are transfused, they are immediately destroyed. Nursing actions for the patient who is at risk for injury from bleeding are outlined in Table 31-7.

Thrombotic Thrombocytopenic Purpura (TTP)

TTP is an exaggerated immunologic response to vessel injury that results in extensive clot formation and decreased blood flow to the site. These patients become critically ill, developing fever, thrombocytopenia, hemolytic anemia, renal impairment, and neurologic symptoms.

The main treatment for TTP is plasmapheresis, which presumably removes the immunologic agent that triggered the TTP from the plasma. The patient's blood is centrifuged in an apheresis machine that separates the blood components so that the plasma can be selectively removed. The patient's own white blood cells, red blood cells, and platelets are reinfused during the treatment. Critically ill patients can become hemodynamically unstable during this procedure and need close monitoring and timely interventions to maintain cardiac output and blood pressure. Plasmapheresis usually is done daily or every other day for several weeks until the patient's hematologic parameters stabilize. Other treatments include steroids, antiplatelet agents (e.g., aspirin, dipyridamole, or persantine), splenectomy, or all three. Platelet transfusions are usually contraindicated because they may contribute to the abnormal clotting process. Nursing actions for the patient who is at risk for injury from bleeding are outlined in Table 31-7.

Systemic Lupus Erythematosus

Systemic lupus erythematosus (SLE) is an autoimmune disease in which the person's immune system loses its ability to recognize itself and mounts an immune response against its own proteins. Damage results from antibodies and immune complexes directed against one or many organ systems. The cause of SLE is unknown. Ninety percent of cases occur in women, usually of child-bearing age. The disease is much more common in African Americans as compared to Caucasians. Between 82% and 90% of patients with SLE are alive at 5 years, 71% and 80% at 10 years, and 63% and 75% at 20 years. Factors associated with a poor outcome include increased creatinine, hypertension, large amounts of protein excreted in the urine, anemia, and low socioeconomic status.

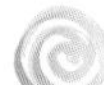

What Does Culture Have to do with Lupus?

Although the cause of SLE is unknown, there may be a genetic predisposition. The disease is more common in women, and is three times more common in African American women than in Caucasian women.

Signs and Symptoms of SLE

Patients with SLE can experience long periods of remission alternating with periods of symptom exacerbation. Almost every organ system can be affected. The most common symptoms, experienced by 95% of patients at some time during the course of their disease, include fatigue, malaise, fever, anorexia, nausea, and weight loss. Musculoskeletal symptoms, also experienced by 95% of patients at some time during the course of their disease, include arthralgias (joint pain) and myalgias (muscle pain). Joints are often swollen, tender, stiff, and painful with movement. Cutaneous symptoms can include a rash and photosensitivity. The classic skin lesion is a butterfly-shaped rash across the bridge of the nose and the cheeks. This rash can extend to the neck, upper trunk, and arms. Life- and organ-threatening symptoms can include inflammation of the kidneys, heart, and/or lungs resulting in organ failure. Inflammation of the retina of the eye can result in sudden-onset blindness, which can be very frightening to patients.

Diagnosis

There is no one test that confirms the diagnosis of SLE. Blood work may detect antinuclear antibody (ANA), but a positive ANA is not specific for SLE. A negative ANA assay makes the diagnosis of SLE unlikely but not impossible. Rather than a blood test, the diagnosis of SLE is based upon the constellation of symptoms the patient is experiencing. Because symptoms come and go, the diagnosis of SLE can be very difficult to make and can take a long time. The American Rheumatism Association has established criteria for the diagnosis of SLE. If a patient experiences any four of the following symptoms, a diagnosis of SLE can be made:

- Characteristic rash
- Photosensitivity with exposure to sunlight
- Oral ulcers
- Arthritis
- Pleuritis or pericarditis (i.e., inflammation of the lungs or heart)
- Renal disorder (e.g., proteinuria)
- Neurologic disorder (e.g., seizures or psychosis)
- Hematologic disorder (e.g., anemia, leukopenia, or thrombocytopenia)
- Immunologic disorder (as evidenced by detection of abnormal antibodies in the blood)
- Positive ANA

Medical Treatment

There is no cure for SLE. The medical treatment of SLE is symptomatic and aimed at minimizing symptoms, preventing organ damage, and maintaining quality of life. Fever, arthralgias, myalgias, and rash are managed with analgesics, nonsteroidal antiinflammatory drugs (NSAIDs), antimalarials, and corticosteroids. If symptoms are not controlled with these drugs or if organ function is threatened, cytotoxic agents (such as azathioprine, chlorambucil, cyclophosphamide, or methotrexate) can be used to suppress the abnormal immune response.

NURSING CARE *of the Patient with SLE*

The nursing care of the patient with SLE varies depending on the severity of the symptoms the patient may be experiencing. Patients are treated primarily as outpatients. Because patients with SLE are frequent consumers of medical care, they often become very knowledgeable about their disease and want to be fully informed of all treatments they are receiving as well as the possible side effects of the treatments. The goal of care is quality of life.

Assessment

The complexity of SLE requires a thorough health history and physical examination. It is critical to do a complete functional assessment to determine the effects of the symptoms on the patient's activities of daily living.

Nursing Diagnoses, Goals, and Outcome Criteria: Systemic Lupus Erythematosus

Nursing goals and diagnoses for the patient with SLE are extremely individualized but may include the following:

Nursing Diagnoses	Goals and Outcome Criteria
Fatigue related to the disease process and treatment	Decreased fatigue: patient manages daily routines without excessive tiring
Acute Pain related to inflammation of joints and muscles	Pain relief: patient states pain is relieved, appears relaxed
Disturbed Body Image related to skin rash	Improved body image: patient makes positive statements about self, employs measures to improve appearance
Ineffective Coping related to stress of chronic illness	Effective coping: patient employs positive coping skills to reduce stress
Ineffective Therapeutic Regimen Management related to lack of knowledge about disease process and treatment	Patient resumes self care: patient accurately describes disease process, treatments, and side effects of treatment

Interventions

Fatigue

Almost all patients with SLE report experiencing fatigue. Causes of fatigue in these patients can include a low red blood cell count from both the disease and treatment, chronic pain, disrupted sleep, and the psychological stress of the disease and treatment. A detailed discussion of the nursing management of fatigue is presented in Chapter 24.

Acute Pain

Pain can be caused by inflammation of muscles and joints as well as inflammation of various organs. Closely monitor the patient's pain level and medication usage. Keeping a flow sheet of patient reports of pain on a 10-point scale can be helpful, especially as different nurses care for the patient throughout the day. A 0 represents no pain, whereas a 10 represents the worst pain a patient has ever experienced. The patient report of pain coupled with the amount of pain medication he or she is receiving can guide the nurse and physician as to the appropriate type and amount of pain medication. Pharmacologic and nonpharmacologic pain management strategies are presented in Chapter 14.

Disturbed Body Image

Encourage the patient to avoid prolonged exposure to the sun and to use sunscreen with an SPF rating of >15 to prevent the skin rash and exacerbation of symptoms.

Ineffective Coping

A diagnosis of SLE is always a shock to patients and their families. Patients must deal not only with the disease and treatment but also with the emotions of facing a chronic illness. Encourage patients to ask questions and to talk about their feelings. A referral to a social worker, chaplain, or mental health counselor may be indicated if the patient and family are having difficulty in coping.

Ineffective Therapeutic Regimen Management

It is very important that the patient receive accurate, consistent information from all members of the health care team. A clinical nurse specialist or other specially trained nurse can usually provide comprehensive information about the disease and its treatment to the patient and family and answer questions as they arise during hospitalization. It is important for you to know what the patient has been told about the disease, the treatment, and the prognosis so that correct information can be reinforced. Most important, the patient's interpretation and understanding of the information is essential. There are several resources available about SLE for patients, families, and health care providers, including the Lupus Foundation of America (1300 Piccard Drive, Suite 200; Rockville, MD 20850-4303; website: http://www.lupus.org; telephone: 1-301-670-9292 and 1-800-558-0121) and the American Lupus Society (260 Maple Court, Suite 123; Ventura, CA 93003-3511; telephone: 1-805-339-0443 and 1-800-331-1802). These organizations provide excellent free literature on SLE and can help locate support groups in specific regions of the country.

PATIENT TEACHING PLAN
Systemic Lupus Erythematosus

- Know the names, dosages, schedule, and side effects of your drugs.
- Avoid prolonged exposure to the sun and use sunscreen with an SPF rating of >15.
- You can get additional information from the Lupus Foundation of America and the American Lupus Society.

HUMAN IMMUNODEFICIENCY VIRUS INFECTION

Human immunodeficiency virus (HIV) is a retrovirus that infects cells expressing CD4 on their cell membranes, primarily T_H cells. The HIV copies its RNA into the host cell's DNA and then remains quiescent until the host cell is activated to mount an immunologic response. Activation of the host T_H CD4 cells also initiates replication and production of the HIV RNA, which is released into the circulation. This newly made HIV then infects other T_H CD4 cells. HIV is transmitted via intimate sexual contact, contaminated needles, and contaminated blood products; from mother to fetus; and from mother to breast-feeding infant.

The initial stage of HIV infection lasts 4 to 8 weeks. High levels of virus are in the blood. The patient experiences generalized flulike symptoms. The virus then enters a latent stage in which it is inactive in infected, resting T_H CD4 host cells. When the resting CD4 host cell is activated for an immune response, the virus begins to replicate. Levels of virus are high in the lymph nodes where T_H CD4 cells reside but low in the blood. T_C cells and B cells attempt to destroy the T_H CD4 cells harboring virus. However, the T_C cells and B cells are crippled without adequate T_H CD4 support. This latent stage can last 2 to 12 years, during which time the patient is asymptomatic. During this time the number of T_H CD4 cells declines. During the third stage of HIV infection, the patient begins to experience opportunistic infections. Levels of T_H CD4 cells are usually below 500 cells/mm^3 and declining while levels of virus in the blood are increasing. This stage can last 2 to 3 years. Once the CD4 cell levels drop below 200 cells/mm^3, the patient is considered to have acquired immunodeficiency syndrome (AIDS). Virus levels in the blood are high. This stage ends in death, usually within 1 year.

The major complications of HIV infection are opportunistic infections, wasting, secondary cancers, and dementia. Patients with AIDS are at very high risk for opportunistic fungal, parasitic, and viral infections. Infections these patients commonly experience include oral candidiasis, *Pneumocystis carinii* pneumonia, herpes simplex, cytomegalovirus retinitis, *Cryptosporidium* enteritis, *Cryptococcus neoformans* meningitis, and toxoplasmosis. Almost all patients with HIV experience a wasting syndrome characterized by weight loss and malnutrition. Reduced food intake, malabsorption of nutrients, and altered metabolic pathways all contribute to this wasting syndrome. Cancers such as Kaposi's sarcoma, non-Hodgkin's lymphoma, anal cancer, and cervical cancer occur in 40% of patients with HIV infection. Presumably this increased incidence of cancer is due to the inability of the patient's crippled immune system to identify and destroy cells that undergo malignant changes. The virus can affect the central nervous system, causing encephalopathy, cognitive impairment, and dementia.

Signs and Symptoms of HIV Infection

Patients in the initial stage of HIV infection may only experience generalized flu-like symptoms. During the second, latent stage of the disease, patients may not experience any symptoms. Eventually, patients begin to experience frequent and persistent infections. Patients may present for medical care complaining of fever, night sweats, swollen lymph nodes, or other symptoms specific to the site of infection such as headache, skin lesions that do not heal, sore throat, dyspnea, burning with urination, or diarrhea. Patients also may report extreme fatigue and weight loss. Any of these symptoms coupled with a history of unprotected sexual contact with persons possibly infected with HIV, a history of intravenous drug abuse using shared needles, or a history of a blood transfusion before 1989 warrants consideration of a diagnosis of HIV infection.

Diagnosis

HIV infection is diagnosed with a positive result on an enzyme-linked immunosorbent assay (ELISA) and confirmed with a positive result on a Western blot test. The ELISA is a less expensive screening test for HIV antibody. If the ELISA is positive, a Western blot should be done to confirm the results because false positives do occur with ELISA. Once HIV infection is diagnosed, other blood tests (i.e., T cell counts and viral load) and skin testing help determine the stage of infection and the treatment approach and establish baseline values to evaluate the patient's response to treatment. Table 32-2 describes the procedures for collecting blood for these tests and for performing skin tests.

Medical Treatment

There is no cure for HIV. The medical treatment of HIV infection is symptomatic and is aimed at reducing the viral load, preventing and treating infections, and treating malignancies. Table 32-6 outlines drugs used to treat the HIV infection. Patients also are encouraged to maintain a balanced diet, exercise regularly, maintain good dental hygiene, stop smoking and using illicit drugs, limit alcohol intake, minimize stress, and practice safe sexual habits.

NURSING CARE *of the Patient with HIV Infection*

The nursing care of the patient with HIV infection varies depending on the stage of infection the patient is experiencing (see Nursing Care Plan: The Patient with HIV Infection). During the early stages of the disease patients are treated primarily as outpatients. Because patients with HIV infection are frequent consumers of medical care, they often become very knowledgeable about their disease and treatment options and want to be actively involved in all treatment decisions. In the later states of HIV infection, nursing care is much more intensive as the patient becomes more debilitated. Throughout the trajectory of this disease, the goal of all treatments is quality of life.

Assessment

Infection is the leading cause of death in patients with HIV infection. Therefore it is important to frequently assess the patient for any signs or symptoms of infection. The most common sites of infection are the lungs, mouth, gastrointestinal tract, skin, blood, and central nervous system. Any change in the physical examination findings or any change in function should be reported to a registered nurse or physician. While doing a physical assessment, assess how much the patient knows about the disease and treatment and how the patient is coping with this life-threatening disease.

Nursing Diagnoses, Goals, and Outcome Criteria: HIV Infection

Nursing Diagnoses	Goals and Outcome Criteria
Ineffective Therapeutic Regimen Management related to lack of knowledge about disease process and treatment, denial, fear	Effective self-care management: patient correctly describes and demonstrates self-care measures
Anxiety related to the disease and treatment	Reduced anxiety: patient reports anxiety is lessened, more relaxed manner
Risk for Injury related to infection (lung, mouth, gastrointestinal tract, skin, blood, central nervous system, eye)	Patient remains free of infection: no fever, signs of inflammation, lesions
Impaired Oral Mucous Membranes related to the disease and oral infections	Intact oral mucous membranes: normal color of mouth tissues, no lesions
Imbalanced Nutrition: Less than Body Requirements and Deficient Fluid Volume related to the disease, diarrhea, and gastrointestinal infections	Adequate intake of nutrients and fluids: stable weight, intake and output approximately equal, moist mucous membranes
Disturbed Thought Processes related to disease-induced dementia	Improved thought processes: patient remains oriented Patient safety: absence of injuries associated with confusion
Pain related to the disease and treatment	Pain relief: patient states pain in relieved, appears relaxed

Interventions

Ineffective Therapeutic Regimen Management

It is very important that the patient receive accurate, consistent information from all members of the health care team. A clinical nurse specialist or other specially trained nurse can usually provide comprehensive information about the disease and its treatment to the patient and family and answer questions as they arise during hospitalization. You can reinforce this teaching. Excellent sources of current information about HIV and AIDS for patients, families, and health care providers are on the Internet (e.g., http://www.thebody.com and http://www.hivinsite.ucsf.edu).

Anxiety

A diagnosis of HIV infection is always a shock to patients and their families. Patients must deal not only with the disease and treatment but also with the emotions of facing a life-threatening illness. Encourage patients to ask questions and to talk about their feelings. Many times a patient's fears are due to a lack of knowledge about the disease and treatment. The clinical nurse specialist or other specially trained nurse can answer many of the patient's and family's questions. Many times information will help the patient and family deal with their anxiety. A referral to a social worker, chaplain, or mental health counselor may be indicated if the patient and family are having continued anxiety and difficulty in coping. It is important for you to

NURSING CARE PLAN

The Patient with HIV Infection

ASSESSMENT

Health History: Darla Hughes is a 25-year-old divorced mother of two children. She works as a freelance accountant and lives with her parents, who provide financial and emotional support. She was diagnosed with HIV infection during the pregnancy with her daughter, Lindsay. Lindsay, now 3, has shown no signs of HIV infection. Darla's husband divorced her when the infection was diagnosed. His HIV status is not known. Darla reports tiring easily but most days is able to work about 6 hours and care for her children. She is seen monthly by a nurse practitioner at a local neighborhood clinic. Her medications are indinavir (Crixivan), stavudine (Zerit), and didanosine (Videx). She reports bouts of depression and anxiety about her own and her children's future. Her most recent blood studies show a decline in the number of T helper (CD4) cells. The CD4 cell level today is 480 cells/mm^3. Darla has been treated twice this fall for upper respiratory tract infections. She does not sleep well. She has experienced a 10-pound weight loss in the past 3 months and reports poor appetite and frequent diarrhea.

Physical Examination: Healthy-looking young woman. Alert. Converses easily. Vital signs WNL. No fever. Lungs clear on auscultation. No lymphadenopathy. Abdomen soft. Bowel sounds present in all 4 quadrants. Normal reflexes. Full range of motion in all joints.

Nursing Diagnosis	*Goals and Outcome Criteria*	*Interventions*
Ineffective therapeutic regimen management related to lack of knowledge about disease process and treatment, denial, and fear.	Patient will effectively manage self-care, as evidenced by correctly taking prescribed medications, following medical advice for rest and protection from infection.	Provide written and verbal instructions for prescribed drug(s). Advise her of the kinds of side and adverse effects that she might experience. Explain the importance of continuing the drugs under medical supervision. Discuss ways to conserve energy and to promote restful sleep at night. Explore options to obtain assistance with child care.
Anxiety related to disease and treatments.	Patient will verbalize decreased anxiety and will appear more relaxed.	Encourage her to ask questions and talk about her feelings. Be accepting of feelings she may express (fear, anger, depression are common). Provide information or refer to a social worker, chaplain, or mental health counselor if needed.
Risk for injury related to infection associated with impaired resistance.	Patient will remain free of infection, as evidenced by absence of fever, lesions, or signs of inflammation.	Encourage her to immediately report any signs of infection. If antibiotics are ordered, encourage her to take them as prescribed. Explain the need to avoid people with infections and crowded public places during seasons when upper respiratory tract infections are common.
Impaired oral mucous membranes related to HIV infection and oral opportunistic infections.	Patient will have intact oral mucous membranes with normal color and no lesions.	Teach importance of regular dental care. Advise her to use a soft toothbrush and to avoid traumatizing oral tissues. Explain how maintaining good fluid intake keeps mucous membranes moist and reduces oral complications.
Imbalanced nutrition: less than body requirements and deficient fluid volume related to HIV infection, diarrhea, and gastrointestinal infections.	Patient's intake of food and fluids will be adequate, as evidenced by stable body weight, moist mucous membranes, and normal blood pressure and pulse.	Suggest addition of Carnation Instant Breakfast to daily diet to increase calorie intake. Weigh weekly. Talk to nurse practitioner about prescribing antinausea medication, appetite stimulant, and antidiarrheal agent.

know what the patient has been told about the disease, the treatment, and the prognosis so that correct information can be reinforced. Most important, the patient's interpretation and understanding of the information are essential.

Infection

Patients with HIV are at high risk for opportunistic infections. Early detection and prompt treatment of infection are vital. Many patients take anti-infective drugs (e.g., trimethoprim-sulfamethoxazole, pentamidine) prophylactically to prevent infection. Educate the patient about the importance of taking drugs exactly as prescribed. If a patient does develop an infection, he or she must take the antibiotics exactly as prescribed. Stopping antibiotic therapy early can result in incomplete treatment and the development of resistant organisms. Many of the antibiotics must be administered intravenously and require nursing coordination for intravenous access and either clinic or home administration.

Impaired Oral Mucous Membranes

Patients with HIV can experience altered oral mucous membrane integrity due to both the disease and oral infections. Encourage patients to regularly clean their teeth and mouth with dental floss and a soft toothbrush. Debilitated patients may need assistance with mouth care. Encourage fluids to maintain hydration and to keep oral mucous membranes moist. Topical anesthetics to control pain can be applied before eating. Prescribed topical antibiotics should be reapplied after eating and routine mouth care. Regular dental evaluations can help prevent and manage oral disease and infections in these patients.

Imbalanced Nutrition: Less than Body Requirements

A referral to a dietician for nutrition education and counseling should be made as soon as the patient is diagnosed with HIV. Strategies to maximize calorie and nutrient intake can be discussed. Oral supplements with Carnation Instant Breakfast, Ensure, Sustacal, or Resource can be added as indicated. Administer medications to improve appetite (e.g., megestrol, dronabinol), relieve nausea (e.g., prochlorperazine, metoclopramide), and control diarrhea (e.g., diphenoxylate hydrochloride with atropine sulfate) as prescribed.

Disturbed Thought Processes

Patients with HIV encephalopathy may experience both cognitive and motor impairment. Patients may withdraw from social activities because of embarrassment. Patients may become angry and hostile with the onset of yet another disability. Many patients with HIV-induced encephalopathy improve with zidovudine therapy. Both in the hospital and at home, patient safety needs to be constantly reevaluated based on the patient's mental and physical capabilities.

Pain

Pain has been an under-recognized problem for patients with HIV infection. Pain can be caused by opportunistic infections, viral invasion into the nerves and muscles, malignant tumors, and diagnostic procedures. Closely monitor the patient's pain level and medication usage. Keeping a flow sheet of patient reports of pain on a 10-point scale can be helpful, especially as different nurses care for the patient throughout the day. A 0 represents no pain, while a 10 represents the worst pain a patient has ever experienced. The patient's report of pain coupled with the amount of pain medication he or she is receiving can guide the nurse and physician as to the appropriate type and amount of pain medication. Pharmacologic and nonpharmacologic pain management strategies are presented in Chapter 14.

NON-HODGKIN'S LYMPHOMA

Non-Hodgkin's lymphoma is a cancer of the lymph system. The American Cancer Society estimated that 53,900 new cases of non-Hodgkin's lymphoma would be diagnosed in 2002, accounting for about 4% of all new cases of cancer diagnosed. Patients of any age and either sex may develop non-Hodgkin's lymphoma, although the disease is more commonly seen in older people. Non-Hodgkin's lymphomas are staged as low-grade, intermediate-grade, and high-grade. The higher the grade of lymphoma, the more aggressive is the cancer. Medical treatment of non-Hodgkin's disease can include either radiation therapy or chemotherapy, depending on the stage of the disease. High-dose therapy with bone marrow transplantation or peripheral blood stem cell transplantation is an option for some patients who suffer disease recurrence after standard treatment. Again, survival rates vary widely, depending on the grade of the disease at diagnosis. The overall 5-year survival rate for patients with non-Hodgkin's lymphoma is 52%.

HODGKIN'S DISEASE

Hodgkin's disease is a type of lymphoma characterized by Reed-Sternberg cells in the lymph nodes. The American Cancer Society estimated that 7,000 new cases of Hodgkin's disease would be diagnosed in 2002, accounting for less than 1% of all new cases of cancer diagnosed. The incidence of the disease is highest in people in their twenties and in their fifties. Men are more likely than women to have the disease. The medical treatment of Hodgkin's disease can include either radiation therapy or chemotherapy, depending on the stage of the disease. High-dose therapy with bone marrow transplantation or peripheral blood stem cell transplantation is an option for patients who suffer disease recurrence after standard treatment. Survival rates vary widely, depending on the stage of the disease at diagnosis. The overall 5-year survival rate for patients with Hodgkin's disease is 82%.

MULTIPLE MYELOMA

Multiple myeloma is a cancer of the plasma cells in the bone marrow that causes abnormally high levels of immunoglobulins. Multiple myeloma is most commonly seen in people over the age of 60. There is no known cause for multiple myeloma; however, radiation exposure and genetic factors may play a role. Patients with multiple myeloma usually seek medical care because of bone pain. Other symptoms of the disease can be hyperuricemia if the myeloma proteins become trapped in the kidneys, anemia, hypercalcemia from bone destruction, bone fractures, and spinal cord compression. Multiple myeloma is diagnosed with radiographs, serum protein electrophoresis, 24-hour urine protein electrophoresis, and a bone marrow biopsy. Tables 32-2 and 31-4 describe the procedures for doing these studies. There is no cure for multiple myeloma. Radiation therapy and chemotherapy are given to control symptoms.

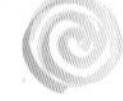

What Does Culture Have to do with Multiple Myeloma?

Multiple myeloma affects African Americans twice as often as whites.

TRANSPLANT REJECTION

Patients who undergo kidney, heart, liver, or other organ transplantation risk that their own healthy immune system will recognize the transplanted organ (or allograft) as foreign and try to destroy it. Rejections occur through various mechanisms. T_C lymphocytes can directly attack the allograft, resulting in acute transplant rejection within hours of the transplant. B lymphocytes can make antibodies against the allograft. Fibrin accumulates on the transplanted tissue, causing ischemia. In this way the allograft is slowly rejected over months to years. Tissue matching of donor to recipient minimizes the chance of the recipient's immune system attacking the allograft after transplantation.

Various combinations of drugs are also given to suppress the recipient's immune system and minimize the immune response to the allograft. However, these drugs also suppress the patient's ability to fight bacteria, viruses, fungi, and parasites, putting the patient at increased risk for infection. Combinations of steroids (which inhibit the inflammatory response by inhibiting the production of prostaglandins), cyclosporine (which inhibits T lymphocytes), and azathioprine (which inhibits B cell and T cell proliferation) are commonly used to chronically suppress the immune system after an organ transplant. Table 32-6 describes the nursing care of patients taking these drugs. There are also several newer drugs that target the T cells while preserving B cell function and thus more of the patient's immune function. Examples of these drugs include tacrolimus (Prograf), antilymphocyte globulin, antithymocyte globulin, and murine monoclonal antibody to CD3 (OKT3). Patients who have undergone organ transplantation must take immunosuppressive therapy the rest of their lives to preserve the allograft. These immunosuppressive drugs, which are needed to preserve the allograft, paradoxically put patients at an increased risk of infection from environmental bacteria, viruses, fungi, and parasites.

Put on your THINKING CAP!!

Explain what would happen physiologically if transplant recipients did not take immunosuppressant drugs to prevent organ rejection.

Consider the Alternative!

Herbs such as echinacea that stimulate immune function may interfere with the actions of immunosuppressants.

The views of this author are her own and do not purport to reflect the position of the Army Medical Department, Department of the Army, or the Department of Defense.

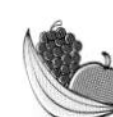

Nutrition Concepts

1. Because food contains microorganisms, patients with low white blood cell counts are discouraged from eating raw fruits and vegetables and from drinking milk.
2. Management of nausea and vomiting is essential to maintain good nutrition in patients having chemotherapy.
3. Patients with HIV require high calorie and nutrient intake to combat wasting.

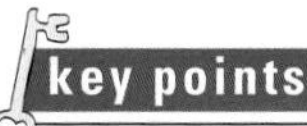

key points

- The immune system is the body's defense network against infection; it provides the body with resistance to invading organisms and enables it to fight off invaders once they have gained access.
- Body organs that are part of a functioning immune system include the bone marrow, lymph nodes, spleen, and thymus.
- Antigens are foreign substances that stimulate a response from the immune system, whereas antibodies are proteins that are produced by the immune system to help eradicate antigens.
- Innate immunity is present in the body at birth, whereas acquired immunity develops after birth as a result of the body's immune response to specific antigens.
- Many types of leukocytes act as nature's cleanup mechanism by migrating to infected or inflamed areas and engulfing and destroying antigens through a process known as phagocytosis.
- The two types of acquired immunity are antibody-mediated and cell-mediated.
- Acquired immunity depends on the proper development and functioning of specific white blood cells called B and T lymphocytes.
- Immunodeficiency occurs when the body is unable to launch an adequate immune response, resulting in an increased risk of infection.
- Because the bone marrow becomes less productive with age, the older person's immune response may be inadequate under stressful situations.
- The patient with a low white blood cell count is at risk for infection.
- Bone marrow transplantation and peripheral blood stem cell transplantation are procedures that reconstitute the hematologic and immunologic systems after certain cancer therapies.
- The two main types of leukemia are myelogenous and lymphocytic.
- Infection is the leading cause of death in patients with leukemia.
- Drugs used to suppress the immune response after organ or tissue transplants also put the patient at risk for infection.
- Allergy or hypersensitivity occurs when a normally inoffensive foreign substance stimulates an atypical or exaggerated immune response.
- Systemic lupus erythematosus is considered an autoimmune disorder.

- Systemic lupus erythematosus can affect multiple body systems.
- Human immunodeficiency virus infection inactivates T helper (CD4 cells) lymphocytes, resulting in opportunistic infections and secondary cancers.
- Once the CD4 cell level drops below 200 cells/mm^3, the patient is considered to have acquired immunodeficiency syndrome (AIDS).

REVIEW QUESTIONS

1. A patient has a neutrophil count that is 70% of his total WBC count. You should suspect:
   1. bacterial infection.
   2. viral infection.
   3. parasitic infestation.
   4. allergic reaction.
2. Mr. B had chickenpox as a child. When he was exposed to chickenpox years later, he did not become infected. His resistance was most likely due to:
   1. passive acquired immunity.
   2. innate immunity.
   3. active acquired immunity.
   4. idiopathic immunity.
3. Which statement best describes the effects of age-related changes in the immune system?
   1. The older person has little resistance to infection.
   2. The immune system functions well under normal circumstances.
   3. Lymphatic tissue enlarges to compensate for decreased activity.
   4. Older people have better immune function than most young adults.
4. Which of the following is an autoimmune disorder?
   1. Type 2 diabetes mellitus
   2. Hypothyroidism
   3. Leukemia
   4. Systemic lupus erythematosus
5. A priority when assessing the patient with an immune disorder is:
   1. signs and symptoms of infection.
   2. unexplained changes in weight.
   3. increased blood pressure.
   4. characteristics of urine.
6. During report, it is noted that there is a shift to the right on your patient's CBC. You know that this could mean that:
   1. your patient has a mild infection.
   2. your patient's infection is resolving.
   3. your patient has an overwhelming infection.
   4. your patient is producing excess neutrophils.
7. A patient with leukemia is on compromised host precautions, which include:
   1. visitors and staff should wash their hands before patient contact.
   2. the patient can have only fresh, raw fruits and vegetables.
   3. staff should always wear masks when in the patient's room.
   4. monitor vital signs at least every 8 hours.
8. Shortly after receiving an antibiotic, a patient experienced a type 1 immediate hypersensitivity reaction. Signs and symptoms would include:
   1. mental confusion.
   2. difficulty breathing.
   3. hypertension.
   4. nausea and vomiting.
9. Pain management during the acute phase of a sickle cell crisis usually requires:
   1. nonsteroidal anti-inflammatory agents.
   2. physical therapy.
   3. nerve blocks.
   4. opioid analgesics.
10. A patient with HIV infection has recently become confused. You should explain to the patient's partner that:
    1. confusion with HIV is rare and irreversible.
    2. the patient's confusion is probably related to something other than HIV.
    3. the patient's mental status may improve with drug therapy.
    4. confusion usually occurs shortly before death.

CHAPTER 33 Cardiac Disorders

JUDY L. MALTAS

objectives

1. Label the major parts of the heart.
2. Describe the flow of blood through the heart and coronary vessels.
3. Name the elements of the heart's conduction system
4. State the order in which normal impulses are conducted through the heart.
5. Explain the nursing considerations for patients having procedures to detect or evaluate cardiac disorders.
6. Identify nursing implications for common therapeutic measures, including drug, diet, or oxygen therapy; pacemakers and cardioverters; cardiac surgery; and cardiopulmonary resuscitation.
7. For selected cardiac disorders, explain the pathophysiology, risk factors, signs and symptoms, complications, and treatment.
8. List the data to be obtained in assessing the patient with a cardiac disorder.
9. Assist in developing nursing care plans for patients with cardiac disorders.

key terms

Afterload (p. 559)
Arteriosclerosis (ăr-tē-rē-ō-sklĕ-RŌ-sĭs, p. 579)
Atherosclerosis (ăth-ĕr-ō-sklĕ-RŌ-sĭs, p. 579)
Bradycardia (brăd-ĕ-KĂR-dē-ă, p. 560)
Dysrhythmia (dĭs-RĬTH-mē-ă, p. 560)
Hemodynamics (hē-mō-dī-NĂM-ĭks, p. 587)
Infarction (ĭn-FĂRK-shŭn, p. 580)
Murmur (MŬR-mĕr, p. 561)
Palpitation (păl-pĭ-TĀ-shŭn, p. 560)
Perfusion (pĕr-FŪ-zhŭn, p. 576)
Preload (p. 559)
Regurgitation (rē-gŭr-jĭ-TĀ-shŭn, p. 594)
Syncope (SĬN-kō-pē, p. 560)
Tachycardia (tăk-ē-KĂR-dē-ă, p. 560)
Thromboembolism (thrŏm-bō-ĔM-bō-lĭsm, p. 580)

The cardiovascular system carries oxygenated blood and nutrients to the cells and transports carbon dioxide and wastes from the cells. It requires a reservoir for blood coming from the tissues, pumping action to send blood to the lungs and the body, and an intact vascular system to transport the blood. A malfunction in any of these components may affect other body systems and may threaten the life and health of the person.

The heart is a hollow muscular pump located in the mediastinum (Fig. 33-1). The right and left sides of the heart receive blood from and send blood to different parts of the body. The heart is covered and protected by the sternum and the ribs anteriorly and flanked by the lungs laterally. The esophagus, the descending aorta, and the fifth through the eighth thoracic vertebrae are directly behind the heart. The heart rests on the diaphragm, with two thirds of it to the left of the sternum. The right side of the heart is located under the sternum. The heart is approximately the size of the person's fist, weighs 10 to 14 ounces in the adult, and is covered by membranes called the visceral and parietal pericardium. The space between the pericardial membranes contains fluid that lubricates the membranes and decreases friction.

ANATOMY AND PHYSIOLOGY OF THE HEART

CHAMBERS

The heart is divided into four chambers: two upper atria (right and left) and two lower ventricles (right and left). The four chambers are separated by septa (walls) with two chambers on the right (right atrium and ventricle) and two chambers on the left (left atrium and ventricle). Valves separate the atria from the ventricles.

The right atrium (RA) is a thin-walled reservoir and conduit for systemic blood. It receives blood from the inferior and the superior venae cavae and from the coronary sinuses. The right ventricle (RV) has thicker walls than the RA and receives blood from the RA through the tricuspid valve. Blood moves rather passively from the RA to the RV. When the RV contracts (systole), blood is ejected through the pulmonic valve into the pulmonary artery. The pulmonary artery carries the blood to the lungs, where it releases carbon dioxide as waste and picks up oxygen to be taken to the tissues. Pulmonary veins carry the blood from the lungs to the left atrium (LA).

The blood passes from the LA through the mitral valve into the left ventricle (LV), the chamber with the thickest, strongest muscle. The LV is cone-shaped and contains the apex of the heart located at the midclavicular line at the fourth or fifth intercostal space. An apical pulse is taken by auscultating the heartbeat at this location.

When the LV contracts (systole), blood is ejected through the aortic valve into the aorta and the systemic circulation. The systemic circulation carries oxygen and nutrients to all

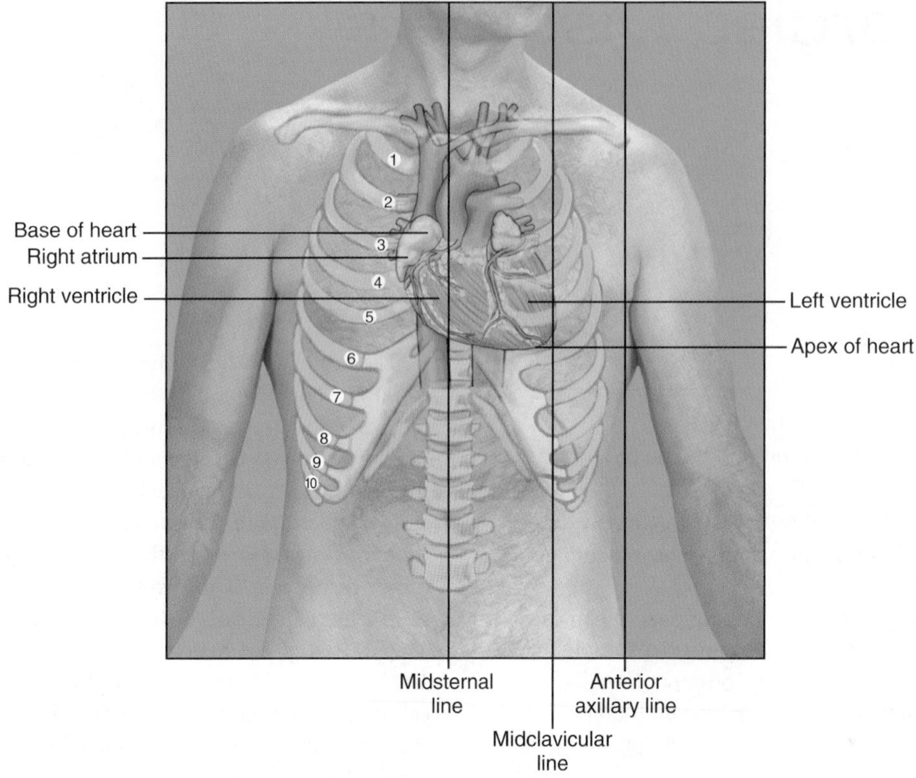

FIGURE **33-1** Anatomic location of the heart.

active cells and transports wastes to the kidneys, liver, and skin for excretion (Fig. 33-2).

The pressures in the RA and RV are very low compared with the pressures in the LA and LV. This is because the LV pumps blood out into the systemic circulation. The pressure in the LV is the highest of all of the chambers.

MUSCLE LAYERS

There are three layers of cardiac muscle tissue: the endocardium, the myocardium, and the epicardium. The endocardium is the inner layer that lines the heart chambers. The middle layer, the myocardium, is made of muscle fibers. It is responsible for the pumping action of the heart. The thickness of the myocardium varies with each chamber. The outer layer, the epicardium, is also the visceral pericardium. The coronary arteries are embedded in the epicardium.

VALVES

There are four valves in the heart: the mitral, the tricuspid, the aortic, and the pulmonic. Their purpose is to retain blood in one chamber until the next chamber is ready to receive it. The valves keep blood flowing in one direction. The valves open and close passively in response to changes in pressure and volume. A valve opens when the pressure behind it is greater than the pressure ahead of it. A valve closes when the pressure ahead of it is greater than the pressure behind it.

Atrioventricular Valves

The mitral and tricuspid valves are called atrioventricular (AV) valves because they separate the atria from the ventricles. The mitral valve is between the LA and the LV. The tricuspid valve separates the RA from the RV. The cusps, or leaflets, are attached by chordae tendineae to the papillary muscles that line the floor of the ventricles. These valves are closed during systole and open in diastole.

Semilunar Valves

The semilunar valves, called aortic and pulmonic, separate the ventricles from the aorta and the pulmonary artery, respectively. These valves are open during systole and are closed during diastole. The semilunar valves have three cusps (cup-shaped structures) each.

Heart Sounds

Closure of the valves produces the heart sounds auscultated over the heart. The first heart sound (S_1), referred to as "lub," occurs when the ventricles contract during systole and when the mitral and tricuspid valves close. The second heart sound (S_2), called "dub," occurs during ventricular relaxation or diastole and is caused by the closing of the aortic and pulmonic valves.

CORONARY BLOOD FLOW

The coronary arteries are the first branches of the systemic circulation. These arteries supply blood to the myocardium

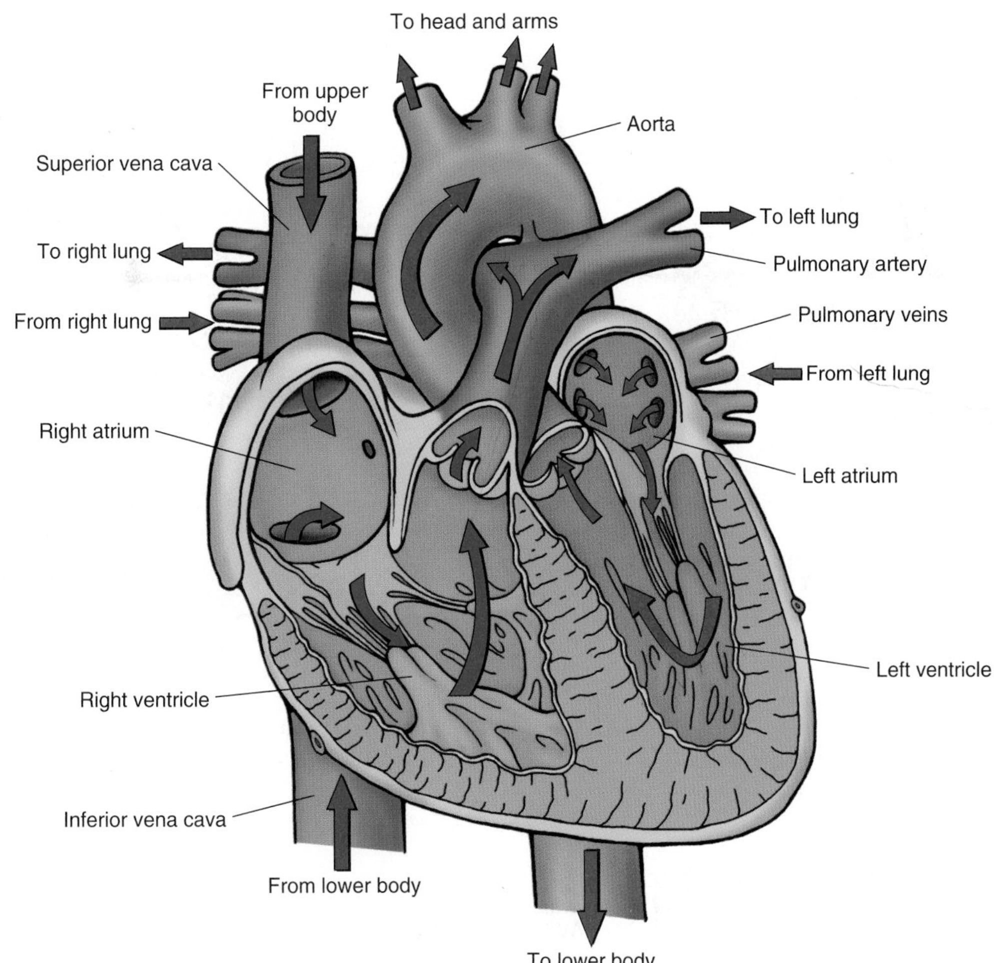

FIGURE **33-2** Normal circulation through the heart.

and the conductive tissue of the heart. The two major coronary arteries, the left coronary artery and the right coronary artery, arise from the aorta just beyond the aortic valve. Blood flow through the coronary arteries occurs during diastole. The left coronary artery, which branches into the left anterior descending and circumflex arteries, supplies blood to the LA, most of the LV, and most of the septum between the two ventricles (interventricular septum). The right coronary artery branches to supply the sinoatrial (SA) and the atrioventricular (AV) nodes, the RA and RV, and the inferior part of the LV. Variations in the pattern of arterial branching are common.

Collateral arteries are connections between two branches of arteries. They are more common in certain areas of the heart. It is not known whether they protect the heart or develop in response to ischemia.

In general, the venous system parallels the arterial system: the great cardiac vein follows the left anterior descending artery and the small cardiac vein follows the right coronary artery. The veins meet to form the coronary sinus (the largest coronary vein), which returns deoxygenated blood from the myocardium to the right atrium (Fig. 33-3).

CONDUCTION SYSTEM

For the heart to pump blood through the chambers, nerves must stimulate muscle contractions in an orderly fashion. The conduction pattern follows a particular route. The SA node, also called the pacemaker, initiates the impulse. The impulse is carried throughout the atria to the AV node, located on the floor of the RA. The impulse is delayed in the AV node, then transmitted to the ventricles through the bundle of His. The bundle is made up of Purkinje cells and is located where the atrial and ventricular septa meet. The bundle of His divides into the left and right bundle branches. The left bundle branch divides into anterior and posterior branches called *fascicles.* The terminal ends of the right and left branches are called the *Purkinje fibers.* When the impulse reaches the Purkinje fibers, the ventricles contract (Fig. 33-4).

The impulse produces a change in the movement of electrically charged ions across the membrane of cardiac cells. Cardiac cells at rest are electrically polarized, with the inside of the cell negatively charged and the outside of the cell positively charged. When stimulated, cardiac cells lose their internal negativity by a process called *depolarization.* Depolarization

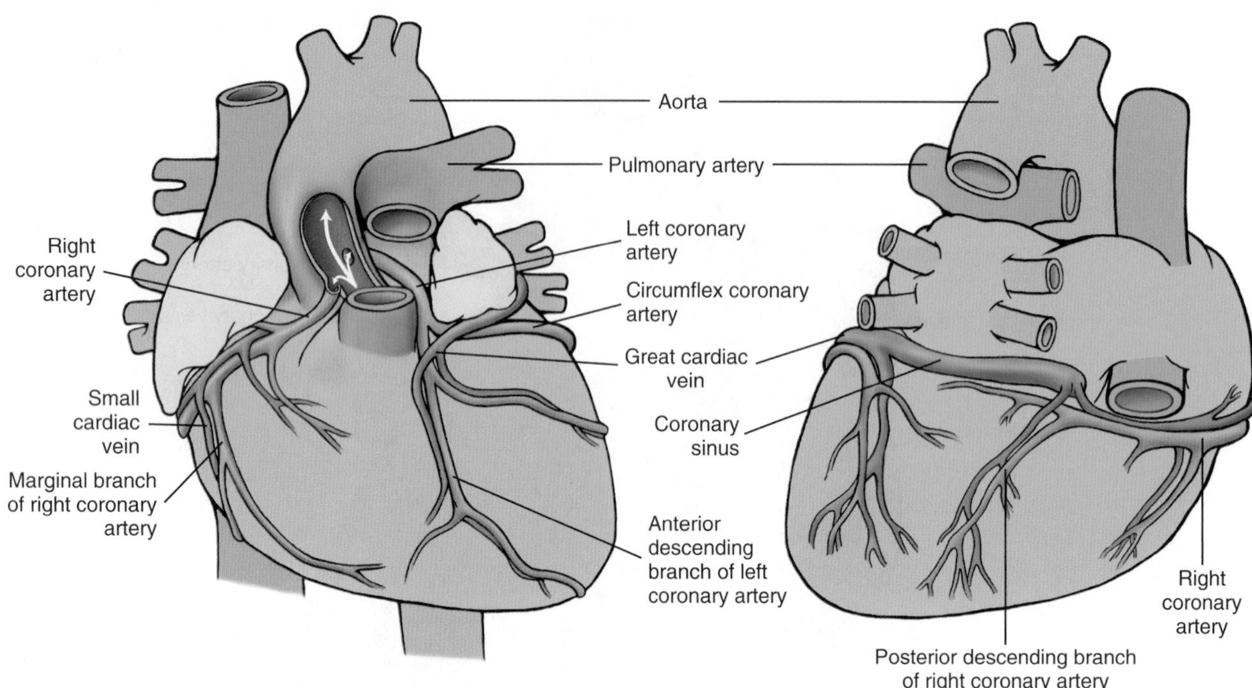

FIGURE **33-3** Coronary arteries and veins.

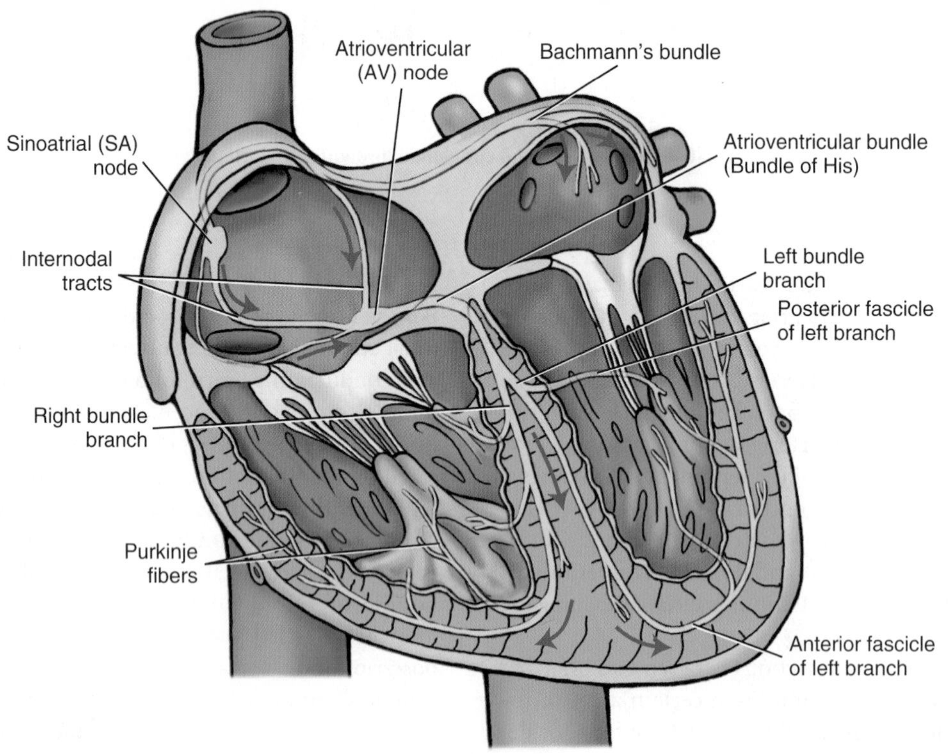

FIGURE **33-4** The conduction system of the heart.

table 33-1 ***Intrinsic Heart Rates***

INITIATION OF IMPULSE	RATE
Sinoatrial node	60-100 bpm
Atrioventricular node	40-60 bpm
Ventricle	15-40 bpm

moves from cell to cell, producing a wave of electrical activity that is transmitted throughout the heart. Once depolarization is complete, the resting state (i.e., inside of the cell more negative than the outside) is restored through a process called *repolarization.*

The SA node normally generates these impulses at a rate between 60 and 100 beats per minute (bpm). The SA node is called the pacemaker of the heart. The AV node is also capable of generating an impulse if the SA node should fail. The AV node rate is 40 to 60 bpm. The Purkinje network also can generate an impulse, but at less than 40 bpm, which could prevent cessation of heart function for a short time (Table 33-1).

Cardiac Innervation

The heart is innervated by sympathetic and parasympathetic fibers of the autonomic nervous system. Sympathetic fibers are distributed throughout the heart. Sympathetic stimulation results in increased heart rate, increased speed of conduction through the AV node, and more forceful contractions. Parasympathetic fibers, which are part of the vagus nerve, are found primarily in the SA and AV nodes and the atrial tissue. Parasympathetic stimulation results in slowing of the heart rate, slowing of conduction through the AV node, and decreased strength of contraction.

CARDIAC FUNCTION

The primary function of the heart is to pump blood through the pulmonary and systemic circulations. This is accomplished by a continually repeating pattern of contraction and relaxation.

Cardiac Cycle

Contraction and relaxation of the heart make up one heartbeat and are called the *cardiac cycle.* When the ventricles are at rest (relaxation phase), they are filling up with blood coming from the atria. This is called *diastole.* At the end of diastole, the atria contract to eject more blood into the ventricles (called the atrial kick). Once the ventricles have filled with blood and the electrical impulse has reached the terminal fibers of the conduction system, the ventricles contract and eject blood into the pulmonary artery from the RV and into the aorta from the LV. This is called *systole.* In a person with a heart rate of 60 bpm, there would be 60 cardiac cycles per minute.

Cardiac Output

The volume of blood ejected by the heart each minute is determined by the stroke volume and the heart rate. Stroke volume is the amount of blood ejected with each ventricular contraction. The normal stroke volume is 60 to 100 ml. Cardiac output is the amount of blood (in liters) ejected by the heart per minute. It is calculated by multiplying the heart rate by the stroke volume (CO = HR × SV). The normal cardiac output is 4 to 8 L/min. In the normal heart, cardiac output responds to the increased demands for oxygen and nutrients that occur with exercise, infection, or stress.

Three factors affect stroke volume: preload, contractility, and afterload.

Preload

Preload is the amount of blood remaining in a ventricle at the end of diastole or the pressure generated at the end of diastole. Increased preload results in increased stroke volume and, therefore, increased cardiac output. Factors that increase preload include increased venous return to the heart and overhydration. Factors that decrease preload include dehydration, hemorrhage, and venous vasodilation.

Contractility

Contractility is the ability of cardiac muscle fibers to shorten and produce a muscle contraction. *Inotropy* is a term used to refer to the contractile state of the cell. Factors that increase contractility are said to have a positive inotropic effect and factors that decrease contractility create a negative inotropic effect.

Afterload

Afterload is the amount of pressure the ventricles must overcome to eject the blood volume. It is determined primarily by the pressure in the arterial system. Afterload is decreased by vasodilation and increased by vasoconstriction.

Myocardial Oxygen Consumption

Myocardial tissue routinely needs 70% to 75% of the oxygen delivered to it by the coronary arteries. Skeletal muscles, by contrast, need 35% at rest and up to 75% during exercise. The only ways to increase oxygen supply to the myocardium are to (1) increase the coronary blood flow by coronary artery vasodilation or to (2) increase the oxygen in the blood by administering supplemental oxygen.

AGE-RELATED CHANGES

It is difficult to separate the normal age-related changes in the heart and blood vessels from the changes caused by disease. In general, age-related changes progress slowly, whereas pathogenic changes are more likely to be sudden.

HEART

Changes in the heart muscle include increased density of connective tissue and decreased elasticity. Cardiac contractility may decline, making the heart less able to adapt to changes in circulating blood volume. The valves may thicken and stiffen. If they do not close properly, the patient may have a murmur. The valves may also partially block the path of blood flow, causing incomplete emptying of the chambers.

The number of pacemaker cells in the SA node decreases, as does the number of nerve fibers in the ventricles. The aging heart takes longer to respond to stress and then responds less dramatically. It also takes longer to return to normal after exercise or stress. Cardiac dysrhythmias are more common in older people but should still be evaluated because they can be dangerous.

BLOOD VESSELS

Changes in connective tissue and elastic fibers in arteries cause them to become stiffer. Pulse pressure (the difference between the systolic and diastolic pressures) and systolic blood pressure generally increase. Experts disagree about what exactly constitutes hypertension in the elderly. The veins stretch and dilate, leading to venous stasis and sometimes impaired venous return. Thrombophlebitis and varicosities are more common in older people.

The cardiovascular system adapts more slowly to changes in position; therefore postural hypotension may occur.

NURSING ASSESSMENT OF CARDIAC FUNCTION

HEALTH HISTORY

A complete assessment is important for the cardiac patient. If the patient is having acute symptoms, however, a detailed assessment must be deferred until the patient is stable.

The Chief Complaint and History of Present Illness

Assess the patient's reason for seeking medical care. Common symptoms that may be related to cardiac disorders include fatigue, edema, palpitations, dyspnea, and pain. Note when symptoms occur, what aggravates them, and what relieves them.

Medical History

Ask whether the patient has had specific conditions that may be related to cardiac disease. These include hypertension, kidney disease, pulmonary disease, stroke, rheumatic fever, streptococcal sore throat, and scarlet fever. Document previous cardiac disorders and hospitalizations. List recent and current medications and note allergies in appropriate records. It is also important to ask whether the patient is taking any vitamins, herbs, or homeopathic remedies. It may be easier to ask something such as "What are you doing to stay healthy or to help you feel better?"

Family History

Because cardiovascular problems are often familial or hereditary, assess whether immediate relatives have had hypertension, coronary artery disease (CAD), other cardiac disorders, or diabetes mellitus.

Review of Systems

Systematically assess whether the patient has experienced the following specific symptoms: weight gain, fatigue, dyspnea (shortness of breath), cough, orthopnea (difficulty breathing in a supine position), paroxysmal nocturnal dyspnea (sudden dyspnea during sleep), palpitations, chest pain, syncope (fainting), concentrated urine, or leg edema.

If the patient has had dyspnea or orthopnea, determine when it occurred and whether the onset was gradual or sudden. Pain also requires detailed descriptions. The pain of heart problems may radiate or be referred to other areas. The pain may radiate down either arm, to the jaw, or to just below the sternum. The severity may range from mild, intermittent discomfort to severe, crushing chest pain. Ask the patient to rate the severity of the pain on a scale of 1 (mildest) to 10 (worst possible). Chest pain may be different in women and may be described as indigestion, as a feeling of anxiety, as nausea, or as a feeling of fatigue. Document the exact description, location, and severity, whether there is radiation, events causing the pain, and what relieves the pain.

Functional Assessment

Determine how this illness has affected the patient's ability to carry out usual activities. Describe activity and rest patterns and usual diet. It is especially important to record salt and fat intake. Ask the patient about sources of stress and coping strategies.

PHYSICAL EXAMINATION

Begin the physical examination with measurement of height and weight and recording of vital signs.

Vital Signs

Blood Pressure

The correct-sized blood pressure cuff must be used. Position the arm at the heart level and check the blood pressure in both arms. Note the pulse pressure (difference between the systolic and diastolic pressures) because it is a noninvasive measure of cardiac output. Next, measure blood pressures and pulse rates in the lying, sitting, and standing positions. A blood pressure decrease of 20 mm Hg or more with a position change indicates decreased blood volume or an autonomic response. As blood pressure decreases, the pulse should increase as a compensatory mechanism.

Pulses

Assess the radial pulses for rate, rhythm, quality, and equality. Auscultate the apical pulse for rate and rhythm. Apical and radial pulses may be taken simultaneously to detect a pulse deficit. The normal heart rate is 60 to 100 bpm. A rate of less than 60 bpm is considered to be bradycardia; tachycardia is characterized by a heart rate in excess of 100 bpm. The rhythm is assessed as regular, irregular, or regularly irregular. The quality of the pulse is graded on a four-point scale: 0, absent pulse (not palpable); 1, weak or thready pulse (pulse easily obliterated by slight finger pressure, returning as pressure is released); 2, normal pulse (easily palpable); and 3, bounding pulse (forceful, not easily obliterated by finger pressure). With a stethoscope, listen at the fifth intercostal space at the midclavicular line to assess the apical pulse. In addition to the radial pulse, assess the carotid, brachial, femoral, popliteal, posterior tibial, and dorsalis pedis pulses at appropriate times in the physical examination (see Fig. 34-4).

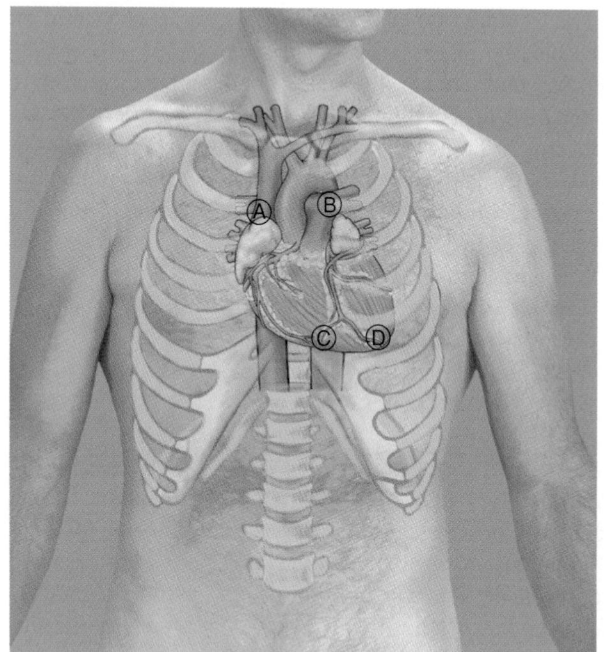

FIGURE 33-5 Auscultation of the heart. *A,* Aortic valve at the second intercostal space to the right of the sternum. *B,* Pulmonic valve at the second intercostal space to the left of the sternum. *C,* Tricuspid valve at the fifth intercostal space to the left of the sternum. *D,* Mitral valve at the fifth intercostal space in the midclavicular line.

Respirations

Observe the patient's respiratory effort and skin color. Count the respiratory rate and auscultate the breath sounds for crackles and wheezes. If the patient produces sputum, describe the color, amount, and appearance.

Skin

Inspect the skin for color, hair distribution, and capillary refill and palpate the temperature. Skin color and temperature should be relatively the same over the entire body.

Heart Sounds

The heart sounds are systole (lub) and diastole (dub). To auscultate heart sounds, place the diaphragm of the stethoscope firmly on the anterior chest. Avoid auscultating heart sounds through clothing. Figure 33-5 shows where the heart sounds, made by closing of the valves, may be heard best. With practice, you can learn to distinguish these. The following pattern of auscultation is recommended:

1. Listen to the aortic area first and then the pulmonic. As the aortic and the pulmonic valves close, the dub should be louder than the lub in the aortic and pulmonic areas.
2. Listen to the tricuspid and mitral valves in the areas indicated. In these areas, the lub should be louder than the dub.
3. After listening to each area with the diaphragm, repeat the pattern with the bell of the stethoscope. Note additional sounds of S_3 and S_4. The S_3 and S_4 sounds are heard best with the bell of the stethoscope placed at the apex when the patient is positioned on the left side. S_3, also called a *ventricular gallop,* occurs early in diastole. S_3 is normal in children and young adults and may be pathologic after age 30. S_4, also called an *atrial gallop,* occurs late in diastole. S_4 is an abnormal heart sound.

table 33-2 ***Grading of Heart Murmurs***

GRADE	DESCRIPTION
I	Very faint
II	Faint, but recognizable
III	Loud, but moderate in intensity
IV	Loud and accompanied by a palpable thrill
V	Very loud, accompanied by a palpable thrill, and audible with the stethoscope partially off the client's chest
VI	Extremely loud, may be heard with the stethoscope slightly above the client's chest

From Ignatavicius, D. D., Workman, M. L., & Mishler, M. A. (1999). *Medical-surgical nursing across the health care continuum* (3rd ed., p. 735). Philadelphia: Saunders.

Heart Murmurs

A heart **murmur** is the sound produced by turbulent blood flow across the valves. Murmurs are recorded as having high, low, or medium pitch and they are located using the anatomic landmarks where they are heard best. The timing of a murmur relates to when it is heard in the cardiac cycle: systole or diastole. Murmurs are graded according to intensity or loudness (Table 33-2).

A rub is heard when the pericardium is inflamed. A scratchy or muffled sound may be heard best by having the patient sit upright and lean forward. This position brings the pericardium closer to the chest wall. A pericardial friction rub is best heard along the left sternal border throughout the cardiac cycle. It may help to ask patients to hold their breath briefly. If a rub is heard during this brief time, it is a pericardial rub rather than pleural.

table 33-3 ASSESSMENT *of Patients with Cardiac Disorders*

HEALTH HISTORY

Present Illness: Fatigue, edema, palpitations, pain; aggravating and relieving factors
Past Medical History: Hypertension, kidney disease, pulmonary disease, diabetes mellitus, stroke, rheumatic fever, streptococcal sore throat, scarlet fever, previous cardiac diseases or conditions, previous hospitalizations, recent and current medications, allergies
Family History: Hypertension, coronary artery disease or other cardiac conditions, diabetes mellitus
Review of Systems: Weight gain, fatigue, dyspnea, cough, orthopnea, palpitations, chest pain, fainting, concentrated urine, leg edema
Functional Assessment: Effects of illness on usual activities, activity and rest pattern, lifestyle, diet, sodium and fat intake, sources of stress, coping strategies

PHYSICAL EXAMINATION

General Survey: Apparent distress
Height and Weight
Vital Signs: Blood pressure in both arms and while supine, sitting, standing; apical heart rate and rhythm; peripheral pulses: rate, rhythm, quality, equality; respiratory effort and rate
Skin: Color, hair distribution, capillary refill, temperature
Thorax: Heart sounds, heart murmurs, rubs; breath sounds, crackles, wheezes; presence and appearance of sputum
Extremities: Pulses, color, warmth, edema, hair distribution

Extremities

Inspect and palpate the extremities for color, edema, warmth, temperature, pulse quality, and hair distribution.

Assessment of the cardiac patient is summarized in Table 33-3.

DIAGNOSTIC TESTS AND PROCEDURES

A number of tests or procedures may be employed to assess cardiac structure and function. More common tests are described here. Patient preparation and postprocedure care are detailed in Table 33-4.

ELECTROCARDIOGRAM

The electrocardiogram (ECG) allows study of the electrical activity (conduction system) through the heart muscle. An electrical impulse causes contractions as it passes through the heart muscle. Electrodes placed on the surface of the skin pick up the electrical impulses of the heart. Moving electrodes to various positions permits detection of conduction disturbances in specific areas of the heart.

The ECG is graphed on standardized paper or viewed on an oscilloscope. Each cardiac cycle is represented by a series of P, Q, R, S, and T waves. The activity represented by each wave is explained later in this chapter in the section Interpretation of Electrocardiograms on p. 597. The ECG is interpreted to detect abnormalities in rate, rhythm, or impulse conduction. The normal finding is called a *normal sinus rhythm,* which is characterized by:

1. A rate of 60 to 100 bpm
2. A regular rhythm
3. A P wave preceding each QRS complex
4. A PR interval that is within 0.12 to 0.20 second
5. A QRS complex that is 0.10 second or less

AMBULATORY ECG (HOLTER MONITOR)

An ambulatory ECG uses a portable ECG machine with a memory to provide continuous cardiac monitoring for 24 to 48 hours. A complete record of the heart rhythm is stored and analyzed later. This type of monitoring is used to detect dysrhythmias that occur infrequently, to determine if symptoms correlate with any underlying cardiac disease, to assess the effects of medications, and for research purposes. The patient records in a diary all activity that occurs during the monitoring, such as walking, stair climbing, sleeping, and engaging in sexual activity. The monitor strip is computer scanned and then interpreted by a physician.

Even more sophisticated monitoring is accomplished by transtelephonic means. An audio signal is sent over telephone lines to a station operated by personnel trained to recognize potentially dangerous dysrhythmias.

ECHOCARDIOGRAM (HEART SONOGRAM)

The echocardiogram visualizes and records the size, shape, position, and behavior of the heart's internal structures, especially the valves. Ultrasonic waves are beamed into the heart, and their echoes are recorded. This painless test may be performed at the bedside or in a laboratory. Gel is applied to the skin and a special device called a transducer is moved over the precordium. The transducer picks up sound waves and converts them to electrical impulses that are recorded as waveforms on an oscilloscope, a videotape, or a strip chart.

TRANSESOPHAGEAL ECHOCARDIOGRAM (TEE)

At times the echocardiogram is not diagnostic and a transesophageal echocardiogram (TEE) is used. A flexible endoscopic probe with an ultrasound transducer is passed down the back of the throat into the esophagus. A local anesthetic to the throat decreases the gag reflex. Occasionally, an intravenous sedative is needed to reduce patient anxiety. Images are obtained from behind the heart as the probe moves down into the stomach. The probe is down for approximately 15 to 20 minutes. The TEE provides information useful in the evaluation of ventricular wall motion and function and possible heart valve disorders.

table 33-4 **DIAGNOSTIC TESTS AND PROCEDURES | *the Heart***

TEST	PURPOSE/PROCEDURE	PATIENT PREPARATION	POSTPROCEDURE NURSING CARE
Electrocardiogram (ECG)	Electrodes are placed on the skin to detect electrical activity of the heart. Detects abnormalities in conduction of impulses, including changes caused by heart damage.	Tell the patient what to expect and that the procedure is painless. No special preparation is required.	Remove gel from skin. No special care needed.
Echocardiogram	Uses ultrasound to create images of the heart. Gel is placed on the patient's skin and a transducer moved over the area. Detects valve abnormalities, left ventricular hypertrophy, hypertrophic cardiomyopathy.	Tell the patient what to expect and that the procedure is painless. No special preparation is required.	Remove gel from skin. No special care needed.
Transesophageal echocardiogram	Used when conventional echocardiogram not diagnostic. Probe inserted through esophagus into stomach (behind heart). Same purpose as echocardiogram.	Tell patient what to expect: throat will be anesthetized, may have IV. Signed consent required.	Monitor vital signs, gag reflex, and, if sedated, level of consciousness.
Magnetic resonance imaging	Creates images of body structures without radiation. The patient lies on a firm pad that rolls into a circular device. "Open MRI" better tolerated by claustrophobic patients because machine does not surround patient. Clanging sounds are heard as the machine works.	All metal must be removed. Sedation may be ordered if patient is very anxious or unable to be still.	No special care needed. Safety precautions if sedative has been given.
Multiple-gated acquisition scanning	Radioactive material is injected intravenously and the heart scanned to evaluate function. May be done at rest or during exercise.	Tell patient what to expect. Nothing by mouth (NPO) for 2 hr before procedure, Start intravenous infusion as ordered. Signed consent required.	No special care needed.
Stress test (exercise tolerance test)	Assesses presence and severity of coronary artery disease by having the patient exercise during ECG monitoring. Blood pressure is monitored and the test stopped if symptoms of coronary artery disease occur.	Tell the patient what to expect. NPO for 2 hr before test. Give beta blocker if prescribed. Have patient wear loose clothing and comfortable shoes. Signed consent required.	No special care needed.
Thallium imaging	Thallium-201 is given intravenously and the heart scanned to assess blood flow. Scanning may be done at rest or after exercise.	Same as stress test. Tell patient intravenous injection will be given and that radiation dose is small and quickly eliminated.	No special care needed.
Holter monitor	Provides continuous ECG monitoring for a 24- to 48-hour period. Detects occasional dysrhythmias that may be correlated with specific activities noted in patient's diary.	Tell patient to wear loose clothing, take only sponge bath, avoid magnets and metal detectors, and monitor placement of electrodes. Emphasize keeping accurate diary of activities and to push "event button" if symptoms occur.	Return at scheduled time. ECG recording will be retrieved for interpretation.

Continued

table 33-4 DIAGNOSTIC TESTS AND PROCEDURES | *the Heart—cont'd*

TEST	PURPOSE/PROCEDURE	PATIENT PREPARATION	POSTPROCEDURE NURSING CARE
Cardiac catheterization	A catheter is passed through a vein or artery and dye is injected. Radiographs are taken to visualize heart structures and blood vessels. The procedure is done in a special room. Blood pressure, pulse, and ECG are monitored throughout test.	Tell patient what to expect. Assess allergies to seafood or iodine and inform radiologist. NPO for specified time before procedure. Tell patient to expect flushing sensation when dye is injected. Give sedative if ordered. Signed consent required.	Check puncture site. Maintain pressure per protocol if a vascular sealing device is not used. Monitor vital signs and peripheral pulses on affected extremity. Enforce bed rest as ordered.
Electrophysiology study (EPS)	A catheter with multiple electrodes is passed into the right side of the heart through the femoral vein. The electrodes record electrical activity of the conduction system and may be used to stimulate the patient's dysrhythmia.	Tell the patient what to expect. NPO for 6 hr before procedure. Premedicate with prescribed sedatives. Signed consent required.	Similar to cardiac catheterization (above).
Complete blood count (CBC)	Counts white and red blood cells, hemoglobin and hematocrit, red blood cell indices, and sometimes platelets. (See Normal Values in Table 32-7.)	Tell patient a blood sample will be drawn. No special preparation.	Check venipuncture site. Apply pressure if oozing.
Cardiac enzymes	Measure creatine phosphokinase, lactate dehydrogenase, and aspartate aminotransferase to detect elevation associated with heart damage.	Same as CBC. To detect acute myocardial infarction, draw specimen before other invasive procedures.	Check venipuncture site. Apply pressure if oozing.
Troponin	Measures protein released after myocardial injury. Troponin T (TnT) & Troponin I (TnI).	Tell patient a blood sample will be drawn. No special preparation.	Check venipuncture site. Apply pressure if oozing.
Myoglobin	Measures myoglobin levels in the blood.	Tell patient a blood sample will be drawn. No special preparation.	Check venipuncture site. Apply pressure if oozing.
Arterial blood gases	Assesses acid-base balance by measuring pH, PCO_2, PO_2, HCO_3, and base excess.	Tell patient about arterial puncture. Prepare heparinized syringe and obtain blood sample.	Remove air bubbles from sample. Place tube on ice and send for immediate analysis. Apply pressure to puncture site for 5 min. Report results.
Lipid profile	Measures common serum lipids (cholesterol, triglycerides, phospholipids). Used to evaluate risk of coronary artery disease.	Tell patient to expect venipuncture. NPO for 12 hr before sample drawn. Usual diet for 2 weeks before test.	Check venipuncture site. Apply pressure if oozing.

MAGNETIC RESONANCE IMAGING (MRI)

A magnetic resonance imaging (MRI) scan provides high-resolution, three-dimensional images of body structures. Cardiac tissue is imaged without lung or bone interference. The patient is enclosed in a chamber for approximately 5 minutes for an MRI scan of the heart. No loose metallic objects are permitted in the chamber during the procedure. Patients with intracranial aneurysm clips, intraocular metal foreign bodies, heart valves manufactured before 1964, and some middle-ear prostheses should not have MRI scans because the devices may be affected by the magnetic field or may interfere with the MRI. Other implanted devices that contraindicate MRI include pacemakers, automatic implantable cardioverter-defibrillators

(AICDs), and implanted infusion pumps. For patients who are claustrophobic, an open MRI may be available.

MULTIPLE-GATED ACQUISITION SCAN (MUGA)

In a multiple-gated acquisition scan, the patient is injected with technetium 99m, which concentrates in acutely necrotic myocardial tissue. The heart is then scanned to assess left ventricular structure and function, to evaluate myocardial wall motion, to detect intracardiac shunting, to assess valvular disease, and to identify location and size of an acute myocardial infarction (AMI). Assessment of ventricular function can be done while the patient is resting or exercising. Sublingual nitroglycerin may be administered to assess its effect on ventricular function.

STRESS TEST (EXERCISE TOLERANCE TEST)

The stress test is a noninvasive method of assessing the presence and severity of CAD by recording a person's cardiovascular response to exercise. It is also used to measure functional capacity for work, sport, or participation in a rehabilitation program. The stress test is not flawless, as false-positive and false-negative results are common. A negative test result does not absolutely exclude CAD. It is, however, the best noninvasive screening procedure available. The alternative is the much more invasive cardiac catheterization.

For the stress test, a continuous ECG is monitored while the patient uses a treadmill or a stationary bicycle. The speed and incline angle of the treadmill are increased until (1) the patient cannot continue for whatever reason, (2) the patient's maximum heart rate is achieved (220 − patient's age = maximum heart rate), (3) symptoms intervene, or (4) significant changes are detected on the ECG. The target heart rate is 85% of the predicted maximum heart rate for the patient's age and sex.

Significant CAD limits blood flow to the myocardium. The increased demands of exercise may cause the patient to have symptoms of CAD, which are angina, dizziness, dyspnea, dysrhythmias, a falling blood pressure, and certain ECG findings. If these symptoms occur, the test must be stopped immediately.

Contraindications for the test include acute systemic illness, severe aortic stenosis, uncontrolled congestive heart failure (CHF), severe hypertension, angina at rest, and significant dysrhythmia. Although the mortality rate for test participants is very low, cardiopulmonary resuscitation equipment must be available.

Thallium Imaging

Thallium-201 may be administered to assess myocardial blood flow during stress testing. Thallium, which is taken up by normal myocardial cells, is used to detect old or new myocardial ischemia and to evaluate patency of coronary artery bypass grafts. After thallium-201 is injected intravenously, the heart is scanned to assess the areas of concentration. The scan takes approximately 1 hour to complete and is repeated in 2 to 4 hours to assess for redistribution.

Thallium does not enter infarcted or scarred areas and, therefore, shows "cold spots" in areas without blood flow. Exercise-induced ischemia resolves with rest. Scar-induced ischemia, such as that caused by AMI, does not resolve with rest.

For patients who are physically not able to exercise, the heart can be stressed with medications such as dipyridamole (Persantine). These medications mimic the effects of exercise by causing vasodilation of the coronary arteries, which increases blood flow to well-perfused areas, thereby stealing blood from ischemic areas. These differences in flow will show up on the scan.

CARDIAC CATHETERIZATION (CARDIAC ANGIOGRAPHY, CORONARY ARTERIOGRAPHY)

Cardiac catheterization is a procedure in which a catheter is inserted into a vein or artery and is threaded into the heart chambers, coronary arteries, or both, under fluoroscopy (Fig. 33-6). A contrast dye is injected through the catheter and films are made of the visualized heart structures. Vital signs and ECG are monitored during the procedure.

In a catheterization of the right side of the heart, the catheter is inserted into a vein and threaded into the vena cava, RA, RV, and pulmonary artery. Pressures in the RA, RV, and pulmonary artery may be determined. The function of the pulmonic and tricuspid valves may be assessed.

In a catheterization of the left side of the heart, the catheter is inserted into an artery and threaded against the flow of blood into the coronary arteries or the LV. The femoral vein and artery are the preferred insertion sites. The function of the coronary arteries and the aortic and mitral valves may be assessed. Blood samples may be drawn, and pressures in the various structures are measured.

Complications of cardiac catheterization include bleeding, hematoma formation, infection, and embolus or thrombus formation. Nursing care before and after the procedure is very important. See Table 33-5.

ELECTROPHYSIOLOGY STUDY (EPS)

The electrophysiology study (EPS) is used to record the heart's electrical activity from within the heart using catheters with multiple electrodes inserted through the femoral vein into the right side of the heart. The electrodes record the electrical activity of the heart's conduction system. In addition, the electrodes can be used to stimulate dysrhythmias that will help to locate the source of the patient's dysrhythmia.

LABORATORY TESTS

Arterial Blood Gases

Arterial blood gases are analyzed to determine the body's ability to maintain the acid-base balance. Acidity or alkalinity is determined by pH. If the serum pH is less than 7.35, the blood is acidic; greater than 7.45 indicates alkalinity. Carbonic acid dissociates into carbon dioxide and water. The lungs regulate carbon dioxide. The partial pressure of carbon dioxide in the blood is abbreviated P_{CO_2}. A P_{CO_2} greater than 45 with

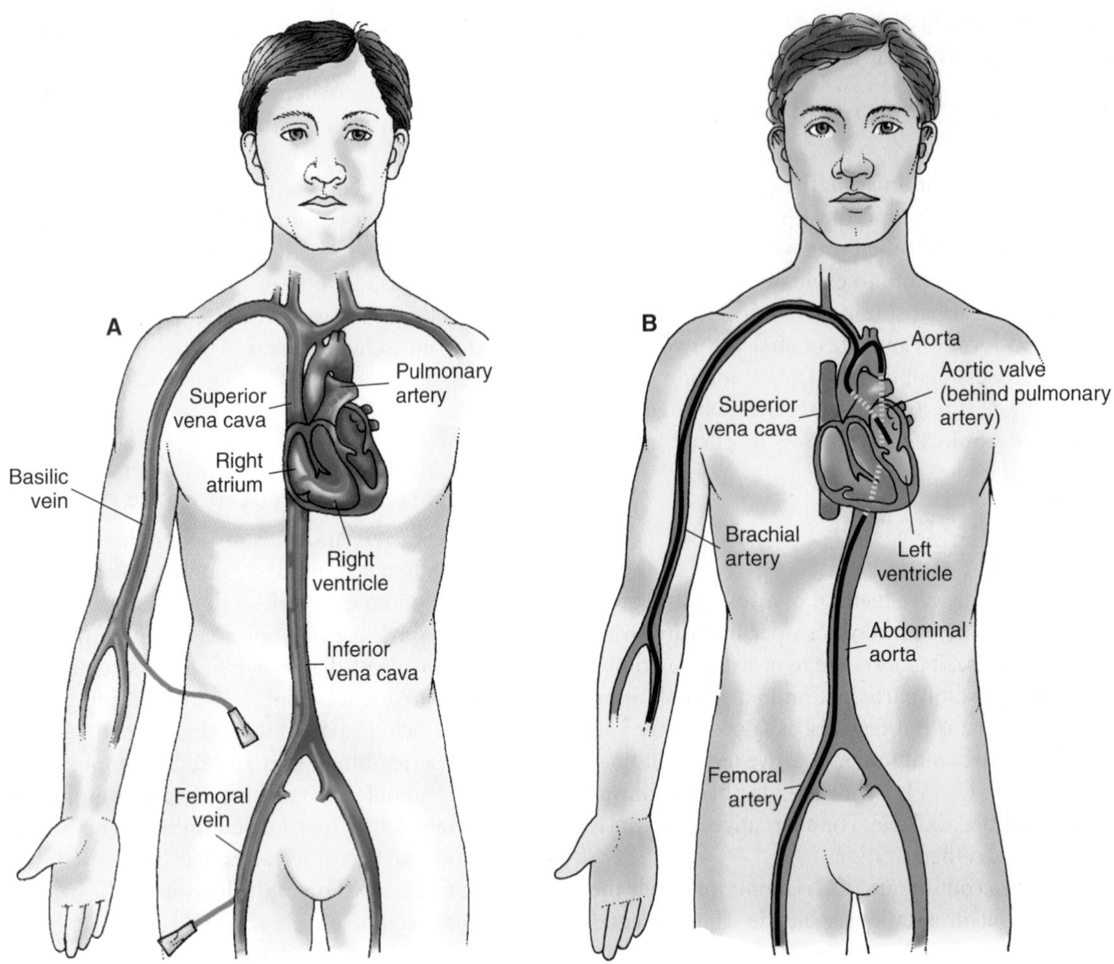

FIGURE **33-6** Right-sided *(A)* and left-sided *(B)* heart catheterization.

table 33-5 ***Interpreting Arterial Blood Gases***

CONDITION	PH	P_{CO_2}	HCO_3
Normal range	7.35-7.45	35-45	22-26
Respiratory acidosis	↓	↑	Normal
Respiratory alkalosis	↑	↓	Normal
Metabolic acidosis	↓	Normal	↓
Metabolic alkalosis	↑	Normal	↑

↑, Elevated; ↓, decreased. If the arrows are in the same direction, a metabolic problem exists; if arrows are in opposite directions, a respiratory problem exists.

an acidic pH is a respiratory acidosis and indicates that the body is unable to excrete the excess carbon dioxide through the lungs. With a pH in excess of 7.45 and a P_{CO_2} of less than 35, a respiratory alkalosis is present.

The kidneys regulate bicarbonate (HCO_3) through excretion and retention. The HCO_3 (or base excess—a combination of all serum bases) is assessed to determine metabolic causes of imbalance. If the pH is less than 7.35 and the HCO_3 is less than 22, the body is in metabolic acidosis. With a pH greater than 7.45 and an HCO_3 greater than 26, the interpretation is metabolic alkalosis (Table 33-5).

PULSE OXIMETRY

A pulse oximeter noninvasively measures arterial oxygen saturation. Light is passed through a pulsating artery and interpreted mechanically to determine the oxygen saturation. The transdermal clip or patch may be applied to a digit (finger or toe), the ear, or the nose (Fig. 33-7).

Cardiac Enzymes

Cardiac enzymes are released when heart cells die as a result of damage. These enzymes are measured in the serum, and their values rise as indicators of damage to the heart cells. Table 33-6 lists normal cardiac enzyme levels.

Creatine Phosphokinase

The creatine phosphokinase enzyme is found in high concentration in three tissues: the brain, the heart, and the skeletal muscle. The type of creatine phosphokinase (CPK) specific to heart tissue is CPK-MB. Elevation of the CPK-MB level indicates damage to the myocardial cells. The CPK-MB can be expected to rise 4 to 6 hours after an AMI, peak in 12 to 24 hours at more than 6 times the normal value, and return to normal within 2 to 3 days if no new damage occurs. Serial trends should be observed. The nurse can plot these trends. Musculoskeletal injuries (especially fractures and surgery) and recent excessive athletic activity can also elevate the total CPK level.

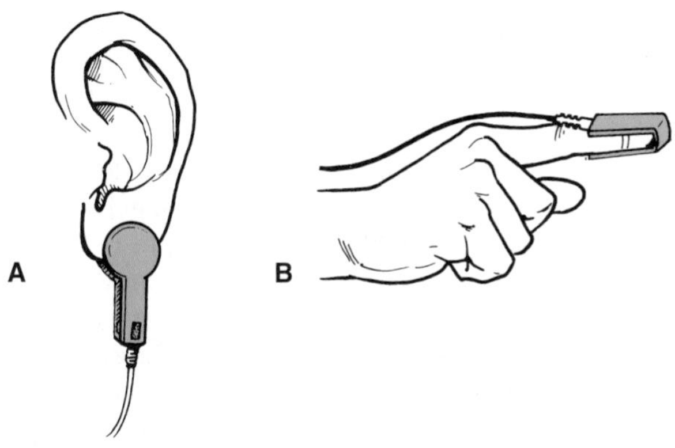

FIGURE 33-7 Pulse oximeter. *A*, Ear probe. *B*, Clip on finger.

table 33-6 ***Cardiac Enzymes***

TEST	NORMAL VALUES
Creatine Phosphokinase (CPK)	
Male	38-174 g/L
Female	96-140 g/L
CPK Isoenzymes	
MM	100%
MB	0%
BB	0%
Lactate Dehydrogenase (LDH)	140-280 U/L
LDH Isoenzymes	
LDH1	17.5%-28.3%
LDH2	30.4%-36.4%
Troponin T (TnT)	<0.1 ng/ml
Troponin I (TnI)	<0.3 ng/ml
Myoglobin	
Male	<92 ng/ml
Female	<76 ng/ml

Values may vary according to the laboratory equipment used.

Lactate Dehydrogenase

Lactate dehydrogenase (LDH) is an intracellular enzyme with highest concentrations in the heart, skeletal muscle, red blood cells (RBCs), liver, kidney, lung, and brain. There are five forms (isoenzymes) of LDH; LDH_1 and LDH_2 are primarily cardiac. In general, LDH_1 is lower than LDH_2. Causes of elevated LDH_1 and LDH_2 are myocardial infarction, infections, liver disease, cancer, and blood transfusions.

Complete Blood Count

The complete blood count is a basic screening test. Included in this test are the white blood cell (WBC) count, the red blood cell (RBC) count, the hemoglobin (Hgb) and hematocrit (Hct) measurements, the RBC indices, and, in some laboratories, the platelet count. Components of the complete blood count are presented in Table 33-7.

White Blood Cell Count

The WBC count indicates the body's ability to defend itself against infection and inflammation. The WBC level usually is elevated with inflammatory processes such as AMI and bacterial infections but it may be below normal with viral infections and bone marrow depression.

table 33-7 ***Complete Blood Count***

TEST	NORMAL VALUES
White Blood Cells	5,000-10,000/ml
Differential:	
Neutrophils	60%-70%
Eosinophils	1%-4%
Basophils	0.5%-1.0%
Lymphocytes	20%-40%
Monocytes	2%-6%
Red Blood Cells	
Male	4,200,000-5,400,000/mm^3
Female	3,600,000-5,000,000/mm^3
Hematocrit	
Male	40%-54%
Female	37%-47%
Hemoglobin	
Male	13.5-17.5 g/dL
Female	12-16 g/dL
Platelets	150,000-350,000/mm^3

Red Blood Cell Count

The RBC count is assessed to determine the ability of the blood to carry oxygen from the lungs to the tissues and carbon dioxide from the tissues to the lungs. The RBC level may be below normal with anemias and malignancies and may be elevated in dehydration.

Hematocrit

The Hct is the percentage of packed RBCs in the total sample of whole blood. With severe dehydration, the plasma portion of the blood decreases and the Hct is elevated. In anemias and hemorrhage, the Hct is below normal. In general, the Hct is three times the Hgb measurement.

Hemoglobin

Hemoglobin is the main component of the RBCs. Its function is to transport oxygen to the cells. The Hgb measurement may be below normal in anemias and hemorrhage. It is elevated in dehydration, chronic obstructive pulmonary disease (COPD), and CHF. An Hgb of less than 5 g/dL leads to heart failure and death if not corrected.

Platelet (Thrombocyte) Count

The platelets (thrombocytes) are the smallest of the formed elements in the blood. They are necessary for coagulation. The platelet count is below normal with anemias, bone marrow depression, and bleeding. The count may be increased in acute infections and some heart diseases. A count of less than 20,000 may result in spontaneous bleeding.

Troponin

Troponin is a protein involved in the contraction of muscles. Two subtypes, troponin T (TnT) and troponin I (TnI) are specific to cardiac muscle and are released into the circulation after an acute myocardial infarction. Troponin I is found only in cardiac muscle, and TnT may also elevate with muscle injury or in renal failure. Troponin levels rise in 3 to 6 hours from onset of symptoms, peak in 24 hours, and remain in the circulation for up to 2 weeks (TnI remains elevated for 5 to 7 days; TnT for 10 to 14 days). This test is done in the emergency department because the results are available more quickly than the cardiac enzymes.

Myoglobin

Myoglobin is another protein found in cardiac and skeletal muscle that is released into the circulation very quickly after myocardial infarction. Myoglobin levels increase in 1 to 4 hours after symptoms. Because it also is found in skeletal muscle, myoglobin levels may be elevated by such things as strenuous exercise, renal failure, and neuromuscular diseases. This makes interpreting myoglobin levels difficult in some circumstances.

Lipid Profile

A lipid profile is a battery of tests that measure the most common serum lipids: cholesterol, triglycerides, and phospholipids.

Cholesterol is a blood lipid produced by the liver. It is used to form bile salts for the digestion of fat and for the production of adrenal, ovarian, and testicular hormones. The normal adult serum cholesterol level is less than 200 mg/dL. Elevated cholesterol levels (hypercholesterolemia) are associated with increased risk of CAD, hypertension, and AMI. The cholesterol accumulates in the arterial lumen and in time results in decreased blood flow and occlusion.

Three forms of cholesterol are identified: (1) high-density lipids (HDLs), (2) low-density lipids (LDLs), and (3) very low-density lipids (VLDLs). The HDLs are desirable because they promote the excretion of LDLs and VLDLs. The normal LDL level is 60 to 160 mg/dL. The risk for CAD is increased if LDL levels are elevated. The risk for CAD is decreased if HDL levels are elevated. Normal HDL levels are 30 to 70 mg/dL. A good way to remember the difference is that HDLs are healthy and LDLs are lethal.

Triglycerides are a major contributor to CAD. They are produced in the liver. Triglyceride levels increase when LDL levels increase. The normal triglyceride level is 40 to 150 mg/dL.

COMMON THERAPEUTIC MEASURES

DRUG THERAPY

Commonly used cardiac drugs are cardiac glycosides, antianginals, antidysrhythmics, and miscellaneous and emergency drugs. Examples of these drugs, their actions and adverse effects, and associated nursing considerations are provided in Table 33-8.

Cardiac Glycosides

The cardiac glycosides are also called cardiotonics or digitalis glycosides. Examples are digoxin (Lanoxin) and digitoxin. These drugs have several important pharmacologic actions on the heart. They slow the heart rate (negative chronotropic effect) and increase the force of myocardial contraction (positive inotropic effect), causing increased stroke volume and cardiac output. Cardiac glycosides are widely used in the treatment of CHF. They are also used to treat some cardiac dysrhythmias.

When rapid effects are needed, a patient can be given a loading dose (called a digitalizing dose) of cardiac glycosides. Once therapeutic blood levels are obtained, a maintenance dose is prescribed to maintain the therapeutic effects. These drugs have high potential for toxicity and require close monitoring. Common practice is to count the apical pulse before giving each dose. If the rate is below 60 bpm in adults, withhold the dose and contact the physician. Because patients are often on cardiac glycosides for long-term therapy, they must be taught to monitor their own pulse and to report symptoms of toxicity (anorexia, nausea, visual disturbances). Other specific nursing considerations are presented in Table 33-8.

Antianginals

Drugs used to treat angina (chest pain related to myocardial ischemia) include calcium channel blockers, vasodilators, and beta-adrenergic blockers. Examples of each classification and nursing considerations are presented in Table 33-8.

Antidysrhythmics

Drugs used to treat abnormal cardiac rhythms are called antidysrhythmics or antiarrhythmics. There are four main classes of antidysrhythmics, each with various actions. In general, they work by slowing the rate of impulse conduction, depressing automaticity, or increasing resistance to premature stimulation. All antidysrhythmics have the potential to cause additional dysrhythmias. Specific drugs and nursing considerations are presented in Table 33-8.

Angiotensin-Converting Enzyme (ACE) Inhibitors

ACE inhibitors work against the renin-angiotensin-aldosterone system to dilate arteries and decrease the resistance to blood flow in the arteries (reduced afterload). In addition, less fluid is retained because aldosterone release is blocked. ACE inhibitors may be prescribed for patients with heart failure and some cases of hypertension. Examples of these medications are captopril (Capoten), enalapril (Vasotec), and quinapril (Accupril). Information about these medications is presented in Table 35-3 in the chapter on hypertension.

Diuretics

Diuretics are often prescribed for cardiac conditions. Many patients with heart problems have fluid retention that is treated with diuretics. The most frequently used diuretics are furosemide (Lasix) and hydrochlorothiazide (Esidrix, HCTZ, and Oretic). Information about these and other diuretics is presented in Table 38-4 in the chapter on urologic disorders.

Anticoagulants

Anticoagulants are used to treat or prevent clot formation. Heparin and warfarin are the most commonly used preventive anticoagulants.

Heparin

Heparin interferes with factor III in the clotting process. It is administered by continuous intravenous drip or subcutaneously. When a patient has a clotting episode, a heparin

Text continued on p. 575

table 33-8 **DRUG THERAPY | *Cardiovascular Drugs***

DRUG	USE/ACTION	NURSING INTERVENTIONS
CARDIAC GLYCOSIDES		
Digoxin (Lanoxin)	Delays impulse conduction through AV node to slow heart rate (negative chronotropic effect). Increases strength or force of myocardial contraction (positive inotropic effect). Increases stroke volume and CO. Used for CHF, atrial fibrillation and flutter, and paroxysmal atrial tachycardia.	Obtain baseline vital signs, ECG, and electrolytes before administering first dose. Assess apical pulse for 1 min; hold and notify MD if <60. Cannot be administered intramuscularly. Monitor K^+ levels; administer K^+ supplements as ordered. Decreased renal function may delay excretion and lead to toxicity. Toxic effects may be indicated by dysrhythmias, pulse <60, anorexia, nausea, syncope, and yellow halos around lights. Therapeutic level: 0.8-2.0 ng/ml Toxic level: >2.0 ng/ml Teach the patient: Take radial pulse for 1 min at the same time each day.
ANTIANGINALS		
Amlodipine (Norvasc)	Calcium channel blocker used to treat angina and hypertension.	Monitor vital signs, ECG. Teach patient to notify physician of irregular heartbeat, dizziness, edema, dyspnea.
Diltiazem hydrochloride (Cardizem) Dosage may need to be reduced in elderly patients.	Calcium channel blocker. Dilates coronary arteries; increases availability of oxygen to the myocardium. Decreases total PVR, afterload, and systolic blood pressure. Slightly decreases myocardial contractility. Prolongs AV node refractory period. Used in chronic stable angina, coronary artery spasm, and hypertension.	Teach the patient: Take radial pulse for 1 min. Limit caffeine intake. Change positions with caution to prevent postural hypotension. Take before meals and at bedtime.
Isosorbide dinitrate (Isordil)	Vasodilator through relaxation of smooth muscles. Decreases preload, afterload, left ventricular end-diastolic pressure, and myocardial oxygen consumption. Used for acute angina and maintenance of chronic angina.	Assess vital signs before administration. Teach the patient: Take 1-2 hr before meals and at bedtime. Sit when taking the sublingual or chewable medications. Change positions slowly to avoid orthostatic hypotension. Avoid hot showers, tubs, saunas. Headache decreases over time. Alcohol potentiates hypotension. If three sublingual or chewable doses do not relieve angina, go to the emergency department.
Nadolol (Corgard) Dosage increased gradually until optimal response is achieved.	Beta-adrenergic blocker. Decreases HR and CO at rest and with exercise. Decreases conduction velocity through the AV node. Used in hypertension and prophylactically for chronic stable angina.	Assess BP and apical pulse before administration. Monitor weight (fluid retention with CHF). Teach the patient: Take radial pulse for 1 min. Hold medication and notify physician if HR <60 or irregular. Weigh daily; report a gain of 3-4 lb. Do not discontinue this drug abruptly; taper off over 1-2 weeks.

AV, Atrioventricular; *BP,* blood pressure; *CBC,* complete blood count; *CHF,* congestive heart failure; *CO,* cardiac output; *ECG,* electrocardiogram; *HR,* heart rate; *IV,* intravenously; *MAP,* mean arterial pressure; *PVC,* premature ventricular contractions; *PVR,* peripheral vascular resistance; *SVR,* systemic vascular resistance.

Continued

table 33-8 **DRUG THERAPY | *Cardiovascular Drugs—cont'd***

DRUG	USE/ACTION	NURSING INTERVENTIONS
ANTIANGINALS—cont'd		
Nifedipine (Procardia)	Calcium channel blocker. Decreases myocardial oxygen consumption. Dilates coronary arteries. Decreases PVR. Increases CO. Used for angina, mild to moderate hypertension, vascular headaches, coronary artery spasms.	Monitor BP during titration (during dosage adjustment). Teach the patient: Smoking is contraindicated (nicotine constricts coronary arteries). Do not discontinue this drug abruptly. Limit caffeine intake.
Nitroglycerin Available as sublingual tablets, ointment, transdermal patch, buccal tablets, mist, and sustained-release oral tablets.	Vasodilator (arteries and veins). Relaxes all smooth muscles, especially vascular smooth muscle. Decreases preload, afterload, BP, CO, and systemic vascular resistance. Used to prevent and treat angina.	Assess BP and pulse before administration. Apply ointment in uniform layer on paper provided; apply to nonhairy skin (chest, back, upper arm); do not touch (causes headache); rotate sites. IV drug is delivered in glass containers with special tubing; use an infusion pump; monitor closely. Teach the patient: Sit or lie down at onset of chest pains. Place tablet under tongue; tablet causing tingling sensation if effective (elderly may not detect this). Repeat q 5 min for total of three dosages; if chest pains not relieved, have someone else drive to emergency department. Keep tablets in containers in which supplied; drug decomposes on exposure to light and air. Headache decreases with tolerance. Drug may be taken before activities likely to cause angina (exercise, sex).
Propranolol (Inderal)	Nonselective beta-adrenergic blocker. Decreases HR, myocardial irritability and contractility. Decreases BP in hypertension. Decreases CO. Used in dysrhythmias, myocardial infarction, hypertension, migraines, and chronic stable angina.	Monitor vital signs. May be administered with diuretic to decrease Na^+ and water retention. May cause bronchial constriction. Use with caution in all patients with obstructive lung disease. Auscultate lungs for crackles and heart for S_3 and S_4 sounds. Monitor weight daily; check for peripheral edema. Monitor blood glucose with diabetes. Teach the patient: Do not discontinue this drug abruptly; taper over 2 weeks. Take at the same time(s) each day. While on this drug, use alcohol only in moderation; no smoking; decrease sodium intake. There is not the normal increase in heart rate with exercise and stress; increase activity slowly. Weigh daily, check for edema.

AV, Atrioventricular; *BP,* blood pressure; *CBC,* complete blood count; *CHF,* congestive heart failure; *CO,* cardiac output; *ECG,* electrocardiogram; *HR,* heart rate; *IV,* intravenously; *MAP,* mean arterial pressure; *PVC,* premature ventricular contractions; *PVR,* peripheral vascular resistance; *SVR,* systemic vascular resistance.

table 33-8 **DRUG THERAPY | *Cardiovascular Drugs—cont'd***

DRUG	USE/ACTION	NURSING INTERVENTIONS
ANTIANGINALS—cont'd		
Verapamil hydrochloride (Calan, Isoptin)	Calcium channel blocker. Slows AV conduction. Dilates peripheral and coronary arteries. Increases oxygen to myocardium. Used to treat supraventricular tachycardias, atrial fibrillation and flutter, angina, hypertension, and vascular headaches.	Assess baseline vital signs, hepatic and renal function. Assess for signs of CHF (pulmonary or peripheral edema). Monitor pulse and BP before each dose. Administer IV bolus more slowly to the elderly. Teach the patient: Take radial pulse for 1 min; report irregular or slow pulse. No caffeine (opposes calcium channel blocking effect). Change position slowly until tolerance develops. Exercise with caution; drug's effects may give false impression of tolerance.
Atenolol (Tenormin) Metoprolol tartrate (Lopressor)	Cardioselective beta-adrenergic blockers used to treat angina and hypertension. Reduces heart rate, BP, cardiac output, and myocardial oxygen consumption.	Monitor vital signs. Continuous ECG monitoring with IV administration. Take apical pulse before each dose. Teach the patient: Take with or after meals. Do not discontinue abruptly. Take pulse and report to physician if below 60. Avoid alcohol and smoking. Avoid over-the-counter cold remedies.
ANTIDYSRHYTHMICS		
Amiodarone hydrochloride (Cordarone)	Antidysrhythmic. Increases action potential duration and effective refractory period. Increases CO. Decreases PVR, coronary artery resistance, and HR. Used for severe tachycardia and supraventricular tachycardias.	Continuously monitor ECG for a decrease in dysrhythmia. Observe for thyroid dysfunction (each 200-mg tablet contains 75 mg of iodine) and neurologic effects (tremors, ataxia, headache, insomnia). Teach the patient: Take radial pulse daily. Photosensitivity and photophobia may occur. Pharmacologic action may have a delayed onset of 5 days to 3 mo. Skin discolorations fade with time.
Bretylium tosylate (Bretylol)	Adrenergic blocker. Suppresses ventricular fibrillation and ventricular tachycardia. Used for short-time treatment of life-threatening ventricular tachycardias in patients who do not respond to conventional therapy, ventricular fibrillation, and cardioversion.	Monitor vital signs, ECG. Have resuscitation equipment available. If nausea and vomiting occur, decrease the rate of infusion.

AV, Atrioventricular; *BP*, blood pressure; *CBC*, complete blood count; *CHF*, congestive heart failure; *CO*, cardiac output; *ECG*, electrocardiogram; *HR*, heart rate; *IV*, intravenously; *MAP*, mean arterial pressure; *PVC*, premature ventricular contractions; *PVR*, peripheral vascular resistance; *SVR*, systemic vascular resistance.

Continued

table 33-8 **DRUG THERAPY | *Cardiovascular Drugs—cont'd***

DRUG	USE/ACTION	NURSING INTERVENTIONS
ANTIDYSRHYTHMICS—cont'd		
Disopyramide phosphate (Norpace)	Reduces the rate of spontaneous diastolic depolarization in pacemaker cells. Increases SVR. Decreases myocardial conductivity. Suppresses ectopic focal activity. Used to suppress and prevent recurrent PVCs and ventricular tachycardia.	Assess apical pulse before administration; hold if <60 or >120 and notify physician. Monitor BP. Monitor intake and output. Urinary retention and constipation may occur. Teach the patient: Take radial pulse daily. Daily weight; observe for edema. Change position slowly. No alcohol (severely decreases BP). Relieve dry mouth with sugarless gum or hard candy. Avoid sunlight (photosensitivity).
Flecainide acetate (Tambocor)	Antidysrythmic. Decreases conduction velocity. Increases ventricular refractory period. Used to treat PVCs, atrial tachycardia, and other dysrhythmias not responsive to other antidysrhythmics.	Monitor ECG.
Lidocaine (Xylocaine)	Increases the electrical stimulation threshold of the ventricular conduction system. Used for rapid control of ventricular dysrhythmias during myocardial infarction, cardiac surgery, cardiac catheterization, and digitalis intoxication.	Administer with an infusion pump. Monitor BP and ECG. May precipitate malignant hyperthermia (tachycardia, tachypnea, elevated temperature). Assess breath sounds for crackles.
Mexiletine hydrochloride (Mexitil)	Antidysrhythmic structurally similar to lidocaine. Used to suppress symptomatic ventricular dysrhythmias.	Administer with food or antacids. Monitor ECG. Mix IV solution immediately before administration.
Phenytoin sodium (Dilantin) May need lower dosage in elderly.	Used to treat paroxysmal atrial tachycardia and ventricular dysrhythmias.	Administer only in normal saline (drug crystallizes in dextrose). Do not exceed 50 mg/min IV. Teach the patient: Alcohol potentiates the action and therefore may precipitate toxicity.
Propranolol (Inderal)	See description under Antianginals.	
Quinidine	Antidysrhythmic. Depresses myocardial excitability, contractility, automaticity, and conduction velocity. Anticholinergic effects increase the ventricular rate. Relaxes muscles. Used for atrial and ventricular dysrhythmias.	If administered with digoxin, may produce toxicity or unpredictable dysrhythmias. Administer with meals to decrease gastric distress. Severe hypotension may occur with large doses. Monitor electrolytes; continuing diarrhea may indicate electrolyte imbalance.
Tocainide hydrochloride (Tonocard)	Antidysrhythmic. Primary analogue of lidocaine. Used for life-threatening ventricular dysrhythmias associated with prolonged QT interval.	Monitor ECG. Administer with food or antacids to decrease gastrointestinal side effects. Monitor CBC for blood dyscrasias (agranulocytosis, leukocytosis, neutropenia).
Verapamil (Calan, Isoptin)	See description under Antianginals.	

AV, Atrioventricular; *BP,* blood pressure; *CBC,* complete blood count; *CHF,* congestive heart failure; *CO,* cardiac output; *ECG,* electrocardiogram; *HR,* heart rate; *IV,* intravenously; *MAP,* mean arterial pressure; *PVC,* premature ventricular contractions; *PVR,* peripheral vascular resistance; *SVR,* systemic vascular resistance.

table 33-8 **DRUG THERAPY | *Cardiovascular Drugs—cont'd***

DRUG	USE/ACTION	NURSING INTERVENTIONS
ANTILIPEMICS		
Cholestyramine (Questran)	Prescribed when diet, exercise, and weight loss fail to bring cholesterol levels in control. Lowers LDL cholesterol. Increases HDL cholesterol.	To get the best effect, teach patients: Continue diet and exercise. Increase fluid intake to counter constipating effects. Interferes with absorption of some other drugs, so check drug-drug interactions before giving.
Gemfibrozil (Lopid)	Decreases synthesis and secretion of VLDL by liver. Decreases triglyceride levels.	For best effect, teach patient: Continue diet and exercise. Take with meals.
Nicotinic acid (Niacin)	Decreases synthesis/secretion of VLDL and LDL by liver. Increases HDL.	For best effect, teach patient: Continue diet and exercise. Take with meals to decrease GI side effects.
Pravastatin (Pravachol) Simvastatin (Zocor) Lovastatin (Mevacor) Atorvastatin (Lipitor)	Increases rate of removal of LDL from plasma. Decreases synthesis of LDL.	For best effect, teach patient: Continue with diet and exercise. Report muscle tenderness. Take as single dose in the evening. Have routine eye exams. Monitor liver function tests.
MISCELLANEOUS AND EMERGENCY DRUGS		
Amrinone lactate (Inocor)	Inotropic agent. Vasodilator. Increases myocardial contractions without increasing HR. Increases blood flow through collateral coronary vessels. Increases stroke volume and CO. Decreases preload and afterload. Used to treat CHF refractory to other medications.	Administer with an infusion pump. Titrate to target BP. Monitor intake and output. Avoid extravasation. Discard solution 24 hr after preparation.
Atropine sulfate	Vagal blocker. Increases HR and CO in heart blocks and severe bradycardia. Used in symptomatic bradycardia and bradydysrhythmias.	Assess HR and rhythm and BP.
Calcium chloride	Necessary for cardiac rhythm, tone, and contraction. Increases muscle tone and force of contraction. Used in cardiac resuscitation and in cardiac irregularities associated with hyperkalemia.	Monitor ECG, BP, and arterial blood gases. Avoid extravasation; causes necrosis. Alkalosis decreases the absorption of calcium. Acidosis increases the absorption of calcium.
Dobutamine (Dobutrex)	Synthetic catecholamine. Beta-adrenergic agonist. Increases CO with less increase in HR and BP than other catecholamines. Used in CHF and after cardiac surgery to increase myocardial contractility, stroke volume, and CO.	Continuous monitoring of ECG, cardiac parameters, and urinary output; titrate to HR and BP. Urinary output should increase with improved CO and renal function. Often used with nitroprusside or dopamine for additive effects. Causes less increase in HR, PVR, and dysrhythmias than dopamine. At a rate <7 μg/kg/min, expect increased myocardial contraction, CO, and renal blood flow. At a rate >7 μg/kg/min, expect peripheral vasoconstriction and increased MAP.
Dopamine hydrochloride (Intropin)	Neurotransmitter; precursor to norepinephrine. Increases CO and BP. Improves renal blood flow and therefore urine output with lower doses. Used for hemodynamic support in shock.	Avoid extravasation; causes necrosis. Monitor vital signs, ECG, urine output, and extremity color. Titrate to target BP; use an infusion pump. Peripheral vasoconstriction is noted with cold upper and lower extremities.

AV, Atrioventricular; *BP*, blood pressure; *CBC*, complete blood count; *CHF*, congestive heart failure; *CO*, cardiac output; *ECG*, electrocardiogram; *HR*, heart rate; *IV*, intravenously; *MAP*, mean arterial pressure; *PVC*, premature ventricular contractions; *PVR*, peripheral vascular resistance; *SVR*, systemic vascular resistance.

Continued

table 33-8 **DRUG THERAPY | *Cardiovascular Drugs—cont'd***

DRUG	USE/ACTION	NURSING INTERVENTIONS
MISCELLANEOUS AND EMERGENCY DRUGS—cont'd		
Epinephrine hydrochloride (Adrenalin Chloride)	Catecholamine. Strengthens myocardial contraction; increases BP, HR, and CO. Dilates bronchial tree. Used in anaphylactic shock and to restore cardiac rhythm in cardiac arrest.	Monitor vital signs and ECG continuously. Avoid extravasation; causes sloughing. Titrate to cardiac response. Caution: available in several concentrations (1:100, 1:1000, 1:10,000); be sure to check for prescribed solution. May be administered by endotracheal tube because drug is rapidly absorbed from the lungs.
Isoproterenol hydrochloride (Isuprel)	Cardiac stimulant (positive inotropic and chronotropic effects). Bronchodilator. Peripheral vasodilator. Increases HR and contractility. Decreases PVR and diastolic BP, resulting in increased CO and systolic BP, decreased MAP, and increased myocardial oxygen consumption. Used as a cardiac stimulant in cardiac arrest, cardiogenic shock, ventricular dysrhythmias, and heart block.	Continuously monitor ECG. Monitor vital signs, urine output, and peripheral blood flow. Titrate to desired HR, BP, and urine output. Avoid extravasation.
Sodium nitroprusside (Nipride)	Vasodilator. Decreases preload and afterload. Used in hypertensive crises.	Light-sensitive preparation; wrap in aluminum foil. Administer with an infusion pump. Titrate to maintain CO. Continuously monitor BP. Discard solution 4 hr after preparation. Assess thiocyanate levels daily for patients on long-term therapy.
Norepinephrine (Levophed)	Catecholamine. Vasoconstriction. Cardiac stimulant: increased BP, myocardial oxygen, and coronary artery blood flow. Used in acute hypertensive states, myocardial infarction, and cardiac arrest.	Mix only with dextrose in water or dextrose in saline. Administer with an infusion pump. Report decreased urine output immediately. Continuously monitor and titrate to BP. Monitor peripheral blood flow. Avoid extravasation.
Sodium bicarbonate	Systemic alkalinizer. Used to correct metabolic acidosis in cardiac arrest.	Do not infuse with calcium. Monitor arterial blood gases. Avoid extravasation; causes severe tissue damage.
Abciximab (ReoPro)	Inhibits platelet aggregation. Given IV to reduce ischemic complications with angioplasty or arthrectomy.	Used only in the hospital. Monitor vital signs, ECG, and level of consciousness. Assess hemoglobin, hematocrit, platelet count, and clotting factors frequently. Watch for bleeding. Protect from trauma.
Ticlopidine (Ticlid)	Decreases platelet aggregation. Prolongs bleeding time. Used to prevent thromboembolic disorders such as stroke and MI.	Monitor liver function studies, CBC, prothrombin time. Teach the patient: Report bleeding. Take with food. Keep appointments for blood work.
Milrinone (Primacor)	Inotropic agent. Increases myocardial contractility and cardiac output. Vasodilation decreases preload and afterload. Used to treat CHF that does not respond to usual therapy.	Monitor vital signs, intake and output, and daily weight during therapy. Monitor ECG continuously. Give potassium as ordered for hypokalemia.

AV, Atrioventricular; *BP,* blood pressure; *CBC,* complete blood count; *CHF,* congestive heart failure; *CO,* cardiac output; *ECG,* electrocardiogram; *HR,* heart rate; *IV,* intravenously; *MAP,* mean arterial pressure; *PVC,* premature ventricular contractions; *PVR,* peripheral vascular resistance; *SVR,* systemic vascular resistance.

bolus is administered and a continuous infusion is started. The infusion rate is set to deliver a prescribed number of heparin units per hour. The physician adjusts the heparin dosage based on the partial thromboplastin time (PTT). When the partial thromboplastin time has stabilized (generally at 1.5 to 2.0 times the control level), the drug can be changed to the subcutaneous route. Because heparin cannot be administered orally, the patient must remain hospitalized during its administration.

Warfarin

The anticoagulant that may be administered orally, warfarin (Coumadin), is started as soon as possible. The warfarin dosage is regulated by the prothrombin time and international normalized ratio (INR). The prothrombin time is kept in a therapeutic range of 1.5 to 2.0 times the normal level. The INR may be kept at 2.0 to 4.5. Patients who have had artificial valve replacements must remain on anticoagulant therapy for life.

PHARMACOLOGY CAPSULE Heparin dosage is adjusted based on the patient's partial thromboplastin time (PTT). Warfarin dosage is adjusted based on the patient's prothrombin time and INR.

Antiplatelet Agents

Antiplatelet therapy is often used after an AMI to prevent additional myocardial infarction and strokes. The dosage of aspirin as an antiplatelet agent in stroke prevention is under investigation. Some studies have shown that one baby aspirin (81 mg) a day is sufficient, and other studies indicate that an even smaller dosage may produce a therapeutic effect. Dipyridamole (Persantine), ticlopidine (Ticlid), and clopidogrel (Plavix) also exhibit antiplatelet effects and may be prescribed for patients who are unable to tolerate aspirin.

Newer antiplatelet agents, Glycoprotein (GP) IIb/IIIa inhibitors, have been developed. These medications block the platelet receptor sites that bind with fibrinogen and lead to platelet aggregation. GP IIb/IIIa inhibitors such as abciximab (ReoPro) and eptifibatide (Integrilin) are used in combination with heparin and aspirin as part of the medical treatment for unstable angina and myocardial infarction. They are also being used in conjunction with thrombolytic therapy and/or percutaneous coronary interventions after acute myocardial infarction.

Thrombolytic Agents

Whereas anticoagulants and antiplatelet agents prevent the continued formation of clots, the thrombolytic agents act to destroy clots that have already formed. Streptokinase, Beteplase, and tissue plasminogen activator are examples of thrombolytics. They are best used as soon as there is evidence of clot formation. They are administered intravenously when certain criteria have been met. Administration is continued until there is evidence of reperfusion or until the maximum dosage has been given.

PHARMACOLOGY CAPSULE Anticoagulants and antiplatelet agents prevent formation of new clots, but thrombolytic agents destroy clots that have already formed.

Information about anticoagulant, antiplatelet, and thrombolytic agents is presented in Table 27-2, the chapter on cerebrovascular accidents, and Table 34-3 , the chapter on vascular disease.

Analgesics

The patient who has an AMI experiences severe chest pain. The first medication administered to a patient with chest pain is nitroglycerin, which is a vasodilator. When this drug does not relieve the pain, morphine is the preferred analgesic. Morphine relieves pain, reduces anxiety, and reduces the workload of the heart by trapping some of the venous blood in the periphery of the body. An alternative to morphine is meperidine hydrochloride (Demerol). Meperidine is less effective in relieving anxiety and cardiac workload than morphine. Morphine and meperidine are most effective when administered intravenously.

DIET THERAPY

Reduction of body weight lessens the workload on the heart. A low-fat, high-fiber diet usually is recommended for cardiac patients. The recommended diet contains less than 30% of the daily calories from fat. Of the 30%, 10% should come from saturated fats and 20% should come from unsaturated fats. High-fiber foods include whole grains, fruits, and vegetables. An exercise program may help the patient achieve optimal weight.

Sodium

If fluid retention accompanies the cardiac problem, the physician may order sodium restriction. A diet containing sodium 2 g/day is most often prescribed. Restrictions greater than this are difficult to achieve, and studies have shown that patients quickly become noncompliant with the dietary regimen. Salt substitutes are available.

Potassium

Patients taking potassium-wasting diuretics (e.g., furosemide and hydrochlorothiazide) need to include adequate potassium in the diet to counteract the depletion. Patients taking large doses of potassium-wasting diuretics need to have potassium supplements prescribed.

PHARMACOLOGY CAPSULE Potassium-wasting diuretics such as furosemide and hydrochlorothiazide may cause hypokalemia, which can lead to dangerous dysrhythmias.

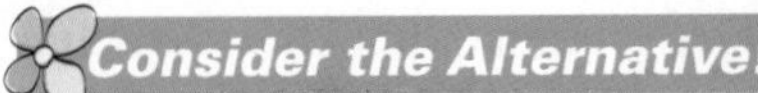

Some people use garlic to reduce plasma lipids and lower blood pressure. The best garlic preparation is an enteric-coated dried preparation that contains adequate allicin and allinase—the "active ingredients" in the preparation. Most of the allicin and allinase are destroyed when garlic is cooked or eaten raw. Garlic irritates the GI tract and increases the effects of anticoagulants and insulin.

OXYGEN THERAPY

The myocardium needs an adequate blood supply to function properly. Any patient complaining of chest pain unrelieved by nitroglycerin should have supplemental oxygen administered. A nasal cannula or face mask should be applied and set to deliver the prescribed liter flow, and the patient's response to this therapy should be monitored.

PACEMAKERS

Pacemakers were first introduced in 1958. Their purpose is to restore regular rhythm and to improve cardiac output and tissue perfusion. Pacemakers may be temporary or permanent and transcutaneous, transvenous, or implantable. A transcutaneous pacemaker has an electrode that delivers an impulse through the skin. A transvenous pacemaker has an electrode that is threaded through a vein to the heart. An implantable pacemaker is surgically placed in the chest. Impulses are conducted from the power source, the pacemaker, to the heart through a lead that stimulates the contraction of the myocardium.

Modes

The pacemaker generator can be set in three modes: chambers paced, chambers sensed, and mode of response. The international code developed for pacemakers is shown in Table 33-9.

The most common setting is DDD because it simulates normal cardiac physiology most closely. This means that both the ventricles and the atria are monitored. If no impulse is generated to initiate a contraction, the pacemaker provides one. Dual mode of response means that the atria are triggered if they do not spontaneously initiate an impulse and the ventricles are inhibited from responding on their own.

Modes are described as fixed rate, demand rate, or AV sequential. The fixed-rate mode delivers a set number, usually 72 or 80, of impulses per minute regardless of the intrinsic cardiac activity. The demand pacemaker delivers impulses when spontaneous beats are less than the minimum number set. This is the most common mode. The AV sequential mode detects activity in both chambers and delivers impulses as needed.

Temporary Pacemakers

A temporary pacemaker is inserted for bradycardia with syncope, tachycardia, AMI, and heart block. The leads are threaded into the RV through the venous system (transvenous) through a closed chest puncture, or during open chest surgery. Pulmonary artery catheters are available with pacemaker capability. Leads may also be applied directly to the chest wall (transcutaneous) for emergency temporary pacing.

Permanent Pacemakers

A permanent implantable pacemaker is inserted under local anesthesia. The batteries, usually lithium, have an 8- to 10-year expected life. Permanent pacemakers are inserted in the operating room, catheterization laboratory, or special procedures area. The electrodes are sutured to the epicardium in the atrial and the ventricular areas, or both. The generator is placed in a subcutaneous pocket, usually under the clavicle or in the abdomen.

NURSING CARE *of the Patient with a Pacemaker*

Patients with inserted pacemakers recover in the postanesthesia care unit and then go to a unit with telemetry capability. Monitor the patient for proper pacemaker functioning.

table 33-9 *NASPE/BPEG Generic Pacemaker Code*

POSITION OR CATEGORY	I (CHAMBERS PACED)	II (CHAMBERS SENSED)	III (RESPONSE TO SENSING)	IV (PROGRAMMABILITY RATE MODULATION)	V (ANTITACHYARRHYTHMIA FUNCTIONS)
LETTER CODES	0 = None	0 = None	0 = None	0 = None	0 = None
	A = Atrium	A = Atrium	T = Triggered	P = Simple programmable	P = Pacing (antitachy-arrhythmia)
	V = Ventricle	V = Ventricle	I = Inhibited	M = Multiprogrammable	S = Shock
	D = Dual (A + V)	D = Dual (A + V)	D = Dual (T + I)	C = Communicating R = Rate modulation	D = Dual (P + S)
MANUFACTURER'S DESIGNATION ONLY	S = Single (A or V)	S = Single (A or V)			

Positions I through III are used exclusively for antibradyarrhythmia function.

NASPE, North American Society of Pacing and Electrophysiology; *BPEG,* British Pacing and Electrophysiology Group.
From Bernstein, A. D., Camm, A. J., Fletcher, R. D., et. al. (1987). The NASPE/BPEG generic pacemaker code for antibradyarrhythmia and adaptive-rate pacing and antitachyarrhythmia devices. *PACE Pacing and Clinical Electrophysiology,* 10:794-799. Reprinted with permission.

Examine the ECG for rhythm, pacemaker spike, and dysrhythmias (premature ventricular contractions and ventricular tachycardia are seen most often). The pacemaker spike is a mark observed on the ECG tracing that represents the impulse generated by the pacemaker. Assess vital signs and inspect the incision frequently. Patients rest for 24 hours after the insertion of a permanent pacemaker. They are ambulated as soon as possible and are encouraged to resume normal activities.

After insertion of a temporary pacemaker, microshock precautions should be followed. Monitor the ECG and transport the patient with a portable cardiac monitor and a nurse in attendance. Assess the pacemaker for misfiring. Plan a gradual increase in activities.

When a permanent pacemaker has been inserted, teach the patient how to count the pulse for 1 full minute daily. Explain wound care and the healing process. Advise the patient to notify the physician of symptoms of decreased cardiac output: dyspnea, dizziness, syncope, weakness, fatigue, and chest pain. Also instruct the patient to carry an identification card describing the type of pacemaker implanted.

CARDIOVERSION

Cardioversion is the delivery of a synchronized shock to terminate atrial or ventricular tachydysrhythmias (rapid abnormal heart rhythms). It may be done as an emergency or elective procedure. The shock is synchronized with the R wave to avoid shocking during the vulnerable period of the T wave. A shock delivered during ventricular relaxation can initiate ventricular fibrillation.

If the patient is receiving digoxin, the drug is withheld for 24 hours before the procedure. Emergency drugs are made available, and the patient has a patent intravenous line in place before the procedure. Explain the procedure and obtain informed consent. A short-acting sedative is usually given. The cardioverter is set to the synchronized mode, and two electrodes are placed on the chest. One electrode is placed to the right of the sternum just below the clavicle and the other is placed at the apex of the heart. The initial impulse varies from 25 to 100 joules depending on the type of dysrhythmia. If the initial impulse does not convert the dysrhythmia to normal sinus rhythm, the impulse energy is increased and the procedure is repeated.

After cardioversion, the patient usually recovers very quickly from the sedation and does not remember the event. Inspect the skin under the electrodes for irritation. Assess the patient's heart rate and rhythm, vital signs, and neurologic status. Transient dysrhythmias and a drop in blood pressure are common. Be especially alert for atrial fibrillation, which can contribute to the formation of atrial wall thrombus and emboli.

CARDIAC SURGERY

The most common surgical procedures involving the heart are pacemaker insertion, heart surgery to repair or replace valves or septa or remove tumors, and coronary artery bypass surgery. Pacemaker insertion is described earlier in this section. Coronary artery bypass surgery is described as a surgical treatment for AMI later in the chapter.

With some of the surgical procedures on the heart, the heart muscle must be at rest during the procedure. This requires placing the patient on a machine to direct the blood away from the heart and lungs and to maintain appropriate oxygen and carbon dioxide levels. The heart's rhythm is interrupted by an electrolyte solution and may be restarted after the surgery by electrical stimulation. During this type of surgery, the patient's core temperature usually is reduced to decrease the oxygen needs of the entire body, especially the brain.

PREOPERATIVE NURSING CARE *of the Cardiac Surgery Patient*

Assessment

Nursing assessment of the patient with cardiac disorders is summarized in Table 33-3. When a patient is facing cardiac surgery, also assess the patient's fears and anxiety. Patients are usually upset and very concerned when heart surgery is recommended. Determine what patients know about the surgery and what more they would like to know.

Nursing Diagnoses, Goals, and Outcome Criteria: Preoperative Cardiac Surgery

Nursing Diagnoses	Goals and Outcome Criteria
Fear related to perceived threat of death or unfamiliarity with setting and procedures	Reduced fear: patient states is less fearful, demonstrates relaxed manner
Anxiety related to threat to health status or uncertain outcome	Reduced anxiety: patient states is less anxious, is calmer

Interventions

Fear and Anxiety

Encourage the patient to identify feelings and then explore the basis of those feelings. Do not assume you know how the patient feels. Accept the patient's feelings and do not give trite reassurance ("Don't worry; everything will be fine."). Accurate information about what to expect helps reduce fear of the unknown. Physical comfort measures such as a massage or back rub may also be soothing. If the patient's anxiety level remains high, notify the physician.

Good patient teaching is essential to address fear and anxiety. The physician reviews necessary diagnostic tests, the surgical procedure itself, and what to expect after surgery. Nevertheless, the nurse must be able to clarify and further explain what the patient will experience. If the surgery is to be done as an emergency, little time is available to do preoperative teaching. Planned cardiac surgery allows time for the patient to accept the need for surgery and to explore why the procedure is necessary. Include the family in the preoperative teaching to decrease their anxiety and allow them to participate in the patient's recovery. The patient teaching plan must be individualized for the type of surgical procedure.

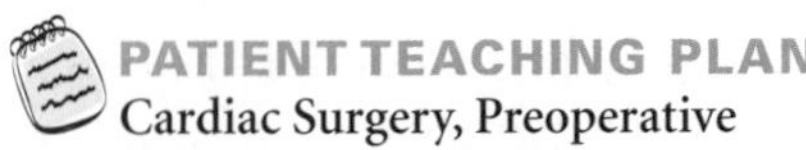

PATIENT TEACHING PLAN
Cardiac Surgery, Preoperative

The specifics of the teaching plan depend on the exact procedure and agency/surgeon procedures. General content of the teaching plan incudes:

- Preoperative routines: NPO, monitoring, diagnostic tests, any special preparation
- Where the patient will be after surgery: in intensive care unit after extensive procedures; to regular units after pacemaker insertion
- The postoperative care setting: the room and the equipment
- Postoperative routines: how to turn, cough, deep breathe, and exercise the leg muscles; monitoring; procedures
- Communication: because most patients are intubated for 4 to 8 hours after surgery, establish a means of communication before surgery

Put on your THINKING CAP!!

A patient is scheduled for extensive cardiac surgery and will be on a ventilator for up to 8 hours postoperatively. What means of communication can you establish in advance? What if the patient is illiterate? What if the patient is deaf?

POSTOPERATIVE NURSING CARE *of the Cardiac Surgery Patient*

Nursing care needs vary considerably depending on the type of surgical procedure. Care specific to certain conditions is discussed with those conditions. In addition, see Chapter 16 for thorough coverage of care of the surgical patient. This section addresses needs common to many patients having cardiac surgery.

Assessment

Assessment of the cardiac patient is summarized in Table 33-3. After surgery, be especially alert to changes in vital signs, breath sounds, urine output, mental alertness, and color. In the intensive care unit, monitor cardiac rhythm, arterial blood gases, and hemodynamic pressures. Assess chest tube function. Frequently inspect all dressings for type and amount of drainage. Examine the surgical wound and insertion sites of tubes and cannulas for increasing redness, swelling, and purulent drainage. Assess urine amount, appearance, and odor.

Nursing Diagnoses, Goals, and Outcome Criteria: Postoperative Cardiac Surgery

NURSING DIAGNOSES	GOALS AND OUTCOME CRITERIA
Ineffective Breathing Patterns related to mechanical ventilation, general anesthesia, pain, or restrictive surgical dressings	Adequate oxygenation: arterial blood gases within normal limits
Acute Pain related to tissue trauma	Pain relief: patient states pain reduced or relieved, relaxed manner
Ineffective Thermoregulation related to cooling during surgery	Normal body temperature: temperature of at least 36.7° C (98° F) orally
Decreased Cardiac Output related to fluid loss or decreased fluid intake	Normal cardiac output: fluid intake equal to output
Risk for Infection related to altered skin integrity	Absence of infection: no fever; decreasing drainage, redness, and swelling of wound
Anxiety related to unfamiliar routines and stressful experience	Reduced anxiety: patient states anxiety is reduced

Interventions

Ineffective Breathing Patterns

Patients with open heart or bypass surgery are unresponsive on arrival in the intensive care unit. Ventilatory assistance is of prime importance. Reassess breath sounds and arterial blood gases frequently. Connect chest tubes to underwater seal drainage. (See Chapter 29 for the care of chest tubes.) Reposition the patient often to promote removal of pulmonary secretions and improve respiratory excursion.

When the patient is extubated, provide an oxygen mask or nasal cannula as ordered to provide supplemental oxygen. Assist the patient to cough and deep breathe frequently. A pillow or a blanket in a pillowcase can be used as an incisional splint during coughing. An incentive spirometer is usually ordered. Monitor its use and remind the patient to use it. Assist with early ambulation, as ordered, to reduce the risk of pulmonary complications.

Pain. Effective pain relief makes it easier for the patient to turn, cough, and deep breathe. Assess the patient's pain: location, severity, aggravating factors, and relieving factors. Administer analgesics as ordered. Intravenous morphine in small doses is most frequently prescribed for analgesia. You may also use independent measures, including position changes, back rubs, relaxation techniques, and imagery. Assess the effectiveness of the interventions in managing pain.

Ineffective Thermoregulation. Warmed blankets, heating blankets, and warming lights may be used to assist rewarming. Monitor body temperature continuously until the patient is stable.

Decreased Cardiac Output. Monitor cardiac pressures continuously in the intensive care unit until they stabilize. Prescribed medications are adjusted based on vital signs, hemodynamic pressures, and cardiac rhythms. Pacing wires are connected to a temporary pacemaker. Monitor fluid and blood administration and assess urinary and other drainage outputs. Volume expanders (albumin, dextran, hetastarch) and vasoactive drugs may be necessary to maintain blood pressure. Oral fluids are ordered shortly after extubation.

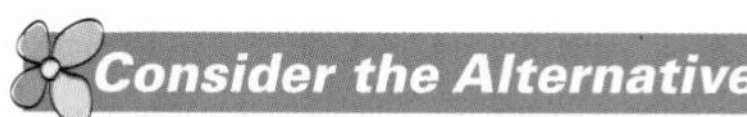

For pain relief, many complementary therapies are used with analgesics. Some examples are massage, relaxation techniques, and imagery.

Risk for Infection. The patient is at risk for incisional, respiratory tract, and urinary tract infections. In addition, the presence of multiple tubes and cannulas provides additional sites for potential nosocomial infection. To reduce the risk of infection, practice a good hand-washing technique and use the aseptic technique when handling dressings and invasive equipment. Provide wound care as ordered or per agency policy. Administer antibiotics as ordered. Before discharge, begin teaching the patient how to care for the surgical wound. Emphasize signs or symptoms that should be reported to the physician: fever, increasing or purulent wound drainage, increasing redness or swelling, and separation of wound margins.

Anxiety. Inform the patient and the family what is being done and how the patient is responding. Remember to talk to the patient and offer reassurance. When the patient is on a ventilator, use the previously established nonverbal means of communication. It is often necessary to repeat instructions because of the effects of pain, medications, and anxiety. As the patient improves, explain the importance of follow-up care and rehabilitation.

CARDIOPULMONARY RESUSCITATION

Cardiopulmonary resuscitation is the restoration of heart and lung function after cardiac arrest. The procedure is used in basic cardiac life support and advanced cardiac life support. The reader is referred to materials prepared by the American Heart Association for current, in-depth coverage of the procedure.

CARDIAC DISORDERS

CORONARY ARTERY DISEASE

Coronary artery disease occurs when the major coronary arteries supplying the myocardium are partially or completely blocked. Blockage of the arteries is caused by coronary artery spasm, arteriosclerosis, or atherosclerosis. Blockage of the coronary arteries results in ischemia and infarction of myocardial tissue.

Arteriosclerosis

Arteriosclerosis is an abnormal thickening, hardening, and loss of elasticity of arterial walls. Smooth muscle cells and collagen migrate into the tunica intima (innermost layer of the artery) and cause the arterial wall to stiffen and thicken and the lumen to decrease in diameter. Lipids, cholesterol, calcium, and thrombi adhere to the damaged arterial wall. This process limits the elasticity of the wall and decreases the flow of oxygen-carrying blood to tissues. Some effects of arteriosclerosis are hypertension, impaired tissue perfusion, and aneurysms.

Atherosclerosis

Atherosclerosis is a form of arteriosclerosis in which thickening and hardening of the vessel wall are caused by soft deposits of intra-arterial fat and fibrin that harden over time. The disease process may take several forms depending on the anatomic location (e.g., coronary or cerebral), age, genetic and physiologic status, and other individual risk factors. LDL deposits occur early when cholesterol accumulates in the arterial wall. Lesions occur primarily within the tunica intima and are of three types: fatty streaks, fibrous plaque, and advanced lesions.

Types of Lesions

Fatty streak. The fatty streak is the earliest lesion to develop in atherosclerosis. Yellow-colored lipids (fat) fill smooth muscle cells, producing streaks of fat that cause no obstruction to the affected vessel. It is commonly found in the aorta by age 10 and in coronary arteries by age 15 regardless of race, sex, or environmental factors. The fatty streak is thought to be reversible. There are no symptoms associated with these lesions.

Fibrous plaque. The fibrous plaque is the characteristic lesion of advanced atherosclerosis. It is rarely found in people younger than age 25. The lipid-laden smooth muscle cells become surrounded by collagen, elastic fibers, and a mucoprotein matrix. The white, raised lesion protrudes into the lumen. The mass fixes itself to the inner wall of the tunica intima and may invade the muscular tunica media. If the lesion enlarges sufficiently, it may occlude the lumen. This lesion occurs most frequently at bifurcations (the points at which blood vessels divide into two smaller vessels), at curves, and where arteries taper.

Advanced lesions. Advanced lesions develop as hemorrhage, calcification, cellular necrosis, and thrombi of the intima alter the fibrous plaques and contribute to the loss of elasticity and resulting occlusion of the vessels.

Collateral Circulation

If plaque formation occurs slowly, collateral circulation may develop. Collateral blood vessels are new branches that grow from existing arteries to provide increased blood flow.

Risk Factors

Factors that increase the risk of atherosclerosis include increased serum lipids, high blood pressure, cigarette smoking (nicotine), diabetes mellitus with elevated blood glucose, obesity, sedentary lifestyle, age, gender, race, and genetics. These risk factors are divided into two categories: risk factors that can be modified and those that cannot be modified. Risk factors that *cannot* be modified are age, gender, genetic predisposition, and race. The focus of patient education is on reducing the risk factors that can be modified. Other factors that may also contribute to the development of coronary heart disease are stress, sex hormones, birth control pills, excessive alcohol intake, and high homocysteine levels.

What Does Culture Have to do with Heart Disease?

Native Americans and African Americans develop CAD at an earlier age than other Americans. The incidence of CAD is highest among middle-aged Causasian males. Hispanics have lower death rates from CAD than non-Hispanics. Nurses can educate high-risk patients about risk factors that can be modified: obesity, hypertension, and stress. Role models from the target population are especially influential.

Signs and Symptoms

Coronary artery disease usually is asymptomatic until the tissue's blood supply is reduced by at least 60%. Then, clinical manifestations depend on the vessels involved and the sites of the lesions. In CAD, the left anterior descending artery is most often affected.

Pain is the most frequent symptom. Pain represents lack of oxygen to tissues. The pain resulting from lack of oxygen to the myocardium is called angina pectoris. It occurs most often with exercise or activity and usually subsides with rest. Other precipitating factors are smoking, physical exertion, emotional stress, and heavy meals. It may be caused by spasms of the coronary arteries, thrombosis, or occlusion of the lumen. The pain is usually substernal and described by the patient as viselike, burning, squeezing, or smothering. The pain may radiate to either arm, the shoulder, the jaw, the neck, or the epigastrium. Accompanying symptoms are diaphoresis, dyspnea, nausea, and vomiting. Angina that is not relieved by drug therapy suggests progressive ischemia that can result in infarction of tissue.

Two less common types of angina are unstable angina and Prinzmetal's angina. Unstable (crescendo) angina indicates acute coronary insufficiency. It may occur at rest or with minimal exertion and is often unrelieved by nitroglycerin. Patients with unstable angina are at increased risk for AMI and sudden cardiac death. Prinzmetal's, or variant, angina occurs at rest and may occur without evidence of atherosclerosis. It is caused by coronary artery spasm.

Medical Treatment

Treatment of CAD includes diet therapy, drug therapy, and reduction of risk factors (smoking, obesity, hypertension). Calcium channel blockers (verapamil, diltiazem, and nifedipine) are used to decrease coronary artery spasm and myocardial oxygen demand.

Diet therapy. Treatment begins with dietary adjustment. The aim of the dietary regimen is to decrease the serum cholesterol and serum triglyceride levels to achieve and maintain ideal body weight. A low-fat, low-cholesterol diet should be encouraged. According to the American Heart Association, fat intake should be decreased to 30% or less of the daily calories and saturated fat should constitute less than 7% of total calories. Daily cholesterol intake should be restricted to less than 200 mg/day.

Drug therapy. Drug therapy may be initiated if dietary control does not reduce cholesterol sufficiently. Antilipemics (agents that reduce serum lipids) include cholestyramine resin (Questran), clofibrate (Atromid-S), gemfibrozil (Lopid), lovastatin (Mevacor), and niacin.

The goals of drug therapy for the patient with CAD may also include reduction of angina. Various forms of nitroglycerin are prescribed for treatment of acute angina. These are administered sublingually or buccally at the onset of pain. They are quickly absorbed and usually effective. Oral, topical, and transdermal nitrates may be ordered to prevent angina attacks. Other drugs used for prophylaxis (prevention) of angina are calcium channel blockers and beta-adrenergic blockers. Low-dose aspirin may also be prescribed to decrease the risk of platelet aggregation and thrombus formation, which can cause an AMI.

Additional information about selected antianginal and antilipemic drugs is presented in Table 33-8.

Surgical intervention. Surgical procedures to treat CAD are discussed in the section on treatment of AMI.

ACUTE MYOCARDIAL INFARCTION

An AMI is the destruction of myocardial tissue as a result of lack of blood and oxygen supply. Approximately 1,100,000 Americans have a new or recurrent myocardial infarction every year; 40% of these result in death. Men predominate in patients younger than age 65; after age 65, the incidence is approximately equal in men and women.

Risk Factors

Risk factors for AMI include obesity, smoking, a high-fat diet, hypertension, family history, male gender, diabetes mellitus, sedentary lifestyle, and excessive stress. Smoking, a high-fat diet, hypertension, sedentary lifestyle, and stress are considered modifiable risk factors. This means that risk can be reduced by cessation of smoking, diet modification, management of hypertension, regular exercise, and stress reduction.

Pathophysiology

An AMI begins with the occlusion of a coronary artery. Over a period of 4 to 6 hours, a process of ischemia, injury, and infarction develops. Ischemia results from a lack of blood and oxygen to a portion of the heart muscle. If ischemia is not reversed, then injury occurs. Deprived of blood and oxygen, the affected tissue becomes soft and loses its normal color. With continued ischemia, an infarction, or death of myocardial tissue, occurs. Ischemia lasting 20 minutes or more is sufficient to produce irreversible tissue damage.

Within 24 hours after an infarction, the healing process begins. By the third day, necrotic tissue has been broken down by enzymes and removed by macrophages. Collateral circulation develops to supply the injured area, and scar tissue begins to form. About 10 to 14 days after the AMI, the myocardium is especially vulnerable to stress because of the weakness of the healing tissue. Complete healing takes about 6 weeks.

Complications

Up to 90% of patients with AMI suffer complications. The major complications are dysrhythmias, cardiac failure, cardiogenic shock, thromboembolism, and ventricular rupture.

Dysrhythmias

Dysrhythmias are disturbances in heart rhythm, including excessively rapid, slow, or irregular heartbeats. They occur in approximately 80% of all patients with AMI. Because some dysrhythmias are life threatening, continuous cardiac monitoring is usually ordered for patients with AMI. This permits early detection and prompt treatment of dysrhythmias. Recognition and treatment of specific dysrhythmias are addressed later in this chapter.

Cardiac Failure

The AMI may cause the heart to fail as a pump if the injured LV is unable to meet the body's circulatory demands. The ventricle fails to empty efficiently. Increased preload leads to systemic and pulmonary edema. Cardiac output and blood pressure fall. Untreated cardiac failure progresses to cardiogenic shock and death. Early symptoms of congestive failure are dyspnea, restlessness, and increasing heart rate.

Cardiogenic Shock

Cardiogenic shock is the most frequent cause of death after an AMI. It is usually related to extensive injury to the LV and is more common when the patient has had a previous infarction. Cardiogenic shock is marked by hypotension; cool, moist skin; oliguria; and decreasing alertness.

Thromboembolism

After an AMI, thrombi may form in the injured heart chambers or in the veins of the legs. The thrombi may break loose, travel through the circulation, and lodge in the lung. Pallor, cyanosis, and heart failure may be caused by pulmonary emboli. Massive pulmonary embolism is characterized by sudden, severe dyspnea. It is usually fatal. Pulmonary emboli are discussed in detail in Chapter 29.

Ventricular Rupture

Weakened areas of the ventricular wall may bulge during contractions. If scar tissue is inadequate to strengthen the wall, an aneurysm may develop and rupture. Ventricular rupture is fatal.

Signs and Symptoms

Pain is the classic symptom of AMI. It is typically a heavy or constrictive pain located below or behind the sternum, as described with CAD. It may radiate to the arms, back, neck, or jaw. The pain may begin with or without exertion. If not relieved by rest and nitroglycerin, it progresses. The patient becomes diaphoretic and lightheaded and may experience nausea, vomiting, and dyspnea. The skin is frequently cold and clammy. The patient experiences great anxiety and often a feeling of impending doom. Dyspnea is sometimes the only symptom experienced by elderly people with AMIs. Anyone with chest pain unrelieved for 30 minutes should go to an emergency department for treatment.

Medical Diagnosis

The diagnosis of an AMI is based primarily on the patient's history and the physical signs and symptoms. The AMI can be confirmed by laboratory evidence and ECG changes.

Troponin

Troponin T (TnT) and troponin I (TnI) are proteins released from cardiac muscle when damaged. TnI is found only in cardiac muscle, and TnT may also elevate with muscle injury or renal failure. Troponin levels elevate as early as 1 hour after myocardial injury, peak in 24 hours, and remain in the circulation for up to 2 weeks (TnI remains elevated for 5 to 7 days; TnT for 10 to 14 days). Troponin levels may be drawn in the emergency room, and results will be back very quickly, helping to establish an early diagnosis.

Myoglobin

Myoglobin is released within 1 hour after an acute myocardial infarction and levels rise before CK-MB levels; therefore, myoglobin levels can be helpful in the early diagnosis of AMI. Myoglobin levels will also be increased after strenuous exercise or renal failure and in the presence of neuromuscular disease.

Cardiac Enzymes

A blood sample is drawn from anyone with prolonged chest pain to measure cardiac enzymes. With sustained ischemia, the cell membrane is impaired and enzymes are released from their intracellular location into the interstitial fluid. These enzymes can be measured in the serum and are assessed at regular intervals to confirm an AMI. CPK and its isoenzyme CPK-MB (myocardial) elevate rapidly with infarction. Beginning 4 to 6 hours after infarction, the CPK rises to 5 or more times the normal level within 12 to 24 hours and returns to normal in 2 to 3 days. LDH elevates 8 to 12 hours after infarction, peaks in 3 to 4 days, and returns to normal in 10 to 14 days. Altered LDH1 and LDH2 are associated with AMI. Normally, LDH2 has a higher value than LDH1. When this is reversed (called a flipped LDH), it confirms an AMI.

Electrocardiogram

Changes in the normal waveform and dysrhythmias can be seen on an ECG. With ischemia, the T wave is inverted. With injury, there is ST segment elevation. With infarction, there is a significant Q wave (Fig. 33-8). A significant Q wave is one that is greater than one third the height of the R wave. The most frequently observed dysrhythmias are premature ventricular contractions, ventricular tachycardia, and ventricular fibrillation.

Medical Treatment

The overall goal of medical therapy is to preserve myocardial tissue. This can best be accomplished by early treatment and risk modification.

Drug Therapy

Sublingual or intravenous nitroglycerin is administered to dilate coronary arteries and increase blood flow to the damaged area. If the nitroglycerin relieves the pain, the infarction may not extend. Morphine sulfate is also used for chest pain. It has many effects in addition to analgesia. Morphine causes peripheral pooling of blood, which decreases the blood returning to the heart and lungs. It also diminishes anxiety, decreases tachypnea, and relaxes bronchial smooth muscles, thereby improving gas exchange. If the patient cannot tolerate morphine, meperidine (Demerol) may be ordered, but it does not have all the nonanalgesic properties of morphine and may increase the heart rate.

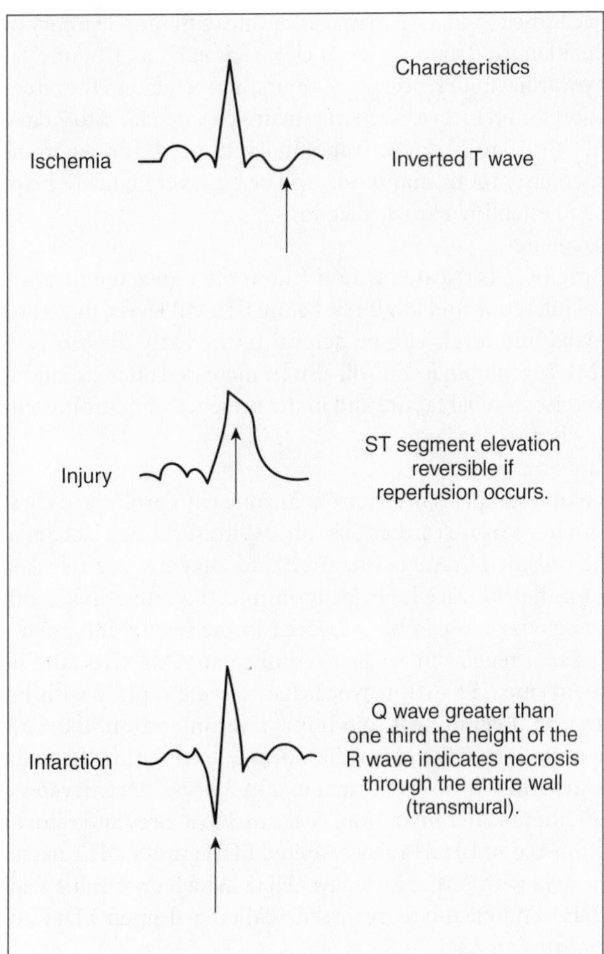

FIGURE 33-8 Electrocardiographic changes with myocardial infarction.

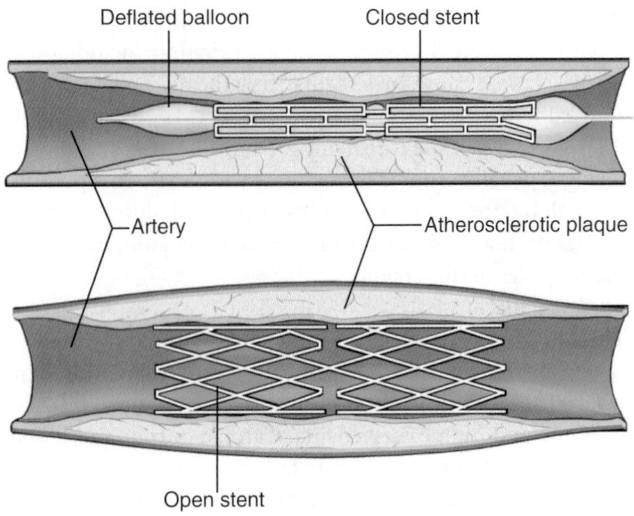

FIGURE 33-9 Intracoronary stent.

Oxygen is administered at 4-6 L/min to assist in oxygenating myocardial tissue to support pumping activity and for repairing damaged tissue.

Thrombolytic therapy is useful for patients whose infarctions are diagnosed early. Streptokinase and tissue plasminogen activator are administered intravenously or into the coronary arteries (during cardiac catheterization) to dissolve thrombi. This treatment is most effective when initiated within 6 hours of the onset of chest pain. The patient must meet strict criteria (no recent surgery or active bleeding; no history of a stroke; no bleeding disorders) and provide informed consent before the administration of thrombolytics. After administration of the thrombolytics, heparin is administered to prevent further clot formation. Once the patient is stable, oral aspirin may be ordered as the anticoagulant of choice.

Lidocaine may be administered for ventricular tachycardia. Digitalis may be ordered to increase myocardial contractility and decrease the heart rate. Beta-adrenergic blockers improve survival rates by decreasing the heart rate, reducing the work of the heart, and lessening the oxygen demand of the myocardium. Calcium channel blockers decrease conduction through the AV node, thereby slowing the heart rate, decrease myocardial oxygen demand, dilate arteries, and decrease systemic vascular resistance. Unstable patients may require dopamine or dobutamine, or both, as inotropic agents. As the myocardium receives blood and oxygen, reperfusion dysrhythmias that require treatment may be noted.

Angioplasty

Percutaneous transluminal coronary angioplasty (PTCA) may be performed if one vessel is occluded. In some cardiac centers, PTCA is being done on multiple vessels as technology improves. The procedure, performed in the cardiac catheterization laboratory, involves passage of a catheter through a peripheral artery into the occluded coronary artery. The tip of the catheter contains a balloon that is inflated to compress the atherosclerotic plaque and dilate the artery.

There are currently many requirements that candidates for PTCA must meet. When appropriate, this procedure is preferred over coronary artery bypass surgery because it can be done under local anesthetic, it is less invasive, and the recovery time is faster. The procedure is safer than bypass surgery but is not without risks. Complications of PTCA include coronary artery rupture, dysrhythmias, coronary spasm, hematoma at the catheter site, restenosis, and death. In approximately 30% of patients, the vessel narrows again within 6 months.

A newer procedure is laser angioplasty. It uses a catheter with a laser on the tip. The laser is used to widen the lumen of the artery by destroying atherosclerotic plaque.

Other procedures performed in the cardiac catheterization laboratory are coronary atherectomy and placement of intracoronary stents. The coronary atherectomy is a procedure that widens the coronary artery by removing the atherosclerotic plaque using a device that shaves the plaque off the vessel walls. Intracoronary stents are devices that are positioned within the blockage through a balloon-tipped catheter, expanded into place, and left to support the arterial wall. Over time, endothelial cells will completely line the inner wall of the stent to produce a smooth inner lining (Fig. 33-9).

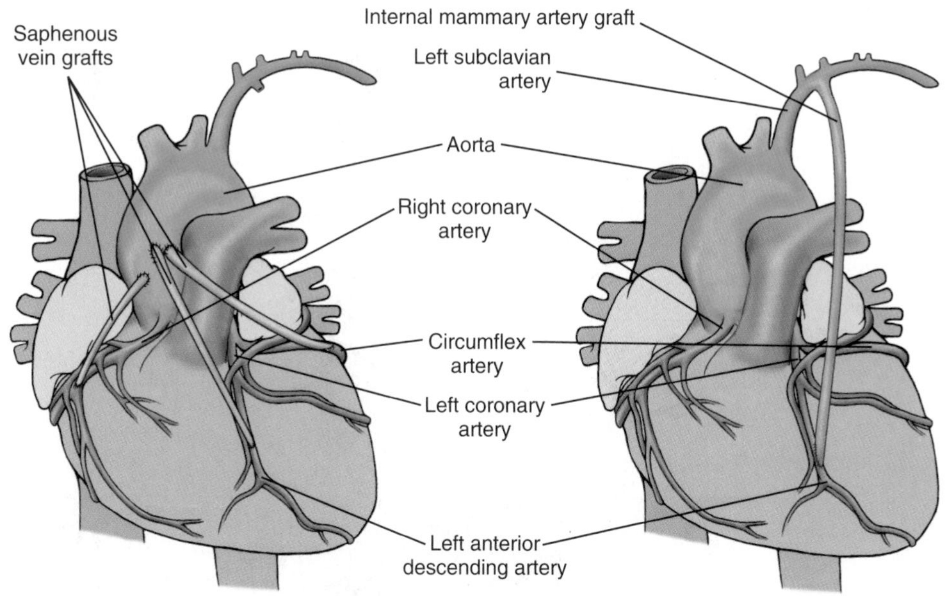

FIGURE **33-10** Coronary artery bypass graft surgery.

Coronary Artery Bypass Graft Surgery

Coronary artery bypass graft surgery may be performed to improve the blood supply to the myocardium. Arterial bypass surgery uses the patient's own vasculature as replacement for occluded coronary arteries. From one to six vessels may be bypassed. The saphenous veins and the internal mammary artery are most commonly used. The saphenous veins are removed from one or both legs, inspected for patency, and reversed so that the valves do not inhibit blood flow. The replacement vessels are attached above and below the occlusions in the coronary arteries and serve as new conduits for oxygenated blood to the myocardium (Fig. 33-10). This is major surgery. The survival rate is higher in patients who are in stable condition.

There is a new approach to surgical revascularization that is being used on patients requiring surgery on the arteries of the anterior heart. This procedure is called *minimally invasive direct coronary artery bypass grafting* and is performed through a small anterior thoracotomy incision. The patient's internal mammary artery is used to bypass the stenosed vessel and the bypass is accomplished on a beating heart. Postoperative care is similar to that of other cardiac surgery, although patients do not require as lengthy ventilatory support and total length of hospital stay is shorter.

Another method of revascularization, used for patients with diffuse coronary vessel disease, is transmyocardial laser revascularization. Tiny holes are drilled in the myocardium using a laser, which helps provide collateral circulation to the ischemic myocardial muscle (Fig. 33-11).

NURSING CARE *of the Patient with Acute Myocardial Infarction*

Assessment

General assessment of the cardiac patient is summarized in Table 33-3. When a patient has AMI, be especially concerned with assessment of pain. When chest pain is present, early evaluation and treatment are paramount. Ask the patient to describe the pain, including type, location, duration, and severity. Record what the patient was doing when the pain started, what action was taken, and the effects of any actions or treatments. Inspect the patient's skin for color and palpate for temperature and moisture. Frequently assess vital signs. Document the mental status and level of anxiety. When cardiac monitoring is initiated, evaluate the rate and rhythm.

Nursing Diagnoses, Goals, and Outcome Criteria: Acute Myocardial Infarction

Nursing Diagnoses	Goals and Outcome Criteria
Anxiety related to feeling of impending doom, lack of understanding of routines	Reduced anxiety: patient statement of lessened anxiety, calm manner and self-care
Pain related to lack of oxygen to the myocardium	Pain relief: patient statement of relieved pain, relaxed manner
Decreased Cardiac Output related to dysrhythmia and abnormal heart rate	Normal cardiac output: normal pulse, blood pressure, and cardiac rhythm

Interventions

Anxiety

Provide as calm an environment as possible. Simply explain procedures and equipment to the patient and family. Keep family members informed of the patient's progress. They can be helpful in calming the patient during the acute episode.

During the acute phase of AMI, provide simple explanations of the procedures and routines. Reinforce information given by the physician about the diagnosis and treatment. Patient teaching is especially important in the rehabilitation phase.

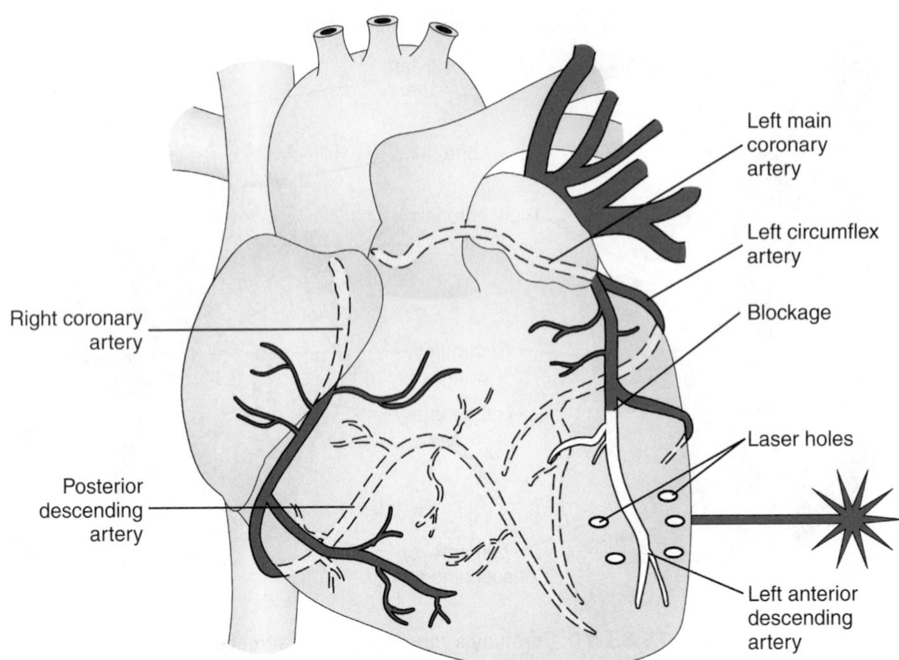

FIGURE **33-11** Transmyocardial laser revascularization.

Pain. Administer analgesics as ordered and monitor for relief of pain. Morphine is usually administered in small amounts (2 to 4 mg) intravenously every few minutes until pain relief is evident. Provide supplemental oxygen as ordered through nasal cannula at 2 to 4 L/min to provide adequate oxygen to the heart muscle. The head of the bed is usually elevated at least 30 degrees. Inform the physician if the patient has an increasing respiratory rate or dyspnea.

Decreased Cardiac Output. Monitor vital signs hourly or more frequently until stable. Monitor the ECG for changes in normal waveform (inverted T wave, ST elevation, and Q wave) and for dysrhythmias. Notify the physician of changes in the rhythm. In an intensive care unit, standing orders prescribe drug therapy for specific dysrhythmias. An intravenous line is usually established so that emergency drugs can be administered quickly and directly. Prompt treatment of dysrhythmias may prevent fatal alterations in rhythm. Monitor the patient for fluid volume excess (crackles, cough, jugular vein distention) and report any such evidence to the physician.

Interventions to decrease demands on the heart include assisting the patient to rest, spacing activities and providing rest periods, providing adequate ventilation and oxygenation, relieving pain, and maintaining a calm, quiet environment.

Cardiac Rehabilitation

As soon as the patient is stable, begin rehabilitation by teaching the patient and family about exercise, medications, and diet. If surgical intervention has been proposed, you may also teach the patient about that procedure.

The purpose of rehabilitation is to minimize the risk of repetition of adverse cardiac events. The goal of rehabilitation is to enable patients to attain the highest level of wellness and work ability.

The program is individualized to the patient for maximal success. The four phases of cardiac rehabilitation are I, inpatient management; II, immediately after discharge, using telemetry monitoring during exercise; III, later rehabilitation, which is unmonitored; and IV, maintenance. A team of medical professionals (e.g., nurse, physician, physical therapist, nutritionist, social worker) plans the individual program. Education during the rehabilitation process should include normal anatomy and physiology of the heart; pathophysiology of coronary artery disease, angina, and AMI; risk factor modification; activity and exercise; medications; and when to seek medical advice.

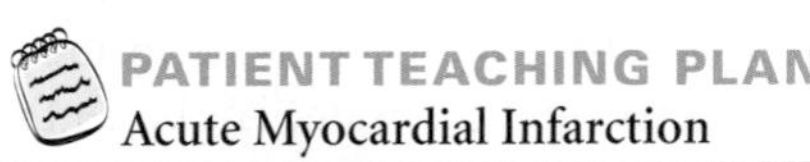

PATIENT TEACHING PLAN
Acute Myocardial Infarction

After AMI, some key points in the discharge teaching plan are:

- It is very important to take your medications as prescribed and to contact the physician if you have any problems. (Provide written information about drug names, dosages, purpose, interactions with other medications and foods, and adverse effects that should be reported.)
- Your physician may prescribe a low-fat, low-sodium diet to decrease weight and to reduce the workload on your heart.
- Participation in cardiac rehabilitation will help you become active again in a safe manner.
- Stop smoking. Smoking stimulates the heart rate and causes blood vessels to constrict, which makes the heart work harder.
- Maintain normal weight (or lose weight if obese) to decrease the work of the heart.

- The local chapter of the American Heart Association is a helpful resource for information and guidance on diet, smoking cessation, and exercise.

 **Put on your THINKING CAP!!**

A new patient is being seen in the doctor's office. Basic information and health history data include: 58 y.o. white male, height 5'9", weight 190 lbs; vital signs: 98° F, 82, 14, 152/84.

SOCIAL HISTORY

Real estate salesman (describes himself as "pretty successful" and able to maintain a good quality of life). Plays tennis 3 times a week; walks 2 miles, 4 times a week. Divorced father of 3 adult children; one son who recently was admitted to rehabilitation for substance abuse has no insurance. Patient has conflict with ex-wife related to son's situation. Enjoys a "few beers" in the evening. Has eggs, bacon, biscuits, coffee for breakfast, has lunch (sandwich, fries) at fast-food restaurant, and cooks dinner (usually "meat and potatoes"). Sleeps 7 to 8 hrs; usually rested on arising. Some recent trouble sleeping because of son's problems. No current significant other.

HEALTH HISTORY

Hypertension for 5 years treated with daily antihypertensive drug; chronic sinusitis; arthritis in left knee related to sports injury.

FAMILY HISTORY

Mother, age 78, living and in moderately good health. Had mild stroke last year without permanent effects. Has diabetes. Father died suddenly at age 66 of acute myocardial infarction. Two living brothers, ages 52 and 49. Both are hypertensive.

1. Based on the data available, identify modifiable and unmodifiable risk factors for coronary artery disease.
2. Identify one strategy to address each modifiable factor.
3. Identify current factors that reduce his risk of coronary artery disease.

CONGESTIVE HEART FAILURE

Congestive heart failure is the inability of the heart to meet the metabolic demands of the body.

Etiology and Risk Factors

Causes of CHF are primarily of two types: disorders that increase the workload of the heart and disorders that interfere with the pumping ability of the heart. Therefore patients at risk for CHF include those with CAD, AMI, cardiomyopathy, hypertension, COPD, pulmonary hypertension, anemia, disease of the heart valves, and fluid volume overload. Other conditions that increase metabolic needs, such as fever and pregnancy, may also precipitate heart failure.

Pathophysiology

The LV, RV, or both fail as pumps. Usually the left side of the heart fails first. In time, the right side fails as a result of the left-sided failure. There is a 50% mortality rate over a 4-year period.

Compensation

Compensation is a term used to describe the cardiac and circulatory adjustments that maintain or restore cardiac output to normal or near normal. Compensation occurs through three mechanisms: sympathetic nervous system stimulation, regulation of blood volume by the kidneys, and enlargement of the ventricular myocardium.

Sympathetic compensation. The sympathetic nervous system responds to decreased cardiac output and blood pressure. Catecholamines are released that increase heart rate, stroke volume, cardiac output, and venous tone. Increased venous tone increases systemic vascular resistance, venous return, and ventricular filling.

Renal compensation. The second mechanism that responds to decreased cardiac output is renal compensation. When cardiac output falls, so does renal perfusion. This initiates the renin-angiotensin mechanism. Renin, secreted by the kidneys, activates angiotensinogen to convert to angiotensin I. Angiotensin I is converted to angiotensin II, which causes vasoconstriction and triggers release of aldosterone. Vasoconstriction raises the blood pressure by increasing peripheral resistance to blood flow. Aldosterone causes the kidneys to retain sodium and water, which increases blood volume.

Ventricular hypertrophy. The third mechanism is enlargement of the ventricular myocardium, called ventricular hypertrophy, which results from strain. The increased blood volume raises the pressure in the ventricles, which can also cause the ventricles to dilate.

After a period, the compensatory mechanisms may no longer be able to meet the increased demands. Contractility decreases; the heart muscle can stretch just so far before becoming inefficient. The force of contraction of the LV decreases. Stroke volume and cardiac output decrease as pumping action fails. Afterload increases with left-sided heart failure. Blood backs up in the LA and then the pulmonary veins. Because of the high pressure in the pulmonary veins (pulmonary hypertension), fluid leaks from the capillaries, causing pulmonary edema. Pulmonary hypertension eventually causes the right side of the heart to fail as well. Then, blood returning to the heart from the body meets resistance, which causes systemic pressure to rise. This results in peripheral edema and enlargement of the liver and spleen. If heart failure is not corrected, death eventually ensues.

With left-sided CHF, there is increased left ventricular end-diastolic pressure, increased left atrial pressure, increased pulmonary pressure, and resulting pulmonary edema as the excess fluid leaks into the lung tissues. In right-sided CHF, right ventricular pressure increases, right atrial pressure increases, and fluid accumulates in the systemic vasculature.

Signs and Symptoms

The patient with left-sided heart failure is typically very anxious, pale, and tachycardic. Consecutive blood pressure readings may show a downward trend. Auscultation of the lung

NURSING CARE PLAN

The Patient with Congestive Heart Failure

ASSESSMENT

Health History: Mrs. Ling is a 73-year-old Chinese-American woman. She is a retired business owner who lives alone and has no immediate family in the area. She began having dyspnea and orthopnea that has become progressively worse over the past 3 days. Her past medical history includes a myocardial infarction 1 year ago and a 10-year history of hypertension treated with diet and verapamil 240 mg daily. In addition to the verapamil, she takes only an occasional laxative. She complains of fatigue, restlessness, nervousness, irritability, insomnia, anorexia, and a productive cough with pink sputum.

Physical Examination: Vital signs: temperature 98° F orally; pulse 104, slightly irregular; respiration 24; blood pressure 168/96. Height 5'2"; weight 152 lbs (a 7-lb increase in 1 week). She is alert but appears anxious. Her skin is pale and diaphoretic. An S_3 is present. Jugular vein distention is noted. Auscultation of the lungs reveals crackles in the lower lobes of both lungs. The abdomen is distended. Bowel sounds are present in all four quadrants. There is 3+ pitting edema in both feet and ankles.

Mrs. Ling is being admitted to the telemetry unit for treatment where she will have continuous electrocardiography and be placed on oxygen.

Nursing Diagnosis	*Goals and Outcome Criteria*	*Interventions*
Decreased cardiac output related to decreased myocardial contractility.	The patient's cardiac output will improve as evidenced by normal heart rate and rhythm, normal blood pressure, normal hemodynamic measures, and breath sounds clear to auscultation.	Monitor vital signs, heart and lung sounds, level of consciousness, electrocardiography. Enforce bed rest with head of bed elevated. Schedule activities to allow rest. Request small, frequent meals. Administer cardiotonics, vasodilators, and ACE inhibitors as ordered.
Fluid volume excess related to decreased glomerular filtration rate, increased aldosterone, sodium and water retention, and increased antidiuretic hormone release.	The patient will have normal fluid balance as evidenced by weight of 145 lbs, absence of edema, absence of crackles and wheezes in the lungs, and ability to participate in activities of daily living without dyspnea.	Monitor for jugular venous distention and peripheral edema. Auscultate heart and lung sounds every 4 hours. Measure weight daily and intake and output accurately. Maintain intravenous lines and correct fluid infusion rate. Administer diuretics as ordered. Teach about sodium restriction and rationale. Protect edematous extremities from pressure or injury.
Impaired gas exchange related to pulmonary congestion.	The patient's gas exchange will be evidenced by pulse oximetry >95%, normal skin color, absence of dyspnea, and clear lung sounds.	Assess lung sounds and respiratory status every 4 hours. Monitor pulse oximetry. Elevate head of bed. Administer oxygen as normal as ordered. Assist to cough and deep breathe every 2 hours. Administer diuretics and morphine sulfate as ordered.
Activity intolerance related to imbalance between oxygen supply and demand.	The patient's activity tolerance will improve as evidenced by performance of activities of daily living without excessive fatigue or dyspnea.	Assess response to activity when permitted. Monitor for dyspnea, changes in vital signs. Limit fatiguing activities. Gradually increase activity as tolerance improves.
Anxiety related to hypoxia, life-threatening situation.	The patient's anxiety will be reduced as evidenced by calm demeanor and statement that she feels less anxious.	Explain procedures and equipment. Tell patient about congestive heart failure and how it is being treated. Point out signs of improvement. Visit often and respond to call light promptly. Offer spiritual counselor if desired.
Deficient knowledge of condition, treatment, self-care, and resources.	The patient will verbalize information about her condition, treatment, self-care measures, and resources.	Provide simple explanation of congestive heart failure, its effects, and its treatment. As discharge nears, discuss diet, exercise, and drug therapy. Explain signs and symptoms that should be reported to physician. Advise of services of American Heart Association for information. Explore sources of support and need for visiting nurse or home health services.

fields may reveal crackles, wheezes, dyspnea, and cough. When assessing heart sounds, S_3 and S_4 may be heard as a result of the backup of fluid and the heart's inability to handle the excess fluids.

With right-sided heart failure, there is increased central venous pressure, jugular venous distention, abdominal engorgement, and dependent edema. Anorexia, nausea, and vomiting may result from the abdominal engorgement. Fatigue, weight gain, and decreased urinary output are common complaints.

Medical Diagnosis

The diagnosis of CHF is made on the basis of the history, physical examination, radiographs, and laboratory test results. A chest radiograph may reveal hazy lung fields, distended vasculature, and cardiomegaly. An echocardiogram may reveal heart enlargement and ineffective ventricular contraction. Laboratory tests indicative of CHF are decreased serum sodium and Hct from hemodilution and decreased saturated arterial oxygenation from poor pulmonary perfusion. The blood urea nitrogen (BUN) and creatinine are elevated with decreased renal function. Liver function test results are elevated with hepatomegaly (liver enlargement). The patient who is critically ill with CHF may require more intensive monitoring of **hemodynamics.**

Medical Treatment

Medical treatment includes management of the underlying cause, drug therapy to improve cardiac output and eliminate excess fluid, and conservative measures to decrease demands on the heart.

Treatment of the underlying problem may involve such interventions as correction of dysrhythmias, management of hypertension, and valve replacement or repair.

Drug Therapy

The primary drugs used to treat CHF are cardiac glycosides or inotropic agents, diuretics, and vasodilators. Digoxin, an inotropic agent, is prescribed to improve pump function by increasing contractility and decreasing heart rate. Dopamine, dobutamine, and amrinone are other inotropic agents that may be prescribed to improve cardiac contractility, improve renal perfusion, and decrease fluid retention. Diuretics are prescribed to decrease circulating fluid volume and decrease preload. Morphine may be used to decrease anxiety, dilate the vasculature, and reduce myocardial oxygen consumption in the acute stage. Table 33-8 provides additional information about drugs used to treat CHF.

Decreasing cardiac workload and increasing oxygenation to the myocardium are accomplished by using vasodilators such as angiotensin-converting enzyme inhibitors and nitrates, the intra-aortic balloon pump, the semi-Fowler's position, and mechanical ventilation. The intra-aortic balloon pump is a temporary device used in the intensive care unit to increase cardiac output and coronary artery perfusion.

Surgery

Cardiomyoplasty is a surgical procedure used to treat end-stage heart failure. The procedure involves wrapping a skeletal muscle (the latissimus dorsi) around the heart and stimulating it to contract the heart muscle. This assists the heart's contractility and improves cardiac output. The procedure involves a thoracotomy incision to bring the latissimus dorsi muscle through to the mediastinum and a mediastinal incision to access the heart so that the skeletal muscle can be wrapped around the heart. A sensing electrode is placed on the heart, and pacing electrodes are placed on the latissimus dorsi muscle. These are attached to a cardiostimulator implanted subcutaneously. The cardiostimulator senses the heart's electrical activity (depolarization) and stimulates the latissimus dorsi to contract at the same time as the heart. The muscle must be trained to contract effectively with the heart muscle contraction. Training begins approximately 2 weeks after surgery and takes up to 3 months to reach maximum effectiveness. Postoperative nursing care is similar to that with other open-heart surgery.

Complications

Dysrhythmias, renal failure, and ventricular aneurysm with potential rupture of the aneurysm are possible complications of CHF.

NURSING CARE *of the Patient with Congestive Heart Failure*

Assessment

Complete assessment of the cardiac patient is outlined in Table 33-3 (see also Nursing Care Plan: The Patient with Congestive Heart Failure). It is especially important to assess heart sounds, rate, and rhythm. The point of maximum impulse is noted. Assess the apical and radial pulses frequently. Inspect for jugular vein distention. A baseline respiratory assessment of rate, rhythm, and breath sounds is vital. Measure weight and blood pressure accurately. Inspect the skin and palpate for turgor and edema. Intake and output records and daily weights may be done to evaluate fluid retention or loss. If ordered, take central venous pressure and hemodynamic readings as well. If cardiac monitoring is done, observe for dysrhythmias. Nurses who work in intensive care units routinely interpret ECGs. Interpretation is discussed later in this chapter.

Put on your THINKING CAP!!

1. Explain why Mrs. Ling's congestive heart failure caused her to: (1) feel anxious and (2) gain weight.
2. Before discharge, Mrs. Ling's physician advises her to try to lose 30 pounds. What nursing strategies would help her achieve this goal?
3. You suspect that Mrs. Ling is not taking her blood pressure medication regularly as prescribed when she is at home. She confirms that she sometimes forgets. What strategies might improve her compliance?

PHARMACOLOGY CAPSULE Before each dose of digitalis, the apical pulse is counted for 1 full minute. If the heart rate is less than 60 bpm, the drug is withheld and the physician is notified.

Nursing Diagnoses, Goals, and Outcome Criteria: CHF

Nursing Diagnoses	Goals and Outcome Criteria
Fluid Volume Excess related to ineffective cardiac pumping	Normal fluid volume: no edema or dyspnea, blood pressure consistent with patient norms
Impaired Gas Exchange related to decreased pulmonary perfusion	Adequate oxygenation: clear breath sounds, respiratory rate 12 to 20 without dyspnea
Anxiety related to edema and difficulty breathing	Reduced anxiety: patient statement of reduced anxiety, calm manner
Decreased Cardiac Output related to mechanical failure	Improved cardiac output: normal heart rate and rhythm, fluid intake and output equal
Activity Intolerance related to inability to meet oxygen demands	Increase activity tolerance: performance of activities of daily living without fatigue

Interventions

Fluid Volume Excess

Fluid retention is a response to CHF, an attempt to maintain normal cardiac output. Unfortunately, it compounds the problem by increasing the workload on the heart. Therefore measures are taken to reduce the fluid volume to normal while improving the function of the heart. Administer diuretics as ordered and monitor the patient for adverse effects. The most common adverse effects of diuretic therapy are fluid and electrolyte disturbances. Signs and symptoms that may indicate fluid or electrolyte disturbances include cardiac dysrhythmias, muscle weakness or twitching, cramps, changes in mental status, and abdominal distention. Frequent serum electrolyte measurements are usually ordered. Note the results and notify the physician of abnormal findings. If hourly urine output is being measured, report an output of less than 30 ml/hr to the physician as well.

An intravenous catheter is usually placed to provide a line for drug administration. If intravenous fluids are administered, monitor the rate of administration very carefully. If fluid retention is not relieved by other means, fluid restriction may be instituted. All staff should know the exact amount of fluid allowed and must record all intake. Fluid restriction can be very uncomfortable for the patient. Even with fluid volume excess, the patient may feel thirsty because of electrolyte imbalances. Present oral fluids in small containers and offer them at reasonable intervals. Frequently provide mouth care. The patient and family must understand why fluids are restricted so that the patient does not exceed the prescribed intake.

The most common therapeutic dietary measure for CHF is sodium restriction. The patient may be limited to 2 g of sodium/day. In severe cases, a limitation of 500 to 1,000 mg/day may be prescribed. Reduced sodium intake decreases fluid retention, thereby reducing the cardiac workload. For a 2-g sodium diet, advise the patient to avoid foods high in sodium (a list should be provided), not to add salt before or after cooking, and to use no more than 2 cups of milk products daily. Patients often have difficulty changing their use of seasonings. Acknowledge the difficulty and explain how sodium limitation contributes to improvement of cardiac function.

It is best to identify the type of diet to be prescribed on discharge as early as possible. This allows time for a dietary consultation to be arranged, which should be followed by reinforcement by the nurse. The person who prepares the patient's meals at home must be included in the teaching sessions.

PHARMACOLOGY CAPSULE The most common adverse effects of diuretic therapy are fluid and electrolyte imbalances.

Impaired Gas Exchange. Hypoxia is a common finding with left-sided heart failure because of pulmonary edema. It is common with right-sided heart failure because of decreased blood flow to the lungs. The patient with CHF usually breathes more easily in a semi- or high-Fowler's position. Elevation of the upper body facilitates breathing by reducing pressure of the abdominal organs on the diaphragm. Supplemental oxygen is usually prescribed at 4 to 6 L/min per nasal cannula. The flow rate is reduced to 2 L/min for patients with chronic hypoxia. Assess respiratory status and blood gases frequently.

Prescribed bedrest can lead to other pulmonary complications related to immobility: hypostatic pneumonia and pulmonary emboli. Teach the patient to cough and deep breathe at least every 2 hours to promote respiratory excursion and to mobilize secretions. Other interventions to prevent complications of immobility are detailed in Chapter 20.

On discharge, the physician may order portable oxygen for use at home. The nurse or a respiratory therapist instructs the patient in the use of the equipment and the safety precautions to take when using oxygen (see Chapter 29).

Anxiety. Factors that may cause the patient to become anxious are dyspnea, unfamiliar setting and routines, and uncertainty about what is happening. Acknowledge the patient's anxiety and attempt to identify the basis. While taking immediate measures to relieve dyspnea, calmly explain what is being done. It may be helpful to tell the patient how specific measures help relieve symptoms. The presence of family members may have a calming effect if the relatives understand that they, too, must remain calm.

Decreased Cardiac Output. Give inotropic drugs, such as digitalis, vasodilators, and diuretics as ordered, and monitor the patient for therapeutic and adverse effects. Elderly patients are more susceptible to adverse drug effects because they may metabolize and excrete drugs more slowly. This is especially true when the older patient is taking digitalis. Advise the patient to report early signs of digitalis toxicity: anorexia, nausea, and visual disturbances. Bedrest and stress reduction decrease the cardiac workload. When the patient is acutely ill, eliminate unnecessary activity. Give partial baths rather than complete bed baths. Assist the patient to change positions at least every 2 hours so that the skin can be inspected for signs of pressure. Visitors may be permitted, but advise them to sit quietly with the patient for short periods.

Activity Intolerance. Frequent rest periods, pacing of activities, and relaxation techniques help the patient conserve energy. As the fluid volume is decreased and the cardiac output is increased, the patient can expect to be less fatigued.

The patient may be referred to a rehabilitation facility for exercise training. In general, the patient is advised to plan rest periods before and after tiring activities. Activity should be increased gradually, with rest periods taken when fatigue or dyspnea occurs. The physician may prescribe vasodilators for patients who experience chest pain with some activities. If monitoring is indicated after discharge, request a referral to a home nursing agency.

Instruct the patient to notify the physician if the following problems develop: increasing dyspnea or edema, excessive fatigue, or pain that is not relieved by rest or prescribed medications. In addition, advise the patient to avoid smoking and smoky environments and to refrain from wearing constricting clothing on the lower extremities.

PHARMACOLOGY CAPSULE Elderly people are more susceptible to adverse drug effects because they metabolize and excrete drugs more slowly.

PATIENT TEACHING PLAN
Chronic Congestive Heart Failure

- Reducing sodium in your diet will help control swelling and reduce the workload on your heart.
- Excess weight makes your heart work harder. Your physician may prescribe a weight-loss diet for you.
- Take your medications as prescribed to improve your heart function. (Provide written information about drug names, actions, dosage, schedule, side and adverse effects, special aspects of administration, and interactions with other medications and food.)
- Gradually increase your activity. Avoid activity that causes shortness of breath or severe fatigue.
- Weigh yourself each morning, before breakfast, on the same scale and with the same amount of clothing.
- Contact your physician if you gain 2 or more pounds in a week, develop a persistent cough, or have shortness of breath or chest pain.
- Resources:
  The American Heart Association provides information about diet and exercise.
  The Visiting Nurses Association or a home health agency can monitor your condition and help you in your home.

INFLAMMATORY DISORDERS

Inflammation of the heart most often results from systemic infections. The endocardium, myocardium, and pericardium may be affected.

Infective Endocarditis

Etiology and Risk Factors

Microbial infections of the endocardium primarily affect the valves. Organisms present in the blood easily colonize valves damaged by rheumatic heart disease or congenital defects, or a mitral valve that is prolapsed.

Although the incidence of infective endocarditis (IE) has decreased with the use of antibiotics, there has been a resurgence of the problem in intravenous drug abusers. The more frequent use of invasive intravascular catheters for severely compromised patients has also contributed to the frequency with which IE occurs.

Patients with known valvular disease are also at risk for IE. They should be treated with prophylactic antibiotics before dental or invasive procedures. Immunosuppression or any source of bacterial contamination (lacerations, pneumonia, invasive procedures, or intravenous drug use with contaminated needles) places patients at risk.

Pathophysiology

Pathogens, usually bacteria, enter the bloodstream by any of the previously mentioned means. The pathogen accumulates on the heart valves and/or the endocardium and forms vegetations. The mitral valve is the most common site for these vegetations. The turbulence of the blood flow through the heart weakens the vegetations and causes pieces to break off. These emboli can then obstruct circulation and impair tissue perfusion in the lungs, brain, kidneys, and heart.

Complications

Complications of IE include ventricular septal defect, CHF, and embolization. CHF is the most frequent cause of death with IE.

Signs and Symptoms

Patients usually present with fever, chills, malaise, fatigue, and weight loss. The fever may be low grade (37.2° to 38.9° C [99° to 102° F]) or higher (38.9° to 40.6° C [102° to 105° F]). The fever is accompanied by chills and night sweats. Chest or abdominal pain may be reported, possibly indicating embolization.

Medical Diagnosis

The diagnosis of IE is based on the history, physical examination, and results of laboratory studies. A history of recent dental or surgical procedures may precede IE. Auscultation may reveal a heart murmur. Echocardiography helps to visualize lesions and valvular regurgitation. Right-sided or left-sided heart failure may be evident. Serial blood cultures may give clues to the causative organism or organisms. The WBC count may be elevated.

Medical Treatment

Antimicrobials, rest, and limitation of activities are the primary therapeutic measures for IE. Antimicrobials are given intravenously for 2 to 6 weeks, depending on the organism. The patient is usually hospitalized for at least 1 week and then receives home intravenous therapy if that is available. Prophylactic anticoagulants may be necessary. Surgery may be necessary to replace an infected prosthetic valve.

NURSING CARE *of the Patient with Infective Endocarditis*

Assessment

Complete assessment of the cardiac patient is summarized in Table 33-3. With IE, review the patient's history for risk factors, recent invasive procedures, known pathologic cardiac conditions, and onset of symptoms. Assess for temperature elevation, heart murmur, evidence of CHF (cough, peripheral edema), and embolization.

Nursing Diagnoses, Goals, and Outcome Criteria: Infective Endocarditis

Nursing Diagnoses	Goals and Outcome Criteria
Decreased Cardiac Output related to impaired valve function	Normal cardiac output: normal pulse and blood pressure
Impaired Physical Mobility related to fatigue and prolonged intravenous therapy	Resumption of usual physical activities without symptoms: performance of activities of daily living without fatigue
Ineffective Tissue Perfusion related to embolization	Normal tissue perfusion: absence of dyspnea or signs of circulatory obstruction

Interventions

Administer prescribed antibiotics. Throughout the course of the illness, continue to assess cardiac output and monitor for complications. Teach the patient about the medications prescribed and any restrictions imposed. Encourage adequate rest, which is necessary during the healing process. Range-of-motion exercises may be necessary during the acute stage and until the patient is ambulatory.

Pericarditis

Etiology and Risk Factors

Pericarditis is an inflammation of the pericardium. It may be a primary disease or associated with another inflammatory process. The disease may be acute or chronic. Acute pericarditis is caused by viruses, bacteria, fungi, chemotherapy, or AMI (Dressler's syndrome). Chronic pericarditis is caused by tuberculosis, radiation, or metastases.

Pathophysiology

In acute pericarditis, the inflammatory process causes an increase in the amount of pericardial fluid and inflammation of the surrounding tissues. With effusion, clear or turbid fluid accumulates in the pericardial space. In effusive-constrictive pericarditis, adhesions occur. In constrictive pericarditis, scarring of the pericardium fuses the visceral and parietal pericardia together. Loss of elasticity results from the scarring. This constrictive process prevents adequate ventricular filling.

Complications

The major complication of pericarditis is pericardial effusion or accumulation of fluid in the pericardial space. This may lead to cardiac tamponade when sufficient fluid accumulation decreases ventricular filling. The resulting drop in cardiac output is an emergency. It is treated with pericardiocentesis to remove the accumulated fluid.

Signs and Symptoms

Chest pain is the hallmark symptom of pericarditis. The pain is most severe on inspiration. It is most often sharp and stabbing but may be described as dull or burning. It is relieved by sitting up and leaning forward. Dyspnea, chills, and fever accompany pericarditis. A pericardial rub may be present. Slowly progressing pericardial effusion does not result in hemodynamic compromise until 400 to 500 ml of fluid have accumulated. Rapidly accumulating fluid may precipitate sudden symptoms with only 250 ml of fluid.

Medical Diagnosis

The diagnostic challenge is to differentiate pericarditis from AMI. The WBC count is elevated with pericarditis. Serial ECGs show that the ST segment elevation resolves in several weeks. QRS voltage may decrease because of the accumulated fluid in the pericardial space. An echocardiogram may show pericardial thickening and effusion. Atrial fibrillation may occur because of the irritation. The CPK-MB may be elevated. Blood cultures may identify the causative organism or organisms.

Medical Treatment

The patient is treated with analgesics, antipyretics, anti-inflammatory agents, and antibiotics. With constrictive pericarditis, the patient would be treated as for CHF. Surgical creation of a pericardial window (removal of a segment of parietal pericardium to allow continuous drainage of pericardial fluid) may be necessary for treating chronic pericarditis with effusion.

NURSING CARE *of the Patient with Pericarditis*

Assessment

General nursing assessment of the cardiac patient is summarized in Table 33-3. With pericarditis, assessment of heart sounds is especially important.

Nursing Diagnoses, Goals, and Outcome Criteria: Pericarditis

Nursing Diagnoses	Goals and Outcome Criteria
Pain related to pericardial inflammation	Pain relief: patient statement that pain is reduced, relaxed manner

Decreased Cardiac Output related to pericardial constriction	Improved cardiac output: normal pulse and blood pressure
Anxiety related to illness	Decreased anxiety: patient statement that anxiety is reduced, calm manner

Interventions

Rest and reduction of activity decrease the workload of the heart. Administer medications and teach the patient about the medications. Emotional support from the nursing staff and significant others is vital. The patient can be instructed in relaxation techniques. Monitor vital signs and auscultate for a pericardial friction rub. The rub is heard during inspiration with the diaphragm of the stethoscope placed between the second and the fourth intercostal spaces at the left sternal border. It is heard when there is no fluid accumulation. Distant heart sounds may be heard when there is fluid accumulation. Note pain characteristics and response to analgesics and anti-inflammatory agents. Monitor the ECG for dysrhythmias.

CARDIOMYOPATHY

Etiology and Risk Factors

Cardiomyopathy is disease of the heart muscle. Its cause is unknown. The disease usually leads to heart failure. Three types of cardiomyopathy are recognized: dilated, hypertrophic, and restrictive (Fig. 33-12). Dilated cardiomyopathy is the most common type and is found primarily in men 40 to 60 years of age. There is an increased incidence in African-American males. A relatively poor prognosis exists for dilated cardiomyopathy, with a 50% mortality rate in 5 years. Hypertrophic cardiomyopathy is usually of genetic origin. People with hypertrophic cardiomyopathy usually die by age 40, and the incidence of sudden cardiac death with this diagnosis is high. Restrictive cardiomyopathy is the least common type and occurs in young men and women.

Three risk factors are associated with dilated cardiomyopathy: excessive use of alcohol, pregnancy, and infections. The genetic predisposition with hypertrophic cardiomyopathy is known to skip generations. Amyloidosis, sarcoidosis, and other immunosuppressive disorders may predispose young people to restrictive cardiomyopathy.

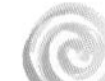
What Does Culture Have to do with Cardiomyopathy?

African-American males are at increased risk for dilated cardiomyopathy. Be alert to complaints of decreasing exercise tolerance and dyspnea in this population.

Pathophysiology

With dilated cardiomyopathy, there is an interference with calcium uptake. This causes decreased cellular contractility, decreased ejection fraction and stroke volume, and increased left ventricular end-diastolic pressure. Pressure backup results in dilation of all four chambers and is most pronounced in the ventricles. Left ventricular failure and resulting CHF are seen as the result of excessive back pressure (see Fig. 33-12A).

In hypertrophic cardiomyopathy, the LV hypertrophies and there is thickening of the ventricular septum and the mitral valve. The left ventricular capacity decreases and narrows the left ventricular outflow. The size of the LA increases as a result of the back pressure. Ventricular dysrhythmias are common (see Fig. 33-12B).

In restrictive cardiomyopathy, the myocardium becomes rigid and less distensible systole. This reduces ventricular filling and cardiac output. Pulmonary and systemic congestion result. The exterior heart size remains normal, but all four chambers decrease in size (see Fig. 33-12C).

Signs and Symptoms

Dilated cardiomyopathy is a progressive, chronic disease. The onset is gradual, with dyspnea, fatigue, left-sided heart failure,

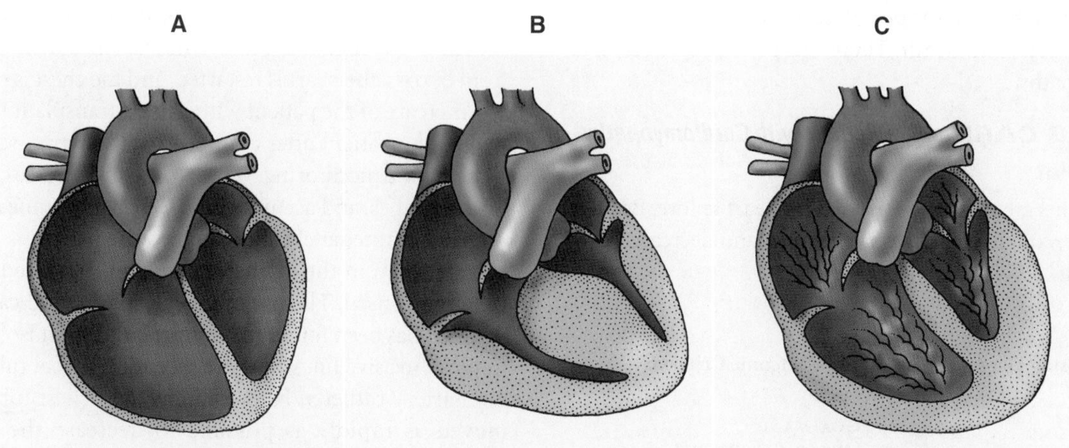

FIGURE 33-12 Cardiomyopathy. *A,* Dilated cardiomyopathy. *B,* Hypertrophic cardiomyopathy. *C,* Restrictive cardiomyopathy.

and moderate-to-severe cardiomyopathy. Mitral valve regurgitation and S_3 and S_4 sounds are evident.

With hypertrophic cardiomyopathy, the progression of symptoms is slow. Dyspnea, orthopnea, angina, fatigue, syncope, palpitations, ankle edema, and S_4 sounds are found.

With restrictive cardiomyopathy, the primary symptom is exercise intolerance. Dyspnea, fatigue, right-sided CHF, S_3 and S_4 sounds, and mitral valve regurgitation are also noted.

Medical Diagnosis

Diagnosis of dilated cardiomyopathy is made primarily on the basis of echocardiography results. Cardiac enlargement may be noted on chest radiography. The echocardiogram and chest radiograph are also used to diagnose hypertrophic cardiomyopathy. Other findings include an aortic murmur and atrial and ventricular dysrhythmias. An enlarged LV may be accompanied by left atrial enlargement. The diagnosis of restrictive cardiomyopathy is demonstrated by decreased cardiac output and CHF. It must be differentiated from pericarditis. An echocardiogram may show thickened ventricular walls and small ventricular cavities.

Medical Treatment

Supportive measures are used for dilated cardiomyopathy. Positive inotropic drugs to improve cardiac output, diuretics and nitrates to decrease preload, and vasodilators to decrease afterload provide this type of therapy. Anticoagulants may be used to prevent thrombi. If all other measures fail, the patient needs a heart transplant. Surgery, in the form of a myomectomy, ventriculomyomectomy (incision of the hypertrophied septal muscle and resection of some of the hypertrophied muscle), or mitral valve replacement are considered for hypertrophic cardiomyopathy. Medical treatment for hypertrophic cardiomyopathy includes antidysrhythmics, antibiotics, anticoagulants, calcium channel blockers, and beta blockers. Positive inotropic drugs, diuretics, and nitrates are contraindicated with hypertrophic cardiomyopathy. Treatment of restrictive cardiomyopathy is similar to that of CHF therapy. Heart transplantation may be considered. Complications observed with all types of cardiomyopathy are dysrhythmias, CHF, and death. There is a poor prognosis with cardiomyopathy.

NURSING CARE *of the Patient with Cardiomyopathy*

Assessment

These patients are primarily assessed for heart failure. Be alert for dyspnea, cough, edema, dysrhythmias, and decreased cardiac output.

Nursing Diagnoses, Goals, and Outcome Criteria: Cardiomyopathy

Nursing Diagnoses	Goals and Outcome Criteria
Decreased Cardiac Output related to ventricular failure	Improved cardiac output: normal pulse and blood pressure
Activity Intolerance related to poor tissue perfusion	Increased activity tolerance: performance of daily activities without excessive fatigue
Hopelessness related to poor prognosis	More positive outlook: patient's expression of feelings about condition and hopeful statements

Interventions

The care of these patients is similar to that of patients with CHF. In addition, a hopeful atmosphere and a careful explanation of care requirements are necessary. Encourage the family to support the patient. The teaching plan guides the patient to make lifestyle changes. Encourage the patient to make decisions and choices.

CARDIAC TRANSPLANTATION

The first heart transplantation was performed in 1967 in South Africa by Dr. Christiaan Barnard. Today, heart transplantations in the United States, approximately 1,800 per year, are done for end-stage heart disease. Most of the cases of end-stage heart disease that require transplantation are caused by cardiomyopathy. Psychological makeup is carefully assessed before transplantation. Patients with a history of depression, noncompliance, and inability to cope with stress are poor candidates. In the United States, there are federal regulations that prohibit the sale of human organs.

The donor must meet the criteria for brain death, have no malignancies outside the central nervous system, be free of infection, and not have experienced severe chest trauma. Prolonged advanced life support measures are avoided. The donor and recipient organs must be carefully matched. The donor heart size must be sufficient to meet the needs of the recipient. The donor heart may be preserved for 4 to 6 hours before transplantation.

The recipient must be free of infection at the time of transplantation. The patient is prepared for surgery as with any open-heart procedure. Cardiopulmonary bypass is initiated and the recipient's heart is removed except for the posterior portions of the atria (Fig. 33-13). The donor heart is trimmed and anastomosed to the remaining native heart. The patient is removed from bypass, the heart is restarted, and the chest is closed.

Aftercare of the patient with a heart transplant is similar to that of the patient after coronary artery bypass surgery. Hemodynamic monitoring, ventilation, cardiac assessment, care of chest tubes, and accurate intake and output measurements are vital. Immediately after surgery, the patient is placed in a private room in the intensive care unit. Modified protective isolation is used. The use of gowns, masks, and careful hand washing has been found to be superior to strict isolation techniques. Invasive lines/tubes (e.g., endotracheal tube, pulmonary artery catheter, Foley catheter, and chest tubes) are removed as rapidly as possible to decrease the chance of infection. The prevention of postoperative infection is a major goal. Pulmonary infections are most frequently found after heart transplantations. Moving the patient from the intensive care unit to a private room and to home as soon as

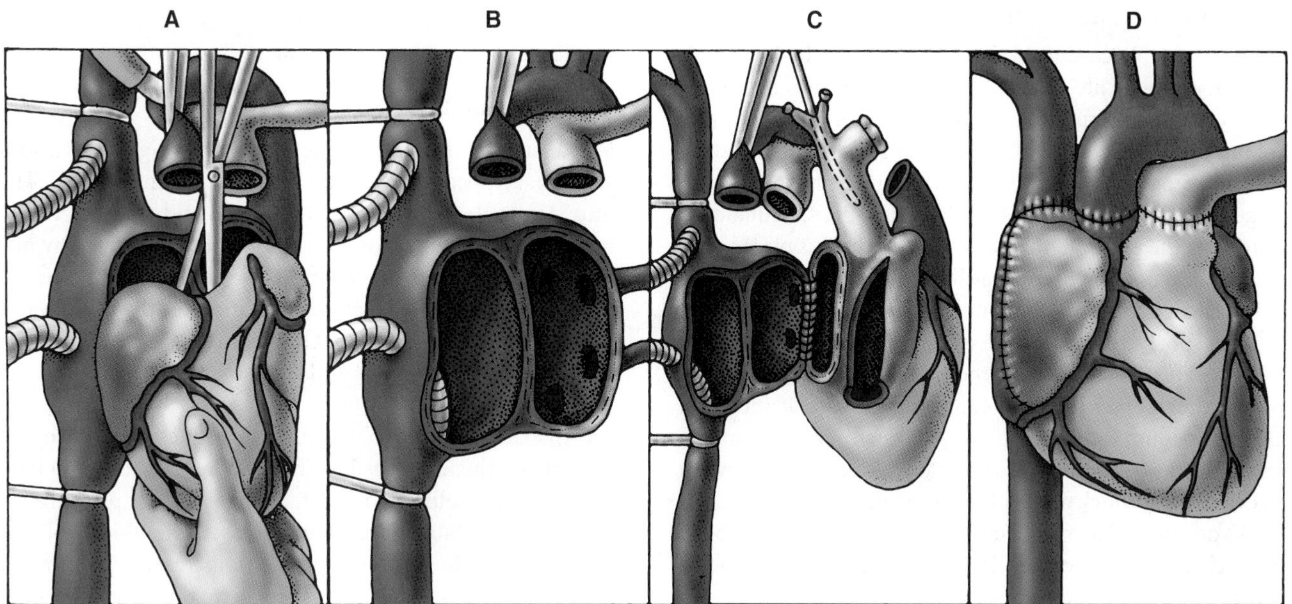

FIGURE **33-13** Heart transplantation. *A,* After the recipient is placed on cardiopulmonary bypass, the heart is removed. *B,* The posterior walls of the recipient's left and right atria are left intact. *C,* The left atrium of the donor heart is anastomosed to the recipient's residual posterior atrial walls, and the other atrial walls, the atrial septum, and the great vessels are joined. *D,* Postoperative result.

possible decreases the incidence of nosocomial infections. Patients and families are taught the signs and symptoms of infection and to avoid crowds and others with infections.

In addition, the patient with a transplant receives immunosuppressive medications. Lifelong immunosuppression is administered to prevent the body from rejecting the donated heart, which it recognizes as foreign tissue. Initially, large doses of corticosteroids are administered, and the dose is decreased over time. At the first indication of rejection (increased temperature, infection, dyspnea, malaise, fatigue, dysrhythmia), the steroid dose usually is increased. Other drugs used to prevent and treat rejection are azathioprine (Imuran), cyclosporine (Sandimmune), the monoclonal antibody OKT-3, antithymocytic globulin, antilymphocytic globulin, FK-506, and rapamycin. Protocols using several immunosuppressive agents are considered most effective. Reduced dosages of each drug provide for a lower incidence of toxicity.

Rejection is monitored through endomyocardial biopsies. These are performed frequently in the immediate period after transplantation and less frequently over time. Patients are taught to monitor their own progress and to report problems promptly. Patients are followed closely by the transplant team and are observed for infection, rejection, quality of life, and complications. Common complications noted after heart transplantation are hypertension, elevated cholesterol, obesity, and malignancies.

PHARMACOLOGY CAPSULE Patients taking immunosuppressive drugs to prevent rejection of transplanted tissue have reduced resistance to infection.

SUDDEN CARDIAC DEATH

Sudden cardiac death occurs when heart activity and respirations cease abruptly. The most common underlying reason for sudden cardiac death is coronary heart disease.

The sudden cardiac death event usually occurs during ordinary activity. It is often preceded by ventricular tachycardia or ventricular fibrillation and occasionally by severe bradydysrhythmias (slow, abnormal cardiac rhythms). An episode of sudden cardiac death may be the first indication of CAD. Other causes include left ventricular dysfunction, cardiomyopathy, hypokalemia, antidysrhythmics, liquid protein diets, and high alcohol consumption.

Those who survive an episode of sudden cardiac death need to have extensive testing done to determine the nature and cause of the sudden cardiac death. Many of these people will need treatment of CAD (medical therapy, PTCA, or coronary artery bypass grafting). Most of these patients have a lethal dysrhythmia that requires intervention. Diagnostic tests include 24-hour Holter monitoring, stress testing, and electrophysiology study. During the electrophysiology study, pacing electrodes are placed in the heart and electrical stimuli are used to elicit the dysrhythmia. This helps the physician determine appropriate medical therapy. In some patients, the dysrhythmia may be treated during the electrophysiology study with catheter ablation. The ablation (removal or "burning") of abnormal conduction pathways or irritable sites in the heart can prevent the dysrhythmia from recurring. Still other patients are treated effectively with antidysrhythmics. If these therapies are ineffective, the patient may be considered a candidate for an implantable cardioverter/defibrillator (ICD).

Implantable Cardioverter/Defibrillator

The implantable cardioverter/defibrillator (ICD) is used to treat patients with life-threatening recurrent ventricular fibrillation who are unresponsive to medications or pacemakers. Its use has greatly decreased the mortality from sudden cardiac death. The device senses heart rate and interprets waveform shape. The ICD generator is implanted in the subcutaneous tissue over the pectoral muscle. The lead system is placed via a subclavian vein into the endocardium. The cardioverter recognizes ventricular fibrillation and ventricular tachycardia and uses the shocks to convert the dysrhythmia to normal sinus rhythm. When the ICD senses these lethal dysrhythmias, it delivers a shock of 25 joules or less to defibrillate. If the heart rhythm does not return to normal, the device can continue to deliver shocks. The patient is instructed to sit or lie down when experiencing a shock and to keep a record of the number of shocks delivered. Patients report that the shocks feel like a blow to the chest. In addition to defibrillation, the newest generation of ICDs are also able to function as antitachycardia and antibradycardia pacemakers.

Complications

Complications associated with the ICD are inappropriate shocks, broken or displaced leads, and failure to deliver shocks as a result of battery failure or failure to recognize a dysrhythmia.

NURSING CARE *of the Patient with an Implantable Cardioverter/Defibrillator*

Nurses can promote psychosocial adaptation in patients with ICDs. The patient may be concerned with body image change and a fear of shocks. It is important to decrease anxiety about being shocked. Some patients become very dependent on the machine. These patients and families need much teaching and support. People who touch the patient during a shock will feel a tingling sensation, which is not harmful. An established support group for the patient and family is very helpful. The family must be instructed in cardiopulmonary resuscitation. An identification bracelet and a card with instructions about the ICD setting are carried at all times. Advise patients to avoid strong magnetic fields (metal detectors, power plants, and MRI). Batteries should be checked every 2 months.

VALVULAR DISEASE

The purpose of the heart valves is to maintain blood flow in one direction. If the valves are damaged through a congenital defect or acquired disease, their function is compromised. Stenosis and regurgitation are the two major valve problems. Stenosis is narrowing of the valvular opening. A stenotic valve limits the amount of blood ejected from one chamber to the next. Regurgitation, the inability of the valve to close completely, allows the blood to flow backward when a valve does not close efficiently. The left side of the heart is most often affected, and the mitral valve is the most frequently affected of all the valves. The pulmonic valve is infrequently affected. Only left-sided valvular disease is discussed here.

Antibiotics have decreased the incidence of valvular disease from rheumatic fever, but the incidence of nonrheumatic valvular disease has increased. Longer life span and intravenous drug abuse are the primary causes of the increasing incidence of nonrheumatic valvular disease.

Mitral Stenosis

Mitral stenosis is a narrowing of the opening in the mitral valve that impedes blood flow from the LA into the LV. The mitral valve leaflets become thickened and fibrotic. Young women, 20 to 40 years of age, are most often affected by mitral stenosis. Rheumatic heart disease is the leading cause of mitral stenosis. Congenital malformations of the mitral valve occur but are not common. Other causes are calcium accumulation on valve leaflets and atrial myxomas (tumors).

Pathophysiology

The thickening of the valve structures reduces the outflow of blood from the LA to the LV. The LA dilates to accommodate the amount of blood not ejected and left atrial pressure increases. As left atrial pressure increases, the blood volume backs up into the pulmonary system, increasing pulmonary pressures. This increases the workload on the right side of the heart, leading to right ventricular hypertrophy. Eventually, the RV fails, and cardiac output decreases because less blood is delivered to the LV.

Signs and Symptoms

Symptoms may begin soon after the disease process or may be delayed for many years. Dyspnea, fatigue, cough, chest pain, and activity intolerance are the most frequent symptoms. Exertional dyspnea and pulmonary edema occur as blood backs up in the pulmonary system and serous fluid leaks into the pulmonary tissues. Because stenosis causes turbulent blood flow through the valve, a murmur is present during diastole (best heard at the apex of the heart).

Medical Diagnosis

Diagnosis is made on the basis of the patient history, physical examination, and results of diagnostic procedures. The chest radiograph shows left atrial, right ventricular, and pulmonary vascular enlargement. Echocardiography is used to visualize the mitral valve. Cardiac catheterization is used to confirm the diagnosis and determine the extent of the disease process.

Medical Treatment

When symptomatic, the patient with mitral stenosis is treated as for CHF with drug therapy, sodium and fluid restrictions, and activity restriction. Digoxin, diuretics, beta blockers, and antidysrhythmics may be prescribed. If the patient has atrial fibrillation, anticoagulants also may be prescribed. Prophylactic antibiotics are prescribed before any invasive procedure for patients with mitral stenosis because bacteria tend to cluster on the damaged valves.

Surgical Treatment

Surgical treatment includes commissurotomy, mitral valve replacement, and balloon valvuloplasty. Commissurotomy is excision of parts of the leaflets to enlarge the opening. The mitral valve may be replaced with a biologic or synthetic valve (Fig. 33-14). Both commissurotomy and mitral valve replacement require major surgery with cardiopulmonary bypass.

Balloon valvuloplasty is a procedure done in the cardiac catheterization laboratory that has been very successful in dilating stenosed heart valves. It is less invasive than valve replacement or commissurotomy. To dilate the mitral valve, a

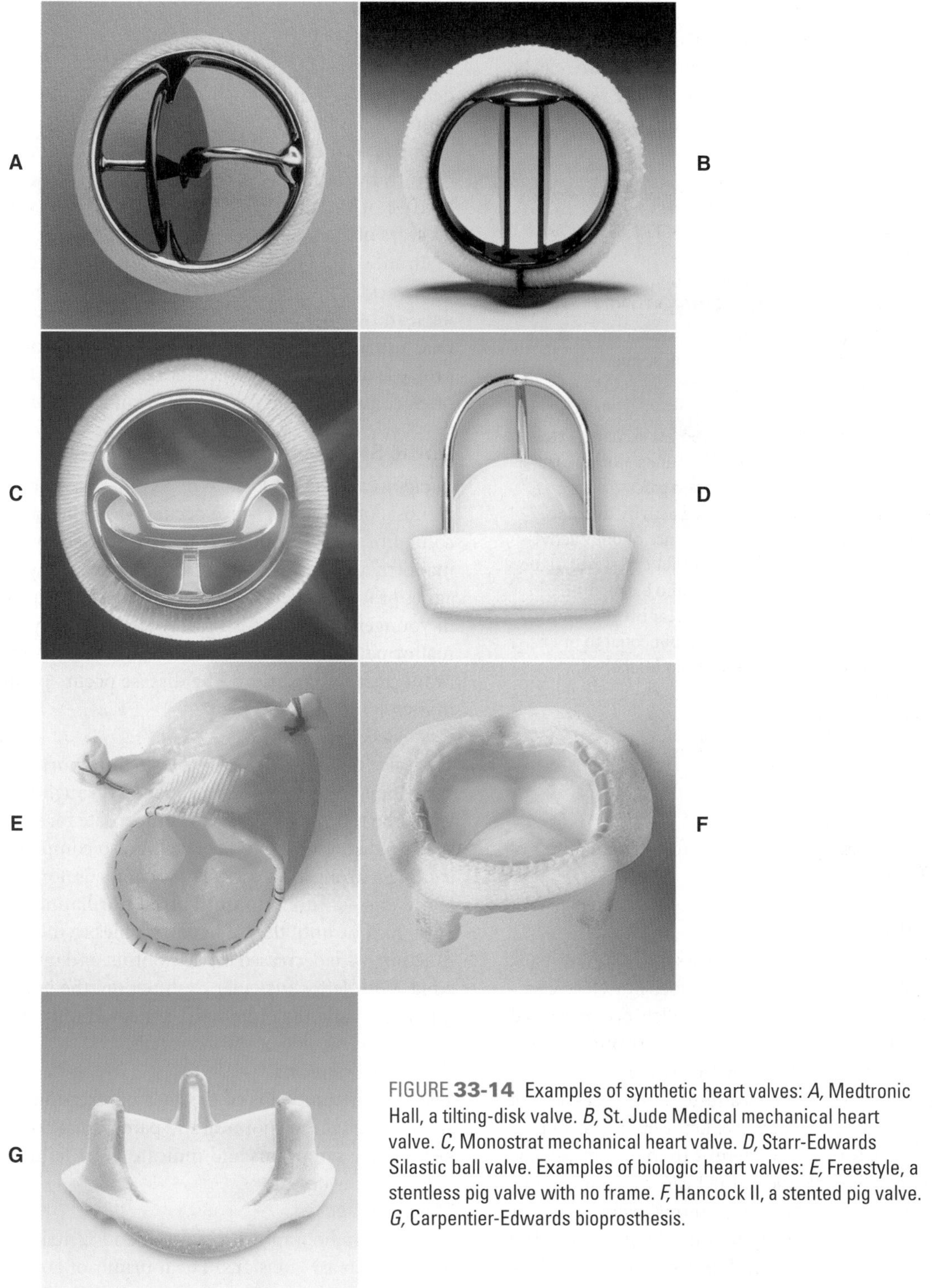

FIGURE **33-14** Examples of synthetic heart valves: *A,* Medtronic Hall, a tilting-disk valve. *B,* St. Jude Medical mechanical heart valve. *C,* Monostrat mechanical heart valve. *D,* Starr-Edwards Silastic ball valve. Examples of biologic heart valves: *E,* Freestyle, a stentless pig valve with no frame. *F,* Hancock II, a stented pig valve. *G,* Carpentier-Edwards bioprosthesis.

balloon catheter (like the one used for PTCA) is threaded from the femoral artery to the mitral valve. The balloon is positioned in the valve and inflated until the valve opens sufficiently. After the procedure, the patient is observed closely in an intensive care unit for dysrhythmias and complications. Complications include valve regurgitation, restenosis, perforation of the myocardium, and, rarely, systemic embolization.

NURSING CARE *of the Patient with Mitral Stenosis*

Assessment

It is most important to obtain a complete history as summarized in Table 33-3 and a record of signs and symptoms being experienced. Take the vital signs and auscultate for heart murmurs. The murmur of mitral stenosis is described as rumbling and low pitched. It is heard best at the apex of the heart. The

ECG may show a notched P wave, indicating left atrial enlargement. Atrial fibrillation is frequently seen. Tachycardia and tachypnea are common signs. The pulse pressure may be decreasing, indicating low cardiac output. Jugular venous distention and crackles are found with pulmonary congestion.

Nursing Diagnoses, Goals, and Outcome Criteria: Mitral Stenosis

The nursing diagnoses and goals for mitral stenosis are the same as those for CHF and for all valvular diseases:

Nursing Diagnoses	Goals and Outcome Criteria
Decreased Cardiac Output related to narrowing or insufficiency of valvular competence	Increased cardiac output: normal pulse and blood pressure
Impaired Gas Exchange related to pulmonary congestion	Improved gas exchange: clear breath sounds, normal arterial blood gases
Activity Intolerance related to imbalance between oxygen supply and demand	Improved activity tolerance: performance of daily activities without excessive fatigue
Fluid Volume Excess related to decreased glomerular filtration rate, increased aldosterone, sodium and water retention, and increased antidiuretic hormone release	Normal fluid balance: no edema, clear breath sounds, fluid output equal to or exceeds fluid intake

Interventions

See the section on nursing care for CHF for the remainder of the nursing process.

Mitral Regurgitation

Mitral regurgitation (insufficiency) allows blood to flow back into the LA during diastole. The valve does not close completely because one or both of the valve leaflets becomes rigid and shortens. Mitral regurgitation occurs more often in men when the cause is other than rheumatic disease.

The LA and LV hypertrophy as a result of the backflow of blood against the incompetent valve. Left ventricular hypertrophy is compensatory in an attempt to maintain cardiac output. Eventually, the left side of the heart fails, and symptoms are then the same as those with mitral stenosis.

The murmur of mitral regurgitation is high pitched and blowing and occurs during systole. It is best heard at the apex and may radiate to the axilla. With severe disease, S_3 and S_4 sounds may be auscultated. Atrial fibrillation occurs as the LA enlarges.

Mitral regurgitation is treated with vasodilators to decrease the afterload and therefore the regurgitation. Other medical treatment includes activity restriction, dietary sodium limitation, diuretics, and digitalis. Surgical treatment includes annuloplasty and mitral valve replacement. Annuloplasty is reconstruction of the leaflets and the annulus.

Mitral Valve Prolapse

The mitral valve prolapses when one or both leaflets enlarges and protrudes into the LA during systole. It has a tendency to run in families and may be caused by heart infections, rheumatic fever, or a wide variety of congenital anomalies. The disease is usually benign but may progress to mitral insufficiency. Mitral valve prolapse occurs in 5% to 10% of the population. Most victims are women 20 to 55 years of age.

In most patients, symptoms do not occur or may occur with stress. Symptoms include chest pain, palpitations, dizziness, and syncope. Some patients exhibit dysrhythmias. The ECG usually shows normal findings. Evidence of mitral valve prolapse may be found on echocardiography. The problem is often controlled with stress-reduction techniques.

Aortic Stenosis

Etiology and Risk Factors

Stenosis of the aortic valve occurs when the valve cusps become fibrotic and calcify. It may be caused by a congenital malformation or result from rheumatic fever, syphilis, or the aging process (atherosclerosis and calcification). When seen in younger patients, it is most often caused by a congenital malformation. The aortic valve is most commonly diseased in the aging population. The disease occurs predominantly in men.

Pathophysiology

The valve opening decreases to one-third normal size before symptoms occur. As flow is impeded through the narrowed valve, the LV hypertrophies to compensate for the extra pressure needed to eject blood. The LA also compensates by delivering a strong atrial kick. These compensatory mechanisms allow normal function until atrial fibrillation disrupts the atrial kick or until the LV hypertrophies to the point of dysfunction, with decreased cardiac output and myocardial ischemia. With left ventricular dysfunction, the blood backs up into the LA and the pulmonary system. If uncorrected, eventually the right side of the heart fails.

Signs and Symptoms

The patient complains of dyspnea on exertion, angina, and syncope. Fatigue, orthopnea, and paroxysmal nocturnal dyspnea are late symptoms and indicate heart failure. A systolic murmur may occur.

Medical Diagnosis

The chest radiograph shows atrial and ventricular enlargement, which are late signs. The murmur of aortic stenosis is heard best in the aortic area, the second intercostal space to the right of the sternum. The echocardiogram shows left ventricular wall thickening. An exercise tolerance test may be ordered to evaluate heart function.

Medical Treatment

Prophylactic antibiotics are prescribed to prevent IE with dental and invasive procedures. Heart failure is treated with digoxin, diuretics, a low-sodium diet, and activity restriction. Surgical treatment includes balloon valvuloplasty and aortic valve replacement.

NURSING CARE *of the Patient with Aortic Stenosis*

Monitor for a bounding arterial pulse and widened pulse pressure. The nursing process is the same as for CHF (see Nursing Care Plan: The Patient in Congestive Heart Failure).

AORTIC REGURGITATION

Fibrosis and thickening of the aortic cusps progress until the valve no longer maintains unidirectional blood flow. Aortic regurgitation (insufficiency) is caused primarily by rheumatic fever. Other causes include IE, blunt chest trauma, calcification of the valve, and chronic hypertension. Approximately 75% of the patients with aortic regurgitation are men. However, when both the aortic and the mitral valves are diseased, women predominate.

Regurgitation of blood into the LV during diastole increases the amount of blood in the LV. The LV dilates and hypertrophies. Myocardial ischemia and left ventricular failure occur. Blood backs up into the pulmonary system and eventually right ventricular failure occurs.

The murmur of aortic regurgitation is high pitched and blowing and occurs in diastole. It is auscultated best at the aortic area. The point of maximal impulse may be shifted to the left and down. Tachycardia and palpitations are compensatory mechanisms. Later signs of CHF such as fatigue, dyspnea, and ascites develop. A widened pulse pressure (increased difference between systolic and diastolic pressures) results from a low diastolic pressure. S_3 and S_4 sounds are often auscultated.

Left atrial and ventricular dilation are noted on chest radiography. The echocardiogram shows left ventricular dilation. Cardiac catheterization is used to determine the extent of incompetence.

As with other patients with valve disease, these patients have prophylactic antibiotics prescribed before invasive procedures. Digoxin and diuretics are prescribed for left ventricular hypertrophy. Aortic valve replacement provides long-term correction.

ELECTROCARDIOGRAM MONITORING

Nurses working in critical care areas are responsible for monitoring and interpreting ECGs. Patients usually are monitored continuously at the bedside and have intermittent monitoring through a 12-lead ECG.

12-LEAD ELECTROCARDIOGRAM

A 12-lead ECG looks at the heart from 12 directions or perspectives. This permits more precise evaluation of the heart's electrical activity. Three leads are placed on the limbs, three leads are augmented, and there are six chest, or precordial, leads. Electricity flows from the negative to the positive lead. If the depolarization wave flows toward the positive pole (electrode), the deflection is upright. If the wave flows away from the positive pole, the deflection is negative.

CONTINUOUS MONITORING

For continuous ECG monitoring, only one or two single leads are used. Three to five electrodes are applied to the chest. The electrodes are held in place by adhesive pads. Thoroughly clean the electrode sites before applying the pads. Change the pads according to agency policy. Monitor the skin for irritation or breakdown. Lead II is the most commonly monitored lead. In that lead, the P wave, QRS complex, and T wave are upright.

INTERPRETATION OF ELECTROCARDIOGRAMS

To interpret an ECG strip, the reader is referred to Figure 33-15. The graph paper consists of horizontal and vertical small and large squares. The horizontal axis measures time; the vertical axis measures voltage. Each small square represents 0.04 second on the horizontal axis and 1 mm on the vertical axis. Each large square, bounded by heavy lines, is made up of five small squares, and represents 0.20 second and 5 mm. The electrical activity of the heart is represented by deflections, positive and negative, from the baseline. A deflection is an upward or downward movement from the baseline. The baseline is called the isoelectric line. The first positive deflection (upward movement) is the small, rounded P wave that represents atrial depolarization. The second positive deflection is the peaked QRS complex that represents ventricular depolarization. The Q is the first negative deflection, meaning the line moves below the isoelectric line. The R wave corresponds to the patient's pulse. Atrial repolarization occurs during ventricular depolarization and is obscured by the QRS complex. The third deflection is the rounded T wave, which represents ventricular repolarization. The fourth deflection, if present, is the U wave. It is small, rounded, and usually indicates electrolyte imbalance (hypokalemia).

The PR interval represents the time it takes the impulse to travel from the atria through the AV node to the ventricles. The PR interval is measured from the beginning of the P wave to the Q wave. The normal PR interval is from 0.12 to 0.20 second. The QRS complex is measured from the point at which the Q leaves the isoelectric line to the point at which the S returns to the isoelectric line. The normal QRS complex is 0.06 to 0.10 second. The ST segment represents the time from ventricular depolarization to ventricular repolarization. The ST segment should be along the isoelectric line. The QT segment represents ventricular refractory time. It is measured from the beginning of the QRS complex to the end of the T wave. The normal QT segment time range is 0.36 to 0.44 second. The QT segment is affected by age, sex, and heart rate.

Criteria for Interpreting Electrocardiograms

Criteria have been established for interpreting an ECG strip. The ECG is evaluated for rate, regularity, P waves, PR interval, and QRS complexes (Table 33-10).

Rate Calculation

Most ECG strips have tic marks indicating 3-second time periods. There are several ways to calculate heart rate from the

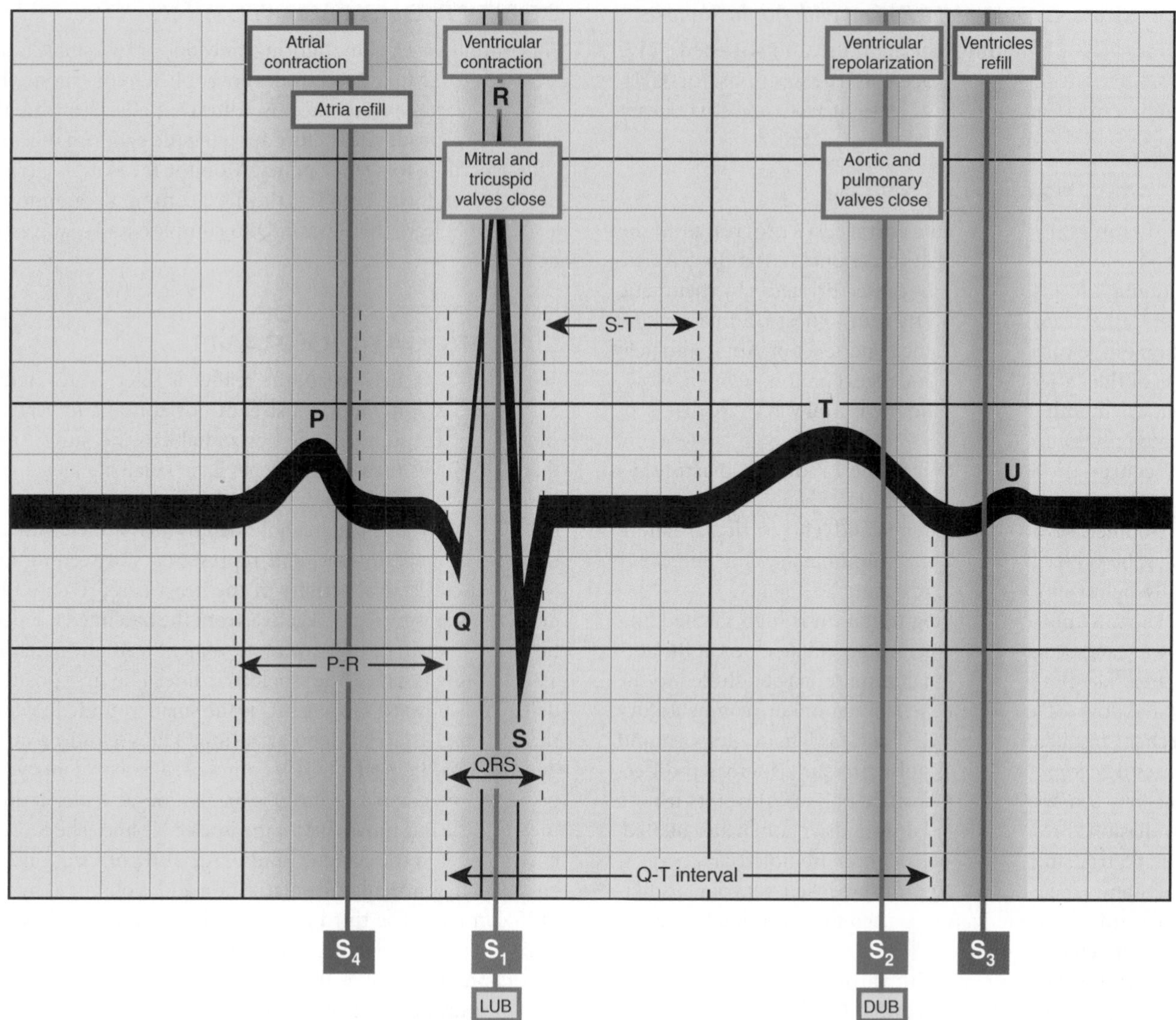

FIGURE **33-15** Relationship between the cardiac cycle and the heart sounds.

table 33-10 ***Criteria for Electrocardiogram Interpretation***

Rate	Are the atrial and ventricular rates the same as measured by the P-P and R-R intervals?
Rhythm	Is the rate regular or irregular? If irregular, is there a pattern? Are these ectopic beats? Where do they occur?
P waves	Is there a P wave before every QRS complex? Does each P wave have the same size and shape?
PR interval (PRI)	Are all the PRIs the same length? If not, is there a pattern to the irregularity? Are the PRIs within normal range?
QRS complexes	Do all the QRS complexes look alike? Are all the QRS complexes within the normal range (0.06-0.10 sec)?
T waves	Do all the T waves look alike? Are the T waves upright or inverted?

ECG strip. The quickest but least accurate method is to count the number of R waves in a 6-second strip (between 3 tic marks or 30 large squares) and multiply by 10 for the estimate of the number of beats per minute. For example, if there are six R waves in a 6-second strip, the heart rate is 60 bpm.

Another method is to find an R wave on a heavy line. Count the number of heavy lines until the next R as 300, 150, 100, 75, 60, 50, 43, and 37. For example, if there are three heavy lines between two consecutive R waves, the heart rate would be 100 bpm. A third method, the most accurate, uses the number of small squares between two R waves. Divide 1,500 by the number of small squares. For example, if there are 25 small squares between two R waves, the rate is 60 bpm (1,500 divided by 25). The atrial rate is determined by the number of P waves and the ventricular rate by the number of QRS complexes. The normal rate is from 60 to 100 bpm.

Regularity

The consecutive R-R intervals are measured for consistency. Using calipers or a blank piece of paper, note the distance between R waves. If the distances do not vary more than one

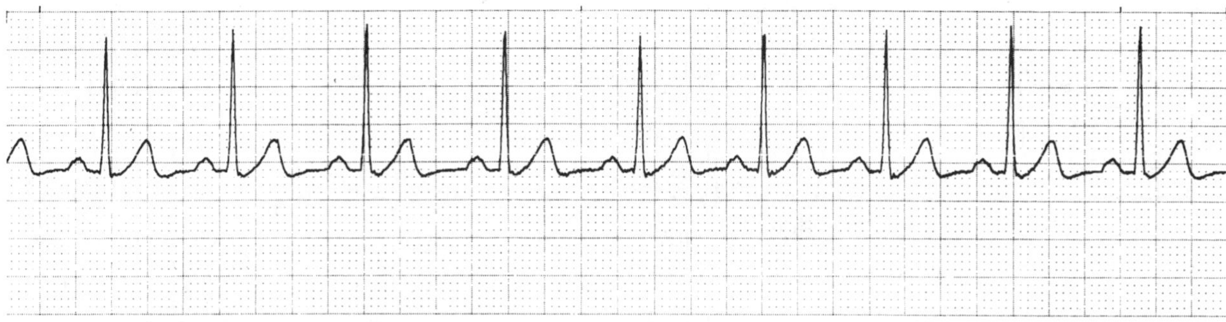

FIGURE **33-16** **Normal sinus rhythm.** Each segment between the dark lines (above the monitor strip) represents 3 seconds, when the monitor is set at a speed of 25 mm/sec. *Characteristics:* **Rate**—60 to 100 bpm; **Regularity**—essentially regular (P-to-P and R-to-R intervals are regular with only minor variation); **P wave, PR interval**—there is a P before every QRS; each P wave is the same size and shape; PR interval is between 0.12 and 0.20 sec; **QRS**—falls between 0.06 and 0.10 sec; **T wave**—rounded, all the same shape. *Interpretation:* Normal sinus rhythm.

small square, the rhythm is considered regular. If the distances are greater than one small square, the rhythm is irregular.

P Waves

The next evaluation is of P waves. Is there a P wave before each QRS complex? If so, the rhythm originates in the SA node. Do all the P waves appear the same size and shape? If so, the impulse originates in the SA node.

PR Interval

Does the PR interval fall within the normal range of 0.12 to 0.20 second? If so, there is no interference in conduction from the SA to the AV node.

QRS Complex

Does the QRS complex fall within the 0.06- to 0.10-second range? If the QRS is prolonged (0.12 second or greater), there is a delay in conduction through the ventricles.

T Waves

Are the T waves rounded and the same size and shape? Do the T waves follow the QRS complexes?

Normal Sinus Rhythm

The most common cardiac rhythm is sinus in origin because the impulse originates in the SA node, is conducted normally, and meets all of the criteria established earlier. Normal sinus rhythm is displayed in Figure 33-16.

Common Dysrhythmias

A dysrhythmia is a disturbance of the rhythm of the heart caused by a problem in the conduction system. Dysrhythmias are categorized according to the site of the origin of the impulse formation. Dysrhythmias originating in the atria are called atrial dysrhythmias. Dysrhythmias originating in the AV node are called junctional or escape rhythms. Dysrhythmias originating below the AV node are called ventricular. Blocks are interruptions in impulse conduction. Dysrhythmias and blocks have characteristics that are noted on the ECG. See Figures 33-17 through 33-30 for examples. Antidysrhythmic drugs are used to treat dysrhythmias and restore normal sinus rhythm.

HEMODYNAMIC MONITORING

In addition to noninvasive cardiac assessment and ECG monitoring, more sophisticated measures may be needed to determine what is going on within the heart itself. Nurses who work in intensive care areas frequently work with patients who have central venous catheters, pulmonary artery catheters, or arterial lines.

CENTRAL VENOUS CATHETER

The central venous catheter is placed through the skin, into a venous access (brachial, femoral, subclavian, or jugular sites), and threaded into the RA. The catheter may have one to three lumens. With this catheter, the pressure in the RA (called right atrial pressure [RAP] or central venous pressure [CVP]) can be measured. This measurement is used as an indication of fluid volume. The normal CVP or RAP is 2 to 6 mm Hg. Measurements below normal indicate hypovolemia, and measurements above normal indicate hypervolemia. This catheter may also be used to infuse fluids, blood and blood products, and medications as well as to withdraw blood for analysis.

PULMONARY ARTERY CATHETER

The pulmonary artery catheter, frequently called a Swan-Ganz catheter, is longer than the central venous catheter. It is inserted like the central venous catheter and is threaded through the RA, the tricuspid valve, the RV, the pulmonic valve, and into the pulmonary artery. The catheter is balloon tipped and flows with the blood. Different waveforms are seen on an oscilloscope as the catheter moves through the different areas of the heart. Pulmonary artery catheters have multiple lumens and are approximately 110 cm (44 inches) long. Various lumens are used to measure the pulmonary capillary wedge pressure, inflate the balloon, measure RAP, determine cardiac output, and administer fluids and drugs. Newer catheters incorporate fiberoptics for continuous monitoring of saturated venous oxygenation (SVO_2), a measure of tissue perfusion.

Text continued on p. 607

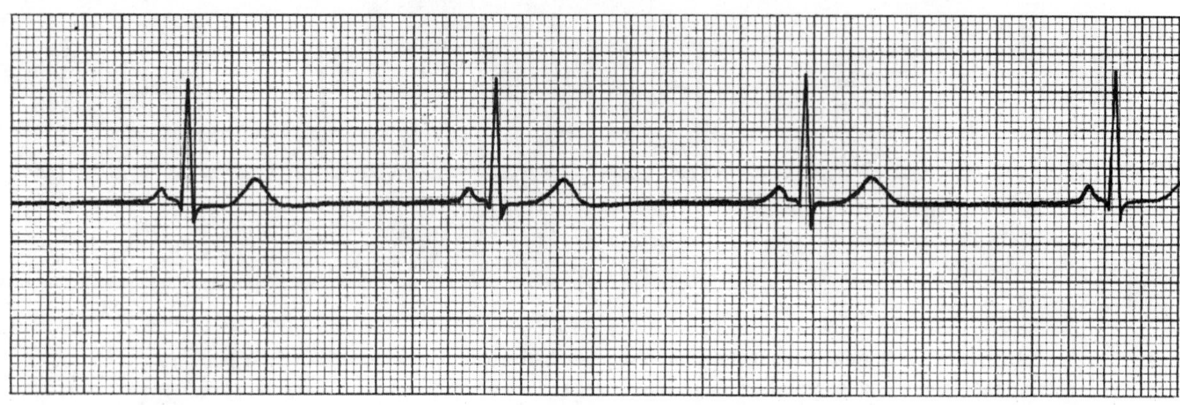

FIGURE **33-17** **Sinus bradycardia.** *Characteristics:* **Rate**—less than 60 bpm; **Regularity**—normal; **P wave, PR interval**—normal; **QRS**—normal; **T wave**—normal. *Interpretation:* All characteristics are within normal ranges except for the rate, which is slow. Causes: Drugs, including digitalis and beta blockers, vagal stimulation (Valsalva maneuver), severe pain, hyperkalemia, infection, and myocardial infarction. Frequently seen in athletes as a result of conditioning. Symptoms: Dizziness, syncope, chest pain, hypotension, sweating, nausea, dyspnea, and disorientation; sometimes no symptoms. Treatment: Not treated unless the patient is symptomatic. The underlying cause is treated. Atropine may be given to increase the heart rate. Isoproterenol is used with extreme caution. A pacemaker may be needed.

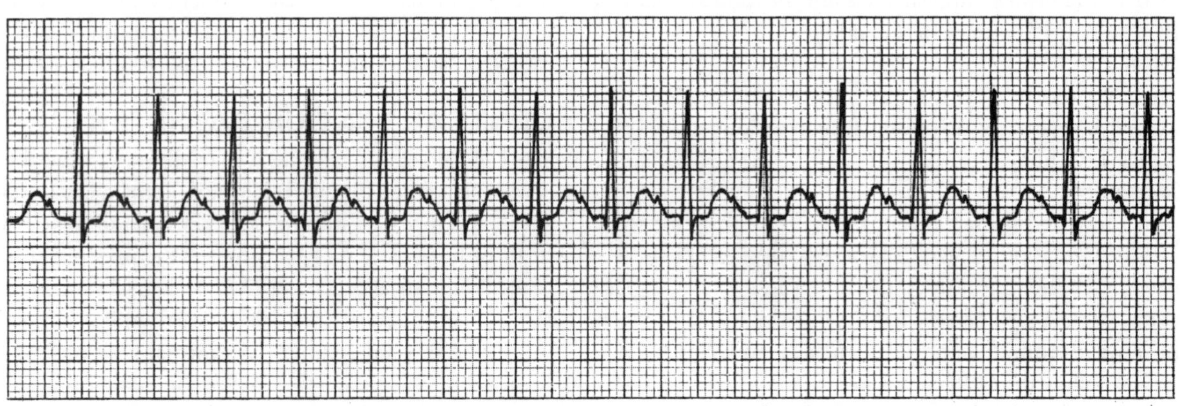

FIGURE **33-18** **Sinus tachycardia.** *Characteristics:* **Rate**—greater than 100; usually less than 150 bpm; **Regularity**—regular; **P wave, PR interval**—P waves may be buried in T wave of preceding beat with very rapid rates, more than 140 bpm; **QRS**—normal; **T wave**—normal. *Interpretation:* All characteristics are within normal range except for the rate, which is excessive. Causes: Fever, dehydration, hypovolemia, increased sympathetic nervous system stimulation, stress, exercise, and acute myocardial infarction. Symptoms: Palpitations most common. Angina and decreased cardiac output from the decreased ventricular filling time may also occur. Treatment: Correction of underlying cause. Elimination of caffeine, nicotine, and alcohol. Vagal stimulation may decrease the rate but does not treat the cause. Beta blockers.

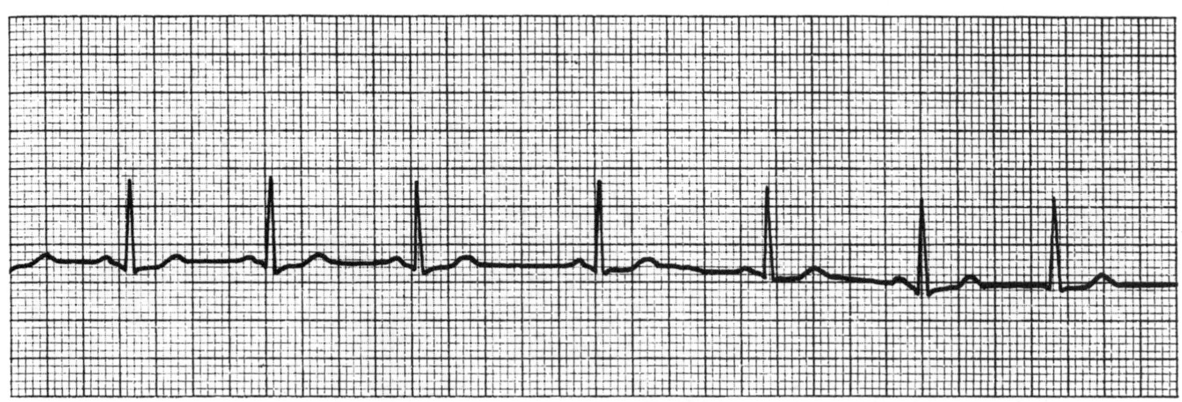

FIGURE **33-19** **Sinus dysrhythmia.** *Characteristics:* **Rate**—normal; **Regularity**—slightly irregular, varies with respirations; **P wave, PR interval**—P-to-P intervals vary, the difference between the shortest and longest P-to-P interval is greater than 0.12 sec; the PR interval is normal; **QRS**—normal; **T wave**—normal. *Interpretation:* The rate varies with respirations. Considered normal when the rhythm varies in relation to the respiratory cycle: The R-to-R interval is shorter during inspiration; therefore the rate is increased; the R-to-R interval is longer during expiration; therefore the rate is decreased. Causes: When unrelated to respirations, is often the result of digoxin toxicity, increased intracranial pressure, or inferior wall myocardial infarction. In the elderly, marked variation may indicate a condition known as sick sinus syndrome. Symptoms: Usually none. Treatment: If treatment is necessary, atropine is used and the underlying problem is treated.

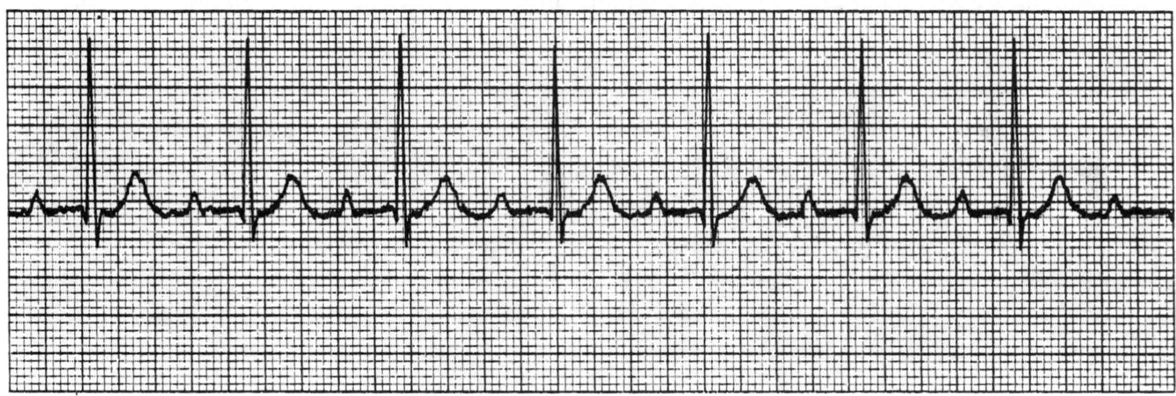

FIGURE **33-20** **First-degree atrioventricular (AV) block.** *Characteristics:* **Rate**—normal; **Regularity**—regular; **P wave, PR interval**—all P waves are conducted to the ventricles, but AV conduction is prolonged through the AV node; PR interval is greater than 0.20 sec and constant; **QRS**—normal; **T wave**—normal. *Interpretation:* The PR interval is prolonged. Causes: Increased vagal tone, coronary artery disease, digoxin toxicity, heart infections, and quinidine. Symptoms: Usually none, may be bradycardic. Treatment: Correction of underlying cause.

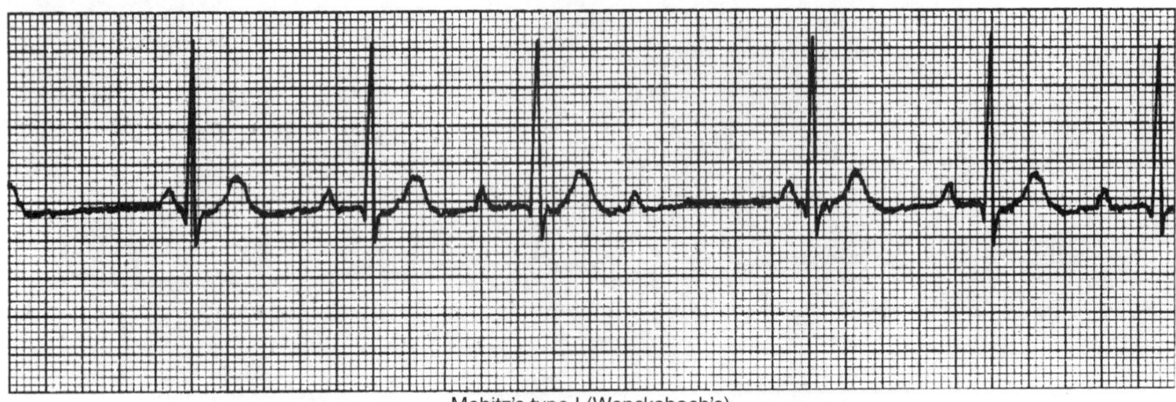

FIGURE **33-21** **Second-degree atrioventricular block: type I (Mobitz I; Wenckebach).** *Characteristics:* **Rate**—atrial rate is greater than ventricular rate; **Regularity**—atrial rate is regular; ventricular rate is irregular; **P wave, PR interval**—there are more P waves than QRS complexes; the PR interval increases until a P wave is not followed by a QRS; **QRS**—some are absent; **T wave**—absent when the QRS is dropped. *Interpretation:* Progressively lengthening PR interval and a dropped beat. Causes: Myocardial ischemia with progressive increase in conduction time through the sinoatrial node, inferior wall myocardial infarction, digoxin toxicity, and electrolyte imbalance. Symptoms: Decreased blood pressure and syncope, if any. Treatment: Atropine, pacemaker.

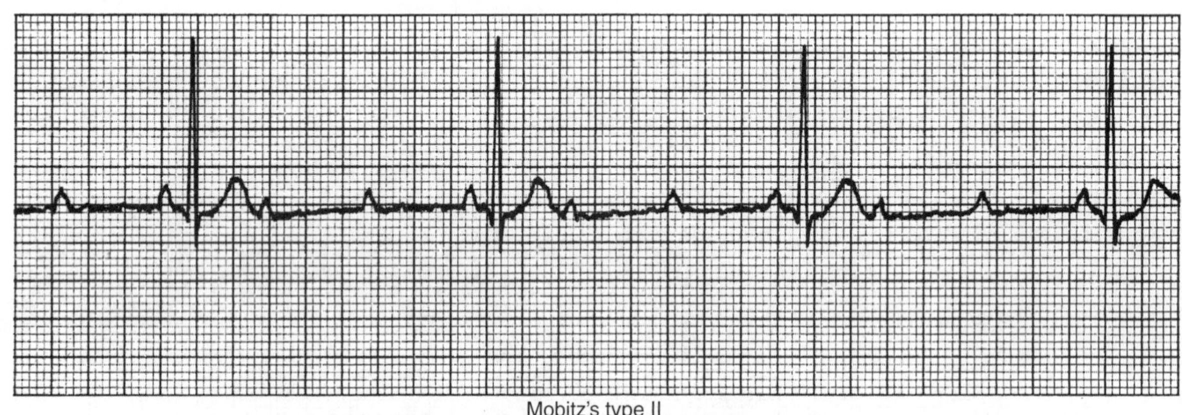

FIGURE **33-22** **Second-degree atrioventricular (AV) block: type II (Mobitz II).** *Characteristics:* **Rate**—atrial rate regular; ventricular rate may be less than atrial; **Regularity**—irregular; **P wave, PR interval**—P-to-P intervals are regular; PR interval is fixed at normal or greater than 0.2 sec; **QRS**—QRS complexes do not always follow P waves; the QRS may be normal or widened; **T wave**—normal after completed conduction. *Interpretation:* Sudden blocking of a QRS. Causes: Conduction abnormalities in the ventricles, acute myocardial infarction. Symptoms: Hypotension, bradycardia; decreased cardiac output with frequent blocks. Treatment: Pacemaker may be necessary to prevent third-degree AV block or asystole.

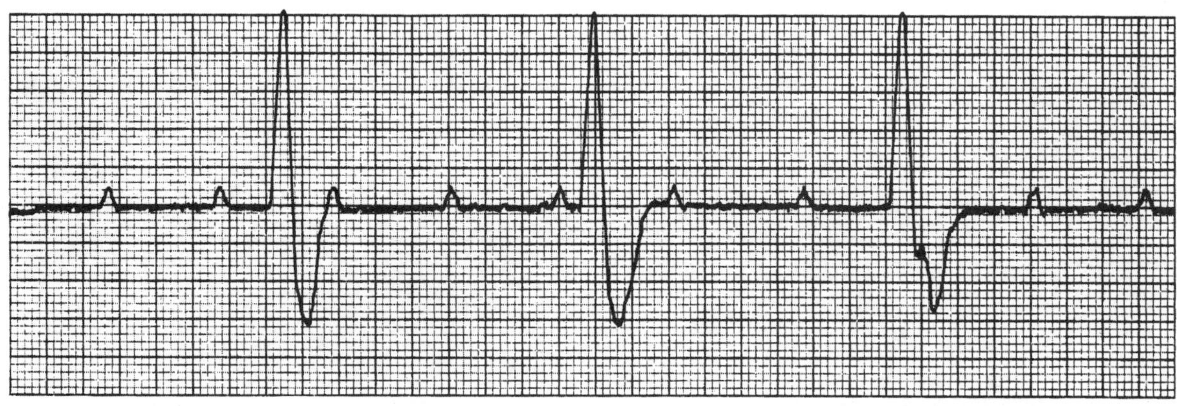

FIGURE **33-23** **Third-degree atrioventricular (AV) block.** *Characteristics:* **Rate**—atrial rate is faster than ventricular rate; ventricular rate is generally less than 45 bpm; **Regularity**—irregular; **P wave, PR interval**—no relationship exists between the P waves and the QRS complexes; **QRS**—atria and ventricles are beating independently; the QRS is ventricular in origin; **T wave**—normal. *Interpretation:* Impulses originating in the sinoatrial node are blocked at the AV node. The ventricles respond to a secondary pacemaker. Causes: Digoxin toxicity, conduction damage during mitral valve replacement, hypoxia, and rheumatic fever. Symptoms: Hypotension, syncope, decreased cardiac output. The underlying cause is treated. Treatment: Atropine, pacemaker, isoproterenol with extreme caution. *Do not* administer lidocaine, which could suppress ventricular response.

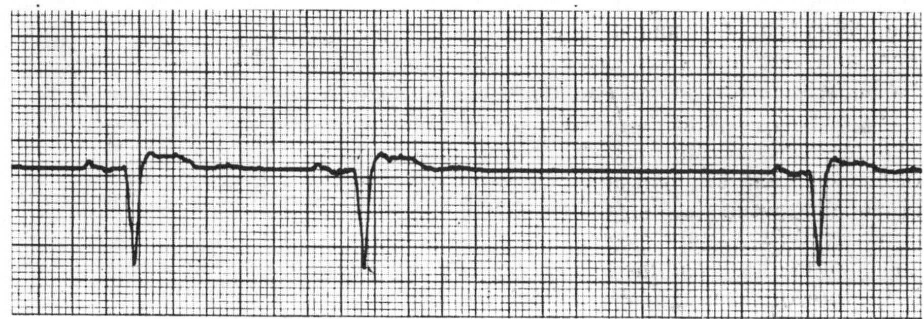

FIGURE **33-24** **Sinus arrest.** *Characteristics:* **Rate**—normal or slow before arrest; **Regularity**—regular except when interrupted by a dropped beat; **P wave, PR interval**—normal when present; absent during pause; **QRS**—normal to absent during pause; **T wave**—normal to absent during pause. *Interpretation:* A pause in the cardiac cycle as the sinoatrial node fails to generate an impulse. Causes: Degenerative heart disease, myocardial infarction, digoxin toxicity. Symptoms: Bradycardia, decreased cardiac output. Treatment: Pacemaker if the patient experiences repeated episodes.

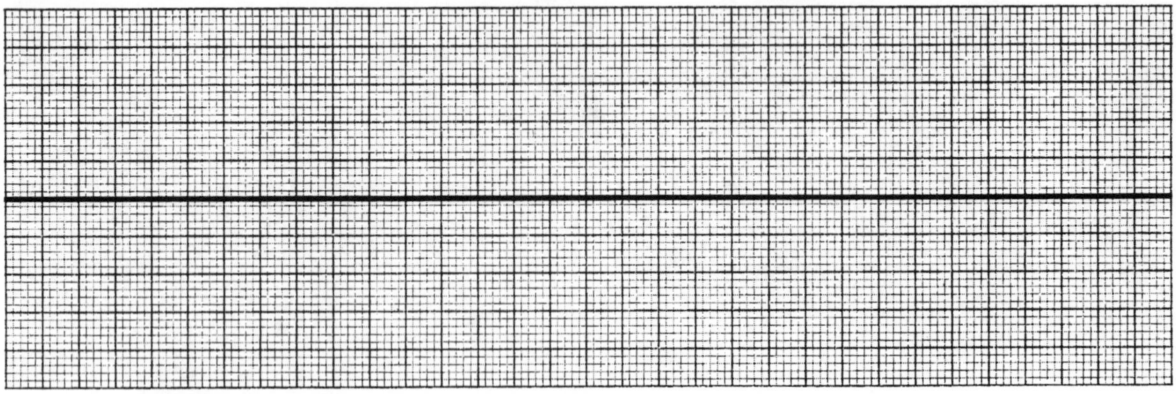

FIGURE **33-25** **Asystole.** *Characteristics:* **Rate**—none; **Regularity**—none; **P wave, PR interval**—there may be P waves but none is conducted; the PR interval is not measurable; **QRS**—absent; **T wave**—absent. *Interpretation:* Straight or only slightly wavy baseline. Causes: Severe metabolic deficit, acute respiratory failure, and myocardial damage. Symptoms: Loss of consciousness, no pulse. Treatment: Immediate response with cardiopulmonary resuscitation and advanced cardiac life support; epinephrine, atropine; transcutaneous pacemaker.

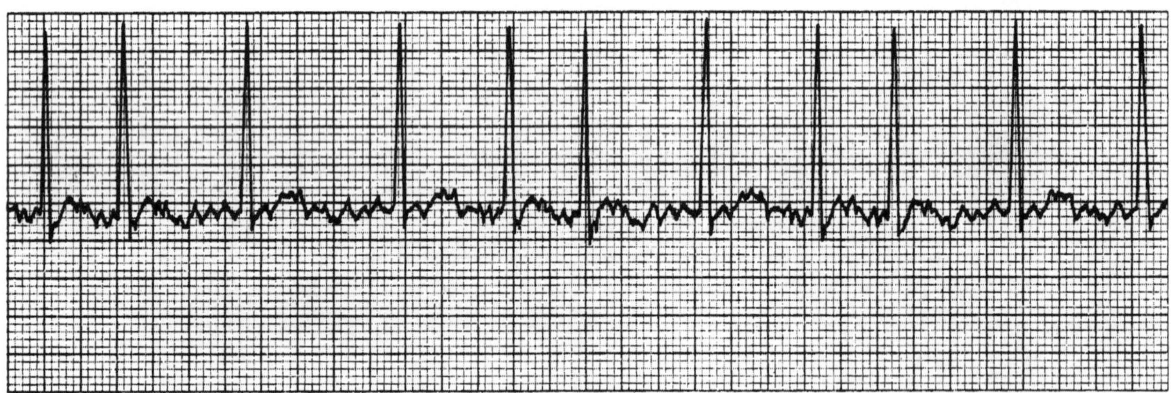

FIGURE **33-26** **Atrial fibrillation.** *Characteristics:* **Rate**—atrial rate is greater than 400 bpm if it can be determined at all; the ventricular rate is 100 to 150 bpm; **Regularity**—very irregular; **P wave, PR interval**—no P waves; PR interval unmeasurable; **QRS**—normal; **T wave**—undeterminable. *Interpretation:* The baseline between QRS complexes is wavy. Causes: Rheumatic fever, mitral valve stenosis, coronary artery disease, hypertension, cardiomyopathy, myocardial infarction, hyperthyroidism, chronic obstructive pulmonary disease, and congestive heart failure. It is frequently seen in the elderly after the administration of anesthesia. Symptoms: May have palpitations, angina, and decreased cardiac output. The concerns with atrial fibrillation are development of an atrial thrombus and loss of atrial kick from ineffective atrial function. Treatment: calcium channel blockers or beta blockers to reduce a rapid ventricular response; anticoagulants to prevent embolization; synchronized cardioversion or drug therapy (amiodarone or ibutilide) to restore a normal rhythm.

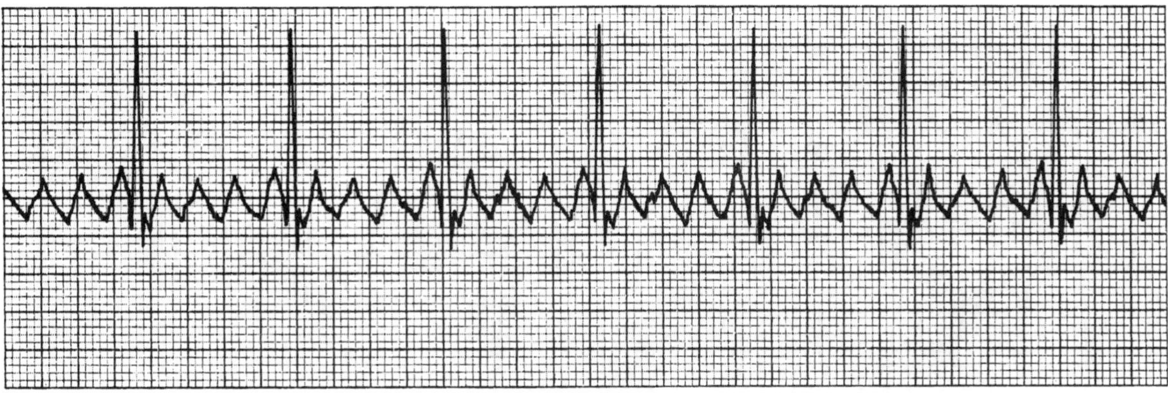

FIGURE **33-27** **Atrial flutter.** *Characteristics:* **Rate**—atrial rate 250 to 350 bpm; ventricular rate 60 to 100 bpm; **Regularity**—atrial rate regular; ventricular regular or irregular; **P wave, PR interval**—P waves are rounded "F" or flutter waves; PR interval unmeasurable; **QRS**—usually normal; **T wave**—undeterminable. *Interpretation:* The sawtooth P waves are characteristic; there may be a pattern to the number of flutter waves and ventricular response: 4 to 1, 3 to 1, or 2 to 1. Causes: Coronary artery disease, myocardial damage, valvular disease, heart infections, and digoxin toxicity. Symptoms: Palpitations, decreased cardiac output. Treatment: Harder to treat than atrial fibrillation. Calcium channel blockers or beta blockers to control the rate. Synchronized cardioversion or drug therapy (amiodarone or ibutilide) to convert the rhythm.

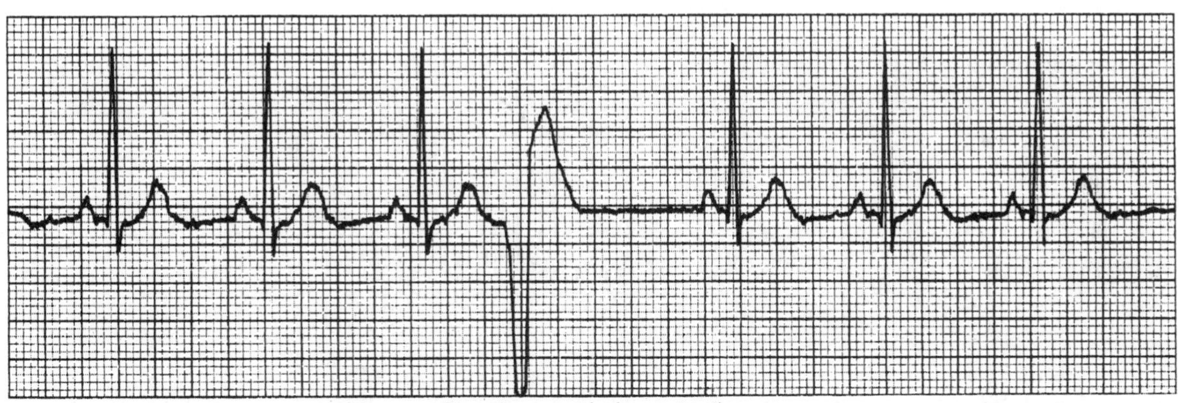

FIGURE **33-28** **Premature ventricular contractions (PVCs).** *Characteristics:* **Rate**—normal; **Regularity**—irregular because of PVCs; **P wave, PR interval**—no P wave with the PVC; inverted P wave may follow a PVC; there is no PR interval with the PVC; **QRS**—wide and bizarre in the PVC; **T wave**—opposite deflection to the PVC. *Interpretations:* Wide QRS. Unifocal PVCs originate from one site. Multifocal PVCs arise from different ventricular sites and have a poorer prognosis. Causes: Digoxin toxicity, hypokalemia, hypercalcemia, sympathetic nervous system stimulation (stress, caffeine, nicotine), and excess catecholamine release. Symptoms: The patient may or may not note a "skipped" beat. The PVCs are not palpable at peripheral pulse sites, but a pause may be observed. Cardiac output diminishes with frequent PVCs. Treatment: No treatment necessary for infrequent PVCs, which probably occur undetected in most people; treat the cause and administer antidysrhythmics for symptomatic or frequent PVCs.

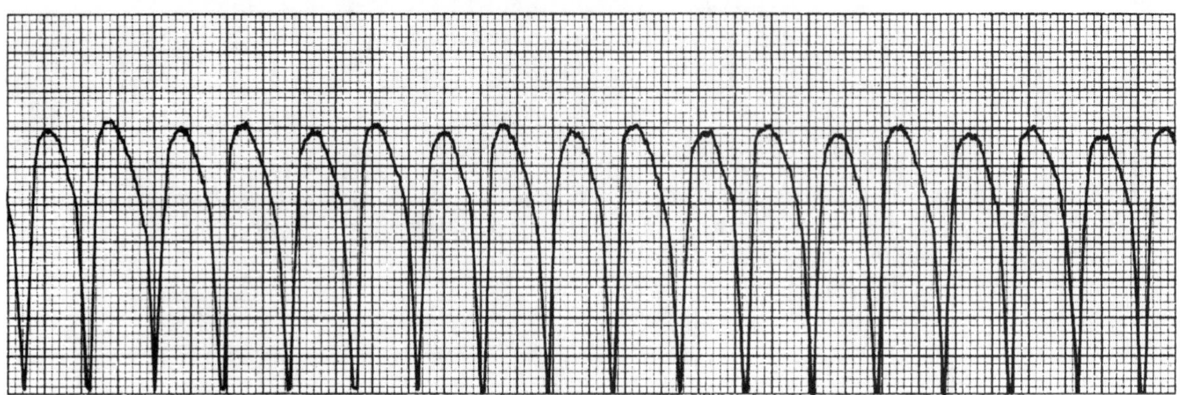

FIGURE 33-29 **Ventricular tachycardia.** *Characteristics:* **Rate**—100 to 250 bpm; there is no relationship between the atrial and the ventricular contractions; **Regularity**—ventricular rhythm usually regular; **P wave, PR interval** —absent; **QRS**—wide, bizarre; greater than 0.12 second; may look like PVCs; **T wave**—opposite deflection to QRS. *Interpretation:* This is a life-threatening dysrhythmia that often precedes ventricular fibrillation. Causes: Myocardial irritation, myocardial infarction, coronary artery disease, rheumatic heart disease, hypokalemia, and digoxin toxicity. Symptoms: Initially palpitations, dizziness, and chest pain progressing to decreased cardiac output and loss of consciousness. Treatment: Assess for pulse, signs and symptoms. If ventricular tachycardia without pulse, defibrillate up to three times and follow advanced cardiac life support algorithm. With pulse but unstable: Synchronized cardioversion. If stable, with pulse: Lidocaine, procainamide, bretylium; then synchronized cardioversion.

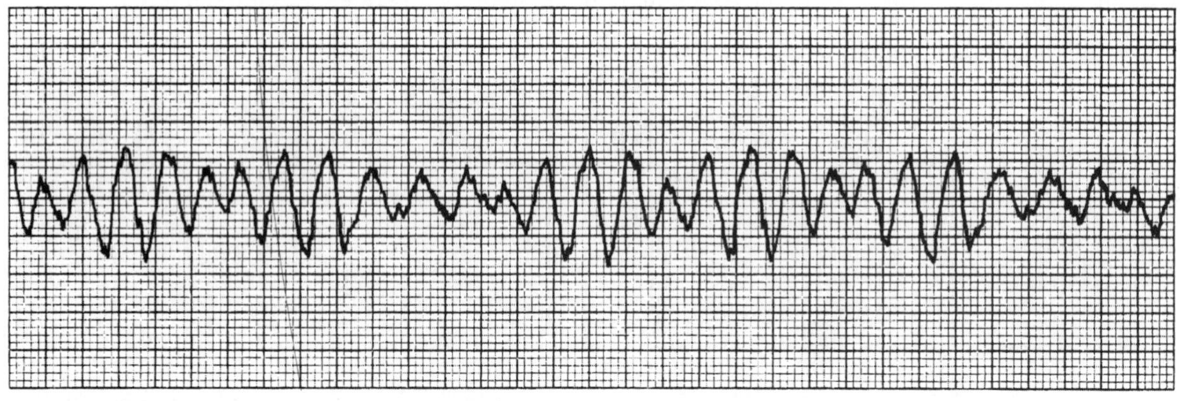

FIGURE 33-30 **Ventricular fibrillation.** *Characteristics:* **Rate**—undeterminable; **Regularity**—chaotic, wavy baseline; **P wave, PR interval**—undeterminable; **QRS**—undeterminable; **T wave**—undeterminable. *Interpretation:* This life-threatening dysrhythmia must be terminated quickly if the patient is to resume useful function. Causes: Coronary artery disease, acute myocardial infarction, untreated ventricular tachycardia, electrolyte and acid-base imbalances, electric shock, and hypothermia. Symptoms: Loss of consciousness, cessation of heartbeat and respirations, dilation of pupils. Treatment: Cardiopulmonary resuscitation, defibrillation, and advanced cardiac life support measures are used to treat ventricular fibrillation.

The purpose of a pulmonary artery catheter is to measure right-sided heart pressures and pulmonary artery pressures and to assess left-sided heart function. The proximal port is used to measure the RAP or CVP (normal value, 2 to 6 mm Hg). The distal port measures the pulmonary artery pressure (normal value, 20 to 30/0 to 10). The lungs are low-pressure organs unless the patient has COPD.

The pulmonary capillary wedge pressure is used to assess the function of the left side of the heart. To determine the pulmonary capillary wedge pressure, the balloon is inflated with up to 1.5 ml of air. This allows the tip of the catheter to float into a pulmonary capillary until it occludes the capillary. This measures the pressure ahead of the catheter; therefore the left ventricular heart function. The normal pulmonary capillary wedge pressure is 4 to 12 mm Hg. Once the pressure is recorded, the balloon is deflated. This pressure is lower when fluid is restricted, when diuretics are being administered, and when patients are receiving vasodilators such as nitroglycerin or morphine. The pressure is elevated with excess fluid, when fluid volume expanders such as albumin, dextran, or hetastarch are being administered or in left heart dysfunction.

Cardiac Output

With a pulmonary artery catheter in place, cardiac output can be measured continuously or by the thermodilution method. The normal cardiac output is 4 to 8 L/min. Stress increases the cardiac output. Cardiac output may decrease with AMI, CHF, bradycardia, tachycardia, and some drugs. It is important for the nurse to use consistent technique in measuring cardiac output.

ARTERIAL LINE

An arterial line may be inserted (most often in the radial artery) to provide a direct measurement of systolic and diastolic blood pressures. Once the line is inserted, it is connected to a pressurized solution to keep the catheter patent and to a transducer to assess pressure. The mean arterial pressure is an indication of tissue perfusion. This pressure is elevated with sympathetic stimulation and increased heart rate.

Nutrition Concepts

1. A major part of treatment for people with heart disease is reduction of fat and cholesterol in the diet.
2. When fats are used in cooking or eating, unsaturated fats (vegetable oil such as corn oil, canola oil, or olive oil) should be substituted for saturated fats (animal fat such as butter or lard).
3. Fats and oils used in cooking or eating should be limited to five to eight servings daily in normal adults.
4. Saturated fat can be limited by eating only 5 to 7 ounces of meat daily.
5. Foods that contain omega-3 fatty acids (certain fish, walnuts, and soybeans) lower serum triglycerides and decrease the number of deaths resulting from heart disease.

key points

- The primary function of the heart is to pump blood through the pulmonary and systemic circulation.
- The heartbeat has two phases: systole (contraction) and diastole (relaxation).
- Cardiac output is the amount of blood ejected per minute by each ventricle; stroke volume is the amount of blood ejected by a ventricle in a single contraction.The factors that affect stroke volume are preload, contractility, and afterload.
- The heart sounds are "lub," heard during systole, and "dub," heard during diastole.
- The most common cardiac surgical procedures are pacemaker insertion, valve repair or replacement, septal repair, and coronary artery bypass surgery.
- Nursing concerns after cardiac surgery include ineffective breathing patterns, pain, ineffective thermoregulation, decreased cardiac output, risk for infection, and anxiety.
- Pacemakers are electronic devices that deliver impulses to stimulate contraction of the myocardium.
- Coronary artery disease is treated with drug therapy, diet modifications, lifestyle modifications, surgical intervention, or a combination of these.
- Risk factors for atherosclerosis are age, gender, genetic predisposition, diabetes mellitus with elevated blood glucose, decreased serum high-density lipoproteins, nicotine, hypertension, obesity, sedentary lifestyle, and stress.
- Angina pectoris is the pain that results from myocardial ischemia. It is treated with vasodilators and rest.
- Procedures used to improve myocardial blood flow include percutaneous coronary balloon angioplasty, laser angioplasty, atherectomy, stent placement, coronary artery bypass grafts, and transmyocardial laser revascularization.
- Acute myocardial infarction, caused by occlusion of a coronary artery, can lead to dysrhythmias, cardiac failure, cardiogenic shock, thromboembolism, and ventricular rupture.
- Nursing care of the patient with myocardial infarction addresses anxiety, pain, and decreased cardiac output.
- Patients with acute cardiac conditions often have continuous cardiac monitoring to detect potentially fatal dysrhythmias for prompt treatment.
- Cardiac rehabilitation begins with a cardiac incident, lasts throughout life, and includes the patient and family in teaching about exercise, diet, and medications.
- Congestive heart failure, the inability of the heart to meet the metabolic demands of the body, may be caused by disorders that increase the heart's workload or interfere with its pumping action.
- The cornerstone of treatment of congestive heart failure is cardiotonic glycosides, also called inotropic agents, which increase the pumping effectiveness of the heart.
- Treatment of congestive heart failure may include correction of underlying causes, drug therapy to improve cardiac function and eliminate excess fluid, and measures to decrease demands on the heart.
- Complications of congestive heart failure are dysrhythmias, cardiac failure, and ventricular aneurysms and rupture.

- Nursing care of the patient with congestive heart failure focuses on fluid volume excess, impaired gas exchange, anxiety, decreased cardiac output, and activity intolerance.
- Cardiac inflammatory conditions (endocarditis, myocarditis, and pericarditis) are treated with drug therapy and rest.
- Cardiomyopathy is a disease of the heart muscle that is treated with supportive measures but may lead to cardiac failure that eventually requires cardiac transplantation.
- Patients who have received heart transplants require immunosuppressive drugs for the remainder of their lives to prevent rejection of the foreign tissue.
- Signs and symptoms of cardiac transplant rejection are fever, dyspnea, fatigue, and dysrhythmias.
- Sudden cardiac death, the abrupt cessation of heart activity and respirations, is fatal in 80% of all cases.
- An implantable cardioverter/defibrillator is an implanted device that monitors cardiac activity, detects life-threatening dysrhythmias, and delivers a shock to convert the rhythm to a normal one.
- The primary disorders of the heart valves are stenosis, which interferes with blood movement from one chamber to the next, and regurgitation, which allows blood to flow backward.
- Valve disease may be treated with drug therapy to improve cardiac function, with balloon valvuloplasty to dilate stenosed valves, with commissurotomy to enlarge the opening, and with valve replacement using a biologic or synthetic valve.
- General measures to maintain perfusion of vital organs are modified Trendelenburg's position, oxygen, intravenous fluids, and drugs to maintain or restore blood pressure.
- A dysrhythmia (also called an arrhythmia) is a disturbance of the heart rhythm caused by a problem in the conduction system.

REVIEW QUESTIONS

1. Normally, the impulse that stimulates a myocardial contraction begins in the:
   1. AV node.
   2. bundle of His.
   3. Purkinje cells.
   4. SA node.
2. Which statement correctly describes one of the three factors that affects stroke volume?
   1. Contractility is the ability of cardiac muscle fibers to shorten and produce a muscle contraction.
   2. Preload is the amount of blood remaining in the atria at the end of diastole.
   3. Cardiac output is the amount of blood ejected by the heart with each ventricular contraction.
   4. Afterload is the amount of blood remaining in the ventricles at the end of systole.
3. Which of the following age-related changes in the circulatory system can cause heart murmurs?
   1. Decreased elasticity of connective tissue in the heart muscle
   2. Arterial stiffening caused by changes in connective tissue and elastic fibers
   3. Heart valves that are stiff and do not close properly
   4. Stretching and dilation of veins resulting in impaired venous return
4. Before administering digoxin, you count a patient's apical heart rate and find that it is 62 bpm. The patient's usual rate ranges from 65-75 bpm. What should you do?
   1. Withhold the digoxin and notify the physician.
   2. Administer the digoxin and document the heart rate.
   3. Hold the drug and recheck the heart rate in an hour.
   4. Give half of the prescribed dose of digoxin.
5. An adverse effect common to all antidysrhythmic drugs is:
   1. fluid and electrolyte imbalance.
   2. drowsiness.
   3. diarrhea.
   4. additional dysrhythmias.
6. The usual dietary recommendations for cardiac patients include:
   1. no more than 10% saturated fats.
   2. low fiber and carbohydrates.
   3. sodium restricted to 1 g/day.
   4. 20% or less of total fat intake.
7. Risk factors for atherosclerosis that can be modified include:
   1. gender.
   2. race.
   3. genetic predisposition.
   4. sedentary lifestyle.

8. Characteristics of angina pectoris include that it:
   1. most often occurs at rest.
   2. is accompanied by drop in blood pressure.
   3. is usually substernal but may radiate.
   4. is commonly treated with digitalis.

9. Which of the following drugs may be administered after acute myocardial infarction to dissolve thrombi?
   1. Heparin
   2. Tissue plasminogen activator
   3. Aspirin
   4. Lidocaine

10. When cardiac output falls, compensatory mechanisms include:
    1. elimination of excess fluid by the kidneys.
    2. dilation of blood vessels in the extremities.
    3. stimulation of the parasympathetic nervous system.
    4. enlargement of the ventricular myocardium.

11. Discharge teaching for a patient with congestive heart failure should include instructions to:
    1. immediately begin a vigorous program of exercise.
    2. inform the physician if you gain more than 2 pounds in a week.
    3. weigh yourself before going to bed each night.
    4. expect to continue having shortness of breath, chest pain, and cough.

12. Before invasive procedures including dental work, patients with valvular heart disease usually are prescribed antibiotics to prevent:
    1. pericarditis.
    2. abscess formation.
    3. infective endocarditis.
    4. cardiomyopathy.

13. A patient who has had heart transplantation comes into the doctor's office complaining of fever, fatigue, shortness of breath, and an irregular heart beat. You should suspect:
    1. infection in the surgical wound.
    2. congestive heart failure.
    3. rejection of the transplanted heart.
    4. postoperative anxiety and depression.

14. Which of the following findings would you expect in a patient with mitral stenosis?
    1. Increased left atrial pressure
    2. Decreased pulmonary pressure
    3. Increased cardiac output
    4. Decreased right ventricular pressure

CHAPTER

34 Vascular Disorders

objectives

1. Identify specific anatomic and physiologic factors that affect the vascular system and tissue oxygenation.
2. Indicate appropriate parameters for assessing a patient with peripheral vascular disease, aneurysm, and aortic dissection.
3. Discuss tests and procedures used to diagnose selected vascular disorders and the nursing considerations for each.
4. State the pathophysiology, signs and symptoms, complications, and medical or surgical treatments for selected vascular disorders.
5. Assist in developing a plan of care for patients with selected vascular disorders.

key terms

Aneurysm (ĂN-ū-rĭzm, p. 610)
Bruit (BRŪ-ē, p. 615)
Embolism (ĔM-bō-lĭzm, p. 620)
Hemoconcentration (p. 613)
Ischemia (ĭs-KĒ-mē-ă, p. 613)
Paresthesia (păr-ĕs-THĒ-zē-ă, p. 613)
Phlebitis (flĕ-BĪ-tĭs, p. 632)
Phlebothrombosis (flĕb-ō-thrŏm-BŌ-sĭs, p. 632)
Poikilothermy (poi-kĕ-lō-THĔR-mē, p. 613)
Thrombophlebitis (thrŏm-bō-flĕ-BĪ-tĭs, p. 632)
Thrombosis (thrŏm-BŌ-sĭs, p. 610)
Vasoconstriction (văz-ō-kŏn-STRĬK-shŭn, p. 612)
Viscosity (vĭs-KŎS-ĭ-tē, p. 612)

The delivery of oxygen and nutrients to the tissues is dependent on adequate perfusion (blood flow), which requires a functionally intact cardiovascular system. When the cardiovascular system is compromised by vascular disease, the homeostasis of the body is affected. Risk factors for vascular disease include advanced age, heredity, smoking, obesity, physical inactivity, hypertension, and diabetes mellitus. Vascular diseases can affect both the arterial and the venous components of the circulation. Nearly 1 million people in the United States are affected by atherosclerotic peripheral vascular disease (PVD). Especially among older adults, PVD can lead to functional impairment. Each year, approximately 500,000 people are diagnosed with deep vein **thrombosis** (DVT), and nearly 140,000 die as a result of complications. Although peripheral **aneurysms** are less common, abdominal aortic aneurysms are present in 5% to 7% of American males over age 60. Of aneurysms larger than 6 cm in diameter, half rupture within one year, often with fatal consequences.

Atherosclerosis is covered in Chapter 33. Other peripheral vascular disorders as well as aortic aneurysm and aortic dissection are presented here.

ANATOMY AND PHYSIOLOGY OF THE VASCULAR SYSTEM

The peripheral vascular system comprises arteries, capillaries, veins, and the lymph vessels (Fig. 34-1). The function of this system is to maintain blood flow to supply adequate oxygen and nutrients to all tissues. Any interruption of the blood flow results in tissue hypoxia, which can lead to tissue necrosis (death) if untreated.

ARTERIES

Arteries are the vessels that carry the blood away from the heart toward the tissues. These vessels are normally elastic and have greater tensile strength than the veins. The aorta, which is the largest artery in the body, transports oxygenated blood from the heart. Arteries that branch from the aortic arch supply the head and arms. The thoracic branch of the descending aorta supplies intercostal muscles, the esophagus, and some respiratory passages. The abdominal branch of the descending aorta supplies the GI organs, the kidneys, the gonads, the lumbar area of the back, and the legs. Arteries branch into progressively smaller vessels as they travel away from the aorta. The smallest branches of the arteries are called arterioles.

Arteries and arterioles are thick-walled structures with three layers: the intima, the media, and the adventitia (Fig. 34-2). The *intima* is composed of endothelial cells that form the smooth inner surface of the arteries, allowing the blood to flow with little resistance. The middle layer is the *media,* the primary structure of the artery. The media is composed of smooth muscle, elastic fibers, and connective tissue fibers.

Smooth muscles encircle and control the diameter of arteries and arterioles. Contraction of the muscles constricts the vessels, whereas relaxation of the muscles results in vessel dilation. Smooth muscle contraction and relaxation are governed by the autonomic nervous system and other chemical and hormonal factors.

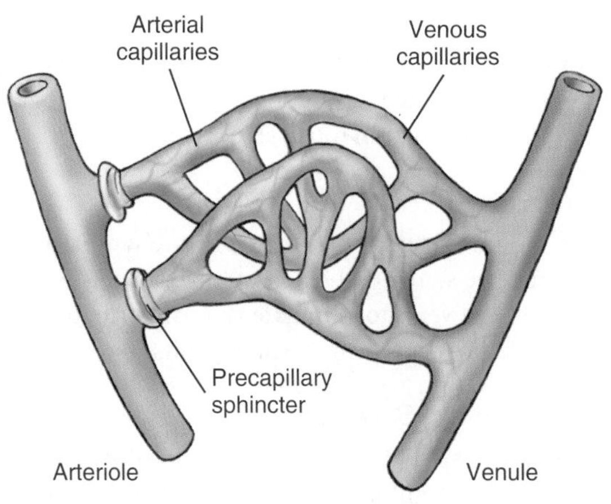

FIGURE **34-1** Capillary bed. Foods, nutrients, and oxygen are delivered to tissues through the capillaries, and wastes are collected from the capillaries for recycling or excretion. Precapillary sphincters help regulate the flow.

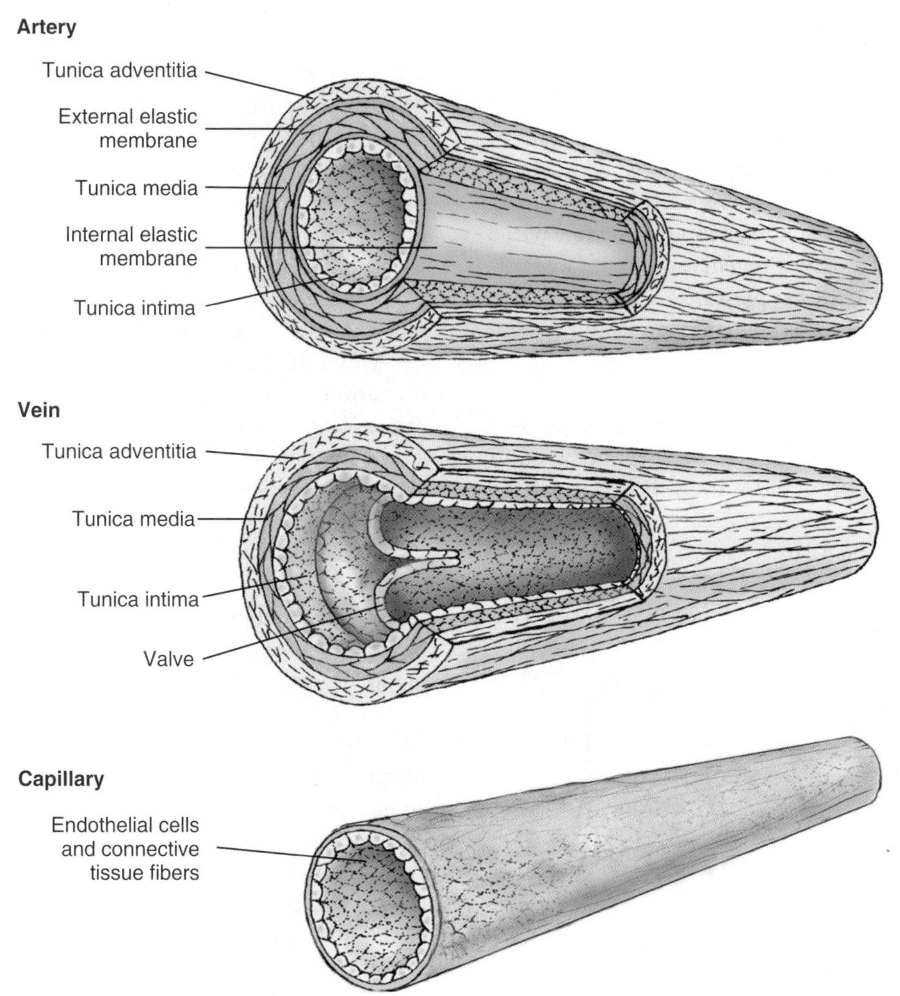

FIGURE **34-2** Tissue layers of veins and arteries.

The outer layer of the arteries and arterioles is the *adventitia.* This layer, which is composed mostly of connective tissue, secures the artery or arteriole to the surrounding structures.

CAPILLARIES

Arterioles branch into progressively smaller and smaller vessels, until they form the capillaries. Capillaries consist of a single layer of endothelial cells that allow the efficient delivery of nutrients and oxygen into the tissues and the removal of metabolic wastes from the tissues. Transfer of oxygen and nutrients between the blood and the tissue cells occurs in the capillaries. Red blood cells have to conform to the size of the capillaries by changing their shape to fit through the small diameter.

The tiny vessels that receive blood from the capillaries are venules, which are the smallest veins. The distribution of capillaries is determined by the metabolic activity occurring in the tissue. Tissues such as skeletal muscles and digestive tract lining have a rich capillary network, whereas tissues such as bone and cartilage have a scanty capillary network.

Because capillaries have less smooth muscle than the arteries, the amount of blood in the capillary is controlled by sphincters on the arteriolar side of the capillary. Other factors such as chemical stimulation and hormonal changes also influence blood flow and fluid shifts in the capillaries. For example, histamine causes the capillary permeability to increase, allowing more fluid to shift into the tissues.

VEINS

The blood is returned to the heart by way of the venules and veins. These vessels are formed as the capillaries organize into larger and larger vessels. The venous system is less sturdy and more passive than the arterial system. The walls of veins and venules are composed of the same three layers as the walls of the arteries and arterioles, but the layers are less defined (see Fig. 34-2). Because the walls of the veins and venules are thinner and less muscular, they can stretch more than those of the arterial system. Thus the venous system can store a large volume of blood under relatively low pressure. As much as 75% of the body's total blood volume is housed in the venous system.

Valves

The venous system is equipped with valves that are composed of endothelial leaflets (Fig. 34-3). Valves allow the blood to move in only one direction and prevent backflow of the blood in the extremities. Skeletal muscle contractions compress the veins, forcing blood back toward the heart. This action reduces venous pooling and increases the circulating blood volume. As deoxygenated blood moves toward the heart, carbon dioxide and other metabolic wastes are carried to the lungs and kidneys for elimination.

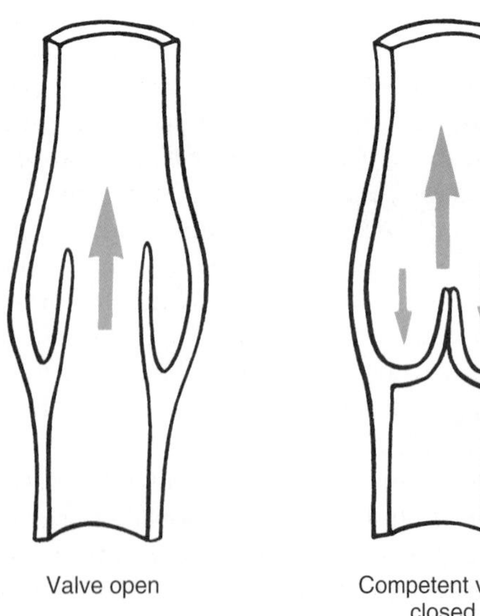

FIGURE 34-3 Veins contain bicuspid valves that open in the direction of blood flow but prevent regurgitation of flow when pockets become filled and distended.

Innervation

The venous system is innervated by the sympathetic nervous system. The sympathetic nervous system acts on the musculature of the veins to stimulate venoconstriction. Blocking of sympathetic nerve stimulation permits venodilation.

LYMPH VESSELS

The lymph system is an organization of small, thin-walled vessels that resemble the capillaries. These vessels accommodate the collection of lymph fluid from the peripheral tissues and the transportation of the fluid to the venous circulatory system. Because the lymph system interacts with the venous system, it is classified as part of the cardiovascular system. The lymph system comprises two main trunks: the thoracic duct and the right lymphatic duct. Each of these trunks is responsible for collecting and draining fluid from specific areas of the body. (See Chapter 32 and Figure 32-1 for additional information.)

Lymph fluid is composed of plasma-like fluid, large protein molecules, and foreign substances. Because these protein molecules are too large to enter the capillaries or the venules, the lymph fluid carries them to the lymphatic ducts, where they are emptied into the subclavian and the internal jugular veins. The movement of lymph fluid is accomplished by the contraction of muscles that encircle the lymphatic walls and surrounding tissues.

FACTORS THAT AFFECT BLOOD FLOW

The body has multiple homeostatic mechanisms to control the systemic and local blood volume. The mechanisms work by changing resistance within the vessels or by changing the blood viscosity.

Resistance

Resistance within the vascular system is controlled by the diameter of the vessels. When vascular diameter increases, peripheral resistance falls and blood flow increases. When vascular diameter decreases, however, peripheral resistance increases, thereby reducing blood flow. As previously noted, the diameter of blood vessels is controlled by the central nervous system, hormones, some ions, and blood pH.

The sympathetic nervous system plays a major role in adjusting vascular resistance. The diameter of peripheral blood vessels is regulated by the vasomotor center located in the medulla and the pons. Stimulation of the sympathetic nervous system by either physiologic or psychological stressors also triggers the adrenal glands to release norepinephrine and epinephrine, which cause vasoconstriction.

Other factors that cause changes in vascular resistance are angiotensin, serotonin, histamine, the kinins, and the prostaglandins. Angiotensin is a potent chemical released by the kidneys that causes intense vasoconstriction and retention of salt and water by the kidneys. The kinins, histamine, and prostaglandins cause vasodilation, which decreases peripheral resistance. Serotonin, a chemical that is liberated from platelets when vessel walls are damaged, can cause vasoconstriction or vasodilation, depending on tissue conditions.

Blood Viscosity

In addition to changes in peripheral resistance, modification of blood viscosity also helps regulate blood flow to peripheral tissues. Viscosity describes the thickness of the blood. The blood viscosity is usually constant, but can be affected by changes in the proportions of the solid or liquid components. An increase in red blood cells or a decrease in body water produces **hemoconcentration,** which increases blood viscosity. When blood is concentrated, the kidneys usually begin to retain water, and the movement of fluid out of the capillaries is restricted.

An important factor that affects blood viscosity is capillary permeability. Hydrostatic and osmotic pressures normally maintain balanced movement of fluids in and out of the capillaries. Any mechanism that alters capillary permeability changes the amount and direction of fluid movement, resulting in a change in blood viscosity. Factors that increase capillary permeability include histamine, bradykinin, leukotrienes, and prostaglandins. Certain muscle metabolites, hypoxemia, malnutrition, and pH imbalances can also increase capillary permeability. When the proportion of serum to solid components in the blood is higher than normal, blood is less viscous and the kidneys excrete excess fluid.

AGE-RELATED CHANGES

The primary age-related change in peripheral vessels is stiffening of the vessel walls, called arteriosclerosis. As arteriosclerosis develops, the delivery of oxygen and nutrients to the tissues is compromised, and there is a buildup of waste products in the tissue.

The stiffening of the peripheral vessels associated with aging occurs in both the intima and the media of the vessel wall. The intima is thickened and hardened by the proliferation of cells. It becomes roughened, which increases the risk of thrombus formation and emboli. The connective and elastic tissue fibers in the media become calcified. This process produces a thinner and fragmented layer within the peripheral vessels. Loss of elasticity in the peripheral vessels increases peripheral resistance, which impairs blood flow and results in increased left ventricular workload. As a result, the transportation of oxygen and nutrients to and the removal of wastes from the tissues are affected adversely. The same changes that affect peripheral blood vessels also occur in the aorta of the older adult. The aorta stiffens, thickens, and loses distensibility, which causes increased resistance to blood flow.

The transportation of oxygen also may be compromised by the decrease of hemoglobin seen in some older adults. A reduction of hemoglobin in the blood produces a decline in the oxygen-carrying capacity of the blood. Because the stiffening blood vessels result in decreased blood flow and because a decrease in hemoglobin compromises the oxygen-carrying capacity, peripheral circulation can be substantially affected.

Overall, aging in the vascular system may cause a slowing of the heart rate and a decrease in the stroke volume, which may result in a 30% to 40% decrease in cardiac output. If cardiac output is altered, the older adult may adapt more slowly to changes in the peripheral vascular system.

NURSING ASSESSMENT OF THE VASCULAR SYSTEM

HEALTH HISTORY

Chief Complaint and History of Present Illness

The nursing assessment of a patient who may have a vascular disorder requires a thorough cardiovascular assessment, as described in Chapter 33. Assessment of the peripheral circulation focuses on the six classical "P's" characteristic of peripheral vascular disease: pain, pulselessness, **poikilothermy,** pallor, **paresthesia,** and paralysis. Each of these characteristics needs to be evaluated.

Pain

A thorough pain history provides invaluable information for diagnosing vascular disease. Describe the nature of any pain or discomfort in the calf, thigh, hip, or buttock areas. Document the nature of the pain (e.g., sharp, throbbing, continuous, intermittent), the location and duration of the pain, the precipitating factors (e.g., exercise, lying down in bed), and alleviating factors (whatever brings relief). Acute pain is associated with acute arterial obstruction. Intermittent claudication and pain at rest are considered chronic pain.

When pain is caused by a venous disorder, patients typically describe it as tenderness, heaviness, or fullness in the extremity. Note whether the pain was alleviated by elevating the extremity or by wearing support stockings. Pain associated with an aortic aneurysm varies with the location of the aneurysm.

Intermittent claudication. Intermittent claudication is pain associated with decreased perfusion that is aggravated by exercise and relieved by rest. Intermittent claudication can affect any major muscle group distal to (beyond) the point of arterial occlusion. The pain is described as a feeling of tightness, burning, fatigue, aching, or cramping. Exercise causes the muscle group to become ischemic because blood flow is inadequate to supply nutrients and oxygen and to remove wastes. This results in the development of pain. When the exercise is stopped, the muscle tissue's metabolic demands decrease, wastes are removed from the tissues, and the pain is relieved.

Rest pain. Rest pain reflects the presence of a severe arterial occlusion. As a result of the occlusion, tissue **ischemia** develops in the extremity. Patients who have rest pain experience severe, burning pain in the affected foot after lying flat for a period of time. The pain is relieved when the extremity is dangled in a dependent position that promotes blood flow by gravity. Frequently, the patient sleeps best in a chair or with the feet in a dependent position.

Pulselessness

Assess the peripheral pulses for rate, rhythm, and quality. Compare pulses bilaterally to detect any differences.

Poikilothermy and Pallor

Document the presence or absence of poikilothermy and pallor. Poikilothermy is decreased temperature at an ischemic site. The rest of the extremity is warmer than the poikilothermic area. Pallor is paleness over an area of reduced blood supply.

Paresthesia and Paralysis

Note any paresthesia and paralysis. Paresthesia is an abnormal sensation such as numbness, tingling, a "pins and needles" sensation, or a crawling sensation. Paralysis is impairment of motor function. These symptoms may be associated with impaired conduction of nerve impulses caused by the reduction of oxygen and nutrients to the nerve tissues and the accumulation of waste materials.

Past Medical History

The past medical history includes the cardiovascular assessment, as described in Chapter 33. Document a history of hypertension, coronary artery disease, myocardial infarction, or atherosclerosis. Because atherosclerosis affects the cerebral, renal, and respiratory blood vessels, include each of these areas in the discussion of past medical problems. Note the presence of diabetes because peripheral vascular disease is a common complication of diabetes.

Family History

The family history determines any cardiovascular disorders in the immediate family members. Relevant cardiovascular diseases include hypertension, coronary artery disease, myocardial infarction, atherosclerosis, and aneurysm. Document a family history of diabetes.

Review of Systems

Changes in the integument provide important clues to the presence and severity of peripheral vascular disease. Changes that may be associated with PVD are thick and brittle nails; shiny, taut, scaly, and dry skin; skin temperature variations; skin ulcerations; muscle atrophy; localized redness and hardness; and hair loss on the extremities.

Another component of the review of systems is the assessment for chest pain and dyspnea. These symptoms are important because a pulmonary embolus develops in 10% of people with deep vein thrombosis.

Aneurysms are often asymptomatic. Depending on the location of the aneurysm, the patient may report hoarseness, dysphagia, dyspnea, abdominal or back pain, or swelling of the head and arms.

Functional Assessment

The functional assessment determines the impact of the disease process on the patient's life. The pain associated with the disease can interfere with work and recreation. Inactivity can reduce the patient's stamina. If limb amputation is necessary because of tissue necrosis, explore the effect of the limb loss on all aspects of the patient's functioning. Other aspects of the functional assessment that are relevant to vascular disease are smoking history and dietary habits. Smoking causes vasoconstriction, and a high fat intake can contribute to arteriosclerosis. Both are associated with peripheral vascular disease.

PHYSICAL EXAMINATION

The physical examination findings help determine whether the disease process is arterial or venous in nature. In general, arterial complications involve multiple areas, whereas venous complications remain more localized, usually in the lower extremities. Inspect the skin for color and lesions. Paleness suggests peripheral vasoconstriction or inadequate arterial blood flow. A reddish-brown discoloration called *rubor* in a dependent lower extremity suggests the presence of arterial occlusive disease. In venous disorders, the affected areas of the skin may have a brownish discoloration and be cyanotic when the extremity is dependent. Be alert for open ulcers and for scars around the ankles that may be associated with either arterial or venous disease. Note the presence of stasis dermatitis, a brown pigmentation with flaky skin over the edematous areas of the ankles. It may take on a bluish cast when the ankle is in a dependent position. Arterial stasis dermatitis begins as ulcerations in the toes. The ulcers are painful, pale, crusty, and located over bony prominences. Venous stasis dermatitis starts as ulcers in the ankle area. They develop very slowly, are usually painless, and are difficult to heal.

Assess capillary refill time in the nail beds to determine the adequacy of peripheral perfusion. Press the nail bed until it blanches (turns pale). Then release the pressure and note the number of seconds it takes for the color to return. Capillary refill time greater than 3 seconds denotes a reduction in peripheral perfusion.

Palpate the affected areas to evaluate the temperature, detect edema, and assess peripheral pulses. Palpate skin temperature bilaterally, moving proximally to distally (toward the feet), to detect any ischemic areas. A cool limb suggests an arterial problem, and a warm limb suggests a venous problem. Abdominal palpation may detect an aneurysm as a pulsating mass.

Dependent edema develops as a result of systemic disorders, lymphatic dysfunction, deep vein thrombosis, or chronic venous insufficiency. To assess the severity of edema, press the thumb into the edematous area for approximately 5 seconds. The severity is graded from 1+ to 4+, depending on the depth of depression: less than ¼ inch = 1+; ¼ to ½ inch = 2+; ½ to 1 inch = 3+; and more than 1 inch = 4+. If the depression of the thumb remains in the edematous area, the edema is said to be pitting. Compare the same area on both extremities.

Another aspect of the assessment is the evaluation of peripheral pulses (Fig. 34-4). Assess pulses for presence, symmetry, volume, and rhythm. The peripheral pulses assessed in the upper extremities include the brachial, ulnar, and radial arteries. The peripheral pulses appraised in the lower extremities are the femoral, popliteal, dorsalis pedis, and posterior tibial arteries. Compare pulses bilaterally. Document

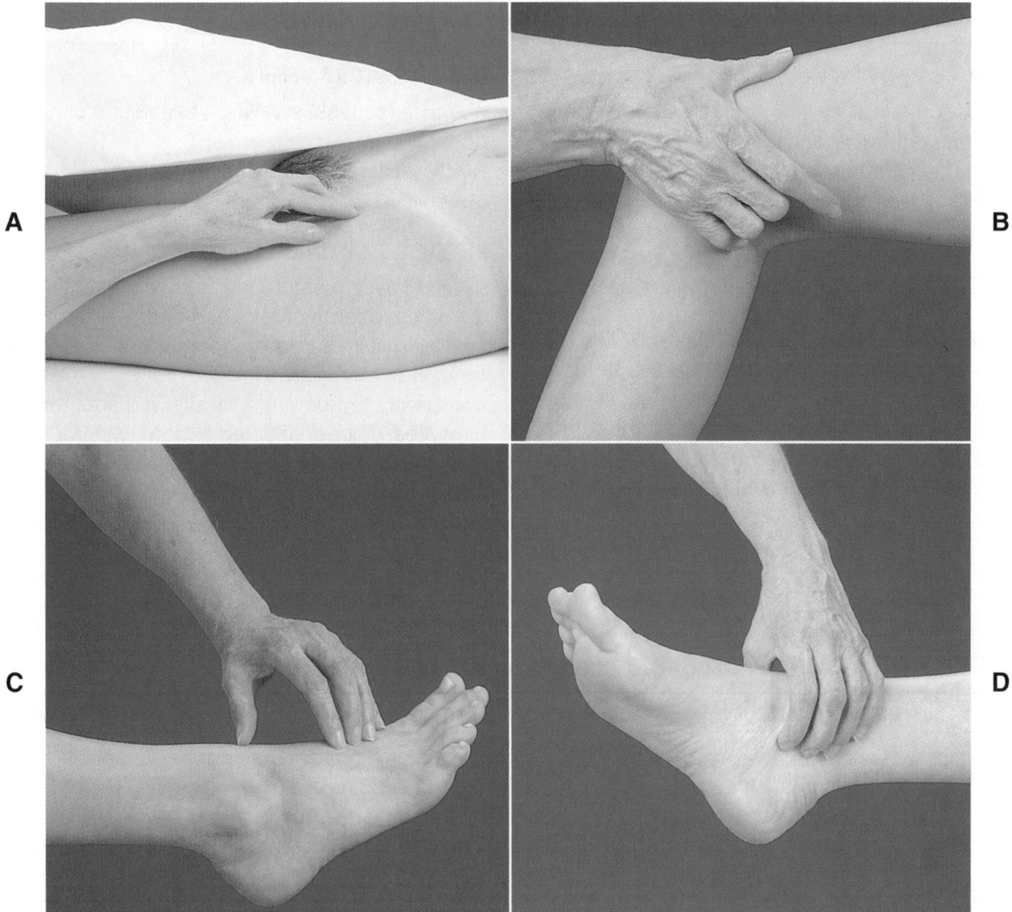

FIGURE 34-4 Palpating distal pulses. *A,* Femoral. *B,* Popliteal. *C,* Dorsalis pedis. *D,* Posterior tibial.

absent or asymmetric pulses. The palpation of the arteries provides valuable information concerning the condition of the vessels. A sclerotic vessel feels stiff and cordlike, whereas a normal vessel can be palpated as soft and springy.

When peripheral vascular disease is suspected, Homans' sign should be evaluated. With the knee slightly flexed, sharply dorsiflex the patient's foot. If dorsiflexion causes pain in the calf area or behind the knee, the test is said to be positive for venous thrombosis. Approximately 50% of patients with venous thrombosis experience deep calf pain during the testing process. However, many patients with a positive Homans' sign prove not to have venous thrombosis.

Another test that can be beneficial in the assessment of the peripheral vascular system is Allen's test. Allen's test is used to determine the adequacy of arterial circulation to the hand. Ask the patient to clench the fist tightly while you occlude the radial and ulnar arteries. Tell the patient to open the fist, and release pressure on the ulnar artery. If the ulnar artery is patent, the palm should promptly return to a normal color. A persistence of pallor in the palm area indicates an occlusion of the ulnar artery. The test can be repeated with the ulnar artery being occluded instead of the radial artery to detect occlusion within the radial artery (see Fig. 29-7).

The nurse with advanced education can further evaluate peripheral vascular function by auscultating the sounds of blood flow through the arteries. Bruits sound like turbulent, fast-moving fluid. The presence of bruits can signal the presence of an aneurysm or the development of chronic arterial occlusive disease long before other signs appear.

Nursing assessment of the patient with peripheral vascular disease is summarized in Table 34-1.

DIAGNOSTIC TESTS AND PROCEDURES

Based on findings of the physical examination, selected diagnostic studies are ordered by the physician to confirm the disease process and to determine the severity of the condition. The procedures and tests commonly used to diagnose peripheral vascular disease are Doppler ultrasound, plethysmography, pressure measurement, stress testing, and angiography, which includes arteriography and venography (Table 34-2). Imaging procedures include magnetic resonance imaging, computed tomography scanning, and venous duplex scanning, which aid in the determination of the severity of the disease process. Procedures that are useful in the diagnosis of

table 34-1 **ASSESSMENT** ***of the Patient with Peripheral Vascular Disease or Aneurysm***

HEALTH HISTORY

Present Illness: Complaints of pain, pulselessness, poikilothermia, pallor, paresthesia, and paralysis

Past Medical History: Hypertension, coronary artery disease, myocardial infarction, amputations, atherosclerosis, diabetes mellitus

Family History: Hypertension, coronary artery disease, myocardial infarction, atherosclerosis, diabetes mellitus, aneurysm

Review of Systems: Hairlessness on lower extremities; peripheral edema; discoloration of dependent areas; temperature changes in compromised areas; ulcerations on lower extremities; limb pain; thick, brittle toenails; temperature variation over involved area; muscle atrophy; localized redness and induration in affected extremity; chest pain; dyspnea. Hoarseness, swelling of head and/or arms, back or abdominal pain.

Functional Assessment: Mobility restricted by pain, decreased stamina

PHYSICAL EXAMINATION

General Survey: Posture, gait, presence of pain in affected extremities, edema of face and/or arms

Cardiovascular: Symmetric peripheral pulses, capillary refill time, Homans' sign

Integument: Temperature of affected area, edema in dependent area, color of affected extremity, rubor in lower extremities, stasis dermatitis or ulcers

Abdomen: Palpable pulsatile mass

table 34-2 **DIAGNOSTIC TESTS AND PROCEDURES** | ***Peripheral Vascular Disease (PVD)***

TEST	PURPOSE/PROCEDURE	PATIENT PREPARATION	POSTPROCEDURE NURSING CARE
Doppler ultrasound	Uses sound waves to facilitate diagnosis of PVD; monitor changes in blood flow associated with vascular disease	Tell patient test is painless and has no risks. Patient may be asked to change position of extremity being evaluated and perform breathing exercises.	No special care
Plethysmography	Used to detect deep vein thrombosis, to screen patients who are at risk for PVD, to investigate the possibility of pulmonary emboli	Tell patient procedure is safe, painless, and takes about 30-45 min. Leg will be elevated and pressure cuff placed on the thigh. Electrodes record information about blood flow in the veins.	No special care
Pressure measurement	Types: segmental limb pressures and pulse volume measurements	Tell patient blood pressures will be measured in multiple sites over the extremities to assess the blood vessels. Pressures are measured during activity and while at rest. The test is noninvasive, painless, and safe.	No special care
Exercise (treadmill) test	Evaluates the functional abilities of patients with PVD by measuring pulse volumes before, during, and after exercise	Tell patient test is noninvasive; will be asked to walk for approximately 5 min on a treadmill. The test will be stopped if the patient has pain or dyspnea.	Carefully monitor for any complications that may develop as a result of the test.
Angiography (venography, arteriography, and radiographs)	Taken to identify venous obstruction, confirm PVD, detect clots, or identify suitable vessel for grafting	Tell patient dye will be injected and radiographs taken. May briefly feel burning sensation when dye is injected. Signed consent required. NPO 4 hr before test. Inform radiologist if allergic to iodine or seafood. Risks: hemorrhage at insertion site, dye-induced allergic reaction, thrombosis/embolism, renal insufficiency, pseudoaneurysm.	Bedrest for several hours; monitor vital signs and pulses hourly for 6 hr. Assess injection site for bleeding, hematoma, and pulsating mass (pseudoaneurysm); neurovascular checks (pulses, sensation, movement, color, warmth).

aneurysms include chest radiography, abdominal ultrasound, computed tomography, and transthoracic echocardiography.

DOPPLER ULTRASOUND

Doppler ultrasound is used to facilitate the diagnosis of peripheral vascular disease and to monitor the changes in blood flow associated with vascular diseases. It a noninvasive, inexpensive, highly reliable diagnostic tool. Low-intensity, high-frequency sound waves are directed toward the artery or vein being tested. These sound waves strike the moving blood cells and are reflected back to the receiver. Arteries reflect a high-pitched sound, whereas veins produce sounds that vary with respirations and have a "blowing" tone. In the presence of an occlusion or narrowed vessel, the sounds are diminished. The primary vessels examined are the posterior tibial, popliteal, and common femoral veins. The test takes 10 to 20 minutes. Abdominal ultrasound may be used to screen for abdominal aneurysms.

PLETHYSMOGRAPHY

Plethysmography is a noninvasive study used to measure blood volume and outflow of blood through the veins. There are various types of plethysmography. The type used to assess peripheral vascular disease is impedance plethysmography.

With the patient in a supine position, the leg being tested is raised to a 30- to 35-degree angle to promote venous drainage of the area. A pressure cuff is placed on the thigh and inflated to allow for full venous distention. Pressure readings are taken and the cuff is rapidly deflated. Electrodes measure electrical resistance and provide information about venous volume changes that is printed as waveforms on a strip chart. When a thrombus is present, the tracings reflect reduced venous volume and venous volume changes.

Both legs are tested to allow for comparison of the readings. Because the test may require three to five tracings per leg, the test usually takes 30 to 45 minutes.

PRESSURE MEASUREMENT

Pressure measurements can be completed as segmental limb pressures (sometimes called segmental plethysmography) and pulse volume measurements. The pulse volumes are recorded as waveforms. These waveforms provide information about the elasticity of blood vessels. Blood pressure is measured at multiple sites over the extremities to be examined. Pressure readings are reduced at the location of a narrowed or occluded vessel. Measurements are taken while the patient is at rest.

EXERCISE (TREADMILL) TEST

The exercise test is sometimes referred to as a stress test. This noninvasive procedure helps to evaluate the patient's tolerance for physical activity. Signed consent is required.

The patient is asked to walk for approximately 5 minutes at a rate of 1.5 miles per hour on a treadmill. Continuous EKG and BP monitoring is done. The patient is monitored for any signs of distress such as cardiac dysrhythmias, claudication, or dyspnea. If distress occurs, the test is stopped immediately. After the test, the patient should be monitored until vital signs return to normal.

ANGIOGRAPHY

The purposes of angiography are to confirm the diagnosis of peripheral vascular disease, to distinguish clot formation from venous obstruction, and to locate a suitable vessel for grafting. Angiography is an invasive procedure that requires the injection of dye into the vascular system, which makes the vessels visible on radiographs. The two types of angiography are arteriography, which examines arteries, and venography, which examines veins. Abnormalities can be visualized and assessed during the procedure. The risks that are associated with these tests are hemorrhage at the IV insertion site, dye-induced allergic reactions, thrombosis at the insertion site, and emboli. The patient is exposed to relatively high doses of radiation.

COMMON THERAPEUTIC MEASURES

The primary goals for the patient with peripheral vascular disease are to increase the arterial blood supply to the extremities, reduce venous congestion, dilate blood vessels to increase arterial blood flow, prevent vascular compression, provide relief from pain, attain or maintain tissue integrity, and encourage adherence to the treatment plan.

Exercise programs, stress management, pain management, smoking cessation, elastic stockings, intermittent pneumatic compression units, body positioning, drug therapy, surgical interventions, and patient education are used in the management of the disease process.

EXERCISE

The simple act of walking stimulates the movement of blood from the dependent areas of the extremities toward the heart. Walking contracts the muscles of the lower extremities, pushing venous blood upward toward the heart and promoting the development of collateral circulation. For patients with vascular disease, any exercise program must be prescribed by the physician. Patients who display leg ulcers, gangrene, or acute thrombotic occlusion may be restricted to bedrest until the condition improves.

A specific type of exercise program that is effective in the management of peripheral vascular disease is the use of Buerger-Allen exercises or active postural exercises (Fig. 34-5).

PATIENT TEACHING PLAN
Buerger-Allen Exercises

- These exercises allow gravity to fill and empty the blood vessels.
- Lie flat on your back and raise your legs above the level of your heart for 2 minutes or until they become very pale.

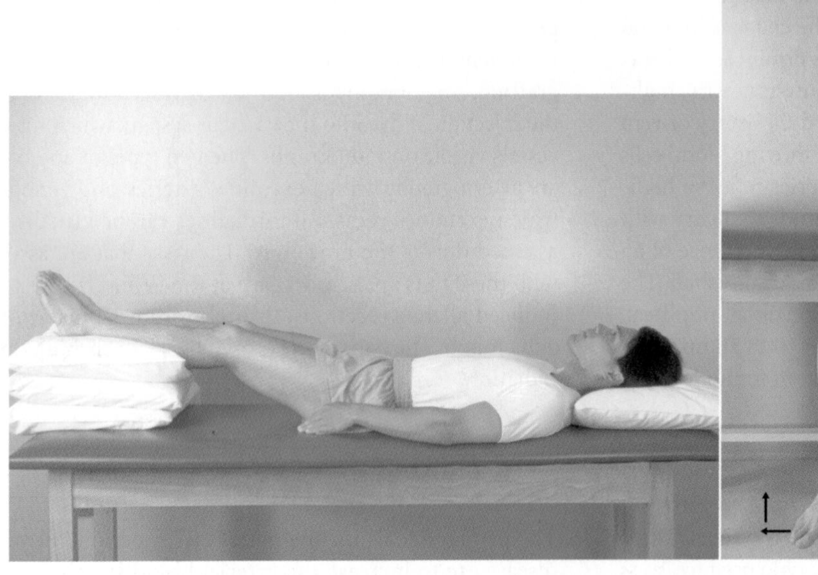

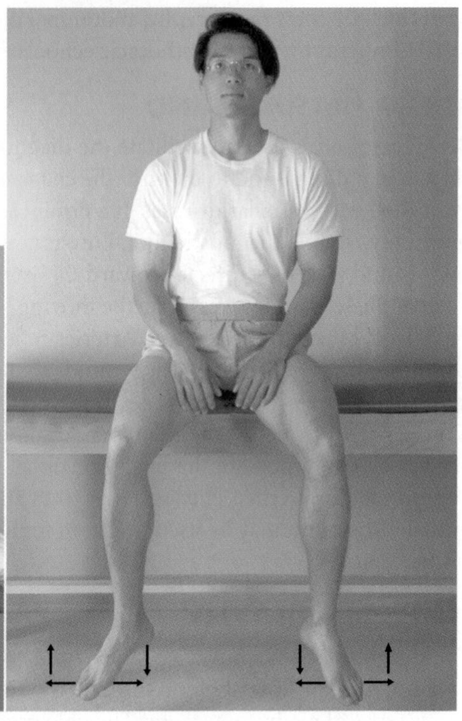

FIGURE **34-5** *A,* Elevate and support the legs at a 45- to 90-degree angle, or until the skin blanches, for 2 to 3 minutes. *B,* Sit with feet in a dependent position so the skin turns red. Support the legs in this position for 5 to 10 minutes. Then flex, extend, pronate, and supinate each foot three times. Finally, lie flat in a supine position for 10 minutes.

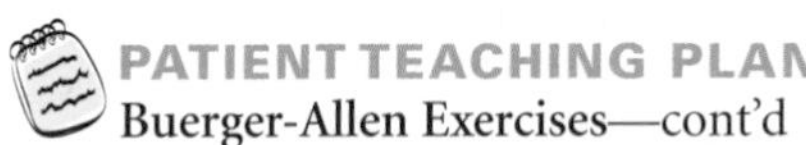

PATIENT TEACHING PLAN
Buerger-Allen Exercises—cont'd

- Lower the legs to a dependent position, flex and extend your feet for 3 minutes or until color returns to your legs.
- Keep your legs flat for 5 minutes.
- Go through the entire process six times in each session if you can tolerate it. Three to four sessions a day provide the best results.
- Stop the exercises immediately if you have pain or severe skin color changes.

STRESS MANAGEMENT

Emotional stress causes peripheral vasoconstriction, which is detrimental to a patient whose circulation is already compromised. Resistance to blood flow is increased, which reduces blood flow to the tissues. Emotional stress cannot be avoided entirely but can be reduced with a stress management plan, which may include lifestyle changes, massage, relaxation, or other stress-reducing activities.

PAIN MANAGEMENT

The patient with peripheral vascular disease often limits ambulation because of pain. However, immobility tends to worsen circulatory problems. Therefore, pain management is an important aspect of care. Pain can be managed by promoting circulation to the affected area, by administering prescribed analgesics, or both. When intermittent claudication occurs, the patient should stop the exercise. Rest decreases circulatory demands and alleviates the pain. Once the pain is relieved, the activity may be resumed. Advise the patient to avoid constrictive garments such as girdles, garters, belts, and tight pantyhose that can cause pain by obstructing blood flow.

SMOKING CESSATION

Smoking cessation is critical to effective management of peripheral vascular disease because smoking causes vasoconstriction (constriction of the blood vessels). Vasoconstriction can be documented for up to 1 hour after a cigarette has been smoked. In addition, the nicotine in tobacco causes vasospasms, which drastically restrict the peripheral circulation. Measures to help the patient include encouragement; reinforcement; teaching about the nature of tobacco addiction, the harm of smoking, and the benefits of stopping; self-help materials or "Quit Kits" that are available from various agencies; and pharmacotherapy. Nicotine (patches, spray, gum, inhalers) and bupropion, individually or together, greatly enhance the chance of success. Even though the best smoking cessation programs have about a 25% to 30% success rate, that rate is significant when you realize that 45 million Americans smoke cigarettes and that smoking is responsible for about 430,000 preventable deaths in the U. S. annually.

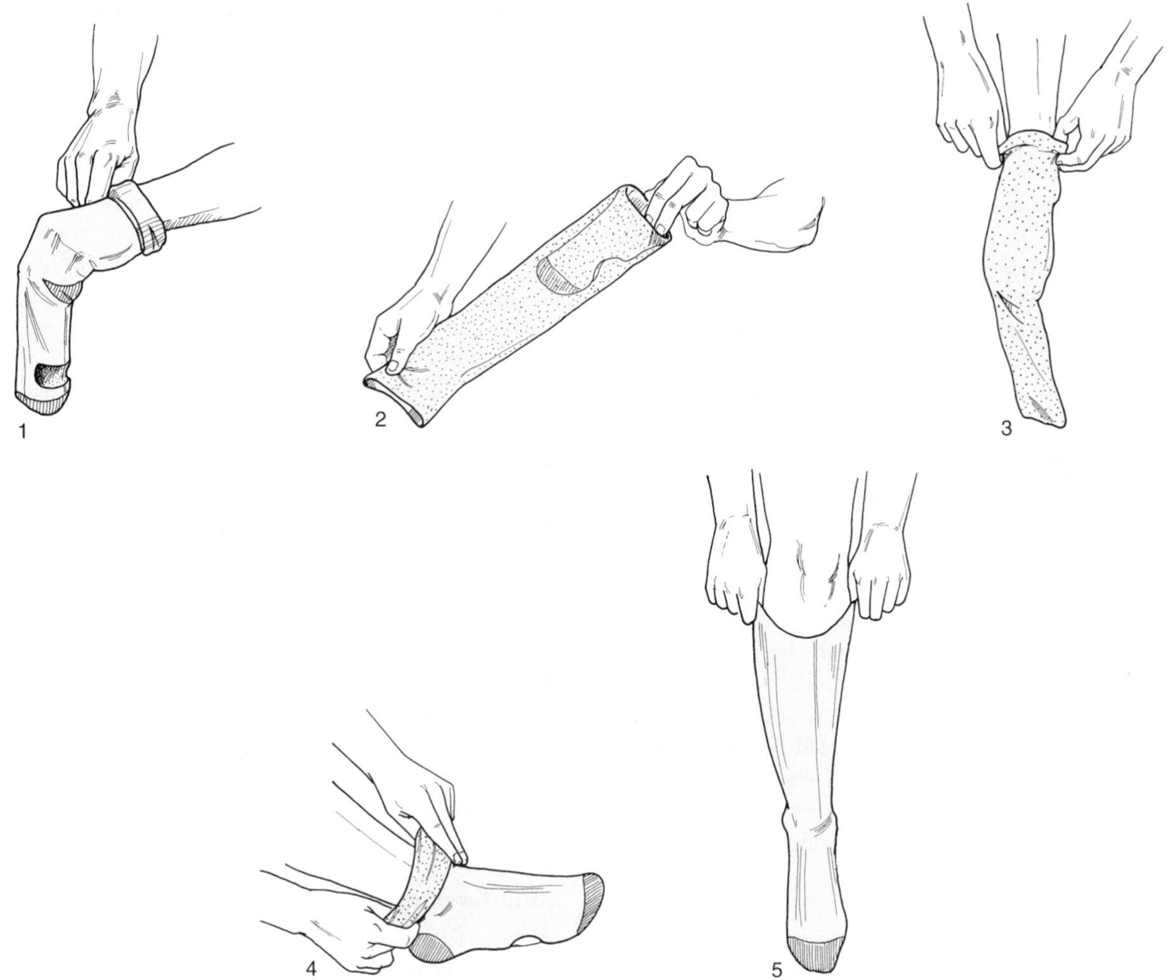

FIGURE **34-6** Elastic stockings provide sustained, consistently distributed pressure over the entire surface of the calves and thighs to promote venous return

PHARMACOLOGY CAPSULE Drugs that help some people who are trying to quit smoking are nicotine and bupropion.

ELASTIC STOCKINGS

Another therapy that is useful in the management of peripheral vascular disease is the use of elastic stockings or antiembolism hose. These stockings provide sustained, evenly distributed pressure over the entire surface of the calves and thighs. The correct placement of elastic stockings compresses superficial veins, resulting in improved blood flow to the deeper veins. Take care when applying these stockings because they can become tourniquets if applied incorrectly. The proper size of elastic stockings must be determined for each patient by using the instruction sheet provided by the manufacturer. Elastic stockings are best applied in the morning before rising from bed because swelling is usually at its lowest level at this time of the day. With the stockings inside out, start the placement by pulling the stocking onto the foot with firm, even support (Fig. 34-6). Once the elastic stocking is positioned over the heel, pull from the sides so it distributes evenly over the entire length of the leg. The stockings should be smooth when the application process is completed. If the top is allowed to roll or turn down, circulatory stasis occurs. Remove the stockings for 10 to 20 minutes twice a day. While the stockings are off, it is best for the patient to be resting in bed or with the extremities in a nondependent position. When the elastic stockings are removed, inspect the skin for any signs of irritation, pressure, or tenderness, which could reflect developing complications.

INTERMITTENT PNEUMATIC COMPRESSION

Intermittent pneumatic compression or a pulsatile antiembolism system may be used for patients who are confined to bed after surgery or a traumatic injury. The primary function of these devices is to prevent deep vein thrombosis. With intermittent pneumatic compression, elastic stockings are applied that are sequentially inflated from the ankles, calves, and thighs and then deflated. This expansion and contraction mimics the muscle pumping of the lower extremities, prevents venous pooling, and stimulates the circulation.

POSITIONING

Body positions play an important part in the management of peripheral vascular disease. Frequently, patients are restricted to bed during the acute phases of the disease process. It is important to use different positions to mobilize the blood volume that has become stagnant in the dependent areas. Lowering the extremities below the level of the heart enhances arterial blood supply. Elevating the lower extremities above the level of the heart promotes venous return and reduces venous stasis. For patients who are not restricted to bed, prolonged standing puts strain on the venous system. Instruct the patient to sit down and elevate the extremity to a nondependent position whenever possible.

THERMOTHERAPY

Thermotherapy with either warm or cold can be used for its effects on the circulatory system. Heat, whether dry or moist, works as a vasodilator that promotes arterial flow to the peripheral tissues. Use heat cautiously, however, because patients with peripheral vascular disease may have impaired sensation as a result of tissue ischemia. Blood vessels constrict in response to cold. Clothing can be used effectively to promote warmth and to prevent vasoconstriction due to chilling.

PROTECTION

Affected extremities must be protected from trauma because the healing process is usually impaired with peripheral vascular disease. To prevent injury to poorly perfused tissues, the patient must avoid scratching and vigorous rubbing. Caution the patient to wear properly fitting shoes and clean socks or hose, to keep fingernails and toenails trimmed and smooth, and not to walk about barefoot. Inform the physician of ingrown toenails, blisters, or skin injuries so prompt treatment can be initiated.

PATIENT TEACHING

Patient education is important in the management of peripheral vascular disease. The patient must understand the disease process and the prescribed therapies. The teaching plan should include cleanliness, warmth, safety, comfort measures, prevention of constricting blood flow, exercise, signs and symptoms that should be reported to the health care provider, drug therapy, and the importance of smoking cessation.

SURGICAL PROCEDURES

As peripheral vascular disease progresses, surgical intervention may become necessary. Embolectomy, percutaneous transluminal angioplasty, endarterectomy, sympathectomy, ligation and vein stripping, and sclerotherapy are procedures that may be used.

Embolectomy

Embolectomy is the removal of a blood clot located in a large vessel. An incision is made into the vessel and the clot is removed under direct visualization of the site or through a catheter. This procedure is used when an arterial **embolism** is present and the patient has complicating factors that restrict the use of thrombolytic agents. Another method for performing an embolectomy is the use of a Fogarty embolectomy catheter. The catheter, which has a soft, inflatable balloon near the tip, is positioned in the artery. The tip of the catheter is passed through the embolus and inflated. Once the balloon is inflated, a steady tension is placed on the catheter to withdraw the entire embolus and catheter from the vessel.

Percutaneous Transluminal Angioplasty

Percutaneous transluminal angioplasty is used to gain access to the arteries in the lower extremities in people who are poor surgical risks. The primary purpose of this technique is to relieve arterial stenosis in such areas as the superficial femoral and iliac arteries. Under local anesthesia, a balloon catheter is passed into the vessel to the stenotic area. Once the catheter is maneuvered into the optimal position, the balloon is inflated. The inflated balloon presses outwardly against the vessel walls, dilating the lumen of the artery and improving blood flow. Heparin is injected through the catheter at the time of removal to prevent clot formation. Pressure must be applied to the catheter insertion site for approximately 10 to 20 minutes to prevent hemorrhage from the site. Complications of percutaneous transluminal angioplasty are hematoma formation, embolus, arterial dissection, and allergic reactions.

Endarterectomy

An endarterectomy requires an incision into the obstructed vessel. The emboli and atherosclerotic plaque are stripped away from the intima of the vessel, and the vessel is surgically closed.

Sympathectomy

A sympathectomy may be done to improve vascular circulation when the patient has intermittent claudication. The process involves the excision of the sympathetic ganglia, which results in arteriolar dilation and increased blood flow. When poor circulation is related to atherosclerotic vessels, a sympathectomy is not the treatment of choice because the hardened blood vessels have limited ability to dilate. To evaluate the capacity for vascular dilation, a lumbar sympathetic block may be done and the temporary effects monitored.

Vein Ligation and Stripping

Vein ligation and stripping are used primarily to treat varicose veins. The greater or lesser saphenous systems, or both, are the vessels removed in this manner. The surgeon must be certain the deeper veins are patent before the varicosities are removed. Pressure and elevation are used during the procedure to reduce the bleeding. A disadvantage to this procedure is that removal of the saphenous vein means it would not be available if the patient required coronary artery bypass graft surgery in the future.

Sclerotherapy

Sclerotherapy is another method for managing varicose veins, primarily for cosmetic treatment of small, prominent varicosities. Sclerotherapy requires the injection of a chemical that irritates the venous endothelium, causing localized inflammation and fibrosis. The vein becomes thrombosed and eventually closes. Sclerotherapy may be used in conjunction with vein ligation and stripping. The protocol followed after the procedure depends on the physician but usually involves wearing compression stockings or support stockings for a specified period of time. An exercise program of walking is emphasized to encourage and facilitate the blood flow to the extremity. Potential complications include pulmonary embolism, thrombosis, injection site necrosis, vasospasm, hemolysis, and allergic reactions.

NURSING CARE *Related to Surgery*

Preoperative Nursing Care

General preoperative care is covered in Chapter 16. The patient with severe cardiovascular disease may have activity restrictions to reduce the demands on the circulatory system until the surgical procedure is done. The affected extremity should be maintained in a level or slightly dependent position as ordered. To optimize peripheral circulation, keep the extremity warm. Protect the limb from further injury.

Postoperative Nursing Care

The primary goal of the postoperative period is to stimulate circulation by encouraging movement and preventing stasis within the extremity. Closely monitor tissue perfusion in the postoperative period. Evaluate tissue perfusion by assessing the affected extremity for color, temperature, complaints of pain or tenderness, capillary refill time, presence of edema, quality of peripheral pulses, and exercise tolerance. Anticoagulants are usually continued after surgery to prevent the formation of a thrombus at the operative site. If a peripheral pulse disappears, suspect a thrombus. During the recovery period, emphasize that the patient should not cross the legs or place the affected extremity in a dependent position for long periods of time. Elevating the extremity helps prevent edema.

DRUGS

Drugs most often used to treat peripheral vascular disease include anticoagulants, thrombolytics, platelet aggregation inhibitors, vasodilators, nonsteroidal anti-inflammatory drugs, and analgesics (Table 34-3).

Anticoagulants

Anticoagulant therapy is used to prolong the clotting time, hinder the extension of a thrombus, and inhibit the formation of a thrombus during the postoperative period. The primary anticoagulant medications used are heparin, low molecular weight heparin (LMWH), and warfarin sodium (Coumadin) derivatives. Heparin is given intravenously for immediate response and subcutaneously for maintenance or prophylaxis. LMWH is given only SC, and warfarin is given orally. The clinical indications for anticoagulant treatment are venous thrombosis, pulmonary embolism, and risk for embolism. When anticoagulant therapy is used, regular coagulation tests are done to assess the effectiveness of the treatment regimen. The effective range for the activated partial thromboplastin time during heparin treatment is 1.5 to 2.5 times the control. Warfarin dosage is based on the patient's prothrombin time (PT) and INR (international normalized ratio). The target PT and INR depend on the condition being treated. LMWH has advantages over heparin because a fixed dose can be administered, laboratory monitoring is not necessary, and one or two doses daily are sufficient.

The fundamental complication of anticoagulant therapy is spontaneous bleeding that can occur anywhere in the body and may be evident in the urine, stool, emesis, or integument. Because of the risk of bleeding, the antidotes for each type of anticoagulant should be accessible. The antidote for heparin and LMWH is protamine sulfate; for warfarin sodium it is vitamin K.

Medications such as antibiotics, mineral oil, NSAIDs, aspirin, and tolbutamide can intensify the anticoagulant effects of warfarin sodium. Some drugs that decrease the effectiveness of warfarin are antacids, barbiturates, oral contraceptives, and adrenal corticosteroids.

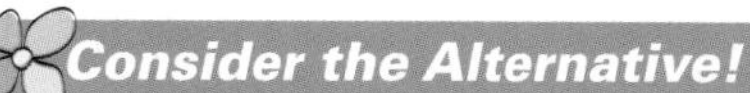

Many herbal remedies interact with conventional drugs. Feverfew, garlic, ginger root, and ginkgo enhance the effects of antiplatelet drugs. St. John's wort can decrease the effectiveness of warfarin. Caution patients against using herbal remedies while on prescribed anticoagulants.

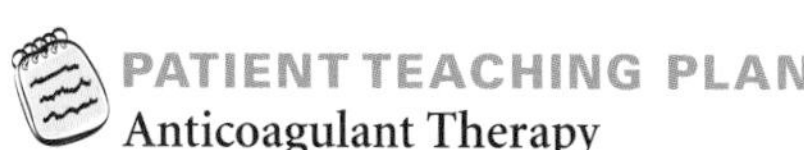

Anticoagulant Therapy

- Anticoagulants help prevent blood clots from forming. Take your medications exactly as prescribed.
- Because these drugs can interfere with normal blood clotting, notify your physician of excessive bruising, bleeding gums, or blood in stools or urine.
- Consult your physician before taking any additional medications because some drugs affect the action of your anticoagulant.
- Keep appointments for regular blood tests to monitor the blood level of your drugs. Test results are used to ensure your dosage is safe and effective.
- Wear a medical alert bracelet noting anticoagulant therapy.

PHARMACOLOGY CAPSULE Patients taking anticoagulant drugs must be monitored for bleeding.

Thrombolytics

Thrombolytic therapy is given intravenously to dissolve an existing clot. Examples of thrombolytic medications are streptokinase (Kabikinase), urokinase (Abbokinase), tissue plasminogen activator (Activase), reteplase (Retavase), and anistreplase (Eminase). Thrombolytic therapy is used to treat

table 34-3 **DRUG THERAPY** | ***Peripheral Vascular Diseases***

DRUG	USE/ACTION	SIDE EFFECTS	NURSING INTERVENTIONS
ANTICOAGULANTS			
Heparin Sodium (Liquaemin Sodium)	Interferes with blood clotting; prevents formation of new clots; does not affect existing clots	Thrombocytopenia, bleeding, hemorrhage, nausea and vomiting, local irritation at injection site	Blood tested regularly to monitor effects on clotting. Check APTT before each dose. Goal is APTT 1.5 to 2.5 times normal. Monitor for bleeding. Avoid trauma. Heparin given IV or subq. After subq injection, apply pressure but do not massage. Rotate injection sites.
Low molecular weight heparin Enoxaparin (Lovenox) Dalteparin (Fragmin) Ardeparin (Normiflo)	Prevents formation of fibrin and thrombin	Thrombocytopenia, anemia, edema, nausea, fever, confusion, cardiac toxicity, bruising	Given SC only! Do not aspirate. Rotate sites. Leave bubble in syringe when administered. Administer at same time each day. Avoid IM injections. Teach patient to report any bleeding and to use soft toothbrush and electric razor. Do not take aspirin.
Warfarin sodium (Coumadin)	Interferes with blood clotting; may prevent extension of existing clots and formation of new clots	Bruising, hemorrhage, nausea, anorexia	Check prothrombin time/INR before each dose. May be required to notify physician before each dose. Monitor for bleeding. Teach patient not to take aspirin with warfarin.
PLATELET AGGREGATION INHIBITORS/ANTIPLATELETS			
Cilostazol (Pletal)	Inhibits platelet aggregation; used to treat intermittent claudication	Cardiac dysrhythmias, CHF, MI, cerebral infarct Hemorrhage, dizziness, back pain, cough, diarrhea	Monitor for bleeding, signs of heart failure. Blood work must be done during therapy. May take up to 12 weeks for effects.
Aspirin	Inhibits platelet aggregation; decreases inflammation and fever; reduces pain	GI irritation, tinnitus, pruritus, headache, bleeding	Assess for bruising, bleeding. Give with milk or food if GI irritation occurs.
Ticlopidine (Ticlid)	Inhibits platelet aggregation	Rash, diarrhea, hepatitis, cholestatic jaundice, bleeding, blood dyscrasias	Tell patient importance of having regular blood tests done and to report any bleeding. Taking with food decreases GI symptoms.

THROMBOLYTICS			
Streptokinase (Kabikinase) Urokinase (Abbokinase) Alteplase (Activase, t-PA)	Dissolves existing clots	Minor to major bleeding; transient thrombocytopenia and alopecia; hypersensitivity rare; cardiac dysrhythmias	Monitor blood tests of clotting activity. Monitor electrocardiogram and vital signs. Assess for bleeding. Protect from trauma.
VASODILATORS **Calcium Channel Blockers**			
Nifedipine (Procardia) Amlodipine (Norvasc) Diltiazem (Cardizem)	Dilates peripheral and coronary arteries	Drowsiness, dizziness, cardiac dysrhythmias, CHF, MI, hypotension, polyuria	Monitor BP and P. Assess for edema. Tell patient to limit caffeine, avoid alcohol, swallow extended release and caps whole. Teach patient how to manage postural hypotension.
Alpha-Adrenergic Blockers			
Prazosin (Minipres) Terazosin (Hytrin)	Decreases vascular resistance; lowers BP	Dizziness, headache, drowsiness, nausea, orthostatic hypotension, edema, palpitations	Teach patient to manage orthostatic hypotension, take safety precautions if dizzy, monitor weight daily. Take first dose or any increased dose at bedtime because of potential hypotension. Monitor BP and P.
ANTIANGINAL			
Nitroglycerin (topical patch, ointment)	Dilates coronary arteries; reduces peripheral resistance	Headache, flushing, dizziness, orthostatic hypotension	Transdermal patches can be removed at night to decrease development of tolerance. Patches are waterproof. Rotate sites. Apply to hairless areas on trunk or upper arms. Remove patch or ointment from one site before applying it to another site. Do not touch ointment with bare hands or rub ointment into skin. Cover ointment with occlusive dressing if ordered.
HEMORRHEOLOGIC AGENT			
Pentoxifylline (Trental)	Decreases blood viscosity, fibrinogen, and platelet aggregation; increases flexibility of RBCs to allow passage through small vessels; used to treat intermittent claudication	Dyspepsia, epistaxis, dizziness, nausea, vomiting, angina, tachycardia, cardiac dysrhythmias, leukopenia, headache, tremors, rash	Assess vital signs. Administer with meals to decrease GI upset. Take safety precautions if dizzy. Tell patient to report rapid or irregular pulse. Explain how to manage epistaxis if it occurs. Monitor WBC count.

APTT, Activated partial thromboplastin time; *GI*, gastrointestinal.

acute myocardial infarction, pulmonary embolism, deep vein thrombosis, and arterial thrombosis or embolism. Uncontrolled bleeding can result from thrombolytics; therefore the patient must be assessed continuously during the treatment regimen.

PHARMACOLOGY CAPSULE Anticoagulants prevent the formation of blood clots; thrombolytics dissolve existing blood clots.

Other Medications

Many other types of medications are used to treat peripheral vascular diseases. Vasodilators are used to relax the vascular smooth muscle, which reduces resistance in the vessels and results in increased blood flow. Commonly used vasodilators are calcium channel blockers and alpha adrenergic inhibitors. Analgesics including nonsteroidal anti-inflammatory agents are used to relieve the pain caused by ischemia. With less pain, a patient can participate more in exercises. Platelet aggregation inhibitors (antiplatelets) such as aspirin are used to prevent clot formation by making the platelets less likely to clump together. Pentoxifylline is used to treat peripheral vascular disease by improving the passage of red blood cells through small vessels.

In addition to drugs that prevent clot formation, patients also may be taking medications such as hypoglycemics and antihypertensives to control conditions that contribute to the development of peripheral vascular disease.

PHARMACOLOGY CAPSULE Monitor patients taking vasodilators for hypotension. Teach them how to manage orthostatic hypotension.

DIETARY INTERVENTIONS

The dietary interventions used with peripheral vascular disease are like those recommended for cardiovascular health. Atherosclerotic plaques create rough vessel walls and contribute to peripheral vascular complications. Low-fat diets reduce serum cholesterol levels, thereby reducing the risk of atherosclerotic plaque formation. A weight reduction diet may be prescribed if the patient is obese because obesity causes a strain on the heart, increases venous congestion, and reduces peripheral circulation. Adequate vitamin B, vitamin C, and protein are needed to promote healing and improve tissue integrity.

DISORDERS OF THE PERIPHERAL VASCULAR SYSTEM

ARTERIAL EMBOLISM

Pathophysiology

The development of an arterial embolism is a potentially life-threatening event. The arterial embolus usually forms in the heart. However, a roughened atheromatous plaque in any artery can lead to thrombus formation. If a thrombus breaks loose, it becomes an embolus traveling through the circulatory system until it lodges in a vessel, blocking blood flow distal to the occlusion. The effects of arterial occlusion depend on the size of the embolus formed, the organs involved, and the extent to which collateral circulation can maintain sufficient blood supply to affected tissues.

Signs and Symptoms

Whereas some patients with arterial obstruction have no pain, others experience severe pain and other symptoms of tissue ischemia. When the collateral circulation cannot compensate for the compromised blood flow, the patient has distinct symptoms of reduced blood flow to the tissues. Signs and symptoms of inadequate blood supply are the following:

1. Severe, acute pain
2. Gradual loss of sensory and motor function in the affected areas
3. Pain aggravated by movement or pressure
4. Absent distal pulses
5. Pallor and mottling (irregular discoloration)
6. A sharp line of color and temperature demarcation: tissue beyond the obstruction is pale and cool

Medical and Surgical Treatment

Arterial embolism is managed with intravenous anticoagulants and thrombolytic agents. These medications cannot be used with active internal bleeding, cardiovascular accident, recent major surgery, uncontrolled hypertension, and pregnancy. Patients who cannot be treated with medications may be prepared for embolectomy—surgical removal of the thrombus.

NURSING CARE *of the Patient with Arterial Embolism*

Assessment

The assessment of the patient with peripheral vascular disease is outlined in Table 34-1.

Nursing Diagnoses, Goals, and Outcome Criteria: Arterial Emboli

Nursing Diagnoses	Goals and Outcome Criteria
Ineffective Tissue Perfusion related to compromised circulation	Improved tissue perfusion: normal skin color, palpable pulses, capillary refill time less than 3 seconds in affected extremity
Fear related to the treatments, environment, and risk of death	Reduced fear: patient calm, states fear reduced or relieved
Impaired Physical Mobility related to the surgical procedure and compromised circulation	Improved physical mobility: patient increases activity without discomfort
Impaired Skin Integrity related to ischemic changes from the impairment of peripheral circulation	Healthy skin in affected areas: skin intact

Ineffective Therapeutic Regimen Management related to lack of knowledge of self-care	Patient knows and practices prescribed self-care measures: patient correctly describes and demonstrates self-care measures

Interventions

Nursing interventions are designed to improve circulation and prevent further damage to the affected tissue.

Ineffective Tissue Perfusion

To promote circulation, maintain the affected extremities at or slightly below the horizontal, administer prescribed medications, and perform range of motion exercises as ordered.

Fear

To decrease fear, orient the patient to the environment and the expected therapies using simple statements to explain the disease process and procedures. Encourage the expression of feelings of helplessness and anxiety, and help the patient identify coping mechanisms that have worked in other situations.

Impaired Physical Mobility

Improved physical mobility requires instruction in range-of-motion exercises and the development of a progressive exercise plan. This exercise plan usually is limited to 15 minutes, three times a day, for the initial days after surgery or treatment. The progression of exercise is determined by the individual patient's response.

Impaired Skin Integrity

With arterial embolism, the affected tissue is highly susceptible to injury. Protect the limb from pressure, trauma, and extreme heat or cold. Edematous tissue is equally susceptible to injury and must be protected.

Ineffective Therapeutic Regimen Management

Patient teaching enables the patient to participate in the plan of care during and after hospitalization. If the patient is on anticoagulant therapy, also see Patient Teaching Plan: Anticoagulant Therapy.

PATIENT TEACHING PLAN
Arterial Embolism

Discharge teaching should include:

- Protect affected limbs from pressure, trauma, and temperature extremes.
- Exercise improves blood flow; gradually increase your activity as you are able to tolerate it.
- Report pain, numbness, coolness, or pale or bluish skin color to your physician.

PERIPHERAL ARTERIAL OCCLUSIVE DISEASE

Pathophysiology

Peripheral arterial occlusive disease is called *atherosclerosis obliterans, arterial insufficiency,* and *peripheral vascular disease.* It is characterized by pathologic changes in the arteries, typically plaque formations that arise where the arteries branch, veer, arch, or narrow (Fig. 34-7). The most common sites for arterial occlusion are the distal superficial femoral and the popliteal arteries. Occlusions prevent the delivery of oxygen and nutrients to the tissues. Hypoxia affects all tissues distal to the occlusion. Peripheral nerves and muscles are more susceptible to harm from hypoxia than the skin and subcutaneous tissues. Severe oxygen deprivation may lead to ischemia and then to necrosis (tissue death).

Because peripheral arterial occlusive disease develops gradually, compensatory mechanisms attempt to maintain circulation. These compensatory mechanisms include the development of collateral blood vessels, vasodilation, and anaerobic metabolism. Collateral blood vessels are small, new vessels that branch out to supply blood to poorly perfused tissues. The extent of collateral circulation determines the severity of symptoms.

Peripheral arterial occlusive disease is most common in men older than 50 years of age. Factors that contribute to the development of this disease include atherosclerosis, embolism,

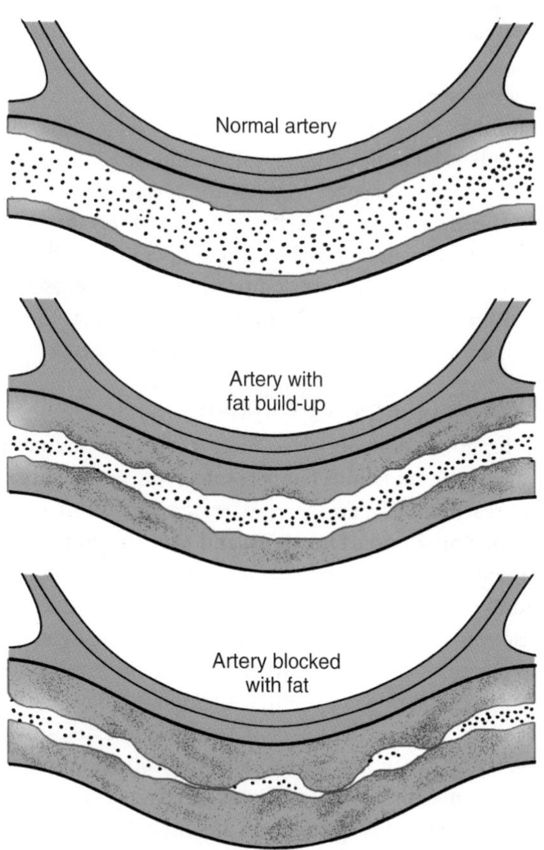

FIGURE **34-7** Development of atherosclerosis.

thrombosis, trauma, vasospasm, inflammation, and autoimmune responses. Other risk factors that are more controllable are hyperlipidemia, diabetes mellitus, hypertension, cigarette smoking, and stress.

Signs and Symptoms

The clinical manifestations of peripheral arterial occlusive disease develop gradually. Intermittent claudication is the classic sign. It is experienced as the aching, cramping, tiredness, and weakness in the legs that occurs with walking and is relieved by rest. Another manifestation of peripheral arterial occlusive disease is the absence of peripheral pulses below the occlusive area. Rest pain, pain that develops during rest, is common. Rest pain is described as persistent and aching. Complaints of tingling or numbness or both in the toes are common. The affected extremity is cold and numb owing to the reduction in the flow of blood to the area. Muscle atrophy may be evident. The skin of the affected area is pale because of reduced blood flow. When the extremity is in a dependent position, the color becomes red. Reduced blood supply to toenails can cause the nails to thicken. Other signs of arterial occlusion are shiny, scaly skin; subcutaneous tissue loss; hairlessness on the affected extremity; and ulcers with a pale gray or yellowish hue, especially at the ankles. If one extremity is affected more than the other, size differences between the extremities may be apparent.

Medical Diagnosis

The diagnostic tests used to confirm a diagnosis of peripheral arterial occlusive disease are Doppler ultrasonography, plethysmography, angiography, segmental limb pressures, pulse volume measurements, and exercise testing.

A lumbar sympathetic block is used at times to evaluate the peripheral circulation. A local anesthetic is injected into the lumbar epidural space to block the sympathetic innervation to the lower extremities. Blocking the nerves should produce vasodilation and an increase in temperature to the lower extremities. Vessels that are compromised by atherosclerotic changes are unable to dilate, a finding that supports the diagnosis of peripheral arterial occlusive vascular disease.

Medical and Surgical Treatment

Drug therapy may include vasodilators and the hemorrheologic agent pentoxifylline. Surgical interventions that are used in the treatment of peripheral arterial occlusive disease are sympathectomy, endarterectomy, and percutaneous transluminal angioplasty. A sympathectomy is used to increase the collateral circulation. An endarterectomy with a graft is the surgical replacement of a diseased segment of an artery with a graft of some type—either synthetic or from another blood vessel. Percutaneous transluminal angioplasty may be used to enlarge the interior diameter of the blood vessel. Possible complications with percutaneous transluminal angioplasty are hematoma formation, embolus, arterial dissection, and allergic reaction. These procedures are discussed earlier in this chapter.

NURSING CARE *of the Patient with Peripheral Arterial Occlusive Disease*

Assessment

Complete assessment of the patient with peripheral vascular disease is summarized in Table 34-1. When the patient has had surgical intervention, it is especially important to assess the pulses distal to the surgical site and compare them with the same pulses in the unaffected extremity. Cessation of a pulse suggests possible arterial occlusion, and the surgeon must be notified immediately. Other important aspects of the postoperative assessment are vital signs, color and temperature of the affected extremity, fluid intake and output, central venous pressure, and mental status. If the patient has pain, document the location, severity, and nature of the pain.

Nursing Diagnoses, Goals, and Outcome Criteria: Peripheral Arterial Occlusive Disease

Nursing Diagnoses	Goals and Outcome Criteria
Activity Intolerance related to impaired blood flow to extremities	Improved activity tolerance: patient states he or she is increasingly able to perform activities without pain
Chronic Pain related ischemia	Reduced pain: patient states his or her pain reduced, relaxed manner
Impaired Skin Integrity related to inadequate circulation	Healthy skin: skin intact with normal color and warmth
Disturbed Body Image related to muscle atrophy, stasis ulcers, and skin discoloration	Positive body image: positive patient statements about self, patient makes effort to maintain good physical appearance
Ineffective Tissue Perfusion related to vascular occlusion	Adequate tissue perfusion: palpable peripheral pulses, extremity warm with normal skin color
Ineffective Therapeutic Regimen Management related to lack of knowledge of disease process, treatment, and self-care	Patient carries out proper self-care measures: patient describes and demonstrates self-care

If surgical intervention is performed, additional diagnoses and goals may include the following:

Nursing Diagnoses	Goals and Outcome Criteria
Risk for Infection related to surgical incision, graft placement	Absence of infection: normal body temperature, decreasing wound redness and drainage
Decreased Cardiac Output related to hemorrhage, diuresis, fluid shifts	Normal cardiac output: pulse and blood pressure consistent with patient norms

Ineffective Tissue Perfusion related to graft thrombosis	Patent graft: operative extremity warm, with improved color and palpable pulses
Acute Pain related to surgical incision	Pain relief: patient relaxed, states that pain is relieved
Impaired Physical Mobility related to weakness, fear, surgical procedure	Increased physical mobility: increasing activity without pain

Interventions

Activity Intolerance

To monitor the patient's activity tolerance, assess the patient before, during, and after planned activities. Then monitor progress as treatment progresses. When planning an exercise regimen, use the following guidelines:

1. Work with the patient to plan the activity schedule and goals.
2. Gradually increase the exercise time as tolerance increases.
3. Discontinue activity if the patient has chest pain, bradycardia, dyspnea, or intermittent claudication. After rest relieves the pain of intermittent claudication, the patient may resume activity.
4. Reduce the intensity of the activity if the pulse takes longer than 3 to 4 minutes to return to the baseline rate or if the patient has severe dyspnea.
5. For patients confined to bed, start exercises with range-of-motion exercises twice daily.
6. Patients should *not* exercise when they have leg ulcers, cellulitis, deep vein thrombosis, or gangrene.

Chronic Pain. The chronic pain associated with ischemia is exhausting and greatly reduces the patient's quality of life. Therefore pain management must be a priority. The most direct interventions are those that increase circulation or decrease metabolic demands of ischemic tissues. Resting the extremities in a dependent position may help relieve the pain of arterial occlusive disease. Administer analgesics as prescribed, along with other comfort measures. Nonpharmacologic pain relief measures include relaxation techniques, warm baths, breathing exercises, and backrubs. See Chapter 14 for a detailed discussion of pain management.

Impaired Skin Integrity. The nursing interventions for maintaining skin integrity are the same as those for patients with arterial embolism. To maintain skin integrity, take measures to improve circulation and avoid tissue trauma. If ulcers develop, bedrest is usually prescribed. Keep the ulcerated area clean and free of pressure. Treatment protocols vary but may include wet to damp dressings, whirlpool therapy, and surgical debridement followed by the application of occlusive dressings.

The feet are especially susceptible to injury and require special care. Advise the patient not to go barefoot, to wear only shoes that fit properly, to inspect the feet daily for signs of pressure or lesions, and to keep the toenails neatly trimmed. Because of the risk of ingrown nails, nails should not be trimmed too short. Toenails should always be cut straight across rather than in a curved shape. The patient should see a peripheral vascular specialist promptly if any foot problems develop.

Ineffective Therapeutic Regimen Management. To cope with peripheral arterial occlusive disease, the patient must understand the disease process and treatment. Include the family in patient teaching because their fears and concerns can have an enormous impact on the patient's perception of the situation. The patient teaching plan is the same as for the patient with arterial embolism.

Disturbed Body Image. Encourage the patient to express feelings that result from problems associated with peripheral arterial occlusive disease, such as activity intolerance, stasis ulcers, discoloration of the extremities, and, for some, amputations. Be supportive and help the patient identify coping strategies to deal with the feelings.

Ineffective Tissue Perfusion. Administer vasodilators and other drugs that improve blood flow as ordered. Encourage exercise according to the individualized exercise plan. Maintain adequate warmth, and discourage smoking. Elevation of the extremities usually is *not* recommended with arterial disease.

Additional interventions are indicated for the postoperative patient.

Risk for Infection. After surgery, patients are at risk for infection of the surgical incision and the grafts (especially synthetic grafts) that are used to replace the diseased blood vessel. An infected synthetic graft is very serious because it necessitates removal of the graft and often amputation. Monitor the patient's temperature and report fever to the surgeon. Inspect the incision for increasing redness, edema, and drainage that suggest infection. Antimicrobials are usually ordered before surgery and may be continued after surgery.

Decreased Cardiac Output. Monitor for signs and symptoms of deficient fluid volume: tachycardia, restlessness, decreased urine output, pallor, and hypotension. Provide intravenous and oral fluids as ordered, and keep records of fluid intake and output. Monitor daily weights. Inspect the surgical dressing for bleeding, which must be reported immediately to the surgeon.

Ineffective Tissue Perfusion. Thrombus formation can occur in the graft, causing occlusion and impaired blood flow. Monitor the pulses, warmth, and color of the operative extremity and promptly inform the surgeon of diminishing pulses, coolness, and pallor or cyanosis. Some patients are given anticoagulants or thrombolytics to decrease the risk of graft occlusion. Edema for 4 to 8 weeks is common after bypass surgery. The leg is usually wrapped in a light dressing or vascular boot and kept flat initially. Elastic stockings are not used immediately after a vein graft.

Consider the Alternative!

Relaxation, warm baths, breathing exercises, and backrubs can help the patient with chronic pain.

Pain. Acute postoperative pain is treated with analgesics, positioning, and relaxation techniques as described in Chapters 14 and 16.

Impaired Physical Mobility. After surgery, the patient's activities are increased gradually. A specific program of exercises may be prescribed. Assist the patient and assess muscle strength and tolerance of activity.

THROMBOANGIITIS OBLITERANS

Thromboangiitis obliterans, also called Buerger's disease, is an inflammatory thrombotic disorder of arteries and veins in both the lower and upper extremities. It is not an atherosclerotic process. The exact cause is unknown, but it occurs only in smokers. Signs and symptoms may include intermittent claudication, rest pain, skin color and temperature changes in affected areas, cold sensitivity, abnormal sensation, ulceration, and gangrene. Diagnosis is based on physical findings and arteriography.

The most important aspect of treatment is smoking cessation. Palliative treatments include sympathectomy and drugs such as calcium channel blockers, antibiotics, and anticoagulants. If gangrene develops (most commonly below the knee), amputation is the only option. Forty percent of patients who continue tobacco use eventually require amputations. Nursing care is similar to that of patients with peripheral arterial occlusive disorders. Emphasis is on smoking cessation measures (see Chapter 30) and protection of the affected extremities.

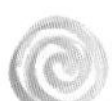

What Does Culture Have to do with Buerger's Disease?

Buerger's disease is very common in India, Korea, and Japan. It is relatively uncommon in the U.S. When assessing patients, especially those of Indian, Korean, or Japanese heritage, be alert for related signs and symptoms.

RAYNAUD'S DISEASE

Pathophysiology

Raynaud's disease and phenomenon are forms of an intermittent constriction of arterioles that affects the hands primarily, although it can affect the toes and tip of the nose. Increased or unusual sensations of coldness, pain, and pallor reflect temporary constriction of the arterioles in the affected areas. Gangrene is not common but can develop in the skin on the tips of the digits. The cause of this condition is unknown, but it may be related to hypersensitivity to cold or release of serotonin. Women from the ages of 16 to 40 years are primarily affected, especially during the winter months or in northern areas where cold weather is more common. Stress seems to aggravate the disease process. Raynaud's phenomenon follows the same general pattern but is typically secondary to connective tissue or collagen vascular disease. The term primary Raynaud's phenomenon is synonymous with Raynaud's disease; secondary Raynaud's phenomenon is also called simply Raynaud's phenomenon.

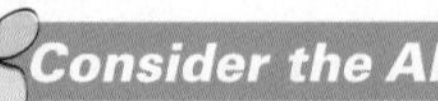

Consider the Alternative!

Biofeedback is sometimes helpful in controlling vasospastic episodes with Raynaud's disease.

Signs and Symptoms

The cardinal signs and symptoms of Raynaud's disease are chronically cold hands, numbness, tingling, and pallor. Finger involvement is not symmetric, and the thumb is not usually affected. During an arterial spasm the skin color changes from pallor to cyanosis to redness. Pallor is the result of sudden vasoconstriction. Cyanosis reflects inadequate oxygenation. As the spasm resolves, vasodilation allows blood flow to return, which produces a red color.

Medical Diagnosis

The diagnosis of Raynaud's disease is usually based on the signs and symptoms and on the absence of evidence of occlusive vascular disease.

Medical and Surgical Treatment

The goals of the medical treatment plan for Raynaud's disease are to prevent pain and to promote vasodilation in the extremities. The primary drugs used are vasodilators, including calcium antagonists, angiotensin-converting enzyme inhibitors, alpha-adrenergic blockers, and sympatholytic agents. Intravenous prostacyclin and topical nitroglycerin have also been used with good results in some patients. Recently, liothyronine has been used to induce hyperthyroidism, which results in vasodilation in the skin. At times the physician may resort to sympathectomy to interrupt the sympathetic nerves. This surgical procedure aids some patients but tends to have temporary effects and is not used routinely.

NURSING CARE *of the Patient with Raynaud's Disease*

Assessment

Assessment of the patient with peripheral vascular disease is summarized in Table 34-1. With Raynaud's disease, assessment of the hands is the priority.

Nursing Diagnoses, Goals, and Outcome Criteria: Raynaud's Disease

Nursing Diagnoses	Goals and Outcome Criteria
Acute Pain related to the ischemia that develops from vasoconstriction	Reduced pain: patient states that his or her pain has decreased, appears relaxed
Ineffective Tissue Perfusion related to vasoconstriction	Improved oxygenation of peripheral tissues: improved warmth and color of affected areas
Fear related to the potential loss of work, difficulty performing activities of daily living	Relief from fear: patient states fear is reduced, appears more relaxed

Interventions

Pain and Ineffective Tissue Perfusion

Nursing interventions to reduce pain and improve tissue perfusion focus on teaching the patient to avoid the stimuli that cause the vasoconstriction: exposure to cold, smoking, and excessive stress. Encourage the patient to take part in a smoking cessation program and to dress warmly when going out in cold weather. Mittens are better than gloves for maintaining warmth. Sometimes the patient can interrupt an acute attack by placing the affected parts in warm water or by using a hair dryer or hand- and foot-warming devices.

Pain can be managed by carefully warming the area when vasoconstriction occurs. However, the affected areas must be protected from trauma. Do not use hot water to warm affected tissue because the lack of sensation during the period of vasoconstriction could result in serious burns.

Fear. Fear can be addressed in much the same manner as anxiety. Attempt to determine the actual cause of fear, which might be loss of work, loss of limb, or pain. Accept and explore the patient's feelings, provide factual information, encourage problem solving, and help the patient learn to live with the condition and to manage the prescribed therapy.

ANEURYSMS

Pathophysiology

An aneurysm is a dilated segment of an artery caused by weakness and stretching of the arterial wall. Aneurysms can be congenital or acquired. Conditions associated with congenital aneurysms are Marfan's syndrome and Ehlers-Danlos syndrome. Acquired aneurysms can be caused by arteriosclerosis, trauma, or infection. The most common cause of aneurysms is atherosclerosis. Hypertension is apparently a contributing factor. The effect of atherosclerosis on the media, the middle layer of the arterial wall, is to weaken elastic fibers, which allows a segment of the vessel to balloon out. Infections, including syphilis, can also damage the media and result in the formation of aneurysms. The abdominal aorta is the most common site of aneurysm formation.

Signs and Symptoms

Signs and symptoms, if any, vary with the location of the aneurysm. People with thoracic aneurysms usually have no symptoms, though some report deep, diffuse chest pain. If the aneurysm puts pressure on the recurrent laryngeal nerve, the patient may complain of hoarseness. Pressure on the esophagus may cause dysphagia (difficulty swallowing). If the superior vena cava is compressed, the patient may have edema of the head and arms. Signs of airway obstruction may be present if the aneurysm presses against pulmonary structures.

Abdominal aneurysms are usually detected during routine physical examinations or radiologic studies. The aneurysm may be palpated as a pulsating mass in the area slightly left of the umbilicus. Although most abdominal aneurysms are asymptomatic, pressure on abdominal organs and nerves may cause back pain, epigastric pain, or constipation.

Complications

Complications of aneurysms include rupture, thrombus formation that obstructs blood flow, emboli, and pressure on surrounding structures.

Medical Diagnosis

Diagnosis is made on the basis of physical findings and radiologic studies. Studies performed to obtain better visualization of the aneurysm include echocardiography, ultrasonography, computed tomography, and aortography.

Medical and Surgical Treatment

Repair of aneurysms may be done by replacing the dilated segment of the artery with a synthetic graft or, in some cases, by suturing or patching the defective area. Repair is usually done as soon as possible but may be delayed until the patient is evaluated for other problems that increase surgical risk.

Decisions to attempt repair of aneurysms are based on the size of the defect and the patient's general status. For example, an abdominal aortic aneurysm smaller than 5 cm is usually monitored with periodic ultrasound studies. If it begins to enlarge, surgical repair may then be recommended.

Complications of aneurysm surgery vary with the location of the defect. Complications of aortic abdominal aneurysm surgery include myocardial infarction, sexual dysfunction, renal failure, emboli, spinal cord ischemia with paralysis, bowel and bladder incontinence, and impaired sensation.

PREOPERATIVE NURSING CARE

When surgical repair of an aneurysm is planned, prepare the patient physically and emotionally as described in Chapter 16. It is important to document chronic conditions such as emphysema or heart disease that increase the risk of postoperative complications.

POSTOPERATIVE NURSING CARE

After aortic aneurysm repair, the patient is usually kept in a critical care area for 24 to 48 hours. Mechanical ventilation may be used initially to maintain good oxygenation status.

Assessment

General postoperative assessment is outlined in Table 16-4. Assessment after repair of an aortic aneurysm focuses on vital signs, hemodynamic monitoring, renal function, and fluid balance. Assess the extremities for color, warmth, and peripheral pulses.

Nursing Diagnoses, Goals, and Outcome Criteria: Aortic Aneurysm Repair

In addition to the routine problems of the postoperative patient (see Chapter 16), nursing diagnoses for the patient who has had an aortic aneurysm repair may include the following:

Nursing Diagnoses	Goals and Outcome Criteria
Impaired Urinary Elimination related to interrupted blood flow	Normal urinary function: urine output approximately equal to fluid intake

Nursing Diagnoses, Goals, and Outcome Criteria: Aortic Aneurysm Repair—cont'd

Nursing Diagnoses	Goals and Outcome Criteria
Risk for Injury related to ileus	Absence of injury related to ileus: wound margins intact, no abdominal distention, bowel sounds present
Ineffective Breathing Patterns related to abdominal incision or splinting	Effective breathing patterns: regular respirations, 12 to 20/min, clear breath sounds
Decreased Cardiac Output related to myocardial infarction, occlusion of blood vessels, graft leakage	Adequate cardiac output: pulse and blood pressure consistent with patient norms
Ineffective Tissue Perfusion related to vascular occlusion	Normal peripheral circulation: warm extremities with palpable pulses

Interventions

Impaired Urinary Elimination

During repair of an abdominal aneurysm, the aorta is clamped for a period of time. This poses a risk of renal damage and subsequent renal failure. Therefore you must measure and record fluid intake and urine output hourly. Report declining urine output to the physician. Blood urea nitrogen, creatinine, and electrolyte levels are usually assessed daily to detect increases associated with renal failure. Assess for edema, which may be caused by fluid retention or by circulatory obstruction. Administer intravenous fluids as ordered.

Risk for Injury

After abdominal surgery, peristalsis ceases temporarily. A nasogastric tube is usually inserted and attached to suction to prevent gaseous distention of the bowel, which is uncomfortable and places stress on the abdominal incision. Be sure the suction is working properly and monitor for distention and the return of bowel sounds.

Ineffective Breathing Patterns

Whether the patient has an abdominal or a thoracic incision, there is a risk of poor lung expansion. After thoracic surgery, patients are at especially high risk for atelectasis and pneumonia. Mechanical ventilation in the immediate postoperative period maintains adequate ventilation until the patient is able to breathe effectively. Thereafter, assist the patient to turn, deep breathe, and cough frequently. An incentive spirometer may be used to encourage lung expansion. Support the patient's incision during the breathing exercises. Administer analgesics and use other pain relief measures. The patient can breathe more effectively if good pain relief is achieved. Monitor lung sounds frequently to assess for abnormalities.

Decreased Cardiac Output

Cardiac output may fall as a result of myocardial infarction, cardiac dysrhythmias, heart failure, or hemorrhage. Hemorrhage may occur in the incision or by separation of the graft. Closely monitor the patient's vital signs and hemodynamics. Assess the wound dressing and drains for increasing bleeding. Early signs of circulatory failure are restlessness and tachycardia. Later signs are hypotension, cyanosis, and decreased alertness. Immediately notify the physician if there is evidence of decreasing cardiac output.

Ineffective Tissue Perfusion

There is a risk of impaired blood flow below the level of the aneurysm. Monitor peripheral pulses and the color and warmth of the extremities. This assessment is especially important when a patient has had a femoral or popliteal aneurysm repair. Signs and symptoms of occlusion include pain, pallor or cyanosis, and coldness distal to the repair. If these manifestations occur, they must be reported to the physician at once.

AORTIC DISSECTION

Aortic dissection is different from an aneurysm. A small tear in the intima permits blood to escape into the space between the intima and the media. Blood accumulates between the layers, possibly causing the media to split lengthwise. The split may extend up and down the aorta, where it can occlude major arteries. If no complications occur, the patient may be managed with antihypertensives and drugs to decrease the strength of cardiac contractions. Otherwise, the affected area is replaced with a synthetic graft. A key aspect of postoperative care is keeping the blood pressure at the lowest possible level. In other respects, the care is similar to that of a patient who has had an aneurysm repair.

VARICOSE VEIN DISEASE

Pathophysiology

Varicose veins are referred to as *varicosities.* Varicosities are dilated, tortuous, superficial veins, often the saphenous veins in the lower extremities (Fig. 34-8). The dilation of the vessels results from incompetent valves in the veins—that is, the valves cannot prevent backflow of blood. Vein incompetence is a result of hereditary weakness, aging, pregnancy, obesity, occupations requiring prolonged standing, or a combination of these. Restrictive clothing aggravates the condition. Varicose veins are classified as primary (only superficial veins are affected) and secondary (characterized by deep vein obstruction). In addition to peripheral veins, varicosities can occur in other areas such as the esophageal and hemorrhoidal veins. Incompetent valves cannot be repaired.

Signs and Symptoms

The onset of varicose vein disease is gradual, but the condition is progressive. When only the superficial veins are involved, the signs and symptoms are minimal except for the cosmetic changes that occur. The dilated veins are seen as oversized, discolored (purplish), and tortuous. Symptoms typically include dull aching sensations when standing or walking, a feeling of heaviness in the affected legs, muscle cramps, especially at night, increased muscular fatigue in the

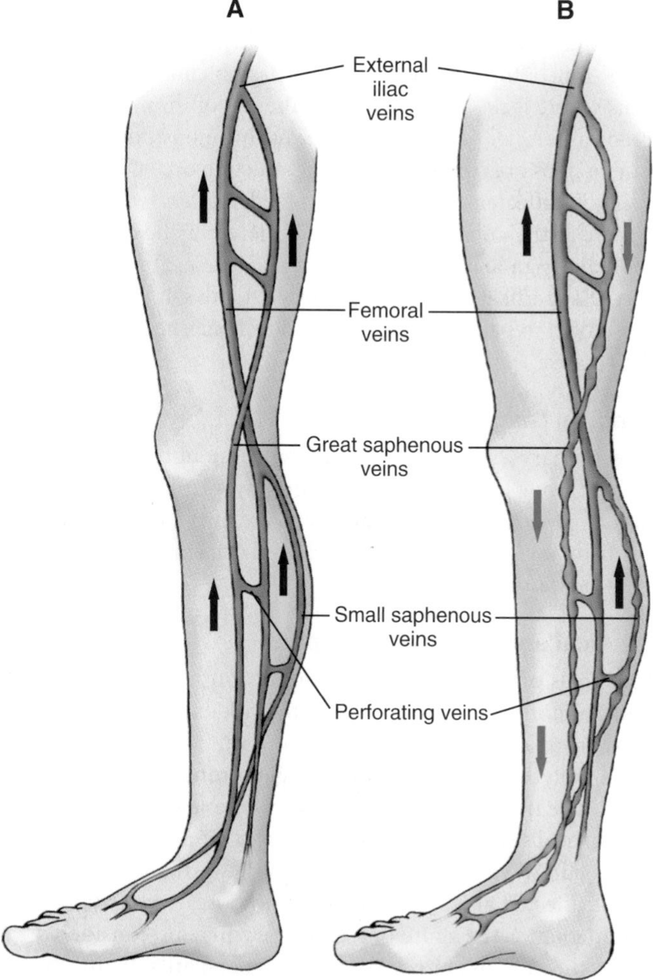

FIGURE 34-8 Venous return from the legs. *A,* Normal flow. *B,* Varicosities and retrograde venous flow.

affected area, and ankle edema. Over time, some people develop postphlebitic syndrome, which is evidenced by persistent edema, brownish skin discoloration, and ulcers most commonly on the inner aspect of the ankle.

Medical Diagnosis

The diagnosis of varicose veins may be based on plethysmography, lower limb venography, Doppler ultrasonography, and the Brodie-Trendelenburg test. The Brodie-Trendelenburg test demonstrates the backward flow of blood in the venous system. The patient is asked to lie down with the affected leg elevated to accommodate emptying of the blood from the vessels. A soft tourniquet is positioned around the upper thigh to restrict the veins. The patient is asked to stand and walk around. The response of the vessels before and after the release of the tourniquet demonstrates to the health care provider the extent of the incompetent valves located in the deep veins and the superficial vessels. Information about other diagnostic tests and procedures is presented in Table 34-2.

Medical and Surgical Treatment

Conservative treatments of varicosities are used whenever possible. Encourage the patient to avoid restrictive garments, prolonged standing or sitting, crossing the legs or knees, and injury to the compromised areas. Inform the obese patient that weight reduction usually reduces pressure on the lower extremities. If the physician recommends support stockings, help the patient learn how to put them on correctly.

When surgery is necessary, sclerotherapy, ligation and stripping, or both are done. Surgery may be recommended for cosmetic reasons or if stasis ulcers develop.

NURSING CARE *of the Patient with Varicose Vein Disease*

Assessment

When a patient has varicose veins, the health history determines the presence of pain, edema, cramps, and muscle fatigue. Note a family history of varicose veins. Document the patient's occupation and usual activities. When taking a pain and discomfort history, determine what measures the patient has used for pain control. The physical examination focuses on inspection of the legs for color, edema, turgor, and capillary refill. Palpate the legs for tenderness. Postoperative assessment is especially concerned with monitoring peripheral circulation and tissue perfusion.

Nursing Diagnoses, Goals, and Outcome Criteria: Varicose Veins

NURSING DIAGNOSES	GOALS AND OUTCOME CRITERIA
Pain related to engorgement of the veins	Reduced pain: patient states that pain with activity has decreased
Activity Intolerance related to feelings of heaviness and fatigue	Improved activity tolerance: gradual increase in activity with less discomfort
Ineffective Therapeutic Regimen Management related to management of the varicosities	Patient carries out appropriate self-care: patient correctly verbalizes and demonstrates self-care

Interventions

The primary nursing role in the care of the patient with varicose veins is teaching self-care. Interventions to improve activity tolerance and to manage pain are outlined in the patient teaching plan. In general, measures that improve venous return also decrease pain.

For the surgical patient, patient teaching also is of paramount importance because the procedure is often done as a same-day surgical procedure. While the patient is still in the surgical suite, pressure bandages are placed on the extremities. The surgeon orders specific aspects of postoperative care such as when the pressure bandages should be removed, what types of stockings are recommended afterwards and how long they should be worn, activity restrictions, and positioning of the legs (usually 15-30 degrees for the first 24 hours).

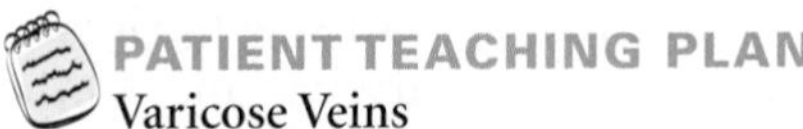

PATIENT TEACHING PLAN
Varicose Veins

- Wear antiembolism hose or support hose as recommended by your physician.
- Exercise regularly to promote circulation.
- Avoid prolonged standing, sitting, crossing your legs.
- Avoid restrictive clothing.
- Elevate extremities whenever possible.
- Obesity contributes to the development of varicose veins. People who are overweight usually see improvement with weight loss.
- Nonprescription analgesics and frequent position changes usually control pain.

VENOUS THROMBOSIS

Pathophysiology

The terms *phlebitis, thrombophlebitis, phlebothrombosis,* and *deep vein thrombosis* are often used interchangeably. Each term in reality describes a slightly different process. Phlebitis is an inflammation of the vein wall. With thrombophlebitis, a clot has formed at the site of inflammation within a vein. Phlebothrombosis describes the presence of a thrombus in a vein as a result of stasis, deviation of the intima, or hypercoagulability (an abnormally increased tendency of blood to clot). Deep vein thrombosis (DVT) refers to the presence of a clot in one of the deep veins rather than in the superficial vessels. The deep veins commonly involved with thrombi are the femoral, popliteal, and small calf veins. A grave complication of deep vein thrombosis is a pulmonary embolism. The superficial vein that is most often the site of thrombus formation is the saphenous vein.

Risk Factors

Some of the risk factors that may predispose a person to the development of thrombi are the following:

1. Prescribed bedrest
2. Surgery under general anesthesia for people older than 40 years of age
3. Leg trauma resulting in immobilization from casts or traction
4. Previous venous insufficiency
5. Obesity
6. Use of oral contraceptives
7. Malignancy

Research has identified three factors (called *Virchow's triad*) that contribute to venous thrombus formation: (1) stasis of the blood, (2) damage to the vessel walls, and (3) hypercoagulability. At least two of the three factors must be present for a thrombus to form.

Signs and Symptoms

The signs and symptoms of each of the disease processes are slightly different, depending on the diagnosis, the size and location of the thrombus, the amount of obstruction, the collateral circulation, and the existence of other medical problems. Phlebothrombosis frequently has no clinical signs because there is no inflammation at the site of thrombosis. As many as 50% of patients with venous thrombosis display no visible signs or symptoms. When obstruction occurs in a deep vein, the affected extremity may be edematous, warm, and tender at the area of compromise; there may be a positive Homans' sign and prominent superficial veins. In comparison, if superficial vessels are obstructed, the symptoms may be limited to pain, redness, warmth, or tenderness in the affected area.

Medical Diagnosis

The primary diagnostic examinations used in the detection of thrombus formation are venography, plethysmography, and Doppler ultrasound. These tests are instrumental in the confirmation of the disease process and determination of the treatment plan.

Medical and Surgical Treatment

The goals of treatment are to prevent thrombus extension and pulmonary emboli, to reduce the risk of further thrombus formation, and to reduce discomfort. Anticoagulant or thrombolytic therapy, or both, is begun promptly after diagnosis. The treatment plan typically includes patient teaching about the disease; the ongoing assessment for pulmonary emboli; bedrest; elevation of the extremity; warm, moist soaks to the affected area; and antiembolism hose. Ambulation is initiated after the acute phase. Surgery may be considered when the patient cannot receive anticoagulants or thrombolytic therapy or when the possibility of pulmonary emboli is high.

NURSING CARE *of the Patient with Venous Thrombosis*

Assessment

Assessment of the patient with peripheral vascular disease is summarized in Table 34-1.

Nursing Diagnoses, Goals, and Outcome Criteria: Phlebitis, Thrombophlebitis, Phlebothrombosis, and Deep Vein Thrombosis

Nursing Diagnoses	Goals and Outcome Criteria
Impaired Skin Integrity related to venous stasis	Intact skin: absence of redness, rash, pallor, lesions
Acute Pain related to impaired circulation and tissue ischemia	Pain relief: patient verbalizes pain relief, relaxed manner
Anxiety related to hospitalization and uncertainty of disease process	Reduced anxiety: patient states that anxiety is reduced, calm manner
Activity Intolerance related to leg pain or swelling	Improved activity tolerance: increasing activity without pain
Ineffective Tissue Perfusion related to impaired peripheral circulation	Adequate tissue perfusion: pulses present and symmetric, normal skin color and warmth

Impaired Gas Exchange related to pulmonary emboli	Normal gas exchange: respiratory rate consistent with patient norms, no dyspnea or chest pain
Ineffective Therapeutic Regimen Management related to the developing disease process, treatment, self-care	Patient adheres to prescribed plan of care: correctly describes and demonstrates self-medication, exercises, and precautions

Interventions

Impaired Skin Integrity

Maintaining intact skin is a priority. Carefully inspect the skin to detect early signs of breakdown. Compare the extremities for symmetry in color, warmth, pulses, and circumference. Elevate affected extremities to promote venous return and improve circulation to the area. Because edematous tissue is easily injured and heals poorly, it must be protected from trauma, including pressure.

Pain. The patient's pain must be reduced before activity tolerance can improve. Administer analgesics as prescribed. Implement other prescribed comfort measures such as warm, moist soaks and elevation of the extremity. Massage is contraindicated because it may dislodge a thrombus. A "traveling" blood clot is called an embolus. It is very dangerous because it can obstruct blood flow with serious effects including a potentially fatal pulmonary embolism.

Anxiety. Anxiety may be related to lack of knowledge about the disease and its treatment and by concerns about the effects of the condition on employment, activities of daily living, and quality of life. The patient may even restrict activities out of fear of pain. The relief of anxiety can help the patient move toward an acceptable level of activity. Anxiety can be reduced by helping the patient understand the condition and how it best can be managed.

Activity Intolerance. Because inactivity aggravates venous thrombosis, make an effort to get the inactive patient mobile again as soon as permitted. Work with the patient to establish a realistic exercise or activity plan. The plan should begin at the patient's current level and slowly add activities over a period of several weeks. Instruct the patient to stop any activity temporarily if pain occurs. Once the pain subsides, the activity may be continued.

Ineffective Tissue Perfusion. Improved peripheral circulation aids in tissue perfusion, which decreases pain, improves skin integrity, reduces anxiety, and increases physical activity. Administer prescribed anticoagulants or platelet aggregation inhibitors to prevent new clots or thrombolytics to dissolve existing clots and reestablish blood flow to the affected area. Check blood test results before giving anticoagulants and take action according to agency policy. Apply warm, moist packs to the affected area as ordered to improve circulation. Assist the patient in the placement of antiembolism hose to prevent stasis and improve circulation. Explain how stress reduction and smoking cessation also improve tissue perfusion by reducing vasoconstriction.

Impaired Gas Exchange. The possibility of a pulmonary embolus developing during the treatment of venous thrombosis is an ever-present threat. When an embolus lodges in the lung, the affected blood vessels can no longer exchange gases. Pressure builds in vessels behind the embolus. Symptoms of pulmonary embolism depend on the amount of tissue affected. Small emboli may produce no symptoms. Larger emboli can cause dyspnea, chest pain, tachycardia, cough, fever, anxiety, and a change in mental status. A massive embolus can cause heart failure and shock. Sixty percent of people do not survive massive emboli.

To improve oxygenation when a patient has a pulmonary embolism, elevate the head of the bed to a 45-degree angle and administer oxygen as ordered. Monitor and document any changes in the patient's respiratory pattern, address anxiety, teach the patient deep breathing and coughing techniques, and assist with position changes every 2 hours. Administer drugs as ordered to dissolve existing clots and prevent future clots. Surgical removal of the clot, called pulmonary embolectomy, is sometimes indicated.

Ineffective Therapeutic Regimen Management. To follow the long-term plan of care, the patient must understand the condition and how it best can be managed. Once the acute process has resolved, discharge planning must include patient teaching as outlined below. If the patient is on anticoagulant therapy, also see Patient Teaching Plan: Anticoagulant Therapy.

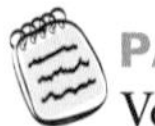

PATIENT TEACHING PLAN
Venous Thrombosis

- Protect your legs from pressure and trauma.
- Elevate your legs when sitting to improve circulation.
- Do not massage or rub affected areas.
- Gradually increase your activity; slow down or stop if you have pain during activity.
- Avoid prolonged standing and crossing your legs.
- Notify your physician if you have any chest pain or shortness of breath.

CHRONIC VENOUS INSUFFICIENCY

Pathophysiology

Chronic venous insufficiency is the culmination of longstanding venous hypertension that stretches the veins and damages the valves. Elevated venous pressure causes edema, primarily around the ankles. Red blood cells seep into the tissues and combine with metabolic wastes to impart a brownish color, called stasis dermatitis, around the ankles. Ulcers may form because of the pressure exerted by edema or as a result of trauma. The ulcers most often develop on the medial malleolus (the prominent bone on the inner aspect of the ankle). Because of the poor circulation, the ulcers are very resistant to healing and susceptible to infection. Some ulcers eventually necessitate amputation.

Signs and Symptoms

Signs and symptoms of chronic venous insufficiency include edema around the lower legs, pain, brownish skin discoloration (stasis dermatitis), and stasis ulcerations. Patients often describe pain as "heaviness" or "dull ache" in the calf or thigh. The skin temperature is cool, and nails are normal. Peripheral pulses are present but may be difficult to palpate because of the edema. The feet and ankles often are cyanotic when in a dependent position.

Medical Diagnosis

Noninvasive screening is done with Doppler ultrasonography and plethysmography to confirm the diagnosis of chronic venous insufficiency. A culture may be ordered to determine the infectious agent if the stasis ulcer is draining.

Medical and Surgical Treatment

The medical management of stasis ulcerations is constantly changing. Among the many options you may see ordered to promote venous return are elastic or compression stockings and pneumatic compression devices. If the patient has an ulcer, treatment may include special dressings, systemic antibiotics, topical debriding agents such as Elase, and Unna boots. There is disagreement as to whether oxygen-permeable (e.g., Op Site) or oxygen-impermeable dressings (e.g., DuoDerm) are superior, so you may see either used. Unna boots are medicated dressings used to allow the patient to be ambulatory while protecting the ulcer in a sterile environment. Infected ulcers are treated with systemic antibiotics, which are more effective than topical ointments. Surgery is rarely employed with chronic venous stasis because it is seldom successful. Hyperbaric oxygen therapy may be prescribed in an attempt to promote healing of the ulcer by reducing capillary pressure and hyperoxygenating the blood. The overall goal for medical management of ulcerations is to preserve the extremity by stimulating granulation tissue in the ulcer.

NURSING CARE *of the Patient with Chronic Venous Insufficiency*

Assessment

The complete general assessment of peripheral vascular status is summarized in Table 34-1. When the patient has chronic venous insufficiency, it is especially important to inspect the lower extremities for rubor and stasis dermatitis, palpate skin temperature, assess for Homans' sign, and determine the presence of pain in the affected extremity (see Nursing Care Plan: The Patient with a Venous Stasis Ulcer).

Nursing Diagnoses, Goals, and Outcome Criteria: Chronic Venous Insufficiency

Nursing Diagnoses	Goals and Outcome Criteria
Ineffective Tissue Perfusion related to reduced vascular circulation	Improved peripheral circulation and venous return: absence of edema and lesions, improved skin color
Disturbed Body Image related to chronic, open stasis ulcerations	Patient adapts to changes in appearance: patient expresses concerns about changes, makes effort to maintain/improve appearance
Risk for Infection related to compromised circulation and impaired skin integrity	Absence of infections: normal body temperature, absence of local redness or drainage
Impaired Skin Integrity related to stasis dermatitis and ulcerations	Restored skin integrity: skin intact in affected areas

Interventions

Ineffective Tissue Perfusion

To improve circulation in areas of compromised vascular function, the patient should elevate the legs whenever sitting and should wear antiembolism stockings. The patient should avoid standing still, crossing the legs, and wearing restrictive clothing, especially socks or hose with tight, narrow bands.

Disturbed Body Image

Encourage the patient to share feelings about body image changes. Be accepting and supportive. Encourage the patient to pay attention to grooming. Discuss strategies for concealing ulcers and discolored extremities.

Risk for Infection

Carefully monitor for signs of infection such as elevated temperature, chills, general malaise, and localized redness, pain, and purulent drainage. Teach the patient thorough hand washing, good hygiene, and appropriate wound care. The fragile edematous tissue also must be protected from trauma to avoid creating portals for pathogens.

Impaired Skin Integrity

Assess for dermatitis and ulcerations. Patient education is critical because these ulcerations are frequently treated on an outpatient basis. Instruct the patient and family in the management of the ulcerations while in the home setting. A referral for home health care may be appropriate.

LYMPHANGITIS

Pathophysiology

Lymphangitis is acute inflammation of the lymphatic channels. The inflammation is the result of an infectious process in the lower extremities. Streptococcus is an infectious agent commonly implicated in lymphangitis.

Signs and Symptoms

The primary characteristic of lymphangitis is enlargement of the lymph nodes along the lymphatic channel. Each node can be palpated along the course of the channel. The patient complains of tenderness as these nodes are assessed. A red streak from the infected wound extends up the extremity along the path of the lymphatics, as each node drains into the lymphatic system and the cardiovascular system. These nodes are located in the groin, the axilla, and the cervical regions. The symptoms of a generalized infection—elevated temperature and chills—are present. The infectious material can localize into an abscess with necrotic, suppurative discharge from the area.

NURSING CARE PLAN

The Patient with a Venous Stasis Ulcer

ASSESSMENT

Health History: DeWayne Barry is a 75-year-old man who is being seen in the community clinic for an ulcer on the medial malleolus of the right ankle. The ulcer is shallow and measures 1.5 × 2.5 cm. He describes a "heavy" burning sensation in the lower legs. He worked for many years as a toll booth attendant and has had chronic venous insufficiency for 5 years. He reports having had hypertension in the past but is taking no medication for it. Otherwise he has been in good health and remains active. He is the caregiver for his wife, who has been disabled for 3 years because of a stroke. He has a daughter who helps with her care and who has been dressing the leg ulcer.

Physical Examination: Vital signs: temperature, 97° F orally; pulse, 64; respiration, 16; blood pressure, 194/102. Alert and oriented. Walks with slight limp. 1+ edema both ankles. Varicosities noted in both legs. Stasis dermatitis in ankles and calves. Ulcer is 1.5 × 2.5 cm and shallow. The ulcer is slightly moist, pink, with no drainage or odor. Ankles and feet are cooler than calves. Pedal pulses faint but palpable, slightly stronger in left foot.

Nursing Diagnosis	*Goals and Outcome Criteria*	*Interventions*
Altered tissue perfusion related to compromised circulation.	Tissue perfusion will improve as evidenced by reduced pain, redness, and edema; skin warm to touch.	Instruct the patient in measures to improve circulation: exercise moderately each day, elevate the legs above the level of the heart when resting, avoid smoking, use support stockings as ordered, avoid prolonged periods of walking or standing still. Teach wound care as ordered. At each visit, assess condition of ulcer, peripheral pulses, skin color and warmth, pain, and edema.
Risk for infection related to open wound.	The patient will remain free of signs and symptoms of infection: fever, increasing redness, purulent drainage.	Teach hygienic techniques of hand washing and wound care. Encourage diet with adequate protein and vitamins. Teach signs and symptoms of infection that should be reported to physician. Instruct in antimicrobial therapy if prescribed.
Chronic pain related to circulatory impairment.	The patient will report pain relief.	Encourage the patient to increase movement and maintain warmth to improve circulation. Teach pain relief measures including relaxation, deep breathing techniques, cutaneous stimulation, and behavior modification. Explain the use of prescribed analgesics. Assess effectiveness of measures.
Impaired skin integrity related to circulatory impairment.	The patient's wound will heal completely.	Assess and document the condition of the ulcer during each clinic visit. Advise the patient to use gentle soaps for bathing, to avoid trauma, and not to rub the ulcer. Encourage good nutrition and adequate fluid intake. Discuss wound care with physician or clinical nurse specialist in wound care.
Ineffective management of therapeutic regimen related to lack of knowledge of chronic venous insufficiency and treatment of stasis ulcer.	The patient will correctly explain chronic venous insufficiency and demonstrate correct care of ulcer.	Assess the patient's understanding of condition and self-care. Advise to avoid restrictive clothing, smoking, and weight gain. Explore sources of stress and coping strategies.
Ineffective therapeutic regimen management related to lack of knowledge of importance of treating hypertension.	The patient will verbalize understanding of need to have blood pressure evaluated and will make an appointment for evaluation.	Explain importance of detecting and treating hypertension. Refer to physician or blood pressure clinic for evaluation.

Medical Diagnosis

The classic signs and symptoms, supported by wound culture results, are usually adequate to confirm lymphangitis. Lymphangiography, which uses a contrast medium for the radiologic visualization of the lymphatic system, will also provide evidence of lymphangitis.

Medical and Surgical Treatment

Antimicrobials are used to treat lymphangitis. When an abscess develops, the area is incised to drain the suppurative material. Other supportive measures that may be ordered are rest and elevation of the limb, warm, wet dressings; and elastic support hose.

NURSING CARE *of the Patient with Lymphangitis*

Assessment

Assessment of the patient with lymphangitis includes inspection of the skin for open wounds, signs of inflammation (redness, warmth, edema), and presence of red streaks along the paths of lymphatic channels. Palpate the lymph nodes in the groin and underarm areas for any enlargements.

Nursing Diagnoses, Goals, and Outcome Criteria: Lymphangitis

Nursing Diagnoses	Goals and Outcome Criteria
Acute Pain related to the inflammatory process in the lymphatic system	Pain relief: patient verbalizes less pain, appears relaxed
Activity Intolerance related to the pain with movement	Improved activity intolerance: patient increases activity without increased pain
Risk for Injury related to infection	Resolution of infection: absence of fever, normal white cell count, decreasing swelling and pain

Interventions

Pain

Nursing interventions to relieve pain include the administration of the prescribed analgesics and antimicrobials and elevation of the extremity to reduce lymphedema. Nonpharmacologic measures should be used as well as analgesics. The application of warm, moist soaks to the infected areas as prescribed improves the circulation to the area. As the circulation is improved, white blood cells, nutrients, and oxygen are delivered, which aids in the recovery of the healthy tissue. Elastic support hose are used for several months after an acute attack of lymphangitis to prevent the formation of lymphedema.

Activity Intolerance and Risk for Injury

Nursing care of the patient with lymphangitis is essentially the same as that for chronic venous insufficiency.

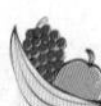

Nutrition Concepts

1. Edema frequently is treated with a low-sodium diet, and sodium-restricted diets vary from 4 g (least restrictive) to 250 mg (severe sodium restriction) daily.
2. Foods high in sodium include salt, monosodium glutamate (MSG), smoked or processed meats (ham, bacon, frankfurters, cold cuts), salted foods (potato chips, pretzels, salted nuts, popcorn), prepackaged frozen foods, and canned foods.
3. Older adults taking diuretics are not generally encouraged to restrict sodium intake because they are at risk for low-sodium syndrome.
4. Salt substitutes are a source of potassium, which is desirable in patients receiving potassium-wasting diuretics; however, salt substitutes should always be approved by a physician before using.

key points

- The peripheral vascular system comprises arteries, capillaries, veins, and lymph vessels, each of which plays a critical role in the oxygenation and nourishment of body tissues.
- Risk factors for peripheral vascular disease include older age, heredity, smoking, obesity, physical inactivity, hypertension, and diabetes mellitus.
- Common age-related changes in the vascular system include arteriosclerosis (stiffening of blood vessel walls), decreased hemoglobin, slower heart rate, and decreased cardiac output.
- The six P's characteristic of peripheral vascular disease are pain, pulselessness, poikilothermia, pallor, paresthesia, and paralysis.
- Intermittent claudication is pain in any major muscle group that is precipitated by exercise and relieved by rest.
- Poikilothermia describes an area of the body that is cooler than the rest of the body owing to local ischemia.
- Tests and procedures used to diagnose peripheral vascular disease include Doppler ultrasound, plethysmography, pressure measurement, exercise testing, angiography, and venography.
- Common therapeutic measures used in the management of peripheral vascular disease are exercise programs, stress management training, pain management, smoking cessation, elastic stockings or intermittent pneumatic compression devices, positioning, thermotherapy, protection, and patient teaching.
- Surgical interventions for peripheral vascular disease include embolectomy, percutaneous transluminal angioplasty, endarterectomy, sympathectomy, vein ligation and stripping, and sclerotherapy.
- Blood flow may be improved with drug therapy using anticoagulants, thrombolytics, platelet aggregation inhibitors, and vasodilators. NSAIDs and other analgesics may be needed for pain and inflammation.
- A low-fat diet is usually prescribed, and a weight reduction program may be advised if appropriate.
- An arterial embolus, an unattached clot or other material in an artery, can lodge in an artery and obstruct blood

flow; it may be dissolved with thrombolytic therapy or may be removed surgically.

- Nursing care of the patient with an arterial embolus focuses on ineffective tissue perfusion, fear, impaired skin integrity, impaired physical mobility, and ineffective therapeutic regimen management
- Peripheral arterial occlusive diseases impair blood flow and may be treated surgically.
- Nursing care of the patient with peripheral arterial occlusive disease focuses on activity intolerance, chronic pain, impaired skin integrity, disturbed body image, ineffective tissue perfusion, and ineffective therapeutic regimen management.
- Thromboangiitis obliterans (Buerger's disease) is an inflammatory thrombotic disorder of arteries and veins in upper and lower extremities of smokers; atherosclerosis is not a factor.
- Raynaud's disease and phenomenon are characterized by intermittent arteriolar vasoconstriction that is usually treated with vasodilators.
- An aneurysm is a dilated segment of an artery, most often the aorta, that can rupture, serve as a site for thrombus formation, and compress surrounding tissues.
- Aortic dissection results from a tear in the intima that allows blood to escape into the space between the intima and the media that causes the media to split lengthwise.
- Varicose veins are dilated, tortuous, superficial veins that result from incompetent venous valves; they may lead to chronic venous insufficiency and are treated with conservative measures to improve venous return and sometimes with surgical intervention.
- Phlebitis is inflammation of a vein wall, whereas thrombophlebitis describes clot formation in an inflamed vein.
- Thrombosis is clot formation, and deep vein thrombosis indicates the clot is located in deep veins—a condition that poses a high risk for pulmonary emboli.
- Risk factors for thrombus formation are bedrest, surgery in people older than 40 years of age, leg trauma and immobilization, previous venous insufficiency, obesity, oral contraceptives, and malignancy.
- Nursing care of the patient with venous thrombosis addresses impaired skin integrity, acute pain, anxiety, activity intolerance, ineffective tissue perfusion, impaired gas exchange, and ineffective therapeutic regimen management.
- Chronic venous insufficiency causes edema and stasis dermatitis around the ankles.
- Lymphangitis is an inflammation of the lymphatic channels that is treated with antimicrobials, analgesics, heat therapy, and rest.

REVIEW QUESTIONS

1. The exchange of oxygen and nutrients occurs at the level of the:
   1. arteriole.
   2. capillary.
   3. venules.
   4. lymphatics.
2. Thickening and hardening of the intima put the older adult at risk for:
   1. anemia.
   2. bradycardia.
   3. emboli.
   4. hypotension.
3. A patient complains of pain and cramping in the legs that occurs when walking and is relieved by rest. This complaint is typical of:
   1. intermittent claudication.
   2. venous thrombosis.
   3. pulmonary embolism.
   4. poikilothermy.
4. When assessing a patient's legs, you press your thumb into an edematous area around the ankles. When you remove your thumb, a depression ¼ inch remains on both ankles. You would document:
   1. 1+ edema noted
   2. Pitting edema, both ankles
   3. Mild edema, both ankles
   4. 2+ edema, both ankles
5. Which of the following is an invasive diagnostic procedure used to assess the vascular system?
   1. Ultrasound
   2. Plethysmography
   3. Angiography
   4. Exercise test
6. For the patient with peripheral vascular disease, the common purpose of exercise, elastic stockings, and elevation of extremities is to:
   1. improve venous return.
   2. stimulate arterial blood flow.
   3. reduce vasoconstriction.
   4. strengthen venous valves.
7. The dosage of low molecular weight heparin is based on:
   1. activated partial thromboplastin time.
   2. international normalized ratio.
   3. prothrombin time.
   4. fixed recommended dosage.
8. Discharge teaching for the patient with peripheral arterial occlusive disease affecting both legs includes:
   1. Advise the patient to elevate the feet when sitting.
   2. Tell the patient that exercise is contraindicated.
   3. Promptly report any injury to the feet or legs.
   4. Explain how to take prescribed vasoconstrictors.

9. Following repair of an abdominal aneurysm, it is especially important to monitor:
   1. reflexes in the lower extremities.
   2. intake and output.
   3. mental status.
   4. electrocardiogram.

10. The most serious complication of venous thrombosis is:
    1. pulmonary embolism.
    2. stasis dermatitis.
    3. ankle ulceration.
    4. pitting edema.

CHAPTER

35 Hypertension

objectives

1. Define hypertension.
2. Explain the physiology of blood pressure regulation.
3. Discuss the risk factors, signs and symptoms, diagnosis, treatment, and complications of hypertension.
4. Identify the nursing considerations when administering selected antihypertensive drugs.
5. List the data to be obtained in the nursing assessment of a person with known or suspected hypertension.
6. Identify the nursing diagnoses, goals, and outcome criteria for the patient with hypertension.
7. Describe the nursing interventions for the patient with hypertension.

key terms

Epistaxis (ĕp-ĭ-STĂK-sĭs, p. 641)
Hyperlipidemia (hī-pĕr-lĭp-ĭ-DĒ-mē-ă, p. 641)
Hypertension (hī-pĕr-TĔN-shŭn, p. 639)
Hypertrophy (hī-PĔR-trō-fē, p. 641)
Orthostatic hypotension (ōr-thō-STĂT-ĭk hī-pō-TĔN-shŭn, p. 645)
Syncope (SĬN-kō-pē, p. 648)
Thrombus (*pl.* thrombi) (THRŎM-bŭs) (THRŎM-bī, p. 641)

Hypertension (high blood pressure) is considered the most common cardiovascular problem in the United States today. Approximately 50 million people have hypertension that requires monitoring, treatment, or both. The condition is usually detected in people aged 30 to 50 years; however, it is being found with increasing frequency in children.

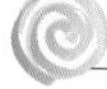

What Does Culture Have to do with Blood Pressure?

Hypertension occurs twice as often in African Americans as in whites and is more common in women than in men. Screening needs to take in all segments of the population and education should be sensitive to cultural differences.

Hypertension is called "the silent killer" because it often has no symptoms and is not discovered until a serious complication develops. In the past, it was estimated that 50% of those with hypertension do not know they have it, but public education is improving the detection rates for this condition. More recent figures estimate that the percentage of people who do not know they have hypertension has fallen to 27%.

Complications of hypertension, including damage to the heart, blood vessels, kidneys, brain, and eyes, increase after age 50 years. Men, especially African Americans, suffer serious complications more often than women. Cardiac disease is the leading cause of death in hypertensive people. Improved management of hypertension has significantly reduced the death rate from stroke in women age 50 and older.

DEFINITIONS

The Joint National Committee on Prevention, Detection, Evaluation, and Treatment of High Blood Pressure defines normal blood pressure as systolic pressure of less than 120 mm Hg and diastolic pressure of less than 80 mm Hg. Patients with systolic pressures between 120 and 139 and with diastolic pressures between 80 and 89 are said to have prehypertension. The stages of hypertension are specified in Table 35-1. If the systolic and diastolic pressures fall into different stages, the higher measurement is used to classify the stage of hypertension. Complications and death increase directly with the stage of hypertension.

In addition to staging, hypertensive patients are classified as Risk Group A, B, or C. Individuals in Risk Group A have no major risk factors, no target organ damage, and no clinical cardiovascular disease. Individuals in Risk Group B have one or more risk factors, not including diabetes, no target organ damage, and no clinicial cardiovascular disease. Individuals in Risk Group C have target organ damage/clinical cardiovascular disease and/or diabetes, with or without other risk factors.

Some people have only occasional elevations in blood pressure and normal readings at other times. These findings are called isolated pressure elevations. Isolated systolic blood pressure elevations of 160 mm Hg or more frequently occur in the elderly. The elevations are most often due to atherosclerosis.

TYPES OF HYPERTENSION

Hypertension is classified as primary (essential) or secondary. Primary hypertension accounts for 90% to 95% of all cases of hypertension. Its cause is unknown. Secondary hypertension is caused by underlying factors such as kidney disease, certain arterial conditions, some drugs, and occasionally pregnancy.

table 35-1 Classification of Blood Pressure for Adults 18 Years of Age and Older*

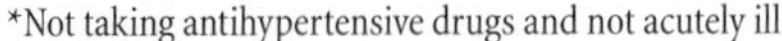

CATEGORY	SYSTOLIC (mm Hg)		DIASTOLIC (mm Hg)
Normal†	<120	and	<80
Prehypertension	120-139	and	80-89
Hypertension‡			
Stage 1	140-159	or	90-99
Stage 2	= or >160	or	= or >100

*Not taking antihypertensive drugs and not acutely ill.
†Optimal blood pressure with respect to cardiovascular risk is below 120/80 mm Hg. However, unusually low readings should be evaluated for clinical significance.
‡Based on the average of two or more readings taken at each of two or more visits after an initial screening.
From Joint National Committee on Prevention, Detection, Evaluation, and Treatment of High Blood Pressure (2003). *The seventh report of the Joint National Committee on Prevention, Detection, Evaluation, and Treatment of High Blood Pressure.* Bethesda, MD: National Institutes of Health, National Heart, Lung, and Blood Institute.

ANATOMY AND PHYSIOLOGY OF BLOOD PRESSURE REGULATION

Two factors determine blood pressure: cardiac output and peripheral vascular resistance. Blood pressure (BP) equals cardiac output (CO) times peripheral vascular resistance (PVR)—that is, BP = CO × PVR.

CARDIAC OUTPUT

Cardiac output is the volume of blood pumped by the heart in a specific period of time (usually 1 minute). It is determined by the strength, rate, and rhythm of the contraction of the left ventricle and by the blood volume.

PERIPHERAL VASCULAR RESISTANCE

Peripheral vascular resistance is the force in the blood vessels that the left ventricle must overcome to eject blood from the heart. Resistance to blood flow is primarily determined by the diameter of the blood vessels and blood viscosity (thickness). Increased peripheral vascular resistance results from a narrowing of the arteries and arterioles or an increased fluid volume in the blood vessels that results from sodium and water retention. Increased peripheral vascular resistance is the most prominent characteristic of hypertension.

The diameter of blood vessels is regulated largely by the vasomotor center. The vasomotor center is located in the medulla of the brain. Sympathetic nervous system tracts from the medulla extend down the spinal cord to the thoracic and abdominal regions. Stimulation of the sympathetic nervous system causes release of the hormones norepinephrine and epinephrine. These hormones, called catecholamines, are vasoconstrictors, meaning that they cause the blood vessels to constrict, making the diameter smaller. By constricting blood vessels, norepinephrine increases peripheral vascular resistance and raises blood pressure. Epinephrine constricts

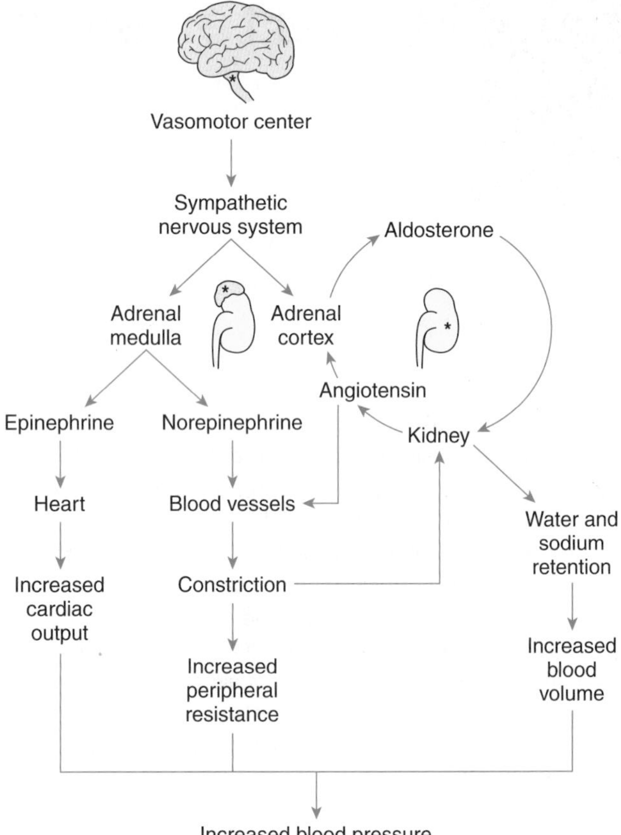

FIGURE **35-1** Factors that increase blood pressure.

blood vessels and increases the force of cardiac contraction, causing blood pressure to rise.

Vasoconstriction decreases blood flow to the kidneys, which then release renin. Renin leads to the formation of angiotensin, another potent vasoconstrictor. Angiotensin stimulates the adrenal cortex to secrete aldosterone, a hormone that promotes sodium and water retention. This results in an increased blood volume. Vasoconstriction, cardiac stimulation, and retention of fluid all contribute to hypertension. Figure 35-1 illustrates how various factors raise blood pressure.

AGE-RELATED CHANGES AFFECTING BLOOD PRESSURE

Some age-related changes affect blood pressure. With aging, atherosclerotic changes reduce the elasticity of the arteries, causing a decrease in cardiac output and an increase in peripheral vascular resistance. After age 60 years, peripheral vascular resistance increases by approximately 1% per year. Systolic pressure rises in response to increased peripheral vascular resistance. In addition, pulse pressure (the difference between the systolic and diastolic pressures) widens in response to a decreased ability of the aorta to distend (stretch).

In the past, elevated blood pressure was considered normal in the older person and was often untreated. Because research has shown that older people do benefit from controlling hypertension, age is no longer considered a barrier to aggressive treatment.

PRIMARY (ESSENTIAL) HYPERTENSION

RISK FACTORS

The most significant risk factors for primary (essential) hypertension are dyslipidemia, atherosclerosis, diabetes mellitus, cigarette smoking, age over 60 years, male gender (and postmenopausal females), family history (for people under age 55), and sedentary lifestyle. Obesity, defined as weight 20% over ideal body weight, is also a risk factor. The additional weight and fat cause increases in the number of blood vessels, circulating blood volume, and cardiac workload. Atherosclerosis decreases the elasticity of the arteries and arterioles, causing increased systemic and peripheral vascular resistance. Nicotine in cigarettes constricts blood vessels and causes the release of epinephrine and norepinephrine. These hormones, as already mentioned, also constrict blood vessels and raise heart rate and blood pressure. Lack of physical activity leads to pooling of blood in the extremities and increases the workload of the cardiovascular system.

Other risk factors include stress, overstimulation, and a family history of obesity, hypertension, or hyperlipidemia. Hyperlipidemia is excess insoluble fats in the blood, a factor that contributes to atherosclerosis. Stress caused by such factors as a high-pressure job, financial worries, or family problems increases secretion of catecholamines. Stimulants that may contribute to or aggravate hypertension include caffeine, nicotine, and amphetamines. Caffeine is found in tea, coffee, and chocolate. Nicotine is obtained by smoking or chewing tobacco products.

SIGNS AND SYMPTOMS

Many people who are hypertensive have no symptoms. Symptoms that may accompany hypertension include occipital headaches that are more severe on arising, lightheadedness, and epistaxis (nosebleed). If hypertension has damaged blood vessels in the heart, kidneys, eyes, or brain, the patient may have symptoms of impaired function of those organs.

COMPLICATIONS

The long-term effect of prolonged hypertension is replacement of elastic arteriolar tissue with stiffer, fibrous collagen tissue. Thickening of the arteriolar wall decreases its ability to distend, resulting in increased peripheral vascular resistance and decreased blood flow to various organs. The effects are most significant in the eyes, heart, kidneys, and brain. Patients with hypertension must be assessed frequently for damage to these sensitive ("target") organs (Fig. 35-2).

Eyes

Damage to the eyes may include narrowing of the retinal arterioles, retinal hemorrhages, and papilledema (edema of the optic nerve). These changes may lead to blindness.

Heart

Coronary artery disease develops in patients with hypertension two to three times more frequently than in people with normal blood pressures. Coronary artery disease reduces blood supply to the myocardium, which can result in angina, myocardial infarction, and congestive heart failure. Myocardial infarction, commonly called a heart attack, results when the blood supply to the heart muscle is inadequate and the myocardium is deprived of oxygen.

Sustained hypertension requires the left ventricle to work harder to overcome increased peripheral resistance. The increased workload may cause the left ventricle to hypertrophy (enlarge), and it may eventually fail.

Kidneys

Narrowing of the renal arteries may decrease renal function and lead to chronic renal failure. Initial indicators of renal failure are nocturia (need to urinate during the night) and azotemia (accumulation of nitrogen waste products in the blood). In addition, urinalysis may reveal protein (proteinuria) or blood (hematuria), or both, in the urine.

Brain

Prolonged hypertension constricts and damages cerebral arteries, putting the patient at risk for transient ischemic attacks and cerebrovascular accidents. A transient ischemic attack, sometimes called a TIA or "little stroke," is a temporary neurologic dysfunction caused by cerebral ischemia.

A cerebrovascular accident (CVA, or stroke) results from interrupted blood flow in the brain caused by a rupture of a blood vessel or a thrombus (clot) occluding the vessel. People with hypertension have a sevenfold greater incidence of cerebrovascular accidents than those with normal blood pressures.

DIAGNOSTIC TESTS AND PROCEDURES

Diagnosis of hypertension is based on direct and indirect data. Hypertension is confirmed by repeated findings of average pressures equal to or greater than 140/90. When elevations are found in clinics or in screenings, the physician might have patients monitor their own BP at home for comparison. Also, ambulatory blood pressure monitors, which are commonly programmed to record readings every 15-30 minutes for 24 hours, typically provide readings lower than clinic readings. These readings provide a better foundation for the diagnosis of hypertension than a few isolated readings. The process would not be cost-effective for all patients but is appropriate in selected situations.

On finding an elevated blood pressure, the physician examines the patient for effects of hypertension on the heart, eyes, kidneys, and brain. Blood samples are usually drawn

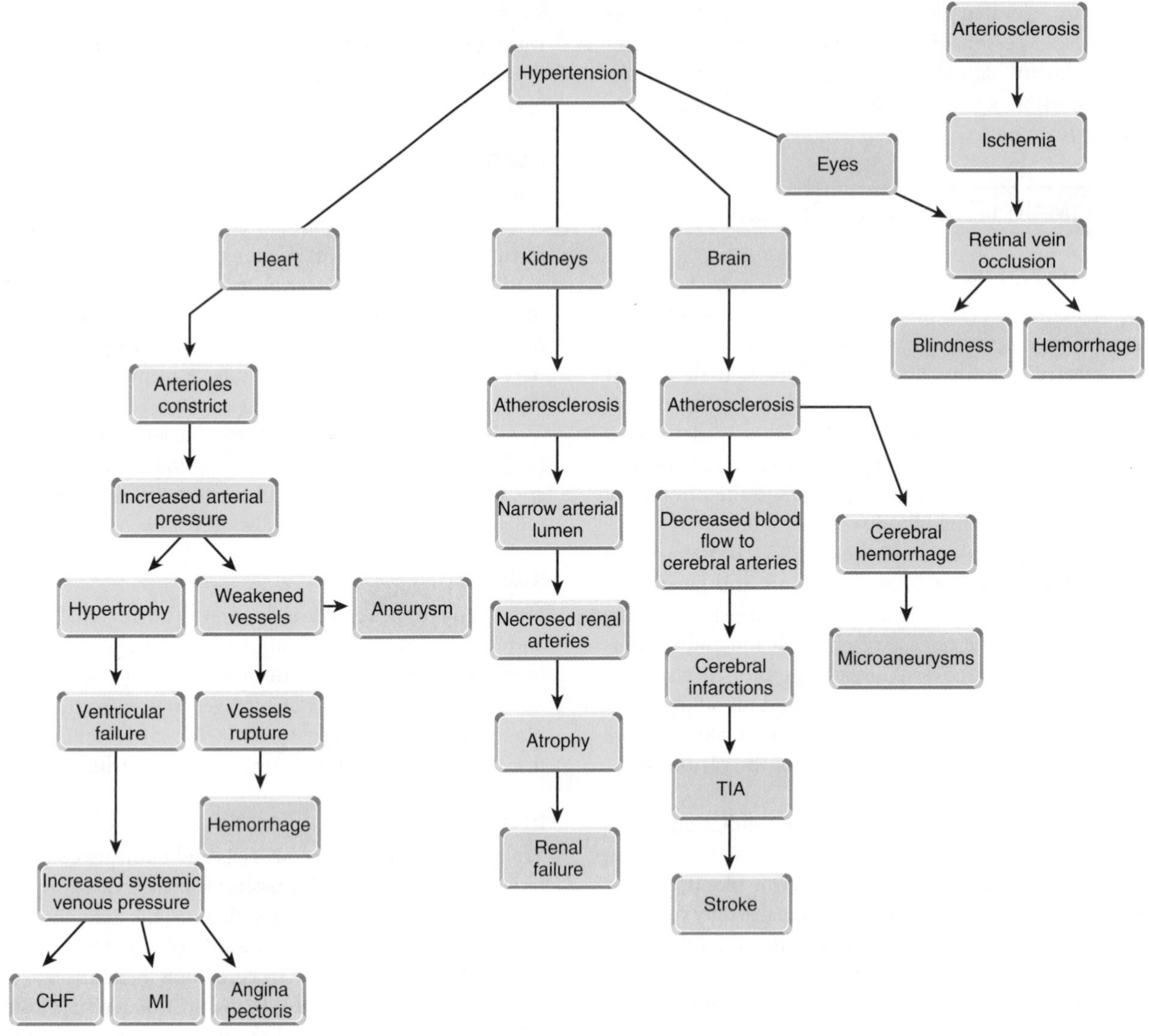

FIGURE **35-2** How hypertension affects major target organs.

for a complete blood count and assessment of liver and kidney function. If there is kidney damage, the blood urea nitrogen and serum creatinine levels are elevated. Elevated serum cholesterol may indicate atherosclerosis. A chest radiograph may show enlargement of the heart or pulmonary blood vessels.

Physicians disagree about the need for trying to determine the cause of hypertension. If there is no evidence to suggest an underlying disease process, the general consensus is to limit diagnostic tests to those that are most significant. This reduces patient care costs.

MEDICAL TREATMENT

The goal of therapy for hypertension is to gradually reduce peripheral vascular resistance and blood pressure. Optimal blood pressure is usually defined as a diastolic pressure of less than 80 mm Hg and systolic pressure less than 120 mm Hg. Treatment of underlying conditions may lower the blood pressure in people with secondary hypertension.

For treatment of primary hypertension, a conservative, nonpharmacologic method (without drugs) usually is tried first. Drug treatment may be added if needed.

Lifestyle Modifications

A nonpharmacologic approach includes weight reduction, smoking cessation, sodium and alcohol restriction, exercise, and relaxation techniques. Reduction of weight can reduce blood pressure by reducing the cardiac workload. Stopping smoking eliminates vasoconstriction caused by nicotine. Reduction of sodium in the body reduces water retention and decreases the blood volume.

A planned program of exercise improves cardiac efficiency by increasing cardiac output and decreasing peripheral vascular resistance. Exercise also decreases the patient's blood glucose and cholesterol levels and promotes a sense of well-being. Isotonic exercises such as walking, bicycling, and swimming help to reduce weight and promote relaxation.

Consider the Alternative!

Complementary therapies such as relaxation, biofeedback, and behavior modification may be used along with traditional medical treatment of hypertension.

Relaxation therapy, biofeedback, and behavior modification techniques also may be used to reduce stress and lower blood pressure. Alcohol intake should not exceed 2 ounces per day because alcohol can increase blood pressure and can alter the effects of some antihypertensive drugs.

Lifestyle modifications are recommended for individuals with high-normal and all stages of hypertension regardless of the risk group.

Pharmacologic Therapy

Drug therapy is indicated if the blood pressure is very high initially (SBP = or >160, DBP = or >100) or if conservative therapies for less severe hypertension are not effective within 3 to 6 months. Drug therapy must be individualized for each patient and may be recommended at earlier stages. The goal of drug therapy is to normalize blood pressure using the smallest number of the safest drugs at the lowest effective dosages. A single agent is preferred if good control can be achieved because patients are more likely to take one drug as prescribed than multiple agents. Antihypertensive drugs are listed in Table 35-2.

Stepped-Care Approach

The stepped-care approach (Table 35-3) is a plan for selecting drugs to treat hypertension. It begins with administration of a single, relatively safe drug. The physician progresses to the next step until good control is achieved.

Step one. The first step recommends starting the patient on a low dose of either a thiazide diuretic or a beta-adrenergic receptor blocker (beta blocker). If thiazide diuretics and beta blockers are contraindicated, the first choice may be an angiotensin-converting enzyme (ACE) inhibitor or a calcium antagonist (calcium channel blocker).

Step two. If the first drug is not effective, step two is to increase the dosage of the first drug or add a second drug from step one. An alternative drug also might be selected.

Step three. The third step is implemented if the patient does not respond to the step one or two drugs. In step three, there are three options: increase the dosage of those drugs prescribed in step two, add a third drug, or try a different drug from step one.

Monotherapy

The stepped-care approach is used less often now than in the past. At this time, it is common for the physician initially to select a single drug that is compatible with a patient's condition. The patient is then monitored for several weeks. If blood pressure remains elevated, the dosage may be increased, or another single drug may be tried.

Specific Antihypertensive Drugs

Diuretics. Diuretics lower blood pressure by: (1) reducing blood volume by promoting renal excretion of sodium and water; and (2) decreasing the sensitivity of blood vessels to catecholamines, thereby reducing vascular resistance. There are several types of diuretics: thiazide, loop (high ceiling), and potassium-sparing. Among the diuretics that may be used to treat hypertension are hydrochlorothiazide (HydroDIURIL), furosemide (Lasix), and amiloride (Midamor). Diuretics are especially effective in treating hypertensive African American patients.

Patients taking diuretics must be monitored for fluid and electrolyte imbalances, especially hypovolemia and potassium imbalances. Intake and output records may be kept on hospitalized patients who are taking diuretics.

Hypokalemia is a potentially serious problem except with potassium-sparing diuretics. Older patients are especially susceptible to hypokalemia. Monitor for signs of hypokalemia: confusion, irritability, muscle weakness, and anorexia. To prevent hypokalemia, encourage the patient to consume additional dietary potassium. Sources of potassium include bananas and orange juice. Some patients require supplementary potassium.

PHARMACOLOGY CAPSULE When patients are taking diuretics, monitor for signs and symptoms of hypokalemia: cardiac dysrhythmias, muscle weakness, and diminished bowel sounds.

Beta-adrenergic receptor blockers. These agents, commonly called beta blockers, reduce blood pressure by blocking the beta effects of catecholamines. Examples of beta blockers used to treat hypertension are atenolol (Tenormin), labetalol (Normodyne), metoprolol (Lopressor), and propranolol (Inderal). When beta receptors are stimulated, they stimulate the heart and relax bronchial smooth muscle. Beta blockers prevent this stimulation, resulting in decreased heart rate, decreased strength of cardiac contraction, and bronchial constriction. There are a number of beta blockers that have slightly different effects. Some affect cardiac function more; others have a greater effect on the bronchi. Except for labetalol, beta blockers are less effective for African American patients than other types of antihypertensive drugs.

Common side effects of beta blockers include bradycardia and hypotension, hypoglycemia, and increased low-density lipoprotein in the blood. Beta blockers usually are not recommended in patients with asthma, chronic obstructive pulmonary disease, heart block, or congestive heart failure. When a patient is taking a beta blocker, the nurse should monitor for bradycardia and hypotension. People with diabetes should be watched carefully for hypoglycemia because beta blockers lower blood glucose and suppress the usual signs of hypoglycemia. Diaphoresis (excessive perspiration) may be the only sign of hypoglycemia when people with diabetes are taking beta blockers. Elderly patients are at greater risk than young patients for hypotension and bradycardia associated with beta blockers. Therefore they should be started on low doses that are cautiously increased if needed.

table 35-2 DRUG THERAPY | *Antihypertensive Drugs and Nursing Interventions*

GENERAL CONSIDERATIONS

1. Monitor blood pressure (BP) regularly with patient in supine, sitting, and standing positions.
2. Encourage patients to take medications and keep follow-up appointments even when they are feeling well.
3. Teach patients with orthostatic hypotension to rise slowly, avoid prolonged standing, and avoid hot baths and showers.
4. Advise patients to consult physician or pharmacist about safety of over-the-counter drugs.
5. Do not stop drugs abruptly because rebound hypertension may occur.

DRUG CLASSES/EXAMPLE	USE/ACTION	SIDE EFFECTS	NURSING INTERVENTIONS
CENTRALLY ACTING DRUGS (ALPHA$_2$ AGONISTS)			
Clonidine (Catapres) Methyldopa (Aldomet)	Act on central nervous system to block vasoconstriction, which lowers BP; also reduces anxiety	Drowsiness, dry mouth, weakness, depression, retention of sodium and water. Orthostatic hypotension with some drugs.	Monitor BP. Safety precautions. Oral hygiene. Assess for edema. Teach patient to manage orthostatic hypotension.
GANGLIONIC BLOCKERS			
Mecamylamine (Inversine)	Block transmission of nerve impulses that constrict blood vessels; vessels dilate, reducing BP	Sodium and water retention, bradycardia, impaired ejaculation, nasal stuffiness, gastrointestinal disturbances. Some drugs cause orthostatic hypotension.	Monitor pulse and BP. Assess for edema, sexual dysfunction. Give with meals to reduce gastrointestinal distress. Teach patient to manage orthostatic hypotension.
ALPHA-ADRENERGIC BLOCKERS			
Phentolamine (Regitine) Prazosin (Minipress) Terazosin (Hytrin)	Block effects of norepinephrine, causing vasodilation	Reflex tachycardia, palpitations, headache, dizziness, drowsiness, nausea. Potentially severe orthostatic hypotension with first or increased dose of prazosin.	Monitor pulse and BP. Advise patient that most side effects diminish over time. Give first or increased dose of prazosin at bedtime. Advise of possible orthostatic hypotension.
BETA-ADRENERGIC BLOCKERS			
Propranolol (Inderal) Atenolol (Tenormin)	Decrease cardiac stimulation	Bradycardia, fatigue, drowsiness, depression, hypoglycemia, bronchial constriction.	Monitor pulse, BP, and respiration. Assess emotional status. Monitor patients with asthma for dyspnea; patients with diabetes for low blood glucose.
DIRECT VASODILATORS			
Hydralazine (Apresoline)	Relax vascular smooth muscle, causing vasodilation	Reflex tachycardia, headache, dizziness, nausea and vomiting, anorexia, hypotension.	Monitor pulse and BP.
CALCIUM CHANNEL BLOCKERS			
Verapamil (Calan) Nifedipine (Procardia) Diltiazem (Cardizem)	Decrease force of cardiac contraction and dilate peripheral blood vessels	Bradycardia, flushing, dizziness, headache.	Monitor pulse. Elevate legs when sitting to reduce edema.
ANGIOTENSIN-CONVERTING ENZYME INHIBITORS			
Captopril (Capoten) Enalapril (Vasotec)	Reduce aldosterone secretion and prevent formation of angiotensin II, thus decreasing peripheral resistance and fluid volume	Skin rash, neutropenia. Renal failure in patients with renal artery stenosis. Cough.	Monitor blood cell counts. Report changes in urine output.
DIURETICS			
Hydrochlorothiazide (HCTZ) Furosemide (Lasix)	Reduce fluid volume; may cause vasodilation; sodium loss may reduce vasoconstriction	Fluid volume deficit, hyponatremia, hypokalemia (except with potassium-sparing diuretics).	Monitor fluid balance: hydration, urine output, mental status, muscle tone. Recommend foods high in potassium (bananas, orange juice) unless on potassium-sparing diuretics.
ANGIOTENSIN II RECEPTOR ANTAGONISTS			
Losartan (Cozaar) Valsartan (Diovan)	Block action of angiotensin II; vasodilation; reduce blood volume by excretion of water and salt	Dizziness.	Safety precautions.

BP, Blood pressure.

table 35-3 Stepped-Care Approach

STEP ONE
Low dose of one of the following:
Thiazide diuretic
Beta-adrenergic receptor blocker
In selected situations:
Angiotensin-converting enzyme inhibitor
Calcium antagonist
STEP TWO
Increased dosage of the first drug or addition of another Step One drug
STEP THREE
Increased dosage of Step Two drug
OR
Addition of a third drug
OR
Prescription of a different drug from Step One

PHARMACOLOGY CAPSULE Monitor people with diabetes for low blood glucose if they are taking beta blockers.

What Does Culture Have to do with Antihypertensive Drugs?

Your genes affect the way you metabolize drugs. Therefore ethnicity and race explain some variations in effects of antihypertensive drugs. For example, Asians respond better to beta blockers than whites do. Whites respond better than African Americans to beta blockers and ACE inhibitors.

Calcium antagonists. Calcium antagonists are called calcium channel blockers because they block the movement of calcium into cardiac and vascular smooth muscle cells. This action reduces the heart rate, decreases the force of cardiac contraction, and dilates peripheral blood vessels. Because dilated vessels present less resistance to blood flow, blood pressure is reduced. Diltiazem (Cardizem), isradipine (DynaCirc), nicardipine (Cardene), nifedipine (Procardia), and verapamil (Calan) are examples of calcium channel blockers used for hypertension.

Common side effects of calcium channel blockers are flushing, dizziness, and headache. The nurse should also monitor for hypotension, bradycardia, and edema.

Angiotensin-converting enzyme inhibitors. These drugs prevent the conversion of angiotensin I to angiotensin II, a potent vasoconstrictor. Blocking the production of angiotensin II decreases peripheral resistance. ACE inhibitors also decrease fluid retention by decreasing the production of aldosterone. Examples of ACE inhibitors are captopril (Capoten) and enalapril (Vasotec). ACE inhibitors with diuretics are often effective for African American patients. Adverse effects can include a chronic cough, dizziness, headache, fatigue, angioedema, hyperkalemia, and hypotension.

Angiotensin II receptor antagonists. These drugs prevent vasoconstriction in response to angiotensin. They also prevent the release of aldosterone, which increases excretion of salt and water, thereby reducing blood volume. Examples of angiotensin II receptor antagonists are losartan (Cozaar) and valsartan (Diovan). Unlike the ACE inhibitors, the only significant adverse effect of these drugs has been dizziness in some patients.

Other Antihypertensive Drugs

Other drugs used to treat hypertension include central adrenergic blockers, alpha-adrenergic blockers, and direct vasodilators.

Central adrenergic blockers. Central adrenergic blockers inhibit impulses from the vasomotor center in the brain that maintain the muscle tone in blood vessels. The effect of this type of drug is to reduce peripheral resistance and lower blood pressure. Examples of centrally acting adrenergic blockers are clonidine (Catapres) and methyldopa (Aldomet).

Alpha-adrenergic receptor blockers. Stimulation of alpha receptors produces constriction of arterioles. Drugs such as prazosin (Minipress) and doxazosin (Cardura) block alpha receptor stimulation and lower blood pressure by reducing peripheral resistance. The most important adverse effect is orthostatic hypotension, which is most severe with initial or increased dosages. Patients should lie down for 2 hours after taking a first or increased dose of this drug. For this reason, it is best given at bedtime. Alpha blockers can also cause dizziness, headache, and drowsiness.

Direct vasodilators. Direct vasodilators lower blood pressure by relaxing arteriolar smooth muscle. Examples of direct vasodilators are fenoldopam (Corlopam), minoxidil (Loniten), hydralazine (Apresoline), diazoxide (Hyperstat IV), and sodium nitroprusside (Nipride). Fenoldopam, nitroglycerin, sodium nitroprusside, hydralazine, and diazoxide are used to treat hypertensive crisis. Most emergency vasodilators are diluted in intravenous fluids and administered at the rate needed for the desired results. Diazoxide is given by direct intravenous injection (IV push), usually in small, repeated doses until the blood pressure reaches the target reading.

Nursing Implications. You need to be familiar with the drugs commonly prescribed for hypertension. Nursing responsibilities include administering the drugs to inpatients, monitoring for therapeutic and adverse effects, and teaching patients about their drugs. Additional information about antihypertensive drugs and nursing interventions is presented in Table 35-4.

The elderly respond differently to drug therapy. Older patients are at greater risk for adverse effects of medications because of reduced liver and kidney function. They are especially susceptible to orthostatic hypotension because their blood vessels respond more slowly to position changes. This creates increased risk for falls.

Older people may respond differently to beta blockers and to diuretics. The effectiveness of beta blockers may be reduced because beta receptor activity is lessened in the elderly. In

table 35-4 ASSESSMENT *of the Patient with Known or Suspected Hypertension*

HEALTH HISTORY

Present Illness: Description of reason for seeking care
Past Medical History: Hypertension; last blood pressure reading; renal, cardiac, or endocrine disorders; pregnancy; current medications
Family History: Hypertension, myocardial infarction, cerebrovascular accident
Review of Systems: Headache, dizziness, epistaxis, visual disturbances, dyspnea, angina, nocturia
Functional Assessment: Occupation, activity and exercise, sleep and rest, nutrition, interpersonal relationships, current stressors

PHYSICAL EXAMINATION

General Appearance: Distress
Height and Weight
Vital Signs
Blood Pressure: Supine, sitting, standing
Pulse
Respiration
Temperature
Extremities: Edema
Neuromuscular: Abnormalities

addition, diuretics may produce a more profound decrease in blood volume in these patients. Elderly patients often also are taking medications for other diseases. Drug interactions can alter therapeutic effects or enhance side effects. Dosages for antihypertensive medications may need to be reduced or adjusted depending on what diseases the patient has.

Put on your THINKING CAP!!

You have been asked to give a talk on hypertension to members of a senior center. The members are low income and have minimal education. Some speak limited English.

1. How might you explain the effects of hypertension on the body?
2. Select one lifestyle modification and explain how it reduces risk of hypertension.

SECONDARY HYPERTENSION

Secondary hypertension, which has a specific known cause, is less common than primary hypertension. Examples of causes are renal disease, excess secretion of adrenal hormones, narrowing of the aorta, and increased intracranial pressure, as well as some drugs such as vasoconstrictors.

NURSING CARE *of the Patient with Hypertension*

Assessment

Early detection, education, and promotion of adherence are the keys to blood pressure control. Periodic blood pressure checks detect new or unknown hypertensive people and provide data to evaluate the effect of therapy in known hypertensive people.

The nursing assessment of the known or suspected hypertensive person begins with a complete history and physical examination.

Health History

Record the patient's reason for seeking health care. Because hypertension often has no symptoms, the visit may be related to some other problem. Explore the past medical history to determine whether the patient has ever had hypertension or renal, cardiac, or endocrine disorders. Note the date and readings of the last blood pressure measurement. If the patient is female and if appropriate, ask about pregnancy and about hormone replacement therapy. List current medications, including over-the-counter drugs. In the family health history, assess the presence of hypertension, myocardial infarction, or cerebrovascular accidents among relatives.

Review the body systems for significant signs and symptoms, particularly headaches, epistaxis, dizziness, visual disturbances, dyspnea, angina, or nocturia. The functional assessment may detect some potential risk factors for hypertension. It includes occupation, exercise and activity, sleep and rest, nutrition, interpersonal relationships, and stressors.

Physical Examination

While taking the health history and beginning the physical examination, observe the patient's general appearance, noting any obvious distress. Measure height and weight and vital signs. The nurse may be the first to detect elevated pressure, so accurate measurement of blood pressure is very important. The proper cuff size is essential. Too small a cuff may give a false high reading, whereas a cuff that is too large may give a false low reading. For a more accurate reading, determine the systolic pulse first by palpation. Then deflate the cuff and take the pressure by auscultation, being careful to reinflate it above the palpated systolic pressure.

The blood pressure should be assessed in both arms in the supine, sitting, and standing positions. Begin blood pressure assessment with the patient resting supine for at least 10 minutes. After supine blood pressure assessment, take the sitting and then the standing readings after 1 to 3 minutes in each position. When body position is altered from supine to standing, the systolic pressure normally falls approximately 10 mm Hg, and the diastolic pressure rises approximately 5 mm Hg. Assess the apical and peripheral pulses for rate, rhythm, and quality or character in each position.

If blood pressure is elevated initially, reassess it after 1 to 5 minutes. If the pressure remains elevated, refer the patient for medical evaluation. Remember that a single elevated reading does not mean that the patient has hypertension. If the blood pressure is severely elevated (diastolic pressure of 115 mm Hg or more), the patient is in imminent danger of a stroke and immediate medical care is needed.

In general, blood pressure readings obtained in the home are more valid measures because patients are more relaxed there than in a clinic or office.

In addition to blood pressure and pulses, assess respiratory rate and effort. Inspect extremities for edema and color. Note any abnormalities in neurologic or muscular function.

Nursing assessment of the patient with known or suspected hypertension is summarized in Table 35-4.

Nursing Diagnoses, Goals, and Outcome Criteria: Hyptertension

Nursing Diagnoses	Goals and Outcome Criteria
Ineffective Therapeutic Regimen Management related to lack of knowledge about management of hypertension, drug side effects, difficulty maintaining lifestyle changes	Effective patient management of prescribed treatment: patient correctly explains hypertension and its treatment. Patient adheres to prescribed treatment plan: lowered blood pressure, evidence of positive lifestyle changes (weight loss, cessation of smoking)
Risk for Injury related to orthostatic hypotension secondary to antihypertensive drug therapy, sedation	Lack of injury: no falls or other incidents associated with orthostatic hypotension or sedation
Ineffective Coping related to depression secondary to drug side effects	Effective coping: patient reports positive emotional state
Sexual Dysfunction related to drug side effects	Satisfactory sexual function: patient's statement of ability to manage effects of drug therapy on sexual function

Interventions

Ineffective Therapeutic Regimen Management

Adherence to therapy requires commitment and active participation on the part of the patient. Lifestyle changes may be required, and pharmacologic side effects may be unpleasant. Failure to follow the prescribed regimen is often referred to as *noncompliance.* Some people prefer the term *nonadherence* as being less judgmental. In counseling the patient, it must be stressed that hypertension is a chronic disease requiring long-term management. Lack of symptoms or reduction of blood pressure often prompts patients to discontinue drug therapy inappropriately.

Patient education is critical for effective management of hypertension. Education begins as soon as the condition is diagnosed and continues throughout life. As with any patient teaching, begin by finding out what the person already knows and is most interested in learning. Addressing the patient's immediate concerns first builds trust that should facilitate further teaching. Do not present measures to manage hypertension as a long list of "don'ts," but rather as health practices that are beneficial to everyone. Include members of the patient's household, especially a spouse, in the teaching. Their understanding and cooperation can be very supportive to the patient.

Teaching patients about their medications will, it is hoped, promote adherence. Information in writing and a chart with times for medication administration may be helpful. Patients who do not take their medications as prescribed often cite the adverse side effects as reasons for noncompliance. It is important to teach patients to report unpleasant drug side effects to the physician promptly. A change in dosage or in the medication itself may reduce undesirable effects, but the patient should not make changes unless advised to do so by the physician. Common side effects of antihypertensive drugs that may affect adherence are orthostatic hypotension, sedation, sexual dysfunction, and depression.

Diet Therapy

The goals of diet therapy for the person with hypertension are to maintain ideal body weight and to prevent fluid retention. Total calorie intake may need to be adjusted to achieve these goals. A diet low in saturated fats with no more than 2 g of sodium is often prescribed. Sodium restriction is more effective for some patients than for others. The National Research Council recommends a maximum daily sodium intake of 2400 mg.

If the patient is taking a potassium-wasting diuretic, dietary potassium intake may need to be increased or potassium supplements may be recommended.

The nurse and the dietitian should cooperate in teaching patients about their prescribed dietary alterations. If someone other than the patient prepares the food at home, that person should be included during the dietary teaching.

What Does Culture Have to do with Diet?

Cultural dietary practices affect the types of foods eaten and how they are prepared. These practices must be considered and incorporated when teaching patients about healthier dietary practices.

Exercise

Nutrition and exercise go hand in hand. It is very difficult to maintain or lose weight without engaging in some form of exercise. Walking is highly recommended as an exercise that increases cardiovascular functioning, burns calories, relieves stress, and promotes a sense of well-being. An exercise program can benefit people of all ages, even the elderly. Advise patients to ask their physicians before beginning new exercise programs. Instruct them to increase their activities gradually over a period of time.

When people engage in a program of good nutrition and exercise, it is often possible to decrease or eliminate medications used to control hypertension. This information may be motivating to some people.

Stress Management

Patients need to understand that stress can raise blood pressure. Help patients identify stressors in their lives and explore ways to reduce them. Referrals to professional counselors may be in order for patients with complicated or multiple stressors. Some agencies or community centers offer classes in stress management or relaxation techniques.

Drug Therapy

Patients need to be well informed about their medications. Review with the patient the name, dosage, purpose, and side effects of any prescribed medications. Advise patients not to discontinue their drugs or change the dosage without consulting with the physician even if they feel well. Blood pressure can be very high with no symptoms. Suddenly stopping antihypertensive drugs may produce adverse effects, including rebound hypertension (sudden return of elevated blood pressure), myocardial infarction, and cerebrovascular accident. Also, explain that many over-the-counter drugs such as cold remedies contain vasoconstrictors that can counteract blood pressure medications.

PHARMACOLOGY CAPSULE Advise patients not to discontinue antihypertensive therapy simply because they feel well. Blood pressure can be very high with no symptoms.

Risk for Injury

The patient taking antihypertensive medications may be at risk for injury because of drug side effects. The effects that pose the greatest potential for injury are orthostatic hypotension and sedation.

Orthostatic Hypotension

Orthostatic or postural hypotension is a sudden drop in systolic blood pressure, usually 20 mm Hg, when going from a lying or sitting position to a standing position. Monitor for lightheadedness, dizziness, and syncope (fainting) in patients who are at risk for orthostatic hypotension. Instruct patients who are prone to orthostatic hypotension to exercise their legs and then to rise slowly from a lying or sitting position. They should avoid activities that cause blood pressure to fall, such as prolonged standing in one place and taking very hot baths or showers.

Sedation

Sedation may be dealt with by taking medications at bedtime to promote sleep. Advise patients if drowsiness is likely so that dangerous activities or those requiring alertness can be avoided during times of peak drug effect.

Ineffective Coping

If depression occurs as a side effect of an antihypertensive drug, consult the physician so that another drug may be substituted. This side effect should be taken very seriously. Refer patients with severe depression to a mental health professional.

Sexual Dysfunction

A common side effect of many antihypertensive medications is sexual dysfunction. Dysfunctions may take the form of decreased libido, inability to achieve an erection, or delayed ejaculation. Many patients consider sexual function to be a very personal subject, so it must be handled in a sensitive manner. Some patients volunteer information about sexual changes. Others may fail to relate the problem to their medications and not report it to the nurse or the physician. You can introduce the subject by saying, "Some people taking this medication have changes in sexual function. Has this been a problem for you?" If it is a problem for the patient, advise the physician so that an alternative medication or other intervention can be considered.

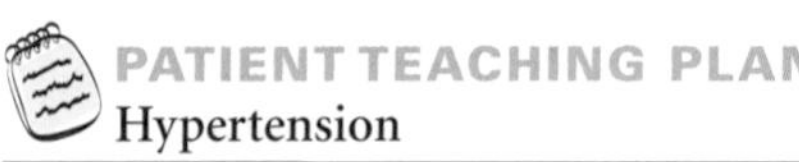

- Good control of hypertension reduces the risk of heart attack and stroke.
- A diet low in saturated fats and sodium may help to lower blood pressure.
- Regular exercise as advised by your physician helps with weight control and reduction of blood pressure.
- Smoking aggravates hypertension; the American Heart Association has programs to help you quit smoking.
- Relaxation techniques lower blood pressure.
- Do not stop taking your medications unless instructed by your physician. Suddenly stopping these drugs may cause blood pressure to rise rapidly.
- Keep appointments for follow-up care; feeling better does not necessarily mean your hypertension is under control.

OLDER PATIENTS

Planning nursing care for older hypertensive patients requires some additional considerations. Response to drug therapy is more difficult to predict, and side effects are more common. Orthostatic hypotension and sedation are especially problematic for the older person, who is prone to fall and suffer serious injuries. Depression also must be taken very seriously because it lowers motivation, impairs quality of life, and can lead to suicide.

Health care providers tend to assume that the elderly are not sexually active. Therefore they often fail to assess sexual function or dysfunction in older people. This is a real disservice to the older person whose sexual functioning is impaired as a result of antihypertensive drugs. The older patient should be treated just like a younger patient in the assessment and management of distressing drug effects.

HYPERTENSIVE EMERGENCIES

Hypertensive crisis is a life-threatening medical emergency. The patient presents with severe headache, blurred vision, nausea, restlessness, and confusion. Along with a very elevated diastolic blood pressure (130 mm Hg or more), the heart and respiratory rates are increased. This episode may result from having stopped taking antihypertensive drugs or may be caused by malignant hypertension, hypertensive encephalopathy, eclampsia, pheochromocytoma (adrenal tumor), or a cerebrovascular accident. Malignant hypertension is a specific type of hypertensive emergency in which the diastolic pressure exceeds 140 mm Hg. It has a sudden onset and is seen most often in African American men aged 30 to 40 years.

Without appropriate treatment, the patient in hypertensive crisis may incur cardiac and renal damage. Death may ensue as a result of a cerebrovascular accident, renal failure, or cardiac failure.

MEDICAL DIAGNOSIS

Assessment in the emergency room reveals elevated blood pressure, pulse, and respiratory rate. Retinal hemorrhage or papilledema, or both, can be observed in the fundus (back, interior portion) of the eye.

The physician may order blood drawn for arterial blood gases, complete blood count, electrolytes, blood urea nitrogen, creatinine, and cardiac enzymes. A chest radiograph may be requested. Direct blood pressure monitoring through an arterial catheter is preferred.

MEDICAL TREATMENT

The goal of drug therapy is to rapidly reduce the pressure to a non–life-threatening level and then to bring it slowly within normal range. This is done with diuretics and potent vasodilators. Examples of drugs that may be ordered include fenoldopam, nitroglycerin, diazoxide, hydralazine, phentolamine, labetalol, and nitroprusside. An intravenous line is usually established because many drugs are given by that route. Oral options for the management of hypertensive crisis include captopril, clonidine, and nifedipine. Drugs used to treat hypertensive crisis are listed in Table 35-5.

NURSING CARE *of the Patient in Hypertensive Crisis*

Assessment

The patient in hypertensive crisis must be closely monitored. Frequently assess the patient's blood pressure, pulse, respiration, and level of consciousness. Some drugs are given in intravenous fluids, requiring continuous monitoring and adjustment. Maintain a careful record of fluid intake and output. Nausea and vomiting may indicate an impending seizure or coma.

Interventions

The nurse's role in caring for the patient in hypertensive crisis includes administering prescribed drugs, monitoring vital signs before and after each drug dose, assessing cardiac and renal function, starting and maintaining intravenous therapy and oxygen as ordered, and comforting the patient.

Take appropriate safety measures if the patient shows signs of seizure activity or a decreasing level of consciousness. Bed siderails should be raised and padded if necessary. Elevate the head of the bed to facilitate breathing. Place an oral airway and suction equipment at the bedside. Offer brief explanations or words of encouragement to allay some of the patient's anxiety. As the patient's condition improves, it is important to explain how to manage hypertension and to prevent future crises from developing.

Nutrition Concepts

1. Diet and lifestyle changes, including weight reduction, exercise, and stress management, are important in the treatment of hypertension.
2. Weight loss in obese people lowers blood pressure at a rate of 1 mm Hg per kg (2.2 pounds) of body weight.
3. Sodium-restricted diets help lower blood pressure in many people with hypertension.
4. A high potassium intake may help lower blood pressure as well as replace potassium lost with potassium-wasting diuretics. Foods particularly high in potassium are fresh fruits and vegetables.
5. An adequate calcium intake may help in preventing and treating hypertension. Two to three cups of milk or yogurt per day, 4 ounces of low-sodium cheese, or calcium supplements (calcium carbonate, 1 to 2 g/day) can provide adequate calcium intake.

table 35-5 ***Emergency Antihypertensive Drugs***

VASODILATORS
Sodium nitroprusside (Nipride)
Nitroglycerin
Fenoldopam (Corlopam)
Diazoxide (Hyperstat)*
CALCIUM CHANNEL BLOCKER
Nifedipine (Procardia)
ADRENERGIC BLOCKER
Labetalol (Normodyne)
ACE INHIBITORS
Captopril (Capoten)
ALPHA$_2$ AGONISTS
Clonidine (Catapres)

*Obsolete when no intensive monitoring is available.
From Lehne, R. A. (2001). *Pharmacology for nursing care* (4th ed). Philadelphia: Saunders.

Put on your THINKING CAP!!

Albert Smith, a 34-year-old African American male, arrives at the emergency room complaining of severe headache and blurred vision. His BP is 220/146. The physician diagnoses malignant hypertension. Mr. Smith is anxious and says his father died of a stroke at age 39. Mr. Smith is a carpenter who reports no history of serious illness except thyroid deficiency. What is Mr. Smith's primary risk factor for malignant hypertension?

key points

- Hypertension is called "the silent killer" because it often has no symptoms and is not discovered until a serious complication develops such as damage to the blood vessels in the kidneys, eyes, heart, or brain.
- Hypertension is defined as a persistent elevation of arterial blood pressure of 140/90 mm Hg or greater.

- Primary (essential) hypertension has no known cause, whereas secondary hypertension is caused by an underlying factor such as kidney disease.
- The two factors that determine blood pressure are cardiac output and peripheral vascular resistance.
- The primary risk factors for primary hypertension are family history of hypertension, obesity, atherosclerosis, cigarette smoking, and sedentary lifestyle.
- Blood pressure tends to rise as people age, but age is not a barrier to aggressive treatment of hypertension.
- Hypertension often has no symptoms, but some people experience occipital headaches, lightheadedness, and epistaxis.
- A diagnosis of hypertension is usually based on multiple readings and is accompanied by tests to rule out possible correctable causes.
- Conservative measures to treat hypertension include weight reduction, smoking cessation, sodium restriction, exercise, relaxation techniques, and modified alcohol intake.
- Pharmacologic treatment is based on the stepped-care approach, which begins with the prescription of a single, relatively safe drug and advances through specific steps until good control is achieved.
- Types of drugs used to treat hypertension include diuretics, beta-adrenergic receptor blockers, calcium channel blockers, angiotensin-converting enzyme inhibitors, angiotensin II receptor antagonists, central adrenergic blockers, alpha-adrenergic blockers, and direct vasodilators.
- Ethnicity affects response to many antihypertensive drugs.
- Nursing care of the hypertensive person addresses ineffective therapeutic regimen management, risk for injury, ineffective coping, and sexual dysfunction.
- Hypertensive crisis, defined as a diastolic blood pressure of 130 mm Hg or more, is a life-threatening medical emergency that is usually treated with diuretics and potent vasodilators.
- Complications of hypertensive crisis include stroke, heart failure, and kidney failure.

REVIEW QUESTIONS

1. A consistent blood pressure of 144/100 is considered:
   1. normal.
   2. high normal.
   3. stage 1 hypertension.
   4. stage 2 hypertension.
2. Individuals at greatest risk for severe complications of hypertension are:
   1. white males.
   2. white females.
   3. African American males.
   4. African American females.
3. The cause of primary (essential) hypertension is:
   1. kidney disease.
   2. unknown.
   3. arteriosclerosis.
   4. pregnancy.
4. Complications associated with prolonged hypertension include:
   1. glaucoma.
   2. damage to heart valves.
   3. chronic renal failure.
   4. Alzheimer's disease.
5. A patient who is taking hydrochlorothiazide for hypertension complains of weakness, feeling grouchy, and loss of appetite. You should suspect:
   1. hypotension.
   2. hypokalemia.
   3. hyponatremia.
   4. hypocalcemia.
6. Beta blockers lower blood pressure by:
   1. eliminating excess body fluid.
   2. inhibiting cardiac stimulation.
   3. blocking the movement of calcium into myocardial cells.
   4. preventing the formation of angiotensin II.
7. To obtain the most accurate blood pressure reading, you should:
   1. determine the diastolic pressure first by palpation, then by auscultation
   2. take readings in sequence: supine, sitting, and standing positions
   3. have the patient rest supine for at least 10 minutes before taking BP
   4. assess the pressure only in the patient's dominant arm.
8. A patient on antihypertensive drugs complains of feeling dizzy when first getting up. What should you advise the patient to do when this occurs?
   1. Change positions slowly and exercise the legs before standing.
   2. Discontinue all antihypertensive drugs immediately.
   3. Go back to bed and call the physician.
   4. Increase salt intake to bring blood pressure up to normal.
9. An 80-year-old patient who has been diagnosed with hypertension is not taking her prescribed medications. She says, "Wouldn't you expect my blood pressure to be up a bit at my age?" The nurse's most appropriate reply is:
   1. "Blood pressure tends to increase with age, but treatment reduces the risk of complications regardless of your age."
   2. "As long as you are feeling well, it will not hurt for you to skip your medication."
   3. "High blood pressure medications probably offer little benefit to someone your age."
   4. "Your doctor is going to be pretty upset if you don't follow medical orders."

CHAPTER 36 Digestive Tract Disorders

objectives

1. Identify the nursing responsibilities in the care of patients undergoing diagnostic tests and procedures for disorders of the digestive tract.
2. List the data to be included in the nursing assessment of the patient with a digestive disorder.
3. Describe the nursing care of patients with gastrointestinal intubation and decompression, tube feedings, total parenteral nutrition, digestive tract surgery, and drug therapy for digestive disorders.
4. Describe the pathophysiology, signs and symptoms, complications, and medical treatment of selected digestive disorders.
5. Assist in developing nursing care plans for patients receiving treatment for digestive disorders.

key terms

Anorexia (ăn-ŏ-RĔK-sē-ă, p. 665)
Caries (KĂ-rē-ēz or KĂR-ēz, p. 672)
Cathartic (kă-THĂR-tĭk, p. 665)
Dyspepsia (dĭs-PĔP-sē-ă, p. 654)
Dysphagia (dĭs-FĀ-jē-ă, p. 676)
Emesis (ĔM-ĕ-sĭs, p. 670)
Eructation (ĕ-rŭk-TĀ-shŭn, p. 680)
Flatulence (FLĂT-ū-lĕns, p. 654)
Flatus (FLĀ-tŭs, p. 663)
Gingivitis (jĭn-jĭ-VĪ-tĭs, p. 672)
Laxative (LĂK-să-tĭv, p. 695)
Peritoneum (pĕ-rĭ-tō-NĒ-um, p. 651)
Peritonitis (pĕr-ĭ-tō-NĪ-tĭs, p. 689)
Regurgitation (rē-gŭr-jĭ-TĀ-shŭn, p. 678)
Stomatitis (stō-mă-TĪ-tĭs, p. 671)

To remain healthy, the human body must have a steady supply of nutrients and fluids. The primary role of the digestive tract is to extract the molecules essential for cellular function from food and fluids. Disorders of the digestive tract can threaten the patient's nutritional status, leading to disorders in the structure and functioning of other body systems.

ANATOMY AND PHYSIOLOGY OF THE DIGESTIVE TRACT

The functions of the digestive tract are ingestion, digestion, and absorption of nutrients, and elimination of wastes. Digestion is the breakdown of food into simple nutrient molecules that can be used by the cells. The process of digestion requires (1) the adequate intake of food and fluids, (2) the mechanical and chemical breakdown of food, and (3) the movement of food through the digestive tract. Absorption is the transfer of digested food molecules from the digestive tract into the bloodstream. Elimination is the removal of solid food wastes from the body.

The digestive tract is also called the gastrointestinal tract (or GI tract) and the alimentary tract (Fig. 36-1). It is a muscular tube about 30 feet long. The main parts of the digestive tract are the mouth, pharynx, esophagus, stomach, small intestine, large intestine, and anus.

Other organs that are outside the digestive tract but are considered part of the digestive system are called accessory organs. Accessory organs include the salivary glands, liver, gallbladder, and pancreas. Each of these secretes fluid, containing specialized enzymes, into the digestive tract. These enzymes play a part in the breakdown or metabolism of foodstuffs (Table 36-1).

A two-layer membrane, the **peritoneum,** lines the abdominal cavity and covers the surfaces of the abdominal organs. Lubricating fluid between the two layers permits the organs to move without friction during breathing and digestive movements.

MOUTH

Food is taken into the mouth, where the teeth, tongue, and salivary glands begin the process of food digestion. As the teeth cut and grind the food, the salivary glands secrete saliva, a watery solution that contains amylase (ptyalin). Amylase is an enzyme that initiates the breakdown of carbohydrates. The tongue helps by mixing saliva with the food and pressing it against the teeth. When the bolus is to be swallowed, the tongue forces the food into the pharynx.

PHARYNX

The pharynx is a muscular structure that is shared by the digestive and respiratory tracts. It joins the mouth and nasal

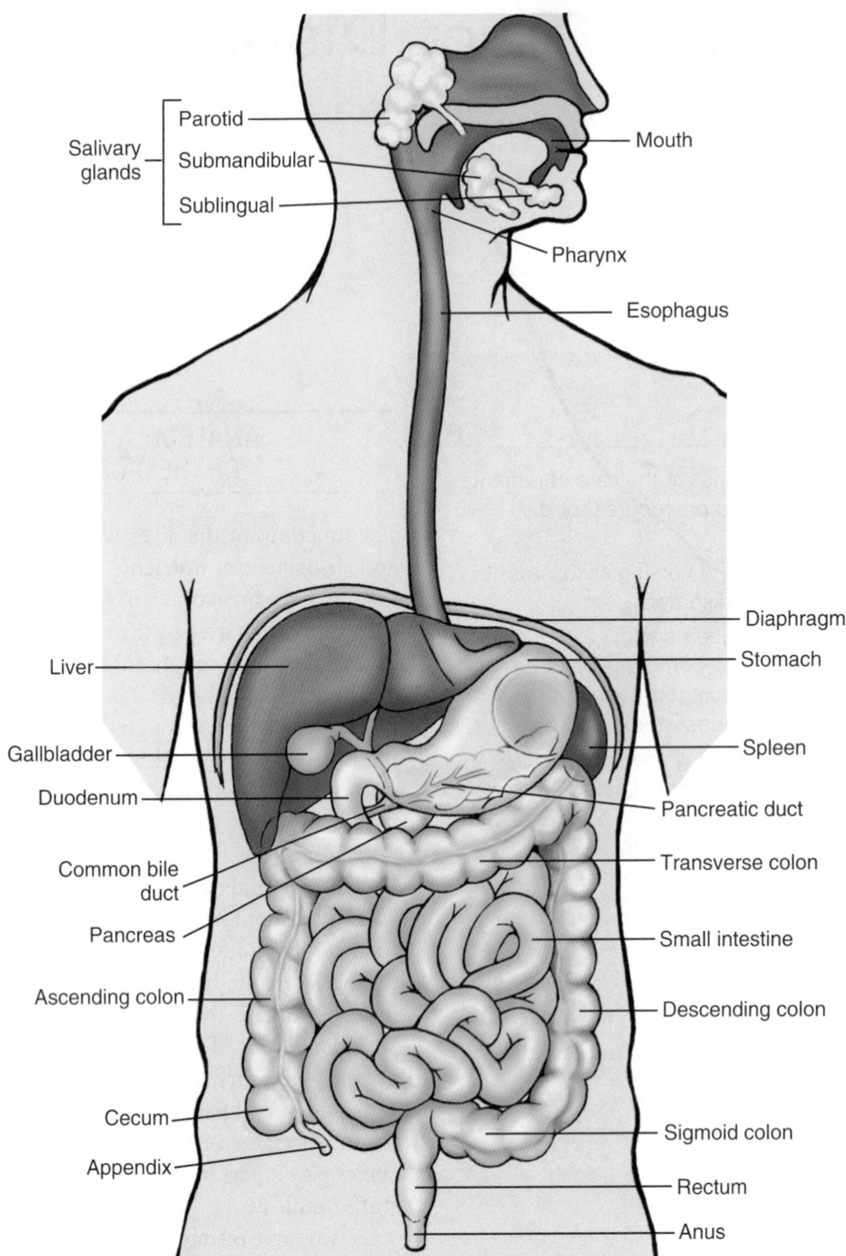

FIGURE **36-1** The digestive tract and associated structures.

passages to the esophagus. During swallowing, the epiglottis covers the airway like a trapdoor to prevent food from entering the respiratory tract.

ESOPHAGUS

Food moves from the pharynx into the esophagus, a long muscular tube that passes through the diaphragm into the stomach. Gravity helps but is not essential for the movement of food through the esophagus. Circular, wave-like contractions of the muscles of the digestive tract propel food down the tract. This movement is called peristalsis.

STOMACH

The stomach is the widest section of the digestive tract. It is separated from the esophagus by the cardiac sphincter. The stomach is not very large when empty, but it expands considerably when food is present. It consists of three sections: the fundus, the body, and the pylorus. A unique arrangement of muscle layers allows the stomach to churn the food, mixing it with gastric secretions until it becomes a semiliquid mass called chyme. Gastric secretions include rennin, pepsin, hydrochloric acid, and lipase. Rennin starts to break down milk proteins, lipase breaks down fats, and pepsin and hydrochloric acid partially digest proteins. The pyloric sphincter between the stomach and the small intestine keeps food in the stomach until it is properly mixed.

SMALL INTESTINE

Chyme leaves the stomach and enters the small intestine, where chemical digestion and absorption of nutrients take

table 36-1 ***Digestive Enzymes and Substrates***

SITE	ENZYME	SUBSTRATE: CARBOHYDRATES	SUBSTRATE: PROTEIN	SUBSTRATE: FATS
Mouth	Ptyalin	X		
Stomach	Rennin		X	
	Pepsin		X	
	Lipase			X
Small intestine	Pancreatic enzymes:			
	Trypsin		X	
	Chymotrypsin		X	
	Carboxypolypeptidase		X	
	Ribonuclease		X	
	Deoxyribonuclease		X	
	Elastase		X	
	Lipase			X
	Cholesterase ester			X
	α-Amylase	X		
	Small intestine enzymes			
	Carboxypeptidase		X	
	Aminopeptidase		X	
	Dipeptidase		X	
	Nucleosidase		X	
	Enterokinase		X	
	Lipase			X
	Sucrase	X		
	α-Dextrinase	X		
	Maltase	X		
	Lactase	X		

place. The small intestine is approximately 20 feet long and consists of three sections: the duodenum, the jejunum, and the ileum.

Liver and pancreatic secretions enter the digestive tract in the duodenum. Bile, produced in the liver and stored in the gallbladder, breaks down large fat globules. Pancreatic enzymes further reduce the fat to glycerol and fatty acids, which can easily be absorbed. The functions of the liver, gallbladder, and pancreas are discussed in greater detail in Chapter 37.

Three layers of tissue make up the walls of the small intestine. The mucous membrane layer secretes the digestive enzymes sucrase, lactase, maltase, carboxypeptidase, aminopeptidase, dipeptidase, nucleosidase, lipase, and enterokinase. Enzymes and their substrates are listed in Table 36-1. The inner layer is lined with thousands of microscopic projections called villi. Digested food molecules are absorbed through the villi into the bloodstream. Muscle layers contract to continue mixing the chyme, moving it toward the large intestine.

LARGE INTESTINE AND ANUS

Chyme enters the large intestine through the ileocecal valve. The first section of the large intestine is the cecum, where the appendix is located. The large intestine goes up the right side of the abdomen (the ascending colon), across the abdomen just below the waist (the transverse colon), and down the left side of the abdomen (the descending colon). The part of the descending colon between the iliac crest and the rectum is called the sigmoid colon. The last 6 to 8 inches of the large intestine is the rectum, which ends at the anus, where wastes leave the body. The presence of sphincters in the anus allows wastes to be stored until voluntary elimination occurs.

Unlike the small intestine, the large intestine has no villi and secretes no digestive enzymes. Its function is to absorb water from the chyme and eliminate the remaining solid wastes in the form of feces.

AGE-RELATED CHANGES

Normal aging generally does not significantly impair ingestion, digestion, absorption, or elimination. When acute or chronic illnesses occur, however, the older person is at increased risk for problems with digestion and elimination.

The teeth are mechanically worn down with age. They appear darker and somewhat transparent. The gingiva (gum) tends to recede. Although tooth loss is not a normal effect of aging, about 40% of all Americans aged 65 years and older are edentulous. The main reasons for tooth loss are caries and periodontal disease. Many older people have complete or partial dentures. There is a significant loss of taste buds with age. Xerostomia (dry mouth) is common but may be caused by poor hydration and drug side effects rather than aging.

The walls of the esophagus and stomach become thinner with aging, and secretions lessen. The production of hydrochloric acid and digestive enzymes decreases. Gastric motor activity slows; thus, gastric emptying is delayed and hunger contractions diminish. There are no significant changes in the small intestine with age. In the large intestine, the muscle layer and mucosa atrophy. Smooth muscle tone and blood flow decrease, and connective tissue increases.

Constipation is a frequent complaint among the elderly, and they use laxatives more often than young people. Many experts believe that constipation is not a normal age-related change but rather is caused by such factors as low fluid intake, lack of dietary fiber, inactivity, drugs, depression, and hypothyroidism.

NURSING ASSESSMENT OF THE DIGESTIVE TRACT

HEALTH HISTORY

Chief Complaint and History of Present Illness

Begin the health history with a detailed description of the present illness. Complaints may include weight changes, problems with food ingestion, symptoms of digestive disturbances, or changes in bowel elimination.

Past Medical History

The past medical history may disclose recent surgery, trauma, burns, or infections. Note serious illnesses such as diabetes, hepatitis, anemia, peptic ulcers, gallbladder disease, and cancer. Also identify any alternative methods of feeding or fecal diversion (ileostomy, colostomy). If feedings are given via nasogastric, gastrostomy, enterostomy, or esophagogastrostomy tubes, record the type and amount of feedings as well as the feeding schedule. The past history also includes a list of recent and current medications, both prescription and over the counter. Use of antacids and laxatives is especially important to note. Record any food allergy or intolerance, with a description of the reaction that occurs when the offending food is eaten.

Family History

Inquire whether the patient has a family history of diabetes, cancer of the digestive tract, peptic ulcers, gallbladder disease, hepatitis, alcoholism, intestinal polyps, or obesity.

Review of Systems

The review of systems begins with an assessment of the patient's general health state. Ask about changes in the skin, including jaundice (yellow color) and pruritus (itching). Assess for mouth problems, specifically dental caries, lesions, bleeding, increased or decreased salivation, abnormal tastes or odors, and pain. Note any difficulties with chewing or swallowing. Also inquire about changes in appetite, food intake, and weight. If nausea, vomiting, **dyspepsia** (indigestion), heartburn, flatus, abdominal distention, or pain is present, identify factors that seem to be related to the symptoms. Describe pain location, along with precipitating factors, relationship to meals, and measures that relieve the pain. Assessment of elimination includes usual bowel habits and recent changes, **flatulence** (gas), change in stool characteristics (frequency, amount, color, consistency), bleeding, and painful defecation.

PHARMACOLOGY CAPSULE Many drugs affect gastrointestinal function, causing anorexia, nausea, vomiting, and diarrhea or constipation.

Functional Assessment

The functional assessment focuses on nutrition, activity, and stressors. Information about general dietary habits should include the daily pattern of food intake (mealtimes, food eaten in a typical day, food likes and dislikes, and use of food supplements), attitudes and beliefs about food, and changes in dietary habits related to health problems. Describe the effects of the chief complaint on usual functioning.

PHYSICAL EXAMINATION

Begin the physical examination with the measurement of height, weight, and vital signs. Observe the patient's general appearance and then begin the head and neck examination.

Head and Neck

Inspect the mouth to determine the condition of the lips, teeth, gums, tongue, and mucous membranes. Describe moisture, color, and lesions. Note any unpleasant or unusual odors of the mouth. If the patient has dentures, examine the mouth with and without the dentures in place. A tongue blade is needed to depress the tongue and examine the pharynx. Instruct the patient to say *ah* while observing the movement of the uvula and soft palate. Normally, the uvula and soft palate move upward, with the uvula remaining in the midline.

Abdomen

For the abdominal examination, the patient should be supine, with the head raised slightly and the knees slightly flexed. The areas of the abdomen are commonly described as quadrants. An imaginary line is drawn horizontally across the abdomen at the level of the umbilicus. A second imaginary line extends from the sternum to the pubic bone. This creates the four quadrants: the right upper quadrant, the left upper quadrant, the right lower quadrant, and the left lower quadrant. Findings can then be documented by anatomic location (Fig. 36-2).

Inspection

Inspect the skin of the abdomen for color, texture, scars, striae, rashes, lesions, and dilated blood vessels. Describe the general contour of the abdomen. Contour is described as flat, convex (rounded), concave (sunken), protuberant, or distended. Note the location and contour of the umbilicus. Aortic pulsations and peristalsis are sometimes observed, especially in thin people.

Auscultation

After inspecting the abdomen, auscultate the abdomen to assess bowel sounds. Auscultation is done before palpation because palpation can alter normal bowel sounds. The diaphragm of the stethoscope should be warmed and used to

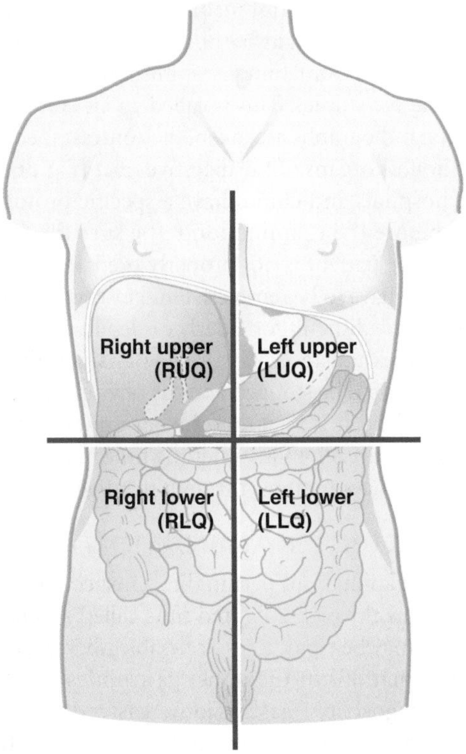

Right upper (RUQ)
Left upper (LUQ)
Right lower (RLQ)
Left lower (LLQ)

Quadrants of the abdomen and their underlying organs*

Right upper quadrant (RUQ)	Left upper quadrant (LUQ)
Adrenal gland (right)	Adrenal gland (left)
Colon (hepatic flexure and portions of ascending and transverse)	Colon (splenic flexure and portions of transverse and descending)
Duodenum	Kidney (portion of left)
Kidney (portion of right)	Liver (left lobe)
Liver (right lobe)	Pancreas (body)
Gallbladder	Spleen
Pancreas (head)	Stomach
Pylorus	

Right lower quadrant (RLQ)	Left lower quadrant (LLQ)
Appendix	Bladder (if distended)
Bladder (if distended)	Colon (sigmoid and portion of descending)
Cecum	Kidney (lower pole of left)
Colon (portion of ascending)	Ovary (left)
Kidney (lower pole of right)	Salpinx (uterine tube; left)
Ovary (right)	Spermatic cord (left)
Salpinx (uterine tube; right)	Ureter (left)
Spermatic cord (right)	Uterus (if enlarged)
Ureter (right)	
Uterus (if enlarged)	

*Small intestine loops in all quadrants.

FIGURE **36-2** The abdomen is divided into four quadrants.

listen to each quadrant. Normal bowel sounds include clicks and gurgles that occur 5 to 30 times per minute. Listen for at least 2 minutes in each quadrant. If no sounds are heard, listen for a full 5 minutes before recording bowel sounds as absent. Bowel sounds may be described as present, absent, increased, decreased, high-pitched, gurgling, tinkling, or gushing. Loud gurgling sounds are called borborygmi. Record the presence or absence of bowel sounds in each quadrant.

Percussion

Nurses with advanced training in physical examination use percussion and palpation to collect additional data. Percussion is tapping on the skin to detect the presence of air, fluid, or masses in the underlying tissues. It also can be used to locate the margins of internal organs. Percussion over an air-filled organ produces a high-pitched, hollow sound called tympany. Tympany is similar to the sound made by a kettle drum. Percussion over a solid or fluid-filled structure sounds dull and flat. Normally, tympany is heard more often than dullness. All four quadrants of the abdomen should be percussed.

Palpation

Palpation is done to detect tenderness, sensitivity, masses, swelling, and muscular resistance. Hold your fingers together and depress the abdomen gently in all four quadrants. Light palpation depresses the abdominal wall only about 1 cm. Deep palpation uses more pressure. To assess for rebound tenderness, the abdomen is depressed and then quickly released. Deep palpation and tests for rebound tenderness should be done only by people who are trained in these techniques.

Rectum and Anus

Wear gloves to examine the anus and perianal area. Inspect the perianal skin for color, rashes, and lesions. Note the presence of any external hemorrhoids. The rectal examination is performed by a trained examiner. You may help position, drape, and comfort the patient. The examiner inserts a gloved, lubricated finger into the rectum and points it toward the umbilicus. The patient is instructed to bear down as if to have a bowel movement. This relaxes the anal sphincter. The examiner palpates for lumps and tenderness in the rectum.

Assessment of the patient with a digestive tract disorder is summarized in Table 36-2.

DIAGNOSTIC TESTS AND PROCEDURES

Diagnostic tests for digestive disorders include radiographic studies, endoscopic examinations, and laboratory studies. Always advise patients about the tests and procedures. Be sure required consent forms are signed.

- For radiographs and imaging procedures, follow agency protocol regarding NPO orders and any other

table 36-2 **ASSESSMENT *of the Patient with a Disorder of the Digestive Tract***

HEALTH HISTORY

Present Illness: Weight changes, problems with food ingestion, symptoms of digestive disturbances, alterations in bowel elimination
Past Medical History: Recent surgery, trauma, infections; history of diabetes mellitus, hepatitis, anemia, peptic ulcers, gallbladder disease, cancer; alternative methods of feeding: type, amount, schedule; fecal diversion: type; allergies: food, drugs
Family History: Diabetes mellitus, cancer of the digestive tract, peptic ulcers, gallbladder disease, hepatitis, alcoholism, intestinal polyps, obesity
Review of Systems:
Skin Color, Pruritus
Oral Cavity: Presence and condition of teeth, condition of gums, moisture, pain, abnormal tastes or odors, difficulty chewing
Appetite
Dysphagia
Digestive Disturbances: Nausea, vomiting, dyspepsia, heartburn, pain
Bowel Elimination: Changes, pain, flatulence, bleeding, stool characteristics
Functional Assessment: Dietary pattern, attitudes and beliefs about food, activity, stressors

PHYSICAL EXAMINATION

Height and Weight
Vital Signs
General Appearance
Head and Neck: Condition of teeth, gums, tongue, mucous membranes, odors, uvula position
Abdomen: Skin color, texture, scars, striae, rashes, lesions, dilated blood vessels; abdominal contour, distention; umbilicus location and contour; bowel sounds; abdominal tenderness, masses, swelling, muscular resistance, rebound tenderness
Perianal Skin: Color, rash, lesions; hemorrhoids

preparation. If contrast media will be used, assess for allergy to the "dye," iodine, and shellfish. If the patient is allergic to any of these, notify the radiologist.

- For laboratory blood tests, tell the patient a blood sample will be taken and whether NPO is required.
- For a urine specimen, instruct the patient in the collection procedure.

Studies are described briefly in Table 36-3.

RADIOGRAPHIC STUDIES

Radiographic studies include the upper gastrointestinal (UGI or GI) series (barium swallow), small bowel series, and barium enema examination. Radiographs of the gallbladder are obtained as well and are discussed in Chapter 37. These studies allow the radiologist to study the structure and function of the digestive tract. A contrast medium is used in some studies. This is a substance, such as barium sulfate, that can be given orally or by enema. Sometimes air is introduced into the bowel for radiographic studies. This is called an air contrast procedure. When radiographs are taken, the contrast medium outlines the hollow organs of the digestive tract (Fig. 36-3).

Most hospitals and clinics have a specific protocol to be followed before the examination to be sure the GI tract is cleansed. If the patient is not properly prepared for the procedure, it may have to be repeated. Fluid restriction and bowel cleansing can be difficult for elderly or debilitated patients. If they become exhausted or if their vital signs change, the preparation should be stopped and the physician notified. After the procedure, it is vital that the barium be cleared from the GI tract. Figure 36-4 illustrates the time required for food or other substances to move through the digestive tract.

ENDOSCOPIC EXAMINATION

Endoscopic examinations permit direct inspection of hollow, interior organs through a lighted tube called an endoscope. Endoscopes may be rigid tubes or flexible fiberscopes. Endoscopic examinations of the upper gastrointestinal tract include esophagoscopy, gastroscopy, gastroduodenoscopy, esophagogastroduodenoscopy, and endoscopic retrograde cholangiography. Endoscopic examinations of the lower digestive tract include colonoscopy, proctoscopy, and sigmoidoscopy. The names of these examinations sound complicated but can easily be broken down to determine what structures are being studied. Table 36-4 lists prefixes for parts of the digestive system that can be combined with the suffix *-scopy,* meaning *to examine.*

Prior to endoscopic examinations, signed consent may be required. Patients are usually not permitted food or fluids for 6 to 8 hours prior to the examination. Bowel cleansing may be very thorough or may just require enemas. A sedative may be ordered before the procedure to reduce anxiety. The most serious complication of endoscopy is perforation, or puncture, of the digestive tract.

LABORATORY STUDIES

The most common laboratory studies are performed on gastric secretions and stool specimens.

Gastric Analysis

Gastric analysis is performed to determine the hydrochloric acid content of the gastric fluid. A nasogastric tube is inserted, and gastric secretions are withdrawn every 15 minutes for 1 hour. This enables measurement of basal gastric secretions. If a gastric acid stimulation test is ordered as well, a drug that stimulates acid secretion (e.g., pentagastrin [Peptavlon]) is administered to the patient. Once again, specimens are collected at 15-minute intervals, labeled, and sent for analysis.

Tubeless gastric analysis detects the presence of gastric hydrochloric acid. A gastric stimulant is given, followed an hour

table 36-3 **DIAGNOSTIC TESTS AND PROCEDURES | *the Digestive Tract***

TEST/PURPOSE	PATIENT PREPARATION	POSTPROCEDURE NURSING CARE
RADIOGRAPHIC TESTS		
Upper gastrointestinal (UGI or GI) series. Barium swallow detects abnormalities of esophagus and stomach.	Inform patient he will need to drink a solution containing contrast media. Radiographs will be taken of the esophagus, stomach, and duodenum via fluoroscope. Films will be repeated 6 hr later to see how much barium has passed through the stomach. NPO 6-8 hr before procedure, per agency protocol.	Monitor stools at least 2 days for passage of white stools that show that barium is being eliminated (normal stool color returns in 3 days). Laxatives may be ordered to promote elimination. Provide food, extra fluids, and rest.
Small bowel series detects abnormalities of small intestine.	Patient drinks a contrast solution. Films are taken at 20-30 min intervals as solution passes through small intestine. Patient will be asked to assume various positions for x-rays. Procedure may take several hours. Preparation same as UGI series.	Same as for UGI series.
Barium enema detects abnormalities of large intestine.	Contrast solution is administered by enema, and radiographs are taken with patient in a variety of positions. May take as long as 1¼ hr. Patient may be restricted to clear liquids day or evening before procedure. Laxative and enemas are given on previous day. Usually NPO after midnight. Enemas are given until intestine is clear on morning of procedure.	Same as for UGI series.
ENDOSCOPIC TESTS		
Upper Digestive Tract		
Esophagoscopy visualizes esophagus. Gastroscopy visualizes stomach. Gastroduodenoscopy visualizes stomach and duodenum. Esophagogastroduodenoscopy visualizes esophagus, stomach, and duodenum. Endoscopic retrograde cholangiography visualizes bile ducts and gallbladder.	Upper digestive tract examinations: NPO for 6-8 hr. If ordered, give sedative shortly before examination.	NPO until gag reflex returns. Monitor for signs of trauma: bleeding from the throat or rectum. Monitor for signs of perforation: fever, abdominal distention, cramping pain, vague discomfort.
Lower Digestive Tract		
Colonoscopy visualizes colon. Proctoscopy visualizes rectum.	NPO for 6-8 hr before examination. May be restricted to liquids previous day or evening. Bowel cleansing may be done with cathartics, suppositories, and enemas.	Monitor for signs of perforation: fever, abdominal distention, cramping pain. Assess for rectal bleeding.
Sigmoidoscopy visualizes rectum and sigmoid colon.	Cathartics and suppositories are usually given the evening before the test. Enemas until colon is clear may be ordered on morning of test.	
LABORATORY TESTS		
Blood Tests		
Serum electrolytes measure electrolytes in the blood to detect imbalances.	Medications that affect results may be held until blood is drawn.	Resume medications.

NPO, Nothing by mouth; *NG*, nasogastric.

Continued

table 36-3 **DIAGNOSTIC TESTS AND PROCEDURES | *the Digestive Tract—cont'd***

TEST/PURPOSE	PATIENT PREPARATION	POSTPROCEDURE NURSING CARE
LABORATORY TESTS—cont'd		
Blood Tests—cont'd		
Serum protein electrophoresis measures serum protein, which may be decreased with peptic ulcers, acute cholecystitis, malabsorption.	Medications that can alter test results (aspirin, isoniazid, neomycin, bicarbonate, sulfonamides) may be withheld until blood sample is drawn.	Resume medications.
Carcinoembryonic antigen (CEA); presence in the blood may indicate GI malignancy, although test is not specific. Also used to monitor response to cancer therapy.	No special preparation. Note whether patient smokes; if smokes, normally will have a positive CEA test.	No special care.
Gastric Analysis		
Basal secretion test measures HCl and pepsin secreted in the stomach.	NPO for 12 hr. Tell patient an NG tube will be inserted and the stomach contents aspirated and discarded. At 15-min intervals for 1 hr, contents are aspirated again. Collect specimens separately.	Remove tube. Resume meals and medications. Offer comfort measures.
Gastric acid stimulation test; secretions increase with ulcers and decrease with gastric cancer.	Same as basal secretion test. Then, a drug will be given to stimulate secretions and additional specimens aspirated at 15-min intervals for another 1-2 hr.	Same as basal secretions test.
Stool Analysis		
Stool occult blood detects GI bleeding when blood is not readily seen.	Advise patient of need for specimen. See text guidelines for collecting specimen. Instruct patient of need for specimen. If test done at home, explain procedure.	No special care.
Stool ova and parasite detects parasitic infections.	Same as stool occult blood.	No special care.
Fecal fat; increased fat in stools occurs with Crohn's disease, malabsorption, and pancreatic disease.	Instruct patient in a 60-gm fat diet to be followed for 3-6 days, followed by collection of a stool specimen. No laxatives, enemas, or suppositories may be used for 3 days before the test. See text guidelines for specimen collection.	Resume normal diet.

NPO, Nothing by mouth; *NG,* nasogastric.

later by a resin dye. The dye is given orally. It reacts with gastric hydrochloric acid to release the dye, which is excreted in the urine. If hydrochloric acid is present in the stomach, the dye appears in the urine 2 hours later.

Occult Blood Test

One test that is done often on the nursing unit detects occult blood in body fluids. Occult blood is blood that is not visible with the naked eye. Specimens most often tested for occult blood are vomitus, gastric secretions, and stool. To test for occult blood, a small sample of the body fluid or stool is placed on a special type of paper that is then treated with a chemical. If blood is present, specific color changes are observed on the paper.

Stool Examination

Stool specimens are examined most often for blood, bile, pathogenic organisms, and parasite ova (eggs). Fecal fat and the white blood cell count may be determined in certain circumstances. Several important points must be remembered when stool examinations are ordered:

1. Collect the specimen in a clean, dry container. Urine should not be in the container because it destroys parasites. Bathroom tissue should not be discarded in the container because the paper contains bismuth, which interferes with some tests.
2. It is best to deliver stool specimens to the laboratory immediately. If temporary storage is necessary, specimens for ova and parasites must be kept warm. Specimens for pathogens should be refrigerated.
3. When a stool specimen is being tested for occult blood, the patient should not eat red meat for 2 to 3 days before the specimen is collected. Red meat interferes with the test results.
4. Examples of drugs that may interfere with results are salicylates, ascorbic acid, anticoagulants, and steroids.

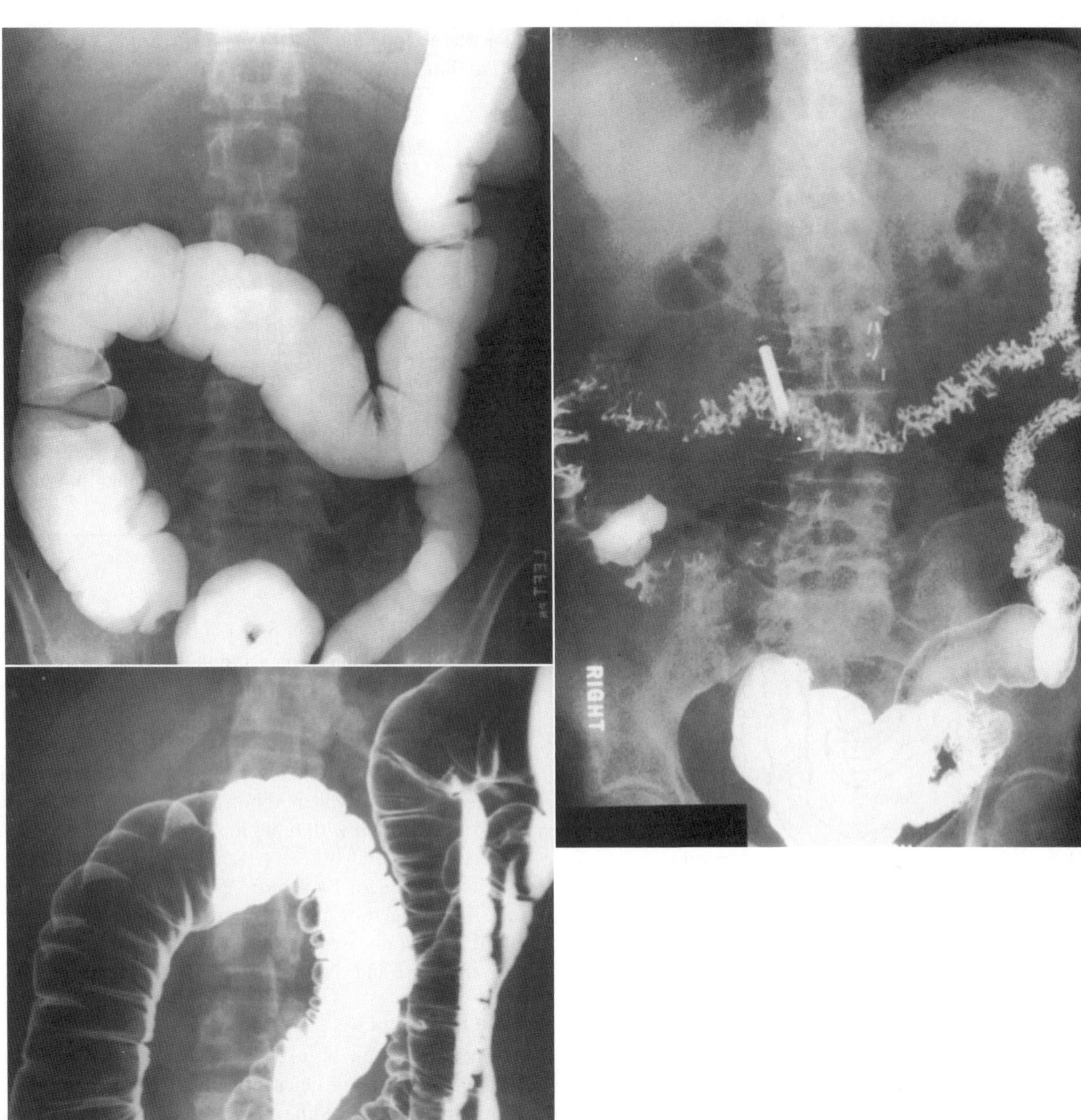

FIGURE **36-3** Contrast medium outlines the hollow organs of the digestive tract.

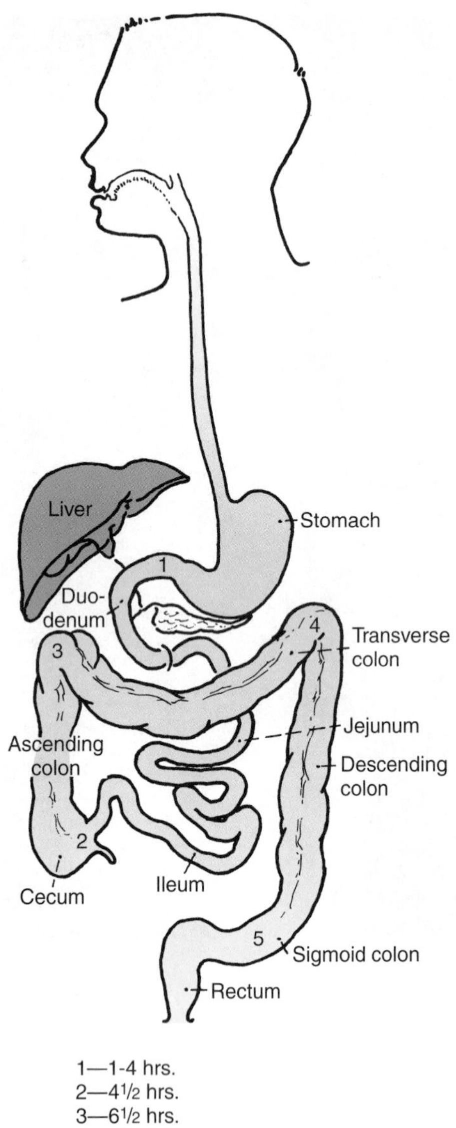

FIGURE **36-4** Time required for the passage of substances through the digestive tract.

5. If visible blood or mucus is present in the stool, include it in the specimen sent to the laboratory.

COMMON THERAPEUTIC MEASURES

GASTROINTESTINAL INTUBATION

Tubes are inserted most often into the stomach or intestines to deliver feedings or to keep the digestive tract empty (decompression). Tubes that are passed through the nose are called nasogastric, nasoduodenal, or nasoenteric tubes, depending on whether the end is located in the stomach or the small intestine.

There are a variety of tubes for special purposes (Fig. 36-5). Levin and gastric sump tubes are nasogastric tubes and may be used for feedings or decompression (Fig. 36-6). Gastrostomy tubes, used for feedings, are placed in the stomach through an opening (stoma) in the abdominal wall. Smaller nasoduodenal tubes, such as the Dobbhoff feeding tube, are weighted so that they pass through the stomach into the duodenum.

table 36-4 ***Terminology for Diagnostic Studies of the Digestive Tract***

ROOT	REFERS TO
Esophag-	Esophagus
Gastro-	Stomach
Duoden-	Duodenum
Sigmoid-	Sigmoid colon
Proct-	Rectum
Cholangi-	Gallbladder
Pancreat-	Pancreas

How to interpret new terms:
scopy = "to examine"
Proctoscopy = *Proct* + *scopy*
Proctoscopy = to examine the rectum
Esophagogastroduodenoscopy = *esophag* + *gastr* + *duoden* + *scopy*
Esophagogastroduodenoscopy = to examine the esophagus, stomach, and duodenum

Nasoenteric tubes used for decompression of the small intestine include the Miller-Abbott, Cantor, and Harris tubes. Care of the patient with tubes for feeding or decompression is discussed separately.

The Sengstaken-Blakemore esophageal-gastric balloon tube is a special tube used to control bleeding in the esophagus. It is generally used in patients with severe complications of liver disease and is therefore discussed in Chapter 37.

Tube Feedings

Patients who are unable to eat or swallow normally may have feeding tubes inserted. Once the tube is in place, exact feeding orders are written. Feedings may be delivered by gravity flow or by infusion pump. Without a pump, use a syringe barrel or a packaged delivery set to put the feeding into the tube. Regardless of the method used, several key points must be remembered about this procedure:

1. Assist the patient into the Fowler's position to reduce the chance of aspiration (regurgitation and passage of fluids into the respiratory tract). Keep the head and chest elevated for about 30 minutes after the feeding is completed.
2. It is critical to confirm that the tube is in the stomach or the duodenum before administering feedings. Radiographic confirmation is the most reliable. This is usually required before feedings when small-bore tubes are used, but are not routinely required with large-bore tubes. Various other methods of checking placement have been used. Currently, observation of aspirated material and assessment of pH are thought to be the most reliable. Stomach contents are grassy green, clear

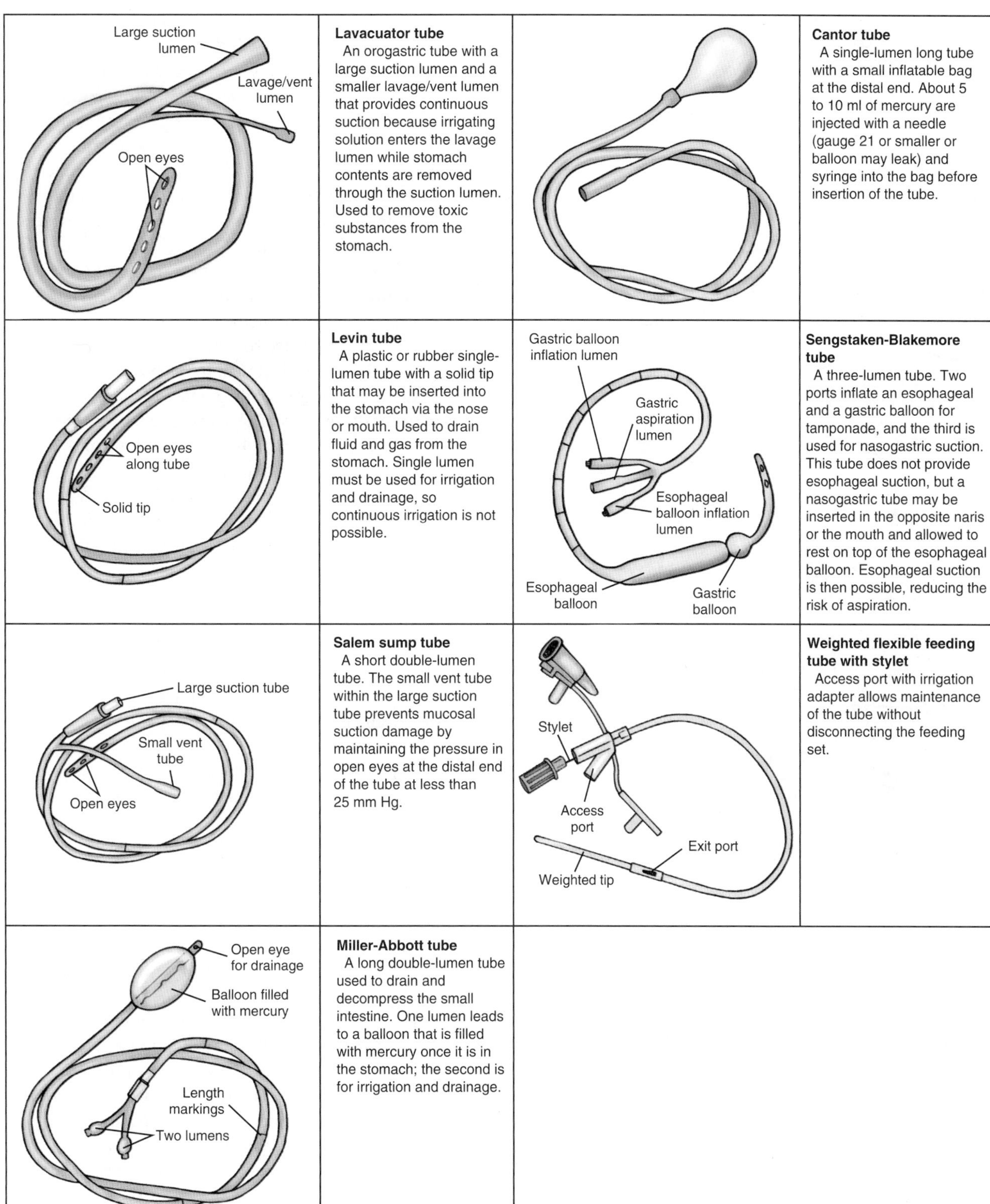

Large suction lumen
Lavage/vent lumen
Open eyes
Lavacuator tube
An orogastric tube with a large suction lumen and a smaller lavage/vent lumen that provides continuous suction because irrigating solution enters the lavage lumen while stomach contents are removed through the suction lumen. Used to remove toxic substances from the stomach.
Cantor tube
A single-lumen long tube with a small inflatable bag at the distal end. About 5 to 10 ml of mercury are injected with a needle (gauge 21 or smaller or balloon may leak) and syringe into the bag before insertion of the tube.
Open eyes along tube
Solid tip
Levin tube
A plastic or rubber single-lumen tube with a solid tip that may be inserted into the stomach via the nose or mouth. Used to drain fluid and gas from the stomach. Single lumen must be used for irrigation and drainage, so continuous irrigation is not possible.
Gastric balloon inflation lumen
Gastric aspiration lumen
Esophageal balloon inflation lumen
Esophageal balloon
Gastric balloon
Sengstaken-Blakemore tube
A three-lumen tube. Two ports inflate an esophageal and a gastric balloon for tamponade, and the third is used for nasogastric suction. This tube does not provide esophageal suction, but a nasogastric tube may be inserted in the opposite naris or the mouth and allowed to rest on top of the esophageal balloon. Esophageal suction is then possible, reducing the risk of aspiration.
Large suction tube
Small vent tube
Open eyes
Salem sump tube
A short double-lumen tube. The small vent tube within the large suction tube prevents mucosal suction damage by maintaining the pressure in open eyes at the distal end of the tube at less than 25 mm Hg.
Stylet
Access port
Exit port
Weighted tip
Weighted flexible feeding tube with stylet
Access port with irrigation adapter allows maintenance of the tube without disconnecting the feeding set.
Open eye for drainage
Balloon filled with mercury
Length markings
Two lumens
Miller-Abbott tube
A long double-lumen tube used to drain and decompress the small intestine. One lumen leads to a balloon that is filled with mercury once it is in the stomach; the second is for irrigation and drainage.

FIGURE **36-5** Examples of tubes used in the digestive tract.

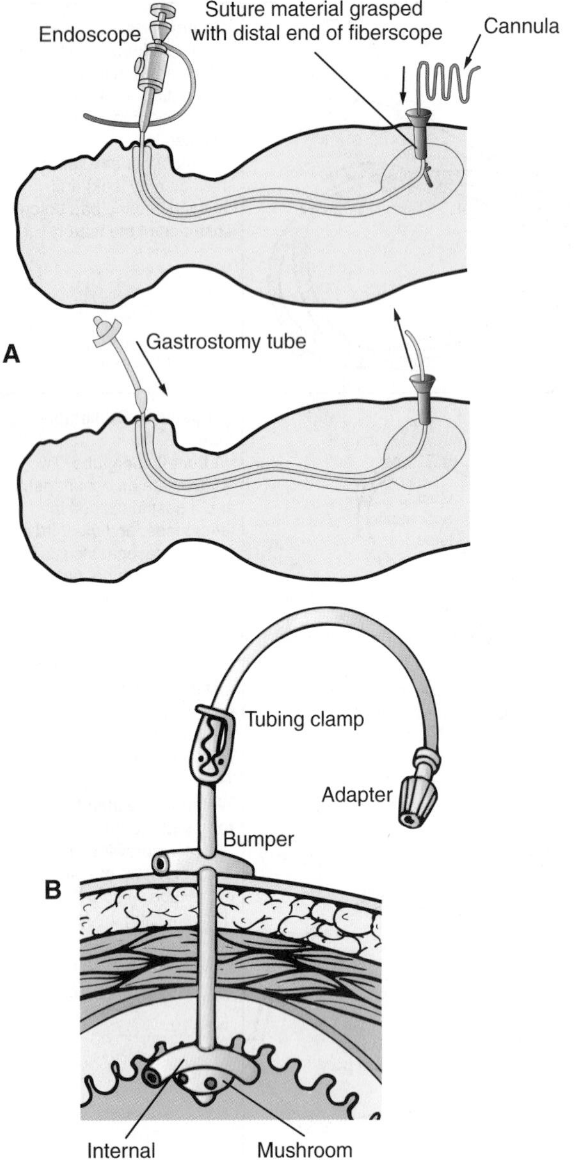

FIGURE **36-6** Percutaneous endoscopic gastrostomy (PEG). *A,* Placement of PEG tube. Using endoscopy, a gastrostomy tube is inserted through the esophagus into the stomach. A cannula is inserted through the abdominal wall into the stomach. The fiberscope grasps the cannula, and the cannula and tube are pulled out through the abdominal wall. *B,* A retention disk and bumper keep the tube in place.

and colorless, or brown; and normally have a pH of 5 or less. The intestinal pH is normally 6 or higher. Other measures that are being evaluated are checking the aspirated fluid for enzymes and bilirubin. Methods that *lack scientific support* are listening over the stomach area with a stethoscope while injecting air through the tube, placing the end of the tube in water to see if bubbles appear, testing the patient's ability to speak, and observing for respiratory symptoms. When a patient has continuous feedings, placement is usually checked at least once each shift.

3. Residual is monitored to help prevent overfilling of the stomach. Check for residual (formula remaining in the stomach from the previous feeding) before each feeding or according to agency procedure. Use a syringe to withdraw and measure the formula. Agency policies dictate what action should be taken based on the amount of residual formula. The physician may need to be notified. The amount of the residual may be subtracted from the next feeding, or feedings may be discontinued for a specified period of time. The residual formula should be returned through the tube to prevent loss of electrolytes.
4. Obtain the correct formula. In the hospital setting, feedings are commercially prepared. There are many varieties of formulas. Be sure to give the right formula, in the right amount, at the right dilution, on the right schedule, to the right patient.
5. When tube feedings are first started, they often are diluted to one-half or one-fourth strength. If the patient tolerates the formula well, the concentration is gradually increased.
6. Stop the feeding and notify the physician if the patient has nausea or pain.
7. Rinse the tube by flushing it with at least 30 ml of water after each bolus feeding. Extra water may be ordered.
8. If diarrhea occurs, contact the physician regarding decreasing the concentration or the rate of delivery, or both, of the formula.
9. Dumping syndrome may occur with rapid feedings of concentrated formula. Signs and symptoms are cold sweat, abdominal distention, dizziness, weakness, rapid pulse rate, nausea, and diarrhea.
10. If using a syringe to give the feeding, do the following:
    - Remove the plunger from the barrel of the syringe.
    - Attach the barrel to the feeding tube.
    - Pinch or kink the tube while the syringe barrel is filled with formula to prevent air from being forced into the stomach.
    - Hold the barrel about 12 inches above the level of the stomach, and allow the fluid to flow by gravity.
    - Flush tubing with water per agency protocol.
11. If an infusion pump is used to deliver the feeding, fill the tubing with formula before connecting it to the feeding tube to reduce the amount of air forced into the digestive tract. Continuous feedings are usually given at a rate of 80 to 150 ml per hour. No more than 6 hours' worth of formula should be hung because it can become contaminated. Bolus feedings are given at specified intervals. They usually consist of 200 to 300 ml over 30 to 45 minutes for each feeding. Oral drugs can usually be given through a nasogastric tube, but some drugs should not be crushed. Consult a drug reference. The tubing and bag must be changed every 24 hours.

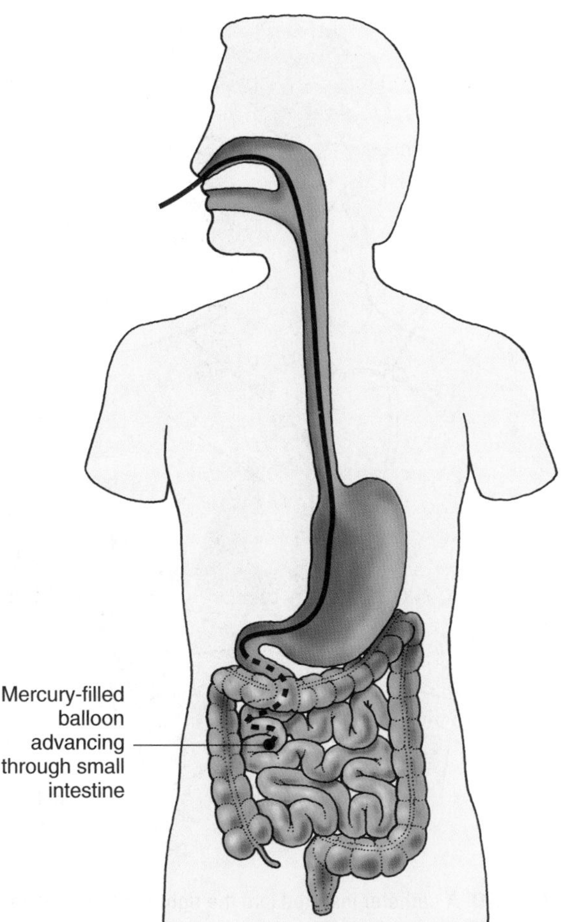

FIGURE 36-7 A nasointestinal tube has a mercury-filled balloon that stimulates peristalsis and advances the tube through the intestines.

Gastrointestinal Decompression

Gastrointestinal decompression is used for the relief or prevention of distention. A tube is passed through a nostril and into the stomach or intestines (or both) and attached to suction. The suction removes fluid and gases that accumulate when gastrointestinal motility is impaired. Conditions that slow motility include peritonitis, obstruction, and any type of surgery performed while the patient is under general anesthesia. Handling of the bowel in abdominal surgery often causes a temporary loss of peristalsis. Decompression may be ordered until bowel activity returns, usually in 3 to 5 days.

Several types of tubes are used for gastrointestinal decompression. As mentioned earlier, the Levin and gastric sump tubes can be used for gastric decompression (often called GI suction). Miller-Abbott, Cantor, and Harris tubes are weighted and are used for intestinal decompression (Fig. 36-7). The patient may return from surgery with the tube in place, or it can be inserted on the nursing unit. The following are key points to remember when caring for the patient with gastrointestinal suction:

1. Attach the tube to a suction apparatus as ordered. Generally, low, intermittent suction pressure is used with single lumen tubes; low, continuous suction is used with double lumen tubes.
2. Monitor the patency of the tube. Observe for the movement of fluids through the tubing into the suction container. If the tube does not seem to be draining, change the patient's position. Gently rotate the tube or pull it out very slightly. (*Exception:* Do not reposition tubes after gastric surgery.) Notify the physician if drainage does not resume.
3. Irrigations should not be done routinely, but they may be ordered occasionally as needed. Frequent irrigations cause acid-base disturbances. For adults, irrigations are usually done with 20 to 30 ml of normal saline. Check the physician's order or the agency procedure manual.
4. Monitor the suction output. Record the amount, color, and characteristics every shift. When blood is present, the drainage may be bright red, dark red, brown, or black. Dark brown or green fluid suggests that there is an obstruction below the point where bile enters the digestive tract.
5. Monitor the patient for successful decompression. If distention is not being effectively relieved, the patient may have nausea and vomiting, shortness of breath, a feeling of fullness, and enlargement of the abdomen.
6. Assess for the return of peristalsis, indicated by the presence of bowel sounds and passage of flatus (gas) through the rectum.
7. Provide comfort measures. The nasopharynx and throat are often very tender. Because the patient is allowed nothing by mouth, mouth dryness is another source of discomfort. Handle the tubing gently. Cleanse the nostrils and apply a water-soluble lubricant to reduce drying and irritation. Provide mouth care frequently. Moisturize the lips. Offer oral spray or lozenges as ordered to provide temporary relief of sore throat.
8. Once the tube is in place, tape it to keep it from being pulled out unless it is the type of tube intended to move through the digestive tract. Tape should secure the tube to the upper lip and cheek or nose (Fig. 36-8). Do not tape the tubing to the forehead because this puts excessive pressure on the nasal tissues. During activity, move the tube carefully to avoid trauma to the nasopharynx. Wrapping the tube with a piece of tape that is pinned to the patient's gown may prevent accidental traction on the tube.

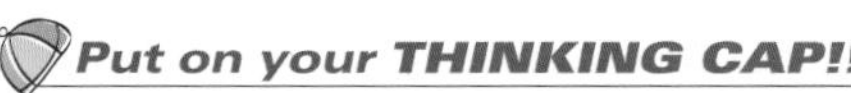
Put on your THINKING CAP!!

What type of acid-base imbalance could result from frequent irrigations of nasogastric tubes? Explain why.

TOTAL PARENTERAL NUTRITION

Sometimes the digestive tract cannot be used for feedings. Total parenteral nutrition (TPN) bypasses the digestive tract by delivering nutrients directly to the bloodstream. A catheter

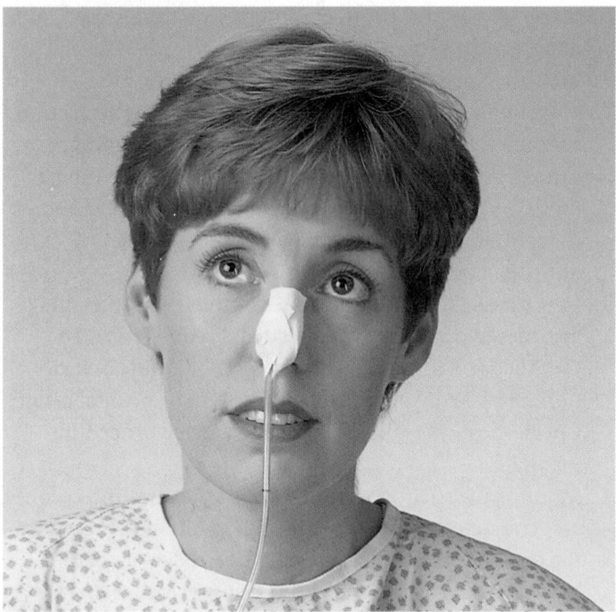

FIGURE **36-8** This method of taping a nasogastric tube anchors it securely, while avoiding trauma to the nose.

inserted into a large vein such as the subclavian is used for the feedings (Fig. 36-9). The feeding passes directly into the superior vena cava and the right atrium. This placement allows for rapid dilution of the concentrated feeding. If the solution were given in a smaller vein, it would cause thrombophlebitis (inflammation of the vein).

When the catheter is inserted, it is sutured to the skin and the insertion site is covered with a sterile dressing. A radiograph is ordered to check placement before the catheter is used for feedings.

Regular intravenous feedings can provide only water, glucose, electrolytes, minerals, and vitamins. This is adequate for short-term problems but does not provide all the nutrients necessary to maintain health or promote healing.

Two types of solutions are used for TPN therapy. The first is a concentrated solution of glucose, amino acids, vitamins, and minerals. It is administered using a special filter. A lipid solution also can be given through a peripheral vein. The lipids are not mixed with the TPN solution.

Important points to remember when caring for the patient receiving TPN include the following:

1. Take great care to prevent infection at the insertion site. Always use sterile technique for site care. The exact procedure should be ordered or written in the agency procedure manual. With each dressing change, inspect the site for signs of infection (redness, swelling, foul odor, or purulent drainage). Monitor the patient's temperature for an elevation.
2. Monitor the flow rate. If given too rapidly, the patient may have circulatory overload, changes in blood glucose, or excessive diuresis (urine output). If the feeding falls behind schedule, do not speed up the rate to catch up.

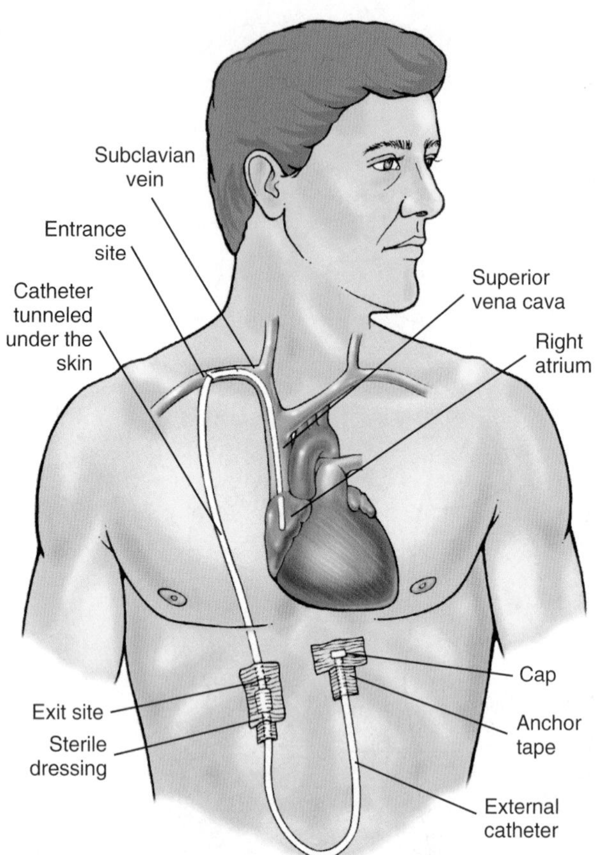

FIGURE **36-9** A catheter inserted into the right subclavian vein for total parenteral nutrition. A transparent waterproof dressing allows vapor to escape while maintaining sterility.

3. Monitor the patient for signs and symptoms of blood glucose changes. The concentrated glucose solution can raise the blood glucose excessively (hyperglycemia). Elevated glucose stimulates the pancreas to produce more insulin, which may then cause a drop in blood glucose (hypoglycemia). Blood should be monitored to detect abnormal glucose levels.
4. Label TPN lines, and do not use the TPN catheter to administer drugs.
5. Be sure that all staff who give medications differentiate TPN lines from small-bore enteral feeding tubes. Patient deaths have occurred as a result of oral medications being administered through a TPN line.
6. Be alert for depression, which often occurs with illnesses requiring TPN. Talk to the patient about his or her feelings. Report sadness and discouragement to the nursing team and the physician.

PHARMACOLOGY CAPSULE Never use a total parenteral nutrition (TPN) line to administer drugs

GASTROINTESTINAL SURGERY

Many conditions of the digestive tract require surgical treatment. Surgery on the mouth and esophagus may be needed to correct defects or to treat cancer. Surgical conditions of the stomach include bleeding ulcers, hiatal hernia, and cancer. Less commonly, surgery is done to decrease the capacity of the stomach for the treatment of extreme obesity. Conditions of the large intestine that may require surgery include cancer, diverticulosis, appendicitis, polyps, obstruction, and ulcerative colitis. General care of the surgical patient is covered in Chapter 16.

PREOPERATIVE NURSING CARE *of the Patient Having Gastrointestinal Surgery*

Radiographic examinations of the digestive tract often are done before surgery. These may be done on an outpatient basis or after admission to the hospital.

The digestive tract is usually cleansed before gastrointestinal surgery. The extent of the cleansing depends on the exact site of the surgery. Oral preparations such as magnesium citrate or large-volume cathartic (laxative) solutions may be prescribed. Use of enemas until the returning fluid is clear also may be ordered. This process is tiring and may exhaust the very ill or elderly patient. The nurse should offer assistance with toileting and hygiene. Changes in vital signs (abnormal heart rate or rhythm, hypotension) or mental state during the bowel cleansing process should be reported to the physician.

Diet is usually limited to liquids for 24 hours before the surgery. The patient should have nothing to eat or drink for a specified period before surgery. Intravenous fluids may be ordered, especially if gastrointestinal suction is being used. Oral antibiotics may be given to reduce the bacterial flora in the bowel, thereby decreasing the risk of contamination of the peritoneal cavity during surgery.

General anesthesia and abdominal surgery cause a temporary loss of peristalsis. Therefore, before or during surgery, a nasogastric tube may be inserted and attached to suction. This prevents the accumulation of fluid and gas in the digestive tract until peristalsis returns.

POSTOPERATIVE NURSING CARE *of the Patient Who Has Had Gastrointestinal Surgery*

Usual postoperative care, discussed in Chapter 16, includes measures to relieve pain, detect complications (hemorrhage, infection), and prevent adverse effects of immobility, anesthesia, and drug therapy. Immediately after surgery on the digestive tract, be especially concerned with preventing gastric or abdominal distention, replacing lost fluids, and maintaining urine elimination. The patient usually has a nasogastric tube in place for decompression. The continuous removal of fluids and gas decreases the stimulation of the digestive tract and reduces pressure on the internal incisions. Monitor gastrointestinal suction to be sure it is draining. Inspect, describe, and measure the drainage. Assess the abdomen for distention and bowel sounds. Check the physician's orders regarding irrigation. After gastric surgery, do *not* irrigate or reposition the tube because of the possibility of traumatizing healing tissue. If the tube is not draining properly or if distention is noted, notify the physician.

Intravenous fluids are given until gastrointestinal suction is discontinued and oral intake is adequate. Keep strict intake and output records. The patient is at risk for fluid and electrolyte imbalances when gastrointestinal suction is used. Because patients often have difficulty voiding after abdominal surgery, an indwelling catheter is usually inserted during the procedure. If there is no catheter, nursing measures may be needed to promote voiding. These measures are discussed in Chapter 38.

DRUG THERAPY

Drugs that are used for their effects on the digestive tract include emetics, antiemetics, laxatives, cathartics, antidiarrheals, antacids, anticholinergics, mucosal barriers, histamine-2 (H_2)-receptor blockers, prostaglandins, and antibiotics. These drugs are discussed with the conditions for which they are prescribed. In addition, Table 36-5 summarizes these drugs, their actions, and nursing interventions.

DISORDERS OF THE DIGESTIVE TRACT

DISORDERS AFFECTING INGESTION

Anything that interferes with the ability to eat a balanced diet can cause nutritional deficiencies. Problems can be as basic as anorexia, inability to feed oneself, or dysphagia, or they may occur secondary to other problems such as oral infection and inflammation, dental problems, oral cancer, and parotitis.

Anorexia

The intake of food is largely dependent on having an appetite. Lack of appetite is called anorexia.

Causes

Anorexia can occur with many physical and emotional disturbances. Nausea, a decreased sense of taste or smell, mouth disorders, and medications are some physical factors that may decrease one's appetite. Emotional problems such as anxiety, depression, or unpleasant thoughts also may cause anorexia. The environment can influence appetite as well. Unpleasant odors or sights can quickly dampen a patient's enthusiasm for a meal. Therapeutic diets such as pureed, low-salt, and low-fat diets are unappetizing to some people. Older people often report decreased appetite. This may be attributed to diminished senses of taste and smell, drug effects, decreased activity, and social isolation.

Medical Diagnosis

The physician assesses the patient for evidence of malnutrition. Weight may be monitored over several weeks. A complete history and physical examination are done to detect underlying problems and the effects of inadequate intake. Initial diagnostic tests that are likely to be ordered include measurements of serum hemoglobin, iron, total iron-binding capacity, transferrin, calcium, folate, B_{12}, and zinc. Tests of thyroid function may be ordered to detect metabolic disorders, and skin tests may be ordered to evaluate allergic responses. A stool specimen may be tested for occult blood. If indicated,

Text continued on p. 670

table 36-5 **DRUG THERAPY** | ***Disorders of the Digestive Tract***

DRUG	USE/ACTION	SIDE EFFECTS	NURSING INTERVENTIONS
ANTACIDS			
Magnesium hydroxide Aluminum hydroxide Calcium carbonate Sodium bicarbonate	Reduce pain of peptic ulcers by neutralizing acid in stomach, decreasing irritation of stomach lining, and inhibiting production of pepsin.	Calcium and aluminum salts tend to cause constipation. Magnesium salts tend to cause diarrhea. Combinations may be used to neutralize these effects.	Teach patients that antacids are nonprescription drugs, but they still have side effects, interact with other drugs, and can be abused. Shake liquids before pouring. Follow dose with water or milk to deliver antacid to stomach. Antacids interfere with absorption of oral drugs if given within 1-2 hr of each other. Tablets should be chewed before swallowing.
H_2 RECEPTOR ANTAGONISTS			
Cimetidine (Tagamet) Ranitidine (Zantac) Famotidine (Pepcid) Nizatidine (Axid)	Reduce secretion of gastric acid and promote healing of ulcers.	Diarrhea, muscle pain, rash, confusion, drowsiness. Cimetidine can cause impotence and gynecomastia and impairs metabolism of many common drugs. Other drugs have fewer side effects; do not cause impotence or gynecomastia.	Give with or after meals. Do not give ranitidine at same time as antacids.
MUCOSAL BARRIER			
Sucralfate (Carafate)	Interacts with acid to form protective gel that coats ulcer surface to permit healing.	Constipation, dry mouth, drowsiness, rash, itching.	Give on empty stomach: 1 hr before meals and at bedtime. Do not give within 30 min of antacids. Interferes with absorption of some other drugs.
SYNTHETIC PROSTAGLANDINS			
Misoprostol (Cytotec)	Decreases gastric acid secretion and protects gastric mucosa. Often used to prevent gastric ulcers caused by NSAIDs.	Contraindicated during pregnancy. Side effects: diarrhea, abdominal pain, miscarriage, headache, flatulence, nausea/vomiting.	Usually given with meals and at bedtime.
ANTICHOLINERGICS			
Atropine Pirenzepine (Gastrozepine)	Block action of acetylcholine. Decrease salivary and gastric secretions. Reduce pain by reducing smooth muscle tone in GI tract.	Dry mouth, constipation, visual disturbance, urine retention. Much milder side effects with pirenzepine than with atropine. Elderly may become confused, agitated, or drowsy.	Contraindicated with narrow-angle glaucoma, renal disease, prostatic hypertrophy, or intestinal obstruction. Best given ½ to 1 hr before meals and at bedtime. Provide oral hygiene. Monitor stools and urine output. Report changes in behavior.

LAXATIVES	Facilitate bowel elimination.		
Stimulants Bisacodyl (Dulcolax) Senna (Senokot) *Cascara sagadra* Castor oil	Stimulate GI tract by irritating mucosa. Tend to produce diarrhea-like stool. Castor oil too harsh for routine use.	Bisacodyl suppositories can irritate the anus. Cascara and senna can make urine pink or brownish. Castor oil rapidly produces watery stool.	Monitor stools. Encourage adequate fluids and fiber to reduce need for laxatives. Laxatives are intended for temporary, occasional relief of constipation and are contraindicated with undiagnosed abdominal pain and inflammatory conditions of GI tract. Chill castor oil and follow with fruit juice.
Bulk-Forming Laxatives Psyllium (Metamucil) Methylcellulose (Citrucel)	Retain water in stool to increase bulk and fluid, which stimulates peristalsis with passage of formed, soft stool.	One of safest laxatives for long-term therapy and during pregnancy. Obstruction can occur if not taken with adequate fluids or if passage through the intestine is arrested.	Patient must take adequate fluids, or mass can harden. May take up to 3 days before effect evident, so used primarily for prevention of constipation.
Saline (Osmotic) Laxatives Magnesium citrate Magnesium hydroxide (milk of magnesia) Sodium phosphate (Fleet Phospho-Soda)	Draw water into bowel to distend and stimulate evacuation. Short-term use only.	Risk of dehydration with prolonged use.	Contraindicated with kidney disease, heart failure, hypertension, and edema.
Lubricants Mineral oil	Lubricate feces for easier passage.	Risk of lipid pneumonia if aspirated.	Impair absorption of fat-soluble drugs and nutrients, so should be given on an empty stomach.
Fecal Wetting Agents Docusate calcium (Surfak) Docusate sodium (Colace)	Soften fecal mass. May take up to 3 days before effects evident, so used primarily for prevention of constipation.		Liquid forms can be given in milk or juice to mask taste.
Suppositories Glycerin Bisacodyl (Dulcolax)	Stimulate evacuation by irritating or distending bowel. Usually act within an hour.		
Other Lactulose (Cephulac)	Increases fecal water content to stimulate evacuation. Promotes passage of ammonia through rectum. Used in hepatic encephalopathy.	Cramps, flatulence, diarrhea, hyperglycemia with diabetes.	Can be mixed with full glass of water, milk, or juice to disguise taste. More effective on empty stomach.
Polyethylene glycol–electrolyte solution (GoLYTELY)	Rapidly causes diarrhea by allowing a large volume of water to be retained in colon. Four liters given over approximately 3 hr; cleans bowel in about 4 hr. Most often used to prepare GI tract for diagnostic procedures or surgery.		Rapid, dramatic effect, so be sure toilet is convenient.

GI, Gastrointestinal; *CNS*, central nervous system.

Continued

table 36-5 **DRUG THERAPY** | ***Disorders of the Digestive Tract—cont'd***

DRUG	USE/ACTION	SIDE EFFECTS	NURSING INTERVENTIONS
ANTIDIARRHEAL AGENTS			
Opiates Morphine Diphenoxylate HCl (Lomotil) Loperamide HCl (Imodium)	Decrease intestinal motility so that liquid portion of feces is reabsorbed.	CNS depression, drowsiness dizziness, constipation, nausea, dry mouth.	Sometimes given after each stool for acute diarrhea, but do not exceed maximum dosage. Use safety precautions. Oral hygiene.
Adsorbents Kaolin Aluminum hydroxide	Bind to substances that may cause diarrhea.		Shake suspension before pouring. Do not administer with other oral drugs because adsorbents will interfere with absorption.
***Lactobacillus* Products**	Replace normal bacterial flora of bowel.		May require refrigeration.
EMETICS			
Ipecac syrup	Cause vomiting. Used to treat some types of poisoning and oral drug overdose.	CNS depression (use cautiously with other CNS depressants).	Follow ipecac with water according to age: <1 yr: ≤1 glass. Older children: 1-2 glasses Adults: 3-4 glasses Emetic action inactivated by charcoal. Milk interferes with action of ipecac.
ANTIEMETICS	Prevent and treat nausea.		
Antihistamines Promethazine (HCl) (Phenergan) Dimenhydrinate HCl (Dramamine)	Decrease sensitivity of vestibular apparatus of inner ear. Suppress vomiting center.	Drowsiness and confusion, especially if given with other CNS depressants.	Use cautiously with asthma, glaucoma, prostatic hypertrophy.
Sedatives Hydroxyzine	Decrease sensitivity of vestibular apparatus and suppress vomiting center. Often used to prevent motion sickness.		

Anticholinergics			
Scopolamine (Transderm Scop)			Transderm Scop is a medicated adhesive disk that is placed behind ear.
PROKINETIC AGENT			
Metoclopramide (Reglan)	Speeds up gastric emptying into small intestine.	CNS depression, GI upset, Parkinson-like symptoms.	Contraindications: GI perforation, obstruction, or hemorrhage; epilepsy.
ANTI-INFECTIVES			
Sulfasalazine (Azulfidine)	Treatment of ulcerative colitis.	Orange-yellow color to urine and skin, photosensitivity.	Contraindication: allergy to aspirin. Adequate fluid intake needed to prevent crystalluria and urinary stone formation. Avoid direct sunlight.
Olsalazine (Dipentum)	Treatment of ulcerative colitis.	Abdominal pain, diarrhea, headache, nausea.	Discontinue if hives, rash, wheezing occur. Encourage fluids.
Amoxicillin (Amoxil)	Combined with omeprazole, prostaglandins, and/or bismuth subsalicylate to treat *H. pylori.*	Rash, diarrhea, anaphylaxis, superinfections (colitis).	Instruct patient to take full course of treatment.
ANTIFUNGALS			
Nystatin (Mycostatin)	Effective against *Candida albicans* (yeast) infections.	Nausea, vomiting, diarrhea with nystatin.	Instruct patient to dissolve lozenges in mouth. Shake suspensions well. Swish nystatin in mouth before swallowing.
Clotrimazole (Mycelex)		Nausea, vomiting, itching with clotrimazole.	Vaginal preparations are available.

GI, Gastrointestinal; *CNS*, central nervous system.

the physician may perform additional procedures to detect possible cancers of the digestive system, lungs, and breasts.

Medical Treatment

Correctable causes of anorexia are treated, but sometimes no physical cause is found. Nutritional supplements may be ordered. The oral route is preferred, but, in extreme cases, enteral feedings or TPN may be indicated.

NURSING CARE *of the Patient with Anorexia*

Assessment

The general assessment of the patient with digestive disturbances is summarized in Table 36-2. In assessing the patient with anorexia, explore factors that may be affecting appetite. Record chronic and recent illnesses, hospitalizations, medications, and allergies. Obtain the female patient's obstetric history as well. The review of systems may provide clues to anorexia. Significant symptoms include pain, nausea, dyspnea, and extreme fatigue. The functional assessment reveals patterns of activity and rest, usual dietary patterns, current stressors, and coping strategies—all factors that can affect appetite. During the physical examination, be especially alert for signs of malnutrition: glossitis (inflammation of the tongue), cheilosis (cracked lips), edema, jaundice, and muscle wasting. The examination also should assess for inflammation or lesions of the mouth and dental problems. If the patient has dentures, evaluate the fit. It is very important to have the patient remove the dentures before the gums are assessed.

Nursing Diagnosis, Goal, and Outcome Criteria: Anorexia

Nursing Diagnosis	Goal and Outcome Criteria
Imbalanced Nutrition: Less than Body Requirements related to anorexia	Improved appetite and adequate food intake: patient states appetite is better, increased intake of food, and stable or increased body weight

Interventions

It is helpful if you can identify factors that contribute to the patient's anorexia. Depending on the reason for the anorexia, a number of interventions may be successful in improving the patient's appetite. If the patient has a dry mouth or bad taste in the mouth, assist with oral hygiene before and after meals. If the teeth or gums are in poor condition, teach proper oral hygiene and refer the patient for dental care. Poorly fitting dentures need to be relined for a tighter fit or to be replaced.

When a patient is nauseated, institute measures to relieve the nausea before presenting a meal tray. Nausea and anorexia both can be related to unpleasant stimuli in the environment. Before serving a meal tray, remove bedpans and emesis basins from sight, conceal drains and drainage collection devices, and deodorize the room if necessary.

Many people enjoy meals more when they are in the company of others. Socialization during mealtime can greatly improve a person's appetite. Encourage a family member to visit during meals or accompany the patient to a dining facility so that they can eat together. Some facilities provide guest trays for patients' family members. In long-term care facilities, a central dining room is usually available for those who enjoy company during meals. On nursing units, small groups of patients often enjoy having their meals together in a sunroom or lounge.

Even people with good appetites eat some foods more willingly than others. For the patient with anorexia, it is especially important to respect food likes and dislikes. If the food being served is unappealing, ask the dietitian to discuss the diet with the patient. Sometimes food from home is a special treat. Before food is brought in by family or friends, advise them of any dietary restrictions. Small servings are more acceptable than large ones to the anorexic person. Additional nutrients can be provided by between-meals snacks. In the inpatient setting, the nurse has little control over the specific food served, but in the home, the meal preparer can be encouraged to provide foods that vary in color, texture, and taste.

Position the patient comfortably and with easy access to the food. If the patient cannot cut food or open packages, be sure to do this. Do not schedule tiring activities immediately before mealtime.

Fortunately, anorexia is a temporary problem for most people. For others, however, it is a chronic problem. Teach the patient the importance of adequate nutritional intake. When they understand how nutrition is related to their health goals, most patients will make an effort to eat. If the patient seems to be anxious or depressed, ask about concerns that he or she may have. Consult the physician about possible counseling if emotional distress persists.

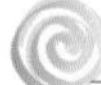

What Does Culture Have to do with Anorexia?

Food preferences, including seasoning and methods of preparation, have a strong cultural basis. When a patient is not accustomed to traditional American food, inquire about whether more familiar foods can be provided or brought in by the family.

Feeding Problems

Patients may require assistance with meals because of temporary impairments or long-term disabilities. Those likely to need assistance include patients with paralysis, arthritis, neuromuscular disorders, confusion, weakness, or visual impairment. Thorough assessments and individualized interventions are needed to ensure adequate nutrition despite disability.

Medical Diagnosis and Treatment

The medical diagnosis is directed at identifying the basic problems and prescribing treatment as appropriate. Patients often are referred to physical therapy and occupational therapy to help them regain basic self-care skills.

NURSING CARE *of the Patient with Feeding Problems*

Assessment

Assess each patient's ability to feed himself or herself independently. Determine the nature of the patient's difficulty and identify remaining abilities. Some patients are temporarily impaired because they are immobilized or confined to restricted positions as part of their medical treatment. Important aspects of the physical examination are visual acuity, range of motion and muscle strength in both arms, and range of motion and grip strength in both hands. Evaluate the patient's ability to follow instructions as well.

Nursing Diagnoses, Goals, and Outcome Criteria: Feeding Problems

NURSING DIAGNOSES	GOALS AND OUTCOME CRITERIA
Feeding Self-Care Deficit related to paralysis, weakness, poor coordination, confusion, visual impairment	Improved self-feeding: patient participates in feeding within his or her capabilities
Imbalanced Nutrition: Less than Body Requirements related to inability to feed self	Adequate food intake: stable body weight or attainment of ideal body weight

Interventions

Encourage patients to be as independent in feeding as possible. For some, proper positioning and arrangement of the meal tray are all that is needed. Assistive devices designed for paralyzed and arthritic patients are available. These can be obtained through the physical therapy or occupational therapy department. Simple adaptations such as padding the handles of utensils may enable the patient with limited grasping ability to feed himself or herself.

When patients need only partial assistance, open milk cartons, cut meat, butter bread, and season food. Sometimes the patient can hold finger foods while you provide food that requires utensils. Before seasoning food or sweetening drinks, ask about patient preferences. Most people feel very strongly about these preferences. Confused patients often can feed themselves if the task is made simple. They may require occasional reminders to continue eating. Sometimes a group dining situation works well for these patients because they may imitate the behavior of others who are eating.

The term *feeder* is sometimes used to refer to patients who must be fed. This label is demeaning and threatens the patient's self-esteem. The patient should be addressed as an adult. Engage the patient in pleasant conversation while he or she is being fed. Remember the following points when feeding a patient:

1. Check the diet and patient's name for accuracy.
2. Seat the patient upright, with the head tilted slightly forward.
3. Tuck a napkin or towel at the patient's chin to catch spills.
4. If the patient is able to communicate, ask in what order the food should be offered. The practice of mixing all food together to make sure the patient gets a little of everything is unappetizing and not recommended.
5. Some patients do not open their mouths voluntarily. Touch the lips with the spoon or gently press just below the lower lip with a finger to encourage them to do so.
6. Pacing is important, so observe that the patient has swallowed before offering more food.
7. In stroke patients, food may accumulate in the affected side of the mouth. Check the mouth at intervals for accumulated food.
8. Offer fluids periodically.

At the completion of the meal, provide mouth care and record the amount of food taken.

Put on your THINKING CAP!!

Practice feeding a classmate a simple meal. Then reverse roles and permit the classmate to feed you. Assume the person being fed is unable to speak clearly, but understands what is said. Immediately afterward write down (1) the steps you went through when feeding another person; (2) how you felt while being fed; and (3) what you learned from the experience that you could apply in patient care.

Oral Inflammation and Infections

Stomatitis

Stomatitis is a general term for inflammation of the oral mucosa. It may result from the mechanical trauma of poorly fitting dentures, the irritation of excessive tobacco or alcohol use, poor oral hygiene, inadequate nutrition, pathogenic organisms, radiation therapy, or drug therapy. Disorders of the kidney, liver, or blood also can cause stomatitis. Emotional tension and excessive fatigue seem to make people more susceptible to some types of stomatitis. Medical treatment is directed toward determining the cause and eliminating it. If specific pathogenic organisms are identified, appropriate antibiotics (usually topical) or antiviral agents may be prescribed. A soft, bland diet may be ordered.

Vincent's Infection

Vincent's infection is caused by bacteria. It has been called trench mouth because it often developed among soldiers in the field in World War I. It is a bacterial infection that causes bleeding ulcers and a metallic taste in the mouth, foul breath, and increased salivation. The patient also may have signs of a general infection, such as fever, enlarged lymph nodes, and anorexia. Topical antibiotics and mouthwashes are used to treat the infection. Rest, a nutritious diet, and good oral hygiene are helpful.

Herpes Simplex

Herpes simplex is caused by the herpes simplex virus, type 1. Ulcers and vesicles develop in the mouth and on the lips. People commonly refer to these lesions as cold sores or fever blisters. They tend to occur in people who have upper respiratory tract infections, have had excessive sun exposure, or are under stress. Spirits of camphor, topical steroids, and antiviral agents may be prescribed as treatment.

Aphthous Stomatitis

Aphthous stomatitis ("canker sore") may be caused by a virus. It is characterized by ulcers of the lips and mouth that recur at intervals. Topical or systemic steroids may be used to treat this chronic condition.

Candida Albicans

Candida albicans, a yeast-like fungus, causes the oral condition known as thrush or candidiasis. Bluish white lesions can be seen on the mucous membranes of the mouth. Patients at high risk for candidiasis include those on steroid or long-term antibiotic therapy. Oral medications are usually prescribed to treat candidiasis. Chronic candidiasis may be treated with topical antifungal agents. Vaginal nystatin tablets can be used like lozenges and allowed to dissolve in the mouth.

NURSING CARE *of the Patient with Oral Inflammation or Infection*

Patients with only oral inflammation or infections are usually treated as outpatients, so the nurse's role is limited to reinforcing medical instructions. These conditions, however, may develop in patients who are hospitalized for other reasons. The nurse then has a more active role in treating the condition and teaching patients.

Assessment

The nursing history includes a thorough description of the patient's symptoms. Describe pain location, onset, and precipitating factors. Note measures that have helped relieve the pain as well. Record any known illnesses and treatments, including drugs and radiation therapy. Describe habits, including diet, oral care practices, alcohol intake, and use of tobacco. Assess the patient's stress level. Inspect the lips and oral cavity for redness, swelling, and lesions.

Nursing Diagnoses, Goals, and Outcome Criteria: Stomatitis

Nursing Diagnoses	Goals and Outcome Criteria
Acute Pain related to tissue trauma, irritation, infection	Pain relief: relaxed appearance, patient statement that pain is reduced or relieved
Impaired Oral Mucous Membranes related to trauma, ineffective oral hygiene, infection, adverse drug effects	Healthy oral mucous membranes: membranes intact, without redness or lesions
Imbalanced Nutrition: Less than Body Requirements related to inflamed or infected oral tissue	Adequate nutrition: usual food intake, stable body weight

Interventions

When acute inflammation is present, gentle oral hygiene and the use of prescribed mouthwashes are soothing. The teeth and tongue can be cleansed with a soft-bristle toothbrush, sponge, or cotton-tipped applicator. Medications must be given as ordered. It is important to read the directions for these medications carefully. Instead of just swallowing the medication, the patient may need to swish liquid medication in the mouth or to permit tablets to dissolve in the mouth. If the patient is discharged while taking a medication, emphasize the importance of completing the entire prescription. Teach the patient proper techniques for brushing and flossing the teeth. Emphasize the importance of daily oral hygiene and good nutrition in preventing recurrences.

PHARMACOLOGY CAPSULE When drugs are given for stomatitis, the directions may be to "swish and swallow" the medication. Be sure to instruct patients appropriately and evaluate their understanding of directions.

Disorders of the Teeth and Gums

Dental Caries

The term *dental caries* refers to a destructive process of tooth decay. Dental decay starts with the presence of plaque on the teeth. Plaque is a substance made up of bacteria, saliva, and cells that sticks to the surface of the teeth. Bacteria produce acids that destroy the protective tooth enamel, permitting decay. Untreated decay erodes into the canal of the tooth, causing intense pain and death of the pulp. The only treatment for dental caries is removal of the decayed part of the tooth, followed by filling the cavity with a restorative material.

Tooth decay can be prevented largely by good oral hygiene and nutrition. Fluoride is so effective in strengthening tooth enamel that many cities add it to the public water supply. In addition, a dentist may apply fluoride directly to tooth surfaces. Toothpastes containing fluoride are recommended by the American Dental Association to reduce the risk of tooth decay. Patients are encouraged to limit sugar intake as well. Be aware that some mouthwashes contain sugar and others contain alcohol, which are inappropriate for some patients.

Periodontal Disease

Periodontal disease begins with gingivitis (inflammation of the gums) and progresses to involve the other structures that support the teeth. In gingivitis, the gums are typically red, swollen, painful, and bleed easily. Gingivitis results primarily from inadequate oral hygiene. Food particles accumulate between the teeth and the gums, causing irritation. Gingivitis is more common in people who are missing some teeth or whose bite does not close properly. Other contributing factors are poor general health, anemia, vitamin deficiencies, and some blood dyscrasias.

Early detection and treatment of gingivitis can stop the progression. Treatment in the early stage consists of professional dental care for teeth cleaning and correction of contributing problems. If the condition is not treated, abscesses develop around the roots, the teeth loosen, and extraction becomes necessary. In more advanced cases, treatment may include not only removing calculus (hardened plaque) but also smoothing root surfaces and surgical removal of the soft, diseased gum tissue. Abnormalities of the teeth and gums are illustrated in Figure 36-10.

NURSING CARE *of the Patient with a Tooth or Gum Disorder*

Assessment

In the health history, determine the presence of oral pain or soreness. Note the patient's usual diet, frequency of dental examinations, and mouth care practices. When examining the mouth, observe the condition of the teeth and gums. Document missing or broken teeth, caries, redness or lesions of the gums, and gum recession. It is especially important for nurses in long-term care to assess patients' mouths at frequent intervals. Oral problems often are overlooked until they are quite advanced.

Nursing Diagnoses, Goals, and Outcome Criteria: Disorders of the Teeth and Gums

NURSING DIAGNOSES	GOALS AND OUTCOME CRITERIA
Acute Pain related to dental caries, tissue inflammation	Pain relief: relaxed appearance, patient statement that pain is reduced or relieved
Imbalanced Nutrition: Less than Body Requirements related to oral pain	Adequate nutrition: stable body weight

Interventions

Most patients are treated for dental and gum conditions in dentists' offices. Sometimes, however, dental problems develop when the patient is receiving nursing care for some other reason. In that case, interventions may be directed at minimizing pain until the problem can be corrected by a dentist. The physician or dentist may order analgesics for acute pain. Gentle mouth care should be performed several times daily.

Provide oral care for patients who cannot do it themselves. Nurse aides and attendants need to understand the importance of regular mouth care and know how to provide it. Clearly include this care in the aide's daily instructions.

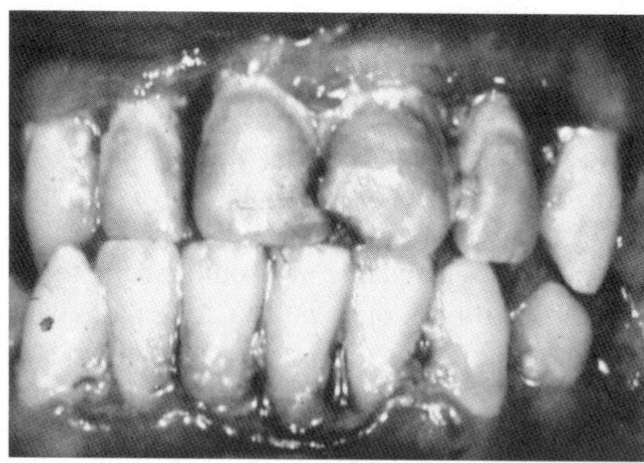

FIGURE **36-10** Acute gingivitis.

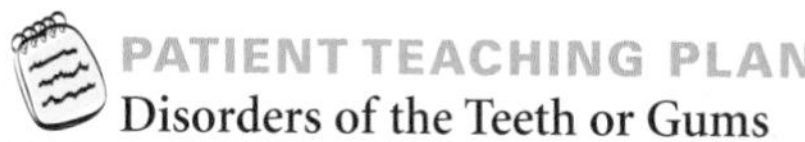

PATIENT TEACHING PLAN
Disorders of the Teeth or Gums

You are in a position to teach patients how to prevent dental caries and gingivitis. Include the following in your instructions:

- Seek periodic dental examinations so that problems can be detected early and expert instruction in mouth care may be obtained.
- Brush your teeth at least twice daily and floss every day.
- Eat a balanced diet with limited sugar intake.

Oral Cancer

The most life-threatening disorder affecting the mouth is cancer. Two types of malignant tumors develop in the mouth: squamous cell carcinoma and basal cell carcinoma. Squamous cell carcinomas occur on the lips, buccal mucosa, gums, floor of the mouth, tonsils, and tongue. The most common site for basal cell carcinoma is the lip.

Risk Factors

Cancer of the lip is related to prolonged exposure to irritants, including sun, wind, and pipe smoking. Factors that increase the risk of cancers inside the mouth include tobacco and alcohol use (especially in combination), poor nutritional status, and chronic irritation.

Signs and Symptoms

Symptoms of oral cancer include tongue irritation, loose teeth, and pain in the tongue or ear. Malignant lesions may appear as ulcerations, thickened or rough areas, or sore spots. The presence of hard, white patches in the mouth is called leukoplakia. Leukoplakia is considered a premalignant condition.

Medical Diagnosis and Treatment

A biopsy of suspicious lesions is done to make a medical diagnosis. When a malignancy is confirmed, the physician often orders endoscopic examinations and radiographs of the upper digestive and respiratory tracts to see whether there is evidence of metastases. Depending on the extent of the cancer, treatment may include surgery, radiation, or chemotherapy, or a combination of these. Small lesions simply may be excised and sutured. Larger lesions that are more invasive usually require more extensive surgery. An incision can be made along the jawbone for access to the oral cavity. Grafts are sometimes needed to close large defects caused by the surgical procedures. The donor site is usually the patient's anterior thigh. Surgical procedures are illustrated in Figure 36-11.

NURSING CARE *of the Patient with Oral Cancer*

Assessment

Assessment of the patient with a disorder of the digestive tract is summarized in Table 36-2. When a patient is being evaluated for possible oral cancer, it is especially important to note a history of prolonged sun exposure, tobacco use, or alcohol consumption. Ask whether the patient or immediate family members have a history of cancer. Significant signs and symptoms to be recorded include difficulty swallowing or chewing, decreased appetite, weight loss, change in fit of dentures, and

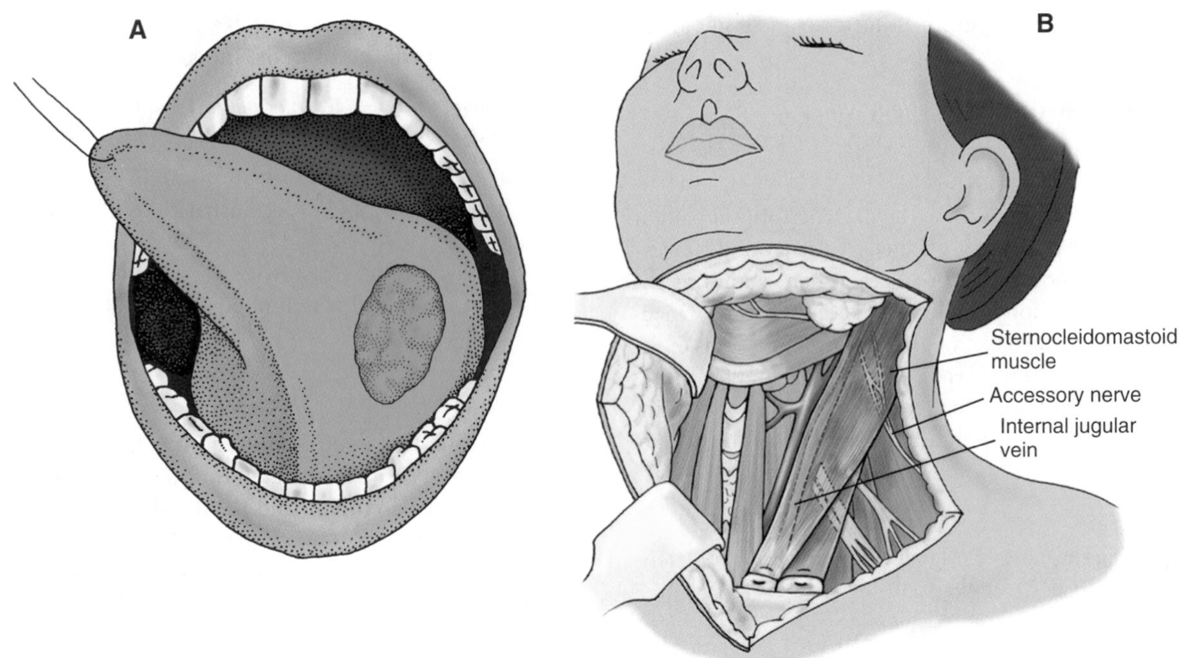

FIGURE **36-11** Approaches to surgery of the oral cavity for cancer. *A,* Peroral (through the mouth). *B,* Radical neck dissection for advanced oral and pharyngeal cancers.

hemoptysis. The physical examination should focus on examination of the mouth for lesions. In addition, assess the neck for limitation of movement and enlarged lymph nodes.

Nursing Diagnoses, Goals, and Outcome Criteria: Oral Cancer

Nursing Diagnoses	Goals and Outcome Criteria
Impaired Oral Mucous Membranes related to tumor, edema, secretions	Healthy oral mucosa: membranes intact without lesions, healed surgical incisions
Ineffective Breathing Patterns related to tumor, tissue trauma	Effective breathing patterns: normal respiratory rate and effort

When surgery is performed, additional nursing diagnoses may include the following:

Nursing Diagnoses, Goals, and Outcome Criteria: After Surgery for Oral Cancer

Nursing Diagnoses	Goals and Outcome Criteria
Acute Pain related to tissue trauma	Pain relief: relaxed appearance, patient statement that pain is reduced or relieved
Imbalanced Nutrition: Less than Body Requirements related to pain, edema, medical restrictions on oral intake	Adequate nutrition: caloric intake sufficient to maintain body weight
Impaired Verbal Communication related to edema, tissue trauma	Effective communication: patient communicates needs verbally or nonverbally
Disturbed Body Image related to surgical or radiation treatment	Adjustment to altered appearance or function: patient statement of acceptance of changes, positive statements about self
Risk for Infection related to broken skin, traumatized tissue	Absence of infection: no fever, normal white blood cell count, incision free of excessive swelling and redness, no purulent drainage
Ineffective Tissue Perfusion of graft related to inadequate blood flow	Adequately perfused graft: warm tissue with normal color

Interventions

Impaired Oral Mucous Membranes

Mouth care varies with the type of lesion and the treatment performed. Surgical incisions can be extensive, with considerable tissue trauma. Radiation therapy causes edema. Dry mouth is often a problem after radiation of the mouth. Consult with the physician before doing any mouth care for the patient who has had oral surgery or radiation. Temperatures are usually taken by the tympanic or rectal route after oral surgery. The physician may order specific solutions for rinsing the mouth. One solution that soothes and cleans is half hydrogen peroxide and half normal saline. Another is made by mixing 12 teaspoons of baking soda in 8 ounces of water. Good hydration keeps the oral mucosa moist and thins secretions.

Ineffective Breathing Patterns

Edema, secretions, and an enlarging tumor can cause obstruction of the airway. Monitor respiratory status frequently and report signs of inadequate oxygenation (dyspnea, restlessness, tachycardia). If edema is present, elevate the head of the bed. Steroids may be ordered to decrease inflammation and production of secretions. Oral suction may be ordered to remove secretions that might be aspirated. A tracheotomy may be performed to prevent or treat airway obstruction. Care of the patient with a tracheostomy is covered in Chapter 51.

Pain

Patients with oral cancer may have pain as a result of the lesion, surgical trauma, or the effects of radiation. Patients who have had grafts often report more pain in the donor site than in the grafted site. Administer analgesics as ordered to manage pain. Inform the physician if the medication is not controlling the patient's pain. In addition to drug therapy, use relaxation, imagery, and other strategies, as described in Chapter 14.

Imbalanced Nutrition: Less than Body Requirements

If the patient is able to swallow, a soft or liquid diet may be prescribed. Mouth care before and after meals may improve appetite and keeps the mouth free of food particles. If the patient cannot or should not take oral nutrition, a feeding tube (nasogastric or gastrostomy) will probably be needed. Another option is TPN. Monitor intake and output records and daily weights to assess adequate intake. With large tumors that cannot be completely removed, or following extensive oral surgery, the feeding tube may be needed indefinitely. See the section on common therapeutic measures earlier in this chapter for care of the patient with a feeding tube. When the patient is able to take oral fluids, assess swallowing and monitor the amount of food taken. Therapy may be needed to help the patient learn to swallow again. Speech therapists are experts in evaluating and managing swallowing disorders.

Impaired Verbal Communication

A large tumor or one that interferes with movement of the tongue is likely to affect speech. In addition, surgical procedures can damage structures involved in normal speech. Assess the patient's ability to read and write. Devise a system to enable the patient to communicate with others. Provide a Magic Slate or pen and pad and keep it within the patient's reach. The call button also must be within reach at all times. Mark the intercom system at the nurse's station so that staff will know to go to the patient's room rather than asking what is needed over the intercom. If the speech organs are intact, the patient may need speech therapy to regain clear oral communication. The nurse and others need to realize how traumatic it is for the patient who is unable to express thoughts verbally. Be patient and do not rush the patient. Compliment successful communication.

Disturbed Body Image

Patients with oral cancer may have body image disturbances as a result of impaired speech, inability to eat, and altered physical appearance. Sometimes external incisions are extensive and disfiguring. Patients need to feel accepted by caregivers and family. Demonstrate acceptance by attentive care, patience, touching, and listening. Assure patients that edema related to surgery will resolve. Some disfigurement, however, may be permanent. Encourage the patient to resume grooming and explore ways to improve appearance. Professional counseling may be needed to help the patient learn to cope with body image changes.

Risk for Infection

Patients with open lesions or surgical incisions are at risk for infection. If a graft has been done, the patient's donor site is also a potential site for infection. Be alert for signs and symptoms of infection (fever, redness, swelling, purulent drainage), and advise the physician if they are present. Prophylactic antibiotics may be ordered. Provide care of external incisions according to physician's orders and agency policy.

Ineffective Tissue Perfusion

When living tissue is grafted, the primary concern is maintaining adequate blood supply so that the tissue remains alive. Monitor graft color and warmth and protect the graft from pressure. Report coolness or darkness to the physician.

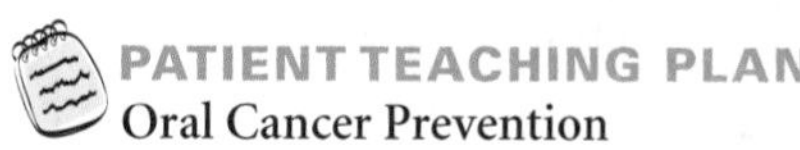

PATIENT TEACHING PLAN
Oral Cancer Prevention

- Avoid known risk factors: tobacco and alcohol use, excessive sun exposure.
- Report any dental problem or pain in the mouth to a dentist or physician for early evaluation.
- Good nutrition and mouth care are essential for oral health and wound healing.

If the patient is discharged with a feeding tube or tracheostomy, begin teaching for self-care as soon as the patient is well enough to participate. If the patient and family need assistance, contact the physician about a referral to a home health agency.

Parotitis

Parotitis is inflammation of the parotid glands. This condition causes painful swelling of the salivary glands below the ear next to the lower jaw. Pain increases during eating. Parotitis may develop in patients who are unable to take oral liquids for a long time, especially if their oral hygiene is poor. Patients who are very weak and have little resistance to infection also are at risk for parotitis.

The condition is treated with antibiotics, mouthwashes, and warm compresses. If chronic inflammation develops, surgical drainage or removal may be necessary. Otherwise, the infected gland can rupture, spreading infection into surrounding tissues. Parotitis might be prevented in susceptible patients by providing chewing gum or citrus-flavored hard candy (if allowed) to stimulate saliva production. Assess the patient's temperature and comfort level and monitor swelling of the infected gland. Provide antibiotics and mouth care as ordered.

Achalasia

Achalasia is characterized by progressively worsening dysphagia (difficulty swallowing). It is caused by failure of the lower esophageal muscles and sphincter to relax during swallowing. The cause is unknown but is thought to be a neuromuscular defect affecting the esophageal muscles. Treatment includes drug therapy, dilation, and surgical measures. Isosorbide dinitrate and nifedipine may provide short-term improvement. Botulinum toxin, when injected into the sphincter via endoscopy, may improve achalasia for several months. The procedure, however, is controversial. Esophageal dilation is done on an outpatient basis. The main complication is perforation of the esophagus. Symptoms of perforation are chest and shoulder pain, fever, and subcutaneous emphysema. Esophagomyotomy is a surgical procedure that cuts the esophageal sphincter. Either a thoracic or an abdominal approach may be used. Hospitalization is expected for several days. The success rate for this procedure is very high. Nursing care is more complex than with dilation. See Chapter 29 for care of the patient after thoracic surgery. Care of the patient having abdominal surgery is addressed in this chapter.

Measures to decrease symptoms are usually determined through patient experimentation. The patient can eliminate foods that seem to cause problems, find the eating position that works best, and avoid restrictive clothing. Elevating the head of the bed at night helps control esophageal reflux.

Esophageal Cancer

Pathophysiology

Cancer of the esophagus is not common, but when it does occur, it has a very poor prognosis. Most esophageal cancers are located in the middle or lower portion of the esophagus. There is no known cause, but predisposing factors are cigarette smoking, excessive alcohol intake, chronic trauma, poor oral hygiene, and eating spicy foods.

Cancer of the esophagus often has begun to metastasize by the time it is diagnosed. The liver and lung are common sites of metastasis. The lesion also can extend to the aorta, causing erosion and hemorrhage. Other complications are esophageal obstruction and perforation.

What Does Culture Have to do with Esophageal Cancer?

In the United States, the incidence of esophageal cancer is higher among African-American males than among white males and is related to tobacco use and dietary factors. The incidence is higher in areas of the world where food and soil contamination and nutritional deficiencies are common.

Signs and Symptoms

Progressive dysphagia (difficulty swallowing) is the primary symptom of esophageal cancer. The patient has difficulty with meat first, then with soft foods, and eventually with liquids. Pain associated with swallowing may be substernal, epigastric, or located in the back and radiating to the neck, jaws, ear, or shoulder. Some patients report sore throats and choking. Obstruction is a late sign of esophageal cancer. Weight loss may be dramatic.

Medical Diagnosis

Radiologic studies used to diagnose cancer of the esophagus include barium swallow and computed tomography. Esophagoscopy may be done to permit the physician to visualize and biopsy the lesion. Endoscopic ultrasonography also may be used to assess the lesion and surrounding tissue. Additional information about common diagnostic tests and procedures is summarized in Table 36-3.

Medical and Surgical Treatment

Esophageal cancer may be treated with surgery, radiation, chemotherapy, or various combinations of these. Three surgical procedures can be done to treat this type of cancer (Fig. 36-12):

- Esophagectomy—removal of all or part of the esophagus and replacement of the resected part with a Dacron graft
- Esophagogastrostomy—resection of the diseased part of the esophagus and attachment of the remaining esophagus to the stomach
- Esophagoenterostomy—replacement of the diseased part of the esophagus with a segment of colon

Patients who are considered poor surgical risks may receive palliative treatment such as:

- Dilation of the esophagus to decrease dysphagia
- Placement of a stent (a rigid tube) in the esophagus to keep it open
- Laser treatment through an endoscope
- Radiation therapy, usually a 6- to 8-week course of therapy
- Chemotherapy
- Photodynamic therapy in which the patient is given a light-sensitive drug. Two days later, a special fiberoptic probe placed in the esophagus activates the drug, which destroys only cancer cells.

Because maintaining good nutrition is a major challenge, the physician may insert a feeding tube, often a gastrostomy tube, to provide adequate nourishment.

NURSING CARE *of the Patient with Esophageal Cancer*

Assessment

Assessment of the patient with a digestive tract disorder is summarized in Table 36-2. When caring for the patient with cancer of the esophagus, key data in the health history are dysphagia, pain, and choking. Obtain a thorough description of the patient's pain, including location, severity, precipitating factors, and measures that bring relief. The nursing assessment of dysphagia includes the patient's description of the problem and observations of the patient while eating. Note the conditions under which the patient has dysphagia, as well as the temperature and texture of foods that cause problems. Assess for the presence of hoarseness, cough, anorexia, weight loss, and regurgitation. The functional assessment documents the use of alcohol and tobacco and dietary practices.

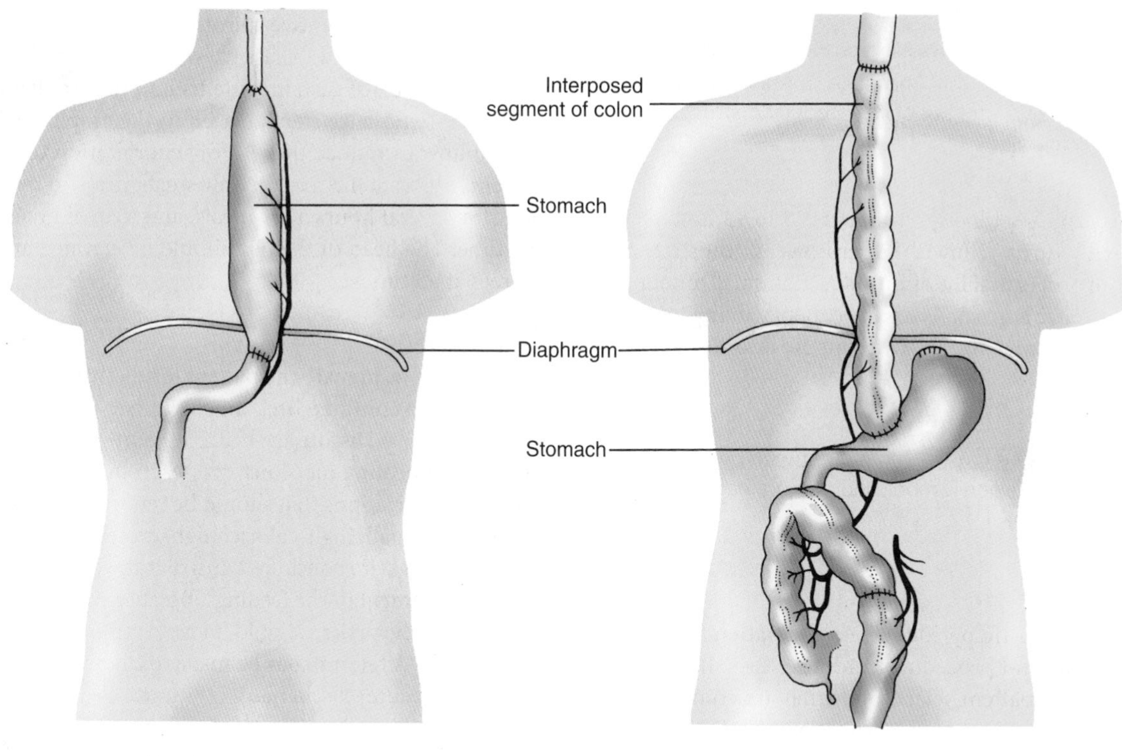

FIGURE 36-12 Surgical approaches to the treatment of esophageal cancer.

General physical appearance and height and weight are important aspects of the physical examination. It is helpful to observe the patient eating. Note body position, size of bites, chewing efforts, and speed of eating.

Nursing Diagnoses, Goals, and Outcome Criteria: Esophageal Cancer

Nursing Diagnoses	Goals and Outcome Criteria
Acute Pain related to esophageal lesion, effect of radiation therapy	Pain relief: relaxed manner, patient statement of pain reduction or relief
Imbalanced Nutrition: Less than Body Requirements related to dysphagia	Adequate nutritional intake: stable or increased body weight
Anxiety related to diagnosis, therapy, uncertain outcome	Decreased anxiety: calm manner, patient statement of lessened anxiety
Risk for Injury related to leakage at anastomosis sites	Reduced risk for injury: healed incisions; no signs of complications such as tarry stools, abdominal pain, or distention
Impaired Gas Exchange related to incisional pain, splinting	Adequate gas exchange: normal respiratory effort and rate, clear breath sounds
Deficient Knowledge of wound care and maintenance of nutrition	Adequate knowledge for self care: patient cares for wounds properly and employs measures to maintain nutrition

Interventions

Pain

Monitor the patient's comfort level. Asking the patient to rate pain on a scale of 1 to 10 is helpful in documentation and in assessing the effects of interventions. Administer analgesics as ordered. Independent measures to reduce or relieve pain are discussed in Chapter 14.

Imbalanced Nutrition: Less than Body Requirements

Nutrition is a major problem for the patient with esophageal cancer. Daily weights, intake and output measurements, and calorie counts all may be kept to monitor adequacy of intake. A high-calorie, high-protein diet is recommended. The texture of food is adjusted as needed (e.g., soft, semisolid), depending on the patient's ability to swallow.

Some general interventions may be helpful in managing dysphagia. A quiet, relaxed environment helps the patient concentrate on effective swallowing. An erect position is preferred. The head should be tilted slightly forward. Some patients think that they can swallow better with the head thrown back. In reality, that position actually makes swallowing more difficult and increases the risk of aspiration. If dysphagia prevents adequate nutritional intake, an alternative feeding method must be used. Options include nasogastric and gastrostomy feedings and TPN.

Postoperatively, patients usually have nasogastric tubes in place and attached to suction. Do not irrigate or reposition nasogastric tubes in patients who have had esophageal surgery. Notify the physician if the tube is not draining properly.

Consider the Alternative!

Yoga, tai chi, music therapy, massage, meditation, and imagery all have been found effective in reducing stress.

Drainage is typically bloody for the first 8 to 12 hours and then gradually turns yellowish. After bowel sounds return, the physician orders oral fluids introduced in small amounts. At first, only water is given. Assess the patient's ability to swallow. Intake and output and daily weights are recorded to evaluate nutrition.

PHARMACOLOGY CAPSULE The patient with dysphagia may be able to take liquid medications more easily than capsules or tablets.

Anxiety

During the diagnostic period, assess the patient's understanding of tests and procedures and offer explanations as needed. Help the patient select foods that are comfortably swallowed. A diagnosis of cancer evokes many questions and fears. It is important to know what the patient has been told about the treatment and the prognosis so that correct information can be reinforced. Preoperative teaching emphasizes the importance of turning, coughing, and deep breathing after surgery. Tell the patient to expect a nasogastric tube, chest tube, and intravenous fluids. Unfortunately, esophageal cancer is often fatal. Encourage patients to ask questions and talk about fears. Be accepting of the patient's feelings and avoid using trite phrases and false reassurance. A referral to a spiritual or mental health counselor may be indicated.

Risk for Injury

Depending on the surgical procedure, the patient may have multiple incisions and wound drains. Assist the patient in supporting the wounds during coughing and position changes. Like any surgical patient, the patient who has undergone surgery for esophageal cancer must be monitored for signs and symptoms of hemorrhage (restlessness, tachycardia, hypotension) and infection (fever, increased white blood cell count, erythema, purulent wound drainage). In addition to the risk of infection, the patient is at risk for leakage at anastomosis sites. If the anastomosis is not secure, digestive fluids leak into the thoracic or abdominal cavity. The risk of leakage is greatest 5 to 7 days after surgery. Signs and symptoms of leakage are fever, tachycardia, tachypnea, and fluid accumulation. The physician should be notified immediately if leakage is suspected.

Impaired Gas Exchange

Immediately after surgery, the patient may be artificially ventilated to maintain adequate oxygenation. Chest tubes are needed to remove fluid from the thoracic cavity. When the ventilator is discontinued, you must encourage and support the patient in turning, coughing, and deep breathing. Chest physiotherapy or incentive spirometry may be ordered. Elevate the patient's head to ease chest expansion and to reduce the risk of reflux of gastric contents into the esophagus.

Patients who have stents placed in the esophagus should be told how to reduce the risk of regurgitation of stomach contents. Instruct them to eat only small meals, to remain upright for several hours after meals, and to avoid lying flat at any time. The head of the bed should be elevated at least 30 degrees at all times.

Deficient Knowledge

Postoperatively, prepare the patient for discharge. Encourage the patient to continue breathing exercises and to gradually increase activity. Discourage bedrest. Point out the characteristics of the healing incisions and teach the patient signs of wound complications that should be reported. Stress the importance of small, high-calorie, high-protein meals. If nasogastric feedings are continued, instruct the patient and family in management of the feedings. Because esophageal cancer often recurs, the patient should know to report increased pain or dysphagia. A referral may be made to a home health agency for assistance after discharge.

DISORDERS AFFECTING DIGESTION AND ABSORPTION

Nausea and Vomiting

Nausea is a feeling of discomfort sometimes referred to as queasiness. It may or may not be accompanied by abdominal pain, pallor, perspiration, and cold, clammy skin. Causes of nausea include irritating foods, infectious diseases, radiation, drugs and other chemicals, hormonal changes and imbalances, and distention of the digestive tract. It is common after surgery and in patients with motion sickness and inner ear disorders.

Nausea and vomiting often occur together. Vomiting is the forceful expulsion of stomach contents through the mouth. It occurs when the vomiting reflex in the brain is stimulated. Very forceful ejection of stomach contents is called projectile vomiting. **Regurgitation** is the gentle ejection of food or fluid without nausea or retching. Just before vomiting occurs, a person usually senses what is about to happen. Tachycardia and increased salivation are common just before vomiting.

Complications

Prolonged or severe vomiting can lead to significant losses of fluids and electrolytes. In addition to dehydration, metabolic alkalosis may develop due to loss of stomach acids. Patients who are very weak or unable to move are at risk for aspirating the vomited stomach contents. Therefore, nausea and vomiting must be treated to relieve patient discomfort and to prevent complications.

Medical Treatment

Drugs that prevent or treat nausea and vomiting are classified as antiemetics. Most antiemetic drugs have multiple uses. They may have local effects (adsorbents), or they may act on the central nervous system. Centrally acting antiemetics include anticholinergics, antihistamines, phenothiazines, and marijuana derivatives. Examples of these drugs are listed in

Table 36-5. A common side effect of most centrally acting antiemetics is drowsiness. They also may cause tachycardia, hypotension, constipation, urinary retention, and dry mouth. Antiemetics are generally contraindicated in patients with glaucoma, myocardial infarction, bowel or urinary obstruction, and pregnancy.

Intravenous fluids may be ordered to prevent dehydration. Oral fluids may be limited to clear liquids or withheld completely until the vomiting stops. At times, a nasogastric tube is inserted and attached to suction to keep the stomach empty. Severe or prolonged vomiting may necessitate TPN to meet the patient's metabolic needs.

PHARMACOLOGY CAPSULE A common side effect of most antiemetics is drowsiness, so take necessary safety precautions.

NURSING CARE *of the Patient with Nausea and Vomiting*

Assessment

The nursing assessment plays an important part in the management of nausea and vomiting. The health history should elicit a description of the onset, frequency, and duration of the present illness. Note the conditions under which nausea and vomiting occur. For example, is it before or after meals, at a certain time of day, or after taking a certain medication? If vomiting occurs, record the amount, color, odor, and contents of the vomitus. Contents might include undigested food or medications. Vomitus containing bile has a characteristic green color. A bright red color suggests recent bleeding in the esophagus or stomach, although it could be due to recently ingested red food or liquid. When blood has been in the stomach long enough to be acted on by stomach secretions, it turns dark brown and resembles wet coffee grounds.

Obtain a complete health history when the patient is able to participate. Record surgeries, chronic illnesses, allergies, and medications. Inquire about pregnancy because many drugs are contraindicated in the pregnant woman.

In the physical examination, describe the patient's general appearance and record vital signs and height and weight. Evaluate hydration status on the basis of pulse and blood pressure, tissue turgor, mental status, and muscle tone. Evaluate respiratory rate, effort, and breath sounds. Assess the abdomen for distention, the presence or absence of bowel sounds, and tenderness.

Nursing Diagnoses, Goals, and Outcome Criteria: Nausea and Vomiting

Nursing Diagnoses	Goals and Outcome Criteria
Imbalanced Nutrition: Less than Body Requirements related to inability to consume or retain food	Adequate nutrition: stable body weight, retention of food and fluids
Deficient Fluid Volume related to loss of fluids by vomiting	Normal hydration: pulse and blood pressure consistent with patient norms, urine output equal to fluid intake, moist mucous membranes
Risk for Aspiration related to decreased level of consciousness, impaired swallowing, wired jaws, depressed gag reflex, vomiting	Absence of aspiration: respiratory rate 12-20 without dyspnea, clear breath sounds

Interventions

Imbalanced Nutrition and Deficient Fluid Volume

When a patient complains of nausea, assist him or her in assuming a still, comfortable position. Maintain a cool room temperature, and remove any unpleasant stimuli. Provide an emesis basin. Apply a cool, damp cloth to the face and neck for comfort. Advise the patient that taking deep breaths and swallowing may be effective in suppressing the vomiting reflex. Unless the episode passes promptly, administer an antiemetic drug as ordered. In situations in which nausea can be anticipated, antiemetics are best given before nausea occurs. It is easier to prevent nausea than to treat it.

If the patient does vomit, remain close by and offer reassurance. Empty the emesis basin as promptly as possible and return it to the bedside in case it is needed again. Replace soiled clothing and linen. Offer mouth care to remove unpleasant tastes when the urge to vomit subsides.

Severe or prolonged vomiting puts the patient at risk for deficient fluid volume. Infants and the elderly are especially susceptible to deficient fluid volume because their kidneys are less efficient in conserving body fluids. Monitor intake and output, vital signs, and other measures of hydration. Signs of deficient fluid volume include tachycardia, hypotension, oliguria, confusion, and poor tissue turgor.

When the patient is ready to resume oral intake, he or she is usually started on clear liquids. Tea, broth, flat carbonated liquids, and gelatin generally are tolerated best. Other liquids may be added if nausea and vomiting do not recur. If permitted, offer dry toast or crackers to help relieve nausea. Advise the patient to eat slowly.

When regular meals are resumed, encourage the patient to take fluids between meals rather than with meals. As mentioned earlier, alternative methods of feeding will be necessary if nausea and vomiting threaten the patient's fluid or nutritional status.

Risk for Aspiration

The patient who is unconscious or has impaired swallowing or a depressed gag reflex is at risk for aspiration. This risk is much greater when the patient is vomiting. Position the patient on the side so that vomitus can drain from the mouth. Keep the suction apparatus on hand and use it as needed to clear the mouth and upper airway. Monitor the patient's respiratory rate and effort and breath sounds. Notify the physician of increasing respiratory rate, dyspnea, and abnormal breath sounds.

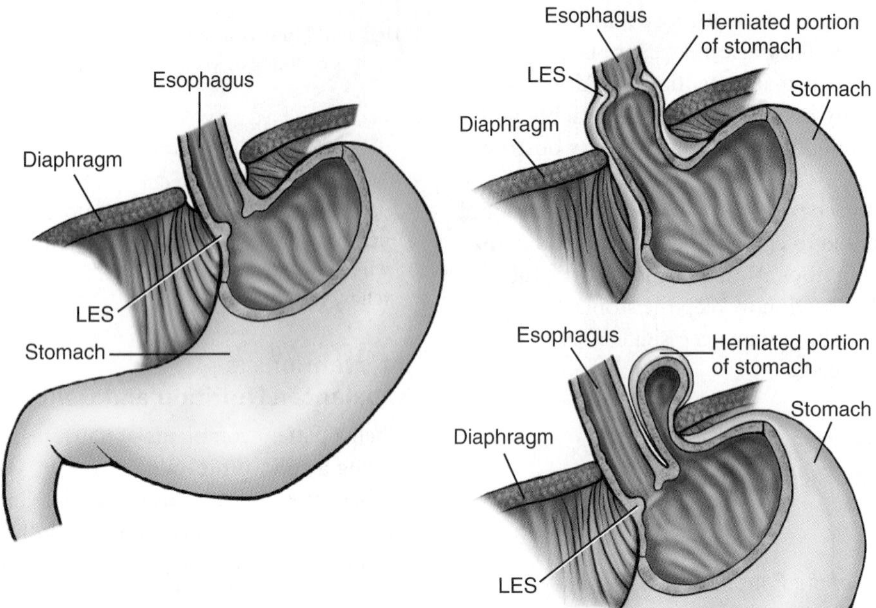

FIGURE **36-13** Hiatal hernia.

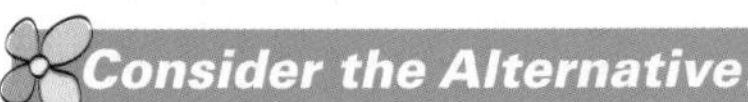

Ginger root is effective in calming upset stomach, reducing flatulence, and preventing motion sickness. Be aware that it enhances anticoagulants and antiplatelet agents.

Hiatal Hernia

Pathophysiology

The esophageal hiatus is the opening in the diaphragm through which the esophagus passes. A hiatal hernia is the protrusion of the lower esophagus and stomach upward through the diaphragm and into the chest. Figure 36-13 illustrates the two types of hiatal hernias, sliding hernia and paraesophageal (rolling) hernia. In a sliding hernia, the gastroesophageal junction is above the hiatus. The stomach slides into the thoracic cavity when the patient reclines. It slides back into place when the patient stands or sits up. Sliding hernias are commonly associated with gastroesophageal reflux disease (GERD). Weakness of the esophageal sphincter permits gastric fluids to flow backward into the esophagus. Acidic gastric fluids can cause inflammation of the esophagus. However, not all patients with hiatal hernias have GERD, and not all patients with GERD have hiatal hernias. GERD is discussed later in this chapter after hiatal hernias.

In a rolling hernia, the gastroesophageal junction remains in place but a portion of the stomach herniates up through the diaphragm through a secondary opening.

Complications of hiatal hernia include ulcerations, bleeding, and aspiration of regurgitated stomach contents. The paraesophageal hernia can also result in strangulation of the hernia, a situation in which the herniated tissue becomes trapped and deprived of blood flow.

Causes

Possible causes of hiatal hernia include weakness of the muscles of the diaphragm in the area where the esophagus and the stomach join (the lower esophageal sphincter [LES]) and an unusually short esophagus. Factors that contribute to development of hiatal hernia include excessive intra-abdominal pressure, trauma, and long-term bedrest in a reclining position. Intra-abdominal pressure is increased by obesity, pregnancy, abdominal tumors, ascites, and repeated heavy lifting or strain. Hiatal hernia develops in about half of all people over 60 years of age.

Signs and Symptoms

Many patients with hiatal hernias have no symptoms at all. Others report feelings of fullness, dysphagia, eructation (belching), regurgitation, and heartburn. Heartburn is a feeling of burning and tightness rising from the lower sternum to the throat. It is triggered by foods and drugs that decrease LES pressure and by lying down or bending over.

Medical Diagnosis

When hiatal hernia is suspected, several tests and procedures may be ordered. A barium swallow examination with fluoroscopy outlines the esophagus and demonstrates esophageal peristalsis. A CT scan helps to visualize the abnormality. In the patient with hiatal hernia, the reflux of gastric contents is evident. Esophagoscopy is direct examination of the esophagus with an endoscope. Structural abnormalities and tissue inflammation may be detected. Tissue specimens can be taken for biopsy during endoscopy.

Esophageal manometry measures the pressures in the stomach and the esophagus. With the patient sitting up, a

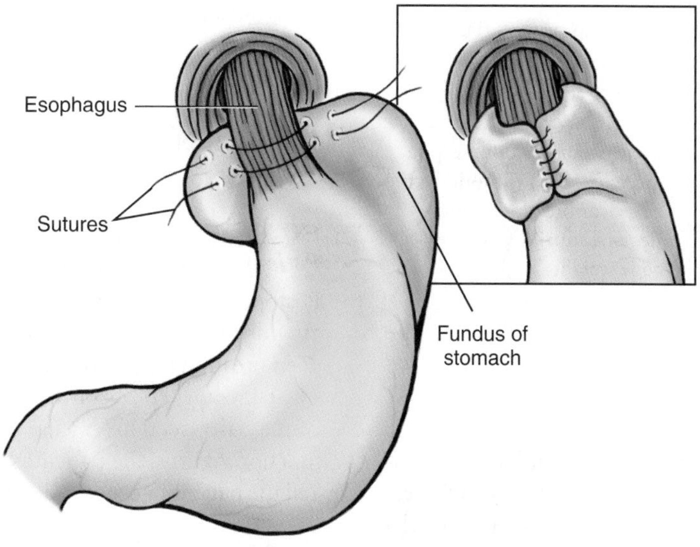

FIGURE **36-14** Nissen fundoplication for hiatal hernia repair.

small tube is inserted through the nose into the stomach. The patient is then placed in a supine position. Small amounts of water or gelatin are given to the patient to swallow. Pressure measurements are taken in the stomach and esophagus. For acid reflux testing, a second probe that is sensitive to acid is inserted through the nose into the esophagus. The detection of acid in the esophagus is consistent with esophageal reflux.

Medical Treatment

In many cases, hiatal hernia can be managed with drug therapy, diet, and measures to avoid increased intra-abdominal pressure. Drug therapy includes antacids and, sometimes, drugs such as H_2-receptor blockers (e.g., ranitidine [Zantac]) to reduce gastric acid secretion. Bethanechol chloride (Urecholine) may be ordered to increase the tone of the LES.

Surgery may be necessary if severe bleeding or narrowing of the esophagus occurs. Surgical options to treat hiatal hernia include fundoplication and placement of the synthetic Angelchik prosthesis. Fundoplication (Fig. 36-14) strengthens the LES by suturing the fundus of the stomach around the esophagus and anchoring it below the diaphragm. The Angelchik prosthesis, illustrated in Figure 36-15, is a C-shaped silicone device. It is tied around the distal esophagus, anchoring it below the diaphragm. For these procedures, incisions may be made in either the abdomen or the chest. Either way, there is a risk of postoperative respiratory complications.

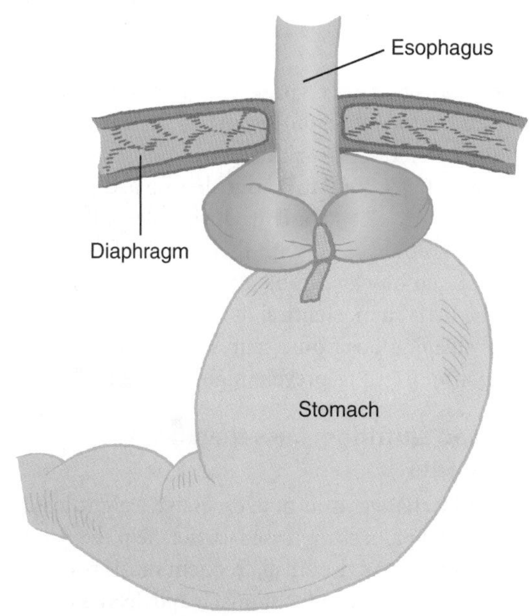

FIGURE **36-15** Placement of the Angelchik prosthesis.

NURSING CARE *of the Patient with Hiatal Hernia*

Assessment

Assessment of the patient with a digestive tract disorder is summarized in Table 36-2. When a patient has hiatal hernia, assess the symptoms (pain, dysphagia, eructation). Record factors that trigger the symptoms as well as measures that aggravate or relieve them. Note any abdominal trauma in the past medical history. Describe the patient's dietary habits, use of alcohol and tobacco, and medication history. Inquire about activities requiring lifting or intense physical exertion. In the physical examination, measure the patient's height and weight.

Nursing Diagnoses, Goals, and Outcome Criteria: Hiatal Hernia

Nursing Diagnoses	Goals and Outcome Criteria
Chronic Pain related to esophageal inflammation	Pain relief: patient statement of less or no pain, relaxed manner

Nursing Diagnoses, Goals, and Outcome Criteria: Hiatal Hernia—cont'd

NURSING DIAGNOSES	GOALS AND OUTCOME CRITERIA
Risk for Aspiration related to regurgitation of gastric contents	Absence of aspiration: respiratory rate 12-20 without dyspnea, clear breath sounds
Imbalanced Nutrition: Less than Body Requirements related to dysphagia	Adequate nutrition: stable body weight

Interventions

Chronic Pain

Pain is caused by the reflux of acid into the inflamed esophagus. Therefore, pain can be reduced by increasing LES pressure, which keeps gastric contents from passing into the esophagus. Drugs that increase LES pressure, neutralize acid, and reduce acid secretion are administered as ordered. Evaluate the effects of drug therapy. Dietary alterations, discussed later, are helpful in reducing the symptoms of hiatal hernia.

Risk for Aspiration

Gastric contents that are regurgitated into the esophagus may be aspirated into the respiratory tract, causing aspiration pneumonia. To reduce the risk of aspiration, food and fluids should not be taken for 2 to 3 hours before bedtime. This reduces reflux of stomach contents during sleep. Patients with hiatal hernia should sleep with their heads elevated 6 to 12 inches. Wooden blocks can be placed under the legs of the head of the bed if a mechanical or electrical bed is not available. This sleeping position requires a period of adjustment but is very important to prevent nighttime reflux.

Imbalanced Nutrition: Less than Body Requirements

Assess weight changes and note excessive weight loss. Measures to control pain, as discussed earlier, help the patient eat more comfortably. Advise small, frequent meals because large meals increase pressure in the stomach and delay gastric emptying. Encourage the patient to avoid foods that are known to decrease LES pressure: fatty foods, coffee, tea, cola, chocolate, and alcohol. Also, acidic and spicy foods may be irritating when the esophagus is inflamed. Counsel the obese patient about the relationship between obesity and increased intra-abdominal pressure.

PATIENT TEACHING PLAN
Hiatal Hernia

- Drug therapy: know the drugs you take, their dosages, schedule, and adverse effects.
- Eat small, frequent meals. Avoid foods that aggravate the condition (fatty foods, caffeine, alcohol).
- Maintain normal weight to decrease intra-abdominal pressure.
- Elevate the head of your bed to discourage reflux.
- Avoid smoking.
- Learn stress management techniques.
- To prevent increased intra-abdominal pressure, avoid bending forward, lifting, or straining, and avoid clothing that is tight around the waist or abdomen.

POSTOPERATIVE NURSING CARE *of the Patient with Hiatal Hernia Repair*

Postoperative care after hiatal hernia repair is similar to that after any major abdominal surgery. Turning, coughing, and deep breathing are particularly important for these patients. The patient will probably have a nasogastric tube in place and connected to suction for a day or two after surgery. Until bowel function returns, the patient is given only intravenous fluids. Tell the patient to expect mild dysphagia for several weeks.

Gastroesophageal Reflux Disease

Gastroesophageal reflux disease (GERD) is the backward flow of gastric contents from the stomach into the esophagus. A key finding is inappropriate relaxation of the lower esophageal sphincter (LES). GERD is often associated with a sliding hernia, although the two are not always found together.

Pathophysiology

Factors that contribute to the development of GERD include abnormalities around the LES, gastric or duodenal ulcer, gastric or esophageal surgery, prolonged vomiting, and prolonged gastric intubation. The acidic stomach contents flow backwards into the esophagus and eventually cause esophagitis (inflammation of the esophagus).

Signs and Symptoms

The onset of GERD symptoms may be sudden or gradual. Patients typically report a painful burning sensation that moves up and down, commonly occurs after meals, and is relieved by antacids. If severe, the pain may radiate to the back, neck, or jaw. Acid regurgitation, intermittent dysphagia, and belching are common. Symptoms are likely to occur after activities that increase intra-abdominal pressure such as lifting, straining, and lying supine.

Medical Diagnosis

A diagnosis of GERD is based on signs and symptoms, radiographic studies, endoscopy, biopsy, gastric analysis, esophageal manometry, 24-hour monitoring of esophageal pH, and acid perfusion tests.

Medical Treatment and Nursing Care

Medical treatment and nursing care are like those described earlier for hiatal hernia. In brief, drug therapy may include:

- H_2-receptor blockers (e.g., ranitidine [Zantac])
- Prokinetic agents (e.g., metoclopramide [Reglan])
- Proton pump inhibitors (omeprazole [Prilosec])

If medical care is unsuccessful, surgical fundoplication may be done.

Put on your THINKING CAP!!

Draw pictures or create a model to illustrate what a sliding hiatal hernia is and how it causes heartburn.

Gastritis

Pathophysiology

Gastritis is an inflammation of the lining of the stomach. The area of the inflammation and the depth of stomach tissue affected vary with different types of gastritis. Gastritis is commonly classified as acute, chronic type A, and chronic type B. Despite a variety of causes, the pathophysiology is common to all. The muscosal barrier that normally protects the stomach from auto-digestion breaks down. Hydrochloric acid, histamine, and pepsin act to cause tissue edema, increased capillary permeability, and possible hemorrhage.

Among the many causes of gastritis, *Helicobacter pylori* is thought to be the prime culprit. Gastritis induced by *H. pylori* affects primarily the superficial tissues. The type associated with NSAIDs, stress, and alcohol tends to affect deeper tissue and is more prone to hemorrhage. Large quantities of hot, spicy, irritating foods can have equally damaging effects. Other related factors are reflux of bile salts from the duodenum, prolonged vomiting, intense stress, and CNS lesions. Chronic gastritis type A probably is induced by immune mechanisms. The changes in the stomach lining with chronic atrophic gastritis result in decreased production of acid and intrinsic factor. Intrinsic factor is needed for the absorption of vitamin B_{12}, which is essential for the maturation of red blood cells. Without intrinsic factor, a serious condition called pernicious anemia develops. The management of pernicious anemia is discussed in Chapter 31.

PHARMACOLOGY CAPSULE Only the parenteral form of vitamin B_{12} is effective in pernicious anemia.

Signs and Symptoms

Symptoms of acute gastritis usually include nausea, vomiting, anorexia, a feeling of fullness, and pain in the stomach area. In people who abuse alcohol, hemorrhage may be the only symptom. Symptoms of chronic gastritis may be the same as acute gastritis. Some patients, however, have only mild indigestion or no symptoms at all unless they develop pernicious anemia.

Medical Diagnosis

The best means of diagnosing gastritis is gastroscopy. The physician is able to visualize the interior of the stomach and biopsy any suspicious areas. Laboratory studies may be done to detect occult blood in the feces, low blood hemoglobin and hematocrit, and low serum gastrin levels. The presence of *H. pylori* can be confirmed by breath, urine, or serum tests, or by gastric tissue biopsy. Because *H. pylori* has been associated with gastric and duodenal ulcers and with gastric cancer, cytologic examination of a tissue specimen commonly is done.

Medical Treatment

The medical management of acute gastritis is concerned with treatment of the symptoms and fluid replacement. If hospitalization is considered necessary, oral fluids and foods usually are withheld until the acute symptoms subside. Intravenous fluids can be ordered to prevent or treat dehydration. Medications to reduce gastric acidity (antacids and H_2-receptor blockers) and to relieve nausea may be given. Analgesics may be ordered for pain relief and antibiotics for *H. pylori*. When nausea and vomiting stop, oral fluids are gradually increased. Typically, the patient progresses from clear liquids to full liquids and then to a soft, bland diet.

The medical management of chronic gastritis focuses on elimination of the cause (e.g., *H. pylori*, alcohol, drugs) and treatment of pernicious anemia. Treatment of *H. pylori* usually requires a combination of omeprazole (Prilosec), which reduces gastric acid secretion, and one or two antibiotics (amoxicillin and/or clarithromycin). Prepackaged combinations are available. Corticosteroids also may be used to reduce inflammation. Vitamin B_{12} injections must be given regularly to prevent long-term complications. A bland diet given in six small feedings per day is usually prescribed, with antacids ordered after meals when reflux is most common.

Surgical intervention may be needed if conservative measures fail to correct or control gastritis or if the patient is hemorrhaging. Specific procedures and nursing implications are the same as for peptic ulcer disease, which is discussed later in this chapter.

NURSING CARE *of the Patient with Gastritis*

Assessment

In taking the health history, first describe the patient's present illness. Patients often complain of pain, indigestion, nausea, and vomiting. Determine the onset, duration, and location of pain. Note factors that trigger or relieve the symptoms. Document chronic illnesses, as well as current and recent medications. Ask whether the patient has had any unexplained weight loss, and if stools have been bloody or black. The functional assessment provides information about dietary practices, use of alcohol and tobacco, and activity and rest patterns. Ask if there are significant sources of stress at present.

In the physical examination, observe the patient's general appearance for signs of distress. Measure vital signs and height and weight for comparison to previous readings. Assess skin color and turgor. Inspect the abdomen for distention and palpate for tenderness and guarding. Auscultate the abdomen for increased bowel sounds.

Nursing Diagnoses, Goals, and Outcome Criteria: Gastritis

Nursing Diagnoses	Goals and Outcome Criteria
Pain related to inflammation of the gastric mucosa	Pain relief: patient states less or no pain, relaxed manner
Imbalanced Nutrition: Less than Body Requirements related to anorexia, pain, nausea and vomiting	Adequate nutrition: stable weight
Deficient Fluid Volume related to vomiting, bleeding	Normal hydration: pulse and blood pressure within patient norms, moist mucous membranes, urine output equal to fluid intake Absence of bleeding: normal stool color, no blood in emesis

Nursing Diagnoses, Goals, and Outcome Criteria: Gastritis—cont'd

Nursing Diagnoses	Goals and Outcome Criteria
Ineffective Coping related to chronic illness	Effective coping strategies: patient employs stress management techniques and resources

Interventions

Pain

Give medications as ordered, including antacids, H_2-receptor blockers, other anti-ulcer agents, analgesics, and antibiotics. Assess drug effectiveness and inform the physician if pain is not relieved. Nonpharmacologic methods of pain control as described in Chapter 14 may be employed as well.

Imbalanced Nutrition: Less than Body Requirements

Encourage the patient to identify foods that seem to aggravate the symptoms and to eliminate them from the diet. Teach the patient that a soft, bland diet taken in small meals may decrease symptoms. Caffeine is usually eliminated from the diet. Note the patient's dietary intake. Daily weights may be appropriate to determine whether the patient is receiving adequate nourishment.

Deficient Fluid Volume

Deficit fluid volume may result from dehydration or from hemorrhage. The patient may become dehydrated because of poor oral intake or severe vomiting. Be alert for signs of deficient fluid volume (oliguria, tachycardia, dry skin and mucous membranes, poor tissue turgor, and hypotension). Record intake and output. Inspect vomited fluids for bright red blood or dark brown particles that indicate bleeding in the stomach. Inspect the stool for the maroon or tarry black appearance characteristic of bleeding from the stomach. Give intravenous fluids as ordered, monitoring the rate of infusion.

Ineffective Coping

Chronic illness drains the patient physically and emotionally. Explore how the patient is dealing with gastritis and what additional supports are needed. Professional counseling may be needed to help the patient learn relaxation and stress management techniques. When alcohol abuse contributes to gastritis, provide information about community resources such as Alcoholics Anonymous.

PATIENT TEACHING PLAN
Gastritis

- Adjust your diet to include soft, bland, small meals; avoid irritants.
- You need to know the name, dosage, schedule, and adverse effects of your drugs.
- Some stress reduction techniques that you might find helpful are exercise, soft music, and regular leisure activities.
- Notify your physician if you have bloody vomitus or dark, tarry stools.
- It is vital that you avoid using tobacco because it stimulates acid secretion.
- Do not take aspirin or NSAIDs because they aggravate gastritis and increase the risk of hemorrhage.

Consider the Alternative!

Alternative therapies for stress reduction include acupuncture, therapeutic massage, guided imagery, progressive relaxation, meditation, yoga, and aromatherapy with chamomile, lavender, citronella, and mandarin.

Peptic Ulcer

Pathophysiology

A peptic ulcer is a loss of tissue from the lining of the digestive tract. Normally, a mucous barrier protects the lining from the digestive fluids. When that barrier fails, pepsin and hydrochloric acid cause injury to the unprotected tissue.

Peptic ulcers may be acute or chronic, depending on the layers of tissue affected. Acute ulcers affect only the superficial layers of the digestive lining, whereas chronic ulcers extend into the muscle layer. Acute ulcers are sometimes called acute gastric lesions.

Peptic ulcers are classified as gastric or duodenal, depending on their location. Gastric and duodenal ulcers differ in depth of injury, amount of gastric secretions, incidence, and signs and symptoms. These differences are presented in Table 36-6.

Gastric ulcers occur most often in men and in the elderly. Women who have ulcers are more likely to have gastric ulcers than duodenal ulcers. The incidence rate of gastric ulcers is higher among people with type A blood than among people with other blood types. Although people think of ulcers as a condition of the rich and powerful, gastric ulcers are actually more common among unskilled laborers.

Eighty percent of peptic ulcers occur in the duodenum. Duodenal ulcers are more common in younger men and in people with type O blood. There is an increase in the secretion of gastric acid. Duodenal ulcers are found among people in all occupations and income levels.

Causes

Factors that contribute to the development of ulcers are thought to include drugs, infection, and stress. Drugs that are associated with ulcer disease include aspirin and nonsteroidal anti-inflammatory drugs (NSAIDs) such as ibuprofen. However, there is considerable evidence that most ulcers are caused by the microorganism *Helicobacter pylori.* Also, extremely stressful events such as shock, burns, and trauma are thought to cause a temporary decrease in blood flow to the gastric mucosa. Inadequate blood flow interferes with the mucosal barrier, permitting breakdown of the stomach lin-

table 36-6 ***Comparison of Gastric and Duodenal Ulcers***

CHARACTERISTIC	GASTRIC ULCER	DUODENAL ULCER
Incidence	More common in older men, working class, those with blood type A, substance abusers, and people under severe stress.	More common in younger men, all social classes, those with blood type O, people with chronic illnesses.
Ulcer depth	Shallow	Deep
Gastric secretions	Unchanged or decreased	Increased
Signs and symptoms	Burning and pressure in upper left abdomen below rib cage and in back. Pain 1-2 hr after meals. Relieved by food or fluids.	Burning and pressure in upper middle abdomen and back. Pain 2-4 hr after meals. Relieved by antacids or foods.
Complications	Hemorrhage, perforation, obstruction.	Hemorrhage, perforation, obstruction.

ing. Ulcers attributed to this process are called stress ulcers. Spicy foods often have been blamed for ulcers, but this link has not been proved. With gastric ulcers, gastric acid production is usually normal or decreased.

Conditions that cause excessive gastric acid secretion seem to contribute to the development of duodenal ulcers. Examples of such conditions are chronic obstructive pulmonary disease, cirrhosis of the liver, chronic pancreatitis, and hyperparathyroidism. Heavy alcohol and tobacco use also is associated with duodenal ulcers, as well as with gastric ulcers.

Signs and Symptoms

Gastric ulcers typically produce burning pain in the epigastric area 1 to 2 hours after meals. Nausea, anorexia, and weight loss are sometimes present. Some patients have no pain at all until serious complications develop.

Although some patients with duodenal ulcers have no pain, others experience a burning or cramping pain 2 to 4 hours after meals. The pain is located in the area just beneath the xiphoid process. It is often relieved by antacids or food. The patient commonly reports pain that lasts for several weeks or months, disappears, and returns.

Complications

Peptic ulcers can lead to serious, even life-threatening complications. Intractability is the term used to describe symptomatic peptic ulcer disease that does not respond to treatment. Hemorrhage is more common in the elderly and in people with gastric ulcers. If the hemorrhage is not brought under control, the patient can bleed to death.

A perforation is a break in the wall of the stomach or the duodenum that permits digestive fluids to leak into the peritoneal cavity, causing inflammation of the peritoneum (peritonitis).

The pylorus is the opening between the stomach and the duodenum. With peptic ulcer disease, pyloric obstruction may develop as a result of edema and scarring. Pyloric obstruction causes persistent vomiting that can lead to severe fluid and electrolyte imbalances.

Medical Diagnosis

Tests and procedures used to detect peptic ulcers include barium swallow examination, gastroscopy, and esophagogastroduodenoscopy. These studies, including patient preparation and aftercare, are described in Table 36-3.

Gastric analysis may be done to determine the acidity of stomach secretions. However, the value of this test is in doubt. The test may be more accurate if pentagastrin is given to stimulate gastric secretions prior to collection of the specimens.

Medical Treatment

The goals in treating peptic ulcer are to relieve symptoms, promote healing, prevent or detect complications, and prevent recurrence. Interventions include drug therapy, diet, and stress management.

PHARMACOLOGY CAPSULE Antacids are drugs and can have adverse effects if taken excessively!

Drug therapy. Drug therapy is intended to relieve symptoms, heal the ulcer, cure *H. pylori* infections, and/or prevent recurrence. Anti-secretory drugs decrease gastric acid secretion, which relieves symptoms and allows the ulcer to begin healing. H_2-receptor blockers, proton pump inhibitors, and prostaglandins are examples of anti-secretory drugs. H_2-receptor blockers, which are the most commonly used antiulcer drugs, include cimetidine (Tagamet), famotidine (Pepcid), ranitidine (Zantac), and nizatidine (Axid). If *H. pylori* infection is confirmed, it is treated with various combinations of antibiotics, bismuth preparations, proton pump inhibitors, and H_2-receptor blockers. Multiple antibiotics are needed to prevent the development of resistant strains.

Antacids were once considered the first line treatment for peptic ulcer disease. They do neutralize acid and prevent the formation of pepsin. However, they are no more effective than H_2-receptor blockers, which are more convenient and have fewer side effects in most patients. When used, antacids are usually ordered 1 and 3 hours after meals and at bedtime. Because antacids are available without a prescription, patients may think they can do no harm. In fact, they can have serious side effects. They also impair the absorption of many other drugs if they are taken at the same time. The patient should be cautioned to take the exact amount prescribed and not to adjust it on his or her own.

There are some other drugs that you may see prescribed to treat ulcers. Pirenzepine (Gastrozepine) is a unique anticholinergic drug that reduces acid secretion without serious

table 36-7 ***Complications of Peptic Ulcer Disease***

COMPLICATION	SIGNS AND SYMPTOMS	TREATMENT	NURSING CARE
Hemorrhage	Thready pulse, restlessness, diaphoresis, chills, oliguria, hematemesis, tarry stools, hypotension.	Saline lavage, vasopressin, arterial embolization.	Assist with procedure. Monitor effects of treatment. Monitor for water intoxication: headache, coma, tremor, sweating, anxiety. Monitor vital signs, intake and output. Maintain patent NG tube. IV fluids as ordered.
Perforation	Sudden, sharp midepigastric pain that spreads over entire abdomen. Rigid abdomen. Absence of bowel sounds. Shock.	NG suction, IV fluids, antibiotics.	Monitor vital signs, intake and output. Enforce NPO order. Give fluids and blood as ordered. Keep NG tube patent.
Obstruction	Feeling of fullness, nausea after eating, persistent vomiting.	NG suction.	Monitor vital signs, intake and output. Keep NG tube patent.

NG, Nasogastric; *IV,* intravenous; *NPO,* nothing by mouth.

side effects. Metoclopramide (Reglan) is a prokinetic agent that causes the stomach to empty more quickly, removing food and drugs that stimulate acid production. Sucralfate (Carafate) is a mucosal barrier. It clings to the surface of the ulcer and protects it so that healing can take place. It is used less often now than in the past.

In special cases, anti-secretory therapy may be continued as a preventive measure after the ulcer has healed. Misoprostol (Cytotec) and the proton pump inhibitor omeprazole (Prilosec) may be used to prevent ulcers in patients who take NSAIDs. Antacids, sucralfate, and H_2-receptor blockers are not recommended for this purpose.

Diet therapy. The recommended diet therapy for ulcer patients has changed over the years. The current approach is to permit the patient almost any foods that do not produce discomfort. The patient is usually discouraged from taking in foods that stimulate acid secretion but do not neutralize acids. These foods include coffee, tea, meat broth, and alcohol. The effect of spicy foods is debated, but they should be excluded if they cause pain. Symptoms occur more often when the stomach is empty. Therefore, frequent small feedings throughout the day are recommended. The ulcer patient should be advised not to skip meals.

Managing complications. Complications may be treated medically or surgically. If hemorrhage is suspected, a nasogastric tube is inserted and attached to suction to remove and measure blood in the stomach. After the stomach has been suctioned, the physician may use saline lavage to control bleeding. The patient is placed on the left side, and 50 to 200 ml of saline (traditionally, iced saline has been used to cause vasoconstriction) is instilled in the stomach through the nasogastric tube. The saline is then suctioned out, and the procedure is repeated until the returning fluid is clear and free of clots. Some experts now recommend that room-temperature saline be used to decrease the risk of damage to the gastric mucosa and to avoid stimulation of the vagal nerve. Vasopressin may be given intravenously to control hemorrhage. Arterial embolization is a procedure that uses the patient's own blood and other substances to seal bleeding arteries. Once bleeding is controlled, antacids and H_2-receptor blockers are usually ordered at frequent intervals.

Perforation is treated initially with gastric decompression and intravenous fluids and antibiotics. A small perforation may close spontaneously. Otherwise, surgical repair is needed.

Obstruction may be due to edema and spasm, which often respond to medical treatment. A nasogastric tube is inserted to decompress the stomach, and intravenous fluids are provided. The nasogastric tube is clamped after 72 hours. If there is no evidence of continued obstruction, oral fluids are introduced. Continued obstruction requires surgical intervention.

Complications of peptic ulcer disease, signs and symptoms, related treatments, and nursing care are summarized in Table 36-7.

Surgical intervention is indicated to reduce acid secretion or for treatment of complications that do not respond to conservative treatment. Procedures that decrease acid secretion include vagotomy, pyloroplasty, gastroenterostomy, antrectomy, and subtotal gastrectomy. In extreme cases, total gastrectomy is necessary. Some of these procedures are described in Table 36-8 and illustrated in Figure 36-16.

NURSING CARE *of the Patient with Peptic Ulcer Managed Medically*

Nursing care of the patient with peptic ulcer disease can be quite complicated, depending on the severity of the condition and the medical or surgical treatment. Therefore, nursing care of the medical patient and the surgical patient is discussed separately (see also Nursing Care Plan: The Patient with a Peptic Ulcer).

Assessment

Complete assessment of the patient with a disorder of the digestive tract is summarized in Table 36-2. When a patient has peptic ulcer disease, describe the symptoms that caused the patient to seek medical care. Document the presence of pain, including location, aggravating factors, and measures that bring relief. Note the relationship between pain and food intake.

table 36-8 Surgical Treatment of Peptic Ulcer Disease

OPERATION	PROCEDURE	PURPOSE	ADVERSE EFFECTS
Vagotomy Truncal	Vagus nerve that supplies stomach is severed.	Decreases stimulation of gastric acid secretion.	May have delayed gastric emptying. Feeling of fullness, dumping syndrome, diarrhea.
Selective or superselective	Severs that part of vagus nerve that stimulates acid production. Spares nerve supply to pyloric sphincter.	Decreases stimulation of gastric acid secretion.	Delayed gastric emptying.
Pyloroplasty	Widens pylorus.	Improves passage of stomach contents into duodenum. Usually done with vagotomy to prevent gastric stasis.	Dumping syndrome due to rapid emptying of stomach into duodenum.
Simple gastroenterostomy	Creates passage between body of stomach and jejunum.	Permits passage of alkaline intestinal secretions into stomach to neutralize gastric acid.	May actually increase gastric acid secretion.
Antrectomy	Removal of antrum of stomach.	Reduces gastric acid by removing source of acid secretion.	Diarrhea, feeling of fullness after eating, dumping syndrome, malabsorption, anemia.
Subtotal gastrectomy Gastroduodenoscopy (Billroth I)	Part of distal portion of stomach, including antrum, is removed. Remaining stomach is anastomosed to duodenum.	Reduces acid by removing source of acid secretion.	Dumping syndrome (less often than with other procedures), anemia, malabsorption, weight loss, bile reflux.
Gastrojejunostomy (Billroth II)	Part of distal portion of stomach, including antrum, is removed. Remaining stomach is anastomosed to jejunum.	Removes source of acid secretion.	Dumping syndrome, weight loss, malabsorption, duodenal infection, pernicious anemia, afferent loop syndrome (obstruction of duodenal loop).
Total gastrectomy	Removal of entire stomach. Esophagus anastomosed to duodenum.	Removes source of gastric acid secretion.	Can only consume small, frequent meals of semisolid foods. Pernicious anemia; dumping syndrome.

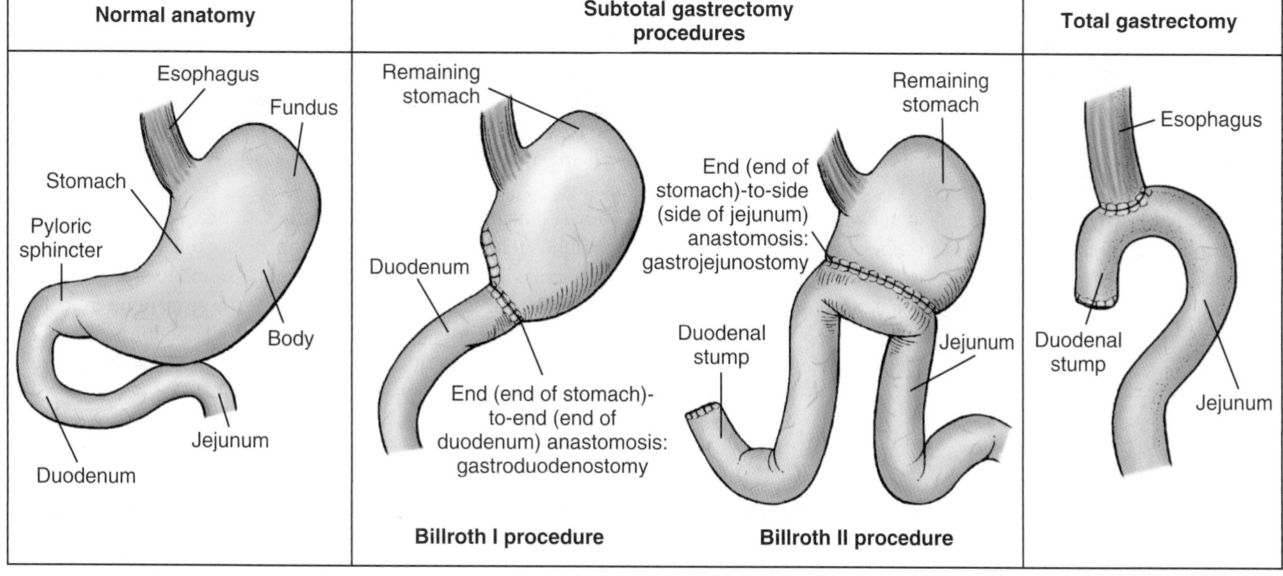

FIGURE 36-16 Gastric surgical procedures: *A,* Normal anatomy. *B,* Subtotal gastrectomy procedures (Billroth I and Billroth II). *C,* Total gastrectomy.

NURSING CARE PLAN

The Patient with a Peptic Ulcer

ASSESSMENT

Health History: Mr. Louis Kennon is a 47-year-old man who has recently been diagnosed as having duodenal ulcers. He has a history of burning pain 2 to 3 hours after meals. The pain is located just beneath the xiphoid process and is relieved by antacids. Symptoms are sometimes accompanied by nausea but not vomiting. He noticed that his stools have been darker than usual this week. Mr. Kennon describes his health as good but is being treated for hypertension. He states that he rarely drinks alcoholic beverages but smokes 1½ packs of cigarettes daily. He is a truck driver who usually eats only two meals each day, at irregular hours.

Physical Examination: Vital signs: temperature, 97.6° F; pulse, 76; respiration, 16; blood pressure, 136/82 mm Hg. Height, 5'10"; weight, 210 lb. Alert and oriented. Abdomen soft. Bowel sounds present in all 4 quadrants.

Nursing Diagnosis	*Goals and Outcome Criteria*	*Interventions*
Pain related to ulceration of duodenum.	Patient will verbalize pain relief and appear relaxed.	Administer drugs that decrease acid secretion, neutralize acid, or coat ulcer surfaces as ordered. Promote a restful environment and explain importance of rest to patient. Teach relaxation techniques.
Imbalanced nutrition: less than body requirements, related to nausea, vomiting, anorexia, dietary restrictions.	Patient will maintain adequate nutrition, as evidenced by stable body weight.	Provide diet as ordered: often bland, low-fat diet given in six small feedings. Administer antiemetics for nausea and vomiting. Monitor weight. Consult dietitian if patient is losing weight.
Risk for injury related to hemorrhage, perforation, and obstruction.	Patient will remain free of complications, as evidenced by normal vital signs and no vomiting, hematemesis, or tarry stools.	Monitor for signs and symptoms of bleeding: hematemesis, tarry stools, weakness, tachycardia, pallor, and hypotension. If hemorrhage occurs, notify physician and monitor vital signs. Perform lavage via nasogastric tube as ordered. Keep patient quiet and enforce nothing-by-mouth order. Maintain intravenous lines to ensure venous access in emergency. Monitor for signs and symptoms of perforation: sudden, sharp pain in midepigastric region that spreads across abdomen, patient drawing knees up toward chest. If perforation occurs, notify physician and monitor vital signs. Withhold oral fluids. Anticipate need for nasogastric suction and intravenous fluids. Monitor for signs and symptoms of pyloric obstruction: persistent vomiting. Carry out orders, including nasogastric suction, intravenous fluids, and antibiotics.
Ineffective coping related to prescribed alterations in lifestyle.	Patient will express intent to implement lifestyle alterations.	Identify behaviors such as use of alcohol and tobacco that aggravate peptic ulcer disease. Explain effects of behaviors on disease. Offer information about resources (American Cancer Society, American Lung Association) that provide services to help patients give up tobacco.
Deficient knowledge of self-care to manage peptic ulcer disease.	Patient will correctly describe self-care measures to promote healing of duodenal ulcers and prevent recurrence.	Advise patient to avoid substances that stimulate release of gastrin: alcohol, tobacco, caffeine. Stress importance of taking drugs as prescribed. Explain side and adverse effects and their management. List drugs that are contraindicated: aspirin, nonsteroidal anti-inflammatory drugs, and corticosteroids. Supplement verbal instruction with written information. Encourage follow-up care.

Important aspects of the past medical history include recent serious illnesses, previous peptic ulcer disease, and a medication history. Inquire about a family history of ulcers as well. Significant symptoms include nausea, vomiting, and indigestion. Ask if blood has been noted in vomitus and if stools have changed color or consistency. The functional assessment records the patient's usual diet, use of alcohol and tobacco, activities, sleep patterns, and stressors.

Begin the physical examination with general observations of the patient. Take vital signs to detect tachycardia and hypotension, which may indicate complications in the acutely ill patient. Measure height and weight. Assess the skin and mucous membranes for turgor and moisture. Inspect the abdomen for distention and palpate for tenderness. Auscultate for bowel sounds.

Nursing Diagnoses, Goals, and Outcome Criteria: Peptic Ulcer

Nursing Diagnoses	Goals and Outcome Criteria
Pain related to ulceration of stomach or duodenum	Pain relief: patient states pain reduced or relieved, relaxed manner
Imbalanced Nutrition: Less than Body Requirements related to nausea, vomiting, anorexia, dietary restrictions, nothing by mouth status	Adequate nutrition: stable body weight
Risk for Injury related to hemorrhage, perforation, obstruction	Absence of complications: vital signs within patient norms; no vomiting, hematemesis, or tarry stools
Ineffective Coping related to prescribed alterations in lifestyle	Effective coping: adjustment to prescribed changes in lifestyle, adherence to treatment regimen

Interventions

Pain

The most important means of reducing pain associated with peptic ulcer disease are drug therapy, rest, and diet. Drugs reduce pain by neutralizing acid, decreasing acid secretion, or coating the ulcer surface. For maximum effect, give the medications at the recommended times. For example, antacids are most effective when given 1 hour after meals and at bedtime. Know the side effects of these drugs and monitor for them. Notify the physician if pain persists or worsens despite drug therapy. Rest reduces symptoms of peptic ulcer disease because physical activity stimulates gastric secretions. The environment should be as restful as possible. Encourage relaxation techniques and stress management strategies as described in Chapter 14.

Imbalanced Nutrition: Less than Body Requirements

Dietary restrictions have long been part of the treatment of peptic ulcer disease. Many experts now question the impact of special diets on ulcers. When the patient has acute symptoms, a bland low-fiber diet often is given in six small feedings. The patient is advised to avoid any foods that have caused gastric distress in the past. In general, alcohol, tobacco, and beverages that contain caffeine are discouraged because they stimulate release of gastrin. The physician may advise the patient to adhere to a low-fiber diet with limited protein and calcium. Some patients tolerate decaffeinated coffee, but it contains peptides that also can stimulate gastrin release.

When nausea and vomiting are present, oral fluids may be restricted to clear liquids, or the patient may be allowed nothing by mouth. Administer antiemetics as ordered. Promptly remove emesis basins and measure vomited fluid. If necessary, help the patient to wash and replace soiled clothing.

Risk for Injury

Monitor the patient for signs and symptoms of complications. Signs of bleeding are hematemesis (vomiting blood) and the presence of blood in the feces. Blood that has passed through the digestive tract is maroon to black and causes the stool to have a sticky or tarry quality. Stools and vomited fluid may be tested for occult blood. When blood loss is significant, the patient may go into shock. Early signs of shock are weakness, tachycardia, and pallor. Hypotension is a relatively late sign.

If hemorrhage occurs, notify your supervisor or the physician and continue to monitor the patient's vital signs. Anticipate insertion of a nasogastric tube and saline lavage. Assist with the procedures and reassure the patient. Keep the patient quiet; give nothing by mouth. Maintain intravenous lines and record fluid intake and output. The patient may have to be prepared for transfer to intensive care or to surgery.

Perforation is characterized by sudden, sharp pain starting in the midepigastric region and spreading across the entire abdomen. Digestive fluids in the abdomen cause peritonitis (inflammation of the peritoneum). With peritonitis, the abdomen is rigid and tender. The patient tends to draw the knees up toward the chest.

When perforation is suspected, the nursing care is much like that provided for hemorrhage. Notify the physician, and monitor the patient's vital signs. Give nothing by mouth. Anticipate the need for nasogastric intubation and decompression and for intravenous fluids. The patient may be prepared for surgery.

The most prominent symptom of pyloric obstruction is persistent vomiting. The patient also may have signs and symptoms of fluid deficit and electrolyte imbalances. Insert a nasogastric tube for decompression as ordered. Administer intravenous fluids and antibiotics. When the nasogastric tube is removed, monitor the patient's tolerance of fluids.

Ineffective Coping

During periods of acute discomfort, patients are often receptive to measures that bring relief. Once acute symptoms resolve, however, many patients return to behaviors such as use of alcohol and tobacco that aggravate peptic ulcer disease. Explore what the patient thinks about prescribed treatments and how they will affect his or her lifestyle. Resources to help patients who have difficulty giving up alcohol or tobacco are available.

PATIENT TEACHING PLAN
Peptic Ulcer

- It is important for you to know the name, dosage, schedule, and adverse effects of each drug you take.
- Avoid aspirin, NSAIDs, alcohol, and smoking because they aggravate peptic ulcer disease.
- Your physician may recommend a specific diet that will decrease irritation to your stomach.

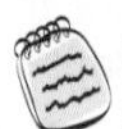

PATIENT TEACHING PLAN
Peptic Ulcer—cont'd

- Follow-up care is important to assure that your ulcer is healing or has not recurred.
- Resources for stress management techniques and alcohol abuse (if appropriate) are available.

NURSING CARE *of the Patient with Peptic Ulcer Managed Surgically*

Preoperative nursing care is like that outlined in Chapter 16 for any patient having major surgery. This section emphasizes the special postoperative needs of the patient who has undergone gastric surgery for peptic ulcer disease.

Assessment

Postoperatively, assess the patient for pain, nausea, and vomiting. If the patient has pain, describe the severity (using a scale of 1 to 10), location, and related factors. Measure vital signs at frequent intervals until the patient is stable. Note the amount and type of intravenous fluids, and check the infusion site for swelling or redness. If a nasogastric tube is present, assess patency of the tube as well as the color and amount of drainage. Inspect the skin around the nostril where the tube is located for irritation. Auscultate for breath sounds. Inspect the wound dressing for bleeding. Once the dressing is removed, examine the wound for increased redness, swelling, drainage, and incomplete closure. Describe any drainage from the wound or from drains. Inspect the abdomen for distention and auscultate for bowel sounds. Monitor urine output and assess for bladder distention.

Nursing Diagnoses, Goals, and Outcome Criteria: Gastric Surgery

Nursing Diagnoses	Goals and Outcome Criteria
Risk for Injury related to gastric dilation, obstruction, perforation	Absence of complications: vital signs within patient norms, minimal vomiting
Imbalanced Nutrition: Less than Body Requirements related to decreased capacity for intake of nutrients	Adequate nutrition: maintains/attains ideal body weight
Decreased Cardiac Output related to hypovolemia secondary to dumping syndrome	Normal cardiac output: no decrease in blood pressure after meals

Interventions

Risk for Injury

Potential complications of gastric surgery include gastric dilation, obstruction, and perforation. Gastric dilation results from accumulation of fluid in the stomach. The patient complains of feeling full and having epigastric pain. Tachycardia, hypotension, and hiccups may develop. Obstruction can result from edema at the surgical site, causing pain and vomiting.

A nasogastric tube is usually inserted preoperatively and remains in place after surgery. Specific orders for suction will be written. It is very important to maintain suction and drainage as ordered. Excessive fluid and gas in the stomach put pressure on the incision that could cause perforation. Perforation could result in hemorrhage and peritonitis.

Following gastric surgery, *do not* irrigate or reposition the tube. To do so may cause the suture line in the stomach to tear. Nasogastric drainage is usually bright red immediately after surgery. The color darkens over the first 24 hours and then turns yellow or green. The tube is removed when peristalsis returns, usually on the third to fifth postoperative day. Document the presence of bowel sounds and the passage of flatus through the rectum.

Imbalanced Nutrition: Less than Body Requirements

After the tube is removed, the diet is gradually advanced from clear liquids to full liquids and then to solid foods. As the diet is progressed, assess for nausea, vomiting, or abdominal distention. Special dietary needs depend on the type of surgery. After subtotal gastrectomy, small frequent meals are given until the stomach stretches enough to tolerate three regular meals a day. After total gastrectomy, small, frequent meals of semisolid foods are usually necessary for the rest of the patient's life.

Gastric surgery can have serious effects on the patient's nutritional status. The absorption of vitamin B_{12}, folic acid, iron, calcium, and vitamin D may be impaired, so supplements will be needed. Without vitamin B_{12}, the patient develops pernicious anemia. Pernicious anemia is more common after a total gastrectomy but can follow a subtotal gastrectomy. As discussed earlier, the parietal cells in the stomach produce intrinsic factor, a substance that is needed to absorb vitamin B_{12}. Vitamin B_{12} is essential for the production of red blood cells. When all or part of the stomach is removed, the patient develops a vitamin B_{12} deficiency and, eventually, severe anemia. The condition is easily treated with regular injections of vitamin B_{12}.

Decreased Cardiac Output

Some patients experience dumping syndrome after gastric surgery. This occurs because the absence or decreased size of the stomach prevents normal pacing of chyme movement into the intestine. Within 15 to 30 minutes after the patient eats, the concentrated liquid chyme moving into the intestine draws fluid out of the blood. The patient's blood volume falls, causing weakness, dizziness, diaphoresis, and palpitations. The increased fluid in the intestines causes cramps, loud bowel sounds, and the urge to defecate. Symptoms may last as long as an hour after meals.

Dumping syndrome usually disappears within a few months. Meanwhile, the following directions for the patient will help:

1. Consume a diet low in carbohydrates and refined sugar, moderate in fat, and moderate to high in protein. It should be divided into six meals daily.

2. Drink fluids between meals, not with them.
3. Lie down for about 30 minutes after meals.

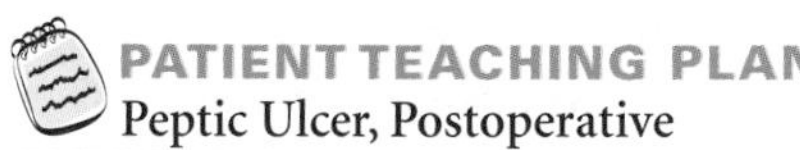

PATIENT TEACHING PLAN
Peptic Ulcer, Postoperative

- For each of your drugs, know the name, dosage, schedule, and adverse effects.
- After subtotal gastrectomy, eat small, frequent meals until your stomach capacity expands. After total gastrectomy, you will probably need to eat small, frequent meals for the rest of your life.
- Promptly inform your physician if you have nausea, vomiting, abdominal pain, or dark, tarry stools.
- Reduce the risk of recurrence by avoiding caffeine, alcohol, aspirin, and NSAIDs.
- If you are very stressed, try stress management techniques like relaxation exercises or seek personal counseling

Stomach Cancer

Pathophysiology

Cancer of the stomach is diagnosed in more than 25,000 people in the United States each year. The incidence is highest among males, African Americans, people over age 70, and people of lower socioeconomic status.

Stomach carcinoma begins in the mucous membranes, invades the gastric wall, and spreads to the regional lymphatics, liver, pancreas, and colon. Distant metastases are found in the lungs and bones. Unfortunately, there are no signs or symptoms in the early stages. Late signs and symptoms are vomiting, ascites, liver enlargement, and an abdominal mass. By the time late signs appear, the cancer is advanced and the patient's chance of 5-year survival is only about 10%.

Risk Factors

No specific cause of gastric cancer is known. Risk factors include pernicious anemia, chronic atrophic gastritis, and achlorhydria (lack of hydrochloric acid). Other factors that seem to be related to stomach cancer are cigarette smoking and a diet high in starch, salt, pickled foods, salted meats, and nitrates. Patients who have had the Billroth II procedure (gastrojejunostomy) also have increased incidence of stomach cancer.

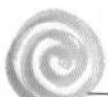

What Does Culture Have to do with Stomach Cancer?

The incidence of stomach cancer in African-American males is higher than in whites. Also, culturally based dietary patterns (high intake of starch, salt, pickled foods, salted meats, and nitrates) increase the risk of stomach cancer.

Medical Diagnosis

Gastroscopy is used to examine the interior of the stomach and to take specimens for microscopic study. The physician also may order an upper GI series to detect masses and obstructions. Laboratory studies include hemoglobin and hematocrit, serum albumin, liver function tests, and carcinoembryonic antigen. Stool specimens may be tested for occult blood.

Medical Treatment

Stomach cancer may be treated with surgery and chemotherapy. Radiation therapy has limited usefulness. If the cancer is detected early, surgical options include subtotal gastrectomy with lymph node dissection and total gastrectomy. Sometimes part of the esophagus or duodenum is resected. In more advanced cancer, the surgeon may remove as much of the tumor as possible to relieve or prevent obstruction without removing the entire stomach. Gene therapy and immune-based therapy are in early phases of study and may someday prove useful.

PREOPERATIVE NURSING CARE *of the Patient with Stomach Cancer*

In the preoperative period, assess the patient's understanding of the condition and what to expect after surgery. It is important to know what the physician has told the patient so that conflicting messages are not sent.

Nursing care focuses on patient teaching. Inform the patient about the nasogastric tube and intravenous fluids and teach coughing, deep breathing, and leg exercises. Identify and support the patient's usual coping methods. Include sources of support such as family members or a spiritual counselor in the preoperative care.

POSTOPERATIVE NURSING CARE *of the Patient with Stomach Cancer*

General nursing care for the postoperative patient is covered in Chapter 16. Special needs of patients having surgery for gastric cancer are discussed here. Chapter 24 presents general care of the patient who has cancer.

Assessment

Data that are especially important after surgery for stomach cancer are comfort, appetite, and nausea and vomiting. Monitor weight changes and determine dietary preferences. Identify the patient's support system and coping strategies.

Nursing Diagnoses, Goals, and Outcome Criteria: Stomach Cancer

Nursing Diagnoses	Goals and Outcome Criteria
Pain related to tumor or surgical trauma, or both	Pain relief: patient states less or no pain, relaxed manner
Imbalanced Nutrition: Less than Body Requirements related to anorexia, pain, nausea and vomiting	Adequate nutrition: maintains or attains ideal body weight
Ineffective Coping related to diagnosis of cancer, poor prognosis	Effective coping: patient verbalizes concerns, seeks and utilizes resources as needed, makes realistic plans

Interventions

Pain

Give analgesics as ordered, but also employ other nursing measures to manage pain. Massage, relaxation techniques, and mental imagery are examples of measures to treat pain.

Imbalanced Nutrition: Less than Body Requirements

Nutritional needs are much like those of the patient who has undergone surgery for peptic ulcer disease. When nasogastric suction is discontinued, oral fluids are introduced. If the patient tolerates clear liquids, the diet is gradually advanced. Small servings of bland foods are tolerated best. If dumping syndrome is a problem, it is managed with a diet that is low in carbohydrates and refined sugar, moderate in fat, and moderate to high in protein. Food is served in six small meals, and fluids should be taken between meals, not with them. Advise the patient to lie down for 30 minutes after eating. Monitor the patient's weight carefully. If weight is not maintained with oral intake, TPN may be instituted.

Ineffective Coping

The patient and family may need help in coping with this life-threatening illness. Encourage the patient to talk. Be accepting of the thoughts and feelings expressed. Guide the patient to think about changes that may be necessary in daily routines after discharge. If chemotherapy or radiation therapy is planned, the patient needs to know what to expect. Share information about community resources such as home health agencies or the American Cancer Society.

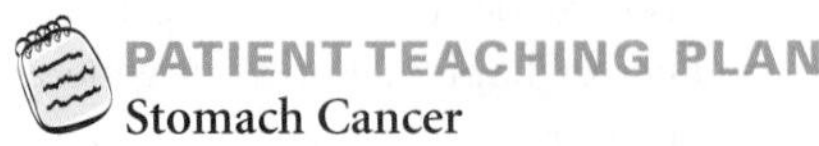

- For each of your drugs, know the name, dosage, schedule, and adverse effects.
- Eat six small meals a day and drink fluids between meals rather than with meals.
- Notify your physician if your wound shows increasing redness, swelling, pain, or drainage.

If the patient is scheduled for chemotherapy or radiation therapy, explain what the patient can expect.

Obesity

Obesity is defined as increased body weight caused by excessive body fat. The term is used to describe body weight that is greater than 20% higher than ideal. The term *morbid obesity* is used when a person weighs twice as much as his or her ideal weight.

Causes

Factors related to obesity include heredity, body build and metabolism, and psychosocial factors. Although many factors may contribute to obesity, the basic problem is that caloric intake exceeds metabolic demands. Excess food energy is converted to fat cells, which are capable of great expansion. When fat cells reach a certain size, they divide to form new fat cells. Fat cells decrease in size, but not in number, when a person loses weight.

Many attempts have been made to explain why some people become obese. There may be a mechanism in the hypothalamus that regulates weight within a certain range. When a person's nutrient intake falls below the level required to maintain the set weight, the body conserves energy to maintain that weight. This may explain why some people always seem to return to a certain weight despite strict dieting and temporary weight loss.

Complications

Complications of obesity include cardiovascular and respiratory problems, polycythemia, diabetes mellitus, cholelithiasis (gallstones), infertility, endometrial cancer, and fatty liver infiltration. Obesity also aggravates degenerative joint disease. In addition, obesity can take its toll on the patient's emotional and social well-being. Very obese people may be ostracized and experience discrimination. Even health care providers sometimes treat obese patients as uncooperative and unmotivated.

Medical Diagnosis

Obesity may be defined on the basis of comparison to standard weight tables. The amount of body fat can be estimated by measuring skinfold thickness at selected body sites. The physician may order tests of endocrine function to rule out correctable causes of obesity. Additional diagnostic tests and procedures may be done to detect complications associated with obesity.

Medical and Surgical Treatment

The primary treatment of obesity is a weight reduction diet accompanied by a planned exercise program. The ideal diet consists of foods from the basic four food groups and takes individual preferences into account. The calorie allowance may be as low as 800 calories a day. Amphetamines are effective in suppressing appetite but are not widely prescribed because their effects are temporary and they aggravate cardiac disease and hypertension. Selective serotonergic agonists have been marketed as weight loss agents, but dexfenfluramine (Redux) was withdrawn from the market when some patients experienced serious adverse effects. Other drugs that are available include benzphetamine (Didrex), phendimetrazine (Adipost, et al), mazindol (Sanorex), Orlistat (Xenical), and sibutramine (Meridia). To be effective, drugs must be used in combination with diet and exercise. The antidepressant bupropion (Wellbutrin) is being studied for usefulness in weight loss.

When morbid obesity persists over a period of years despite conservative treatment, surgical intervention may be recommended. One approach, the *Roux-en-Y gastric bypass,* decreases the size of the stomach by creating a small pouch that receives food from the esophagus, and then connects the pouch directly to the jejunum. This decreases the stomach capacity for food and bypasses much of the absorptive section of the GI tract. The patient eats less and absorbs less. The *biliopancreatic diversion,* which involves removal of part of the stomach and gallbladder, closure of the duodenum, and anastomosis of the jejunum to the ileum, may be used if other procedures fail. Both the Roux-en-Y bypass and the biliopancreatic diversion cause some malabsorption. In the vertical banded gastroplasty, which is not used much now, the stomach is banded to reduce its capacity. The opening be-

Consider the Alternative!

Ephedra sinica (Ma Huang) is an herbal product that many people use as an over-the-counter (OTC) weight loss product. Caution patients that it stimulates the body, especially the heart and central nervous system. The side effects can be most dangerous for people with hypertension, diabetes, prostate enlargement, and seizure disorders.

tween the stomach and the duodenum also is banded to slow emptying of the stomach. "Plain" *gastroplasty* is what people often call "stomach stapling." The stomach is divided into two compartments with staples, which decreases the capacity of the portion that receives food from the esophagus and empties into the duodenum.

Each of these procedures carries the risk of some complications. The Roux-en-Y bypass can cause dumping syndrome because food passes too rapidly into the jejunum. Deficiencies of iron, calcium, and cobalamin may require supplements. The biliopancreatic diversion is more likely to cause metabolic and nutritional complications. Vertical banded gastroplasty can cause persistent vomiting if solids are consumed too rapidly, distention of the walls of the functional pouch, rupture of the staple line, and erosion of the band into the stomach tissue. Gastroplasty does not cause dumping syndrome or malabsorption, but weight loss is often less impressive.

Procedures that usually are done for cosmetic reasons include *liposuction*—the removal of adipose tissue through a suction cannula; and *lipectomy*—the surgical excision of flabby folds of adipose tissue.

NURSING CARE *of the Obese Patient*

Assessment

Assessment of the obese patient identifies factors that may contribute to obesity and explores the physical and psychosocial effects. Record the patient's reason for seeking care. The past medical history documents pertinent chronic illnesses such as cardiac, respiratory, and orthopedic problems and diabetes mellitus. Assess usual dietary practices. Identify factors that trigger overeating and reactions to overeating. Inquire about interpersonal relationships, stresses, and coping strategies. In addition, collect data about previous efforts to lose weight and current interest in losing weight.

During the assessment, it is essential to convey an attitude of respect and concern. Be aware of your personal feelings about obese people and consider how these feelings affect the nurse-patient relationship.

Nursing Diagnoses, Goals, and Outcome Criteria: Obesity

Nursing Diagnoses	Goals and Outcome Criteria
Imbalanced Nutrition: More than Body Requirements related to excessive calorie intake for metabolic needs	Appropriate nutrient intake: patient attains ideal body weight
Ineffective Tissue Perfusion related to increased workload on heart	Adequate tissue perfusion: pulse and blood pressure within normal ranges
Ineffective Breathing Patterns related to restricted lung expansion	Effective ventilation: respiratory rate 12-20 without dyspnea
Disturbed Body Image related to excessive weight, perceived unattractiveness	Improved body image: positive patient statements about self, good grooming

Interventions

Imbalanced Nutrition: More than Body Requirements

Before nutrition teaching begins, determine what the patient already knows and what he or she is motivated to learn.

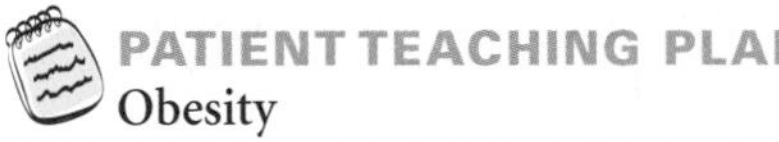

PATIENT TEACHING PLAN
Obesity

- A balanced, low-calorie diet is more effective over time than a faddish, quick weight loss program.
- Eating habits must be changed or the weight loss will be temporary.
- Goal weight should be determined with the physician and the dietitian. Realistic goals for weight loss should be set at 1 or 2 pounds per week.
- A list of foods to include and those to avoid will be provided.
- Weighing food portions at the beginning of the diet makes you more aware of portion sizes.
- Physical activity is important for weight loss. With your physician's approval, gradually increase your activity as tolerance increases.

Ineffective Tissue Perfusion

Monitor the patient's tolerance of physical activity. Tachycardia and dyspnea suggest that the patient's tolerance has been exceeded. When an obese patient is hospitalized for a medical or surgical condition, take extra precautions to maintain circulation and respirations. Position changes, deep breathing, and leg exercises reduce the risk of cardiopulmonary complications.

Ineffective Breathing Patterns

Monitor the patient's respiratory rate, effort, and breath sounds. During hospitalization, position changes and breathing exercises are especially important. The patient often breathes easier with the head of the bed elevated.

Disturbed Body Image

Demonstrate acceptance of obese patients by spending time with them, avoiding judgmental comments, and touching. Encourage the patient to identify solutions for overcoming perceived limitations imposed by weight. Acknowledge and compliment good grooming and attention to appearance and attributes other than physical size.

DISORDERS AFFECTING ABSORPTION AND ELIMINATION

Malabsorption

Malabsorption is a term used to describe a condition in which one or more nutrients are not digested or absorbed. Among the many causes of malabsorption are bacteria, deficiencies of bile salts or digestive enzymes, alterations in the intestinal mucosa, and absence of all or part of the stomach or intestines. The specific effects of malabsorption depend on the type of deficiency that is present. Likewise, treatment is directed at replacing deficient enzymes or avoiding substances that cannot be absorbed. Two examples of malabsorption are sprue and lactase deficiency.

There are two types of sprue: celiac (nontropical) and tropical. Celiac sprue is caused by a genetic abnormality. It is characterized by severe changes in the intestinal mucosa and impaired absorption of most nutrients. Tropical sprue is caused by an infectious agent and results in malabsorption of fats, folic acid, and vitamin B_{12}.

People with lactase deficiency do not have adequate lactase to metabolize lactose. These people are said to have lactose intolerance. Lactase deficiency may be inherited or acquired. Causes of acquired lactase deficiency include inflammatory bowel disease, gastroenteritis, and sprue syndrome.

What Does Culture Have to do with Malabsorption?

Inherited lactase deficiency is most prevalent among African Americans, Asians, and South Americans. The dietitian should be contacted to help the patient design an appropriate, culturally appropriate diet.

Signs and Symptoms

A common sign of malabsorption is steatorrhea, the presence of excessive fat in the stool. Stools are large, bulky, foamy, and foul smelling. Patients also may have weight loss, fatigue, decreased libido, easy bruising, edema, anemia, and bone pain.

Bloating, cramping, abdominal cramps, and diarrhea are symptoms of lactase deficiency that commonly occur within several hours of consuming milk products.

Medical Diagnosis

The diagnosis of sprue is based on laboratory studies, endoscopy with biopsy, and radiologic imaging studies. Lactase deficiency is diagnosed on the basis of the health history, the lactose tolerance test, a breath test for abnormal hydrogen levels, and if necessary, biopsy of the intestinal mucosa.

Medical Treatment

Sprue is treated with diet and drug therapy. Foods that aggravate the patient's symptoms are eliminated from the diet. Celiac disease is treated by avoiding products that contain gluten (wheat, barley, oats, and rye). Severe symptoms may be treated with corticosteroids. Tropical sprue is treated with antibiotics, oral folate, and vitamin B_{12} injections.

Lactase deficiency can be treated by the elimination of milk and milk products from the diet, although many adults can tolerate small amounts of lactose without symptoms. Lactase enzyme can be mixed with milk or taken before drinking milk to avoid symptoms. Some milk and milk products that have been treated with lactase also are available. If milk products are limited, the diet must be assessed for adequacy of calcium, vitamin D, and riboflavin. Supplements may be advised.

NURSING CARE *of the Patient with Malabsorption*

Assess the patient's symptoms. Note stool characteristics. In the case of celiac sprue, teach the patient how to eliminate gluten from the diet. Give antibiotics as ordered for tropical sprue. If folic acid therapy is to be continued, instruct the patient in self-medication. The effect of therapy is evaluated by the return of normal stool consistency. Advise the patient with lactase deficiency of dietary restrictions and alternative products.

Diarrhea

Diarrhea is defined as the passage of loose, liquid stools with increased frequency. The patient also may have cramps, abdominal pain, and a feeling of urgency before bowel movements.

Causes

Many factors can cause diarrhea. They include spoiled foods, allergies, infections, diverticulosis, malabsorption, cancer, stress, fecal impactions, and tube feedings. Diarrhea is an adverse effect of some medications.

Complications

Diarrhea is usually temporary and causes no serious problems. It does pose a greater threat, however, to the very old, the very young, and those in poor health. These individuals are more likely to become dehydrated and experience electrolyte imbalances and metabolic acidosis. Chronic diarrhea interferes with absorption of nutrients and can lead to malnutrition and anemia.

Medical Treatment

Acute diarrhea is usually treated by resting the digestive tract and giving antidiarrheal drugs. In the outpatient setting, the patient is advised to consume only clear liquids. A variety of liquids, such as broth, gelatin, and clear fruit juices, provide water, electrolytes, and some calories. Hospitalized patients may be allowed nothing by mouth and be given intravenous fluids. Severe, persistent diarrhea may require TPN. When diarrhea begins to improve, the diet gradually is expanded to include full liquids, bland solids, and then all other foods.

Consider the Alternative!

Natural substances that can help control diarrhea include rice water (made by boiling rice and straining the water), potatoes, and unpeeled apples. An herbal remedy is goldenseal, which is effective for diarrhea caused by some bacteria. High doses of this herb can cause dangerous CNS stimulation and uterine contractions, which contraindicate its use during pregnancy.

NURSING CARE *of the Patient with Diarrhea*

Assessment

Nursing assessment of the patient with diarrhea can help determine possible causes, the severity and progress of the condition, complications, and the effect of treatment. The history should record the presence of diarrhea and detail the onset, severity, precipitating factors, and measures that bring relief. Describe pain that accompanies diarrhea. Ask the patient about stool characteristics, including amount, color, odor, and unusual contents such as blood, mucus, or undigested food. The functional assessment focuses on usual diet, dietary changes, recent and current medications, and recent travel to a foreign country. It is also important to assess the patient's ability to get to the toilet independently or to call for assistance with toileting.

Important aspects of the physical examination include vital signs, weight, and tissue turgor. Tissue turgor is often assessed by gently pinching the tissue on the forearm. If the pinched tissue flattens as soon as it is released, tissue turgor is generally considered good. This test is not a good indicator of hydration in the elderly because their tissue is less elastic, regardless of hydration. Palpate the abdomen for distention or tenderness, and inspect the perianal area for irritation. A rectal examination should be performed as agency policy permits if the nurse suspects fecal impaction.

Diarrhea is a nursing diagnosis, but other related diagnoses, as included in the box below, also may be appropriate for the patient with diarrhea.

Nursing Diagnoses, Goals, and Outcome Criteria: Diarrhea

Nursing Diagnoses	Goals and Outcome Criteria
Deficient Fluid Volume related to fluid loss from diarrhea	Adequate hydration: pulse and blood pressure within patient norms, moist mucous membranes, urine output equal to fluid intake
Imbalanced Nutrition: Less than Body Requirements related to failure to absorb nutrients	Adequate nutrition: attain and maintain normal body weight
Acute Pain related to abdominal cramping and rectal irritation	Pain relief: patient states less or no pain, relaxed manner
Impaired Skin Integrity related to irritation of diarrhea stool	Intact skin: no perianal redness, lesions
Self-Care Deficit: toileting difficulties related to weakness or decreased level of consciousness	Improved self-care ability: patient uses toilet independently and without injury

Interventions

Deficient Fluid Volume and Imbalanced Nutrition: Less than Body Requirements

The prevention of serious fluid and electrolyte imbalances requires careful monitoring and replacement of fluid losses. When patients have severe diarrhea, keep intake and output records. Whenever possible, measure liquid stools. Stool characteristics are also important and should be recorded. Signs and symptoms that suggest possible fluid imbalances include unequal fluid intake and output; decreased blood pressure; changes in pulse rate or rhythm; changes in respiratory rate or depth; confusion; muscle weakness, tingling, or twitching; dry mucous membranes; and poor tissue turgor. These changes may indicate serious imbalances in water and electrolytes. They should be recorded and reported promptly.

If oral fluids are permitted, the patient should take 2,000 to 3,000 ml of various fluids each day. Carefully monitor the flow rates of intravenous fluids. Excessive or rapid fluid replacement can cause heart failure, especially in the elderly.

Impaired Skin Integrity

Liquid stool is very irritating to the anal and perianal areas. With frequent bowel movements, skin breakdown may occur. Assist the patient, if necessary, with perianal care after each stool. Wash the area thoroughly and gently with warm water and mild soap, rinse, then pat dry with a soft towel. Protective creams, sprays, or lotions can be applied.

Pain

Abdominal cramping associated with diarrhea is often relieved by antidiarrheal drugs that reduce intestinal activity. Record the severity, duration, and location of the pain as well as the effects of drug therapy.

Self-Care Deficit

Frail elderly persons or those who are acutely ill may have difficulty with toileting during diarrhea episodes. If possible, place them in rooms close to the nurses' station. Staff should be aware of the need to respond to call lights promptly. A bedside commode is recommended if the toilet is too far from the bed. Patients who are unable to call for help must be checked frequently for the presence of diarrhea stools.

Constipation

The frequency of defecation varies among healthy people. Bowel movements may occur as often as two or three times daily or as seldom as once a week. If the stool is soft and is passed without difficulty, the patient is not constipated. Constipation is a condition in which a person has hard, dry, infrequent stools that are passed with difficulty.

Causes

Many factors can contribute to constipation. When stool is present in the rectum, the urge to defecate occurs. If the urge is ignored, stool remains in the rectum longer than usual and becomes dry. It is then more difficult, and sometimes painful, to have a bowel movement. People who frequently ignore the urge to defecate may become chronically constipated. The frequent use of laxatives or enemas also contributes to chronic constipation. These agents keep the lower digestive tract empty and eventually interfere with the normal pattern of elimination.

Because physical activity promotes normal bowel elimination, people who are inactive are at risk for constipation. Inadequate water intake can lead to constipation because more water will be reabsorbed from the stool in the large intestine. Diet significantly affects the stool. A diet that is low in fiber and high in foods such as cheese, lean meat, and pasta promotes constipation.

Drugs that slow intestinal motility or increase urine output also contribute to constipation. Examples of these drugs are those used for anesthesia, pain relief, and cold symptoms. Medical conditions that may be related to constipation include diseases of the colon or rectum, as well as brain or spinal cord injury. Abdominal surgery causes a loss of intestinal activity, but it should be temporary.

Many people believe that constipation is normal for older people. Normal age-related changes in the large intestine do not explain the frequent complaints of constipation by the elderly. More likely, when constipation does occur, it is related to inactivity, drug therapy, long-term laxative or enema abuse, or some medical condition.

Many elderly people grew up believing that a daily bowel movement was necessary for health. If a day passed without a bowel movement, they used laxatives or enemas to produce one. Over time, this practice fosters laxative or enema dependence. Eventually, the person is unable to have a bowel movement without the laxative or enema. This dependence, established over many years, is very difficult to correct.

Complications

When people are constipated, they have to strain to have bowel movements. Straining occurs when a person attempts to exhale with the glottis closed, causing increased pressure in the chest and abdominal cavities. This is called the Valsalva maneuver. The pressure slows the flow of circulating blood back into the chest, causing a brief drop in pulse and blood pressure. Relaxation allows a rush of blood back into the chest with a resulting rise in pulse and blood pressure. The rapid changes in blood flow can be fatal to a patient with heart disease. Therefore, prevention of constipation and straining is very important in the care of cardiac patients. Chronic constipation contributes to the development of hemorrhoids. Another complication of constipation is fecal impaction, which is discussed later.

Medical Treatment

Treatment of constipation is directed toward immediate relief of the problem and prevention of future episodes. Laxatives, suppositories, enemas, or a combination are ordered to get prompt results. The physician may prescribe stool softeners as well. Stool softeners, as the name suggests, promote normal elimination by allowing more water to be held in the stool so that it is softer and more easily passed. It takes several days for the effects to be seen, so stool softeners are not used for acute constipation. They are relatively safe drugs that are often prescribed over a long period of time. The trade names of some stool softeners are Colace, Surfak, and Metamucil.

Metamucil is an example of a bulk-forming stool softener. In the intestinal tract, it absorbs water to produce a gel-like mass to aid in the passage of a soft stool. If the patient does not take adequate fluids, the mass can harden and cause obstruction in the intestine. Table 34-5 provides additional information about drugs.

PHARMACOLOGY CAPSULE Laxatives, cathartics, enemas, and suppositories usually relieve constipation promptly, but the effects of stool softeners are not seen for several days.

NURSING CARE *of the Patient with Constipation*

Assessment

Assess bowel elimination to detect constipation or risk factors that may cause it. Describe the patient's usual pattern of bowel elimination, including frequency, amount, color, unusual contents (blood, mucus, undigested food), and pain associated with defecation. Note recent changes in any of these factors. Information about diet, exercise, and drug therapy is helpful in revealing potential risk factors for constipation. If any aids to elimination (laxatives, enemas, suppositories) are used, record the type and frequency of use.

Examine the abdomen for distention or visible peristalsis. Auscultate for bowel sounds in all four quadrants of the abdomen. When severe constipation is accompanied by mild diarrhea, a rectal examination should be done to detect a fecal impaction if agency policy permits.

Nursing Diagnosis, Goal, and Outcome Criterion: Constipation

Nursing Diagnosis	Goal and Outcome Criteria
Constipation related to drug therapy, diet, inadequate fluid intake, inactivity, neuromuscular disorders, or laxative abuse	Establishment of normal bowel elimination: regular passage of formed stools without straining

Interventions

Constipation

The first action is directed at relieving the patient's constipation. Sometimes the physician will write an order for a laxative of choice or an enema as needed. An enema or suppository is preferred if the patient is very uncomfortable because it usually acts within an hour. A laxative may take as long as 8 to 10 hours.

When a laxative is truly needed, it should be given. Laxatives are, however, often abused. Frequent use can lead to physical and psychological dependence. Laxatives also can produce diarrhea, which may lead to excessive loss of fluids and electrolytes.

Nurses are often responsible for managing the bowel elimination of severely disabled people. This is especially true in long-term care facilities. It is critical to record and describe all stools so that problems can be found and treated early. Teach nurse's aides the importance of keeping accurate records. If detected early, constipation may be treated easily with a mild laxative or suppository. Severe constipation may require repeated enemas and laxatives for relief.

In most cases, bowel elimination can be maintained with diet, fluids, exercise, and regular toilet habits. Occasional use of elimination aids is not harmful. Some patients, however, require nursing interventions to promote elimination for a long time.

Megacolon. Megacolon is a condition in which the large intestine loses the ability to contract effectively enough to propel the fecal mass toward the rectum. These patients usually need regular enemas for bowel cleansing. Other measures are generally not adequate. Patients who have special problems with constipation are those with neurologic conditions such as spinal cord injuries and cerebrovascular accident (stroke). The management of bowel elimination in these patients and the process of bowel retraining are discussed in Chapter 22.

Fecal Impaction. All nursing staff should understand the possibility of fecal impaction in the physically or mentally impaired person. Fecal impaction refers to the retention of a large mass of stool in the rectum that the patient is unable to pass. Some liquid stool trickles around the impaction and may be mistaken for diarrhea.

Suspect impaction when a patient who has not had a bowel movement for several days has repeated episodes of mild diarrhea. If agency policy permits, assess for impaction by inserting a gloved, lubricated finger into the rectum. The fecal mass is usually easily felt. It may be very hard or soft.

Remove the impaction following agency protocol or specific physician's orders. This process usually requires administration of a mineral oil enema to soften hard stool, followed by a soapsuds enema. It may be necessary to break up and remove the mass manually. This procedure is painful and embarrassing for the patient. With good nursing care, manual extraction should rarely be necessary.

PATIENT TEACHING PLAN
Constipation

- Include high-fiber foods such as fruits, raw vegetables, greens, and whole grains in the diet.
- Drink six to eight 8-ounce glasses of water each day unless the physician has restricted fluid intake for some reason.
- Exercise daily. It need not be strenuous; walking is excellent exercise.
- Go to the bathroom promptly in response to the urge to have a bowel movement.
- Contrary to popular opinion, it is not necessary to have a bowel movement every day. A bowel movement every 2 or 3 days without pain or straining is normal for some people.
- Use a toilet that is comfortable. Feet should touch the floor, causing the hips to bend slightly. Use a footstool if necessary. This helps use of the abdominal muscles.
- Laxatives can be used safely for occasional constipation. If they are used frequently, however, they can interfere with normal elimination. Consult your doctor for a recommended laxative.

Consider the Alternative!

Herbs that have a laxative effect include aloe, *Cascara sagada,* and senna. Other complementary therapies include abdominal massage in a circular pattern with essential oil of rose, marjoram, fennel, or rosemary.

Intestinal Obstruction

Causes

Intestinal obstruction can be caused by many factors, including strangulated hernia, tumor, paralytic ileus, stricture, volvulus (twisting of the bowel), intussusception (telescoping of the bowel into itself), and postoperative adhesions. When the bowel is obstructed, digestive contents cannot progress. Volvulus and intussusception are illustrated in Figure 36-17.

Signs and Symptoms

Symptoms are most acute when an obstruction is located in the proximal portion of the small intestine. Early symptoms of obstruction are vomiting (possibly projectile), abdominal pain, and constipation. Gastric contents are vomited first, followed by bile, then fecal matter. Blood or purulent drainage may be passed rectally. Abdominal distention may develop, especially with colon obstruction.

Complications

Vomiting can lead to fluid and electrolyte imbalances and metabolic alkalosis. If blood supply to the intestine is impaired, gangrene and perforation of the bowel may occur. Untreated obstruction can result in shock and death.

Medical Diagnosis

Intestinal obstruction is suspected on the basis of the history, physical examination, and laboratory studies. It is confirmed by radiologic studies.

Medical Treatment

The initial treatment of obstruction is gastrointestinal decompression. A nasoenteral tube is passed and connected to suction.

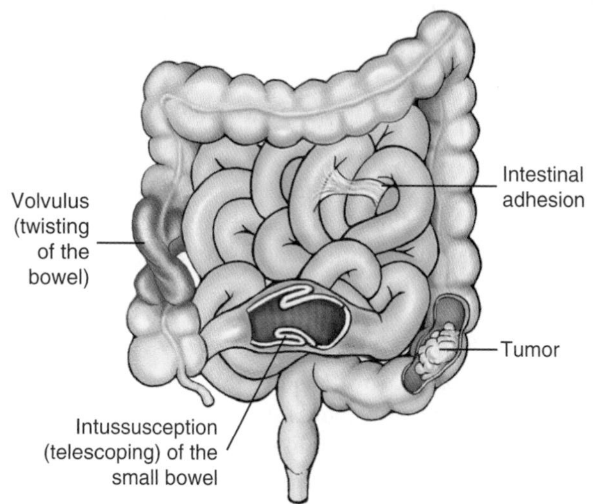

FIGURE **36-17** Mechanical bowel obstruction. *Left,* Volvulus. *Bottom,* Intussusception.

Intravenous fluids are provided. Depending on the cause of the obstruction, surgical intervention may be necessary.

NURSING CARE *of the Patient with Intestinal Obstruction*

Assessment

Assess the patient's symptoms, including pain and nausea. Describe the onset and progression of symptoms. The past medical history should include potentially related conditions, such as hernia, cancer of the digestive tract, and abdominal surgeries. Ask when the patient's last bowel movement was and if the characteristics were normal.

Take vital signs to detect signs of infection (fever, tachycardia) and impending shock (tachycardia, hypotension). Assess skin moisture and tissue turgor, along with moisture of the mucous membranes. Inspect the abdomen for distention and visible peristalsis; auscultate for rapid, high-pitched tinkling bowel sounds; and gently palpate for tenderness and guarding. Note rectal bleeding or drainage.

Preoperative Nursing Diagnoses, Goals, and Outcome Criteria: Intestinal Obstruction

Nursing Diagnoses	Goals and Outcome Criteria
Acute Pain related to distention	Pain relief: patient states less or no pain, relaxed manner
Deficient Fluid Volume related to vomiting, intestinal suction	Normal hydration: pulse and blood pressure within patient norms, moist mucous membranes, equal fluid intake and output
Risk for Infection related to complications of obstruction	Absence of infection: no fever, respiratory rate 12-20, normal white blood cell count
Ineffective Breathing Patterns related to abdominal distention	Effective ventilation: respiratory rate 12-20 without dyspnea
Anxiety related to pain, anticipated surgery	Decreased anxiety: patient states less or no anxiety, calm

Interventions

Acute Pain

Give analgesics as ordered and assess effectiveness. If the physician is withholding analgesics while making a diagnosis, inform the patient of this and use other strategies, such as massage and relaxation.

Deficient Fluid Volume

Promote fluid balance by providing intravenous fluids as ordered. Monitor vital signs and intake and output. If nasoenteral suction is ordered, monitor output and ensure free drainage at all times.

Risk for Infection

Monitor the patient's temperature. Signs of intestinal rupture (increasing tenderness, sudden sharp pain, and abdominal rigidity) are reported to the physician immediately.

Ineffective Breathing Patterns

Elevate the patient's head to relieve pressure on the diaphragm. Encourage deep breathing and coughing. Administer oxygen as ordered. When surgery is planned, carry out preoperative orders, which often include giving an enema and intravenous fluids.

Anxiety

Give simple explanations of what is being done and what the patient should expect postoperatively if surgery is scheduled. Stress the importance of deep breathing, turning, coughing, and leg exercises.

POSTOPERATIVE NURSING CARE *of the Patient Treated Surgically for Intestinal Obstruction*

Postoperative care depends on the surgical procedure performed.

Appendicitis

Pathophysiology

The appendix is a blind pouch in the cecum. Appendicitis is an inflammation of the appendix. Inflammation occurs when the opening of the appendix to the large intestine is blocked by feces, tumors, helminths, or indigestible substances such as seeds. The tissue becomes infected by bacteria in the digestive tract. Pus accumulates, the blood supply is impaired, and the appendix may rupture. A ruptured appendix allows digestive contents to enter the abdominal cavity, causing peritonitis—a life-threatening surgical emergency. Early detection of appendicitis may permit treatment before the appendix ruptures.

Signs and Symptoms

The initial symptom of appendicitis is usually pain in the epigastric region or around the umbilicus, which then shifts to the right lower quadrant. The classic symptom of appendicitis is pain at McBurney's point, which is located midway between the umbilicus and the iliac crest (Fig. 36-18). The patient may have a temperature elevation and nausea and vomiting. Because of the pain, the patient may assume a position of hip flexion. The right leg cannot be straightened without pain. An elevated white blood cell count indicates the presence of infection.

Signs and symptoms of peritonitis are absence of bowel sounds, severe abdominal distention, increased pulse and temperature, nausea, and vomiting. The abdomen may be rigid, although this sign is often absent with peritonitis in older patients. Suspect shock if the patient begins to lose consciousness and is cool and pale.

Medical Diagnosis

A diagnosis of appendicitis is based on classic signs and symptoms and a white blood cell count of 10,000 to 15,000/mm^3.

Medical Treatment

When appendicitis is suspected, the patient is allowed nothing by mouth. A cold pack to the abdomen may be ordered. Laxatives and heat applications should *never* be used for undiagnosed abdominal pain. If the appendix is inflamed, heat or laxatives may cause it to rupture.

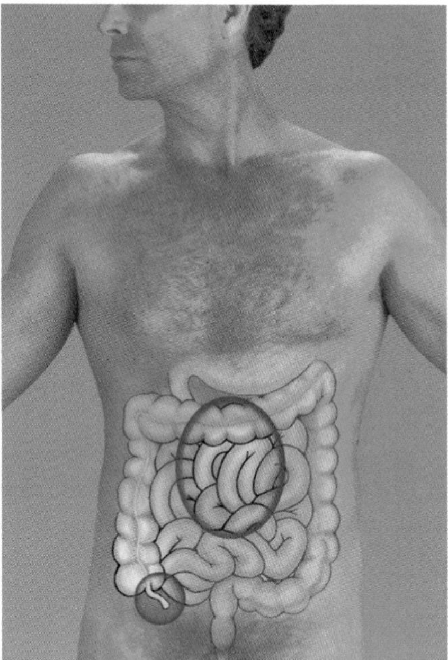

FIGURE **36-18** McBurney's point is located midway between the anterior iliac crest and the umbilicus in the right lower quadrant. Localized tenderness here is typical of appendicitis.

If rupture has not occurred, immediate surgical treatment is indicated. With a ruptured appendix, surgery may be delayed 6 to 8 hours while antibiotics and intravenous fluids are given.

NURSING CARE *of the Patient with Appendicitis*

Assessment

The patient's chief complaint is usually pain. Assess the location, severity, onset, duration, precipitating factors, and alleviating measures in relation to the pain. In the past medical history, note previous abdominal distress, chronic illnesses, and surgeries. Record allergies and medications as well. The presence of nausea and vomiting is determined in the review of systems. Significant data in the physical examination are temperature; abdominal pain, distention, and tenderness; and the presence and characteristics of bowel sounds.

Nursing Diagnoses, Goals, and Outcome Criteria: Appendicitis

Nursing Diagnoses	Goals and Outcome Criteria
Risk for Infection (peritonitis) related to appendix rupture	Absence of infection: normal body temperature and vital signs, bowel sounds present, and abdomen soft
Deficient Fluid Volume related to nausea, vomiting, medical restriction of fluid intake	Normal fluid balance: pulse and blood pressure within patient norms, moist mucous membranes, serum electrolytes within normal limits, fluid intake equal to output
Acute Pain related to inflammation of appendix or surgical tissue trauma	Pain relief: patient states less or no pain, relaxed manner
Ineffective Breathing Patterns related to incisional pain or anesthesia	Effective ventilation: respiratory rate 12-20, clear breath sounds
Fear related to sudden emergency status, minimal preoperative teaching	Reduced fear: patient states less or no fear, calm manner

Preoperative Interventions

Before surgery, the patient will probably be most comfortable in a semi-Fowler or side-lying position with the hips flexed. Until the physician determines the diagnosis, analgesics may be withheld. The location and pattern of the pain are needed to make a diagnosis. Explain this to the patient. If the appendix has not ruptured, surgery is usually done promptly upon diagnosis. With a ruptured appendix, surgery may be delayed while antibiotics and intravenous fluids are given. If rupture is suspected, elevate the patient's head to localize the infection.

Postoperative Interventions

Postoperatively, the patient receives antibiotics, intravenous fluids, and possibly gastrointestinal decompression. Assist the patient in turning, coughing, and deep breathing to promote expansion of the lungs. Incentive spirometry also can be useful. Show the patient how to splint the incision during deep breathing. Early ambulation is usually ordered to reduce the risk of postoperative complications. Assess the abdominal wound for redness, swelling, and foul drainage. Provide wound care as ordered or according to agency policy.

If there are no complications, the patient is usually discharged in a few days. Normal activities can be resumed in 2 to 3 weeks.

Peritonitis

Pathophysiology

Peritonitis is inflammation of the peritoneum caused by chemical or bacterial contamination of the peritoneal cavity. Chemical contamination may follow rupture of a digestive tract structure, including the appendix. Bacterial contamination may be caused by rupture of a digestive tract structure or fallopian tube or from nonsterile, traumatic wounds.

When a chemical or bacterial contaminant is present, the body's defenses attempt to wall off the area to contain the injury. Fluid shifts out of the bloodstream into the peritoneal cavity. Peristalsis slows or stops. If defenses are adequate, the offending fluid remains localized and is eventually eliminated. Complications of peritonitis include abscesses, adhesions, septicemia, hypovolemic shock, paralytic ileus, and organ failure.

Signs and Symptoms

Signs and symptoms of peritonitis include pain over the affected area, rebound tenderness, abdominal rigidity and distention, fever, tachycardia, tachypnea, nausea, and vomiting. The elderly patient may have more subtle symptoms with less pain and the absence of abdominal rigidity.

Medical Diagnosis

A diagnosis of peritonitis is suspected on the basis of the patient's history and physical examination. Diagnostic tests and procedures done to confirm the inflammation include a complete blood cell count, serum electrolyte measurements, abdominal radiography, computed tomography, and ultrasound. Paracentesis may be done to obtain a specimen of fluid for culture.

Medical Treatment

A nasogastric tube is inserted for gastrointestinal decompression. Intravenous fluids, antibiotics, and analgesics are ordered. Surgery may be done to close a ruptured structure and to remove foreign material and fluid from the peritoneal cavity.

NURSING CARE *of the Patient with Peritonitis*

Assessment

Begin by assessing the patient's present illness. Pain is the prominent symptom. Record the onset, location, and severity of the pain and any related symptoms. When peritonitis is suspected, record a history of abdominal trauma, including surgery. Take and record vital signs. Inspect the abdomen for distention and auscultate for the presence of bowel sounds. Note measures of fluid status, including tissue turgor, moisture of mucous membranes, and intake and output.

Nursing Diagnoses, Goals, and Outcome Criteria: Peritonitis

Nursing Diagnoses	Goals and Outcome Criteria
Acute Pain related to inflammation	Pain relief: patient states pain is reduced or relieved, has relaxed manner
Decreased Cardiac Output related to decreased blood volume	Normal cardiac output: pulse and blood pressure within patient norms, skin warm and dry, fluid output equal to intake
Imbalanced Nutrition: Less than Body Requirements related to nausea, vomiting, nothing by mouth status	Adequate nutrition: stable body weight
Anxiety related to threat of serious illness and invasive treatment	Decreased anxiety: patient states anxiety reduced or relieved, calm manner

Interventions

Acute Pain

Administer opioid analgesics as ordered for pain. Position the patient with the head elevated and provide comfort measures such as massage and relaxation techniques. Notify the physician if pain relief is not obtained.

Decreased Cardiac Output

The shift of fluid from the blood into the peritoneal cavity may be so great that the patient develops deficient intravascular fluid volume. Cardiac output falls, and perfusion of vital organs is reduced. Administer intravenous fluids as ordered and monitor fluid intake and output. Monitor vital signs and report increasing pulse, restlessness, pallor, and decreasing blood pressure. In addition to deficient fluid volume, the patient may go into shock because of septicemia (the presence of bacteria in the blood).

Imbalanced Nutrition: Less than Body Requirements

Gastrointestinal decompression usually eliminates nausea and vomiting, but antiemetics may be ordered as needed. Check to be sure that the nasogastric tube is draining at all times.

Anxiety

The patient is likely to be anxious because of pain and uncertainty about what is happening. Even when there is a sense of urgency in caring for the patient, give simple explanations for procedures and tell the patient what to expect. Encourage the patient to ask questions. If surgery is planned, essential preoperative teaching may have to be done quickly. Explain to the patient the importance of breathing and leg exercises after abdominal surgery. The physician may order sedatives to calm the patient.

POSTOPERATIVE NURSING CARE

Postoperative care is like that for any major surgery and is described in Chapter 16.

Abdominal Hernia

Pathophysiology

Muscles play an important role in keeping the abdominal organs in place. Weakness in those muscles may allow a portion of the large intestine to push through the abdominal wall. The bulging portion of intestine is called a hernia. Hernias most often occur in areas where the abdominal wall is already weak. Weak locations include the umbilicus and the lower inguinal areas of the abdomen (Fig. 36-19). Hernias also may develop at the site of a surgical incision.

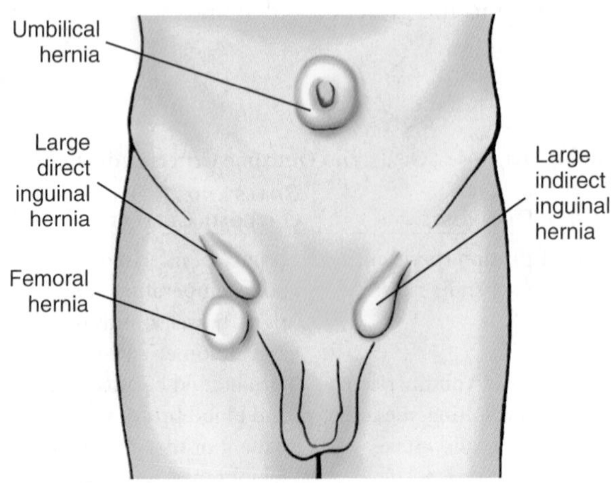

FIGURE **36-19** Abdominal hernias.

Hernias are classified as reducible or irreducible. A reducible hernia slips back into the abdominal cavity with gentle pressure or when the patient lies on his or her back. When the hernia cannot be manipulated back into place, it is said to be irreducible, or incarcerated. An irreducible hernia may impair blood flow to the trapped loop of intestine, causing it to become gangrenous. A hernia that is trapped and deprived of blood is said to be strangulated.

Signs and Symptoms

Hernias are usually diagnosed when a patient reports a smooth lump on the abdomen. The lump may disappear when the patient is lying down or at rest but returns when standing or straining. Heavy lifting or coughing usually causes the hernia to appear.

Hernias usually are not painful unless they become incarcerated. With incarceration, the patient has severe abdominal pain and distention, vomiting, and cramps.

Medical Diagnosis

Hernias are diagnosed on the basis of the health history and physical examination.

Medical Treatment

Surgical repair of hernias is usually recommended even if they are reducible. Repair prevents the possibility of incarceration. Two surgical procedures are used to repair hernias. Herniorrhaphy is the repair of the muscle defect by suturing. If additional measures are needed to strengthen the abdominal wall, a hernioplasty is done. Strong materials are used to cover and reinforce the defect.

Some patients cannot tolerate the stress of surgical hernia repair. For them, a truss may be advised, although trusses are not used as widely as in the past. A truss consists of a pad that is placed over the hernia and a belt that holds it in place. It provides support for the weak muscles.

NURSING CARE *of the Patient with Abdominal Hernia*

Assessment

Begin the assessment with the patient's chief complaint, usually a smooth lump in the abdomen that appears and disappears with various activities and positions. Ask about pain and vomiting, which may be present if the hernia is strangulated. Explore the patient's work and home responsibilities to identify the type of physical exertion required. The most relevant aspect of the physical examination is the assessment of the abdomen. Inspect for abnormalities and listen for bowel sounds in all four quadrants. If the patient wears a truss, inspect the skin underneath it for signs of irritation.

Nursing Diagnoses, Goals, and Outcome Criteria: Abdominal Hernia

Nursing Diagnoses	Goals and Outcome Criteria
Risk for Injury related to hernia strangulation or distention	Absence of injury (strangulation): normal pulse and temperature without abdominal pain
Impaired Skin Integrity related to pressure created by the truss	Absence of complications caused by truss: intact skin without redness under truss

Preoperative Interventions

Risk for Injury

Monitor the patient for signs and symptoms of strangulation (nausea, vomiting, pain, abdominal distention, fever, and tachycardia). If these symptoms develop, immediately notify the physician. It is important for the nonsurgical patient to know that these symptoms should be reported.

Determine what restrictions the patient has in relation to physical exertion and provide verbal and written instructions to the patient.

Impaired Skin Integrity

Teach patients who use a truss what measures to take to avoid injury to the skin.

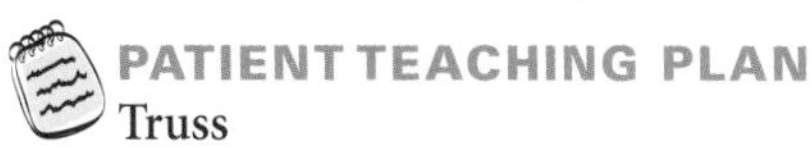

PATIENT TEACHING PLAN
Truss

- Put the truss on before rising each morning.
- Check under the pad and the belt several times daily for skin irritation.
- The truss does not cure a hernia, so you still should avoid straining.

Postoperative Interventions

The general postoperative care of patients who have undergone surgery is discussed in Chapter 16. In addition to the routine postoperative assessments, after hernia repair be especially concerned with assessing bowel and bladder elimination, wound healing, and the patient's knowledge about ways to avoid placing stress on the healing surgical wound.

Nursing Diagnoses, Goals, and Outcome Criteria: Abdominal Hernia Repair

Nursing Diagnoses	Goals and Outcome Criteria
Impaired Urinary Elimination related to abdominal surgery, anesthesia	Normal urinary function: urine output equal to fluid intake, no bladder distention
Constipation related to immobility, effects of anesthesia, and abdominal surgery	Normal bowel elimination: formed stools at regular intervals without pain or straining
Acute Pain related to scrotal swelling	Pain relief: patient states less or no pain, relaxed manner
Risk for Injury related to wound dehiscence	Well-healed wound: margins intact, decreasing redness and swelling

Impaired Urinary Elimination

Many patients have temporary problems with urination after hernia repair surgery. Keep intake and output records, document voiding, and assess for bladder distention.

Constipation

Bowel activity also may cease temporarily in response to the anesthesia and manipulation of the bowel during surgery. Therefore, monitor bowel sounds and note the passage of flatus. Like any other patients having major surgery, hernia repair patients need to keep their lungs clear to prevent complications. Encourage them to turn and deep breathe, but they should not cough or sneeze. Coughing and sneezing put tension on the surgical incision and repaired tissues.

Acute Pain

Scrotal swelling is common after inguinal hernia repair. A scrotal support and an ice pack can greatly reduce the painful swelling.

Risk for Injury

Activities are usually restricted for 2 to 6 weeks. Reinforce the physician's instructions about refraining from exertion and lifting. Advise the patient to report fever or wound drainage to the physician.

Inflammatory Bowel Disease

Pathophysiology

Inflammatory bowel disease (IBD) refers to both ulcerative colitis and Crohn's disease. Crohn's disease is also known as regional enteritis. In both conditions, there is inflammation and ulceration of the lining of the intestinal tract. With ulcerative colitis, the inflammation typically begins in the rectum and gradually extends up the bowel toward the cecum. The progression of Crohn's disease is different in that it can affect any area of the gastrointestinal tract. Although the terminal ileum is most often affected, there may be multiple sites interspersed with healthy segments of bowel.

The two conditions have similar symptoms and are treated much the same way medically. Surgical options, however, are different.

A patient with IBD may have a few isolated attacks or may have a chronic condition. With chronic IBD, attacks may last days or even months, followed by periods of remission lasting several weeks to several years.

What Does Culture Have to do with IBD?

IBD is more common among Caucasians and people of middle Eastern origin than among African Americans and Asian Americans.

Causes

The exact cause of IBD is unknown. Possible causes that are being studied include infectious agents, autoimmune reactions, allergies, and heredity. In the past, it was thought that IBD might be caused by stress. Current thinking, however, suggests that stress is the result of IBD rather than the cause.

Signs and Symptoms

The symptoms of IBD vary with the extent of the disease. When ulcerative colitis affects only the rectum, the patient may be constipated. More commonly, however, patients have diarrhea with frequent bloody stools, and abdominal cramping. In severe cases, the patient also may have fever and weight loss.

Symptoms of Crohn's disease are even more variable, depending on the areas affected. If the stomach and duodenum are involved, symptoms include nausea, vomiting, and epigastric pain. Involvement of the small intestine produces pain and abdominal tenderness and cramping. An inflamed colon typically causes abdominal pain, cramping, rectal bleeding, and diarrhea. Systemic signs and symptoms include fever, night sweats, malaise, and joint pain.

Complications

The local complications of IBD include hemorrhage, obstruction, perforation (rupture), abscesses in the anus or rectum, fistulas, and megacolon. Patients who have had ulcerative colitis for 10 years have a greatly increased risk of cancer of the large intestine. Patients with Crohn's disease also are thought to have an increased risk of colon cancer, although the relationship is less clear.

Systemic complications also may be found with ulcerative colitis. These are conditions outside the intestine but related to the colitis. They include inflammation of the joints and eyes, skin lesions, urinary stones, and liver disease. Of course, severe or prolonged diarrhea can result in malnutrition, anemia, and fluid and electrolyte imbalances.

Medical Diagnosis

Inflammatory bowel disease is suspected on the basis of the history and physical examination. Abdominal radiography may be done to rule out obstruction before additional tests are done. To confirm the diagnosis, the physician may then order a barium enema examination with air contrast and colonoscopy with biopsy, ultrasonography, computed tomography, and cell studies.

Medical Treatment

Treatment of IBD addresses both the local and the systemic effects of the disorders. Intestinal inflammation is treated with drug therapy, diet, and rest. The drugs listed here may be used alone or in combination depending on the specific situation.

- *Corticosteroids* to decrease inflammation in mild to moderately severe episodes
- *Immunosuppressants* to inhibit the immune response
- *Antidiarrheals* to control diarrhea EXCEPT in severe colitis
- *Anticholinergics* to reduce pain and gastrointestinal motility and secretions
- *Antibiotics* to treat mild to moderately severe attacks of Crohn's disease: usually sulfasalazine, mesalamine, olsalazine; sometimes metronidazole, ciprofloxacin, cephalexin, or sulfa-trimethoprim. Antibiotics are not very useful for ulcerative colitis
- *Aminosalicylates,* specifically 5-ASA (mesalamine oral, suppository, or enema; or sulfasalazine), to reduce symptoms
- *Iron supplements* and *vitamin* B_{12} to treat anemia

Patients with ulcerative colitis are usually maintained between acute episodes with aminosalicylates; however, 6-MP is appropriate in some circumstances. Crohn's disease is less responsive to aminosalicylates, so the patient may be maintained on azathioprine or 6-MP.

Research is underway to assess the effects of other drugs including monoclonal antibodies and cytokine interleukin-10. Based on the low incidence of IBD among smokers, therapy with nicotine transdermal patches or gum also is being studied.

A low-roughage diet without milk products is prescribed for mild to moderate IBD. Intravenous fluids or TPN may be needed to provide fluid, electrolytes, and nutrients when symptoms are severe.

Although most patients respond to medical treatment, some require surgery. Removal of the colon (colectomy) is curative for ulcerative colitis. When the colon is removed, an artificial opening from the small intestine through the abdominal wall is needed to allow elimination of digestive wastes. The opening is called an ileostomy. Although good health is usually restored after this surgery, an ileostomy is permanent and requires special care. Therefore, surgery is not usually done unless all other measures have failed. Care of the patient with an ostomy is covered in Chapter 25.

Surgical treatment of Crohn's disease is more likely to be removal of the diseased portion of the intestine. Recurrence is so common that surgery is not usually done unless necessitated by serious complications. Postoperatively, the disease typically reappears at the site of anastomosis within a year. Newly affected areas also may appear in other sections of the intestine.

PHARMACOLOGY CAPSULE Corticosteroids suppress the immune and inflammatory responses, so the patient is more susceptible to infection.

NURSING CARE *of the Patient with Inflammatory Bowel Disease*

The nursing care of a patient during an acute attack of IBD is concerned with ongoing assessment, comfort measures, skin care, emotional support, and administering drugs and monitoring the effects. The nursing needs of the IBD patient who undergoes surgery are like those of other patients who have undergone gastrointestinal surgery, as discussed earlier in this chapter.

Assessment

Assessment of the patient with IBD should identify the symptoms that caused the patient to seek care, usually pain and diarrhea. Record the onset, location, severity, and duration of pain. Note factors that contribute to the onset of pain, such as specific foods or stressors. Also note the onset and duration of diarrhea as well as the presence of blood. Assess the impact of the illness on the patient's life and explore how the patient copes.

Important aspects of the physical examination are vital signs, height and weight, and measures of hydration (tissue turgor, mucous membrane moisture). Inspect the perianal area for irritation or ulceration. Maintain accurate intake and output records. Measure diarrhea stools if possible and count as output.

Nursing Diagnoses, Goals, and Outcome Criteria: Inflammatory Bowel Disease

Nursing Diagnoses	Goals and Outcome Criteria
Acute Pain related to abdominal cramping, perianal irritation	Pain relief: patient states pain is reduced or relieved, manner is relaxed
Diarrhea related to intestinal inflammation	Cessation of diarrhea: stools formed, less frequent
Deficient Fluid Volume related to diarrhea	Adequate hydration: pulse and blood pressure within patient norms, moist mucous membranes
Imbalanced Nutrition: Less than Body Requirements related to malabsorption	Adequate nutrition: stable body weight
Ineffective Coping related to chronic illness	Effective coping: patient reports strategies to deal with IBD; patient sees disease as manageable
Risk for Injury related to adverse drug effects	Absence of adverse drug effects: normal urine output, electrolyte and blood glucose levels within normal limits, no bruising

Interventions

Acute Pain

Perianal pain is treated with gentle cleansing, sitz baths, and skin protectants. Measures to relieve abdominal pain include administration of analgesics and antispasmodics and application of heat to the abdomen as ordered. Positioning, massage, relaxation, imagery, and other strategies described in Chapter 14 also may be used.

Diarrhea

Easy access to a toilet and prompt response to calls for help reduce the chance of episodes of bowel incontinence. Following each stool, gently clean and assess the perianal area. If bedpans or bedside commodes are used, remove and clean them immediately. Use room deodorizers to eliminate odors.

Prescribed drugs for diarrhea usually include antidiarrheals, antispasmodics, anticholinergics, antibiotics, and corticosteroids. The patient may be allowed nothing by mouth or may be given only clear liquids when diarrhea is severe. Bedrest may be prescribed, or the patient may just be encouraged to rest.

Deficient Fluid Volume

Severe diarrhea can quickly deplete the patient's fluid volume. Assess fluid status on an ongoing basis. Signs of fluid volume deficit are dry mucous membranes, hypotension, tachycardia, and decreased urine output. Administer intravenous fluids and TPN as ordered.

Imbalanced Nutrition: Less than Body Requirements

The patient with ulcerative colitis need avoid only foods that worsen symptoms. For the patient with Crohn's disease, total parenteral nutrition and elemental enteral diets (e.g. Ensure) may be prescribed. The patient who is able to take solid food is usually placed on a low-residue diet without caffeine, pepper, or alcohol. Foods that are not allowed include whole grains, nuts, and raw fruits and vegetables. Consult a dietitian to teach the patient about the prescribed diet. Monitor weight on a routine basis.

Ineffective Coping

Inflammatory bowel disease is painful and stressful and can interfere with the patient's everyday life. Try to establish a trusting relationship with the patient. Encourage independence, participation in care and decision making, and realistic goal setting. People who have IBD may benefit from therapy that assists them with stress management. With the patient's approval, initiate a referral to a mental health professional or spiritual counselor. Report sadness and discouragement to the physician.

Risk for Injury

Nursing responsibilities in relation to drug therapy for IBD include administering the drugs, monitoring their effects, and teaching the patient about long-term drug therapy. Sulfasalazine is the antibiotic most often prescribed for patients with ulcerative colitis. It is useful in treating acute attacks and preventing future attacks. After an acute attack has subsided, the drug dosage is gradually reduced. A low-maintenance dose may be given for as long as a year. Teach the patient that discontinuing the drug early may result in another acute attack.

Sulfasalazine can cause crystals to form in the urine (crystalluria), which can damage the kidneys. Therefore, patients taking this drug should take enough fluids to maintain a urine output of 1,500 ml/day. A high urine output reduces the risk of crystalluria.

Corticosteroids are used in IBD for their ability to reduce inflammation. Unfortunately, this action also decreases the ability of the body to resist infection. Patients on steroids must be monitored for any signs and symptoms of infections. Instruct them to avoid unnecessary exposure to others with infectious conditions.

Long-term steroid therapy can have many other serious side effects as well. These effects include fluid and electrolyte imbalances, ulcers, increased blood glucose, weight gain, elevated blood pressure, acne, capillary fragility, and hirsutism (abnormal growth of hair).

PATIENT TEACHING PLAN
Inflammatory Bowel Disease

Topics for patient teaching include:

- Stress reduction measures are recommended to help control your symptoms.
- Because people with IBD have increased risk of cancer, you should have regular colon screening.
- You can facilitate digestion by taking small bites, eating slowly, and chewing well.
- Avoid caffeine and other irritating fluids and foods; consume a high-calorie, low-residue diet.
- You need to know the names, dosages, and schedules of your prescribed drugs and know what effects should be reported to the physician.
- Resources: National Foundation for Ileitis and Colitis (1-212-685-3440); United Ostomy Association, 36 Executive Park, Ste. 120, Irvine, CA 92714.

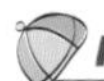

Put on your THINKING CAP!!

Compare and contrast ulcerative colitis and Crohn's disease. How are they similar and how are they different?

Diverticulosis

Pathophysiology

Diverticulosis is a condition characterized by small sac-like pouches in the intestinal wall called diverticula. Diverticula occur when weak areas of the intestinal wall allow segments of the mucous membrane to herniate outward (Fig. 36-20). Most diverticula are found in the sigmoid colon, and there is usually more than one.

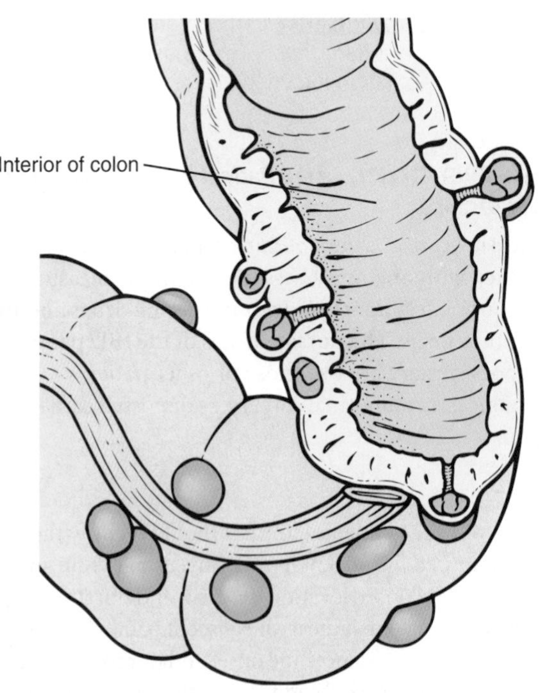

FIGURE **36-20** Diverticula in the sigmoid colon.

Risk Factors

Because diverticulosis is most common in developed countries, it is thought that lack of dietary residue is a contributing factor. Other related factors are age, constipation, obesity, and emotional tension.

Signs and Symptoms

Diverticulosis is often asymptomatic, but many people report changes in bowel habits. The change may be constipation, diarrhea, or periodic bouts of each. Other symptoms might include rectal bleeding, pain in the left lower abdomen, nausea and vomiting, and urinary problems.

Complications

Intestinal contents can lodge in diverticula, causing inflammation or infection. The patient is then said to have diverticulitis. Diverticulitis may be related to irritating foods, alcohol, chronic constipation, and persistent coughing. Symptoms of pain and bleeding are more severe with diverticulitis. The patient also may have a fever.

Possible complications of diverticulitis are severe bleeding, obstruction, perforation (rupture), peritonitis, and fistula formation. A fistula is an abnormal opening. In this case, it is most likely to develop between the colon and the bladder or vagina. The fistula permits bowel contents to pass into these other structures.

Medical Diagnosis

Diverticulosis may be suspected on the basis of the patient's symptoms. The stool is tested for occult blood. Abdominal CT and barium enema examination allow the physician to confirm the presence of diverticula. Because these procedures are invasive, they are delayed if there are signs and symptoms of acute inflammation.

Medical Treatment

Diverticulosis is currently being treated with a high-residue diet without spicy foods. Stool softeners or bulk-forming laxatives are used to treat constipation, and antidiarrheals are prescribed for those who have diarrhea. If pain is severe, it may be treated with analgesics. Opioids, especially morphine, should not be given because they cause constipation and may increase pressure in the sigmoid colon. Broad-spectrum antibiotics are often prescribed. Anticholinergics may be given to decrease spasms in the colon.

During periods of acute inflammation, the patient is placed on bed rest and given nothing by mouth. Intravenous fluids are ordered. Gastrointestinal decompression also may be instituted.

If symptoms persist and complications occur, surgical intervention may be necessary. The affected portion of the colon is removed. A temporary colostomy may be created to rest the colon while the surgical incisions heal. Sometimes elective surgery is recommended because the risk of surgical complications is much lower than it is with emergency surgery.

NURSING CARE *of the Patient with Diverticulosis*

Assess the patient's comfort and stool characteristics. Note any nausea and vomiting. Monitor the patient's temperature. Assess the abdomen for distention and tenderness.

Nursing Diagnoses, Goals, and Outcome Criteria: Diverticulosis

Nursing Diagnoses	Goals and Outcome Criteria
Deficient Fluid Volume related to diarrhea and vomiting	Adequate hydration: pulse and blood pressure within patient norms, urine output equal to fluid intake, moist mucous membranes
Acute Pain related to inflammation	Pain relief: patient states pain is decreased or relieved, has relaxed manner
Risk for Infection related to perforation	Absence of infection: no fever, normal white blood cell count, abdomen soft and not tender

Interventions

Provide fluids as permitted and monitor the patient's intake and output. Give antiemetics as ordered for nausea. Analgesics and anticholinergics may be given as ordered for pain. Be alert for signs of perforation (fever, abdominal distention, and rigidity). Teach the patient about diverticulosis, including the pathophysiology, treatment, and symptoms of inflammation.

If surgery is performed, the nursing care is similar to that described for any major abdominal surgery. General surgical care is included in Chapter 16, and care of the patient with an ostomy is discussed in Chapter 25.

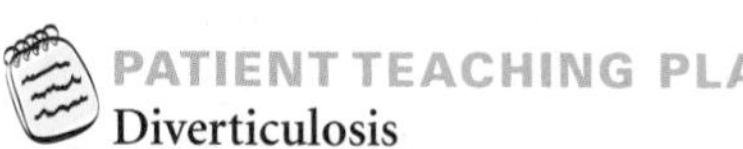

PATIENT TEACHING PLAN
Diverticulosis

- Your diet should be high in fiber. Avoid irritating foods and alcohol.
- For each of your medications, know the drug names, dosages, schedule, and adverse effects.
- Symptoms of inflammation are bleeding, fever, and increased pain; promptly notify the physician if these occur.

Colorectal Cancer

Pathophysiology

Colorectal cancer, or cancer of the large intestine, is the third most common cancer in women. People at greater risk for colorectal cancer are those with histories of inflammatory bowel disease or family histories of colorectal cancer or multiple intestinal polyps. There is some evidence that a high-fat, low-fiber diet and inadequate intake of fruits and vegetables also may contribute to the development of this type of cancer.

Colorectal cancer can develop anywhere in the large intestine. Three fourths of all colorectal cancers are located in the rectum or lower sigmoid colon (Fig. 36-21). These portions of the intestine are easy to examine with a sigmoidoscope.

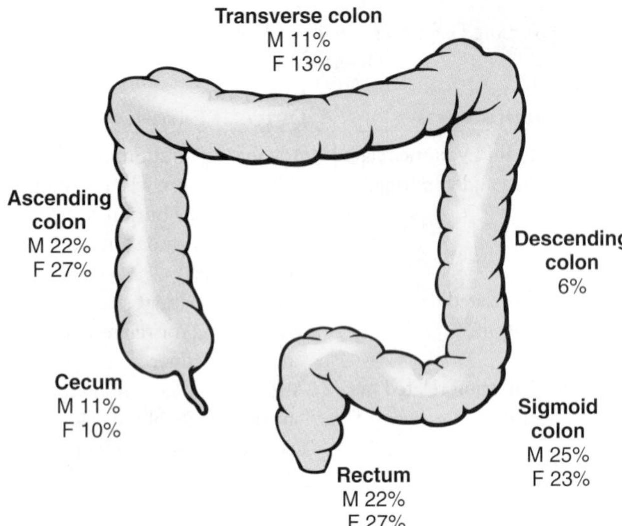

FIGURE **36-21** Sites of colorectal cancer.

Therefore, sigmoidoscopy is often included in the routine physical examinations of older adults.

Signs and Symptoms

Signs and symptoms of colorectal cancer depend on the location of the disease. In the early stages, symptoms are usually mild. If the cancer is located on the right side of the abdomen, the patient may have only vague cramping until the disease is advanced. Unexplained anemia, weakness, and fatigue related to blood loss may be the only early symptoms of right-sided colon cancer.

Cancers on the left side or in the rectum cause more obvious changes in bowel function. Patients may develop diarrhea or constipation and may notice blood in the stool. Stools may become very narrow, causing them to be described as pencil-like. This is due to pressure on the bowel from the growing tumor, which causes a narrowed lumen. The patient may report a feeling of fullness or pressure in the abdomen or rectum. If untreated, obstruction of the bowel eventually occurs regardless of the tumor site.

Medical and Surgical Treatment

Colorectal cancers usually are treated surgically. The exact surgical procedure depends on the location and extent of the cancer. For cancers above the rectum, the diseased portion of the intestine often can be removed. The healthy ends of the remaining intestine are then anastomosed (connected).

Rectal cancers often require more extensive surgery, with incisions in both the abdomen and the perineum (abdominoperineal resection). With removal of the rectum, a permanent colostomy may be created for fecal elimination. However, relatively new procedures may be used to attach the rectal stump to the anus in patients with certain rectal cancers. When this is possible, normal bowel elimination can be maintained and a colostomy can be avoided.

Combination chemotherapy may be recommended postoperatively if the tumor extends through the bowel wall or if lymph nodes are involved. Early stage rectal cancer is sometimes treated with radiation and surgery.

NURSING CARE *of the Patient with Colorectal Cancer*

Because the primary treatment for colon cancer is surgery, nursing care focuses on the surgical patient. Preoperative care includes bowel preparation, hydration, emotional support, and teaching of postoperative routines to prevent surgical complications. Care of the patient with an ostomy is covered in Chapter 25, and care of patients receiving radiation or chemotherapy is covered in Chapter 24.

Assessment

In the postoperative period, assess vital signs, intake and output, breath sounds, bowel sounds, and pain. Describe the appearance of wounds and wound drainage. If there is a colostomy, measure and describe the fecal drainage. Assess the patient's reactions to the surgical procedure and any other anticipated therapies.

Nursing Diagnoses, Goals, and Outcome Criteria: Colorectal Cancer

Nursing Diagnoses	Goals and Outcome Criteria
Risk for Injury related to extensive surgical trauma, open wounds	Wound healing without infection: no fever, intact wound margins without excessive redness
Ineffective Tissue Perfusion related to effects of anesthesia, immobility	Adequate tissue perfusion: vital signs consistent with patient baseline norms
Acute Pain related to tissue trauma	Pain relief: patient states less or no pain, relaxed manner
Sexual Dysfunction related to perineal surgery	Patient understanding of potential sexual dysfunction: patient describes possible problems and corrective measures
Ineffective Coping related to life-threatening illness	Effective coping: patient uses strategies that promote adaptation to illness

Interventions

Risk for Injury

The nursing care of a patient following an abdominoperineal resection is very demanding. The patient has three incisions: one on the abdomen, a second for the colostomy, and a third on the perineum. Check all three for bleeding or drainage. The perineal wound normally drains a large amount of serosanguineous fluid. Serosanguineous fluid is made up of serum and blood. It is a pinkish color and thin in consistency. The wound may be open and packed, partly closed with Penrose drains, or closed and drained with a suction device. An example of a suction drainage system is the Jackson-Pratt drain and fluid collection device. Dressings should initially be reinforced when saturated. Disposable waterproof pads under the patient's hips protect bedding and can easily be changed. A T-binder holds the perineal dressing securely in place.

With so many wounds, especially open ones, these patients are at great risk for infection. Any handling of wound dressings should be done wearing sterile gloves. Always assess the wound for signs of infection (unusual odor, excessive redness or swelling around the wound, and purulent drainage).

If there is packing in a wound, it will be removed gradually. Once the packing has been completely removed, the physician may order the wound to be irrigated on a regular schedule. Gentle irrigations promote healing by keeping the wound clean. Use strict sterile technique during wound irrigations.

Ineffective Tissue Perfusion

Because the abdominoperineal resection requires several incisions and is a lengthy procedure, the patient is at risk for respiratory and circulatory complications. Coughing, deep breathing, and incentive spirometry help prevent fluid accumulation in the lungs. Encourage and help the patient to change positions at least every 2 hours. Leg exercises are important because the pressure on abdominal blood vessels during the long surgery may contribute to the formation of blood clots in the legs.

Acute Pain

Pain is severe for several postoperative days. Give opioid analgesics as ordered. If they do not provide relief, inform the physician. In addition to drug therapy, try comfort measures such as position changes and back rubs. At first, the patient will probably be most comfortable in a side-lying position. Later, he or she will be able to tolerate being supine as well.

When the patient is allowed to be up, sitz baths may be ordered several times a day. The warm water cleans, soothes, and increases circulation to the perineum. Supervise the patient in the sitz bath the first few times in case of dizziness or faintness.

Sexual Dysfunction

Extensive perineal surgery can cause various types of sexual dysfunction. Be open and sensitive to questions that the patient may bring up about sexual function. Refer questions about the specific effects of particular surgical procedures on sexual function to the physician. This is not to say that you should dismiss or ignore patient concerns about sexuality but to stress that the information given must be accurate. Once the correct answers are known, the nurse can reinforce them.

Ineffective Coping

Patients with colorectal cancer and their families often face a difficult period of adjustment. For many people, the thought of having cancer brings up fears of pain, suffering, and a lingering death. These fears may not surface until after the patient recovers from the acute postoperative period. The nurse can help by encouraging the patient to express fears and ask questions and by being a kind listener. Referrals to mental health or spiritual counselors or to support groups can be helpful.

While learning to deal with changes in body image and the threat of a potentially deadly disease, the patient may be faced with receiving chemotherapy as well. Most patients have heard about the side effects of the powerful drugs used in chemotherapy, and they may be justifiably fearful of the treatments. The nursing care of patients receiving chemotherapy is discussed in detail in Chapter 24.

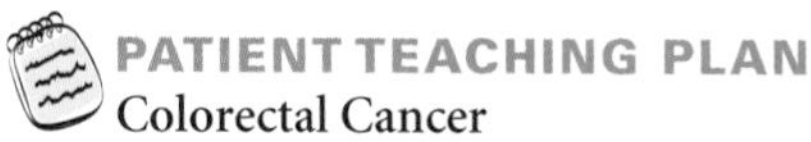

PATIENT TEACHING PLAN
Colorectal Cancer

As the patient improves, the nurse needs to consider long-term needs. The teaching plan should include:

- Wound care
- Colostomy care (see Chapter 24)
- Information about resources of treatment of sexual dysfunction (if appropriate)
- Resources: enterostomal therapist (a nurse who is expert in the care of patients with ostomies); United Ostomy Association, 36 Executive Park, Ste. 120, Irvine, CA 92714.

Polyps

Polyps are small growths in the intestine. Most are benign, but they can become malignant. Two inherited syndromes, familial polyposis and Gardner's syndrome, are characterized by multiple colorectal polyps and almost always lead to cancer. Polyps are usually asymptomatic and are found on routine testing. Potential complications are bleeding and obstruction. Polyps are diagnosed by a barium enema examination or an endoscopic examination. Some of the growths can be removed during the endoscopic examination. Colectomy may be advised for patients with familial polyposis or Gardner's syndrome because of the high risk of malignancy.

Encourage patients who are at risk for cancer to seek medical attention. If the patient has surgery, the postoperative care is similar to that of the patient with cancer of the colon. If a colostomy is created, the patient needs special support and teaching, as described in Chapter 25.

Hemorrhoids

Hemorrhoids are dilated veins in the rectum. They may be above the sphincter muscles of the anus (internal hemorrhoids) or below these muscles (external hemorrhoids) (Fig. 36-22). If blood clots form in external hemorrhoids, they become inflamed and very painful. Hemorrhoids containing clotted blood are said to be thrombosed.

Risk Factors

A key factor in the development of hemorrhoids is increased pressure in the rectal blood vessels. Pressure is increased by constipation, pregnancy, and prolonged sitting or standing.

Signs and Symptoms

The most common symptoms of hemorrhoids are rectal pain and itching. Bleeding may occur with defecation, especially if the hemorrhoids are internal. External hemorrhoids are easy to see and appear red or bluish.

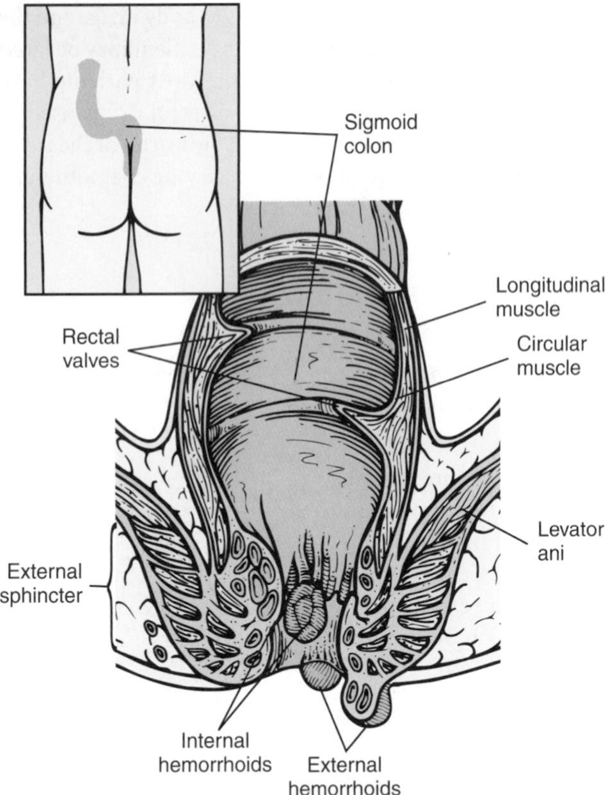

FIGURE **36-22** Internal, external, and prolapsed hemorrhoids.

Consider the Alternative!

Witch hazel compresses applied to the anus after each bowel movement are soothing.

Medical Diagnosis and Treatment

Hemorrhoids are diagnosed upon visual inspection. Nonsurgical treatment of hemorrhoids attempts to relieve pain, swelling, and pressure. Topical medications such as creams, lotions, or suppositories may be ordered to soothe and shrink inflamed tissue. Sitz baths are often comforting. The physician may order heat or cold applications. Sometimes, especially with thrombosed hemorrhoids, ice packs may be applied for a few hours, followed by warm packs.

Outpatient procedures for removing hemorrhoids include:

- Ligation—tying off with rubber bands. The bands cut off the blood supply so that the vessels shrink and die. Dead tissue eventually breaks off and is eliminated.
- Sclerotherapy—the injection of an agent into the tissue around the hemorrhoids that causes them to shrink; results often are temporary.
- Thermocoagulation and electrocoagulation—use of different types of devices to remove the hemorrhoid.
- Laser surgery—effective, but more expensive and risky.

A hemorrhoidectomy is the surgical excision (removal) of hemorrhoids. It is necessary when symptoms are very severe. After the hemorrhoids are removed, the wound may be closed with sutures or packed and left open to heal.

NURSING CARE *of the Patient with Hemorrhoids*

Medical management of hemorrhoids usually does not require hospitalization. Therefore, this section emphasizes the care of the surgical patient. Preoperative care includes bowel preparation and patient teaching of postoperative measures to prevent complications of immobility and anesthesia.

Assessment

After hemorrhoidectomy, monitor vital signs, intake and output, and breath sounds. Assess the perianal area for bleeding and drainage.

Nursing Diagnoses, Goals, and Outcome Criteria: Hemorrhoidectomy

Nursing Diagnoses	Goals and Outcome Criteria
Acute Pain related to tissue trauma	Pain relief: patient states less or no pain, relaxed manner
Impaired Skin Integrity related to surgical procedure	Wound healing: margins intact with decreasing redness, swelling, drainage
Constipation related to delay of defecation	Absence of constipation: soft, formed stools passed at regular intervals without straining or pain

Interventions

Acute Pain

Hemorrhoidectomy patients have severe postoperative pain that requires opioid analgesics for relief. Cold packs over the rectal dressing may be ordered initially. Imagery and relaxation techniques also may help control pain.

Impaired Skin Integrity

The physician removes the wound packing a day or two after surgery. After the packing is removed, assess for rectal bleeding. Sitz baths may then be ordered to soothe and clean the area and to promote circulation. Provide a soft pad or cushion for more comfortable sitting.

Constipation

It is especially important to assess and record any stools passed after rectal surgery. The patient probably will dread the first bowel movement, expecting severe pain. Stool softeners probably will be ordered to reduce the trauma of defecation. Pain medication can be given as ordered before the patient tries to defecate. Someone should stay close by in case the patient feels weak or faint.

PATIENT TEACHING PLAN
Hemorrhoids, Postoperative Care

- Notify your surgeon if you have fever or bleeding.
- To prevent recurrence, avoid constipation, prolonged sitting or standing, or straining to have a bowel movement.

- Ingest a high-fiber diet with plenty of fluids to promote regular, soft stools.
- Use stool softeners if prescribed.
- Follow a regular pattern of bowel elimination, and do not delay defecation when the urge occurs.
- Follow the activity limitations prescribed by your physician.

Anorectal Abscess

An anorectal abscess is an infection in the tissue around the rectum. Signs and symptoms are rectal pain, swelling, redness, and tenderness. The patient often reports a history of diarrhea. If the abscess becomes chronic, it causes bleeding, itching, and discharge.

Anorectal abscess is treated with antibiotics followed by incision and drainage. The procedure may be done under local or general anesthesia, depending on how extensive the abscess is. Preoperatively, pain is treated with ice packs, sitz baths, and topical agents as ordered. Postoperatively, the nursing care is similar to that after hemorrhoidectomy. Pain is treated with opioid analgesics. Patient teaching emphasizes the importance of thorough cleansing after each bowel movement. Advise the patient to consume adequate fluids and a high-fiber diet to promote soft stools.

Anal Fissure

An anal fissure is a laceration between the anal canal and the perianal skin. Fissures may be related to constipation, diarrhea, Crohn's disease, tuberculosis, leukemia, trauma, or childbirth. Sometimes there is no apparent cause. Signs and symptoms include pain before and after defecation and bleeding on the stool or tissue. If the fissure becomes chronic, the patient may experience pruritus, urinary frequency or retention, and dysuria. Fissures usually heal spontaneously, but they can become chronic. Conservative treatment of anal fissures employs sitz baths, stool softeners, and analgesics. Surgical excision may be necessary. Postoperatively, instruct the patient to cleanse the perianal area after defecation. Pain relief measures and stool softeners are continued.

Anal Fistula

An anal fistula is an abnormal opening between the anal canal and the perianal skin. Fistulas can develop from anorectal abscesses or may be related to inflammatory bowel disease or tuberculosis. The patient typically complains of pruritus and discharge. Sitz baths provide some comfort. The surgical treatment is excision of the fistula and surrounding tissue. Sometimes a temporary colostomy is done to allow the surgical site to heal. Postoperative care includes analgesics and sitz baths for pain.

Pilonidal Cyst

A pilonidal cyst is located in the sacrococcygeal area. It appears to result from an in-folding of skin causing a sinus that is easily infected because of its closeness to the anus. Once infected, it is painful and swollen and may form an abscess. Surgical excision is usually recommended. Care is similar to that for the patient having a hemorrhoidectomy.

PATIENT EDUCATION TO PROMOTE NORMAL BOWEL FUNCTION

You often have the opportunity to teach patients how to promote normal bowel function and detect problems early. Acute gastrointestinal disorders can be caused by irritants or infectious agents. Identify and avoid foods that create distress.

Good hand washing and proper food handling reduce the ingestion of infectious agents. Food poisoning can be acquired from food that has been improperly stored, poorly cooked, or exposed to contaminated containers or utensils.

Food poisoning is often a problem for frail elderly who live at home. Poor vision and smell can make food management difficult. It is a good idea for the home health nurse to check the patient's refrigerator and food cabinets to identify potential problems.

People who recognize that stress affects their gastrointestinal function may benefit from relaxation techniques and stress management training.

Signs and symptoms of possibly serious digestive problems should be reported for prompt diagnosis and treatment if indicated. Gastrointestinal symptoms that could indicate gastric cancer include persistent gastric distress, anorexia, and weight loss. Rectal bleeding or a change in bowel habits, or both, often occur with intestinal cancer. As part of the annual physical examination for people over age 40, many physicians do a rectal examination and test the stool for occult blood. For both males and females the American Cancer Society recommends periodic sigmoidoscopy and fecal occult blood tests at intervals beginning at age 50. (See Chapter 24).

Teaching patients what is normal, how to promote normal function, and how to detect problems can help to avoid serious gastrointestinal dysfunction.

Nutrition Concepts

1. People with gastric ulcers experience increased pain after eating.
2. People with duodenal ulcers experience decreased pain after eating.
3. A peptic ulcer diet is individualized and usually consists of small to moderate-sized meals, avoiding foods that cause an increase in gastric acid secretions or consistently cause distress.
4. Diarrhea is caused by pathogenic organisms, diet, intestinal lesions, or irritations associated with various diseases or conditions.
5. The major nutritional goal of therapy for diarrhea is to replace lost fluids.
6. Constipation is caused by insufficient fiber intake, insufficient fluid intake, lack of exercise, some drugs, and the habitual use of laxatives.
7. The dietary treatment of constipation consists of increasing fluid (8-10 glasses of water per day) and fiber intake.
8. A hot drink such as coffee or tea enhances peristalsis and promotes defecation.

key points

- Any disorder of the digestive tract can cause nutritional deficiencies by disrupting one or more of its three functions: digestion, absorption, and elimination.
- Anorexia, or lack of appetite, may be caused by illness, drugs, or emotional factors.
- Oral inflammations and infections can be caused by irritants, bacteria, viruses, and fungi and can interfere with food intake and enjoyment.
- Disorders of the teeth and gums require meticulous oral hygiene and professional dental care to prevent tooth loss.
- Cancers inside the oral cavity are usually squamous cell carcinomas related to poor nutrition, chronic irritation, or combined tobacco and alcohol use.
- Cancers of the lip are usually basal cell carcinomas attributed to prolonged exposure to irritants, including sun, wind, and pipe smoking.
- Nursing care of patients being treated for oral cancers focuses on Acute Pain, Impaired Communication, Imbalanced Nutrition: Less than Body Requirements, Disturbed Body Image, and Impaired Skin Integrity.
- Cancer of the esophagus may be treated with surgery, radiotherapy, chemotherapy, or a combination of these, or by palliative measures to maintain a patent esophagus.
- Vomiting, which can result in fluid and electrolyte imbalances, aspiration, and nutritional deficiencies, is treated with antiemetics, fluid and electrolyte replacement, and sometimes gastrointestinal decompression.
- Treatment of hiatal hernia, the protrusion of the lower esophagus and stomach upward through the diaphragm, may include drug therapy, diet, measures to avoid increased intra-abdominal pressure, or surgery.
- Gastritis is inflammation of the stomach lining caused by excessive intake of food or alcohol, food poisoning, or chemical ingestion.
- Peptic ulcer is loss of tissue from the lining of the stomach or duodenum that can lead to hemorrhage, perforation, and obstruction.
- Nursing care of patients with peptic ulcer focuses on Pain, Imbalanced Nutrition: Less than Body Requirements, Risk for Injury, and Ineffective Coping.
- Dumping syndrome may occur after gastric surgery, causing weakness, dizziness, diaphoresis, and palpitations.
- Nursing care of the patient with stomach cancer, which is often advanced when diagnosed, focuses on Acute Pain, Imbalanced Nutrition: Less than Body Requirements, and Ineffective Coping.
- The term *obesity* denotes body weight more than 20% greater than the person's ideal body weight. Obesity is treated with diet, planned exercise, and, in some cases, drug therapy or surgical intervention.
- There are various types of malabsorption, a condition in which one or more nutrients are not digested or absorbed.
- Diarrhea is the frequent passage of loose or liquid stools. It can lead to fluid and electrolyte imbalances, metabolic acidosis, and malnutrition.
- Constipation is the difficult passage of hard, dry stools. It may be related to inactivity, dehydration, laxative dependence, a low-fiber diet, some drugs, and a variety of medical conditions.
- Fecal impaction is the retention of a large mass of stool in the rectum that the patient cannot pass and that may require removal with enemas and manual extraction.
- Factors that can cause intestinal obstruction include strangulated hernia, tumor, paralytic ileus, stricture, volvulus, intussusception, and postoperative adhesions.
- Appendicitis is inflammation of the appendix that requires surgical treatment to prevent rupture and peritonitis.
- A hernia is a portion of intestine that bulges through a weak area in the muscles of the abdominal wall and can become incarcerated (trapped) and obstructed.
- Inflammatory bowel disease, characterized by inflammation and ulceration of the lining of the intestines, includes ulcerative colitis and Crohn's disease.
- Nursing care of the patient with inflammatory bowel disease focuses on Pain, Diarrhea, Deficient Fluid Volume, Imbalanced Nutrition: Less than Body Requirements, Ineffective Coping, and Risk for Injury.
- Diverticulosis is characterized by small, sac-like pouches in the intestinal wall that can become inflamed, causing obstruction, perforation, peritonitis, and fistula formation.
- Nursing care of the patient with colorectal cancer, which is usually treated surgically, focuses on Risk for Injury, Ineffective Tissue Perfusion, Acute Pain, Sexual Dysfunction, and Ineffective Coping.
- Polyps are small growths in the intestine that are usually benign but may be removed because they may bleed, cause obstructions, or become malignant.
- Hemorrhoids are dilated rectal veins that can become inflamed and thrombosed; they are treated with topical medications, sitz baths, heat or cold, sclerotherapy, or surgical excision.
- Anal disorders include abscesses, fissures, and fistulas, all of which may be treated surgically.

REVIEW QUESTIONS

1. Absorption of nutrients takes place in the:
   1. stomach.
   2. small intestine.
   3. large intestine.
   4. rectum.

2. Assessment of the mouth of an older adult reveals all the data listed below. Which is an *abnormal* finding?
   1. Worn chewing surfaces on the teeth
   2. Recession of the gingiva (gums)
   3. Loss of most of the natural teeth
   4. Teeth appear dark and transparent

3. When assessing the abdomen, the nurse should perform which technique *last?*
   1. Inspection
   2. Auscultation
   3. Percussion
   4. Palpation

4. Other than a radiograph, the *most reliable* way to assess placement of a nasogastric tube is to:
   1. auscultate the epigastrium while injecting air into the tube.
   2. examine and check pH of aspirated stomach contents.
   3. place the end of the tube in water and observe for bubbling.
   4. listen for air movement at the end of the tube.

5. A patient who has had oral surgery complains of dry mouth. Your most appropriate action is to:
   1. tell the patient this is normal after oral surgery.
   2. provide a commercial mouthwash for rinsing the mouth.
   3. contact the physician for mouth care instructions.
   4. suction the mouth after giving the patient sips of water.

6. You are reviewing the admission papers for a new resident in a long term care facility. You note a medical diagnosis of achalasia. A relevant part of the nursing care plan should be:
   1. determine the best position for the patient during meals.
   2. monitor all stools for occult blood.
   3. assess for the presence of bowel sounds in all four quadrants.
   4. maintain strict intake and output records.

7. Which of the following types of antiulcer drugs works by inhibiting the secretion of gastric acid?
   1. Antacids
   2. H_2-receptor blockers
   3. Mucosal barriers
   4. Antibiotics

8. A patient who was admitted with severe abdominal pain is being evaluated for possible appendicitis. You should suspect intestinal rupture if:
   1. the patient's WBC count is 15,000/mm^3.
   2. palpation at McBurney's point causes pain.
   3. the patient keeps both hips flexed.
   4. the patient's abdomen is rigid.

9. Surgery is used to treat Crohn's disease less often than ulcerative colitis because Crohn's disease:
   1. usually returns at the site of the anastomosis.
   2. typically involves the entire small and large intestines.
   3. can usually be cured with combination drug therapy.
   4. is associated with a higher risk of surgical complications.

10. One method of removing hemorrhoids is to use a rubber band to tie off the hemorrhoid. This is called:
    1. sclerotherapy.
    2. photocoagulation.
    3. laser excision.
    4. ligation.

CHAPTER

37 Disorders of the Liver, Gallbladder, and Pancreas

objectives

1. Identify nursing assessment data related to the functions of the liver, gallbladder, and pancreas.
2. Identify the nurse's role in tests and procedures performed to diagnose disorders of the liver, gallbladder, and pancreas.
3. Describe the care of the patient who has an esophageal balloon tube in place.
4. Explain the pathology, signs and symptoms, diagnosis, complications, and medical treatment of selected disorders of the liver, gallbladder, and pancreas.
5. Assist in developing a nursing care plan for the patient with liver, gallbladder, or pancreatic dysfunction.

key terms

Ascites (ă-SĪ-tēz, p. 715)
Cholecystectomy (kō-lĕ-sĭs-TĔK-tō-mē, p. 734)
Cholecystitis (kō-lĕ-sĭs-TĪ-tĭs, p. 733)
Choledocholithiasis (kō-lĕd-ō-kō-lĭ-THĪ-ă-sĭs, p. 733)
Cholelithiasis (kō-lĕ-lĭ-THĪ-ă-sĭs, p. 734)
Cirrhosis (sĭr-RŌ-sĭs, p. 723)
Endocrine gland (ĔN-dŏ-krĭn, p. 738)
Eructation (ĕ-rŭk-TĀ-shŭn, p. 733)
Gluconeogenesis (gloo-kō-nē-ō-JĔN-ĕ-sĭs, p. 712)
Glycogenesis (glī-kō-JĔN-ĕ-sĭs, p. 712)
Glycogenolysis (glī-kō-jĕ-NŎL-ĭ-sĭs, p. 712)
Hepatic (hĕ-PĂ-tĭc, p. 712)
Hepatitis (hĕ-pă-TĪ-tĭs, p. 714)
Hepatomegaly (hĕ-pă-tō-MĔG-ă-lē, p. 715)
Icterus (ĬK-tĕr-ŭs, p. 715)
Jaundice (JĂWN-dĭs, p. 715)

THE LIVER

The liver is the largest internal organ in the body. It is located under the diaphragm in the upper right abdomen, as illustrated in Figure 37-1. The term *hepatic* refers to the liver.

ANATOMY AND PHYSIOLOGY OF THE LIVER

The liver can be divided into four lobes that are made up of many lobules (Fig. 37-2). Blood from the aorta is delivered to the liver via the hepatic artery. The portal vein delivers blood from the intestines to the liver. Portal blood circulates through the liver and is transported to the inferior vena cava by the hepatic veins. Figure 37-3 illustrates hepatic circulation.

Specialized **hepatic** cells allow the liver to carry out many critical functions. Reticuloendothelial cells, called Kupffer cells, ingest old red blood cells and bacteria. Parenchymal cells carry out various metabolic functions, including metabolism of carbohydrates, fats, proteins, and steroids and detoxification of potentially harmful substances.

BILE PRODUCTION AND EXCRETION

Bilirubin is a product of the normal breakdown of old red blood cells in the liver. The initial breakdown product is unconjugated or indirect bilirubin. The liver then converts unconjugated bilirubin into conjugated bilirubin and secretes it into the bile. Bile produced in the liver passes through the cystic duct into the gallbladder for storage.

When fats pass into the duodenum, the gallbladder and the liver respond by delivering bile through the common bile duct into the small intestine. Bile emulsifies fat, meaning that it breaks it into small particles that can easily be absorbed. It also neutralizes the acidic chyme as it leaves the stomach. Bile plays a role in the absorption of fat-soluble vitamins and the removal of some toxins.

Bile travels through the intestines with the chyme. In the large intestine, it is converted to urobilinogen and then to stercobilin. This final breakdown product of bilirubin gives stool its characteristic brown color.

METABOLISM

Glucose Metabolism

The liver helps maintain the blood glucose within a certain range. After a meal, excess glucose molecules are taken up by the liver, combined, and then stored as glycogen. This process is called *glycogenesis.* When the glucose level in the blood falls, the process is reversed by *glycogenolysis,* and the glucose molecules are returned to the blood. *Gluconeogenesis* is the third process by which the liver maintains blood glucose. Fats and protein are broken down in response to low blood glucose levels, and the molecules are used to make new glucose.

Protein Metabolism

Some nonessential amino acids, plasma proteins (albumin and globulin), and clotting factors are synthesized in the liver. Another important liver function in relation to protein metabolism is the conversion of ammonia to urea. Ammonia

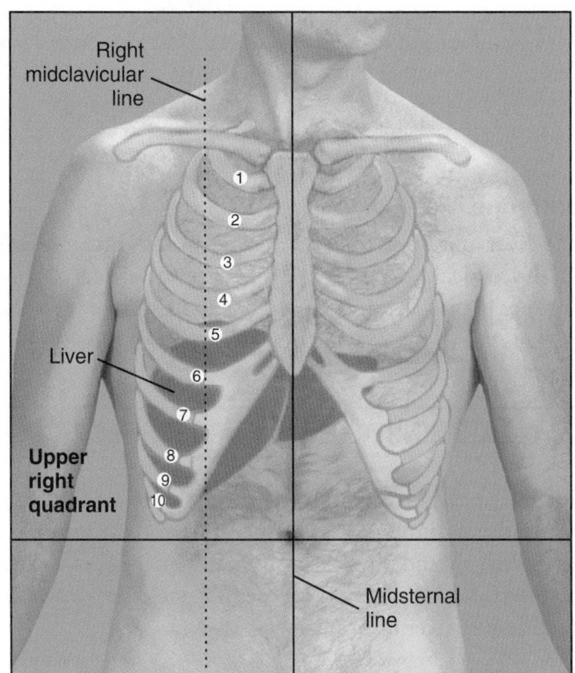

FIGURE 37-1 The liver is located under the diaphragm in the right upper abdomen. Anatomic landmarks are noted.

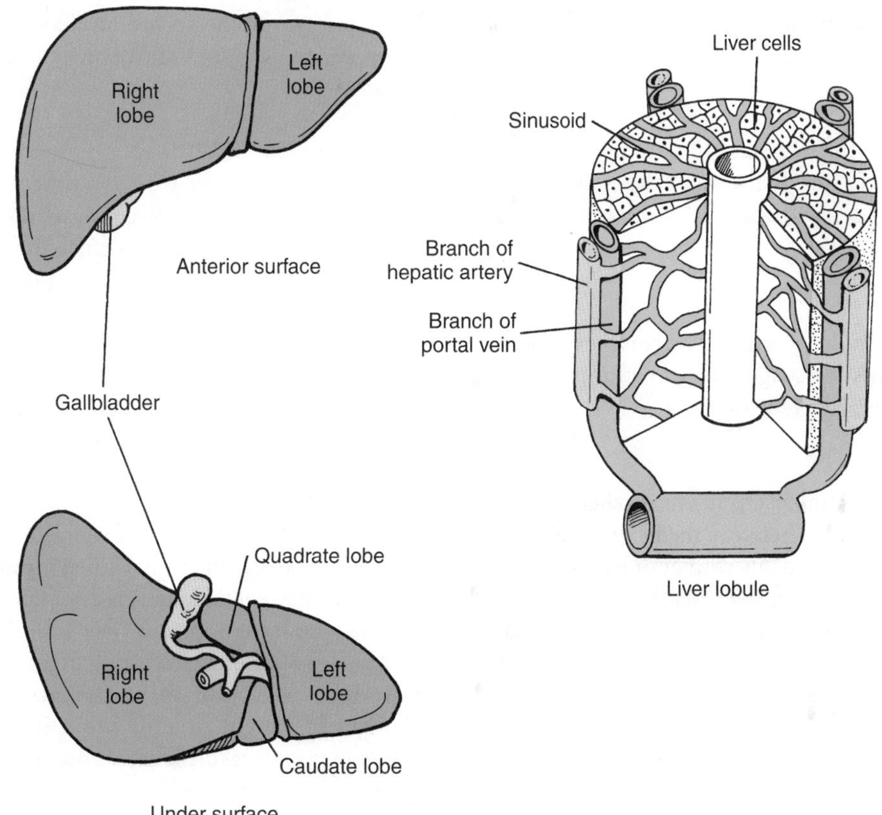

FIGURE 37-2 The liver has four lobes, each made up of many lobules.

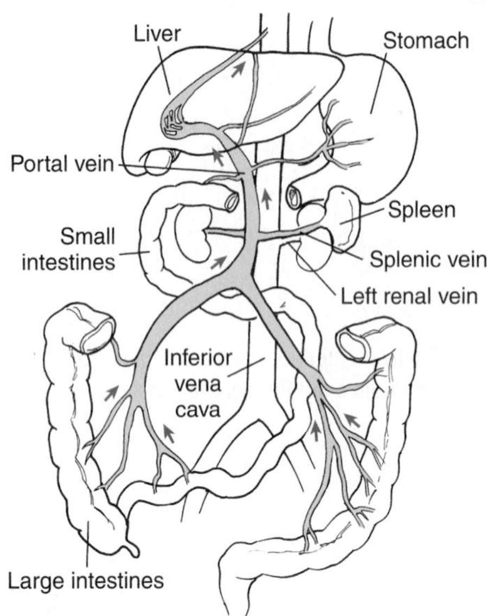

FIGURE 37-3 Hepatic circulation. Venous blood from the spleen, stomach, pancreas, and intestines passes through the liver via the portal vein and is delivered through the hepatic veins to the inferior vena cava.

is a byproduct of the metabolism of amino acids. If ammonia accumulates in the blood, it has toxic effects on brain tissue.

Lipid Metabolism

The liver synthesizes lipids from glucose, pyruvic acid, acetic acid, and amino acids. It also synthesizes fatty acids, breaks down triglycerides, and synthesizes and breaks down cholesterol.

Blood Coagulation

Normal blood coagulation (clotting) is a complex process. Two essential elements for coagulation, prothrombin and fibrinogen, are synthesized by the liver.

Detoxification

The liver filters the blood and inactivates many chemicals, including most medications. Therefore medications are prescribed very cautiously for patients with poor liver function. Patients with liver disease are at increased risk for toxic effects of drugs. With age, there is some decrease in liver function, so lower drug dosages may be adequate. Especially with long-term therapy, the older person should be assessed frequently for signs of toxicity.

PHARMACOLOGY CAPSULE Since many drugs are metabolized in the liver, patients with liver disease are at increased risk for toxic effects of drugs.

Immunity

An important protective mechanism is the development of antibodies to resist pathogens. Antibodies and other substances that help resist infection are produced in the liver.

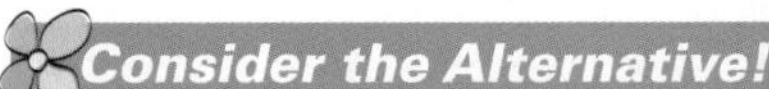

Consider the Alternative!

Inform patients that the following herbs can harm the liver: comfrey, borage, coltsfoot, chaparral, and germander.

Hormone Metabolism

The liver plays an important role in the metabolism of adrenocortical hormones, estrogen, testosterone, and aldosterone. If these hormones are not metabolized, they accumulate, causing an exaggerated effect on target organs.

NURSING ASSESSMENT OF THE LIVER

The liver has so many important functions that alterations may cause a number of systemic signs and symptoms. The health history and physical examination may provide clues to liver dysfunction and may be used to assess responses to the treatment of liver disorders.

HEALTH HISTORY

Begin by asking about the patient's chief complaint. Explore and describe the symptoms that caused the patient to seek medical attention. The patient may report various signs and symptoms, including change in the color of skin, urine, or stools; abdominal pain, nausea, and vomiting; and fatigue.

Past Medical History

The past medical history documents any previous or chronic liver disorders. Record any recent operations, injuries, or blood transfusions since they sometimes expose the patient to the hepatitis virus. Compile a complete list of medications.

Family History

Assess whether any of the patient's family members have had cancer of the liver or colon, hepatitis, or alcoholism.

Review of Systems

Inquire about the patient's general health status and systematically assess for signs and symptoms related to liver dysfunction. General fatigue is a common complaint among people who have impaired liver function. They may have had personality or behavior changes, but the patients are not always aware of these changes. Inquire about any changes in weight or skin color, itching, easy bruising, headaches, enlarged lymph nodes, breast enlargement in men, or dyspnea.

Gastrointestinal symptoms are common with liver disease. Therefore ask about the presence of anorexia, abdominal pain, nausea and vomiting, diarrhea, or gastrointestinal bleeding. Note the color of stools because clay-colored stools are characteristic of bile obstruction, and black stools can indicate GI bleeding. Changes in urine color also may be significant since patients with liver disease often have dark urine.

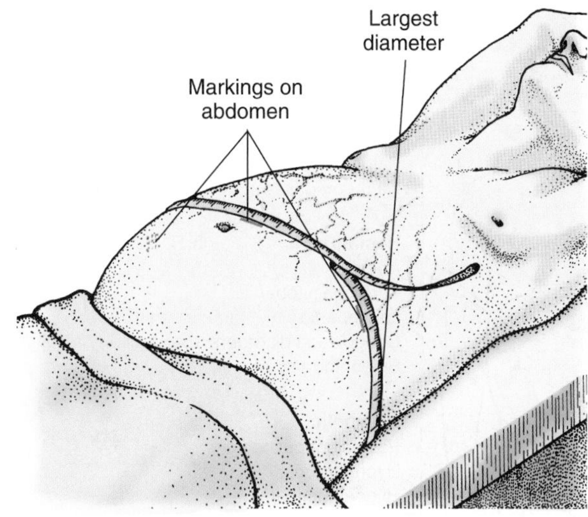

FIGURE **37-4** How to measure abdominal girth. Marks are made on the abdominal midline and both sides so that subsequent measurements can always be made at the same place.

table 37-1 **ASSESSMENT** ***of the Patient with Liver Disease***

HEALTH HISTORY	PHYSICAL EXAMINATION
Present Illness: Fatigue, weight changes, digestive disturbances, skin changes **Past Medical History:** Previous liver disease, hepatitis B immunization, recent and current medications taken **Review of Systems:** Weakness, fatigue, pruritus, dyspnea, anorexia, abdominal pain, nausea and vomiting, diarrhea, bloody stools, changes in urine or stool color, numbness or tingling of extremities **Functional Assessment:** Diet, alcohol intake, occupation, exposure to toxins, stress, coping strategies, interpersonal relationships	**Vital Signs:** Hypertension, tachypnea **Height and Weight** **Skin:** Dryness, scratches, jaundice, bruises **Eyes:** Scleral icterus **Thorax:** Spider angiomas **Breasts:** Gynecomastia **Abdomen:** Distention, prominent veins, girth, liver enlargement

Ask whether the patient has had any numbness, tingling, or edema in the extremities.

Functional Assessment

Explore the patient's daily routines, including dietary intake and patterns of activity and rest. Since liver disease may be associated with exposure to toxins, assess the patient's exposure to chemicals, potentially toxic drugs such as acetaminophen, and alcohol use. Some people are reluctant to discuss alcohol use, so the subject must be handled tactfully. People tend to understate the amount of alcohol they typically consume. Note use of street drugs, especially those taken intravenously.

The last part of the functional assessment is the identification of stressors, usual coping strategies, and sources of support.

PHYSICAL EXAMINATION

Begin the physical assessment with the measurement of vital signs and height and weight and observation of the patient's general appearance. Skin color is especially important in relation to the liver. Jaundice is a golden yellow skin color associated with liver dysfunction or bile obstruction. It is relatively easy to recognize in fair-skinned people.

Inspect the sclera of the eyes. Like the skin, the sclera may turn yellow, a condition called scleral icterus. This sign is especially useful when jaundice cannot be seen elsewhere in dark-skinned people.

Assess for enlargement of breast tissue in men. Such enlargement is called gynecomastia. When inspecting the chest, also look for spider angiomas. Spider angiomas are small, visible vessels shaped like spiders.

The examination of the abdomen is especially important in detecting liver disease. Inspect the shape of the abdomen. Note the presence of prominent veins. If significant ascites (fluid accumulation in the peritoneal cavity) is present, the abdomen appears distended. Measure the abdomen at the largest circumference in order to permit comparative measurements later (Fig. 37-4).

Palpate the abdomen for distention and tenderness. Experienced examiners may be able to palpate the liver, but, unless it is enlarged, it is difficult to locate under the right rib cage. An enlarged, diseased liver may be felt well below the rib margin. Liver enlargement is called *hepatomegaly.*

Examine the extremities for bruising, edema, muscle wasting, and impaired sensation. Inspect the hands for palmar erythema (redness of the palms).

The assessment of a patient with a liver disorder is summarized in Table 37-1. Findings associated with liver disease are illustrated in Figure 37-5.

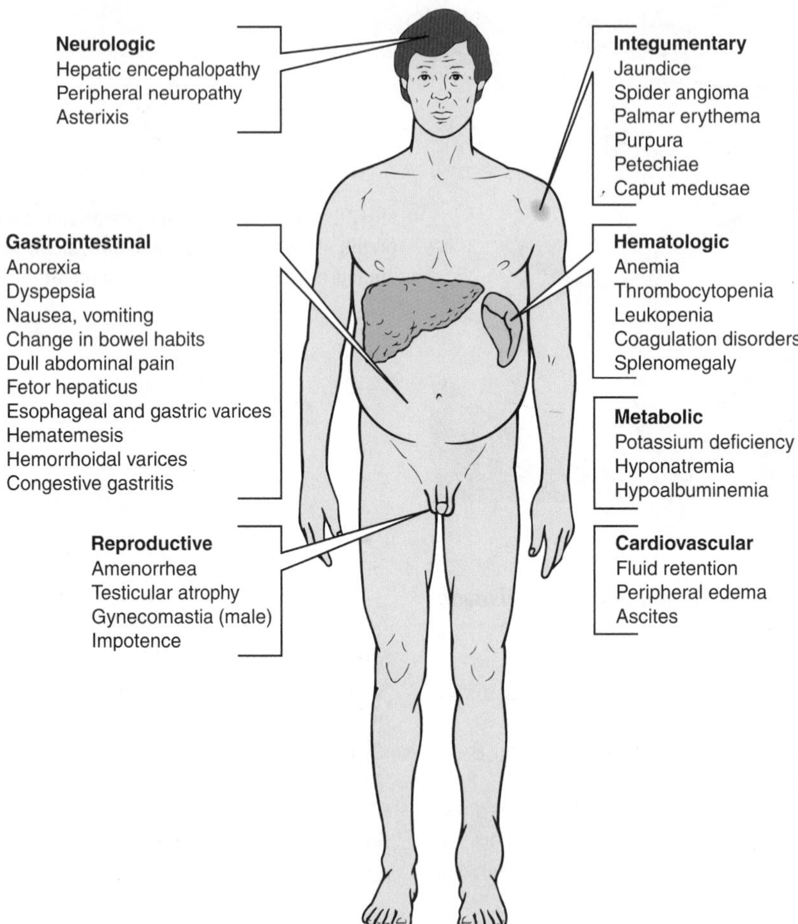

FIGURE **37-5** Findings associated with liver disease.

DIAGNOSTIC TESTS AND PROCEDURES

The physician uses a number of tools to assess liver function, including laboratory studies, imaging studies, and biopsies. Nursing care of patients having specific tests and procedures is presented in Table 37-2.

LABORATORY STUDIES

Laboratory studies of blood specimens are done to measure serum and urine bilirubin, serum proteins, ammonia, prothrombin time, vitamin K production, and serum enzymes. Examples of serum enzymes include alkaline phosphatase (ALP), alanine aminotransferase (ALT), serum glutamic-pyruvic transaminase (SGPT), aldolase (ALS), aspartate aminotransferase (AST), serum glutamic-oxaloacetic transaminase (SGOT), and lactate dehydrogenase (LDH). Table 37-2 explains the significance of these laboratory tests.

Since gastrointestinal bleeding is sometimes a problem with liver disease, gastric fluids and stools may be tested for the presence of occult blood. Urine specimens may also be tested for bilirubin and urobilinogen and stool specimens tested for urobilinogen.

IMAGING STUDIES

Radiographic Studies

Radiographic studies are used primarily to visualize the circulatory and biliary systems in the liver. The liver scan employs a radioactive substance that is injected into a vein. The substance accumulates in the liver. Radiographs are then taken to reveal tumors and abscesses.

Ultrasonography

Ultrasonography uses sound waves to create an image of the liver, spleen, pancreas, gallbladder, and biliary system. It is a noninvasive and painless procedure.

Computed Tomography and Magnetic Resonance Imaging

Computed tomography (CT) and magnetic resonance imaging (MRI) are used to obtain scans of internal organs, including the liver. They are noninvasive, painless procedures.

LIVER BIOPSY

A liver biopsy is a procedure that involves removal of a small specimen of liver tissue for examination. The specimen can

table 37-2 **DIAGNOSTIC TESTS AND PROCEDURES | *Liver and Gallbladder***

General Interventions: Check your agency procedure for diagnostic tests and procedures. Always tell the patient what to expect when tests are ordered. Explain if NPO status is necessary. Document the care provided and relevant assessment data. If venipuncture is done, a dressing should be applied and the site checked for oozing. Apply pressure if patient's blood clotting is impaired. Assess allergy to dyes; monitor for reactions.

TEST	PURPOSE/PROCEDURE	PATIENT PREPARATION	POSTPROCEDURE CARE
LABORATORY STUDIES			
Blood Studies			
Serum bilirubin	Assesses liver function by measuring bilirubin in the blood. Normal values include: Total bilirubin: 0.2-1.0 mg/dl *or* 3.4-17.1 μmol/L Conjugated bilirubin: 0.0-0.2 mg/dl *or* 0.0-3.4 μmol/L Unconjugated bilirubin: 0.2-0.8 mg/dl	Tell patient to fast for at least 4 hrs before blood sample drawn. Avoid yellow foods for 3-4 days before test. Should not be done within 24 hrs after a contrast medium has been given.	No special care.
Alkaline phosphatase	Detects increases associated with liver or bone disease Normal value: Varies with method.	10-12 hr fast may be required. Some drugs may be withheld for 12 hrs.	No special care.
Prothrombin time and INR	Detects prolonged clotting time possibly caused by liver disease or vitamin K deficiency. Normal value: PT: 11.0-12.6 sec INR: 1.0-1.2	No coffee or alcohol for 24 hrs before test. Many natural remedies affect result.	No special care.
Serum enzymes AST (SGOT) ALT (SGPT) LDH	Detects elevations in enzymes related to liver diseases. Normal values: AST: Men 7-21 μ/L Women 6-18 μ/L ALT: Men 6-24 U/L Women 4-17 U/L LDH: Varies with type of test.	Consult agency guidelines to see if fasting is necessary.	No special care.
Serum protein	Electrophoresis helps to diagnose conditions that affect serum proteins.	Avoid high-fat diet for 8 hrs before test. Some medications may need to be withheld for several days before blood sample is drawn.	No special care.

AST, Aspartate aminotransferase; *SGOT,* serum glutamic-oxaloacetic transaminase; *ALT,* alanine aminotransferase; *SGPT,* serum glutamic-pyruvic transaminase; *LDH,* lactate dehydrogenase; *NPO,* nothing by mouth.

Continued

table 37-2 **DIAGNOSTIC TESTS AND PROCEDURES | *Liver and Gallbladder—cont'd***

TEST	PURPOSE/PROCEDURE	PATIENT PREPARATION	POSTPROCEDURE CARE
RADIOGRAPHIC STUDIES			
√Computed tomography (CT)	Creates cross-sectional images of liver and other organs to reveal abnormalities.	Inform radiologist if patient is allergic to contrast media, iodine, or shellfish. Inform patient that the procedure is painless and noninvasive. NPO status may be ordered, but routine drugs can usually be taken. The patient will lie still on a stretcher while a donut-shaped machine moves around him or her. Contrast dye is sometimes injected intravenously. It can create a feeling of warmth, a salty taste, and nausea. Sedation can be ordered if the patient has difficulty lying still.	No special care usually needed. Inform the physician of any signs of allergic response to contrast dye. Give antihistamines as ordered for allergy.
T-tube cholangiography	Evaluates whether bile ducts are open after gallbladder surgery.	Contrast agent is injected into T-tube before radiographs are obtained. Takes about 15 min. Same as for intravenous cholangiography.	A fatty meal helps eliminate dye. Report rash, itching, hive, dyspnea that could be allergic reaction to dye.
Intravenous cholangiography	Permits visualization of bile ducts, usually done when gallbladder is not visualized on cholecystography.	Radiographs are taken before and at intervals after intravenous injection of a contrast agent (if done). Withhold food and fluids as ordered. Takes 4-6 hr. Patient is usually NPO after midnight before study. A laxative also may be ordered night before. Ask about iodine sensitivity, and notify radiologist if patient is sensitive.	Same as for T-tube cholecystography. If solution is given through liver (percutaneous transhepatic cholangiography), watch for signs of bleeding and respiratory distress.
√Percutaneous transhepatic cholangiography	Dye is given and radiography used to visualize the biliary duct system.	Report patient allergies to iodine or seafood before the test. During the procedure, the patient must lie still while a needle is inserted into the liver and dye is injected. Radiography is used to place the needles and observe the outline of the bile ducts or blood vessels.	Bedrest for 8 hr. Check the puncture site for bleeding. Monitor vital signs to detect signs of bleeding. Other care such as T-tube cholangiography.
√Portal venography and hepatic arteriography	Uses intravenous contrast dye followed by radiographs to study blood vessels in liver.		Same as T-tube cholangiography.
√Liver scan	A radioactive substance is given that collects in liver. A scanner maps uptake of radiation, revealing tumors and abscesses. During procedure, the radioactive substance is given intravenously.	The patient should be assured that a small dose of radiation is harmless. The patient is then helped to assume various positions while radiographs are taken. 4-6 hr fast required.	Patient must wash hands thoroughly after voiding for 24 hrs. Report allergic symptoms.

AST, Aspartate aminotransferase; *SGOT,* serum glutamic-oxaloacetic transaminase; *ALT,* alanine aminotransferase; *SGPT,* serum glutamic-pyruvic transaminase; *LDH,* lactate dehydrogenase; *NPO,* nothing by mouth.

table 37-2 **DIAGNOSTIC TESTS AND PROCEDURES | *Liver and Gallbladder—cont'd***

TEST	PURPOSE/PROCEDURE	PATIENT PREPARATION	POSTPROCEDURE CARE
RADIOGRAPHIC STUDIES—cont'd			
Gallbladder scan, hepatobiliary scintigraphy, hepatobiliary imaging, biliary tract radionuclide scan, cholescintigraphy, HIDA scan	A radionuclide is injected and images are taken of the biliary tract to assess patency. Detects cholecystitis.	NPO at least 2 hr before procedure. Explain to patient that scan takes about 90 min. Repeat imaging may be needed 24-48 hr later.	Encourage patient to drink fluids to promote elimination of radionuclide, to wash hands after voiding, and to flush immediately. Caregivers should wear gloves to handle urine. Wash gloved hands before and after removing gloves; dispose of gloves as nuclear waste.
OTHER IMAGING PROCEDURES			
Ultrasonography	Uses high-frequency sound waves to create an image of the liver, spleen, pancreas, gallbladder, and biliary system.	May be NPO for 8-12 hr. Patient teaching: the patient will lie on a table. A technician applies gel to the abdomen and moves an instrument called a transducer over the abdomen. Images are projected onto a screen. Not painful.	No special care needed after the procedure.
Magnetic resonance imaging (MRI)	Creates cross-sectional images of the liver and other organs without radiation.	Advise the patient that MRI is a painless, noninvasive procedure. All metal must be removed before MRI. The patient must be still on a narrow surface. Older MRI is a circular device that surrounds the body like a tunnel. Closing eyes reduces claustrophobia (open MRI eliminates claustrophobia). Machine is noisy.	No special care needed.
TISSUE EXAMINATION			
Liver biopsy	Removes a small specimen of liver tissue for examination.	Baseline vital signs and blood coagulation studies should be obtained.	With *all* liver biopies: Monitor vital signs for indications of bleeding (tachycardia, tachypnea, restlessness, hypotension) and pneumothorax (dyspnea, tachycardia).
Needle biopsy	The specimen is obtained by inserting a special needle into the liver through the abdominal wall.	The patient is positioned supine with the right arm behind the head.	Check pressure dressing for bleeding. Position the patient on the right side as ordered.
Open biopsy	An incision is made under general anesthesia.	Done in the operating room and requires standard preoperative procedures. Informed consent must be obtained from the patient.	
ENDOSCOPY			
Cholangiopancreatography, endoscopic retrograde cholangiopan creatography (ERCP)	A flexible endoscope is passed following injection of dye. Study permits visualization of pancreatic, hepatic, and common bile ducts and ampulla of Vater. Used to diagnose pancreatic disease.	NPO for 8-12 hr. Study takes 30-60 min. May feel flushed when dye injected. Rule out iodine allergy.	Advise warm gargles or ice pack to neck for sore throat. Patient may have belching and bloating. Immediately notify physician of severe pain, fever, dyspnea, hematemesis.

be obtained through an incision under general anesthesia (open biopsy). Another method (needle biopsy) involves the use of a special type of needle inserted through the abdominal wall to obtain the specimen.

Before either procedure, baseline vital signs should be obtained and blood coagulation studies done. Signed consent is required. When preparing for a needle biopsy, tell the patient what to expect during the procedure. For a needle biopsy, position the patient supine with the right arm behind the head. Place a pad under the right chest. The physician instructs the patient to take a deep breath and hold it during the actual puncture.

A pressure dressing is placed over the puncture. It should be checked for bleeding every 15 minutes for the first hour, every 30 minutes for the next hour, and then hourly or according to agency protocol. Monitor vital signs at the same time for signs of blood loss (tachycardia, restlessness, hypotension) or pneumothorax (restlessness, tachypnea). The physician may order the patient kept on the right side for a period of time to maintain pressure on the puncture site.

The primary complications of liver biopsy are hemorrhage and pneumothorax. Bleeding is a possibility because of the liver's rich blood supply and the potential for impaired coagulation in the patient with liver disease. Pneumothorax occurs if the lung is accidentally punctured during the biopsy. Air escapes into the pleural cavity, and the lung on the affected side collapses.

DISORDERS OF THE LIVER

HEPATITIS

Hepatitis is inflammation of the liver. It is estimated that 300,000 cases of viral hepatitis are reported in the United States each year. Although many patients have uneventful recoveries, others develop chronic conditions that can eventually lead to liver failure and death.

Pathophysiology

Hepatitis has both local and systemic effects. Locally, the inflammatory process causes the liver to swell. If swelling is severe, there are two important effects. First, the bile channels are compressed, damaging the cells that produce bile. This results in an elevation in serum bilirubin and jaundice. Second, blood flow through the liver is impaired, causing pressure to rise in the portal circulation (see Fig. 37-3).

Systemic effects are related to altered metabolic functions normally performed by the liver and to the infectious response in viral hepatitis. Systemic signs and symptoms of hepatitis include rash, angioedema, arthritis, fever, and malaise.

Types of Hepatitis

Hepatitis can be classified as infectious or non-infectious. Known causes of infectious hepatitis include viruses, types A, B, C, D, and E. Other viruses that may cause hepatitis include the recently described hepatitis G and hepatitis GB. Noninfectious hepatitis is caused by exposure to toxic chemicals, including drugs. Key features of each type of hepatitis are summarized in Table 37-3.

Hepatitis A

Hepatitis A has been called infectious hepatitis and epidemic hepatitis. It is caused by the hepatitis A virus, which is transmitted from one person to another by way of water, food, or medical equipment that has been contaminated with infected fecal matter. Hepatitis A is the most common type of viral hepatitis. Fortunately, it is rarely fatal and infected persons do not become asymptomatic carriers.

Hepatitis B

Hepatitis B, caused by the hepatitis B virus, is often called serum hepatitis. Since the hepatitis B virus is found in all body fluids of infected persons, modes of transmission include intimate contact with carriers as well as contact with contaminated blood or medical equipment. Some 6% to 10% of these patients develop chronic hepatitis and become carriers, meaning they can transmit the infection to others.

Hepatitis C

Hepatitis C is transmitted by contact with contaminated blood or medical equipment, or by contact with infected body fluids. About 40% to 60% of people with hepatitis C develop chronic infections and become carriers.

Hepatitis D

Hepatitis D is caused by a virus known as the delta agent, which is a defective RNA virus that can only survive in the company of the hepatitis B virus. Hepatitis D is transmitted percutaneously (through the skin or mucous membranes) with the B virus. The presence of hepatitis D greatly increases the risk that the patient will progress to chronic hepatitis and possible liver failure.

Hepatitis E

Hepatitis E only recently has been described. It is similar to hepatitis A and is most commonly transmitted via water contaminated with infected fecal matter. Hepatitis E infection is rare in the United States except among people who have traveled in developing countries where the virus is more common.

Hepatitis G

Hepatitis G has been identified in some blood donors and can be transmitted by blood transfusion. HGV does not appear to cause chronic hepatitis, but its effects may not be fully known at this time.

Noninfectious Hepatitis

Although the cause is not always identifiable, noninfectious hepatitis can be caused by exposure to toxins such as mercury and arsenic and drugs such as alcohol and acetaminophen.

Signs and Symptoms

Regardless of the cause, the signs and symptoms of hepatitis are similar. Differences occur in the number and severity of the symptoms from one person to the next. Many patients have no symptoms at all. For those who are symptomatic, the course of the disease is marked by three phases: preicteric, icteric, and posticteric.

Preicteric Phase

Common findings in the preicteric phase include malaise, severe headache, right upper quadrant abdominal pain,

table 37-3 ***Key Features of Each Type of Viral Hepatitis***

TYPE	CAUSE	TRANSMISSION ROUTE	INCUBATION PERIOD	PREVENTION
Hepatitis A	Hepatitis A virus (HAV)	Fecal-oral route. Often via contaminated water or food.	3-5 wk	Wash hands after toileting. Use clean water and food supplies. Use gloves to handle stool specimens and soiled articles. Immune globulin is given before or within 48 hr after exposure.
Hepatitis B	Hepatitis B virus (HBV)	Introduction of contaminated blood through skin or mucous membranes. Often via contaminated needles or other medical or dental equipment; also by sexual contact. Newborns may be infected before, during, or after birth.	2-5 mo	Vaccine is given to people at risk for exposure. Use disposable needles. Avoid contaminated articles. Screen blood donors. Use caution with body fluids. Hepatitis B immune globulin is given after exposure.
Hepatitis C (non-A, non-B)	Hepatitis C virus (HCV)	Introduction of contaminated blood through skin or mucous membranes, usually by needles or other medical or dental equipment.	7 wk	Use disposable needles. Avoid contaminated articles. Screen blood donors. Use caution with body fluids. No vaccine is available.
Hepatitis D	"Delta agent" hepatitis D virus (HDV)	Transmitted only with HBV via contaminated blood or equipment, or by sexual contact.	1-6 mo	Hepatitis B vaccine.
Hepatitis E	Hepatitis E virus (HEV)	Fecal-oral route often via contaminated water or food.	3-6 wk	Wash hands after toileting. Use clean water and food supplies. Use gloves to handle stool specimens and soiled articles. Immune globulin is given before or within 48 hr after exposure.

anorexia, nausea, vomiting, fever, arthralgia (joint pain), rash, enlarged lymph nodes, urticaria, and enlargement and tenderness of the liver. The preicteric phase lasts 1 to 21 days and is the period when the patient is most infectious.

Icteric Phase

The icteric phase is characterized by jaundice, light or clay-colored stools, and dark urine typical of impaired bile production and secretion. Pruritus may be present and is caused by the accumulation of bile salts under the skin. Gastrointestinal symptoms from the preicteric phase often persist. The icteric phase lasts 2 to 4 weeks. Hepatitis patients in whom jaundice does not develop are said to have anicteric hepatitis.

Posticteric Phase

In the posticteric phase, fatigue, malaise, and liver enlargement persist for several months.

Complications

Most people recover fully from hepatitis A or B, but there can be residual damage and complications. Some patients with hepatitis B or C become carriers. About one fourth of those who become carriers will have chronic active hepatitis, which can lead to cirrhosis. Carriers also are at increased risk for liver cancer. People who have had hepatitis cannot donate blood because of the risk of transmitting the disease to a recipient.

Complications of hepatitis include chronic persistent hepatitis, chronic active hepatitis, and fulminant hepatitis. Chronic persistent hepatitis is characterized by a prolonged recovery with continuing fatigue and liver enlargement that eventually resolves. With chronic active hepatitis, signs and symptoms persist for more than 6 months. Liver damage continues and may lead to cirrhosis. If necrosis of damaged cells occurs without regeneration, fulminant hepatitis results. It is marked by severe liver failure and is often fatal. Hepatitis D virus, which coexists with the hepatitis B virus, can contribute to the development of fulminant hepatitis.

Medical Diagnosis

A diagnosis of hepatitis is supported by abnormal liver function tests. Typical findings consistent with hepatitis include elevated levels of serum enzymes (AST, SGOT, ALT, SGPT, GGT), serum and urinary bilirubin, and urinary urobilinogen. The prothrombin time is prolonged. Albumin may be normal or low, and globulin may be normal or high. The types of viral hepatitis can be identified by the presence of specific viral antigens and antibodies.

Medical Treatment

There is no specific cure for hepatitis. Treatment is designed to promote healing and to manage symptoms. However, alpha-interferon is useful in treating HBV and, to a lesser extent, HCV. Ribavirin (Virazole) enhances the alpha-interferon. Other new antiviral drugs are showing some promise in the treatment of hepatitis. The physician's orders usually include antipyretics for fever and antiemetics for nausea. Corticosteroids, although controversial, may be ordered if the patient is very ill or if fulminant hepatitis is suspected. The selection of drugs is important since hepatotoxic drugs (those that are toxic to the liver) should not be given. Suggested antiemetics are dimenhydrinate (Dramamine) and trimethobenzamide (Tigan). Phenothiazines are contraindicated. If a sedative is needed, chloral hydrate or diphenhydramine (Benadryl) is recommended.

The prescribed diet is usually high-calorie, high-carbohydrate, moderate- to high-protein, and moderate- to low-fat with supplementary vitamins. Recommended activity depends on the patient's signs and symptoms and liver function tests. Bedrest may be ordered during the icteric phase; however, practices vary.

PHARMACOLOGY CAPSULE Hepatotoxic drugs are contraindicated for the patient with hepatitis because they can cause further damage to liver cells.

Prevention

Vaccines are available to immunize people against hepatitis types A and B. At this time there is no vaccine to prevent other types of hepatitis. Immune globulin (IG) can provide temporary passive immunity and prevent hepatitis A if given within two weeks after exposure. Active disease may be averted in patients who have been exposed to HBV by administering the HBV vaccine and hepatitis B immune globulin (HBIG).

NURSING CARE *of the Patient with Hepatitis*

Assessment

Nursing assessment of the patient with liver disease was outlined in Table 37-1. When taking a health history of the person with hepatitis, be sure to include information about general health state, drug and alcohol use, chemical exposure, dietary habits, blood transfusions, recent travel, gastrointestinal disturbances, and changes in skin, urine, or stools.

Ongoing physical assessment includes vital signs, inspection of skin, weight changes, and mental status.

Nursing Diagnoses, Goals, and Outcome Criteria: Hepatitis

Nursing Diagnoses	Goals and Outcome Criteria
Activity Intolerance and **Impaired Physical Mobility** related to fatigue, impaired metabolism, prescribed bedrest	Improved activity tolerance: patient report of less fatigue with activity Absence of complications of immobility: skin intact, breath sounds clear, no calf tenderness
Imbalanced Nutrition: Less than Body Requirements related to anorexia, nausea, and vomiting	Adequate dietary intake: stable body weight
Deficient Fluid Volume related to inadequate intake, vomiting	Normal fluid status: fluid output equal to intake, vital signs consistent with patient norms, moist mucous membranes
Risk for Impaired Skin Integrity related to pruritus and scratching	Intact skin: no abrasions
Disturbed Body Image related to jaundice	Improved body image: patient expresses acceptance of skin discoloration
Anxiety related to hospitalization, unfamiliar procedures, serious illness	Decreased anxiety: patient states that anxiety is decreased or absent, calm manner.

Interventions

Activity Intolerance and Impaired Physical Mobility

When the patient is on bedrest or some other activity limitation, explain that rest allows the liver to heal by regenerating new cells to replace those damaged by hepatitis. Promote rest by planning activities to permit times when the patient is not disturbed. Offer diversions such as reading or television.

Complete bedrest is usually not necessary; however, if it is ordered, the patient is at risk for complications of immobility. Inspect the skin for early signs of pressure (redness, especially over bony prominences). If the patient is unable to turn independently, assist with turning at least every 2 hours. Moisturizing lotions protect the skin and can help relieve itching associated with jaundice.

Teach the patient to cough and deep breathe every 2 hours to reduce the risk of pneumonia. Gentle exercise of the legs promotes circulation and discourages the formation of thrombi. Discourage crossing of the legs.

Inactivity tends to lead to constipation and may cause urinary stasis. Therefore record bowel movements and urine output, and describe any abnormal characteristics of stool and urine. Care of the immobilized patient is discussed in detail in Chapter 20.

Imbalanced Nutrition: Less than Body Requirements

Good nutrition is essential to decrease demands on the liver. Specific dietary orders depend on the extent of liver dysfunction. With uncomplicated hepatitis, protein requirements range from 0.8 to 1.0 gm/kg/day. The recommended daily allowance of protein for healthy adults is 0.75 gm/kg. Fat intake may be restricted. Unfortunately, anorexia is a common symptom of hepatitis. Measures to manage anorexia include small, frequent meals, a pleasant eating environment, frequent oral hygiene, and explanations of the need for a balanced diet. Occasionally, a feeding tube is inserted to increase nutritional intake.

Nausea and vomiting also can contribute to nutritional deficits and fluid and electrolyte imbalances. Best results are usually obtained by administering antiemetics as soon as nausea is reported. A cool, damp cloth applied to the face and neck is sometimes helpful. When the patient vomits, note the amount and contents of vomitus (emesis) as well as any visible or occult blood. Measure emesis and record the volume as output. Remove soiled clothing, linens, and basins promptly and handle according to agency infection control guidelines. Nursing management of nausea and vomiting is discussed in greater detail in Chapter 36.

Deficient Fluid Volume

The patient with hepatitis needs to maintain a fluid intake of 3,000 ml/day unless contraindicated. Maintain intake and output records. Be alert for signs of fluid retention, such as edema, increasing abdominal girth, and rising blood pressure. If the patient's fluid intake is low or if vomiting is present, also monitor for dehydration. Signs of dehydration include dry mucous membranes, tachycardia, concentrated urine, and confusion. Patients who are at risk for dehydration may receive intravenous fluids as prescribed.

Risk for Impaired Skin Integrity

Pruritus, or itching, is an annoying symptom. Patients naturally respond by scratching, which may cause breaks in the skin. Nursing measures are designed to reduce dryness and irritation. Bathe the skin in cool water and then pat dry. Mild soap may be used unless it seems to increase symptoms. Lubricating lotions or topical antipruritics may be applied. Use light strokes in the direction of the heart. Select older, soft sheets. You can suggest that the patient gently pat the skin instead of scratching to reduce the itching sensation. If a patient is confused, trim the fingernails as agency policy permits. Mittens may be needed to prevent excessive scratching. If conservative measures are not effective, consult the physician about ordering an antihistamine.

Disturbed Body Image

The patient may be self-conscious about his or her appearance because of jaundice. Demonstrate acceptance of the patient and explain that the skin color usually returns to normal in 2 to 4 weeks.

Anxiety

Hospitalization and diagnostic tests and procedures can provoke anxiety in the patient with hepatitis. The patient also may be fearful about the expected course of the disease and the risk of complications. Encourage questions and find out what the patient wants to know. Explanations about what to expect reduce the fear of the unknown. Explore how patients usually deal with stress and help them to identify coping strategies.

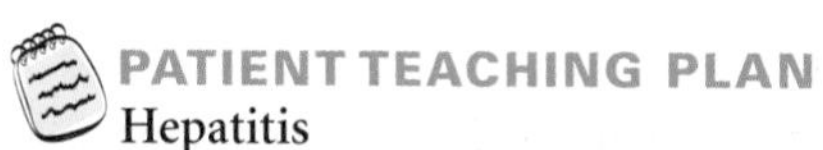

PATIENT TEACHING PLAN
Hepatitis

Take precautions to avoid exposing others to the virus. Precautions vary with the type of hepatitis, but the following guidelines are helpful:

- People who have had close contact with you should be vaccinated with immune globulin to temporarily boost the body's natural resistance to infection.
- Do not share personal items or utensils with others.
- Wash your hands thoroughly after toileting.
- If you have active hepatitis B, use condoms for sexual intercourse; your partner should be vaccinated against HBV.
- Do not expose others to your blood.

Table 37-3 summarizes precautions to be used to prevent the transmission of hepatitis.

Staff Protection

When patients are hospitalized, standard precautions are implemented. Nurses are at risk for exposure to hepatitis because they often handle body fluids. According to the Centers for Disease Control and Prevention, an estimated 15% to 25% of all health care providers contract hepatitis B. For that reason, vaccination for hepatitis B is required by the Occupational Safety and Health Administration for nurses and other health care providers. The vaccine is given in a series of three injections and confers long-term immunity on most people. Follow-up testing may be done to assess the titer level, which is a measure of immunity. If the antibody titer is inadequate, up to three booster doses may be given.

CIRRHOSIS

Pathophysiology

Cirrhosis is a chronic, progressive disease of the liver. It is characterized by degeneration and destruction of liver cells. Fibrotic bands of connective tissue impair the flow of blood and lymph and distort the normal liver structure.

As cirrhosis progresses, there is significant disruption of many physiologic processes. The effects of liver disease include metabolic disturbances, blood abnormalities, fluid and electrolyte imbalances, decreased resistance to infection, accumulation of drugs and toxins, and obstruction of blood vessels and bile ducts in the liver.

Incidence

The highest incidence of cirrhosis is in people between the ages of 40 and 60. It is the fifth leading cause of death in people in that age range in the United States. It is more common in men than in women. The pathology is most often related to alcoholic liver disease or chronic viral infection.

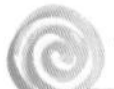

What Does Culture Have to do with Cirrhosis?

Hispanics have the highest rate of deaths from cirrhosis of the liver, followed by African Americans and whites.

Types of Cirrhosis

There are four major types of cirrhosis, classified on the basis of cause: alcoholic cirrhosis, postnecrotic, biliary, and cardiac cirrhosis. Several other types occur infrequently.

Alcoholic Cirrhosis

Alcoholic liver disease progresses in three stages: hepatic steatosis, fatty liver, and cirrhosis. This type of cirrhosis was formerly called Laennec's cirrhosis and is caused by exposure to alcohol. The liver enlarges, becomes "knobby," and then shrinks. Fatty liver is reversible if alcohol intake ceases. Alcoholic cirrhosis is not reversible.

Postnecrotic Cirrhosis

Postnecrotic cirrhosis can be a complication of hepatitis in which there is massive liver cell necrosis.

Biliary Cirrhosis

Biliary cirrhosis is also called obstructive or idiopathic cirrhosis. As the name suggests, it develops as a result of obstruction to bile flow.

Cardiac Cirrhosis

Cardiac cirrhosis follows severe right-sided heart failure. Venous congestion and hypoxia lead to necrosis of liver cells.

Signs and Symptoms

In the early stage, signs and symptoms of cirrhosis are usually subtle. The patient may report slight weight loss, unexplained fever, fatigue, and dull heaviness in the right upper abdomen. These symptoms are probably due to inflammation and enlargement of the liver. The liver may be palpable below the right rib margin.

As the disease progresses, impaired metabolism of carbohydrates, fats, and proteins causes gastrointestinal disturbances such as anorexia, nausea, vomiting, diarrhea or constipation, flatulence, and dyspepsia (heartburn). Resistance to blood flow from the intestines to the liver causes circulation to become congested in the intestines, stomach, and esophagus. Elevated pressure in veins in the gastrointestinal tract causes them to dilate and bulge. Dilated veins in the esophagus are called esophageal varices, and those in the rectum are hemorrhoids. Prominent veins may be visible on the abdomen.

Anemia, leukocytopenia, thrombocytopenia, and prothrombin deficiency are hematologic disorders associated with cirrhosis. As a result, patients tend to tire quickly and are more susceptible to infections. They bruise easily and may bleed excessively from minor trauma. Epistaxis (nosebleed) is common.

Later signs and symptoms of cirrhosis reflect the liver's inability to perform normal functions. Jaundice develops owing to elevated serum bilirubin levels. Two factors contribute to jaundice in the patient with cirrhosis. First, diseased liver cells may be unable to conjugate and excrete bilirubin. Second, structural changes in the liver prevent the normal flow of bile out of the liver. Another effect of impaired bilirubin excretion, as previously mentioned, is the deposition of bile salts under the skin that can cause intense pruritus.

The diseased liver is unable to metabolize estrogen, testosterone, aldosterone, and adrenocortical hormones. The patient, therefore, exhibits signs and symptoms of hormone excesses. Testicular atrophy, impotence, and gynecomastia (breast enlargement) may be noted in men, and amenorrhea may be noted in women. Redness of the palms of the hands, called palmar erythema, and spider angiomas also are attributed to hormone excess. Excess aldosterone contributes to sodium and water retention. The failing liver is also unable to metabolize ammonia, a product of protein metabolism. Excess ammonia affects the central nervous system, leading to confusion and decreasing consciousness.

Cirrhosis impairs the liver's ability to manufacture albumin. Albumin plays a critical role in creating the colloid osmotic pressure that retains water in the vascular compartment. With low serum albumin levels, water leaks from the capillaries, causing decreased blood volume and edema. Ascites is the accumulation of fluid in the peritoneal cavity.

Peripheral neuropathy, characterized by tingling or numbness in the extremities, is common with cirrhosis. This is thought to be caused by dietary deficiencies of vitamin B_{12}, thiamine, and folic acid.

Figure 37-5 illustrates the clinical picture of the patient with liver disease.

Complications

The patient with cirrhosis is at risk for many complications, including portal hypertension, esophageal varices, ascites, hepatic encephalopathy, and hepatorenal syndrome.

Portal Hypertension

The portal vein delivers blood from the intestines to the liver. Changes in the liver with cirrhosis obstruct the flow of incoming blood, causing blood to back up in the portal system. High portal pressure, or portal hypertension, causes collateral vessels to develop. Collateral vessels commonly form in the esophagus, the anterior abdominal wall, and the rectum.

Esophageal Varices

Distended, engorged vessels in the esophagus are called esophageal varices. They are fragile and bleed easily, with the potential for fatal hemorrhage. Circumstances that may trigger bleeding include irritation and increased intra-abdominal pressure. Sources of irritation are alcohol, coarse foods, and stomach acid. Intra-abdominal pressure is increased by vomiting, coughing, heavy lifting, and straining at stool.

Ascites

Ascites is an accumulation of fluid in the peritoneal cavity. Factors that contribute to the development of ascites with cirrhosis include portal hypertension, leaking of lymph fluid and albumin-rich fluid from the diseased liver, low serum albumin levels, increased aldosterone levels, and water retention.

Hepatic Encephalopathy

The failing liver is unable to detoxify ammonia, a breakdown product of protein metabolism. Excessive ammonia in the blood causes neurologic symptoms, including cognitive disturbances, declining level of consciousness, and changes in neuromuscular function. If the condition is not reversed, the patient lapses into unconsciousness, referred to as hepatic coma.

Factors that may precipitate hepatic encephalopathy are infection, fluid and potassium depletion, gastrointestinal bleeding, constipation, and some drugs.

Hepatorenal Syndrome

Hepatorenal syndrome is renal failure in the cirrhosis patient that often follows diuretic therapy, paracentesis, or gastrointestinal hemorrhage. The kidney structure appears unchanged, so the reason for failure is not known.

Medical Diagnosis

When the patient's history and physical examination suggest cirrhosis, tests and procedures may be ordered to confirm or rule out the disease. These studies include blood tests, liver biopsy, liver scan, ultrasonography, computed tomography, and magnetic resonance imaging. Results of blood tests that are consistent with cirrhosis include elevated serum and urine bilirubin, elevated serum enzymes, decreased total serum protein, decreased cholesterol, and prolonged prothrombin time. The complete blood cell count may reveal deficiencies of red and white blood cells and platelets.

The liver biopsy is performed to obtain a tissue specimen for microscopic study. Typical cellular changes occur with cirrhosis. Imaging procedures outline the liver features.

Table 37-2 summarizes tests and procedures used to diagnose liver disorders.

Medical Treatment

The goals of medical treatment for cirrhosis are to limit deterioration of liver function and to prevent complications, but there is no specific medical treatment. The approach is to promote rest so that the liver can regenerate. The earlier the condition is diagnosed and measures are taken to promote healing, the better is the chance of recovery.

Bedrest is usually ordered if the patient is in liver failure. Malnutrition is common, and the specific diet depends on individual patient factors. A diet high in carbohydrates and vitamins with moderate to high protein intake is typically ordered unless the patient's blood ammonia level is elevated. In that case, protein is restricted until the ammonia level falls. Supplementary iron and vitamins also may be ordered. The amount of fat allowed in the diet varies with the patient's condition. Anorexia is frequently a problem with cirrhosis, so small semisolid or liquid meals may be better received. Enteral feedings may be needed to provide adequate nutrients.

Other medical treatments may be ordered to correct the complications of cirrhosis. Intravenous fluids may be needed to correct fluid and electrolyte imbalances. Anemia may require blood transfusions. Water and sodium are likely to be restricted in patients with severe fluid retention.

Ascites

The medical management of ascites aims to promote reabsorption and elimination of the fluid by means of sodium restriction and diuretics. Combinations of various types of diuretics may yield better results than a single diuretic. Salt-poor albumin may be given intravenously to help maintain blood volume and to increase urinary output. Albumin raises the serum colloid osmotic pressure, causing water to be drawn back into the bloodstream. Table 37-4 lists drugs used to treat the patient with ascites.

If ascites does not respond to conservative treatment, fluid can be removed with a needle, a procedure called paracentesis. An alternative is the placement of a peritoneal-venous shunt.

Paracentesis. Paracentesis is the removal of ascitic fluid from the peritoneal cavity. A special instrument called a trocar is inserted through the abdominal wall, and a catheter is placed to allow the fluid to drain. This procedure is indicated only when ascites interferes with the patient's breathing. It is not used frequently because it removes essential protein and electrolytes. In addition, it provides a potential portal of entry for pathogens.

If paracentesis is done to remove ascites, your role is to prepare the patient, assist and support the patient during the procedure, and provide aftercare. The physician should explain what will be done and obtain patient consent. Reinforce explanations and obtain the written consent as agency policy permits. Obtain baseline vital signs, weight, and abdominal girth. Instruct the patient to void.

The procedure is often done at the bedside with the patient in a sitting position. During paracentesis, you should support and encourage the patient. The physician may request monitoring of vital signs during the process. Usually, 2 to 3 L of fluid is removed slowly. Rapid removal of ascitic fluid could result in circulatory collapse. After paracentesis, a sterile dressing is applied to the puncture site. Monitor vital signs every 15 minutes until the patient is stable, and check the dressing for bleeding. Measure the fluid obtained and send a specimen for laboratory analysis. Document the procedure, including the amount and color of the fluid. Monitor for blood in the urine.

Peritoneal-venous shunts. Peritoneal-venous shunts may be implanted permanently to allow ascitic fluid to drain from the abdomen and return to the bloodstream. Advantages to shunting ascitic fluid rather than removing it are 1) protein-rich serum is retained and returned to the vascular compartment; and 2) urine output increases which eliminates excess sodium and water.

The LeVeen peritoneal-venous shunt (Fig. 37-6) is a tube that is placed in the abdomen, running from the peritoneal cavity to the jugular vein or superior vena cava. The tube has a one-way valve that permits excess fluid to drain into the venous circulation when pressure rises in the abdomen. When the patient inspires, intra-abdominal pressure rises, causing the valve to open. The Denver peritoneal-venous shunt involves a manual pump placed under the skin. It can be compressed to cause fluid to flow from the peritoneum to the venous system.

Potential complications of peritoneal-venous shunts are peritonitis, tubing obstruction, circulatory overload, and embolism.

Bleeding Esophageal Varices

Several techniques can be used to control bleeding esophageal varices. These include drug therapy, placement of

table 37-4 **DRUG THERAPY | *Cirrhosis***

GENERAL NURSING IMPLICATIONS

1. No drug can cure cirrhosis.
2. Drug therapy treats symptoms: fluid retention, portal hypertension, encephalopathy, and bleeding.
3. Patients with liver dysfunction may not metabolize drugs normally, so be alert for adverse effects.

DRUG	USE/ACTION	SIDE EFFECTS	NURSING INTERVENTIONS
DIURETICS Spironolactone (Aldactone) Amiloride (Midamor) Furosemide (Lasix) Chlorothiazide (Diuril)	Promote excretion of excess fluid in edema and ascites.	Fluid and electrolyte imbalances, including fluid volume deficit and hyponatremia. Hypokalemia can occur except with potassium-sparing diuretics like spironolactone.	Monitor intake and output, abdominal girth. Check laboratory values for electrolyte imbalances.
PITUITARY HORMONE Vasopressin (Pitressin)	Reduces pressure in portal veins to treat bleeding esophageal varices.	Tissue necrosis with extravasation. Water intoxication, hyponatremia, intestinal and uterine cramping.	Inspect infusion site hourly for blanching; if present, stop infusion and notify charge nurse or physician.
VASODILATORS	Given with vasopressin to decrease side effects.		Follow directions for administration carefully. Monitor vital signs continuously.
Nitroglycerin	Lowers blood pressure.	Tachycardia, hypotension, flushing, and headache.	Dosing titrated based on response.
Nitroprusside (Nipride)	Lowers blood pressure.	Tachycardia, hypotension, acidosis, and fluid retention.	Nitroprusside must be diluted.
BETA-ADRENERGIC BLOCKER Propranolol (Inderal)	Reduces pressure in portal veins to reduce risk of bleeding.	Bradycardia, hypotension, bronchoconstriction. Masks signs of hypoglycemia.	Monitor pulse; if below 60, withhold and notify physician. Monitor blood glucose in people with diabetes.
ANTIBIOTIC Neomycin sulfate	Reduces gastrointestinal bacterial flora, decreasing ammonia production. Used to prevent or treat hepatic encephalopathy.	Toxic to kidney and eighth cranial nerve (hearing and balance). Increases action of neuromuscular blocking agents like anesthetics.	Monitor intake and output. Assess for hearing impairment, tinnitus (ringing in ears), nausea, loss of balance.
LAXATIVE Lactulose (Cephulac)	Promotes elimination of ammonia in feces. Used to prevent or treat hepatic encephalopathy.	Cramps, distention, flatulence, eructation. Hyperglycemia with diabetes.	May be ordered every hour at first. Can be mixed with fruit juice, water, or milk. Monitor diabetics.
DOPAMINERGIC AGENTS Levodopa	Replaces dopamine lost in process of protein breakdown. Used to prevent or treat hepatic encephalopathy.	Nausea, vomiting, orthostatic hypotension.	Teach patient to manage orthostatic hypotension. Provide comfort measures for nausea. Report vomiting. Give antiemetics as ordered.
VITAMINS B complex	Needed for production of red blood cells and for normal growth and development.	Allergic reaction to thiamine (anaphylaxis). Adverse effects rare.	Intradermal test dose may be ordered to detect sensitivity to thiamine. Check site for reaction: redness, swelling. Check reference for incompatibility with other intravenous drugs.
K Menadiol (vitamin K_3) Phytonadione (Aqua-MEPHYTON)	Treats serious bleeding disorders caused by deficiency of prothrombin. Used cautiously with severe liver disease.	Gastric upset (oral route only), rash, urticaria, flushing, hemolytic anemia. Pain and swelling at injection site.	Check lab results for prothrombin time. Report abnormalities. Monitor complete blood cell count. Assess for bleeding. Apply pressure to needle puncture sites for 5 min.

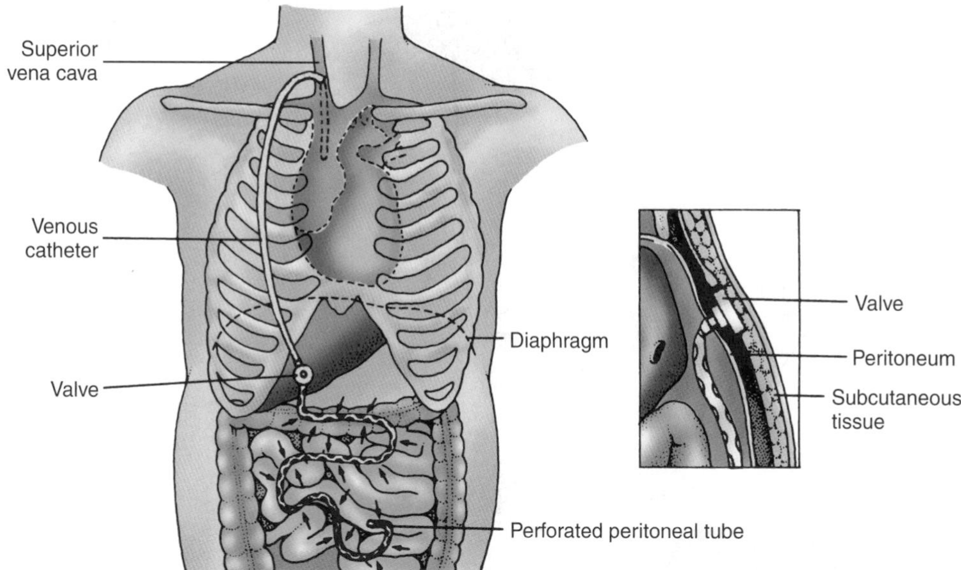

FIGURE **37-6** A peritoneal-venous shunt drains ascitic fluid from the abdominal cavity into the superior vena cava.

an esophageal-gastric balloon tube, surgical ligation, and sclerotherapy.

Acute bleeding episodes may be treated with intravenous vasopressin, which constricts blood vessels and lowers pressure in the hepatic circulation. Nitroglycerin also may be administered to reduce the systemic side effects of vasopressin (hypertension, decreased coronary blood flow). In addition to blood transfusions, vitamin K and H_2 receptor blockers such as ranitidine (Zantac) may be ordered. Neomycin may be administered to prevent the breakdown of blood in the intestines that would release ammonia, contributing to hepatic encephalopathy. Beta-adrenergic blockers may be used to reduce blood pressure in the long-term management of patients following acute bleeding episodes.

Esophageal-gastric balloon tube. Esophageal-gastric balloon tubes may be used to apply direct pressure to bleeding veins in the esophagus and stomach. Examples of tubes used for this purpose are the Sengstaken-Blakemore esophageal-gastric balloon tube and the Minnesota tube. The Sengstaken-Blakemore tube has three ports. One is used to inflate the esophageal balloon, another to inflate the gastric balloon, and the third to suction the stomach. A second nasogastric tube may be inserted with the Sengstaken-Blakemore tube to collect secretions above the esophageal balloon. The Minnesota tube has four lumina that permit inflation of gastric and esophageal balloons and suctioning of both the esophagus and the stomach (Fig. 37-7).

The tube is inserted by a physician. The gastric balloon is inflated first and gently pulled upward to apply pressure to veins in the upper part of the stomach. The esophageal balloon is then inflated. The gastric suction tube is connected to continuous suction. It also may be irrigated to remove clots and maintain patency of the tube. It is important to remove old blood from the stomach so that it will not be digested. Digested blood produces ammonia, which increases the likelihood of hepatic encephalopathy. Gastric suction also reduces the risk of vomiting, which would force the balloons out of place. The tube usually is left inflated for 24 to 48 hours. It then is deflated but left in place so that it can be reinflated if needed.

Surgical treatment of bleeding varices. In an emergency situation, the surgeon may ligate (tie off) bleeding varices directly through an endoscope. The patient can then be stabilized prior to a more extensive corrective procedure. Corrective procedures surgically shunt blood from engorged varices to other veins. A portacaval shunt diverts blood to the vena cava, whereas a splenorenal shunt routes the blood to the splenic vein. The incidence of hepatic encephalopathy is lower with the splenorenal shunt than with the portacaval shunt. A third type of shunt that is placed under fluoroscopy is the transjugular intrahepatic portosystemic shunt. A stent is passed into the right internal jugular vein, through the right atrium and into the vena cava and inserted between the hepatic and portal veins. By shunting the blood in this manner, pressure in the portal venous system and the esophageal varices is reduced.

Sclerotherapy. Sclerotherapy is a procedure in which a solution is injected into the varices or into the veins that supply them, causing the varices to harden and close (Fig. 37-8). The procedure can be done through an endoscope or through a small surgical incision. Sclerotherapy can be done to prevent or to treat bleeding.

After sclerotherapy, patients often report chest discomfort for several days. The physician usually orders a mild analgesic. If it does not relieve the pain, the physician should be notified because persistent pain may indicate perforation of the esophagus. Once a patient has had sclerotherapy, extra care must be taken in the insertion of nasogastric tubes.

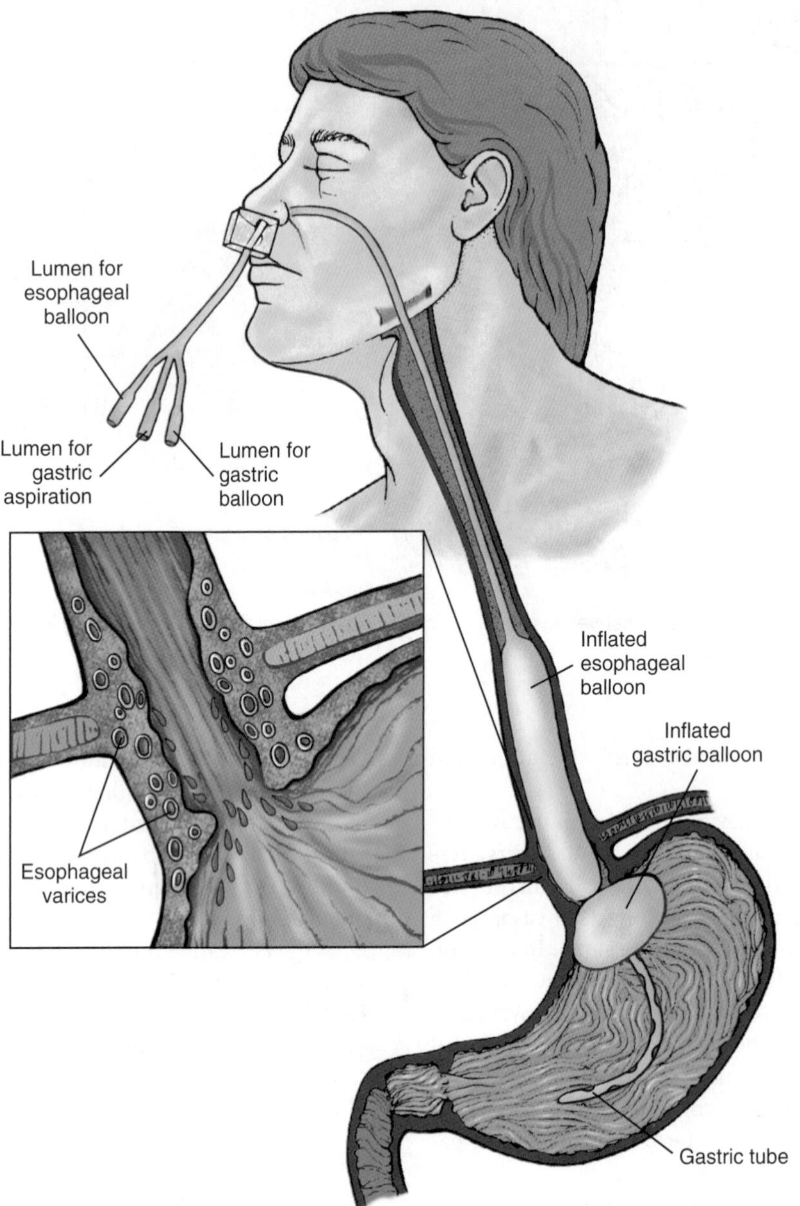

FIGURE **37-7** Sengstaken-Blakemore tube in place to compress bleeding esophageal varices.

Hepatic Encephalopathy

Medical treatment of hepatic encephalopathy is directed toward reducing ammonia formation. This goal is achieved mainly with drug therapy and reduction of protein intake. Lactulose is a cathartic that decreases the absorption of ammonia from the GI tract. Neomycin is an antibiotic that reduces the number of bacteria in the bowel, thereby decreasing ammonia production. However, neomycin is nephrotoxic and can cause superinfections. The use of zinc supplements to reduce ammonia in the blood is under study.

If the patient has been bleeding into the gastrointestinal tract, laxatives and enemas may be ordered to remove old blood and protein. Patients with recurring hepatic encephalopathy may be candidates for liver transplantation. Severe protein restriction should be used only short-term to avoid malnutrition and to provide nutrients for the liver to regenerate.

Hepatorenal Syndrome

Hepatorenal syndrome may be treated with salt-poor albumin, diuretics, and sodium and water restriction. Patients should not receive nephrotoxic drugs like NSAIDs. The prognosis is very poor, however, and liver transplantation may be the only solution.

Drug Therapy

A variety of drugs may be used to treat the effects of cirrhosis. These drugs and nursing implications are summarized in Table 37-4.

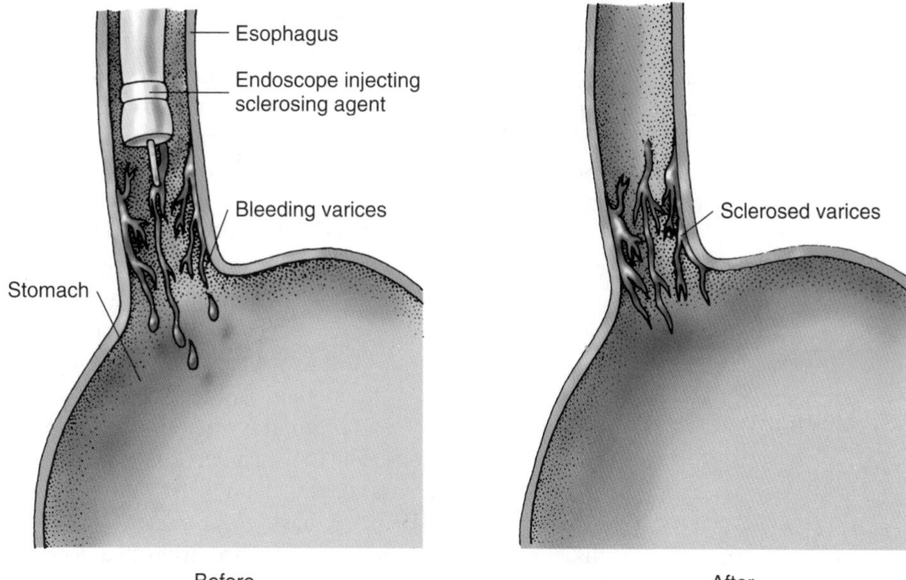

FIGURE 37-8 Injection sclerotherapy.

NURSING CARE *of the Patient with Cirrhosis*

Assessment

Ongoing assessments of the cirrhosis patient should include daily measurement of weight, measurements of intake and output, and measurement of abdominal girth. Patients are monitored for signs and symptoms of complications—bleeding, ascites, encephalopathy, and renal failure.

Nursing Diagnoses, Goals, and Outcome Criteria: Cirrhosis

Nursing Diagnoses	Goals and Outcome Criteria
Imbalanced Nutrition: Less than Body Requirements related to anorexia, metabolic imbalances	Adequate nutrition: stable body weight, consumes meals
Activity Intolerance related to fatigue	Improved activity tolerance: performs activities of daily living without excessive fatigue
Risk for Impaired Skin Integrity related to edema, immobility, pruritus, hypoproteinemia	Intact skin: no redness or breaks in skin. No scratching
Ineffective Breathing Patterns related to ascites	Effective breathing: respiratory rate of 12-20 per minute without dyspnea
Risk for Injury related to impaired coagulation	Absence of bleeding: no blood in emesis or stool, vital signs consistent with patient norms
Disturbed Thought Processes related to elevated blood ammonia	Normal cognitive function: mentally alert, oriented
Deficient Fluid Volume (hypovolemia) and **Excess Fluid Volume** (in third space) related to hypoproteinemia, increased aldosterone	Normal fluid distribution in body fluid compartments: balanced fluid intake and output without edema or ascites; pulse and blood pressure consistent with patient norms
Risk for Infection related to liver dysfunction, impaired response to infection, malnutrition	Absence of infection: oral temperature less than 100° F
Fear related to dyspnea, life-threatening illness	Reduced fear: patient states no or less fear, calm manner

Interventions

Imbalanced Nutrition: Less Than Body Requirements

Good nutrition is essential for regeneration of liver tissue. However, it is a challenge for the cirrhosis patient, who often has anorexia, indigestion, nausea, and vomiting. Furthermore, the diet may be made less palatable by protein or salt restriction.

Explain the need for adequate food intake to the patient and encourage the patient to eat even when he or she is not hungry. Small, frequent meals may be more acceptable to the anorexic patient. Arrange a dietary consult for the patient to report likes and dislikes.

Make mealtimes as pleasant as possible. Put bedpans, emesis basins, and drainage collection devices out of sight. Ventilate the room to reduce odors. Do not schedule tiring activities immediately before meals. Record daily weights as ordered to assess both nutritional and fluid status.

Activity Intolerance

Some activity limitations are usually imposed, depending on the patient's overall status. Schedule nursing care to allow some periods of undisturbed rest. The patient can generally assume any position that is comfortable. If ascites is present, elevate the head of the bed to facilitate breathing. Some patients are more comfortable sitting in a chair with the feet elevated.

If the patient spends all or most of the day in bed, there is a risk of complications related to immobility. Assist the patient to change positions, deep breathe, and exercise extremities regularly.

Risk for Impaired Skin Integrity

The patient with cirrhosis is at risk for skin breakdown for several reasons. Bile salts that are normally processed by the liver may be deposited under the skin, causing intense pruritus. Loss of muscle and fat tissue with advanced disease reduces the padding that normally protects the skin from pressure. Also, many patients have edema, which makes tissue more fragile and impairs healing.

Nursing measures to relieve the itching of pruritus include gentle bathing with mild soap and warm water, thorough rinsing, and application of moisturizing lotions. The patient's nails should be kept short to reduce trauma from scratching. If scratching persists, put soft cotton mittens or gloves on the patient's hands. If itching is severe, consult the physician about ordering a medication to relieve the discomfort. Cholestyramine (Questran) may be ordered to increase the excretion of bile salts.

Ineffective Breathing Patterns

Ascitic fluid can cause the abdomen to become greatly distended. While in bed, the patient breathes easier with the head of the bed elevated. Sitting in a chair with the feet elevated, if allowed, may be even more comfortable.

Risk for Injury

The patient with cirrhosis is at great risk for injury or hemorrhage due to impaired coagulation and fragile varices. Handle the patient gently to avoid trauma. Use a soft toothbrush or swab for mouth care. Apply firm pressure to injection sites to minimize oozing. Pad side rails if the patient is restless.

If the patient has bleeding esophageal varices, an esophageal-gastric balloon tube may be inserted. The patient with this type of tube is usually in an intensive care unit since close monitoring is necessary. The tube is uncomfortable, and the patient is likely to be frightened about both the bleeding and the treatment. When the tube is in place, monitor the patient for signs of continued or renewed bleeding, including restlessness, increasing pulse and respirations, and falling blood pressure. Note stool characteristics. Bleeding from the esophagus or stomach usually produces a sticky (tarry), maroon to black stool. Examine aspirated stomach and esophageal contents for evidence of fresh bleeding. Old blood in the stomach is usually brownish and may be described as resembling coffee grounds. Fresh blood is bright to dark red.

Because the esophagus and the trachea are adjacent to each other, upward movement of the esophageal balloon can cause airway obstruction. Therefore when the balloon tube is in place, monitor the patient for sudden respiratory distress. Should this occur, both balloon ports must be promptly cut and the tubes removed by a properly trained person.

Disturbed Thought Processes

Cognitive changes in the patient with cirrhosis are usually due to hepatic encephalopathy. Nursing care of the patient with hepatic encephalopathy includes monitoring of mental and neurologic status. Inform the physician of changes in status. The patient who is confused or unconscious requires close attention to prevent injury or complications of immobility. Talk to the patient to provide basic information and reassurance. The family also may need an explanation of the patient's behavior. Enforce dietary protein restrictions, and administer prescribed drugs that decrease bacteria in the intestines (for example, lactulose or neomycin). Be alert for adverse effects of drug therapy, which may include diarrhea, vitamin K deficiency, and ototoxicity.

Deficient or Excess Fluid Volume

Fluid needs vary with the patient's condition. Sodium and water are likely to be restricted if there is marked edema or ascites. Despite the excess in total body water, the patient's blood volume may be dangerously low. Adequate water is present, it is just not distributed appropriately. Without adequate albumin in the serum, colloid osmotic pressure falls and water shifts out of the capillaries into the tissues. Administer intravenous fluids and salt-poor albumin as ordered. In addition to monitoring vital signs, evaluate fluid intake and output.

Risk for Infection

The patient with cirrhosis is at risk for infection, for several reasons. The liver is no longer able to filter bacteria from the blood as it comes from the intestines. The function of the spleen also is impaired, which lowers resistance to infection. In addition, these patients tend to be malnourished, so they lack the building materials for tissue repair. Monitor for fever and malaise, which suggest infection. Protect the patient from others with infections. Practice good hand washing and use aseptic technique for invasive procedures.

Fear

Patients with cirrhosis can experience frightening complications, including confusion, dyspnea, and hemorrhage. With advanced cirrhosis, the prognosis is poor, and patients often have repeated emergency admissions. Treatments and diagnostic procedures may be painful and anxiety-producing. The nurse can help by recognizing the patient's fear and acknowledging it.

To provide emotional support to cirrhosis patients, you must be aware of your personal reaction to these patients. There is a stigma attached to cirrhosis because it is often associated with alcohol abuse. Health care providers must treat patients in a nonjudgmental manner. Nurses must realize that alcoholism is a complex chronic disease that is not easily controlled and that cirrhosis can be caused by factors other than alcohol.

Information can help to reduce fear. When the patient is acutely ill, give simple explanations and answer questions. When the patient improves, explore what he or she knows about cirrhosis and determine what additional information is needed. General teaching points are noted here.

PATIENT TEACHING PLAN
Cirrhosis

- A balanced diet will help prevent additional injury to the liver and reduce the risk of complications.
- Avoid specific foods (as advised by the physician and/or dietitian).
- Notify your physician if you have increasing fluid retention, black tarry stools, bloody vomitus, increasing fatigue, or confusion.
- Alcohol is discouraged because of the toxic effects on the liver. Community resources you can use for information and assistance include Alcoholics Anonymous (if appropriate), the American Liver Foundation, and home health nursing services.
- Do not take medications except as approved by your physician. Many drugs, including acetaminophen, can be toxic to the liver.

*Put on your **THINKING CAP!!***

Identify three functions of the healthy liver. Describe how cirrhosis affects those functions. State one nursing implication related to the change with cirrhosis in each function.

CANCER OF THE LIVER

Cancer rarely begins in the liver, but the liver is a frequent site of metastasis. Cirrhosis is a predisposing factor for liver cancer. Signs and symptoms of liver cancer include liver enlargement, weight loss, anorexia, nausea, vomiting, and dull pain in the upper right quadrant of the abdomen. As the disease progresses, the signs and symptoms are essentially the same as those of cirrhosis. Because the early signs and symptoms of liver cancer are vague, the condition is often not diagnosed until it is advanced.

Tests and procedures used to diagnose liver cancer are liver scan and biopsy, hepatic arteriography, endoscopy, and measurement of alpha-fetoprotein levels. If the cancer is confined to one area, a lobectomy may be done; otherwise chemotherapy is the primary treatment. Chemotherapy is generally considered to be palliative, meaning that it may slow the progress of the cancer and increase patient comfort but is unlikely to be curative. In some cases, radiotherapy is prescribed. Transplantation is not generally considered an option with widespread liver cancer.

During the course of the illness, the patient's needs are much like those of the cirrhosis patient, which were covered earlier in this chapter. Additional aspects of nursing care of the patient with cancer are discussed in Chapter 24.

LIVER TRANSPLANTATION

The only possible cure for end-stage liver disease is liver transplantation. Transplantation is also appropriate for patients with cancer that is confined to the liver and for patients with certain congenital disorders.

Patients who are recommended for transplantation are ranked by acuity and need and entered into a national computer network. When a liver becomes available by donation, the best recipient can be identified. Patients awaiting transplantation must be on standby status in case a donor is located. This is a time of alternating hope and fear for patients and families, marked by the recognition that they are waiting for someone else to die.

Following liver transplantation, the patient is cared for in a specialized unit. A transplant patient often has a T-tube, wound drainage devices, a nasogastric tube, and a central line for total parenteral nutrition (TPN). Mechanical ventilation also is used initially.

Nursing assessments focus on neurologic status, vital signs, central venous pressure, respiratory status, and indicators of bleeding. If stable, the patient is moved out of the unit after 3 or 4 days. Continue to monitor vital signs, intake and output, and neurologic status. Provide usual postoperative care, including assistance with turning, coughing and deep breathing, and progressive activity.

Lifelong drug therapy is needed to prevent rejection of the donor liver. Some of the current options include cyclosporine, tacrolimus, and azathioprine and prednisone. All have significant adverse effects. Prednisone usually is given in combination with another drug and can often be discontinued within a year. A monoclonal antibody, OKT3, is a newer agent that may prove to be highly effective and less toxic than other antirejection drugs.

The transplant recipient must be monitored for signs of rejection. These signs include fever, anorexia, depression, vague abdominal pain, muscle aches, and joint pain. Fever is sometimes the *only* sign of rejection. Rejection may be treated with corticosteroids or other immunosuppressants. If this treatment is unsuccessful, retransplantation may be needed.

Before discharge, the patient should know signs and symptoms of transplant rejection and infection, wound care, dietary restrictions (usually sodium restriction), and self-medication.

PHARMACOLOGY CAPSULE Drugs that suppress rejection of transplanted organs reduce the patient's ability to resist infection.

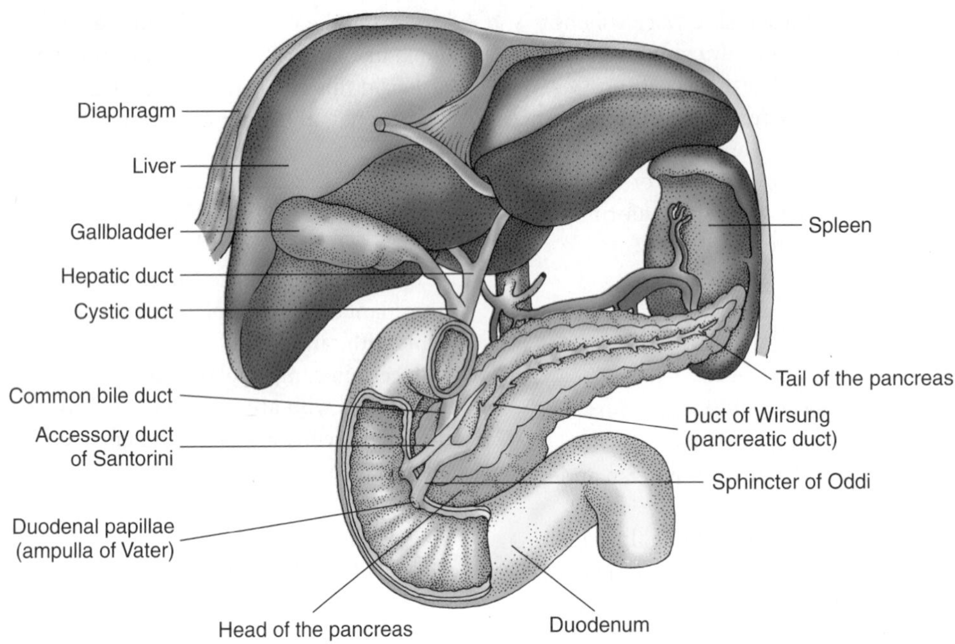

FIGURE **37-9** Anatomy of the liver, gallbladder, and pancreas.

THE BILIARY TRACT

ANATOMY AND PHYSIOLOGY OF THE BILIARY TRACT

Bile is a yellow-green liquid that has several important functions. It contains bile salts, which are essential for the emulsification and digestion of fats. It also provides a medium for the excretion of bilirubin from the liver.

The biliary tract is made up of the gallbladder and the bile ducts. The function of the biliary tract is to deliver bile from the liver to the duodenum. Bile is produced in the liver and channeled into the common hepatic duct. The common hepatic duct joins the cystic duct to form the common bile duct. The cystic duct leads to the gallbladder, a sac-like organ located beneath the liver. Bile flows from the liver to the gallbladder, where it is stored and concentrated (Fig. 37-9).

When fats enter the duodenum, the gallbladder contracts and delivers bile to the intestine through the common bile duct.

table 37-5 **ASSESSMENT *of the Patient with Gallbladder Disease***

HEALTH HISTORY

Present Illness: Digestive disturbances; pain: location, onset, intensity, duration, relationship to meals, aggravating and relieving factors
Past Medical History: Gallbladder disease, pregnancy, surgery, recent and current medications
Family History: Gallbladder disease
Review of Systems: Pruritus, indigestion, fat intolerance, dyspepsia, nausea, vomiting, light-colored stools, dark urine

PHYSICAL EXAMINATION

Vital Signs: Tachycardia, tachypnea, fever
Skin: Dryness, jaundice
Abdomen: Guarding, distention

NURSING ASSESSMENT OF THE BILIARY TRACT

The nursing assessment of the gastrointestinal system was outlined in Table 36-2 of the previous chapter. Data especially important in a patient with known or suspected gallbladder dysfunction are identified here.

HEALTH HISTORY

Common reasons for seeking medical care for biliary problems are digestive disturbances and pain. Obtain a complete description of these symptoms. Note factors that seem to bring on or relieve the symptoms. The relationship between symptoms and meals may be significant. Record the use of estrogen or oral contraceptives. Inquire about factors known to be associated with gallbladder disease: family history, obesity, Native American ancestry, and inactivity. In the review of systems, ask whether the patient has had dry skin, indigestion, fat intolerance, dyspepsia, nausea, vomiting, light-colored stools, or dark urine.

PHYSICAL EXAMINATION

When a patient has gallbladder disease, significant findings on the physical examination include dry skin, fever, jaundice, tachycardia, tachypnea, and abdominal guarding and distention. Assessment of the patient with a biliary tract disorder is summarized in Table 37-5.

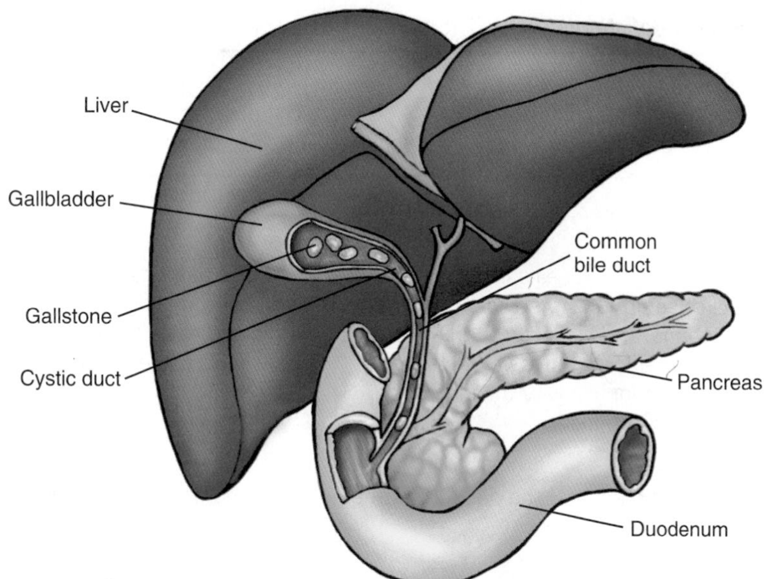

FIGURE **37-10** Gallstones within the gallbladder that could obstruct the common bile duct and the cystic duct.

DIAGNOSTIC TESTS AND PROCEDURES

Tests and procedures used to diagnose gallbladder disorders are ultrasonography, oral cholecystography, intravenous cholangiography, T-tube cholangiography, endoscopic retrograde cholangiopancreatography (ERCP), and percutaneous transhepatic cholangiography. Laboratory studies include liver function tests, serum and urine bilirubin measurements, and a complete blood cell count. Table 37-2 describes common diagnostic tests and nursing implications.

DISORDERS OF THE GALLBLADDER

Gallbladder disease is one of the most common health problems in the United States. The two most common gallbladder disorders are **cholecystitis** and cholelithiasis. Carcinoma of the gallbladder occurs but is unusual.

Risk factors for gallbladder disease include obesity, familial tendency, a sedentary lifestyle, and the use of estrogen or oral contraceptives. Women are at greater risk than men, especially women who have had multiple pregnancies. The "5 F's" are sometimes used to describe those at greatest risk for gallbladder disease: female, fat, fair, forty, and fertile.

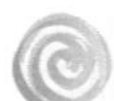

What Does Culture Have to do with Gallbladder Disease?

Native Americans and whites are at increased risk for gallbladder disease.

CHOLECYSTITIS AND CHOLELITHIASIS

Cholecystitis is inflammation of the gallbladder. It most often is caused by the presence of gallstones but can be due to bacteria, toxic chemicals, tumors, anesthesia, starvation, and opioids. The inflamed gallbladder and cystic duct become swollen and congested with blood. The cystic duct may actually become occluded.

When gallstones are present, the patient is said to have *cholelithiasis.* Most gallstones are composed of cholesterol mixed with bile salts, bilirubin, calcium, and protein. It is not known exactly why gallstones form, but the process is associated with high concentrations of cholesterol. The concentration of cholesterol rises when there is stasis of bile (as occurs with pregnancy, immobility, and inflammation of the biliary tract).

Gallstones may be found anywhere in the biliary tract: the gallbladder, the cystic duct, or the common bile duct (Fig. 37-10). The stones may move through the biliary tract with bile flow. If a stone cannot pass through the tract, it lodges and causes an obstruction. Ducts respond to obstruction with spasms in an effort to move the stone. This is responsible for an intense spasmodic pain, called biliary colic.

If the cystic duct is obstructed, bile cannot leave the gallbladder, and inflammation develops. Cystic duct obstruction does not prevent the flow of bile into the duodenum from the liver. However, if the common bile duct is obstructed ***(choledocholithiasis),*** bile is unable to flow into the duodenum.

Signs and Symptoms

Signs and symptoms of cholecystitis vary from one patient to the next. Some have only mild indigestion, whereas others have severe pain, fever, and jaundice. Other symptoms are nausea, **eructation** (belching), fever, chills, and right upper quadrant pain that radiates to the shoulder. Symptoms typically occur about 3 hours after a meal, especially if the food had high fat content.

When bile flow is obstructed, bile production in the liver decreases and the serum bilirubin rises, leading to obstructive

table 37-6 ***Drugs Used to Dissolve Gallstones***

GENRAL NURSING IMPLICATIONS

1. Drugs are effective only against small cholesterol stones.
2. Drug therapy is successful in only about one third to one half of patients treated.

DRUG	SIDE EFFECTS	NURSING INTERVENTIONS
ORAL BILE SALTS		
Chenodeoxycholic acid (Chenix) Ursodeoxycholic acid (UDCA; Actigall)	Diarrhea, cramps, nausea, vomiting, elevated levels of serum enzymes, low-density lipoproteins, and cholesterol. UDCA has milder side effects but is very expensive. Contraindications: biliary tract infection, pancreatitis, pregnancy.	Advise patients not to become pregnant while taking this drug. Stress importance of periodic blood tests to determine liver enzyme and serum cholesterol levels.
DISSOLUTION AGENTS		
Methyl *tert*-butyl ether (MTBE)	Abdominal pain and nausea during treatment.	Oral contrast dye is given the previous evening. Position patient on right side after the procedure to reduce bleeding. Monitor for hemorrhage, shock, and pneumothorax. Measure vital signs every 15 min until stable then 3 times at 4-hr intervals. Bedrest for 24 hr.
Monooctanoin (Moctanin)	Anorexia, nausea, vomiting, diarrhea, abdominal pain. Rarely, acute pancreatitis.	Give antiemetics and antidiarrheals PRN, as ordered. With physician's approval, stop infusion for meals. Keep nasal biliary tube securely anchored. Slowing the rate of infusion may control gastrointestinal distress.

PRN, As needed.

jaundice. Some excess bilirubin is excreted in the urine, creating a dark, amber color. Digestion of fats is impaired, causing intolerance of fatty foods and steatorrhea (excess fat in feces). The absence of urobilinogen in the stool causes it to be a characteristic clay color. The patient is unable to absorb fat-soluble vitamins and may show signs of vitamin deficiencies. Vitamin K deficiency interferes with normal blood clotting, and thus the patient bleeds and bruises easily.

Complications

The most serious complications of cholecystitis and cholelithiasis are pancreatitis, abscesses, cholangitis (inflammation of the biliary ducts), and rupture of the gallbladder.

Medical Diagnosis

A tentative diagnosis of cholelithiasis based on the history and physical examination findings is best confirmed with fluoroscopy using contrast medium injected directly into the biliary tree. Other diagnostic procedures include radiographs, radionuclide imaging, ultrasonography, and oral or intravenous cholangiography.

Blood and urine studies provide additional information. With inflammation or infection, the white blood cell count is elevated. If bile flow is obstructed, levels of serum and urinary bilirubin and serum enzymes may be elevated. Nursing considerations with specific diagnostic tests and procedures are summarized in Table 37-2.

Medical Treatment

Among the options available for the treatment of cholelithiasis are drug therapy, shock wave lithotripsy, endoscopic sphincterotomy, and cholecystectomy. Patients with asymptomatic gallstones usually require no treatment except in special circumstances.

Acute cholecystitis is managed symptomatically. Analgesics and anticholinergics are ordered to relieve pain and muscle spasms. Antibiotics are given to treat infection. Intravenous fluids are selected to maintain fluid balance, especially if the patient has been vomiting. A nasogastric tube may be inserted and attached to suction. This relieves nausea and vomiting and reduces the stimulation of the gallbladder by intestinal contents.

Drug Therapy

Two types of drugs are used to dissolve gallstones: oral bile salts and dissolution agents. Ursodeoxycholic acid (UDCA; Actigall) is the oral bile salt in current use. It may be prescribed when the patient has only small cholesterol stones or for those who are poor surgical risks. However, it is very expensive and requires continuous treatment for 6 months to 1 year.

Methyl *tert*-butyl ether (MTBE) and ethyl proprionate are dissolution agents. The agent MTBE is instilled in the gallbladder through a transhepatic catheter. The physician instills and aspirates the drug repeatedly until fluoroscopy shows that the stones either have dissolved or are not responding to the treatment.

Monooctanoin (Moctanin) is used to treat stones remaining in the common bile duct after cholecystectomy. It is given through a nasobiliary catheter by continuous infusion for 2 to 10 days. The patient is allowed to have a bland diet, and the infusion is stopped during meals. Cholangiograms are obtained periodically to assess the effects of the drug. It is effective about half the time.

Drugs used to treat conditions of the biliary tract are described in Table 37-6.

Extracorporeal Shock Wave Lithotripsy (ESWL)

ESWL uses sound waves to break up gallstones. It has been used for patients with few stones and mild to moderate symptoms. With the advent of laproscopic cholecystectomy, ESWL has been largely abandoned. For general information about lithotripsy, see Renal Calculi in Chapter 38.

Endoscopic Sphincterotomy

Endoscopic sphincterotomy involves the use of endoscopic instruments to incise the sphincter of Oddi and extract stones from the common bile duct, as illustrated in Figure 37-11. The patient is given a sedative but remains conscious during the procedure. Lidocaine spray is used to deaden the gag reflex so that the endoscope can be passed through the mouth. A choledochoscope also can be inserted through a T-tube into the common bile duct. A special basket is used to extract the stones.

After endoscopic sphincterotomy, the patient is usually kept on bedrest for 6 to 8 hours. Nothing is given by mouth until the gag reflex returns. The patient is monitored for signs of complications. Bloody stools and tachycardia may indicate hemorrhage secondary to trauma. Fever and abdominal pain may indicate pancreatitis or perforation of the duodenum.

Cholecystectomy

Cholecystectomy is the most frequently used treatment for cholelithiasis. The two procedures that may be used are via laparoscopy or though a right subcostal incision. For laparoscopic cholecystectomy, the surgeon inserts a laparoscope with a camera through a small abdominal incision. Using the camera, the surgeon guides forceps and a laser toward the gallbladder through other small abdominal incisions. The gallbladder is grasped with the forceps, cut free with the laser, and pulled out through one of the small incisions. Stones remaining in the common bile duct can be removed endoscopically. Complications are rare, and patients usually resume regular activities in 2 or 3 days.

In the classic procedure, an incision is made below the right rib margin. The gallbladder is removed, and the common bile duct is explored for stones. Exploration of the bile duct may cause it to swell and obstruct bile flow from the liver. A T-tube may be placed in the common bile duct to maintain bile flow until swelling in the duct subsides (Fig. 37-12). One part of the tubing is brought through the patient's skin and connected to a closed gravity drainage receptacle. Wound drains also may be present.

When the patient first returns from surgery, the drainage from the T-tube may be bloody, but it should soon become greenish brown. Drainage should gradually decrease as edema subsides in the common bile duct. Measure and record the amount of drainage, and notify the physician if it exceeds 1,000 ml in 24 hours.

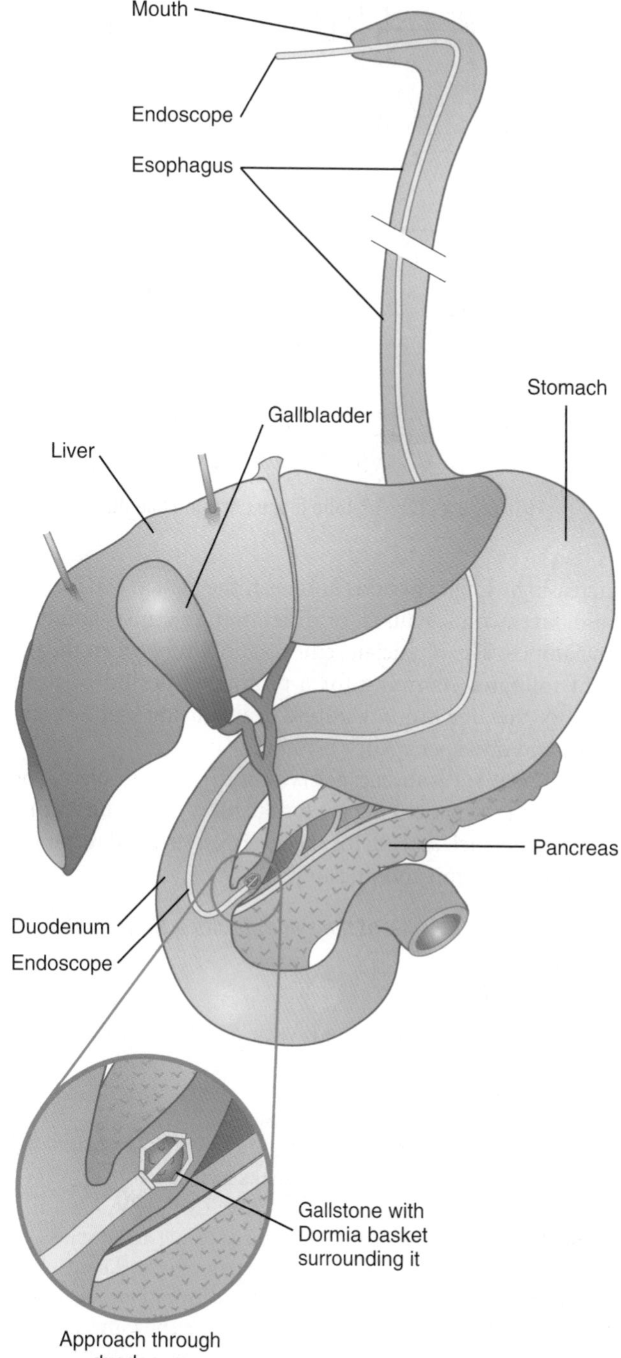

FIGURE **37-11** Choledoscopic removal of gallstones.

Place the patient in a low-Fowler's position with the tube arranged to drain freely. Protect the tube during movement to prevent dislodging it. The physician specifies the level of the drainage bag and when it should be clamped. Orders may call for the tube to be clamped for 1 to 2 hours before meals so that bile is available for digestion. The tube is clamped for

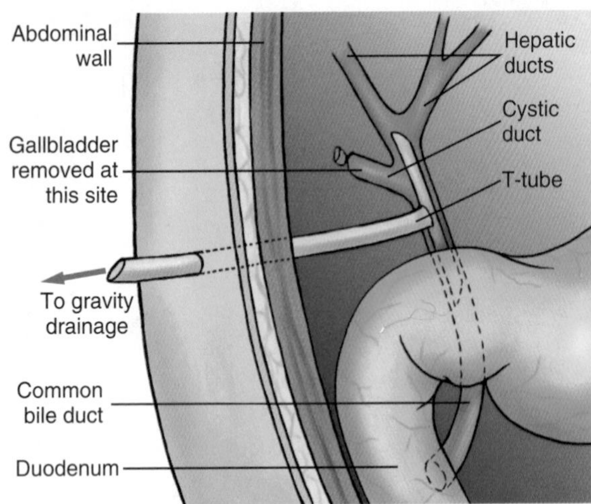

FIGURE **37-12** A T-tube in the common bile duct.

increasingly longer periods of time. If the patient experiences pain, fever, chills, nausea, or distention, the tube should be unclamped. The physician removes the T-tube when the patient tolerates clamping for a prolonged period of time. Cleanse the area around wound drains using aseptic technique and dress per agency protocol.

If the patient is discharged with the T-tube in place, you must teach the patient to care for the tube, including emptying the receptacle, caring for the insertion site, and recognizing when to clamp and unclamp it.

NURSING CARE *of the Patient with a Gallbladder Disorder*

Assessment

General assessment of patients with problems of the biliary tract is outlined in Table 37-5.

Nursing Diagnoses, Goals, and Outcome Criteria: Cholelithiasis

Nursing Diagnoses	Goals and Outcome Criteria
Acute Pain related to biliary colic	Reduced pain: patient states pain reduced or relieved
Deficient Fluid Volume related to vomiting, inadequate intake	Adequate hydration: balanced fluid intake and output; vital signs consistent with patient norms
Risk for Impaired Skin Integrity related to pruritus	Decreased itching: no scratching, patient states less or no itching
Anxiety related to disease, anticipation of invasive procedures	Reduced anxiety: patient states anxiety relieved or reduced, relaxed manner
Risk for Injury (bleeding) related to vitamin K deficiency	Absence of bleeding: no abnormal bruising or bleeding

Interventions

Acute Pain

The degree of pain with cholecystitis varies, but many patients experience severe pain. Atropine and opioid analgesics other than morphine are usually ordered. Morphine is not used because it is believed to cause spasms in the common bile duct, which would increase the patient's pain. Assess comfort often, and medicate the patient as soon as pain is reported instead of waiting for it to become severe. When opioid analgesics are given, take safety precautions because the drugs cause drowsiness. In addition to medications, use position changes, smooth linens, back rubs, and mouth care to promote comfort.

Attacks of biliary colic are caused by stimulation of the gallbladder, most often by fats in the duodenum. A low-fat diet is recommended to decrease the incidence of acute symptoms.

Deficient Fluid Volume

If nausea and vomiting are present, the patient is at risk for fluid and electrolyte imbalances. Administer antiemetics as ordered. Keep intake and output records. Monitor for signs of deficient fluid volume (hypovolemia): tachycardia, hypotension, dry skin, concentrated urine, decreased urine output.

If vomiting is severe, a nasogastric tube may be inserted and attached to suction. Fluids are provided intravenously. Note the amount and characteristics of aspirated fluid. A problem associated with nasogastric decompression is the continuous removal of gastric secretions. When the fluid is continuously drained, the patient loses significant water, electrolytes, and acid. This puts the patient at risk for deficient fluid volume, potassium deficit, sodium excess, and metabolic alkalosis. Serum electrolytes are monitored, and specific intravenous fluids are ordered to maintain or restore balance.

Risk for Impaired Skin Integrity

Patients who have obstructive jaundice due to blockage of the bile ducts often have pruritus caused by accumulated bile salts under the skin. Measures to promote comfort include tepid baths with baking soda or oily lotions, use of soft linens, and maintaining a comfortable room temperature. Patients should be advised not to scratch, but that can be difficult. Short fingernails or even cotton gloves may be suggested to avoid skin injury from scratching. The physician may order a drug such as cholestyramine (Questran) to reduce the discomfort.

Anxiety

Acute pain and unexpected hospitalization can be anxiety-provoking for patients and their families. Provide clear explanations about what is being done and what they can expect. Acknowledge their anxiety and take time to answer questions and offer reassurance.

Risk for Injury

A patient who has obstructed bile flow may have a deficiency of vitamin K because absorption of this vitamin in the digestive tract requires bile salts. Vitamin K is needed for the production of prothrombin, an essential element for clotting. Indications of vitamin K deficiency include bleeding gums and oozing of blood at injection sites. Minimize trauma by using a soft toothbrush or swab for mouth care and by applying gentle pressure to injection sites.

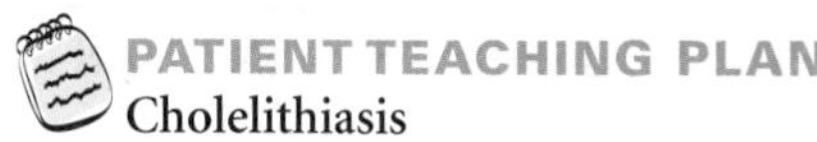

PATIENT TEACHING PLAN
Cholelithiasis

- You need to have a low-fat diet with supplementary fat-soluble vitamins (or as ordered by the physician). The dietitian will explain the details of the diet to you.
- Notify your physician of signs of bile duct obstruction: light stools, dark urine, jaundice, and itching.
- If you are taking bile salts, report gastric upset.
- Keep medical appointments to have blood drawn to monitor liver function.
- Do not rely on oral contraceptives; bile salts interfere with their effectiveness.

PHARMACOLOGY CAPSULE Caution patients that supplementary bile salts interfere with the effectiveness of oral contraceptives.

NURSING CARE *of the Patient Following Surgery for Cholelithiasis*

Common nursing interventions for the patient who has undergone abdominal surgery for cholelithiasis are presented here. Detailed assessment and care of the surgical patient are presented in Chapter 16. Nursing care after laparoscopic cholecystectomy is much simpler because patients usually recover quickly and are discharged the same day or within 24 hours. They usually do not need postoperative nasogastric intubation or T-tubes.

Assessment

Postoperatively, take the patient's vital signs until the patient is stable. Observe chest expansion, and auscultate breath sounds. Inspect the dressing for bleeding. If there is a T-tube present, note the color and amount of drainage. Examine passive drains to be sure that they are functioning properly. Inspect the skin around the incision or the drain for redness or breakdown. If a nasogastric tube is in place, observe the characteristics and amount of the drainage and ensure that the suction is operational. Inspect the patient's nares for irritation or pressure from the tube.

Nursing Diagnoses, Goals, and Outcome Criteria: Cholecystectomy

Nursing Diagnoses	Goals and Outcome Criteria
Acute Pain related to surgical incision, nasogastric tube	Pain relief: patient states pain relieved or reduced, relaxed manner
Ineffective Breathing Patterns related to splinting of the surgical incision	Effective breathing pattern: breath sounds clear on auscultation, respiratory rate of 12-20 per minute
Impaired Skin Integrity related to wound drainage, surgical incision	Wound healing without skin breakdown: clean wound margins without excessive redness
Deficient Fluid Volume related to gastrointestinal suction	Normal fluid and electrolyte status: electrolytes within normal limits, balanced fluid intake and output
Risk for Infection related to surgical incision, invasive procedure	Absence of infection: normal temperature and white blood cell count

Interventions

Acute Pain

When the patient undergoes a procedure that requires a surgical incision, pain is expected. In addition to administering ordered analgesics, reposition the patient for comfort and check to see that any drainage tubes are functioning. Show the patient how to support the incision with the hands or a pillow during coughing and deep breathing. Other pain relief measures are described in Chapter 14. If pain continues despite these measures, notify the physician.

The patient who has a nasogastric tube in place has an additional source of discomfort. The nose and throat may become very sore. Secure the tube to the patient's upper lip or nose so that it is not easily moved or tugged. Gently cleanse the nares, and apply water-soluble lubricant to keep the area moist. Provide frequent mouth care.

Ineffective Breathing Patterns

Potentially ineffective breathing patterns are most likely to be a problem when the patient has a subcostal incision. The incision is located close to the diaphragm, so that full lung expansion is painful. The patient tends to guard the surgical area by not breathing deeply. Explain the importance of deep breathing and coughing to prevent atelectasis and pneumonia. Also demonstrate how splinting the area makes breathing and coughing more comfortable. Adequate pain management enables the patient to breathe more effectively. Monitor respiratory rate and breath sounds.

Impaired Skin Integrity

Patients who have subcostal incisions often have wound drains in place. These drains allow for removal of fluids that collect at the surgical site. A Penrose drain diverts fluids directly onto the wound dressings. This requires frequent dressing changes to prevent skin irritation. It is especially important if bile is present in the drainage because bile contains digestive enzymes, which are even more irritating. A pouch collection device like those used for stomas can be applied if needed to protect the skin. A passive drain such as the Jackson-Pratt drain has a fluid collection device that keeps fluid away from the skin.

Deficient Fluid Volume

Postoperatively, measure fluid intake and output. Until oral fluids are permitted, administer intravenous fluids as ordered.

Blood studies may be ordered to assess serum electrolytes. If nasogastric suction is ordered, check frequently to be sure it is working properly. Otherwise, the patient may have distention that causes vomiting and further loss of fluids and electrolytes.

Risk for Infection

The patient who has undergone gallbladder surgery is at risk for infection of the surgical wound. Draining wounds provide a moist environment for bacterial growth. Meticulous wound care can reduce that risk.

A complication of endoscopic sphincterotomy is pancreatitis caused by accidental entry of the endoscope into the pancreatic duct. Early signs of pancreatitis are pain and fever.

PATIENT TEACHING PLAN
Cholecystectomy

- We will teach you how to care for the T-tube before you go home.
- A low-fat diet is usually recommended for 4 to 6 weeks.
- In general, avoid heavy lifting for 4 to 6 weeks or as prescribed. Other activities, including sexual intercourse, can usually be resumed when you feel well enough.

After laparoscopic cholecystectomy, usual instructions include:

- Avoid fatty foods for several weeks.
- Remove the dressings and bathe or shower normally the next day.
- Notify the physician if there is redness, drainage, or pus from the incision.
- Report any signs of peritonitis: severe abdominal pain, chills and fever, and vomiting.

CANCER OF THE GALLBLADDER

Cancer of the gallbladder is rare and is thought to be related to chronic cholecystitis and cholelithiasis. The diagnosis is often delayed because early signs and symptoms are essentially the same as those of cholecystitis and cholelithiasis.

Treatment options include surgery, chemotherapy, and radiation therapy, but the prognosis is generally poor. Often only supportive, symptomatic care is given. Nursing care is similar to that for other patients with gallbladder disease. You also need to focus on the needs of the cancer patient, as discussed in Chapter 24.

THE PANCREAS

The pancreas is a gland that has both endocrine and exocrine functions. As an **endocrine gland**, it secretes into the blood hormones that regulate the blood glucose level. The exocrine function is the production of digestive enzymes that are secreted into the duodenum through a duct. This section focuses on disorders of the pancreas, with the exception of diabetes mellitus, which is covered in Chapter 44.

ANATOMY AND PHYSIOLOGY OF THE PANCREAS

The pancreas is a fish-shaped organ located in the upper left quadrant of the abdomen behind the stomach. The head of the pancreas lies against the duodenum, and the tail lies next to the spleen. The pancreatic ducts connect the pancreas to the duodenum. One duct goes directly to the duodenum, and the other merges with the common bile duct, as shown in Figure 37-10.

EXOCRINE FUNCTION

The exocrine function of the pancreas is carried out by acinar tissue. Acinar tissue is composed of tiny grape-like clusters of cells that produce pancreatic fluid. Pancreatic fluid contains enzymes needed for the digestion of proteins, fats, and carbohydrates. It is secreted into the duodenum through the pancreatic duct.

The pancreatic enzymes trypsin, amylase, and lipase act on partially digested foods in the small intestine. Trypsin plays a role in the digestion of protein by breaking proteases and peptones into small polypeptides. Normally, trypsin is not activated until it enters the duodenum. Otherwise, it would digest the protein tissue of the pancreas itself. Amylase acts with intestinal enzymes to reduce starch, sucrose, and fructose to glucose, fructose, and galactose. Lipase acts on emulsified fats to yield fatty acids, glycerides, and glycerol.

ENDOCRINE FUNCTION

The endocrine function of the pancreas is carried out by clusters of specialized cells scattered throughout the pancreas. These cells are called islets of Langerhans. The islets contain alpha, beta, delta, and PP cells. Alpha cells produce and secrete glucagon. Beta cells produce and secrete insulin. Delta cells produce somatostatin, which inhibits the release of glucagon and insulin. PP cells secrete pancreatic polypeptide, a hormone of uncertain function.

Glucagon is secreted when the blood glucose level falls. It stimulates the liver to convert glycogen into glucose. Insulin is secreted when the blood glucose rises, as after a meal. It stimulates the use of glucose by the cells so that a normal blood glucose level is maintained. The endocrine function of the pancreas is covered more thoroughly in Chapter 44.

NURSING ASSESSMENT OF THE PATIENT WITH A PANCREATIC DISORDER

Assessment of the patient with a pancreatic disorder is outlined in Table 37-7. The assessment focuses on digestive and metabolic functions.

Health History

Inquire about the patient's general health status because pancreatic disorders are often accompanied by weakness and fatigue. The past medical history may reveal previous disorders of the biliary tract or duodenum, abdominal trauma or surgery, and metabolic disorders such as diabetes mellitus. The medication history should be detailed and specifically include

table 37-7 ASSESSMENT *of the Patient with a Pancreatic Disorder*

HEALTH HISTORY

Present Illness: General well-being, digestive disturbances, pain
Past Medical History: Disorders of the biliary tract or duodenum, abdominal trauma or surgery, metabolic disorders; medication history, especially thiazides, furosemide, estrogens, corticosteroids, sulfonamides, opiates
Family History: Pancreatic disorders
Review of Systems: Pruritus, respiratory distress, nausea and vomiting, abdominal pain
Functional Assessment: Dietary habits, alcohol intake

PHYSICAL EXAMINATION

General Survey: Restlessness, flushing, diaphoresis
Vital Signs: Low-grade fever, tachycardia, tachypnea, hypotension
Skin: Jaundice, dryness, scratches
Abdomen: Distention, tenderness, diminished bowel sounds, discoloration

the use of thiazides, furosemide, estrogens, corticosteroids, sulfonamides, and opiates. Note a family history of pancreatic disorders. In the review of systems, obtain a complete description of any pain in the upper abdomen or epigastric area. Symptoms that may be important in relation to pancreatic disorders are dyspnea, nausea, and vomiting. The functional assessment includes data about the patient's dietary habits and use of alcohol.

Physical Examination

Note any restlessness, flushing, or diaphoresis during the examination. Vital signs may disclose low-grade fever, tachypnea, tachycardia, and hypotension. Inspect the skin for jaundice. Assess the abdomen for distention, tenderness, discoloration, and diminished bowel sounds.

DIAGNOSTIC TESTS AND PROCEDURES

Tests and procedures used to diagnose pancreatic disorders include laboratory analyses of blood, urine, stool, and pancreatic fluid, and imaging studies (CT scan, endoscopic ultrasonography, MRI, PET, and ERCP).

Specific blood studies used to assess pancreatic function include measurements of serum amylase, lipase, glucose, calcium, and triglycerides. Urine amylase and renal amylase clearance tests also may be ordered. Stool specimens may be analyzed for fat content.

The secretin stimulation test measures the bicarbonate concentration of pancreatic fluid after secretin is given intravenously to stimulate the production of pancreatic fluid.

If cancer is suspected, blood levels of CA 19-9, carcinoembryonic antigen, pancreatic oncofetal antigen, and others that are considered "markers" for cancer may be measured. Unfortunately, levels of these antigens are elevated with many types of cancer, so their presence does not specifically indicate pancreatic cancer.

Additional information about diagnostic tests and procedures for the pancreas is provided in Table 37-8.

DISORDERS OF THE PANCREAS

PANCREATITIS

Pancreatitis is inflammation of the pancreas. It may be acute or chronic. Chronic pancreatitis may follow the acute condition but often develops independently.

Pancreatitis is most often caused by biliary tract disorders or alcoholism. Other causes include viral infections; peptic ulcer disease; cysts; metabolic disorders (renal failure, hyperparathyroidism); and trauma from external injury, surgery, or endoscopic procedures. In addition, chronic pancreatitis is sometimes associated with cancer of the duodenum or pancreas.

Normally, pancreatic enzymes are activated in the small intestine. With pancreatitis, digestive enzymes (trypsin, elastase, and phospholipase A) are activated by some unknown mechanism and begin to digest pancreatic tissue (a process called autodigestion), fat, and elastic tissue in blood vessels. Pancreatic fluid may leak into the surrounding tissues. The effect of this escaped fluid has been compared to an internal chemical burn, and the effects can be devastating.

Chronic pancreatitis is often related to alcohol abuse. It is usually characterized by obstruction of the pancreatic duct, leading to progressive destruction of the pancreas.

Put on your *THINKING CAP!!*

The term *autodigestion* is used to describe the effects of pancreatitis. Explain what this means.

Signs and Symptoms

Abdominal pain is the most prominent symptom of pancreatitis. The pain is typically severe, with a sudden onset, and is centered in the upper left quadrant or the epigastric region and radiates to the back. Severe vomiting, flushing, cyanosis, and dyspnea often accompany the pain. Other signs and symptoms are low-grade fever, tachypnea, tachycardia, and hypotension.

The abdomen may be tender and distended. Bowel sounds may be absent, suggesting an ileus. Trypsin may damage blood vessels, causing pancreatic hemorrhage and discoloration of the abdomen. You may observe cyanosis or greenish discoloration of the abdominal wall, the flanks, and the area around the umbilicus. Enzymes released into the abdominal cavity increase capillary permeability, permitting protein-rich serum to leak from blood vessels. Bleeding and shifting of fluid reduce blood volume and may lead to shock. Early signs and symptoms of shock are restlessness and tachycardia. Hypotension is a late sign.

table 37-8 **DIAGNOSTIC TESTS AND PROCEDURES | *the Pancreas***

TEST	PURPOSE/PROCEDURE	PATIENT PREPARATION	POSTPROCEDURE NURSING CARE
LABORATORY STUDIES			
Amylase	Increases with pancreatitis, parotitis, cholecystitis.	For all laboratory studies, advise patient that a blood sample will be drawn and inform him or her whether fasting is required by agency protocol.	For all laboratory studies, check venipuncture site for bleeding. Apply pressure if necessary.
Serum Enzymes	Decreases with liver disease, burns, thyrotoxicosis. Normal value: 50-150/L. Lipase increases with pancreatic inflammation, carcinoma. Normal values vary with type of test used.		
Serum Calcium	Decreases with many conditions, including pancreatic disorders.		
Serum Triglycerides	Increase with pancreatitis and many other conditions.		
Tumor Markers			
Carcinoembryonic antigen (CEA); pancreatic oncofetal antigen (POA)	Increases with many types of cancer, including pancreatic; pancreatitis, cirrhosis, hepatitis, and chronic cigarette smoking.		
SECRETIN STIMULATION TEST	Secretin is given intravenously. Gastric and duodenal fluids are aspirated through a double-lumen tube. Fluid is analyzed. Decreased volume of secretions and bicarbonate is consistent with pancreatitis.	Tell patient that a medication will be given in a vein and that a tube will be passed through nose into stomach so that fluid can be removed from stomach for study.	Remove tube unless instructed otherwise. Provide comfort measures.

URINE AMYLASE	Increases with acute pancreatitis, peptic ulcer, and choledocholithiasis. Test may be ordered for a 1-, 2-, or 24-hr specimen.	Advise patient of time for collection of specimens. Encourage fluids during test if not contraindicated.	
IMAGING STUDIES			
Abdominal ultrasound	Uses sound waves to visualize pancreas directly. Is noninvasive.	Some labs require patient to be NPO before procedure. Study cannot be done if barium or excessive gas is in digestive tract. Tell patient that he or she will lie on back on an examination table. A gel or oil is applied to skin, and an instrument is moved over upper abdomen. Images are seen on a screen and recorded.	No special care.
Computed tomography (CT)	Uses radiographs with a special scanner to provide detailed information about internal organ position and structure. Contrast medium may be given orally or intravenously.	NPO is needed before some CT scans. Tell patient to expect to lie on a narrow stretcher. Scanner is a donut-shaped machine that moves back and forth and around stretcher. It makes clicking noises. Contraindicated during pregnancy. Assess allergies to dye and inform radiologist.	No special care.
Endoscopic retrograde cholangiopancreatography (ERCP)	Uses an endoscope to examine gallbladder and pancreas to evaluate bile obstruction and to confirm pancreatic disease. Contrast medium is injected into bile duct.	A consent form must be signed. Patient will be NPO as long as 12 hr. Physician may order patient to gargle with a topical anesthetic. An intravenous line may be started to administer sedatives.	Monitor vital signs for 4 hr. Check gag reflex before giving fluids or food. Monitor for urinary retention. Report temperature elevation that may indicate inflammation.

NPO, Nothing by mouth.

Symptoms of chronic pancreatitis are similar to those of the acute disease but usually appear as periodic attacks that become more and more frequent. In addition, patients with chronic pancreatitis may develop diabetes mellitus and malabsorption with steatorrhea.

Complications

Complications of pancreatitis include pseudocyst, abscess, hypocalcemia, and pulmonary, cardiac, and renal complications.

A pseudocyst is a fluid-filled pouch attached to the pancreas. It contains products of tissue destruction and pancreatic enzymes. The fluid can leak into the digestive tract or the abdominal cavity. Symptoms of pseudocyst include abdominal pain, nausea, vomiting, and anorexia. Sometimes a mass can be palpated in the epigastric area. Necrosis within the pancreas can lead to pancreatic abscess, a fluid-filled cavity in the pancreas. Symptoms are similar to those of pseudocyst. Patients usually run a high fever.

Hypocalcemia (low serum calcium) is caused by the action of fatty acids on calcium and increased loss of calcium in the urine. The pulmonary complications of pancreatitis are pneumonia and atelectasis. Pancreatitis can be fatal. In the early stage of acute pancreatitis, causes of death are usually cardiovascular, renal, or pulmonary failure. Later, sepsis and abscesses are the leading causes of death.

A person may recover completely from an attack of acute pancreatitis, have repeated acute episodes, or experience chronic pancreatitis.

Medical Diagnosis

The most important diagnostic findings in acute pancreatitis are elevated serum amylase, serum lipase, and urinary amylase levels. When the kidneys clear amylase more rapidly than they clear creatinine, acute pancreatitis is strongly suspected. Other findings with acute pancreatitis are elevated white blood cell count, elevated serum lipid and glucose level, and decreased serum calcium level. Ultrasonography and ERCP may reveal the presence of gallstones, cysts, or abscesses and help to rule out other disorders that might be causing the patient's symptoms.

Tests for chronic pancreatitis include the secretin stimulation test and fecal studies in addition to the tests used for acute pancreatitis. Findings consistent with chronic pancreatitis are decreased volume and bicarbonate concentration of pancreatic fluid and high fecal fat content.

Medical Treatment

The patient is usually allowed nothing by mouth. This removes the stimulus for secretion of pancreatic fluid. If the patient is vomiting or if an ileus is suspected, a nasogastric tube is inserted and connected to suction. Sometimes peritoneal lavage or laparoscopy is used to remove toxic fluid from the peritoneum.

Intravenous fluids are ordered to restore and maintain fluid balance. Total parenteral nutrition may be needed to provide adequate nutrients. Blood or plasma expanders are given if the blood volume is low. Urine output is monitored and should be at least 40 ml/hour. Since the inflamed pancreas is susceptible to infection, some physicians order prophylactic antibiotics.

Drug Therapy

Pain control is a major problem with pancreatitis. Meperidine (Demerol) has traditionally been the analgesic of choice, although opiates (such as morphine) have been avoided because they are thought to cause more spasm in the pancreatic ducts. Researchers are now studying the opiates to see if this concern is warranted. With chronic pancreatitis, there is concern about addiction to opioid analgesics. Anticholinergics decrease secretions, which can reduce spasms and pain. Antispasmodics such as nitroglygerin also are used.

The patient with chronic pancreatitis needs to take pancreatic enzymes in order to digest food. The enzymes can be taken with meals or snacks. The effect of the enzymes can be determined by examining the stools. Steatorrhea (bulky, frothy stools with a high fat content) results from inadequate enzymes. If diabetes mellitus develops, insulin or oral hypoglycemic drugs are needed.

The patient requires diabetes education. Other drugs that may be needed are antacids, anticholinergics, and histamine blockers to decrease hydrochloric acid in the stomach. Bile salts also may be needed to enhance absorption of fat-soluble vitamins. Drugs used to treat pancreatitis are described in Table 37-9.

Surgical Intervention

If an abscess, pseudocyst, or severe peritonitis develops, surgical intervention is indicated. Débridement involves resection of necrotic tissue and irrigation of the cavity to remove harmful fluid. The procedure may have to be repeated more than once. Following surgical débridement, multiple sumps are placed in the abdomen for continuous postoperative irrigation. Each sump tube is connected to a separate suction apparatus. Irrigations may be alternated as ordered.

NURSING CARE *of the Patient with Pancreatitis*

Assessment

General nursing assessment of the patient with a pancreatic disorder is outlined in Table 37-7 (see also Nursing Care Plan: The Patient with Pancreatitis). When a patient has acute pancreatitis, it is especially important to assess for signs of hypovolemic shock: restlessness, tachycardia, tachypnea, hypotension, decreased urinary output, and discoloration of the abdomen and flanks. In addition, the patient's mental status should be assessed. Alterations may be due to metabolic imbalances. The alcoholic patient may develop confusion and agitation due to alcohol withdrawal.

If the patient has surgery, general postoperative assessment should include data covered in Chapter 16.

Nursing Diagnoses, Goals, and Outcome Criteria: Pancreatitis

Nursing Diagnoses	Goals and Outcome Criteria
Acute Pain related to inflammation, infection, biliary obstruction, autodigestion	Pain relief: patient states pain reduced or relieved, relaxed manner

table 37-9 ***Drugs Used to Treat Pancreatitis***

DRUG	USE/ACTION	SIDE EFFECTS	NURSING INTERVENTIONS
ACUTE PANCREATITIS			
Opioid analgesics Meperidine (Demerol)	Pain relief.	Sedation, confusion, hypotension, nausea, vomiting, constipation.	Monitor BP, P, R. Assess bowel elimination. Observe safety precautions. Give antiemetics as ordered.
Smooth muscle relaxants Nitroglycerin	Relieve spasm, reduce pain.	Headache, dizziness, flushing, tachycardia, hypotension.	Monitor BP and P. Use special containers and tubing for IV administration.
Antispasmodics Propantheline bromide (Pro-Banthine)	Decrease bicarbonate and pancreatic enzyme secretion.	Tachycardia, dry mouth, constipation, urinary retention and hesitancy, drowsiness.	Administer 30 min before meals. Don't give within 1 hr of antacids or antidiarrheals. Observe safety precautions if patient is drowsy. Provide mouth care. Monitor stools.
Antacids	Neutralize gastric acid; indirectly decrease production of pancreatic secretions.	Constipation with aluminum; diarrhea with magnesium.	Monitor electrolytes. Give 1 hr apart from other oral drugs. Give on empty stomach. Have patient chew tablets and follow with full glass of water. Shake liquids well.
Carbonic anhydrase inhibitors Acetazolamide (Diamox)	Reduce bicarbonate concentration in pancreatic secretions.	Rash, drowsiness, nausea, vomiting, renal calculi, hypercalcemia, aplastic anemia, leukopenia, seizures, hypokalemia.	Encourage 2,000-3,000 ml fluid/day unless contraindicated. Give with food to decrease GI distress. Observe safety precautions. Monitor electrolytes and blood cell counts.
Somatostatin	Inhibits secretion of pancreatic enzymes.		
Histamine-2 receptor blockers Cimetidine (Tagamet) Ranitidine (Zantac) Famotidine (Pepcid)	Decrease production of HCl so that pancreatic enzymes cannot be activated.	Confusion, nausea, diarrhea, constipation, drowsiness, headache, rash, agranulocytosis.	Administer with or immediately after meals. Discourage smoking, which counteracts these drugs. Observe safety precautions. Report sore throat or fever.
Vitamin and mineral supplements	Supplement poor dietary intake or impaired absorption. Calcium treats hypocalcemia.	Potential for overdose of fat-soluble vitamins and calcium. Calcium potentiates cardiac glycosides.	
Adrenocortical steroids	Decrease inflammation.	Fluid retention, hypokalemia, hyperglycemia, hypocalcemia, decreased resistance to infection, mood swings.	Monitor BP, P, and blood glucose. Assess for edema. Protect from infection. Explain that emotional/personality changes are temporary.
CHRONIC PANCREATITIS			
Pancreatic enzymes Pancreatin Pancrelipase (Cotazym, Viokase, Pancrease)	Supplement normal pancreatic enzyme secretion; aid in digestion of fats, carbohydrates, and proteins. Goal is less frequent stools with lower fat content.	Diarrhea, nausea, stomach cramps, abdominal pain.	Give with meals or snacks. Capsule contents can be sprinkled on food but should not be chewed. Mix powders with fruit juice or applesauce to mask taste. Do not mix with protein foods. Have patient wipe lips with wet cloth to prevent skin irritation. Evaluate drug effect by noting number and consistency of stools.
Hypoglycemic agents Insulin Oral hypoglycemics	Needed when pancreas is unable to produce sufficient insulin.	Hypoglycemia.	See Chapter 44 for details on hypoglycemic drug therapy.

BP, Blood pressure; *P*, pulse; *R*, respiration; *IV*, intravenous; *GI*, gastrointestinal; *HCl*, hydrochloric acid.

NURSING CARE PLAN

The Patient with Pancreatitis

ASSESSMENT

Health History: Mrs. Sanchez is a 57-year-old Latina admitted with repeated attacks of severe pain in the upper left quadrant that radiates to her back. She reports having vomited repeatedly over the past 24 hours. When the pain is severe, she reports feeling flushed, faint, and short of breath. She has no other related symptoms. Mrs. Sanchez reports having had a gallbladder attack several months ago that resolved without surgery. She is a high school teacher who lives with her husband.

Physical Examination: The patient appears to be in acute distress, but she is alert and oriented. Vital signs: temperature, 100.2° F orally; pulse, 92; respiration, 24; blood pressure, 144/84. Abdomen tender and distended, with hypoactive bowel sounds in all four quadrants.

Nursing Diagnosis	*Goals and Outcome Criteria*	*Interventions*
Acute pain related to inflammation, biliary obstruction, autodigestion.	The patient will report decreased pain and will appear more relaxed.	Document painful episodes and treat promptly with analgesics and antispasmodics as ordered. Use distraction, imagery, and relaxation techniques to enhance drug therapy. Advise physician if pain is unrelieved.
Deficient fluid volume related to vomiting, bleeding, fluid shift from bloodstream to abdominal cavity.	The patient's fluid status will stabilize, as evidenced by stable blood pressure and pulse, normal skin color, urine output equal to fluid intake.	Insert nasogastric tube and connect to low suction as ordered. Initiate intravenous fluid therapy and administer as ordered. Monitor vital signs, intake and output, weight, and electrolyte studies. Report signs of fluid volume deficit: tachycardia, hypotension, dry skin, concentrated urine.
Risk for infection related to tissue necrosis.	The patient will be free of signs and symptoms of infection: fever, tachycardia, increased white blood cell count.	Monitor vital signs and blood cell counts. Report signs of infection. Administer antimicrobials as ordered. Use standard precautions for invasive procedures.
Impaired gas exchange related to pain, pulmonary complications.	The patient will remain free of pulmonary complications, as evidenced by absence of dyspnea, tachypnea, and abnormal breath sounds.	Assess respirations and breath sounds. Assist to change positions, cough, and deep breathe at least every 2 hours. Use semi-Fowler's position to promote lung expansion.
Imbalanced nutrition: less than body requirements related to anorexia, vomiting, digestive disturbances.	The patient's body weight will remain stable.	Administer total parenteral nutrition if ordered. Monitor for hyperglycemia and administer insulin as ordered. Take daily weights. When oral intake is permitted, monitor patient tolerance. Discourage spicy foods, caffeine, and alcohol.
Anxiety related to acute symptoms.	The patient will report decreased anxiety and will be calm.	Check on patient often. Respond to her needs promptly. Ask what questions she has and provide explanations of the condition and the treatment she is receiving.

Nursing Diagnoses, Goals, and Outcome Criteria: Pancreatitis—cont'd

Nursing Diagnoses	Goals and Outcome Criteria
Deficient Fluid Volume related to vomiting, bleeding, fluid shift from the blood to the abdominal cavity	Normal fluid balance: balanced fluid intake and output, pulse and blood pressure consistent with patient norms
Risk for Infection related to tissue necrosis	Absence of infection: normal body temperature and white blood cell count
Impaired Gas Exchange related to pain, pulmonary complications	Adequate gas exchange: breath sounds clear to auscultation, respiratory rate 12-20 per minute
Imbalanced Nutrition: Less than Body Requirements related to anorexia, vomiting, digestive disturbance	Adequate nutrition: stable body weight
Anxiety related to unfamiliar setting and procedures; acute illness	Reduced anxiety: patient states anxiety lessened, calm manner

Interventions

Acute Pain

Assess the patient's pain and provide ordered analgesics and antispasmodics promptly. Reposition the patient for comfort. Other nursing measures for pain are described in Chapter 14

Consider the Alternative!

Distraction, imagery, relaxation, and cutaneous stimulation can enhance the effects of analgesics to promote pain relief.

and include distraction, imagery, and cutaneous stimulation. Evaluate and record the effectiveness of pain control measures. Consult the physician if pain is not relieved.

Deficient Fluid Volume

If ordered, insert a nasogastric tube and connect it to suction. Administer prescribed intravenous fluids. Assess the patient's fluid status by monitoring vital signs, intake and output, and weight. Signs of fluid volume deficit include tachycardia, hypotension, dry skin, concentrated urine, and decreased urine output. The physician should be informed if the urine output falls below 40 ml/hour. Depletion of blood volume causes hypovolemic shock and leads to death if not corrected. Other potential fluid imbalances are metabolic alkalosis from severe vomiting, hypokalemia, hyponatremia, hypocalcemia, and hypochloremia.

Risk for Infection

Necrosis of the pancreas and surrounding tissue provides a site for infection. If a surgical procedure is done, there also is risk for wound infection. Inform the physician of fever, purulent drainage, or separation of wound margins—all signs of infection. Take special care to maintain asepsis during wound care.

Impaired Gas Exchange

Fluid accumulation in the peritoneal cavity puts upward pressure on the diaphragm, thereby limiting lung expansion. Because the acutely ill patient is inactive, secretions may pool in the lungs. Poor lung expansion and inactivity combine to invite pneumonia and atelectasis. Monitor for tachypnea, dyspnea, and abnormal breath sounds.

Measures to prevent pulmonary complications in the patient with pancreatitis include frequent turning, coughing, and deep breathing. The semi-Fowler's position promotes lung expansion.

Imbalanced Nutrition: Less than Body Requirements

Initially, the patient will be NPO because food and fluids stimulate pancreatic fluid secretion. When oral intake is resumed, small feedings of a bland, high-carbohydrate, low-fat, high-protein diet are provided. Spicy foods, caffeine, and alcohol should be avoided. Total parenteral nutrition (Chapter 36) is usually only needed with severe malnourishment. Daily weights are used to evaluate the adequacy of the nutrition plan.

Anxiety

Attempt to determine the reasons for the patient's anxiety. Some concerns can be alleviated by telling the patient what is happening and what to expect. Respond promptly to the patient's needs and offer comforting reassurance by checking on the patient frequently. Anxiety can be related to pain or hypoxia as well as to emotional distress, so assess comfort and oxygenation status and take appropriate corrective actions. During acute attacks, answer questions and give simple explanations. As the patient improves, implement your teaching plan.

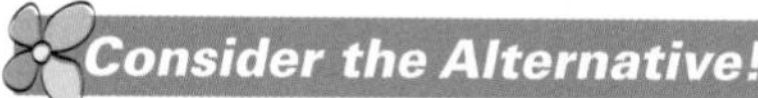

Consider the Alternative!

Some patients have found acupuncture helpful for treatment of alcoholism.

PATIENT TEACHING PLAN
Pancreatitis

- Your prescribed diet (usually bland, high-protein, high-carbohydrate, low-fat) will avoid stimulating your pancreas and will promote healing.
- At first, you may tolerate small, frequent meals better than large meals.
- Abstaining from alcohol decreases your risk of recurrence.
- Community resources such as Alcoholics Anonymous can assist if it is hard for you to abstain from drinking alcohol (website: http://www.alcoholics-anonymous.org; telephone: 1-212-686-1100).

CANCER OF THE PANCREAS

Cancer of the pancreas is extremely serious. Pancreatic cancer quickly spreads to the duodenum, stomach, spleen, and left adrenal gland. About 29,000 new cases are diagnosed each year in the United States. Most of these people die within a year. Among the risk factors for pancreatic cancer are chronic pancreatitis and smoking. Other probable risk factors are a high-fat diet and exposure to certain toxic chemicals. Tumors may develop in the head, body, or tail of the pancreas.

Signs and Symptoms

Signs and symptoms of pancreatic cancer vary with the stage and location but often include pain, jaundice with or without liver enlargement, weight loss, and glucose intolerance. When located in the head of the pancreas, tumors typically obstruct the common bile duct, causing jaundice. In the early stage of the disease, jaundice may be the only sign present. If the patient seeks medical care early, the chance of survival is somewhat better. Other signs and symptoms may be weight loss, upper abdominal pain, anorexia, vomiting, weakness, and diarrhea.

When the tumor is in the body or the tail of the pancreas, the patient may not have any symptoms until the disease is advanced. Then the liver, gallbladder, and spleen may be enlarged. Pressure on the portal veins may cause esophageal and gastric varices (dilated veins) that bleed easily into the gastrointestinal tract. Pressure on nerves may cause back pain.

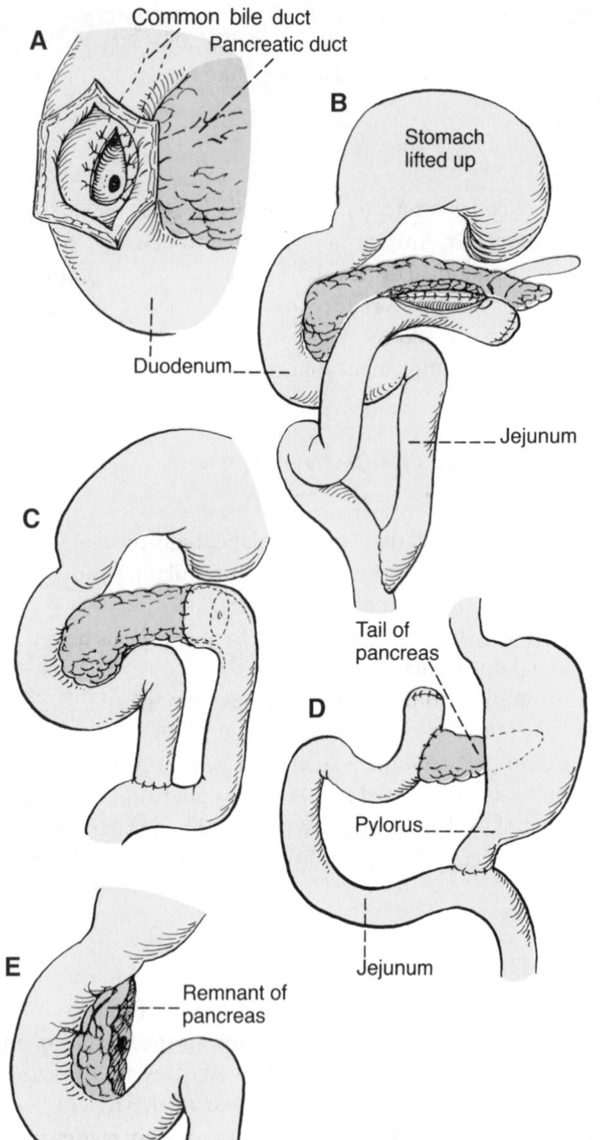

A. **Sphincteroplasty (ampullary)**
Indicated for stenosis of sphincter of Oddi with dilation of pancreatic duct. This procedure has limited application in pancreatitis, and its use is decreasing.

B. **Side-to-side pancreaticojejunostomy (ductal drainage)**
Indicated when gross dilation of pancreatic ducts is associated with septa and calculi. The most successful procedure, with rates of 60% to 90%.

C. **Caudal pancreaticojejunostomy (ductal drainage)**
Indicated for the uncommon cases of isolated proximal pancreatic ductal stenosis not involving the ampulla.

D. **Pancreaticoduodenal resection (ablative) (with preservation of pylorus) (Whipple procedure)**
Indicated when major changes are confined to head of pancreas. Preservation of pylorus avoids usual sequelae of gastric resection.

E. **Subtotal pancreatectomy (ablative)**
Indicated when other operations fail and when ducts are unsuitable for decompression. Because metabolic sequelae are significant, this procedure is declining in popularity.

FIGURE **37-13** Surgical procedures for pancreatic cancer.

Medical Diagnosis

The most useful diagnostic tests and procedures when pancreatic cancer is suspected are computed tomography and endoscopic ultrasonography. Blood studies and other imaging procedures can be helpful as well. Blood values associated with pancreatic cancer include elevated serum amylase, lipase, bilirubin, and enzyme levels. Carcinoembryonic antigen and CA 19-9 titers are usually elevated, although CA 19-9 is more specific for pancreatic cancer than is carcinoembryonic antigen.

Percutaneous transhepatic cholangiography and ERCP allow the physician to detect obstructed pancreatic ducts and to take samples of pancreatic fluid and tissue. The patient is allowed nothing by mouth for at least 4 hours before either of these procedures. A sedative is given. Afterward, monitor vital signs for indications of bleeding. After percutaneous transhepatic cholangiography, the patient should lie on the right side for 4 hours to prevent bleeding. During ERCP, medication is used to suppress the gag reflex. Therefore do not give fluids or food to the patient who has undergone ERCP until the gag reflex returns.

Medical Treatment

Treatment depends on the location and extent of the malignant tissue. If the tumor is confined to the head of the pancreas, surgery may be an option. A variety of procedures may be used for pancreatic cancer as well as for pancreatitis. The most common are side-to-side pancreaticojejunostomy, caudal pancreaticojejunostomy, and pancreaticoduodenal resection (Whipple procedure) as illustrated in Figure 37-13. Potential complications of the Whipple procedure are listed in Table 37-10.

Sometimes surgical procedures are done primarily to relieve obstruction and improve patient comfort. Opioid anal-

table 37-10 Potential Complications of the Whipple Procedure

COMPLICATION	NURSING INTERVENTIONS
Hemorrhage	Monitor vital signs for tachycardia, falling blood pressure. Assess for restlessness. Check dressings and drains for excess or bright bleeding.
Fluid and electrolyte imbalances	Assess for cardiac dysrhythmias, muscle weakness or twitching, changes in mental status. Monitor intake and output, tissue turgor. Check laboratory reports and notify physician of abnormalities.
Respiratory failure	Monitor respiratory rate and effort, skin color, breath sounds.
Circulatory failure	Monitor for dysrhythmias, tachycardia, falling blood pressure.
Renal failure	Measure intake and urine output. Report output of less than 30 ml/hr. Assess for edema. Maintain prescribed fluid intake.
Hepatic failure	Assess for jaundice, fatigue, confusion, digestive disturbances.
Wound infection, dehiscence, and fistulas	Assess dressing and drains for excess bleeding, foul odor, purulent drainage. Check temperature for fever. Note elevation in white blood cell count.
Hyperglycemia	Monitor blood glucose as ordered. Note drowsiness, thirst, polyphagia, polyuria.

gesics are ordered for pain management. At times, a jejunostomy tube is placed below the obstruction so that the patient can be given tube feedings.

Postoperative radiation therapy and chemotherapy may prolong survival. The use of preoperative chemotherapy is also being studied. These therapies are discussed in detail in Chapter 24.

NURSING CARE *of the Patient with Pancreatic Cancer*

Assessment

General assessment of the patient with a pancreatic disorder is outlined in Table 37-7. With pancreatic cancer, pay particular attention to assessment of gastrointestinal function, pain, and emotional state. If surgery is planned, assess the patient's knowledge about pre- and postoperative care.

Nursing Diagnoses, Goals, and Outcome Criteria: Cancer of the Pancreas

Nursing Diagnoses	Goals and Outcome Criteria
Acute Pain related to obstruction, extensive malignancy	Pain relief: patient states pain reduced or relieved, more relaxed
Fear and Anticipatory Grieving related to diagnosis or poor prognosis	Reduced fear: patient states is less fearful, calm manner Family coping: family and patient make realistic plans, support each other
Imbalanced Nutrition: Less than Body Requirements related to anorexia, nausea, vomiting	Adequate nutrition: stable body weight
Impaired Skin Integrity related to pruritus, inactivity, nutritional deficiencies	Healthy skin: skin intact without reddened area or abrasions
Disturbed Body Image related to jaundice, weight loss	Effective coping with physical changes: patient makes effort to improve appearance, attends to grooming and dress
Deficient Knowledge of symptom management, self-care, and sources of support	Adequate knowledge: patient and family demonstrate understanding of patient care and resources

Interventions

In many ways, the care of the patient with pancreatic cancer is like that of the patient with pancreatitis, as discussed earlier. Chapter 24 also provides details of caring for the patient with cancer. Areas requiring special attention with pancreatic cancer are discussed here.

Acute Pain

Assess and record pain severity, nature, and location. Opioid analgesics are usually needed for severe pain management; however, non-opioids may be effective for mild to moderate pain. Radiation therapy and chemotherapy can reduce pain by shrinking the tumor. A celiac plexus nerve block can be done during surgery or percutaneously and provides excellent pain control. Other options for intolerable pain are patient-controlled analgesia (PCA) and epidural opioids. The effectiveness of drug therapy may be enhanced by distraction, imagery, and cutaneous stimulation, as discussed in Chapter 14.

Fear and Anticipatory Grieving

You can help the patient by assessing and acknowledging fear, showing compassion, teaching, and providing attentive care. A referral to a mental health professional or spiritual counselor can be made with the patient's consent.

Imbalanced Nutrition: Less than Body Requirements

Monitor the patient's dietary intake and weight. If intake is poor, consult the dietitian. Small, frequent meals may be ordered. Pancrealipase tablets are needed if the patient has malabsorption. Sometimes a jejunostomy tube is placed, and feeding is delivered by pump. Feedings are usually started with dilute formula given at a slow rate. Both the concentration and the rate are gradually increased. Inform the physician if the patient develops diarrhea. Some patients require total parenteral nutrition for adequate nourishment.

Impaired Skin Integrity

If pruritus is a problem, special skin care and protection are needed. Eliminate bath soaps and apply emollient lotions. Keep the fingernails short to reduce trauma from scratching. Supply mittens if the patient is unable to avoid scratching. The physician may order diphenhydramine (Benadryl) to reduce pruritus. If a patient has drains or fistulas, irritating digestive fluids may come in contact with the skin. Carefully cleanse the exposed skin. Skin barriers and pouches may be effective in protecting the skin. An enterostomal therapist may be consulted for advice on skin care.

Disturbed Body Image

Weight loss and jaundice alter the patient's appearance and may be distressing. Assist patients with grooming and encourage them to look their best.

Deficient Knowledge

People under stress retain only part of what they hear, so information often must be repeated and reinforced. Provide written material in addition to verbal instruction. The patient's family also may need information and support when dealing with a diagnosis of pancreatic cancer. Refer questions about medical decisions and prognosis to the physician. The specific teaching plan will depend on the diagnostic and therapeutic measures prescribed. You should advise the patient of community resources, including the American Cancer Society and home health nursing services.

Surgical Complications and Postoperative Nursing Care

In general, the postoperative care of the patient with pancreatic cancer is like that of any patient undergoing major abdominal surgery. If the Whipple procedure is performed, the patient is at risk for many complications. These include hemorrhage; fluid and electrolyte imbalances; respiratory, circulatory, renal, and hepatic failure; wound infection and dehiscence; fistulas; and hyperglycemia. Therefore ongoing nursing assessments are critical. Closely monitor vital signs, intake and output, and blood glucose values. Assess the wound for bleeding, infection, and separation of margins. Evaluate mental status to detect changes associated with electrolyte imbalances, poor circulation, and hepatic or renal failure.

Nutrition Concepts

1. People with gallbladder disease should follow a low-fat diet because fat intake usually causes pain.
2. For a person with hepatitis, the diet should be high in calories and vitamins with moderate to high protein and moderate to low fat.
3. When the liver is damaged by cirrhosis, protein may be restricted to lower blood ammonia.
4. In both hepatitis and cirrhosis, carbohydrates should provide most of the calories.
5. A bland, high-carbohydrate, high-protein, low-fat diet is recommended for pancreatitis.
6. Pancreatitis patients must avoid alcohol and spicy foods that stimulate the pancreas.

key points

- The liver plays an important role in bile production and excretion; glucose, protein, and lipid metabolism; blood coagulation; detoxification; immunity; and hormone metabolism.
- Signs of liver dysfunction include jaundice (a golden yellow skin color) and scleral icterus (yellowing of the sclera of the eyes).
- Hepatitis is liver inflammation caused by a viral infection or exposure to toxic substances; it can lead to hepatic failure.
- Nursing care of the patient with hepatitis addresses activity intolerance and impaired physical mobility, imbalanced nutrition: less than body requirements, pain, impaired skin integrity, deficient fluid volume, disturbed body image, and anxiety.
- Health care providers should be vaccinated against hepatitis B since it can be spread through contact with body fluids.
- Cirrhosis is chronic, progressive liver failure that disrupts metabolism and causes blood abnormalities, fluid and electrolyte imbalances, decreased resistance to infection, accumulation of drugs and toxins, and obstruction of blood vessels and bile ducts in the liver.
- Cirrhosis may be caused by nutritional deficiencies, toxins (including alcohol), hepatitis, biliary obstruction, and heart failure.
- Complications of cirrhosis include portal hypertension, esophageal varices, ascites, hepatic encephalopathy, and hepatorenal syndrome.
- Nursing care of the patient with cirrhosis addresses imbalanced nutrition: less than body requirements, activity intolerance, risk for impaired skin integrity, pain, ineffective breathing patterns, risk for injury, ineffective tissue perfusion, disturbed thought processes, deficient fluid volume, risk for infection, and fear.
- The only cure for end-stage liver disease is liver transplantation, which requires lifelong treatment with antirejection drugs that suppress the immune system and put the patient at risk for infection.
- Signs and symptoms of transplanted organ rejection are fever, anorexia, depression, vague abdominal pain, muscle aches, and joint pain.
- Bile is produced in the liver, stored in the gallbladder, and delivered to the intestine, where it is essential for emulsification and digestion of fats.
- Cholecystitis is inflammation of the gallbladder, usually caused by gallstones; the gallstones may obstruct bile

flow, causing symptoms from mild indigestion to nausea, chills and fever, and right upper quadrant pain that radiates to the shoulder.

- Cholelithiasis (stones in the bile) may be treated with cholecystectomy, oral bile salts, dissolution agents, lithotripsy, or endoscopic sphincterotomy.
- Nursing care of the patient with cholecystitis and cholelithiasis focuses on acute pain, deficient fluid volume, risk for impaired skin integrity, pruritus, anxiety, risk for injury, and for surgical patients, ineffective breathing patterns, and risk for infection.
- The pancreas has both an endocrine function (insulin secretion) and an exocrine function (secretion of digestive enzymes).
- Pancreatitis is inflammation of the pancreas; it can lead to pseudocyst, abscess, hypocalcemia, and pulmonary, cardiac, and renal complications.
- Nursing care of the patient with pancreatitis addresses acute pain, deficient fluid volume, risk for infection, impaired gas exchange, imbalanced nutrition: less than body requirements, anxiety, and deficient knowledge.
- Most patients with pancreatic cancer die within a year, especially if the cancer is in the body or the tail of the pancreas.
- Nursing care of the patient with pancreatic cancer usually focuses on acute pain, fear, anticipatory grieving, imbalanced nutrition: less than body requirements, impaired skin integrity, and disturbed body image.

REVIEW QUESTIONS

1. Your assessment of a hepatitis patient reveals jaundice, light-colored stools, and dark urine. These findings are typical of which phase of hepatitis?
   1. Preicteric phase
   2. Icteric phase
   3. Posticteric phase
   4. Recovery phase
2. Measures to control pruritus include:
   1. application of lubricating lotions.
   2. assisting with hot baths twice daily.
   3. vigorous massage of affected areas.
   4. administration of prescribed antibiotics.
3. Health care providers are routinely vaccinated against which of the following?
   1. Hepatitis A
   2. Hepatitis B
   3. Hepatitis C
   4. Hepatitis D
4. In the cirrhosis patient, esophageal varices and hemorrhoids are caused by which of the following?
   1. Blood vessels weakened by malnutrition
   2. Inability to conjugate and excrete bilirubin
   3. Elevated pressure in gastrointestinal blood vessels
   4. Fluid retention associated with excess aldosterone
5. A patient comes to the clinic for follow-up one month after liver transplantation. Which of the following assessment findings would concern you *most?*
   1. Heartburn
   2. Constipation
   3. Pale urine
   4. Fever
6. Which option reflects the correct sequence of bile flow from the liver to the gallbladder?
   1. Common bile duct, common hepatic duct
   2. Cystic duct, common bile duct
   3. Common hepatic duct, common bile duct
   4. Common hepatic duct, cystic duct
7. The purpose of a T-tube following cholecystectomy is to:
   1. maintain bile flow in the common bile duct.
   2. relieve pressure on the liver.
   3. divert intestinal contents from the surgical site.
   4. prevent bile leakage into the abdomen.
8. The exocrine function of the pancreas is which of the following?
   1. Storage and secretion of insulin in response to high blood glucose levels
   2. Conversion of excess blood glucose to glycogen for storage
   3. Breakdown of excessive fats and carbohydrates in the intestine
   4. Production and secretion of digestive enzymes into duodenum through a duct
9. In a patient with chronic pancreatitis, the effects of pancreatic enzyme tablets can be assessed by:
   1. monitoring daily weights.
   2. examining the stools for steatorrhea.
   3. recording urine intake and output.
   4. asking whether pain is relieved.
10. The risk of pancreatic cancer can be reduced by which of the following?
    1. Smoking cessation
    2. Increased dietary protein
    3. Regular exercise
    4. Moderate alcohol intake

CHAPTER 38 Urologic Disorders

objectives

1. List the data to be collected when assessing a patient who has a urologic disorder.
2. Describe the diagnostic tests and procedures for patients with urologic disorders.
3. Explain the nursing responsibilities for patients having tests and procedures to diagnose urologic disorders.
4. Describe the nursing responsibilities for common therapeutic measures used to treat urologic disorders.
5. Explain the pathophysiology, signs and symptoms, complications, and treatment of disorders of the kidneys, ureters, bladder, and urethra.
6. Assist in developing a nursing care plan for patients with urologic disorders.

key terms

Anuria (ă-NŪ-rē-ă, p. 755)
Azotemia (ă-zō-TĒ-mē-ă, p. 783)
Calculus (*pl.* Calculi) (KĂL-kŭ-lŭs) (KĂL-kŭ-lī, p. 755)
Cystectomy (sĭs-TĔK-tō-mē, p. 762)
Diuretic (dī-ŭr-RĒ-tĭc, p. 763)
Dysuria (dĭs-Ū-rē-ă, p. 755)
Hematuria (hĕm-ă-TŪ-rē-ă, p. 755)
Incontinence (ĭn-KŎN-tĭ-nĕns, p. 754)
Lithotomy (li-THOT-o-me, p. 772)
Lithotripsy (LĬTH-ō-trĭp-sē, p.772)
Nephrotoxic (nĕf-rō-TŎK-sĭk, p. 755)
Nocturia (nŏk-TŪ-rē-ă, p. 754)
Oliguria (ŏl-ĭ-GŪ-rē-ă, p. 755)
Polyuria (pŏl-ē-U-rē-ă, p. 755)
Uremia (ū-RĒ-mē-ă, p. 783)

The urinary tract plays a vital role in maintaining homeostasis and removing metabolic wastes. Because body systems are interdependent, disease processes in other body systems may have a direct and harmful effect on the urinary system. Similarly, urinary system diseases may affect significantly the respiratory and circulatory systems. Serious alterations in urinary function eventually affect all other systems. A person can live with one functioning kidney, but the body cannot support life with the loss of both kidneys.

ANATOMY AND PHYSIOLOGY OF THE URINARY SYSTEM

ANATOMY

The urinary system consists of two kidneys, two ureters, the bladder, and the urethra (Fig. 38-1).

Kidneys and Ureters

The kidneys are bean-shaped organs located just under and below the 12th rib near the waist in an area of the body trunk called the flank (Fig. 38-2). They each are surrounded by fibrous capsules and layers of fat. They are tightly wedged between the peritoneum, a membrane that separates them from the digestive system, and a layer of muscle in the back.

The hilus, or entry, to the kidney is located on the concave surface of the kidney near the spine (Fig. 38-3). The right and left renal arteries branch off from the abdominal artery and enter the kidneys at the hilus. The entire blood supply circulates through the kidneys every 4 to 5 minutes. Each renal vein returns filtered blood directly to the inferior vena cava. The kidney is divided into an outer layer called the cortex and an inner layer called the medulla. The cortex receives a large blood supply and is very sensitive to changes in blood pressure and blood volume. The medulla is organized into 8 to 18 pyramid-shaped structures that concentrate and collect urine and drain it into the calices. The calices then drain urine into the renal pelvis. The renal pelvis is at the center of the kidney and forms the funnel-shaped proximal end of the ureter. The ureter carries urine from the renal pelvis to the bladder.

The nephron is the functional unit of the kidney. There are 1 to 1.25 million nephrons in each kidney. The nephron is a vascular tubular system consisting of a glomerulus, a Bowman's capsule, and a tubule. The glomerulus is a mass of blood vessels tucked into the cuplike Bowman's capsule. Each tubule consists of a proximal tubule, the loop of Henle, a distal tubule, and a collecting duct (Fig. 38-4). The nephron is located mostly in the cortex of the kidney, with the loop of Henle dipping into the medulla and the collecting ducts traveling through the medulla to the calices (see Fig. 38-4).

Bladder and Urethra

The bladder is a muscular sac that readily stretches to store urine. The bladder rests on the floor of the pelvic cavity behind

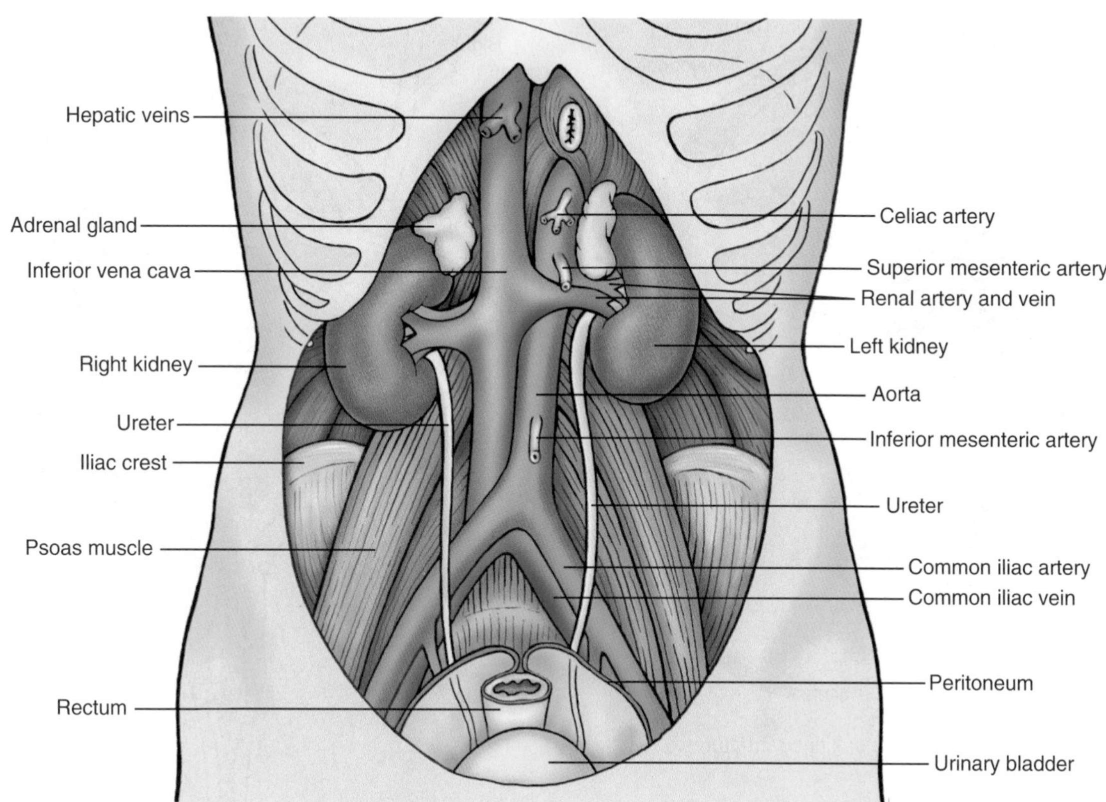

FIGURE 38-1 The kidney and related structures.

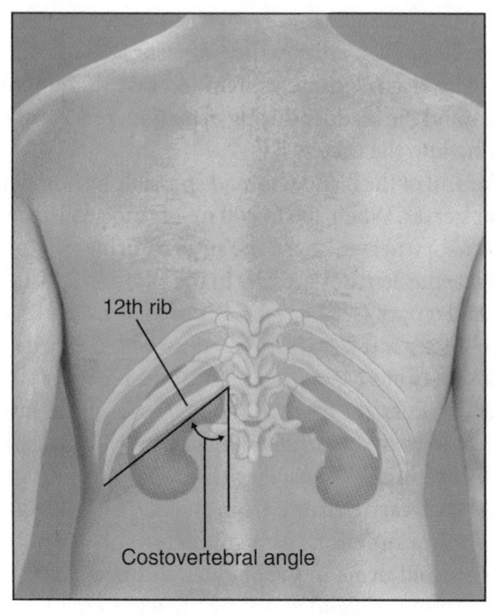

FIGURE 38-2 The kidneys are located just under and below the 12th rib. The costovertebral angle is illustrated here.

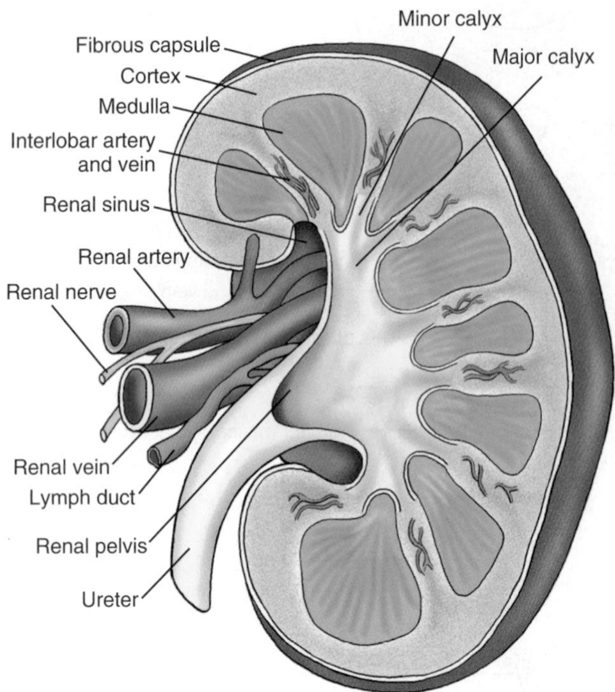

FIGURE **38-3** View of interior kidney structures.

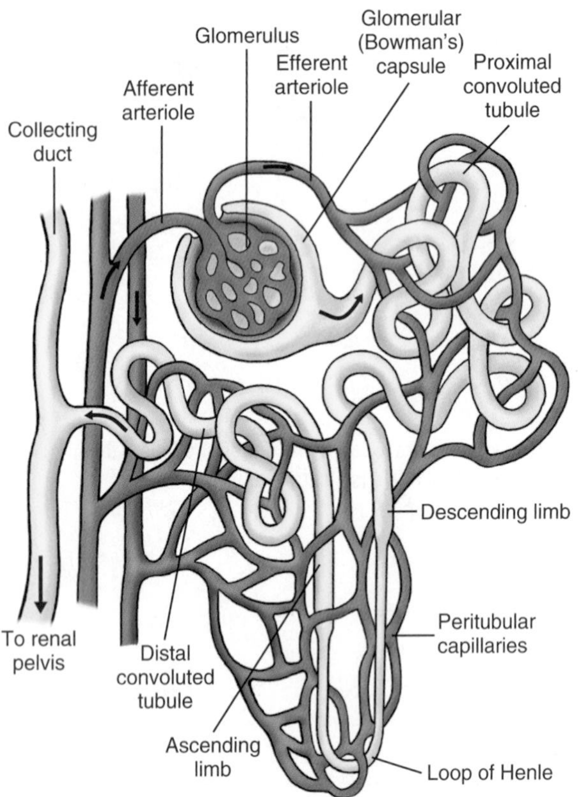

FIGURE **38-4** Details of a nephron.

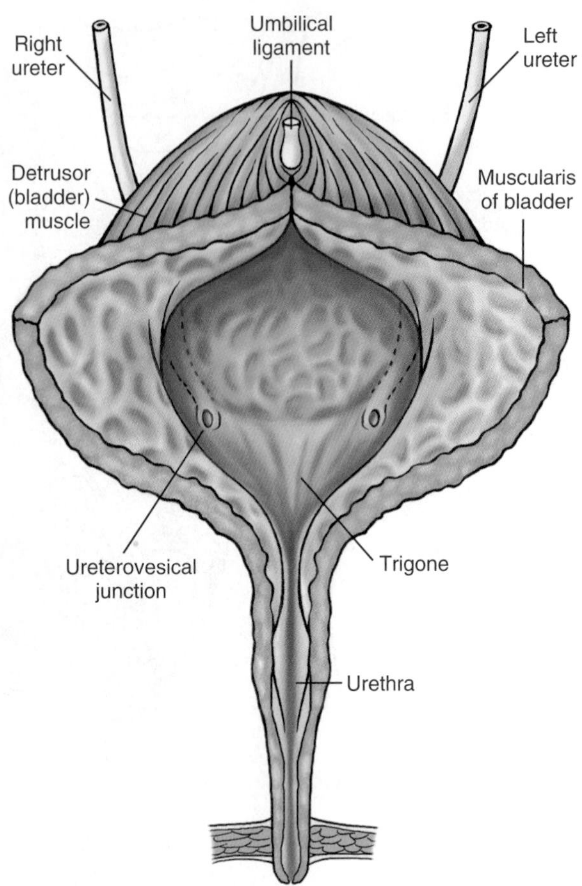

FIGURE **38-5** The urinary bladder cut to reveal the interior.

the peritoneum. It is located in front of the rectum in men and in front of the vagina and uterus in women. The upper portion of the bladder is called the apex, and the base, or fundus, is close to the pelvic floor. The bladder neck, containing the internal sphincter, is the most inferior portion. The trigone is a triangular-shaped area on the posterior wall as seen in Figure 38-5. The trigone muscles help to close the junction of the ureters and the bladder during urination, preventing backflow of urine into the ureters.

Control of the bladder is made possible by both sensory and motor nerves. When 200 to 400 ml of urine collect in the bladder, sensory nerves cause the urge to urinate. Motor nerves stimulate the detrusor muscles in the base of the bladder to contract and empty (see Fig. 38-5). Pelvic floor muscles and external sphincter muscles can be contracted voluntarily to control outflow of urine. Meanwhile, back at the junction of the ureters and the bladder, the trigonal and ureteral muscles involuntarily contract to prevent backflow of urine into the ureters.

The urethra is a muscular tube lined with mucous membranes that carries urine from the bladder out of the body. The urethra functions as a sphincter, meaning that it contracts to hold urine in the bladder and relaxes to allow urine to flow from the bladder. Approximately 3 cm of the proximal male urethra is encircled by the prostate gland. The urethra is about 20 cm long in men and 3 to 5 cm long in women. The short length and proximity of the urethra to the female anus are two reasons for the higher incidence of bladder infections in women.

PHYSIOLOGY

The functions of the urinary system are regulatory, excretory, and hormonal. Regulatory functions are performed by the formation of urine and by the secretion of renin, which affects blood pressure. Regulatory processes maintain fluid balance, keep electrolytes in normal range, and maintain acid–base balance. The excretory function of the kidney is the elimination of urine. The hormonal function is to stimulate red blood cell production.

Regulation and Excretion

Urine Production

Three processes occur in urine production: glomerular filtration, tubular reabsorption, and tubular secretion.

Glomerular filtration. Glomerular filtration is an ultrafiltration process in the glomerular capsule. Fluids, electrolytes, and other substances are filtered out of the blood as it passes through the glomerulus. Plasma proteins are too large to pass through the glomerulus and, therefore, remain in the blood. The ultrafiltration process requires adequate blood volume and blood pressure. The product of glomerular filtration is called the glomerular filtrate. It contains water, electrolytes (sodium, potassium, calcium, magnesium, chloride, bicarbonate, phosphate, and other anions), glucose, urea, creatinine, uric acid, and amino acids. Glomerular filtrate and blood plasma are essentially the same except that the filtrate does not have proteins. Most of the filtrate is returned to the blood from the tubules by reabsorption.

Tubular reabsorption. Water, some electrolytes, and nonelectrolytes are reabsorbed from the tubules of the kidney back into the blood as needed to maintain normal fluid balance. Reabsorption occurs through diffusion, active transport, and osmosis. Some nonelectrolytes (urea, creatinine, and uric acid) are not readily reabsorbed and are excreted in the urine. The reabsorption of water reflects the ability of the kidney to concentrate or dilute urine as necessary. The amount of water reabsorbed is influenced by antidiuretic hormone and aldosterone. Antidiuretic hormone, stored in the posterior pituitary, affects the amount of water reabsorbed in the distal tubules and the collecting ducts. If blood volume decreases or blood osmolality (concentration) increases, antidiuretic hormone is secreted from the posterior pituitary. The distal tubules and collecting ducts of the kidney become more permeable to water, so that reabsorption back into the circulating blood increases and urine becomes more concentrated.

Tubular secretion. Potassium and hydrogen ions are secreted into the tubules from the blood. This secretion process regulates serum potassium levels and is the basis for the kidney's acid–base regulating mechanism. The normal pH of urine is 4.5 to 8.0.

The kidneys and lungs work together to maintain the acid–base balance of the body. The lungs excrete CO_2, a volatile acid, and the kidneys excrete fixed acids produced by normal metabolism. Base levels are maintained by renal conservation of bicarbonate, excretion of sodium for hydrogen, and excretion of ammonia.

The end product of glomerular filtration, tubular reabsorption, and tubular excretion is urine. Urine is composed mostly of water, sodium, potassium, chloride, urea, creati-

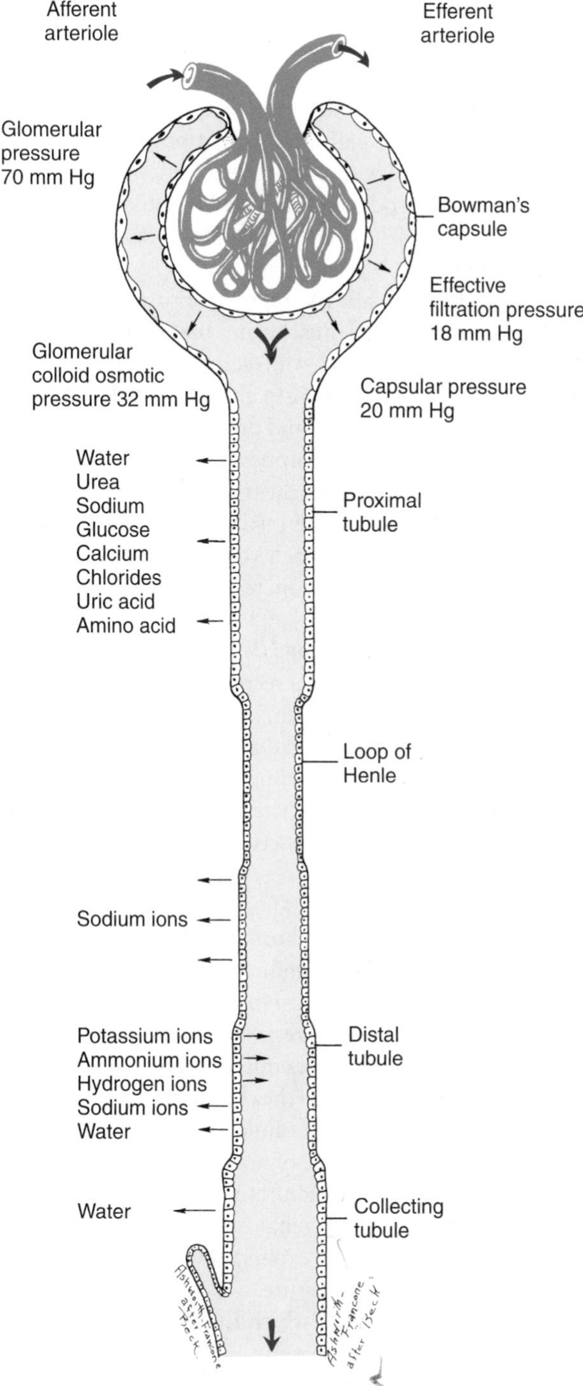

FIGURE **38-6** Urine production.

nine, and uric acid. The body normally excretes 1 to 2 L of urine each day, which is approximately 1% of the blood filtered by the glomeruli in the same period of time. Glucose and proteins are substances present in blood but not normally present in the urine. Normally, glucose is completely reabsorbed in the tubules. The presence of proteins in urine indicates glomerular damage. Urine is delivered to the renal pelvis, where it flows into the ureter. The production of urine is illustrated in Figure 38-6.

Urine Elimination

Peristaltic waves move urine from the kidney through the ureter to the bladder. The presence of 200 to 400 ml of urine in the bladder causes the urge to urinate, although the bladder can distend to hold several times that amount. Urination is a complex process that is under a variety of neural controls and is voluntary for the toilet-trained person with intact motor and sensory nerve pathways. Urination generally occurs five to six times a day and may occur once at night. The amount of urine produced is affected by fluid intake, temperature, diaphoresis, vomiting, diarrhea, and medications such as diuretics.

A series of events allows the release of urine from the bladder. The pelvic floor muscles and the urethral sphincter relax. The trigonal muscles contract, closing the ureters to prevent backflow of urine into the ureters. The bladder muscle (detrusor) contracts, and urine is forced through the urethra. After the bladder empties, the bladder muscle relaxes, the bladder neck closes, the trigonal muscles relax, and the perineal muscles resume resting tone. Voiding is primarily an involuntary reflex act. Voluntary control of voiding is exhibited in the initiation, restraint, and interruption of urine flow.

Regulation of Serum Calcium and Phosphate

Parathormone is a hormone secreted by the parathyroid glands to maintain serum calcium levels. When serum calcium is low, parathormone is secreted and acts on the tubules to promote reabsorption of calcium ions. At the same time, tubular reabsorption of phosphate is decreased. This mechanism helps to maintain normal serum calcium and phosphate levels.

Regulation of Blood Pressure

Blood pressure is regulated through fluid volume maintenance and release of the hormone renin from the kidneys. One way to raise or lower blood pressure is to change blood volume. This can be done by retaining additional fluid or by eliminating excess fluid. For example, suppose a patient has had severe vomiting and diarrhea resulting in dehydration and low blood pressure. Hypertonic plasma caused by dehydration stimulates the release of antidiuretic hormone from the posterior pituitary. Antidiuretic hormone causes reabsorption of water from the renal tubules, decreasing urine volume. The retained fluid expands blood volume, with a subsequent rise in blood pressure.

A second mechanism by which the kidneys affect blood pressure is the secretion of renin. Renin is released in response to inadequate renal blood flow or low arterial pressure. Renin acts on angiotensinogen, a hormone produced by the liver, and converts it to angiotensin I. A lung enzyme converts angiotensin I to angiotensin II. Angiotensin II is a powerful peripheral vasoconstrictor. Also, angiotensin II triggers the release of aldosterone from the adrenal cortex. Aldosterone stimulates tubular reabsorption of sodium and water, and plasma volume is expanded.

With severely decreased cardiac output, as seen in hemorrhage and shock, the renal arteries constrict to prevent fluid loss and to shunt blood to more vital organs (heart, lungs, brain). This vasoconstriction limits renal blood flow. If blood flow is not restored, death of renal tissue may occur.

Hormonal Stimulation of Red Blood Cell Production

Erythropoietin is secreted in the kidneys and stimulates the bone marrow to produce red blood cells. This process is triggered by decreased oxygen in renal blood. Patients in renal failure have a deficiency of erythropoietin, which causes them to become anemic.

AGE-RELATED CHANGES IN THE URINARY SYSTEM

As people age, significant changes occur in the urinary system. Fortunately, the kidneys have enough reserve that normal function is usually maintained. When older people are stressed, however, the kidneys do not adapt as well as they do in younger people.

Structural changes in the kidney include loss of nephrons, thickening of membranes in nephrons, and sclerosis of renal blood vessels. As a result of these changes, renal blood flow and glomerular filtration decline. In addition, plasma renin and aldosterone levels fall and tubules are less responsive to antidiuretic hormone. As a result of all these changes, the older person's kidneys are less able to concentrate and dilute urine in response to changes in serum osmolality (concentration).

Creatinine clearance decreases with age. This means that the rate at which the kidneys are able to remove creatinine from the blood is diminished. Creatinine clearance is a better indicator of kidney function than serum creatinine. There also is some decline in erythropoietin, a factor that may contribute to anemia. In an older person, serum glucose may be considerably elevated before it is detected in the urine.

In younger people, urine production peaks during waking hours. This pattern is lost with age such that urine production does not decrease at night. Therefore, older people often have **nocturia**, meaning that they awaken from sleep to void.

The bladder also undergoes changes with age. Bladder muscles weaken, and connective tissue increases. The effect is decreased capacity and incomplete emptying. The mechanism that prevents the reflux of urine from the bladder into the ureters is less effective and can contribute to kidney infections.

Incontinence is not a normal consequence of age, but it is common. Female urinary incontinence is often caused by relaxed pelvic muscles related to childbirth trauma and lack of estrogen after menopause. For detailed information on incontinence, see Chapter 22. In men, urethral obstruction is more often a problem. It is often caused by the enlarged prostate closing in on the urethra. Prostate enlargement is discussed in Chapter 46.

NURSING ASSESSMENT OF THE URINARY SYSTEM

Elimination is considered to be a very personal activity, and people are not accustomed to discussing it with others. Assessment of urinary function and problems, therefore, may be embarrassing to the patient. Privacy and a calm, accepting manner help put the patient at ease.

HEALTH HISTORY

Chief Complaint

Begin the assessment by exploring what caused the patient to seek health care. Patients with urinary problems most often report changes in urine quality or quantity, pain, or changes in urination.

History of Present Illness

Assess the patient's normal or usual pattern of urination. Important data include volume of urine, frequency of voiding, and appearance of urine. The patient may have difficulty estimating the amount of urine voided but usually can recognize an increase or decrease from normal. If intake and output records are available, note the recent pattern. Terms used to describe urine volume are *polyuria, oliguria,* and *anuria.* **Polyuria** refers to a large urine output, **oliguria** to a low output, and **anuria** to the absence of output. Urine characteristics to record include color, clarity (clear or cloudy), presence of particles, and odor. *Hematuria* is the presence of blood in the urine.

Pain may or may not occur, but it is more common with acute conditions. Painful urination is called *dysuria.* Assess the presence of pain or discomfort. Describe the characteristics of the pain: intensity, location, distribution, onset, duration, frequency, relationship to urination, precipitating factors, and measures that provide relief. Urologic conditions also may cause pain in the flank, abdomen, pelvic area, and genitalia. The pain may be so severe that it causes nausea and vomiting.

Include questions about any problem the patient has had initiating or controlling urination. Document circumstances under which these problems occur. For example, involuntary loss of urine with laughing or sneezing is typical of stress incontinence. Urge incontinence is the inability to hold urine when feeling the urge to void.

Past Medical History

After the present illness has been fully described, explore the patient's past medical history. Significant findings include a history of streptococcal infections, recurrent urinary tract infections (UTIs), renal **calculi** ("stones"), gout, or hypercalcemia. Ask if the patient has had urologic surgery, catheterization, examination (e.g., cystoscopy or radiography), or trauma, and if the patient uses any type of urinary diversion or collection device. Document recent and current medications, including prescription and over-the-counter drugs and herbal remedies, because some medications are **nephrotoxic** (harmful to the kidneys). Assess exposure to toxic chemicals in the home or the workplace.

PHARMACOLOGY CAPSULE Nephrotoxic drugs are harmful to the kidneys.

Family History

Assess the patient's family medical history. Important conditions to note are congenital kidney problems such as polycystic kidneys or urinary tract malformations, diabetes mellitus, and hypertension.

Review of Systems

Review the body systems to detect other problems that may be related to the urinary tract complaints. Ask if the patient has had changes in skin color, respiratory distress, edema, fatigue, nausea, vomiting, chills, and fever.

Functional Assessment

The functional assessment includes information about habits and practices that might affect or contribute to urinary tract disorders. Assess daily fluid intake because urine production varies with fluid intake. It is also helpful to determine the patient's usual exercise pattern because excessive exercise or prolonged immobility affects the urinary system. Determine the effects of the chief complaint on daily life as well.

PHYSICAL EXAMINATION

Begin the physical examination with inspection of the skin for color (ashen, yellow) and the presence of crystals on the skin (uremic frost). Evaluate tissue turgor to detect dehydration or edema. Examine the area around the eyes for periorbital edema, which suggests fluid retention. Inspect the mouth for moisture and odor. Patients in renal failure may have an odor of urine on their breath.

Observe respiratory rate, pattern, and effort. Respirations may be rapid with metabolic acidosis, infection, and fluid overload. Kussmaul respirations, seen with metabolic acidosis, are rapid and deep. Dyspnea may be evident with fluid overload. Auscultate the lungs for crackles or rhonchi that may indicate fluid overload. Heart rhythm irregularities may be noted with potassium imbalances.

Inspect the abdomen for scars and contours and palpate for tenderness and bladder distention. Auscultate the kidney area over the costovertebral angle (see Fig. 38-2) to detect renal bruits (swishing sounds caused by turbulent blood flow). Renal bruits indicate renal artery stenosis (narrowing). Then percuss the abdomen. A dull sound may be heard over a full bladder. Pain may be elicited over one or both kidneys.

Observe for edema throughout the examination. With renal failure, edema is generalized, not dependent. The skin may be dry, flushed, and shiny over the edematous area.

The last part of the physical examination is inspection of the genitalia. Standard precautions should be observed. Examine the penis for lesions, scars, or discharge. If there are penile lesions or urethral discharge, smears should be obtained for culture. A nurse with advanced skills or the physician also may perform rectal and pelvic examinations, especially if symptoms suggest problems of the reproductive system. The pelvic examination may reveal gynecologic rather than urologic problems. The male rectal examination helps

table 38-1 ASSESSMENT *of Urologic Function*

HEALTH HISTORY

Present Illness: Changes in urine quality or quantity, voiding pattern, pain
Past Medical History: Streptococcal infections, urinary tract infections or calculi, gout, hypercalcemia, urologic surgery or instrumentation, urinary diversion, recent and current medications
Family History: Urinary disorders, diabetes mellitus, hypertension
Review of Systems: Fatigue, pruritus, dyspnea; urine quantity: polyuria, oliguria, anuria; urine quality: color, odor, components; frequency of voiding; pain: onset, intensity, frequency, location, duration, precipitating and relieving factors
Functional Assessment: Fluid intake, diet, activity

PHYSICAL EXAMINATION

General Appearance: Level of consciousness, orientation
Vital Signs
Height and Weight
Skin: Color, moisture, turgor, crystals
Respirations: Rate, pattern, effort, breath sounds
Circulation: Dysrhythmias, blood pressure alterations
Abdomen: Scars, contour, tenderness, bruits
Genitalia: Lesions, scars, discharge

detect prostate enlargement, which often creates problems with voiding. Nursing assessment of urologic function is outlined in Table 38-1.

DIAGNOSTIC TESTS AND PROCEDURES

Diagnostic tests and procedures for urinary disorders are described here. Related nursing care is presented in Table 38-2.

URINE TESTS

Urinalysis

A urine specimen is examined for color, pH, specific gravity, glucose, protein, blood, ketones, and bilirubin. Normal urine is straw colored and slightly acidic. Microscopic examination is used to assess for cells, casts, bacteria, and crystals. Chemical examination to assess electrolytes and osmolality (concentration) of the urine determines the ability of the kidneys to excrete or conserve electrolytes and water. By comparing the osmolality of urine with serum osmolality, it is possible to know if the kidneys are functioning appropriately. If serum osmolality is elevated, the kidneys should reabsorb or conserve water to dilute the serum and excrete more concentrated urine (i.e., urine with high osmolality). If serum osmolality is low (urine is dilute), the kidneys should reduce reabsorption of water to increase serum concentration and produce more dilute urine (i.e., urine with low osmolality). Specific gravity is a measure of osmolality. Data reported from a routine urinalysis are summarized in Table 38-3.

Urine Culture and Sensitivity

Normal urine is sterile. A urine culture permits identification of microorganisms present in the urine. Sensitivity testing determines which antibiotics will be effective against the specific organisms. The specimen can be obtained by the patient, if able, or the nurse. Instructions are given in Table 38-2.

Creatinine Clearance

Creatinine clearance, the rate at which the kidney removes creatinine from the blood, is the best test of overall kidney function. It serves as an estimate of glomerular filtration rate. This test requires collection of all urine for 12 or 24 hours, as ordered. Normal levels vary for men and women. Because values depend on muscle mass, they are usually lower in women. Urine and serum creatinine levels are compared to determine kidney function. If serum creatinine rises and urine creatinine falls, it is an indication of decreased kidney function and glomerular filtration rate.

BLOOD TESTS

Blood Urea Nitrogen

The blood urea nitrogen test is a general indicator of the kidneys' ability to excrete urea, an end product of protein metabolism. In addition to renal failure, factors that increase blood urea nitrogen (BUN) are a high-protein diet (especially with renal disease), gastrointestinal bleeding, dehydration, and some drugs (aspirin, chemotherapeutic agents, diuretics, gentamicin, lithium carbonate, morphine, steroids, sulfonamides, and tobramycin).

Serum Creatinine

Creatinine is a waste product of skeletal muscle breakdown. The level of creatinine in the blood is an indication of the kidneys' ability to excrete wastes. Serum creatinine is elevated only in renal disorders and is a better measurement of kidney function than BUN. Unlike BUN, creatinine is not influenced by diet, hydration, nutritional status, or liver function. With normally functioning kidneys, the serum creatinine level is very low and the urine level is high. The normal ratio of BUN to creatinine is 10:1.

Serum Electrolytes

Serum electrolytes must be monitored in the renal patient because imbalances can have very serious consequences. In renal failure, sodium and potassium levels are elevated and calcium levels are decreased.

RADIOGRAPHIC TESTS AND PROCEDURES

Flat Plate

A flat plate radiograph of the abdomen, or KUB (for kidneys, ureters, and bladder), provides a general outline of the kidneys, revealing their approximate size and contour. Tu-

table 38-2 **DIAGNOSTIC TESTS AND PROCEDURES | *Urinary Disorders***

TEST/PURPOSE	PATIENT PREPARATION	POSTPROCEDURE NURSING CARE
LABORATORY STUDIES		
General Considerations: Check agency manual for specific instructions. Tell the patient that a sample (blood, urine, etc) is needed and why. Determine whether the patient needs to fast before the sample is obtained. Urine specimens should be sent to the lab promptly; refrigerate if there is a delay. For blood studies, apply small dressing to venipuncture site. Apply pressure if oozing persists or if patient's blood does not clot normally. For urine samples, instruct patient or assist in sample collection.		
Urine culture and sensitivity: Culture identifies microorganisms in urine. Sensitivity determines which antibiotic will be effective. Normal: no growth. Results in 24-36 hr.	Collect specimen of first voided urine of day. Instruct patient in midstream, clean-catch technique: Cleanse penis or vulva thoroughly, void a small amount, stop the urine stream, and then void into a sterile container. If catheterization is necessary, collect the specimen after discarding a small amount of urine. Cap the container and immediately send it to the laboratory. If delivery is delayed, refrigerate the specimen.	Cap specimen and refrigerate or send to laboratory.
Blood urea nitrogen: Indicates kidneys' ability to excrete urea, an end product of protein metabolism. Increases with renal failure, GI bleeding, dehydration, and some drugs. Decreases with alcohol abuse, acromegaly, inadequate protein, hemodialysis, and some drugs.	No special preparation.	
Urine creatinine clearance: Estimates glomerular filtration rate. Decreases with renal disease. Normal value: varies with patient gender and age (usually lower in women).	Provide specimen container. Document first void and save all urine for next 12 or 24 hr as ordered. Keep specimen refrigerated. If patient has a Foley catheter, place drainage bag in basin of ice and empty into refrigerated container hourly.	
Serum creatinine: Measures kidneys' ability to excrete waste based on amount of creatinine in blood. Normal values: varies with method used; should be small. Increased with impaired renal function, urinary obstruction, muscle disease. Decreased with muscular dystrophy.	Patient should avoid strenuous exercise for 8 hours and excessive red meat for 24 hours before the test.	
Serum electrolytes: Detects alterations reflecting inability of kidney to retain or excrete electrolytes. Sodium and potassium elevated and calcium decreased in renal failure. Normal values: see Chapter 13.	No special preparation.	Check laboratory reports and notify physician of abnormalities. Electrolyte imbalances can be life threatening. See Chapter 13 for details on specific electrolytes.

Continued

table 38-2 **DIAGNOSTIC TESTS AND PROCEDURES | *Urinary Disorders—cont'd***

TEST/PURPOSE	PATIENT PREPARATION	POSTPROCEDURE NURSING CARE
ULTRASOUND (US)		
Abdominal and renal US: Uses sound waves to detect cysts, tumors, urinary calculi, urinary tract malformations or obstructions. Can be used to guide needle insertion for closed biopsy.	Patient may have to drink a specified amount of water (typically 3-4 8-oz glasses of water within 2 hr of the procedure) so that bladder will be full during ultrasound. Tell patient that procedure is painless except for discomfort of full bladder. Takes about 15 min. Enema usually given if transrectal route used. For transabdominal route, gel is applied to skin, and an instrument is moved over the lubricated skin surface. Images are recorded for study. Patient instructions will vary if other routes are used.	Wash gel off skin if transabdominal route used.
RADIOGRAPHIC STUDIES		
General Interventions: Explain the test to the patient. Radiation exposure is generally contraindicated during pregnancy. If the contrast medium contains iodine, ask whether the patient is allergic to iodine or shellfish. Inform the radiologist of such allergies. Some patients who are allergic react to contrast medium because they are allergic to iodine. Patients who are allergic to seafood, which is high in iodine, also may be allergic to contrast medium. Itching, hives, wheezing, and respiratory distress are symptoms of an allergic reaction. Allergic reactions are treated by discontinuing the administration of the contrast, giving antihistamines, and administering cardiopulmonary resuscitation if necessary. The patient can expect a flushed, warm feeling, a salty taste in the mouth, and maybe nausea when the contrast medium is injected. The procedure takes about 45 minutes.		
Flat plate (KUB [kidneys/ureters/bladder]): Provides radiographic view of kidneys, ureters, and bladder.	No special preparation. Schedule before studies that use contrast media.	No special care.
Intravenous pyelogram (IVP): Uses x-rays and fluoroscope to outline kidneys. Uses contrast medium to show urine flow and obstructions. Detects urinary abnormalities, calculi, ureters, and bladder.	Tell patient that "dye" will be injected and radiographs taken to study urinary tract. Give laxatives and enemas as ordered before test. NPO 8-10 hr.	Encourage fluids to flush contrast medium from body. Monitor for signs of iodine allergy: urticaria, rash, nausea, swollen parotid glands. Check injection site for inflammation.
Angiogram: Uses radiographs and contrast medium to examine blood vessels of kidney.	Tell patient that physician will insert catheter into blood vessel (usually in groin) and inject "dye." Radiographs are then taken as dye circulates through kidneys. Usual preparation: NPO for 8-12 hr, laxatives and enemas. Anticoagulant drugs withheld before test to reduce risk of bleeding. Signed consent required. Premedicate if ordered. Have patient void before sedation.	Assess for signs of bleeding: tachycardia, dyspnea, restlessness, abdominal or flank pain. Check injection site for bleeding. A pressure dressing should be in place. Monitor respiratory status if sedated. EKG monitoring may be ordered. Monitor pulse, color, warmth and sensation of extremity in which catheter was inserted. Maintain bedrest as ordered. Encourage fluids to eliminate dye. Measure intake and output.

NPO, Nothing by mouth.

table 38-2 **DIAGNOSTIC TESTS AND PROCEDURES | *Urinary Disorders—cont'd***

TEST/PURPOSE	PATIENT PREPARATION	POSTPROCEDURE NURSING CARE
RADIOGRAPHIC STUDIES—cont'd		
Renal scan: Uses radioisotopes and x-rays to study renal blood flow. Detects infarctions, trauma, atherosclerosis, transplant rejection, some renal diseases.	Tell patient that isotope will be injected and radiographs taken. Takes about 1 hr. Radiation dose is small and quickly eliminated.	No special care unless patient is incontinent. Then, wear gloves to handle urine and change linens. Discard per agency protocol. Continent patients can use toilet. Pregnant caregivers should avoid these patients for 24 hr.
INVASIVE PROCEDURES		
Renal biopsy: Excision of small amount of kidney tissue for examination. May be obtained through incision (open biopsy) or with special needle (closed biopsy).	Physician explains procedure selected. For closed biopsy, patient is positioned prone with rolled blanket under abdomen for approximately 45 min. Be sure reports of clotting studies (prothrombin time, partial thromboplastin time, platelets) are on chart. Report elevated blood pressure, which increases the risk of bleeding. NPO 6 hr or as ordered. Signed consent required.	Check pressure dressing for bleeding. Monitor vital signs for hemorrhage: tachycardia, restlessness, flank pain radiating to abdomen. Position supine with blanket roll or sandbag under flank area. Bedrest for 24 hr. Advise patient to do no heavy lifting, exercise, or sports for 1-2 wk. Hemoglobin and hematocrit are checked at 6 and 24 hr after the biopsy.
Cystoscopy: Uses lighted cystoscope inserted through the urethra to see urethra, bladder, and ureteral openings. Allows diagnosis of problems, removal of bladder calculi, biopsy, some treatments. Local or general anesthesia may be used. Dye may be injected into kidneys through ureters (retrograde pyelography).	Signed consent required. Tell patient that procedure is done in operating room or special room under sterile conditions. For local anesthesia, liquids may be allowed; NPO before general anesthesia. Laxatives or enemas as ordered. Give medications as ordered to reduce anxiety and bladder spasms. Antibiotics may be ordered 2-3 days before procedure and continued several days afterwards.	Safety precautions first time up, because orthostatic hypotension is common. Monitor intake and output, vital signs, urine color; urine may be pink tinged to wine colored; lightens to usual color in 24-48 hr. Report severe pain. Give prescribed analgesics or antispasmodics as ordered or assist with sitz baths for pain or urinary frequency. Encourage 2-3 L of fluids daily. Tell patient that pink-tinged urine is expected for 1-2 days.
URODYNAMIC STUDIES		
Cystogram and cystourethrogram: Uses dye injected into bladder through catheter followed by radiographs to outline bladder and demonstrate reflux of urine from bladder to ureters.	For voiding cystourethrogram, bladder and urethra are radiographed during urination. Rate of urine flow is measured. Tell patient that catheter will be inserted and dye instilled into bladder.	Monitor urine output and vital signs. Encourage increased fluids unless contraindicated. Observe for allergic reaction to dye. Assess for urinary retention.
Cystometrogram: Evaluates bladder tone.	Tell patient fluid will be instilled into bladder through urethral catheter. When patient feels urge to void, catheter will be removed. Patient voids, and residual urine is measured. Drugs may be given to test bladder response.	Encourage increased fluids unless contraindicated. Monitor intake and output. Administer drugs as ordered for bladder spasms.

table 38-3 Urinalysis Data

COMPONENTS	NORMAL VALUES	IMPLICATIONS OF ABNORMAL VALUES
Color	Light yellow to amber	Dilute, colorless: overhydration, diabetes insipidus, diabetes mellitus, chronic renal failure Concentrated dark amber: dehydration, some medications or foods Bright red: gross hematuria in acid urine Tea colored: gross hematuria in alkaline urine
Appearance	Clear	Cloudy, hazy: bacteria, pus, small amount of blood
pH	4.5-8.0	<5.0: acidosis, starvation, diarrhea >7.0: alkalosis, bacteriuria, UTI
Specific gravity	1.010-1.025	<1.005: diabetes insipidus, overhydration, renal disease, severe hypokalemia >1.030: dehydration, diabetes mellitus
Protein	Up to 8 mg/dL; reagent strip negative	>8 mg/dL: exercise, severe stress, fever, renal disease, malignancy
Glucose	Negative	Positive: diabetes mellitus, stroke, Cushing's syndrome, anesthesia, severe stress
Ketones	Negative	Positive: diabetes mellitus, starvation, excessive protein ingestion
Bilirubin	Negative	Positive: liver disease (jaundice)
MICROSCOPIC EXAMINATION		
RBCs	0-2.0	>2.0 (hematuria): kidney trauma, renal disease, anticoagulants
WBCs	0-4.0	>4.0: UTI, strenuous exercise
Casts	Negative to occasional hyaline casts	Positive: fever, renal disease, heart failure
Crystals	Negative	Positive: renal stone formation
Bacteria	Negative	Positive: UTI

RBCs, Red blood cells; *UTI*, urinary tract infection; *WBCs*, white blood cells.

mors, malformations, and calculi may be found with this type of radiograph. This procedure requires no special preparation or aftercare. It is not done on pregnant patients, and it should be done before any other studies that require contrast media.

Intravenous Pyelogram

An intravenous pyelogram (IVP) is a diagnostic procedure in which a radiographic contrast medium ("dye") is injected intravenously. Radiographs of the kidneys, ureters, and bladder are taken at 5- to 15-minute intervals. As the contrast is concentrated by the kidneys and excreted through the ureters into the bladder, kidney function and structures, ureter size and patency, bladder size and shape, and presence of calculi (stones) or other obstructions can be assessed. The procedure is contraindicated in elderly patients with known renal insufficiency and in patients with diabetes mellitus or multiple myeloma.

Angiogram

A renal angiogram permits study of the renal blood vessels. It is used to diagnose renal artery stenosis, aneurysms, vascular tumors, renal cysts, and renal infarctions. In angiography, a catheter is inserted through the femoral artery and threaded into the aorta. A contrast medium is injected into each renal artery, and radiographs are taken as the contrast passes through the kidneys.

Renal Scan

A renal scan indicates the size, shape, and location of the kidneys; detects renal infarction, atherosclerosis, trauma, or rejection of a transplant; and identifies primary renal disease. An intravenous radioisotope is injected, and radiographs are taken to demonstrate blood flow to each kidney. The test is not done on pregnant women but can be used for patients who are allergic to contrast containing iodine.

ULTRASONOGRAPHY

Ultrasonography (ultrasound) uses high-frequency sound waves to create images of the bladder. It is used to detect urinary tract malformations and obstructions, tumors, renal calculi, perineal fluid accumulation, and cysts. Ultrasound also may be used to guide a needle inserted to aspirate specimens from cysts or tumors. The bladder should be full for visualization of organs and tissues. The procedure may be done through the abdominal wall (transabdominal), the rectum (transrectal), the urethra (transurethral), or the vagina (transvaginal). Preparation and patient instructions are specific for each approach.

INVASIVE PROCEDURES

Renal Biopsy

A renal biopsy is performed to obtain a specimen of renal tissue for direct microscopic examination. It is usually done to evaluate conditions leading to renal failure. The procedure may be done through open or closed methods. The open method is a surgical procedure in which an incision is made in the flank, and a specimen of kidney tissue is removed. The closed procedure involves insertion of a needle under fluoroscopy or ultrasonography to aspirate the tissue specimen. For the closed procedure, the patient must be able to lie in the prone position with a blanket roll under the lower abdomen for up to 45 minutes. Patients with breathing problems may not be able to tolerate this position or alter their breathing patterns as needed during the procedure.

The most serious complication of a renal biopsy is hemorrhage. If bleeding is suspected, the patient is given intravenous fluids to restore fluid volume. Persistent bleeding may require surgery.

Cystoscopy

Cystoscopy is the direct visualization of the interior of the urethra, bladder, and ureteral orifices. The procedure may be done in the physician's office for diagnostic reasons, or in an outpatient facility for diagnostic or treatment purposes under local or general anesthesia. As a diagnostic procedure, the cystoscopy allows the physician to observe lesions, locate sources of bleeding, and take biopsy samples. Treatments that can be done with this procedure include cauterization of lesions; removal of calculi, tumors, or foreign materials; implantation of radium seeds; insertion of ureteral catheters; and control of bleeding. A lighted tube called a cystoscope is inserted through the urethra into the bladder under sterile conditions. Retrograde pyelography, which involves injecting contrast into the ureters, also can be done during cystoscopy.

Back pain, bladder spasms, urinary frequency, and burning on urination are common following cystoscopy. Mild analgesics may bring relief. Belladonna and opium suppositories may be ordered to reduce bladder spasms. Bladder perforation is rare but should be suspected if the patient has severe abdominal pain.

URODYNAMIC STUDIES

Urodynamic studies are performed to determine the physiology of urination. The studies assess innervation of the bladder, incontinence, and other variations in urinary patterns. Urodynamic studies measure the rate and volume of urine flow during voiding. The rate of flow is decreased with obstruction or decreased innervation.

Cystogram and Voiding Cystourethrogram

The cystogram outlines the contour of the bladder and shows reflux or backflow of urine from the bladder into the ureters. Cystograms are useful in diagnosing neurogenic bladders, fistulas, tumors, and ruptured bladders. For a cystogram, a catheter is inserted into the bladder, contrast is injected, then radiographs are taken.

A voiding cystourethrogram gives the physician additional information on urethral disorders during voiding. The bladder is filled with contrast, and radiographs are taken during and after urination. This procedure may be embarrassing for the patient. Explain the need for the test and provide as much privacy as possible during the procedure.

Cystometrogram

The cystometrogram is used to evaluate bladder tone in the patient with incontinence or with a neurogenic bladder. A catheter is inserted into the bladder, and fluid is instilled until the patient reports the urge to void. When the patient feels urgency, the catheter is removed, the patient voids, and residual urine is measured. Drugs may be given to see if they effectively enhance or relax bladder tone in the individual patient.

COMMON THERAPEUTIC MEASURES

CATHETERIZATION

Catheterization is the introduction of a catheter through the urethra into the bladder for the purpose of draining urine. Catheters are inserted when patients are unable to void as a result of the effects of anesthesia, paralysis, trauma, unconsciousness, certain surgical procedures, and other factors that inhibit voiding. The major concern with catheterization is the potential for introduction of bacteria into the normally sterile bladder. Catheterization is the primary cause of nosocomial (hospital acquired) infections. Therefore, it is essential that strict aseptic techniques be followed when catheterization is necessary.

Urinary catheters are available in a variety of sizes for adults (generally from the small 12 French to the larger 20 French) and may be of a retaining or nonretaining design. Examples of retaining catheters are the coudé, Foley, Malecot, and Pezzer. A retaining catheter is one that has a device, like an inflatable balloon, that anchors the catheter in the bladder. Robinson and whistle-tip catheters are nonretaining or straight catheters. Nurses are most familiar with Foley catheters that have either double or triple lumina. Malecot and Pezzer catheters are used most often as suprapubic catheters.

Occasionally, patients are catheterized to measure residual urine. This procedure may be diagnostic, but it is often part of a bladder training program for patients who have lost control over bladder function. To measure residual volume, the patient must be catheterized immediately after voiding. Less than 50 ml of residual urine is considered normal.

The reader should refer to a fundamentals textbook for detailed information on the insertion and care of urethral catheters. Key points to remember when catheterization is necessary are:

1. Catheterize only after other noninvasive measures have failed or when absolutely necessary for diagnostic purposes.
2. Use sterile technique and equipment to insert the catheter.
3. With an indwelling catheter, do the following:
   a. Secure the tubing to the female patient's inner thigh, or to the male patient's abdomen.

b. Handle the catheter gently to avoid trauma to the urethra.
c. Keep the urine collection bag below the level of the patient's bladder and the tubing in a circular fashion *on* the bed.
d. Keep the drainage system closed as much as possible.
e. Provide perineal care twice daily (*Note:* Antibiotic ointments are not recommended).
f. Use standard precautions before and after handling the catheter.

URETERAL CATHETER

A ureteral catheter is threaded through a ureter into the renal pelvis. It can be inserted through the bladder during cystoscopy or through an abdominal incision. A ureteral catheter permits urine to flow through the swollen ureter after traumatic surgery. The catheter is connected to a drainage system, and output is measured frequently. Record output from this catheter separately from other urine output. Make certain that the catheter is not kinked or clamped because pressure would build up in the kidney, causing tissue damage. The capacity of the renal pelvis is only 3 to 5 ml. If irrigation is ordered, slowly instill no more than 5 ml (or less as ordered) of lukewarm, sterile normal saline. Use strict aseptic technique for the irrigation. Unless both ureters are completely obstructed, urine continues to drain into the bladder. Remember to record urine from each source on the output record.

The patient with a ureterostomy tube is usually kept on bedrest unless a double-j catheter is used. The double-j catheter has one coiled end in the renal pelvis and the other coiled end in the bladder.

NEPHROSTOMY TUBE

When a ureter is completely obstructed, the physician may insert a nephrostomy tube through a flank incision directly into the kidney pelvis. The tube is connected to a drainage system and assessed frequently. You must ensure that the tube is not kinked or clamped at any time because drainage must be continuous. Some urine usually leaks around the tube and flows through the flank incision. Perform sterile dressing changes and skin care are as needed. Irrigation with a small amount of sterile normal saline may be ordered. Because of the small capacity of the renal pelvis, no more than 5 ml of irrigating fluid is used. You must use strict aseptic technique.

URINARY STENT

A stent is a hollow tube that is placed in a structure to give it support and allow fluid to flow through. A urinary stent may be placed in the ureter to maintain alignment or to provide a route for urine drainage. The stent is inserted by the physician. It may be completely internal or it may extend through the urethra or skin. Several types of stents are available.

UROLOGIC SURGERY

Urologic surgery may be done on any part of the urinary tract. *Nephrectomy* is removal of the kidney because of cancer, massive trauma or bleeding, severe chronic failure with infection, polycystic kidney disease, or for donation. Many types of surgery are used to remove calculi, depending on their location. A surgical opening may be made in the renal tissue, renal pelvis, ureter, or bladder. *Lithotripsy* is a noninvasive procedure used to break up calculi, but patient care is similar to that of the surgical patient. Bladder surgery may be necessitated by bleeding, functional problems, or cancer. Removal of the bladder is a *cystectomy;* an incision in the bladder is a *cystotomy.* Some surgical procedures can be done through a cystoscope, so there is no external incision. Surgical procedures that reroute the flow of urine are called *urinary diversions.* A *cystostomy* is the formation of an opening or stoma on the abdomen for catheterization or to enable the collection of urine in an external reservoir.

Preoperative Care

Preparation for urologic surgery includes a complete diagnostic workup to rule out other medical problems. Fluid status is evaluated, and any imbalances are corrected. Usual preoperative care measures are taken as described in Chapter 16. Bowel cleansing may be ordered before some procedures. If the patient will have a stoma for urine drainage, an enterostomal therapist is usually consulted for patient counseling and teaching.

Postoperative Care

After surgery, particular attention is given to urine output, respirations, and bowel function. Output is closely monitored, with drainage from various tubes recorded separately. Urine output of less than 30 ml/hr should be reported to the physician. Flank or abdominal incisions cause pain on deep breathing. Adequate pain management and support of the patient for coughing and deep breathing decrease the risk of atelectasis and pneumonia. Auscultate lungs frequently to assess breath sounds. Urologic surgery often involves manipulation of the bowel, which can lead to paralytic ileus. Therefore, food and fluids are usually withheld until bowel sounds are present.

DRUG THERAPY

A number of drugs are available to treat urinary tract disorders. Major classifications of commonly used drugs are diuretics, antihypertensives, phosphate binders, hormones, vitamin and mineral supplements, and immunosuppressants. These classifications, specific drugs, their actions and adverse effects, and nursing interventions are summarized in Table 38-4. Immunosuppressant drugs are addressed separately in Table 38-5.

Consider the Alternative!

Herbal remedies, like medications, can be harmful to the kidney. For example, aloe can cause nephritis, and ephedra (ma huang) can cause kidney stones. Teach patients to always include alternative remedies in their medication histories.

Text continued on p. 767

table 38-4 DRUG THERAPY | *Urinary Disorders*

GENERAL CONSIDERATIONS

1. Drugs are selected carefully because many drugs are nephrotoxic.
2. Drug dosages need to be reduced if renal function is impaired and the drug is excreted in the urine.

DRUGS	USE/ACTION	SIDE EFFECTS	NURSING INTERVENTIONS
DIURETICS AND ANTIHYPERTENSIVES			
Diuretics	Cause kidneys to excrete water and sodium. Lower blood pressure.	Dehydration, electrolyte imbalances.	Monitor intake and output, blood pressure, weight. Administer in morning to avoid nocturia. Assess for electrolyte imbalances. Monitor serum potassium level. Potassium supplements may be ordered except with potassium-sparing drugs.
Osmotic diuretics (mannitol, urea)		Dehydration, electrolyte imbalances.	Monitor infusion site for extravasation. Administer only freshly prepared solutions.
Thiazide diuretics (hydrocholorothiazide [HydroDiuril], metolazone [Zaroxolyn])		Hypokalemia, hypercalemia.	Monitor patients with diabetes for hyperglycemia. Encourage potassium-rich foods.
Loop diuretics (furosemide [Lasix])		Orthostatic hypotension, hypokalemia, hyponatremia.	Monitor patients with diabetes for hyperglycemia. Encourage potassium-rich foods. Teach patients to cope with orthostatic hypotension.
Potassium-sparing diuretics (spironolactone [Aldactone])		Hyperkalemia, drowsiness. Gynecomastia in men on long-term therapy.	Safety measures. Assess for hyperkalemia: diarrhea, muscle twitching, dysrhythmias.
Antihypertensives	Lower blood pressure.	Orthostatic hypotension. Reflex tachycardia and fluid retention with some types. Rebound hypertension if stopped suddenly.	Monitor blood pressure. Do not discontinue suddenly. For orthostatic hypotension, teach patients to change position slowly and avoid prolonged standing.
Centrally acting antiadrenergics (methyldopa [Aldomet], clonidine [Catapres])		Drowsiness, hemolytic anema, liver damage.	Administer at bedtime. Safety precautions. Advise patient to discontinue drug only under medical direction.
Peripherally acting antiadrenergics (prazosin [Minipress])		Hypotension (especially with initial dose).	Give first dose or increased dose at bedtime. Teach patient to manage orthostatic hypertension.
Beta-adrenergic blockers (propranolol [Inderal])		Bronchoconstriction, bradycardia, hypoglycemia, heart failure.	Monitor respirations in asthmatics and patients with chronic obstructive pulmonary disease. Masks symptoms of low blood glucose. Assess for edema.
Vasodilators (hydralazine [Apresoline])		Tachycardia, palpitations, headache, lupus-like syndrome.	Report lupus-like signs: fever, sore throat, skin rash.

Continued

table 38-4 **DRUG THERAPY | *Urinary Disorders—cont'd***

DRUGS	USE/ACTION	SIDE EFFECTS	NURSING INTERVENTIONS
PHOSPHATE BINDERS			
Aluminum hydroxide gel (Amphojel)	Binds with phosphate in intestines to prevent absorption. Given to prevent renal osteodystrophy. Raises serum calcium.	Hypophosphatemia: muscle weakness, anorexia, bone pain. Constipation.	Monitor for hypophosphatemia. Record bowel movements. Give laxatives and stool softeners as ordered.
VITAMIN AND MINERAL SUPPLEMENTS			
Ferrous sulfate	Treats iron deficiency anemia.	Constipation or diarrhea, dark stools.	Administer on empty stomach with water. Can give liquid with water or fruit juice to disguise taste.
Folic acid	Supplements dietary intake.	Few adverse effects.	Occasional hypersensitivity.
Calcium gluconate	Treats hypocalcemia.	Hypercalcemia. Constipation.	Monitor blood studies. Administer in divided doses with or after meals. Do not take with other drugs.
HORMONES			
Recombinant human erythropoietin (epoetin alfa)	Improves red blood cell formation. Reverses anemia. Requires adequate serum iron and ferritin to be effective.	Headache, tachycardia, hypertension, dyspnea, diarrhea, hyperkalemia, nausea, vomiting, clotted vascular access, seizures.	Monitor blood pressure. Contraindicated in uncontrolled hypertension. Dosage is adjusted to maintain hematocrit between 30% and 33%.
ANTIBIOTICS			
Sulfonamides			
Sulfisoxazole* (Gantrisin)	Treats UTIs.	Drowsiness, dizziness, agranulocytosis, anemia, thrombocytopenia. Nausea, vomiting, diarrhea. Liver dysfunction. Crystalluria leading to renal tubular damage. Photosensitivity. Allergy. Infertility.	Tell patient urine will be orange. Monitor blood cell counts. Give with full glass of water. Maintain urine output of 1,500 ml/day to prevent crystalluria. Have patient avoid excessive sun exposure. Do not give if patient has history of sulfonamide allergy.
Trimethoprim* (Trimpex)	Used to treat acute or chronic UTIs. Especially effective against recurrent UTIs in men.	Nausea, vomiting, glossitis. Skin rash.	Tell patient to report skin rash—may be allergic response.

Aminoglycosides (gentamicin [Garamycin])	Effective against gram-negative bacilli.	Ototoxicity, hepatotoxicity.	Assess hearing. Drug should be stopped if patient has tinnitus or subjective hearing loss. Monitor intake and output. Check BUN and creatinine.
Penicillins (ampicillin)	Effective against most gram-positive and some gram-negative pathogens.	Anaphylaxis, GI distress, rash, blood dyscrasias.	Monitor for allergic reaction: rash, itching, wheezing. Report immediately.
Fluoroquinolones (ciprofloxacin)	Broad spectrum. Effective against many gram-positive and gram-negative pathogens.	Drowsiness, headache, agitation, seizures, cardiac dysrhythmias, hepatotoxicity, pseudomembranous colitis. Anaphylaxis, severe skin reactions, crystalluria.	Observe closely for allergic reaction: rash, pruritus, urticaria, wheezing. Notify physician immediately. Monitor liver function tests. Advise patient to drink 1,500-2,000 ml each day to prevent crystal formation. Do not take within 2 hr of antacids, iron, or zinc. Check for many other drug-drug interactions. Safety measures for drowsiness.
URINARY ANTISEPTICS			
Methenamine (Mandelamine)	Antibacterial. Effective only in acid urine. Used to prevent or suppress recurrent UTIs.	Nausea, vomiting, diarrhea.	Give with meals to reduce gastrointestinal effects. Encourage adequate fluids. Discourage large intake of milk products.
Nalidixic acid (NegGram)	Antibacterial. Used for chronic UTIs.	Headache, malaise, vertigo, syncope, confusion, peripheral neuritis, vision disturbances. Nausea and vomiting. Photosensitivity.	Advise patient to avoid prolonged sun exposure. Administer 1 hr before meals unless gastrointestinal upset occurs. Encourage adequate fluids.
Nitrofurantoin (Furadantin, Macrodantin)	Used to treat acute and chronic UTIs.	Dyspnea. Nausea and vomiting. Numbness and tingling of legs.	Administer with food or milk to reduce gastric distress.
OTHERS			
Pentosan polysulfate sodium (Elmiron)	Increases bladder defense mechanisms or detoxifies irritants that harm the bladder lining.		

**NOTE:* Trimethoprim/sulfamethoxazole is a combination drug. Trade names: Bactrim, Septra, and others.
UTIs, Urinary tract infections; *BUN,* blood urea nitrogen.

table 38-5 **DRUG THERAPY | *Immunosuppressants***

GENERAL CONSIDERATIONS

1. Patients on immunosuppressants have reduced resistance to infection, so they must be monitored for subtle signs of infection.
2. Protect patients from infections.
3. Teach patients the importance of taking drugs as prescribed and keeping follow-up appointments.
4. Immunosuppressants increase the risk of malignancies.

DRUGS	USE/ACTION	SIDE EFFECTS	NURSING INTERVENTIONS
CORTICOSTEROIDS			
Prednisone (Deltasone) Methylprednisolone (Medrol) Methylprednisolone sodium succinate (Solu-Medrol)	Anti-inflammatory: Prevent movement of leukocytes into transplanted tissue.	Retention of water and sodium; loss of potassium, elevated blood glucose, hypertension, gastrointestinal bleeding, mood swings, psychosis, infections, impaired healing.	Monitor intake and output. Assess for fluid and electrolyte imbalances: edema, increased blood pressure, cardiac dysrhythmias, muscle weakness, confusion. Antacids are often ordered to protect stomach.
CYTOTOXIC DRUGS			
Azathioprine (Imuran) Cyclophosphamide (Cytoxan) Mycophenolate mofetil (CellCept)	Used with cyclosporine and corticosteroids to inhibit proliferation of B and T lymphocytes.	Diarrhea, bone marrow suppression, vomiting, sepsis, sterility. Azathioprine and mycophenolate are teratogenic.	Be sure pregnancy has been ruled out before starting drugs. Assess for decreased platelets (bruising, bleeding), and decreased white blood cells (frequent infections). Check CBC reports.
MONOCLONAL ANTIBODIES			
Muromonab-CD3 (Orthoclone OKT3) Basiliximab (Simulect) Daclizumab (Zenapax) Lymphocyte immune globulin (Atgam)	React with T-cell antigens and destroy them. Used to treat acute rejection in renal transplant recipients.	Fever, chills, headache, tremor, dyspnea, flushing, anaphylaxis, nausea, vomiting, diarrhea, chest pain. Potentially fatal anaphylaxis.	Monitor closely for anaphylaxis, especially with first dose. Monitor for fluid overload. Check infusion site. Have site changed if evidence of extravasation.
T-CELL SUPPRESSORS			
Cyclosporine (Sandimmune and Neoral are NOT interchangeable!)	Interferes with T-lymphocyte activity. Enhances transplant survival with less risk of infection.	Nephrotoxicity (elevated serum creatinine), fluid retention, hypertension, hyperkalemia, hirsutism, venous thrombosis, gingival hyperplasia, tremors, infections, anemia, leukopenia, thrombocytopenia. Anaphylaxis with intravenous administration. Hepatoxic.	Monitor serum creatinine and electrolytes. Check for edema. Monitor blood pressure. Have epinephrine available during intravenous administration. Monitor liver function studies. Mix oral form with food or chocolate to disguise unpleasant oiliness.

DISORDERS OF THE URINARY TRACT

URINARY TRACT INFLAMMATION AND INFECTIONS

Urinary tract infections (UTIs) are common, especially among women. They can involve any part of the urinary tract and can be acquired through the blood or lymph or may enter through the urethra. Infections are called ascending when pathogens move from the urethra to the bladder and descending when pathogens travel from the kidney to the bladder. UTIs are the most common nosocomial infections (infections acquired while hospitalized). Most UTIs are bacterial, but they can be caused by viruses, yeasts, and fungi. It is important to treat UTIs to prevent renal scarring that can lead to failure. Risk factors for UTI are listed in Table 38-6.

Urethritis

Urethritis is inflammation of the urethra. Inflammation may be caused by microorganisms, trauma, or hypersensitivity to chemicals in products such as vaginal deodorants, spermicidal jellies, or bubble bath detergents. The most frequently identified causative microorganisms are *Escherichia coli, Chlamydia, Trichomonas, Neisseria gonorrhoeae,* and herpes simplex virus type 2.

Signs and Symptoms

Signs and symptoms of urethritis include dysuria, frequency, urgency, and bladder spasms. A urethral discharge may be noted.

Medical Diagnosis

Urethritis is diagnosed based on patient signs and symptoms, urinalysis, and urethral smear. Cystitis may be present at the same time.

Medical Treatment

Antimicrobials are used to treat the condition when it is caused by microorganisms. If the patient is sexually active, both the patient and the sexual partner may be treated with antimicrobials to prevent reinfection.

NURSING CARE *of the Patient with Urethritis*

Assessment

Assessment of the urology patient is outlined in Table 38-1. Important aspects of assessment when a patient has urethritis are comfort, possible causative factors, and understanding of treatment and prevention.

Nursing Diagnoses, Goals, and Outcome Criteria: Urethritis

Nursing Diagnoses	Goals and Outcome Criteria
Acute Pain related to tissue inflammation	Pain relief: patient states pain relieved, relaxed manner
Ineffective Management of Therapeutic Regimen related to lack of knowledge of cause, treatment, and prevention of urethritis	Patient manages treatment plan effectively: patient accurately describes treatment and preventive measures, has no recurrence

table 38-6 *Risk Factors for Urinary Tract Infections*

- Female gender
- Vaginal infections
- Bubble baths and vaginal deodorant sprays
- Dehydration
- Tight-fitting, synthetic undergarments
- Infrequent voiding
- First trimester of pregnancy
- Trauma during delivery

Interventions

Sitz baths are soothing and may reduce the pain of urethritis. Instruct female patients to wipe from front to back after toileting and to void before and after sexual intercourse as a means of preventing urethritis. Discourage bubble baths and vaginal deodorant sprays. Instruct uncircumcised male patients to clean the penis under the foreskin regularly.

Cystitis

Cystitis is inflammation of the urinary bladder. The most common cause is bacterial contamination. Other factors that increase the incidence of cystitis are prolonged immobility, renal calculi, urinary diversion, and indwelling catheters. Women are more susceptible than men to cystitis because the female urethra is shorter and closer to the vagina and rectum. The longer urethra and antibacterial substances in prostatic fluid are thought to decrease the incidence of UTIs in men. Cystitis in the absence of other pathology of the urinary tract is said to be *uncomplicated. Recurring* UTIs are more likely to be associated with urinary tract pathology.

Signs and Symptoms

Symptoms of cystitis include urgency, frequency, dysuria, hematuria, nocturia, bladder spasms, incontinence, and low-grade fever. Urine may be dark, tea-colored, or cloudy. Fever, fatigue, and pelvic or abdominal discomfort are common. Bladder spasms may be manifested by pain behind the symphysis pubis. Spasms may occur during or after urination. Some patients have bacteria in the urine, but no symptoms at all.

Medical Diagnosis

A urine specimen is obtained for urinalysis, culture, and sensitivity. The presence of bacteria does not mean the patient has an infection, unless the patient also has white blood cells (WBCs) in the urine. The presence of WBCs reflects bacterial tissue invasion—an indicator of infection. Other diagnostic procedures may be indicated to rule out pathology that might be responsible for the infection.

Medical Treatment

Cystitis is treated with antibiotics that concentrate in the urine. The physician may order an antibiotic while awaiting the results of the culture and sensitivity. The order is changed if the results show that another antibiotic would be more effective. For uncomplicated cystitis, treatment may be given in a single dose or in a 1- to 3-day regimen. Patients with recurrent cystitis may be placed on continuous prophylactic antibiotics. A mild analgesic such as acetaminophen is useful for relieving discomfort. Phenazopyridine (Pyridium) may be ordered for 2 to 3 days to decrease discomfort and bladder spasms. Hyoscyamine (Cystospaz) and flavoxate (Urispas) also may be ordered to decrease bladder spasms.

NURSING CARE *of the Patient with Cystitis*

Assessment

The general assessment of the patient with a urinary tract disorder is outlined in Table 38-1. The nursing assessment of the patient with cystitis focuses on patient symptoms, possible causative factors, and understanding of treatment and prevention.

Nursing Diagnoses, Goals, and Outcome Criteria: Cystitis

Nursing Diagnoses	Goals and Outcome Criteria
Acute Pain related to tissue inflammation	Pain relief: patient states pain relieved, relaxed manner
Ineffective Management of Therapeutic Regimen related to lack of knowledge of cause, treatment, and prevention of urethritis	Patient effectively manages treatment plan: patient accurately describes treatment and preventive measures; has no recurrence

Interventions

Administer analgesics as ordered for pain. Warm sitz baths also are comforting. Patient teaching emphasizes the need for a high fluid intake, instructions about prescribed drugs, and measures to avoid future infections. The patient needs to consume at least 30 ml/kg of fluid per day and void frequently. Fluids should be consumed during the day and at night so that the urinary tract is continually flushed. Instruct the patient to complete the entire course of prescribed antibiotics. Also advise the patient taking phenazopyridine, a drug that relieves burning on urination, that the drug causes an orange-red urine color that may stain clothing.

Put on your THINKING CAP!!

Using the recommended fluid intake for a person with cystitis, calculate how much fluid you would need to take in 24 hours based on your body weight.

PHARMACOLOGY CAPSULE Instruct patients to complete the entire course of antimicrobial therapy to ensure that the infection is eradicated.

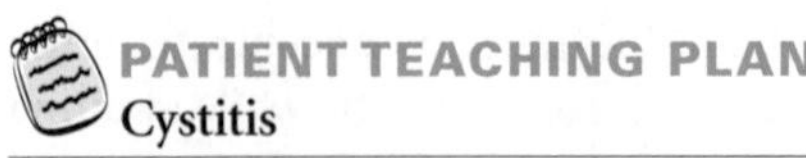

PATIENT TEACHING PLAN
Cystitis

To reduce the risk of future infections:

- Wear cotton undergarments because they keep the perineum drier than synthetic materials. Moisture encourages bacterial growth.
- Avoid tight-fitting clothing in the perineal area.
- Showers are preferred over tub baths.
- Avoid coffee, tea, carbonated beverages with caffeine, and apple, grapefruit, orange, and tomato juices because these irritate the bladder.
- Maintain a high fluid intake and empty your bladder often.
- Cranberry juice is sometimes recommended to make the urine more acidic and discourage bacterial growth. Although there is some disagreement about the value of the juice and the amount needed to be effective, it is a safe, simple measure to try.
- Women should wipe from front to back after bowel movements or voiding.
- Drink a glass of water before and after intercourse to "flush" the urethra.
- It is important to keep appointments for follow-up urinalyses to be sure the infection has been eliminated.

Interstitial Cystitis

Pathophysiology and Diagnosis

Interstitial cystitis is a chronic inflammatory disease of the bladder. The cause of the disease, which usually affects females, is unknown. The patient typically reports severe bladder and pelvic pain and urinary frequency and urgency. Chronic inflammation can cause the bladder to become scarred and stiff, which reduces its capacity. Ulcers may form in the bladder lining, and bleeding may occur. The condition is diagnosed by cystoscopy. Other diagnostic measures may be done to rule out other pathology such as cancer.

Medical Treatment

Treatment is directed toward symptom management and attempts to treat possible causes. Initial treatments often employ tricyclic antidepressants, antispasmodics, bladder anesthetics, and NSAIDs. A newer drug that is bringing symptomatic relief to many is pentosan polysulfate (Elmiron). Other treatments include stretching the bladder under anesthesia, instillation of various medications including dimethyl sulfoxide into the bladder, and electrostimulation. Some sources advise dietary and activity changes and heat application. Cystectomy (surgical removal of the bladder) is an extreme measure that is necessary in some cases.

NURSING CARE *of the Patient with Interstitial Cystitis*

Patients are usually treated as outpatients, so you are more likely to encounter them in clinic or home settings than in hospitals. It is important for you to show acceptance of the patient and empathy for the disruption of lives caused by this disease. It is a physiologic illness, not a psychologic one. Your primary role is teaching and support.

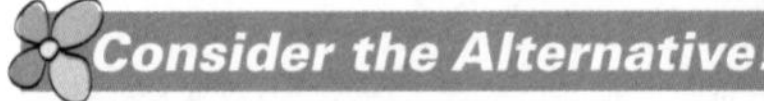

Consider the Alternative!

Biofeedback may help some patients deal with the symptoms of interstitial cystitis.

Pyelonephritis 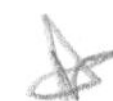

Pyelonephritis is inflammation of the renal pelvis. It may affect one or both kidneys. Acute pyelonephritis most often is caused by an ascending bacterial infection, but it may be blood borne. Chronic pyelonephritis may be persistent or recurrent and results in damage to the renal parenchyma (functional tissue). It most often is the result of reflux of urine from inadequate closure of the ureterovesical junction during voiding. Progressive scarring results in atrophy of the affected kidneys, and hypertension and renal ischemia develop.

Chronic pyelonephritis, usually caused by longstanding UTIs with relapses and reinfections, may lead to chronic renal failure. If the patient progresses to renal atrophy and end-stage renal disease, dialysis or transplantation are the only means of keeping the patient alive.

Signs and Symptoms

Signs and symptoms of acute pyelonephritis include high fever, chills, nausea, vomiting, and dysuria. Severe pain or a constant dull ache occurs in the flank area. The patient with chronic pyelonephritis often complains of bladder irritation, chronic fatigue, and a slight aching over one or both kidneys.

Medical Treatment

The goal of treatment for pyelonephritis is to prevent further damage. Antibiotics, urinary tract antiseptics, analgesics, and antispasmodics may be ordered. Long-term antibiotic therapy may be prescribed for patients who have repeated acute infections or chronic infection. Additional medications may be needed to treat hypertension. Dietary salt and protein restriction may be imposed on the patient with chronic disease. If an obstruction or congenital anomaly is present, it should be treated. Urine samples must be obtained for follow-up cultures to determine whether the infection has been resolved.

NURSING CARE *of the Patient with Pyelonephritis*

Assessment

The general assessment of the patient with a urinary tract disorder is outlined in Table 38-1. When assessing the patient with pyelonephritis, record the presence of related signs and symptoms, a history of previous urinary tract disorders, any predisposing factors, and the effects of the infection on daily activities.

Nursing Diagnoses, Goals, and Outcome Criteria: Pyelonephritis

Nursing Diagnoses	Goals and Outcome Criteria
Acute Pain related to inflammation	Pain relief: patient states pain relieved, relaxed manner
Activity Intolerance related to fatigue	Improved activity tolerance: completes activities of daily living without excessive fatigue
Deficient Fluid Volume related to vomiting, anorexia	Adequate hydration: fluid intake and output equal; pulse and blood pressure consistent with patient norms
Imbalanced Nutrition: Less than Body Requirements related to anorexia, nausea, vomiting	Adequate nutrition: stable body weight
Ineffective Management of Therapeutic Regimen related to lack of knowledge of treatment and future prevention of pyelonephritis	Patient effectively manages treatment plan: patient accurately describes prescribed treatment and preventive measures; has no recurrence

Interventions

Acute Pain

Administer analgesics as ordered when the patient reports pain. Antibiotics and antiseptics do not provide direct pain relief but eventually help by eliminating the cause of the inflammation.

Activity Intolerance

The pain and systemic symptoms of infection contribute to fatigue and activity intolerance. Assist with activities of daily living and schedule activities to allow for periods of uninterrupted rest. If the patient is being treated at home, advise family members of the patient's need for additional rest. Encourage the family to relieve the patient of some responsibilities until recovered.

Deficient Fluid Volume and Imbalanced Nutrition

Adequate food and fluids are very important for the patient with pyelonephritis. If nausea and vomiting occur, inform the physician and administer antiemetics as ordered. Record food and fluid intake and fluid output. If the patient is unable to take the recommended 2 to 3 L of fluid daily, intravenous fluids may be prescribed. Be careful when forcing fluids to avoid circulatory overload. In the older patient, a sudden increase in fluid volume may result in congestive heart failure. Possible signs of this complication are bounding pulse, rising blood pressure, dyspnea, and edema.

Ineffective Management of Therapeutic Regimen

If the patient will be taking medications at home, review the drugs and stress the importance of taking them as prescribed. Explain the importance of follow-up evaluation to assess effects of treatment and the need to report suspected recurrence to the physician immediately. Patients with chronic pyelonephritis must be adequately prepared for self-care.

PATIENT TEACHING PLAN
Pyelonephritis

- Take your medications exactly as prescribed. Report adverse effects (for specific drugs) to your physician. Be sure to complete the course of therapy.
- Limit your physical activity and exercise as advised by your physician.
- Even after this infection has been treated, drink at least eight (8-ounce) glasses of fluids each day to dilute urine and to reduce the risk of recurrence.

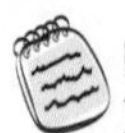

PATIENT TEACHING PLAN
Pyelonephritis—cont'd

- If advised, follow dietary protein and sodium restrictions.

Polycystic Kidney Disease

Polycystic kidney disease is a hereditary disorder. There are two types: childhood and adult. In adults, it usually is manifested by age 40 years. It is characterized by grapelike cysts in place of normal kidney tissue (Fig. 38-7). The cysts enlarge, compress functional renal tissue, and eventually result in renal failure. They also may create pressure on nearby organs. As the kidneys lose the ability to concentrate urine, hypertension and congestive heart failure develop. Often, cystic lesions are found on other organs. Chronic infection contributes to progressive loss of function.

Signs and Symptoms

This slowly progressive disorder begins with various types of pain: dull, aching abdominal, lower back or flank pain, or colicky pain that begins abruptly.

Medical Treatment

Supportive treatment is recommended to preserve kidney function, treat UTI, and control hypertension. Infections should be treated promptly with appropriate antibiotics. As the disease progresses, kidney function decreases and end-stage renal disease develops. Dialysis, nephrectomy, and transplantation are then treatment options. Genetic counseling is advised for these patients because each of their children has a 50% chance of having the condition.

NURSING CARE *of the Patient with Polycystic Kidney Disease*

See sections on nursing care of patients having renal surgery, dialysis, and transplantation.

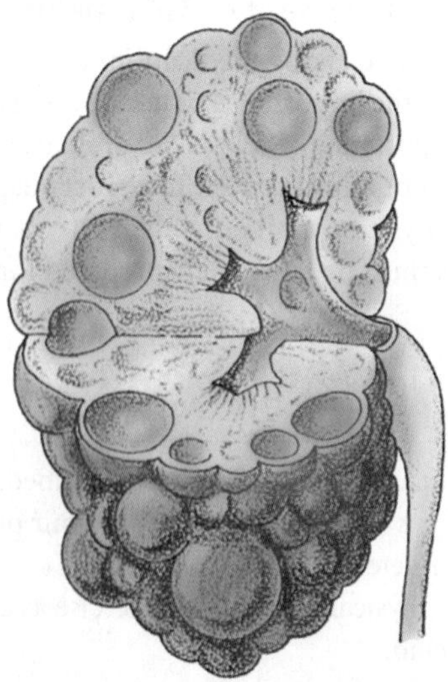

FIGURE **38-7** Polycystic kidney.

Acute Glomerulonephritis

Pathophysiology

Glomerulonephritis is an immunologic disease characterized by inflammation of the capillary loops in the glomeruli. There are several immunologic mechanisms that can cause acute glomerulonephritis. For example, the patient may develop antibodies against antigens in the glomeruli. A common type of glomerulonephritis follows an infection of the respiratory tract caused by group A–negative hemolytic streptococcus. An antigen–antibody reaction results in inflammation of the glomeruli, and scar tissue forms. Glomerular permeability increases, allowing proteins to leak into the urine. The glomerular filtration rate decreases and nitrogenous wastes accumulate in the blood. Both BUN and serum creatinine rise. Acute glomerulonephritis usually resolves completely, but some patients develop chronic glomerulonephritis or progress to irreversible renal failure.

Signs and Symptoms

Urine becomes tea colored as output decreases. Peripheral and periorbital (around the eyes) edema is evident. As glomerular filtration decreases, mild to severe hypertension occurs and hypervolemia (increased blood volume) results.

Medical Diagnosis

Diagnosis is based on patient assessment and laboratory tests. A urinalysis is done to detect proteinuria and red blood cell casts. Blood studies measure BUN, creatinine, and albumin. Streptococcal antibody tests indicate whether the patient has had a streptococcal infection. Findings in blood and urine studies tend to vary from one patient to another. Renal ultrasound, renal biopsy, or both also may be ordered.

Medical Treatment

Acute glomerulonephritis is treated with diuretics and, for severe hypertension, antihypertensive medications. Antibiotics are indicated if there is evidence of current streptococcal infection. In the acute phase, bedrest is ordered to prevent or treat heart failure and severe hypertension from fluid overload. Activity restriction usually is continued as long as urine tests show blood or protein, or blood pressure is elevated. Fluids, sodium, potassium, and protein may be restricted until there is sufficient recovery of kidney function. When fluid overload has been corrected, moderate activity is permitted, but the patient still needs sufficient rest to allow the kidneys to heal.

Because some patients with acute glomerulonephritis develop renal insufficiency, follow-up is very important. If renal failure develops, dialysis is necessary. Patients who progress to chronic glomerulonephritis acquire end-stage renal disease in 1 to 30 years. (See chronic renal failure later in this chapter.)

NURSING CARE *of the Patient with Acute Glomerulonephritis*

Assessment

Assessment of patients with urinary tract disorders is outlined in Table 38-1. For the patient with acute glomerulonephritis, it is especially important to note signs and symptoms, recent infections (especially sore throat or skin lesions), and changes in urine characteristics.

During the physical examination, inspect the area around the eyes, the extremities, and the abdomen for fluid accumulation. Assess tissue turgor. Evaluate respiratory and cardiac function for evidence of excess fluid volume: dyspnea, tachycardia, hypertension. Accurate intake and output records and daily weights help to assess the kidneys' ability to excrete excess fluid.

Nursing Diagnoses, Goals, and Outcome Criteria: Acute Glomerulonephritis

Nursing Diagnoses	Goals and Outcome Criteria
Excess Fluid Volume related to renal dysfunction	Restoration of normal fluid balance: balanced fluid intake and output, vital signs consistent with patient norms; no edema
Activity Intolerance related to retention of chemical wastes, fatigue, prescribed bedrest	Improved activity tolerance: patient reports less fatigue with physical activity
Self-Care Deficit related to prescribed bedrest, lack of knowledge of treatment measures	Patient adheres to plan of care: self-care is accomplished within activity restrictions, patient adheres to plan of care
Anxiety related to possibility of chronic illness	Reduced anxiety: patient states anxiety is lessened, appears calm

Interventions

Excess Fluid Volume

Administer diuretics as ordered. Maintain careful records of fluid intake and output. Instruct patients and family members in the importance of accurate records. If fluids are restricted, explain the need for the restriction and help the patient plan the timing and amounts of allowed fluids. Fluid restriction can be very distressing. It helps to present fluids in small containers rather than serving an ounce or two in a large glass. If the patient has edema, special skin care is needed. Handle the patient gently because taut, swollen tissue is easily damaged and heals slowly.

Activity Intolerance

Activity intolerance may be due to infection, accumulated toxins, or anemia. During the acute illness, discourage activity to allow the kidneys to heal. Explain the importance of rest for recovery. Schedule activities to allow for periods of uninterrupted rest. Of course, the patient on bedrest is at risk for complications of immobility: skin breakdown, pneumonia, muscle weakness, joint stiffness, constipation, and thrombus formation. Therefore, have the patient change positions, cough and deep breathe, and gently exercise joints periodically. Nursing measures to prevent the complications of immobility are described in Chapter 20.

Self-Care Deficit

Provide assistance with activities of daily living. The patient needs to understand that rest, dietary restrictions, and medications promote recovery. Emphasize the need for follow-up care. When the patient is discharged, reinforce the importance of reporting any signs of recurrence such as changes in urine characteristics or edema. Instruct the patient to increase activities gradually as the edema and fatigue resolve.

Anxiety

The patient with acute glomerulonephritis may be very concerned about the possibility of developing a chronic, life-threatening condition. Give the patient an opportunity to ask questions and share concerns. Helpful interventions may include empathetic listening, providing factual information, or referrals to other professionals.

URINARY TRACT OBSTRUCTIONS

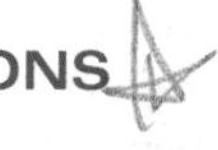

Renal Calculi

Urolithiasis is the formation of calculi (stones) in the urinary tract. It affects 500,000 people in the United States each year, is most common among males, and has a high incidence of recurrence.

Pathophysiology

Most calculi are precipitations of calcium salts (calcium phosphate or calcium oxalate), uric acid, magnesium ammonium phosphate (struvite), or cystine. All these substances are normally found in the urine. Factors that foster the development of calculi are:

- Concentrated urine
- Excessive intake of calcium, vitamin D, protein, oxalates, calcium-based antacids
- Familial tendency
- Hyperparathyroidism
- Immobility, urinary stasis
- Sedentary lifestyle
- Altered urine pH
- Lack of kidney substance that inhibits calculi formation

Urine is normally acidic, with a pH ranging from 4.5 to 8.0. Some substances tend to precipitate in acid urine, causing calculus formation; others precipitate in alkaline urine. UTIs, particularly those caused by *Proteus, Klebsiella,* and *Pseudomonas,* are associated with calculi because these organisms cause the urine to become alkaline. The kidneys excrete substances that are believed to inhibit calculi formation, so a decrease in these substances may contribute to calculus formation.

Most calculi originate in the kidney (nephrolithiasis) and travel through the ureters into the bladder (urolithiasis).

What Does Culture Have to do with Urinary Calculi?

The incidence of uric acid stones is high among Jewish males. Caucasians have a greater risk of urinary calculi than do African Americans. Cultural factors such as diet as well as genetic factors probably explain some of these differences.

Signs and Symptoms

The patient's chief complaint is usually pain. The location and characteristics of the pain may provide clues to the site of the calculus. Dull flank pain suggests a calculus in the renal pelvis or stretching of the renal capsule from urine retention (hydronephrosis). If a calculus lodges in a ureter, the patient usually has excruciating pain in the abdomen that radiates to the groin or the perineum. The ureter goes into spasm (colic) in an attempt to move the calculus along and relieve the obstruction. Nausea, vomiting, and hematuria may accompany the pain. The patient also may show signs and symptoms of UTI.

Medical Diagnosis

The presence and location of calculi in the urinary tract may be confirmed by KUB, IVP, retrograde pyelogram, or ultrasound. A CT scan can help to rule out other pathology. A routine urinalysis and culture and sensitivity usually are ordered as well. If a calculus can be obtained, its composition can be determined by laboratory analysis.

Medical Treatment

Most calculi are passed spontaneously. Ambulation and adequate hydration facilitate the passage of many calculi. Opioid analgesics and antispasmodics are ordered to relieve the intense, colicky pain. Antibiotics are ordered if infection is present or if internal manipulation of the calculus is necessary. If the calculus does not pass and symptoms continue, several procedures may be used to destroy or remove it.

Lithotripsy. Lithotripsy (shattering of the calculus) may be accomplished by a variety of means. Extracorporeal shock wave lithotripsy (ESWL) uses a device called a lithotriptor to deliver a series of shock waves to disintegrate the calculi. The patient is placed in a tank of water, or a water-filled cushion is placed on the abdomen or flank. General anesthesia or preoperative sedation and analgesics may be given because the series of 1,000 to 1,500 shocks is painful. The procedure is monitored with a fluoroscope (Fig. 38-8).

With extracorporeal piezoelectric lithotripsy (EPL), the patient lies over a bath of degassed, preheated water that is contained in a closed bath. Only the patient's loin area is in contact with the water. Ultrasound is used to locate the calculus, which is then broken up with a series of shocks. Unlike ESWL, EPL can be used without general anesthesia. Sedatives may be ordered for patients who are very anxious. Unfortunately, EPL is not effective for cystine calculi, for large calculi, or for the initial treatment of staghorn calculi. Lithotripsy usually takes approximately 45 minutes. The pulverized calculus is excreted in the urine over 1 to 4 weeks. Stents may be placed in the ureter before treatment to facilitate passage of the stone fragments. The stent is usually removed in several weeks. Bruising and hemorrhage are possible complications of lithotripsy. However, most patients are able to resume normal activities the next day after the procedure.

Following lithotripsy, the urine is often bright red at first, gradually turning dark red or smoky. Antibiotics are generally given for about 2 weeks to prevent urinary tract infection.

Lasertripsy. With lasertripsy, a scope is passed into the urethra and the calculus is visualized and destroyed with a laser. Fragments are usually passed in the urine. General anesthesia is used, but premedication is commonly omitted because of the need to obtain radiographs immediately before the procedure.

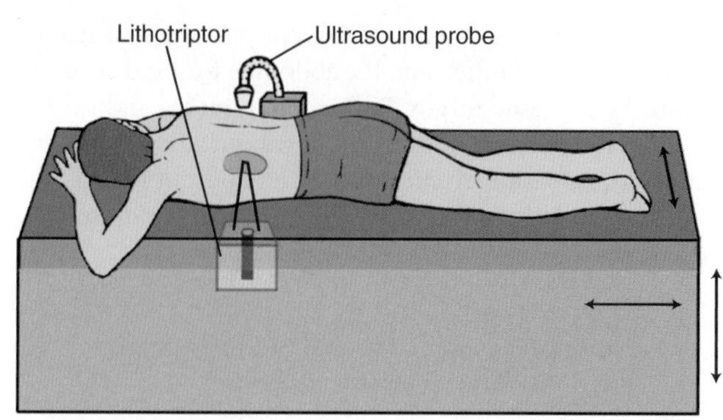

FIGURE **38-8** Extracorporeal lithotripsy.

Lithotomy. If calculi are not passed spontaneously or crushed with a lithotriptor, surgery may be necessary. The incision of an organ or a duct to remove a calculus is a lithotomy. A nephrolithotomy is the surgical procedure used if the calculus is in the kidney. The removal of a calculus from the renal pelvis is a pyelolithotomy. A ureterolithotomy is removal of a calculus from a ureter (Fig. 38-9).

Prevention

An important medical goal is to prevent recurrence of renal calculi. Long-term medical management of these patients includes a high fluid intake to keep urine dilute, dietary restrictions for specific elements (i.e., calcium and purines), regular exercise, and occasionally medications to alter the urine pH. Medications are less effective than dietary management.

NURSING CARE *of the Patient with Renal Calculi*

Assessment

Assessment of the patient with a urinary tract disorder is discussed earlier in this chapter (see also Nursing Care Plan: The Patient with Renal Calculi). When the patient has known or suspected urinary calculi, pay particular attention to a personal or family history of calculi. Describe the patient's usual fluid intake and diet, including vitamin and mineral supplements. If pain is present, describe the location, severity, and nature of the pain. Also record any changes in urine amount or characteristics. Take the temperature to detect fever. A nurse who is trained in physical examination palpates and percusses the flanks and the abdomen, noting the presence of pain, tenderness, or a distended bladder.

Nursing Diagnoses, Goals, and Outcome Criteria: Urinary Calculi

Nursing Diagnoses	Goals and Outcome Criteria
Acute Pain related to obstruction, trauma, and renal colic	Pain relief: patient states pain has been relieved; relaxed manner
Impaired Urinary Elimination related to obstruction	Unobstructed urine elimination: urine output equal to fluid intake

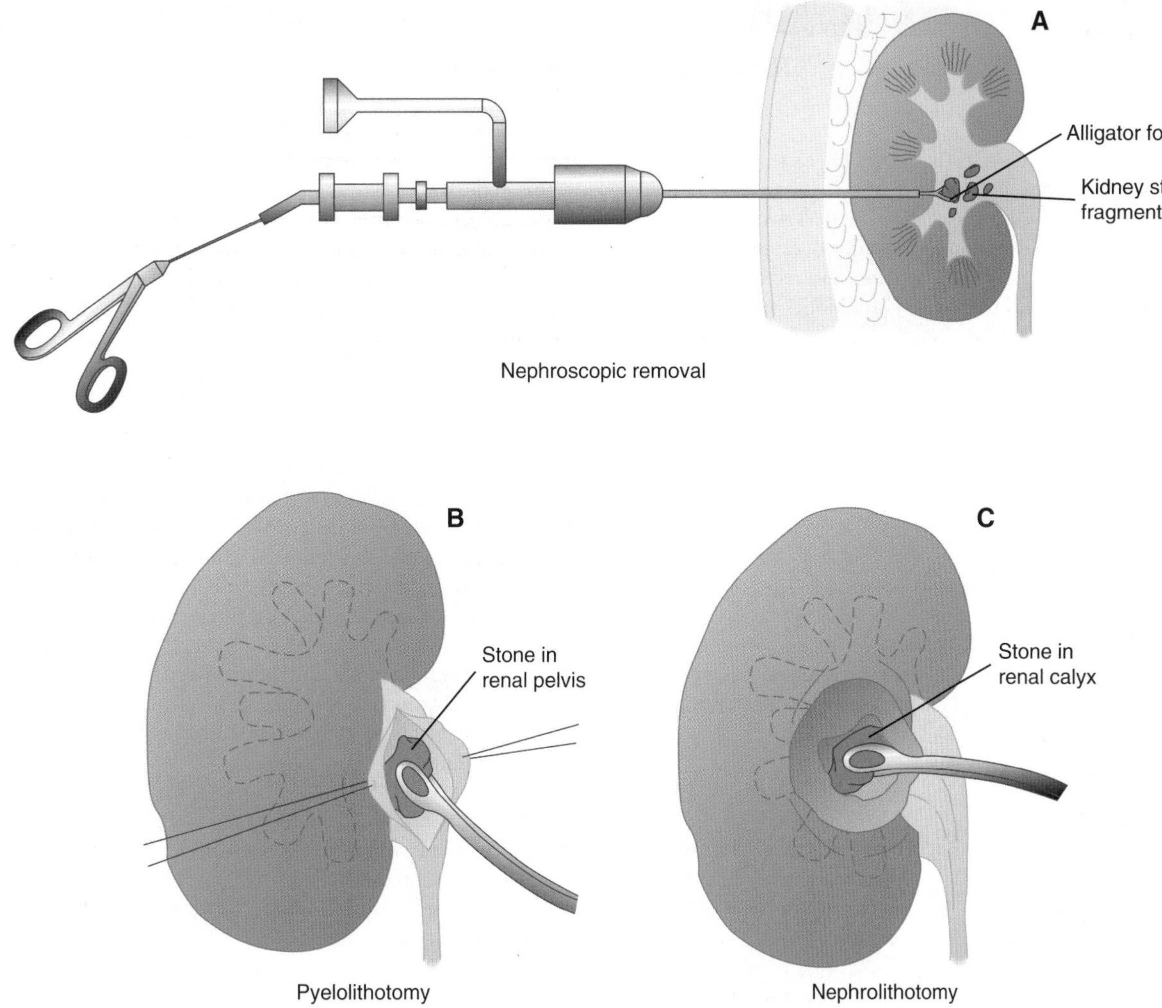

FIGURE 38-9 Surgical procedures for renal calculi. *A*, Nephroscopy. *B*, Pyelolithotomy. *C*, Nephrolithotomy.

Risk for Deficient Fluid Volume related to anorexia, nausea, and vomiting	Normal fluid balance: fluid intake and output approximately equal, pulse and blood pressure consistent with patient norms
Ineffective Management of Therapeutic Regimen related to lack of knowledge of prevention and treatment of calculi	Patient effectively manages treatment plan and takes preventive measures: patient accurately describes prevention and treatment, adheres to preventive measures; has no recurrences

If surgery is performed, additional nursing diagnoses and goals are the following:

Nursing Diagnoses	Goals and Outcome Criteria
Risk for Infection related to invasive procedures	Absence of infection: normal body temperature and white blood cell count, clear urine
Decreased Cardiac Output related to blood loss	Adequate cardiac output: pulse and blood pressure consistent with patient norms
Ineffective Breathing Patterns related to splinting of painful incision	Effective breathing patterns: clear breath sounds throughout lung fields, respiratory and depth consistent with patient norms

Interventions

Acute Pain

Because calculi in the urinary tract can cause excruciating pain, pain relief is a major nursing concern. Initially, it may be necessary to administer opioid analgesics intravenously to relieve the pain. Antispasmodics are usually ordered to reduce the smooth muscle spasms in the ureters. If pain is intermittent, the patient may be permitted to ambulate when comfortable. Ambulation may actually help the calculus move through the urinary tract. Of course, safety precautions are needed if opioids have been given. The pain may resolve

NURSING CARE PLAN

The Patient with Renal Calculi

ASSESSMENT

Health History: Mr. Frank Scarpino, age 43 years, was admitted with excruciating abdominal pain radiating to the groin. He experienced nausea and vomiting with the pain. Review of systems revealed a history of hypertension controlled with captopril. He also has had repeated urinary tract infections, most recently 1 month ago. At that time, he was treated with antibiotics and the symptoms subsided. Radiologic studies detected a calculus lodged in the right ureter. EPL was done to shatter the calculus. Mr. Scarpino returned to his hospital room 3 hours ago. He is complaining of soreness in the right lower abdomen.

Physical Examination: Mr. Scarpino is fully oriented but drowsy. Vital signs: temperature, 100° F orally; pulse, 88; respiration, 20; blood pressure, 138/74. His abdomen is soft but tender. There is no bladder distention. He voided 350 ml pink-tinged urine. Intravenous fluids are infusing at 150 ml/hr.

Nursing Diagnosis	*Goals and Outcome Criteria*	*Interventions*
Acute pain related to obstruction, trauma, renal colic.	Patient will report pain relief and will appear more relaxed.	Assess pain characteristics. For severe pain, administer morphine as ordered. Administer antispasmodics as ordered. Assist with ambulation when permitted to promote passage of calculus fragments. Milder pain may be treated with non-opioid analgesics. Position changes, back rubs, relaxation, and imagery may be used to enhance analgesia. Document effects of pain relief interventions.
Impaired urine elimination related to obstruction.	Patient's urine output will be approximately equal to fluid intake.	Measure all fluid intake and output. Report low output to physician. Strain all urine to collect calculi fragments. Send fragments to laboratory for analysis. Maintain intravenous fluids.
Risk for deficient fluid volume related to NPO (nothing by mouth) status, nausea, and vomiting.	The patient will be adequately hydrated as evidenced by moist mucous membranes, dilute urine, and vital signs consistent with patient's norms.	Administer intravenous fluids as ordered. Assess for deficient fluid volume: hypotension, tachycardia, sticky mucous membranes, concentrated urine. Encourage oral fluids when permitted. Administer antiemetics as ordered for nausea and vomiting.
Ineffective breathing patterns related to abdominal pain, splinting.	Patient's breath sounds will be normal throughout the lung fields.	Assess respiratory status: rate, effort, breath sounds. Encourage deep breathing and coughing every 2 hours until fully ambulatory.
Decreased cardiac output related to blood loss.	Patient's cardiac output will remain normal as evidenced by vital signs consistent with patient's norms and by absence of tachycardia, hypotension, or restlessness.	Assess the abdomen and groin area for bruising—some is expected. Note red color and increased viscosity of urine associated with bleeding. Report increased redness. Monitor vital signs to detect decreasing cardiac output: tachycardia, restlessness, hypotension.
Ineffective management of therapeutic regimen related to lack of knowledge of prevention and treatment of calculi, self-care after lithotripsy.	Patient will effectively manage self-care: as evidenced by correct description of self-care after EPL and measures to prevent recurrence of calculi.	Tell the patient that the fragments are usually passed in the urine over a period of several weeks and may cause some pain. Administer antibiotics as ordered and emphasize importance of treating any new UTIs to reduce the risk of calculi formation. Advise patient to consume 3 to 4 L of fluid daily unless the physician prescribes less. Fluids should be taken around the clock to prevent concentration during the night. If any dietary restrictions are imposed, request a dietary consult to explain them to the patient.

suddenly if the calculus moves into the bladder or is passed through the urethra.

Impaired Urine Elimination

Depending on its size and location, a calculus may obstruct urine flow. If urine backs up into the kidney, hydronephrosis may develop. Hydronephrosis is distention of the kidney with urine, a condition that can cause permanent damage (Fig. 38-10). Maintain accurate records of fluid intake and output and report low output to the physician. In addition, urine is usually strained and examined for calculi. If any calculi are recovered, send them to the laboratory for analysis.

Risk for Deficient Fluid Volume

Renal colic is often accompanied by nausea and sometimes vomiting. Give antiemetics promptly as ordered. The physician will probably order intravenous fluids to maintain dilute urine and to flush the urinary tract. A fluid intake of as much as 4 L/day may be recommended. Large volumes of fluids like this must be given carefully to the older patient, in whom fluid volume excess can easily develop. Vital signs must be monitored for signs of circulatory overload (tachycardia, bounding pulse, dyspnea, edema, hypertension).

Postoperative Care. Before surgery, explain the expected procedure to the patient and answer any questions. Goals of postoperative care are maintenance of urine drainage, prevention of UTI, and prevention of pulmonary and circulatory complications.

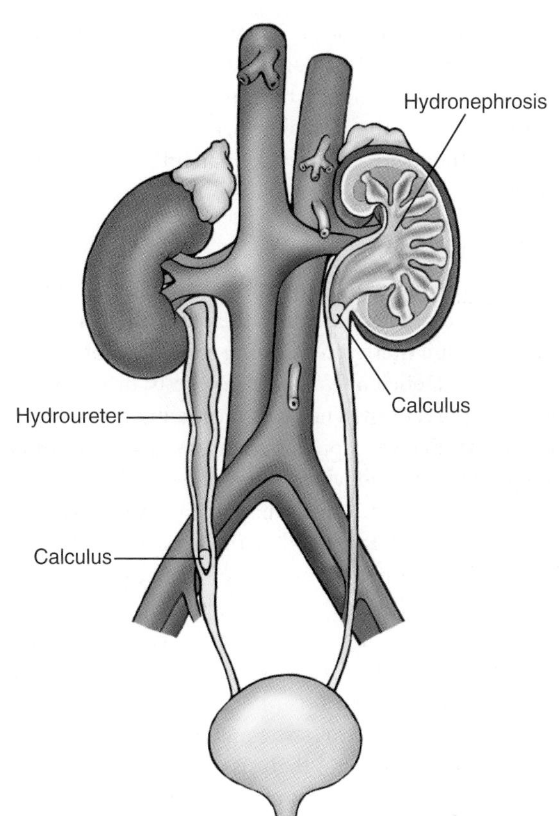

FIGURE **38-10** Hydronephrosis caused by obstruction of the upper portion of the ureter; hydroureter caused by obstruction of the lower portion of the ureter.

Risk for Infection

To maintain alignment and urine flow, the patient is apt to have drains, catheters, a ureteral stent, or a combination of these. Each tube is connected to its own closed drainage system. Position tubes for free flow of urine at all times. Keep accurate accounts of drainage from each tube. If the patient has a flank incision, frequently check the area around the dressing for drainage because urine tends to leak from the incision. A large amount of serosanguineous drainage is normal immediately after surgery. In approximately 2 days, the drainage changes to serous. Frequent dressing changes using sterile technique may be required. In some cases, an ostomy appliance is used to collect drainage and to permit accurate measurement of the drainage.

Some patients have nephrostomy tubes placed directly in the kidney. The tube is placed for drainage or for instillation of irrigating fluid. It also diverts urine flow from the ureter until adequate healing has occurred. If irrigations are ordered, use strict aseptic technique and not more than 5 ml of warm, sterile normal saline at a time.

Decreased Cardiac Output

The patient is at risk for the same postoperative complications as any surgical patient. Be especially alert for any signs of excessive bleeding, infection, or pulmonary complications. To detect bleeding, inspect the dressing and drainage hourly for the first 24 hours. Immediately report bright bleeding, excessive serosanguineous drainage, increasing pulse, restlessness, or decreasing blood pressure to the physician. Indications of infection such as odor, cloudy drainage, or temperature above 100° F also should be reported. Measures to reduce the risk of infection include maintaining closed drainage systems, changing wet dressings promptly, and use of strict aseptic technique when handling tubes or dressings.

Ineffective Breathing Patterns

Monitor the patient's pulmonary status carefully. A flank incision makes taking a deep breath very painful. Assist the patient to turn, cough, and deep breathe at least every 2 hours. An incentive spirometer helps determine how much the patient is able to inflate the lungs. When the patient coughs, the incision needs to be splinted with pillows or folded blankets. For the first 1 or 2 postoperative days, administer analgesics before turning, coughing, and deep breathing to make these activities more comfortable. Adequate fluid intake thins respiratory secretions and makes them easier to expectorate. Early and frequent ambulation promotes improved respiratory function. All of these efforts help prevent atelectasis and pneumonia, a primary treatment goal.

Prevention. When the patient is discharged, reinforce the need to continue to consume 4 L of fluid daily unless contraindicated. The fluid needs to be consumed over the 24-hour period so that urine does not become concentrated at night.

Advise the patient to drink two glasses of water before bed and another two glasses when awakening at night to void. This pattern should be followed for life to reduce the risk of calculus formation in the future. If the physician has prescribed a special diet or dietary restriction, provide instructions or have the dietitian do so.

UROLOGIC TRAUMA

The kidneys sustain 50% of all urologic injuries. Trauma may be penetrating or blunt. Penetrating injuries most often result from knives or guns. Blunt trauma occurs when a force is applied to the abdominal wall and the energy is diffused into the abdominal cavity. Examples of blunt force are motor vehicle accidents, contact sports injuries, falls, and intentional injuries. Blunt injuries to the kidneys produce lacerations or contusions. The ureters are rarely injured with blunt trauma. They are most often disrupted by penetration and require surgical anastomosis. The bladder may rupture from blunt trauma if full, but, if empty, it is rarely harmed. The urethra is most apt to be injured in men because of its unprotected anatomic location.

When blunt trauma is suspected, the patient is observed for bruising on the abdomen or in the flank area. Assess for signs of shock (tachycardia, restlessness, hypotension, pallor), pain, and a palpable abdominal or flank mass. The presence of bruises over the flank and lower back that occur with retroperitoneal bleeding is called Grey Turner's sign.

The physician may order a KUB, urography, computed tomography, or ultrasound to determine the extent of injury. Diagnostic peritoneal lavage may be performed to determine whether there is bleeding in the peritoneal cavity. A positive finding necessitates surgery to find and eliminate the source of bleeding.

The most common indication of urologic trauma is hematuria. It is best if the patient can void, but this may not be possible with other injuries. Before catheterizing a patient with suspected trauma, carefully inspect the urethral meatus. If there is blood in or around the meatus, a urologist should perform the catheterization or insert a suprapubic catheter.

If the injury is not severe, if there is little bleeding, and if there are no signs of shock, monitor the patient closely. More severe injuries most likely require surgery to repair damage. Postsurgical care of these patients is similar to the care of the patient with a nephrectomy, urinary calculi, or cystectomy.

CANCERS OF THE URINARY SYSTEM

Care of the patient with cancer is covered in Chapter 24. This section focuses on the specific needs of the patient with cancer of the urinary tract.

Renal Cancer

Malignancies of the kidney account for 3% of all reported cancers. Eighty percent of renal malignancies are adenocarcinomas, which primarily affect men 55 to 60 years of age. Less common squamous cell carcinomas of the renal pelvis affect men and women equally.

A renal tumor may reach considerable size before it is detected. Renal malignancies metastasize to the liver, lungs, long bones, and the other kidney. Direct extension of the tumor may be found in the ureter. Early symptoms are anemia, weakness, and weight loss. Painless, gross hematuria is the classic sign, but it usually occurs in the advanced stage. A dull ache in the flank area also is a late symptom.

Medical Diagnosis

The physician may be able to palpate a mass in the flank area. Diagnostic tests and procedures to study the mass may include excretory urography, retrograde pyelography, ultrasound, arteriography, computed tomography, magnetic resonance imaging, and renal biopsy. Care of the patient undergoing these procedures is detailed in Table 38-3.

Medical Treatment

Removal of a kidney is called a nephrectomy. Radical nephrectomy is the treatment of choice for renal cancer and involves removal of the kidney and its adjacent tissue, adrenal gland, renal artery and vein, and local lymph glands. Before nephrectomy, the renal artery may be occluded to reduce the blood supply to the tumor. In general, renal tumors are not responsive to radiation or chemotherapy, but radiation is sometimes used as a palliative measure for inoperable cancer. Immunotherapy and chemotherapy have had positive results in only a small percentage of patients.

NURSING CARE *of the Patient with Renal Cancer*

Assessment

Nursing assessment of the patient with a urologic disorder is outlined in Table 38-1. When a patient has a suspected or confirmed renal malignancy, there may be very few signs and symptoms. Inquire about weakness, fatigue, and any changes observed in the urine. Explore the patient's emotional state, usual coping strategies, and support systems.

Preoperative Care

General preoperative nursing care is discussed in detail in Chapter 16. Before nephrectomy, the patient's primary nursing diagnoses are **Ineffective Coping** related to potentially fatal disease and **Deficient Knowledge** of tests, procedures, and effects of nephrectomy. The goals of nursing care are for the patient to use effective coping mechanisms and to understand what is being done and what to expect.

Thorough explanations of diagnostic tests and preoperative teaching provide needed information. Assure the patient that one functioning kidney can sustain adequate kidney function. Tests are done to confirm that the unaffected kidney functions adequately before a nephrectomy. Serum and urine laboratory tests are usually ordered to serve as baseline data for postoperative comparison. Older patients are more likely to have renal insufficiency, and they may eventually need renal dialysis after nephrectomy. The teaching plan includes what to expect in the postoperative period and how to turn, cough, and deep breathe. Other preoperative care is the same as that for any other major surgery.

Postoperative Care

Common aspects of postoperative care are covered in Chapter 16. After nephrectomy, monitor vital signs to detect fluid volume alterations related to blood loss or fluid retention. Record intake and output as another measure of fluid balance and renal function. Routinely check drains and tubes to ensure proper function. Monitor dressings for drainage. Once the dressings have been removed, assess the wound for intactness and signs of infection (excessive redness or swelling, purulent drainage). Assess the patient's comfort level. Auscultate breath sounds and bowel sounds. Anticipate some emotional distress and encourage the patient to express thoughts and feelings about having cancer.

Nursing Diagnoses, Goals, and Outcome Criteria: Renal Cancer, Postoperative

Nursing Diagnoses	Goals and Outcome Criteria
Acute Pain related to incisional tissue trauma	Pain relief: patient states pain is relieved, relaxed manner
Risk for Deficient Fluid Volume related to dehydration, blood loss	Normal hydration and blood volume: pulse and blood pressure consistent with patient norms, normal skin turgor
Ineffective Breathing Patterns related to proximity of incision to diaphragm	Effective breathing patterns: clear breath sounds throughout lung fields
Risk for Injury related to decreased peristalsis caused by bowel manipulation during surgery	Absence of abdominal distention: active bowel sounds, abdomen soft
Risk for Infection related to break in skin	Absence of infection: normal body temperature and white blood cell count
Ineffective Coping related to diagnosis of cancer	Effective coping: patient practices strategies that reduce anxiety but do not interfere with therapeutic plan
Deficient Knowledge of postoperative limitations	Patient understands postoperative restrictions: accurately describes and adheres to activity limitations

Interventions

Acute Pain

Obtain a complete description of the patient's pain. Incisional pain is intense at first and deserves prompt administration of prescribed analgesics. Because of the patient's position in surgery, there may be muscle aches in the opposite side and flank area. Medication can be supplemented with position changes and back rubs. Other comfort measures are described in Chapter 14.

Risk for Deficient Fluid Volume

Intravenous fluids are given initially. The physician normally orders approximately 3 L of fluid daily. Maintain accurate intake and output records. At first, the urine may be measured every 1 to 2 hours. Notify the physician if less than 30 ml is produced in an hour. When the patient is able to be weighed, daily weights are an even better measure of fluid balance than intake and output. BUN, serum creatinine, serum electrolytes, and urine specific gravity are assessed and compared with preoperative values.

Also monitor the nephrectomy patient for bleeding. Frequently check the dressing for drainage. Be careful to check *under* the patient because blood flows to the most dependent area. Sometimes, the dressing is dry and intact but the patient is lying in a pool of blood.

Ineffective Breathing Patterns

The location of the flank incision causes pain with expansion of the thorax. Patients tend to protect the area by not breathing deeply. This may lead to pneumonia and atelectasis. It is especially important to have the patient turn, cough, and deep breathe every 1 to 2 hours. You can help by supporting the incision during respiratory exercises. Supervise use of an incentive spirometer to encourage deeper inspiration. As soon as ambulation is permitted, assist the patient out of bed. Be careful not to place tension on tubes and drains. Gradually increase the time and distance walked.

Risk for Injury

Anesthesia and manipulation of abdominal organs cause temporary cessation of peristalsis in the intestines. Until peristalsis returns, the patient is not permitted to take anything by mouth. If peristalsis does not return within 3 to 4 days, the patient is said to have paralytic ileus. Because paralytic ileus is fairly common after nephrectomy, a nasogastric tube may be inserted and attached to suction during surgery. Suction keeps the stomach empty, reducing the risk of nausea and abdominal distention. The return of peristalsis is detected by active bowel sounds and the passage of flatus (gas). Auscultate the abdomen for bowel sounds and observe for abdominal distention. Ambulation promotes the return of peristalsis.

Risk for Infection

During dressing changes, use strict aseptic technique. Montgomery straps may decrease irritation from the adhesive tape if frequent dressing changes are required.

Ineffective Coping

The patient facing cancer fears the possibility of death, mourns the loss of an organ, and may dread additional cancer therapy. You can help by encouraging the patient to talk and clarify concerns, listening empathetically, providing requested information, and referring the patient to expert counselors. Explore usual coping strategies and sources of support. Chapter 24 provides additional detail on nursing care of the cancer patient.

Deficient Knowledge

Before discharge, caution the patient not to lift or participate in strenuous activities for 8 weeks. Contact sports are prohibited for life because trauma to the remaining kidney could eliminate all kidney function.

Bladder Cancer

Cancer of the bladder is the most common malignancy of the urinary tract. It occurs most often in men 50 to 70 years of age. The ureteral orifices and the bladder neck are the most common sites of bladder cancer. Over the years, chemical agents have been suspected as carcinogens. The tars found in smoking tobacco, aniline dyes found in industrial compounds, and tryptophan all have been implicated in the development of bladder cancer.

What Does Culture Have to do with Bladder Cancer?

Risk factors for bladder cancer include cigarette smoking and exposure to chemicals used in the rubber and cable industries. Historically, men have been more likely than women to smoke and to work in industry, which might help explain why this cancer is three times as common among men as among women.

Signs and Symptoms

The most common sign of bladder cancer is painless, intermittent hematuria. Other signs and symptoms include bladder irritability; infection, with dysuria, frequency, and urgency; and decreased stream of urine.

Medical Diagnosis

When the patient's signs and symptoms suggest bladder cancer, the physician may order a urinalysis, IVP, and CT scan. Cystoscopy is done to visualize the bladder and permit biopsy of any observable lesions. Details of these tests and procedures and nursing implications are provided in Table 38-3.

Medical Treatment

Bladder malignancies respond more favorably to chemotherapy than do kidney tumors, but surgery is the treatment of choice. The type of surgery depends on whether the cancer is superficial, invasive, or metastatic. Superficial cancers involve only the bladder mucosa or submucosa, or both. Superficial lesions with low recurrence rates may be treated with cystoscopic resection and fulguration or with laser photocoagulation. Cystoscopic resection is the removal of tissue through a cystoscope with a special cutting instrument. Fulguration is the use of electric current to burn and destroy tissue. Laser photocoagulation is the use of an intense beam of light (argon laser) to destroy tissue.

Two other surgical procedures for bladder cancer are segmental bladder resection and radical cystectomy. A segmental bladder resection is done for a single, primary tumor too large to remove by cystoscopic resection. It involves removal of the tumor and adjacent bladder muscle, a procedure that decreases the size of the bladder. A radical cystectomy is removal of the entire bladder and adjacent structures with diversion of the ureters. This procedure is reserved for malignancies that are untreatable with less conservative measures. This is very extensive surgery, and an optimal state of health before surgery is desirable. Radiation and/or chemotherapy may be done before or after surgery depending on the extent of the malignancy.

In some situations, pharmacologic interventions may be used. Intravesical chemotherapy is the instillation of drugs such as thiotepa, doxorubicin (Adriamycin), and mitomycin-C into the bladder. Bacille Calmette-Guérin (BCG) also may be used in intravesical immunotherapy.

Urinary diversion. When the bladder and urethra must be removed completely, urine must be allowed to drain through another route, called urinary diversion. There are several types of urinary diversions: ileal and sigmoid conduits, ureterostomy, and nephrostomy. These diversions are illustrated in Figure 38-11.

To form an ileal conduit, a portion of the ileum is resected from the small bowel. The ureters are implanted in the ileum, one end of the ileum is closed, and the open end is implanted on the abdominal surface as a stoma. Urine is excreted through the ileal conduit rather than the urethra. A urinary drainage pouch is attached to the skin to collect the urine. A sigmoid conduit is formed by the same procedure except that a section of sigmoid colon instead of ileum is used. A ureterostomy brings the ureter to the abdominal surface, where urine is eliminated through a stoma. A nephrostomy is the placement of a tube in the kidney so that urine may drain through the tube into an external collection device. Detailed information about urinary diversion is presented in Chapter 25.

NURSING CARE *of the Patient with Bladder Cancer*

Assessment

Assessment of the patient with possible or confirmed bladder cancer includes a complete description of urinary signs and symptoms. Fatigue and weight loss are significant and should be noted. The health history may reveal use of tobacco or exposure to carcinogenic chemicals. Assess the patient's emotional state, coping strategies, and sources of support.

Preoperative Care

In addition to the common nursing care described in Chapter 16, important preoperative nursing diagnoses for the patient facing segmental resection for cancer may be **Fear** related to life-threatening diagnosis and **Ineffective Coping** related to lifestyle change. The goals of nursing care are reduced fear and effective coping strategies. To accomplish these goals, explore the patient's fear and provide information and encouragement. The thought of having cancer is frightening, and nurses must educate the public that it is often curable. Assess coping strategies and provide resources as needed. The patient needs support to accept the diagnosis and follow through with the treatment.

The patient having radical cystectomy faces a more difficult adjustment—that of permanent urinary diversion. The patient needs to be prepared psychologically as well as physically to deal with a change in body image. The enterostomal therapist is a valuable resource to both you and the patient in preparing for this surgery. The therapist selects the stoma site with the patient. The patient may be advised to wear a water-filled pouch for several days before surgery to

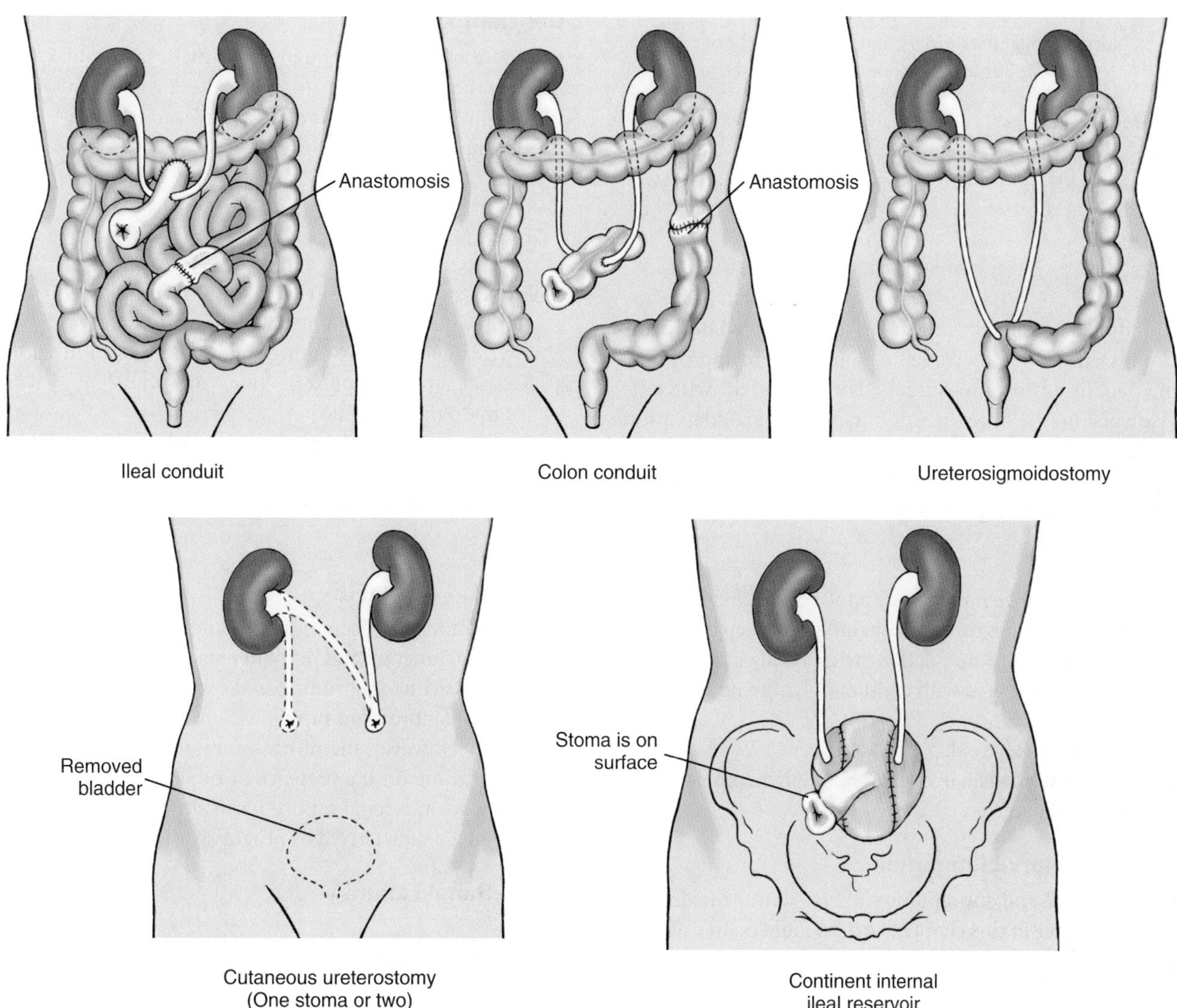

FIGURE 38-11 Types of urinary diversion procedures.

help ensure proper stoma placement. If the patient would like to talk to someone who has had a cystectomy, this often can be arranged through a local Ostomy Club chapter of the American Cancer Society.

Preoperative care for an ileal or sigmoid conduit includes thorough preparation of the intestinal tract. Bowel preparation requires several days. The patient begins with a low-residue diet and then a clear-fluid diet. Oral neomycin, an antibiotic that is not absorbed from the intestinal tract, is ordered to reduce bacteria in the bowel. Enemas also are ordered before surgery.

The patient who has received effective preoperative nursing interventions demonstrates reduced fear and realistic problem solving.

Postoperative Care

Postoperative assessment includes vital signs, intake and output, patency of tubes, bowel sounds, comfort, and appearance of the drainage, stoma, and wound.

Nursing Diagnoses, Goals, and Outcome Criteria: Bladder Surgery, Postoperative

Nursing Diagnoses	Goals and Outcome Criteria
Acute Pain related to tissue trauma	Pain relief: patient states pain relieved, relaxed manner
Impaired Urinary Elimination related to urinary diversion	Unobstructed urine drainage: urine clear, flows freely, output equal to fluid intake
Impaired Skin Integrity related to surgical incision	Well healed incision: wound margins intact, decreasing redness and swelling
Risk for Infection related to tissue trauma	Absence of infection: normal body temperature and white blood cell count
Risk for Injury related to absence of peristalsis secondary to bowel manipulation during surgery	Normal peristalsis: active bowel sounds, soft abdomen

Nursing Diagnoses, Goals, and Outcome Criteria: Bladder Surgery, Postoperative—cont'd

Nursing Diagnoses	Goals and Outcome Criteria
Deficient Knowledge of postoperative self-care	Patient understands self-care after discharge: patient accurately describes and demonstrates care

Additional nursing diagnoses such as **Disturbed Body Image** and **Deficient Knowledge** of stoma care are appropriate if the patient has ostomy surgery. For the patient with urinary diversion, the outcomes of nursing care are adaptation to disturbed body image, patient demonstration of stoma care, and patient knowledge of significant signs and symptoms that should be reported to the physician.

Interventions

Routine postoperative nursing care aimed at the prevention of complications includes turning, coughing, and deep breathing. Leg exercises and early ambulation are especially important to prevent edema associated with excision of lymph nodes.

Acute Pain

Administer prescribed analgesics and use other comfort measures to control pain.

Impaired Urinary Elimination

Inspect urethral and suprapubic catheters and provide care as detailed earlier in this chapter. Urine should be free of sediment, blood, or casts. Once the catheters are removed, encourage frequent voiding in the patient who has had a segmental resection. Bladder capacity will increase up to 250 to 300 ml over several months.

If a patient has had a radical cystectomy, inspect the stoma for inflammation and irritation. Details of stoma care are provided in Chapter 25.

Impaired Skin Integrity

Monitor the surgical incision to ensure that it is healing without increasing redness or swelling or purulent drainage. Provide wound care as ordered or per agency protocol. Sites of urine drains and the stoma also must receive care to prevent skin irritation and breakdown.

Risk for Infection

These patients are at risk for infections in the surgical incisions, drain sites, and urinary tract. Monitor the patient's vital signs, blood work, and wounds for evidence of infection (fever, elevated white blood cell count, and foul odor). Use strict aseptic technique when providing wound care.

Risk for Injury

Withhold oral fluids as ordered until bowel sounds provide evidence that peristalsis has returned. Administer intravenous fluids as ordered. When oral intake is permitted, encourage an adequate fluid intake (2,500 to 3,000 ml/day).

Deficient Knowledge

Patient teaching must begin in the early postoperative period because the patient needs to learn self-care before discharge. Allow time for the patient or a caregiver to practice self-care procedures.

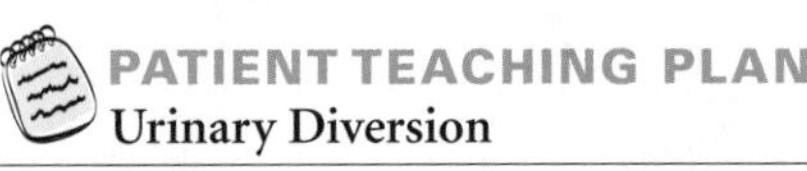

Urinary Diversion

- Proper stoma care reduces the risk of complications.
- Notify your physician of signs of infection: fever; increasing redness, swelling, and tenderness of incisions.
- Restrict activity as prescribed by your physician to avoid strain on the surgical site.
- Resources include the enterostomal therapist, American Cancer Society, United Ostomy Association (telephone, 1-800-826-0826 or e-mail, uoa@deltanet.com).

RENAL FAILURE

Any condition that decreases blood flow to the kidneys may impair renal function and result in renal failure. Renal failure is classified as acute or chronic based on onset and reversibility. Acute renal failure has a rapid onset (1 to 7 days) and may be reversible. However, the mortality rate ranges from 35% to 65% depending on the presence of other diseases or complications. Chronic renal failure has a slow onset (months to years) and is characterized by progressive, irreversible damage.

Acute Renal Failure

Causes

Causes of renal failure can be prerenal, intrarenal, or postrenal. Prerenal failure results from decreased blood flow to the glomeruli. A systolic blood pressure of 70 mm Hg or greater is necessary to sustain glomerular filtration. If the systolic pressure drops below 70 and is not corrected, renal failure may develop.

Intrarenal failure may be caused by nephrotoxic agents, kidney infections, occlusion of intrarenal arteries, hypertension, diabetes mellitus, or direct trauma to the kidney. Antibiotics (particularly the mycins), heavy metals (lead and mercury), cleaning compounds, pesticides, and poisonous mushrooms may be toxic to the kidneys. Pyelonephritis, glomerulonephritis, renal tuberculosis, and polycystic kidney disease are examples of kidney conditions that may lead to kidney failure. The arteries in the renal parenchyma may become narrowed as a result of atherosclerosis, hypertension, nephrosclerosis, or blood components (sickled red cells, hemoglobin, or myoglobin). Trauma from motor vehicle accidents, contact sports injuries, and other direct blows also may be intrarenal causes of failure.

PHARMACOLOGY CAPSULE Nephrotoxic antibiotics can lead to acute renal failure.

Postrenal causes of renal failure are obstructions beyond the kidneys that cause urine to back up. Ureteral calculi and benign prostatic hypertrophy are examples of postrenal causes of failure.

Patients at risk for acute renal failure include those having major surgery, experiencing major trauma, or receiving large doses of nephrotoxic drugs. These patients should have their blood pressure and fluid balance assessed more frequently than usual. Older people also are at risk for acute renal failure because they are less able to adapt to alterations in fluid balance or cardiac output. Renal function should always be assessed with any acute condition in the older patient. Early detection and treatment may significantly decrease the risk of death from acute renal failure.

Stages of Acute Renal Failure

The four stages of acute renal failure are onset, oliguria, diuresis (increased production of urine), and recovery.

Onset stage. The onset stage is short (1 to 3 days) and characterized by increasing BUN and serum creatinine with normal to decreased urine output. The primary treatment goal during this stage is reversal of failing renal function to prevent further damage.

Oliguric stage. During the oliguric stage, the urine output decreases to 400 ml/day or less. The serum values for BUN, creatinine, potassium, and phosphorus increase. Serum calcium and bicarbonate decrease. The oliguric stage follows the onset stage and continues for up to 14 days. Urine specific gravity becomes fixed at 1.010 (normal range, 1.010-1.025), indicating the inability of the tubules to concentrate urine. The patient becomes hypervolemic, meaning that the blood volume is greater than normal. Urine osmolality decreases and serum osmolality increases as waste products are retained.

Diuretic stage. The diuretic stage begins when urine output exceeds 400 ml/day and may rise above 4 L/day. Despite the production of large quantities of urine, few waste products are excreted, and wastes accumulate in the blood. Toward the end of the diuretic stage, the kidneys begin to excrete BUN, creatinine, potassium, and phosphorus and retain calcium and bicarbonate. This is an indication of return of kidney function.

Recovery stage. As renal tissue recovers, serum electrolytes, BUN, and creatinine return to normal. This recovery stage lasts 1 to 12 months. If complete recovery does not occur, renal insufficiency or chronic renal failure may develop. Renal insufficiency is indicated by loss of approximately 80% of function. It is possible to lead a relatively normal life with renal insufficiency unless there are other illnesses that place an additional burden on kidney function.

Medical Treatment

The primary goal of treatment for acute renal failure (ARF) is to prevent further damage. Supportive measures aim to control symptoms and to prevent complications. Support measures include fluid and dietary restrictions, restoration of electrolyte balance, and dialysis if needed. Nephrotoxic drugs and drugs that reduce renal blood flow must be avoided. Additional treatment depends on the cause of the failure. For pre-renal ARF, blood pressure and blood volume must be restored. Treatment of intrinsic ARF is based on efforts to stimulate urine production with IV fluids, dopamine, furosemide, or both. Post-renal ARF is treated by removal of the cause (typically an obstruction).

Drug therapy. Oliguria is treated with diuretics, most often an osmotic diuretic like mannitol or a loop diuretic like furosemide (Lasix) or ethacrynic acid (Edecrin). Hyperkalemia, which typically accompanies oliguria, is treated aggressively because it can be life threatening. Drugs given intravenously to lower serum potassium include hypertonic glucose and insulin, sodium bicarbonate, and calcium gluconate. Sodium polystyrene sulfonate (Kayexalate), given orally or rectally, also lowers serum potassium.

PHARMACOLOGY CAPSULE Oliguria may be treated with diuretics such as mannitol or furosemide.

Diet. Dietary modifications for acute renal failure are based on consideration of serum electrolytes and urea. Sodium and potassium allowances are individually determined. Adequate carbohydrates are provided to prevent the breakdown of fat and protein. Essential amino acid supplements may be ordered. If the patient's nutritional needs are not being met by oral intake, enteral nutritional support is instituted. If the GI tract is not functioning, total parenteral nutrition is necessary.

Fluids. Daily fluid needs usually are calculated by adding 500 ml to the previous day's fluid output. The extra 500 ml represents the daily insensible loss (through breathing and perspiration). For example, an oliguric patient who has an output of only 400 ml today would be allowed 400 plus 500 ml, for a total of 900 ml, tomorrow.

Hemodialysis and peritoneal dialysis. Conditions that warrant hemodialysis when conservative measures fail include hyperkalemia, severe metabolic acidosis, pulmonary edema, and rising blood urea nitrogen. A cannula placed in the femoral vein can be used for temporary hemodialysis. If the cannula is left in place between dialysis treatments, the patient must be immobile. If the cannula is removed and replaced repeatedly, however, there is a risk of hematoma formation. An alternative is to use a subclavian cannula that can be left in place between treatments. The disadvantage of leaving the cannula in place is that the risk of infection increases. Peritoneal dialysis is also an option, especially for the patient in congestive heart failure. The section on Chronic Renal Failure describes these procedures in more detail.

Continuous renal replacement therapy. Continuous renal replacement therapy (CRRT) offers additional options for treating the patient in acute renal failure. A cannula placed in an artery and a vein or two veins is connected to tubing that contains a blood filter and a collection device. The patient's blood flows through the tubing, and excess fluids, electrolytes, and wastes are filtered into the collection device. The blood is then returned to the patient. This procedure does not require dialysate, has little effect on cardiovascular stability, and is continuous. It can be used alone or with hemodialysis.

NURSING CARE *of the Patient in Acute Renal Failure*

Assessment

Complete assessment of the patient with a urinary disorder is summarized in Table 38-1. For the patient in acute renal failure, monitoring fluid status is critical. Intake and output records must be kept carefully. Daily weights are an effective means of assessing changes in fluid status (500 ml of fluid weighs approximately 1 pound). To be useful, daily weights must be done at the same time each day, using the same scale, and with the patient wearing the same amount of clothing. Because hypervolemia (fluid volume excess) is a major problem during the oliguric stage, assess for signs and symptoms of impending heart failure: hypertension, bounding pulse, edema, cough, dysrhythmias.

Electrolyte imbalances can include alterations in serum potassium, sodium, calcium, phosphate, and magnesium. Signs and symptoms of each of these imbalances are discussed in Chapter 13. General assessment of electrolyte balance includes cardiac rate and rhythm, neuromuscular status, edema, and mental status. The acutely ill patient also must be monitored for signs and symptoms related to immobility: pressure sores, impaired circulation, constipation, and atelectasis.

One final area of assessment is the patient's understanding of the condition and its treatment. Identify fears, anxiety, coping strategies, and sources of support.

Nursing Diagnoses, Goals, and Outcome Criteria: Acute Renal Failure

NURSING DIAGNOSES	GOALS AND OUTCOME CRITERIA
Excess Fluid Volume related to impaired kidney function (oliguric stage) OR **Deficient Fluid Volume** related to high-output renal failure (diuretic stage)	Normal fluid and electrolyte balance: normal tissue turgor, absence of dyspnea, normal serum electrolyte values
Decreased Cardiac Output related to fluid and electrolyte imbalances	Normal cardiac output: pulse and blood pressure consistent with patient norms
Anxiety related to life-threatening illness	Decreased anxiety: patient states anxiety reduced, calm manner
Disuse Syndrome related to immobility	Absence of complications associated with immobility: intact skin, regular bowel movements without difficulty, breath sounds clear to auscultation
Deficient Knowledge of condition, treatment, and self-care	Patient understands condition, treatment, and self-care: patient accurately describes and participates in self-care as allowed

Interventions

Excess Fluid Volume

Assess and document fluid status on an ongoing basis. In the oliguric stage, fluid is likely to be restricted. Explain and reinforce fluid restrictions. The fluid allowance during the oliguric stage may be very limited. Measures to help the patient cope with fluid limitations include considering patient preferences in fluid selection and carefully planning fluid intake throughout waking hours. Remember to plan for fluids needed to take medications. When only a few ounces of fluids are allowed at a time, a small juice cup should be used rather than a large glass that is only one quarter full. This creates an illusion of volume that may make the patient feel less deprived. To obtain patient cooperation, it is essential for the patient and family to understand the importance of adhering to the fluid restriction.

Give diuretics as ordered, and monitor the patient for adverse effects. A fluid challenge of normal saline may be rapidly infused while diuretics are given to promote improved renal perfusion.

Decreased Cardiac Output

In the diuretic stage, patients produce large volumes of dilute urine. Fluid volume deficit becomes a possibility. The heart rate must increase to make up for the diminished blood volume. Because eventually the heart may fail, it is important to monitor for cardiac dysrhythmias, changes in blood pressure, and shortness of breath. Give oral and intravenous fluids as ordered with careful monitoring of output at the same time.

Anxiety

Anxiety is understandable when a vital organ fails. The patient may fear death or chronic illness, with the potential for financial ruin, loss of vitality, and dependence on medical care. Provide honest responses to questions about renal failure and its treatment. Refer specific questions about the patient's prognosis to the physician.

The patient in acute renal failure may have a complete recovery. This may take up to 1 year. Unfortunately, some patients do not recover but instead progress to chronic renal failure. Those who do not improve need special support to help them learn to accept and deal with this major health deviation.

Disuse Syndrome

The patient with acute renal failure is very ill and may be immobilized. Therefore, you must attend to prevention of complications of immobility as well as to the acute renal problem. This includes skin care, turning, coughing, deep breathing, leg exercises, and measures to promote bowel elimination. Care of the immobilized patient is described in Chapter 20.

Deficient Knowledge

When the patient is acutely ill, provide basic information about the disease, diagnostic tests and procedures, and treatments. Explain the reasons for interventions such as fluid restrictions, turning, deep breathing, and leg exercises. As the patient improves, patient teaching should include management of fluids, diet, drug therapy, activity, and signs and symptoms that should be reported to the physician (dyspnea, edema, fever).

Chronic Renal Failure

When 90% to 95% of kidney function is lost, the patient is considered to be in chronic renal failure. Chronic renal failure is characterized by **azotemia** (increased nitrogenous waste products in the blood). *Uremia* is the term used when the condition advances to the point that the kidneys are unable to maintain fluid and electrolyte or acid–base balance. Uremia is also called end-stage renal disease. All of the causes of acute renal failure listed earlier may lead to chronic renal failure. In addition, chronic renal infections may predispose the patient to progressive renal failure. The most common causes, however, are hypertension, diabetes mellitus, and atherosclerosis.

Signs and Symptoms

Azotemia. The first function lost in chronic renal failure is the ability to concentrate urine. This results in an increase of waste products in the blood, despite producing large amounts of dilute urine. As the disease progresses, urine output typically declines until very little to no urine is produced.

Blood urea nitrogen is an approximate estimate of the glomerular filtration rate. It is affected by protein breakdown. Normal BUN ranges from 10 to 20 mg/dL. When BUN reaches or exceeds 70 mg/dL, dialysis is needed to reduce it.

Serum creatinine is a waste product of skeletal muscle breakdown. It is a more reliable measure of kidney function than BUN. It is not affected by diet, hydration, hepatic function, or metabolism. Normal serum creatinine is 0.5 to 1.5 mg/dL. A serum creatinine level that is twice the normal level reflects a 50% loss of function. When the value reaches or exceeds 10 times normal or greater, 90% of function has been lost. The kidneys are able to adapt to a loss of up to 80% of function. The kidneys increase in size in an attempt to maintain function.

Creatinine clearance (a urine test) is the best indicator of renal function. It is ordered less often than serum creatinine, however, because it requires collection of all urine in a 12- or 24-hour period. Normal creatinine clearance exceeds 100 ml/min.

Hyperkalemia. The primary means of potassium excretion is through the kidneys. As kidney function fails, potassium is retained, which results in hyperkalemia, the most life-threatening effect of renal failure. The normal range for serum potassium is 3.5 to 5.0 mEq/L. Elevated serum potassium interferes with normal cardiac function, causing cardiac dysrhythmias. Dysrhythmias are potentially fatal. The patient becomes apathetic and confused and may have nausea, abdominal cramps, muscle weakness, and numbness of the extremities. Serum potassium greater than 6 mg/dL requires cardiac monitoring. If the serum potassium is not reduced, bradycardia (pulse 50 beats per minute or less) or asystole (no heartbeat) may develop.

Hyperkalemia is treated with intravenous glucose and insulin or with sodium bicarbonate. These drugs drive potassium back into the cells, reducing the serum potassium level. They are used as temporary emergency measures. Kayexalate, given orally or rectally, causes potassium to be drawn into the bowel and eliminated in the feces. The method of reducing elevated serum potassium used most often is dialysis.

Hypocalcemia. Diseased kidney tissue lacks the enzyme that activates vitamin D. Without active vitamin D, calcium absorption from the bowel decreases. The body tries to compensate by shifting calcium from the bones into the blood. Serum phosphate binds with calcium, further depleting calcium levels. The normal serum calcium level is 9 to 11 mg/dL or 4.5 to 5.5 mEq/L. Abnormally low serum calcium is called hypocalcemia. Patients with hypocalcemia experience tingling sensations, muscle twitches, irritability, and tetany. Tetany is sustained, painful muscle contraction. Hypocalcemia is treated with calcium supplements, active vitamin D, and phosphate binders. Phosphate binders such as aluminum hydroxide gel should be administered with meals but not with other medications. Side effects of phosphate binders include hypophosphatemia and constipation. Antacids with magnesium, such as milk of magnesia, magnesium carbonate, magnesium oxide, and magnesium trisilicate, should be avoided.

Metabolic acidosis. Failure of the renal tubules to excrete acid ions and acid waste products causes the body's acid level to rise. Decreased bicarbonate reabsorption renders the body unable to neutralize the excess acid. Excess acid leads to metabolic acidosis. The lungs attempt to compensate by eliminating more carbon dioxide through hyperventilation. Manifestations of metabolic acidosis are headache, lethargy, and delirium.

Fluid balance. Most patients with chronic renal failure retain sodium and water, causing hypernatremia and hypervolemia. Elevated blood pressure and edema are signs of hypervolemia. Congestive heart failure may develop in the hypervolemic patient because the patient's heart cannot handle the high fluid volume. Prevention and treatment of hypervolemia include fluid restriction, diuretics, and dialysis if necessary. A few patients are sodium wasters. These patients lose excess sodium and water in the urine and become hyponatremic and hypovolemic.

Insulin resistance. With renal failure, cells become resistant to the action of insulin. As a result, blood insulin and glucose levels rise. Hyperinsulinemia (high blood insulin) stimulates the liver to produce triglycerides. Patients in chronic renal failure have high serum levels of very low-density lipoproteins. Elevated lipids in the blood (hyperlipidemia) contribute to accelerated atherosclerosis.

Anemia. Kidneys of patients in chronic renal failure produce less erythropoietin, a hormone necessary for red blood cell production. Even the red blood cells that are produced have a shorter life span than usual because of the toxic environment in which they live. Therefore, patients in chronic renal failure have anemia. Iron supplements and folic acid may be ordered. Transfusions may be required if the hematocrit drops below 20% (normal values, 35% to 45% for women and 45% to 55% for men). A genetically engineered erythropoietin (epoetin alfa) can be administered intravenously after hemodialysis or subcutaneously for patients on peritoneal dialysis. This product improves red blood cell formation and has reversed anemia and the need for transfusions in some patients in chronic renal failure.

Immunologic function. Because the inflammatory response diminishes with chronic renal failure, fewer white blood cells gather at the site of an infection or injury. The general immune response is suppressed, and antibody production declines. Therefore, the patient has reduced ability to resist infections.

Cardiovascular system. The cardiovascular system is affected by hypervolemia, hyperkalemia, and hypocalcemia. Hypervolemia increases the workload of the heart, possibly leading to congestive heart failure. Manifestations of congestive heart failure are moist breath sounds, bounding pulse, dependent edema, and dyspnea. Dysrhythmias may be caused by hyperkalemia or hypocalcemia.

Neurologic system. Neurologic effects of chronic renal failure are mental status changes (lethargy, irritability, confusion) and peripheral neuropathy. Peripheral neuropathy may be evident initially as a restless feeling and later as footdrop, loss of feeling in the legs, or paralysis of the legs. Many physicians treat the development of peripheral neuropathy as a signal to begin dialysis.

Disequilibrium syndrome may occur with hemodialysis. The rapid removal of urea from the blood leaves a higher concentration of solutes in the brain and the cerebrospinal fluid (CSF). The solutes increase the osmotic pressure, which draws fluid from the bloodstream into the CSF and brain tissue. Confusion, lethargy, headache, nausea, and vomiting may progress to coma or seizures if not treated. Disequilibrium is corrected with the administration of hypertonic glucose.

Integumentary system. The integumentary system is also affected by the accumulation of waste products. Calcium phosphate crystals and urea accumulate in the skin, causing itching. Dryness results from decreased oil gland production and decreased perspiration. A pale gray to yellow color may result from anemia and from unexcreted bilirubin and uremic pigments. Hair and nails become dry and brittle. Uremic frost is the term used when whitish crystals composed of urea and other salts precipitate on the skin. Uremic frost is most often noted around the mouth. It is a very late sign in chronic renal failure.

Gastrointestinal system. Ammonia is a breakdown product of urea. When ammonia accumulates in the gastrointestinal tract, it causes irritation, nausea, vomiting, a metallic taste in the mouth, and bleeding. Antacids administered every 2 hours help to relieve the irritation. A diet high in carbohydrates and low in protein is prescribed to reduce the accumulation of urea. Other common gastrointestinal disturbances with chronic renal failure are stomatitis (inflammation of the mouth), anorexia, nausea, vomiting, constipation, and diarrhea.

Musculoskeletal system. Renal osteodystrophy refers to the skeletal changes characteristic of chronic renal failure. The three major changes are metastatic calcification, bone demineralization, and osteitis fibrosa. Metastatic calcification is deposition of calcium phosphate complexes in blood vessels and in joints, lungs, muscles, and eyes. Deposits in blood vessels can impair blood flow so severely that fingers and toes may become gangrenous. Bone demineralization is directly related to hypocalcemia. Low serum calcium triggers increased production of parathormone by the parathyroid glands. Parathormone mobilizes calcium from the bone and shifts it into the blood. Over time, there can be significant loss of bone mass. When calcium is lost from bones, it is replaced with fibrous tissue. This condition is called osteitis fibrosa.

Reproductive system. Chronic renal failure affects both the male and female reproductive systems. The production of sex hormones declines and libido is diminished. Ovulation and menstruation usually cease in women. Men typically have low sperm counts and erectile dysfunction. The general effects of a chronic illness undoubtedly affect sexual desire and function as well.

Endocrine function. Patients with chronic renal failure usually appear hypothyroid. Hyperparathyroidism occurs in response to the chronically low serum calcium and high serum phosphates. Patients with diabetes require less exogenous insulin because the enzyme that normally breaks down insulin (renal insulinase) is reduced. Oral hypoglycemics also place the patient at risk for hypoglycemia because the drugs are normally excreted by the kidneys.

Emotional and psychological effects. Emotional and psychological effects of chronic renal failure include emotional lability, depression, anxiety, and slowed intellectual functioning.

Medical Treatment

Treatment of chronic renal failure aims to promote elimination of wastes, maintenance of fluid balance, and management of the systemic effects of the disease. Conservative treatment of the systemic effects of chronic renal failure is provided in the preceding section. To summarize, these treatments include:

- Intravenous glucose and insulin, sodium bicarbonate, or sodium polystyrene sulfonate to treat hyperkalemia
- Calcium, active vitamin D, and phosphate binders to treat hypocalcemia
- Fluid restriction and diuretics to treat hypervolemia
- Iron supplements, folic acid, blood transfusions, and synthetic erythropoietin to treat anemia
- Hypertonic glucose to treat disequilibrium syndrome
- High-carbohydrate, low-protein diet to prevent excess urea

Dialysis. When kidney failure can no longer be managed conservatively, dialysis is required to sustain life. Dialysis is the passage of molecules through a semipermeable membrane into a special solution called dialysate solution. Dialysis operates like the kidney. Small molecules like urea, creatinine, and electrolytes pass out of the blood, across a membrane, and into a solution.

The goals of dialysis are to:

- Remove the end products of protein metabolism from the blood
- Maintain safe concentrations of serum electrolytes
- Correct acidosis and replenish the body's bicarbonate buffer system
- Remove excess fluid from the blood

Dialysis enables many patients to maintain or regain self-esteem and to be productive members of society. However, initial positive feelings about dialysis sometimes turn to depression as the reality of "being tied to a machine" is recognized. Two primary means of dialysis are hemodialysis and peritoneal dialysis.

Hemodialysis. Hemodialysis is a process by which blood is removed from the body and circulated through an "artificial kidney" for removal of excess fluid, electrolytes, and wastes. The dialyzed blood is then returned to the patient (Fig. 38-12). Hemodialysis requires vascular access (access to the patient's bloodstream). This may be accomplished by catheter, cannula, graft, or fistula. Subclavian or femoral catheters can be used for temporary access for dialysis during acute renal failure while a graft or fistula matures (dilates and toughens) or for patients on peritoneal dialysis who need immediate access for hemodialysis. The catheters may be used for up to 1 week.

Internal connections between veins and arteries do not require dressings. An internal fistula between the patient's artery and vein requires approximately 2 weeks to mature and may be used 3 to 5 years. Connections may be made by using bovine or synthetic grafts that require 1 to 2 weeks to heal before use and last 7 to 9 years.

An arteriovenous shunt or cannula is an external connection between an artery and a vein (Fig. 38-13). By connecting the external ends of the synthetic tubing for dialysis, venipuncture is not necessary. However, because the cannula is external, there is danger of hemorrhage, risk of skin breakdown, restriction of activities, and risk of site infection. The arteriovenous shunt may be used for temporary vascular access but is very rarely used for chronic treatment because of the potential complications.

All vascular access sites must be assessed for patency. Check pulses below the shunt to be sure circulation is adequate. Palpate the venous side of the shunt for a "thrill" or rippling sensation caused by movement of blood through a changed pathway. A bruit or "swoosh" may be heard through a stethoscope with each heartbeat. Absence of these signs may indicate occlusion of the vessel, making it unsuitable for hemodialysis.

Once vascular access is established, the patient may be hemodialyzed. Blood flows from the artery through the vascular access device, circulates through the dialyzer, and returns through the venous line. Heparin is used as an anticoagulant to prevent blood from clotting. Hemodialysis requires specially trained personnel and expensive equipment. Although dialysis for chronic renal failure is usually performed in a dialysis center, home dialysis is available. The hemodialysis process takes approximately 4 hours and is usually done three times weekly. Certain medications such as antihypertensives may be withheld.

Advantages of hemodialysis include its usefulness in emergencies and the rapid removal of wastes, electrolytes, and fluid. Disadvantages include the need for vascular access, the use of an anticoagulant, and the potential for hemorrhage, anemia, rapid fluid and electrolyte shifts (dialysis disequilibrium syndrome), muscle cramps, nausea and vomiting, and air emboli.

Complications of hemodialysis include atherosclerotic cardiovascular disease, anemia, gastric ulcers, disturbed calcium metabolism, and hepatitis. The leading causes of death for hemodialysis patients are cerebrovascular accident and myocardial infarction, followed by infection.

Peritoneal dialysis. Peritoneal dialysis uses the patient's own peritoneum as a semipermeable dialyzing membrane. Fluid is instilled into the peritoneal cavity. Waste products are drawn into the fluid, which is then drained from the peritoneal cavity (Fig. 38-14).

Peritoneal dialysis may be done on either a temporary or a permanent basis. For temporary use, a catheter in inserted into the peritoneal cavity through the abdominal wall. For long-term use, a catheter is implanted into the peritoneal cavity. Over time, a bacterial barrier forms at the insertion site and provides some protection against infection.

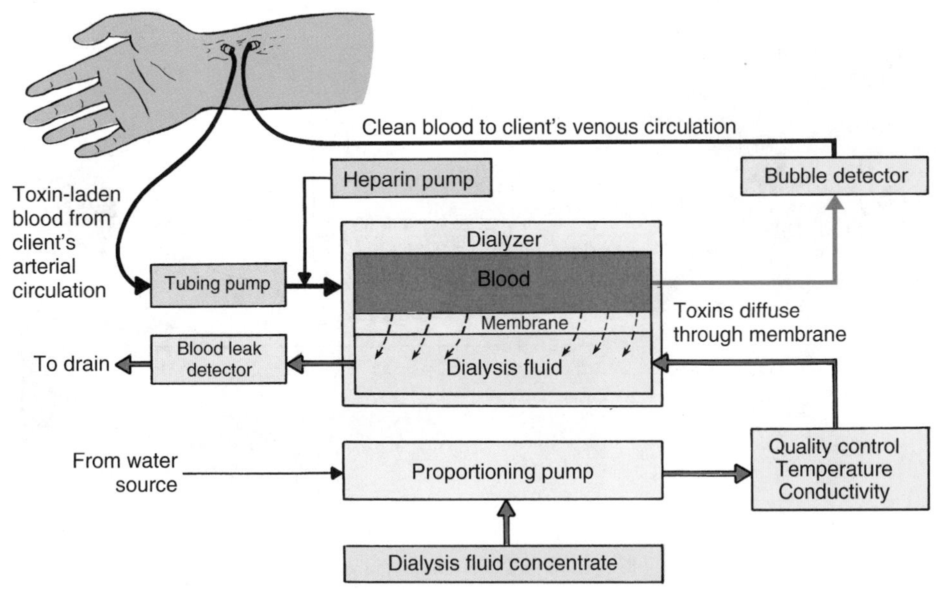

FIGURE **38-12** Schematic diagram of hemodialysis. As the patient's blood passes through the dialyzer, toxins diffuse into the dialysis fluid.

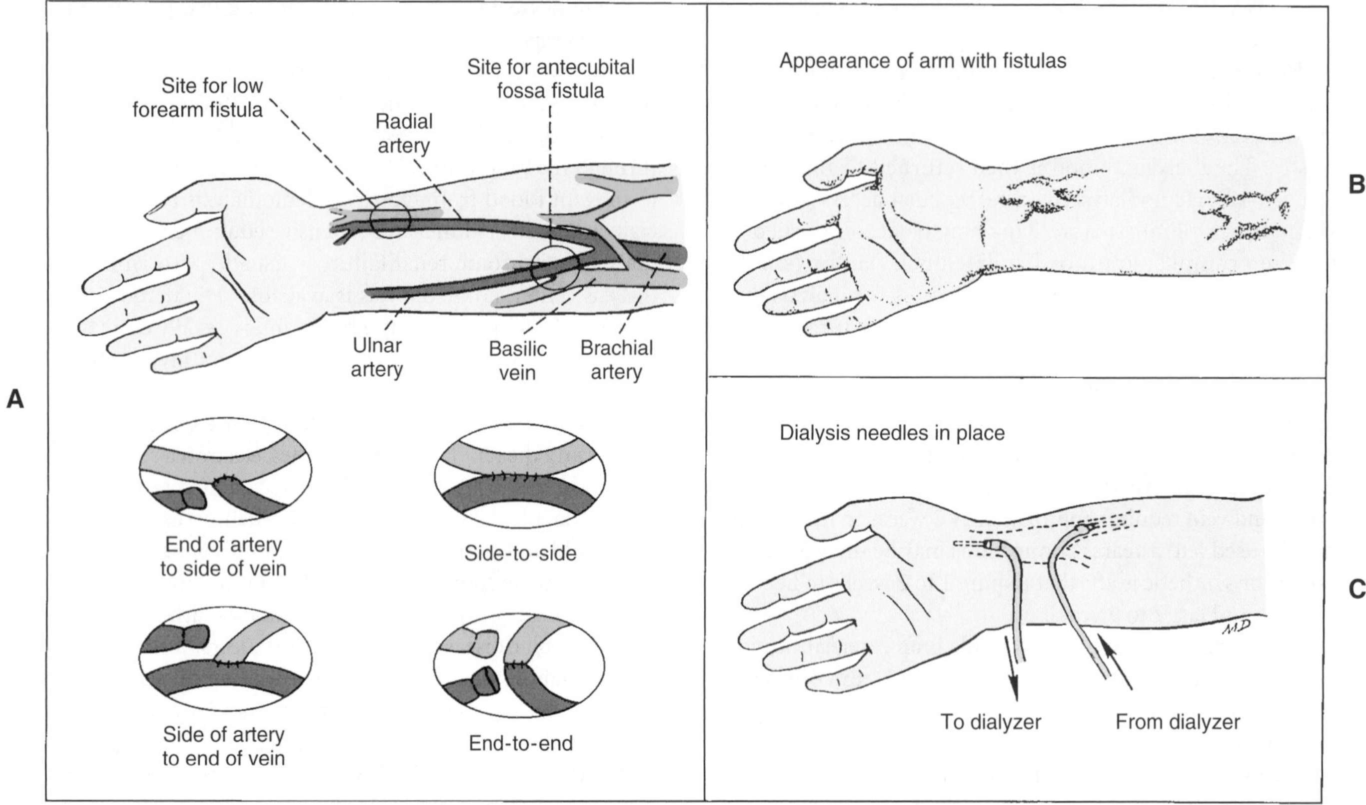

FIGURE **38-13** An internal arteriovenous fistula created by joining an artery and a vein. The fistula will be used for hemodialysis. *A,* Types of fistulas. *B,* The appearance of the arm with fistulas. *C,* Dialysis needles in place in the fistula.

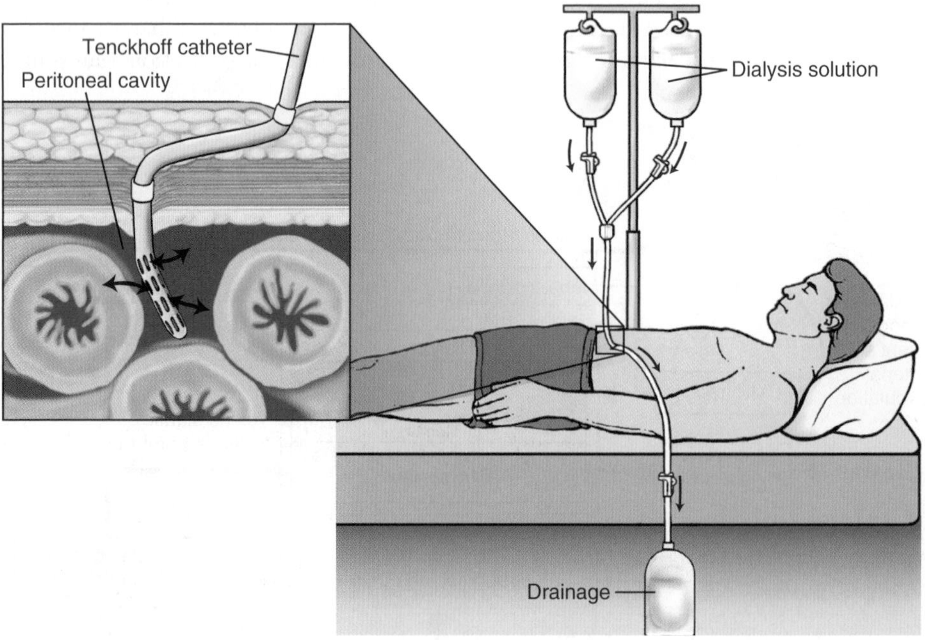

FIGURE **38-14** Peritoneal dialysis.

Advantages of peritoneal dialysis over hemodialysis include less anemia, reduced cost of equipment, fewer dietary and fluid restrictions, independence, and closer resemblance to normal kidney function. Also, it can be initiated in almost any hospital. Disadvantages include the risk of peritonitis (the major complication) and catheter site infection, hyperglycemia, elevated serum lipids, and body image disturbance. Also, peritoneal dialysis cannot be used for patients with recent abdominal surgery, extensive abdominal trauma, or open abdominal wounds.

Peritoneal dialysis has three phases: inflow, dwell, and drain. The three phases comprise one exchange. During inflow, fluid (commonly 2 liters) is allowed to drain into the peritoneal catheter through an established catheter over about 10 minutes. During the dwell time, fluid remains in the cavity for a specified period of time while ultrafiltration, osmosis, and diffusion occur. The fluid bearing wastes and excess water is then drained from the cavity over 20 to 30 minutes.

Continuous ambulatory peritoneal dialysis (CAPD) allows the patient freedom from a machine and the independence to perform dialysis alone. The exchange process usually is repeated four times each day by out-patients. It may be done more often in acutely ill hospitalized patients. Strict aseptic technique must be used with the initiation of the process and with each exchange. The patient or a reliable caregiver must be taught the process by someone who understands it well.

Automated peritoneal dialysis uses a device called a cycler to perform the exchanges during the night. This allows the patient freedom during the day. It also reduces the risk of infection because the system is interrupted less often. There are several variations of this procedure, which may be done from five to seven times a week and may or may not leave the fluid in the abdomen during the waking hours.

Peritonitis, infection of the peritoneum, is the most serious complication of peritoneal dialysis. Infections also may develop at the catheter exit site and tunnel where the catheter is placed under the skin. Cloudiness and particles in the fluid in the outflow container are evidence of infection. Redness, swelling, and purulent drainage are signs of infection at the exit site. Immediately report any signs of infection to the physician. Peritonitis is usually treated with antibiotics administered through the peritoneal catheter. Other complications include bleeding, abdominal pain, hernias, low back pain, respiratory distress, and decreased serum albumin. Encapsulating sclerosing peritonitis is a condition in which a thick membrane develops around the bowel. The thickened membrane can obstruct the intestines and interferes with ultrafiltration.

NURSING CARE *of the Patient in Chronic Renal Failure*

Assessment

The general nursing assessment of the patient with a urologic disorder is outlined in Table 38-1. For the patient in chronic renal failure, frequent monitoring for changes in status is especially important. Fluid balance is evaluated closely. During hospitalization, accurate intake and output records must be kept. Be alert for signs and symptoms of fluid volume excess that can lead to cardiac failure. Warning signs include increasing edema, dyspnea, tachycardia, bounding pulse, and rising blood pressure.

Serum electrolytes are measured frequently, but you must still be alert for signs and symptoms of electrolyte imbalances. With chronic renal failure, the nurse is most concerned with detecting hyperkalemia, hypocalcemia, and metabolic acidosis. Hyponatremia and hypovolemia are less common. Assessment of fluid and electrolyte imbalances includes characteristics of pulse and respirations, blood pressure, mental status, and neuromuscular activity.

Assessment of nutrition includes appetite, usual daily intake, weight gain or loss pattern, and prescribed diet. Determine how well the patient understands and follows the prescribed diet.

Do not overlook mental and emotional status when assessing the patient with renal failure. Increasing confusion or loss of consciousness can be due to accumulated toxins or electrolyte imbalances. Emotional responses to a diagnosis of chronic renal failure vary. Determine the patient's perceptions of the situation and identify usual coping strategies. Anxiety, fear, disturbed body image, depression, and lowered self-esteem are common.

The long-term effects of chronic renal failure and its treatment put the patient at risk for many complications. Assess bowel elimination for either constipation or diarrhea. Monitor for signs and symptoms of local or systemic infections (redness, swelling, foul drainage, fever, increased white blood cell count). Inspect the skin for bruising, bleeding, or trauma. Evaluate sensation in the extremities. Ask if sexual dysfunction has been a problem and obtain a description of the difficulty.

Assess patient understanding about chronic renal failure, its treatment, and self-care measures. Document the patient's ability to perform activities of daily living.

Specific nursing diagnoses and goals vary based on the individual patient assessment. Many diagnoses and interventions discussed in the section on acute renal failure also apply to the patient with chronic renal failure. The emphasis in this section is on the common problems experienced by the patient in chronic failure.

Nursing Diagnoses, Goals, and Outcome Criteria: Chronic Renal Failure

Nursing Diagnoses	Goals and Outcome Criteria
Excess Fluid Volume related to fluid retention	Reduced fluid volume and absence of symptoms of heart failure: normal tissue turgor, blood pressure within patient norms, no dyspnea
Imbalanced Nutrition: Less than Body Requirements related to anorexia, nausea, vomiting, stomatitis, dietary restrictions	Adequate nutrition: consumption of prescribed diet, serum albumin and total protein within acceptable limits.

Nursing Diagnoses, Goals, and Outcome Criteria: Chronic Renal Failure—cont'd

Nursing Diagnoses	Goals and Outcome Criteria
Disturbed Sensory Perception related to effects of uremia on the nervous system	Normal sensory perception: alert and oriented
Ineffective Coping related to multiple life changes	Effective coping: patient uses coping strategies that decrease anxiety without compromising care
Situational Low Self-Esteem related to self-worth, change in appearance, loss of kidney function, venous access devices, inability to fulfill usual roles and responsibilities	Improved self-esteem: positive statements of confidence
Risk for Infection related to impaired immune response, malnutrition, break in skin integrity	Absence of infection: normal body temperature and white blood cell count
Risk for Injury related to coagulation disorder, impaired wound healing, bone demineralization, peripheral neuropathy	Absence of injury: no bruises, bleeding, fractures
Constipation related to inactivity, drug side effects, fluid restriction, electrolyte imbalances	Normal bowel elimination: regular formed stools passed without straining
Diarrhea related to electrolyte imbalances, drug side effects	Normal bowel elimination: formed stools
Sexual Dysfunction related to fatigue, drug side effects, hormone deficiencies, altered self-image	Satisfactory sexual function: patient states intimate relationship is satisfactory
Self-Care Deficit related to lack of knowledge, confusion, anemia, fatigue	Accomplishment of self-care: patient performs activities of daily living within limitations imposed by renal failure and treatments

Interventions

Excess Fluid Volume

As renal failure progresses, the patient's ability to excrete excess fluids continually declines. In the early stages, diuretics may be used to treat fluid retention, but they are not used once dialysis is begun. Fluid intake may be restricted. If intravenous fluids are ordered, closely monitor the rate of infusion. Antihypertensives may be needed to control blood pressure, and digitalis may be given to support cardiac function. Dosage adjustments often are needed because kidney failure affects the ability to excrete these drugs. Administer medications, monitor for side effects, and teach the patient how to take them after discharge and what adverse effects to report.

Patients with fluid volume excess require comfort and safety measures. Edematous legs are easily injured and heal slowly. Protect them from pressure or trauma. If cardiac failure and dyspnea develop, position the patient with the head elevated to ease breathing. Cerebral edema causes confusion and decreasing consciousness. Implement safety measures to protect the confused or semiconscious patient from injury.

PHARMACOLOGY CAPSULE Because most drugs are excreted in the urine, people with impaired renal function are at risk for drug toxicity.

Imbalanced Nutrition: Less than Body Requirements

Adequate nutrition can be a real challenge for the patient in chronic renal failure. Anorexia, nausea, vomiting, and stomatitis interfere with food intake. In addition, sodium, protein, and sometimes fat restrictions make the diet less appealing. Measures to encourage food intake include frequent mouth care and small feedings. Explain the importance of good nutrition to the patient and family. The dietitian can help the patient learn to cope with the diet. The person who prepares the patient's food at home should be included in dietary instructions. Vitamin supplements are routinely ordered because of dietary restrictions. Monitor weight to evaluate both fluid and nutritional status. Teach the patient and the caregivers about medications and status monitors.

Disturbed Sensory Perception

Renal failure affects both the central and the peripheral nervous systems. Cerebral edema and elevated metabolic wastes in the blood can cause confusion, slowed thought processes, lethargy, and loss of consciousness. Protect confused patients and orient them to person, place, and time. Present information simply and repeat as needed. Avoid sensory overload by reducing environmental stimuli and demands on the patient. For safety reasons, assign the patient to a room close to the nurse's station. Put the bed in low position and keep the call button within reach.

The effects of renal disease on the peripheral nerves can lead to loss of sensation in the extremities (peripheral neuropathy). These patients are at risk for injury. Inspect the affected areas daily for any signs of injury. Pressure, ill-fitting shoes, or external heat or cold can cause serious injury before the patient is aware of it. Teach the patient about peripheral neuropathy and how to prevent injuries.

Ineffective Coping

Patients with chronic renal failure often experience anxiety and fear. They face life-threatening illness, endure invasive treatments and procedures, and undergo radical changes in lifestyle. Explore the patient's coping strategies and identify factors that interfere with adjustment to renal disease. It helps for the patient to have a regular primary nurse so that a therapeutic relationship can develop. Nurses can help by talking to patients and helping them focus on the sources of their distress. It is important to be accepting of the patient's thoughts and feelings. Do not give false reassurance or tell patients not to worry! Explain routines and procedures and provide practical advice on the management of everyday problems. Many patients benefit from talking to a mental health professional or attending support groups with people with similar problems. While encouraging patients to accept treatment, respect their rights to be informed and to refuse treatment.

Dialysis patients typically go through stages of adjustment. When dialysis is first started, they usually feel much better. They feel encouraged and view dialysis positively. This might be described as a honeymoon period. At this stage, the patient is most receptive to teaching. It is wise to take advantage of this opportunity to educate the patient.

After several months of treatment, patients tire of the routine. Depression and disappointment are common. Some cope by denying the need for treatment. They may omit medications or fail to keep appointments for follow-up. Be accepting of the patient but not the behavior at this stage. Confront the patient when ineffective coping behaviors are identified.

Eventually, most dialysis patients accept the need for ongoing treatment. They may try to resume their former levels of activity. At this point, you may need to guide them in realistic goal setting.

Situational Low Self-Esteem

The patient's self-esteem may suffer because of changes in body image and role performance. Encourage patients to talk about the changes they are experiencing and what they mean. Therapeutic communication and touch convey acceptance to patients. Help the patient with grooming to enhance appearance.

Encourage patients to examine their daily routines and look for ways to conserve time and energy. Sources of help and support need to be identified. Family functions may have to be redistributed. It is important for the patient to continue to have roles in the family and to be seen as a contributing family member.

Risk for Infection

Patients in chronic renal failure must avoid exposure to others with infections. Be sure they know how to take their own temperatures. Instruct them to report fever or other signs of infection to the physician. Practice good hand washing and aseptic technique for invasive procedures.

Risk for Injury

The patient is susceptible to injury because of impaired coagulation and wound healing, bone demineralization, and peripheral neuropathy. Calcium, vitamin D, and phosphate binders are ordered to reduce loss of calcium from the bones. Encourage ambulation, which helps to strengthen bones. Assess and protect body parts that lack sensation. Provide an environment with adequate support equipment and few obstacles that might cause bruises or falls.

Constipation

Constipation is a common problem with chronic renal failure because of inactivity, fluid restriction, electrolyte imbalances, and drug side effects. Encourage activity within the patient's tolerance level. Stool softeners often are ordered to prevent constipation.

Diarrhea

Diarrhea may be caused by drugs or by anxiety. Measure liquid stools and count as fluid output. Give antidiarrheals as ordered. Provide perianal care after each stool.

Sexual Dysfunction

Sexual dysfunction is attributed to both physical and emotional causes. At first you may feel uncomfortable discussing sexual function with patients, but patients need to know that it is acceptable to express concerns. Explain how kidney disease affects sexual function and explore what this means to the patient. Referral to a counselor who specializes in treatment of sexual dysfunction may be appreciated. Alternative means of sexual expression may enable the patient to continue to feel loved and to be intimate with another person.

Self-Care Deficit

Patients in chronic renal failure spend more time at home than they do in the hospital. Nurses need to prepare them for self-care.

RENAL TRANSPLANTATION

Kidney Donation

A healthy kidney may be obtained from a live donor (usually a relative) or from a cadaver. The tissues of the donor and the recipient must match or the recipient will reject the new kidney. Matching is based on ABO blood groups and human leukocyte antigens. Crossmatching between the blood of the prospective donor and recipient reveals any cytotoxic preformed antibodies that would certainly result in organ rejection. When a kidney is obtained from a living related donor, the 1-year survival rate for transplantation is approximately 95% to 97%. Ninety percent of patients who receive transplants from cadavers are alive 1 year later. A national network maintains lists of people awaiting donor kidneys. When a cadaver kidney is available, the network tries to locate the best match for the kidney to improve the chances of success.

Kidney donors must be at least 18 years of age, free of systemic disease or infection, have no history of cancer or renal disease, have normal renal function, and be without major medical problems. People older than 60 years of age may be considered as candidates for donation on an individual basis. Unfortunately, many older people have advanced cardiac or respiratory disease that makes them ineligible.

Consider the Alternative!

Patients with irreversible chronic diseases are vulnerable to claims of miracle cures. Caution patients to discuss alternative therapies with the physician to prevent potentially harmful outcomes.

Cadavers must meet the same criteria as living donors. Many people carry signed donor cards indicating willingness to have organs used for transplantation in the event of brain death. If brain death does occur, written permission is still sought from the family of the potential donor before organs are removed. The vital organs of the brain-dead person must be kept functioning until the kidney is removed.

PREOPERATIVE NURSING CARE *of the Renal Transplant Recipient*

In some respects, preoperative care of the renal transplant recipient is similar to that of any other patient facing major surgery (see Chapter 16). The patient must be prepared mentally and physically for the procedure. The unique aspect of this situation is that the patient awaits an organ from another human being. If a relative is the donor, the surgery can be planned and both people emotionally prepared. Counseling is advised for both the donor and the recipient. The patient may be ambivalent about receiving a relative's organ. The gift of a kidney can restore health, but the recipient may feel guilty about asking a loved one to endure surgery and to give up an organ. The donor also faces the stress of surgery and a future with only one kidney. The donor also has to accept that the kidney could be rejected. Both recipient and donor face the threat of surgical complications.

If awaiting a cadaver kidney, the patient must face the idea that someone must die for a kidney to be available. These potential recipients are on call and must be ready to report to the hospital at any time. In a given year, only about 1 in 4 of the 35,000 patients on waiting lists receive a kidney.

The recipient and the live donor have complete diagnostic workups to rule out other medical problems and to evaluate the function of the urinary tract. Normal function of both of the donor's kidneys must be affirmed. The recipient is given medications to bring blood pressure within normal limits. Immunosuppressant drugs are started to control the body's response to foreign tissue (i.e., the donated kidney; see Table 38-5). The recipient also may be given a transfusion of the donor's blood, a measure that has been found to reduce rejection. If the recipient has severe hypertension or a UTI, bilateral nephrectomies may be done before transplantation. The patient is dialyzed shortly before transplantation.

Assessment

In the preoperative period, a complete assessment is done as outlined in Chapter 16. Before renal transplantation, assess the patient's understanding of the surgery. Record baseline vital signs. Identify any specific fears or questions that need to be addressed.

Nursing Diagnoses, Goals, and Outcome Criteria: Renal Transplantation, Preoperative

NURSING DIAGNOSES	GOALS AND OUTCOME CRITERIA
Fear related to perceived threat of death	Reduced fear: patient states fear is lessened
Deficient Knowledge of surgical routines	Patient understands surgical routines: patient verbalizes accurate information, cooperates in care

Interventions

To achieve these goals, acknowledge and encourage the patient to discuss concerns. Accept fear as understandable and natural. Factual information helps the patient cope by reducing the fear of the unknown. Involve the patient in planning and in self-care. When patients are active participants in their care, they feel less helpless and less anxious. Preoperative teaching begins when the patient is identified as a candidate for transplantation. Reinforce information when the actual surgery is imminent. It is somewhat more difficult to teach the patient who is awaiting a cadaver kidney because one never knows when, or if, the transplantation will take place.

Surgical Procedure

The donor kidney is removed from the live donor in an operating room and taken to an adjacent room where the recipient has been prepared to receive it. A cadaver kidney is removed under sterile conditions and transported to the hospital where the recipient is waiting. The donor kidney is placed in the recipient's abdomen and anastamosed (attached) to the bladder and to blood vessels (Fig. 38-15).

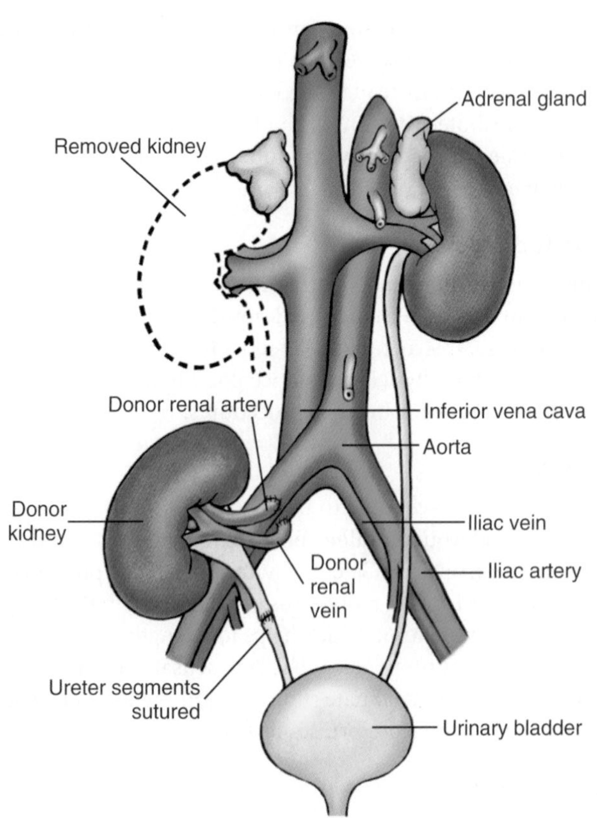

FIGURE **38-15** Placement of a transplanted kidney.

Complications

Complications after renal transplantation include rejection, renal artery stenosis, hematomas, abscesses, and leakage of ureteral or vascular anastomoses. Rejection of the new organ by the recipient is a major problem with most tissue transplants. Rejection is characterized by fever, elevated blood pressure, and pain over the location of the new kidney. Three types of rejection can occur: hyperacute, acute, and chronic. Hyperacute rejection occurs within 48 hours after transplantation. It is not reversible, and the kidney must be removed. Acute rejection develops between 1 week and 2 years after transplantation and is treated with increased immunosuppressant drugs. Chronic rejection develops and progresses slowly. Eventually, chronic rejection mimics chronic renal failure, and dialysis may become necessary.

Immunosuppressant drugs, begun before surgery, are continued in the postoperative period to reduce the risk of rejection. These drugs include (1) T-cell suppressors: cyclosporine, tacrolimus, or sirolimus; (2) cytotoxic drugs: mycophenolate mofetil, azathioprine, or cyclophosphamide; and (3) corticosteroids. Antibodies are drugs that are used primarily for short periods to prevent or reverse acute rejection. Those used for transplant patients include polyclonal antibodies (antithymocyte globulin, antilymphocyte globulin) and monoclonal antibodies (muromonab-CD3). Examples of immunosuppressants, their actions and adverse effects, and nursing interventions are provided in Table 38-5. They are called *immunosuppressants* because they inhibit the body's immune response to foreign tissue. This action is intended to prevent the donor kidney from being destroyed by the recipient's defenses. Unfortunately, the action of immunosuppressants also reduces the body's response to pathogens. Therefore, patients who take these drugs are at increased risk for infection.

POSTOPERATIVE NURSING CARE *of the Renal Transplant Recipient*

Assessment

General postoperative care is described in Chapter 16. This section emphasizes care that is unique to the renal transplant recipient. Assessment of the renal transplant recipient is similar to that of any surgical patient. It is especially important to monitor fluid intake, urine output, weight changes, and vital signs. Patients are usually in critical care for at least the first 24 hours because circulatory status requires constant monitoring including central venous pressure readings.

Nursing Diagnoses, Goals, and Outcome Criteria: Renal Transplantation, Postoperative

Nursing Diagnoses	Goals and Outcome Criteria
Impaired Urinary Elimination related to rejection of transplanted kidney, renal failure	Adequate urine elimination: fluid intake and output equal
Deficient Fluid Volume related to diuresis, blood loss	Normal fluid volume: pulse and blood pressure consistent with patient norms
Risk for Infection related to suppression of immune response	Absence of infection: normal body temperature and white blood cell count
Ineffective Management of Therapeutic Regimen of immediate and long-term postoperative care	Effective management of self-care: patient accurately describes and carries out plan of care
Anxiety related to possibility of organ rejection	Reduced anxiety: patient states anxiety is lessened, calm manner

Interventions

Immediately after surgery, the patient is taken to a special care unit for close monitoring. As with any surgical patient, the transplant recipient is monitored for circulatory and respiratory complications. Assist the patient with turning, coughing, deep breathing, and leg exercises. Institute pain control measures.

Impaired Urinary Elimination

The patient has an indwelling catheter for up to a week to permit constant observation of urine output. Urine is pink to bloody initially, then gradually clears. Maintain catheter patency at all times. Closely monitor the patient for signs that the transplanted organ is functioning: increasing urine output, normal blood pressure, decreasing BUN and serum creatinine, and stable weight. Commonly, the patient begins to diurese as soon as blood flow to the donor kidney is established. The output may be as high as 1 L/hr until BUN and serum creatinine return to normal.

If the patient is oliguric, a fluid challenge and diuretics are prescribed. In addition to the possibilities of renal failure and rejection, be alert for signs and symptoms of cardiac failure related to fluid volume excess: dyspnea, edema, bounding pulse, and cardiac dysrhythmias.

Put on your THINKING CAP!!

What are some measures you can take to maintain catheter patency in the post-transplant patient?

Deficient Fluid Volume

Massive postoperative diuresis causes fluid volume deficit in some patients. With excessive fluid loss, the patient is at risk for electrolyte imbalances and decreased cardiac output. A thready pulse, low blood pressure, and poor tissue turgor suggest dehydration. Serum electrolyte studies are ordered to identify specific imbalances. Intravenous fluid orders must be carefully individualized.

Risk for Infection

Because the immunosuppressant drugs that protect the new kidney also inhibit the body's ability to resist pathogens, you must monitor the transplant recipient carefully for signs and symptoms of infection: fever, elevated white blood cell count, cough, and purulent wound drainage. Signs and symptoms may be very subtle despite a major infection. Use good hand washing and aseptic technique when working with the patient. Separate the patient from others who have infections. Teach the patient and family members the importance of protecting the patient from exposure to infections. Give prophylactic antibiotics as prescribed. The physician prescribes any restrictions on diet, fluids, and activity. Clarify and reinforce these orders. It is critical that the patient knows how to recognize signs and symptoms of infection, rejection, and renal failure.

Ineffective Management of Therapeutic Regimen

Ideally, patient teaching begins before the transplant, so it can be reinforced after the procedure.

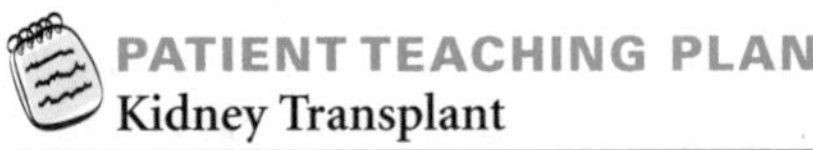

PATIENT TEACHING PLAN
Kidney Transplant

- Take your medication exactly as prescribed to control rejection and prevent other complications.
- Report adverse effects (specific to the patient's drugs) to the physician.
- Follow the diet prescribed by your physician.
- Avoid people with infections because your resistance is lowered.
- Increase activity as allowed by your physician.
- Immediately notify your physician of signs and symptoms of infection (fever, cough, increasing wound drainage) and rejection (fever, pain in kidney area).

Anxiety

Anxiety may lessen as renal function improves, but the patient always lives with the possibility of rejection. It is helpful for the patient to talk about feelings and explore ways to deal with them. Some patients find comfort in a support group of people who have had similar experiences or in spiritual resources. Others may need referral to a mental health professional to help them deal constructively with their stress.

THE KIDNEY DONOR

In the excitement over the patient finally receiving a kidney, never forget the role of the donor at this dramatic time. Physical care of the donor is similar to that described earlier for nephrectomy. The nephrectomy may be conventional or laparoscopic. Pain is considerably worse with the conventional approach, so be sure to provide good pain control measures. With the conventional approach, the patient will be hospitalized 3 to 5 days and return to work in 4 to 6 weeks. With the laparoscopic approach, the donor is hospitalized 2 to 3 days and can return to work in 2 to 3 weeks.

Emotionally, the donor usually feels very good about the experience because of the value of the kidney to the recipient. If the kidney fails, however, the donor may be very disappointed. Be sensitive to the emotional needs of the donor.

Nutrition Concepts

1. Renal failure results in an inability of the kidneys to excrete wastes and maintain fluid and electrolyte balance.
2. In renal failure, the nutritional goal is to modify the diet so that the work of the kidneys is reduced.
3. Fluid intake may be restricted to 1,000 to 1,500 ml/day for patients with renal disease.
4. Sodium and potassium intake is restricted (including medications) in patients who require dialysis to maintain electrolyte balance.
5. Protein is restricted in patients with renal disease, and any protein ingested should be high in essential amino acids. Examples of these proteins are eggs, meat, poultry, fish, and milk products.
6. People with renal calculi should increase fluid intake to maintain at least 2 L of urine output daily and avoid foods leading to the formation of calculi.
7. Calcium restriction is limited to certain types of renal calculi.

key points

- The urinary system eliminates metabolic wastes in urine, stimulates red blood cell production, and maintains fluid, electrolyte, and acid–base balance.
- Age-related changes in the urinary system include reduced ability to concentrate or dilute urine, nocturia, and decreased bladder capacity.
- Untreated or repeated urinary tract infections can result in renal scarring and lead to renal failure.
- Inflammatory conditions of the urinary tract include cystitis (bladder inflammation), urethritis (urethral inflammation), glomerulonephritis (glomerular inflammation), and pyelonephritis (inflammation of the renal pelvis).
- Risk factors for urinary tract infection include prolonged immobility, renal calculi, urinary diversion, and indwelling urinary catheters.
- Urinary tract infections are treated with antibiotics, urinary tract antiseptics, analgesics, and antispasmodics.
- Acute glomerulonephritis commonly follows a streptococcal respiratory infection and results in an immune response that scars the glomeruli.
- Patients with renal disorders are at risk for excess fluid volume, hypertension, and heart failure.
- Management of renal disorders requires attention to pain management, fluid balance, activity intolerance, and patient education.
- Urinary obstructions anywhere in the urinary tract can lead to hydronephrosis and kidney damage.
- Urinary calculi (stones) form in the urinary tract and may move through the tract with the flow of urine.
- Although most calculi pass spontaneously, some require surgical removal or disintegration by lithotripsy.
- Nursing care of the patient with renal calculi focuses on Acute Pain, Impaired Urinary Elimination, Risk for Deficient Fluid Volume, and Ineffective Management of Therapeutic Regimen.

- Complications of urinary tract surgery include urinary tract and wound infection, atelectasis, paralytic ileus, and hemorrhage.
- Renal tumors are often large before they are detected because early symptoms are subtle.
- Cystectomy (bladder removal) requires urine to be diverted to an alternate drainage or collection system. Types of urinary diversion used now are ileal and sigmoid conduits, ureterostomy, and nephrostomy.
- Nursing care after bladder surgery focuses on pain management, unobstructed urine flow, skin integrity, bowel function, and self-care.
- Renal failure can result from hypotension, toxins, infections, impaired blood flow, trauma, and obstructions.
- The four stages of acute renal failure are onset, oliguria, diuresis, and recovery.
- Management of acute renal failure emphasizes fluid and dietary restrictions, restoration of fluid balance, waste elimination, and maintenance of cardiac output.
- When 90% to 95% of kidney function is lost, the patient is considered to be in chronic renal failure.
- Effects of chronic renal failure include excess fluid volume, hyperkalemia, hypocalcemia, hyperuricemia, and anemia.
- Dialysis uses a semipermeable membrane to draw excess water, electrolytes, and wastes into a special solution called dialysate.
- Renal transplantation is the only alternative to dialysis for the patient in end-stage renal disease.
- Signs and symptoms of rejection of a transplanted kidney are fever, increased blood pressure, and pain over the location of the new kidney.

REVIEW QUESTIONS

1. An 88-year-old female was seen in the clinic 3 times last year for kidney infections. Age-related factors that may be contributing to these frequent infections include:
   1. relaxed pelvic muscles related to lack of estrogen.
   2. renal blood flow and glomerular filtration decline.
   3. decreased creatinine clearance by the kidneys.
   4. weak, ineffective contraction of trigonal muscles.
2. A patient tells you she has a painful, burning sensation during urination. You should record this symptom as:
   1. dysuria.
   2. dysphagia.
   3. dysmenorrhea.
   4. dystrophy.
3. The first time a patient voids after cystoscopy, you notice the urine is pink-tinged. You should:
   1. promptly notify the physician.
   2. encourage additional fluids.
   3. recognize that this is normal.
   4. assess the patient's blood pressure.
4. The primary cause of hospital-acquired infections is:
   1. wound contamination.
   2. catheterization.
   3. tracheal suctioning.
   4. diagnostic procedures.
5. Patient teaching to reduce the risk of cystitis in women should include:
   1. Tub baths are recommended over showers.
   2. Drink a glass of water before and after intercourse.
   3. Cleanse the perineum from back to front after elimination.
   4. Wear synthetic undergarments that serve as a barrier to moisture.
6. Glomerulonephritis is caused by:
   1. bacteria.
   2. viruses
   3. urinary obstruction.
   4. immunologic processes.
7. A procedure that uses sound waves to break up renal calculi is:
   1. lithotripsy.
   2. lithotomy.
   3. nephrolithotomy.
   4. ureterolithotomy.
8. The maximum amount of fluid that can be used to irrigate a nephrostomy tube is:
   1. 1 ml.
   2. 5 ml.
   3. 30 ml.
   4. 100 ml.
9. Following a nephrectomy, a patient's urine output was 25 ml in the past hour. You should:
   1. have the patient change positions.
   2. give the patient an 8-ounce glass of water every 2 hours.
   3. increase the flow rate of the patient's intravenous fluids.
   4. notify the physician that the patient's urine output is too low.
10. A patient in chronic renal failure becomes confused. He complains of nausea, abdominal cramps, and lack of sensation in his legs. His heart rhythm is irregular. You should suspect:
    1. increased blood urea nitrogen.
    2. hyperkalemia.
    3. metabolic acidosis.
    4. hypocalcemia.

CHAPTER

39 Connective Tissue Disorders

LAURIE J. SINGEL

objectives

1. Define connective tissue.
2. Describe the function of connective tissue.
3. Describe the characteristics and prevalence of connective tissue diseases.
4. Describe the diagnostic tests and procedures used for assessing connective tissue diseases.
5. Discuss the drugs used to treat connective tissue diseases.
6. Describe the pathophysiology and treatment of basis for osteoarthritis (degenerative joint disease), rheumatoid arthritis, osteoporosis, gout, progressive systemic sclerosis, polymyositis, bursitis, carpal tunnel syndrome, ankylosing spondylitis, polymyalgia rheumatica, Reiter's syndrome, Behçet's syndrome, and Sjögren's syndrome.
7. Identify the data to be collected in the nursing assessment of a patient with a connective tissue disorder.
8. Assist in developing a nursing care plan for a patient whose life has been affected by a connective tissue disease.

key terms

Ankylosis (ăng-kĭ-LŌ-sĭs, p. 809)
Arthroplasty (ĂR-thrō-plăs-tē, p. 804)
Bouchard's node (boo-SHĂRZ, p. 803)
Crepitus (KRĔP-ĭ-tŭs, p. 796)
Goniometer (gō-nē-ŎM-ĕ-tĕr, p. 796)
Heberden's node (HĒ-bĕr-dĕnz, p. 803)
Hyperuricemia (hī-pĕr-ŭr-ĭ-SĒ-mē-ă, p. 814)
Intra-articular (ĭn-tră-ăr-TĬK-ū-lăr, p. 803)
Rheumatoid nodule (RŪŪ-mă-toyd NŎD-ūl, p. 810)
Tophi (TŌ-fī, p. 814)
Vasculitis (văs-kū-LĪ-tĭs, p. 810)

More than 37 million people in the United States have one or more connective tissue diseases. Often called rheumatoid disorders, these conditions affect women more frequently than men but have no particular racial prevalence. Most are chronic and are characterized by alternating exacerbations and remissions, with progressive deterioration. Many have no known cause or cure. Rheumatoid disorders challenge the spirit and body of the patient. They can dramatically alter the patient's lifestyle, self-image, employability, and hope for the future.

A number of the conditions discussed in this chapter are classified as autoimmune disorders. They are included here because their primary effects are on connective tissue. For a thorough explanation of autoimmunity, see Chapter 32.

ANATOMY AND PHYSIOLOGY OF CONNECTIVE TISSUES

Connective tissues bind structures together, providing support for individual organs and a framework for the body as a whole. They also store fat, transport substances, provide protection, and play a role in repair of damaged tissue. The types of connective tissue are loose (areolar, adipose, reticular), dense (tendons, fascia, dermis, gastrointestinal tract submucosa, fibrous joint capsules), elastic (aortic walls, vocal cords, parts of trachea and bronchi, some ligaments), hematopoietic (blood), and strong supportive (cartilage, bone, ligaments).

This chapter is primarily concerned with disorders that affect bone, cartilage, ligaments, and tendons. Although selected autoimmune disorders that significantly affect the musculoskeletal system are included in this chapter, see Chapter 32 for a detailed discussion of autoimmune disorders. Blood disorders are addressed in Chapter 31, and skin disorders other than scleroderma are discussed in Chapter 48.

BONE

Bone is the hard tissue that makes up most of the skeletal system. The functions of the bones are support, protection, movement, storage of calcium and other ions, and manufacture of blood cells.

CARTILAGE

Cartilage is a specialized fibrous connective tissue. It provides firm but flexible support for the embryonic skeleton and part of the adult skeleton. Cartilage differs from bone in that its matrix has the consistency of a firm plastic or gristle-like gel. Cartilage cells are called chondrocytes and are located in tiny spaces that are distributed throughout the matrix.

LIGAMENTS

Ligaments are strong and flexible fibrous bands of connective tissue that connect bones and cartilage and support muscles. Yellow ligaments and white ligaments have distinctively different functions. Yellow ligaments, located in the vertebral column, are elastic and allow for stretching. White ligaments, found in the knee, do not stretch but provide stability.

TENDONS

Tendons are composed of very strong and dense fibrous connective tissue. They are in the shape of heavy cords and anchor muscles firmly to bones. One of the most prominent tendons is the Achilles tendon, which can be felt at the back of the ankle just above the heel.

JOINT STRUCTURE AND FUNCTION

Connective tissue disorders are often manifested as joint disorders since joint mobility is dependent on functional connective tissue. A joint is the site at which two or more bones of the body are joined. Joints permit motion and flexibility of the rigid skeleton. The only bone in the human body that does not articulate with at least one other bone is the hyoid bone, to which the tongue is attached.

Classified on the basis of the extent of movement, joints include synarthroses (fixed joints), amphiarthroses (slightly movable joints), and diarthroses (freely movable joints). Synarthroses, such as those in the skull, allow no movement at all. An example of a slightly movable joint, an amphiarthrosis, is the juncture of the ulna and radius in the forearm. Diarthroses, such as those in the elbows, shoulders, fingers, hips, and knees, allow considerable movement. Diarthroses are sometimes called synovial joints. They are encased in a fibrous capsule made of strong cartilage and lined with synovial membrane.

The synovial membrane is very smooth, thus permitting structures to move without friction. Ligaments are tough fibrous cords that bind the capsule. A smooth layer of cartilage also covers the ends of the bones, where it serves as a type of shock absorber. Synovial fluid fills and lubricates the space in the middle of the joint. Bursae are sacs of synovial fluid found in joints that also promote smooth articulation of joint structures. The bursae permit tendons to slide easily with movement of the bones.

AGE-RELATED CHANGES

Age-related changes in connective tissue can significantly impact function. There is a loss of bone mass and bone strength. The progressive loss of bone density during later adult life accounts for the decline in bone strength. Significant bone loss, called osteoporosis, is more common in women but affects men as well. These changes put the older patient at risk for fractures.

Age-related joint changes are primarily related to the changes in cartilage. With age, cartilage gradually loses elasticity, then becomes soft and frayed. Water content decreases, and cartilage may ulcerate, leaving bony joint surfaces unprotected and promoting the growth of osteophytes (bony spurs). These joint changes result in pain and limited mobility and can contribute to a loss of independence.

NURSING ASSESSMENT OF CONNECTIVE TISSUE STRUCTURES

HEALTH HISTORY

The nursing assessment requires a detailed health history, because many of the signs and symptoms of connective tissue disorders are insidious. Also, patients with chronic conditions may come to accept their symptoms as a way of life and fail to report them to the nurse. Therefore it may be helpful to have a family member present to assist the patient as historian. The family member may provide a clearer picture of how the changes in health have evolved.

Chief Complaint and History of Present Illness

Determine why the patient is seeking health care. Complaints that suggest possible problems related to connective tissue disorders are aches, pain, joint swelling or stiffness, generalized weakness, a change in ability to work or to enjoy leisure activities, a change in appearance that is significant to the patient, and a change in ability to carry out activities of daily living.

Past Medical History

The past medical history provides information about the patient's prior state of health. Inquire about major childhood and adult illnesses, operations, and current medications and allergies. Ask whether there is a history of tuberculosis, poliomyelitis, diabetes mellitus, gout, arthritis, rickets, infection of bones or joints, autoimmune diseases, and neuromuscular disabilities. Record the dates of immunizations for polio and tetanus, because postpolio syndrome and tetanus are characterized by musculoskeletal symptoms.

Accidents and Injuries

Accidents and injuries, even in the distant past, may be significant because they could be related to the patient's current problem. For example, low back pain in the present may be the result of an injury sustained several years ago. Inquire about participation in sports and the type of work the patient did. Many types of sports injuries result in osteoarthritis later in life.

Current Medications

Record the use of prescription and over-the-counter drugs. Self-medication is common with musculoskeletal pain, and patients may fail to report it unless specifically asked. Inquire about the use of alternative therapies, including the use of herbal supplements and home remedies. Many herbal supplements interact with traditional medications and have significant side effects. List all medications prescribed previously and identify their effectiveness. Note any problems associated with the medication and whether the patient thinks the medication is effective. Record any allergies.

Family History

Ask whether the patient or any relative has had osteoporosis, osteoarthritis, rheumatoid arthritis, gout, or scoliosis, because these conditions appear to have some genetic basis. Inquire about any history of other autoimmune diseases such as thyroid disorders.

Review of Systems

Assess each body system for significant symptoms. Assessment of general health status determines the patient's perception of well-being. Specifically, ask whether the patient has had fatigue, malaise, anorexia, weight loss, pain, stiffness, dysphagia, or dyspnea. With joint pain and stiffness, it is especially helpful to determine whether the symptoms are present on arising in the morning and how long they persist. Be aware that many cultures react differently to pain and disability; some may be stoic, while others are very expressive. The loss of ability to perform certain daily functions can have a significant impact on the role in the family and therefore cause emotional distress and frustration. For example, a husband crippled with arthritis, who can no longer work to support his family, will be greatly affected, both physically and psychologically.

Functional Assessment

The following questions may be used to assess the patient's functional status and the significance of any changes to the patient:

How does this problem affect the way you live?
Have you had to change your everyday activities?
How do you feel about any changes that you have had to make?
What have you found helpful in adapting to these changes?
How do you carry out the treatment program prescribed by your physician?
Has your treatment plan been effective for you?
What kind of support systems do you have at home?

PHYSICAL EXAMINATION

Begin the physical examination by recording the patient's vital signs and height and weight. Be aware that many patients with arthritis have limited physical abilities to stand, step up, or get onto an examination table. A scale-chair has been very useful for these patients. Compare findings with the patient's norms, if available. Be alert for fever, tachycardia, tachypnea, weight loss, and loss of height.

Inspect the skin for color, rashes, lesions, scars, or any signs of injuries. Palpate the skin for warmth, edema, and moisture. Palpate lymph nodes for enlargement and tenderness. Inspect joints for swelling and deformity and palpate for warmth, swelling, and tenderness. Assess joint pain and range of motion by asking the patient to move each extremity through the normal range of motion. Be very careful not to extend joints beyond their range/point of comfort. Inflamed joints are extremely sensitive to movement and pressure. During the movement, watch for signs of pain and listen for the crackling sound called crepitus. A more precise assessment of joint motion may be done by the physician or other advanced health care provider by using an instrument called a goniometer, which measures the range of movement of the joints. Measurement of limb length and muscle strength also may be done.

The nursing assessment of the patient with a connective tissue disorder is outlined in Table 39-1.

table 39-1 ASSESSMENT *of the Patient with a Connective Tissue Disorder*

HEALTH HISTORY

Present Illness: Changes in movement, activities of daily living; areas of pain, swelling, or tenderness, fatigue
Past Medical History: Tuberculosis, poliomyelitis, diabetes mellitus, gout, arthritis, rickets, neuromuscular disabilities
Family History: Rheumatoid arthritis, degenerative arthritis (need for joint replacement surgery), gout, scoliosis, other autoimmune disorders
Review of Systems: Pain or swelling in joints, limitation of movement, weakness, malaise, change in general appearance of skin
Functional Assessment: Past or recent injuries due to accidents or falls, use of assistive devices

PHYSICAL EXAMINATION

General Survey: Posture, balance, gait, skin condition
Joints: Warmth, redness, swelling, tenderness, nodules, range of motion, crepitus, function of hands
Skin: Color, scars, bruising, warmth, swelling
Upper Extremities:
Symmetry, swelling, tenderness, pain, range of motion, posture
Lower Extremities: Movement of hips, knees, and ankles; pain; skin condition

DIAGNOSTIC TESTS AND PROCEDURES

Diagnostic procedures used to diagnose connective tissue diseases are mainly laboratory studies of blood and urine and radiologic imaging studies of the bones and joints.

Routine blood studies that are useful in diagnosing connective tissue disorders include a complete blood cell count, the erythrocyte sedimentation rate (ESR), and C-reactive protein determination. These studies help determine whether a disorder is inflammatory or noninflammatory. Other blood studies are the Venereal Disease Research Laboratory (VDRL), rheumatoid factor (RF), creatinine, and antinuclear antibody (ANA) tests. Urine may be tested for creatinine and uric acid levels. Fluids aspirated from joints may be studied to detect uric acid crystals or white blood cells. Most laboratory tests are not diagnostic for a single condition—that is, many factors could cause measures of inflammation to increase. The physician may rely on multiple diagnostic procedures along with the patient assessment to reach a diagnosis.

Radiologic imaging studies include radiography, ultrasonography, arthrography, nuclear scintigraphy, magnetic resonance imaging, diskography, tomography, and computed tomography. Other useful measures are biopsy and arthroscopy. Table 39-2 summarizes commonly used diagnostic studies

table 39-2 **DIAGNOSTIC TESTS AND PROCEDURES | *Connective Tissue Disorders***

COMMON NURSING IMPLICATIONS: Always tell the patient what to expect before, during, and after the test/procedure. When blood samples will be needed, inform the patient that blood will be drawn.

TEST/PURPOSE	PATIENT PREPARATION	POSTPROCEDURE NURSING CARE
BLOOD STUDIES		
Antinuclear Antibodies (ANA)		
Positive in SLE, RA, systemic sclerosis, Raynaud's disease, Sjögren's syndrome, and necrotizing arteritis.	Fast 8 hr before test.	Apply pressure to venipuncture site. Assess site for bleeding.
C-Reactive Protein		
Detects active inflammation as in RA and disseminated lupus erythematosus.	Restrict food and fluids for 4 hr.	Apply pressure to venipuncture site. Assess site for bleeding.
Creatinine		
Assesses renal function. Increased with SLE, PSS, polyarteritis.	Fasting *not* required.	Apply pressure to venipuncture site. Assess site for bleeding.
Erythrocyte Sedimentation Rate (ESR)		
Determines presence of inflammation. Increased with RA, rheumatic fever. Decreased with osteoarthritis.	Fasting *not* required.	Apply pressure to venipuncture site. Assess site for bleeding.
Red Blood Cell (RBC) Count		
Detects and differentiates blood dyscrasias. Decreased in RA, SLE.	Fasting *not* required.	Apply pressure to venipuncture site. Assess site for bleeding.
Rheumatoid Factor (RF)		
Detects antibodies often present with RA.	Fasting *not* required.	Apply pressure to venipuncture site. Assess site for bleeding.
Venereal Disease Research Laboratory (VDRL) Test		
Measures antibodies to syphilis. Sometimes decreased in SLE.	Fasting *not* required.	Apply pressure to venipuncture site. Assess site for bleeding.
White Blood Cell (WBC) Count		
Increased in infection, tissue necrosis, inflammation; may decrease in SLE.	Fasting *not* required.	Apply pressure to venipuncture site. Assess site for bleeding.
URINE STUDIES		
24-Hour Urine for Creatinine		
Measures renal function and status of muscle diseases.	Instruct the patient to collect a 24-hr urine specimen. Discard the first morning specimen. Save rest of urine voided over 24-hr period in a clean, refrigerated 3-L container with or without preservative. Include urine voided at end of 24-hr period. Fasting *not* required.	None.
Urinary Uric Acid (24-Hr Collection)		
Measures uric acid metabolism; increased in gout, liver disease, chronic myelogenous leukemia, fever.	Requires 24-hr urine specimen (as described above). Fasting *not* required.	None.

See agency laboratory manual for specific preparation and norms. Results vary with different types of tests and may be reported in different units of measurement.

Continued

table 39-2 **DIAGNOSTIC TESTS AND PROCEDURES | *Connective Tissue Disorders—cont'd***

TEST/PURPOSE	PATIENT PREPARATION	POSTPROCEDURE NURSING CARE
RADIOLOGIC STUDIES		
Arthrography		
Use contrast medium to show soft-tissue joint structures.	Question patient about allergy to contrast agent, seafood, iodine. If yes, notify radiologist. Tell patient that needle insertion may cause discomfort. May cause swelling that lasts several days.	Assess and document discomfort, swelling. Instruct patient to avoid strenuous activity 12-24 hr after test. Joint may be wrapped.
Computed Tomography (CT)		
Detects tumors and some spinal fractures.	Tell patient that procedure may be lengthy (up to 30 min per body part). Patient lies on stretcher while a machine scans area being studied.	None
Diskography		
Visualizes vertebral disk after contrast medium injected into disk.	Same as for arthrography.	Same as for arthrography.
Magnetic Resonance Imaging (MRI)		
Visualizes soft tissue. May detect avascular necrosis, disk disease, tumors, osteomyelitis, and torn ligaments.	Tell patient that procedure is painless; must lie still for 30 min or more. Some equipment has videos that patient can view to reduce anxiety. Ask whether patient is claustrophobic. Give sedation if ordered for agitated or anxious patients. Remove any metallic objects such as jewelry. Inquire whether patient has any implanted devices such as cardiac pacemaker or intracranial aneurysm clips and notify radiologist. Procedure is contraindicated with some implants. Metal may not be a problem with some newer equipment.	No special postprocedure care. Safety precautions if sedated.
Nuclear Scintigraphy (Bone Scan)		
Detects bone malignancies, osteoporosis, osteomyelitis, and some fractures.	Contraindicated during pregnancy. Tell patient that a small amount of radioactive material will be injected intravenously, then a scanner will move slowly back and forth over the body as the patient lies on a stretcher. May take 1 hr. Procedure is painless except for venipuncture. Radioactive isotopes are not harmful except to fetus. Empty bladder immediately before procedure for comfort and to prevent blocked view of pelvis.	No special precaution required for handling urine or stool.

and related nursing care. Agency procedure manuals will provide more specific preparation and postprocedure care.

COMMON THERAPEUTIC MEASURES

Management of the patient with a connective tissue disorder often requires the services of a team that includes the patient, nurse, physician, social worker, physical therapist, and occupational therapist. The goals of therapy are to reduce inflammation and pain and to promote adaptation to the condition. Therapeutic measures may include physical and occupational therapy, modification of activities of daily living, patient education and support, drug therapy, and surgical intervention. Although none of these measures is curative, they can greatly enhance the patient's function and quality of life.

PHYSICAL AND OCCUPATIONAL THERAPY

Physical therapy employs exercise and positioning to help preserve functional capability and minimize disability. For many patients, braces and splints will be ordered to help sup-

table 39-2 **DIAGNOSTIC TESTS AND PROCEDURES | *Connective Tissue Disorders—cont'd***

TEST/PURPOSE	PATIENT PREPARATION	POSTPROCEDURE NURSING CARE
Radiography		
Shows density, texture, and alignments of bones; reveals soft tissue involvement	Tell patient to expect to lie on an x-ray table or to stand next to a special device while films are taken. Remove any radiopaque objects (jewelry, etc.) that can interfere with results. Advise radiology of patient's physical limitations r/t moving, turning, climbing.	None.
Tomography		
Provides details of structures otherwise hidden by bone.	Requires lying in a cylindric scanner; assess for claustrophobia and inform radiologist.	None.
Ultrasonography		
Reveals masses or fluid in soft tissue.	None.	None.
SPECIAL TESTS		
Arthroscopy		
A surgical procedure to visualize a joint cavity and structure and to obtain fluid and/or tissue for study.	Inform patient that procedure is performed in operating room under local or general anesthesia.	The patient will have a sterile dressing applied, then wrapped with compression dressing. Report any drainage of blood or fluid. Instruct patient to limit activity for a few days.
Joint Aspiration		
Examination of fluid taken from a joint to diagnose inflammation.	Procedure is usually done at bedside or in examination room. Tell patient that a local anesthetic agent is used to minimize discomfort.	Apply pressure dressing to joint. Instruct patient to rest joint for 8-24 hr. Record on patient's charts and report to physician or nurse supervisor any leakage of blood or fluid. Apply pressure dressing to affected area and keep immobilized for 12-24 hr.
Muscle Biopsy		
A sample of muscle tissue is taken to detect inflammation reaction, as in polymyositis or myopathic disease.	May be performed under local or general anesthesia.	Apply pressure dressing to affected area and keep immobilized for 12-24 hr.
Skin Biopsy		
Studies excised skin to confirm inflammatory connective tissue diseases such as SLE and PSS.	Tell patient a local anesthetic will be injected; there may be slight discomfort when skin sample is obtained.	Keep biopsy site clean and dry with small adhesive bandage until scab develops. Patients who are taking aspirin or NSAIDs are at risk for bleeding and/or bruising at the biopsy site.

port inflamed joints, protect from further injury, and relieve discomfort. Occupational therapy assists the patient in making adaptations in work and personal life that allow maximal possible function.

EDUCATION AND SUPPORT

Education emphasizes the treatment plan and how it will benefit the patient. Team members must be sensitive to the inconvenience and discomfort the disease has caused and must also help the patient identify ways to cope with the condition. Patients and their families need information about community support groups that can offer encouragement, information, and resources. A patient's attitude toward the disease is very important in the successful treatment and management, and psychological support should be provided. Many research studies have shown the connection between a patient's positive attitude and a successful outcome with chronic diseases.

DRUG THERAPY

Drug therapy for connective tissue disorders has traditionally included glucocorticoids and nonsteroidal anti-inflammatory drugs (NSAIDs) to reduce inflammation (Table 39-3). When

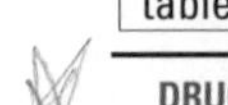

table 39-3 DRUG THERAPY | *Drugs Used to Treat Connective Tissue Disorders*

DRUG USE/ACTION	SIDE EFFECTS	NURSING INTERVENTIONS
FIRST-GENERATION NONSTEROIDAL ANTI-INFLAMMATORY DRUGS (NSAIDS)		
Aspirin Diclofenac sodium (Voltaren) Ibuprofen (Motrin, Rufen) Naproxen (Naprosyn) Nabumetone (Relafen) Analgesic Antipyretic Anti-inflammatory (inhibits prostaglandin synthesis) Decreases pain and deformity. Inhibits platelet aggregation (clumping).	Gastrointestinal (GI) upset, GI bleeding may be silent in elderly. Ototoxicity. Bleeding because of anticoagulation. Some may cause drowsiness. Increased blood pressure because of fluid retention.	Instruct patient to take with food or to take enteric-coated aspirin and report ringing in ears (tinnitus), abdominal pain, dark stools. Assess for bruising and bleeding. Caution patients not to take aspirin and NSAIDs concurrently and not to drive if drowsy.
SECOND-GENERATION NONSTEROIDAL ANTI-INFLAMMATORY DRUGS: COX-2 INHIBITORS		
Celecoxib (Celebrex) Rofecoxib (Vioxx) Analgesic Antipyretic Anti-inflammatory (inhibits prostaglandin synthesis)	GI bleeding (less risk than first-generation NSAIDs), fatigue, dependent edema, nausea, increased blood pressure because of fluid retention. Dizziness.	Administer with food or full glass of water. Remain in upright position 15-30 min after taking. Safety precautions if dizzy. Do not confuse with Celexa (antidepressant) or Cerebyx (injectable fosphenytoin to treat seizures). Do not use with aspirin, alcohol, or acetaminophen concurrently.
INDOLE ANALOGUES		
Indomethacin (Indocin) Sulindac (Clinoril) Analgesic Anti-inflammatory (inhibits prostaglandin synthesis) Indicated for severe ankylosing spondylitis, painful shoulders.	Gastric bleeding, headaches, dizziness, psychiatric disturbances.	Administer with food. Report any signs of bleeding (tarry stools, hematemesis) to physician.
GLUCOCORTICOIDS		
Hydrocortisone (Cortef, Hydrocortone) Hydrocortisone sodium succinate (Solu-Cortef, cortisol) Cortisone acetate (Cortone) Prednisone (Deltasone) Prednisolone (Delta-Cortef) Suppress normal immune response and inflammation. Used in inflammatory and allergic conditions.	Muscular weakness, nausea, anorexia, hypotension; sodium retention, hypokalemia; insomnia; nervousness; euphoria; rise in serum glucose. Osteoporosis. Increased susceptibility to infections.	Highest dose usually given in early morning; lowest dose given later in day to mimic normal secretion in body. Stress to patient need to adhere to prescribed schedule. Remember that glucocorticoids mask signs of infection. Observe for any unusual drainage, odors, and elevated temperatures. Must be tapered off rather than stopped abruptly.
DISEASE-MODIFYING ANTIRHEUMATIC DRUGS (DMARDS)		
Methotrexate (Folex) Treats rheumatoid arthritis.	Anorexia, nausea, vomiting, diarrhea. Toxic effects on oral tissues, liver, lungs, bone marrow, skin, and kidneys. Hemorrhage; hair loss.	Monitor periodic mild immunosuppressant blood and urine studies to detect abnormalities because of toxicity. Encourage fluid intake. Tell patient to avoid trauma because of risk of bleeding; to avoid people with infections; and to report bruising, bleeding, or signs of infection promptly.
Hydroxychloroquine sulfate (Plaquenil, Sulfate) Basis of antirheumatic effects unknown; may suppress antigens that trigger hypersensitivity reactions.	Headache, nausea, vomiting, anorexia. Ocular toxicity. With prolonged therapy: bone marrow suppression, psychosis.	Ask about known allergy to drug. Tell patient to report visual or hearing disturbances promptly. Monitor complete blood cell count and liver function studies.

table 39-3 | DRUG THERAPY | *Drugs Used to Treat Connective Tissue Disorders—cont'd*

DRUG USE/ACTION	SIDE EFFECTS	NURSING INTERVENTIONS
DISEASE-MODIFYING ANTIRHEUMATIC DRUGS (DMARDS)—cont'd		
Sulfasalazine (Azulfidine) Antimicrobial, anti-inflammatory. Used to treat rheumatoid arthritis.	Anorexia, nausea, vomiting, headache, oligospermia. Toxic effects on bone marrow, liver, kidneys. Rarely: anaphylaxis.	Monitor liver and kidney function. Ensure urine output of at least 1,500 ml/day. Assess for bruising, jaundice, fever, sore throat. Tell patient to avoid direct sunlight.
Leflunomide (Arava) Treats active rheumatoid arthritis, retards structural damage. Slows disease progression.	Diarrhea, liver toxicity, hair loss. Teratogenic.	Monitor liver studies. Tell patient to report severe diarrhea. Known to cause fetal harm; women of childbearing age should avoid conception. Avoid alcohol consumption while on medication.
ANTIARTHRITIC, BIOLOGIC RESPONSE MODIFIERS		
Etanercept (Enbrel) Used to treat severe rheumatoid arthitis in adults who do not respond to other DMARDs. Binds tumor necrosis factor, which is involved in immunity and inflammation.	Injection site reaction, abdominal pain, heartburn, headache, dizziness, upper respiratory infections, cough.	Reconstitute supplied diluent, add to powder, swirl to mix (do not shake), and administer immediately. Use only clear, colorless solution. Do not mix with other drugs. Administer subq in upper arm, abdomen, or thigh. Rotate sites. Check injection site for redness, itching. Caution in people with recurring infections or people at risk for infections.
Infliximab (Remicade) A monoclonal antibody that neutralizes activity of tumor necrosis factor, which decreases inflammation. Used to treat RA, Crohn's disease.	Anaphylaxis, anemia, tachycardia, GI distress, skin rash, headache, dizziness, depression, upper respiratory infections, muscle aches, painful urination, chest pain, hypotension, hypertension.	Given IV q 1-2 months in combination with methotrexate. 2 hr infusion. Reconstitute and use immediately. Monitor for signs of infection, especially upper respiratory tract infections. Cannot be infused in IV line with other agents.
ANTIGOUT AGENTS		
Allopurinol (Xyloprim) Inhibits synthesis of uric acid.	Drowsiness. Toxicity: maculopapular rash, fever, chills, joint pain. Rarely: bone marrow depression, nausea, diarrhea.	Tell patient to drink 8-10 glasses of fluid daily to maintain output of at least 2,000 ml/day. Assess urine for abnormal characteristics. Safety precautions if drowsy. Tell patient it takes several weeks for full effects. Assess and record response.
Probenecid (Benemid) Increases urinary excretion of uric acid.	Headache, urinary frequency, GI distress. Rarely: anaphylaxis. Toxicity: maculopapular rash, fever, joint pain, leukopenia, GI distress. Urinary calculi (stones).	Assess allergies. Do not give with penicillin. Use caution with renal impairment. Encourage fluid intake to maintain output of at least 2,000 ml/day. Tell patient it takes several weeks for full therapeutic effect.
BONE RESORPTION INHIBITORS		
Alendronate sodium (Fosamax) Increases bone mineral density by impairing bone resorption.	Abdominal pain, muscle pain, diarrhea, constipation, severe GI disturbances with overdose, hypocalcemia.	Take with 6-8 oz water on arising in AM, nothing else by mouth for 30 min. Patient should not lie down for 30 min after taking.
Calcitonin (Miacalcin) Impairs bone resorption. Given parenterally, orally, or per nasal spray.	With injections: hypotension, flushing, nausea, vomiting, sweating. With oral form: Constipation, edema.	Monitor for hypercalcemia (dry mouth, constipation, headache, depression, weakness). Take tablets with full glass of water ½ to 1 hr after meals. Not to be taken with other oral medications, alcohol, or foods with fiber. Patient must avoid excess tobacco use and caffeine.
Raloxifene (Evista) Prevents bone loss and lowers cholesterol without stimulating endometrium. Used to prevent osteoporosis in postmenopausal women.	Frequent side effects: infection, flu syndrome, nausea, hot flashes, weight gain, joint pain, sinusitis, thrombosis.	Check for Homans' sign. Seek medical care for chest pain, dyspnea, changes in vision. Should not be taken during pregnancy, before menopause, or during periods of immobility.

glucocorticoids are indicated, occasional local injections are preferred over systemic therapy. For many patients already on NSAIDs, acetaminophen is often prescribed as a safe analgesic. Other, less safe drugs are gold salts, azathioprine, penicillamine, and cyclosporine.

Recent advances in the treatment of various connective tissue diseases, including rheumatoid and osteoarthritis, include the development of biologic response modifiers (BRMs), disease-modifying antirheumatic drugs (DMARDs), and cyclooxygenase-2 (Cox-2) inhibitors. BMRs target certain features of the immune system specifically involved in inflammatory disease. Two new BMR drugs are etanercept (Enbrel) and infliximab (Remicade). They work by blocking the action of tumor necrosis factor (TNF), a chemical involved in inflammation.

Disease-modifying antirheumatic drugs (DMARDs) may retard the progression of some diseases. They include leflunomide (Arava), minocycline (Minocin), methotrexate, hydroxychloroquine, and sulfasalazine.

The cyclooxygenase-2 (Cox-2) inhibitors work much like older NSAIDs but are less likely to cause stomach ulcers and bleeding. The first two drugs developed in this new category are celecoxib (Celebrex) and rofecoxib (Vioxx).

SURGICAL TREATMENT

Surgical intervention may be indicated in some musculoskeletal disorders, such as degenerative joint disease and arthritis. Specific surgical interventions are discussed with the particular conditions.

A device used after some types of joint replacement surgery is the continuous passive motion (CPM) machine. This device moves the joints through a set range of motion at a set rate of movements per minute. The movement prevents formation of scar tissue and promotes flexibility of the new joint. The affected extremity may be placed in the continuous passive motion machine in the postanesthesia care unit or on the first postoperative day. The CPM machine is used for specific intervals, and the time and degree of flexion and extension are gradually increased. The part of the machine that cradles the limb is padded to prevent pressure or abrasions. Be sure the machine settings are correct as ordered and the limb is properly aligned. Keep the machine clean since it could be a possible source of contamination. Several types of continuous passive motion machines are illustrated in the section on total joint replacement.

DISORDERS OF CONNECTIVE TISSUE STRUCTURES

OSTEOARTHRITIS

Osteoarthritis is the most common form of arthritis. Although the condition is sometimes called degenerative joint disease (DJD), not all agree this term is appropriate. Osteoarthritis is classified as a noninflammatory condition; however, tissue breakdown may result in inflammation of the surrounding synovium.

Osteoarthritis may be classified as primary or secondary, depending on the cause. In primary osteoarthritis some unknown factor triggers the release of chemicals that break down joint cartilage. Osteoarthritis that occurs with aging is generally considered to be primary and may have a genetic basis. Secondary osteoarthritis may be associated with trauma, infection, congenital deformities, or corticosteroid therapy. The incidence of osteoarthritis increases with age, with persons over 50 most often affected. It is estimated that more than 100,000 people in the United States are unable to walk independently to and from the bathroom because of osteoarthritis.

Osteoarthritis generally affects joints under pressure, especially the spine, fingers, knees, hips, and shoulders. People who are obese, who have poor posture, or who experience occupational stress are at greatest risk for the disease. The most common source of major disability is osteoarthritis of the knee.

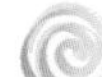

What Does Culture Have to do with Osteoarthritis?

The sites affected most often by osteoarthritis vary with ethnic background. For example, osteoarthritis of the hips is more common among people who live in Japan and Saudi Arabia than among whites in the United States.

Pathophysiology

Osteoarthritis is characterized by the degeneration of articular cartilage with hypertrophy of the underlying and adjacent bone. Normally, the articular cartilage provides a smooth surface for one bone to glide over another (Fig. 39-1). The cartilage transfers the weight of one bone to another so the bones

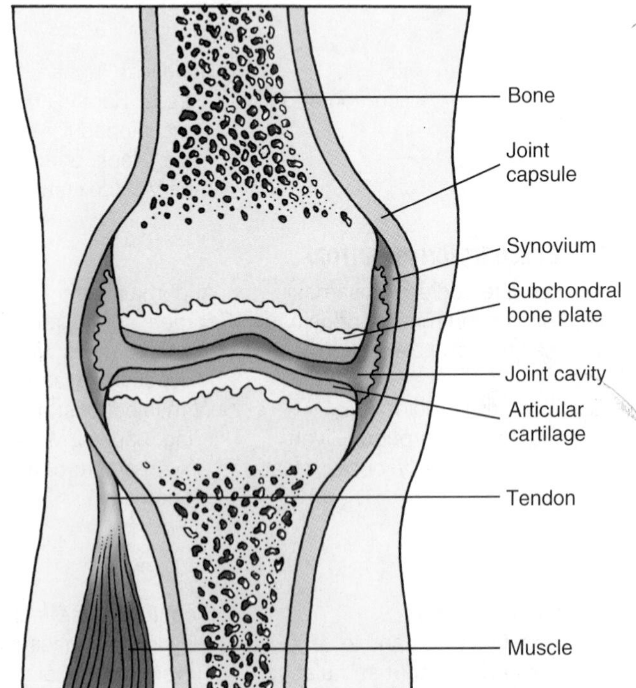

FIGURE **39-1** The structure of a diarthrodial joint. Synovium lines the joint capsule but does not extend into the articular cartilage.

do not shatter. In osteoarthritis, deterioration of the articular cartilage means the shock-absorbing protection is gradually lost. New bone growth is stimulated by exposed bone surfaces, causing bone spurs to develop. Although osteoarthritis is generally classified as a noninflammatory condition, inflammation of the joint is common in advanced conditions due to tissue breakdown.

Signs and Symptoms

Many people with osteoarthritis have no symptoms, but others have pain ranging from mild to severe. The pain is what usually brings the patient to the physician. Pain is commonly associated with activity but relieved by rest. Along with pain in the affected joint, the patient with osteoarthritis may complain of stiffness, limitation of movement, mild tenderness, swelling, and deformity or enlargement of the joint (Fig. 39-2). Sometimes the symptoms subside for long periods of time and then return. The disease usually affects a single joint or only a few joints.

Medical Diagnosis

The diagnosis of osteoarthritis is usually based on the health history and radiographic studies. In the early stages of the disease, the patient may have no symptoms, even though radiographs reveal classic joint changes. From radiographic evidence, 68% of women over age 65 have osteoarthritis. The incidence is slightly lower for men of the same age. The extent of the disease process is not necessarily related to the severity of symptoms.

Because plain radiographs do not always reveal cartilage abnormalities, arthroscopy and magnetic resonance imaging may be employed as well. Synovial fluid may be aspirated to assess the presence of leukocytes. A normal ESR, negative RF assay, and synovial fluid with few or no leukocytes are expected. However, it is not unusual for a healthy older person to have a slightly elevated ESR and low titers of RF and ANA.

Medical Treatment

There is no known cure for osteoarthritis, but much can be done to make the patient more comfortable. The goals of patient therapy are to reduce the pain to a manageable level, maintain as much mobility as possible, and minimize disability.

The medical treatment regimen can include drug therapy, surgery, education, and physical therapy. For some patients, diet and counseling are indicated. Referral to a pain specialist may be indicated if conservative measures are not effective. The course of the treatment is dictated by the individual patient's condition and response.

Drug Therapy

Although drug therapy is not curative, the pain in osteoarthritis can usually be controlled with nonopioid analgesics such as acetaminophen, NSAIDs, disease-modifying drugs, Cox-2 inhibitors, or a low dose of salicylates (aspirin). NSAIDs may decrease pain and improve mobility in patients with osteoarthritis, but their side effects are more dangerous than those of acetaminophen. NSAIDs are especially effective when the patient shows signs of inflammation, such as warmth, swelling of joints, and erythema (redness). Similar to NSAIDs, indomethacin (Indocin) is effective in reducing inflammation but may cause serious adverse effects (see Table 39-3).

Salicylates are relatively inexpensive, but there is a risk of toxicity. The symptoms of salicylate intoxication in the elderly may be atypical. Instead of the common gastrointestinal complaints or ototoxicity, the older person may exhibit confusion, slurring of speech, agitation, or seizures. Although systemic glucocorticoids are not indicated for the treatment of osteoarthritis, intra-articular injections can be beneficial. These injections can be given only three or four times a year, because the drug may cause breakdown of cartilage with frequent use.

PHARMACOLOGY CAPSULE Most NSAIDs and indomethacin (Indocin) can cause gastrointestinal irritation and bleeding.

PHARMACOLOGY CAPSULE Salicylate toxicity may be manifested by tinnitus or, in the elderly, by confusion, agitation, slurred speech, or seizures.

Two new herbal supplements have recently been heralded as a new treatment for the damage caused by osteoarthritis: glucosamine and chondroitin. Although both supplements have received great attention as over-the counter supplements to repair damaged cartilage and tissues, there is no valid research confirming these claims at this time.

Surgical Management

Surgical management is usually reserved for persons with severe disease who respond poorly to conservative treatment.

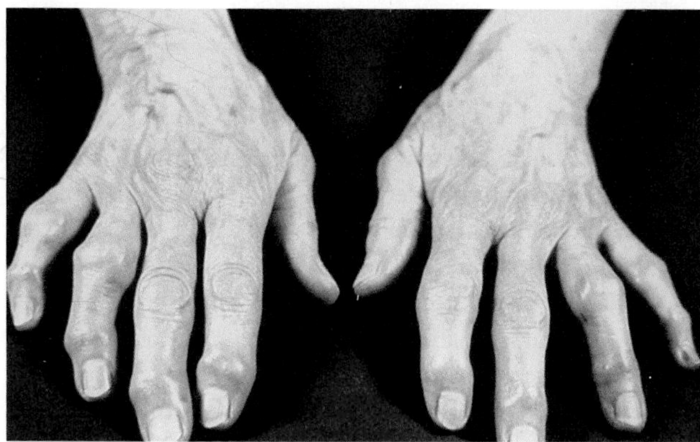

FIGURE **39-2** Degenerative joint disease; Heberden nodes at the distal interphalangeal joints and Bouchard nodes at the proximal interphalangeal joints.

Consider the Alternative!

Some people use glucosamine and chondroitin to treat osteoarthritis. Both are sold as dietary supplements and are under study to determine safety and effectiveness.

NURSING CARE PLAN

The Patient with a Total Hip Replacement

ASSESSMENT

Health History: A 74-year-old homemaker has had osteoarthritis for 10 years, with progressive loss of function in both hips. She had a left total hip replacement (arthroplasty) 2 days ago. Her past medical history reveals no other major health problems except poor vision. She lives with her daughter and helps with household chores, which gives her some satisfaction. Postoperatively she is alert and participates in her exercises. The physical therapist assisted her out of bed for the first time this morning. She was somewhat weak but was able to walk a short distance.

Physical Examination: Vital signs: temperature, 98° F orally; pulse, 82; respiration, 16; blood pressure, 148/66 mm Hg; height, 5'9"; weight, 162 lb. She is positioned on her right side with an abductor cushion in place. Breath sounds are clear on auscultation. Abdomen is soft, and bowel sounds are present. There is no bladder distention and no redness over bony prominences on back and left side. Warmth, color, and peripheral pulses are symmetric in both legs. She has good sensation in affected leg. The dressing on the surgical incision is dry and intact.

Nursing Diagnosis	*Goals and Outcome Criteria*	*Interventions*
Risk for impaired tissue perfusion related to deep vein thrombosis, decreased mobility, and surgical trauma.	The patient will have adequate circulation in the affected extremity, as evidenced by warmth, normal color, and palpable pulses.	Assess neurologic and circulatory status. Check vital signs at least every 4 hr. Report and record any abnormalities. Observe for excess swelling or bleeding at operative site. Assist with exercises as prescribed by physical or occupational therapist. Record and report any change in condition of skin at operative site and pressure areas.
Risk for injury related to unsteady gait	The patient will experience no falls during hospitalization.	Assist patient in and out of bed. Place call light in easy reach. Check frequently for patient's need to toilet and need for change of position. Provide assistive devices as ordered.
Risk for injury related to subluxation (dislocation) of joint prosthesis because of improper position, movement, or activity.	The patient will maintain proper body alignment and hip positioning and will not exhibit signs of prosthesis dislocation: sudden severe pain, abnormal position.	Instruct patient to keep legs slightly abducted. May place pillows between legs to achieve abduction while supine and during turning. Turn only to unaffected side. Tell patient not to cross legs or put on own shoes, socks, or stockings for 2 months. Assess for pain and loss of function. Make home health referral if needed to facilitate transition to home setting.
Risk for infection related to break in skin integrity from surgical hip replacement procedure.	The patient will be free of infection during hospitalization as evidenced by orientation to person, place, and time; normal body temperature, intact wound with decreasing redness, minimal edema, and no purulent drainage.	Encourage fluids and activity when appropriate. Observe for change in mental status or confusion, which may be first signs of infection in elderly. Keep in mind that previous administration of prednisone may mask symptoms of infection. Turn at least every 2 hr from back to unaffected side only. Use aseptic technique for wound care. Offer fluids at least every 2 hr.

The surgical treatment of choice for osteoarthritis is total joint replacement (**arthroplasty**) (see Nursing Care Plan: The Patient with a Total Hip Replacement). The primary indication for total joint replacement is intractable pain that disrupts sleep and daily activities. Total hip or knee arthroplasty usually relieves pain and restores function to the joint (Fig. 39-3). For some patients, arthroscopic surgery with removal of cartilage debris brings pain relief.

Physical Therapy

The physical therapy program employs measures to improve range of motion and to strengthen muscles. Most patients with osteoarthritis benefit from such a program. Isometric exercises are recommended over isotonic exercises because isotonic movements place greater strain on the joints. Exercise should be followed by periods of rest during the day.

Moist heat and occasionally cold can be used to help relieve pain. Heat also prepares the muscles and joints for exercise. Heat may be contraindicated, however, in patients who have had arthroplasty or have metal prostheses because it may lead to deep thermal burns. Transcutaneous nerve stimulation (TENS) devices are especially effective for treating back pain.

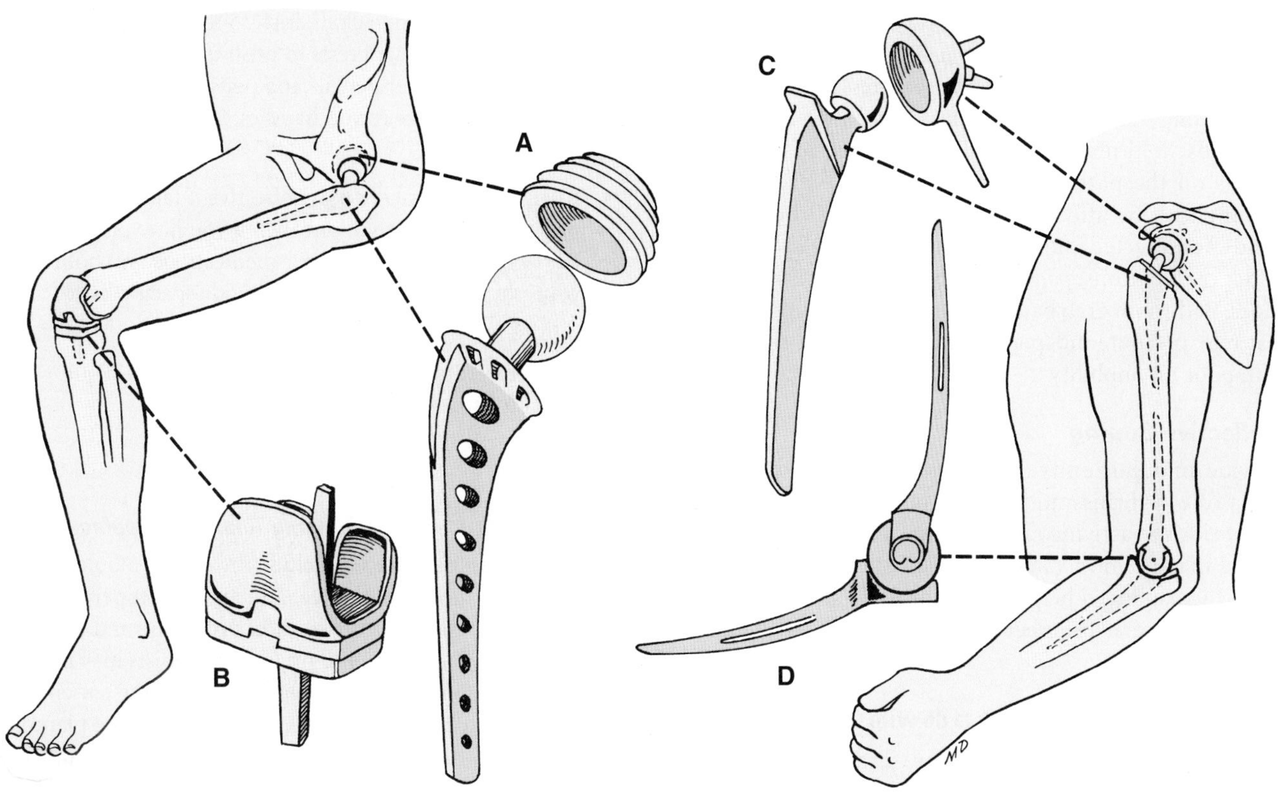

FIGURE 39-3 Total joint replacements. *A,* Hip. *B,* Knee. *C,* Shoulder. *D,* Elbow.

NURSING CARE *of the Patient with Osteoarthritis*

Assessment

The general nursing assessment of the patient with a connective tissue disorder is summarized in Table 39-1. When a patient has osteoarthritis, focus on assessing affected joints for crepitus, tenderness, enlargement, deformity, limitations of movement, and decreases in range of motion compared with unaffected joints. Gently support joints during the examination to minimize the patient's discomfort. Observe the patient's movements and gait, noting abnormalities. Record the location and severity of any problems. Determine how the disease affects the patient's mobility and ability to perform activities of daily living.

Nursing Diagnoses, Goals, and Outcome Criteria: Osteoarthritis

Nursing Diagnoses	Goals and Outcome Criteria
Chronic Pain with motion related to loss of smooth joint surfaces	Pain relief: patient states pain reduced or relieved, relaxed manner
Impaired Physical Mobility related to pain, limited range of motion	Improved functional mobility: patient accomplishes activities of daily living with minimal discomfort
Ineffective Coping related to pain, discomfort, disability	Effective coping: patient states is able to make adaptations to cope with condition, makes positive comments about ability to manage
Ineffective Therapeutic Regimen Management related to lack of understanding of osteoarthritis management and self-care	Patient manages disease appropriately: patient demonstrates self-care measures and describes prescribed regimen

Interventions

Chronic Pain

With good pain management a patient can be more active and have a better quality of life. Administer prescribed analgesics and anti-inflammatory drugs or instruct the patient in self-medication. Carry out heat or cold treatments as ordered. Monitor and record the effects of interventions designed to relieve pain. Be sure the physician is aware whether the pain relief measures are ineffective. Measures that protect the joint, discussed next under impaired physical mobility, also help reduce chronic pain.

Impaired Physical Mobility

Impaired physical mobility can significantly interfere with the patient's ability to carry out usual activities in the home or work setting. Modification of daily activities and joint protection measures can help to maintain function. Recommend a regular program of exercise. Stress the importance of balancing rest and activity to avoid becoming overly tired. The household may need to be reorganized to reduce demands on the patient. Everyday tasks like dressing and bathing may be affected by the disorder. If the patient's hands are affected, suggest clothing with Velcro closures rather than buttons, pants with an elastic waist, and slip-on shoes. Bathroom grab bars, a shower seat, and a raised toilet seat may promote independence and safety for the patient with poor hip mobility.

Ineffective Coping

Provide an opportunity for the patient to discuss concerns about osteoarthritis and its effects on lifestyle. Help the patient prioritize activities and plan how to continue those activities that are most valued. Practical suggestions for managing the condition help the patient feel a sense of control and confidence in his or her ability to live with the condition.

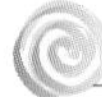

What Does Culture Have to do with Osteoarthritis?

How people react to chronic illness, disability, and dependence is related to their cultural values and beliefs. Consider the elderly Japanese American patient who values family interdependence over independence, the Mexican American patient who accepts illness as God's will, or the person of German heritage who faces pain stoically. Each of these may handle osteoarthritis differently. Nurses must consider these factors when planning patient care.

Ineffective Therapeutic Regimen Management

Determine what the patient already knows about osteoarthritis and correct any misconceptions. Design and implement an individualized teaching plan.

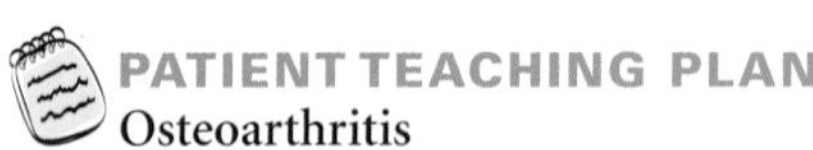

PATIENT TEACHING PLAN
Osteoarthritis

To reduce joint strain and pain:

- Maintain proper posture and body alignment.
- Identify activities that take a long time to do or for which you need assistance.
- Plan activities when help is available or when time is not a major concern, and take periodic rest breaks.
- Wear splints or support devices that rest or relieve painful, unstable joints.
- Push or slide heavy objects rather than pull them.
- Wear low heels to help decrease stress on the knee joints.
- Avoid stairs whenever possible.
- Sit rather than stand.
- Use high stools when sitting at a counter.
- Use higher chairs rather than low sofas.
- When arising from a chair, inch to the edge of the seat and then use the arm rests to push up from the seat.
- Use large-diameter pencils and pens, and use eating utensils with large round handles.

Self-medication:

- Analgesics are usually more effective if taken routinely as prescribed, rather than only when you have pain.
- Know the side effects of your medications and notify your physician if they occur (provide specific list).

Resources:

- Arthritis Foundation (telephone, 1-800-283-7800; website, http://www.arthritis.org).

NURSING CARE *following Total Joint Replacement*

Joints that can be replaced include the elbow, shoulder, phalangeal finger joints, hip, knee, and ankle. Preoperative care prepares the patient for the surgical procedure and the postoperative period. Nurses and physical therapists may instruct the patient in postoperative exercises. Advise the patient and family of postoperative limitations and encourage planning to adapt the home and work environment as needed. General nursing care of the surgical patient is discussed in Chapter 16. This section describes the postoperative nursing care needs of the patient who has had a joint replacement. Surgical orders or protocols are usually very specific for each type of joint surgery and may vary somewhat among surgeons. Common postoperative measures for specific procedures are presented in Table 39-4.

Assessment

Routine postoperative care includes assessment of vital signs, level of consciousness, intake and output, respiratory and neurovascular status, urinary function, bowel elimination, wound condition, and comfort. After total joint replacement, it is especially important to monitor circulation and sensation in the affected extremity. Determine the need for assistance with activities of daily living.

Nursing Diagnoses, Goals, and Outcome Criteria: Total Joint Replacement, Postoperative

Nursing Diagnoses	Goals and Outcome Criteria
Acute Pain related to tissue trauma	Pain relief: patient states pain reduced, relaxed expression
Risk for Injury related to improper alignment, dislocated prosthesis, weakness	Decreased risk for injury: patient maintains proper alignment of operative joint
Impaired Physical Mobility related to immobilization, pain, weakness	Physical mobility without complications of immobility: patient is increasingly mobile without excess fatigue or injury

table 39-4 Guidelines for Nursing Care after Replacement of Specific Joints

HIP REPLACEMENT

1. Do not flex hip more than 90 degrees.
2. Avoid flexion, adduction, and internal rotation.
3. Place a large pillow between patient's legs when turning patient, when patient is supine, and when patient is lying on unaffected side.
4. Advise patient not to cross legs or feet and not to put on own shoes, socks, or stockings for 6 weeks to 2 months, as directed by surgeon.
5. Apply leg abductor splints as ordered.
6. Do not turn onto operative side unless specifically ordered by surgeon.
7. Have patient sit in a chair that has arms to facilitate rising without extreme hip flexion.
8. Arrange for a raised toilet seat to allow toileting without extreme hip flexion.
9. Permit weight bearing as ordered, depending on type of prosthesis used and whether cement was used.
10. Encourage patient to exercise unaffected extremities to maintain strength.

KNEE REPLACEMENT

1. Encourage quadriceps-setting exercises and straight leg lifts beginning postoperative day 2-5, as ordered.
2. Use passive motion machine as ordered; check alignment and settings.
3. Monitor weight bearing with walker or crutches as ordered.

FINGER JOINT REPLACEMENT

1. Instruct patient to elevate affected hand.
2. Assess sensation and warmth in affected fingers.
3. Instruct patient to use splints during sleep as ordered.
4. Reinforce exercises taught by physical therapist—must be continued for 10-12 weeks.
5. Advise patient not to lift heavy objects with affected hand.

Impaired Tissue Perfusion related to trauma, hemorrhage, thrombi, compression of blood vessels	Normal circulation to affected extremity: symmetric color and warmth of extremities, palpable pulse in affected limb, negative Homans' sign
Risk for Infection related to invasive procedure, prosthesis placement	Absence of infection: normal body temperature, decreasing wound redness, normal white blood cell count
Anxiety or Fear related to outcome of procedure	Reduced anxiety/fear: patient states anxiety/fear reduced, calm manner
Deficient Knowledge related to postoperative self-care	Patient understands self-care: patient describes and demonstrates self-care

Interventions

Acute Pain

Assess the patient's pain, describing its location, nature, and severity. Surgical pain is expected, but the patient with osteoarthritis may also have pain in other joints. Administer analgesics as ordered, and assess and record their effects. Reposition the patient as permitted by physician's orders. Use massage, relaxation techniques, imagery, or other strategies described in Chapter 14 to help the patient deal with the pain. Notify the surgeon of sudden, severe pain in the surgical area, which may signal prosthesis dislocation. Uncontrolled pain may make the patient reluctant to participate in rehabilitation measures. Administer analgesics 30 minutes to 1 hour before painful exercises to improve patient participation.

Risk for Injury

Prosthetic joints can become dislocated if they are not maintained in proper alignment. For example, after hip replacement, the affected leg must be kept in a position of abduction to prevent dislocation. Instruct patients not to cross the legs or flex the hip more than 90 degrees. Splints or traction may be used if ordered to maintain the desired position. Progressive exercises are usually prescribed and may be done by the physical therapist. As the patient's activity is increased, teach and reinforce precautions. Teach the patient to recognize signs and symptoms of dislocation, including pain in the affected joint, loss of function, and shortening or deformity of the extremity.

Impaired Physical Mobility

The degree of mobility impairment depends on which joints are affected as well as on the patient's general physical state. In general, early mobility is encouraged. When mobility is severely impaired, the patient is at risk for pulmonary and circulatory complications, urine retention, constipation, and skin breakdown. In addition, unused muscles weaken, and unused joints stiffen. Reposition the patient as allowed, carefully assessing pressure areas for redness caused by circulatory impairment. Coach and support the patient during coughing and deep breathing exercises and use of the incentive spirometer. Auscultate for breath sounds to detect atelectasis or retained secretions. Assess the abdomen for bladder or bowel distention. Administer intravenous fluids as ordered until the patient takes adequate oral fluids. Give stool softeners and laxatives as ordered.

The patient may have self-care deficits related to mobility impairments or restrictions. Identify activities the patient

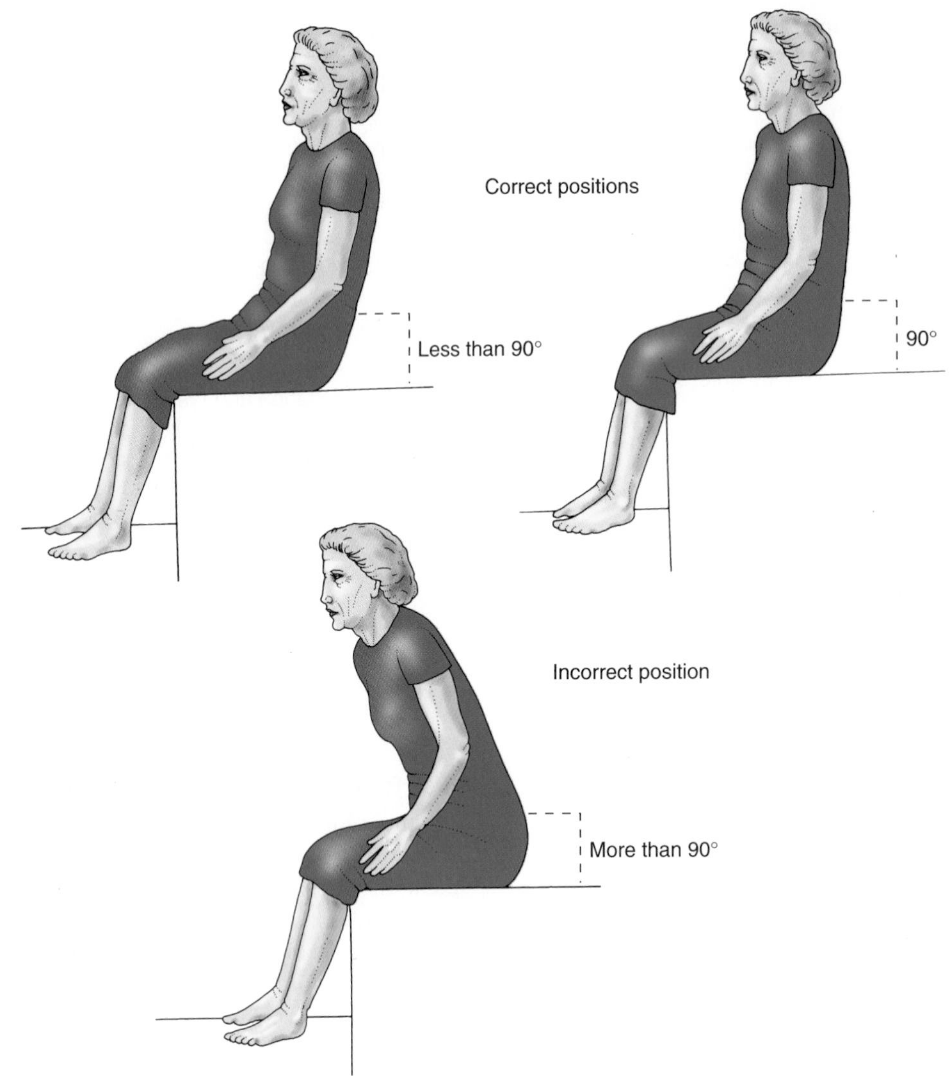

FIGURE 39-4 Correct and incorrect hip flexion after a total hip replacement.

cannot do alone and provide appropriate assistance. As the patient progresses, encourage increasing independence. Rehabilitation requires patient participation in the prescribed exercise program. The patient may need reassurance that the joint can and should be exercised (Fig. 39-4). A patient generally exercises better if there is adequate pain control. A continuous passive motion machine may be used to reduce scar tissue formation and improve range of motion (Fig. 39-5).

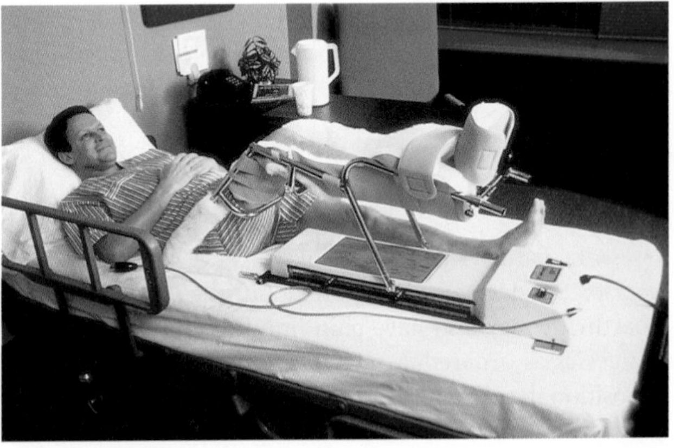

FIGURE 39-5 A continuous passive motion exerciser in use.

Impaired Tissue Perfusion

Monitor body areas distal to the operative joint for circulatory adequacy by assessing warmth, color, and peripheral pulses. Splints, dressings, and antiembolic stockings also can restrict circulation and must be checked for proper positioning. To reduce the risk of deep vein thrombosis in the legs, do not place pillows or pads under the legs. Signs and symptoms of deep vein thrombosis include tenderness, swelling, redness, warmth, firm palpable blood vessels called cords, and a positive Homans' sign (pain behind the knee or in the calf when the foot is dorsiflexed). Determine the specific exercises that may be done, based on the physician's orders and protocols. For example, after hip replacement, the patient should flex and extend the toes, feet, and ankles hourly to promote venous return.

The patient is at risk for hemorrhage after joint replacement. Check the dressings and wound drainage for increasing bleeding; monitor vital signs for tachycardia and hypoten-

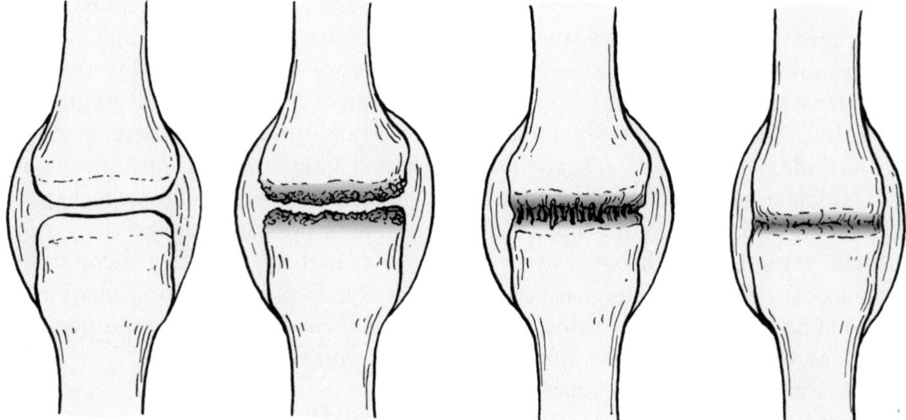

FIGURE 39-6 The four phases of joint damage in rheumatoid arthritis.

sion; and observe for restlessness and anxiety. Inspect and measure wound drainage in suction devices at least every 8 hours. There is also a risk of fat embolus, which can produce signs of local or cerebral blood vessel occlusion: petechial (pinpoint) hemorrhage of the upper chest and conjunctiva, fat globules in the urine, headache, irritability, confusion, and loss of consciousness.

Pressure caused by edema or constrictive dressings can cause nerve damage, which may be manifested by anesthesia (lack of sensation) or paresthesia (abnormal sensation). Therefore monitor sensation distal to the joint and report symptoms of impairment to the surgeon. Check dressings, stockings, and splints to be sure they are not too tight.

Supervise ambulation until the patient is steady and clearly understands the limitations. Keep the environment free of clutter.

Risk for Infection

Monitor the patient's temperature for elevations that may indicate infections. Assess the surgical wound for redness, swelling, warmth, and foul-smelling drainage. Use strict sterile technique when handling the wound, drains, or dressings. Keep wound dressings clean and dry. Administer antimicrobials as ordered. Instruct the patient in hand washing and wound care.

Anxiety or Fear

Total joint replacement is usually done after conservative treatments have failed to maintain joint mobility. The patient is typically hopeful but anxious about the outcome of the surgery. Tell the patient what to expect, explain procedures and equipment, and offer to answer questions. Responding promptly to the patient's needs and checking on him or her frequently are reassuring.

Deficient Knowledge

From admission through discharge, teach the patient about self-care, wound care, and signs of possible infection. Ensure understanding by having patients repeat back important information in their own words. Before teaching, assess for pain, fatigue, or communication barriers. Recognize cultural differences in lifestyle, diet, and care issues. Assist patients in planning for care at home, and involve family members in teaching sessions.

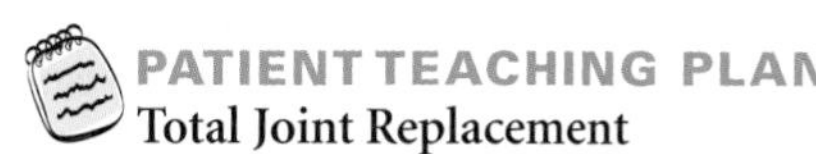

PATIENT TEACHING PLAN
Total Joint Replacement

Specifics of the teaching plan depend on which joint was replaced, but all patients need to know the following:

- What activities are permitted
- What activities are contraindicated
- Directions for drug therapy
- Wound care
- Signs and symptoms to be reported to the surgeon
- When to return for follow-up care
- Sources of assistance such as home health care

RHEUMATOID ARTHRITIS

Rheumatoid arthritis (RA) is a chronic, progressive inflammatory disease. Although it is a systemic disorder, the most notable effect of RA is on diarthroses (synovial joints). The disease has a peak onset in people 30 to 60 years of age and is more common in females than in males. It affects an estimated 1% to 3% of the population in the United States. The course of the disease is variable, ranging from minimal symptoms to severe debilitation.

Pathophysiology

There is no single known cause for RA, but it is considered an autoimmune disorder. Proposed causes include an unknown antigen in the patient's system, one or more viruses, genetic predisposition, and hormonal factors. While research to determine the exact cause continues, many recent discoveries have improved the lives of RA patients.

The onset of the disease is characterized by inflammation of the synovial tissue (the tissues that hold the lubricating fluid of the joints). In RA, the synovium thickens, and fluid accumulates in the joint space. Vascular granulation tissue, called pannus, forms in the joint capsule and breaks down cartilage and bone. Fibrous tissue invades the pannus, converting it first to rigid scar tissue and finally to bony tissue. These changes result in ankylosis (loss of joint mobility) (Fig. 39-6).

Signs and Symptoms

The most common symptom of RA is pain in the affected joints that is aggravated by movement. Morning stiffness lasting more than 1 hour is almost always a feature of RA, unlike the stiffness of osteoarthritis, which is relieved within minutes. Other symptoms include weakness, easy fatigability, anorexia, weight loss, muscle aches and tenderness, and warmth and swelling of the affected joints. Joint changes are usually symmetric, meaning the same joints in both extremities are affected simultaneously. The distal interphalangeal and metacarpophalangeal joints are most often affected. The wrist, elbow, knee, and ankle are other possible areas affected. **Rheumatoid nodules,** which are subcutaneous nodules over bony prominences, also may be present (Fig. 39-7).

Any organ of the body may be affected by RA. If blood vessels are affected, they become inflamed, a condition called **vasculitis.** With vasculitis, the blood supply to body organs is impaired, with possible ischemia or infarction of affected organs. Ischemic lesions of the skin are brownish spots most often seen around the nail beds. Large lesions that tend to ulcerate may appear on the legs. Secondary effects on bone can cause osteoporosis, making the bones susceptible to fractures. The disease may produce inflammatory changes in the tissues of the heart, lungs, kidneys, and eyes. Pleural effusions and pulmonary fibrosis can lead to respiratory impairment or pulmonary hypertension and eventual heart failure.

Some patients with RA develop clusters of symptoms, including Sjögren's syndrome, Felty's syndrome, or Caplan's syndrome. Sjögren's syndrome is characterized by dryness of the mouth, eyes, and vagina. Felty's syndrome, characterized by liver and spleen enlargement and neutropenia, is less common. Caplan's syndrome, marked by rheumatoid nodules in the lungs, occurs most often in coal miners and asbestos workers.

Medical Diagnosis

The diagnosis of RA is based on the health history and physical examination, laboratory findings, and radiographic changes. There is no single test to diagnose RA, but groups of tests and radiographic findings may help to confirm the disorder. See Table 39-2 for common studies for connective tissue disorders.

The presence of RF does not establish the diagnosis of RA; however, its presence may support a diagnosis in persons who

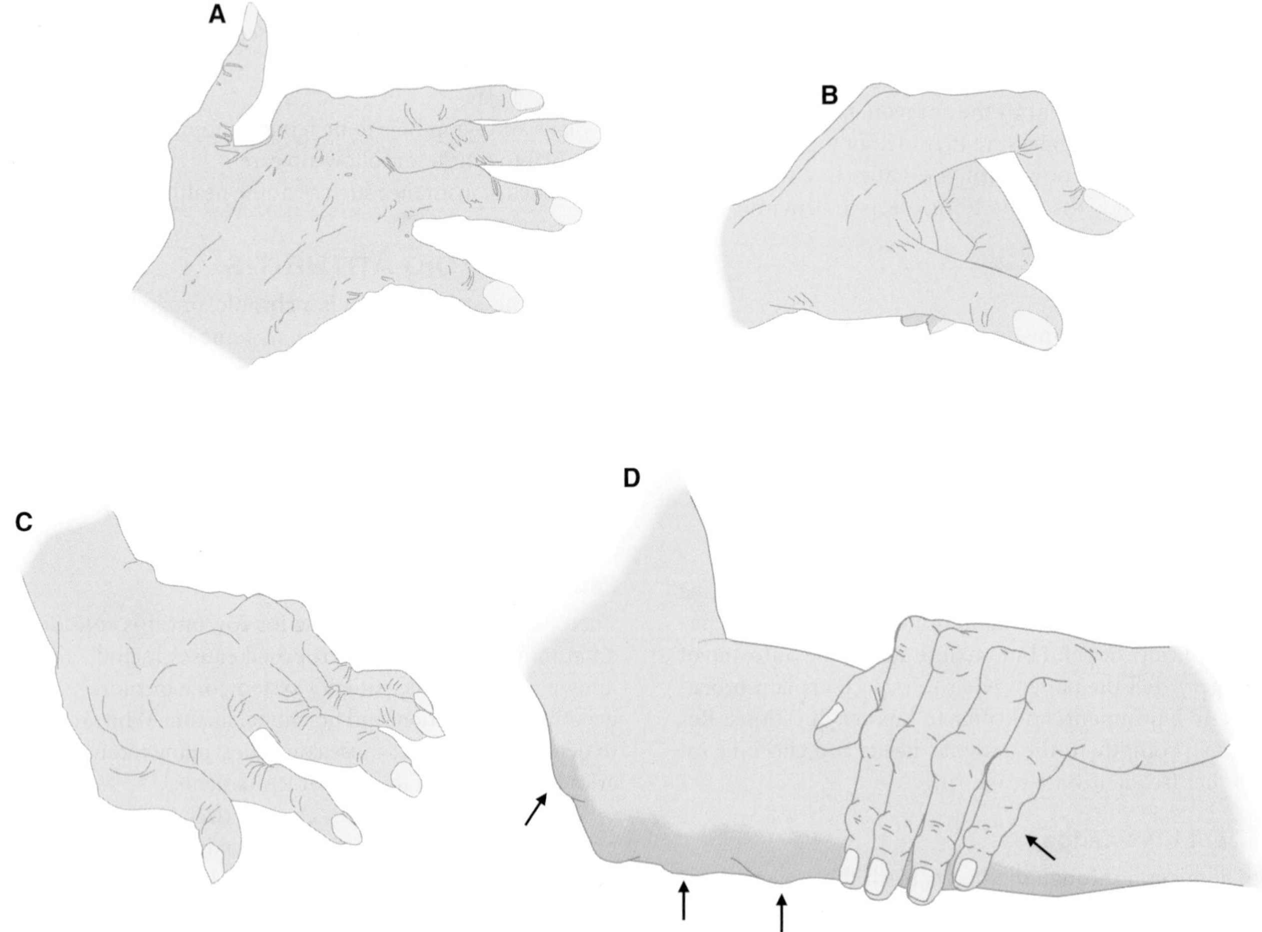

FIGURE **39-7** Four types of hand deformity characteristic of clients with rheumatoid arthritis. *A,* Ulnar drift. *B,* Boutonnière deformity. *C,* Swan-neck deformity. *D,* Rheumatoid nodules.

have other signs and symptoms. The C-reactive protein level and ESR, although not specific, also help support the diagnosis in patients with other suggestive symptoms. Synovial fluid is analyzed for viscosity, white blood cells, and glucose and is subjected to a mucin clot test.

The primary purpose of radiographs is to detect changes brought about by RA and to determine the potential usefulness of disease-modifying drugs or surgery.

Medical Treatment

The treatment of RA involves medicine, nursing, physical therapy, occupational therapy, and social services.

Drug therapy is aimed at controlling the local inflammatory process and providing symptomatic relief. Traditional agents used for symptomatic relief included aspirin and other NSAIDs for several months, with the addition of gold compounds, *d*-penicillamine, antimalarials, or sulfasalazine if needed. These agents could provide significant clinical improvement for weeks or even months at a time. More aggressive therapies now are used to relieve inflammation within a 3-month period and to prevent deformities. Combinations of NSAIDs, analgesics, COX-2 inhibitors, and DMARDs are prescribed to meet the individual patient's therapeutic goal. Leflunomide (Arava) is a newer DMARD that reportedly can slow the progression of the disease. Etanercept (Enbrel) and infliximab (Remicade) are BRMs that have shown great success in rheumatoid patients, with some patients having a remission of the disease. Joint injections of corticosteroids can also be given two to three times a year and may provide significant symptomatic relief. Cytotoxic drugs such as methotrexate sodium (Folex) or cyclophosphamide (Cytoxan) are often very effective in the symptomatic treatment of RA. Systemic glucocorticoids, although effective in reducing the inflammatory process, are the last choice, owing to their adverse side effects (see Table 39-3).

In addition to drug therapy, supportive treatments may be employed—including rest, splinting joints to reduce motion that aggravates the inflammation, orthotic devices to support deformed joints, and assistance in modifying activities of daily living.

Surgical management of RA is reserved for those patients with severe pain and deformities. Arthroplasties, including total joint replacements, can be done. The most successful procedures are those performed on the knees and hips (see the discussion of osteoporosis).

PHARMACOLOGY CAPSULE Aspirin and NSAIDs prolong bleeding time; thus patients must be monitored for bruising and bleeding.

NURSING CARE *of the Patient with Rheumatoid Arthritis*

Assessment

The general assessment of the patient with a connective tissue disorder is summarized in Table 39-1. When a patient has RA, include assessment for pain, symmetric bilateral joint swelling, tenderness, limitation of movement, decreased ability to perform activities of daily living (dressing, grooming, eating, toileting), fatigue, and joint deformities.

Nursing Diagnoses, Goals, and Outcome Criteria: RA

Nursing Diagnoses	Goals and Outcome Criteria
Chronic Pain related to swelling and tenderness	Reduced pain: patient reports decreased pain, relaxed manner
Activity Intolerance related to fatigue	Improved activity tolerance: performance of small tasks without needing a rest period
Ineffective Coping related to frustration, embarrassment, inability to do activities independently	Effective coping: patient identifies ways to deal with physical changes
Social Isolation related to physical impairment and poor body image	Increased social activity: patient resumes as least one social activity that had been abandoned, has realistic view of physical abilities
Ineffective Therapeutic Regimen Management related to lack of understanding of RA, its treatment, and self-care	Patient effectively manages self-care: patient describes and demonstrates correct self-care

Interventions

Chronic Pain

Chronic pain imposes a terrible burden on the patient. Measures to control pain include application of heat or cold and administration of medications as ordered. A warm shower on arising may relieve morning pain and stiffness. Maintaining a program of exercise and rest also can help to manage joint pain and relieve stress. Care of the patient with pain is discussed in Chapter 14.

Activity Intolerance

With the patient, develop a plan of activities around periods of rest and activity. Provide assistance as needed with getting in and out of bed and going to the bathroom. Patients who are severely disabled may need help with all activities of daily living. If needed, help the patient change positions and provide assistance with meals. Physical and occupational therapy may be ordered. Encourage the patient to follow the prescribed therapy program.

Ineffective Coping

A trusting, collaborative relationship is a prerequisite to providing therapeutic care. Visit the patient often to explore

Consider the Alternative!

Nonpharmacologic approaches to pain management include application of heat or cold, balanced exercise and rest, relaxation exercises, meditation, imagery, and music.

concerns, answer questions, teach, and plan care. Emphasize the patient's strengths and explore previously used coping skills. Some patients respond to their physical and functional losses with demanding behavior that others see as manipulative. Patients from other cultures may deal with the pain and disability differently; some may be more stoic and reserved, while others may be demanding or helpless. Caregivers must recognize this as an attempt by the patient to maintain some control in his or her life. An important part of coping is learning to maintain maximal possible independence despite the crippling effects of RA. Adaptations in the home and workplace and the use of appropriate assistive devices can promote independence and an improved sense of well-being.

Because a chronic illness affects the family as well as the patient, reach out to the family, offering information, encouragement, problem solving, and resources. Recognize that the family structure differs from one culture to another, and the patient's role in the family plays an important part in how they view the effects of the disease. Provide information about community resources such as the local chapter of the Arthritis Foundation. If indicated, make a referral to a home care agency to help the patient learn to manage better at home.

What Does Culture Have to do with Pain?

The way people deal with pain is culturally based. For example, people of German, Japanese, and Irish heritage try to be stoic and are reluctant to express pain, whereas people from Italy and the Dominican Republic are more likely to express pain openly. Nurses should not make assumptions about a patient's pain based only on their behavior.

Social Isolation

Physical deformities that alter appearance and impair function evoke a great sense of loss in the RA patient. The resulting depression, irritability, and feelings of helplessness can have a devastating effect on the patient's interpersonal relationships. In addition, patients who take glucocorticoids often have mood swings, which make their behavior unpredictable. These emotional changes may discourage visits from staff and from family, which increases the patient's isolation. Visit the patient often so he or she does not feel isolated and lonely. Explain the patient's irritability and mood swings to family and friends. Emphasize the importance of their continued support to the patient. Encourage the patient to identify social activities that are appropriate and to remain involved to the extent possible.

Ineffective Therapeutic Regimen Management

The teaching plan should include information about the disease process, drug therapy, and the need for balanced rest and activity.

PATIENT TEACHING PLAN
Rheumatoid Arthritis

- Take your medications exactly as prescribed, and notify your physician of any adverse effects (provide drug names, dosage, schedule, side and adverse effects).
- Keep follow-up appointments; the effects of many drugs need to be monitored with periodic blood studies.
- You must balance your activity and rest.
- Avoid prolonged bedrest, which can lead to further loss of function.
- Use assistive devices as needed to maintain safe mobility.
- Support your joints in functional positions to reduce the risk of contractures.
- Continue to do as much as you can for yourself, but don't hesitate to ask for help with difficult tasks.
- Avoid straining your joints with heavy lifting.

Put on your THINKING CAP!!

A 30-year-old mother of a 6-month-old infant and a 5-year-old child has just been diagnosed with rheumatoid arthritis. She is married and works full time as a teacher. Identify ways she can modify strain on her joints in the home setting and the work setting.

OSTEOPOROSIS

Pathophysiology

Bone is constantly being formed and absorbed. Until adolescence, bone formation exceeds bone absorption. The processes remain equal through the twenties, but, beginning around age 30, bone absorption surpasses bone formation. Loss of trabecular bone, the innermost layer, occurs first. The loss of cortical bone, the hard outer shell, begins later in life. The loss of cortical bone begins earlier and progresses faster in women than in men. The net result is loss of bone mass, which makes the patient susceptible to fractures. Common sites of fractures due to osteoporosis are the wrist, vertebrae, and hip. Age-related loss of bone mass without apparent underlying medical causes is called primary osteoporosis. Secondary osteoporosis is loss of bone mass due to factors other than age, such as hyperparathyroidism or long-term therapy with corticosteroids or heparin.

Risk Factors

Many factors appear to increase the risk of osteoporosis. At greatest risk are elderly women who have small frames, who are white or of northern European heritage, and who have fair skin and blond or red hair. Other risk factors are removal of both ovaries, physical inactivity, inadequate calcium or vitamin D intake, and excessive use of cigarettes, caffeine, and alcohol. A number of disorders, such as Cushing's disease and type 2 diabetes mellitus, also seem to be associated with osteoporosis.

Signs and Symptoms

Signs and symptoms of osteoporosis may include back pain, fractures, loss of height due to vertebral compression, and kyphosis. Bone deterioration in the jaw can cause dentures to fit poorly.

Medical Diagnosis

Bone mass can be measured using a technique called absorptiometry. Absorptiometry is a quick, painless radiologic procedure that measures the amount of bone tissue in the hip and spine. Blood studies are usually normal with primary osteoporosis, but a battery of tests may be ordered to rule out possible causes of secondary osteoporosis. Radiographs show bone fractures but do not reveal decreased bone density until there is loss of 30% to 50% of the bone mass. A bone specimen may be obtained for study from the iliac crest.

Medical Treatment

It is generally accepted that calcium supplementation and estrogen replacement for postmenopausal women slow bone loss. The recommended elemental calcium intake is 1,000 mg/day for premenopausal women and for postmenopausal women who are on estrogen replacement therapy. Postmenopausal women who are not on estrogen replacement therapy need 1,500 mg/day of calcium. The only contraindications to supplementary calcium are hypercalcemia, hypophosphatemia, or a history of kidney stones. Estrogen replacement is controversial, but if it is not contraindicated, it may have beneficial effects on the bones for up to 15 years after the onset of menopause. The patient should discuss the issue with her physician. A physical therapist may be consulted to develop an appropriate exercise program for the patient.

Medical treatment has long aimed at preventing fractures and stimulating bone formation, but until recently there were no drugs that actually reversed the progression of osteoporosis. Alendronate sodium (Fosamax) is a promising drug that inhibits bone resorption without retarding mineralization.

It is believed that regular exercise promotes bone formation and improves strength, balance, and reaction time, thereby reducing the risk of falls and fractures. Aerobic exercise at least three times a week is encouraged. The incidence or severity of the disorder may be reduced by identifying high-risk people and taking steps to promote healthy bone development.

Patients who have spinal fractures caused by osteoporosis may benefit from percutaneous vertebroplasty, which requires a needle to be inserted into the vertebra so that a special type of cement can be injected directly into the vertebra. This procedure is reported to prevent additional compression of the vertebra and to relieve pain caused by compression. Because percutaneous vertebroplasty is minimally invasive, risks are minimized and the recovery time is short.

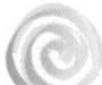

What Does Culture Have to do with Osteoporosis?

Small fair-skinned women of northern European heritage are at greatest risk for osteoporosis. These women should be targeted early for bone-building dietary and exercise programs.

NURSING CARE *of the Patient with Osteoporosis*

Assessment

The nursing assessment of the patient with a connective tissue disorder is summarized in Table 39-1. When a patient has osteoporosis, specifically assess the patient's diet, calcium intake, and exercise plan. In the reproductive history, note whether the patient is menopausal or has had an oophorectomy (surgical removal of the ovaries). Measure the patient's height and compare with previous measurements. Describe the patient's posture, clearly noting the presence and degree of deformity. Assist the patient with changes in position during the examination for safety and comfort.

Nursing Diagnoses, Goals, and Outcome Criteria: Osteoporosis

Nursing Diagnoses	Goals and Outcome Criteria
Risk for Trauma related to loss of bone strength	Absence of trauma: performance of daily activities without falls or other injuries
Chronic Pain related to fractures, pressure on nerves due to vertebral compression	Pain relief: patient states pain relieved, relaxed manner
Ineffective Therapeutic Regimen Management related to lack of understanding of measures to promote bone formation and prevent bone loss	Effective patient management of condition: patient describes and demonstrates activities to improve bone mass

Interventions

Risk for Trauma

Monitor the patient's ability to carry out activities of daily living. Provide assistance if necessary. Advise ambulatory patients to wear good supportive shoes. Provide canes or walkers to improve balance if needed. Keep the environment free of hazards that might cause the patient to fall. Place personal articles within the patient's reach. In the home setting, assess possible hazards and take steps to provide a safer environment. Also assess the patient's gross visual acuity. In order to maneuver safely, the patient must be able to see. If indicated, recommend an eye examination.

Chronic Pain

Obtain a complete description of the patient's pain. Administer analgesics as ordered, but consider nonpharmacologic interventions as well (see Chapter 14). Some patients, especially those with vertebral compression, may have chronic pain that is difficult to manage. You may suggest referral to a clinic that specializes in pain management. Document the effects of pain management strategies.

Ineffective Therapeutic Regimen Management

Patient teaching is key to helping the patient learn to manage osteoporosis.

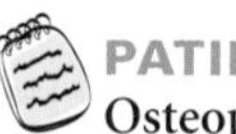

PATIENT TEACHING PLAN
Osteoporosis

- Before menopause and while on hormone replacements, you need 1,000 mg of calcium daily.
- After menopause, if you do not take hormone replacements, you need 1,500 mg of calcium daily.
- There are about 300 mg of calcium in each of the following: 1 cup of milk, 1 cup of yogurt, 1 ounce of Swiss cheese.

PATIENT TEACHING PLAN
Osteoporosis—cont'd

- Nonfat and skim milk have as much calcium as whole milk.
- If you take calcium supplements, increase your fluid intake unless advised not to do so by your physician.
- You need 400 IU vitamin D every day (300 IU for men).
- Limit your intake of alcohol and caffeine.
- If Fosamax is prescribed, take it in the morning with a full glass of water on an empty stomach, and sit or stand for 30 minutes after taking it.
- Regular weight-bearing exercise helps maintain bone strength.
- Avoid activities that might lead to falls and fractures.

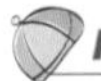

Put on your THINKING CAP!!

List two different ways a premenopausal woman can obtain her recommended daily calcium intake without supplements.

GOUT

Gout is a systemic disease characterized by the deposition of urate crystals in the joints and other body tissues. There are two forms of gout: primary gout, in which uric acid is elevated because of a metabolic disorder, and secondary gout, in which uric acid is elevated owing to another disease process. Primary gout is more prevalent among men than women, with a peak incidence in men in their forties and fifties. Women are rarely affected before menopause. Although the cause of most cases of gout is unknown, genetic and environmental factors appear to contribute to the development of this condition. The risk increases with hyperuricemia, obesity, alcohol consumption, and diuretic use.

Pathophysiology

Gout is characterized by **hyperuricemia** (excess uric acid in the blood) and is related either to an excessive rate of uric acid production or to decreased uric acid excretion by the kidneys. Features of gout may include (1) increased serum urate levels, (2) recurring acute attacks of arthritis, (3) the clumping of urate clusters around the joints of the extremities, causing crippling deformities, (4) renal disease involving blood vessels and interstitial tissues, and (5) uric acid kidney stones.

There are four stages of gout: asymptomatic hyperuricemia, acute gouty arthritis, asymptomatic intercritical period, and chronic tophaceous gout. Infection may develop if the skin breaks open. Kidney stones develop in about 20% of patients with gout.

Signs and Symptoms

In the first stage, the patient's blood uric acid level is elevated, but there are no other symptoms. Many people with asymptomatic hyperuricemia never progress to the next stage. The onset of stage 2, acute gouty arthritis, is abrupt, usually occurring at night. The patient is suddenly afflicted with severe, crushing pain and cannot bear even the light touch of bedsheets. The joint commonly affected is that of the great toe. The attack may be precipitated by trauma, diuretics, increased alcohol consumption, or a high-purine diet (food high in proteins). The symptoms usually disappear within a few days, and joint function is completely restored until the next attack. Patients with advanced gout have **tophi,** which are deposits of sodium urate crystals under the skin (Fig. 39-8).

Medical Diagnosis

Gout is usually suspected on the basis of the history and physical examination and confirmed by the finding of urate crystals in synovial fluid. A 24-hour urine specimen may be ordered to measure urinary uric acid, and a fasting blood sample may be drawn to measure the blood uric acid level.

Medical Treatment

Asymptomatic hyperuricemia usually requires no medical treatment. Colchicine is used to abort impending attacks of acute gouty arthritis and to treat initial acute episodes. It may be given hourly until the acute symptoms ease or until the patient develops nausea and vomiting. For subsequent attacks, other drugs effective in abating symptoms are indomethacin and NSAIDs (see Table 39-3). Some sources recommend these drugs instead of colchicine in elderly patients. If the patient does not respond to colchicine or NSAIDs, parenteral glucocorticoids or adrenocorticotropin may be prescribed. When a single joint is affected, prednisone may be injected into the joint. Drugs used to inhibit uric acid synthesis during the asymptomatic period include allopurinol

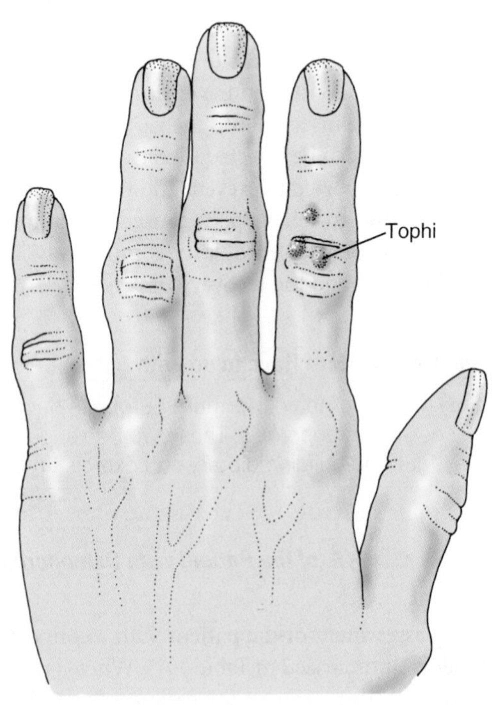

FIGURE **39-8** Typical appearance of tophi, which may occur in chronic gout, on an index finger.

(Zyloprim) and probenecid (Benemid). These same agents may be used to treat chronic tophaceous gout.

PHARMACOLOGY CAPSULE Patients taking antigout drugs need to maintain urine output of at least 2,000 ml/day to reduce the risk of urinary calculi formation.

NURSING CARE *of the Patient with Gout*

Assessment

Complete assessment of the patient with a connective tissue disorder is summarized in Table 39-1. The patient with gout should be specifically assessed for pain, joint swelling, tophi, uric acid stones, fever, and a history of trauma, injury, or surgery.

Nursing Diagnoses, Goals, and Outcome Criteria: Gout

NURSING DIAGNOSES	GOALS AND OUTCOME CRITERIA
Acute Pain related to joint inflammation	Pain relief: patient states pain reduction/relief, appears relaxed
Impaired Physical Mobility related to painful joint movement	Improved mobility: patient gradually resumes activities without unbearable pain
Impaired Urinary Elimination related to urate kidney stones	Normal urine output without symptoms of urinary obstruction: fluid intake and output equal; no flank or abdominal pain; no hematuria
Ineffective Therapeutic Regimen Management related to lack of knowledge of gout, its treatment, and self-care measures	Patient effectively manages condition: correctly describes and follows plan of care

Interventions

Acute Pain

Nursing care to decrease discomfort includes elevating the affected extremity, administering prescribed medications, and avoiding pressure on the area. Because even bedsheets may cause pain, a bed cradle should be used. Hot or cold packs may be ordered. Splints or bandages may be used to immobilize the affected joint.

Impaired Physical Mobility

Bedrest is usually recommended during the acute period. Provide assistance with activities of daily living as needed. When ambulation is permitted, advise the patient to protect affected joints from trauma by wearing supportive, firm shoes and by keeping walking pathways clearly lighted and free of obstacles that might cause falls.

Altered Urinary Elimination

When the serum uric acid level is elevated, the excess acid is excreted in the urine, where it may form uric acid stones. Urinary stones can obstruct urine flow from the kidney, causing renal damage. To prevent this complication, advise the patient to drink at least eight 8-ounce glasses of fluid daily unless contraindicated. Drugs may be prescribed to make the urine alkaline since uric acid stones precipitate in acid urine. During hospitalization, intravenous fluids may be given. Monitor intake and urine output. Promptly report signs and symptoms of urinary stones (pain in the flank, lower abdomen, or genitals; fever; hematuria; decreased urine output) to the physician.

Ineffective Therapeutic Regimen Management

Instruct the patient in measures to prevent or decrease future attacks.

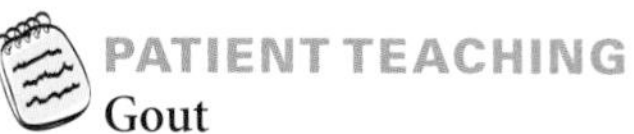

PATIENT TEACHING PLAN
Gout

Consult a dietitian to help the patient plan a well-balanced diet, and give the patient the following instructions:

- Your diet should be high in carbohydrates, moderate in protein, and low in fat. Limited purine intake is often advised (Table 39-5). Your doctor will advise you of dietary restrictions when you have no symptoms.
- Occasional, moderate alcohol intake may be permitted.
- Maintain a fluid intake of at least eight 8-ounce glasses daily to reduce the risk of uric acid stone formation in the urinary tract.
- Take your drugs as prescribed (provide specific dosage, schedule, list of side effects).
- To prevent severe attacks, report early joint or urinary symptoms to the physician. Severe attacks may be averted if treatment is begun soon after symptoms develop.
- If you are overweight, weight loss may help by reducing stress on joints.

table 39-5 ***Purine Content of Selected Foods***

HIGH PURINE CONTENT

Avoid these foods during both acute and remission stages of gout:

Anchovies	Bouillon	Brains	Broth
Consommé	Goose	Gravy	Heart
Herring	Kidney	Mackerel	Meat extracts
Mincemeat	Mussels	Partridge	Roe
Sardines	Scallops	Sweetbreads	Yeast (baker's and brewer's as supplement)

MODERATE PURINE CONTENT

One serving (2-3 oz) meat, fish, or fowl or 1 serving (½ cup) of vegetable from these groups is allowed daily (depending on condition) during remissions:

Fish, Poultry, Meat, Shellfish
Vegetables: Asparagus, dried beans, lentils, mushrooms, dried peas, spinach

Modified with permission from Mahan, L. K., & Escott-Stump, S. (1996). *Krause's food, nutrition, and diet therapy* (9th ed., p. 895). Philadelphia: Saunders.

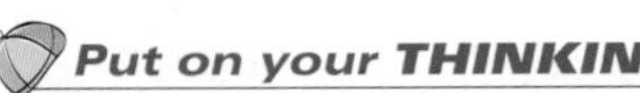
Put on your THINKING CAP!!

Explain how increased fluid intake will help prevent kidney stones in the patient with gout.

PROGRESSIVE SYSTEMIC SCLEROSIS (PSS or SCLERODERMA)

Progressive systemic sclerosis is commonly called scleroderma. It is a chronic, multisystem autoimmune disease of unknown origin that takes its name from the characteristic hardening of the skin. Other organs affected include the blood vessels, gastrointestinal tract, lungs, heart, and kidneys. The course of the disease varies among individuals, depending on the severity of involvement of the internal organs. The onset of disease is usually between 30 and 50 years of age, with more women than men affected. Death may occur due to infection or cardiac or renal failure. There are approximately 100,000 to 200,000 cases of PSS in the United States.

There are two types of PSS: progressively fatal sclerosis and the CREST syndrome. Progressively fatal sclerosis is characterized by thickening of the skin and systemic effects. The CREST syndrome consists of five symptoms: *c*alcinosis (calcium deposits in the tissues), *R*aynaud's phenomenon (vascular spasms), *e*sophageal dysfunction, *s*clerodactyly (scleroderma of the digits), and *t*elangiectasis (dilated superficial blood vessels).

Pathophysiology

Progressive systemic sclerosis is thought to be the result of primary vessel injury or dysfunction of the immune system. The manifestations of the disease follow a chain of events, from inflammation to degeneration of tissues, that results in decreased elasticity, stenosis, and occlusion of vessels.

Signs and Symptoms

The signs and symptoms of PSS reflect problems of the blood vessels, skin, joints, and internal organs. Common manifestations are Raynaud's phenomenon, symmetric painless swelling or thickening of the skin, taut and shiny skin, morning stiffness, frequent reflux of gastric acid, difficulty swallowing, weight loss, dyspnea, pericarditis, and renal insufficiency.

Medical Diagnosis

A complete history and physical examination may lead the physician to suspect fibrotic changes typical of PSS in the skin, lungs, heart, or esophagus. A positive ANA assay result, elevated ESR, and increased serum muscle enzyme levels support the diagnosis.

Medical Treatment

Even though there is no cure for PSS, treatment with high doses of steroids or other immunosuppressants may bring about remission. Additional aims of treatment are management of symptoms and prevention of complications. Treatment includes physical therapy to maintain joint mobility and preserve muscle strength. Esophageal reflux may be treated with drugs to decrease the acidity of gastric secretions and periodic dilation of the esophagus and other measures, such as small, frequent feedings and elevation of the head of the bed.

The management of Raynaud's phenomenon is aimed at elimination of anything that causes vasospasm: smoking, cold environmental temperature, and vasoconstricting drugs. Topical nitroglycerin ointment and oral alpha-blockers such as prazosin or calcium channel blockers such as nifedipine are often effective.

Various drugs can be used to treat the symptoms of PSS. *d*-Penicillamine is used to decrease skin thickening and reduce the severity of visceral organ involvement. Antihypertensives are used to control hypertensive crisis, with ACE inhibitors being most effective in averting kidney complications, and anti-inflammatory drugs can be used to control joint pain and stiffness.

NURSING CARE *of the Patient with Progressive Systemic Sclerosis*

Assessment

The general assessment of the patient with a connective tissue disorder is summarized in Table 39-1. When a patient has PSS, you should specifically seek information about pain and stiffness in the fingers and intolerance for cold in the health history. In the review of systems, identify signs and symptoms suggestive of cardiovascular, respiratory, renal, and gastrointestinal problems.

During the physical examination, inspect for skin rash, loss of wrinkles on the face, limitations of joint range of motion, muscle weakness, and dry mucous membranes. Carefully examine the hands for contractures of the fingers and for color changes or lesions on the fingertips. Palpate to determine warmth of the fingers.

Nursing Diagnoses, Goals, and Outcome Criteria: PSS

The nursing diagnoses and goals for patients with PSS are similar to those of patients with other connective tissue diseases. The following are the major diagnoses:

Nursing Diagnoses	Goals and Outcome Criteria
Impaired Skin Integrity reltated to thickening of tissues	Optimal skin integrity: warm, intact skin with normal color and texture
Self-Care Deficits related to pain, contractures of fingers, discomfort	Independent self-care: patient performs activities of daily living without excessive discomfort
Chronic Pain related to swelling and stiffness, vasospasm	Pain relief: patient states pain relieved, relaxed manner
Social Isolation related to poor self-concept, changes in physical appearance	Decreased social isolation: patient maintains or increases social interactions
Imbalanced Nutrition: Less than Body Requirements related to esophageal dysfunction	Adequate nutrition: stable body weight, maintains weight within standards recommended for height

Ineffective Therapeutic Regimen Management related to lack of understanding of PSS, medical management, and self-care	Effective management of condition: patient correctly describes and follows plan of care

Interventions

Impaired Skin Integrity

Keep the skin clean and dry. Encourage the patient to wear protective clothing as needed to maintain warmth and reduce skin discomfort. Cool baths with mild soaps followed by skin lotions may be soothing. Meticulous mouth care is warranted to prevent oral lesions. Administer anti-inflammatory drugs as ordered. Advise the patient to avoid practices that trigger vasospasm, such as exposure to cold and smoking.

Self-Care Deficits

Encourage the patient to participate in self-care as much as possible. Monitor the patient's tolerance for activity and provide assistance as needed. Schedule rest periods after activities to prevent overtiring. Permit the hospitalized patient to maintain independence in activities within abilities.

Chronic Pain

The patient with PSS usually has chronic joint pain and episodes of severe pain in the hands and feet associated with Raynaud's phenomenon. Measures to treat joint pain are like those described for rheumatoid arthritis. During acute episodes of Raynaud's phenomenon, the patient may be unable to tolerate anything touching the affected skin. A bed cradle can be used to keep the linens off the body. Adjust the room temperature to prevent chilling, which could provoke vasospasm. Be sure the patient is aware that smoking and severe stress can also trigger vasospasm.

Social Isolation

Swelling of the hands and facial changes can create a bird-like appearance that may cause the patient to withdraw from social interactions (Fig. 39-9). Explore the patient's concerns about the altered appearance and help the patient anticipate how to deal with various social situations. Demonstrate acceptance of the patient by expressing concern and using touch.

Imbalanced Nutrition: Less than Body Requirements

If the patient has esophageal involvement, suggest smaller, more frequent meals, which may be better tolerated. A relaxing environment before and after meals is helpful. Spicy foods, alcohol, and caffeine are discouraged because they stimulate gastric secretions. Give antacids and histamine-2 receptor blockers as ordered to neutralize gastric acid and reduce the risk of esophagitis and ulceration caused by esophageal reflux. After meals, the head of the bed should remain elevated for 1 to 2 hours to discourage reflux. Monitor and assess the adequacy of nutritional intake.

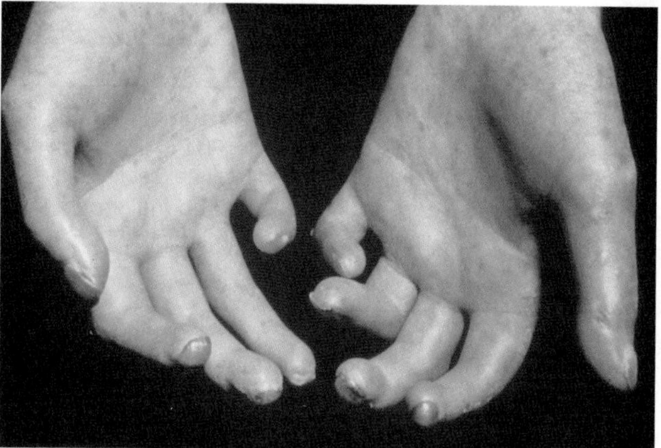

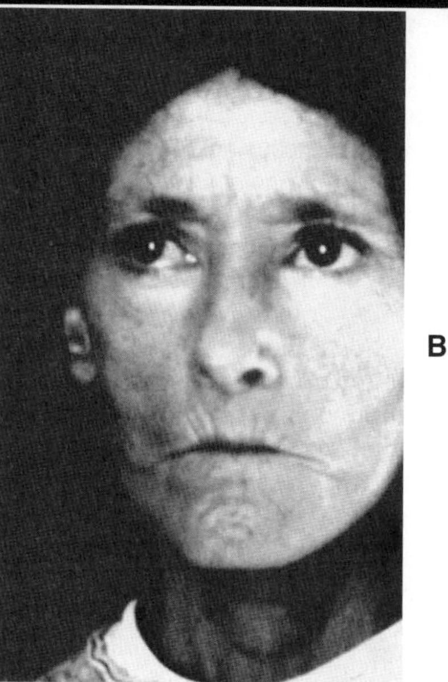

FIGURE **39-9** Late-stage skin changes seen in clients with progressive systemic sclerosis. *A,* Edema of the hands and fingers. *B,* Typical facial appearance.

Ineffective Therapeutic Regimen Management

As with other chronic illnesses, the patient must learn to implement the medical plan and manage the signs and symptoms of the condition. Patient teaching with PSS includes the nature of the disease, measures to prevent episodes of Raynaud's phenomenon, measures to maintain good nutrition and prevent esophageal reflux, signs and symptoms that should be reported to the physician, and self-medication. Key points are listed in the teaching plan.

PATIENT TEACHING PLAN
Progressive Systemic Sclerosis

- To prevent vasospasm, keep your hands warm and reduce stress and exhaustion.
- Take drugs as prescribed and report adverse effects to your physician (provide specific information about drug names, dosage, schedule, and adverse effects).

table 39-6 ***Other Connective Tissue Disorders***

DISORDER	PATHOPHYSIOLOGY	MANAGEMENT
Bursitis	*Description:* Acute or chronic inflammation of the bursae caused by trauma, strain, or infection. Calcification of bursae may occur. *Etiology:* Usually excessive use of joint. *Signs and symptoms:* Pain and limited movement in affected joints. Shoulder and hip most often affected.	NSAIDs, rest, splinting. Cold compresses first 24 hr, heat thereafter. Lidocaine injections for temporary pain relief. Once pain resolves, progressive range of motion such as "walking" the fingers of the affected arm up the wall.
Carpal tunnel syndrome	*Description:* Common condition in which the median nerve in the wrist becomes compressed, causing pain and numbness. *Etiology:* Caused by pressure on median nerve as it passes through structures of the wrist. People who do repetitive wrist movements like typing are at risk. *Signs and symptoms:* Pain and numbness in palmar side of fingers, weakness of thumb.	Splinting to prevent flexion and hyperextension. Glucocorticoid injections. Surgical release of transverse carpal ligament. Postoperatively, assess color and temperature of hand. Notify surgeon of pallor, cyanosis, or numbness.
Ankylosing spondylitis	*Description:* Inflammatory disease that affects vertebral column, causing spinal deformities. Chronic but not usually disabling. *Etiology:* Unknown but appears to be linked to HLA-B27 antigen. *Signs and symptoms:* First symptom usually dull, aching pain in buttocks. Also, low back morning stiffness of several hours' duration that improves with activity. Fatigue. *Complications:* Spinal fractures, iritis (inflammation of the iris of the eye), arthritis.	NSAIDs, physical therapy.
Polymyalgia rheumatica	*Description:* Rheumatic disease. *Etiology:* Unknown but likely has hereditary link. *Signs and symptoms:* Aching and morning stiffness in neck, shoulders and hips, proximal extremities, and torso. Symptoms resolve in 1-2 hr and return after a period of inactivity. Fatigue, weight loss, low-grade fever, anemia.	Prednisone: 30 days or less, NSAIDs.
Reiter's syndrome	*Description:* Connective tissue disease. *Etiology:* Often follows venereal disease or dysentery; incidence higher in people with certain familial tendencies. *Signs and symptoms:* Triad of arthritis, urethritis, conjunctivitis. Fever, malaise, fatigue, anorexia, weight loss, conjunctivitis, heel pain, skin lesions.	NSAIDs, physical therapy.
Behçet's syndrome	*Description, signs and symptoms:* Chronic syndrome characterized by oral and genital ulcers, skin lesions, uveitis, joint pain, phlebitis, and GI ulcers. *Etiology:* Not considered hereditary, but there seems to be a familial link.	Treatment varies, based on specific manifestations. May include anticoagulants, glucocorticoids, cyclosporine, chlorambucil, azathioprine, methotrexate, and retinal protein S.
Sjögren's syndrome	*Description:* Inflammatory disease that obstructs secretory ducts in the eyes, mouth, and vagina. *Etiology:* Autoimmune disorder; often seen with rheumatoid arthritis, polymyositis, scleroderma, or systemic lupus erythematosus. *Signs and symptoms:* Dry eyes, mouth, and vagina.	Artificial tears and lubricant ointments; artificial saliva, pilocarpine hydrochloride to stimulate salivary flow, dental care; perineal hygiene. Glucocorticoids.
Periarteritis nodosa	*Description:* A form of systemic necrotizing vasculitis; also called *polyarteritis nodosa.* Inflammation of small and medium-sized arteries; can result in thrombosis, infarction, hemorrhage. *Signs and symptoms:* Onset insidious. Fever, weight loss, skin lesions, hypertension, joint swelling, malaise, abdominal pain, change in urinary pattern, anemia, ischemia of fingers, pleuritis. Symptoms of renal, GI, and cardiac involvement.	Glucocorticoids, methotrexate, cyclophosphamide, antihypertensive, diuretics. Other drugs are prescribed for specific manifestations of the disorder.

NSAIDs, Nonsteroidal anti-inflammatory drugs; *GI,* gastrointestinal.

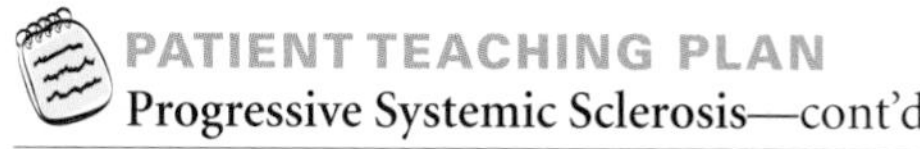

- Esophageal reflux can be managed with drug therapy; relaxing meals; avoiding spicy foods, caffeine, and alcohol; and maintaining an upright position for 1 to 2 hours after eating.

DERMATOMYOSITIS/POLYMYOSITIS

Dermatomyositis and polymyositis are relatively rare acute or chronic inflammatory diseases that primarily affect the skeletal muscle. The term *polymyositis* is applied to the condition when there is no skin involvement, and *dermatomyositis* is used when there is a characteristic skin rash. There is no known cause for these conditions, but they are frequently seen in patients with scleroderma, rheumatoid arthritis, vasculitis, systemic lupus erythematosus, or Sjögren's syndrome.

Pathophysiology

The major activity producing pathology in polymyositis is infiltration of inflammatory cells, causing destruction of muscle fibers. Inflammation of tissues surrounding blood vessels is an outstanding pathologic feature of the disease. The condition is sometimes associated with malignancy.

Signs and Symptoms

The primary symptom of polymyositis is muscle weakness, reflected in inability to do normal activities like climbing stairs, raising the arms over the head, and turning over in bed. Other symptoms are Raynaud's phenomenon and joint pain and inflammation. Patients with dermatomyositis typically have periorbital edema (swelling around the eyes) as well. The onset may be abrupt or slow.

Medical Diagnosis

The diagnosis is based on the presence of proximal muscle weakness, a muscle biopsy positive for muscle degeneration, elevated muscle enzymes, and myopathic electromyographic changes.

Medical Treatment

Drug therapy includes high-dose glucocorticoids such as prednisone and chemotherapeutic agents such as methotrexate. Supportive treatment centers on the balancing of rest and exercise to prevent contractures. This goal is difficult, because range-of-motion exercises may aggravate the condition.

NURSING CARE *of the Patient with Polymyositis*

Because polymyositis is seen in conjunction with other connective tissue diseases, the reader should refer to earlier sections of the chapter for applicable nursing interventions.

OTHER CONNECTIVE TISSUE DISORDERS

Other connective tissue disorders described in Table 39-6 are bursitis, carpal tunnel syndrome, ankylosing spondylitis, polymyalgia rheumatica, Reiter's syndrome, Behçet's syndrome, Sjögren's syndrome, and periarteritis nodosa.

Nutrition Concepts

1. A diet high in calcium (1,000 to 1,500 mg/day) and vitamin D (400 IU/day) is important for the prevention of osteoporosis.
2. Eight ounces of milk (whole, low-fat, or skim) provides 300 mg of calcium.
3. A well-balanced diet, including foods high in vitamin E and zinc, is recommended for persons with rheumatoid arthritis.
4. A weight loss program for persons with osteoarthritis helps reduce stress on weight-bearing joints.
5. Patients with gout may be advised to limit purine intake.
6. The patient with esophageal involvement of progressive systemic sclerosis needs small, frequent meals and limited spicy foods, alcohol, and caffeine.

key points

- The major connective tissues are bone, blood, cartilage, ligaments, skin, and tendons.
- Age-related changes in connective tissue can have a significant effect on function and quality of life.
- Osteoarthritis is characterized by degeneration of articular cartilage, hypertrophy of underlying and adjacent bone, and inflammation of surrounding synovium that leads to pain with joint movement.
- Osteoarthritis may be treated with drug therapy, education, physical therapy, modification of daily activities, and surgery.
- Nursing care of the patient with osteoarthritis focuses on chronic pain, impaired physical mobility, ineffective coping, and ineffective therapeutic regimen management.
- Total joint replacements can be done on the elbow, shoulder, phalangeal finger joints, hip, knee, and ankle.
- Nursing care after total joint replacement addresses pain, risk for injury, impaired physical mobility, impaired tissue perfusion, risk for infection, anxiety and fear, and ineffective therapeutic regimen management.
- Rheumatoid arthritis, a chronic, progressive inflammatory disease that leads to deformity and loss of joint mobility, is treated with drug therapy, supportive treatments, and modification of activities of daily living.
- Gout, a systemic disease characterized by the deposition of urate crystals in the joints and other body tissues, usually responds to drug therapy that lowers the serum uric acid level.
- Progressive systemic sclerosis, commonly called scleroderma, is characterized by thickening of the skin and may affect the blood vessels, gastrointestinal tract, lungs, heart, and kidneys.
- Nursing care for the patient with progressive systemic sclerosis addresses impaired skin integrity, self-care deficits, pain, social isolation, imbalanced nutrition, and ineffective therapeutic regimen management. Less common connective tissue disorders are polymyositis, ankylosing spondylitis, polymyalgia rheumatica, Reiter's syndrome, Behçet's syndrome, Sjögren's syndrome, and periarteritis nodosa.
- Most connective tissue disorders are chronic and, although they are not specifically curable, can be improved with symptomatic treatment.

REVIEW QUESTIONS

1. The joints between the bones of the skull are classified as:
   1. synarthroses.
   2. amphiarthroses.
   3. diarthroses.
   4. synovial.
2. Age-related changes in connective tissue include:
   1. hardening of bone tissue.
   2. increased water content.
   3. loss of cartilage elasticity.
   4. decreased osteophytes.
3. A patient who has gout calls the clinic to report having flank pain and blood in her urine. You should:
   1. recognize signs and symptoms of urinary stones and notify the physician immediately.
   2. tell her these symptoms are normal with gout and that they will improve soon.
   3. make an appointment for her to see the physician within one week.
   4. document her complaints in her record and ask her to call the next day if symptoms continue.
4. A continuous passive motion machine (CPM) has been ordered for a patient after a total joint replacement. The primary purpose of the CPM machine is to:
   1. prevent postoperative boredom.
   2. prevent scar tissue formation.
   3. restore muscle strength.
   4. test the prosthetic joint.
5. One week after total hip replacement surgery, a patient complains of sudden severe pain in the affected hip and inability to bear weight on that leg. You should suspect:
   1. wound dehiscence.
   2. prosthesis rejection.
   3. a new hip fracture.
   4. prosthesis dislocation.
6. Common nursing diagnoses for a patient with rheumatoid arthritis (RA) include:
   1. activity intolerance related to fatigue.
   2. risk for injury related to sensory losses.
   3. impaired tissue perfusion related to vasoconstriction.
   4. risk for aspiration related to esophageal dysfunction.
7. What is the recommended daily calcium intake for a patient who is postmenopausal and not taking hormone replacement therapy?
   1. 100 mg
   2. 500 mg
   3. 1,000 mg
   4. 1,500 mg
8. When probenecid (Benemid) is prescribed for a patient with gout, patient teaching should include which of the following pieces of advice?
   1. You must be careful to avoid people who have infections because your immune system is depressed.
   2. Drink at least eight 8-ounce glasses of fluid each day to prevent urinary stones.
   3. You can expect to feel the results of this medication within 72 hours.
   4. Remain in an upright position for at least 30 minutes after taking this medication.
9. Which statement should be included in the teaching plan for a patient with progressive systemic sclerosis (PSS/scleroderma)?
   1. Keep the temperature in your home below 70 degrees.
   2. Remain upright for 1-2 hours after meals.
   3. This is an acute condition that will improve over time.
   4. PSS affects only the skin.
10. A disorder in which the eyes, mouth, and vagina become dry because of obstructed secretory ducts is:
    1. Behçet's syndrome.
    2. Periarteritis nodosa.
    3. Reiter's syndrome.
    4. Sjögren's syndrome.

CHAPTER

40 Fractures

objectives

1. Identify the types of fractures.
2. Describe the five stages of the healing process.
3. Discuss the major complications of fractures, their signs and symptoms, and their management.
4. Compare the types of medical treatment for fractures, particularly reduction and fixation.
5. Describe common therapeutic measures for fractures, including casts, traction, crutches, walkers, and canes.
6. Discuss the nursing care of a patient with a fracture.
7. Describe specific types of fractures, including hip fractures, Colles' fractures, and pelvic fractures.

key terms

Bone remodeling (p. 822)
Closed reduction or manipulation (p. 825)
Comminuted fracture (KŎM-ĭ-nūt-ĕd, p. 825)
Compartment syndrome (p. 823)
Complete fracture (p. 821)
Delayed union (p. 824)
Fat embolism (ĔM-bō-lĭzm, p. 823)
Fixation (fĭx-SĀ-shŭn, p. 825)
Fracture (p. 821)
Greenstick fracture (p. 821)
Incomplete fracture (p. 821)
Malunion (măl-ŪN-yŏn, p. 824)
Nonunion (nŏn-ŪN-yŭn, p. 824)
Open or compound fracture (p. 821)
Open reduction (p. 825)
Reduction (p. 825)
Stress fracture (p. 821)

A **fracture** is defined as a break or disruption in the continuity of a bone. With a fracture, injury to surrounding soft tissue also occurs. The severity of soft-tissue injury depends on the location and severity of the break.

All fractures are either complete or incomplete. A **complete fracture** is one in which the break extends across the entire bone, dividing it into two separate pieces. An **incomplete fracture** is one in which the bone breaks only part way across, leaving some portion of the bone intact. The term **greenstick fracture** has been used to describe the incomplete fractures most commonly seen in children. In this case, the bone is broken on one side, but only bent on the other.

CLASSIFICATION OF FRACTURES

Fractures may be classified as open or closed, depending on the type and extent of soft tissue damage. A closed or simple fracture is one in which the broken bone does not break through the skin. In an **open or compound fracture,** the fragments of the broken bone break through the skin. Open fractures have three grades of severity:

Grade I: least severe injury, with minimal skin damage
Grade II: moderately severe injury, with skin and muscle contusions (bruises)
Grade III: most severe injury (wound larger than 6 to 8 cm), with skin, muscle, blood vessel, and nerve damage

Fractures also may be classified as stress or pathologic fractures, depending on their cause. A **stress fracture** is caused by either sudden force or prolonged stress. Stress fractures are often related to sports such as track or basketball. A pathologic fracture occurs because of a pathologic condition in the bone such as a tumor or disease process that causes a spontaneous break. Figure 40-1 illustrates common types of fractures.

ETIOLOGY AND RISK FACTORS

Fractures are most commonly caused by trauma to the bone, especially as a result of automobile accidents and falls. Bone disease such as bone cancer also can lead to a fracture. Hip fractures in the elderly usually are associated with falls. Risk factors for hip fractures include osteoporosis, advanced age, white race, use of psychotropic drugs, and being female.

In adults, the bones most commonly fractured are the ribs. Fractures of the femur are most common in young and middle-aged adults, whereas hip and wrist fractures are most common in the elderly. More than 250,000 hip fractures occur each year in the United States, and the number is rising. Most people with fractured hips must be hospitalized, resulting in an overall estimated annual cost of more than $7 billion.

What Does Culture Have to do with Fractures?

Because older white women have a high incidence of osteoporosis, they are at greater risk for fractures. The risk can be reduced by targeting these women for preventive measures throughout life. Osteoporosis is easier to prevent than to treat.

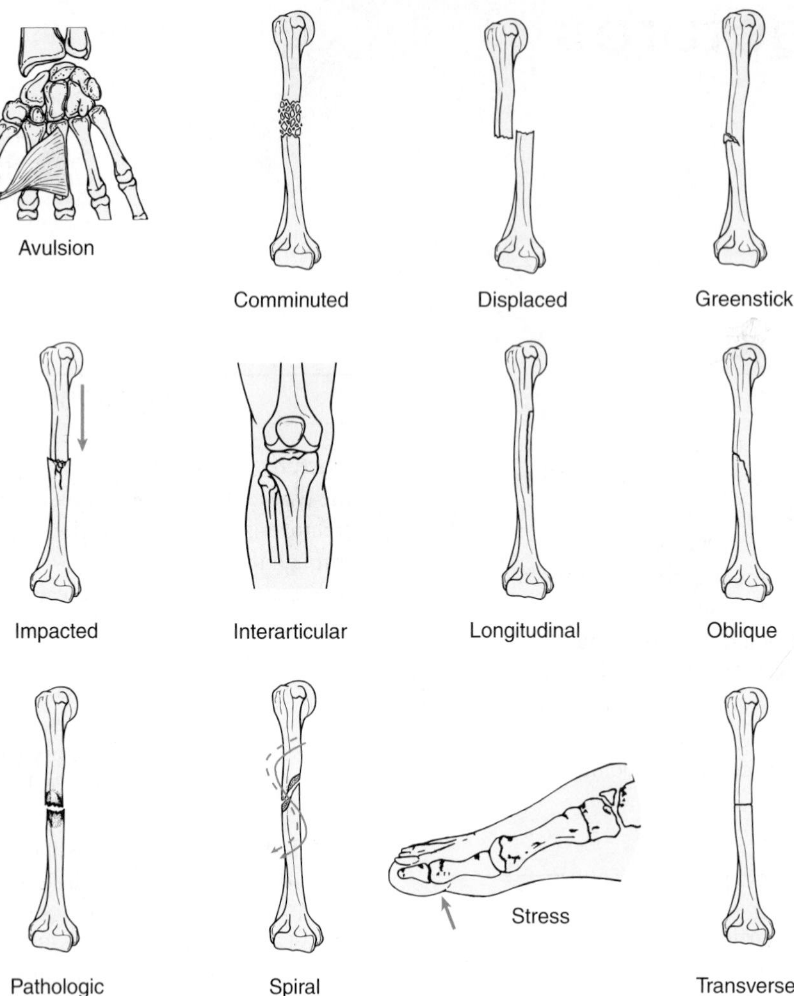

FIGURE **40-1** Common types of fractures.

FRACTURE HEALING

A bone begins to heal as soon as an injury occurs. New bone tissue is formed to repair the fracture, resulting in a sturdy union between the broken ends of the bone. Healing occurs in the following five stages:

STAGE 1: *Hematoma formation.* Immediately after a fracture, bleeding occurs, along with edema. In 48 to 72 hours, a clot or hematoma forms between the two broken ends of the bone.

STAGE 2: *Fibrocartilage formation.* The hematoma that surrounds the fracture does not resorb, as does a hematoma in other parts of the body. Instead, other tissue cells enter the clot, and granulation tissue forms. The granulation tissue then forms a collar around each end of the broken bone, gradually becoming firm and forming a bridge between the two ends.

STAGE 3: *Callus formation.* By the end of the first week after injury, the granulation tissue changes into a callus formation. Callus is made up of cartilage, osteoblasts (bone cells that form new bone), calcium, and phosphorus. The callus is larger than the diameter of the bone and serves as a temporary splint.

STAGE 4: *Ossification.* Within 2 to 3 weeks after the break, a permanent bone callus, known as woven bone, forms. It is during this stage that the ends of the broken bone begin to knit.

STAGE 5: *Consolidation and remodeling.* Consolidation occurs when the distance between bone fragments decreases and eventually closes. During bone remodeling, the immature bone cells are gradually replaced by mature bone cells. The excess bone is naturally chiseled away by stress to the affected part from motion, exercise, and weight bearing. The bone then takes on its original shape and size (Fig. 40-2).

Healing is affected by many factors, including the location and severity of the fracture, the type of bone, other bone pathology, circulatory adequacy, and the adequacy of immobilization. Other factors that affect healing include age, endocrine disorders, and some drugs. The healing time for fractures increases with age, and it may take six times as long for the same type of fracture to heal in an older adult as in an in-

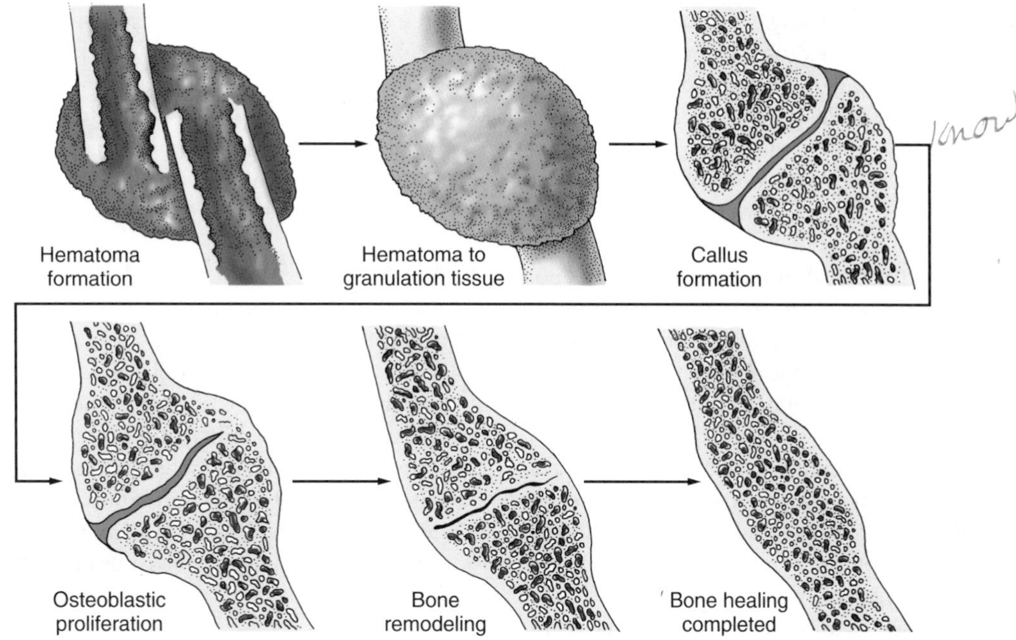

FIGURE **40-2** Stages of fracture healing.

fant. In the absence of bone disease, most older adults eventually heal as well as younger adults. However, many older adults, especially women, have a loss of bone mass.

COMPLICATIONS

Complications of a fracture can delay or impede healing and may even be life threatening. Short-term complications include shock, fat embolism, deep vein thrombosis, compartment syndrome, and infection. Long-term complications include joint stiffness and contractures, post-traumatic arthritis, malunion, nonunion, delayed union, avascular necrosis, and reflex sympathetic dystrophy.

SHOCK

After a fracture, there is a risk of excessive blood loss. Tissue trauma may rupture local blood vessels, and vascular internal organs may be punctured, with resultant internal bleeding. Loss of blood leads to shock, which is evidenced by tachycardia, anxiety, pallor, and cool, clammy skin. Careful immobilization of fractures reduces the risk of hemorrhage. If severe external bleeding is evident, external pressure should be applied and medical assistance summoned immediately. Management of hypovolemic shock is discussed in Chapter 18.

FAT EMBOLISM

Fat embolism is a condition in which fat globules are released from the marrow of the broken bone into the bloodstream. Once the fat droplets enter the circulation, they migrate to the lungs. Because they are too large to pass through the pulmonary circulation, they lodge in the capillaries and obstruct blood flow. The fat particles break down into fatty acids, which inflame the pulmonary blood vessels, leading to pulmonary edema.

Fat embolism syndrome is most commonly associated with fractures of the long bones, multiple fractures, and severe trauma. It occurs 24 to 48 hours after injury, most often in young men aged 20 to 40 and in older adults aged 70 to 80. An older patient with a hip fracture is at highest risk.

Respiratory distress is the first sign of a fat embolism, followed by tachycardia (rapid heartbeat), tachypnea (rapid breathing), fever, confusion, and decreased level of consciousness. Another characteristic feature is petechiae, a measles-like rash over the neck, upper arms, chest, or abdomen. Treatment of fat embolism consists of bedrest, gentle handling, oxygen, ventilatory support, and fluid restriction and diuretics for pulmonary edema. Though controversial, corticosteroids sometimes are used. The prognosis is generally good; however, the condition can be fatal.

DEEP VEIN THROMBOSIS

Venous stasis, vessel damage, and altered clotting mechanisms all contribute to the formation of blood clots (thrombi), most commonly in the deep veins of the legs. Like fat particles, thrombi can break off and travel to the lungs, causing a pulmonary embolism. The prevention and treatment of deep vein thrombosis and pulmonary embolism are covered in Chapter 29.

COMPARTMENT SYNDROME

Compartment syndrome is a serious complication that results from internal or external pressure on the affected area. Compartments are located in the muscles of the extremities. They are enclosed spaces made up of muscle, bone, nerves, and blood vessels wrapped by a fibrous membrane. Internal pressure can be caused by bleeding or edema into a compartment; external pressure can be caused by a cast or tight dressing. When there is bleeding or edema into a compartment, there is nowhere for the drainage to go because it is trapped in the space. The increased fluid puts pressure on the tissues, nerves, and blood vessels, so that blood flow is decreased, resulting in pain and tissue damage. External pressure also can decrease blood flow to the area.

Although compartment syndrome is relatively rare, it is a serious condition and can create an emergency situation. Within 4 to 6 hours after the onset of compartment syndrome, irreversible muscle damage can occur. Paresis (partial paralysis) can result if the condition is not treated within 24 hours. In 24 to 48 hours, the limb can become useless.

A primary symptom of compartment syndrome is pain, especially with touch or movement, that cannot be relieved with opioid analgesia. Other signs and symptoms are edema, pallor, weak or unequal pulses, cyanosis, tingling, numbness, paresthesia, and, finally, severe pain.

The goal of treatment is to relieve pressure. When there is internal pressure, a surgical fasciotomy, which entails making linear incisions in the fascia, may be done to relieve pressure on the nerves and blood vessels. For external pressure, the cast or dressings are removed and replaced.

INFECTION

Infection of the bone, called osteomyelitis, can result from contamination of the open wound associated with a fracture or from contamination of the indwelling hardware used to repair the broken bone. Any infection can interfere with normal healing. Osteomyelitis most commonly occurs after an open fracture and surgical repair and may become chronic. In deep, grossly contaminated wounds, gas gangrene may develop.

Signs and symptoms of bone infection are local pain, redness, purulent wound drainage, chills, and fever. With gas gangrene, there is a foul-smelling watery drainage with significant redness and swelling of affected tissue.

Osteomyelitis requires aggressive antibiotic therapy. Intravenous antibiotics may be given for 4 to 8 weeks, followed by an additional 4 to 8 weeks of oral drug therapy. Wound care may include irrigation, treatment with antibiotic cement or beads, and surgical removal of dead bone tissue.

***Put on your* THINKING CAP!!**

A 16-year-old male was admitted after a motorcycle accident. He had a compound fracture of the thigh with severe soft tissue injury. Following surgery, he has an external fixation device on the affected leg. A Jackson-Pratt drain is in place. Daily wound care is ordered. List all potential sources of bone infection that you can.

JOINT STIFFNESS AND CONTRACTURES

Joint fractures or dislocations may be followed by stiffness or contractures, especially in older people. Prevention requires appropriate positioning and progressive exercise programs as prescribed. Treatment may employ splints, traction, casts, surgical manipulation, and aggressive physiotherapy.

POST-TRAUMATIC ARTHRITIS

Weight-bearing joints are most vulnerable to post-traumatic arthritis. Excessive stress and strain on the joint or fracture must be avoided to reduce the risk of this complication.

AVASCULAR NECROSIS

A variety of factors can interfere with the blood supply after a bone injury. Once bone cells are deprived of oxygen and nutrients, they die and their cell walls collapse. This condition is called avascular necrosis. Signs and symptoms include increasing pain, instability, and decreased function in the affected area. Among the conservative treatment measures are relief of weight bearing and removal of part of the bone to decrease pressure. If conservative measures fail, a variety of surgical procedures may be recommended. Sometimes amputation is necessary.

MALUNION, NONUNION, AND DELAYED UNION

Malunion is improper alignment of bone ends resulting in external deformity. *Nonunion* occurs when a fracture never heals. Failure of a fracture to heal in the expected time is called *delayed union.* These complications may be caused by inadequate immobilization or excess movement, poor alignment of the bone fragments, infection, or poor nutrition.

When there is nonunion of a fracture, a variety of methods may be used to stimulate fracture healing. The implantation of bone grafts is an *osteogenic method. Osteoconductive methods* employ synthetic materials to provide a matrix for bone growth. The use of substances such as platelet-derived growth factor is called *osteoinduction.* In addition, several types of electric stimulation devices may be used to stimulate bone growth. The stimulation may be internal or external and is done up to 10 hours a day for 3 to 6 months. Although the procedure is time-consuming, it can prevent further surgery and bone grafts.

REFLEX SYMPATHETIC DYSTROPHY

Reflex sympathetic dystrophy, also called complex regional pain syndrome, is usually precipitated by minor trauma. It is characterized by severe pain at the injury site, edema, muscle spasm, stiffness, vasospasms, increased sweating, atrophy, contractions, and loss of bone mass. The condition is treated with nerve blocks, physical therapy, transcutaneous electrical stimulation, and drugs including analgesics, muscle relaxants, and antidepressants.

SIGNS AND SYMPTOMS

The signs and symptoms of a fracture depend on the type and location of the break. Some fractures have so few clinical manifestations that they can be detected only radiologically. The most common signs and symptoms are swelling, bruising, pain, tenderness, loss of normal function, abnormal po-

table 40-1 *Signs and Symptoms of Fractures and Their Causes*

DEFORMITY

Strong muscle pull may cause bone fragments to override; therefore, alignment and contour changes occur, such as (1) angulation, rotation, and limb shortening; (2) bone depression; or (3) altered curves in the injured site, especially when compared with the opposite site. Swelling (edema) may appear rapidly from localization of serous fluid at the fracture site and extravasation of blood into adjacent tissues. Bruising (ecchymosis) may result from subcutaneous bleeding. Muscle spasms—involuntary muscle contractions near the fracture—may occur.

TENDERNESS

Tenderness over the fracture site is due to underlying injuries.

PAIN

There is immediate, severe pain at the time of injury. After injury, pain may result from muscle spasm, overriding of the fractured ends of the bone, or damage to adjacent structures.

IMPAIRED SENSATION (NUMBNESS)

Sensation may be impaired as a result of nerve damage or nerve entrapment from edema, bleeding, or bony fragments.

LOSS OF NORMAL FUNCTION

Normal function may be lost because of instability of the fractured bone, pain, or muscle spasm.

PARALYSIS

Paralysis may be caused by nerve damage.

ABNORMAL MOBILITY

Movement of a part that is normally immobile is due to instability when the long bones are fractured.

CREPITUS

Crepitus results from broken bone ends rubbing together. Grating sensations or sounds are felt or heard if the injured part is moved.

HYPOVOLEMIC SHOCK

Hypovolemic shock may result from blood loss or other injuries.

Modified from Black, J. M., Hawks, J. H., & Keene, A. M. (2001). *Medical-surgical nursing: Clinical management for positive outcomes.* (6th ed., pp. 588, 590). Philadelphia: Saunders.

sition, and decreased mobility. Table 40-1 lists various signs and symptoms of fractures and their causes.

DIAGNOSTIC TESTS AND PROCEDURES

The most common diagnostic tests used to confirm the presence of a fracture are radiologic studies. Standard radiographs are used first to reveal bone disruption, deformity, or malignancy. Computed tomography (CT) may be used to detect fractures of complex structures, such as the hip and pelvis, or compression fractures of the spine. A bone scan may be useful for detecting small bone fractures or fractures caused by stress or disease. Diagnostic tests for fractures are the same as those for connective tissue disorders described in Table 39-2.

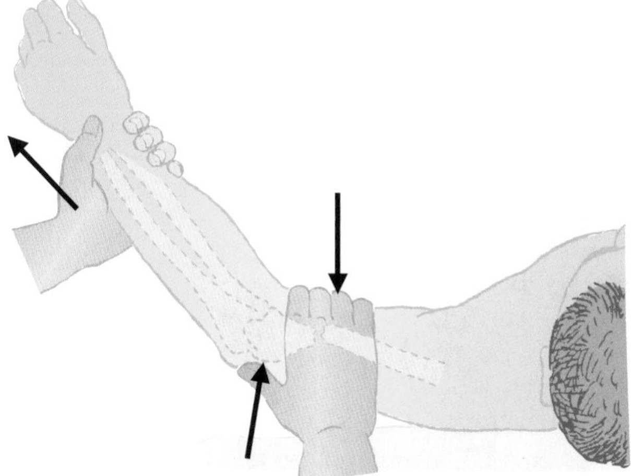

FIGURE **40-3** Closed (manipulative) reduction to realign a fracture of the arm.

MEDICAL TREATMENT

The goals of medical treatment for a fracture are to realign the bone fragments, establish a sturdy union between the broken ends of the bone, and restore function. The most common therapeutic techniques to accomplish these goals are closed and open reduction and internal and external fixation.

REDUCTION

Reduction is the process of bringing the ends of the broken bone into proper alignment. **Closed reduction or manipulation** is the nonsurgical realignment of the bones that returns them to their previous anatomic position. No surgical incision is made; however, general or local anesthesia is given. Closed reduction may be done by using traction, angulation, or rotation, or a combination of these (Fig. 40-3). After reduction of a fracture, a radiograph is taken and a cast is usually applied.

Open reduction is a surgical procedure in which an incision is made at the fracture site. It is usually done for open (compound) or **comminuted fractures** (bone is broken or crushed into small pieces) to clean the area of fragments and debris.

Effective pain management of a fracture is essential for mobilization and healing. Once the fracture is aligned, immobilization is necessary for healing to occur.

FIXATION

Fixation is an attempt to attach the fragments of the broken bone together when reduction alone is not feasible because of

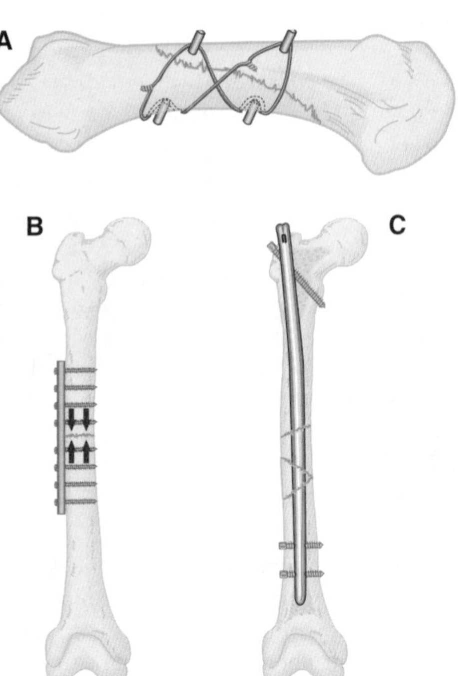

FIGURE 40-4 Examples of different types of internal fixation devices. *A,* Tension band wiring technique using Kirschner wires for fracture of a phalanx. *B,* Compression plate applied to the lateral aspect of the femur. *C,* Intramedullary nail fixed to both proximal and distal fragments of the femur.

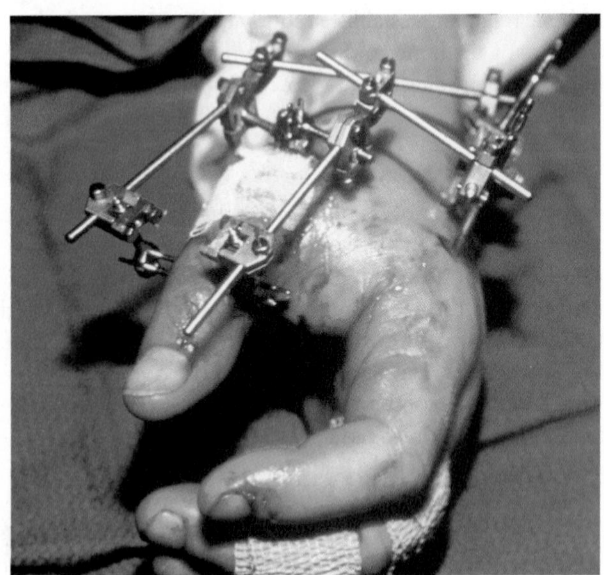

FIGURE 40-5 External fixators. Mini Hoffman system in place on hand.

the type and extent of the break. Fixation is done during the open reduction surgical procedure. Internal fixation includes the use of rods, pins, nails, screws, or metal plates to align bone fragments and keep them in place for healing (Fig. 40-4). Figure 40-4C illustrates an open reduction and internal fixation of a

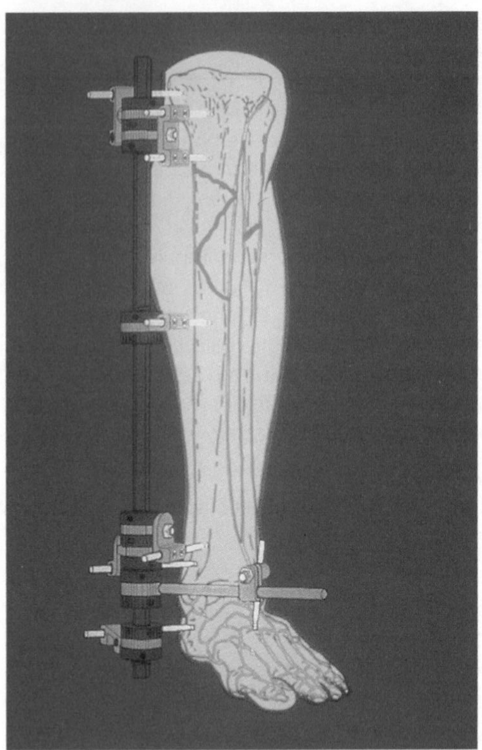

FIGURE 40-6 The Hex-Fix external fixation system for tibial fractures.

fractured femur in which a nail was used to maintain alignment. Internal fixation promotes early mobilization and is often preferred for older adults who have brittle bones that may not heal properly, or who may suffer the consequences of immobility.

External fixation is similar to internal fixation, but the pins in the bone are attached to an external frame (Figs. 40-5 and 40-6). When there is extensive soft tissue damage or infection, external fixation allows easier access to the site and facilitates wound care. In addition, the device allows for early ambulation and mobility while relieving pain. Pin track infection occurs in approximately 10% of patients with external fixation. Pin care is extremely important to prevent the migration of organisms along the pin from the skin to the bone. Patients should be taught to do their own pin care and to recognize signs of infection.

COMMON THERAPEUTIC MEASURES

CASTS, SPLINTS, AND IMMOBILIZERS

Casts, splints, and other immobilizers are used to secure the position of the body parts being treated. They hold the bone in alignment while allowing enough movement of other parts of the body to carry out activities of daily living. Types of materials used for a cast are plaster of Paris, fiberglass, thermoplastic resins, thermolabile plastic, and polyester-cotton knit impregnated with polyurethane. A variety of materials are used to make splints and immobilizers.

Plaster of Paris consists of anhydrous calcium sulfate embedded in gauze. It is the least expensive type of cast to use.

After a well-fitting stockinette has been applied, the gauze is immersed in water and wrapped around the affected part. The stockinette must not be too tight because it may impair circulation. A stockinette that is too loose can wrinkle and result in pressure sores. The strength of the cast is determined by the number of layers of wrapped gauze and the technique of application.

Initially the wet cast is hot, and the heat may cause edema of the underlying tissues from the increased circulation. The cast quickly becomes damp and cool. It dries after about 24 to 72 hours, depending on the size and location. When the cast is dry and strong, it can withstand weight bearing and other stresses. The underlying stockinette covers the edges of the cast to prevent scratching and irritation from the rough plaster. Short pieces of tape are sometimes placed over the edges of the casts to prevent skin irritation by rough edges and to protect the cast from moisture and soiling. This is referred to as "petaling."

Fiberglass is a synthetic material used for casts that is lighter and has a shorter drying time than plaster of Paris. Drying time is 10 to 15 minutes, and the cast can withstand weight bearing 30 minutes after application. Sometimes physicians use plaster of Paris casts on lower extremities for heavier weight bearing and fiberglass casts on upper extremities.

Other types of synthetic materials are thermolabile plastic (Orthoplast) and thermoplastic resins (Hexcelite). They are heated in warm water and molded to fit the torso or extremity. Polyurethane is formed from chemically treated polyester and cotton fabric. The fabric is immersed in cool water to start the chemical process for wrapping.

Sometimes the cast is split down the front to allow the casting material and padding to spread. This is referred to as a univalved cast. A bivalved cast is cut down both sides so that the front portion can be removed while the back portion maintains immobilization. When an opening is cut into the cast to allow inspection of the body area or to relieve pressure, it is said to be a windowed cast. Always save the cut out "window," because it may be reinserted later.

The four main groups of casts are (1) upper extremity, (2) lower extremity, (3) cast brace, and (4) body or spica cast. Examples of various types of casts are shown in Table 40-2. An upper extremity cast is used for breaks in the shoulder, arm, wrist, and hand. A patient who is wearing an arm cast should keep the arm elevated above the heart when lying in bed to prevent swelling. The arm is kept in a sling for support when the patient is up.

Lower extremity casts are used for breaks in the upper and lower leg, ankle, and foot. A leg cast is used to allow mobility and may be used with crutches. A cast shoe or rubber walking pad protects the cast and prevents falls. The affected leg should be elevated on several pillows during the first few days after the break to prevent swelling.

After an adequate amount of healing has taken place and edema has subsided, cast braces may be used for injury to the knee. A cast brace supports the affected part while allowing the knee to bend. This is accomplished by applying a cast above and below the knee and connecting them with a hinge.

Body or spica casts are used when a fracture is located somewhere in the trunk of the body. A body cast encircles the trunk, whereas a spica cast encases the trunk plus one or two extremities. Body or spica casts severely limit mobility and may cause complications related to lack of movement, such as skin breakdown, respiratory problems, constipation, and joint contractures. In addition, a condition known as cast syndrome is caused by compression of a portion of the duodenum between the superior mesenteric artery and the aorta and vertebral column. Signs and symptoms of cast syndrome include nausea and abdominal distention.

The cast is removed only on physician's orders. A special device called a cast cutter is used to cut the plaster. Blunt scissors are then used to cut the padding. Tell the patient that the cutter blade is noisy but will not cut the skin. However, when the cast is removed the skin that had been under the cast will be tender and dry and may have crusts of dry skin. Gently wash the area and explain that the skin will regain its normal appearance after a few days. Muscle atrophy may be apparent. Assure the patient that muscle mass will be restored with use of the limb.

PATIENT TEACHING PLAN
Cast Care

- Keep plaster casts dry; follow physician's instructions regarding wetting synthetic casts.
- Do not remove any padding.
- Do not insert any foreign object inside the cast.
- Do not bear weight on a new plaster cast for 48 hours (with synthetics, may be less than an hour).
- Do not cover the cast with plastic for prolonged periods.
- *Do* report swelling, discoloration of toes or fingers, pain during motion, and burning or tingling under the cast to a health care provider.

TRACTION

Traction exerts a pulling force on a fractured extremity to provide alignment of the broken bone fragments. It also is used to prevent or correct deformity, decrease muscle spasm, promote rest, and maintain the position of the diseased or injured part.

Traction may be applied directly to the skin (skin traction) or attached directly to a bone (skeletal traction) by means of a metal pin or wire. Examples of skin traction such as Buck's traction are shown in Figure 40-7. It is used for hip and knee contractures, muscle spasms, and alignment of hip fractures. Skin traction weight is no more than 5 to 10 pounds to prevent injury to the skin.

Skeletal traction provides a strong, steady, continuous pull and can be used for prolonged periods of time. Examples of skeletal traction are Gardner-Wells, Crutchfield, and Vinke tongs and a halo vest, in which pins are inserted into the skull on either side (see Fig. 27-8). Heavier weights can be used with skeletal traction, usually from 15 to 30 pounds. Crutchfield's traction and a halo vest are used for reduction

table 40-2 ***Cast Types and Common Uses***

TYPE	ILLUSTRATION	COMMON USES
Short leg cast	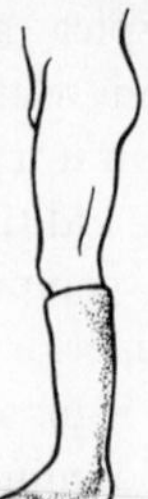	Fracture of foot, ankle, or distal tibia or fibula Severe sprain or strain Postoperative immobilization following open reduction and internal fixation Correction of deformity, such as talipes equinovarus
Long leg cast	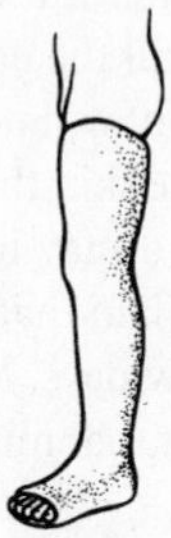	Fracture of distal femur, knee, or lower leg Soft tissue injury to knee or knee dislocation Postoperative immobilization following open reduction and internal fixation
Bilateral long leg hip spica cast	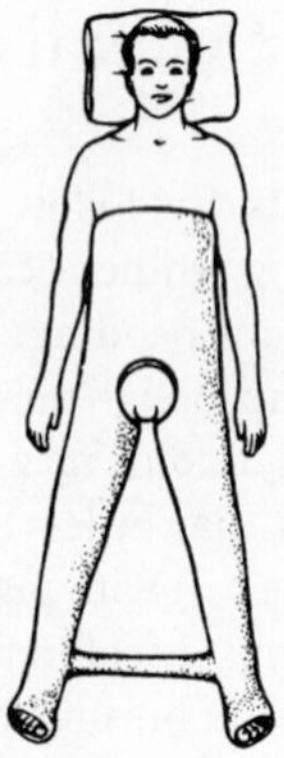	Fractures of femur, acetabulum, or pelvis Postoperative immobilization following open reduction and internal fixation
Body jacket cast	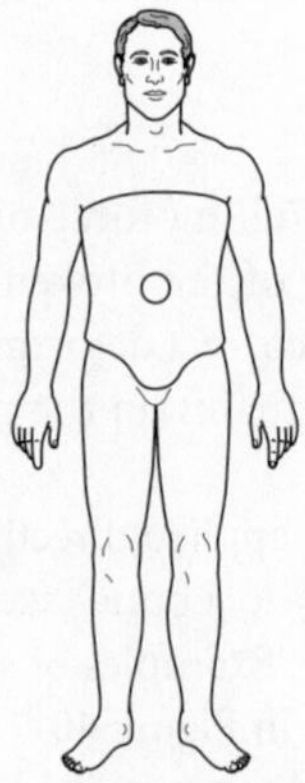	Stable spine injuries of the thoracic or lumbar spine

Drawings from Maher, A. B., Salmond, S. W., & Pellino, T. A. (1994). *Orthopedic nursing* (pp. 279-280). Philadelphia: Saunders. Body jacket cast drawing from Lewis, S. M., Heitkemper, M. M., & Dirksen, S. R. (2000). *Medical-surgical nursing: Assessment and management of clinical problems.* (5th ed., p. 1776). Philadelphia: Saunders.

table 40-2 ***Cast Types and Common Uses—cont'd***

TYPE	ILLUSTRATION	COMMON USES
Short arm cast		Fracture of hand or wrist Postoperative immobilization following open reduction and internal fixation
Long arm cast		Fracture of forearm, elbow, or humerus Postoperative immobilization following open reduction and internal fixation Can be weighted to create traction

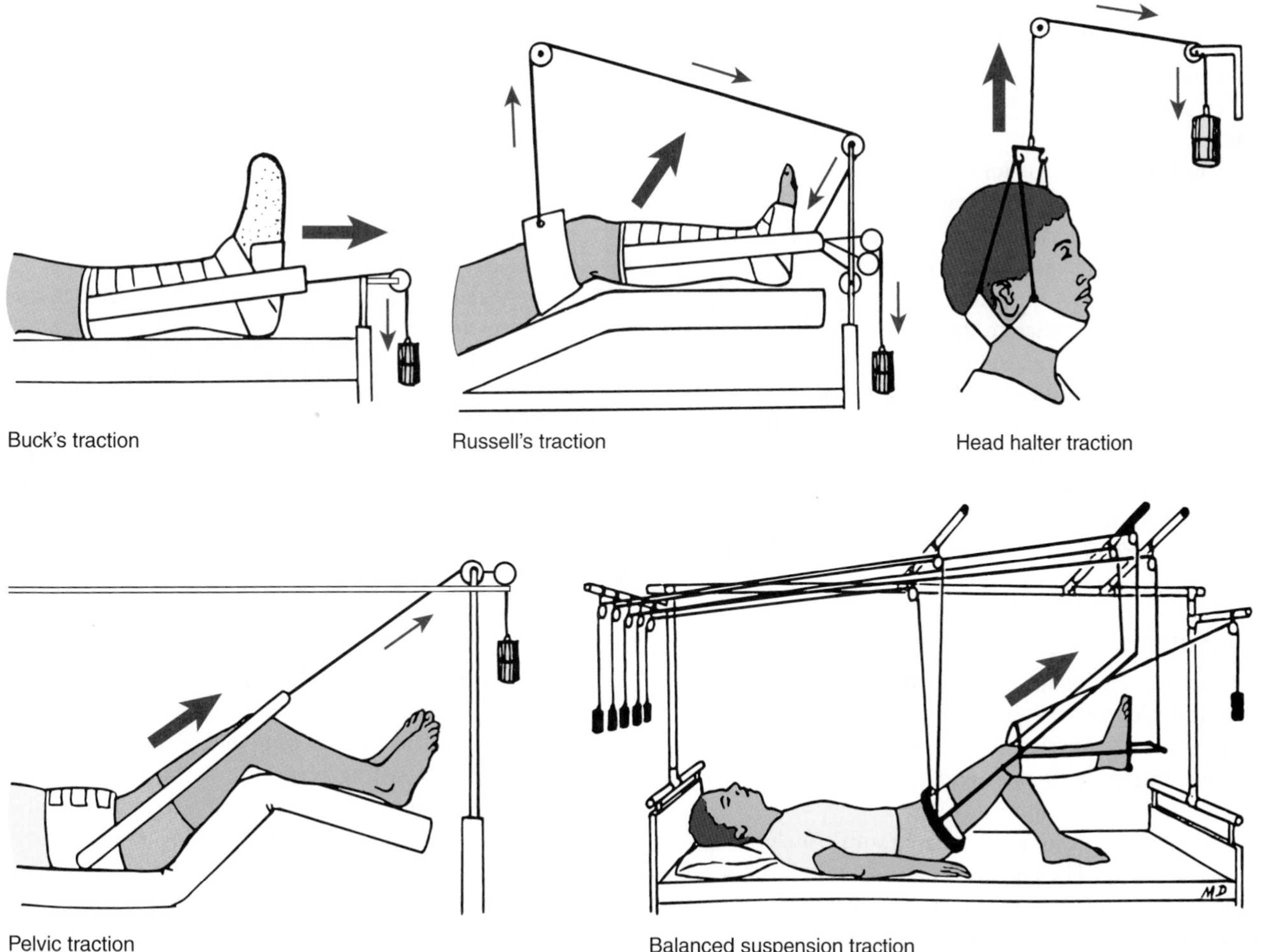

FIGURE **40-7** Examples of skin traction.

and immobilization of fractures of the cervical or high thoracic vertebrae.

Traction may involve complications such as impaired circulation, inadequate fracture alignment, skin breakdown, and soft tissue injury. As noted earlier, pin track infection and osteomyelitis can occur with skeletal traction. Important points to remember when patients are in traction are:

1. Weights always must hang freely.
2. Be sure the amount of weight used is correct as ordered, clamps are tight, and ropes move freely over pulleys.
3. Maintain good body alignment so the line of pull is correct.
4. Use padding to prevent trauma to skin where traction is applied. Report skin breakdown or irritation to physician.
5. Assess affected extremities for temperature, pain, sensation, motion, capillary refill time, and pulses.
6. With skeletal traction, assess pin sites for redness, drainage, or odor, which may indicate infection.

CRUTCHES

Crutches increase mobility and assist with ambulation after a fracture of the lower extremity. Success in crutch walking depends on many factors, including the patient's motivation, age, interests and activities, and ability to adjust to the crutches. Crutch use requires good upper body strength, so it may not be appropriate for elderly or frail patients.

In most cases, a physical therapist measures the patient for proper fit and instructs the patient in crutch-walking techniques. The nurse reinforces the instructions and evaluates whether the crutches are being used properly. A properly fitted crutch should reach to three fingerbreadths below the axilla to avoid pressure on the axilla when walking (Fig. 40-8). Axillary pressure could result in temporary or permanent numbness in the hands. When walking, the patient's weight should be put on the hand grips. The hand grips are adjusted so that the elbow is flexed no more than 30 degrees when the patient is standing in the tripod position, which is the basic crutch stance: feet parallel, crutches 6 inches in front of and 6 inches to the side of each foot.

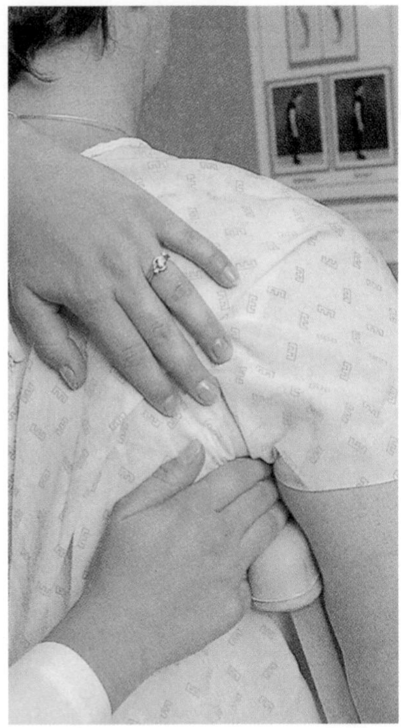

FIGURE **40-8** The distance between the crutch pad and the patient's axilla should be 3 to 4 fingerbreadths.

Gait Patterns

Several types of gait patterns are used with crutches. The type of gait used depends on the severity of the patient's disability and the patient's physical condition, trunk strength, upper and lower extremity strength, and balance. All of the gaits begin with the tripod position.

The five types of gait patterns used with crutches are:

1. *Two-point gait:* The crutch on one side and the opposite foot are advanced at the same time. This gait is used with partial weight-bearing limitations and with bilateral lower extremity prostheses.
2. *Three-point gait:* Both crutches and the foot of the affected extremity are advanced together, followed by the foot of the unaffected extremity. This gait requires strength and balance. It is used for partial weight bearing or no weight bearing on the affected leg.
3. *Four-point gait:* The right crutch is advanced, then the left foot, then the left crutch, then the right foot. This gait is used if weight bearing is allowed and one foot can be placed in front of the other.
4. *Swing-to gait:* Both crutches are advanced together, then both legs are lifted and placed down again on a spot behind the crutches. The feet and crutches form a tripod.
5. *Swing-through gait:* Both crutches are advanced together, then both legs are lifted through and beyond the crutches and placed down again at a point in front of the crutches. This gait is used when there is adequate muscle power and balance in the arms and legs.

To sit down after walking with crutches, the patient walks up to a chair, turns using the crutches, and backs up until the unaffected leg touches the seat of the chair. One hand then grips both crutches by the hand grips, and the crutches are placed to the unaffected side. The patient bends at the waist, places the hand on the affected side on the seat, moves the affected leg forward, and lowers onto the seat slowly (Fig. 40-9). To get up from a sitting position, the patient pushes off against the chair with the hand of the affected side and pushes down with the other hand, which is holding both crutches by the hand grips.

Going up and down stairs on crutches is challenging. For stair climbing, the unaffected leg goes up the step first while the body is supported by the crutches. The full body weight is transferred to the unaffected leg, followed by movement of the crutches and the affected leg to the step. To descend stairs, the affected leg and the crutches move down one step first, then the unaffected leg. So, when climbing stairs, the good leg goes first, and when descending stairs, the bad leg goes first. ("The good leads up, and bad leads down").

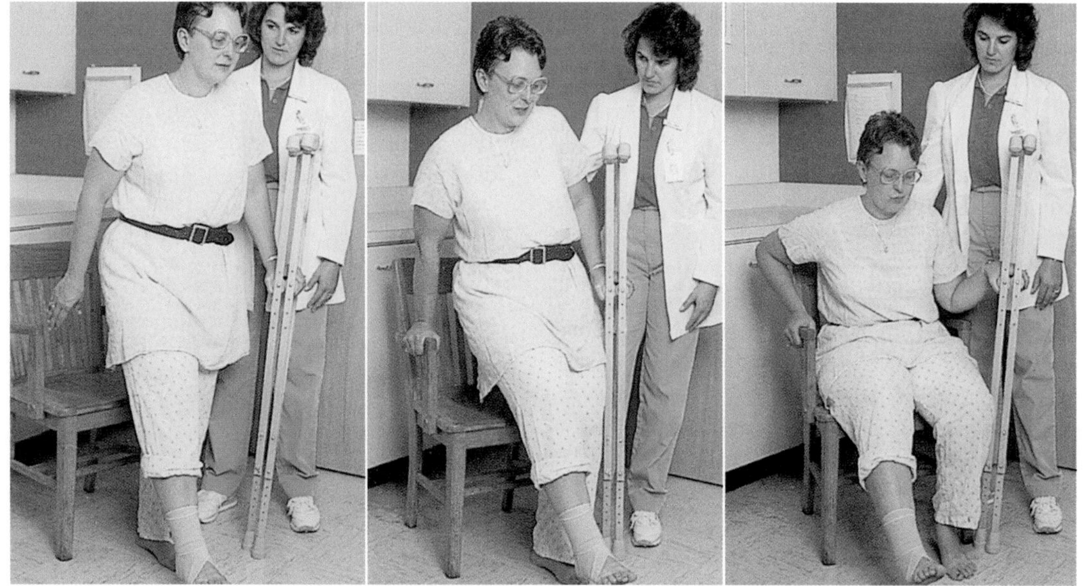

FIGURE 40-9 Standing to sitting with crutches.

WALKERS

A walker is used for support and balance, usually by older clients. A modified swing-to gait is used with a walker so that the walker is pushed or lifted forward, then the legs are brought up to it. Rather than lifting both legs forward together, as with crutch walking, one foot is brought forward at a time.

CANES

Canes are used to provide minimal support and balance and to relieve pressure on weight-bearing joints. The cane is placed on the unaffected side with the top of the cane even with the patient's greater trochanter. The elbow should be flexed to approximately 30 degrees (Fig. 40-10). Two-point or four-point gaits are used with a cane. The cane should be held close to the body on the unaffected side and advanced with the affected leg. When walking, it is better to lift the cane rather than slide it along to prevent catching the cane tip and tripping or falling.

ELECTRICAL STIMULATION

Electrical stimulation may be used to promote bone healing by promoting bone growth. An electrical current is delivered through one of three methods: a surgically implanted device, a device with pins that are inserted through the skin to the fracture site, and a pack of electrical coils that is applied to the skin around the fracture site. Electrical bone stimulators are successful in approximately 80% of cases, with an average healing time of 16 weeks.

NURSING CARE *of the Patient with a Fracture*

Once the initial emergency treatment and medical management of a patient with a fracture have been provided, nursing care becomes very important. The focus of nursing care is on preventing complications and restoring the patient to independent

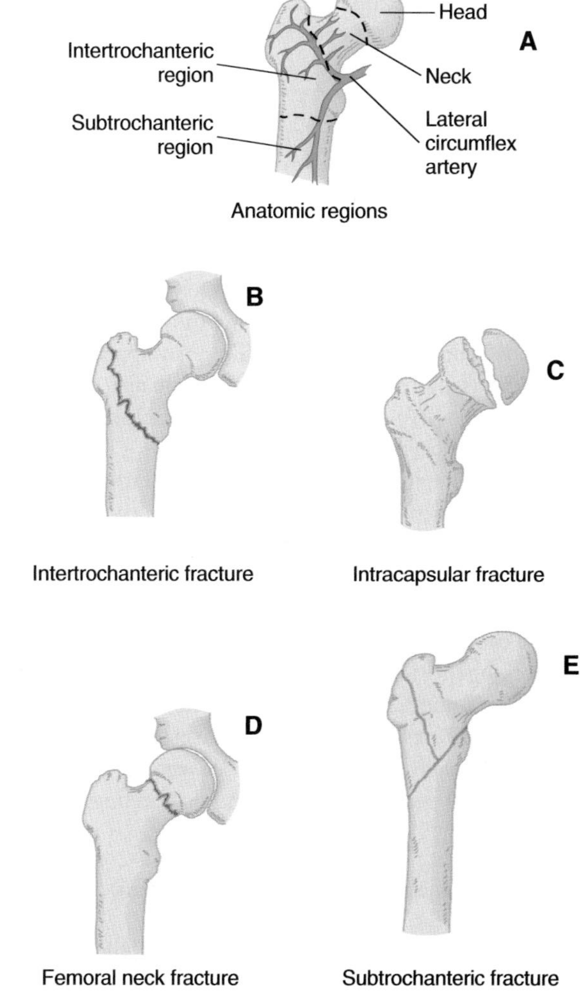

FIGURE 40-10 Femoral fractures. *A,* Anatomic regions of the proximal end of femur. *B,* Intertrochanteric fracture. *C,* Intracapsular fracture. *D,* Femoral neck fracture. *E,* Subtrochanteric fracture.

function. (See Nursing Care Plan: The Patient with a Fracture, and Chapter 15 for a discussion of emergency care.)

Assessment

Health History

Even after the initial medical care has been given and the fracture has been set, it is helpful to gather information on the cause, type, and extent of the injury. This information is important because it allows you to observe for complications or other injuries that may have been overlooked during the emergency situation. Ask the patient, family members, or witnesses about the events leading up to the accident and exactly what happened during the accident. In addition, describe symptoms associated with the injury, including the type and extent of pain, the presence of numbness or tingling or both, the loss of motion and sensation, and the complaint of muscle spasms.

Assess the number and types of prescription and over-the-counter medications taken by the patient to determine whether they played any role in the development of the fracture or will affect the recovery and rehabilitation. It is also helpful to find out about other medical problems that either may have been related to the cause of the fracture, such as a pathologic fracture, or that may affect healing. Determine the patient's occupation and usual roles and responsibilities, and discuss with the patient and family the effects of the injury on usual activities.

Physical Examination

Because fractures usually involve some type of accidental injury, be alert for signs of serious complications, such as head, thoracic, or abdominal injuries. In addition, examine the patient for associated tissue trauma, such as bleeding, bruising, and lacerations.

When inspecting the suspected fracture area, observe for deviations in bone alignment. The limb may appear to be deformed. The length of the extremity may change, usually becoming shorter. Inspect the skin over the fracture for lacerations, bruising, or swelling.

Compare the affected extremity with the unaffected extremity. Do neurovascular checks (pulse, skin color, capillary refill time, sensation) in the areas distal to the wound to compare circulation and sensation. Assess pulse rate and volume, as well as capillary refill time in the nails distal to the injury. Observe capillary refill time by applying pressure to the nail and checking the time required for color to return to the area. Skin color is a good indication of circulation to the extremity, and pallor indicates poor circulation. Determine sensation by pinprick, especially in the web space between the first and the second toes or between the thumb and the forefinger.

Nursing Diagnoses, Goals, and Outcome Criteria: Fracture

Nursing Diagnoses	Goals and Outcome Criteria
Acute Pain related to bone fracture, edema, soft tissue damage, or muscle spasm	Pain relief: relaxed manner, patient statement of pain relief
Ineffective Tissue Perfusion related to tissue trauma or pressure caused by edema, bone fragments, hemorrhage, or therapeutic devices	Adequate circulation: affected tissue warm, normal pulses, normal skin color, minimal edema
Risk for Infection related to break in skin, bone trauma, soft tissue damage	Absence of infection: normal body temperature and white blood cell count, clear wound drainage, decreasing edema and redness
Impaired Physical Mobility related to pain and immobilization	Improved physical mobility: patient performs daily activities as permitted while protecting fracture
Risk for Impaired Skin Integrity related to injury, immobility, and immobilizing devices	Intact or healing skin: absence of open wounds, redness or pallor due to pressure; skin warm
Activity Intolerance related to prolonged immobilization	Improved activity tolerance: performance of daily activities without fatigue

Additional nursing diagnoses may include **Imbalanced Nutrition: Less than Body Requirements** related to additional metabolic needs of healing bone and soft tissues; **Constipation** related to prolonged immobility; **Self-Care Deficit** related to pain and immobility; **Ineffective Coping** related to prolonged immobility, hospitalization, or altered lifestyle; **Disturbed Sleep Pattern** related to pain or immobility; and **Deficient Diversional Activity** related to immobility.

Interventions

Acute Pain

Fractures are painful. The degree of pain experienced depends on the extent and type of injury and the pain tolerance of the patient. The primary method of pain relief is immobilization of the affected part. Analgesic medications and muscle relaxants also are used. Other methods of pain relief include repositioning, massage, and diversion. General pain management is discussed in more detail in Chapter 14.

Ineffective Tissue Perfusion

Factors that cause impaired peripheral tissue perfusion are soft tissue injury resulting from trauma, fracture fragments, hemorrhage, edema, compartment syndrome, and positioning. The treatment of the fracture also can interfere with peripheral circulation, including moving or splinting the fracture, manipulation during reduction, and application of a cast, a splint, traction, or a brace.

Frequent neurovascular checks determine whether circulation is adequate and detect signs of pressure on nerves. For patients at risk for circulatory impairment, elevate the affected part above the level of the heart, apply cold packs as ordered to minimize edema, and encourage finger and toe movement. Evidence of impaired circulation includes abnormal coolness or warmth, weak or absent pulses, and pale or bluish skin color. Pressure on a nerve can cause pain or

NURSING CARE PLAN

The Patient with a Fracture

ASSESSMENT

Health History: Mrs. Jacobson, age 80, was admitted for a Colles' fracture in the left wrist 2 days ago. Before the injury, she lived alone and cared for herself. She was active, alert, and independent. Since the fracture repair, she has complained of pain over the area of the break but has had no signs of infection. Her physician is ready to discharge her to her home.

Physical Examination: Vital signs: temperature, 97.4° F orally; pulse, 98 with slight irregularity; respiration, 20; blood pressure, 165/95 mm Hg. Height, 5'3". Weight, 132 lb. Alert and oriented to time, place, and person. Needs assistance with activities of daily living, particularly bathing, dressing, and toileting. Cast on left arm from above her elbow to her fingers.

Nursing Diagnosis	*Goals and Outcome Criteria*	*Interventions*
Acute pain related to bone fracture, edema, soft tissue damage, muscle spasm.	The patient's pain will be relieved as evidenced by absence of verbal complaints, anxiety, and moaning or wincing; patient confirms pain relief.	Provide adequate pain relief using medications and other comfort measures such as positioning and massage.
Ineffective tissue perfusion related to decreased blood flow caused by injury.	The patient will have adequate tissue perfusion, as evidenced by normal skin color in areas distal to the fracture, adequate capillary refill, and adequate sensation.	Relieve edema by elevating the affected limb above the level of the patient's heart while she is lying in bed and applying cold for brief periods of time; encourage patient to wiggle fingers to increase circulation to the area.
Impaired physical mobility related to pain and treatment modalities for fracture.	The patient will maintain as much mobility as possible as evidenced by independence in activities of daily living (ADL) and absence of secondary complications.	Encourage regular movement, including passive or active range-of-motion exercises. Reinforce activity and exercise program for the patient. Seek referral to home health for assistance at home.
Risk for impaired skin integrity related to cast.	The patient will maintain skin integrity, as evidenced by intact skin.	Inspect the skin around cast edges for pressure or irritation. Monitor circulation and sensation in fingers.
Deficient knowledge related to lack of experience with immobilization devices (e.g., casts).	The patient will demonstrate understanding of immobilization and mobilization device's description of proper care and complications that should be reported.	Teach the patient interventions that promote bone and tissue healing; teach patient to recognize signs and symptoms of complications that should be reported to a physician. Instruct patient in cast care.
Self-care deficit related to immobilization of wrist.	The patient performs activities of daily living independently or with assistance.	Assess ability to do ADL and to perform tasks such as cooking and grocery shopping. Determine whether she has anyone to assist her if needed. If not, request a home health or social work evaluation so that home care or assistance can be provided.

numbness. Immediately report signs of impaired circulation to the physician. If a cast is too tight, it may have to be cut or replaced.

Risk for Infection

Disruption of skin may occur with a fracture, and when there is open reduction with external fixation, the potential for infection always exists. Infection can delay healing and rehabilitation. Bone infections are especially difficult to treat. Use strict aseptic technique for dressing changes, wound irrigations, and pin care. Observe wounds and pin sites for signs of infection, such as drainage, redness, swelling, and warmth, and monitor the patient's temperature for fever. If an infection develops, employ standard infection control precautions and administer antibiotics as prescribed. The management of infection is discussed more completely in Chapter 12.

Impaired Physical Mobility

Interventions for immobility are aimed at promoting independence and preventing related complications. Patients may experience anxiety and powerlessness when their activity is restricted because of the enforced immobilization related to traction, casts, or other equipment. In addition, they may experience secondary complications of immobility such as deep vein thrombosis, pulmonary embolism, contractures or muscular atrophy, skin breakdown, and gastrointestinal problems, especially constipation. Older individuals are particularly vulnerable to the effects of immobility.

Encourage all patients with fractures to engage in regular movement of some kind. Passive or active range-of-motion exercises are helpful for both bedridden and ambulatory patients. Support the joints above and below the injury in functional positions. Periodic elevation of the affected limb promotes venous return and reduces edema. Gait training with crutches, walkers, and canes promotes mobility and independence. A physical therapist usually works out an activity and exercise program for patients recovering from fractures, and the role of the nurse is to reinforce and encourage patients to carry out the program. More discussion of immobility appears in Chapter 20.

If patients are unable to care for themselves independently at home, assistance from formal agencies such as home health services or social services may be needed. Areas to be assessed for home care needs include ability to carry out activities of daily living, mobility, mental status, and skilled nursing needs. If you think home care will be needed, consult the case manager or social worker about the appropriate referral.

Put on your THINKING CAP!!

Assume you are going home with a walker. Assess the barriers in your home and modifications that would be needed for you to get around safely.

Risk for Impaired Skin Integrity

Skin integrity may be impaired as a result of the injury itself or the treatment of the injury. A compound fracture causes a break in the skin, and soft tissue injury occurs with almost every kind of fracture. Treatment measures such as immobilization or devices such as casts or traction may cause pressure on areas of the skin and result in pressure sores. In addition, the improper use of equipment can cause pressure on certain areas of the skin. Individuals who are at highest risk for skin breakdown are older adults, people with preexisting conditions such as diabetes mellitus, and people whose general condition was poor before the injury.

To prevent skin breakdown, patients should begin moving around as soon as possible after the fracture has been treated. Proper positioning and frequent turning are essential for the prevention of skin breakdown. Guidelines for proper positioning are listed in Table 40-3. Good nutrition and fluid intake help to maintain healthy tissues.

Activity Intolerance

With prolonged immobility, people become weaker and their ability to participate in activities diminishes. Encourage patients to keep their strength up by carrying out range-of-motion exercises, resistance exercises of the unaffected extremities, and, when possible, ambulation. Participation in activities of daily living and recreational activities also is helpful. Rest periods between activities help to preserve strength.

Teaching should take place in the hospital immediately after the fracture is treated to prepare for the patient's discharge home. Assess the patient and family members for their readiness and ability to learn. Patient teaching after fractures should include the types of medical and nursing interventions that will be carried out to promote bone and tissue healing, signs and symptoms of complications that should be reported to a physician, how to use equipment and assistive devices, and techniques for managing activities of daily living.

PHARMACOLOGY CAPSULE Patients who administer their own pain medications are more in control and better able to manage their pain successfully.

table 40-3 ***Tips on Positioning***

FRACTURE	POSITIONING
Cervical	Before treatment: with victim supine, immobilize neck with sandbags or Philadelphia collar If patient *must* be turned, be sure head and neck alignment is maintained
Thoracic spine	Position of comfort
Lumbar spine	Avoid high sitting positions, log roll
Pelvis	Stable fracture or after fixation: turn to side opposite fracture Unstable: do not turn
Hip	Before surgical treatment: turn toward fracture (avoid dislocation or further displacement of fragments) with pillows between legs Postoperatively: turn away from fracture until comfortable enough to turn on operative side, with pillows between legs Arthroplasty: maintain abduction at all times with abduction pillow or regular pillows between legs
Shoulder/humerus	Elevate head of bed to comfort Turn to side opposite fracture
Forearm/foreleg	Elevate distal portion of extremity higher than heart

From Maher, A. B., Salmond, S. W., & Pellino, T. A. (1994). *Orthopedic nursing* (p. 281). Philadelphia: Saunders.

MANAGEMENT OF SPECIFIC FRACTURES

FRACTURE OF THE HIP

By age 90, 17% of men and more than 30% of women sustain hip fractures. Most hip fractures are in the femoral neck and intertrochanteric regions. The most common direct cause is a fall on a hard surface; however, it is thought that many fractures in older individuals result from decreased bone mass or brittle bones associated with osteoporosis. Signs and symptoms of a hip fracture are a history of a fall, severe pain and tenderness in the region of the fracture site, evidence of soft tissue trauma, the affected leg shorter than the unaffected leg, and the hip on the affected side rotated externally.

Medical Diagnosis

The diagnosis of hip fracture is confirmed by radiography. Other studies may be done in preparation for surgery, such as a complete blood cell count, a urinalysis, and electrocardiography.

Medical Treatment

Traction and surgical repair (internal fixation, femoral head replacement, or total hip replacement) are the standard treatments for hip fracture. For older patients, surgical repair of the fracture is often the treatment of choice because it allows them to move around sooner and results in fewer complications related to immobility. Traction may require 12 to 16 weeks of immobilization for healing.

Postoperatively, patients may begin physical therapy as early as 1 day after surgery, depending on the type of repair. They may begin by sitting in a chair and then progress to walking with a walker. Following internal fixation, weight bearing on the affected side is limited initially and then gradually increased as tolerated. After total hip replacement, weight bearing can begin almost immediately.

NURSING CARE *of the Patient with a Hip Fracture*

Assessment

Assess patients with a hip fracture in the same way as patients with other types of fractures. Assess for pain, impaired peripheral circulation on the affected side, complications of immobility, skin breakdown, and ability to carry out activities of daily living. Older patients are particularly prone to developing delirium after a broken hip; therefore, note mental status and problem behaviors related to confusion.

Nursing Diagnoses, Goals, and Outcome Criteria: Hip Fracture

General nursing diagnoses, goals, and outcome criteria for the patient with a fracture were presented earlier in this chapter. The special needs of the patient with a hip fracture are discussed here.

Interventions

Nursing interventions are geared toward relieving pain, promoting mobility and independence, and preventing complications. Older patients have special nursing care needs because they are vulnerable to complications of immobility and confusion. Pain management is of utmost importance. Confused patients may not be able to tell you the extent or degree of their pain, and many times they may be undermedicated. Problem behaviors such as agitation, trying to climb out of bed, pulling out intravenous tubes or other tubes, and alterations in sleep patterns may be related to pain. Employ comfort measures such as repositioning, body massage, and diversional activities to enhance the effect of medications.

Proper body alignment is extremely important in preventing injury to the fracture area after it has been treated. Turn patients from side to side as ordered. Following total hip replacement, the affected hip must not be adducted and must not be flexed more than 90 degrees because excessive flexion or adduction can dislocate the prosthesis. Instruct these patients to use elevated toilet seats, sit in supportive chairs with straight backs and seats, and avoid crossing their legs. Care of the patient who has undergone joint replacement surgery is detailed in Chapter 39.

COLLES' FRACTURE

Colles' fracture is a break in the distal radius (wrist area). Colles' fractures often occur in older adults, particularly older women, when an outstretched hand is used to break a fall. The major signs and symptoms are pain and swelling in the area of the injury and a characteristic displacement of the bone in which the wrist has the appearance of a dinner fork. The most common complication is impaired circulation in the area resulting from edema.

Medical Diagnosis

The diagnosis is confirmed by the characteristic bone deformity of the wrist and by radiography.

Medical Treatment

Colles' fractures are managed by closed reduction or manipulation of the bone and immobilization in either a splint or a cast. The elbow is immobilized as well to prevent misalignment.

NURSING CARE *of the Patient with a Colles' Fracture*

Assessment

Assess patients for pain and swelling following medical treatment of the fracture.

Nursing Diagnoses, Goals, and Outcome Criteria: Colles' Fracture

General nursing diagnoses, goals, and outcome criteria for the patient with a fracture were presented earlier in this chapter. The special needs of the patient with a Colles' fracture are discussed here.

Interventions

Interventions are aimed at relieving pain and preventing or reducing edema. The extremity should be supported and protected and can be elevated on a pillow during the first few days. Encourage patients to move their fingers and thumb to promote circulation and reduce swelling, and to move their shoulders to prevent stiffness and contracture. In addition, teach proper cast care.

FRACTURE OF THE PELVIS

Although pelvic fractures account for a small percentage of total fractures (3%), they are the second leading cause of death from trauma, after head injury. Motor vehicle accidents are the most common cause of pelvic fractures in young adults, and falls are the main cause in older adults. The extent of the injury can range from minimal in a non–weight-bearing fracture to severe in a weight-bearing fracture. Internal trauma, such as laceration of the colon, hemorrhage, or rupture of the urethra or bladder, often accompanies a pelvic fracture. The patient may have local swelling, tenderness, bruising, and deformity. Pelvic fractures typically heal within 6 to 8 weeks.

Medical Diagnosis

As with other fractures, the diagnosis and severity of the injury are confirmed by radiography.

Medical Treatment

Medical treatment depends on the severity of the fracture. A less severe non–weight-bearing fracture is usually treated with bed rest on a firm mattress or bed board for a few days to 6 weeks. A more severe weight-bearing fracture may require a pelvic sling, skeletal traction, a double hip spica cast, or external fixation. Because of the high risk of internal trauma, monitor the patient so that specific injuries can be treated immediately. Check for the presence of blood in the urine and stool and watch the abdomen for any signs of rigidity or swelling.

NURSING CARE *of the Patient with a Pelvic Fracture*

Assessment

Observe for signs of bleeding, swelling, infection, thromboembolism, and pain. Assess urine output because the absence of urine may indicate a perforated bladder.

Nursing Diagnoses, Goals, and Outcome Criteria: Pelvic Fracture

General nursing diagnoses, goals, and outcome criteria for the patient with a fracture were presented earlier in this chapter. The special needs of the patient with a pelvic fracture are discussed here.

Interventions

Interventions are designed to alleviate pain, promote mobility, and prevent complications. When handling patients, take extreme care to prevent displacement of the fracture fragments. Turn the patient only on the order of a physician. Provide back care when the patient is raised from the bed using the trapeze or with adequate assistance from others. Because of the potentially severe consequences of immobility, ambulation may be encouraged even though painful. Follow the physician's orders regarding ambulation.

Nutrition Concepts

1. Calcium in the diet and calcium supplements are recommended to help *prevent* fractures due to osteoporosis in older age.
2. Prolonged immobilization, which often is required after multiple fractures, contributes to the loss of calcium and protein.
3. Essential nutritional elements for optimal bone healing are protein, calcium, and vitamins D, B, and C.
4. Supplemental feedings that are high in calories, protein, and calcium, such as milkshakes, may be served between meals to promote healing.
5. During periods of immobilization, a daily fluid intake of 2,000 to 3,000 ml is recommended to promote bowel and bladder function.
6. Advise the patient in a hip spica that overeating may cause abdominal pressure and cramping.

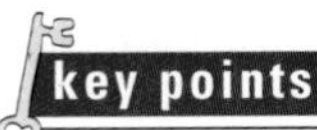

key points

- A fracture is a break or disruption in the continuity of a bone, usually causing injury to surrounding soft tissue.
- Open or compound fractures have three grades of severity, ranging from least severe injury, with minimal skin damage, to most severe injury, with skin, muscle, blood vessel, and nerve damage.
- Fractures of the femur are most common in young and middle-aged adults, and hip and wrist fractures are most common in the elderly.
- Fractures are usually caused by trauma to the bone, especially as a result of automobile accidents and falls.
- Risk factors for hip fractures include osteoporosis, advanced age, white race, use of psychotropic drugs, and being female.
- The most common signs and symptoms of a fracture are swelling, bruising, pain, tenderness, loss of normal function, and abnormal mobility.
- Bone healing occurs in five stages: (1) hematoma formation, (2) fibrocartilage formation, (3) callus formation, (4) ossification, and (5) consolidation and remodeling.
- Healing time for fractures increases with age, and it may take six times as long for the same type of fracture to heal in an older person as it does in an infant.
- Complications of a fracture include infection, fat embolism, deep vein thrombosis and pulmonary embolism, joint stiffness and contractures, post-traumatic arthritis, compartment syndrome, malunion, nonunion, delayed union, avascular necrosis, and reflex sympathetic dystrophy.
- The goals of medical treatment for a fracture are to realign the bone fragments, establish a sturdy union between the broken ends of the bone, and restore function.
- The most common therapeutic techniques used to treat a fracture are closed and open reduction and internal and external fixation.
- Casts are used for external fixation of extensive fractures and fractures of the extremities.
- Traction provides alignment of the broken bone fragments, prevents or corrects deformity, decreases

muscle spasm, promotes rest and exercise, and maintains the position of a diseased or injured part.
- Crutches increase mobility and assist with ambulation after a fracture of the lower extremity.
- A walker is used for support and balance, usually by older patients.
- Canes provide minimal support and balance and relieve pressure on weight-bearing joints.
- The focus of nursing care for a patient with a fracture is on prevention of complications, pain relief, and restoration to independent function.

REVIEW QUESTIONS

1. A patient is brought to the ER with an injury to his arm that was incurred in a fall. A bone end protrudes from his forearm. The surrounding skin is bruised and swollen. Exposed muscle tissue is also swollen. The patient has normal sensation in his fingers. His injury is best described as:
   1. Closed complete fracture.
   2. Grade III incomplete open fracture.
   3. Grade I complete closed fracture.
   4. Grade II complete open fracture.
2. During which stage of bone healing do the ends of the broken bone begin to knit?
   1. Stage II
   2. Stage III
   3. Stage IV
   4. Stage V
3. A patient with a femoral fracture suddenly complains that he can't catch his breath. His pulse is 106, respirations 30. You notice a measles-like rash on his neck and chest. You should suspect:
   1. shock.
   2. fat embolism.
   3. avascular necrosis.
   4. compartment syndrome.
4. Methods used to stimulate bone growth include:
   1. traction.
   2. thermoplastic resins.
   3. fixation.
   4. electrical stimulation.
5. A patient is being discharged with a plaster of Paris cast on her arm. Patient teaching should include:
   1. Notify the physician if your fingers become discolored.
   2. Use a cotton-tipped applicator to scratch underneath the cast.
   3. After the cast dries, you can take a shower without damaging it.
   4. Loss of sensation is normal; it will return when the cast is removed.
6. Crutches are properly fitted when the:
   1. patient says they are comfortable.
   2. elbows are bent at 45-degree angles.
   3. crutch is 75% of the patient's height.
   4. crutch pad is 3 fingerbreadths from the axilla.
7. The main advantage of surgery over traction for older patients with hip fractures is:
   1. traction is more expensive because a longer hospitalization is required.
   2. surgery allows earlier mobilization, which results in fewer complications.
   3. after a few days, surgical treatment is generally less painful than traction.
   4. bones of older people heal better with surgery than with traction.
8. The most common cause of Colles' fracture is:
   1. using an outstretched hand to break a fall.
   2. jumping from a high place onto a hard surface.
   3. landing in a sitting position after falling.
   4. falling with the leg in a position of outward rotation.
9. The diet for a patient with a serious fracture should include:
   1. reduced fat and calories to prevent weight gain.
   2. increased protein and calcium to build new bone.
   3. large doses of vitamin A and zinc for healing.
   4. decreased fluid intake to prevent bladder distention.
10. A grating sound heard when fractured bone ends rub together is called:
    1. crackling.
    2. bruits.
    3. crepitus.
    4. ecchymosis.

CHAPTER

41 Amputations

objectives

1. Identify the clinical indications for amputations.
2. Describe the different types of amputations.
3. Discuss the medical and surgical management of the amputation patient.
4. Identify appropriate nursing interventions during the preoperative and postoperative phases of care.
5. Assist in developing a nursing care plan for the amputation patient.

key terms

Amputation (ăm-pū-TĀ-shŭn, p. 838)
Amputee (ăm-pū-TĒ, p. 838)
Closed amputation (p. 840)
Congenital amputation (kŏn-JĔN-ĭ-tăl ăm-pū-TĀ-shŭn, p. 838)
Gangrene (găng-GRĒN, p. 838)
Guillotine amputation (GĬL-ō-tēn ăm-pū-TĀ-shŭn, p. 840)
Open amputation (p. 840)
Phantom limb (p. 840)
Replantation (rē-plăn-TĀ-shŭn, p. 838)
Residual limb (rē-ZĪ-dū-ăl lĭm, p. 840)
Staged amputation (p. 840)
Stump (p. 845)

Derived from the Latin word meaning "cutting around," the term *amputation* refers to the removal of body limbs or parts of limbs. Amputations have been performed since the beginning of mankind, according to findings by archaeologists. Ancient amputations were originally performed to remove gangrenous or damaged limbs; they also were performed for ritual sacrifice, punishment, exorcism of evil spirits, and, in some cases, beautification.

In the past two decades, many advances have been made in surgical amputation and **replantation** (limb reattachment) techniques, prosthetic devices (artificial limbs), and rehabilitation programs. This has allowed many **amputees** (people with amputations) to remain active and productive despite their disabilities. In the United States, the vast majority of amputees have had lower extremity amputations.

AMPUTATION

Amputation can occur through a joint (between the bones) or through a bone itself. Disarticulation is the term for an amputation through the joint. The general site of the amputation is described by the joint nearest to it. For example, removal of the lower leg at the middle of the shin or calf is called a below-knee amputation. Some of the most common sites of amputation are shown in Figure 41-1.

INDICATIONS AND INCIDENCE

Conditions or situations that lead to the need for an amputation can generally be grouped into four categories: trauma, disease, tumors, and congenital defects.

Trauma

In some serious accidents, part or all of a limb may be removed. This often is referred to as a *traumatic amputation.* In other situations, the limb may be damaged so severely that it must be removal surgically. Common types of accidents and injuries leading to amputation include those involving motorcycles and automobiles, farm machinery, firearms and explosives, electrical equipment, power tools, and frostbite. Trauma tends to be the most common reason for upper extremity amputations. Because these accidents are typically occupational hazards, the victims are usually young men.

Disease

Vascular diseases account for the majority of the estimated 30,000 lower extremity amputations performed in the United States each year. In these cases, blood supply to the tissues is inadequate, and the tissues become deprived of oxygen and other important nutrients. Without these nutrients, necrosis or death of the tissue occurs. Some examples of diseases leading to impaired circulation are peripheral vascular disease, diabetes mellitus, and arteriosclerosis. These problems also can be complicated by infection because wounds sustained by limbs without a good blood supply do not heal well and **gangrene** can set in quickly. Circulation problems are more common among the elderly and in the lower extremities.

Tumors

Amputations also may be performed for bone tumors that are very large and invasive. Treatment may require amputation and disarticulation of an entire limb. Primary bone tumors occur most frequently in adolescents but can occur at any age. Approximately one third of these individuals are 11 to 20 years of age.

Congenital Defects

In some situations, a limb or part of a limb may be absent or deformed at birth. These are sometimes called **congen-**

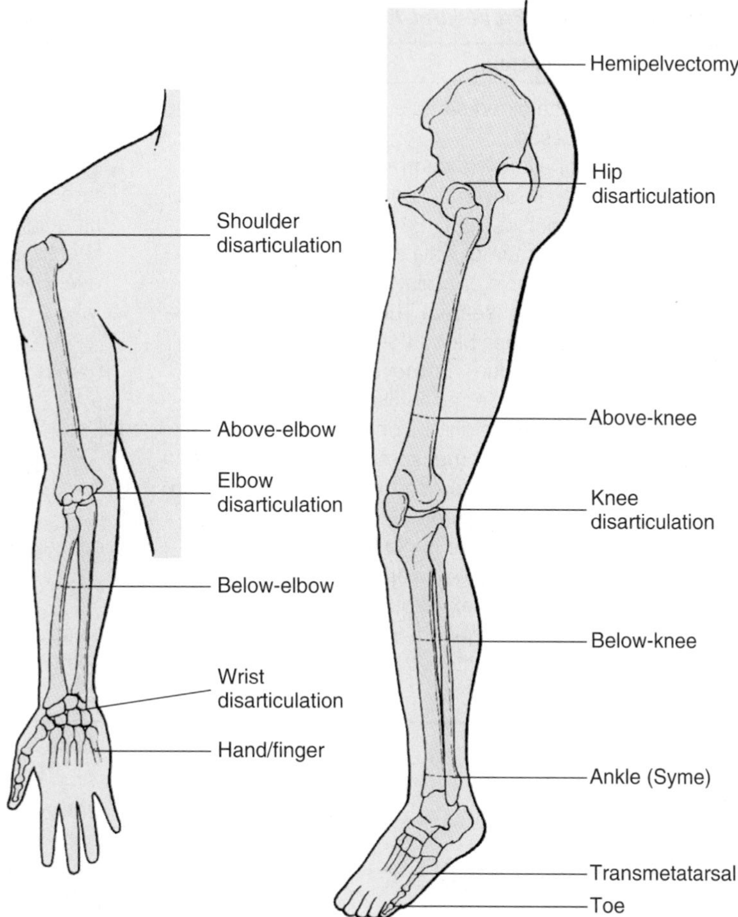

FIGURE **41-1** Common sites of amputation in the upper and lower extremities.

ital amputations. They result from factors that affect the developing fetus in such a way that the infant is born with a missing, deficient, or abnormal limb. Sometimes surgery is performed in order to convert a deformed limb into a more functional one that can be fitted with a prosthetic device.

DIAGNOSTIC TESTS AND PROCEDURES

The types of diagnostic studies done for a patient requiring amputation depend on the underlying disease or injury. For example, in a patient with vascular disease, tests to assess circulation are indicated. An elevated white blood cell count is consistent with infection. Table 41-1 lists examples of diagnostic findings associated with some of the contributing factors in amputations.

Vascular Studies

Vascular studies may be done for a patient with compromised circulation, such as in trauma or vascular disease. Angiography is a procedure that involves the injection of a radiopaque dye into blood vessels, which are then viewed radiographically to determine their patency.

Pulse Volume Recording

Pulse volume recording uses a noninvasive device that gives general information about the volume of blood flow to an extremity. Another name for this procedure is plethysmography.

Thermography

Thermography involves the use of a device that detects and records heat in various parts of the body. Relatively hot or cold spots are revealed, indicating the amount of blood flow to that part of the body. Cool areas generally indicate a decreased blood flow as compared to warm areas.

Doppler Ultrasound

Doppler ultrasound uses sound waves to determine the presence of pulses in the extremities. This technology is much more sensitive than using the fingertips to try to palpate a pulse.

Biopsy

In patients with tumors, a biopsy is often done to determine the nature of the tumor. A biopsy involves removing a small portion of tissue, which is then examined for malignancy.

table 41-1 *Nursing Care Related to Diagnostic Procedures Associated with Indications for Amputation*

TEST/PURPOSE	PATIENT PREPARATION	POSTPROCEDURE CARE
WBC count detects elevation associated with infection	Tell patient a blood sample will be drawn. Fasting not necessary.	Apply small dressing to site. Assess for bleeding.
Arteriography detects arterial occlusion	Assess for allergy to contrast medium, iodine, shellfish. Inform radiologist if allergic. Mark peripheral pulses. NPO 8 hours before. Signed consent required. Tell patient "dye" will be injected into arm or groin; may briefly feel flushed or nauseated. Then radiographs will be taken to assess blood flow. Should void just before procedure. Remove jewelry and metal objects. Must remain still during test.	Maintain pressure dressing on puncture site as ordered. Assess for bleeding. Frequent neurovascular checks on extremity used to inject dye. Encourage increased fluid intake if permitted.
Pulse volume recording (plethysmography) used to evaluate arterial blood flow to an extremity	Pressure cuffs are placed on extremities and arterial pressure is measured during inflation and deflation. Explain procedure to patient. Signed consent not required.	No special care.
Doppler ultrasound used to assess pulses, patency of blood vessels	Tell patient procedure is noninvasive and painless. Conductive gel is applied and a sensor passed over the extremity to detect pulses.	Cleanse gel from skin.
Bone biopsy usually done after imaging procedures reveal suspicious lesions	Signed consent required. Sample of bone surgically excised for study.	Assess site for bleeding. Administer analgesics as ordered.

MEDICAL AND SURGICAL TREATMENT

The management of amputations requires both medical and surgical approaches by the physicians involved in the care of the patient.

Medical Treatment

The medical care of the patient undergoing amputation must include the appropriate treatment and control of any underlying diseases or injuries. For example, diet, medication, and exercise are used to help patients with diabetes and poor peripheral circulation attain good control of their diabetes. Patients with peripheral vascular disease are encouraged to stop smoking because nicotine causes vasoconstriction. The patient who has experienced trauma may have to be stabilized with measures that will maintain his or her heart rate and blood pressure within a normal range.

Surgical Treatment

Amputation is recommended only when other options are not possible or have failed. In an effort to avoid amputation, the physician may perform angioplasty or surgical bypass of obstructed vessels.

Surgical management of the patient aims for amputation at the lowest level that will still preserve healthy tissue and favor wound healing. The surgeon chooses one of two basic types of surgical procedures, depending on the condition of the extremity and the reason for the surgery. These two types are closed amputations and open amputations.

Closed Amputations

Closed amputations are usually performed to create a weight-bearing residual limb, which is especially important for lower extremity amputations. In this procedure, a long skin flap with soft tissue and muscle is positioned over the severed end of the bone and sutured in place. The sutures are usually placed so that they do not bear the full weight of the patient. This technique has many variations.

Open Amputations

In open amputations, the severed bone or joint is left uncovered by a skin flap. This type of amputation is required when an actual or potential infection exists, as may occur with gangrene or trauma. The wound is left open for 5 to 10 days, sometimes longer, and is closed surgically when infection no longer poses a problem. Another term for this procedure is a staged or guillotine amputation.

Prostheses

Prostheses are artificial substitutes for missing body parts. A prosthetist creates and supervises the use of a prosthesis. He or she explains the type of device to be used as well as the process of fitting the patient and instructing the patient in its use. In some situations, a limb prosthesis may be placed while the patient is still in the operating room. This requires placement of a rigid dressing to accommodate the temporary prosthesis. In other cases, fitting of the prosthesis is delayed until the residual limb has healed adequately. Various prostheses are depicted in Figures 41-2 and 41-3.

COMPLICATIONS

Many complications are associated with amputations, including hemorrhage and hematoma, necrosis, wound dehiscence, gangrene, edema, contracture, pain, infection, phantom limb sensation, and phantom limb pain. Factors contributing to each of these complications are listed in Table 41-2.

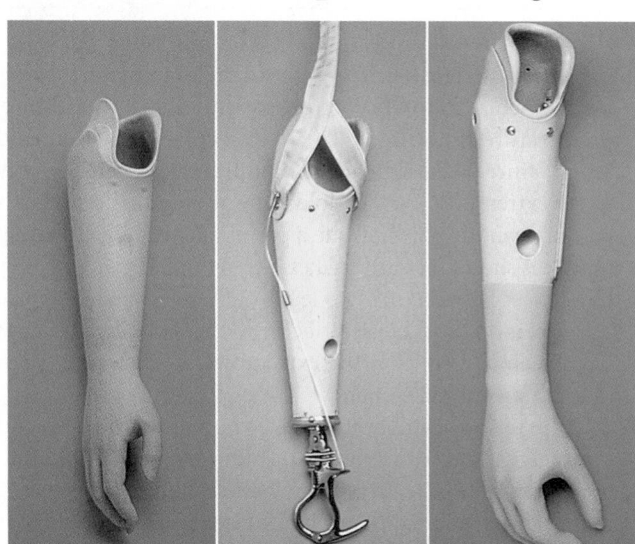

FIGURE **41-2** Upper extremity prostheses. *A,* Cosmetic. *B,* Cable-activated. *C,* Myoelectrically controlled.

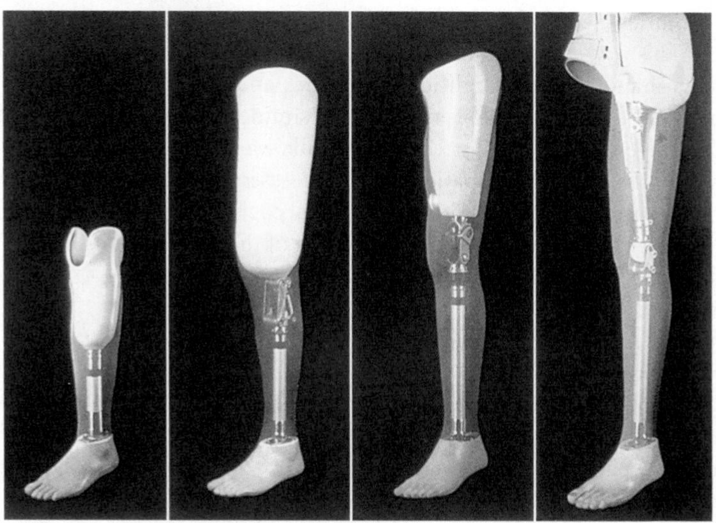

FIGURE **41-3** Lower extremity prostheses.

table 41-2 ***Complications of Amputation***

COMPLICATION	DESCRIPTION AND CONTRIBUTING FACTORS
Hematoma and hemorrhage	Bleeding into tissue in and around residual limb due to inadequate hemostasis
Necrosis	Tissue destruction and death due to ongoing disease; requires surgical debridement or revision, or both
Wound dehiscence	Opening of suture line due to early removal of sutures or trauma; requires reclosure
Gangrene	Death of tissue associated with inadequate blood supply and bacterial destruction of tissue; requires reamputation
Edema	Swelling and discomfort in residual limb due to dependent position or incorrect wrapping; requires elevation and rewrapping
Contracture	Flexion of joints with loss of range of motion due to prolonged elevation or immobilization of extremities; may be prevented by frequent position changes and range-of-motion exercises
Pain	Extreme, sharp pain at incision site due to scar formation on nerve fibers (neuroma); may require surgical treatment
Infection	Redness, warmth, swelling, and exudate formation at residual limb site due to invasion of tissues by pathogens; may require antibiotics and surgical drainage
Phantom limb sensation	Patient experiences sensations (tingling, numbness, itching, warmth/cold) as if the limb were still present; caused by stimulation along a nerve pathway in which sensory endings were in the amputated part
Phantom limb pain	Patient experiences pain as if the limb were still present. More common when patient had pain in limb before amputation. Pain may be enhanced by anxiety and depression. Usually diminishes over time but may become chronic.

NURSING CARE *of the Patient having Amputation Surgery*

PREOPERATIVE NURSING CARE

Nursing care of the amputation patient is based on a preoperative phase and postoperative phase. Routine preoperative and postoperative care are detailed in Chapter 16. This section focuses on the specific needs of the patient having an amputation (see also Nursing Care Plan: The Patient with an Upper Extremity Amputation). Preoperative nursing assessment of the patient having an amputation is summarized in Table 41-3. The patient needs to prepare both physically and psychologically for an impending amputation.

Assessment

Health History

Record the conditions that resulted in the need for an amputation (diseases such as diabetes mellitus or peripheral vascular insufficiency, traumatic injuries, neoplasms, and birth defects). Take a complete health history, including information on the patient's past medical and surgical conditions. Note preexisting cardiovascular problems because hypertension, coronary artery disease, congestive heart failure, and cardiac murmurs or defects can affect greatly the patient's ability to tolerate surgery and to recover successfully. Also determine whether the patient has ever had phlebitis, varicosities, thrombosis, emboli, or stasis ulcers in either the affected or the unaffected extremities.

Record relevant disorders in the family history, including diabetes, hypertension, and vascular diseases.

Systematically assess signs and symptoms that relate to the vascular condition or other chronic and acute problems. Significant signs and symptoms are pain (location, severity, type, precipitating factors, alleviating factors), loss of sensation or abnormal sensations, intolerance of local heat or cold, color changes in the extremities, leg ulcers, and sexual dysfunction.

Significant data in the functional assessment are usual diet and fluid intake, intake of salt and alcohol, and use of tobacco. Describe exercise and rest and sleep habits as well as the effects of the current symptoms on the patient's usual activities. Identify the patient's occupation and responsibilities to determine how amputation will affect that aspect of his or her life.

A review of the patient's psychosocial background may offer insight into how the patient will tolerate treatments and procedures. Knowledge of how the patient copes with stress may help in planning care to reduce anxiety and fear. The patient about to undergo an amputation will undoubtedly have a number of fears and concerns about the surgical procedure, the loss of a body part, the potential loss of independence, and pain and disfigurement. Open discussion of these concerns may help alleviate those fears.

Physical Examination

Perform a total physical examination, with special attention to the neurologic, cardiovascular, and integumentary systems. Begin with measurement of height and weight and vital signs to uncover factors that may affect circulation, including obesity and hypertension. Throughout the examination, assess neurovascular status. Record the patient's skin color, texture, temperature, and turgor. The overall color, condition, and temperature of the skin are good indicators of blood supply to the extremities. Cool or cold, clammy, mottled skin that is pale or cyanotic may indicate a poor blood supply. Palpating both legs simultaneously makes it easier to detect circulatory differences between the two legs. Additionally, there may be open areas on the skin. Describe any skin lesions and drainage from them. Wounds to the extremities are common when blood supply is inadequate.

Palpate the peripheral pulses for presence, quality, and symmetry. If pulses are not palpable, a Doppler ultrasound device can be used to assess them. Assess capillary refill by applying pressure to the nail bed of a finger or toe until it blanches (turns white). When the pressure is released, the nail bed normally regains its normal pink color within 3 seconds. In extremities with a diminished supply of blood, capillary refill may take 5 seconds or longer. Assess sensation by asking the patient to identify touch on the extremities. Experienced examiners may evaluate the patient's ability to sense sharp, dull, warm, and cold stimuli.

Assess the patient's mental and emotional status and general cognitive abilities to determine the patient's understanding of the illness and its implications.

Nursing Diagnoses, Goals, and Outcome Criteria: Amputation, Preoperative

Nursing Diagnoses	Goals and Outcome Criteria
Anxiety related to anticipated change in body image and in function	Decreased anxiety: relaxed manner, patient statement that anxiety is reduced
Anticipatory Grieving related to expected loss of body part and function	Progress toward grief resolution: patient expresses feelings about impending losses, demonstrates healthy coping strategies

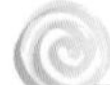

What Does Culture Have to do with Amputations?

Values related to body appearance and function and independence are culturally influenced and will affect the way individuals react to amputation. Also, religious beliefs may dictate the disposal of amputated body parts by burial or cremation. For example, Orthodox Jews require that such body parts be made available for burial.

Interventions

Anxiety

Emotional support is important throughout all phases of care of the patient with an amputation. The patient needs time to prepare psychologically and emotionally for the surgery. Encourage the patient to express thoughts and concerns about the impending amputation. Accept the patient's responses. Allow the patient to express anger or to cry without being

NURSING CARE PLAN

The Patient with an Upper Extremity Amputation

ASSESSMENT

Health History: 32-year-old Frank Blue sustained an injury in an industrial accident that required amputation of his right forearm just below the elbow. Mr. Blue's right hand was his dominant hand. He has had no other serious physical injuries or illnesses. He is a machinist who is a senior employee in his department. He is married and the father of three children. His wife is a housewife who has never worked outside the home.

Physical Examination: Lethargic but responds to commands. Vital signs: temperature, 98.2° F orally; pulse, 80; respiration, 16; blood pressure, 126/28 mm Hg. A bulky dressing is in place on the residual limb of the right arm; dressing is dry and intact. A Jackson-Pratt drain is in place, and the receptacle contains approximately 30 ml of sanguineous fluid. Intravenous fluids are infusing into the left arm.

Nursing Diagnosis	*Goals and Outcome Criteria*	*Interventions*
Decreased cardiac output related to blood loss.	The patient's blood volume will remain normal, as evidenced by stable vital signs, urine output equal to fluid intake, and absence of restlessness or frank bleeding.	Reinforce dressing, apply pressure, and elevate residual limb if bleeding is apparent. Monitor for signs of hypovolemia: tachycardia, restlessness, decreased urine output.
Pain related to surgical incision, trauma, edema.	The patient will state pain is relieved and will appear more relaxed.	Assess pain nature, location, and severity. Administer analgesics as ordered. Provide comfort measures such as back rub, distraction, imagery. Inform surgeon if pain is not relieved.
Risk for infection related to surgical wound, traumatic injury.	The patient will remain free of infection, as evidenced by normal body temperature and absence of foul drainage, excessive redness, warmth, or edema.	Monitor temperature for elevation. Assess dressing for foul drainage. When dressing is removed, inspect residual limb for excessive redness, warmth, or edema. Use standard precautions when handling dressing and residual limb. Teach the patient good hygiene to decrease the risk of infection. Administer antimicrobials as ordered.
Impaired skin integrity related to incision.	The patient's residual limb will heal completely.	Keep the residual limb dressing smooth and snug to mold the residual limb for future prosthesis use. Use caution not to impair blood flow. Check the residual limb for irritation or signs of pressure. Maintain elevation as ordered to minimize edema and pressure on suture line. Apply cold to residual limb dressing as ordered. After the first week, massage the residual limb as ordered to promote circulation.
Disturbed sensory perception related to phantom limb sensation or phantom limb pain.	The patient will report phantom limb sensations or pain if they occur.	Tell the patient that these sensations sometimes follow amputation. Notify the surgeon. Medicate as ordered. Advise the patient that several therapies are available for the treatment of this problem.
Risk for injury related to loss of part of limb, weakness.	The patient will identify activities requiring adaptation and will avoid dangerous activities.	Help the patient identify usual activities that cannot be safely done without the dominant hand. Discuss strategies to adapt activities or to learn to use the left hand. Consult rehabilitation specialist for adaptation in work setting.
Self-care deficit related to loss of part of limb, inability to carry out activities of daily living.	The patient will accomplish self-care with minimal assistance from others.	Assist the patient with self-care but encourage increasing effort on his part. Praise efforts. Organize environment to facilitate self-care (i.e., place bedside objects on the patient's left).
Anxiety related to perceived threat of disability.	The patient will verbalize concerns about injury.	Explore the patient's fears and anxiety. Encourage the patient to talk about the loss. Express concern but not pity. Request services of mental health or spiritual counselor if the patient desires. Include family in care, and explore their needs as well.
Ineffective coping related to overwhelming injury.	The patient will demonstrate realistic goal setting and express intent to participate in rehabilitation program.	Explain the importance of proper residual limb care in preparing for rehabilitation. Consult social worker to assist patient in obtaining rehabilitation services.

Continued

NURSING CARE PLAN—cont'd

Nursing Diagnosis	*Goals and Outcome Criteria*	*Interventions*
Disturbed body image related to loss of body part.	The patient will express feelings about loss of the hand and will consider strategies to improve function and appearance.	Gradually encourage the patient to take more responsibility for care of the residual limb. Counsel family members to demonstrate acceptance of the injury and not to promote excessive dependence. Facilitate meeting with prosthetist to discuss cosmetic and functional options.
Deficient knowledge of therapy, self-care.	The patient will verbalize personal role in recovery and rehabilitation	Teach the patient to care for the residual limb and any prosthesis. 1. Wash residual limb with soap and water daily, rinse, and dry. 2. Inspect residual limb daily for irritation, redness, edema. 3. Keep prosthetic socket and residual limb sock clean and dry. 4. Do not apply lotions, powders, or creams except as prescribed by the physician. 5. If residual limb is red or irritated, temporarily remove the prosthesis; see physician. 6. Prosthesis will require periodic adjustments.

table 41-3 **ASSESSMENT *of the Patient Undergoing an Amputation***

HEALTH HISTORY

Chief Complaint and History of Present Illness: Condition or incident leading to amputation
Past Medical History: Previous illnesses, operations, hospitalizations, trauma, hypertension, coronary artery disease, congestive heart failure, cardiac murmurs or defects, phlebitis, varicosities, thrombosis, emboli, stasis ulcers, diabetes mellitus
Family History: Diabetes mellitus, hypertension, vascular diseases
Review of Systems
Pain: Nature, location, severity, precipitating factors, alleviating factors
Sensation: Loss or change, abnormal perception of heat and cold
Skin: Color, lesions, ulcers
Leg Ulcers
Sexual Dysfunction
Functional Assessment: Usual diet, etc.

HEALTH HISTORY—cont'd

Usual diet and fluid Intake
Intake of salt and alcohol
Use of tobacco
Exercise, rest, and sleep habits
Occupation, roles, and responsibilities
Coping Strategies
Fears and Concerns

PHYSICAL ASSESSMENT

Height and Weight
Vital Signs
Skin: Color, texture, temperature, turgor, lesions
Peripheral Pulses: Presence, quality, symmetry
Capillary Refill
Sensation
Mental Status: Level of consciousness, emotional state
Cognition: Ability to follow directions

judged or given false reassurances. Tell the patient about physical and occupational therapy programs designed to restore maximal independent function.

Anticipatory Grieving

Recognize that the loss of a limb or part of a limb as well as the loss of functional abilities is stressful. Most patients experience a period of grief and mourn over this loss. Grief experienced before the loss actually occurs is called anticipatory grief. The patient may be concerned about altered physical appearance as well as loss of function. Explore the patient's expectations and fears about these changes. Gently encourage the patient to focus on what he or she will be able to do despite physical limitations. Allowing patients to grieve is an important part of their recovery and rehabilitation. Nursing care of the grieving patient is discussed in Chapter 23.

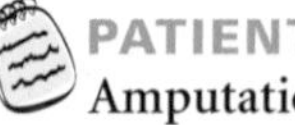

PATIENT TEACHING PLAN
Amputation

- A rehabilitation team, including a prosthetist (if applicable), physical therapist, and occupational therapist, will work with you to help you regain the best function possible.
- If a prosthetic device is appropriate for you, the prosthetist will fit the device and teach you about it.
- Many modern prostheses are nearly lifelike in appearance and function.
- Phantom limb sensations are sensations perceived in the limb that has been removed; they are commonly experienced by amputees.
- Medications and other treatments can be used to treat phantom pain.

- For lower extremity amputation (if applicable): upper body training is important to strengthen your arms.
- If you will be using crutches, we will teach you crutch walking, and you will need to practice.
- We can arrange for a person who has recovered after an amputation like yours to visit, if you would like that.

POSTOPERATIVE NURSING CARE

The postoperative phase begins immediately after the surgical amputation and includes immediate postoperative care as well as the long-term rehabilitation that is necessary for these patients.

Priorities for the postoperative patient are based on three distinct needs: pain relief, restored mobility, and avoidance of complications. The most common problems in the early postoperative period for patients with amputations are hemorrhage, edema, infection, and pain.

Assessment

Assess vital signs frequently in the first 48 hours postoperatively to detect early signs of problems. Inspect the dressing frequently for any bleeding. Some nurses try to monitor the amount of oozing by marking the stained area on the dressing with a pen, although this is a very rough assessment of bleeding. Sometimes the dressing is dry, but blood is draining around the dressing and under the patient. If a drain receptacle is present, note the color and amount of the drainage. The drainage should gradually decrease in amount and lighten in color. Assess the patient's temperature for elevations that may indicate infection. Also note any foul odor from the dressing. After the dressing is removed, inspect the residual limb for edema. Also assess the patient's pain, including type, location, and severity. Other aspects of postoperative assessment are detailed in Chapter 16.

Nursing Diagnoses, Goals, and Outcome Criteria: Amputation, Postoperative

Nursing Diagnoses	Goals and Outcome Criteria
Decreased Cardiac Output related to blood loss	Normal cardiac output: pulse and blood pressure consistent with patient norms; skin warm and dry
Acute Pain related to surgical wound	Pain relief: relaxed manner, patient statement that pain is relieved
Risk for Infection related to surgical disruption of skin integrity	Absence of infection: normal body temperature; decreasing redness and edema of wound margins; drainage that decreases in volume and becomes clear
Impaired Skin Integrity related to incision	Healed wound: incision margins intact
Risk for Impaired Skin Integrity related to advanced age and decreased mobility	Absence of new skin lesions: skin intact, no redness due to pressure
Disturbed Sensory Perception related to phantom limb sensations or phantom limb pain	Patient understanding of phantom limb sensation: patient statement of reduced pain
Risk for Injury related to loss of limb or part of a limb, weakness, debilitation	Absence of injury: no falls or evidence of injury due to weakness or problems with balance
Impaired Physical Mobility related to loss of a limb or part of a limb	Restored mobility: patient performs activities of daily living; gradually returns to preoperative level of functioning
Activity Intolerance related to weakness	Improved activity tolerance: patient carries out daily activities without excessive fatigue, gradual increase in activity level
Self-Care Deficit related to loss of limb or part of a limb, inability to carry out activities of daily living	Resumed self-care: patient performs self-care within limits imposed by limb loss; learns new ways to care for self
Anxiety or Fear related to perceived threat of disability, possibility of death	Decreased anxiety/fear: calm manner, patient statement of lessened anxiety and/or fear
Ineffective Coping related to inadequate support system, use of inappropriate coping mechanisms	Effective coping with loss: patient talks about loss, participates in rehabilitation efforts and self-care
Disturbed Body Image related to loss of a body part	Positive body image: patient accepts limb loss, demonstrates proper care of residual limb, makes positive remarks about self and abilities

Interventions

Decreased Cardiac Output

Hemorrhage is the greatest danger in the early postoperative period. Hemorrhage may be detected by observations of excessive bleeding or changes in vital signs. Check vital signs frequently. Restlessness and increasing pulse and respiratory rates may be early signs of hemorrhage. Hypotension and cyanosis are late signs.

A portable wound suction system, such as a Hemovac or a Jackson-Pratt drain, may be placed to collect drainage. Inspect the dressing and the bed linens under the patient. Bright red bleeding, either from the drains or from the dressing itself, is *not* normal. If this is observed, apply a pressure dressing over the existing dressing, elevate the residual limb (also called a stump), and notify the surgeon immediately. A large blood pressure cuff may be placed at the bedside for emergency use as a tourniquet.

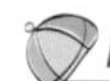
Put on your THINKING CAP!!

Sometimes a cast is applied to the residual limb while the patient is in surgery. The cast makes it difficult to assess the condition of the wound, so you must rely on other assessment

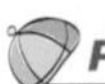

Put on your THINKING CAP!!—cont'd

data. Explain what data would cause you to suspect excessive blood loss in that situation.

Pain

Postoperatively, the patient has incisional pain that is treated with prescribed pain medications, usually opioid analgesics. Sometimes a sympathectomy is done during the amputation to prevent pain. This involves excising sympathetic nerves supplying the area. A second source of pain may be a neuroma, which may develop when severed nerve endings attempt to regenerate. This can cause a great deal of sharp, severe pain and requires excision by the surgeon. Assess and document the effects of analgesics and notify the physician if pain relief is not achieved. Pain management is discussed in detail in Chapter 14.

Risk for Infection

Use aseptic techniques when handling the residual limb, the dressing, and the drains to help reduce the risk of infection. Monitor for signs and symptoms of infection. The incision should be dry, intact, and only slightly red. Suspect infection if a foul or unpleasant odor comes from the dressing, if the patient has a sudden temperature elevation, or if the residual limb is red, excessively warm, or edematous. Laboratory results also may detect an elevated white blood cell count. Treatment for infection may include antibiotics, hot packs, and incision and drainage of the infected residual limb. In severe cases, the infection may cause further tissue damage and require reamputation at a higher level. Therefore it is very important to take measures to prevent infection and to act promptly if there is evidence of infection.

Impaired Skin Integrity and Risk for Impaired Skin Integrity

The care of the residual limb depends on the overall condition of the patient and the type of prosthesis. If the amputation is closed, there is some type of compression dressing with elastic bandages and, in some cases, a cast. The residual limb is bandaged to promote healing and to shrink and shape the residual limb to a tapered, round, smooth end that will fit the prosthesis. Wrap the bandage smoothly with even, moderate tension to all parts of the residual limb. Rewrap the residual limb as needed to maintain pressure. It is very important to avoid a tourniquet-like effect caused by pulling the bandage too tightly or unevenly. Figure 41-4 illustrates the

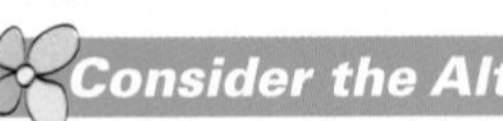

Consider the Alternative!

Many complementary therapies may be used with analgesia to control pain. Examples are imagery, relaxation, meditation, and acupuncture.

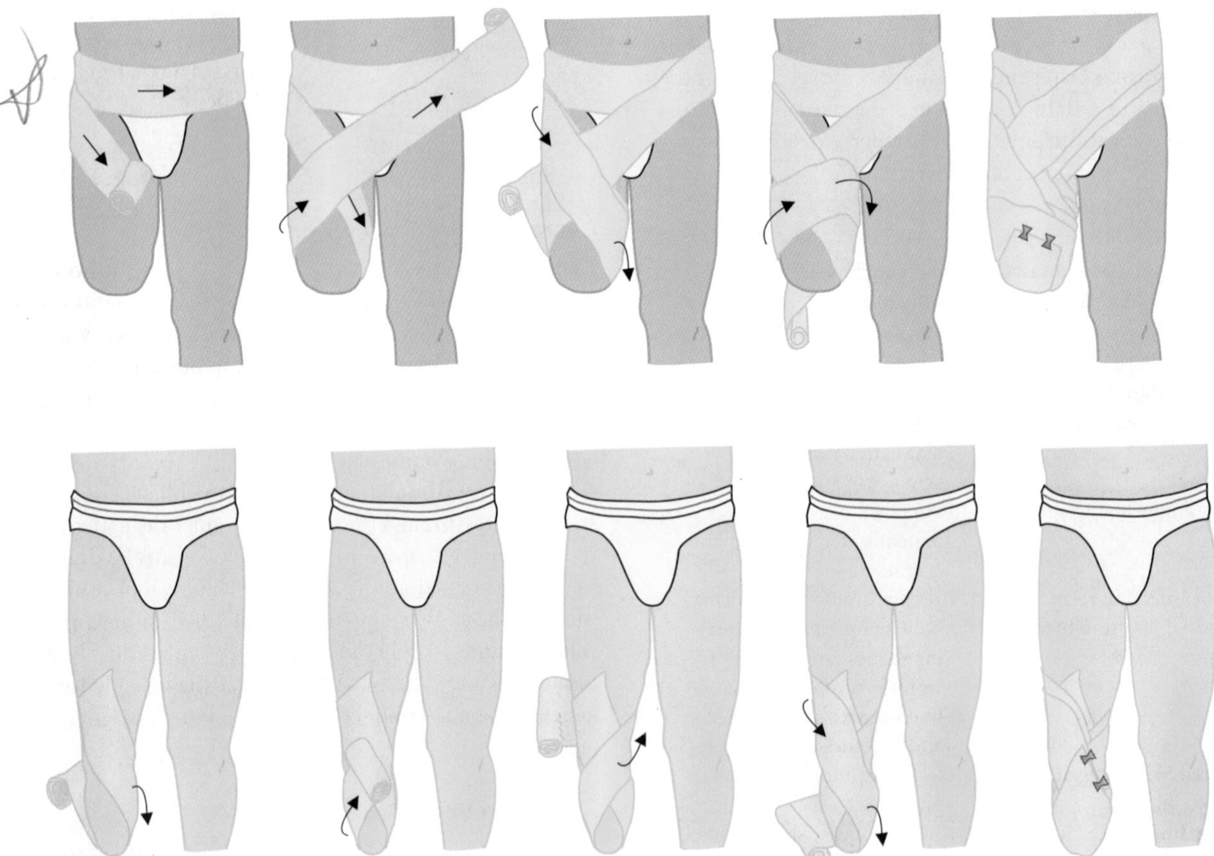

FIGURE 41-4 Proper techniques for wrapping a lower extremity residual limb.

correct bandaging of a residual limb. Commercial "shrinker socks" are available that maintain compression; however, they are expensive and it is difficult to find the right size and length for many patients.

Inspect the residual limb frequently for irritation and edema. Edema in the residual limb is most common during the first 24 hours postoperatively. To minimize this, a heavy cast or pressure dressing is applied in the operating room. Elevate the affected lower extremities by raising the foot of the bed. Pillows can be placed under a below-knee amputation, although the continuous use of pillows is discouraged because it can cause contractures of the hip. For the same reason, position the patient in a low Fowler's rather than high Fowler's position. If ordered, apply ice bags to the residual limb. Ice should be used for only brief periods of time because it can cause cold injury. After the fifth to seventh postoperative day, the residual limb can be massaged to promote circulation. If permitted, a patient with a lower extremity amputation should lie prone part of the day.

Disturbed Sensory Perception

As mentioned earlier, phantom limb sensation is common. It tends to lessen with activity, weight bearing, and exercise. Phantom limb pain, however, is uncommon. It is often described as a burning, stinging, or crushing pain. If the patient reports such pain, notify the surgeon. Treatment for this type of pain may include diversional activities, whirlpool, massage, injection of the residual limb with an anesthetic, or transcutaneous electrical nerve stimulation (TENS). A properly fitting dressing helps some patients. Drugs that are sometimes helpful include beta-blockers, anticonvulsants, neuroleptics, benzodiazepines, and antidepressants.

 ***Put on your THINKING CAP!!***

The home health nurse is visiting an elderly woman who had a lower leg amputation one month ago. The wound appears to be well healed, but the woman complains of pain that is sometimes severe in the amputated limb. She asks if she is going crazy. What would you tell her?

Risk for Injury

The patient must learn to function without the amputated limb. He or she must also learn to compensate for the lost extremity in unexpected ways, such as maintaining balance in sitting and standing positions. After lower extremity amputation, safe mobility is a priority. Reinforce the proper use of assistive devices (crutches, walkers) as taught by the physical therapist. Also encourage and assist the patient to do exercises to strengthen remaining limbs. Keep the environment free of clutter to prevent tripping. Patients with upper limb amputations must learn adaptations to perform activities of daily living. Everyday activities such as cooking may result in injury. The occupational therapist helps the patient learn to perform these tasks safely. Rehabilitation centers typically have demonstration homelike settings that allow patients to practice meal preparation and other daily activities. Occupational therapy services also extend to the home, where the therapist helps the patient and family plan for any needed environmental alterations.

Impaired Physical Mobility

An exercise program is usually initiated by a physical therapist. An important goal is the prevention of contractures. These are most common in the knee, hip, and elbow. The patient with a lower extremity amputation may be instructed to lie prone (if tolerable) with the head turned away from the affected side for 30 minutes three or four times a day. Traction, trochanter rolls, and a firm mattress may keep the body in alignment while the patient is in bed. An overbed trapeze may be ordered to facilitate moving back and forth between the bed and the chair. Avoid prolonged abduction of the hip (as when propped on a pillow). Prolonged sitting can lead to hip and knee contractures. Active and passive range-of-motion exercises also are an important part of maintaining mobility and preventing debilitation. Explain the value of exercises to the patient to encourage cooperation and participation.

The patient may have either an immediate or a delayed prosthetic fitting. An immediate fitting allows the patient to become accustomed to weight bearing, ambulation, and balance shortly after surgery. A delayed fitting is usually performed in above-knee amputations, bilateral extremity amputations, or cases of infection in which an open amputation has been performed. The appropriate time frame for fitting a prosthesis in these situations depends on the healing of the residual limb and the overall condition of the patient. A general goal for weight bearing of a lower extremity amputation is about 3 months. When the residual limb has healed satisfactorily, the patient is fitted for a prosthesis. A suitable choice for a prosthesis is based on the site of the amputation and the age, intelligence, health, motivation, occupation, and financial status of the patient.

Activity Intolerance

Surgery and bedrest may adversely affect the patient's tolerance for any type of sustained activity. It is extremely important to plan care in order to avoid too much patient exertion. Encouraging the patient to resume the preoperative level of activity too soon can impair physical and psychological healing. A typical activity order is for the patient to be assisted out of bed two or three times on the first postoperative day for 1 hour at a time. Over the next few days, the patient with a lower extremity amputation is usually encouraged to remain out of bed for longer periods and to begin to practice ambulation gradually. This may initially involve only a few steps, but these will gradually be increased over time. The patient's level of activity and the rate at which he or she regains endurance depend on many individual factors.

Self-Care Deficit

During the immediate postoperative period, assist the patient in performing activities of daily living as needed. Gradually, guide the patient to adapt to the lost limb and encourage more independence. Patients feel less helpless when they regain the abilities to provide self-care.

Anxiety, Fear, and Ineffective Coping

Provide opportunities for patients to talk about their concerns. It may be helpful to explore how the patient's usual coping strategies can be employed in this situation. Encourage and support effective coping strategies. Identify inappropriate behaviors and attempt to help the patient find alternatives. Referral to a local amputee support group may be helpful. As mentioned earlier, it is important to expect the patient to experience a grieving process, especially if the amputation is traumatic.

Disturbed Body Image

The patient may have difficulty looking at and caring for the affected extremity. It takes time for the patient to incorporate the change into his or her body image. Encourage the patient to talk about the change and what effects it will have. Emphasize ways to adapt to the loss and, if the patient wishes, to conceal it. Gradually encourage the patient to participate more in care of the residual limb. Patient instruction for residual limb care is extremely important. Counsel family and friends to support the patient and not to encourage excessive dependence.

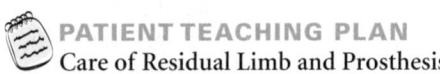

PATIENT TEACHING PLAN
Care of Residual Limb and Prosthesis

Residual Limb

- Wash the residual limb with soap and water every night. Rinse and dry the skin thoroughly.
- Each day use a mirror to inspect the entire residual limb, especially the incision, for irritation, redness, and edema.
- Expose the residual limb to air when possible.
- Residual limb socks should be hand washed, rinsed well, and dried flat. A clean sock should be used every day. Having several socks will allow time for the socks to dry between washings.
- Do not wear mended socks because a seam is irritating and creates pressure.
- Shoes with uneven heels will change the weight distribution of the residual limb and lead to irritation and possible skin breakdown.
- Do not use lotions, ointments, or powders unless prescribed by the physician.
- If redness or irritation develops on the residual limb, discontinue use of the prosthesis until you have the area checked.

Prosthesis

- Keep the prosthetic socket (the opening in which the residual limb is seated) clean.
- The residual limb may shrink in size for up to 2 years after surgery. Annual visits to the prosthetist are recommended for necessary adjustments. (More frequently for children as their residual limb grows in size with them.)
- Each day, wipe the inside of the prosthesis socket with a damp, soapy cloth, then remove the soap with a clean, damp cloth. Dry thoroughly.
- Consult a prosthetist if there are any problems with the prosthesis. Do not attempt to make adjustments yourself.

THE ELDERLY AMPUTEE

The elderly patient with an amputation may have some additional needs that should be taken into consideration when planning and providing care. For example, when constructing a teaching plan for the elderly, keep in mind that the healthy older person is completely capable of learning but often requires smaller units of information, more repetition, and more time. Skip unnecessary details and make sure that during the teaching process patients with glasses or hearing aids have them in place.

It is also important to clearly explain phantom sensations to the elderly. Some may not wish to report phantom sensations or phantom pain for fear of seeming foolish. Reminding the elderly patient that phantom sensations are not uncommon or bizarre can reduce the fear or anxiety that these sensations can cause.

Many elderly have one or more chronic health problems. This factor should be taken into account in choosing a prosthetic device. A patient with diabetes, for example, is prone to circulation problems and poor wound healing and may need a prosthesis with extra padding or support. Poor vision and decreased sensation may keep the older person from recognizing complications.

Because many elderly have decreased appetites, their nutritional status may be poor. Emphasizing high-calorie and high-protein intake is essential to promote healing and to maintain or build strength.

Remembering that the loss of a limb or part of a limb can be especially difficult in the elderly is important in providing psychological support. This is because many elderly individuals have had to deal with other losses in their lives, such as the loss of loved ones, the loss of independence, and the loss of income associated with retirement. Older people may lack confidence that they can adapt and gain strength.

If the patient is unable to participate fully in his or her care, instruct family members along with the elderly patient. Home health nursing services may be arranged to facilitate adaptation in the home setting and to monitor for complications. Empathy, patience, and respect are essential in approaching elderly patients.

REPLANTATION

In some amputation injuries, a type of surgical technique called replantation may be performed. This generally involves the use of a microscope and highly specialized instruments to reanastomose (reconnect) blood vessels and nerve fibers in a severed limb. The limb is then sutured into its correct anatomic position. Advances in microsurgical techniques and preservation of severed limbs have made this technique increasingly successful.

INDICATIONS

A number of factors are taken into consideration by the surgeon before performing replantation surgery—for example, the type of injury and location. Replantation surgery is most likely to be performed for amputations through the hand or wrist. Amputated thumbs are reattached whenever possible because of the thumb's importance in total hand function. In a severely injured hand in which two or more fingers are detached, an attempt is made by the surgeon to restore as many fingers as possible. Amputations above the wrist do not lend themselves as readily to replantation because of the extensive tissue, muscle, and bone damage accompanying the injury. A large muscle mass injury involves a great amount of tissue damage. Severely traumatized tissue can become ischemic, leading to death of the tissues and loss of the replanted limb. Severe crushing injuries or avulsion injuries in which the limb is mutilated also are not appropriate for replantation. In general, the greater the muscle mass injury, the less likely that replantation will be possible.

Another factor that is considered in deciding whether to attempt replantation is the length of warm or cold ischemia time.

EMERGENCY CARE

Proper handling of amputated parts is extremely important for successful replantation. Current preservation techniques include wrapping the amputated parts in a clean cloth saturated with normal saline or Ringer's lactate solution. These parts are then placed in a sealed plastic bag that is placed in ice water. Direct contact between the amputated part and the ice can lead to further tissue damage and cell death. Partially amputated parts should remain attached to the patient and also should be kept cool if possible. Extra care should be taken to avoid detaching any parts since even small connections increase the chances for successful repair.

The patient may require treatment for shock due to blood loss. This may include intravenous fluids and blood products. Blood loss from the residual limb may be minimized by using a clean, dry dressing, which can be reinforced as needed. Tourniquets should not be used unless absolutely necessary, as they can cause ischemia of the residual limb.

NURSING CARE *of the Patient Having Replantation Surgery*

PREOPERATIVE NURSING CARE

Assessment

General preoperative care of the replantation patient includes careful assessment of circulatory status, close monitoring of vital signs, and inspection of the residual limb (or dressing) for bleeding. Assess pain at the site of the injury and at other locations. Measure and record fluid intake and output. Note the patient's emotional status, and assess understanding of the preoperative activities and postoperative routines. Identify sources of support.

Nursing Diagnoses, Goals, and Outcome Criteria: Replantation, Preoperative Care

Nursing Diagnoses	Goals and Outcome Criteria
Decreased Cardiac Output related to decreased blood volume	Normal cardiac output: pulse and blood pressure within patient norms, skin warm and dry
Fear related to severe injury or possible failure of replantation	Reduced fear: calm manner, patient statement of less fear
Anxiety related to lack of knowledge of surgical routines	Decreased anxiety: relaxed manner, patient statement of reduced anxiety
Acute Pain related to tissue trauma	Decreased pain: patient statement of less pain, relaxed manner, pulse and blood pressure within patient norms

Interventions

Administer intravenous fluids and blood as ordered. If the dressing becomes saturated with blood, reinforce the dressing. Report continued or excessive bleeding to the physician. Even though preparations for replantation are hurried, be sensitive to the patient's fear and anxiety. Accept the patient's feelings. Provide brief, simple explanations. Administer analgesics as ordered for pain.

POSTOPERATIVE NURSING CARE

Routine postoperative care is discussed in detail in Chapter 16. This section emphasizes the special needs of the replantation patient.

Assessment

Postoperative assessment includes monitoring vital signs, intake and output, and level of consciousness. An essential aspect of care after replantation is hourly neurovascular assessment of the replanted limb. A Doppler device or pulse oximeter may be used to evaluate circulation. When the patient arrives on the nursing unit, immediately assess and document circulatory status to establish a baseline for comparison. Note and record the limb's color, capillary refill, turgor, temperature, and sensation. Signs of arterial occlusion are pale or blue color, slow capillary refill, shriveled appearance, and coolness. Signs of venous congestion are cyanosis, rapid capillary refill, edema, and warmth. Also assess the limb for edema because massive edema often accompanies replantation.

Nursing Diagnoses, Goals, and Outcome Criteria: Replantation, Postoperative Care

Nursing Diagnoses	Goals and Outcome Criteria
Ineffective Tissue Perfusion related to trauma, edema, compensatory vasoconstriction	Adequate circulation to replanted limb: warmth, normal skin color, arterial pulses

Nursing Diagnoses, Goals, and Outcome Criteria: Replantation, Postoperative Care—cont'd

NURSING DIAGNOSES	GOALS AND OUTCOME CRITERIA
Acute Pain related to tissue trauma	Pain relief: relaxed expression, statement of less pain
Disturbed Body Image related to disfigurement, loss of function	Improved body image: patient touches and looks at affected part, makes positive statements about self

Interventions

Measures to promote circulation to the replanted limb include elevation of the limb and microvascular precautions. Elevation of the limb promotes venous and lymphatic drainage. Take care not to elevate the limb above the level of the heart, as this may impair arterial flow. Several soft pillows or a stockinette connected to an intravenous pole may help to achieve this. Microvascular precautions include avoiding any substances or conditions that contribute to blood vessel spasm or constriction. Encourage the patient to abstain from nicotine- and caffeine-containing products for 7 to 10 days postoperatively. Enforce a strict ban on cigarette smoking. In addition, maintain room temperature at 80° F to prevent compensatory vasoconstriction of the peripheral tissues in response to cold. Loosen tight or restrictive gowns or pajamas. Explain the importance of these measures to the patient and family.

The physician may order intravenous low-molecular-weight dextran (Dextran 40), aspirin, or heparin to reduce the risk of thrombosis. Administer the drugs as ordered and monitor for adverse effects.

Inadequate arterial blood flow to the replanted limb is a medical emergency. If there is evidence of inadequate arterial circulation (no pulse, pallor or cyanosis, cool skin), immediately notify the surgeon, and prepare the patient for a return to the operating suite. In some facilities, venous congestion is treated with leeches. Leeches are attached to a selected area of the replanted limb. The saliva of these worms contains an anticoagulant, a local vasodilator, and a local anesthetic. The leech extracts excess blood, reducing venous congestion.

Provide the patient with an opportunity to discuss thoughts and feelings about the replantation, disfigurement, and loss of function. It may take a while before the patient is able to look at and touch the replanted limb. Support the patient and demonstrate acceptance of him or her. Your comfort with handling the limb can help the patient feel accepted. The rehabilitation team works with the patient to restore maximum possible function.

If the replantation is not successful, the limb is surgically removed. This represents a significant loss to the patient. Recognize this loss and support the patient.

***Put on your* THINKING CAP!!**

What could you do or say to support the patient whose replanted limb must be amputated?

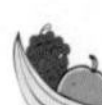

Nutrition Concepts

1. A nutritional assessment should be made preoperatively for patients undergoing surgical amputation, especially for older, immobilized, or chronic alcoholic patients.
2. Patients undergoing surgical amputation should be well hydrated; intravenous fluids may be given if oral fluids are not tolerated.
3. Surgical amputation is accompanied by a stress response, resulting in an increased need for calories and protein for healing.
4. Dietary supplements such as Sustacal or Ensure may be needed for patients whose intake of regular foods is inadequate for healing.
5. Patients are encouraged to become mobile as soon as possible after an amputation to prevent loss of calcium and protein.
6. Dietary choices high in protein, zinc, and vitamin C promote wound healing.

Other essential aspects of care include routine postoperative measures such as frequent position changes, pulmonary toilet, and pain management.

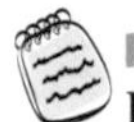

PATIENT TEACHING PLAN
Postoperative Replantation

- Avoid nicotine and caffeine for 7 to 10 days, or as directed by the surgeon.
- Avoid tight clothing that could impair circulation to the replanted limb/digit.
- Keep the limb positioned as instructed.
- A rehabilitation team will teach you proper care to promote improved function.
- Immediately advise your surgeon of changes in the color or warmth of the replanted limb/digit.

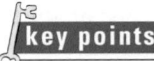

key points

- Amputation is the surgical removal of body limbs or parts of limbs.
- Conditions or situations that can lead to an amputation include trauma, disease, tumors, and congenital problems.
- The medical management of patients who have amputations involves the appropriate treatment and control of underlying diseases such as diabetes mellitus and peripheral vascular disease.
- Complications of amputation include hemorrhage, hematoma, necrosis, wound dehiscence, gangrene, edema, contracture, pain, and infection.
- Preoperatively, the patient needs to prepare physically and psychologically for an impending amputation.
- Postoperative nursing care focuses on decreased cardiac output, acute pain, risk for infection, impaired skin integrity, risk for impaired skin integrity, disturbed sensory perception, risk for injury, impaired physical

mobility, activity intolerance, self-care deficit, anxiety or fear, ineffective coping, and disturbed body image.

- Replantation of severed limbs is sometimes possible.
- Before replantation, nursing and medical care focuses on preserving the severed part and managing the patient's blood loss.
- Priorities after replantation include assessing for and managing ineffective tissue perfusion, acute pain, and disturbed body image.
- If there is evidence of inadequate arterial circulation in a replanted limb, immediately notify the surgeon, and prepare the patient for a return to the operating suite.

REVIEW QUESTIONS

1. The most common cause of lower extremity amputation is:
   1. trauma.
   2. vascular disease.
   3. tumors.
   4. congenital defects.
2. Smoking is contraindicated following replantation because nicotine:
   1. causes vasoconstriction.
   2. increases the risk of bleeding.
   3. impairs the immune system.
   4. causes arteriosclerosis.
3. In which situation would an *open* amputation be most likely?
   1. A teenager with bone cancer
   2. A diabetic patient with vascular disease
   3. A child with a congenital deformity
   4. An accident victim with a crushing injury
4. A patient complains that her amputated foot itches and feels hot. This represents which of the following?
   1. Poor psychological adjustment
   2. Phantom limb sensation
   3. Early symptoms of infection
   4. Denial of the amputation
5. In the early postoperative period, the greatest danger to the patient who has had an amputation is:
   1. infection.
   2. wound dehiscence.
   3. dehydration.
   4. hemorrhage.
6. A compression dressing or a cast is applied after amputation to:
   1. reduce pain.
   2. shape the residual limb.
   3. prevent wound contamination.
   4. prevent stimulation of nerve endings.
7. Measures to prevent contractures in a residual limb after lower extremity amputation include:
   1. Keep the patient up in a chair as much as possible.
   2. Guide the patient through active range-of-motion exercises.
   3. Have the patient lie supine for 30 minutes three or four times a day.
   4. Prop the residual limb on a pillow when the patient is supine.
8. Patient teaching related to care of a residual limb and prosthesis should include which of the following statements?
   1. Clean, rinse, and dry the prosthetic socket every day.
   2. Always powder the residual limb before putting on the sock.
   3. Redness and irritation of the residual limb are normal.
   4. Wash the residual limb with soap and water once a week.
9. The best way to preserve an amputated body part for possible replantation is to:
   1. cover the part with ice.
   2. wrap the part in a clean, dry cloth.
   3. wash the part carefully, dry, and wrap in plastic.
   4. seal the part in a plastic bag and put in ice water.
10. When you assess a patient's replanted hand, it is slightly bluish, swollen, and warm. These findings indicate:
    1. arterial occlusion.
    2. rejection of the replanted hand.
    3. venous congestion.
    4. that the replantation was successful.

CHAPTER 42 Pituitary and Adrenal Disorders

objectives

1. Identify nursing assessment data relevant to the function of the adrenal and pituitary glands.
2. Describe the tests and procedures used to diagnose disorders of the adrenal and pituitary glands.
3. Describe the pathophysiology and medical treatment of adrenocortical insufficiency, excess adrenocortical hormones, hypopituitarism, diabetes insipidus, and pituitary tumors.
4. Assist in developing nursing care plans for patients with selected disorders of the adrenal and pituitary glands.

key terms

Acromegaly (ăk-rō-MĔG-ă-lē, p. 857)
Addison's disease (ĂD-ĭ-sŏnz dĭ-ZĒZ, p. 868)
Adrenalin (ă-DRĔN-ă-lĭn, p. 866)
Androgens (ĂN-drō-jĕnz, p. 868)
Catecholamines (kăt-ĕ-KŌL-ă-mēnz, p. 866)
Cushing's disease (KŬSH-ĭng dĭ-ZĒZ, p. 874)
Cushing's syndrome (KŬSH-ĭng SĬN-drōm, p. 874)
Diabetes insipidus (DI) (dī-ă-BĒ-tēz ĭn-SĬP-ĭ-dŭs, p. 864)
Endocrine gland (ĔN-dŏ-krĭn, p. 852)
Estrogens (ĔS-trō-jĕnz, p. 868)
Gigantism (JĪ-găn-tĭzm, p. 857)
Glucocorticoid (gloo-kō-KŎR-tĭ-koyd, p. 867)
Hypophysectomy (hī-pō-fĭ-SĔK-tō-mē, p. 860)
Mineralocorticoid (mĭn-ĕr-ăl-ō-KŎR-tĭ-koyd, p. 867)
Syndrome of inappropriate antidiuretic hormone (SIADH) (ăn-tĭ-dī-ū-RĔT-ĭk HŎR-mōn, p. 865)

Virtually every cell in the human body is affected by the endocrine system. The endocrine system is a complex communication network composed of glands and glandular tissue that make, store, and secrete chemical messengers called *hormones.* Hormones are delivered to target organs and body tissues by the bloodstream. The **endocrine glands** are depicted in Figure 42-1.

Another class of glands includes the exocrine glands. The exocrine glands pass secretions through ducts or tubes that empty outside the body or into the lumen or opening of other organs. Examples of this type of gland are sweat glands and the portion of the pancreas that secretes digestive enzymes.

HORMONE FUNCTIONS AND REGULATION

The term *hormone* was coined in 1905. It is derived from the Greek word meaning "I arouse to activity." This definition is appropriate because hormones are usually released in response to the body's needs. Hormones are responsible for important functions related to reproduction, fluid and electrolyte balance, host defenses, responses to stress and injury, energy metabolism, and growth and development. The overall mission of the endocrine system is to maintain homeostasis. Homeostasis is the maintenance of physiologic stability despite the constant changes that occur in the environment. A hormone is a substance composed of amines, peptides, or steroids. These substances bind to receptors located inside the cell nucleus or on the cell membranes of target organs or tissues. Receptors are specific for certain kinds of hormones. Once the hormones bind with their receptors, they exert their effects on the organ or tissue.

Regulation of endocrine activity is controlled by mechanisms, called feedback mechanisms, that either stimulate or inhibit hormone synthesis and secretion. Feedback mechanisms are triggered by blood levels of specific substances. These substances may be hormones or other chemical compounds regulated by hormones. Feedback may be either positive or negative (Fig. 42-2).

In negative feedback, high levels of a substance inhibit hormone synthesis and secretion, whereas low levels stimulate hormone synthesis and secretion. A simple example of this is the household thermostat. As the environmental temperature rises, the production of heat is decreased or stopped; however, as the temperature drops, heat production increases. In positive feedback, high levels of a substance stimulate hormone synthesis and secretion, whereas low levels inhibit additional hormone synthesis and secretion.

Regulation of hormone production and activity varies with the time of day. Humans and most other animals have a circadian or diurnal rhythm. This rhythm is based on a 24-hour cycle, during which hormone synthesis and secretion are at their slowest rate during the early morning hours and at their highest rate during the evening hours.

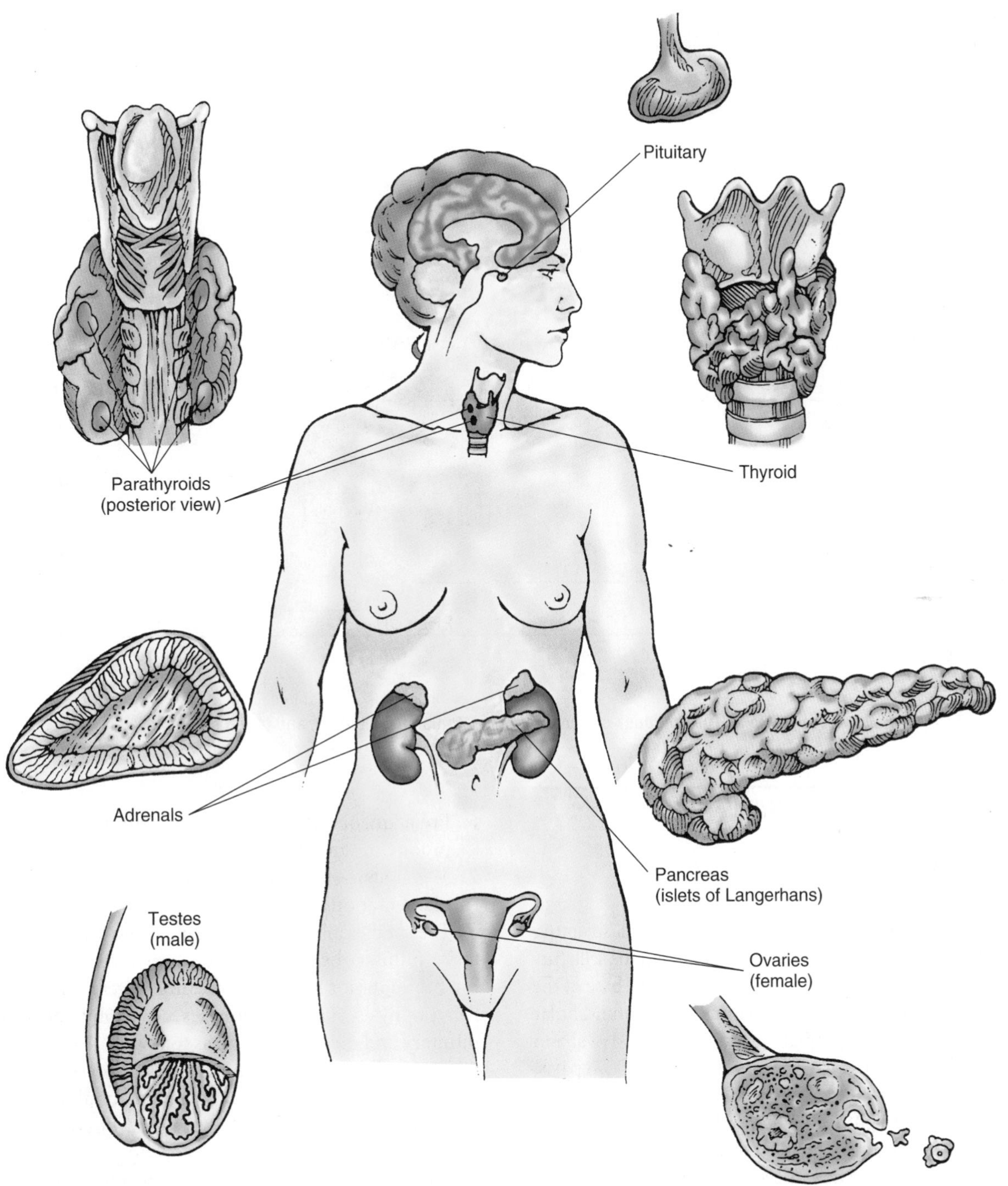

FIGURE **42-1** The endocrine system. The organs of the endocrine system include the pituitary gland, thyroid gland, parathyroid glands, adrenal glands, pancreas, testes (in the man), and ovaries (in the woman).

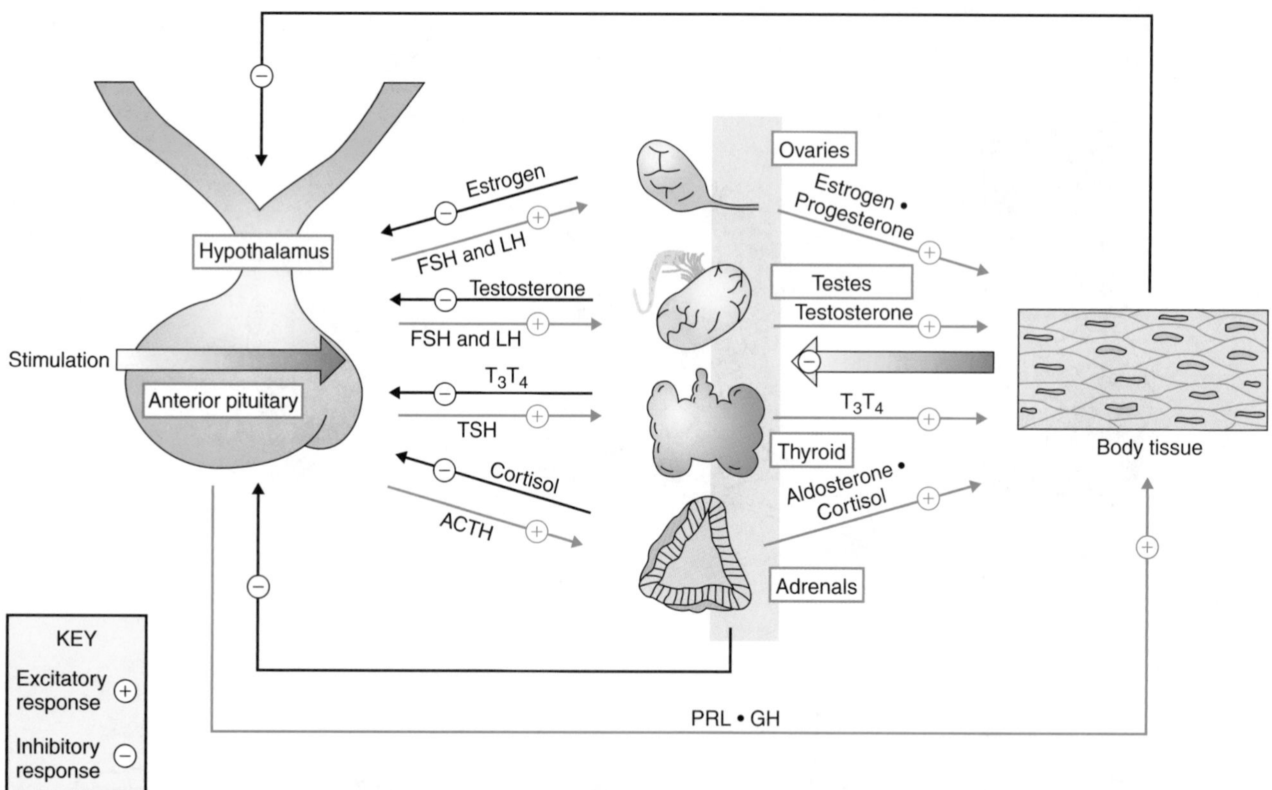

FIGURE 42-2 The feedback system of the hypothalamus, pituitary, and target glands.

THE PITUITARY GLAND

ANATOMY AND PHYSIOLOGY OF THE PITUITARY GLAND

The pituitary gland, also called the hypophysis, is a structure that weighs approximately 0.6 gm and is located in the sella turcica, a small indentation in the sphenoid bone at the base of the brain. It is connected to the hypothalamus by the infundibular (hypophyseal) stalk. The pituitary gland is small and oval and has a diameter of approximately 1 cm. It consists of two parts, or lobes. The larger of the two lobes, which accounts for 70% to 80% of the gland's weight, is the anterior lobe. The anterior lobe is also called the adenohypophysis. The hormones of the anterior pituitary and their actions are as follows:

1. Growth hormone (GH), or somatotropic hormone: stimulates the growth and development of bones, muscles, and organs.
2. Adrenocorticotropic hormone (ACTH): controls the growth, development, and function of the cortex of the adrenal glands; controls release of glucocorticoids and adrenal androgens; necessary for secretion of aldosterone but does not control rate of aldosterone secretion.
3. Thyroid-stimulating hormone or thyrotropic hormone: controls the secretory activities of the thyroid gland.
4. Follicle-stimulating hormone: stimulates the development of the eggs in the ovary of the woman and sperm production in the man.
5. Luteinizing hormone: controls ovulation or egg release in the woman and testosterone production in the man.
6. Prolactin, or lactogenic hormone: stimulates breast milk production in the woman.
7. Melanocyte-stimulating hormone: promotes pigmentation.

The smaller lobe of the pituitary also is known as the posterior pituitary because of its location in the sella turcica behind the anterior lobe. It is sometimes referred to as the neurohypophysis. The hormones secreted by the posterior pituitary and their actions are as follows:

1. Antidiuretic hormone (ADH), or vasopressin: causes the reabsorption of water from the renal tubules of the kidney. By doing so, water excretion from the body in the form of urine is decreased.
2. Oxytocin: causes contractions of the uterus in labor and the release of breast milk.

NURSING ASSESSMENT OF THE PITUITARY GLAND

Health History

Present Illness

Some problems related to pituitary function that may bring the patient to seek medical care are slowed or accelerated growth, visual disturbances, headache, and changes in urine output, appearance, skin, and secondary sex characteristics.

Past Medical History

Inquire about a history of brain tumors, pituitary surgery, head trauma, central nervous system infection, vascular disorders, chronic renal failure, hypothyroidism, and disease of the pancreas, liver, or bone.

Family History

Document a family history of diabetes insipidus (DI).

Review of Systems

Ask about the patient's general health state and note fatigue, weakness, restlessness, or agitation. Inquire about skin moisture and changes in body hair distribution. Note reports of significant sensory changes such as blurred vision and diplopia (double vision). For both men and women, ask about changes in the breasts. Also assess the presence of chest pain, constipation, polyuria, changes in genitalia, sexual dysfunction, joint pain, abnormal sensations, edema, seizures, and intolerance of heat or cold.

Functional Assessment

In the functional assessment, determine whether the patient has had sleep disturbances. Obtain a description of usual diet, and assess the effects of symptoms on the person's self-concept and usual activities.

Physical Examination

Measure vital signs and height and weight. Palpate the skin for moisture and edema. Inspect the head and face for thickened lips, broad nose, and prominent forehead and jaw. Test visual acuity. Inspect the breasts for enlargement in men, atrophy in women, and discharge. Inspect and palpate the extremities for edema. Assess joint range of motion, noting any crepitus. Test reflexes for slowness of response. Inspect the male genitalia for loss of hair and palpate for testicular atrophy. The nursing assessment of the patient with a pituitary disorder is outlined in Table 42-1.

table 42-1 ASSESSMENT *of the Patient with a Pituitary Disorder*

HEALTH HISTORY

Chief Complaint/Present Illness: Slowed or accelerated growth; change in appearance, urine output, and/or secondary sex characteristics

Past Medical History: Brain tumors, pituitary surgery, head trauma, central nervous system infection, vascular disorders, chronic renal failure, hypothyroidism, diseases of the pancreas, liver, or bone

Family History: Diabetes insipidus

Review of Systems: Fatigue, restlessness, agitation, skin moisture and hair distribution, vision disturbances, changes in breasts, chest pain, constipation, polyuria, changes in genitalia, sexual dysfunction, joint pain, abnormal sensations, edema, seizures, intolerance of heat or cold

Functional Assessment: Sleep pattern, usual diet, effects of disease on self-concept and daily life

PHYSICAL EXAMINATION

General Survey: Body proportion, behavior, mental-emotional state

Vital Signs

Height and Weight

Skin: Moisture and edema

Head and Face: Thickened lips, broad nose, prominent forehead and jaw

Neck: Jugular venous distention

Eyes: Visual acuity

Breasts: Enlargement, discharge

Extremities: Edema, range of motion, crepitus

Neurologic: Slow reflexes

Genitalia: Loss of pubic hair, testicular atrophy

AGE-RELATED CHANGES

In healthy older adults, pituitary function remains adequate. Increased ADH secretion impairs the ability to concentrate urine, increasing the risk of dehydration.

DIAGNOSTIC TESTS AND PROCEDURES

Radiographic Studies

Conventional radiographs and computed tomographic (CT) scans may indicate the presence of a pituitary or cranial tumor. Cerebral angiography, in which a radiopaque dye is injected into the cerebral arteries, may indicate the presence of aneurysms or arteriovenous malformations. Vascular anomalies can interfere with the supply of blood in the brain and lead to pituitary damage.

Laboratory Studies

Because hormones are circulated in very small quantities, tests to identify normal levels must be sensitive and precise. The radioimmunoassay is a commonly performed test that identifies whether adequate levels of hormones are present.

A similar type of test is the enzyme-linked immunosorbent assay (or ELISA). This is also thought to be an accurate test for levels of hormones in the blood.

Hormone reserve activity also can be measured using a number of "suppression" or "stimulation" tests. In these cases, an agent that stimulates or suppresses hormonal function is introduced into the body and hormone levels are measured. The response of target glands to stimulation helps the physician determine whether a deficiency is caused by failure of the target organ or dysfunction of the hypothalamic-pituitary regulatory mechanisms.

A glucose tolerance test for GH suppression may be done by administering a standard amount of glucose (100 gm or 0.5 gm/kg body weight) intravenously and measuring serial blood glucose levels for 120 minutes. The rationale is that the glucose will suppress GH levels through a negative feedback process. In normal patients, GH levels fall less than 5 mg/ml. In patients with hyperpituitarism, large decreases in GH occur. This constitutes a positive result.

Additional information about nursing care of patients having diagnostic tests and procedures for pituitary disorders is presented in Table 42-2.

DISORDERS OF THE PITUITARY GLAND

Dysfunction of the pituitary gland can result from a problem in the gland itself or from a problem in the hypothalamus. The hypothalamus is an organ in the brain that secretes factors that can directly inhibit or stimulate the pituitary (see Fig. 42-2). Pituitary disease is usually manifested by excess or deficient production and secretion of a specific hormone.

table 42-2 **DIAGNOSTIC TESTS AND PROCEDURES | *Pituitary Disorders***

TEST/PURPOSE	PATIENT PREPARATION	POSTPROCEDURE NURSING CARE
Cerebral computed tomography scan: Uses radiographs to create images of internal structures; detects tumors, edema, structural abnormalities.	Tell patient he/she will lie still on a stretcher while circular scanner moves around the head. Clicking sounds are heard, but no sensations are felt. Remove jewelry and hairpins. If contrast medium is to be used, assess sensitivity to iodine and shellfish and inform radiologist if allergic.	If contrast medium used, assess for side effects: nausea, vomiting, headache, delayed allergic reaction.
Cerebral angiogram: Radiographs are taken to study cerebral blood flow and blood vessels.	Signed consent required. General anesthesia needed for patients who cannot cooperate. Tell patient there may be a burning sensation when contrast medium in injected. Stress importance of lying still. Remove jewelry and hairpins from head. Assess for sensitivity to contrast medium.	Apply pressure to arterial puncture site for 15 min. Assess for bleeding afterward. Record V.S. per agency protocol. Immobilize extremity as ordered. Bedrest 12-24 hr. Neurologic checks hourly 4 times, then every 4 hr 20 times.
Glucose tolerance test: Evaluates response to glucose dose to detect diabetes mellitus and hyperpituitarism.	Tell patient fasting blood glucose will be measured; then intravenous or oral glucose solution given, and blood samples taken to measure glucose levels at specified intervals. Enforce NPO.	Check venipuncture site. Apply bandage if needed. Provide ordered diet.
Dexamethasone suppression tests: Measure cortisol, which increases with adrenal hyperplasia, Cushing's syndrome, oat cell carcinoma; decreases with histoplasmosis and tuberculosis.	Tell patient that baseline serum and urine cortisol will be measured. For overnight test, a dose of dexamethasone is given, usually around 11 P.M., and a blood sample is drawn for cortisol level at 8 A.M. Alternative tests are the low-dose test and high-dose test with various schedules for obtaining blood and urine specimens. Explain 24-hr urine collection, if ordered.	Send blood samples to lab within 30 min. Apply dressing to venipuncture site. Check for bleeding.
Pituitary hormone levels (luteinizing hormone, follicle-stimulating hormone, growth hormone, adrenocorticotropic hormone, thyroid-stimulating hormone, prolactin): Serum levels are measured to detect elevations or deficiencies of pituitary hormones.	Tell patient a blood sample will be required. Check agency manual for any special preparation.	Check venipuncture site. Apply dressing and check for bleeding.
Hypertonic saline test: An infusion of hypertonic saline is given to stimulate release of ADH to detect DI.	Tell patient IV fluids will be given. Urine output and specific gravity will be measured hourly. Explain urine collection process.	No special care.
Fluid deprivation: Detects changes in specific gravity and osmolality after aqueous vasopressin is given subcutaneously. Specific gravity and osmolality decrease with primary and secondary DI. No response with nephrogenic DI.	NPO for specified time. Tell patient vital signs will be taken; urine specimens collected; body weight measured hourly. A medication will be given and additional measurements done. Administer ordered medication and collect designated specimens.	No special care.

NPO, Nothing by mouth; *ADH,* antidiuretic hormone; *DI,* diabetes insipidus.

These hormone imbalances lead to disorders that can be manifested in a variety of ways, including changes in physical appearance, emotional state, mental status, metabolism, and homeostatic mechanisms essential for survival. The pituitary disorders that are discussed in this chapter are hyperpituitarism, hypopituitarism, diabetes insipidus (DI), and syndrome of inappropriate ADH (SIADH).

Hyperpituitarism

Etiology

Hyperpituitarism is a pathologic state caused by excess production of one or more of the anterior pituitary hormones. GH and prolactin are the hormones most often produced in excess. GH is responsible for the growth and development of the body's muscles, bones, and other tissue. Overproduction of GH can lead to gigantism or acromegaly. Overproduction of prolactin causes hyperprolactinemia.

The most common factor in hyperpituitarism is the presence of a pituitary adenoma. An adenoma is a benign tumor composed of epithelial tissue. It may vary in size and invasiveness. Those that are larger than 10 mm are called macroadenomas; those that are smaller than 10 mm are called microadenomas. Adenomas tend to occur most commonly in young women in their teens through early thirties. Pituitary adenomas that secrete hormones may cause amenorrhea, galactorrhea (abnormal milk secretion), hyperthyroidism, and Cushing's syndrome, in addition to gigantism or acromegaly.

Growth hormone, in addition to regulating tissue growth, mobilizes stored fat for energy. As a result of lipolysis of body adipose, excess levels of GH elevate free fatty acids in the bloodstream. This can stimulate the development of atherosclerosis, which causes coronary artery disease and cerebrovascular disease over time. Excess GH also antagonizes insulin and interferes with its effects, thus leading to hyperglycemia and possibly diabetes.

Prolactinemia. Excess prolactin can cause prolactinemia characterized by abnormal lactation (galactorrhea), amenorrhea, decreased vaginal lubrication, impotence and decreased libido in men, depression, anxiety, and visual loss.

Gigantism. Gigantism occurs in early childhood or puberty while the long bones of the body are still growing. The long bones consist of epiphyses, which are the end portions of the bone, and a diaphysis, which is the middle or shaft of the bone. Toward the end of puberty or in early adulthood, the line between these structures seals or closes, thus preventing further growth. Before the epiphyseal plates on the ends of these bones close, the diaphysis or long shaft of the bone may continue to grow to great lengths when stimulated by excess GH. The growth in these bones is usually proportional and may cause affected people to reach heights of up to 8 feet and weights of over 300 pounds. These people tend to have multiple health problems and often die in early adulthood. Figure 42-3 illustrates gigantism.

Acromegaly. Acromegaly, although rare, is more common than gigantism. Most patients with acromegaly are found to have pituitary macroadenomas that secrete excess GH. Symptoms usually appear in the fourth or fifth decades of life and affect men and women equally. In these people, excess GH production occurs after epiphyseal closure. The closed epiphyses prevent longitudinal growth of the bones; instead, bones increase in thickness and width.

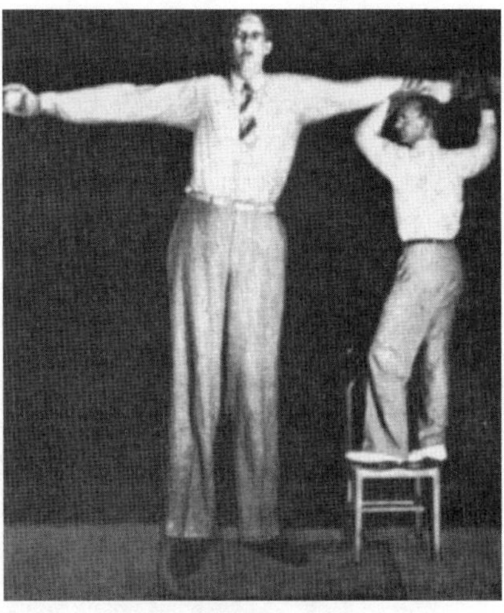

FIGURE **42-3** Clinical features of growth hormone excess. Robert Wadlow, nicknamed "The Alton Giant," weighed 9 pounds at birth but grew to 32 pounds by 6 months of age. By his first birthday, he weighed 62 pounds. He died at age 22 because of complications from cellulitis of the feet. At the time of his death, he was 8 feet, 11 inches tall and weighed 475 pounds.

Signs and Symptoms

Visual deficits are common in hyperpituitarism and may be the first symptoms of a problem. Visual problems are most often a result of pressure on optic nerves where they are joined near the pituitary gland. Physical features of the disease include enlargement of the hands, feet, and paranasal and frontal sinuses and deformities of the spine and mandible. In addition, soft tissues may become enlarged, especially the tongue, skin, liver, and spleen. This may in turn lead to speech impediments, coarse or distorted facial features, and abdominal distention. People with acromegaly also may experience diaphoresis, oily skin, peripheral neuropathies, degeneration of the joints, and proximal muscle weakness.

In addition to the features described above, patients with gigantism and acromegaly initially present with increased strength, progressing rapidly to complaints of weakness and fatigue. The examiner also may detect organomegaly (enlargement of internal organs), hypertension, dysphagia, and a deep voice due to hypertrophy of the larynx. Those patients who also have elevated levels of prolactin may present with galactorrhea in women and hypogonadism in men. A dramatic example of acromegaly is presented in Figure 42-4.

Medical Diagnosis

The diagnosis of hyperpituitarism is based on a number of data sources, including physical assessment, radiographic studies, and laboratory findings.

Radiographic studies. Radiographic films of the skull may show a large sella turcica and increased bone density. Enhanced CT scans using a water-soluble dye or magnetic resonance imaging may be performed to locate and evaluate potential

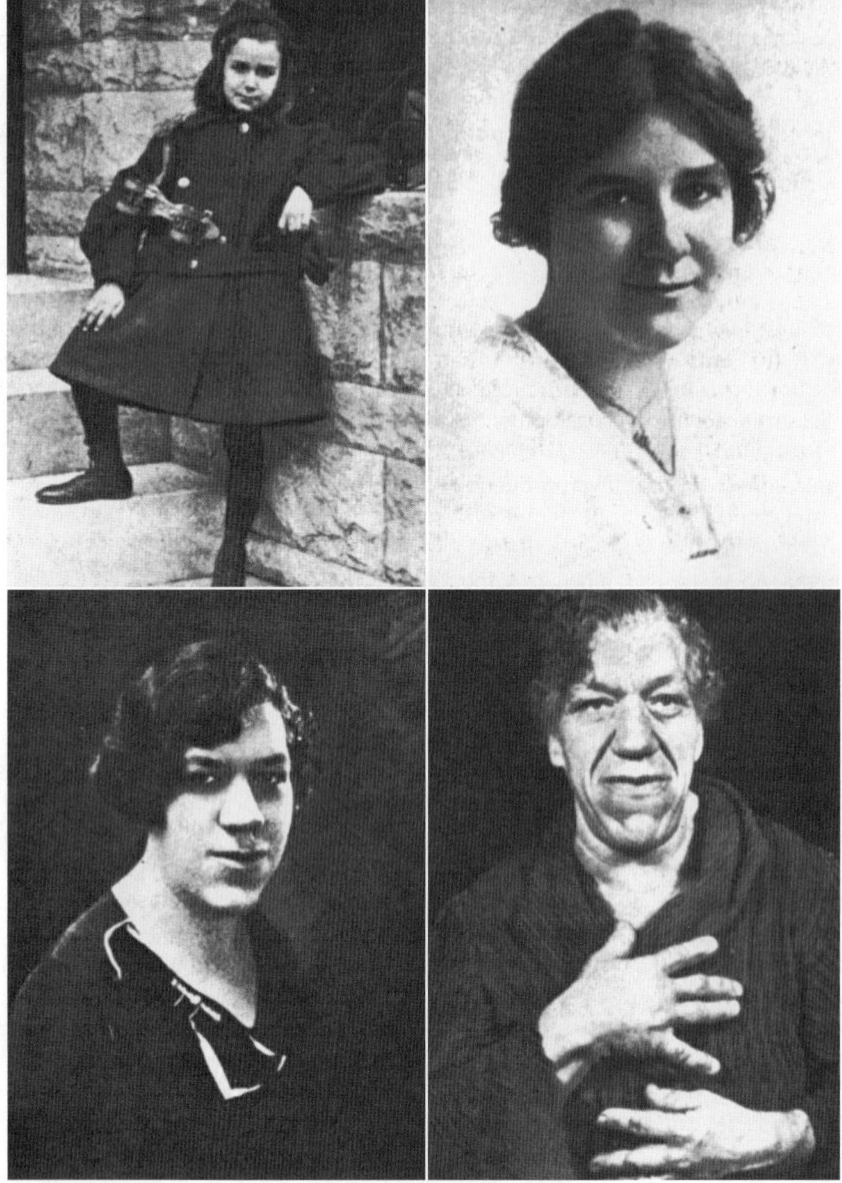

FIGURE **42-4** The progression of acromegaly. A series of photographs of the same person over the course of her lifetime depicts the physical changes that occurred. The woman was affected after reaching maturity.

intracellular or extracellular lesions or tumor formation. Angiography also may be of use to rule out any vascular abnormalities such as aneurysms or arteriovenous malformations.

Laboratory studies. As mentioned earlier, in hyperpituitarism only one pituitary hormone is usually produced in excess, such as GH or prolactin. Pathologic conditions producing elevated levels of luteinizing hormone or follicle-stimulating hormone are extremely rare. In suspected cases of hyperpituitarism, levels of anterior pituitary hormones are measured. Elevation of any hormone level requires further evaluation and follow-up. It is normal for luteinizing hormone and follicle-stimulating hormone to be slightly elevated in postmenopausal women. The glucose tolerance test is the most reliable test for acromegaly.

Dexamethasone suppression tests are used to rule out problems related to dysfunction of the adrenal glands (discussed in detail in the section on Disorders of the Adrenal Glands).

Medical Treatment

Typically, the patient with hyperpituitarism that is manifested as acromegaly or gigantism has skeletal changes and disfigurement that cannot be reversed with treatment. Radiation therapy is sometimes used to treat tumors that produce excess GH, but overall response is slow, and numerous complications, such as hypopituitarism, optic nerve damage, and visual defects, can occur. Gamma knife radiotherapy may prove to be the best radiotherapy for acromegaly.

Drug therapy. One drug commonly prescribed for patients with hyperpituitarism is bromocriptine (Parlodel). Bromocrip-

table 42-3 **DRUG THERAPY | *Pituitary***

DRUG	USE/ACTION	SIDE EFFECTS	NURSING INTERVENTIONS
ADH HORMONE PREPARATIONS	All promote conservation of water.	All can cause water intoxication, inadequate tissue perfusion due to vasoconstriction.	Monitor for early signs and symptoms of water intoxication: drowsiness, listlessness, headache. Patient should reduce fluid intake first few days of treatment.
Lypressin (Diapid) nasal spray	Treats diabetes insipidus (DI).	Rhinorrhea, nasal irritation and congestion. Rarely, dyspnea, hypertension, coronary vasoconstriction.	Teach patient use of intranasal inhaler: hold bottle upright, place nozzle in nostril, spray prescribed number of times, do not inhale. Explain how to monitor intake and output. With DI, stress need for lifelong therapy. Monitor BP, pulse.
Desmopressin (DDAVP) nasal spray, parenteral, oral preparations	Treats DI, hemophilia (increases production of clotting factor VIII), nocturnal diuresis, headache.	Same as lypressin.	Same as lypressin.
Vasopressin (Pitressin) Synthetic for SC and IM	Treats DI, postoperative abdominal distention, used to dispel gas before abdominal radiography. Powerful vasoconstrictor.	May cause angina, MI in patients with coronary artery disease.	Same as lypressin. Also, assess cardiac and peripheral circulation. Extreme caution with cardiac disease.
PITUITARY HORMONE SUPPRESSANTS			
Bromocriptine (Parlodel)	Inhibits release of prolactin from anterior pituitary. Suppresses lactation. Restores ovulation. Treats acromegaly.	Nausea, vomiting, constipation, hypotension, drowsiness, MI, pulmonary infiltrates, nasal stuffiness, vasoconstriction, anorexia, headache. Rarely, visual disturbances, confusion.	Safety measures if dizzy. Monitor BP. Record bowel movements and stool consistency. Assess effects. Teach patient to report chest pain and/or dyspnea immediately, to rise slowly to standing position, that driving may be dangerous because of drowsiness and dizziness, and that the drug may restore fertility.
Octreotide acetate (Sandostatin)	Suppresses secretion of growth hormone. Most effective drug for acromegaly.	Nausea, vomiting, diarrhea, headache, flushing, edema, dizziness, altered blood glucose, drowsiness, orthostatic hypotension, visual disturbances, cholelithiasis.	Monitor weight, BP, pulse, respirations, urine output. Assess for edema. Refrigerate ampules. Discard if discolored or contains visible particles. Teach patient to give self-injections; advise to take exactly as prescribed and never take double doses. Assess for changes in blood glucose. Caution about drowsiness and dizziness. Very expensive.

SC, Subcutaneously; *IM*, intramuscularly; *MI*, myocardial infarction; *BP*, blood pressure.

tine activates dopamine receptors in the central nervous system and inhibits the release of GH and prolactin, thus decreasing serum levels of these substances. Bromocriptine may be used in conjunction with radiation therapy or alone. Bromocriptine is usually administered on a daily basis, with gradual increases in dosage until an optimum response is attained and serum levels of GH or prolactin, or both, decrease. Some of the most common side effects of this drug are headache, dizziness, drowsiness, confusion, nausea, vomiting, dry mouth, and urticaria.

Octreotide acetate (Sandostatin) also may be prescribed to suppress the secretion of GH. Common side effects of octreotide acetate are nausea, vomiting, diarrhea, abdominal pain, and pain at the injection site. Because this drug also suppresses insulin secretion, the patient's blood glucose must be monitored. Blood pressure and weight are monitored to detect fluid retention. Sometimes bromocriptine and octreotide are used together to achieve therapeutic effects with fewer side effects of each drug.

Table 42-3 provides additional information about drugs used to treat hyperpituitarism.

PHARMACOLOGY CAPSULE Drugs used to treat gigantism and acromegaly decrease hormone secretion but do not reverse the existing skeletal effects of the condition.

Surgical Management

For patients diagnosed with pituitary tumors, the surgical removal of the adenoma or of the pituitary itself (hypophysectomy) is the treatment of choice. A transsphenoidal approach is the most commonly used surgical method. A transsphenoidal hypophysectomy is a microsurgical procedure performed under general anesthesia with the patient in the semi-Fowler position. An incision is made at the inner aspect of the upper lip through the maxillary bone, and the sella turcica is entered through the sphenoid sinus (Fig. 42-5). After the gland or a portion of it is removed, a small piece of adipose tissue is harvested from the abdomen and is used to pack the dura mater (one of the meningeal layers) to prevent leakage of cerebrospinal fluid (CSF). An absorbent gauze or similar dressing is used to pack the nasal passages, and an external nasal dressing is applied to keep the packing in place.

An earlier surgical approach, called a transfrontal craniotomy, is sometimes used if a tumor is especially large or is invading other structures. This is a more invasive procedure that involves the removal of a portion of the frontal bone of the skull. The cranial vault is then entered, and structures superior to the pituitary gland are displaced to reach it. This involves manipulation of the meningeal layers and the frontal and temporal lobes of the cerebrum, as well as the optic nerve. As a result, the risk of complications and brain damage is great.

NURSING CARE *of the Patient with Hyperpituitarism*

Education and emotional support are vital components in the nursing care of the patient with hyperpituitarism. Patients presenting with hyperpituitarism need to know that many body changes, such as visual disturbances and visceral enlargement, are not reversible. Surgical treatment is aimed only at preventing further symptoms and complications.

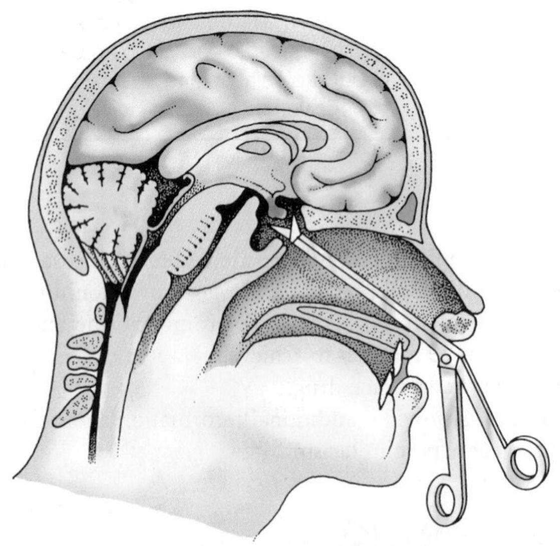

FIGURE **42-5** The transsphenoidal surgical approach to the pituitary gland.

Assessment

Assessment of the patient with a pituitary disorder is summarized in Table 42-1. When a patient has gigantism or acromegaly, areas that merit special attention are energy level, height and weight, vital signs, contours of the face and skull, visual acuity, speech, voice quality, and abdominal distention. If surgical intervention is planned, determine what the patient knows and expects.

Nursing Diagnoses, Goals, and Outcome Criteria: Hyperpituitarism

Nursing Diagnoses	Goals and Outcome Criteria
Disturbed Body Image related to changes in physical appearance	Adjustment to physical changes: patient verbalizes feelings about body and indicates acceptance of changes
Activity Intolerance related to fatigue	Improved activity tolerance: accomplishment of daily activities without excessive tiring
Chronic Pain related to musculoskeletal overgrowth, headache	Pain relief: patient verbalizes relief of pain, appears relaxed
Ineffective Therapeutic Regimen Management related to lack of knowledge of condition, treatment, and expected outcomes	Patient manages own treatment with realistic expectations: patient correctly describes self-medication, therapeutic effects and drug adverse effects

Interventions

Disturbed Body Image

Demonstrate acceptance of the patient and provide opportunities for the patient to share feelings and concerns. Encourage the patient to pay attention to grooming. If he or she has difficulty adjusting, a referral to a support group or mental health professional may be appropriate.

Activity Intolerance

Because the patient with acromegaly tires quickly, plan activities to allow for adequate rest periods. Help the patient develop a daily schedule that permits achievement of necessary activities balanced with rest requirements.

Chronic Pain

Assess and document pain. Teach relaxation techniques as discussed in Chapter 14. Administer prescribed analgesics and evaluate effects.

Consider the Alternative!

Imagery, relaxation exercises, and massage all can be used with analgesia to manage pain.

Ineffective Therapeutic Regimen Management

Advise patients on bromocriptine or octreotide to take drugs exactly as prescribed and not to take double doses if a dose is missed. Other nursing implications are in Table 42-3.

If the patient has surgery (in this case, hypophysectomy), general preoperative and postoperative care is provided, as described in Chapter 16. This section describes specific nursing care of the patient having pituitary surgery. The patient may be admitted to a critical care unit for the first 24 hours after surgery because of the risk of a number of complications.

POSTOPERATIVE NURSING CARE *of the Patient with Hyperpituitarism*

Assessment

During the postoperative period, frequent and thorough assessment of neurologic status and vision is important. Give particular attention to level of consciousness, pupil size and equality, vital signs, and intake and output. Ask the patient to place his or her chin to the chest to assess for nuchal rigidity (severe head or neck pain associated with meningeal inflammation). Changes in assessment findings that may reflect edema due to the manipulation of tissues or intracranial bleeding are decreasing alertness, slow pupil response to light, and decreased or asymmetric muscle strength.

Strict documentation of intake and output and measurement of specific gravity are important because these patients are at risk for DI or possibly SIADH. These disorders are discussed in detail later in this chapter.

Inspection of nasal packing for drainage is important because CSF leaks may sometimes occur. Document clear, colorless drainage and notify the surgeon. A bedside test using a testing strip may be done in an effort to determine whether drainage is CSF. Because CSF has a high glucose content, a positive glucose reading is thought to confirm that the fluid is CSF. It should be noted that the reliability of this test has been questioned, so it is no longer recommended. CSF leaks are often resolved with rest; however, severe, persistent headaches may be treated with a spinal tap to reduce CSF pressure. A return to surgery is rarely indicated.

Monitoring the patient for signs and symptoms of infection also is an important aspect of nursing care. Elevations in white blood cell counts, sudden rises in temperature, headache, or nuchal rigidity may be indications of meningitis (inflammation of the meninges, the protective layer of membranes that cover the brain and spinal cord).

Nursing Diagnoses, Goals, and Outcome Criteria: Hypophysectomy, Postoperative

Nursing Diagnoses	Goals and Outcome Criteria
Anxiety related to lack of knowledge of surgical postoperative care and routines	Reduced anxiety: patient calm; states he or she feels less anxious
Disturbed Sensory Perception (visual) related to tissue trauma and swelling	Absence of visual disturbances: patient reports no change in vision
Acute Pain related to tissue trauma	Pain relief: patient statement of pain relief, relaxed manner
Impaired Oral Mucous Membrane related to surgical incision	Healed surgical incision: incision closed, minimal swelling and redness
Excess Fluid Volume or **Deficient Fluid Volume** related to abnormal ADH production	Normal fluid balance: fluid intake and output approximately equal, normal tissue turgor
Risk for Infection related to impaired tissue integrity	Absence of infection: normal white blood cell count; no neck stiffness, fever, or headache
Risk for Injury related to disruption of packing	Absence of CSF drainage: no clear nasal drainage

Interventions

Anxiety

Orient the patient to the environment and explain all procedures. Give drugs as ordered to replace pituitary hormones. When the patient is well enough, provide information about drug therapy and self-medication. The patient who has a complete hypophysectomy requires hormone replacements for the rest of his or her life. Replacement therapy typically includes glucocorticoids and thyroid medication (see the section on Disorders of the Adrenal Glands for a more detailed discussion of glucocorticoids).

Impaired Sensory Perception

Be aware of existing visual disturbances, and assess for new disturbances that might indicate increased intracranial pressure. Treatment usually does not correct existing disturbances, but can prevent further harm.

Acute Pain and Impaired Oral Mucous Membranes

The immediate postoperative period is uncomfortable because the nasal packing remains in place for 2 to 3 days and the patient is forced to breathe through the mouth. Administer analgesics as ordered, and assess the effects. The presence of a "moustache" dressing also may make the patient feel uncomfortable or embarrassed. Frequent mouth care with moistening of the lips increases comfort. Tooth brushing is not permitted until the incision heals.

Risk for Injury

To prevent dislodgment of the fat pad or adipose graft at the surgical site, instruct the patient to avoid any activities that can cause a Valsalva maneuver. Coughing, straining, vomiting, or sneezing can create enough intracranial pressure to disrupt the surgical site and cause CSF leakage or even bleeding. Stool softeners and laxatives may be ordered to prevent straining. Instead of coughing, incentive spirometry and deep-breathing exercises help maintain pulmonary function without increasing intrathoracic and intracranial pressure. Advise the patient to avoid lifting heavy objects and bending from the waist. Instruct patients to avoid these activities at home as the physician directs (usually 2 to 3 months after surgery).

Excess Fluid Volume or Deficient Fluid Volume

Provide intravenous fluids as ordered, and monitor pulse, BP, and intake and output. Monitor for transient diabetes insipidus (large volume of dilute urine). Notify the physician of excessive fluid retention or diuresis. Changes in vital signs, mental status, and neuromuscular status suggest fluid and electrolyte imbalances.

Risk for Infection

Administer antibiotics as ordered. Monitor body temperature. Be especially alert for stiffness of the neck and headache because these are symptoms of meningitis.

PATIENT TEACHING PLAN
Hypophysectomy, Postoperative

- If the anterior pituitary is removed, you will need hormone replacements for the rest of your life.
- For 3 months (or as advised by your physician), avoid any activities that cause straining, heavy lifting, and bending from the waist.
- It is important to prevent constipation because straining increases intracranial pressure.
- Numbness of the incision area and decreased sense of smell are temporary.
- Follow-up care is essential to monitor for any signs of tumor recurrence.

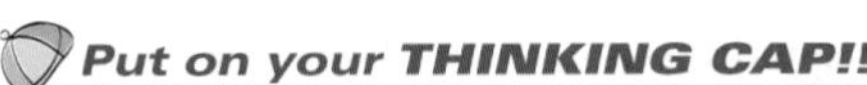

Put on your THINKING CAP!!

Explain why some people with excess growth hormone (GH) develop gigantism and other people with excess GH develop acromegaly.

Hypopituitarism

Etiology and Pathophysiology

When inadequate secretion of GH occurs during preadolescence, a syndrome called dwarfism may result. Dwarfism is defined as attainment of a maximum height that is 40% below normal. In addition, chronic diseases associated with inadequate growth may be present. The causes of dwarfism may be hereditary or may be related to damage to the anterior portion of the pituitary gland. The anterior pituitary may be damaged by necrosis after hemorrhage, trauma, infection, radiation, or autoimmune disorders. Inadequate secretion of GH or an inability of the target organs to respond to GH is usually considered to be the major cause. In rare instances, hypothalamic dysfunction can lead to dwarfism as well. It is important to note that although an actual or relative deficiency of GH may exist, other anterior pituitary hormones also may be deficient.

If growth has been completed and some pathologic process impairs the function of the pituitary, a syndrome known as panhypopituitarism can occur. In this situation, all hormones of the anterior pituitary are usually affected. There are a number of causes for panhypopituitarism, which are identified as follows:

1. Sheehan's syndrome: shock and hypotension during the postpartum period leading to infarction of the pituitary gland
2. Tumors of the pituitary gland itself or cranial tumors that impinge on the pituitary
3. Chronic recurrent infections
4. Total or subtotal destruction or removal of the pituitary as a result of trauma, surgery, or radiation therapy
5. Suppression of pituitary tropic hormones by excess target gland hormones (such as is seen in patients on prolonged corticosteroid therapy)

Signs and Symptoms

The manifestations of hypopituitarism depend on the stage of life when the deficiency occurs and which hormones are deficient. In dwarfism, which occurs early in life, the person is remarkably short in stature, sometimes as short as 36 inches, but with proportional physical characteristics. These people often have delayed or absent sexual maturation. There is a greater frequency of mental retardation than in the population at large. Dwarfs also have an accelerated pattern of aging and thus have a shorter life span than the general population, by as much as 20 years.

When a state of panhypopituitarism exists, a syndrome called Simmonds' cachexia is present. The patient has muscle and organ wasting and disruptions of both digestion and metabolism. Decreased muscle and organ size is attributed to decreased GH. An absence of ACTH affects the person's ability to cope effectively with stress. (See the section on Adrenal Hypofunction later in this chapter.) This in turn affects the person's ability to metabolize glucose, and hypoglycemia may result. Because thyroid-stimulating hormone is depleted, the thyroid is unable to produce thyroid hormone. A lack of thyroid hormone produces a state referred to as *hypothyroidism.* In hypothyroidism, insufficient thyroid hormone is available for normal metabolism and thermogenesis, or heat production. Consequently, people who are hypothyroid may be unable to maintain a normal basal metabolic rate or body temperature.

If there is a lack of melanocyte-stimulating hormone, decreased pigmentation of the skin occurs. This results in extreme pallor. Finally, with the absence of gonadotropins, gonads may become atrophied. In both men and women, there may be loss of libido, decreased body hair, and sexual dysfunction, and in women, amenorrhea (absence of menstruation).

General signs and symptoms may include fatigue, weakness, malaise, cold intolerance, and lethargy. Again, the type and degree of symptoms depend on specific hormones affected.

Medical Diagnosis

A diagnosis of dwarfism or panhypopituitarism is based on the health history, physical examination, and diagnostic tests. In cases of dwarfism, the physical examination findings are fairly diagnostic. Diagnostic tests and procedures may include conventional radiographs and CT scans to detect pituitary or cranial tumors. Cerebral angiography may be ordered to detect malformed blood vessels. Serum levels of pituitary hormones may be measured as well.

Medical Treatment

Deficient hormones are replaced as needed depending on the specific deficiencies of the patient. Deficiency of thyroid-stimulating hormone necessitates thyroid replacement with drugs such as levothyroxine (Synthroid) or liothyronine (Cytomel), usually for the rest of the person's life. Gonadotropin deficiency requires lifelong therapy. To produce or maintain libido, secondary sexual characteristics, and well-being, men also should receive testosterone and women should receive estrogen. In patients for whom childbearing is desirable, follicle-stimulating hormone and luteinizing hormone are administered to both men and women. GH replacement is necessary in children but not in adults. In most instances, GH is administered until the person reaches a height of 5 feet. The use of human GH produced by bacteria through recombinant DNA technology such as somatrem (Protropin) is considerably safer than products used previously. The annual cost of therapy with GH is very expensive. If a tumor is causing hypopituitarism, surgery is the treatment of choice. (See the section on Surgical Management under Hyperpituitarism, earlier in this chapter). Table 42-3 provides additional information about drug therapy for hypopituitarism.

NURSING CARE *of the Patient with Hypopituitarism*

Assessment

The general assessment of the patient with a pituitary disorder is summarized in Table 42-1. When assessing the patient with hypopituitarism, be especially aware of mental acuity, emotional stability, and affect. Document the patient's general sense of well-being, energy level, and appetite. In reviewing the systems, ask the patient about changes in skin texture, body temperature, hair, and libido. Determine the patient's usual activities and whether there has been any difficulty carrying out those activities.

In the physical examination, measure height and weight and compare with previous measurements. Inspect the hair for distribution, texture, and thickness. Inspect and palpate the skin and nails for color, texture, and moisture. Document the development of secondary sex characteristics, including axillary and pubic hair, genital maturity, breast development, and onset of menarche.

Nursing Diagnoses, Goals, and Outcome Criteria: Hypopituitarism

Nursing Diagnoses	Goals and Outcome Criteria
Disturbed Body Image related to lack (or loss) of secondary sex characteristics	Improved body image: patient makes positive statements about self and takes measures to improve appearance
Sexual Dysfunction related to hormone deficiency	Enhanced sexual development and function: secondary sex characteristics and satisfying sexual function
Imbalanced Nutrition: More or Less than Body Requirements related to hormone imbalance	Adequate nutrition: body weight normal for height
Deficient Fluid Volume related to hormone deficiency, impaired homeostasis	Normal fluid balance: normal tissue turgor, pulse, and blood pressure
Ineffective Therapeutic Regimen Management related to lack of understanding of condition, treatment, and self-care	Patient follows prescribed treatment regimen: correctly demonstrates self-care, diminishing signs and symptoms of hormone deficiency

Interventions

Patient education is the most important aspect of nursing care because disturbances in body image, sexual function, nutritional status, and fluid balance all can be improved if the patient understands and follows the prescribed therapy. Meanwhile, acknowledge the patient's feelings and encourage expression of concerns. Referral to a mental health counselor is appropriate if the patient has difficulty dealing with the effects of the disease. Good teaching is essential for patients and families to understand hypopituitarism and to participate in the treatment plan.

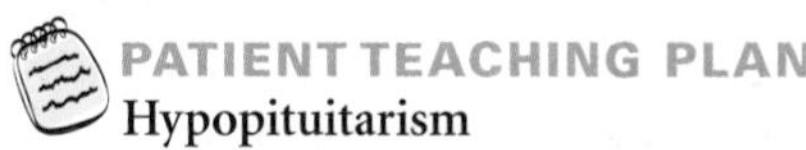

PATIENT TEACHING PLAN
Hypopituitarism

- It will be necessary for you to take medications for the rest of your life to replace the pituitary hormones.
- You must become familiar with the signs and symptoms of inadequate or excessive hormone replacement (provide written descriptions) and appropriate actions.
- You must have periodic follow-up care.
- Wear a medical alert bracelet or necklace so that your condition can be quickly recognized in an emergency.
- Carry a card that lists prescribed drugs and dosages and your physician's name and phone number.

POSTERIOR PITUITARY DISORDERS

Disorders of the posterior pituitary or neurohypophysis are characterized by deficient or excess ADH production. Another name for ADH is *vasopressin.* ADH helps to maintain fluid balance by promoting reabsorption of water in the renal tubules when body water is decreased or very concentrated. The amount of ADH secreted is reflected in the amount of water retained by the kidney. Increased ADH release causes increased water retention. This results in increased intravascular volume and decreased urine output.

Two disorders are associated with dysfunction of the neurohypophysis: DI and SIADH. DI is the more common of the two disorders.

Diabetes Insipidus

Etiology

Diabetes insipidus (DI) is characterized by excessive output of dilute urine. It can be caused by a number of factors. Thus, DI is classified as nephrogenic, hypothalamic (central), or primary polydipsia. Nephrogenic DI is an inherited defect in which the renal tubules of the kidney do not respond to ADH, resulting in inadequate water reabsorption by the kidneys. In this case, ADH is produced in sufficient amounts, but the kidneys do not respond to it appropriately. In hypothalamic DI, there is a defect in either the production or secretion of ADH. Hypothalamic DI can result from hypothalamic tumors, head trauma, infection, surgical procedures (hypophysectomy), or metastatic tumors originating in the lung or breast. It also can be triggered by a cerebrovascular accident, aneurysm, or intracranial hemorrhage. Some cases are caused by drugs such as lithium carbonate (Eskalith-CR) or demeclocycline (Declomycin), which affect the kidney by inhibiting its response to ADH. Primary polydipsia is a disorder of thirst stimulation. When the patient ingests water, serum osmolality decreases, which causes reduced vasopressin secretion. Other factors that may be associated with primary polydipsia are habitual excessive water intake and psychiatric conditions. The severity of symptoms in primary polydipsia varies.

Pathophysiology

Antidiuretic hormone deficiency or an inability of the kidneys to respond to ADH results in the excretion of large volumes of very dilute urine, a symptom referred to as *polyuria.* The distal tubules and collecting ducts do not reabsorb excess water. Massive diuresis occurs, resulting in increased plasma osmolarity, which stimulates the osmoreceptors. The osmoreceptors in turn relay information to the cerebral cortex, causing the person to feel thirsty. Increased thirst serves as a compensatory mechanism in that it causes the person to increase water ingestion. Unfortunately, this compensatory mechanism cannot keep up with the demand for water, and diuresis continues. Massive dehydration ensues, which leads to decreased intravascular volume, hypotension, and circulatory collapse. This is accompanied by neurologic changes such as a decreased level of consciousness and severe electrolyte imbalances. Electrolyte imbalances contribute to circulatory collapse by causing arrhythmias and impaired contractility of the heart. If left untreated, severe cases of DI can lead to cardiac arrest and death.

Signs and Symptoms

Common signs and symptoms of DI are massive diuresis, dehydration, and thirst. Dehydration is characterized by hypotension, tachycardia, dizziness, decreased skin turgor, weakness, and possible fainting episodes. Additional findings include malaise, lethargy, and irritability. An irregular heartbeat may be detected.

Medical Diagnosis

The diagnosis of DI is made primarily on the basis of the health history, physical examination, and laboratory findings. A history of any known etiologic factors, such as surgery, infection, injury, or medication ingestion, should be noted.

The loss of free water is apparent in laboratory studies of blood and urine. An initial diagnosis of DI is made on the basis of a 24-hour urine output of greater than 4 L of fluid, without food or fluid restrictions. Patients with DI can excrete up to 30 L/day, depending on the severity of the ADH deficiency or relative deficiency. Because the urine is very dilute, the specific gravity is also extremely low and the osmolarity of the urine is decreased. Additional studies used to diagnose DI are listed in Table 42-2.

Medical Treatment

The management of DI is geared to controlling the signs and symptoms of the disease and possibly reversing the cause of the syndrome. Intravenous fluid volume replacement and vasopressors often are required to maintain adequate blood pressure. Treatment also includes a variety of pharmacologic therapies. A list of these agents can be found in Table 42-3. Most of these agents act by augmenting existing ADH or replacing it. Short-term therapy is usually managed with subcutaneous injections of aqueous vasopressin. This is usually indicated in situations in which the cause of DI is reversible, such as infection- or medication-related DI. Patients on long-term therapy are placed on nasal spray (lypressin), which may be required for life. This long-term therapy may be necessary after hypophysectomy or other surgical procedures. Patients with primary polyuria related to a psychiatric condition may require ADH supplementation while psychotherapy is used to treat the underlying disorder.

Sodium intake may be restricted and thiazide diuretics prescribed for nephrogenic DI. This depletes sodium and decreases the glomerular filtration rate, which increases the reabsorption of water in the proximal tubules.

PHARMACOLOGY CAPSULE Adverse effects of vasopressin administered as a nasal spray are mucous membrane ulcers, chest tightness, and upper respiratory infections.

NURSING CARE *of the Patient with Diabetes Insipidus*

Assessment

A complete history of the patient's symptoms, medical history, and drug history should be obtained. Monitor for thirst, change in urine appearance or volume, dizziness, weakness, fainting, and palpitations. The physical examination focuses on the symptoms of DI. Assess hydration, including skin turgor, moisture of mucous membranes, pulse rate and quality, blood pressure, and mental status. Maintain records of intake and output, daily weights, and urine specific gravities.

Nursing Diagnoses, Goals, and Outcome Criteria: Diabetes Insipidus

Nursing Diagnoses	Goals and Outcome Criteria
Anxiety related to physical symptoms and diagnosis	Decreased anxiety: patient states anxiety is reduced; appears calm

Disturbed Body Image related to altered function	Adaptation to physical changes: patient adjusts routines to minimize symptoms
Deficient Fluid Volume related to excessive urine output	Normal fluid balance: fluid intake approximately equal to fluid output
Activity Intolerance related to fatigue and weakness	Improved activity tolerance: patient performs activities of daily living without tiring
Ineffective Therapeutic Regimen Management related to lack of understanding of symptom management and treatment of DI	Appropriate self-care: patient describes and demonstrates self-care and self-medication

Interventions

The patient with a pituitary disorder may be experiencing mild to moderate symptoms or may be critically ill. Specific nursing care largely depends on the type of DI, the severity of the symptoms, and the needs identified in the nursing assessment.

Anxiety and Disturbed Body Image

The patient who is able must be allowed adequate time to ventilate feelings and discuss the disorder. Changes in body function can be very disturbing. Assure the patient that some changes can be controlled with proper treatment. Be alert to the patient's emotional status and provide support and make referrals as necessary.

Deficient Fluid Volume

Carefully measure intake and output. When the urine output is excessive, as in DI, the physician may order measurement of output at 15- to 30-minute intervals. Because adequate hydration is essential, administer intravenous fluid replacements as ordered. Encourage oral intake, with the prescribed amount based on the volume of urinary output. In addition, weigh the patient at least once daily to identify significant weight loss secondary to water loss.

In situations in which the patient is experiencing an excessive fluid loss, administer exogenous ADH as ordered (see Table 42-3). Be familiar with routes of administration, side effects, and contraindications associated with the use of these agents. Be aware that reversal of the fluid volume deficit with ADH can result in water intoxication. Continued monitoring of urine output and osmolality is essential.

Activity Intolerance

Extreme fatigue or muscle weakness can interfere with the patient's ability to participate in activities of daily living, such as hygiene and grooming. Frequently assess the functional ability of these patients, and address the amount of assistance required in the patient's care plan.

Ineffective Therapeutic Regimen Management

Patients who require long-term treatment of DI must learn to manage their symptoms and medications. If the patient has difficulty doing this, a family member or friend may be included in the teaching sessions. Some patients are taught to adjust dosages based on urine output, specific gravity (using a hydrometer), and thirst. If the patient's self-care abilities are in doubt, initiate a referral to a home nursing service.

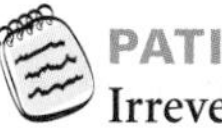

PATIENT TEACHING PLAN
Irreversible Diabetes Insipidus

- Continue your prescribed drug therapy, and notify your physician of any side or adverse effects (provide written details).
- Notify your physician if you have increased urine output, thirst, weight loss, and general feelings of malaise or weakness. You may need additional treatment.
- Prolonged use of nasal sprays can cause ulceration of mucous membranes, chest tightness, upper respiratory infections, and respiratory problems.
- Keep office or clinic appointments to identify any changes in pituitary function.
- Schedule activities and regular rest periods to avoid excessive fatigue.
- Wear a medical alert bracelet.
- Drowsiness, listlessness, and headache are signs of water intoxication, which may result from vasopressin therapy.

Syndrome of Inappropriate Antidiuretic Hormone

Etiology

The syndrome of inappropriate antidiuretic hormone (SIADH) is characterized by a water imbalance related to an increase in ADH synthesis or secretion, or both. Factors that may cause or contribute to the development of SIADH include brain trauma, surgery, tumors, and infection; some drugs, including vasopressin, general anesthetic agents, oral hypoglycemics, and tricyclic antidepressants; some pulmonary diseases; hypothyroidism; lupus erythematosus; and some types of cancer, including oat cell bronchiogenic carcinoma, duodenal cancer, and pancreatic cancer.

Pathophysiology

When ADH is elevated despite normal or low serum osmolality, the kidneys retain excessive water. Plasma volume expands, causing the blood pressure to rise. Body sodium is diluted (hyponatremia), and water intoxication develops. There are several types of SIADH with various patterns of abnormal ADH secretion.

Signs and Symptoms

The main symptoms of SIADH initially reflect the effects of dilutional hyponatremia and water retention: weakness, muscle cramps or twitching, anorexia, nausea, diarrhea, irritability, headache, and weight gain without edema. When the central nervous system is affected by water intoxication, the level of consciousness deteriorates. The patient may have seizures or lapse into a coma.

Medical Diagnosis

The diagnosis of SIADH is confirmed by laboratory tests of serum and urine electrolytes and osmolality. Major characteristics include hyponatremia, hypouricemia, normal or reduced serum creatinine, increased urine sodium, and fluid volume excess without edema. Urine osmolality may be high considering the level of serum osmolality or it may be extremely dilute. Radiographic studies of the brain and lungs also may be done to detect causative factors.

Medical Treatment

The treatment is intended to correct the cause, if possible, and promote elimination of excess water. Acutely ill patients (those with neurologic symptoms and serum sodium of <120 mEq/L) are treated with hypertonic saline given over a 4- to 6-hour period. Once neurologic symptoms resolve, principles of chronic therapy are instituted. One approach is to restrict fluids to 1000 ml/day with a high intake of dietary sodium. Another approach is administration of normal saline with loop diuretics. Patients who cannot adhere to fluid restriction with high sodium intake may be given demeclocycline or lithium carbonate, which block the effects of ADH on the renal tubules thereby increasing water excretion. Adverse effects of these drugs can cause complications (see Table 42-3).

NURSING CARE *of the Patient with Syndrome of Inappropriate Diuretic Hormone*

Assessment

The health history assesses the presence of anorexia, nausea, vomiting, diarrhea, headache, irritability, and muscle cramps and weakness. Record a history of cancer, pulmonary disease, nervous system disorders, hypothyroidism, or lupus erythematosus. Note any prescription drugs the patient is taking. Assess the patient's vital signs, weight, intake and output, and urine specific gravity. Palpate the skin for moisture and edema. Test muscle strength by having the patient grip your hands and push and pull against resistance. Document seizures and muscle weakness, twitching, or cramps. Assess mental status (level of consciousness and orientation) at least every 4 hours in the alert, oriented patient and hourly if there is evidence of impairment.

Nursing Diagnoses, Goals, and Outcome Criteria: SIADH

Nursing Diagnoses	Goals and Outcome Criteria
Risk for Injury related to confusion associated with water intoxication, cerebral edema	Absence of injury: no seizures or associated trauma
Excess Fluid Volume related to excess ADH secretion	Normal fluid balance: normal tissue turgor, fluid intake and output approximately equal
Ineffective Therapeutic Regimen Management related to lack of understanding of management of chronic SIADH	Patient effectively manages prescribed therapy: takes drugs correctly, monitors for and reports adverse effects

Interventions

Risk for Injury

If the patient becomes confused, take measures to ensure safety, including putting the bed in low position and checking on the patient frequently. With cerebral edema, position the patient with the head elevated 30 to 45 degrees or as specified by the physician.

Excess Fluid Volume

Advise the physician of declining neurologic status or weight gain in excess of 2 lb/day. Enforce fluid restrictions, which may be as little as 500 ml/24 hr. Explain the restriction to the patient and family. Remove the large water pitcher. Space fluids over waking hours to reduce thirst and feelings of deprivation. Serve oral fluids in small containers to create the illusion of volume. Encourage frequent mouth care.

Ineffective Therapeutic Regimen Management

Although SIADH is usually temporary, it may not resolve during hospitalization, and the patient may need to learn how to manage the condition at home. Provide verbal and written information about prescribed drugs, dosages, and adverse effects. Be sure the patient has a scale at home.

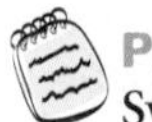

PATIENT TEACHING PLAN
Syndrome of Inappropriate Diuretic Hormone

- Weigh daily and notify the physician if you gain 2 lb or more in one day.
- In addition to weight gain, signs and symptoms of excessive water retention (water intoxication) are drowsiness, listlessness, and headache.
- Do not take any nonprescription drugs without consulting your physician or pharmacist.
- See your physician on a regular basis.
- If taking demeclocycline or lithium carbonate, report adverse effects to your physician (provide specifics).

THE ADRENAL GLANDS

ANATOMY AND PHYSIOLOGY OF THE ADRENAL GLANDS

The adrenal glands are a pair of small, highly vascularized, triangular-shaped organs. They are located in the retroperitoneal cavity on the superior poles of each kidney, lateral to the lower thoracic and upper lumbar vertebrae. Each gland weighs approximately 4 gm and measures 3.3 cm in length. The adrenal gland itself is composed of two parts: an outer portion called the cortex and an inner portion called the medulla. The cortex and medulla have very different, independent functions.

Medulla

The medulla constitutes 10% of the gland and contains sympathetic ganglia (groups of nerve cell bodies) with secretory cells. Stimulation of the sympathetic nervous system causes the medulla to secrete two types of catecholamines: norepinephrine (noradrenaline) and epinephrine (adrenalin). Both of these substances act as neurotransmitters. They are released into the circulation and transported to target organs or tissues, where they exert their effects by binding to adrenergic receptors. Catecholamine effects vary depending on the specific receptor in the cell membrane of the target organ. There are multiple adrenergic receptors including $alpha_1$, $alpha_2$, $beta_1$, and $beta_2$ receptors. Norepinephrine binds to alpha-adrenergic receptors, whereas epinephrine affects primarily beta-adrenergic receptors. Table 42-4 lists the specific effects of these catecholamines and the types of receptors with which they bind. The major function of these substances is adaptation to stress, as characterized by the "fight-or-flight response," and maintenance of homeostasis.

Cortex

The adrenal cortex, which comprises 90% of the adrenal gland, is the outer portion of the gland. This is the portion that is considered to be a part of the endocrine system. The cortex is essential for maintenance of many life-sustaining physiologic activities. The cells of the cortex are organized into three distinct layers or zones. Proceeding from the outermost to innermost layers, they are the zona glomerulosa, zona fasciculata, and zona reticularis. The hormones synthesized and secreted by the cortex are known as steroids and consist of mineralocorticoids, glucocorticoids, and androgens or estrogens.

FUNCTION OF THE ADRENAL GLANDS

Mineralocorticoids

The zona glomerulosa produces mineralocorticoids, the most abundant of which is aldosterone. Mineralocorticoids play a key role in maintaining an adequate extracellular fluid volume. Aldosterone functions at the renal collecting tubule to promote the reabsorption of sodium and the excretion of potassium by the kidney. The secretion of aldosterone is regulated by several factors: serum levels of potassium, the renin-angiotensin mechanism, and ACTH.

Renin, Angiotensin, and Aldosterone

Renin is produced by the juxtaglomerular cells of renal afferent arterioles. Its release is stimulated by a decrease in extracellular fluid volume. Any factor that can cause this decrease (blood or fluid loss, sodium depletion, or changes in body position or posture) can stimulate renin release. Renin acts on plasma proteins to release angiotensin I, which is catalyzed in the lung to angiotensin II. Angiotensin II stimulates the secretion of aldosterone, which results in sodium and water retention. Retention of sodium and water preserves or increases extracellular fluid volume and subsequently increases blood pressure. This compensatory mechanism plays a very important role in maintaining intravascular volume in shock states.

Glucocorticoids

The glucocorticoids are produced by the zona reticularis and zona fasciculata. The most abundant and potent of the glucocorticoids is cortisol. Approximately 92% of circulating cortisol is bound to a plasma protein. Free cortisol (8%) binds with receptors in the cytoplasm and nuclei of target cells. Cortisol has a permissive effect on other physiologic processes, meaning that the glucocorticoid must be present for other processes, such as catecholamine activity and excitability of the myocardium, to occur. Glucocorticoid functions include control of carbohydrate, lipid, and fat metabolism, regulation of anti-inflammatory and immune responses, and control of emotional states by:

- Increasing hepatic gluconeogenesis and inhibiting peripheral glucose use to maintain glucose levels
- Increasing lipolysis and release of glycerol and free fatty acids
- Increasing protein catabolism
- Degrading collagen and connective tissue
- Increasing polymorphonuclear leukocytes released from bone marrow
- Decreasing capillary permeability, movement of white blood cells into the injured tissue, phagocytosis
- Stabilizing lysosomal membranes
- Suppressing lymphocyte reproduction
- Maintaining behavioral and cognitive functions

table 42-4 *Receptors and Effects of Adrenal Medullary Hormones on Selected Organs and Tissues*

ORGAN OR TISSUE	RECEPTOR	EFFECT
Heart	β_1	Positive inotropic action (increases myocardial contractility) Positive chronotropic action (increases heart rate)
Blood vessels	α	Vasoconstriction (except in cardiac and skeletal muscles)
	β_2	Vasodilation
Gastrointestinal tract	α, β	Increased sphincter tone, decreased motility
Kidney	β_2	Increased renin release
Bronchioles	β_2	Relaxation, dilation
Bladder	α	Sphincter contractions, urinary retention
	β_2	Relaxation of detrusor muscle
	α	Increased sweating, piloerection
Adipose tissue	β	Increased lipolysis
Liver	α	Increased gluconeogenesis and glycogenolysis
Pancreas	α	Decreased glucagon and insulin release
	β	Increased glucagon and insulin release
Eyes	α	Dilation of pupuils

Sex Hormones

Adrenal androgens are another class of steroids produced in the zona fasciculata and zona reticularis of the adrenal cortex. Their primary function is masculinization in men. Other sex hormones include estrogen and progesterone. In men, these substances contribute little to reproductive maturation. In women, however, estrogens are supplied by both the ovaries and the adrenal glands. In postmenopausal women, the adrenal cortex is the primary source of endogenous estrogen.

NURSING ASSESSMENT OF THE PATIENT WITH AN ADRENAL DISORDER

Health History

Present Illness

Symptoms of adrenal dysfunction that may cause the patient to seek medical attention include decreased energy, mental changes (depression, anxiety, nervousness, confusion), sexual dysfunction, gastrointestinal disturbances, and abnormal skin pigmentation.

Past Medical History

Aspects of the past medical history that may be significant include radiation to the head or abdomen, intracranial surgery, and recent and current medications. Tuberculosis is the most common cause of primary adrenal insufficiency.

Review of Systems

Assess the patient's perception of his or her general state of health. Ask about changes in skin color, especially bronzed or smoky pigmentation, and increased facial hair in women. Note changes in weight and appetite. Symptoms that may be related to adrenal dysfunction are headache, lightheadedness with position changes, muscle weakness, nausea, vomiting, abdominal pain, anorexia, menstrual dysfunction, and erectile dysfunction.

Functional Assessment

Document usual dietary and activity patterns and disruptions in lifestyle.

Physical Examination

Measure the patient's height, weight, and vital signs. Take the blood pressure when the patient is reclining and after the patient has moved to an upright position to detect a significant drop. Note patient responses and ability to follow instructions. Inspect the skin for a bronzed or smoky pigmentation (especially in surgical scars, the skin over the knuckles, in skinfolds, and the areola), bruising, petechiae, vitiligo (loss of pigmentation), and pallor. Inspect the face of the female patient for excess facial hair. Examine the oral mucous membranes for color changes. Inspect the anterior thorax for fat pads under the clavicles, and the posterior thorax for the "buffalo hump." Note obesity of the trunk. Examine the breasts for striae and darkening of the areola. Inspect the abdomen for striae, and the extremities for muscle wasting and edema. During examination of the external genitalia assess for atrophy, hair loss, and appropriateness for age.

Assessment of the patient with an adrenal disorder is summarized in Table 42-5.

table 42-5 ASSESSMENT *of the Patient with an Adrenal Disorder*

HEALTH HISTORY

Present Illness: Decreased energy, mental changes, sexual dysfunction, gastrointestinal disturbances, abnormal skin pigmentation

Past Medical History: Radiation to head or abdomen, intracranial surgery, recent and current medications

Review of Systems: General well-being, bronzed or smoky skin color, increased facial hair in women, headache, lightheadedness with position changes, muscle weakness, nausea, vomiting, abdominal pain, anorexia, menstrual dysfunction, erectile dysfunction

Functional Assessment: Changes in height and weight, changes in diet, salt craving, disruption of lifestyle by symptoms

PHYSICAL EXAMINATION

Height and Weight

Vital Signs

Mental Status

Skin: Smoky or bronzed pigmentation prominent on surgical scars, knuckles, in skin folds, areola; bruising, petechiae, vitiligo, pallor

Head and Face: Excess facial hair

Mouth: Color change of oral mucous membranes

Thorax: Supraclavicular fat pads, "buffalo hump"

Trunk: Obesity

Breasts: Striae, darkening of areola

Abdomen: Striae

Extremities: Muscle wasting, edema

Genitalia: Atrophy, loss of hair, appropriate development for age

AGE-RELATED CHANGES

Under normal circumstances, adrenal function remains adequate in the older person. Some patients have a decline in cortisol secretion, but this is balanced by a decrease in cortisol metabolism such that blood levels remain normal. Secretion of aldosterone and plasma renin activity decline with age, and thus the abilities to conserve sodium and adapt to position changes become less efficient.

DIAGNOSTIC TESTS AND PROCEDURES

Because only two deviations from normal adrenal function are covered here, the appropriate diagnostic tests and procedures are discussed with each condition.

DISORDERS OF THE ADRENAL GLANDS

Adrenal Hypofunction

Etiology

Adrenal insufficiency may be classified as either primary or secondary. Primary adrenal insufficiency, which is also called *Addison's disease,* is frequently due to a destructive disease process affecting the adrenal glands that results in deficiencies of cortisol and aldosterone. The most common cause of Ad-

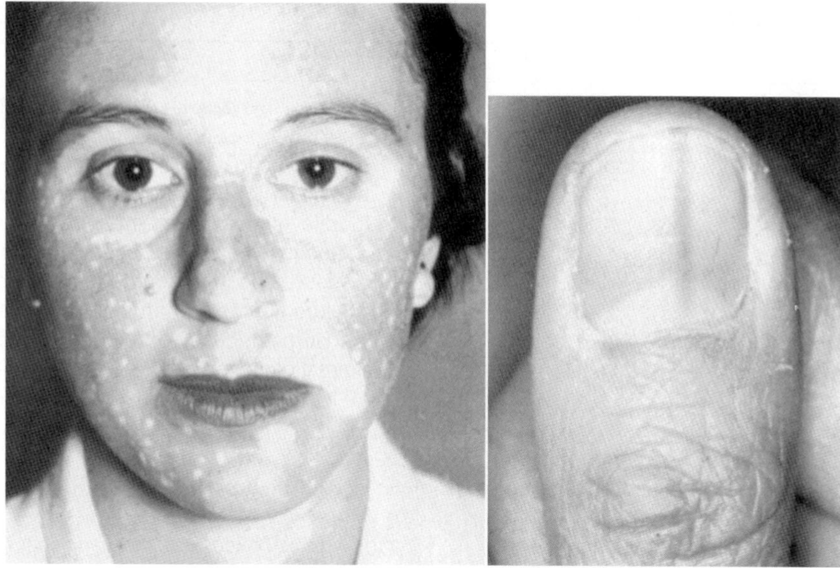

FIGURE **42-6** The increased pigmentation seen in primary adrenocortical insufficiency.

dison's disease is idiopathic atrophy, an autoimmune disease in which adrenal tissue is destroyed by antibodies formed by the patient's own immune system. Other causes of Addison's disease are tuberculosis, hemorrhage related to anticoagulant therapy, fungal infections (histoplasmosis, coccidioidomycosis), acquired immunodeficiency syndrome, metastatic cancer, gram-negative sepsis (Waterhouse-Friderichsen syndrome), adrenalectomy, adrenal toxins, and abrupt withdrawal of exogenous steroids.

Secondary adrenal insufficiency is a result of dysfunction of the hypothalamus or pituitary (decreased corticotropin, ACTH), which leads to decreased androgen and cortisol production. Unlike primary adrenal insufficiency, in which all steroids are affected, aldosterone may or may not be affected. Causes of secondary adrenal insufficiency include pituitary tumors, postpartum necrosis of the pituitary (Sheehan's syndrome), hypophysectomy, radiation therapy, pituitary or intracranial lesions, or high-dose, long-term glucocorticoid treatment, which suppresses the adrenal glands' intrinsic activity.

Pathophysiology

Insufficiency of adrenocortical steroids causes defects associated with the loss of mineralocorticoids and glucocorticoids. Impaired secretion of cortisol results in decreased gluconeogenesis and decreased liver and muscle glycogen. This in turn decreases supplies of available glucose, causing hypoglycemia. In addition, the glomerular filtration rate of the kidneys and gastric acid production by the parietal cells of the stomach both slow significantly. The cumulative effects of these processes cause decreased urea nitrogen excretion, irritability, anorexia, weight loss, nausea, vomiting, and diarrhea.

Decreased levels of aldosterone alter the clearance of potassium, water, and sodium by the kidney. Potassium excretion is decreased, and hyperkalemia may occur. Because hyperkalemia promotes hydrogen ion retention, metabolic acidosis also can occur. Hypovolemia and hyponatremia may result from accelerated sodium and water excretion.

Other manifestations of adrenal insufficiency are progressive weakness, lethargy, unexplained abdominal pain, and malaise. Skin hyperpigmentation, particularly in sun-exposed areas, pressure points, joints, and creases of the body, is another possible sign. It is most likely due to increased secretion of a beta-lipoprotein or a melanocyte-stimulating hormone, which is released by a part of the pituitary. This is a direct result of hypocortisolism and a lack of negative feedback (Fig. 42-6).

If adrenal androgen levels are lowered, there may be a decrease or loss of body, axillary, and pubic hair. In prepubescent people, facial, pubic, and axillary hair may fail to grow entirely. The severity of these symptoms is linked to the degree of hormone deficiency. This lack of secondary sex characteristics tends to be seen in primary adrenal insufficiency rather than in secondary adrenal insufficiency.

Symptoms of chronic insufficiency are generally less dramatic and life-threatening than symptoms presented during acute adrenal crisis. Acute adrenal crisis is discussed later in this section.

Put on your THINKING CAP!!

Explain how a pituitary disorder could cause adrenal insufficiency.

Acute adrenal crisis (addisonian crisis). Patients with either primary or secondary adrenal insufficiency are at risk for episodes of acute adrenal crisis, also called addisonian crisis, which is a life-threatening emergency. This usually results from a sudden marked decrease in available adrenal hormones. Precipitating factors are adrenal surgery, pituitary destruction, abrupt withdrawal of steroid therapy (often a result of a patient unwittingly stopping medications), and stress. Any factor that causes stress in the person can initiate a crisis. Examples of stressors include infection, illness, trauma, and emotional or psychiatric disturbances.

table 42-6 ***Emergency Medical Care: Acute Adrenal Crisis***

INTERVENTION	RATIONALE
1. Complete blood count, electrolytes, blood urea nitrogen, plasma cortisol levels.	1. To establish a baseline and obtain data for diagnosis and treatment.
2. Initial dose of hydrocortisone (Solu-Cortef) IV push, followed by infusion over 8 hr.	2. To provide a loading dose and maintenance infusion. The half-life of IV hydrocortisone is 60-90 minutes so blood level must be maintained by continuous infusion. If blood level falls, the patient may have a relapse.
3. Concomitant doses of hydrocortisone IM every 12 hr as ordered by physician.	3. To ensure constant source of glucocorticoids in case of IV failure (infiltration infusion phlebitis).
4. After resolution of crisis, medications and dosage adjusted to include: a. Oral glucocorticoids started. b. Decreased dosage of oral glucocorticoids over several days as maintenance levels are reached. c. Supplemental mineralocorticoids as glucocorticoid dosage is tapered.	4. To ensure adequacy of mineralocorticoid activity with minimal glucocorticoid dose.
5. Provide emotional support to patient and family.	5. To minimize excess anxiety and fear during a crisis period

Modified from Ignatavicius, D. D., Workman, M. L., & Mishler, M. (1999). *Medical-surgical nursing across the health care continuum* (3rd ed., p. 1602). Philadelphia: Saunders.
IV, Intravenous; *IM,* intramuscular.

PHARMACOLOGY CAPSULE When steroid therapy is discontinued, the drug is tapered gradually. An abrupt decline in adrenal hormones could precipitate acute adrenal crisis.

Manifestations of an addisonian crisis include symptoms of mineralocorticoid and glucocorticoid deficiency but are more severe: hypotension, tachycardia, dehydration, confusion, hyponatremia, hyperkalemia, hypercalcemia, and hypoglycemia. If left untreated, fluid and electrolyte imbalances can lead to circulatory collapse, cardiac arrhythmias, cardiac arrest, coma, and death. The management of an addisonian crisis is outlined in Table 42-6.

Medical Diagnosis

Laboratory studies. In addition to the presence of various clinical signs and symptoms, the diagnosis of Addison's disease is made on the basis of a variety of laboratory findings, including a low serum cortisol level, decreased fasting glucose, decreased sodium, and increased potassium and blood urea nitrogen. In addition, 24-hour urine tests may be performed. This type of testing reflects steroid secretion over a 24-hour period and is the most accurate measurement of steroid secretion, which varies with the diurnal rhythm. Urinary 17-hydroxycorticosteroids also are sometimes measured as an indicator of glucocorticoid metabolites and are specific for this category of steroids. Androgen metabolites can be determined by measurement of 17-ketosteroids. Both of these substances are low or borderline low in adrenal hypofunction. See Table 42-7 for a list of drugs that interfere with urine tests for 17-hydroxycorticosteroids and 17-ketosteroids.

table 42-7 ***Drugs that Interfere with Urine Tests for 17-Hydroxycorticosteroids and 17-Ketosteroids***

Acetaminophen	Medroxyprogesterone
Acetazolamide	Meperidine
Acetylsalicylic acid	Metyrapone
Amphetamines	Mitotane
Ascorbic acid	Morphine
Barbiturates	Nalidixic acid
Calcium gluconate	Oral contraceptives
Carbon disulfide	Paraldehyde
Chloral hydrate	Penicillin
Chlordiazepoxide	Pentazocine
Chlorthalidone	Perphenazine
Colchicine	Phenobarbital
Corticotropin	Phenothiazines
Cortisone	Phenylbutazone
Dexamethasone	Phenytoin
Diazepam	Promazine
Digoxin	Propoxyphene
Diphenhydramine	Quinidine
Erythromycin	Quinine
Estrogens	Reserpine
Fructose	Secobarbital
Glutethimide	Spironolactone
Hydralazine	Testosterone
Iodides	Vitamin K

Modified from Ignatavicius, D. D., Workman, M. L., & Mishler, M. (1999). *Medical-surgical nursing: A nursing process approach* (3rd ed., p. 1604). Philadelphia: Saunders.

Measurement of plasma ACTH concentration before treatment is begun helps to define the basis of the patient's symptoms. If the plasma ACTH level is low, the pituitary is at fault for not producing adequate ACTH. An increased plasma ACTH level suggests that the adrenals are at fault because they are unable to respond to stimulation to produce corticoids. An ACTH stimulation test is necessary for a definitive diagnosis of hypoadrenalism. One common technique used in this test is the administration of a dose of synthetic ACTH (cosyntropin), which is given intramuscularly. Plasma cortisol levels are measured at onset of administration and at 30 and 60 minutes after administration. In primary adrenal insufficiency, the cortisol response is absent or markedly decreased. In secondary insufficiency, there is a decrease in serum cortisol levels; however, it is not as significant a decrease as in cases of primary insufficiency. An eosinophil count may be performed during ACTH stimulation. The eosinophil count drops significantly after ACTH administration in normal people. Patients with Addison's disease show little or no change in the number of circulating eosinophils. If a glucose fasting test is performed, the serum glucose does not rise as high as it would in normal people and returns to a fasting level more rapidly.

Electrocardiogram. Alterations in electrolyte levels often are reflected as deviations in the normal electrocardiogram. For example, hyperkalemia results in peaked T waves, a widened QRS interval, and an increased PR interval.

Radiographic studies. Skull films, arteriograms, and CT scans may be performed to rule out causative factors in secondary adrenal insufficiency. They may reveal intracranial lesions that impinge on the pituitary, aneurysms, or other defects. An abdominal CT scan may detect atrophy of the adrenal glands and identify a possible cause of primary insufficiency.

Medical Treatment

The mainstay of treatment of patients with Addison's disease is replacement therapy with glucocorticoids and mineralocorticoids. Glucocorticoids, such as cortisone, are typically divided into doses: two thirds of a daily dose is taken in the morning and one third in the evening. This dosage schedule is based on human hormonal variations. Glucocorticoids normally peak in the early morning and are at their lowest level in the evening. A mineralocorticoid (fludrocortisone), if needed, is typically given in the afternoon or evening. See Table 42-8 for drug therapy details. Some glucocorticoids have mineralocorticoid effects also.

Secondary adrenal insufficiency is treated with glucocorticoids, but mineralocorticoids are usually unnecessary.

PHARMACOLOGY CAPSULE Addison's disease is treated with glucocorticoids given in divided doses to mimic the body's normal hormonal cycles.

NURSING CARE *of the Patient with Addison's Disease*

Assessment

Assessment of the patient with an adrenal disorder is summarized in Table 42-5 (see also Nursing Care Plan: The Patient with Addison's Disease). Details of the health history that are especially relevant to Addison's disease are weight loss, salt craving, nausea and vomiting, abdominal cramping and diarrhea, muscle weakness and aches, poor stress response, decreased libido, and amenorrhea. The patient may be irritable or confused. The physical examination may reveal pale skin with bronzed areas, emaciation, sparse body hair, poor skin turgor, hypotension, and muscle wasting. The patient with acute episodes of Addison's disease requires frequent reassessment, monitoring of fluid and electrolyte levels, and measurement of daily weights.

Nursing Diagnoses, Goals, and Outcome Criteria: Addison's Disease

Nursing Diagnoses	Goals and Outcome Criteria
Ineffective Tissue Perfusion related to electrolyte imbalance, hypovolemia, cardiac dysrhythmias	Improved tissue perfusion: warm, dry skin with strong peripheral pulses
Risk for Injury related to acute adrenal insufficiency, postural hypotension, impaired physiologic response to stress	Decreased risk for injury: blood pressure within patient norms, absence of faintness with position changes
Imbalanced Nutrition: Less than Body Requirements related to impaired metabolism, inability to ingest sufficient nutrients, lack of interest in eating	Adequate nutrition: weight within 5 pounds of patient's baseline
Fatigue related to fluid, electrolyte, and glucose imbalances	Improved stamina: patient states fatigue is lessened, performs activities of daily living without tiring
Disturbed Body Image related to changes in appearance and function	Adaptation to physical changes: patient efforts to improve appearance, positive comments about self
Ineffective Therapeutic Regimen Management of long-term glucocorticoid and mineralocorticoid replacement therapy	Patient manages self-care and prescribed treatment: patient explains disease process and treatment with stated intent to adhere to prescribed regimen

Interventions

Ineffective Tissue Perfusion

Monitor for signs and symptoms of inadequate tissue perfusion: confusion, disorientation, tachycardia, apical-radial pulse deficit, general weakness and malaise, and hypotension (including postural changes). Administer prescribed intravenous normal saline, plasma expanders, and vasopressors to maintain blood volume. The patient whose fluid output is greater than intake is at risk for hypovolemia. Because the patient is at risk for hyperkalemia, monitor serum electrolytes and assess for weakness, paresthesia, dizziness, and electrocardiogram changes. Promptly report these signs and symptoms of hyperkalemia to the physician.

Risk for Injury

Assess the patient for postural hypotension and other signs of hypovolemia. Instruct the patient who has dizziness with position changes to call for help when getting out of bed and to rise slowly to prevent falls. Exercising the legs before standing promotes venous return and may minimize the drop in blood pressure.

table 42-8 **DRUG THERAPY | *Adrenal Disorders***

DRUG	USE/ACTION	SIDE EFFECTS	NURSING INTERVENTIONS
GLUCOCORTICOIDS			
Cortisone acetate (Cortone Acetate) Prednisolone (Delta-Cortef, Prelone) Prednisolone acetate (Econopred) Hydrocortisone (Cortef)	All stimulate formation of glucose, promote storage of glucose as glycogen, affect fluid and electrolytes, increase hemoglobin, suppress inflammation. Used to treat adrenal insufficiency. Some have mineralocorticoid effects also.	All: hypokalemia, hypocalcemia, nausea and vomiting, edema, hypertension, increased risk of infection, hyperglycemia, muscle wasting, osteoporosis, ulcer development, acne, pathologic fractures. May cause death if suddenly discontinued.	Monitor weight, intake and output, BP, blood glucose. Assess for edema. Protect from sources of infection. Report signs of infection even if subtle. Assess for hypocalcemia: muscle weakness and twitching. Assess for hypokalemia: muscle weakness and tingling, cardiac dysrhythmias, irritability. Protect from falls and possible fractures. Give oral drugs with food or milk. Many patients with adrenal insufficiency manage with only glucocorticoids.
MINERALOCORTICOIDS			
Fludrocortisone (Florinef Acetate)	Stimulate reabsorption of sodium and excretion of potassium and hydrogen ions in renal tubules. Used to treat adrenal insufficiency.	Hypokalemia, nausea and vomiting, edema, hypertension, muscle weakness, dizziness, tendon contractures, congestive heart failure.	Monitor weight, intake and output, BP, heart rate and rhythm, serum electrolytes. Assess for hypokalemia-prescribed sodium intake. Do not discontinue suddenly. Tell patient to carry drug identification card.
ADRENOCORTICAL CYTOTOXIC AGENTS			
Mitotane (Lysodren)	Suppress adrenocortical function.	Nausea and vomiting, diarrhea, lethargy, dizziness, hypouricemia, hearing and vision disturbances, BP changes, dyspnea.	Monitor BP. Report infections or trauma so drug can be temporarily discontinued. Tell patient not to have immunizations without physician approval and to avoid contact with people who have recently had polio vaccine. Increase fluid intake and monitor uric acid.
ANTIFUNGAL AGENTS			
Ketoconazole (Nizoral)	Fungistatic. Suppresses adrenocortical function.	Nausea and vomiting, pruritus, diarrhea or constipation, GI bleeding, lethargy, headache, dizziness, adrenocortical insufficiency. Occasionally, thrombocytopenia, hemolytic anemia, hepatotoxicity.	Monitor stools. Administer antipruritics or apply topical agents as ordered. Safety measures if dizzy or drowsy. Monitor liver function tests and assess for pale stools, dark urine, fatigue, and anorexia. Avoid alcohol.

BP, Blood pressure; *GI,* gastrointestinal.

Sudden profound weakness with postural hypotension is characteristic of acute addisonian crisis and leads to shock and death if not corrected. Administer fluid replacement and hormones as ordered to treat addisonian crisis.

Imbalanced Nutrition: Less than Body Requirements

Weigh the patient daily to monitor fluid balance. Weight changes also provide information about the adequacy of the patient's diet. If nutrition is a problem, consult the dietitian. The prescribed diet is usually high protein, low carbohydrate. Salt may be used liberally because patients with Addison's disease tend to lose sodium. Respect the patient's food preferences as much as possible. The mealtime atmosphere should be conducive to eating.

Hypoglycemia may develop as a result of decreased cortisol secretion. Encourage frequent rest periods to avoid depletion of glycogen stores. Meals should be taken regularly, and between-meal snacks may be needed to maintain blood glucose. Monitor for and teach the patient symptoms of hypoglycemia: headache, tachycardia, trembling, sweating. Periodic laboratory studies are done to assess nitrogen balance,

NURSING CARE PLAN

The Patient with Addison's Disease

ASSESSMENT

Health History: A 52-year-old white man is admitted with Addison's disease. He considers himself healthy but has had some joint pain in his knees. He had an appendectomy 20 years ago. The patient complains of weight loss, anorexia, weakness, and darkening of the skin on his face and arms. His usual weight is 170 pounds. He has had bouts of nausea, vomiting, and diarrhea accompanied by vague abdominal pain. The patient is a salesman and reports that his symptoms are making it difficult for him to keep up with his work. He is embarrassed about the change in his skin color.

Physical Examination: Vital signs: blood pressure, 110/80 (sitting) and 88/42 (standing); pulse, 102 with slight irregularity; respiration, 20; temperature, 98° F orally. Height, 5'8". Weight, 155 lb. The patient is oriented but somewhat lethargic. The skin on his face and arms and his abdominal scar is darkly pigmented. His body hair is sparse. The patient's oral mucous membranes are slightly dry.

Nursing Diagnosis	*Goals and Outcome Criteria*	*Interventions*
Ineffective tissue perfusion related to electrolyte imbalance, fluid volume deficit, and cardiac dysrhythmias.	The patient will have improved tissue perfusion as evidenced by warm, dry skin, strong peripheral pulses, and fluid output equal to fluid intake.	Monitor for signs and symptoms of inadequate tissue perfusion: confusion, disorientation, tachycardia, hypotension, apical-radial pulse deficit, fluid output exceeding intake. Administer intravenous fluids (normal saline, plasma expanders) and vasopressors, as ordered. Monitor for hyperkalemia: weakness, paresthesia, and dizziness. Report evidence of inadequate tissue perfusion or hyperkalemia to physician.
Risk for injury related to acute adrenal insufficiency, impaired stress response, postural hypotension.	The patient will remain free of injury due to hypotension, shock, or falls.	Monitor for postural hypotension. If the patient has dizziness with position changes, instruct him to exercise his legs before rising, to rise slowly, and to call for help when getting out of bed. Administer fluids and hormones as ordered.
Imbalanced nutrition: less than body requirements related to impaired metabolism, inability to ingest sufficient nutrients, and lack of interest in eating.	The patient will be adequately nourished as evidenced by weight within 5 pounds of baseline.	Weigh daily to monitor fluid balance and nutritional status. Request dietary consult for patient education and so that food preferences can be respected. Provide high-protein, low-carbohydrate diet as ordered. Tell the patient salt may be used freely. Provide a pleasant atmosphere for meals. Report signs of hypoglycemia: headache, trembling, tachycardia, sweating.
Fatigue related to fluid, electrolyte, and glucose imbalances.	The patient will report improved stamina.	Explain medically prescribed activity limitations. Plan care to allow for periods of rest. Discuss energy conservation after discharge.
Disturbed body image related to changes in appearance and function.	The patient will adapt to altered physical appearance and function as evidenced by efforts to improve appearance and positive comments about self.	Explore how the patient feels about skin changes. Discuss strategies to deal with changes: long sleeves, avoidance of excess sunlight. Advise to arrange work with rest periods. Encourage attention to grooming. Compliment efforts.
Ineffective therapeutic regimen management related to lack of understanding of long-term glucocorticoid therapy.	The patient will manage self-care and prescribed treatment; correctly explain the disease, its treatment, and medication therapy; will state intent to adhere to prescribed regimen.	Implement teaching plan, to include the following: Patient Teaching Plan: Addison's Disease • Wear a medical alert tag and carry emergency kit with dexamethasone. • Take glucocorticoid in divided doses in morning and afternoon with food. • Increase medication dosage as ordered when under stress. • Notify physician or go to emergency room if unable to take oral medications for more than 24 hours. • Lifelong therapy and monitoring are needed. • Report signs and symptoms of inadequate and excessive hormone replacement.

liver function, and serum albumin, glucose, electrolytes, blood urea nitrogen, and creatinine.

Fatigue

Explain any prescribed activity limitations to the patient. Plan specific rest periods to conserve energy. Provide assistance with activities of daily living as needed. If the patient is on bedrest, intervene to prevent complications of immobility as described in Chapter 20.

Disturbed Body Image

Explore the patient's reaction to the physical changes experienced. Discuss strategies to cope with changes. When the patient's condition has stabilized, encourage attention to grooming and compliment the patient's efforts.

Ineffective Management of Treatment Regimen

Care of the patient with a chronic disease requires in-depth education and information about stress management. It is critical for the patient to understand Addison's disease and to know how to recognize the effects of the disease as well as those of overmedication. Provide written material to supplement the teaching sessions.

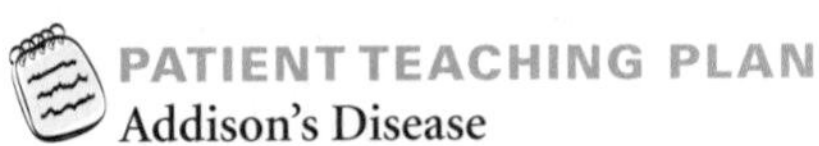

PATIENT TEACHING PLAN
Addison's Disease

- *Never* stop taking prescribed medications unless advised and monitored by your physician; you will need lifelong cortisol replacement therapy.
- Take glucocorticoids as ordered in divided doses, one dose in the morning and the other in the afternoon.
- Take glucocorticoids with food.
- Increase the dosage as directed by the physician if you have severe emotional stress or increased physical demands, including pregnancy, surgery, or an acute illness.
- If you are unable to take your oral medicine for more than a day, notify your physician or go to an emergency room so that you can be given your medication by injection.
- Always wear a medical alert tag and carry an emergency kit with a dose of dexamethasone to be administered in the event of acute addisonian crisis.

Adrenal Hypersecretion (Cushing's Syndrome)

Etiology

Hypersecretion of the adrenal cortex may result in the production of excess amounts of corticosteroids, particularly glucocorticoid. The condition that results from excessive cortisol is called *Cushing's syndrome.* The overproduction of adrenocortical hormones may result from endogenous (internal) as well as exogenous (external) causes.

Endogenous causes include corticotropin-secreting pituitary tumors, a cortisol-secreting neoplasm within the adrenal glands, and excess secretion of corticotropin by a carcinoma of the lung or other tissues. Excessive production of ACTH because of a pituitary tumor is called *Cushing's disease.* The incidence of Cushing's syndrome caused by disease is infrequent, affecting women eight times more often than men. Approximately 25% of cases of Cushing's syndrome are due to adrenal tumors.

The single exogenous cause of Cushing's syndrome is prolonged administration of high doses of corticosteroids. This is also the most common cause of Cushing's syndrome.

Pathophysiology

Clinical manifestations of Cushing's syndrome affect most body systems and are related to excess levels of circulating corticosteroids. In some instances, signs and symptoms of mineralocorticoid and androgen excess may appear; however, signs and symptoms of glucocorticoid excess usually predominate.

Hyperadrenalism produces marked changes in the personal appearance of the affected person, including obesity, facial redness, hirsutism (excess hair), menstrual disorders, hypertension of varying degrees, and muscle wasting of the extremities (Fig. 42-7). Additional findings can be delayed wound healing, insomnia, irrational behavior, and mood disturbances such as irritability and anxiety. The hallmark findings that lead to a diagnosis of Cushing's syndrome are:

Truncal obesity (excess adipose in body trunk)

Protein wasting (slender extremities and very thin and friable skin)

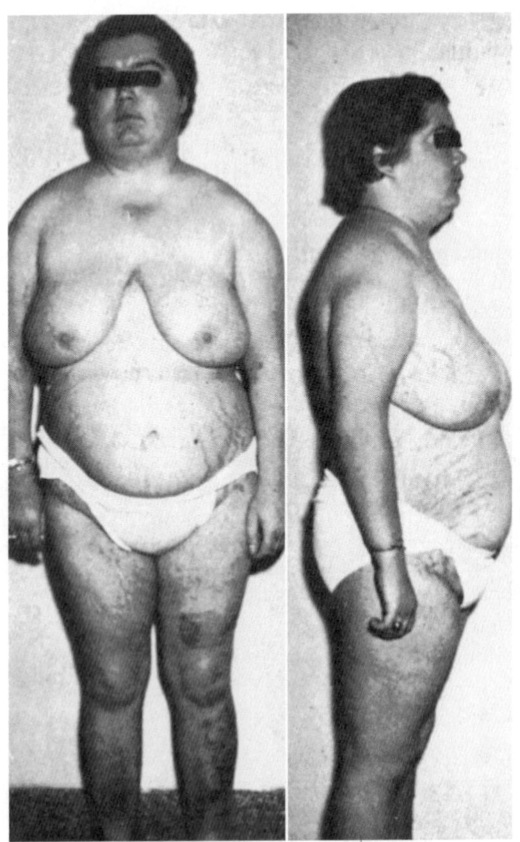

FIGURE **42-7** Clinical manifestations in the patient with Cushing's syndrome.

Facial fullness, often called a "moon face"
Purple striae on the abdomen, breasts, buttocks, or thighs
Osteoporosis (a significant finding in premenopausal women)
Hypokalemia of uncertain etiology

Medical Diagnosis

In addition to physical signs and symptoms, some laboratory, radiographic, and imaging results may be useful in determining a diagnosis.

Laboratory studies. Abnormal laboratory findings include polycythemia, hypokalemia, hypernatremia, hyperglycemia, leukocytosis, glycosuria, hypocalcemia, and elevated plasma cortisol. ACTH may be high or low depending on whether the basic problem lies in the adrenals or in the pituitary. In some cases, malignant tumors, especially small cell cancer of the lung, can secrete ACTH, which stimulates excess cortisol secretion.

The overnight dexamethasone test is used as an initial screening for Cushing's syndrome. Patients are instructed not to take any medications for 2 days because some drugs can interfere with results. At midnight on the first day of testing, the patient receives oral dexamethasone. The following morning, the plasma cortisol levels are measured. A normal finding is a serum level of less than 5 mg/dL. If the level is higher, a dexamethasone suppression test using a low dose may be given. For this test, the patient is again instructed to avoid certain medications (see Table 42-7) and to avoid excess stress. On day 1 of the test, a baseline 24-hour urine sample is collected. Dexamethasone is then administered every 6 hours, and 24-hour urine collections are taken on day 2 and again on day 3. The urine is tested for 17-ketosteroids, 17-hydroxycorticosteroids, creatinine, and free cortisol. In normal people, the cortisol and 17-hydroxycorticosteroid levels are suppressed. If these levels are not suppressed (compared with the baseline sample), the test is repeated using a higher dose of dexamethasone.

Radiographic studies. If a tumor is suspected as a causative factor in Cushing's syndrome, a CT scan and magnetic resonance imaging may be done to localize the site of the tumor. Radiographic films also may reveal osteoporosis of the spinal column, especially in women.

Medical Treatment

Depending on the specific patient and the etiology of the disease, a combination of therapies may be used. These include drug therapy, radiation, and surgery. If Cushing's syndrome is caused by administration of synthetic glucocorticoids, the physician may gradually withdraw them. Most patients affected with hyperadrenalism due to a single benign adrenal tumor undergo surgical intervention. Bilateral benign tumors more often are treated with an aldosterone antagonist, that is, a drug that reduces aldosterone secretion or blocks its effects. An example of an aldosterone antagonist is the potassium-sparing diuretic spironolactone (Aldactone). Patients with metastatic adrenal cancer are usually treated with surgery and chemotherapy. However, a cure for metastatic adrenal cancer is yet to be found. When Cushing's syndrome is caused by a pituitary tumor, removal of part of the pituitary may reduce ACTH secretion without disturbing other pituitary functions. If this fails, the remaining pituitary tissue may be removed.

Drug therapy. In situations in which it is not feasible for the patient to undergo surgery, certain agents that interfere with ACTH production or adrenal hormone synthesis may be administered. One example is mitotane (Lysodren), a cytotoxic substance that is used as a palliative treatment for inoperable adrenal tumors. Agents that interfere with cortisol production include ketoconazole (Nizoral), aminoglutethimide (Cytadren), and metyrapone (Metopirone). Metyrapone is also used in combination with mitotane for enhanced effects. There is a risk of acute adrenal crisis when patients are on drugs that suppress adrenal function. In addition, the drugs must be promptly discontinued if trauma or shock occurs because the patient's ability to adapt is diminished. Table 42-8 provides additional information about drug therapy.

PHARMACOLOGY CAPSULE Drugs that suppress adrenal function can lead to acute adrenal crisis and must be promptly discontinued if shock or trauma occurs.

Radiation. In cases in which a pituitary adenoma causes excessive secretion of ACTH, the adenoma may be treated with radiation therapy. Radiation can be administered either externally or internally. Internal radiation involves the transsphenoidal implantation of a radioactive material that remains in place for a specified period of time. Radiation therapy is not always effective and can destroy healthy tissue. If radiation therapy is being used to treat a patient with a pituitary adenoma, you must be alert for any significant changes in the patient's neurologic status, such as a complaint of headache or a change in mentation or pupillary responses. In addition, the patient may experience side effects associated with radiation therapy. These include alopecia (hair loss) and dry, red, or irritated skin. The patient must be educated about these drug effects.

Surgical Management

The surgical treatment of hyperadrenalism depends on the specific cause of the disorder. For example, if adrenal hypersecretion is due to a pituitary adenoma that is producing ACTH, a transsphenoidal hypophysectomy is performed (see Surgical Management in the section on Hyperpituitarism, earlier in this chapter). If adrenal adenoma or carcinoma is the cause of the adrenal hypersecretion, an adrenalectomy (removal of the adrenal gland) is performed. If only one gland is removed, the procedure is referred to as a unilateral adrenalectomy; the removal of both of the glands is called a bilateral adrenalectomy. An adrenalectomy may be performed in situations in which drug and radiation therapy are unsuccessful. Patients who are undergoing a unilateral adrenalectomy can expect to require replacement therapy for up to 2 years after surgery. A bilateral adrenalectomy necessitates lifelong replacement of both glucocorticoid and mineralocorticoids. Depending on the tumor size, a laparoscopic procedure may be an option. Surgery and chemotherapy are indicated for metastatic adrenal cancer. These treatments may induce remission but are not curative.

NURSING CARE *of the Patient with Cushing's Syndrome*

Assessment

Initial assessment of the patient with Cushing's syndrome includes a detailed history and physical examination. Obtain specific information about the onset of symptoms, prior treatments, drug allergies, and current medications. The complete nursing assessment of the patient with an adrenal disorder is summarized in Table 42-5.

Nursing Diagnoses, Goals, and Outcome Criteria: Cushing's Syndrome

Nursing Diagnoses	Goals and Outcome Criteria
Risk for Infection related to high serum cortisol levels	Absence of infection: normal body temperature and white blood cell count
Disturbed Thought Processes related to fluid and electrolyte imbalance	Normal thought processes: stable mood, patient denial of depression
Risk for Impaired Skin Integrity related to changes in skin and connective tissue and edema	Absence of injury to skin: skin intact with minimal or no bruising
Risk for Injury (fracture) related to osteoporosis	Absence of fractures: no skeletal trauma or fractures
Disturbed Body Image related to changes in physical appearance and function	Adaptation to altered body image: patient attends to appearance, grooming; makes positive comments about self
Ineffective Therapeutic Regimen Management related to lack of understanding of disease, drug therapy, diet, and self-care	Patient follows prescribed treatment: verbalizes and demonstrates self-care; condition stabilizes

Interventions

Risk for Infection

Exposure to people with infections should be avoided because of the patient's decreased resistance to infection. Minor symptoms, such as a low-grade fever (99.5° F or higher), sore throat, or aches, can indicate the onset of a potentially serious infection. Any symptoms indicative of a cold or other problem should be brought to the attention of the physician.

Disturbed Thought Processes

Personality changes often accompany adrenal disorders. When they do occur, discuss them with the patient and the family. Understanding that mood swings are a part of this disorder may help the patient and family cope more effectively. If the emotional changes, particularly depression, become severe, carefully monitor the patient. A psychiatric referral may be necessary.

Risk for Impaired Skin Integrity

The skin of the patient with Cushing's syndrome is extremely fragile. Inspect the skin daily to detect early signs of pressure or injuries. Assist the patient with limited mobility to change positions at least every 2 hours. Keep bed linens clean and dry. Advise the patient to wear shoes when out of bed to reduce the risk of foot injuries. During transfers and position changes, be careful to prevent trauma to the skin.

Risk for Injury

Because fractures occur very easily, protect the patient with Cushing's syndrome from falls or trauma. Keep the bed in low position and the call button within reach. If the patient is very weak or confused, raise the side rails. Instruct the patient to call for assistance when getting in and out of bed.

Disturbed Body Image

Bruises, abnormal fat distribution, and hirsutism may cause embarrassment to the patient. Provide an opportunity for the patient to share thoughts and concerns about these changes. If they are distressing, suggest clothing to conceal them. Encourage and assist patients to be well groomed. Women may choose to shave or to use depilatories to remove unwanted hair. Reassure the patient that physical changes usually improve gradually after medical or surgical treatment.

Ineffective Therapeutic Regimen Management

To manage Cushing's syndrome, the patient must understand the condition, complications, treatment, and self-care. Provide written information to supplement verbal teaching about drugs, including drug names and dosages, schedules, and adverse effects. A referral may be made to the dietitian for nutritional counseling. The diet is typically low in calories with sufficient protein and calcium. The following patient teaching plan includes the key patient teaching points.

PATIENT TEACHING PLAN
Cushing's Syndrome

- Avoid people with infections because you have increased risk of infections; report any temperature elevation to your physician.
- Mood swings and changes in appearance are usually corrected with treatment.
- Avoid activities that could result in trauma because you have increased risk of bleeding and fractures.
- It is critical that you continue drug therapy under medical supervision.

Consider the Alternative!

Patients with Cushing's syndrome should be cautioned that long-term use of some herbs, including celery, juniper, licorice, and parsley, can cause hypokalemia.

NURSING CARE *of the Adrenalectomy Patient*

General nursing care of the surgical patient is discussed in Chapter 16. This section addresses the specific needs of the adrenalectomy patient.

PREOPERATIVE NURSING CARE

Preoperative care of the patient undergoing an adrenalectomy involves assessing for and correcting any existing electrolyte imbalances. The prevention of infections in these susceptible patients is maintained through strict hand washing and observance of asepsis. Preoperative education involves a discussion of glucocorticoid replacement therapy, including dosage, side effects, and complications.

POSTOPERATIVE NURSING CARE

After adrenalectomy, patients are sent to a critical care unit for at least 1 to 2 days for close observation and assessment. During this period, monitor the vital signs for signs and symptoms of impending shock, which may be evident as hypotension, a weak or thready pulse, decreased urinary output, and changes in level of consciousness. Pulse and blood pressure may be unstable for 24 to 48 hours after surgery, and vasopressors may be needed to maintain blood pressure in the immediate postoperative period.

A nursing diagnosis specific to the adrenalectomy patient is **Risk for Injury** related to addisonian crisis as a result of the sudden decrease in adrenal hormone secretion. Assess for signs and symptoms of acute adrenal insufficiency: vomiting, weakness, hypotension, joint pain, pruritus, and emotional disturbances. Closely monitor fluid and electrolyte balance. Intravenous fluids may be prescribed to restore or maintain balance. High doses of cortisol are given intravenously during and for several days after surgery to enable the patient to deal with the physical stress of surgery. The dosages are adjusted on the basis of the blood pressure, blood glucose, serum electrolytes, and serum cortisol levels. Later, glucocorticoids are administered orally.

Because the patient's resistance to infection is lowered, be especially careful to protect the patient by using strict aseptic technique for wound care and invasive procedures. Signs of infection may be very subtle.

Assess comfort at frequent intervals and treat pain with opioid analgesics. Document the effects of treatment. To minimize the risk of pulmonary complications, such as stasis of secretions and pneumonia, instruct the patient to turn, cough, deep breathe, or use an incentive spirometer.

Pheochromocytoma

A pheochromocytoma is a tumor, usually benign, of the adrenal medulla that causes secretion of excessive catecholamines. Patients with a pheochromocytoma exhibit episodes of hypertension, hypermetabolism, and hyperglycemia. The classic clinical findings are hypertension with a diastolic pressure of 115 mm Hg or higher; severe, pounding headache; and diaphoresis (profuse sweating). Other signs and symptoms include pallor, dilated pupils, orthostatic hypotension, and blurred vision. Episodes may be triggered by emotional distress, exercise, manipulation of the tumor, postural changes, and major trauma, including surgery.

The condition is treated by surgical removal of the tumor. Before surgery, the surgeon attempts to normalize vital signs with adrenergic antagonists (drugs that block the effects of catecholamines) and stabilize the patient's fluid status. The nurse monitors cardiovascular status and prepares the patient for surgery as detailed in Chapter 16. Postoperative nursing care is generally the same as that described for the patient having an adrenalectomy. However, special postoperative problems in the patient with pheochromocytoma are a greater risk for fluctuations in blood pressure and hypoglycemia. These problems require close monitoring and treatment.

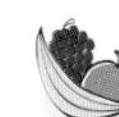

Nutrition Concepts

1. Patients with Cushing's syndrome may experience sodium and water retention.
2. Diet therapy for Cushing's syndrome may include decreased caloric and sodium intake and increased potassium intake.
3. Reducing sodium intake can decrease edema and related weight gain with Cushing's syndrome.
4. Early symptoms of Addison's disease may include anorexia, nausea, vomiting, diarrhea, and weight loss, resulting in impaired nutrition.
5. Patients with diabetes insipidus usually experience excessive thirst or urination, so they must drink liquids almost continuously to avoid dehydration and hypovolemic shock.

key points

- The endocrine system secretes hormones, chemical messengers that affect target organs and body tissues.
- Endocrine activity is regulated by feedback mechanisms that either stimulate or inhibit hormone synthesis and secretion.
- Pituitary hormones affect growth, fluid and electrolyte balance, metabolism, ovulation, milk production, uterine contractions, and skin pigmentation.
- Pituitary and adrenal function usually remain adequate in older people.
- Hyperpituitarism, caused by excess anterior pituitary hormones, leads to gigantism or acromegaly.
- Hyperpituitarism is treated with drugs (bromocriptine, octreotide acetate) or surgery to remove the tumor or the entire pituitary (hypophysectomy).
- Treatment of hyperpituitarism can prevent further changes and complications, but existing body changes are not reversible.
- Dwarfism is the result of inadequate growth hormone.
- Panhypopituitarism is a deficiency of all anterior pituitary hormones and is treated with replacement hormones.
- Diabetes insipidus, caused by a deficit in antidiuretic hormone, results in massive diuresis and is treated with vasopressin.
- Syndrome of inappropriate antidiuretic hormone, caused by excess antidiuretic hormone, results in fluid retention and is treated with diuretics and demeclocycline.

- The adrenal medulla secretes the catecholamines epinephrine and norepinephrine, which promote adaptation to stress.
- The adrenal cortex secretes steroids in the form of mineralocorticoids, glucocorticoids, and androgens or estrogens.
- Primary adrenal insufficiency (Addison's disease) causes hypoglycemia, hyperkalemia, hyponatremia, and hypovolemia and requires lifelong replacement of glucocorticoids and mineralocorticoids.
- Acute adrenal crisis is a life-threatening emergency caused by a sudden marked decrease in adrenal hormones that can lead to circulatory collapse and death.
- Cushing's syndrome results from hypersecretion of cortisol, a glucocorticoid, or from prolonged administration of corticosteroids.
- Cushing's syndrome is characterized by polycythemia, hypokalemia, hyperglycemia, leukocytosis, and glycosuria.
- Cushing's syndrome is treated with drug therapy, radiation, and hypophysectomy or adrenalectomy.
- Nursing care for the patient with Cushing's syndrome is concerned with Risk for Infection, Disturbed Thought Processes, Risk for Impaired Skin Integrity, Risk for Injury, Disturbed Body Image, and Ineffective Therapeutic Regimen Management.
- All chronic pituitary and adrenal conditions require patient teaching to enable the patient to manage the condition by taking medications properly and recognizing the need for medical intervention.
- A pheochromocytoma is an adrenal tumor that increases secretion of catecholamines, causing hypertension, hypermetabolism, and hyperglycemia.

REVIEW QUESTIONS

1. The overall mission of the endocrine system is to:
   1. maintain electrolyte balance.
   2. control metabolic rate.
   3. maintain homeostasis.
   4. resist infection.

2. Hormones secreted by the posterior pituitary include:
   1. antidiuretic hormone.
   2. adrenocorticotropic hormone.
   3. growth hormone.
   4. luteinizing hormone.

3. A patient who has recently started treatment for acromegaly says, "I will be so glad to look like myself again!" The most appropriate response is:
   1. "I know you are looking forward to that."
   2. "The process of reversing the effects of acromegaly is very slow."
   3. "Treatment will keep your symptoms from getting worse but will not reverse them."
   4. "These drugs can slow down the progression of acromegaly, but you will have additional bone enlargement."

4. Following surgery to remove a pituitary adenoma, a patient complains of neck stiffness. You should:
   1. give a gentle neck massage.
   2. administer a prescribed analgesic.
   3. lower the head of the bed.
   4. assess for other signs of infection.

5. Patients with hypopituitarism who wish to have children must be treated with:
   1. follicle-stimulating hormone and luteinizing hormone.
   2. estrogen and progesterone.
   3. testosterone.
   4. prolactin.

6. The main symptom of SIADH is:
   1. increased blood glucose.
   2. water retention.
   3. generalized edema.
   4. hypotension.

7. The patient with diabetes insipidus must maintain records of:
   1. daily diet.
   2. sodium intake.
   3. urine specific gravity.
   4. blood pressure and pulse.

8. Fluid and electrolyte imbalances associated with Addison's disease include:
   1. hypokalemia.
   2. hyponatremia.
   3. hypervolemia.
   4. metabolic alkalosis.

9. A patient who is brought to the emergency room has BP 88/40; pulse 108, thready; and dry skin and mucous membranes. He is confused. A medical alert card in his wallet states that he takes drugs for Addison's disease. You should suspect:
   1. acute adrenal crisis.
   2. Cushing's syndrome.
   3. diabetic ketoacidosis.
   4. Cushing's disease.

10. Nursing care of the patient with Cushing's syndrome should include:
    1. apply moisturizers to dark, toughened areas of skin.
    2. protect the patient from visitors and other patients with infections.
    3. tell the patient that mood swings and irritability will not be tolerated.
    4. encourage the patient to use salt liberally to offset excessive loss in the urine.

CHAPTER 43 Thyroid and Parathyroid Disorders

objectives

1. Identify nursing assessment data related to the functions of the thyroid and parathyroid glands.
2. Describe tests and procedures used to diagnose disorders of the thyroid and parathyroid glands and nursing responsibilities relevant for each.
3. Describe the pathophysiology, signs and symptoms, complications, and treatment of hyperthyroidism, hypothyroidism, hyperparathyroidism, and hypoparathyroidism.
4. Assist in the development of nursing care plans for patients with disorders of the thyroid or parathyroid glands.

key terms

Chvostek's sign (KVŎS-tĕks, p. 893)
Cretinism (KRĒ-tĭn-ĭzm, p. 887)
Exophthalmos (ĕk-sŏf-THĂL-mŏs, p. 880)
Goiter (GOI-tĕr, p. 891)
Goitrogen (GOI-trō-jĕn, p. 888)
Laryngospasm (lă-RĬNG-gō-spăzm, p. 886)
Myxedema (mĭk-sĕ-DĒ-mă, p. 887)
Nodule (NŎD-ūl, p. 879)
Parotiditis (pă-rŏt-ĭ-DĪ-tĭs, p. 883)
Tetany (TĔT-ă-nē, p. 886)
Thyroiditis (thī-roid-Ī-tĭs, p. 883)
Thyrotoxicosis (thī-rō-tŏk-sĭ-KŌ-sĭs, p. 882)
Trousseau's sign (trōō-SŌZ, p. 893)

THE THYROID GLAND

ANATOMY AND PHYSIOLOGY OF THE THYROID GLAND

The thyroid gland is located in the lower portion of the anterior neck. It consists of two lobes, one on each side of the trachea. The lobes are connected in front of the trachea by a narrow bridge of tissue called the isthmus (Fig. 43-1).

The thyroid gland plays a major role in regulating the body's rate of metabolism and growth and development. When the metabolic rate falls, the hypothalamus stimulates the pituitary gland to secrete thyroid-stimulating hormone (TSH). This hormone in turn stimulates the thyroid gland to secrete hormones that affect the production and use of energy.

The hormones produced by the thyroid gland are thyroid hormone, triiodothyronine, and calcitonin. Each of these is known by several names. Thyroid hormone also is called thyroxine, tetraiodothyronine, or T_4. Triiodothyronine is referred to as T_3. Both T_4 and T_3 increase the body's metabolic rate. Calcitonin, or thyrocalcitonin, plays a role in regulating the serum calcium level. It is secreted when serum calcium levels are high to limit the shift of calcium from the bones into the blood.

AGE-RELATED CHANGES IN THYROID FUNCTION

With age, there is an increased incidence of thyroid **nodules.** Serum levels of T_4 remain approximately the same in the healthy older person, but levels of T_3 more often decline. The incidence of hypothyroidism increases with age, especially among women. Thyroid conditions are often overlooked in the elderly because signs and symptoms may be subtle and attributed to the aging process. Weight changes may not occur in the older person as they do with younger people with thyroid disorders. Treatment of thyroid disorders can have a profound positive effect on the patient's quality of life.

NURSING ASSESSMENT OF THE THYROID GLAND

Thyroid disorders may escape detection until they are rather severe because the symptoms are often vague. Periodic assessment of the patient with a thyroid disorder is necessary to evaluate the response to treatment and make adjustments if necessary.

Health History

To elicit information about common symptoms of thyroid disorders, ask if the patient is aware of any changes in energy level, sleep patterns, personality, mental function, or emotional state. Fatigue may be found with both hypothyroidism and hyperthyroidism. Because thyroid hormones affect the metabolic rate, patients may have unexplained weight changes. Hormone deficiency lowers the metabolic rate, so patients may gain weight. At the other extreme, hormone excess increases the metabolic rate, often causing weight loss.

In the review of systems, pay particular attention to changes in menstrual cycles, sexual function, hydration (thirst, changes in urine output, tissue turgor, moisture of

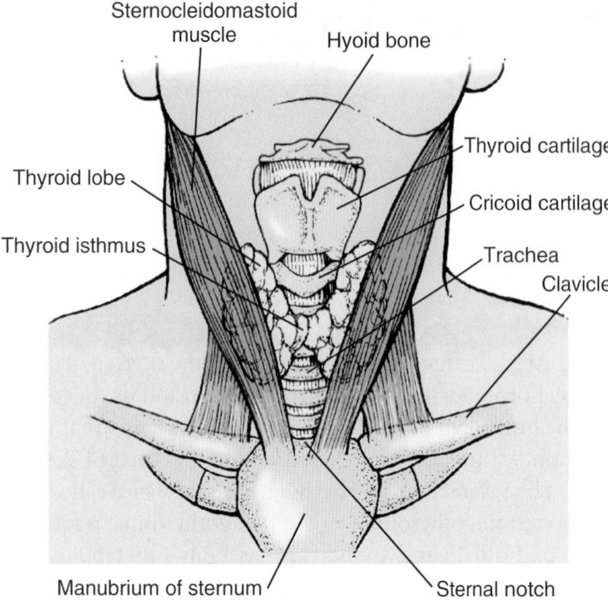

FIGURE **43-1** The thyroid gland.

mucous membranes), bowel elimination pattern, and tolerance of heat and cold.

Physical Examination

Begin the physical examination by taking the patient's vital signs and measuring height and weight. Note the facial expression and characteristics as well as the mental alertness. Vital signs are important because they reflect the metabolic rate. Thyroid disorders may cause increased or decreased heart rate, respirations, blood pressure, and temperature as well as irregular heart rhythms. Inspect and palpate the skin for moisture, temperature, and texture. In the head and neck examination, note the hair texture. Examine the eyes for exophthalmos (bulging). Inspect the neck for enlargement typical of goiter. Observe the hands for tremor. Nurses with advanced physical examination skills may palpate the neck for thyroid enlargement or nodules.

Key components of the nursing assessment of the patient with a thyroid disorder are outlined in Table 43-1.

table 43-1 **ASSESSMENT *of the Patient with a Thyroid Disorder***

HEALTH HISTORY

Present Illness: Fatigue, weight changes, mental-emotional changes
Past Medical History: Recent surgery or trauma, radiation of the head or neck, recent and current medications, history of thyroid or renal disorders
Review of Systems: Fatigue, changes in hair or skin, voice changes, palpitations, edema, constipation or diarrhea, polyuria, nervousness, weight loss, temperature intolerance, excessive perspiration, changes in libido or sexual function
Functional Assessment: Sleep disturbances, usual dietary intake, anorexia, ability to cope with stress

PHYSICAL EXAMINATION

Vital Signs: Abnormal heart rate and rhythm, blood pressure changes, tachypnea
Height and Weight
Skin: Changes in moisture, temperature, and texture
Hair: Changes in texture
Eyes: Exophthalmos
Neck: Enlargement
Hands: Tremor

DIAGNOSTIC TESTS AND PROCEDURES

Diagnostic studies of the thyroid gland include laboratory blood tests and studies employing radioactive iodine. Table 43-2 summarizes the use of each test and identifies nursing implications.

The most useful tests of thyroid function are measurements of serum T_3, free T_4, T_4, and TSH. These tests have become increasingly more sophisticated; thus more specialized tests are rarely needed. The thyroid-releasing hormone (TRH) stimulation test measures the blood level of TSH after administration of TRH. This test shows whether thyroid hormone abnormalities are caused by a disorder of the thyroid gland itself or by altered production of stimulating hormones by the hypothalamus or the pituitary.

The thyroid gland uses iodine to manufacture hormones. Therefore radioactive iodine isotopes (^{131}I, ^{123}I, ^{99m}Tc) are useful for diagnostic purposes because they concentrate in the thyroid. The amount of iodine taken up by the thyroid is measured to assess the activity level of the gland. This test is called a radioactive iodine (RAI) uptake test.

For a thyroid scan, the patient ingests radioactive iodine. Then a specialized instrument is used to scan the area of the thyroid gland. It creates a picture of the gland based on the distribution of the iodine. The picture aids in diagnosing cancer because the patterns of iodine concentration in normal and malignant tissue are different. Because a low dose of radiation is used for diagnostic purposes, the patient poses no danger to the patient or others. However, pregnancy is a contraindication because of possible harm to the fetus.

Thyroid ultrasonography yields very clear images of the thyroid gland and any nodules present. The cytopathologist can use this technology to guide a needle inserted to aspirate material from the nodules. For evaluation of metastatic disease or to image the portion of the thyroid concealed by the sternum, MRI or CT is used.

Put on your THINKING CAP!!

A patient's blood studies show a high level of TSH and a low level of T_4. Explain what this finding means.

table 43-2 **DIAGNOSTIC TESTS AND PROCEDURES | *Thyroid Disorders***

TEST/PURPOSE	PATIENT PREPARATION	POSTPROCEDURE CARE
LABORATORY STUDIES		
Serum T_3 (triiodothyronine) and Serum T_4 measurements of free and total T_4 detect abnormal levels of thyroid hormones. Elevated T_3: Graves' disease, toxic adenoma, and toxic nodular goiter. Elevated T_4: hyperthyroidism, excessive thyroid hormone replacement. T_3 and T_4 decrease with hypothyroidism.	Tell patient that blood sample will be drawn. Nonfasting. Some medications may be withheld before blood is drawn.	After blood sample is drawn, assess for oozing. Apply small dressing.
Serum thyroid-stimulating hormone (TSH) increases hypothyroidism; decreases with hyperthyroidism.	Tell patient a blood sample will drawn.	After venipuncture, assess for oozing. Apply small dressing.
TRH stimulation test assesses response of the pituitary to TRH. Differentiates types of hypothyroidism. TRH normally increases after TRH given intravenously.	Tell patient that a drug will be given intravenously; then several blood samples must be drawn.	Assess venipuncture site for oozing. Apply small bandage.
Radioactive iodine uptake test. After radioactive iodine is given orally, the amount of ^{131}I taken up by thyroid is measured with a special instrument. High uptake with hyperthyroidism; low with hypothyroidism.	Tell patient the procedure is painless. Ask about pregnancy, in which case radiation is contraindicated. Advise patient that radiation dose is small and will not harm others.	For 24 hours after test, patient should wash hands with soap and water after voiding. If caregiver discards urine, gloves should be worn. Then, gloves should be washed, removed, and bare hands washed. Pregnant women should avoid patient contact for 24 hours.
UPTAKE AND IMAGING PROCEDURES		
Thyroid scan ^{131}I, ^{123}I, or ^{99m}Tc is given orally and a scanner used to detect pattern of uptake by the thyroid gland. Can differentiate benign and malignant nodules and detect other abnormalities.	Tell patient about test. If ^{131}I is used, patient will be given isotope in liquid form and will return to radiology 24 hours later for scan. With ^{123}I, scan is done after 3 to 6 hours. Patient will have to lie still on back for 20 minutes during scan. For 1 week before test, patient should not consume iodine. Iodine is in radiographic dyes, some oral contraceptives, weight control drugs, multivitamins, all thyroid drugs, and some food, especially seafood.	Same as for radioactive iodine uptake test.
Thyroid ultrasonography provides high-quality images of thyroid and any nodules.	Advise patient that procedure is painless and noninvasive. An instrument is moved over the neck area and uses sound waves to create an image of the gland.	
Fine needle aspiration biopsy Material from thyroid nodules can be aspirated using a needle and guided by ultrasonography.	Same as thyroid ultrasonography. Also, tell patient the physician will use a small needle to remove a tissue sample.	Assess for any signs of bleeding: swelling in the area of the biopsy site, bleeding from the puncture site, increasing pulse.

DISORDERS OF THE THYROID GLAND

Hyperthyroidism

Hyperthyroidism is characterized by abnormally increased synthesis and secretion of thyroid hormones. Several forms of hyperthyroidism occur. The most common types are Graves' disease (also called *toxic diffuse goiter*) and multinodular goiter (also called *toxic nodular goiter*).

Graves' disease is thought to be an autoimmune disorder. Antibodies activate TSH receptors, which in turn stimulate thyroid enlargement and hormone secretion. Graves' disease most often develops in young women. Regardless of whether the patient has treatment, the condition tends to have periods of remission and exacerbation. Some patients with Graves' disease eventually develop hypothyroidism.

Multinodular goiter occurs most often in women in their sixth and seventh decades. It is most likely to develop in people who have had goiter for a number of years. Hyperthyroidism in this case is caused by small thyroid nodules that secrete excess thyroid hormone. The nodules can be benign or malignant. Symptoms of hyperthyroidism are usually less severe with multinodular goiter than with Graves' disease.

Because all types of hyperthyroidism have many common features and because Graves' disease is the most common form, it will be used as the example of hyperthyroidism.

Signs and Symptoms

Many of the signs and symptoms of hyperthyroidism are caused by an increased metabolic rate and can range from mild to severe. Weight loss and nervousness may be the only symptoms in patients with a mild form of the disease. In more severe cases, the patient's history may reveal restlessness, irritable behavior, sleep disturbances, emotional lability, personality changes, hair loss, and fatigue. Weight loss, even when the patient is eating well, is common. Some patients overcompensate for the increased metabolism, overeat, and gain weight. Many patients report poor tolerance of heat and excessive perspiration. Changes in menstrual and bowel patterns may occur. Examination findings may include warm, moist, velvety skin; fine tremors of the hands; swelling of the neck; and ophthalmopathy including exophthalmos. Exophthalmos is the most apparent effect of hyperthyroidism on the eyes. Tearing, light sensitivity, decreased visual acuity, and swelling occur around the orbit of the eye. Exophthalmos is more common with Graves' disease than with nodular goiter (Fig. 43-2).

Excess thyroid hormones stimulate the heart, causing tachycardia, increased systolic blood pressure, and sometimes atrial fibrillation. The heart rate may be as rapid as 160 beats/min. Even during sleep, the pulse may remain above 80 beats/min.

Complications

If untreated, hyperthyroidism may lead to **thyrotoxicosis** (thyroid storm/crisis). Thyrotoxicosis is excessive stimulation caused by elevated thyroid hormone levels that produce dangerous tachycardia and hyperthermia. There is a risk of heart failure. The patient is restless and agitated and may lapse into a coma. Thyrotoxicosis is a medical emergency. Fortunately, modern treatment of hyperthyroidism makes this complication rare.

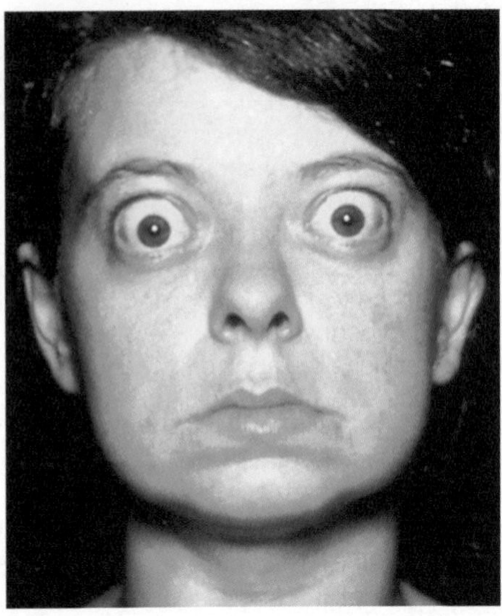

FIGURE **43-2** This patient has exophthalmos, bulging eyes, associated with Graves' disease.

Medical Diagnosis

Elevated serum T_3 is the most common finding with Graves' disease. T_4 measurements may be normal or elevated. TSH can be so low that it cannot be detected in the blood. Measurement of thyroid-stimulating antibodies is useful in specifically diagnosing Graves' disease.

Medical Treatment

Three methods are used to treat hyperthyroidism: drug therapy, surgery, and radiation therapy. In addition, beta-adrenergic blockers like propranolol (Inderal) may be given to relieve some of the cardiovascular symptoms associated with hyperthyroidism.

Drug therapy. Hyperthyroidism may be treated initially with antithyroid drugs. Antithyroid drugs block the synthesis, release, or activity of thyroid hormones. The drugs that may be used as antithyroid agents are thionamides and iodides. These drugs are effective in treating hyperthyroidism; however, they often are used temporarily to lower the level of hormones in the blood before surgery. This process reduces the risk of bleeding and lowers the danger of releasing large amounts of thyroid hormones into the bloodstream during surgery. When a patient is on drugs that interfere with T_4 secretion, monitor for symptoms of hypothyroidism (cold intolerance, edema, and weight gain).

PHARMACOLOGY CAPSULE Patients on antithyroid drugs must be monitored for hypothyroidism.

Thionamides. Examples of thionamides are propylthiouracil and methimazole (Tapazole). It usually takes several weeks before the effects of thionamides are noticeable. The drugs may be given for months or years. The goal is to induce a remission that will allow the drugs to be discontinued. A disadvantage of thionamides is that they can cause agranulocytosis, a condition in which the production of neutrophils is suppressed. Without adequate neutrophils, the patient is unable to resist infection. Any signs of infection, such as sore throat or fever, should be reported to the physician immediately.

Iodides. Iodides are useful because iodine inhibits the synthesis of thyroid hormones. They are used most often after a course of propylthiouracil to suppress hormone secretion before thyroidectomy. The iodides also may be used to treat thyrotoxicosis. Potassium iodide (SSKI) can be given to people who have been exposed to radiation to prevent damage to the thyroid gland.

The iodides most often used to treat hyperthyroidism are Lugol's solution (5% iodine and 10% potassium iodide) and saturated solution of potassium iodide. Iodides may bring some relief within 24 hours, but it takes several weeks for maximum effect. The effect does not last as long as that of thionamides; therefore they are not generally used as the sole treatment for hyperthyroidism.

Iodine solutions can cause discoloration of the teeth and gastric upset. These effects are minimized if the iodine solution is diluted with milk, fruit juice, or some other beverage and sipped through a straw. Signs of iodine toxicity include swelling and irritation of the mucous membranes and increased salivation.

PHARMACOLOGY CAPSULE Iodine solutions can stain the teeth! They should be mixed with a beverage and sipped through a straw.

Radioactive iodine. Radioactive iodine (^{131}I) can be used alone or with antithyroid drugs to treat hyperthyroidism. It quickly accumulates in the thyroid gland, where it causes destruction of thyroid tissue. The resulting decrease in thyroid hormone production is not evident for several months. Meanwhile, beta-adrenergic blockers can be given to control cardiac symptoms.

The radiation dose used to treat hyperthyroidism does not pose a threat to others. It should not be used during pregnancy, however, because it affects the thyroid gland of the fetus. Side effects of the treatment are minimal. Inflammation of the thyroid gland (thyroiditis) and the parotid glands (parotiditis) may occur. Parotiditis causes the mouth to be dry and irritated. Hypothyroidism may develop years after treatment. Drugs used to treat thyroid disorders are summarized in Table 43-3.

Surgical Treatment

Graves' disease is often treated by removing most of the thyroid gland. This procedure is called a subtotal thyroidectomy. As mentioned earlier, patients are commonly given antithyroid drug therapy for several weeks before surgery. Before these drugs were commonly used, patients often had dramatic postoperative responses because of the escape of thyroid hormones into the bloodstream during surgery. This severe episode of hyperthyroidism, called thyroid storm or thyroid crisis, is a medical emergency because it is potentially fatal.

NURSING CARE *of the Nonsurgical Patient with Hyperthyroidism*

Most patients with hyperthyroidism are treated as outpatients. Therefore the nurse in the community or clinic setting may need to help the patient learn to adapt until treatment brings relief.

Assessment

Complete assessment of the patient with a thyroid disorder is summarized in Table 43-1. For the patient with hyperthyroidism, be sure to assess activity tolerance, heat tolerance, bowel elimination pattern, appetite, weight changes, and food intake. Also assess the patient's mental-emotional state, adaptation to the condition, and understanding of the treatment. Measure and record vital signs and height and weight.

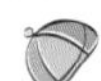

Put on your THINKING CAP!!

Explain why people with hyperthyroidism do not tolerate heat well.

Nursing Diagnoses, Goals, and Outcome Criteria: Hyperthyroidism

Nursing Diagnoses	Goals and Outcome Criteria
Decreased Cardiac Output related to excessive thyroid hormone stimulation	Normal cardiac output: pulse and blood pressure within patient norms: no signs/symptoms of heart failure: edema, dyspnea
Disturbed Sleep Pattern related to metabolic disturbance	Improved sleep pattern: absence of insomnia, patient describes feeling rested on awakening.
Hyperthermia related to increased metabolic energy production	Improved heat tolerance: patient statement of comfort in relation to environmental temperature, no excess perspiration
Imbalanced Nutrition: Less than Body Requirements related to increased metabolic requirements	Adequate nutrition: stable body weight if no significant recent loss, weight gain if underweight
Risk for Injury related to exophthalmos	Decreased risk of eye injury: lids cover eyeball, eyeball is moist, no pain associated with corneal injury
Disturbed Sensory Perception related to ophthalmopathy	Reduced visual disturbance, eye pain, photosensitivity, periorbital edema
Diarrhea related to excessive thyroid hormone stimulation	Normal bowel elimination: formed stools at regular intervals

table 43-3 **DRUG THERAPY | *Thyroid Conditions***

DRUG	USE/ACTION	SIDE EFFECTS	NURSING INTERVENTIONS
THYROID HORMONE REPLACEMENT DRUGS			
Desiccated thyroid (thyroid USP) Levothyroxine (Synthroid) Liothyronine (Cytomel) Liotrix (Euthroid)	Treat hypothyroidism and thyroiditis. Increase metabolic rate.	Overdose: irritability, insomnia, nervousness, tachycardia, diarrhea, weight loss.	Elderly patients more susceptible to toxicity. Low doses of one or more preparations given initially. Dosage gradually increased and patient maintained on one preparation. Hypothyroid patients usually require lifelong therapy. Patient teaching needed. Monitor pluse and blood pressure of elderly patients. Withhold and notify physician if pulse >100. Thyroid preparations interact with many other drugs by affecting metabolic rate.
ANTI-THYROID DRUGS			
Thionamides			
Methimazole (Tapazole) Propylthiouracil (PTU)	Treat hyperthyroidism by interfering with synthesis of thyroid hormones.	Agranulocytosis, rash, thrombocytopenia, skin discoloration, fever, headache, drowsiness, diarrhea, nausea, vomiting.	Avoid use during pregnancy. Monitor patient for bleeding due to decreased platelets and prothrombin, signs of liver toxicity (jaundice, abdominal pain), agranulocytosis (fever, sore throat, malaise), and hypothyroidism (weight gain, fatigue). Teach patient to report any of these signs and symptoms. Safety precautions if drowsy. Encourage patient to adhere to drug prescription and to keep follow-up appointments.
Iodides			
Strong iodine solution (Lugol's solution) Saturated solution of potassium iodide (SSKI)	Reduce size and vascularity of thyroid gland in hyperthyroidism. May be used with other drugs to treat hyperthyroidism or alone before surgery for hyperthyroidism.	Excess iodine: fever, rash, oral lesions, metallic taste, diarrhea, parotitis, hypothyroidism	Dilute liquids in water, fruit juice, or milk. Reduce unpleasant taste and tooth staining by using a straw. Monitor for symptoms of excess iodine. Give SSKI after meals.
Radioactive iodine Sodium iodide ^{131}I and ^{123}I	Concentrates in thyroid tissue for diagnostic scans. Higher therapeutic dose destroys thyroid tissue in hyperthyroidism and thyroid malignancies.	Diagnostic dose: none. Therapeutic dose: nausea, vomiting.	Diagnostic dose usually requires no radiation precautions except precautions with urine for 24 hours after the test (see Table 43-2). Therapeutic dose requires isolation measures. Monitor patient for signs of hypothyroidism (fatigue, weight gain).

Interventions

Decreased Cardiac Output

Monitor the patient's pulse and blood pressure at intervals. Give beta-adrenergic blockers as ordered to counteract the stimulant effects of the elevated thyroid hormones. Signs of heart failure include tachycardia, tachypnea, dyspnea, confusion, and edema. Assess elderly patients often because they are more susceptible to cardiovascular stress with thyroid disease. Immediately report any signs of heart failure to the physician. Medical treatment of heart failure usually includes oxygen, intravenous fluids, sedatives, and cardiac drugs.

Disturbed Sleep Pattern

Despite fatigue and weakness, the hyperthyroid patient often feels restless and has trouble sleeping. Arrange the day to allow periods of rest. Avoid caffeine. Encourage bedtime rituals, which may be helpful in preparing for sleep. Provide a restful environment and a soothing back rub to promote relaxation. Give sedatives as ordered to promote sleep.

In addition to physical rest, patients need emotional rest. The patient and the family may be able to cope better if they understand the reason for the patient's irritability and nervousness. Patients need to recognize stressful situations and avoid them.

Hyperthermia

Owing to their high metabolic rate, hyperthyroid patients usually have some heat intolerance. They tend to feel too warm even when others are comfortable. Only light clothing may be needed. Adjust the environmental temperature as much as possible for comfort. A private room allows the patient more freedom to select the room temperature. If the patient perspires heavily, frequent bathing and clothing changes help promote comfort.

Imbalanced Nutrition: Less than Body Requirements

Despite a normal dietary intake, the patient may not be meeting the increased caloric needs. Weigh daily to monitor nutritional adequacy. A diet high in calories, vitamins, and minerals is recommended. Depending on the severity of the condition, the patient may need additional full meals or between-meal snacks. Some patients require as many as 4,000 to 5,000 calories daily to maintain body weight. The physician may order supplementary vitamins. Additional fluids are recommended to replace fluids lost through increased insensible loss (fluid lost through the skin and the lungs).

Risk for Injury

Exophthalmos is a condition in which deposits of fat and fluid behind the eyeballs make them bulge outward (see Fig. 43-2). Both eyes are usually affected. If the condition is severe, the eyelids do not cover the eyeball. The eyeball is not kept moist and is susceptible to injury. It may be necessary to tape the lids shut. Lubricated eye pads or artificial tears may be used. Raising the head of the bed at night and limiting salt intake may be helpful.

The patient with exophthalmos has a startled appearance. This may make the person self-conscious and embarrassed. Dark glasses help to conceal the eyes. For these patients, disturbed body image is an important additional nursing diagnosis. Reassure the patient that the condition usually goes away after treatment of hyperthyroidism.

Disturbed Sensory Perception

In addition to exophthalmos, the hyperthyroid patient has a variety of eye symptoms that may include double vision, periorbital edema, tearing, photosensitivity, and a feeling of "sand" in the eyes. It helps to elevate the head of the bed, reduce bright lighting, and advise use of tinted glasses. Methylcellulose eye drops and diuretics may be ordered to decrease inflammation and swelling. Severe inflammation is treated with a 2-4 week course of prednisone. After acute inflammation subsides, surgical procedures on the eyeball muscles and the eyelids may be needed to eliminate double vision and to restore coverage of the eye.

Diarrhea

If the patient has diarrhea, electrolyte imbalances and skin irritation may result. Give antidiarrheal medications as ordered, and monitor the effect. Thorough perianal cleansing after each stool reduces the risk of skin breakdown.

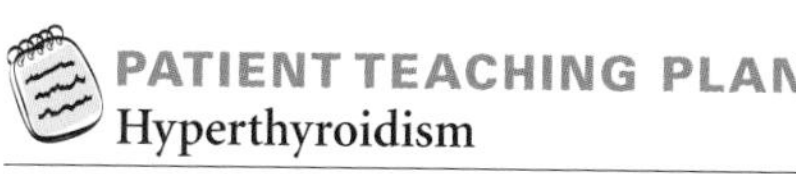

PATIENT TEACHING PLAN
Hyperthyroidism

- This is a chronic condition that requires long-term care.
- You must take your medications exactly as prescribed.
- Notify your physician of excessive fatigue and depression, which may indicate hypothyroidism caused by your antithyroid drug,

NURSING CARE *of the Patient Having a Thyroidectomy*

General care of the surgical patient is discussed in Chapter 16. This section covers the special needs of the thyroidectomy patient.

Assessment

Preoperative

The preparation of the patient undergoing thyroid surgery is essentially the same as for any major surgery. Assess the patient's knowledge about surgery and what to expect before and after the procedure. Nursing diagnoses may include those listed earlier for hyperthyroidism, but the condition is usually brought under control before surgery is scheduled. In addition, identify and address learning needs. Teaching is the primary preoperative nursing intervention. The goals of preoperative teaching are patient understanding of the usual preoperative and postoperative procedures and decreased anxiety. Tell the patient to expect a dressing on the front of the neck. Demonstrate how to avoid straining the neck incision by supporting the head when rising.

To evaluate the effectiveness of preoperative teaching, ask the patient to repeat the information presented. Ask patients to return demonstrations of activities such as deep breathing and supporting the head during position changes.

Postoperative

The patient usually recovers quickly from a thyroidectomy and may be discharged in 2 or 3 days. Rare but serious complications are airway obstruction, recurrent laryngeal nerve damage, hemorrhage, and tetany. One other complication, thyroid crisis, is usually prevented by preoperative treatment with antithyroid drugs.

If part of the thyroid gland is left (subtotal thyroidectomy), it should eventually regenerate and produce adequate hormones. The patient may be somewhat hypothyroid at first, but replacement therapy is not recommended. Giving thyroid hormone interferes with the regeneration of thyroid tissue.

Immediately after thyroidectomy, it is especially important to *assess* and *document* respiratory status, level of consciousness, wound drainage or bleeding, voice quality, comfort, and neuromuscular irritability (a sign of hypocalcemia associated with damage to the parathyroids).

Nursing Diagnoses, Goals, and Outcome Criteria: Thyroidectomy

Nursing Diagnoses	Goals and Outcome Criteria
Ineffective Airway Clearance related to airway obstruction, laryngeal nerve damage, laryngeal spasm	Effective airway clearance: normal breath sounds, respiratory rate of 12 to 20, no dyspnea
Decreased Cardiac Output related to blood loss, heart failure secondary to thyroid crisis	Normal cardiac output: pulse and blood pressure within normal limits; no edema
Disturbed Body Image related to surgical scar	Adaptation to change in appearance: looks at scar, verbalizes acceptance of scar
Acute Pain related to tissue trauma	Pain relief: patient statement of less or no pain, relaxed manner
Risk for Infection related to impaired skin integrity	Absence of infection: wound margins intact, minimal redness, no purulent drainage, normal body temperature

Interventions

Ineffective Airway Clearance

Turning and deep breathing are recommended to prevent respiratory complications, as with any other surgical patient. The surgeon may not want the patient to cough, however, because of possible stress on the suture line.

It is especially important to monitor and document the rate and ease of respirations after thyroidectomy. Respiratory distress can result from compression of the trachea or from a spasm of the larynx due to nerve damage or hypocalcemia. Before the patient returns from surgery, suction equipment, a laryngoscope, an endotracheal tube, oxygen, and an emergency tracheotomy tray must be available. Your agency may require the tracheotomy tray at the bedside. Elevate the head of the bed to decrease edema. Use pillows to prop and support the head to avoid stress on the suture line.

Because of the location of the thyroidectomy incision, edema or bleeding can cause pressure on the trachea. Signs and symptoms of poor oxygenation due to airway obstruction or blood loss include restlessness, increasing pulse and respiratory rates, and dyspnea. Without prompt intervention, the patient with airway obstruction could die.

The laryngeal nerve innervates the vocal cords. If it is damaged during surgery, vocal cord paralysis can occur. Paralysis of both cords may cause spasms **(laryngospasm)** that close the airway. An emergency tracheotomy is needed to restore the airway. Signs of laryngeal nerve damage are hoarseness and inability to speak. This is more severe than the usual hoarseness most people have after general anesthesia. Ask the patient to respond verbally to simple questions to determine voice quality.

Before the function of the parathyroid glands was understood, patients having thyroidectomies often experienced

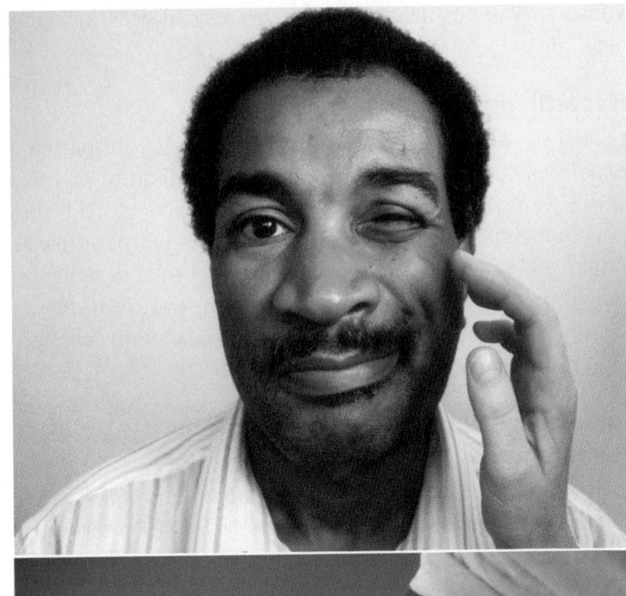

A

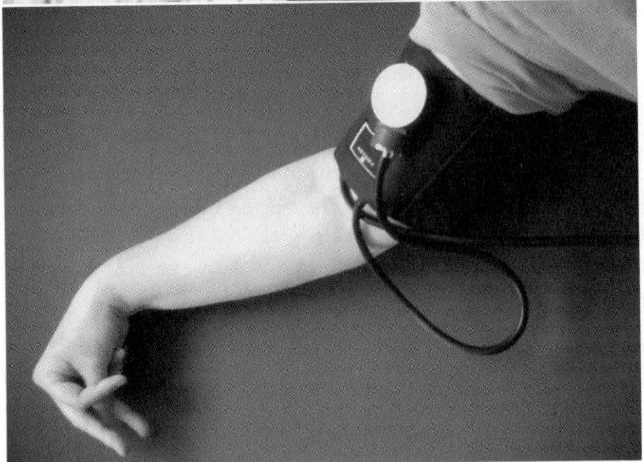

B

FIGURE **43-3** Signs of hypocalcemia: *A,* Chvostek's sign (facial twitch). *B,* Trousseau's sign (carpopedal spasm).

unexplained muscle contractions and respiratory difficulty that sometimes led to death. Eventually, it was determined that the symptoms were caused by a deficiency of parathyroid hormone. Surgeons are now careful to locate and spare the small parathyroid glands. Occasionally, however, the parathyroid glands are injured or accidentally removed during thyroidectomy.

Without parathyroid hormone, the serum calcium level falls, thus causing **tetany.** Muscle contractions begin as twitches around the mouth and eyes. The face, fingers, and toes begin to tingle. The patient may have painful "cramps," including the classic signs depicted in Figure 43-3. The most serious effect of hypocalcemia is spasm of the larynx. As the larynx closes, the patient has difficulty breathing and can suffocate. Cardiac dysrhythmias and seizures also can occur.

Tetany is treated with calcium salts given intravenously or orally. The condition usually improves as the injured parathyroid glands recover. Rarely is hypoparathyroidism permanent. If it is, lifetime treatment is required, as described later in this chapter.

Consider the Alternative!

Position changes and back rubs enhance the effects of prescribed analgesics.

Decreased Cardiac Output

Frequently assess the dressing and the vital signs to detect bleeding. Because the dressing is on the front of the neck, blood might flow under the dressing to the back of the neck. Therefore be sure to check behind the patient's neck and upper back to detect this.

Thyroid crisis can develop when large amounts of thyroid hormone enter the bloodstream during surgery. Approximately 12 hours after surgery, the patient in thyroid crisis shows signs of severe hyperthyroidism (tachycardia, cardiac arrhythmias, vomiting, fever, and confusion). It can also occur in patients with severe hyperthyroidism who develop a severe illness or infection.

If not treated promptly, the patient will die as a result of heart failure. Early detection of thyroid crisis requires careful monitoring of vital signs during the first postoperative day. The risk of thyroid crisis is reduced if serum hormone levels are reduced before surgery with medications.

Treatment of thyroid crisis consists of antithyroid drugs, intravenous sodium iodide, corticosteroids, beta-adrenergic blockers, intravenous fluids, oxygen, and a hypothermia (cooling) blanket or other measures to reduce body temperature.

Disturbed Body Image

The patient may be worried about the appearance of the surgical scar. Thyroidectomy incisions follow the natural contours of the neck. Once the scar fades, it usually is not noticeable. Meanwhile, it is easy to conceal the fresh scar with clothing.

Acute Pain

Frequently assess the postoperative patient's comfort level. Promptly administer prescribed analgesics and evaluate and document effects.

Risk for Infection

Any time the skin is broken, the potential for infection exists. Practice good hand washing and use aseptic technique when handling dressings. Tell the patient to avoid touching the fresh incision and to report any signs and symptoms of infection (fever, increasing wound redness and swelling, and foul drainage). Protect the incision from strain and possible dehiscence by supporting the neck when arising and reclining.

PATIENT TEACHING PLAN
Thyroidectomy

- If all of your thyroid gland was removed, you will need lifelong replacement of thyroid hormones.

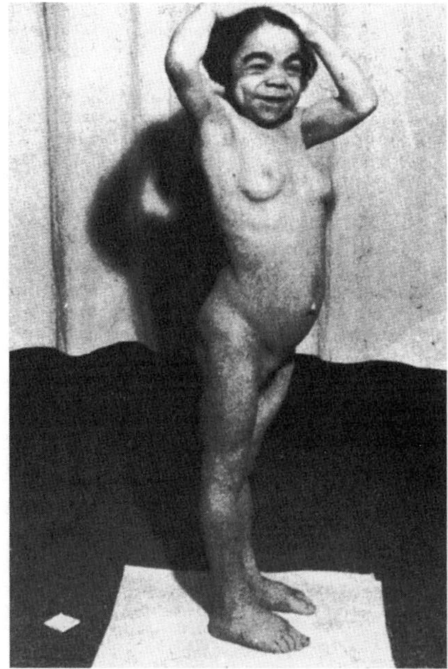

FIGURE **43-4** Cretinism is a condition of permanent physical and mental retardation resulting from untreated hypothyroidism in infancy.

- If only part of your thyroid gland was removed, you may feel tired for a while, but this should improve as the remaining gland increases hormone production
- Thyroidectomy scars usually heal so that they are eventually barely noticeable.
- Take your drugs exactly as prescribed.
- Nervousness and palpitations may be adverse effects of thyroid replacement drugs (hyperthyroidism); notify the physician if they occur.

Hypothyroidism

Hypothyroidism is the result of inadequate secretion of thyroid hormones. It is seen in infants, children, and adults. If not treated early, hypothyroidism during infancy causes permanent retardation of physical and mental development (cretinism) (Fig. 43-4). The effects in adults can be quite serious but usually are reversible with treatment. The term *myxedema* sometimes is used for hypothyroidism. Myxedema actually refers to facial edema that develops with severe, long-term hypothyroidism (Fig. 43-5). Not all hypothyroid patients have myxedema.

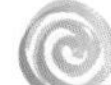

What Does Culture Have to do with Hypothyroidism?

The incidence of hypothyroidism is 10 to 20 times higher in iodine-deficient parts of the world (e.g., Zaire, Nepal) than in the U.S.

Etiology and Risk Factors

Hypothyroidism has many causes—including atrophy of the thyroid gland after years of Graves' disease or thyroiditis,

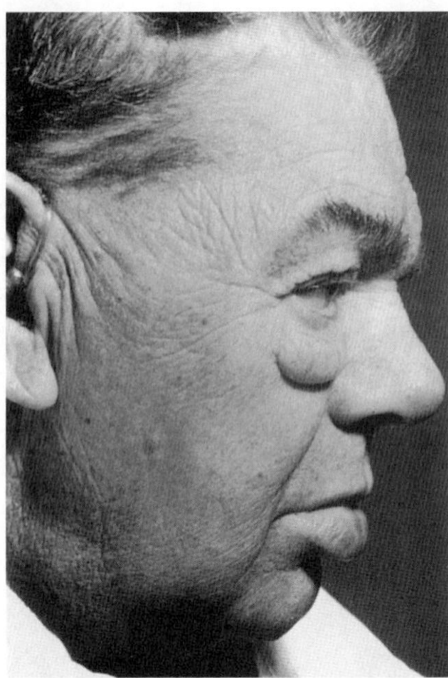

FIGURE **43-5** Typical appearance of the patient with myxedema.

treatment for hyperthyroidism, dietary iodine deficiency, high intake of goitrogens, and defects in thyroid hormone synthesis. These are examples of *primary* hypothyroidism. They account for 90% to 95% of all cases of hypothyroidism. Some foods and drugs act as **goitrogens**, meaning that they suppress thyroid hormone production. Examples of foods that are goitrogens if taken in large quantities are soybeans, turnips, and rutabagas. Goitrogenic drugs that often are used to treat hyperthyroidism are propylthiouracil, methimazole, and iodine.

Hypothyroidism caused by pituitary or hypothalamic disorders is called *secondary* hypothyroidism. Deficiency of TSH lowers the secretion of thyroid hormones even though the thyroid gland itself remains normal. Of course, patients who have had their entire thyroid or pituitary glands surgically removed also will be hypothyroid. Hypothyroidism also can result from tissue resistance to thyroid hormone—that is, the hormone is present, but the body cells are unable to use it normally.

Signs and Symptoms

The signs and symptoms of hypothyroidism in general are the opposite of those of hyperthyroidism (Table 43-4). The onset is usually gradual. The metabolic rate slows, often causing weight gain even with decreased food intake. Hypothyroid patients commonly report lethargy, forgetfulness, and irritability. They may experience frequent headaches, constipation, menstrual disorders, numbness and tingling in the arms and legs, and intolerance to cold. The pulse tends to be slow, and dyspnea may be present.

Examination may reveal swelling of the lips and eyelids; dry, thick skin; bruising; thin, coarse hair; and hoarseness. Generalized nonpitting edema and facial edema may be present. The patient may seem slow, depressed, or apathetic. Pallor may be present, associated with anemia. Signs and symptoms may be more subtle in the elderly or may be masked by signs and symptoms of other acute or chronic disorders. Therefore thyroid function in older adults should be assessed as part of routine checkups.

Medical Diagnosis

Hypothyroidism is diagnosed based on the laboratory determination of free T_4 and TSH. A TRH stimulation test also may be ordered. Free T_4 is low with hypothyroidism except when the problem is tissue resistance to the hormone. TSH level enables the physician to determine whether the basic problem is primary or secondary hypothyroidism.

Complications

Severe, untreated hypothyroidism can progress to myxedema coma. Infection, trauma, excessive chilling, and some drugs (opioids, sedatives, tranquilizers) may precipitate myxedema coma in a hypothyroid patient. The main signs of this life-threatening condition are hypothermia, hypotension, and hypoventilation.

Hypothyroidism is treated with hormone replacement therapy. Natural and synthetic forms of thyroid hormones are available. The natural form is thyroid extract obtained from animal tissue. Examples of the synthetic form are levothyroxine (Synthroid) and liothyronine (Cytomel). Hypothyroid patients usually require lifelong replacement therapy. They should be monitored periodically to evaluate the response to therapy.

A patient with heart disease may have difficulty adapting to a sudden increase in metabolic rate. For that reason, replacement therapy for elderly patients or those with heart disease is usually started with a low dose and gradually increased. If these patients have any chest pain once therapy is started, the physician should be notified immediately.

PHARMACOLOGY CAPSULE Opioids, sedatives, and tranquilizers can precipitate potentially fatal myxedema coma in a severely hypothyroid person.

NURSING CARE *of the Patient with Hypothyroidism*

Hypothyroidism usually does not require hospitalization, but it may be detected when patients are hospitalized for other reasons. Because the onset of symptoms is often subtle, the nurse in the community or long-term care setting must be alert for signs and symptoms of hypothyroidism (see Nursing Care Plan: The Patient with Hypothyroidism).

Assessment

Table 43-1 summarizes the general assessment of the patient with a thyroid disorder. Assessment of the patient with hypothyroidism should include measurement of vital signs, height, and weight. In addition, assess activity and temperature tolerance, voice quality, bowel elimination pattern, and changes in weight and dietary intake. Inspect and palpate the skin for turgor, texture, and moisture. Note level of consciousness and emotional state. Ask if the patient has noticed a change in mental alertness. Also assess the patient's understanding of hypothyroidism and its treatment.

table 43-4 ***Comparison of Signs and Symptoms of Hypothyroidism and Hyperthyroidism***

SYSTEM	HYPOTHYROIDISM	HYPERTHYROIDISM
Integumentary	Coarse, dry skin and hair Thick nails	Smooth, moist skin Silky hair Diaphoresis
Musculoskeletal	Muscle aches and pains Weakness Slow movements	Weakness
Cardiovascular	Bradycardia Dysrhythmias Hypotension Anemia Capillary fragility	Tachycardia Dysrhythmias Palpitations Systolic hypertension Angina
Respiratory	Hypoventilation Dyspnea	Increased respiratory rate Dyspnea
Gastrointestinal	Anorexia Nausea and vomiting Constipation Weight gain	Increased appetite Increased bowel sounds Diarrhea Weight loss
Neurologic	Apathy Lethargy Slowed mental function Depression Slow speech Paresthesias Decreased tendon reflexes	Nervousness and irritability Insomnia Personality change Agitation Inability to concentrate Fine tremor of fingers and tongue Hyperreflexia
Reproductive	Women Amenorrhea or prolonged menses Infertility Decreased libido Men Decreased libido Erectile dysfunction	Women Menstrual irregularities Decreased libido Men Decreased libido Erectile dysfunction Gynecomastia
Other	Cold intolerance Decreased body temperature Facial puffiness or coarseness Thick tongue Nonpitting edema of hands and feet Sensitivity to central nervous system depressants	Increased body temperature Exophthalmos Goiter Sensitivity to central nervous system stimulants

Nursing Diagnoses, Goals, and Outcome Criteria: Hypothyroidism

NURSING DIAGNOSES	GOALS AND OUTCOME CRITERIA
Activity Intolerance related to decreased metabolic energy production	Improved activity tolerance: patient report of less fatigue with daily activities
Imbalanced Nutrition: More than Body Requirements related to intake greater than metabolic needs	Balanced nutrition: stable body weight or gradual return to weight before thyroid disorder
Hypothermia related to cold intolerance	Improved cold tolerance: warm hands and feet, no complaints of coldness
Constipation related to decreased peristalsis	Normal bowel function: regular stools without difficulty
Risk for Impaired Skin Integrity related to dryness and edema	Decreased risk of skin breakdown: skin moist, intact
Decreased Cardiac Output related to cardiovascular changes secondary to hypothyroidism	Normal cardiac output: improved stamina, pulse and blood pressure within normal limits; no dyspnea, edema, dysrhythmias
Disturbed Thought Processes related to decreased cerebral oxygenation	Improved thought processes: oriented to person, place, time; patient reports improved mental function
Disturbed Body Image related to altered physical appearance, disturbed thought processes, lack of energy	Improved body image: patient makes positive statements about appearance, tends to personal appearance

NURSING CARE PLAN

The Patient with Hypothyroidism

ASSESSMENT

Health History: A 53-year-old woman comes to the physician's office complaining of fatigue and irritability. Her symptoms have gradually worsened and are now interfering with her work as an executive secretary. She reports that her health has generally been good, with only one hospitalization for an appendectomy 7 years ago. The review of systems reveals frequent headaches, anorexia, constipation, menstrual irregularity, numbness and tingling in the legs, and intolerance to cold. She has noticed a 10-pound weight gain over the past six months without a change in diet or exercise.

Physical Examination: Vital signs: temperature 97° F orally; pulse, 56; respiration, 18; blood pressure, 90/60. (Her record indicates that her previous blood pressure was 128/76 and that pulse was 74.) Height, 5'5". Weight, 155 lb. She is oriented but lethargic. Her hair is coarse, and her skin is dry.

Nursing Diagnosis	*Goals and Outcome Criteria*	*Interventions*
Activity intolerance related to decreased metabolic energy production.	The patient will report less fatigue with activities of daily living.	Advise patient to schedule additional rest periods until condition improves. Assure her that these symptoms are temporary.
Imbalanced nutrition: greater than body requirements related to intake greater than metabolic needs.	The patient's weight will stabilize within 2 pounds of her usual 145 pounds.	Weigh during each office visit. Encourage balanced diet. Tell her that weight should normalize when condition is corrected.
Hypothermia related to cold intolerance.	The patient will report adequate warmth and increased tolerance of cool temperatures.	Adjust room temperature for patient comfort. Provide adequate covering during physical examination.
Constipation related to decreased peristalsis.	The patient will have regular bowel movements passed without straining.	Encourage increased fluid intake, high-fiber diet with fresh fruits and raw vegetables. Instruct in taking stool softeners if advised by physician. Encourage gradual increase in physical activity as tolerance improves.
Risk for impaired skin integrity related to dryness.	The patient's skin will remain intact, and usual moisture will be restored.	Advise to decrease bathing frequency and to use moisturizing creams or lotions. Advise to avoid scratching.
Decreased cardiac output related to cardiovascular changes secondary to hypothyroidism.	The patient's cardiac output will improve, as evidenced by improved stamina, regular pulse between 60 and 100, blood pressure consistent with patient norms, no dyspnea.	Monitor for tachycardia, hypertension, and dysrhythmias after hormone replacement therapy is begun.
Disturbed thought processes related to decreased cerebral oxygenation.	The patient will report improved mental functioning and will appear less lethargic; is oriented to person, place, and time.	Explain that mental slowness is related to hypothyroidism and that it will improve with treatment. Do not overload patient with information. Teach only critical information initially and supplement with written information. Ask her how her work expectations could be adjusted to accommodate her symptoms temporarily.
Self-care deficits related to fatigue.	The patient's activities of daily living will be accomplished with only normal fatigue.	Ask patient to consider her daily activities and set priorities. Encourage rest periods. Delay difficult or strenuous tasks until condition improves.

Nursing Diagnoses, Goals, and Outcome Criteria: Hypothyroidism—cont'd

Nursing Diagnoses	Goals and Outcome Criteria
Self-Care Deficit related to fatigue	Improved self-care: patient gradually resumes responsibility for personal care, completes care with less fatigue

Interventions

Activity Intolerance

The hypothyroid patient lacks energy and tires easily. Arrange the schedule to allow for rest periods. Sedatives and barbiturates should be avoided because they may cause excessive sedation. If they are given, lower dosages are recommended. Monitor and document the patient's respirations and level of consciousness. Families and employers need to understand the patient's fatigue and make adjustments until the patient recovers. Improvement is gradual but is usually evident after 2-3 weeks.

Imbalanced Nutrition: More than Body Requirements

Despite having a poor appetite, the patient may have had a weight gain. Weekly weights are helpful in evaluating the effects of hormone replacement therapy. Calorie reduction may be prescribed for the patient who is overweight. Encourage a balanced diet.

Hypothermia

Cold intolerance is a very uncomfortable effect of hypothyroidism. Provide extra clothing and blankets as needed. Maintain the room temperature at a level comfortable to the patient. This is easier to manage if the patient has a private room. Once thyroid replacement is initiated, the cold intolerance gradually improves.

Constipation

Constipation is a common problem. Until the hypothyroidism is corrected, take measures to promote normal elimination. Adequate fluids, dietary fiber, and physical activity all help reduce constipation. Bulk laxatives or stool softeners may be indicated if other measures do not solve the problem. Remember that adequate fluids are essential to prevent bowel obstruction with bulk laxatives. Elderly patients should increase activity levels gradually to avoid excessive stress on the heart.

Risk for Impaired Skin Integrity

Dry skin, which is common with hypothyroidism, is prone to breakdown. Liberally apply lotions and creams to help maintain moisture and control itching. Reduce the frequency of bathing to prevent additional drying of the skin.

Decreased Cardiac Output

Atherosclerosis and heart disease develop in patients whose hypothyroidism is uncorrected for a long time. Monitor these patients for any signs and symptoms of heart failure, such as dyspnea and increasing edema. After hormone replacement therapy is begun, there is some risk of excessive cardiac stimulation. Tell the patient that any chest pain should be reported promptly. Monitor the pulse to detect potentially serious changes in rhythm or rate. Remember that the older adult's circulatory system adapts more slowly to increased thyroid hormone.

Disturbed Thought Processes

Mental dullness and depression can significantly affect the patient's life. Explain that these symptoms are related to hypothyroidism and that correction of hypothyroidism usually results in marked improvement. (An exception is the person who has cretinism caused by untreated hypothyroidism during fetal development or early infancy. The mental retardation of cretinism is not reversible.) Until mental function improves, be careful not to demand too much of the patient. Break teaching into small units and reinforce at intervals.

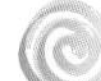
What Does Culture Have to do with Cretinism?

Neonatal hypothyroidism, which causes cretinism if not corrected early, is much more common among whites than blacks.

Disturbed Body Image

The puffy, apathetic look and weight gain associated with hypothyroidism can be very distressing to the patient. Be accepting of the patient's concerns but encourage good grooming and attention to appearance. Tell the patient that treatment will gradually eliminate these changes.

Self-Care Deficit

The hypothyroid patient can expect to need lifelong hormone replacement therapy. Explain this to the patient and stress the need for periodic medical evaluation. Describe the name, dosage, and adverse effects of the prescribed drug therapy. Teach the patient the symptoms of hyperthyroidism that might occur with excessive hormone replacement (tachycardia, weight loss, nervousness). Document patient teaching.

Put on your THINKING CAP!!

A patient who was recently diagnosed with hypothyroidism complains that she has no appetite but has gained 20 pounds over the past few months. How would you explain this to her?

Goiter

Goiter is the term used to describe enlargement of the thyroid gland. Enlargement may be due to simple goiter, thyroid nodules, or thyroiditis.

Simple Goiter

Thyroid enlargement with normal thyroid hormone production is called simple goiter (Fig. 43-6). Causes include iodine deficiency and long-term exposure to goitrogens. The gland

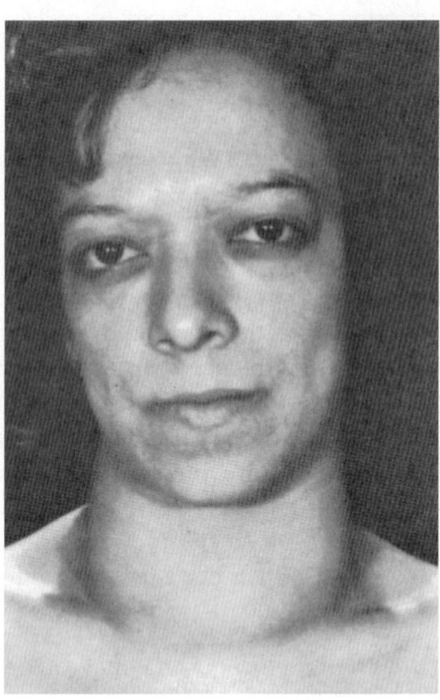

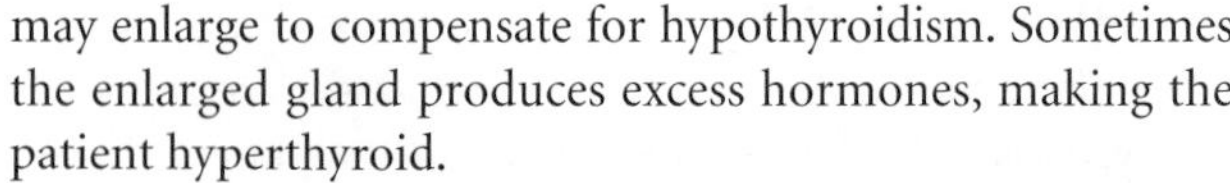

FIGURE 43-6 Goiter.

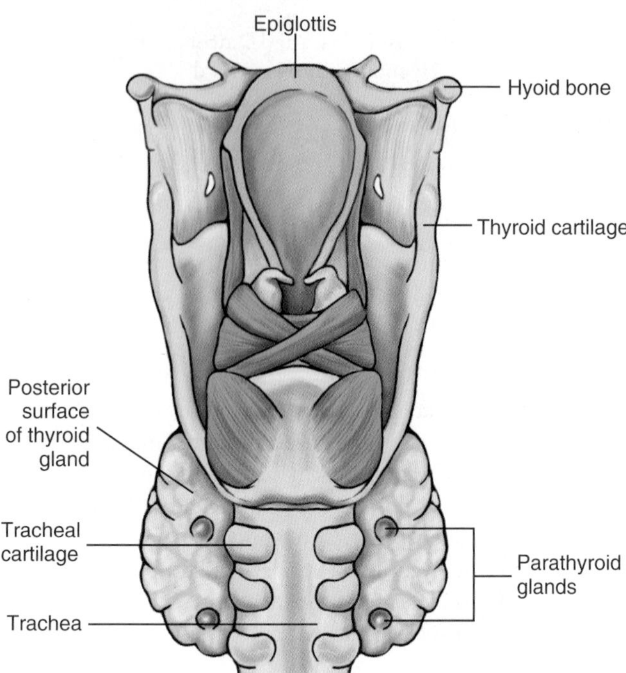

FIGURE 43-7 Posterior view of the neck and thyroid gland, showing the approximate location of the parathyroid glands.

may enlarge to compensate for hypothyroidism. Sometimes the enlarged gland produces excess hormones, making the patient hyperthyroid.

The type of treatment depends on the degree of enlargement and level of thyroid hormone production. If enlargement is mild and hormones are normal, no intervention is required. Some patients need hormone replacement therapy. Surgery is indicated if there is pressure on the trachea or esophagus or if the condition is disfiguring.

Nodules

Multinodular goiter is discussed in the section on hyperthyroidism. As noted, nodules can be benign or malignant. To help determine whether cancer is present, the physician may order a scan that uses radioactive iodine. Nodular goiters are usually surgically removed. In benign conditions, only the nodule may be removed.

Thyroid Cancer

Thyroid cancer is not common, but it is fatal in less than 1% of all cases. In the early stages, the only sign may be a nodule that can be felt on the thyroid gland. Later, if the cancer spreads, enlarged lymph nodes are felt in the neck. The patient may not show dramatic changes in thyroid hormone levels. Total thyroidectomy is the usual treatment. Nursing care of the thyroidectomy patient is covered in the section on hyperthyroidism. If the malignancy has spread beyond the thyroid gland, more radical surgery may be indicated.

Surgery may be followed with radioactive iodine treatment to destroy any remaining tissue that might harbor malignant cells. This is the same type of iodine used in diagnostic studies, but a larger dose is used. The patient needs to be isolated and on radiation precautions. Body fluids must be handled according to radiation precaution guidelines because they are contaminated. The care of the patient receiving internal radiation therapy is discussed in Chapter 24.

The patient will be alarmed at the diagnosis of cancer. He or she may find some comfort in knowing that the 5-year survival rate for thyroid cancer is among the highest of all types of cancer. Long-term care after thyroid cancer includes management of hypothyroidism and monitoring for recurrence. Scans using radioactive iodine are sometimes ordered at intervals to detect the presence of any remaining cancerous tissue. Periodic TSH and thyroglobulin tests may be ordered. Thyroid replacement therapy is based on the TSH level. Thyroglobulin rises if thyroid cancer recurs.

THE PARATHYROID GLANDS

ANATOMY AND PHYSIOLOGY OF THE PARATHYROID GLANDS

The parathyroid glands are small glands usually located on the back of the thyroid gland (Fig. 43-7). Occasionally, some glands are found in the mediastinum as well. Most people have four parathyroids, but some people have more. Even though they are typically embedded in the thyroid, the parathyroids function independently. They secrete only one hormone, but it is a vital one. Parathyroid hormone, or parathormone (PTH), plays a critical role in regulating the serum calcium level.

Calcium is an essential component of strong bones and plays a vital role in the functions of nerve and muscle cells.

table 43-5 ASSESSMENT *of the Patient with a Parathyroid Disorder*

HEALTH HISTORY

Present Illness: Changes in mental-emotional status, neuromuscular symptoms
Past Medical History: Head or neck radiation, renal calculi, chronic renal failure, recent and current medications, including calcium and vitamin D supplements
Review of Systems: Fatigue, irritability, muscle tremors or spasms, bone pain, urinary frequency, polyuria, constipation or diarrhea, depression, personality changes

PHYSICAL EXAMINATION

Vital Signs: Dysrhythmias, hypertension or hypotension
Skin and Hair: Changes in moisture and texture
Urologic: Flank pain
Musculoskeletal: Weakness, tremors
Neurologic: Abnormally active or depressed reflexes, irritability, headache, confusion, positive Chvostek's sign, positive Trousseau's sign

When the serum calcium level falls, PTH is secreted. PTH increases the absorption of calcium from the intestines, transfers calcium from the bones to the blood, and signals the kidneys to conserve calcium. In general, calcium retention by the kidney is balanced by phosphate loss.

NURSING ASSESSMENT OF THE PARATHYROID GLANDS

Health History

When taking the health history, ask if the patient has noticed any change in mental-emotional status, such as memory problems, irritability, or personality changes. Assess a history of musculoskeletal problems, including weakness, skeletal pain, backache, and muscle twitching or spasms. Note if the patient has experienced urinary frequency, polyuria, urinary calculi (stones), or constipation. Document a past medical history of head or neck radiation, renal calculi, or chronic renal failure. List medications, including calcium and vitamin D supplements.

Physical Examination

Important data in the physical examination include heart rate and rhythm, blood pressure, respiratory effort, muscle strength, muscle twitching, and hair and skin texture. Simple tests are used to elicit **Chvostek's sign** and **Trousseau's sign,** which are both indicative of hypocalcemia. Chvostek's sign is a spasm of the facial muscle when the face is tapped over the facial nerve. Trousseau's sign is a carpopedal spasm that occurs when a blood pressure cuff is inflated above the patient's systolic blood pressure and left in place for 2 to 3 minutes (see Fig. 43-3).

Nursing assessment of the patient with a parathyroid disorder is outlined in Table 43-5.

DIAGNOSTIC TESTS AND PROCEDURES

The diagnosis of parathyroid disorders is based on blood and urine studies and skeletal radiographs. Blood tests include measurements of calcium, phosphate, creatinine, uric acid, magnesium, alkaline phosphatase, and PTH. The presence of parathyroid antibodies also may be identified through blood studies. A 24-hour urine specimen may be collected to determine how much calcium is being excreted in the urine.

If excessive calcium has been drawn from bones, demineralization will be apparent on radiographs. Bone cysts and tumors may be found. A dental examination may be done to detect changes in the teeth consistent with parathyroid dysfunction. An electrocardiogram also may be ordered because calcium imbalances can cause alterations in the electrical activity in the heart.

DISORDERS OF THE PARATHYROID GLANDS

Hyperparathyroidism

The secretion of excess PTH is called hyperparathyroidism. It is caused most often by a tumor called an *adenoma.* The tumors can be benign or malignant. Other factors that may stimulate excess PTH secretion are vitamin D deficiencies, malabsorption, chronic renal failure, and elevated serum phosphate. People who receive a kidney transplant after having been on dialysis for a long time also may have hyperparathyroidism.

The most notable effect of hyperparathyroidism is elevation of serum calcium (hypercalcemia). High levels of PTH cause calcium to shift from the bones into the bloodstream. Excess PTH also promotes retention of calcium and loss of phosphate by the kidneys. If untreated, severe demineralization of bone tissue occurs. Bones can become brittle, thus resulting in serious fractures. The high level of calcium in the urine can lead to the formation of urinary calculi. Obstruction of the urinary tubules by calculi can lead quickly to severe kidney damage. The effects of hyperparathyroidism on the heart can cause dysrhythmias and hypertension.

Signs and Symptoms

Because hyperparathyroidism usually develops gradually, symptoms are vague at first. The patient may report weakness, lethargy, depression, anorexia, and constipation. Other findings might include mental and personality changes, cardiac dysrhythmias, weight loss, and urinary calculi. Additional signs and symptoms of hyperparathyroidism are outlined in Table 43-6.

Medical Diagnosis

The diagnosis of hyperparathyroidism is based primarily on blood and urine studies. Typical findings include elevated serum calcium and decreased serum phosphate, elevated PTH, and elevated 24-hour urine calcium. Skeletal radiographs reveal bone demineralization if the condition is severe. Sometimes the condition is not recognized until the patient has a spontaneous fracture. Other procedures that may be employed include CT, MRI, ultrasound, fine needle aspiration, and selective arteriography.

table 43-6 ***Comparison of Signs and Symptoms of Hypoparathyroidism and Hyperparathyroidism***

SYSTEM	HYPOPARATHYROIDISM	HYPERPARATHYROIDISM
Musculoskeletal	Fatigue Weakness Cramps Twitching	Poor muscle tone Weakness Bone pain Demineralization Fractures
Urinary	Frequency	Polyuria Renal calculi
Cardiovascular	Decreased cardiac output Dysrhythmias	Hypertension Dysrhythmias
Nervous	Hyperactive reflexes Memory impairment Depression Anxiety Irritability Personality changes Confusion Numbness and tingling of hands and feet and around mouth Muscle spasms	Depressed reflexes Decreased mental function Depression Mood swings Confusion Coma Poor coordination
Gastrointestinal	Abdominal cramps	Anorexia Nausea and vomiting Constipation
Integumentary	Brittle nails, dry skin	Moist skin

Medical Treatment

If a tumor is causing hyperparathyroidism, it usually is removed surgically. In some cases, more than one gland is removed. The surgeon attempts to leave some parathyroid tissue to prevent hypoparathyroidism. This can be a complicated procedure because some parathyroid glands may be located in the mediastinum. If the condition is mild or the patient is not a good candidate for surgery, medical treatment is aimed at lowering the serum calcium level. The patient is instructed to maintain a high fluid intake to dilute the urine. Calcium intake may be restricted. Sodium and phosphorus replacements may be ordered.

Drug therapy. When it is necessary to lower the calcium level quickly, an infusion of normal saline is often prescribed. Several drugs can be used to treat hypercalcemia. Calcitonin (Calcimar), gallium nitrate (Ganite), biphosphonates (etidronate, pamidronate), and plicamycin (Mithracin) inhibit the release of calcium from bones. Furosemide (Lasix) may be given to promote the excretion of calcium in the urine. Propranolol reduces PTH secretion. Because plicamycin has severe toxic effects, it is usually reserved for patients with metastatic parathyroid cancer. If hypercalcemia is caused by vitamin D intoxication, glucocorticoids are highly effective. Drugs used to treat parathyroid disorders are described in Table 43-7.

PHARMACOLOGY CAPSULE Furosemide (Lasix) is a diuretic that promotes the excretion of calcium in the urine.

NURSING CARE *of the Patient with Hyperparathyroidism*

Assessment

When caring for the hyperparathyroid patient, assess vital signs, urine output, weight, muscle strength, bowel elimination, and digestive disturbances.

Nursing Diagnoses, Goals, and Outcome Criteria: Hyperparathyroidism

NURSING DIAGNOSES	GOALS AND OUTCOME CRITERIA
Activity Intolerance related to weakness and fatigue	Improved activity tolerance: patient reports performing daily activities with less fatigue
Risk for Injury related to weakness and decreased bone mass	Reduced risk for injury: improved muscle strength, no falls
Impaired Urinary Elimination related to urinary calculi	Normal urinary output: urine output equal to fluid intake
Constipation related to altered intestinal motility	Normal bowel elimination: regular stools without straining
Disturbed Thought Processes related to hypercalcemia	Improved mental-emotional state: less irritability, depression
Imbalanced Nutrition: Less than Body Requirements related to nausea and vomiting	Adequate nutrition: stable body weight, no nausea or vomiting

table 43-7 **DRUG THERAPY | *Parathyroid Conditions***

DRUG	USE/ACTION	SIDE EFFECTS	NURSING INTERVENTIONS
CALCIUM SALTS			
Calcium chloride Calcium gluconate Calcium carbonate	Correct calcium deficiency due to hypoparathyroidism.	Overdosage (hypercalcemia): weakness, hypertension, dysrhythmias, polyuria, bone pain	Take with food. Serum calcium levels should be monitored. Notify physician of signs of hypercalcemia.
VITAMIN D			
Calcitrol Dihydrotachysterol Ergocalciferol	Promotes calcium absorption from digestive tract.	Overdosage (hypercalcemia): weakness, hypertension, dysrhythmias, polyuria, bone pain	Serum calcium levels should be monitored. Notify physician of signs of hypercalcemia.
BISPHOSPHONATES			
Pamidronate (Aredia)	Inhibits bone resorption, reduces serum calcium. More effective than etidronate.	Local pain, inflammation at infusion site. Potassium, magnesium, and phosphate deficiencies. GI distress. Fluid overload, hypertension.	Assess infusion site. Do not mix with IV solutions that contain calcium. Monitor P, BP, fluid intake, and urine output.
Etidronate disodium (Didronel)	Reduces serum calcium level in hyperparathyroidism.	Diarrhea, nausea, metallic taste, bone pain, and tenderness. Hypocalcemia: weakness, muscle spasms.	Dividing dose through the day may control diarrhea. Advise that metallic taste is temporary.
OTHER			
Furosemide (Lasix)	Promotes excretion of excess calcium in hyperparathyroidism.	Fluid and electrolyte imbalances: metabolic alkalosis, hypovolemia, dehydration, hyponatremia, hypokalemia. Dizziness, headache, tinnitus, hyperglycemia.	Monitor intake and output, serum calcium and potassium levels, pulse, blood pressure, blood glucose.
Parathormone	Short-term treatment of hypoparathyroidism.	Overdosage (hypercalcemia): dysrhythmias, hypertension, weakness, polyuria, bone pain.	Available only for parenteral use.
Calcitonin (Calcimar, Cibacalcin)	Treats hypercalcemia caused by hyperparathyroidism.	Nausea, vomiting, injection site reactions, facial flushing, anaphylaxis.	Monitor for tachycardia due to hypocalcemia. Have epinephrine, antihistamines, and oxygen available. Sensitivity test should be done before giving. Tell patient that flushing is temporary. Teach self-medication. Encourage adequate fluid intake.
Plicamycin (Mithracin)	Treats hypercalcemia by inhibiting release of calcium from bones.	Hypocalcemia: weakness, muscle spasms. Hypokalemia, thrombocytopenia, leukopenia, bleeding, drowsiness, depression, anorexia, nausea, vomiting.	Reserved for patients with metastatic parathyroid cancer because of severity of toxic effects. Monitor for bleeding. Avoid injections. Apply pressure to venipuncture sites for 10 minutes. Assess for signs of infection. Discontinue infusion if extravasation occurs.
Gallium nitrate (Ganite)	Reduces serum calcium level in hypercalcemia.	Hypotension, nausea, and vomiting, decreased serum calcium and bicarbonate, increased blood urea nitrogen and creatinine.	Administer intravenously with normal saline. Monitor serum electrolytes, blood pressure, complete blood count, and urine output.

Interventions

Activity Intolerance and Risk for Injury

Assess the patient's ability to perform self-care safely and provide help as needed. Move and handle the patient gently. Evaluate the environment for any safety hazards and take corrective measures. Plan care to allow for periods of rest. Assure the patient that weakness and fatigue are caused by the parathyroid disorder and will improve as the condition is corrected.

Impaired Urinary Elimination

Maintain accurate intake and output records because hypercalcemia can cause urinary calculi and serious kidney damage. Decreasing urine output; sharp pain in the flank (kidney area), lower abdomen, or genitalia; and hematuria are consistent with urinary calculi and should be reported to the physician. A high fluid intake, sometimes as much as 4,000 ml/day, may be ordered. Closely monitor urine output and vital signs when large volumes of fluid are administered. The elderly and people with heart disease are at risk for excess fluid volume and congestive heart failure. Patients with cardiac or renal disease may be unable to tolerate this much fluid. Urine may be strained and examined for crystals or calculi. A low-calcium diet and urine acidifiers may be ordered to decrease the risk of calculi formation.

Constipation

Chart bowel movements, including frequency and characteristics of stools. Constipation can often be managed with adequate fluids and fiber in the diet. If these measures are not effective, the physician may order bulk laxatives or stool softeners. It is especially important to monitor bowel elimination in the elderly. Illness, inactivity, and multiple medications combine to increase their risk of constipation and even fecal impaction.

Disturbed Thought Processes

Recognize that irritability, personality changes, and depression are common with hyperparathyroidism. Patients and their families appreciate knowing that these symptoms improve with treatment.

Imbalanced Nutrition: Less than Body Requirements

Take measures to control nausea and vomiting if present. Monitor weight to detect inadequate nutrition if the patient's intake is poor. Small feedings may be better tolerated. Provide a pleasant mealtime environment.

PATIENT TEACHING PLAN
Hyperparathyroidism

- Take drugs exactly as ordered and report adverse effects to the physician.
- Eat a balanced diet.
- Notify the physician of bloody urine or pain in the kidney area or groin.
- Increase fluid intake to the amount recommended by the physician.

Postoperative Care. After parathyroidectomy, the patient requires care like that of any surgical patient, as detailed in Chapter 16. Two potential complications specific to parathyroidectomy are airway obstruction and hypocalcemia. When the patient has a neck incision, accumulated fluid and blood in the surgical site can compress the trachea, thus causing airway obstruction. Monitor and document the respiratory rate and effort and the pulse rate. Increasing pulse and respiratory rates, especially accompanied by restlessness, suggest inadequate oxygenation. Notify the physician of any indications of respiratory distress. Keep an emergency tracheotomy tray at the bedside in the event of acute obstruction.

A second possible cause of airway obstruction is related to severe hypocalcemia. Be alert for tetany, a symptom of hypocalcemia, caused by the postoperative decrease in parathyroid hormones. A tingling sensation around the mouth and in the fingers is an early symptom of tetany. It may progress to severe muscle spasms or cramps and even to laryngospasm. To prevent this happening, calcium and other electrolytes are monitored closely in the postoperative period. Promptly inform the physician of signs of tetany or abnormal electrolyte values. Tetany is treated with oral or intravenous calcium supplements. Treatment of Hypocalcemia is discussed in detail in the section on Hypoparathyroidism.

The patient's incision is on the front of the neck or upper chest, or both, and usually is covered with a bulky pressure dressing. As with the thyroidectomy patient, this patient's suture line should be protected from stress. Show the patient how to support the head when changing positions. Assess the dressing and the back of the patient's neck for bleeding. Elevate the patient's head to help reduce swelling.

Hypoparathyroidism

Hypoparathyroidism is a deficiency of PTH. It is an uncommon condition, most often due to accidental removal of or damage to parathyroid glands during surgery. Primary hypoparathyroidism can be caused by an autoimmune process and by several conditions, including Wilson's disease (copper overload). Inadequate secretion of PTH leads to hypocalcemia. Severe hypocalcemia can progress to convulsions and respiratory obstruction due to spasms of the larynx. Laryngospasm can be fatal.

Signs and Symptoms

Assessment of parathyroid function is most important after thyroid surgery. Trauma or accidental removal of one or more parathyroid glands may lead to symptoms of hypoparathyroidism, as discussed in the section on Nursing Care of the Patient having a Thyroidectomy.

Signs and symptoms of hypocalcemia are painful muscle cramps, fatigue and weakness, tingling and twitching of the face and hands, mental and emotional changes, dry skin, and urinary frequency. With severe hypocalcemia, the patient may have difficulty breathing, convulsions, and cardiac dysrhythmias.

Medical Diagnosis

The diagnosis of hypoparathyroidism is based on patient signs and symptoms and blood studies. Typical findings include low serum calcium, elevated serum phosphate, low urine calcium, and sometimes low serum magnesium. Two classic signs of hypocalcemia that support a diagnosis of hypoparathyroidism are Chvostek's sign and Trousseau's sign.

Medical Treatment

Acute hypoparathyroidism is sometimes treated with parenteral PTH, which is not practical for chronic management. Severe hypocalcemia is treated with intravenous calcium salts.Other electrolyte imbalances must be treated as well.

On a long-term basis, the patient with chronic hypoparathyroidism is treated with oral calcium salts and a form of vitamin D. Aluminum hydroxide also may be ordered with meals to reduce the absorption of phosphates in the intestines. Lowering serum phosphate levels tends to raise serum calcium levels. Chronic hypoparathyroidism that normally is well controlled may be affected when the patient is under severe stress or is very ill. If the patient is unable to take oral calcium, hypocalcemia can develop quickly. Temporary intravenous calcium may be needed.

PHARMACOLOGY CAPSULE Lifelong calcium supplementation is required to treat chronic hypoparathyroidism.

NURSING CARE *of the Patient with Hypoparathyroidism*

Assessment

Assessment of the hypoparathyroid patient is summarized in Table 43-5.

Nursing Diagnoses, Goals, and Outcome Criteria: Hypoparathyroidism

Nursing Diagnoses	Goals and Outcome Criteria
Risk for Injury related to hypocalcemia	Decreased risk for injury: serum calcium level within normal limits; no muscle spasms, convulsions, or respiratory distress; negative Chvostek's and Trousseau's signs
Decreased Cardiac Output related to dysrhythmias and heart failure secondary to hypocalcemia	Normal cardiac output: normal pulse rate and rhythm; normal blood pressure; no dyspnea or edema

Interventions

Administer drugs as ordered for hypoparathyroidism and hypocalcemia. When administering calcium salts intravenously, monitor the infusion site carefully because the leakage of calcium salts into body tissues causes inflammation. The infusion site should be changed if extravasation occurs. Frequently assess the patient for signs and symptoms of calcium imbalances. Hypocalcemia may appear as a result of inadequate calcium supplementation. Hypercalcemia can result from excessive calcium intake.

Nutrition Concepts

1. Hypothyroid and hyperthyroid patients may require adjustments in calorie intake that are appropriate to metabolic needs.
2. Lack of iodine is associated with the development of a goiter (enlargement of the thyroid gland) in adults and cretinism in infants.
3. Iodized salt is the best way to obtain an adequate amount of iodine in the diet.
4. Another important source of iodine is saltwater seafoods.
5. Parathormone, secreted by the parathyroid gland, and thyrocalcitonin, secreted by the thyroid gland, maintain serum calcium levels.

If there has been any recent seizure activity or if the patient shows severe neuromuscular irritability, follow seizure precautions. Any signs of respiratory distress may suggest laryngospasm and should be documented and reported to the physician immediately. Monitor the pulse and blood pressure to detect dysrhythmias and heart failure. Report cardiac irregularities, edema, and dyspnea to the physician.

Teach patients with chronic hypoparathyroidism signs and symptoms of calcium imbalances and provide instructions for self-medication. Advise them to carry medical identification cards to alert health care providers to the disorder in the event of an emergency.

key points

- Thyroxine (T_4), triiodothyronine (T_3), and calcitonin are hormones produced by the thyroid gland that affect metabolic rate, growth and development, and serum calcium regulation.
- Hyperthyroidism is the abnormally increased production of thyroid hormones that may be treated with antithyroid drugs, surgery, or radiation therapy.
- Nursing care of the hyperthyroid patient may address disturbed sleep pattern, hyperthermia, imbalanced nutrition: less than body requirements, decreased cardiac output, risk for injury, and diarrhea.
- Nursing care after thyroidectomy is concerned with ineffective airway clearance, decreased cardiac output, disturbed body image, acute pain, and risk for infection.
- Hypothyroidism is inadequate secretion of thyroid hormones that is treated with hormone replacement therapy.
- Nursing care of the hypothyroid patient addresses activity intolerance, imbalanced nutrition: more than body requirements, hypothermia, constipation, risk for impaired skin integrity, decreased cardiac output, disturbed thought processes, disturbed body image, and self-care deficits.
- Goiter is enlargement of the thyroid gland that may be associated with hypothyroidism or hyperthyroidism.
- The parathyroid glands secrete parathormone, which regulates the serum calcium level.

- Hyperparathyroidism raises the serum calcium level and may cause bone demineralization and obstruction of kidney tubules.
- Nursing care of the patient with hyperparathyroidism focuses on activity intolerance, risk for injury, impaired urine elimination, constipation, disturbed thought processes, and imbalanced nutrition.
- Hypoparathyroidism, a deficiency of parathormone that sometimes follows thyroidectomy, causes the serum calcium level to fall, producing neuromuscular irritability that can progress to seizures, cardiac dysrhythmias, and laryngospasm.
- Nursing diagnoses for the hypoparathyroid patient are risk for injury and decreased cardiac output.

REVIEW QUESTIONS

1. The primary function of thyroid hormones is to regulate:
   1. metabolism.
   2. temperature.
   3. appetite.
   4. thirst.
2. You are notified that a patient with severe hypothyroidism is being admitted to your nursing unit. Which action is appropriate?
   1. Obtain an emergency tracheostomy tray.
   2. Close the blinds to dim the room light.
   3. Have extra blankets put in the room.
   4. Pad the siderails on the bed.
3. Which of the following assessment findings is most likely to be found in a patient with severe hyperthyroidism?
   1. Respiratory rate of 12
   2. Heart rate of 120 bpm
   3. Blood pressure of 110/60
   4. Oral temperature of 96° F
4. During shift report, it is stated that a hyperthyroid patient has exophthalamos. You would expect to see:
   1. enlargement of the patient's neck.
   2. edema of the face and hands.
   3. thin, dry, skin that bruises easily.
   4. prominent, bulging eyeballs.
5. A 6-week course of treatment with propylthiouracil (PTU) is prescribed for a patient who is scheduled for a thyroidectomy. The patient asks why she has to take this medication. Your best response is:
   1. "PTU will help you eliminate excess thyroid hormone."
   2. "It reduces your thyroid activity, which makes surgery safer for you."
   3. "PTU will provide replacement thyroid hormones after your thyroid gland is removed."
   4. "This drug will cause your thyroid gland to shrink, which will reduce pressure on your airway."
6. In the immediate postoperative period following thyroidectomy, the *first* priority is to:
   1. maintain a patent airway.
   2. assess for hemorrhage.
   3. monitor for hypocalcemia.
   4. prevent strain on the suture line.
7. The purpose of measuring serum thyroglobulin in a patient who has had thyroid cancer is to:
   1. assess adequacy of thyroid hormone replacement.
   2. detect any recurrence of the thyroid cancer.
   3. see whether all radioactive iodine has been eliminated.
   4. determine whether parathyroid function is normal.
8. Which statement accurately describes the relationship between parathyroid hormone (PTH) and serum calcium?
   1. The secretion of PTH decreases when serum calcium is low.
   2. Increased secretion of PTH causes the kidneys to retain calcium.
   3. Chronically decreased PTH can lead to bone demineralization.
   4. Decreased serum PTH causes calcium to shift from the bones to the blood.
9. A patient had a parathyroid adenoma removed two days ago. She is now complaining of cramps in her hands and feet. You should suspect:
   1. poor circulation.
   2. thyroid storm.
   3. hypocalcemia.
   4. metabolic acidosis.
10. Nursing implications in administering iodide solutions to a patient include which of the following?
    1. Dilute in milk or juice and provide a straw.
    2. Take the pulse and blood pressure before each dose.
    3. Tell the patient to report any changes in hearing acuity.
    4. Carefully maintain accurate intake and output records.

CHAPTER

44 Diabetes Mellitus and Hypoglycemia

objectives

1. Describe the role of insulin in the body.
2. Explain the pathophysiology of diabetes mellitus and hypoglycemia.
3. Describe the signs and symptoms of diabetes mellitus and hypoglycemia.
4. Explain tests and procedures used to diagnose diabetes mellitus and hypoglycemia.
5. Discuss treatment of diabetes mellitus and hypoglycemia.
6. Explain the difference between type 1 and type 2 diabetes mellitus.
7. Differentiate between acute hypoglycemia and diabetic ketoacidosis.
8. Describe the treatment of a patient experiencing acute hypoglycemia or diabetic ketoacidosis.
9. Describe the complications of diabetes mellitus.
10. Identify nursing interventions for a patient diagnosed with diabetes mellitus or hypoglycemia.
11. Identify nursing interventions for a patient diagnosed with ketoacidosis.

key terms

Endogenous (ĕn-DŎJ-ĕn-ŭs, p. 899)
Euglycemia (ū-glī-SĒ-mē-ă, p. 912)
Exogenous (ĕks-ŎJ-ĕn-ŭs, p. 899)
Glycosuria (glī-kō-SŪ-rē-ă, p. 902)
Hypoglycemia (hī-pō-glī-SĒ-mē-ă, p. 903)
Ketoacidosis (kē-tō-ă-sĭ-DŌ-sĭs, p. 904)
Ketone bodies (KĒ-tōn, p. 905)
Lipoatrophy (lĭp-ō-ĂT-rō-fē, p. 910)
Lipohypertrophy (lĭp-ō-hī-PĔR-trō-fē, p. 910)
Macrovascular (măk-rō-VĂS-cū-lăr, p. 902)
Microvascular (mīk-rō-VĂS-cū-lăr, p. 901)
Nephropathy (nĕ-FRŎP-ă-thē, p. 901)
Neuropathy (nū-RŎP-ĕ-thē, p. 902)
Polydipsia (pŏl-ē-DĬP-sē-ă, p. 900)
Polyphagia (pŏl-ē-FĀ-jē-ă, p. 900)
Polyuria (pŏl-ē-Ū-rē-ă, p. 900)
Retinopathy (rĕt-ĭ-NŎP-ă-thē, p. 901)

DIABETES MELLITUS

Symptoms of diabetes mellitus (DM) have been reported in the literature throughout history, but not until the early 20th century was the cause identified. In an experiment, the pancreata of several sheep were removed, which caused diabetes to develop in the sheep. Through this experiment, insulin and its role in the body were discovered. The search then began for a way to provide insulin to people whose bodies did not produce enough. Before insulin became available for commercial use in 1921, people with diabetes were placed on high-protein diets until they went into acidosis and died, usually a short time after the onset of the disease.

In the United States today, an estimated 16 million people have DM. It is a major health problem and a leading cause of death by disease. People with diabetes are at increased risk for heart disease, renal disease, blindness, amputation, and complications during pregnancy. Fortunately, with early diagnosis and better management, it is possible to reduce the risk of serious complications.

PATHOPHYSIOLOGY

Diabetes mellitus is a chronic disorder characterized by impaired metabolism and by vascular and neurologic complications. A key feature of diabetes is elevated blood glucose, called *hyperglycemia.* The blood glucose level is normally regulated by insulin, a hormone produced by the beta cells in the islets of Langerhans located in the pancreas. In health, small amounts of insulin are secreted continuously into the bloodstream. The ingestion of carbohydrates triggers the secretion of a larger volume of insulin. Insulin that is produced in one's own body is called *endogenous,* meaning it is internally produced. Insulin that is obtained from other sources and administered to a person is called *exogenous,* meaning it comes from an external source.

Diabetes mellitus is classified as type 1 (previously called insulin-dependent DM, or IDDM) or type 2 (previously referred to as non–insulin-dependent DM, or NIDDM). Both types have a genetic component, but most people with diabetes have no genetic predisposition.

Type 1 DM is characterized by the absence of endogenous insulin. It used to be called juvenile-onset diabetes because it most commonly occurs in juveniles and young adults. However, it can also occur in middle-aged and older adults. An autoimmune process, possibly triggered by a viral infection, causes destruction of the beta cells, the development of insulin antibodies, and the production of islet cell antibodies (ICAs). Affected people require exogenous insulin for the rest of their lives.

Type 2 is characterized by inadequate endogenous insulin and the body's inability to properly use insulin. Initially, beta cells respond inadequately to hyperglycemia, resulting in chronically elevated blood glucose. The continuous high glucose level in the blood desensitizes the beta cells so that they become progressively less responsive to the elevated glucose. In relation to the use of insulin, specific receptor sites become insensitive to insulin ("insulin resistance") so that glucose is not admitted to cells. Although type 2 is more common among adults, it is increasingly found in children as well. One inherited form (maturity-onset diabetes of the young) causes type 2 DM among all age groups in affected families.

Type 2 DM may be controlled by diet and exercise alone or may require oral hypoglycemic agents or exogenous insulin. Some patients are treated with insulin initially to normalize blood glucose, then treated with diet, exercise, or oral agents.

Gestational diabetes mellitus (GDM) is diagnosed when a woman is found to have glucose intolerance for the first time during pregnancy. After delivery, the condition resolves. See a maternity nursing text for information on the management of GDM.

Role of Insulin

We usually think of insulin as a critical hormone for glucose metabolism, and that is correct. However, insulin also is needed for the synthesis of fatty acids and proteins (Table 44-1).

Glucose

Insulin stimulates the active transport of glucose into the cells. When insulin is absent, glucose cannot enter most cells, so it remains in the bloodstream. The blood then becomes thick with glucose, which increases its osmolality. Increased osmolality stimulates the thirst center, causing the patient to experience **polydipsia** (excessive thirst) and take in additional fluid. The increased fluid does not pass into body tissues, however, because the high serum osmolality retains the fluid in the bloodstream. As the blood passes through the kidneys, some excess glucose is eliminated. The osmotic force created by the glucose draws extra fluid and electrolytes with it, causing abnormally increased urine volume (**polyuria**).

Because most cells are not able to use glucose without insulin, stored fat is broken down in an effort to provide fuel for heat and energy. Tissue breakdown and loss of lean body mass send hunger signals to the hypothalamus. The patient experiences excessive hunger (**polyphagia**). The patient may take in more food but, unfortunately, cannot use the extra glucose without insulin. Weight loss occurs despite increased appetite and food ingestion.

Insulin is needed to transport glucose into resting muscle cells. During heavy exercise, however, muscle fibers are highly permeable to glucose even in the absence of insulin. Therefore, exercise must be considered in the regulation of serum glucose levels. Other tissues that can use glucose without insulin are the brain, nerves, heart, and the lens of the eye.

Insulin regulates the rate of glucose metabolism. The greater the insulin response to carbohydrate ingestion, the faster the carbohydrates are metabolized.

In a healthy person, when blood glucose falls, insulin production is inhibited and stored glycogen is converted to glucose by a process called *glycogenolysis.* When blood glucose rises, insulin production is stimulated and the conversion of glycogen to glucose is inhibited. This process usually maintains the blood glucose within a normal range. However, when insulin secretion is inadequate, glycogen is converted to glucose in an attempt to nourish glucose-starved tissues, but hyperglycemia occurs because cells cannot use the glucose.

Fatty Acids

Insulin promotes fatty acid synthesis and the conversion of fatty acids into fat, which is stored as adipose tissue. Insulin also spares fat by inhibiting the breakdown of adipose tissue and the mobilization of fat and by inhibiting the conversion of fats to glucose.

Without adequate insulin, fat stores break down and increased triglycerides are stored in the liver. The liver can store up to one third of its weight as fat. Increased fatty acids in the liver can triple the production of lipoproteins, which promotes the development of atherosclerosis. This helps explain why people with DM have a high incidence of cardiovascular disease.

Protein

Insulin enhances protein synthesis in tissues and inhibits the conversion of protein into glucose. Amino acids are admitted into cells, which enhances the rate of protein formation while preventing the degradation of proteins. Without adequate insulin, the storage of proteins halts and large amounts of amino acids are dumped into the bloodstream. High levels of plasma amino acids place people with diabetes at risk for development of gout. Changes in protein metabolism lead to extreme weakness and poor organ functioning.

table 44-1 ***Insulin: Actions and Effects of Deficiency***

INSULIN
Increases the transport of glucose into the resting muscle cell
Regulates the rate at which carbohydrates are used
Promotes the conversion of glucose to glycogen
Inhibits the conversion of glycogen to glucose
Promotes fatty acid synthesis
Spares fat
Inhibits the breakdown of adipose tissue
Inhibits the conversion of fats to glucose
Stimulates protein synthesis in the tissues
Inhibits the conversion of protein into glucose
LACK OF INSULIN
Stimulates the conversion of glycogen to glucose
Permits fat stores to break down
Increases triglyceride storage in the liver
Halts the storage of proteins
Causes protein to be dumped into the bloodstream

ETIOLOGY

Type 1 DM has been attributed to genetic, immunologic, and environmental (viruses, toxins) factors. The tendency toward type 1 DM is found in families with a genetic predisposition.

There is evidence of a strong genetic component in type 2 DM as well.

It is possible that an autoimmune disorder triggers the sudden onset of diabetes in the young (Fig. 44-1). Our bodies are guarded by an elaborate and extensive immune system. When a microbe and its antigen enter the blood, they encounter white blood cells called macrophages that have antigen receptors on their surfaces. These antigen receptors steer the antigens to lymphocytes, which have antigen-specific receptors. When a specific antigen is present, it activates the immune response. The lymphocytes begin producing custom-made antibodies against the antigens, at the same time signaling other types of cells in the immune system to attack the invaders. The lymphocytes and the antibodies are unable to destroy the foreign cells independently without the help of phagocytes and complement cells. This group of cells is selective in identifying and destroying foreign protein. Unfortunately, this part of the immune system can become a renegade faction and turn on its own healthy cells. It is this autoimmune malfunction that may cause complete destruction of the islets of Langerhans in the pancreas, creating type 1 diabetes. In fact, islet cell antibodies are identified in more than 80% of all people with type 1 diabetes at the time of diagnosis.

RISK FACTORS

Risk factors for type 1 DM, other than genetic ones, are not known. According to the American Diabetes Association, risk factors for type 2 DM include:

- Obesity
- Sedentary lifestyle
- Family history of diabetes
- Age 40 years and older
- History of gestational DM
- History of delivering infant weighing more than 10 lbs
- African American (33% higher risk for type 2 DM)
- Latin American/Hispanic (>300% higher risk for type 2 DM)
- Native Americans (33% to 50% higher risk for type 2 DM)

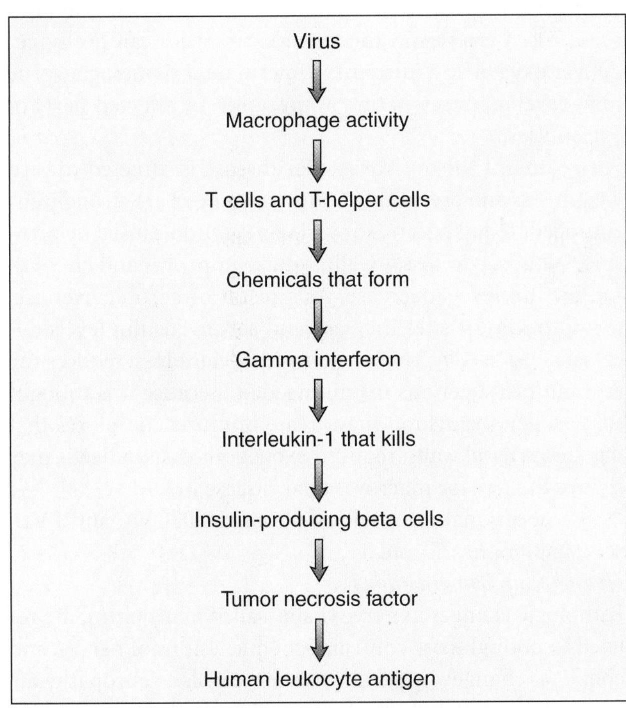

FIGURE **44-1** Possible immunologic cause of diabetes mellitus.

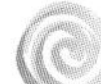**PHARMACOLOGY CAPSULE** Pharmacologic use of glucocorticoids can elevate the blood glucose level. Although unlikely to cause DM in people with normal pancreatic function, glucocorticoid therapy may unmask latent diabetes. It also complicates management of known DM.

What Does Culture Have to do with Diabetes?

The risk of diabetes mellitus among Latin Americans/Hispanic Americans is 300% that of white Americans. Effective measures to decrease this risk must be sensitive to cultural practices and values.

Insulin Resistance Syndrome (Syndrome X)

Syndrome X is the common name used to describe a syndrome that is thought by many to be a precursor to diabetes. This syndrome is also referred to as insulin resistance syndrome and cardiovascular dysmetabolic syndrome. Patients with syndrome X typically have impaired glucose tolerance, high serum insulin, hypertension, elevated triglycerides, low HDL cholesterol, and altered size and density of LDL cholesterol. It is believed that syndrome X represents a chronic low-grade inflammatory process affecting endothelial tissue (the lining of the heart, blood and lymph vessels). The long-term effects include atherosclerosis, ischemic heart disease, left ventricular hypertrophy, and sometimes type 2 DM. Research is now directed at learning how to detect this syndrome early and what interventions might slow or arrest the progress.

COMPLICATIONS

Long-Term Complications

Epidemiologic studies have established that the duration of diabetes and poor glycemic control are the best predictors of the severity of complications. These complications affect almost every organ of the body. They may be classified as microvascular, macrovascular, or neuropathic.

Microvascular Complications

Microvascular complications result from changes in small blood vessels that are unique to diabetes and occur in both type 1 and type 2 disease. The basement membrane of capillaries thickens, which impairs the exchange of nutrients, gases, and wastes. Tissues that are most vulnerable to microvascular complications are the eyes (**retinopathy**) and the kidneys (**nephropathy**). Changes in the capillaries appear to be related to persistent hyperglycemia and are aggravated by hypertension and smoking. Neuropathy is sometimes classified with microvascular complications but is discussed in the section on Macrovascular Complications.

Retinopathy. Among people aged 25 to 74 years, DM is the leading cause of blindness. People with diabetes are at increased risk for retinopathy, cataracts, and glaucoma. Diabetic retinopathy is a term used to describe pathological changes in the retina that are associated with DM. Two types of diabetic retinopathy have been identified: nonproliferative and proliferative. Both types may be present at the same time. Manifestations of nonproliferative disease include small hemorrhages and aneurysms in the retina, hard lipid and protein exudates that leak from the blood vessels, infarcted nerve fibers (described as "cotton wool spots"), and changes in retinal veins. Proliferative disease is characterized by the growth of abnormal capillaries on the retina and the optic disk. These fragile vessels can penetrate the vitreous humor and rupture. When there is hemorrhaging into the vitreous, it becomes cloudy and vision is lost. The blood is eventually reabsorbed, but scars may remain, which places traction on the retina and may result in retinal detachment.

Macular edema occurs with both types of diabetic retinopathy. The macula is the center of vision, and edema causes loss of central vision. To illustrate the effect, imagine this page with only the outer margins clearly visible. The center would be clouded.

Signs and symptoms that suggest impending eye problems are the presence of spots ("floaters") in the field of vision, seeing "cobwebs," or sudden visual changes. Often there are no warning signs of retinal changes. Therefore, patients with diabetes should have eye examinations at least once a year so that early changes in the eye can be detected and measures taken to try to prevent further deterioration and possible blindness. One strategy that may reduce the risk of injury to the eye is control of hypertension. Early laser treatment of macular edema can halt the progression of retinopathy and may even improve vision.

Nephropathy. Renal disease develops in about 20% of people with type 2 DM, compared with 35% to 45% of people with type 1 DM. The leading cause of end-stage renal disease (ESRD) is diabetes. Factors that contribute to nephropathy (kidney damage) include poor control of blood glucose, hypertension, long-standing diabetes, and genetic susceptibility. High concentrations of **glycosuria** (glucose in the urine), along with hypertension, gradually destroy the capillaries that supply the renal glomeruli. Increased permeability of the glomeruli permits serum proteins to be lost in the urine. There are no symptoms in the early stages, but rising microalbuminuria signals the onset of kidney damage. When the level of protein in the urine exceeds 300 mg/day of albumin or 500 mg/day of total protein, the condition will surely progress to ESRD. Signs and symptoms of kidney failure include persistent proteinuria, elevated blood pressure and serum creatinine, hematuria, and oliguria or anuria. Diagnosis is based on laboratory values (see Chapter 38).

What Does Culture Have to do with Nephropathy?

Genetic factors increase the risk for nephropathy among African Americans, Native Americans, and Mexican Americans.

Measures to reduce the risk of damage to the kidneys include good glycemic control, control of hypertension, use of angiotensin-converting enzyme inhibitors, maintaining good hydration, and avoiding nephrotoxic chemicals, including drugs. Modest protein restriction may be recommended. Screening for microalbuminuria can detect early changes that may be amenable to treatment and slow the development of ESRD.

Macrovascular Complications

Atherosclerotic plaque development occurs earlier and is more severe and more extensive in people with diabetes than in other people. Atherosclerosis affects the peripheral, carotid, cerebral, and coronary blood vessels. The accelerated atherosclerotic changes in the person with diabetes are called **macrovascular** complications. Macrovascular complications account for the deaths of 80% of people with type 2 DM.

Chronic hyperglycemia as a result of poor blood glucose control may play an important role in the premature development of atherosclerosis in patients with diabetes. However, there is evidence that the elevated insulin level that occurs with insulin resistance plays a role in the development of atherosclerosis. This is especially apparent in white, middle-aged men. It has been suggested that hyperinsulinemia may affect the endothelium of blood vessels, permitting lipids to be easily deposited on the cell walls of the blood vessels. Other risk factors for macrovascular complications are central obesity, hyperlipidemia, hypertension, genetics, sedentary lifestyle, and smoking.

Macrovascular changes are associated with coronary artery disease (CAD), cerebral vascular accidents (CVA or stroke), and peripheral vascular disease (PVD). Signs and symptoms of PVD may include diminished pedal pulses and claudication (pain in the calf, back, or buttocks while walking). When arteries in the lower extremities can no longer deliver oxygen and nutrients to peripheral tissues, gangrene may develop, necessitating amputation of affected parts of extremities.

Treatment for macrovascular disease is directed toward weight loss and exercise. Patients who smoke are strongly encouraged to quit because of vasoconstriction caused by nicotine. With weight loss, insulin uptake improves and circulating insulin levels decrease. As a result of aerobic exercise, insulin receptor sites increase and serum insulin levels decrease. Exercise, in conjunction with weight loss, reduces the amount of exogenous insulin needed. Because it is thought that exogenous insulin may create immune complexes that damage arterial walls, reduced exogenous insulin needs may reduce the risk for macrovascular disease in DM.

For additional information about CAD, CVA, and PVD, see Chapters 33, 27, and 34.

Neuropathic Complications

Pathologic changes in nerve tissue, called ***neuropathy,*** are related to poor glucose control, ischemic lesions of nerves, and chemical changes in peripheral nerve cells. Neuropathy affects approximately 13% of all people with diabetes. Patients who have had diabetes for more than 25 years have a 50% chance of experiencing neuropathies. Neuropathy can be classified as mononeuropathy, polyneuropathy, or autonomic neuropathy.

Mononeuropathy. Mononeuropathy affects a single nerve or group of nerves. It results from inadequate blood supply and is experienced as sharp, stabbing pain. Pain and atrophy occur in muscles enervated by the affected nerve. Sometimes the pain is relieved by walking.

Polyneuropathy. Polyneuropathy involves both sensory and autonomic nerves. Sensory polyneuropathy commonly affects both legs symmetrically. Symptoms range from tingling, numbness, and burning sensations to complete loss of sensation. Pain is often worse during the night. Sometimes polyneuropathy resolves spontaneously.

Autonomic neuropathy. Autonomic neuropathy affects the sympathetic and parasympathetic nervous systems. It can affect the pupillary response, and functions of the cardiovascular, gastrointestinal, and genitourinary systems. Cardiovascular involvement may be manifested as postural hypotension, resting tachycardia, exercise intolerance, and failure of the heart rate to increase with vigorous exercise. Common gastrointestinal symptoms include constipation or, less commonly, diarrhea, as well as anorexia, nausea, vomiting, gastric reflux, and bloating after meals. The stomach may dilate and lose muscle tone so that gastric emptying is delayed, a condition called *gastroparesis.*

The patient may have urinary problems such as an atonic bladder, in which the bladder capacity increases and eventually causes retention with overflow. Sexual problems in men such as erectile dysfunction and retrograde ejaculation are common. Women may have painful intercourse.

Some areas of the body may cease to sweat (anhidrosis), whereas there is excessive sweating (hyperhidrosis) in other areas. Gustatory sweating (facial sweating after eating) may occur after a meal containing cheese or spicy foods.

Diabetic amyotrophy (loss of muscle mass) causes pain in the muscles of the pelvic girdle and thighs. This pain may be so severe that it interferes with activity and sleep. The muscles look wasted, and fasciculation (involuntary twitching of muscle fibers) may be visible under the skin. These contractions do not produce movement.

Hypoglycemic Unawareness

Normally, patients recognize signs and symptoms of hypoglycemia (abnormally low level of glucose in the blood) so that they can take corrective action. With hypoglycemic unawareness, the usual symptoms of tachycardia, palpitations, tremor, sweating, and nervousness may be absent. Without this "early warning system," the patient may suddenly have changes in mental status as the first sign of hypoglycemia. This phenomenon has been attributed to autonomic neuropathy, but that relationship has not been consistently demonstrated.

Foot Complications of Diabetes

People with diabetes may have foot problems associated with neuropathy, inadequate blood supply, or a combination of both. When neurologic function is impaired but blood flow is adequate, the foot is warm and pink with good pulses, but lacks normal sensation. The patient may have a foot injury but fail to recognize it in the absence of pain.

If the blood supply is impaired but neurologic function is adequate, the foot is cold but sensation is normal. When the foot is raised, it turns pale. When the foot is lowered, it becomes red. Pulses are weak or absent.

Neuropathic ulcers can result from injury to the foot caused by:

- *Mechanical irritation,* such as that caused from rough shoe linings or amateur attempts at shaving calluses or cutting toenails
- *Thermal injury,* such as burns caused from heat exposure such as hot-water bottles and sitting too close to a fire or radiator
- *Chemical irritation* caused by substances such as salicylic acid, found in many corn plasters

Patients who cannot see or feel their feet may fail to notice injuries or dangerous situations. A neglected callus may become inflamed, and blood and fluid may accumulate beneath the lesion, creating a site for infection. An abscess may form that ruptures to create an ulcer. Treatment is difficult and not always effective, so the best treatment is prevention. Listed in Table 44-2 are "dos and don'ts" regarding foot care.

Prevention of Long-Term Complications

The landmark Diabetes Control and Complications Trial (DCCT) found that intensive treatment of type 1 DM delayed the onset or slowed the progress of diabetic retinopathy, nephropathy, and neuropathy. The trial evaluated the effects of tight control of blood glucose levels with multiple daily insulin injections or programmable external insulin pumps. Patients were closely monitored and treated by a team of diabetes experts. The outcomes of the United Kingdom Prospective Diabetes Study (UKPDS) demonstrated similar benefits of tight control with type 2 DM. Tight control means that the blood glucose is maintained in the normal range with carefully balanced drugs, diet, and exercise.

Acute Emergency Complications

Acute Hypoglycemia

Patients being treated with insulin or other hypoglycemic agents are at risk for acute hypoglycemia. Events that may trigger this dangerous drop in blood glucose include taking too much insulin, not eating enough food or not eating at the right time, and an inconsistent pattern of exercise. Other variables that lower blood glucose are gastroparesis, renal insufficiency, and certain drugs including aspirin and beta-adrenergic blockers. Glucose levels between 50 and 70 mg/dL are considered moderate hypoglycemia. However, some people with diabetes have been known to have serum glucose levels below 50 mg/dL without signs and symptoms of hypoglycemia.

The signs and symptoms of hypoglycemia are classified as adrenergic and neuroglucopenic. Adrenergic symptoms appear first and reflect the response of the nervous system to inadequate glucose for cell function. These symptoms are shakiness, nervousness, irritability, tachycardia, anxiety, lightheadedness, hunger, tingling or numbness of the lips or tongue, and diaphoresis.

If treatment is delayed, a second set of symptoms may appear. These symptoms are called neuroglucopenia because they are caused by a shortage of glucose to the brain. If the

table 44-2 ***"Dos and Don'ts" Regarding Foot Care***

DO
Examine your feet daily with a mirror that magnifies images. Look for blisters, cuts, and scratches.
Notify your physician if you notice any blisters, scratches, or cuts.
Check between the toes.
Wear white socks. If there is any drainage, it will show up on white socks.
Wash feet daily, rinse well, and dry carefully, especially between the toes.
Inspect the insides of your shoes for foreign objects, torn linings, and rough or sharp points.
Wear socks to bed if your feet are cold.
Lubricate dry feet with water-soluble lotion after bathing but do not put the oil between the toes.
Buy shoes that are comfortable at the time of purchase. Wear shoes that are supportive, flexible, and do not create pressure on any area of the foot.
See your physician regularly, and ask him or her to examine your feet at each visit.
Wear wool socks and fleece-lined boots to protect your feet from the cold in winter.
DON'T
Smoke.
Take very hot or cold baths or showers.
Soak feet in hot water.
Use heating pads or hot-water bottles.
Walk barefoot, even in the house.
Walk on hot surfaces such as sidewalks or sandy beaches.
Remove corns or calluses yourself. See a podiatrist for their removal.
Secure bandages with adhesive tape.
Wear garters. Instead, wear well fitting pantyhose or socks.
Wear stockings with seams.
Wear stockings that have been darned or mended.
Wear socks or stockings that have not been washed since worn last.
Wear shoes without stockings.
Wear sandals with thongs between the toes.
Cross your legs or ankles.

Modified from Levin, M. E. (1990). Diabetic foot lesions: Pathogenesis and management. *Journal of Enterostomal Therapy, 17*(7), 32.

Consider the Alternative!

Among the many herbal supplements that can lower blood glucose are dandelion, onion, garlic, and ginseng. Patients should consult with their physicians if they consider using these products.

glucose level falls rapidly, however, they may be the first signs of hypoglycemia. These include drowsiness, irritability, impaired judgment, blurred vision, slurred speech, headaches, and mood swings progressing to disorientation, seizures, and unconsciousness. Even more severe hypoglycemia progresses to loss of consciousness, convulsions, coma, and death.

Treatment. To treat hypoglycemia, give the conscious patient 10 to 15 gm of quick-acting carbohydrate such as:

- 4-6 ounces of undiluted orange or apple juice, nondiet soft drink
- 8 ounces skim milk
- 3-4 teaspoons of table sugar
- 4 tablespoons of a light or dark corn syrup, jelly, or jam
- Five or six pieces of hard candy
- Two or three glucose tablets or 15 gm of glucose gel

Repeat every 15 to 30 minutes until the patient's blood glucose is above 60 mg/dL for adults, and 80 to 100 mg/dL for older adults and children.

Any patient on insulin always should have injectable glucagon on hand. If the patient is unable to swallow, an intramuscular or subcutaneous injection of 1 mg of glucagon or an intravenous dose of 50 ml of 50% dextrose should be given as ordered or per protocol. On regaining consciousness, the patient should be given an additional treatment of some form of glucose. If it will be an hour or more until the next meal, give the patient some form of complex carbohydrate and protein such as a slice of cheese or meat with crackers.

Diabetic Ketoacidosis (DKA)

Diabetic ketoacidosis is a life-threatening emergency caused by a relative or absolute deficiency of insulin. This results in disorders in the metabolism of carbohydrates, fats, and proteins. The sequence of events is as follows:

1. Because most tissues cannot utilize glucose without insulin, the serum glucose level rises.
2. The high osmotic pressure created by excess glucose leads to osmotic diuresis. As glucose is eliminated in the kidneys, so are large amounts of water and electrolytes.
3. The patient voids large amounts of dilute urine (polyuria).

4. To make matters worse, the sympathetic nervous system responds to the cellular need for fuel by converting glycogen to glucose and manufacturing additional glucose.
5. As glycogen stores are depleted, the body begins to burn fat and protein for energy.
6. Fat metabolism produces acidic substances called **ketone bodies** that accumulate and lead to metabolic acidosis.
7. Protein metabolism results in the loss of lean muscle mass and a negative nitrogen balance.

Early signs and symptoms of DKA are anorexia, headache, and fatigue. As the condition progresses, the classic symptoms of polydipsia, polyuria, and polyphagia develop. If untreated, the patient becomes dehydrated, weak, and lethargic with abdominal pain, nausea, vomiting, fruity breath, increased respiratory rate, tachycardia, blurred vision, and hypothermia. Late signs are air hunger (seen as Kussmaul's respirations: rapid and deep), coma, and shock. Death can result if prompt medical care is not instituted.

The patient with ketoacidosis has hyperglycemia (300 mg/dL); ketonuria; and acidosis, with a pH of less than 7.3 or a bicarbonate level of less than 15 mEq/L.

The National Diabetes Data Group indicates that 10% of all deaths of people with DM, as recorded on death certificates, result from DKA. It is most likely to occur when diabetes is undiagnosed, when the patient does not take enough insulin, when the patient with uncontrolled type 1 DM exercises too vigorously, or when the patient experiences stress linked to illness, infection, surgery, or emotions. Some drugs such as corticosteroids, sympathomimetics, and thiazide diuretics also can raise serum glucose. In about a quarter of patients with DKA, no cause is identified. Treatment is aimed at correction of the three main problems: dehydration, electrolyte imbalance, and acidosis.

Dehydration. The patient with ketoacidosis may have lost a large volume of fluid as the result of vomiting, polyuria, and hyperventilation. In addition to the risk of shock due to depleted blood volume, the patient is at risk for development of blood clots.

The first need is to replace the fluid, which will aid the kidneys in eliminating excess glucose. The physician usually orders 1,000 ml of normal saline to run over the first hour, followed by an additional 2,000 to 8,000 ml of intravenous fluids for the next 24 hours. If the patient has hypertension or hypernatremia or is at risk for congestive heart failure, the order may be given for 0.45% saline solution instead of normal saline. Also, the rate and total amount of fluid may be decreased in elderly patients who may not tolerate rapid changes in fluid volume.

Electrolyte imbalance. The electrolyte of primary concern in ketoacidosis is potassium. Potassium shifts out of the cells, causing transient hyperkalemia. Once fluid and insulin replacement is started, the patient is at risk for hypokalemia. As the patient is rehydrated and normal urine output is reestablished, potassium is lost in the urine. Also, insulin replacement enhances the movement of potassium from the extracellular compartment back into the cells. Therefore, the patient's extracellular potassium falls, a condition that can cause life-threatening cardiac dysrhythmias.

Replacement of potassium is initiated only after adequate urine output is established. During potassium replacement, you must monitor the patient closely. Large doses of potassium may be required even though the serum potassium level is normal at the onset of treatment because the plasma level will drop during treatment. Because potassium is irritating to the veins and a potassium drip must be carefully regulated, it is better to run the intravenous fluid containing potassium by the piggyback method at a prescribed rate, which is slower than the hydration rate. Remember that potassium must *always* be diluted before intravenous administration.

Sodium deficiency is generally corrected by infusion of normal saline. Phosphate, magnesium, and calcium levels also should be monitored. Once therapy begins, phosphate and magnesium may fall and calcium can rise to dangerous levels.

PHARMACOLOGY CAPSULE When a patient is given insulin to treat diabetic ketoacidosis, monitor for hypokalemia because insulin causes potassium to move from the extracellular fluid into the cells.

Acidosis. Ketoacidosis is primarily a problem with type 1 DM. It occurs when ketone bodies accumulate as the result of the breakdown of fats for energy associated with inadequate insulin.

Ketoacidosis is treated with the slow intravenous infusion of insulin. When the serum glucose level reaches 250 to 300 mg/dL, dextrose solution is added. The intravenous insulin is given continuously or as a bolus until subcutaneous insulin can be given, or else the patient may become ketoacidotic again. The serum glucose level returns to normal several hours before the serum bicarbonate level. As long as the serum glucose level is normal but the serum bicarbonate level remains abnormal, the insulin drip must be maintained and glucose level corrected. More glucose is added to the intravenous fluid to cover the insulin. Normal levels of glucose *do not* mean that the acidosis has been corrected. The insulin drip must be maintained until the serum bicarbonate is 15 to 18 mEq/L. When the patient is able to eat and all laboratory values are normal, subcutaneous insulin can be given and the insulin drip discontinued.

PHARMACOLOGY CAPSULE For continuous IV infusion, insulin is usually diluted in a 100-ml bag of solution. Because insulin binds with plastic, flush plastic tubing with the intravenous solution before adding insulin to the solution.

Hyperglycemic Hyperosmolar Nonketotic Syndrome

Hyperglycemic hyperosmolar nonketotic syndrome (HHNKS) is a condition in which a patient goes into a coma from extremely high glucose levels (>600 mg/dL), but there is no evidence of elevated ketones. Apparently, the patient's pancreas produces just enough insulin to prevent the breakdown of fatty acids and the formation of ketones, but not enough insulin to prevent hyperglycemia.

The basic defect is the lack of effective insulin or the inability to use available insulin. The patient's persistent hyperglycemia causes osmotic diuresis, resulting in the loss of fluid and electrolytes. To maintain osmotic equilibrium, fluid shifts from the intracellular fluid space to the extracellular space. Dehydration and hypernatremia develop. Dehydration and neurologic changes may be more pronounced with HHNKS than with DKA. Patients with HHNKS do not experience gastrointestinal symptoms, nor do they experience Kussmaul's respirations because they lack significant lactic acid levels. These patients often tolerate polyuria and polydipsia for weeks before seeking treatment. For some patients, HHNKS is the first sign of diabetes. Others have been previously diagnosed with borderline diabetes.

Hyperglycemic hyperosmolar nonketotic syndrome may be caused by the same factors that trigger ketoacidosis. It also can be brought about by total parenteral nutrition or dialysis. In both of these procedures, intravenous solutions that contain large amounts of glucose are administered to the patient. Because the digestive system is bypassed, there is no stimulus to trigger the pancreas to release insulin.

MEDICAL DIAGNOSIS

The diagnosis of DM is based on serum glucose levels. The normal fasting serum glucose levels are between 80 and 120 mg/dL. A fasting glucose level of 126 mg/dL or greater merits further investigation. Using the official criteria for a diagnosis of DM published in 1997 by the Expert Committee on the Diagnosis and Classification of Diabetes Mellitus, a patient who meets one or more of the following criteria is considered to have DM:

1. Symptoms of diabetes (polyuria, polydipsia, polyphagia) plus random glucose level of 200 mg/dL or greater. A random reading is based on a blood sample drawn any time of day without regard to mealtimes.
2. Fasting serum glucose level of 126 mg/dL or greater. Patient must fast at least 8 hours.
3. Two-hour postprandial glucose level above 200 mg/dL during oral glucose tolerance test (OGTT) under specific guidelines. Test must use a glucose load of 75 gm of anhydrous glucose dissolved in water. This test is often unnecessary.

Impaired Fasting Glucose

A fasting glucose level between 110 and 125 mg/dL is classified as impaired fasting glucose. Patients with impaired fasting glucose levels are considered at risk for DM.

Impaired Glucose Tolerance

Impaired glucose tolerance is indicated by a glucose tolerance test that shows the presence of moderately high glucose levels; that is, levels that are between normal levels and diabetic levels. These moderately high glucose levels may increase until the patient has overt diabetes, decrease to normal, or remain unchanged. Some classification systems do not recognize impaired glucose tolerance as a separate entity, but as a risk factor for the development of DM and macrovascular disease.

The diagnosis of impaired glucose tolerance is based on (1) fasting serum glucose level between 110 and 125 mg/dL and (2) a 2-hour OGTT result between 140 and 200 mg/dL.

Oral Glucose Tolerance Test

The OGTT is performed when a patient is suspected of having DM. The patient should consume a diet composed of 150 to 300 gm of carbohydrates for 3 days before the test. However, some physicians tell their patients to eat their normal diets. The night before the test, the patient is instructed to fast after midnight. On the morning of the test, a sample of blood is drawn for a fasting serum glucose test. The patient is then given a drink (glucola) containing 75 gm of carbohydrates and instructed to remain quiet. This drink is quite sweet and should be served very cold to make it palatable. In certain situations, the glucose can be given by the intravenous route, but this method is not as accurate as the oral route. Blood is then drawn at 30 minutes and 1 hour after the ingestion of glucose. After these two samples, blood is drawn at hourly intervals until the test is completed. Most physicians order either a 3-hour or a 5-hour OGTT. Because blood must be drawn several times, it may be best to insert a heparin lock into the vein at the time blood is obtained for the fasting blood sugar. This eliminates the need for multiple venipunctures.

MEDICAL TREATMENT

The goals of managing diabetes are to normalize the blood glucose, serum lipids, and body weight while meeting energy needs and achieving healthy body weight.

Nutritional Management

Weight control is an important component of diabetes management. The emphasis has shifted, however, from an ideal body weight to a reasonable body weight. Davidson (1998) defines reasonable body weight as "that level of weight that individuals, both patients and professionals, acknowledge as achievable and maintainable . . . ." Body mass index is a tool used to help people determine their risks for health problems associated with weight.

To maintain weight, a caloric intake of 28 calories/kg of body weight is required. To reduce weight, the caloric intake is calculated based on 15 to 20 calories/kg body weight. To arrive at a person's weight in kilograms, divide the weight in pounds by 2.2. If a woman weighs 110 pounds, her weight in kilograms would be 55 kg. To maintain her weight, she would need to consume 1,540 calories daily.

Several nutrition planning approaches are in use. Carbohydrate counting is particularly useful for people who use intensive insulin therapy or pumps. Insulin doses are based on the total grams of carbohydrate to be ingested. For most patients, the emphasis is on a well-balanced diet within the prescribed distribution of proteins, fats, and carbohydrates using the food pyramid. The American Diabetes Association recommends that the daily calorie intake be distributed as follows:

- Proteins: 10% to 20%
- Carbohydrates and monosaturated fats (peanut oil, olive oil, canola oil, sesame oil, and avocado): 60% to 70%
- Saturated fats (animal fats, egg yolks, coconut oil, palm kernel oil, palm oil, and hydrogenated vegetable oils): less than 10%
- Polyunsaturated fats (corn oil, safflower oil, and most nuts): less than 10%

Sodium should not exceed 3,000 mg/day, which may be modified for medical reasons, and may be restricted further in some clinical situations.

Greater than 20% of the daily intake of calories in protein may be associated with an increase in the glomerular filtration rate. Sustained increases in glomerular filtration rate cause renal and retinal vasodilation, leading to renal damage and retinopathy.

Elevated serum cholesterol and triglyceride levels are often associated with type 2 DM, increasing the risk of cardiovascular disease. Cholesterol should not exceed 300 mg/day. If the patient has elevated low-density lipoprotein levels, saturated fats may be restricted to 7% of the total calories, and dietary cholesterol restricted to less than 200 mg/day. Research in the past several years has indicated that replacing some of the allotted fat calories with calories from carbohydrates and fiber has a positive effect on the lipid profile. The exception is the patient who has glucose intolerance.

The addition of water-soluble fibers in the daily diet may lower total cholesterol and low-density lipoprotein levels. In addition, the lower fat intake permits increased insulin binding to receptor sites, resulting in insulin sparing. Foods containing soluble fibers include oatmeal, rice, dried beans, oat bran, lentils, squash, whole-wheat breads, and some fruits. The potential glucose-lowering effect of fiber in the diet received considerable attention in the past. Research, however, has shown that the effect is minimally significant and requires fiber intake far above that usually recommended. In general, people with diabetes need the same amount of fiber as other adults: 20 to 35 gm/day from soluble and insoluble sources. When fiber is added to the diet, it should be done gradually. A sudden addition of large amounts of fiber to the diet may reduce the amount of glucose available for the exogenous insulin or hypoglycemic agent taken by the patient and may result in hypoglycemic episodes.

A simplified method of planning diets for people with diabetes has been designed by the American Diabetes Association and the American Dietetic Association. Foods are divided into three clusters: carbohydrates, proteins, and fats. Meal planning is presented in a booklet entitled *The Exchange Lists for Meal Planning* that can be ordered by calling 1-800-ADA-ORDER.

Patient teaching should include sample menus that include as many favorite foods as possible. People with diabetes require considerable education and support to learn to manage the dietary guidelines. It is vital to consider their personal and ethnic choices. For help with this aspect of teaching, the registered dietitian is an essential team member. Most nursing care situations do not lend themselves to the in-depth teaching, planning, and reinforcement needed. However, it is important for you to understand and reinforce the dietitian's instructions.

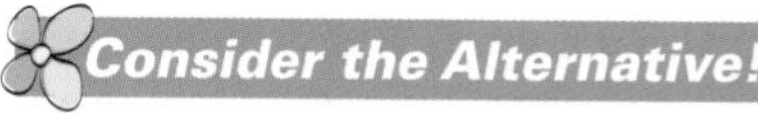

Caution patients who take herbal supplements for diabetes that the supplements should not be used to *replace* conventional therapy. Be sure the physician is aware of supplements being used.

Previously, rigid diabetic diets using exchange lists were recommended for meal planning. Exchange lists are groups of measured foods that represent the same number of calories and the same amount of carbohydrate, fat, and protein. Foods on the same list may be exchanged to add variety to meals. For example, two bread exchanges are equal to a bagel or a plain bun such as a hot dog roll. The patient was taught to select a specific number of foods from each exchange list for the daily meal plan. Exchanges for a variety of foods are published in several books that are available to the public. In addition, food companies often include the exchanges on the packaging of their frozen dinners and other products. Advise patients to read nutrition facts on the labels of prepared foods. Many people, patients, and nurses alike found the original exchange lists difficult to use. You may, however, encounter people who have learned to use them and are reluctant to change their approaches to food selection.

Exercise

Exercise is a very effective treatment adjunct for people with diabetes. It aids in weight loss in obese patients, improves cardiovascular conditioning, improves insulin sensitivity, and promotes a sense of well-being. Exercising muscle uses glucose at 20 times the rate of a muscle at rest and does not require insulin.

Exercise affects patients with type 1 disease differently from those with type 2 disease who do not require insulin. Hyperglycemia may occur with exercise in the patient with type 1 disease whose insulin is inadequate. In patients with type 2 disease, exercise makes insulin receptor sites more sensitive to insulin and lowers plasma glucose levels.

Much of the morbidity and mortality in patients with type 2 disease occurs because of the atherosclerosis that accompanies long-term uncontrolled diabetes and that places the patient at risk for cerebrovascular accident CVA (stroke) and cardiovascular disease. Exercise is known to improve low-density lipoproteins, serum glucose, blood pressure, some blood coagulation parameters, and triglycerides. However, exercise must be accompanied by appropriate nutrition to have long-term beneficial results.

An appropriate combination of aerobic and anaerobic exercises should be determined. Aerobic exercise produces the most therapeutic effect. The patient should exercise for 30 to

60 minutes three to four times a week. Warm-up exercises such as stretching and walking are recommended before exercise, followed by cool-down exercises afterward. The best aerobic exercises are walking, swimming, bicycle riding, and jogging. Anaerobic exercises are done to build muscle mass. These include activities such as weightlifting, yoga, and sit-ups. Very strenuous exercises can raise blood pressure, which is undesirable with retinopathy and nephropathy. Eventually, the patient with type 2 disease who adheres to a sound nutritional plan and exercise regimen may be able to decrease the amount of exogenous insulin or oral hypoglycemic agents needed.

When the patient with type 1 disease exercises, the liver may release more glucose than is metabolized and actually raise the blood sugar. If the pancreas is not producing insulin, the body mobilizes free fatty acids, causing ketone bodies to form. In this manner, exercise increases the hazard of ketosis in patients with type 1 disease.

PATIENT TEACHING PLAN
Exercise and Diabetes

Have a complete medical examination before initiating a new exercise program:

- Because circulating insulin may be inadequate to ensure glucose uptake, avoid exercise when your serum glucose is greater than 250 mg/dL and ketosis is present.
- Exercise with caution if your serum glucose is greater than 300 mg/dL and no ketosis is present.
- Wear comfortable athletic shoes that provide good support.
- Before every exercise session, warm up with 5 to 10 minutes of slow, continuous aerobic exercise and stretching.
- Discuss with your physician whether to alter food or insulin intake before exercise. A general recommendation is to exercise shortly after eating or to have a small snack before exercising if your serum glucose is less than 100 mg/dL.
- Avoid exercise during the peak action of insulin and oral hypoglycemic agents when hypoglycemia is more likely to occur.
- Carbohydrate snacking may be necessary with prolonged or intense exercise.
- If you take insulin, inject it in the abdomen rather than an extremity before a workout because the drug is absorbed much more quickly from the abdomen.
- Some people experience hypoglycemia several hours after exercise; have food available for these situations.

Insulin Therapy

All patients with type 1 disease need insulin injections, and some patients with type 2 disease may eventually need insulin. Insulins are classified by their source and time course of action. For many years, all insulin was obtained from beef and pork. However, beef and pork insulin are not identical to human insulin, and patients could form antibodies against them. The advent of recombinant DNA technology has allowed the manufacture of insulin that is identical to endogenous insulin. This "human" insulin causes fewer problems than that from animal sources. Pork insulin is still available in the United States, but beef insulin is being phased out. Over time, most patients taking insulin from animal sources have been switched to human insulin.

In relation to time course of actions, insulins are classified as rapid acting, short acting, intermediate acting, and long acting. Rapid-acting insulins include insulin lispro (Humalog) and insulin aspart (NovoLog). Regular (Humulin R, Novolin R) insulin is classified as short-acting insulin. Intermediate-acting insulins are NPH (Humulin N) and Lente insulin (Humulin L). Long-acting insulins are Ultralente (Humulin U, Humulin Ultralente), and insulin glargine (Lantus). All rapid-acting and short-acting insulins are clear. Except for insulin glargine (Lantus), which also is clear, the other insulins all are cloudy. Onsets, peaks, and durations are compared in Table 44-3 (Fig. 44-2).

table 44-3 *Insulin Preparations: Time Course of Action*

INSULIN TYPE	ONSET	PEAK	DURATION
RAPID ACTING			
Lispro insulin Insulin aspart	15 min	1 hr	2-4 hr
SHORT ACTING			
Regular insulin	30 min	2-4 hr	6-8 hr
INTERMEDIATE ACTING			
NPH insulin Lente insulin	1-2½ hr	6-12 hr	Up to 18 hr
LONG ACTING			
Ultralente	4-8 hr	Unpredictable	24-36 hr
Insulin glargine	1 hr	None	24 hr

Modified from Lehne, R. A. (2001). *Pharmacology for nursing care* (4th ed., p. 617). Philadelphia: Saunders.

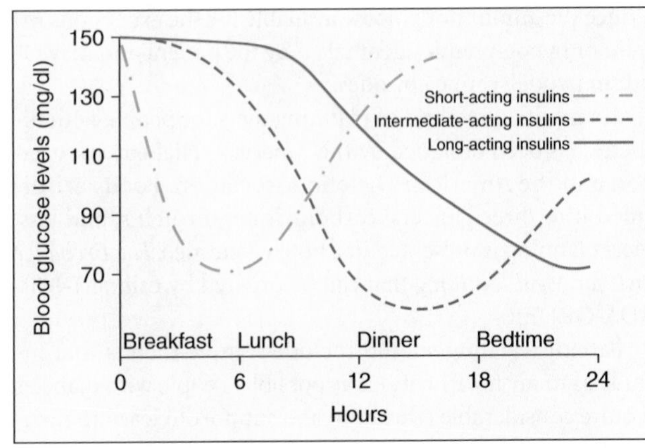

FIGURE **44-2** Effect of insulin on blood glucose levels.

Route

Insulin cannot be given orally because it is rendered useless in the gastrointestinal tract. All insulins can be given subcutaneously, but *only* Regular insulin can be given intravenously. Intranasal insulin is being tested experimentally.

PHARMACOLOGY CAPSULE Insulin lispro and insulin aspart act rapidly. Regular insulin is short acting, NPH and Lente insulins are intermediate acting, and Ultralente insulin is long acting. Be sure to administer the correct type!

Concentrations

Insulins are available in varying concentrations. The U-100 insulin has a concentration of 100 units/ml, and U-500 has 500 units/ml. U-100 is most commonly used. U-500 insulin is used only in emergencies and for patients who are extremely insulin resistant. The insulin with the lowest concentration, U-40, meaning 40 units of insulin per milliliter, is not available in the United States.

Premixed Insulin Products

Premixed insulins that contain both Regular and NPH insulin products are available. There are three mixtures. One contains 70% NPH and 30% Regular insulin; another consists of 50% NPH and 50% Regular insulin and the third contains 75% NPH and 25% Lispro. Premixed solutions are easier to prepare and decrease the risk of errors associated with drawing up two types of insulin in the same syringe.

Dosing Schedules

The pancreas secretes minute amounts of insulin continuously except after the ingestion of a meal, when it secretes a bolus of insulin into the system. Exogenous insulin is administered in an effort to mimic the action of a normal pancreas. Therefore, the person with diabetes requires a bolus of rapid- or short-acting insulin before meals to prevent too rapid a rise in glucose. A long- or intermediate-acting insulin may be prescribed as well in an effort to keep glucose levels even at other times.

Conventional therapy. Conventional therapy uses one of several dosage schedules and typically uses a combination of a short-acting and an intermediate- or long-acting insulin. One example is the one-fifth rule some physicians use for prescribing insulin. In the morning, the patient takes two fifths of the day's supply in an intermediate-acting insulin such as NPH. In addition, the patient takes one fifth of the daily requirement of insulin as Regular insulin. The latter covers breakfast glucose. Because the NPH peaks at lunchtime, the patient does not need Regular insulin for this meal. At suppertime, the patient takes one fifth of the daily insulin requirement in the form of an intermediate-acting insulin and one fifth as rapid-acting insulin to cover supper carbohydrates. For example, a patient who is prescribed 50 units of insulin a day might take it as follows:

A.M.: 20 units of NPH insulin
10 units of Regular insulin
P.M.: 10 units of NPH insulin
10 units of Regular insulin

Another conventional dosage schedule has the patient receive two thirds of the total daily dose in the morning and the remainder late in the day. The doses are fixed so that the patient must maintain a consistent schedule and dietary intake.

Patients on conventional therapy should monitor their blood glucose before meals at least 2 times each day. A major problem with conventional therapy is nocturnal hypoglycemia: blood glucose falls between 3 and 4 A.M.

Intensive therapy. Intensive therapy is designed to achieve tight control (i.e., maintain the blood glucose in the normal range). The patient's regimen may require three or four injections each day. The four-injection regimen requires rapid- or short-acting insulin before each meal and intermediate- or long-acting insulin at bedtime.

The preprandial (before meal) doses are adjusted for the caloric content of the meal. The timing of the injection depends on the type of insulin used. Rapid-acting or short-acting insulins should be taken 30-60 minutes before a meal, and insulin lispro should be taken within 15 minutes before eating. Dosage adjustments also can be made to accommodate physical activity. Home blood glucose monitoring is essential with this program because testing should be done three to five times daily. The intensified program permits more flexibility in meal composition and timing.

Continuous subcutaneous insulin infusion. The last dosing schedule uses continuous subcutaneous insulin infusion. The patient has an indwelling subcutaneous catheter connected to an external portable infusion pump. The pump delivers Regular insulin continuously. Before meals, the patient triggers the pump to provide the appropriate amount of insulin for the meal to be consumed. Patients who use pumps also must do self-blood glucose monitoring.

Insulin Mixing

If the two types of insulin that the patient takes are consistent with available premixed forms, a single injection is needed for each dose. However, many patients have to mix their own insulins to achieve the exact prescribed proportion of the two insulin types. In this case, the two types of insulin can be mixed in one syringe to avoid two injections. Suppose you were to give 20 units of Humulin N and 10 units of Humulin R in a single dose. The following are directions for mixing the two types of insulin:

1. Select vials of the prescribed insulins. The Humulin N is cloudy, and the Humulin R is clear.
2. To mix the Humulin N suspension, roll the vial of intermediate-acting insulin between your hands. Do not shake the vial because this would create bubbles.
3. Wipe tops of both vials with alcohol swabs.
4. Draw 20 units of air into a syringe and inject it into the Humulin N vial.
5. Draw 10 units of air into the syringe and inject the air into the Humulin R vial; withdraw 10 units of Humulin R into the syringe.
6. Wipe the top of the Humulin N, insert the needle, invert the vial, and withdraw 20 units of Humulin N, being careful not to inject the Humulin R insulin into the Humulin N vial.

7. If you draw up too much Humulin N, you must discard the syringe and start over.

PHARMACOLOGY CAPSULE Remember "clear to cloudy!" When mixing short-acting (clear) and longer-acting (cloudy) insulins, draw the short-acting insulin into the syringe first. *Note:* Insulin glargine (Lantus) cannot be mixed with other insulins!

Insulin Injection

The suggested sites for subcutaneous insulin injections are illustrated in Figure 44-3. Site rotation helps prevent lipohypertrophy (swelling or lumps) or lipoatrophy (hollowing or pitting of the subcutaneous tissue). Patients with the latter problem should see a physician about changing the insulin to human insulin (Humulin). In some cases, injecting these sites with their prescribed daily human insulin has resolved the problem. Because lipohypertrophy interferes with the absorption of insulin, affected areas should be avoided as injection sites.

The absorption rate of insulin varies with different body sites. The rate of absorption from the abdomen is approximately 50% faster than from the thighs. For this reason, the American Diabetes Association recommends rotating sites within one anatomic area rather than moving among all areas. Heat and massage increase the absorption rate, as does exercise. As mentioned earlier, if insulin is injected into the thigh before exercise such as jogging, the absorption rate is greatly increased.

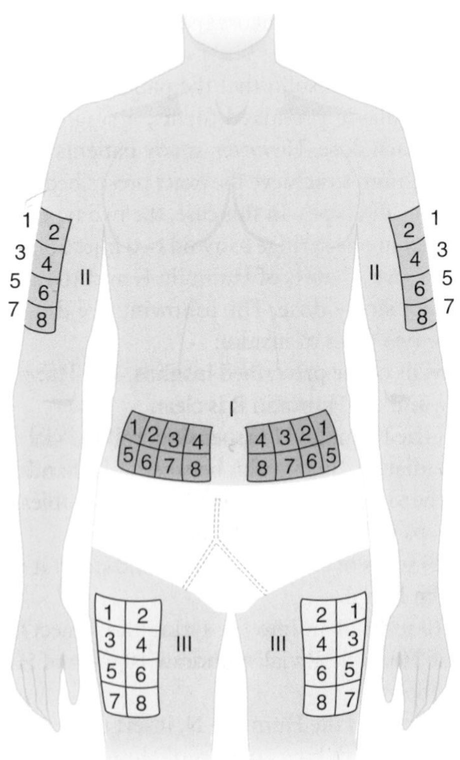

FIGURE **44-3** Insulin injection sites.

Insulin Pump

An external insulin pump looks much like a pager. It consists of a battery-driven syringe with a long piece of tubing (usually made of Teflon) that is attached to a small needle. The needle is inserted subcutaneously in an appropriate part of the anatomy (Fig. 44-4). The syringe usually contains a 2- to 3-day supply of insulin. The pump is programmed to deliver a steady trickle of insulin throughout the day and can provide a bolus of insulin at mealtimes. In this manner, the unit mimics the pancreas. The patient calculates the bolus based on self-monitored blood glucose levels. Every 2 days, the syringe, needle, and tubing are replaced.

One advantage of the external insulin pump is that patients do not have to use intermediate- or long-acting insulins, with their uncertain peaks and valleys. Other advantages are that it gives the patient more flexibility regarding

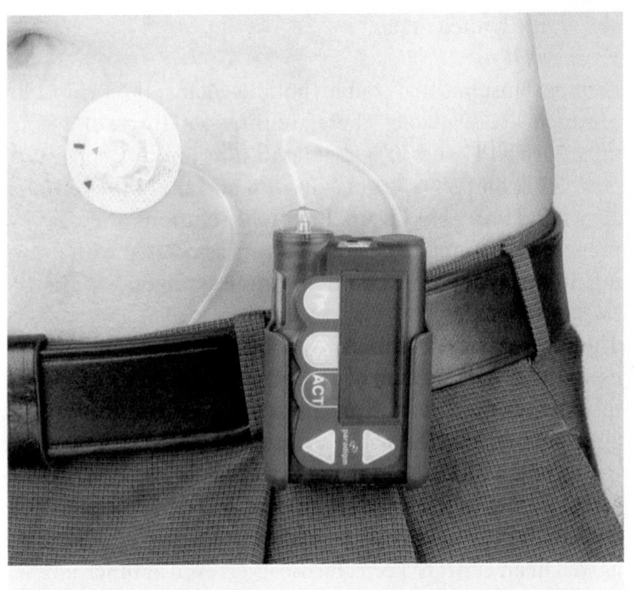

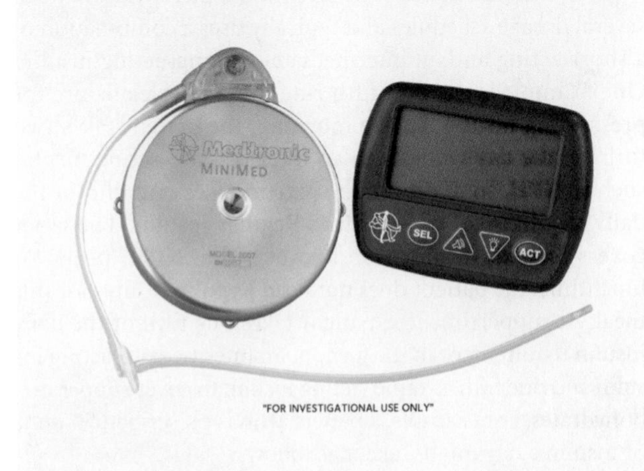

FIGURE **44-4** Insulin pumps. *A,* MiniMed 507 external insulin pump with Quick-Release Infusion Set. *B,* MiniMed 2001 implantable insulin pump and hand-held programmer.

mealtimes, travel, and exercise. Potential problems with the pump are occlusion of the tubing or the needle, and infection at the site of needle insertion. The pump also is a constant reminder that the patient has diabetes, and because it is worn externally, the patient may feel self-conscious about it. To use the pump, the patient must undergo intensive education and be willing to self-monitor blood glucose levels several times a day while on pump therapy. Some medical insurance companies do not cover the cost of the pump or pump therapy, which makes the cost prohibitive to many.

Other less commonly used devices for insulin administration are the jet injector, pen injector, and implanted insulin pump. The jet injector delivers insulin through the skin without a needle. The injection does sting and may bruise thin and elderly people. The high cost of the jet injector is a deterrent to its use. The pen injector looks like a fountain pen and holds preloaded cartridges with the prescribed insulin dose. Implantable pumps work like the portable pump described earlier but are surgically placed under the skin of the abdomen.

Intranasal insulin is being tested experimentally. Only approximately 10% of the drug is absorbed through the nasal mucosa, making it relatively expensive to use. Also, nasal irritation is a frequent side effect. At this time, only Regular insulin is given intranasally, so the patient must still administer longer-acting insulin by injection. Efforts to develop an "artificial pancreas" are underway. The device would be implanted under the skin and would dispense insulin in response to changing blood glucose levels.

Insulin Catheter

Indwelling subcutaneous catheters may be placed in the abdomen to permit repeated insulin injections without repeated needlesticks. The catheter can remain in one location for up to 1 week. With each dose of insulin, the site should be assessed for signs of irritation or infection.

Oral Hypoglycemic (Antihyperglycemic or Antidiabetic) Agents

If patients with type 2 DM are unable to control their blood glucose with a nutrition program and exercise, the physician may prescribe one or more oral hypoglycemic agents. If the serum glucose level rises above 300 mg/dL, insulin may be prescribed temporarily until the blood glucose levels are back below 300 mg/dL. Oral hypoglycemic agents include sulfonylureas (three generations), alpha-glucosidase inhibitors, biguanides, thiazolidinediones, d-phenylalanines, and meglitinides.

Sulfonylureas

Sulfonylureas lower blood sugars by stimulating the pancreas to secrete more insulin and increasing the sensitivity of insulin receptors. First- and second-generation sulfonylureas are equally effective in controlling serum glucose but have some important differences (Table 44-4). Because of the long duration of action, first-generation sulfonylureas are not often used now.

table 44-4 **DRUG THERAPY | *Oral Hypoglycemics for Type 2 Diabetes***

CLASS AND SPECIFIC AGENTS	ACTIONS	MAJOR ADVERSE EFFECTS
SULFONYLUREAS		
Glipizide (Glucotrol) Glyburide (Micronase)	Promote insulin secretion by the pancreas; may also increase tissue response to insulin	Hypoglycemia (more risk with first generation)
MEGLITINIDES		
Repaglinide (Prandin)	Promote insulin secretion by the pancreas	Hypoglycemia Weight gain
D-PHENYLALANINES		
Nateglinide (Starlix)	Promote insulin secretion by the pancreas	Hypoglycemia Weight gain
BIGUANIDES		
Metformin (Glucophage)	Decrease glucose production by liver and increase glucose uptake by muscle	GI symptoms: decreased appetite, nausea, diarrhea Lactic acidosis (rarely)
ALPHA-GLUCOSIDASE INHIBITORS		
Acarbose (Precose) Miglitol (Glyset)	Inhibit carbohydrate digestion and absorption, thereby decreasing the postprandial rise in blood glucose	GI symptoms: flatulence, cramps, abdominal distention, borborygmus
THIAZOLIDINEDIONES		
Rosiglitazone (Avandia) Pioglitazone (Actos)	Decrease insulin resistance, thereby increasing glucose uptake by muscle and decreasing glucose production by the liver	Hypoglycemia, but only in the presence of excessive insulin Weight gain, edema, transient anemia Monitor liver function even though risk of liver damage is thought to be small

Modified from Lehne, R. A. (2001). *Pharmacology for nursing care* (4th ed., p. 624). Philadelphia: Saunders.
GI, Gastrointestinal.

A significant adverse effect of the sulfonylureas is the risk of hypoglycemia. First-generation sulfonylureas also have the potential for interactions with many other drugs, which is problematic in the patient who is taking multiple medications. First-generation drugs are not recommended in patients with liver or renal disease. Because the sulfonylureas are chemically similar to sulfonamide antibacterials, patients who are allergic to one also may be allergic to the other. Be sure to assess for allergy to sulfonamides before a patient starts taking a sulfonylurea.

The second-generation drugs are more potent (so require lower dosage), pose less risk of hypoglycemia, have fewer other side effects, and have fewer drug interactions. Many older people have diminished renal and liver function, which affects metabolism and elimination of drugs, and increases the risk of hypoglycemia. When a sulfonylurea is ordered for the elderly patient, it is usually glipizide (Glucotrol), which must be taken on an empty stomach, or glyburide (DiaBeta, Micronase). Drugs with long durations of action are more likely to accumulate and cause toxic effects in elderly patients.

Alpha-Glucosidase Inhibitors

Examples of alpha-glucosidase inhibitors are acarbose (Precose) and miglitol (Glyset). These drugs delay digestion of complex carbohydrates into glucose and other simple sugars. Sometimes they are given in combination with insulin or a sulfonylurea. Side effects include abdominal cramping and distention, flatulence, and diarrhea. Acarbose does not cause hypoglycemia. However, if the patient becomes hypoglycemic because of another hypoglycemic agent taken in combination with the alpha-glucosidase inhibitor, oral sucrose will not effectively raise the blood sugar because the acarbose will interfere with absorption of the sucrose. The patient will instead require treatment with oral glucose.

Biguanides

Metformin (Glucophage) is a biguanide that decreases glucose production by the liver and increases the use of glucose by muscle cells. Adverse gastrointestinal effects are fairly common. A rare, but potentially fatal, adverse effect is lactic acidosis, which usually occurs in the presence of impaired renal function. Glucophage XR is an extended release form of metformin that is taken only once a day instead of two or three times.

Thiazolidinediones

Thiazolidinediones are a newer class of antihyperglycemic agents that includes rosiglitazone maleate (Avandia) and pioglitazone HCl (Actos). Classified as insulin-sensitizing agents, they increase the uptake of glucose by skeletal muscle and fat tissue. These drugs do not cause hypoglycemia when used alone but may when used with a sulfonylurea. Because the first drug in this class (Rezulin) was found to have serious adverse effects on the liver, liver function must be monitored when this class of drugs is used. To date, Avandia and Actos appear to pose low risk to the liver. Side effects include weight gain, edema, and mild transient anemia. Patients should be aware that these drugs decrease the effectiveness of oral contraceptives. They are contraindicated with class 3 or 4 heart failure and during pregnancy.

Meglitinides and D-Phenylalanines

Repaglinide (Prandin) is a meglitinide, and nateglinide (Starlix) is a d-phenylalanine. Because of the similarity of these two types of drugs, called mealtime insulin secretogogues, they will be discussed together. Meglitinides and d-phenylalanine stimulate the release of insulin from the pancreas. Taken before each meal, they prevent postprandial blood glucose elevations and prolonged hypoglycemia. Patients should omit the medications if they skip a meal. Hypoglycemia may occur with strenuous exercise or alcohol consumption. Weight gain is a side effect. They are used cautiously with moderate to severe liver failure.

Combination Oral Medications

With increasing use of combination therapy, patients must take more medication doses—a factor that often reduces compliance. The first combination drug is glyburide/metformin (Glucovance). The actions and side and adverse effects are the same as for each individual drug.

Approximately 30% to 40% of patients with type 2 diabetes fail to respond to oral agents. Another 10% cease to respond after a period of successful treatment. To maintain optimal glucose control, it is beneficial for these patients to use insulin. Some of them may have to take one dose of insulin, often at night, and then are able to control serum glucose for the rest of the day with oral drugs. A variety of combination regimens (using oral agents and insulin) are being studied.

Newly diagnosed patients with type 2 disease may be placed on insulin to bring their plasma glucose levels within normal limits. They then are placed on a diet and exercise program with or without oral agents to maintain euglycemia (blood glucose within normal range).

Self-Monitoring of Blood Glucose

People with diabetes need to monitor their blood glucose levels so they can regulate their diet, exercise, and medication regimens to remain euglycemic and lead lifestyles as normal as possible.

The self-monitoring of blood glucose levels is seen as the greatest breakthrough in managing diabetes since the advent of insulin. It reduces the complications of long-term diabetes by helping the patient normalize blood glucose levels.

One of several methods of self-monitoring may be used. Visual testing requires a drop of blood taken from the side of the finger and placed on a reagent strip. After a specified length of time, the blood is wiped off and the color change is compared with a color chart provided by the manufacturer that indicates the serum glucose level. If the patient has a problem distinguishing colors, this method is not appropriate.

The use of portable electronic glucose meters has largely replaced other methods of self-monitoring. The patient puts a drop of blood on a special reagent strip and inserts the strip in the meter. In less than a minute, the serum glucose level appears on a monitor. Factors that may affect the use of these meters include cost, comfort with technology, fine motor coordination, intellectual ability, and willingness to use the meter. Self-blood glucose monitoring (SBGM) is a useful tool in managing diabetes during pregnancy, when glucose levels may change hourly. It also is a must in managing unstable diabetes and for patients who are prone to sudden hypoglycemic episodes or ketoacidosis or who have abnormal renal glucose thresholds.

Glycosylated Glucose Levels

Determination of glycosylated hemoglobin (HbA1c) or fructosamine levels every 2 to 3 months is an essential check of glycemic control. The HbA1c reflects glucose levels over the past few months, whereas the fructosamine levels reflect those over several weeks. When the glucose level is elevated, a certain percentage of the glucose molecules bind to the hemoglobin on the red blood cell. The glucose stays on the cell for the life of the cell, which is approximately 3 months. By measuring HbA1c or fructosamine levels, the physician is able to determine how well the blood glucose has been regulated in the recent past. It also allows patients who monitor their own blood glucose levels to evaluate their methods of control. The American Diabetes Association recommends an HbA1c level less than 7% as a treatment goal.

Complications of Therapy

Hypoglycemia

The major complication of insulin therapy is hypoglycemia. If a person injects too much insulin, does not eat enough, eats at the wrong time, or exercises inconsistently, serum glucose levels may suddenly drop. Treatment of hypoglycemia is covered in the section on Emergency Complications, but the main thing to remember is that the patient needs some form of glucose immediately.

Somogyi Phenomenon

Too much insulin can actually cause hyperglycemia. The Somogyi phenomenon is characterized by rebound hyperglycemia occurring in response to hypoglycemia. The phenomenon begins with an episode of hypoglycemia, often during the night. Hypoglycemia triggers the body's stress response in an attempt to restore homeostasis. Epinephrine is secreted, which stimulates the liver to convert stored glycogen to glucose, thereby raising the blood glucose level to the point of hyperglycemia.

The Somogyi phenomenon should be suspected when a patient reports awakening with a headache, and complains of restless sleep, nightmares, enuresis (involuntary voiding during sleep), and nausea and vomiting. The blood glucose records reflect fluctuation between hypoglycemia and hyperglycemia. The patient may have tried without success to correct the hyperglycemia by increasing the insulin.

To confirm suspected Somogyi phenomenon, the patient's blood glucose needs to be measured between 2 and 4 A.M. and again at 7 A.M. The 2 and 4 A.M. levels below 60 mg/dL, and a 7 A.M. level above 180 mg/ support the diagnosis of Somogyi phenomenon.

This vicious cycle can be broken by gradually decreasing the evening dose of exogenous insulin by 2 or 3 units every 3 or 4 days until the rebound hyperglycemia is brought under control. A bedtime snack also may be helpful.

Dawn Phenomenon

Some people with diabetes who are insulin dependent experience an increase in fasting blood glucose levels between 5 and 9 A.M. that is not related to a period of hypoglycemia. The cause is unknown, but it may reflect release of growth hormone and cortisol, which increase blood glucose during early morning rapid eye movement sleep. The blood glucose level is typically normal at 3 A.M., but elevated at 6 or 7 A.M. The condition may be treated with a bedtime snack and delay of the evening intermediate-acting insulin until 10 P.M.

NURSING CARE *of the Patient with Diabetes Mellitus*

Assessment

When a person with diabetes seeks medical care in an emergency situation, a complete assessment must be delayed until the patient is stable. If the patient is in ketoacidosis, your assessment is likely to show ketonuria, Kussmaul's respirations, orthostatic hypotension, hypertension at times, nausea, vomiting, and lethargy or change in level of consciousness. In the hypoglycemic patient, expect to find tachycardia, anxiety, trembling, and decreasing level of consciousness. Be alert for indications of hyperosmolar nonketotic coma (decreased level of consciousness, polyuria, and polydipsia in the absence of ketosis). In each of these situations, attempt to determine the following:

- Type of diabetes
- Hypoglycemic agents: name, dosage, when last dose was taken
- Food and fluid intake for the last 3 days
- Relevant laboratory values: blood glucose, blood pH, bicarbonate levels, electrolytes, and osmolality and urine osmolality

Once the patient is stabilized, a complete health history and physical examination are in order.

Health History

Focus the health history on the signs and symptoms of chronic hyperglycemia and possible complications. Identify physical and psychosocial factors that may have an impact on the patient's capacity to learn and perform self-care activities.

Chief Complaint and History of Present Illness. During the patient interview, ask the patient to describe the signs and symptoms that prompted him or her to seek medical care. The patient might report unexplained weight loss, dryness of skin, vaginal itching, or sores that are slow in healing. Polyphagia, polydipsia, and polyuria, the 3 P's, are classic signs of diabetes mellitus.

Past Medical History. If the patient is known to have DM, inquire about the type and duration. Record the name and dosage of prescribed medications, and note when they were last taken. If the patient monitors blood glucose, ask about the type of equipment used, the testing schedule, and recent test results.

Document a history of circulatory, cardiac, or renal problems. Record previous hospitalizations and surgeries. If the patient is female, take an obstetric history, including number of pregnancies, if any, outcomes of all pregnancies, and birth weights of full-term infants. For patients who had gestational diabetes, determine whether insulin was required or if diet and exercise maintained adequate control. Other important data to collect are immunization records and allergies.

Family History. Assess the patient for family history of diabetes, heart disease, stroke, hypertension, and hyperlipidemia.

Review of Systems. Begin the review of symptoms by asking about the patient's general health. Then ask if the patient has noticed changes in skin moisture or turgor. To detect possible changes in the eyes associated with diabetes, inquire whether the patient has had floaters (dark spots that cross the field of vision), diplopia (double vision), or blurred vision, or has seen white halos around objects. Assess significant abdominal symptoms including diarrhea, abdominal bloating, and gas. Document problems passing or holding urine. Determine whether the patient has any pain in the legs and, if so, when the pain occurs. Describe numbness, tingling, or burning sensations in the extremities. Last, ask if the patient has experienced changes in mental alertness or seizures.

Functional Assessment. The functional assessment explores factors that can affect the patient's ability to perform self-care, including literacy, financial resources such as health insurance, and family support. Ask the patient to describe the usual pattern of activity and rest. Record a typical 24-hour dietary history. Explore the impact of diabetes on the patient's life, including self-concept, social relationships, and employment.

Physical Examination

In the general survey, note the patient's level of consciousness, posture and gait, and apparent well-being. Take vital signs, including blood pressure, and measure height and weight. Throughout the examination, assess the skin for color, warmth, turgor, and lesions.

The trained examiner inspects the eye grounds for evidence of diabetic retinopathy or cataracts. The vision assessment is important because visual defects may affect the patient's ability to read vital medication instructions or labels. Gross visual acuity may be assessed by having the patient read available print. Snellen's test and other more sophisticated measures also may be used to evaluate the function of the eyes. During the examination of the head and neck, assess the patient's breath for a sweet, fruity odor common with ketoacidosis.

The feet receive special attention. Inspect for blisters, lesions, pallor, discoloration, deformities, and edema. Note the condition of the nails, and document thickened or ingrown nails. Palpate both ankles and feet simultaneously for warmth and pedal pulses. Have the patient sit and try to raise and lower each foot while you apply pressure to it. Assess range of motion in the ankles and feet.

Assess neurologic integrity by testing gait, balance, and motor coordination. This is important because patients who have problems walking or feeding themselves have problems manipulating syringes and glucose monitors. Also assess the lower extremities for the ability to perceive hot and cold, sharp and dull sensations, and painful stimuli.

Assessment of the patient with DM is outlined in Table 44-5.

table 44-5 ASSESSMENT *of the Patient with Diabetes Mellitus*

HEALTH HISTORY

Present Illness: Polydipsia, polyuria, polyphagia, unexplained weight loss, dry skin, vaginal itching, delayed healing, blood glucose, urine ketones
Past Health: Established diagnosis of diabetes mellitus, type, onset; cardiovascular or renal disorders; previous hospitalizations; obstetric history: number of pregnancies, outcomes, birth weights, gestational diabetes; immunizations; allergies; and current medications: drug name(s), dosage, schedule, time last dose taken
Family History: Diabetes, heart disease, stroke
Review of Systems: Changes in skin moisture or turgor; changes in vision; diarrhea, abdominal bloating, gas; urine retention or incontinence; pain, tingling, or numbness in extremities; changes in mental status; seizures
Functional Assessment: Literacy, financial resources, usual activity and rest pattern, diet, personal impact of diabetes on life. Self-blood glucose monitoring: Type equipment used, testing schedule, recent test results

PHYSICAL EXAMINATION

General Survey: Level of consciousness, posture and gait, well-being
Vital Signs: Tachycardia, hypertension, hypotension, Kussmaul's respirations
Height and Weight: Current and usual
Skin: Color, warmth, turgor, lesions
Eye: Changes in eye grounds, acuity
Mouth: Sweet, fruity breath odor
Lower Extremities: Blisters, lesions, color, edema, pulses, deformities, strength, range of motion
Neurologic: Gait and balance; motor coordination; perception of temperature, touch, and pain

Nursing Diagnoses, Goals, and Outcome Criteria: Diabetes and Hypoglycemia

NURSING DIAGNOSES	GOALS AND OUTCOME CRITERIA
Ineffective Health Maintenance related to lack of knowledge of dietary management of glucose, faulty metabolism, nausea and vomiting, imbalance between food intake and activity expenditure	Effective health maintenance: patient correctly describes self-care measures, maintains blood glucose within limits of 80 and 120 mg/dL, achieves optimal weight
Ineffective Therapeutic Regimen Management related to financial, personal, family pattern disruption	Effective management of self-care using prescribed treatment regimen: patient verbalizes understanding of and intent to adhere to treatment regimen; patient uses resources needed for DM management

Risk for Deficient Fluid Volume related to hyperglycemia, alterations in urine output	Normal extracellular fluid volume: patient correctly describes fluid needs, recognizes significance of polyuria and oliguria; pulse and blood pressure remain within patient norms
Risk for Injury related to adverse effects of drugs, diminished alertness, increased susceptibility to infection	Decreased risk for injury: blood glucose 80-120 mg/dL, and absence of signs of infection (normal body temperature and white blood cell count)
Activity Intolerance related to impaired tissue perfusion, decreased mobility	Stable or improved activity tolerance: patient performs daily activities without excess fatigue
Chronic Pain related to neuropathy	Pain relief: patient states pain relieved or reduced; appears relaxed
Disturbed Sensory Perception (visual, auditory, tactile) or **Impaired Skin Integrity** related to neurologic and circulatory changes	Absence of injury associated with sensory loss: skin intact, no redness, blisters
Disturbed Thought Processes related to abnormal blood glucose, metabolic imbalances	Normal thought processes: patient is alert and oriented to person, place, and time
Ineffective Coping related to diagnosis, dietary restrictions, disturbed body image, sexual dysfunction, anxiety, fear	Effective coping: patient verbalizes feelings about diabetes and expresses willingness to follow plan of care and to use resources as needed

The diagnoses above are not an exhaustive list because there may be many other nursing diagnoses if a patient has complications associated with DM. The nursing care plan must be individualized based on the assessment. Management of emergencies is discussed in the section on complications.

Interventions

Immediate nursing care of the patient with DM is geared toward urgent needs and complications. After urgent needs are met, nursing care focuses on teaching the patient to manage diabetes.

Ineffective Health Maintenance

Patient education requires that the patient understand the physiology of glucose metabolism and the signs and symptoms of hypoglycemia, ketoacidosis, and hyperglycemic hyperosmolar nonketotic coma. Teach the patient how and when to monitor blood glucose and urine ketone levels, how to interpret the results, and the appropriate actions to take based on the results. If the patient is using a glucose meter, explain and demonstrate calibration and operation of the device, collection of blood samples, and disposal of lancets.

The teaching plan also prepares the patient for self-medication as prescribed. Drug names, dosages, actions, and adverse effects are presented. If insulin is prescribed, demonstrate proper techniques for drawing up and injecting insulin and explain site rotation. Explain how adjustments in insulin or diet and exercise are used to maintain blood glucose levels at 80 to 120 mg/dL. Provide not only verbal instruction but also allow the patient to handle equipment and demonstrate skills multiple times. If the patient cannot correctly draw up insulin, a caregiver can prepare the syringes in advance. If refrigerated, the insulin in the prefilled syringes is stable for 1 week. The syringes should be stored in a vertical or tilted position (needle up) to reduce clogging of the needle. Before administering, tell the patient to pull back the plunger slightly and gently rock the syringe to remix the solution.

Advise the patient to consult the physician or pharmacist before taking new medications because many medications interact with diabetes drugs.

Consult the dietitian regarding diet, and reinforce nutritional information. During hospitalization, record food intake. Details of medical and dietary management are presented earlier in this chapter.

Ideally, you should present small units of content in each teaching session. Unfortunately, there may be time to provide the patient only with "survival skills" during a brief or busy hospitalization. Therefore, verbal instructions should be accompanied by written material and/or videotapes and information about local resources such as the hospital's certified diabetes educator and the local chapter of the American Diabetes Association. Office nurses, community health nurses, and home health nurses also often participate in teaching the patient with diabetes.

PHARMACOLOGY CAPSULE Many drugs can affect blood glucose. For example, beta-adrenergic blockers lower the blood glucose and hydrochlorothiazides raise it.

Ineffective Therapeutic Regimen Management

When a patient has had diabetes education but does not follow the prescribed plan, explore possible barriers to carrying out the plan. Some patients may think the program is too hard to follow and not even try. Others may think complications are inevitable and that treatment will not really make a difference. Another reason for noncompliance is lack of financial resources for drugs, supplies, and a balanced diet. Nursing interventions depend on the barriers identified. They are designed to provide practical help, support, and encouragement.

Teach family members how to support and help the family member with diabetes. Treat the family as integral members of the health care team. It is especially important in the nutrition teaching to include the person who does the shopping and cooking. A referral to social services is necessary if the patient cannot afford syringes and insulin. A referral to a diabetes educator, home health nurse, or community health nurse for follow-up teaching and monitoring also is recommended.

Risk for Deficient Fluid Volume

Teach the patient the relationship between blood glucose and urine output. Explain that abnormally increased output may signal hyperglycemia and may eventually lead to dehydration and ketoacidosis.

Risk for Injury

Advise the patient to keep immunizations current because of increased susceptibility to infection and impaired healing. Teach patients to see a physician promptly if they have signs and symptoms of infection such as fever, cough, painful urination, or lesions with purulent drainage.

On sick days, insulin or oral agents should be taken as usual and blood glucose checked every 2 to 4 hours. If the blood glucose exceeds 250 mg/dL, urine should be tested for ketones. Glucose levels greater than 300 mg/dL or ketonuria should be reported to the physician. Patients with type 1 disease may need additional insulin. To prevent dehydration and ketoacidosis, the patient should eat 10 to 15 gm of carbohydrates every 1 to 2 hours and drink small amounts of fluid every 15 to 30 minutes: 4 ounces of orange or apple juice, non-diet soda, or Jell-O provide approximately 15 gm of carbohydrates. If nausea and vomiting occur, suggest soft foods or liquids instead of solid foods. Tell the patient to report nausea, vomiting, and diarrhea to the physician at once because severe fluid loss may occur. The patient who is unable to retain oral fluids may require hospitalization to restore fluid and electrolyte balance.

Activity Intolerance

An exercise regimen can be designed with the hospital rehabilitation department. "All things in moderation" is the best rule of thumb. Lack of exercise or too vigorous activity just before bedtime may contribute to sleeplessness. Details about the effects of exercise on blood glucose and activity recommendations are discussed earlier in this chapter.

Chronic Pain

Leg pain due to long-term complications may require analgesics. Document pain, administer medications as ordered, and evaluate effects of interventions. If the patient is taking analgesics at home, explain how the medication is to be taken and any significant side effects such as drowsiness.

Disturbed Sensory Perception or Impaired Skin Integrity

Instruct the patient on the importance of having yearly eye examinations. The patient should inform the ophthalmologist of the diagnosis of diabetes. If the patient has impaired vision, audiotapes, special reading materials, and special devices for preparing and administering insulin and for testing blood glucose may be needed.

If the patient has a hearing problem, give directions while facing the patient at eye level and speak clearly. Ask the patient to repeat or demonstrate instructions to make sure that they were heard correctly. Supplement verbal information and demonstrations with written material.

Alterations in tactile sensations may result in burns or frostbite. The patient and the family need to be aware of the danger of impaired sensation. Instruct the patient to avoid injury from heat or cold when outdoors in extreme weather. Caution the patient about the possibility of burns when using heating pads or electric blankets, working around a hot stove, or sitting next to a hot radiator. When taking a bath, measure the temperature of the bath water with a bath thermometer. The temperature should not exceed 43° C (109.4° F). Tissue may be burned before the patient is aware of the excessive heat.

The patient or someone else should examine the patient's feet daily for signs of trauma. Injuries or blisters should be seen promptly by a physician. Foot care for the diabetic is summarized in Table 44-2.

Disturbed Thought Processes

Disturbed thought processes may be due to hypoglycemia, ketoacidosis, or HHNKS. Without treatment, the hypoglycemic patient may be irritable at first, then confused, irrational, lethargic, and eventually comatose. In ketoacidosis, the patient becomes drowsy and the level of consciousness decreases and may progress to coma. HHNKS also is characterized by altered levels of consciousness, progressing from confusion to coma. Emergency and medical treatments are covered earlier in this chapter.

When the patient is confused or disoriented, first initiate actions to determine the cause and seek appropriate medical care. Meanwhile, have someone remain with the patient to ensure safety until the condition improves. Because of the risk of disturbed thought processes, people with diabetes should wear a medical alert tag. The tag identifies the patient as having diabetes so that medical attention will be sought.

Ineffective Coping

Patients may be anxious about the immediate and long-term effects of diabetes and how it will affect their lives. They may be overwhelmed by what they need to learn for self-care. They also may be fearful about lifestyle changes, self-medication, glucose testing, adverse drug effects, and possible complications. Encourage patients to express these concerns so that they can be addressed. Talking with other people who are coping successfully with diabetes can have positive effects.

Encourage patients to express their feelings regarding diabetes and to ask for help or advice when needed. Make every effort to encourage them to resume normal activities and to continue their usual social activities. Help patients identify their strengths and weaknesses and explore coping strategies for managing areas of concern.

One source of stress to some patients is altered sexual function. Listen to the patient's concerns and encourage consultation with the physician on the matter. Altered sexual function may be due to diabetes, but there also may be other causes. Some diagnostic procedures may be done to assess erectile dysfunction. For irreversible erectile dysfunction, the physician can offer the male patient several options (see Chapter 46). Research is ongoing into treatments for female dysfunction. You can explore with the patient the importance of sexual intercourse and his or her willingness to consider alternative means of sexual expression. Patients and their partners may wish to seek counseling from therapists with expertise in sexual dysfunction.

Patient teaching for self-medication cannot be done at the last minute. Supplement teaching with written material and information about outpatient resources.

PATIENT TEACHING PLAN
Diabetes Mellitus

- Learn the names of your prescribed drugs, dosages and schedule, and (if on insulin) technique for injections.
- Take some form of carbohydrate if you have symptoms of hypoglycemia: nervousness, palpitations, hunger.
- Monitoring your blood glucose helps you see how well your diabetes is being controlled.
- We will teach you how to check your blood glucose and interpret the findings, and what actions, if any, to take.
- Nutrition is an important part of managing your diabetes. The dietitian will discuss dietary guidelines with you.
- Regular exercise helps to control your blood glucose and improves circulation.
- Because your feet are susceptible to injury and may not heal well, wear properly fitting shoes, inspect feet daily, and immediately seek medical care for wounds, blisters, and calluses.
- When you are sick, monitor your blood glucose and urine ketones; continue your insulin (if taking), take in carbohydrates that provide 10 to 15 gm of carbohydrates every 1 to 2 hours, and take small amounts of fluids every 15 to 30 minutes.
- Although there is no cure for diabetes at this time, you can reduce your risk of complications with good management.

See Nursing Care Plans for The Patient with Type 1 Diabetes Mellitus and The Patient with Type 2 Diabetes Mellitus.

NURSING CARE PLAN

The Patient with Type 1 Diabetes Mellitus

ASSESSMENT

Health History: A 17-year-old female who has recently been diagnosed with type 1 diabetes mellitus is hospitalized to begin her insulin therapy and stabilize her blood glucose. She sought medical attention because of persistent thirst and increased urination. She has no other health problems but has had frequent upper respiratory infections the past few years. The review of systems reveals periodic blurred vision, itching, increased appetite, weight loss of 7 pounds in 3 months, and fatigue.

Physical Examination: Vital signs: temperature, 98.4° F orally; pulse, 88; respiration, 14; blood pressure, 92/58. Height, 5'2". Weight, 107 lb. Physical findings are all within normal limits.

Nursing Diagnosis	*Goals and Outcome Criteria*	*Interventions*
Ineffective health maintenance related to lack of knowledge of diabetes management.	The patient will correctly describe type 1 diabetes and its treatment. Patient will demonstrate self-medication, meal planning, and understanding of management of exercise and drug effects.	Explain the physiology of glucose metabolism, signs and symptoms of ketoacidosis, and hypoglycemia. Teach to perform self-monitoring of blood glucose and urine ketone testing and how to interpret results. Explain insulin types, actions, and administration. Have patient practice insulin injection. Explain relationship between diet, exercise, insulin, and blood glucose. Obtain dietary consult regarding diet. Monitor food intake and replace food not eaten with substitute identified by dietitian.
Ineffective management of therapeutic regimen related to financial, personal, or family pattern disruption.	The patient will express intent to adhere to prescribed regimen of care.	Request patient education by certified diabetes educator if available. If not, present information in a positive manner and in small units. Identify barriers to self management. Determine resources and sources of support. Have patient repeat aspects of care and consequences of nonadherence to program. Acknowledge difficulty in making major changes in eating and activity patterns and in administering self-injections. Identify community resources such as the local chapter of the American Diabetes Association. Teach the patient and family members to recognize and respond to hypoglycemia and ketoacidosis.
Deficient fluid volume related to altered urine output.	The patient will maintain normal blood volume as evidenced by normal tissue turgor, pulse, and blood pressure.	Stress the importance of drinking at least eight glasses of water daily. Point out that excessive urine output may indicate hyperglycemia. Assess hydration, including tissue turgor, mucous membrane moisture, and vital signs.

Continued

NURSING CARE PLAN—cont'd

Nursing Diagnosis	*Goals and Outcome Criteria*	*Interventions*
Risk for injury related to adverse effects of drugs, increased susceptibility to infection.	The patient's blood glucose will remain within goal range established by physician. The patient will state measures to reduce risk of infection and will identify symptoms that should be reported to physician.	Teach patient to recognize signs and symptoms of hypoglycemia: shakiness, nervousness, irritability, tachycardia, anxiety, lightheadedness, hunger, tingling or numbness of lips and tongue. Instruct to take concentrated sugar if hypoglycemia occurs, followed by a complex carbohydrate (milk, bread) to prevent rebound hypoglycemia. The patient should contact the physician if ill and unable to take food or fluids. Caution the patient that impaired sensation could develop in the extremities and that healing of injuries may be impaired. Encourage to avoid trauma and to inspect the feet daily to detect any injuries.
Activity intolerance related to metabolic imbalance.	The patient will perform usual activities of daily living and carry out planned exercise program without excess fatigue.	An exercise regimen is built into the plan of care. Exercise must be done as part of a regular routine. Tell the patient to avoid injecting insulin into a body area that will be affected by exercise soon after the injection. Patient should not exercise during peak insulin activity and should eat a snack before or during exercise if the blood glucose is <100 mg/dL to avoid hypoglycemia.
Disturbed sensory perception (visual) related to abnormal serum glucose.	The patient will report correction of blurred vision.	Advise the patient that blurred vision may be due to hyperglycemia. Encourage annual ophthalmologic examination to detect vision changes or problems.
Disturbed thought processes related to abnormal serum glucose.	The patient will continue to be alert and fully oriented.	Monitor the patient's mental status. Recognize confusion as a sign of abnormal serum glucose. Tell the patient and family that mental changes are best treated with carbohydrates. If the patient does not improve, the blood glucose should be measured and medical attention must be sought.
Ineffective coping related to diagnosis, dietary restrictions, disturbed body image, anxiety, and fear.	The patient will identify concerns about living with diabetes mellitus and plan strategies for dealing with it.	Encourage the patient to express feelings about diabetes and to ask questions. Assure her that most regular activities can be resumed. Identify the patient's strengths and resources. Explore knowledge about diabetes and any misconceptions. Tell her that pregnancy must be carefully monitored, but that it is a future option. Offer support groups if available.

NURSING CARE PLAN

The Patient with Type 2 Diabetes Mellitus

ASSESSMENT

Health History: An 80-year-old Latina was seen in her physician's office and diagnosed with type 2 diabetes mellitus. A referral has been made to a home health agency. The assessment was done in the patient's home. She is three blocks from a grocery store, which also has a pharmacy. Her physician prescribed glyburide (Micronase), 2.5 mg daily before breakfast. Mrs. Garcia sought medical treatment for fatigue, weight loss (10 lb in 2 months), and symptoms of a urinary tract infection. Mrs. Garcia has a history of hypertension, which is treated with verapamil, and venous insufficiency. When asked, she states she has had some problems with her vision and vaginal pruritus. She reports that her appetite is very good, so she could not understand why she was losing weight. Her usual diet is primarily Mexican-American food, but she reports trying not to eat "too much fat." She expresses concern that a diabetic diet will be too expensive because she has only Social Security income. She said that her father died of a heart attack at age 57, and her mother died at age 73 from kidney failure. One of her brothers has diabetes mellitus, one is deceased from heart disease, and a third is alive and well at age 70. Mrs. Garcia says her symptoms have interfered with performance of usual daily activities and that she is getting up frequently during the night to void, which has affected the quality of her rest. She is a widow who lives alone. She has four adult children, but only one lives in the same city and visits her mother on weekends.

Physical Examination: Vital signs: temperature, 97° F orally; pulse, 86; respiration, 16; blood pressure, 160/95. Patient is alert and oriented. Her skin is dry, and tissue turgor is poor. She has kyphosis and walks slowly. Heart and breath sounds are normal; 2+ edema in both legs. Popliteal pulses are weak; pedal pulses are not palpable. Skin is dark around the ankles. Feet are cool. Capillary return in toenails is 4 seconds. Toenails are unevenly cut. There is a reddened area on one heel, but she says it is not painful.

NURSING CARE PLAN—cont'd

Nursing Diagnosis	*Goals and Outcome Criteria*	*Interventions*
Ineffective health maintenance related to lack of knowledge of dietary management of DM, drug therapy, and self-monitoring.	The patient will demonstrate the ability to adhere to prescribed diet and drug therapy and to monitor blood glucose.	Assess the patient's understanding of her condition and treatment and explore her attitude toward managing type 2 diabetes. Assess gross visual acuity and assist her to get an eye examination and corrective lenses as needed. Contact local Lions Club if she cannot afford prescribed lenses. Design a teaching plan to explain key aspects of care. Emphasize skills needed immediately: how to take medications, what foods to avoid, and how to recognize and treat hypoglycemia. If home blood glucose monitoring is prescribed, practice the process with the patient and evaluate her ability to perform the test and interpret the results. Develop a plan with the patient to cover additional topics. Discuss home health referral with physician.
Ineffective management of therapeutic regimen related to financial limitations and difficulties with transportation for food, drugs, and medical care.	The patient will manage her prescribed diet and drug therapy.	Assess any barriers the patient perceives to managing her prescribed diet and drug therapy. If there are financial problems, consult a social worker or determine what assistance is available. If transportation and shopping are difficult, explore how daughter can help or provide information about public transportation available for the elderly and the disabled. Provide dietary information that incorporates Mexican dishes. Discuss the advantages of using senior nutrition programs or Meals-on-Wheels to provide some meals and ease the burden of food preparation. Monitor weight and blood glucose to assess effects of treatment.
Risk for injury related to adverse effects of drugs, circulatory impairment, decreased sensation, and increased susceptibility to infection.	The patient will take measures to reduce the risk of injury associated with hypoglycemia, inadequate circulation, and diminished sensation; the patient will remain free of fever.	Explain the importance of eating properly while on oral medications that lower the blood glucose. Describe the related signs and symptoms, and advise the patient to consume a glucose source such as sweetened orange juice to reverse hypoglycemia. Stress the importance of contacting the physician if ill and unable to take oral food and fluids. Explain how diabetes affects the blood vessels and nerves, making the extremities especially vulnerable to injury. Emphasize the importance of protecting the feet from injury by wearing properly fitting shoes and keeping the nails trimmed correctly. She should be told to avoid heating pads and to test bath water with a bath thermometer. Advise her to have foot care done by a physician or other specialist (see Table 44-2).
Activity intolerance related to fatigue, venous insufficiency, circulatory impairment.	The patient will resume previous level of activity without excessive fatigue.	Assess energy level. Explore usual day and discuss ways to conserve energy.
Ineffective coping related to diagnosis of serious chronic illness that requires alterations in daily life.	The patient will demonstrate effective coping with management of diabetes.	Encourage patient to share her thoughts and feelings about having diabetes and her ability to deal with it. Assure her that many older people learn to manage quite well and that resources are available to help her. Communicate with her frequently until her confidence increases. Let her know how she can reach ready sources of information.

HYPOGLYCEMIA

PATHOPHYSIOLOGY

Hypoglycemia may result from causes other than the pharmacologic treatment for diabetes. Regulation of blood glucose depends on insulin levels, available glucagon, and the secretion of catecholamines, growth hormone, and cortisol. Hypoglycemia may occur if there are abnormalities in these regulators. Hypoglycemia is defined as a syndrome that develops when the blood glucose level falls to less than 45 to 50 mg/dL. Symptoms can occur at different blood levels according to individual tolerances and how rapidly the level falls. The causes of hypoglycemia may be divided into three categories: exogenous, endogenous, and functional.

Summaries of each of these three categories are presented in Table 44-6. *Exogenous hypoglycemia* results from outside

table 44-6 ***Exogenous, Endogenous, and Functional Causes of Hypoglycemia in Adults***

CAUSES	PREDISPOSING FACTORS	OCCURRENCE
EXOGENOUS CAUSES		
Insulin	Intentional or accidental overdose; may be combined with inadequate food intake, usually increased exercise, decrease in insulin requirement, or potentiating medications	Most frequent cause of hypoglycemia
Oral hypoglycemic agents	Intentional or accidental overdose; may be combined with inadequate food intake, increased exercise, or potentiating medications	Frequent cause of hypoglycemia with sulfonylureas and meglitinides
Alcohol	Particularly likely in chronically malnourished or acutely food-deprived people	Occurs within 6-36 hr of ingesting moderate to large amounts of alcohol
Exercise	Increased duration and intensity of exercise increases glucose uptake and normally decreases insulin secretion	Occurs with both insulin and sulfonylurea administration and intense exercise, but may be unpredictable in onset
ENDOGENOUS CAUSES		
Organic hypoglycemia	Insulinoma (a tumor of the beta cells of the pancreatic Islets of Langerhans)	Uncommon neoplasm of beta cells of islets of Langerhans
Extrapancreatic neoplasms	May be mesenchymal tumors, hepatomas, adrenocortical carcinomas, gastrointestinal tumors, lymphomas, or leukemias	Rare; most common in adults 40-70 yr of age
FUNCTIONAL CAUSES		
Alimentary hypoglycemia	Rapid dumping of carbohydrates into upper small intestine	Postgastrectomy
Spontaneous reactive hypoglycemia	Syndrome with symptoms such as diaphoresis, tachycardia, tremulousness, headache, fatigue, drowsiness, and irritability	Rarely diagnosed throughout the world; widely diagnosed in United States, prompting American Diabetes Association and Endocrine Society to issue statement that entity is probably overdiagnosed
Alcohol-promoted reactive hypoglycemia	Drinking alcohol on an empty stomach	More common with drinks containing both alcohol and glucose or saccharin (e.g., beer; gin and tonic; rum and cola; whiskey and ginger ale)
Posthyperalimentation hypoglycemia	Rapid discontinuation of total parenteral alimentation	Easily prevented
Endocrine deficiency states	Glucocorticoid deficiency	A danger for any person with adrenal insufficiency
Severe liver deficiency	Insufficient glucose output by liver	Fasting hypoglycemia
Lack of body stores for protein, fat, and carbohydrates	Profound malnutrition	Common; also found with relative frequency in kwashiorkor
Prolonged muscular exercise	Metabolism of energy-producing substances	Occurs if exercise is too prolonged or severe or if nutritional intake and carbohydrate stores are insufficient

Modified from Gray, P. D., & Ludwig-Beymer, P. (1990). Alterations of hormonal regulation. In K. L. McCance & S. E. Huether (Eds.), *Pathophysiology: The biologic basis for disease in adults and children* (pp. 594-643). St. Louis: Mosby.

factors acting on the body to produce a low blood glucose. These include insulin, oral hypoglycemic agents, alcohol, or exercise. *Endogenous hypoglycemia* occurs when internal factors cause an excessive secretion of insulin or an increase in glucose metabolism. These conditions may be related to tumors or genetics.

Functional hypoglycemia may result from a variety of causes, including gastric surgery, fasting, or malnutrition. Alimentary hypoglycemia occurs in a patient who has undergone gastric surgery. The gastric contents empty rapidly, resulting in increased glucose absorption. In response to the increased glucose, excessive insulin production occurs, causing the hypoglycemia. In impaired glucose tolerance hypoglycemia, there is an excessive response of insulin to glucose. Spontaneous reactive hypoglycemia has received much publicity by the lay and medical communities alike. Symptoms occur as a result of an extreme insulin response to ingestion of foods containing carbohydrates. Low blood glucose levels need to be verified for the diagnosis to be accepted.

SIGNS AND SYMPTOMS

Signs and symptoms of hypoglycemia vary according to how quickly the blood glucose levels are falling. When the levels fall rapidly, epinephrine, cortisol, glucagon, and growth hormone are secreted by the body in an attempt to increase glucose levels. Symptoms that result from these physiologic responses include weakness, hunger, diaphoresis, tremors, anxiety, irritability, headache, pallor, and tachycardia. The symptoms of a blood glucose level that falls over several hours are attributed to lack of essential glucose to brain tissue. These symptoms include confusion, weakness, dizziness, blurred or double vision, seizure, and, in severe cases, coma.

MEDICAL DIAGNOSIS

The diagnosis of hypoglycemia not associated with diabetes can be based on fasting blood glucose, OGTT, intravenous glucose tolerance test, and 72-hour inpatient fasting. The diagnosis should be based on three criteria known as Whipple's triad: (1) the presence of symptoms, (2) documentation of low blood glucose when symptoms occur, and (3) improvement of these symptoms when blood glucose rises. These criteria must occur in the absence of sulfonylurea treatment or abnormal plasma insulin and C-peptide.

MEDICAL TREATMENT

Treatment of hypoglycemia depends on the cause of the problem and the patient's condition. In an unconscious patient who has diabetes, hypoglycemia should be suspected until it is ruled out. Fifty milliliters of 50% glucose solution should be administered immediately. The patient with a milder form of hypoglycemia is treated with 15 gm of carbohydrate. If the patient's condition does not improve, another 15 gm of carbohydrate should be given after 10 minutes. Giving more than 15 gm initially may lead to rebound hyperglycemia. In terms of food exchanges, one bread exchange contains 15 gm of carbohydrate, one fruit exchange contains 15 gm of carbohydrate, and one milk exchange contains 12 gm of carbohydrate.

Prevention of hypoglycemia by proper food intake is an important treatment component. The diet is directed by the underlying cause. If the cause is related to an overproduction of insulin after carbohydrate ingestion, a low-carbohydrate, high-protein diet is commonly ordered. Restriction of carbohydrates to no more than 100 gm/day is recommended. Simple sugars are avoided, and complex carbohydrates are encouraged. Because no significant increase in blood glucose is noted with protein ingestion, a high-protein diet is recommended. The remaining calories in the diet are obtained from fat. Because carbohydrates are restricted, the calories required from fat are high. Patients may tolerate smaller, more frequent meals. Alcohol should be avoided. Remember, hypoglycemia associated with treatment of diabetes uses different guidelines for treatment.

NURSING CARE *of the Patient with Hypoglycemia*

Assessment

The health history is especially important in the diagnosis of hypoglycemia. Describe the present illness, which may include the following symptoms: shakiness, nervousness, irritability, tachycardia, anxiety, lightheadedness, hunger, tingling or numbness of the lips or tongue, nightmares, and crying out during sleep. Note when the episodes occur in relation to meals and particular food intake. The past medical history documents diabetes, previous gastric surgery, abdominal cancer, or adrenal insufficiency. Record medications, paying particular attention to hypoglycemic agents. Note the names of hypoglycemic agents, prescribed dose, and the time that the last dose was taken. The functional assessment elicits information about current diet, exercise, alcohol intake, and the effects of symptoms on daily activities. Important aspects of the physical examination include general behavior, appearance, pulse, and blood pressure.

Nursing Diagnoses, Goals, and Outcome Criteria: Hypoglycemia

NURSING DIAGNOSES	GOALS AND OUTCOME CRITERIA
Deficient Knowledge of management of hypoglycemia	Patient understands and can manage hypoglycemic episodes: the patient accurately describes and demonstrates self-care measures
Risk for Injury related to episodes of dizziness and weakness	Absence of injury: no falls or injuries as a result of hypoglycemic episodes
Impaired Adjustment related to effects of illness on lifestyles	Adjustment to living with hyperglycemia: patient describes and practices measures to manage hypoglycemia

Interventions

Deficient Knowledge

Patient education is a priority after a confirmed diagnosis to prevent future occurrences. Teach patients to recognize the signs and symptoms and to treat them promptly. Advise the patient of factors that may trigger hypoglycemic episodes, such as foods, medications, alcohol, fasting, and exercise. Basic concepts of the diet described earlier need to be stressed and reinforced. A referral for a consultation with a registered dietitian may be helpful for the patient. As a patient educator, you are very influential in promoting self-monitoring and treatment of hypoglycemia.

Risk for Injury

The hypoglycemic patient is at risk for injury as a result of weakness and dizziness. Be alert for signs and symptoms of hypoglycemia. Monitor serum glucose levels. Administer carbohydrates as prescribed by the physician. Until the episode passes, keep the patient in bed with the side rails up and the call button nearby. Advise the patient not to get up unassisted.

Impaired Adjustment

Emotional support for the patient with hypoglycemia is necessary during both diagnosis and treatment. Prepare the patient for diagnostic tests and tell the patient what to expect. Once the diagnosis is made, explore the patient's feelings and concerns. Support the patient in learning to incorporate management of hypoglycemia into his or her lifestyle. Guide the patient to anticipate problem situations and possible solutions.

Nutrition Concepts

1. Diet is an essential component in the management of both type 1 and type 2 diabetes mellitus.
2. The goal of the diabetic diet is to maintain plasma glucose at as near to the normal physiologic range as possible.
3. A person who requires insulin to control diabetes mellitus should coordinate insulin administration with mealtime patterns.
4. A person with type 2 diabetes can spread food intake throughout the day and eat consistently every day.
5. Diet plans are individualized based on glucose and lipid levels, weight management goals, and what the patient is willing to do.
6. When hypoglycemia is attributed to an overproduction of insulin in response to carbohydrate ingestion, a low-carbohydrate, high-protein diet with smaller meals may control the condition.

key points

- Diabetes mellitus is a condition characterized by impaired metabolism related to tissue resistance to insulin or insulin deficiency.
- Diabetes mellitus is managed with diet, exercise, and insulin and/or oral hypoglycemic agents.
- The major complications of diabetes mellitus are ketoacidosis, hyperosmolar nonketotic coma, vascular changes, and neuropathy.
- Ketoacidosis causes dehydration, electrolyte imbalance, and metabolic acidosis and is treated with fluid and electrolyte replacement and insulin.
- Hyperosmolar nonketotic coma is loss of consciousness due to extremely high serum glucose without ketoacidosis.
- The major complications of insulin therapy are hypoglycemia, insulin shock, and hyperglycemia (Somogyi effect).
- Nursing care of the patient with diabetes mellitus focuses on Ineffective Health Maintenance, Ineffective Therapeutic Regimen Management, Deficient Fluid Volume, Risk for Injury, Activity Intolerance, Chronic Pain, Disturbed Sensory Perception, Disturbed Thought Processes, and Ineffective Coping.
- Hypoglycemia (low serum glucose) in the absence of diabetes mellitus can be caused by pancreatic tumors, adrenal insufficiency, liver disease, and pituitary disorders, but sometimes no specific cause is identified.
- Nursing care of the nondiabetic patient who has hypoglycemia focuses on Deficient Knowledge, Risk for Injury, and Impaired Adjustment.

REVIEW QUESTIONS

1. A function of insulin is to:
   1. serve as an energy source.
   2. help transport glucose into cells.
   3. metabolize glucose for energy.
   4. eliminate excess serum glucose.
2. The incidence of diabetes mellitus is greatest among people of which ethnicity?
   1. Hispanic
   2. African
   3. European
   4. Asian
3. One type of macrovascular complication of diabetes mellitus is:
   1. retinopathy.
   2. end-stage renal disease.
   3. neuropathy.
   4. coronary artery disease.
4. You are assessing a patient who has had type 2 diabetes mellitus for 10 years. He complains of dizziness when rising to a standing position and increasing fatigue with his usual exercise program. His vital signs are normal except for a heart rate of 108. You should suspect:
   1. coronary artery disease.
   2. inadequate control of blood glucose.
   3. autonomic neuropathy.
   4. hyperglycemic episodes.
5. A patient who has just been diagnosed with diabetes and started on oral medications says, "I feel strange and my mouth feels numb. Something is wrong!" You note that his hands are trembling and that he is perspiring. What is your best response?
   1. These are common symptoms of diabetes. They will go away soon.
   2. Let's check your blood sugar. It is probably low.
   3. Your doctor will probably need to increase your medication dose.
   4. This is very unusual. I will call your physician.

6. What is the rationale for limiting protein intake in the patient with diabetes mellitus?
   1. Metabolism of excess protein causes ketoacidosis.
   2. Protein needs are decreased because excess glucose meets metabolic needs.
   3. High protein intake interferes with absorption of other nutrients.
   4. High protein intake indirectly contributes to the development of nephropathy.

7. The advantage of human insulin over beef and pork insulin is:
   1. human insulin is less expensive.
   2. people do not form antibodies for human insulin.
   3. human insulin has a longer duration of action.
   4. human insulin does not cause hypoglycemia.

8. Which type of oral medication is *least* likely to cause hypoglycemia?
   1. Alpha-glucosidase inhibitors
   2. Sulfonylureas
   3. Meglitinides
   4. D-phenylalanines

9. The classic signs and symptoms of diabetes mellitus are:
   1. thirst, tachycardia, tremor.
   2. hyperglycemia, hyponatremia, hyperkalemia.
   3. polyphagia, polydipsia, polyuria.
   4. nephropathy, retinopathy, neuropathy .

10. A patient who was newly diagnosed with diabetes says, "Everyone I know with diabetes has had one or both legs amputated." What is the most appropriate reply?
    1. "Try not to think about that."
    2. "Most people with diabetes eventually have to have amputations."
    3. "The ones who had amputations did not follow their doctor's orders."
    4. "There are many things you can do to reduce your risk of future amputations."

CHAPTER 45 Female Reproductive Disorders

objectives

1. List data to be collected when assessing the female reproductive system.
2. Describe the nursing interventions for women who are undergoing diagnostic tests and procedures for reproductive system disorders.
3. Identify the nursing interventions associated with douche, cauterization, heat therapy, and topical medications used to treat disorders of the female reproductive system.
4. Explain the pathophysiology, signs and symptoms, complications, diagnostic procedures, and medical or surgical treatment for selected disorders of the female reproductive system.
5. Assist in developing a nursing care plan for patients with common disorders of the female reproductive system.
6. Describe the nursing interventions for the patient who is menopausal.

key terms

Cystocele (SĬS-tō-sēl, p. 950)
Dysmenorrhea (dĭs-mĕn-ō-RĒ-ă, p. 945)
Dyspareunia (dĭs-pă-ROO-nē-ă, p. 943)
Dysplasia (dĭs-PLĀ-sē-ă, p. 929)
Endometriosis (ĕn-dō-mē-trē-Ō-sĭs, p. 944)
Hysterectomy (hĭs-tĕr-ĔK-tō-mē, p. 946)
Mastitis (măs-TĪ-tĭs, p. 942)
Menarche (mĕ-NĂR-kē, p. 927)
Menopause (MĔN-ō-păwz, p. 927)
Menorrhagia (mĕn-ō-RĀ-jă, p. 938)
Metrorrhagia (mĕ-trō-RĀ-jă, p. 938)
Rectocele (RĔK-tō-sēl, p. 950)
Retroversion (rĕt-rō-VĔR-zhŭn, p. 953)
Salpingo-oophorectomy (săl-pĭng-gō-ō-ŎF-ō-RĔK-tō-mē, p. 946)
Vaginitis (vă-jĭ-NĪ-tĭs, p. 940)
Vulvitis (vŭl-VĪ-tĭs, p. 940)

The female reproductive system includes external and internal genitalia and the breasts. The term *vulva* refers to the external genitalia, which comprise the mons pubis, labia majora, labia minora, clitoris, and pudendum (Fig. 45-1). Also included in the vulva are mucus-secreting glands. Bartholin's glands are located on both sides of the posterior edge of the vaginal opening, and Skene's glands are located just inside the urethral opening. The perineum is the area between the posterior junction of the labia minora and the anus. The internal genitalia include two ovaries, two fallopian tubes, the uterus, and the vagina (Fig. 45-2).

ANATOMY AND PHYSIOLOGY OF THE FEMALE REPRODUCTIVE SYSTEM

EXTERNAL GENITALIA

The mons pubis is a pad of fatty tissue that covers and protects the symphysis pubis. The labia majora are extensions of the fatty tissue that cover and protect inner vulvar structures. The labia majora extend from the mons pubis to the perineum. The inner folds of the labia majora are smooth and moist.

The labia minora are thin folds of smooth skin that form a hood, called the prepuce, over the clitoris. The clitoris is a small structure that corresponds to the male penis. Like the penis, the clitoris is composed of erectile tissue with sensory nerve endings that are responsive to psychological and physical stimuli. The labia minora are richly endowed with sebaceous glands, nerves, and blood vessels that also respond to psychological and physical stimulation. The labia minora may be entirely covered by the labia majora or may be visible between the outer labia.

The urethral (urinary) meatus is below the clitoris. The openings of Skene's glands are located on both sides of the urinary meatus. The vaginal opening, the introitus, is partially or entirely covered by a thin fold of tissue called the hymen. The hymen may be intact, distended, or ruptured. The size of the introitus varies from very small to large and gaping.

INTERNAL GENITALIA

The vagina is a canal that extends from the vulva to the uterus. This structure has the ability to expand and lengthen to accept an erect penis and to provide an exit for a term fetus. The mucous membranes of the vaginal walls secrete lubricating fluid that cleanses the vagina and interacts with bacteria to maintain an acid pH.

The uterus is a firm, muscular organ that is pear-shaped and hollow. Its lower segment is called the cervix. The end of the cervix extends into the upper aspect of the vagina. The os is the opening of the cervix into the vagina. The inner lining of the uterus is called the endometrium. The upper segment of the uterine body, or corpus, is called the fundus.

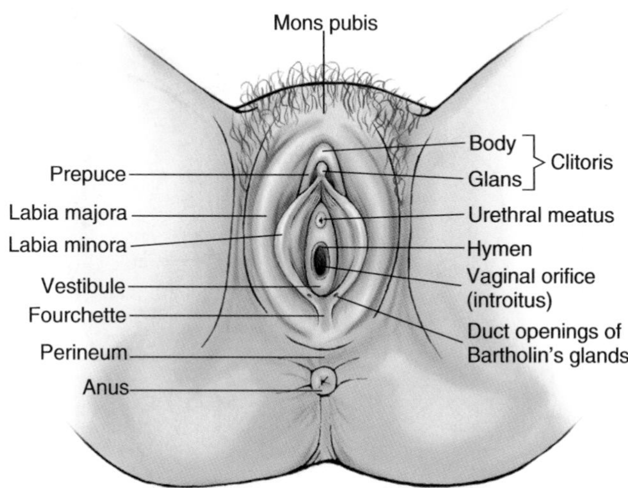

FIGURE 45-1 External female genitalia.

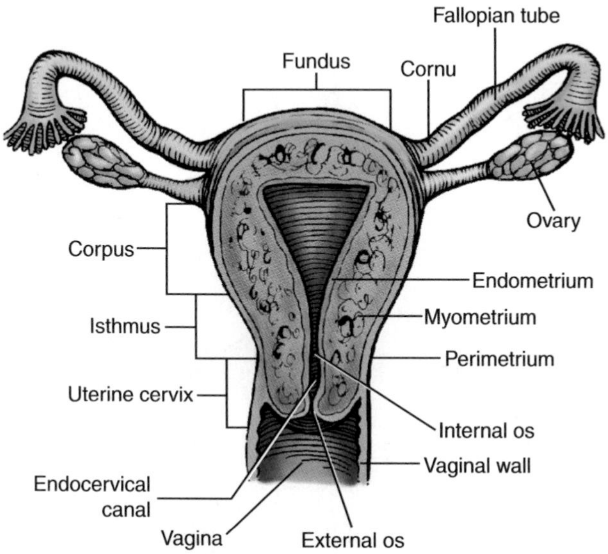

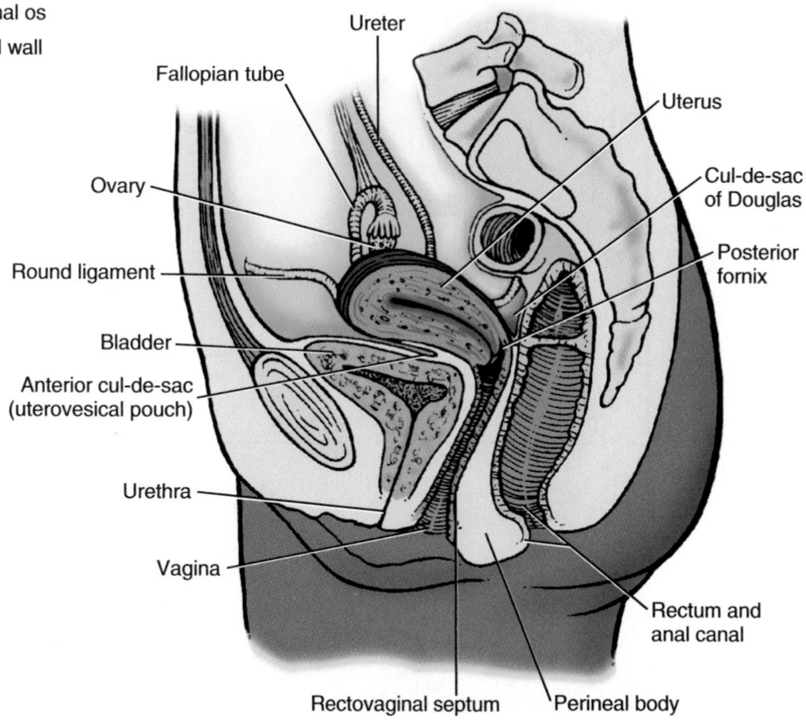

FIGURE 45-2 Internal female genitalia.

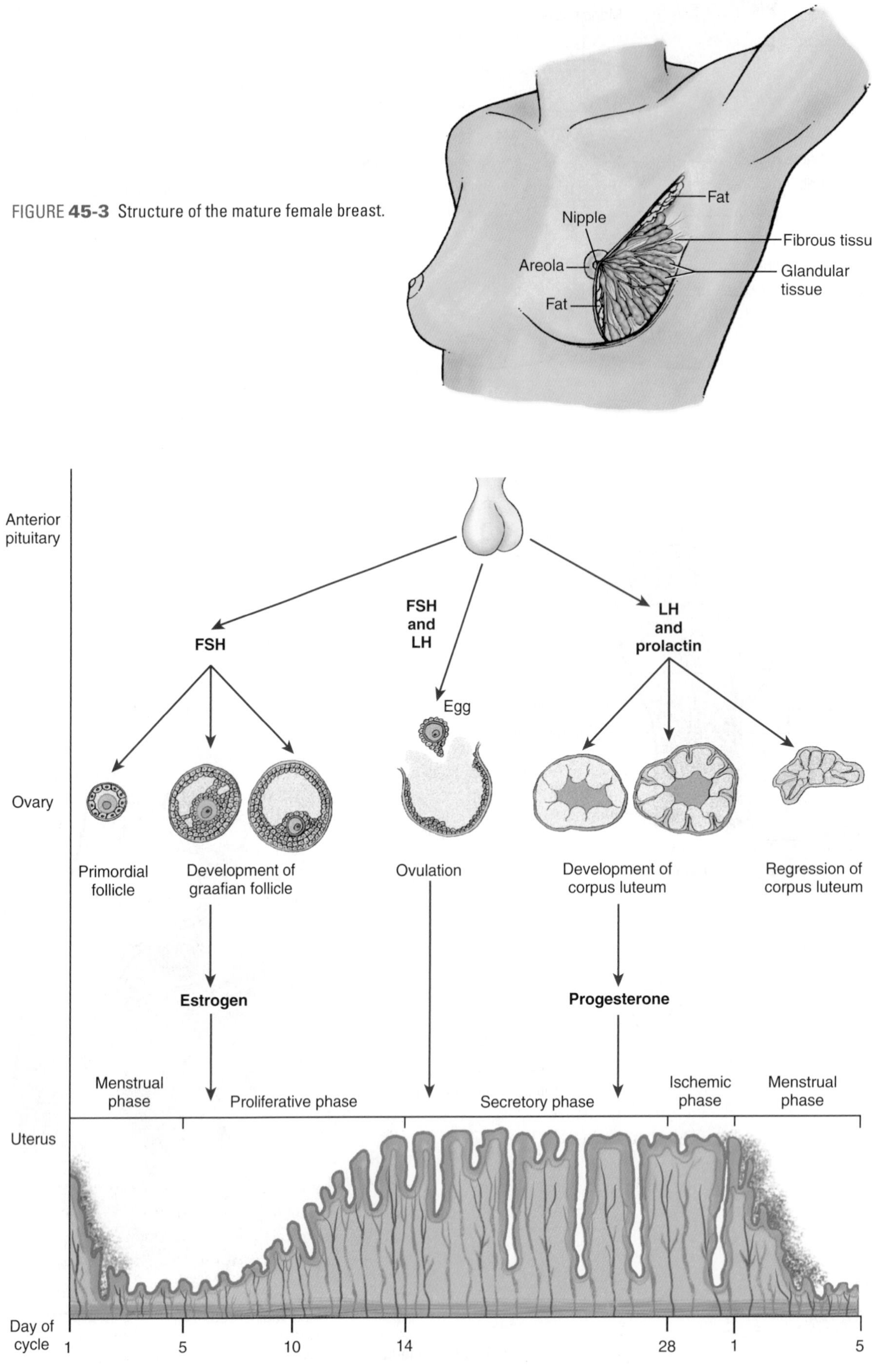

FIGURE 45-3 Structure of the mature female breast.

FIGURE 45-4 Female hormonal cycle.

The two fallopian tubes are thin, hollow, cilia-lined, tubular structures that extend from the uterine fundus. The fallopian tubes have funnel-shaped ends that partially surround the ovaries and that receive the ovum from the ovary. The fallopian tubes serve as passages for ova from the ovaries and for sperm that travel through the vagina and into the tubes. Fertilization, the union of sperm and ovum, takes place in the fallopian tubes.

The two ovaries are almond-shaped structures located on each side of the uterus. They correspond to the male testes. Ovarian functions include maturation and release of ova (ovulation) and secretion of hormones—estrogens, progesterone, androgens, and relaxin.

It is important to note that the pathway through the female reproductive tract, intended to serve as a route for reproduction, also provides a route for infectious organisms to access the pelvic cavity and its organs.

BREASTS

Although the breasts are not directly involved in the reproductive process, they are addressed as accessories to reproduction because of their function: to nourish the infant after birth. Breast structure is illustrated in Figure 45-3. The inner structure is composed of glandular and ductal tissue, fibrous tissue, and fat. (The fat is responsible for most of the variation in breast size and shape.) The breast is divided into several lobes, each divided into lobules. Lobules contain many hollow, grape-shaped alveoli that produce milk when stimulated by the pituitary hormone prolactin. Ducts carry milk from the lobules, through the lobes, to the opening in the nipple.

The nipple with its surrounding areola is a pigmented structure located at the midline of each breast. Breast milk passes through the openings of the lactiferous ducts. Small, round sebaceous glands called Montgomery's tubercules are visible under the skin of the areolae. These glands produce a lubricating secretion that protects nipple tissue. Except during normal lactation, there should be no discharge from the nipple.

MENSTRUAL CYCLE

The menstrual cycle, or female reproductive cycle, consists of the ovarian cycle and the uterine cycle. It results from a complex interaction of the hypothalamus, the anterior pituitary, and the ovary (Fig. 45-4). The interaction causes the ovary to release a mature ovum (ovulation) and prepares the uterine lining to receive and nourish the ovum if it is fertilized. If the ovum is not fertilized, the menstrual cycle begins with the onset of menstruation. Menstruation is the passage through the vagina of a mixture of blood and other fluids and tissue formed in the lining of the uterus to receive the fertilized ovum.

The length of the menstrual cycle averages 28 to 30 days, but the range may be 21 to 40 days and may be affected by various factors such as stress, physical activity, and illness. Regardless of the length of the cycle, the progression is the same:

1. Menstruation (day 1 through days 4 to 7).
2. Maturation of an ovarian follicle, with subsequent rupture and release of an ovum in response to follicle-stimulating hormone and luteinizing hormone from the anterior pituitary (days 1 to 14 in a 28-day cycle).
3. Estrogen production (days 6 to 14) by the maturing follicle; progesterone production (days 15 to 26) by the corpus luteum that is formed from the ruptured follicle.
4. Preparation of the uterine lining for implantation of the fertilized ovum, stimulated by estrogen and progesterone from the follicle and corpus luteum (days 6 to 26).
5. The fertilized ovum implants in the uterine lining and secretes human chorionic gonadotropin, which maintains the corpus luteum and estrogen and progesterone levels; menstruation does not occur (day 14).
6. The unfertilized ovum does not implant. Absence of human chorionic gonadotropin causes the corpus luteum to degenerate, which in turn causes a drop in estrogen and progesterone levels and necrosis of the uterine lining (days 27 to 28). The necrotic lining is shed as menstrual flow and begins another cycle at day 1.

NURSING ASSESSMENT OF THE FEMALE REPRODUCTIVE SYSTEM

HEALTH HISTORY

Whether your responsibility for assessment is limited or extensive, begin the interview with a brief explanation of the purpose for the questions that will be asked.

Chief Complaint and History of Present Illness

Begin the basic assessment with the patient's reason for seeking medical care. "What is the reason for your visit?" is an opening question that allows the patient to describe in her own terms the reason for the visit and to include related information that may guide subsequent questions. If the reason for the visit is an existing problem, include related signs and symptoms and their onset, frequency, and effect on normal functioning. Assess the patient's knowledge about her reproductive health.

Past Medical History

Menstrual History

Record the age at which menstruation began (menarche), the date of the onset of the last menstrual period, the usual number of days between the onset of one period and the onset of the next, the total amount of menstrual flow, the usual number of days of menstrual flow per period, and the use of tampons.

"Many women experience problems with their periods. What problems have you noticed?" is a questioning technique that implies acceptance of a wide variety of problems and invites the patient to provide additional relevant information. Problems commonly reported include spotting or frank bleeding between periods, abdominal pain at the time of ovulation, abdominal cramping or pain before or during periods (or both), and premenstrual mood changes.

For women who have stopped menstruating owing to menopause, record the age at which menstruation ceased as well as related details, such as whether menopause occurred naturally or resulted from surgery, chemotherapy, or radiation therapy. Include information about menopausal symptoms and prescribed or over-the-counter medications taken to relieve menopausal symptoms.

Obstetric-Gynecologic History

"How many times have you been pregnant?" is an appropriate opening question for the obstetric history. If the response indicates that the woman has been pregnant, inquire about the number of term and preterm births, number of living children, number of abortions (spontaneous or induced), and the number of multiple pregnancies (e.g., twins, triplets). Note blood type and Rh factor and a history of rubella or rubella immunization. Terms related to obstetric history are *gravidity* and *parity.* Gravidity refers to the total number of pregnancies. Parity refers to the number of pregnancies that terminated after 20 weeks of gestation, considered the "age of viability." Parity may be recorded according to a number of different codes that use from one- to five-digit numbers. Each institution provides direction on how parity is to be coded for obstetric histories.

The gynecologic history addresses such problems as infections and sexually transmitted diseases, cysts and tumors, structural and functional abnormalities, infertility, and stress incontinence.

Family History

Record a family history of diabetes mellitus, cancer, complications of pregnancy, multiple pregnancies, genetic disorders, or congenital anomalies.

Review of Systems

Record information regarding symptoms and treatment. Commonly reported symptoms are pain, itching, burning, vaginal bleeding between periods or after menopause, heavy or prolonged bleeding with periods, vaginal discharge, and urinary frequency or urgency. Ask questions related to the degree of each reported problem and to any prescribed or self-selected measures taken to relieve each problem.

Functional Assessment

The functional assessment includes a diet history, use of dietary supplements including calcium and iron, exercise pattern, sexual history, occupational exposure to potential teratogens, and effects of symptoms on usual activities.

PHYSICAL EXAMINATION

In the general survey, note the patient's appearance, facial expression, and any obvious signs of distress. Measure vital signs and height and weight. Assess skin color, texture, and moisture. Inspect the breasts for dimpling and abnormal skin texture. Instruct the patient to lean forward and observe for asymmetry when she is leaning forward. Ask the patient about changes from usual contours. Palpate all breast tissue for thickening or lumps (see discussion under Breast Self-Examination in the next section). Inspect the abdomen for distention and palpate for tenderness. Inspect the legs for swelling and palpate for tenderness. Assess for the presence of Homans' sign to detect possible thrombophlebitis. Nurses with advanced training may do the pelvic examination, but it is more commonly performed by the physician. Therefore it is discussed in detail under Diagnostic Tests and Procedures. Basically, the examiner assesses the external genitalia for lesions, lumps, swelling, and discharge. The vagina and uterine cervix are inspected for lesions, growths, discharge, and redness. The vagina, abdomen, and rectum are palpated for abnormalities. Assessment of the female reproductive system is summarized in Table 45-1.

table 45-1 ASSESSMENT *of the Female Reproductive System*

HEALTH HISTORY

Present Illness: Reason for visit, related signs and symptoms, onset and frequency of symptoms, effects on normal functioning

Past Medical History:

Menstrual History: Age at menarche, date of onset of last menstrual period, duration of menstrual period, amount of menstrual flow, use of tampons, pain, bleeding between periods, premenstrual mood changes. If menopausal: age at which menopause occurred, whether menopause was natural or surgical, related symptoms, medications taken to relieve symptoms.

Obstetric and Gynecologic History: Number of pregnancies, number of term and preterm births, number of living children, number of abortions (spontaneous and induced), number of multiple pregnancies, past problems with reproductive organs, fertility, stress incontinence, history of rubella or rubella immunization, frequency of breast self-examination.

Family History: Diabetes, cancer, complications of pregnancy, genetic disorders, multiple pregnancies, congenital anomalies.

Review of Systems: Pain, itching, burning, vaginal bleeding between periods or after menopause, heavy or prolonged bleeding with periods, vaginal discharge, urinary frequency or urgency.

Functional Assessment: Diet, use of dietary supplements—including calcium and iron—exercise pattern, sexual history, occupational exposure to potential teratogens.

PHYSICAL EXAMINATION

General Survey: Appearance, facial expression obvious distress

Vital Signs

Height and Weight

Skin: Texture, moisture, color

Breasts: Dimpling, texture changes in skin, asymmetry when leaning forward, changes from usual contours, changes in texture, lumps, nipple discharge

Extremities: Homans' sign, temperature, swelling, tenderness

Abdomen: Contour, distention, tenderness

Pelvic Examination:

External Genitalia: Appearance, lesions, lumps, swelling, discharge

Vagina and Uterine Cervix: Appearance, lesions, growths, discharge, redness

Rectal Examination

DIAGNOSTIC TESTS AND PROCEDURES

Most diagnostic tests and procedures are performed by the physician or by the nurse practitioner. The responsibilities of the nurse usually focus on patient instruction regarding the procedure, preparation of the patient, support of the patient throughout the tests and procedures, and assistance to the physician or nurse practitioner. Regardless of the test or procedure to be performed, provide anticipatory guidance by telling the patient what to expect. Check the institution's procedure manual for specific preparations and assistants' responsibilities for each test or procedure.

PELVIC EXAMINATION

The pelvic examination allows inspection and palpation of external and internal reproductive structures to identify deviations from normal, to provide information for medical diagnoses, and to collect specimens for laboratory analysis.

The patient assumes the lithotomy position, with her buttocks at the edge of the examination table, her hips and knees flexed, and her feet in stirrups. Many women report that the position is unpleasant because of the sense of vulnerability that they experience. To decrease this effect, delay positioning until just before the examination begins, carefully drape to preserve modesty, and provide verbal and nonverbal support. To decrease physical discomfort associated with use of the stirrups, cover them with thick footlets or encourage the patient to keep socks or shoes on.

The pelvic examination is divided into three parts: (1) visual inspection and palpation of the external genitalia; (2) visual inspection of the vagina and uterine cervix after introduction of a plastic or metal speculum (Fig. 45-5); and (3) bimanual palpation of the vagina and abdomen. The latter procedure may be performed with two fingers of one gloved hand in the vagina or with one finger in the vagina and one finger in the rectum (Fig. 45-6) and the other hand on the abdomen to allow compression of internal structures between the two hands. The final step is a rectal examination with a gloved finger.

Discomfort varies among women. Some women report no discomfort other than feelings of pressure; other women report pain. One common discomfort is related to a cold speculum. You can prevent this by warming the speculum in water or by wrapping the packaged speculum in the folds of a heating pad. Supportive measures include talking to the patient and directing breathing and relaxation techniques to relieve pain and tension.

Following the pelvic examination, assist the patient to sit up and to get off the table. Provide tissues to wipe the perianal area and, if possible, an adhesive panty liner to absorb lubricant as it is expelled from the vagina.

SMEARS AND CULTURES

Collection of specimens for laboratory analysis is one of the purposes of the pelvic examination (Fig. 45-5D). Institutional policy specifies the necessary equipment and the care of slides for each specimen.

Specimens are routinely collected for a Papanicolaou (Pap) smear for detection of cervical cancer and other abnormal cervical cells (**dysplasia**). Additional specimens may be collected for identification of suspected infections such as herpes, *Chlamydia,* and gonorrhea.

ENDOMETRIAL AND CERVICAL BIOPSIES

Endometrial biopsies generally are performed for three reasons: (1) to assess the endometrium for readiness to accept and nourish a fertilized ovum; (2) to indirectly assess corpus luteum function in cases of suspected infertility; and (3) to diagnose uterine cancer. The nurse's responsibilities are similar to those for a pelvic examination and collection of specimens for smears and cultures. The physician or nurse practitioner dilates the cervix and scrapes tissue specimens from the endometrium. The procedure may cause cramping so severe that an anesthetic is necessary.

Cervical biopsies are performed to diagnose suspected cervical cancer. There are two types of biopsy, multiple punch and conization. Multiple punch biopsies are done in a physician's office or an outpatient clinic. Because several specimens are obtained by punching out small samples of cervical tissue, the process is usually painful. The nurse's responsibilities are similar to those for endometrial biopsies. You can support the patient by coaching her to use breathing and relaxation techniques to minimize discomfort.

The cone biopsy is invasive surgery and requires admission to an outpatient surgery facility or a hospital. Under general anesthesia, a large amount of cervical tissue is removed. Although the cone biopsy is rarely used for diagnosing cancer, its advantage lies in its potential both to diagnose and to remove cancerous tissue.

COLPOSCOPY

An instrument called a colposcope is used to inspect the cervix under magnification and to identify abnormal and potentially cancerous tissue. Colposcopy is commonly done before cervical biopsies. Patient preparation and nursing care are similar to those for a pelvic examination.

CULDOSCOPY

A culdoscopy is an invasive surgical procedure usually performed with light sedation and local anesthetic on an outpatient basis. When performed by a skillful physician, culdoscopy is the simplest way to directly visualize the female pelvic cavity. With the patient in the knee-chest position, the culdoscope is inserted through a small incision in the posterior vagina. The culdoscope permits examination of the patient's uterus, ovaries, and fallopian tubes. It is performed to obtain tissue specimens and to identify ectopic pregnancy, pelvic masses, and causes of infertility or pain.

The nurse's responsibilities are similar to those for other outpatient procedures, with details specified by institutional policies. Scrupulous asepsis must be maintained. Many women consider the knee-chest position physically uncomfortable, embarrassing, and humiliating. Assure the patient that she will be draped throughout the procedure, and be conscientious about following through with that assurance. When the procedure is completed, help the patient get out of

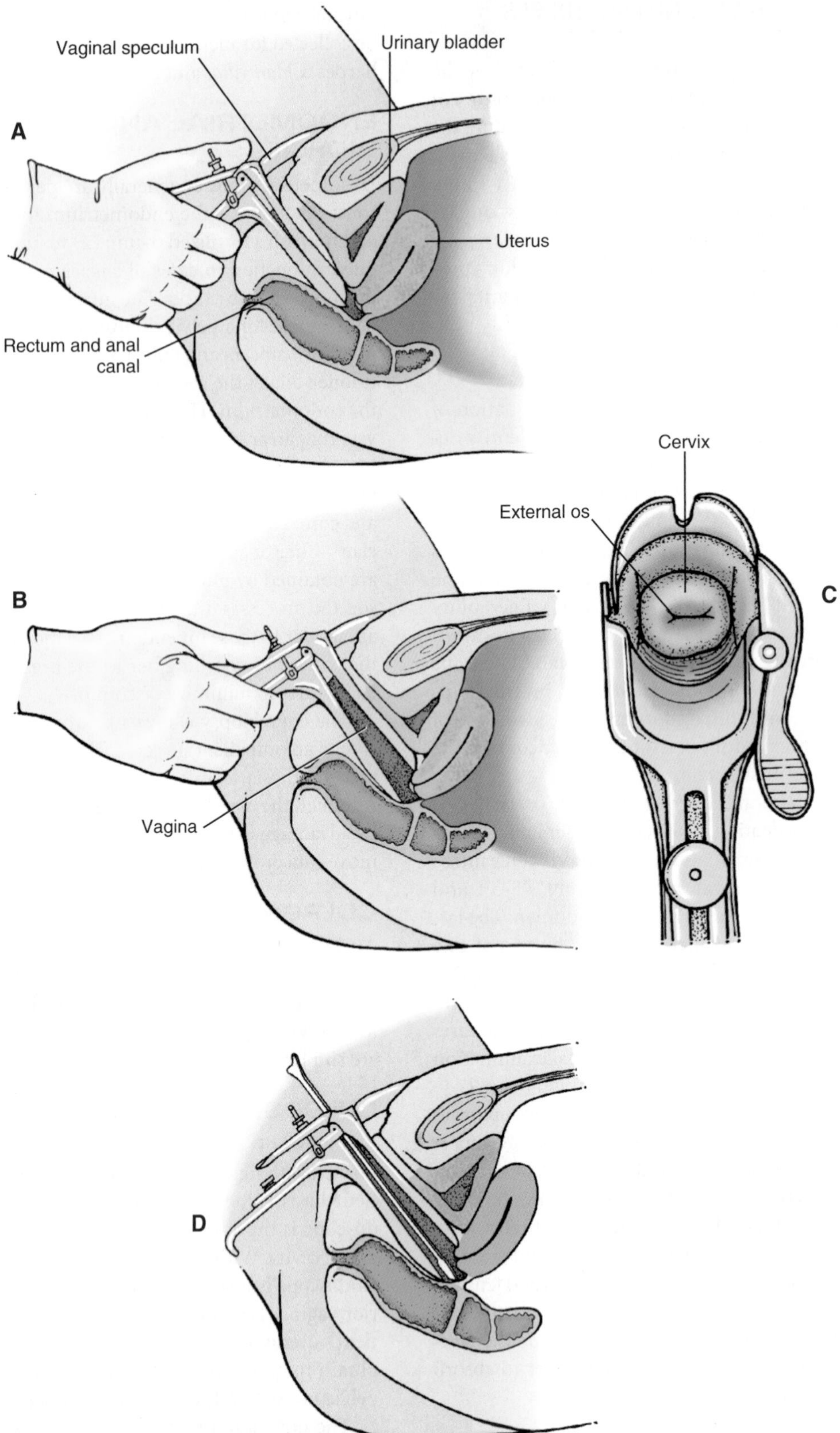

FIGURE **45-5** Internal examination of the cervix. *A,* Insertion of the speculum. *B,* Open speculum within the vagina. *C,* Examiner's view of the cervix through an open speculum. *D,* An instrument called an Ayre spatula is inserted through the speculum to obtain a cervical specimen for a Pap test.

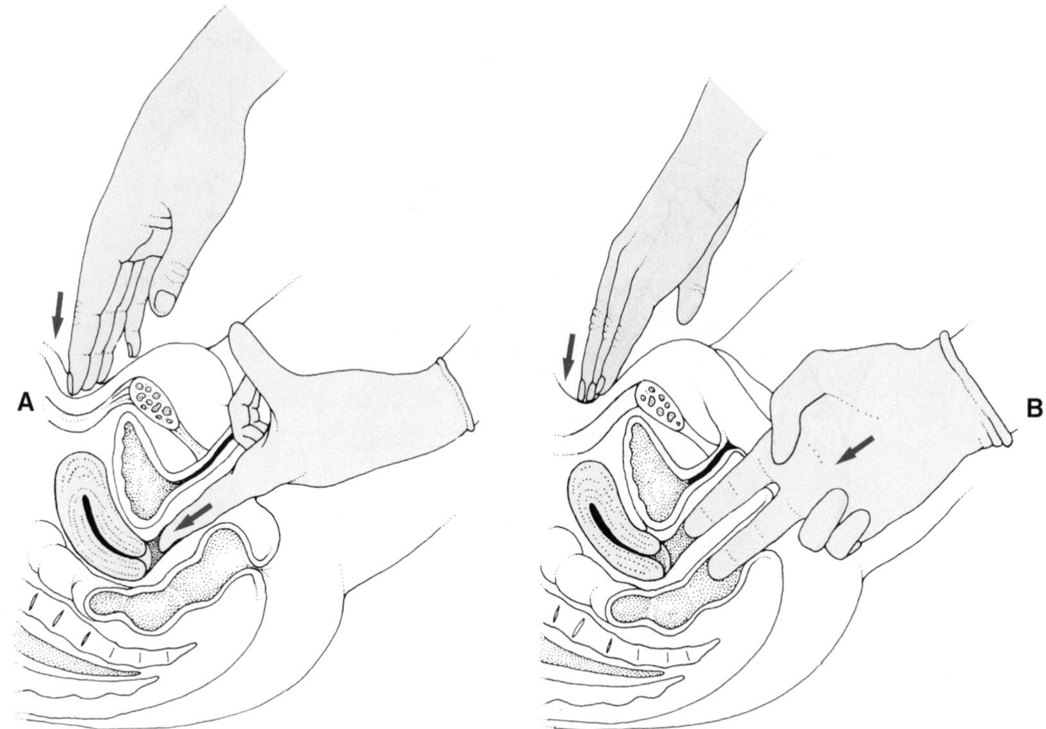

FIGURE **45-6** Bimanual palpation. *A,* Bimanual pelvic examination. *B,* Bimanual rectovaginal examination.

the knee-chest position without exposure. Advise her that she may experience shoulder pain caused by air entering the pelvic cavity during the procedure. Also reassure her that the incision will close and heal without sutures but that nothing should be inserted in the vagina (e.g., no vaginal intercourse, douching, or tampons) for the period of time specified by the physician.

LAPAROSCOPY

Laparoscopy (Fig. 45-7) is a surgical procedure that may be performed under local anesthesia on an outpatient basis or under general anesthesia in an outpatient surgical facility or a hospital. The physician uses an instrument called a laparoscope to visualize abdominal organs and to perform minor surgery such as a tubal ligation. The laparoscope is inserted through a small abdominal incision. Instruments may be inserted through the laparoscope itself or through a small second incision. Before the laparoscope is inserted, a small quantity of gas is injected into the abdomen to create a pocket in which to insert the laparoscope and to allow a clear view of the organs. This gas eventually is absorbed, but in the immediate postoperative period it tends to cause shoulder pain and/or pain below the rib cage. Inform and reassure the patient that the discomfort is expected and is temporary.

DILATION AND CURETTAGE

Dilation and curettage (D & C) is used for diagnostic and treatment purposes. The D & C is used to diagnose uterine cancer and causes of abnormal uterine bleeding. It also may be used to treat some causes of bleeding.

Dilation and curettage is performed in two steps. The first is dilation of the cervix by insertion of a series of progressively larger rods. The second step is endometrial curettage, or scraping of the entire uterine lining. The scraped tissue sample is removed by vacuum aspiration (suction). Tissue samples are prepared for laboratory analysis according to institutional procedures.

Most D & Cs can be performed under local anesthesia in the physician's office or outpatient clinic. Patient preparation and positioning are similar to those used for the pelvic examination. As for all procedures, institutional policy directs the nurse's role and responsibilities.

MAMMOGRAPHY

Mammography is a radiologic test used to detect breast cysts or tumors, especially those not palpated on physical examination. The American Cancer Society recommends that baseline mammograms be obtained in women between the ages of 35 and 39. Subsequent tests should be done every 1 to 2 years for women 40 to 49 years of age and annually for women age 50 and older. The test takes only a few minutes and is performed by a trained technician. For the procedure, each breast is compressed in a mammography machine, and two views are taken of each breast, one from above and one from the side. The film is developed immediately and often is read by a radiologist before the patient leaves the setting.

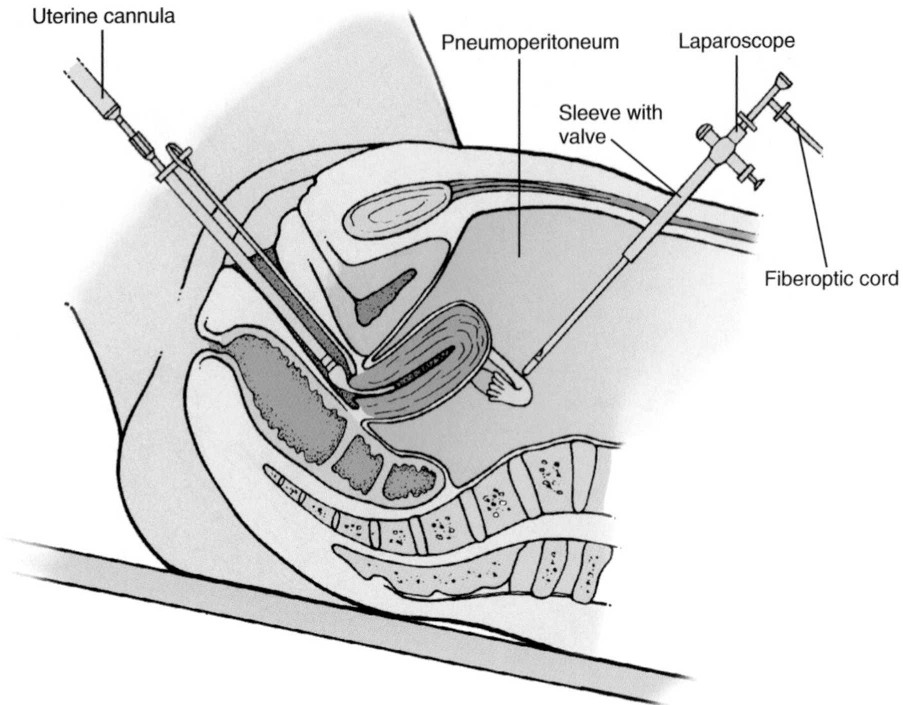

FIGURE **45-7** Laparoscopy.

Most mammograms are obtained in settings that do not routinely employ nurses. However, you need to be familiar with the process so that you can prepare the patient.

Put on your THINKING CAP!!

A 45-year-old woman who has never had a mammogram states that her friends have told her it is extremely painful. What approaches might you use in encouraging her to have a mammogram?

BREAST SELF-EXAMINATION

Through regular monthly breast self-examination (BSE), a woman learns to recognize her normal findings, which helps her detect changes if they occur. Every woman who has begun to menstruate should know the correct way to perform breast self-examination.

The breast self-examination should be done at the same time each month: at the end of the menstrual period for menstruating females or on the same date each month for women who have ceased menstruating. The nurse's responsibilities include teaching the importance of breast self-examination, demonstrating the examination, and evaluating the patient's ability to perform a return demonstration on herself.

The breast self-examination begins with inspection of the breasts while the woman is sitting or standing before a mirror. She looks for changes in her breasts as she assumes each of four positions: (1) with her arms relaxed at her sides, (2) with her arms held straight above her head, (3) with her hands pressed against her waist or hips and her elbows brought forward, and (4) leaning forward. She looks for any changes from the previous examination: for dimpling, puckering, or texture changes of the skin; for elevation or enlargement of one breast when she leans forward or when she brings her elbows forward in the third position; and for other, new differences between the breasts.

The second step of the breast self-examination is palpation of the breasts and the axillary area. The position of choice is for the woman to lie on her back with a folded towel under the shoulder of the breast to be examined. The arm on the same side is raised above her head. Lotion or powder should be applied to the examining hand to help the fingers move smoothly over the skin. The fingers are positioned flat against the skin, and moved to cover the entire breast area in one sliding motion. Firm pressure is used, beginning at the nipple and traveling in a circular track around and around the breast until the breast has been covered. Areas to be covered extend from the midaxillary line, to the sternum, and to the top and bottom boundaries. The process is repeated on the opposite side.

Some practitioners prefer to begin at the midaxillary line and palpate the breast tissue in a vertical pattern. The fingers travel up and down in closely spaced strips without leaving the skin surface until the entire breast has been palpated.

Women with small breasts may examine their breasts while showering. This method is less acceptable for women with larger breasts because it does not allow the breasts to flatten for thorough palpation. Any changes in breast texture, particularly any lumps, and any nipple discharge should be reported as soon as possible to the physician or nurse practitioner.

table 45-2 **DIAGNOSTIC TESTS AND PROCEDURES | *The Female Reproductive System***

TEST/PURPOSE	PATIENT PREPARATION	POSTPROCEDURE NURSING CARE
Pelvic examination includes assessment of external genitalia, vagina, uterine cervix, abdomen, and rectum to identify abnormalities and to collect fluid or tissue specimens.	Explain the examination; then assist the patient into the lithotomy position immediately before the examination. Drape for privacy. Warm the vaginal speculum. Encourage relaxation.	Assist the patient to assume a sitting position and to get down from the examining table. Offer tissues to wipe the perineal area and a panty liner to absorb lubricant as it drains.
Papanicolaou smear: detect abnormalities of cervical cells, including cervical cancer. **Cultures** detect pathogens that cause herpes, *Chlamydia,* gonorrhea, etc.	Obtain appropriate equipment for specimen collection and preparation.	Same as for pelvic examination. Proper handling of specimens is essential for accurate studies. Prepare specimens, label, and send to the laboratory. Properly dispose of used supplies.
Endometrial biopsy: to study fertility, or to detect cancer. **Cervical biopsy:** to detect cancer.	Endometrial and cervical biopsies: assist her to assume the lithotomy position; drape for privacy. Procedure is painful; encourage breathing and relaxation exercises.	Same as for pelvic examination.
Breast biopsy: (or fluid aspiration): to diagnose breast cancer. (Done under local or general anesthesia.)	Recognize patient anxiety about outcome and possible implications. Explain procedure.	Check incision for bleeding. Safety precautions if sedated. Provide opportunity to express fears.
Colposcopy uses a colposcope to inspect the cervix under magnification to identify abnormal tissue. Usually done before cervical biopsy.	Same as for pelvic examination.	Same as for pelvic examination.

Although many women learn to perform breast self-examination from reading magazine articles or pamphlets, it has been observed that women perform the examination more accurately when they have received direct instruction and demonstration and when they have returned the demonstration for correction of technique.

BREAST BIOPSY

When breast changes are discovered, a breast biopsy may be done to determine the reason for the change. A biopsy is the definitive test for diagnosing breast cancer.

The physician decides which diagnostic procedures are appropriate. Breast biopsies for palpable small lumps can be performed under local anesthesia on an outpatient basis (Fig. 45-8). A needle may be used to aspirate fluid from cysts. Solid masses require a surgical approach to obtain a specimen of the questionable tissue or to remove the mass. Biopsies of large masses are performed under general anesthesia in a hospital setting. All removed tissue and aspirated fluid are sent to the laboratory for analysis. Decisions for further treatment are based on biopsy reports.

The patient admitted to the health care setting for a breast biopsy needs a great deal of supportive care. She needs an opportunity to talk about her fears, and she needs a thorough explanation of what she can expect during the preoperative, operative, and postoperative periods.

Information about diagnostic tests and procedures is summarized in Table 45-2.

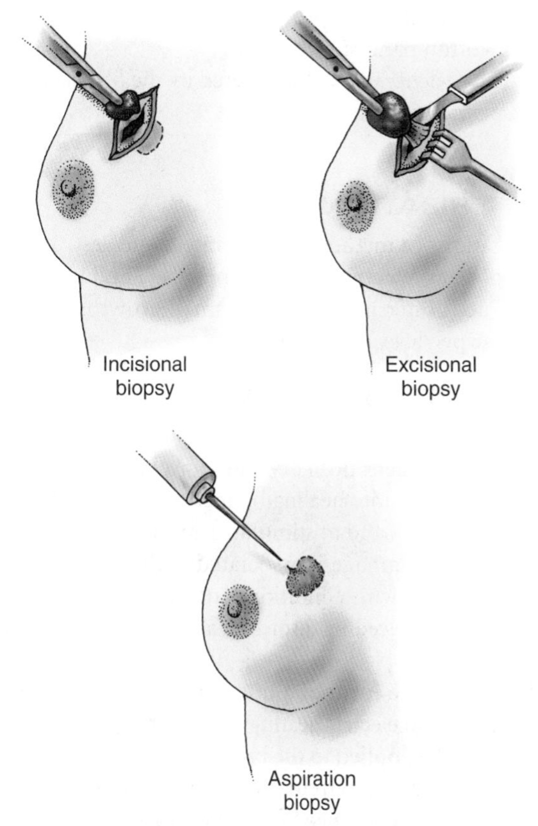

FIGURE **45-8** Breast biopsy techniques.

COMMON THERAPEUTIC MEASURES

DOUCHING

Douching is a procedure in which the vagina is flooded with fluid containing various cleansing or perfumed agents. Douching is not recommended for regular hygiene, because it washes away some of the elements that maintain the normal acidic pH. The acidic environment helps the vagina maintain its self-cleansing properties and fight off pathogenic organisms.

Douching is potentially dangerous, because it may force tissue and microorganisms up into the uterus. In addition, cleansing and perfumed agents may cause allergic or irritant reactions. Contrary to common belief, douching is not an effective contraceptive practice.

Douching may be ordered by the physician or nurse practitioner to wash the vagina with a bactericidal solution in preparation for surgery, radiation therapy, or other treatment. If ordered, prepare the douche solution, using exact measures of prescribed ingredients, and administer the douche according to your institutional procedure.

Because it is also the nurse's responsibility to teach the patient about appropriate vaginal hygiene, you can teach while the douche is administered. Points to be addressed are the following:

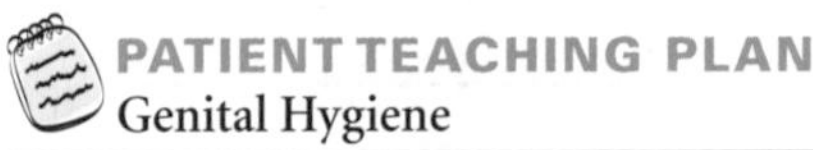

PATIENT TEACHING PLAN
Genital Hygiene

- Wash the external genitalia with plain soap and water at least once a day.
- Keep the genital area clean and dry.
- Wear cotton panties.
- Do not douche unless it is ordered by the physician or nurse practitioner.

CAUTERIZATION

Cauterization is a method of deliberate tissue destruction by means of heat, electricity, or chemicals. The physician or nurse practitioner may cauterize small growths or polyps during the pelvic examination.

APPLICATION OF HEAT

Heat is used as treatment for many reproductive system conditions and disorders. Both dry and moist heat are used to relieve pain, to promote healing by increasing blood flow and tissue metabolism, and to stimulate rupture of abscesses. Because potential damage is associated with excessively high temperature and with conditions such as impaired circulation, edema, and bleeding disorders, any form of heat must be used judiciously.

Dry heat in the form of a hot water bottle, a disposable chemical pack, an electric heating pad, or an aquathermia pad (K-pad) may be applied to the breasts or abdomen to relieve pain and to enhance circulation. The commonly recommended temperature range for most of these devices is 40° to 56° C (104°-130° F). Institutional policy and physician's orders dictate the exact temperature and the duration of application time. Although the exact procedure for each method varies among institutions, key points when applying dry heat are the following:

1. A physician's order is required.
2. Protect the skin by using a barrier between the heating device and the skin.
3. Monitor the patient's response.
4. Maintain the dry heat source temperature in the appropriate range.

Moist heat in the form of hot compresses and sitz baths is employed for the same general purposes as dry heat. Hot compresses are particularly useful for applying heat to small areas such as the vulva or perineum. Depending on the purpose of treatment, the acceptable temperature range for hot compresses is 40.5° to 46.0° C (105°-115° F).

Sitz baths provide heat to the perianal area to relieve pain, to cleanse the area, to promote healing or drainage, or to stimulate urination. The patient sits in warm water that may be in a special tub or in a disposable plastic device that fits on the rim of a regular toilet bowl. A continuous flow of fresh, temperature-controlled warm water is provided by the plumbing apparatus of the sitz bathtub or by a suspended plastic water bag with tubing extended to the disposable device. Water temperature is maintained within the 38° to 46° C (100°-115° F) range; the treatment is employed for a maximum of 25 minutes; and the patient is monitored closely for signs of faintness, shock, or severe pain. Because dilation of large pelvic blood vessels by heat may cause hypotension, the patient should not be left alone. Disposable devices usually are taken home by the patient, so it is your responsibility to give detailed instructions on their use.

TOPICAL MEDICATIONS

Medications for application to the vulva or vagina are in the forms of tablets, creams, and suppositories. Because mucous membranes are both delicate and highly vascular, there is a risk of injury and of excessive drug effects associated with high drug absorption. The application hand should be gloved for protection of both patient and nurse. Whether inserted with a finger or an applicator, tablets and suppositories are positioned with a down and backward motion into the vagina of the supine woman. Cream is administered through an applicator packaged with the cream. Direct the patient to remain supine for at least 15 minutes after application of either medium, to allow the medication to disperse throughout the vagina and be absorbed. The medication will dribble out over time, so advise the patient to use a sanitary pad to protect underclothing from staining. Drugs commonly used to treat disorders of the female reproductive system are listed in Table 45-3.

SURGICAL PROCEDURES

Many disorders of the female reproductive system are treated surgically. Specific examples are given throughout this chapter. Abdominal procedures may be performed through an abdominal incision, vaginally, or endoscopically.

table 45-3 DRUG THERAPY | *Drugs Used to Treat Disorders of the Female Reproductive System*

DRUG	USE/ACTION	SIDE EFFECTS	NURSING INTERVENTIONS
OVARIAN HORMONES			
Conjugated estrogens (Premarin), estradiol (Estrace, Depogen, Dioval, Estinyl)	Replacement of natural hormones after menopause, palliative treatment of advanced breast cancer, treatment of osteoporosis caused by estrogen deficiency. Stimulates endometrial growth and thickening. Enhances bone formation. Depresses beta lipoprotein and cholesterol plasma levels.	Breast tenderness, breakthrough bleeding, vaginal candidiasis, headache, dizziness, depression, elevated blood pressure, thromboembolism, nausea, skin hyperpigmentation, and decreased glucose tolerance. Increased risk of endometrial cancer, especially in postmenopausal women who take estrogens continuously for a year or more.	Advise patients to report signs/symptoms of the following: 1. Thromboembolism: calf pain or swelling, chest pain, numbness, visual disturbances. 2. Cardiovascular problems: weight gain, edema. 3. Liver disorders: abdominal pain, jaundice. 4. Breast lumps. 5. Vaginal bleeding. Discourage smoking, which increases risk of adverse effects. Take with evening meal to reduce nausea. Reinforce physician's instructions.
Oral progestins: medroxyprogesterone acetate (Provera et al), norethindrone (Micronor), norethindrone acetate (Aygestin), micronized progesterone (Prometrium)	Promote secretory function in endometrium. Influence contractile activity of the uterus. Used to treat uterine bleeding, some types of amenorrhea, and premenstrual syndrome (PMS). Palliative treatment of endometriosis and some cancers. Used with estrogens as oral contraceptives.	Breakthrough bleeding, amenorrhea, breast tenderness, edema, pruritus, increased blood pressure, thromboembolism, depression, photosensitivity.	Monitor weight and blood pressure. Assess for pruritus. Tell patient to report signs of circulatory impairment: swelling, numbness, pain in calf or thigh. Advise patient to avoid excessive sun exposure. Assess mental state. Contraindicated with history of thromboembolism, undiagnosed vaginal bleeding, liver dysfunction, cerebral hemorrhage.
Intramuscular progestins: medroxyprogesterone acetate (Depo-Provera), hydroxyprogesterone caproate (Hylutin)			Intravaginal: Use applicator to apply cream or tablet high into vagina.
Intravaginal progestin: progesterone (Crinone)			
Transdermal progestin: norethindrone with estradiol (Combipatch)			Transdermal instructions: Apply to clean, dry skin (not on breast or waistline), press for 10 seconds. Replace once or twice weekly as ordered or if patch falls off. Rotate sites.

Note: Recent research evidence has revealed increased risks of coronary heart disease and invasive breast cancer when combination estrogen and progestin therapy is used in women with intact uteruses.

Continued

table 45-3 DRUG THERAPY | *Drugs Used to Treat Disorders of the Female Reproductive System—cont'd*

DRUG	USE/ACTION	SIDE EFFECTS	NURSING INTERVENTIONS
SELECTIVE ESTROGEN RECEPTOR MODULATORS (SERMS)			
Tamoxifen (Nolvadex) Toremifene (Fareston) Raloxifene (Evista)	Stimulate estrogen receptors in some tissues and block them in other tissues. Intended to provide benefits of estrogen with fewer risks. Tamoxifen and toremifene used to treat breast cancer and to protect against osteoporosis. Raloxifene is approved only to prevent osteoporosis.	Hot flashes,fluid retention, vaginal discharge, nausea, vomiting, blurred vision, bone pain, menstrual irregularities, confusion. Increases risks of endometrial cancer, stroke, thromboembolism. Teratogenic.	Do not double up if a dose is missed. Tell patient to report severe bone pain to physician so analgesics can be prescribed. Pain is evidence of drug effectiveness; resolves over time. Also, report weight gain, edema, or dyspnea. Patient should use nonhormonal barrier method of contraception during and for one month after therapy.
ANDROGENS			
Danazol (Danocrine)	Inhibits production of pituitary gonadotropins. Used to treat endometriosis and fibrocystic breast disease.	Acne, oily skin and hair, hirsutism, edema, weight gain, nervousness, deepening of the voice, decreased breast size, muscle cramps, sleep disorders.	Monitor weight and blood pressure. Assess for signs of liver dysfunction: jaundice, abdominal pain, light-colored stools. Explain side effects to patient. Contraindications: undiagnosed vaginal bleeding; severe cardiovascular, renal, or hepatic disorders.
GONADOTROPIN-RELEASING HORMONE (GnRH) AGONISTS			
Leuprolide acetate (Lupron) Goserelin acetate (Zolodex) Nafarelin acetate (Synarel)	Initially increases, then decreases testosterone levels. Used to treat endometriosis and advanced prostate cancer (see Chapter 46).	Hot flashes, decreased libido, dizziness, headache, nausea, constipation, or diarrhea.	Lupron should be discarded if discolored or if precipitate forms. Use only diluent provided to reconstitute. Administer immediately after reconstituting. Zoladex is gradually dispersed from an implant placed under the skin. Synarel is inhaled nasally. Tell patient to expect hot flashes that usually decrease after time. Pregnancy should be ruled out before giving any of these drugs, because they may cause abortion.

ORAL CONTRACEPTIVES			
Estrogen-progestin combinations (Ortho-Novum, Norinyl, Loestrin, Ovral) Progestin only (Norplant system) Estrogen only (diethylstilbestrol)	Suppress ovulation to prevent pregnancy. Prevent implantation of fertilized ovum. Ovral used as emergency postcoital contraceptive ("morning-after pill"); must be given within 24 hours after intercourse.	Nausea, vomiting, headache, edema, weight gain, breast tenderness. Increased risk of thromboembolism (especially among smokers). Severe nausea and vomiting.	Reinforce instructions for self-medication. Monitor weight. Tell patient to report signs of circulatory impairment: swelling, pain, numbness in an extremity. Contraindicated during pregnancy and in patient with a history of thromboembolism, myocardial infarction, cerebral vascular disease. Follow manufacturer's instructions if a dose is missed.
OVULATORY STIMULANT AND FERTILITY DRUGS			
Clomiphene citrate (Clomid)	All stimulate or mimic actions of natural pituitary gonadotropins. All can result in multiple births.	Hot flashes, breast tenderness, nausea, vomiting, visual disturbances, headache, depression, fatigue, reversible hair loss, weight gain, dizziness, ovarian enlargement.	Contraindicated with liver dysfunction, pregnancy, abnormal bleeding. Safety precautions if patient is dizzy or has visual disturbances. Stop drug and contact physician if visual disturbances occur. Tell patient to report vaginal bleeding or weight gain, signifying ovarian hyperstimulation, in which case monitor fluid status, weight, and possible signs of internal bleeding. Tell patient to avoid sexual intercourse with ovarian enlargement because of possible rupture.
Menotropins (Pergonal)		Pain and irritation at injection site. Ovarian enlargement and abdominal distention. Rarely, flulike symptoms: nausea, vomiting, fever.	Reconstitute with sterile saline and administer immediately.
Urofollitropin (Metrodin)	Stimulates ovarian follicular growth. Used to treat selected patients who have not responded to clomiphene citrate.	Same as with menotropins.	

Note: Recent research evidence has revealed increased risks of coronary heart disease and invasive breast cancer when combination estrogen and progestin therapy is used in women with intact uteruses.

The surgeon selects the specific approach according to the diagnosis and the patient's condition. Nursing care varies with each approach. An abdominal approach results in an external excision that requires assessment and care. You must also assess vaginal discharge in these patients since the vagina provides an exit route for blood and other fluids. Vaginal procedures leave no visible incisions, so the patient must be assessed for excessive bleeding through the vagina or for indications of infection such as purulent or foul-smelling vaginal discharge. Laparoscopic procedures require care similar to that for abdominal incisions, but the incisions are much smaller. Again, the patient may have vaginal discharge that should be assessed after laparoscopic pelvic procedures.

DISORDERS OF THE FEMALE REPRODUCTIVE SYSTEM

UTERINE BLEEDING DISORDERS

Pathophysiology

Normal menstrual patterns vary widely in length of cycles (21 to 40 days), duration of menstruation (2 to 8 days), and amount of blood lost (40 to 100 ml). Bleeding patterns that are irregular in both spacing and amount are common in the first 2 years after the onset of menarche and in the 5-year period before menopause. Deviations from the normal cycles are viewed as uterine bleeding disorders. Two of the most common abnormal bleeding patterns, **metrorrhagia** (bleeding or spotting between menstrual periods) and **menorrhagia** (menstrual periods characterized by profuse or prolonged bleeding), are addressed in Table 45-4. Amenorrhea is the absence of menses.

Etiology and Risk Factors

Both metrorrhagia and menorrhagia are symptoms of underlying factors, rather than being specific definable conditions in themselves. Underlying causes for each vary widely. Common causes include hormonal dysfunction, both benign and malignant tumors, coagulation disorders, systemic diseases, use of some contraceptives, endometrial hyperplasia, inflammatory processes, and systemic diseases. The amount of blood loss varies with the type of disorder. Causes of amenorrhea include pregnancy; excessive weight loss, physical activity, or stress; pituitary, hypothalamic, thyroid, or adrenal disorders; ovarian failure; and uterine abnormalities.

Medical Diagnosis and Treatment

The diagnosis of uterine bleeding is based on the health history and physical examination as well as on the results of various diagnostic tests and procedures. Colposcopy, biopsy, and cauterization as well as laboratory analyses of blood components, hormone levels, and tissue specimens or smears provide diagnostic information. Because anemia may result from excessive bleeding, hemoglobin and hematocrit levels are usually measured as well. The treatment of amenorrhea depends on the cause and whether pregnancy is desired by the patient.

NURSING CARE *of the Patient with Uterine Bleeding*

Assessment

Complete assessment of the female patient with a disorder affecting the reproductive system is summarized in Table 45-1. When a patient has metrorrhagia or menorrhagia, the menstrual history is especially important.

Nursing Diagnoses, Goals, and Outcome Criteria: Metrorrhagia or Menorrhagia

Nursing Diagnoses	Goals and Outcome Criteria
Deficient Knowledge of condition and treatment	Patient understands condition and treatment: patient accurately describes the condition and treatment
Anxiety related to unknown cause of menorrhagia, metrorrhagia	Reduced anxiety: patient states she feels less anxious, calm manner

Interventions

Deficient Knowledge

When the course of treatment has been selected, it may be your responsibility to teach the patient her role in the treatment process and to make sure that she is able to follow through appropriately.

Anxiety

You can be a source of emotional support for the patient, who often is fearful or anxious about the unidentified cause of abnormal bleeding. The underlying causes of abnormal uterine bleeding may be relatively simple and easily treatable or complex and life-threatening. Therefore, you must be prepared to help patients cope with all eventualities. Supportive measures such as encouraging the patient to express her feelings, use of touch, and listening convey concern to the patient. Generally it is your responsibility to provide information regarding procedures to be done. Give explanations in terms the patient can understand.

INFECTIONS

Infections of the female reproductive tract affect patients both physiologically and psychologically. The physiologic effects range from short-term reversible changes to long-term changes that result in infertility. The potential psychological effects are numerous. Changes in relationships, feelings of distrust toward sexual partners, shame, embarrassment, and diminished self-esteem are but a few.

The majority of infections covered in this chapter often are transmitted through sexual intercourse. In addition, the causative organisms often are those associated with sexually transmitted diseases (STDs), as covered in Chapter 47. However, this chapter focuses primarily on the effects of the microorganisms on the female reproductive tract and on subsequent medical and nursing interventions rather than on the specific disease processes.

table 45-4 ***Uterine Bleeding Disorders***

DISORDER	ETIOLOGY	SIGNS AND SYMPTOMS	MEDICAL TREATMENT
Metrorrhagia	Ovulation.	Spotting occurs with regularity 14 days before menses.	None—this is regarded as a normal deviation.
	Intrauterine contraceptive device.	Intermittent spotting between menses.	None if bleeding is not severe and if other causes are ruled out. Monitor serum hemoglobin; if low, iron supplements are prescribed. Remove intrauterine device if bleeding is severe.
	Oral contraceptive use.	Irregular spotting. Early cycle spotting. Late cycle spotting.	Patient is directed to take pill at same time each day. Estrogenic potency of oral contraceptive is increased. Progestational potency of oral contraceptive is increased.
	Trauma; introduction of foreign objects.	Sudden onset of frank bleeding or spotting.	Foreign object is removed. Tissue damage is repaired.
	Vaginitis, cervicitis.	Spotting, combined with vaginal discharge characteristic of infectious organism.	Vaginal examination; culture and Papanicolaou smear to identify underlying cause; cause treated as warranted.
	Ectopic or molar pregnancy.	Spotting or frank bleeding, in addition to symptoms specific to molar pregnancy, ectopic pregnancy.	Ultrasonography and laboratory tests (serum human chorionic gonadotropin level) done. Surgical removal of products of conception.
	Reproductive tract pathology: Endocervical polyps Cervical eversion Cervical dysplasia Endometriosis Salpingitis Ovarian cyst Benign neoplasm Malignant neoplasm	Spotting or frank bleeding, in addition to other symptoms characteristic of specific pathology.	Diagnostic procedures and treatment specific to identified pathologic condition: hormone therapy, antimicrobial or other drug therapy, surgery.
Menorrhagia	Intrauterine contraceptive device.	For all: By definition, profuse or prolonged bleeding during menstruation, in addition to other symptoms characteristic of specific cause.	Substitution of intrauterine device with structural incorporation of progesterone (Progestasert-T) or discontinuation or removal of intrauterine device, with substitution of alternative contraceptive method. Use of PGSIs may be effective in reducing menstrual blood loss. Treatment for remaining causes is specific for each cause.
	Hormonal disturbances.		Determination of hormone status is critically important before hormone therapy or other drug therapy is initiated.
	Endometrial hyperplasia.		Endometrial hyperplasia may be diagnosed and treated by dilation and curettage. For women past childbearing age, hysterectomy may be performed.
	Benign neoplasm.		Benign tumors may be left alone and monitored.
	Malignant neoplasm.		Malignant tumors require a combination of surgical and medical interventions.
	Inflammatory process.		Specific cause is treated.
	Systemic diseases.		Specific cause is treated.

PGSI, Prostaglandin synthesis inhibitor.

Because of their association with sexuality and sexual function, many women view reproductive tract infections as threats or insults to their self-image. They may react with guilt, embarrassment, denial, defensiveness, or a combination of these that cause them to delay seeking diagnosis and treatment. Others are coping with infertility problems that result from infectious processes. When interacting with women who have reproductive tract infections or their effects, you must be sensitive, tactful, and absolutely nonjudgmental.

Vulvitis and Vaginitis

Pathophysiology

Inflammation of the vulva is called vulvitis. Depending on the causative agent, vulvitis may be viewed as an infection, as a local manifestation of a general skin disease, as a reaction to a chemical irritant or allergen, or as a normal consequence of the aging process. Regardless of its cause, the most common characteristics of vulvitis are inflammation and usually intense pruritus of the vulva and perianal region.

Like vulvitis, vaginitis is characterized by a local inflammatory response to various factors. Vaginitis and vulvitis differ in that a significant vaginal discharge is usually present with vaginitis.

Etiology and Risk Factors

Vulvitis and vaginitis are caused by a number of factors that precipitate an inflammatory response. The two most common causes of infection are *Candida albicans* (fungus, or yeast infection) and *Trichomonas vaginalis* (protozoal infection). Both most commonly infect the vagina and produce characteristic vaginal discharges that are irritating to the vulva and vagina. The discharge associated with *C. albicans* has a distinctive odor and a cottage cheese–like appearance; the discharge associated with *T. vaginalis* is profuse, frothy, and yellow-gray in color and has a fishy odor. Both can be transmitted sexually, although yeast infections often are associated with disruption of the normal vaginal flora by antibiotic therapy or with diabetes mellitus. Other common infective microorganisms are streptococci, staphylococci, and intestinal tract organisms.

Generalized skin diseases that may involve the vulva include psoriasis and inflammation of sweat glands. When these conditions affect the vulva, the constant moist state intensifies the inflammation and subsequent itching.

Vulvar reactions to chemical irritants are common. The vulva is exposed to a wide variety of chemicals that may act as irritants and thus elicit an inflammatory response; the response often extends into the vagina. Perfumed soaps, scented toilet tissue and perineal pads, feminine hygiene sprays, laundry detergent residues, and spermicides are a few examples of common irritants.

Estrogen deficiency associated with the aging process frequently results in nonpathogenic vulvitis and vaginitis due to a combination of tissue atrophy and a decrease in the acid vaginal secretions that normally maintain healthy mucous membranes.

Signs and Symptoms

Regardless of the cause, signs and symptoms include local swelling, redness, and itching. Some infectious agents cause characteristic signs and symptoms that aid in their identification.

Complications

Ascending infection (an infection that moves through the vagina to internal structures) is a potential complication of vulvitis and vaginitis. Infection confined to the lower reproductive tract seldom poses a threat to life or fertility.

Medical Diagnosis

The diagnosis is based on the patient's symptoms and on inspection of the vulva and vagina. Discharge specimens may be collected to aid in identification of specific microbes if microbial infection is suspected.

Medical Treatment

Treatment specific to the causative agent may include topical antifungal creams, oral antiprotozoal agents or antibiotics, vaginal suppositories to reestablish normal vaginal flora, topical or systemic estrogen replacement therapy, improved diabetes control, and avoidance of offending chemical agents. Symptoms are managed with frequent cleansing with neutral agents; wearing of cotton panties, cotton-crotched pantyhose, and nonconstricting clothing; and heat in the form of sitz baths and perineal irrigations. Advise the patient not to scratch the itching tissues, which can cause further mechanical trauma and infection. During the course of treatment, she should avoid sexual intercourse or use condoms. The woman's sexual partner or partners may be treated for some infections to avoid reinfection.

NURSING CARE *of the Patient with Vulvitis or Vaginitis*

Vulvitis and vaginitis usually are diagnosed and treated on an outpatient basis. Because patients usually manage their own treatment, you may be responsible for making sure that the patient understands all self-care instructions and for reinforcing other instructions given by the physician or nurse practitioner. General nursing care of patients with reproductive tract infections is addressed in Table 45-5.

Bartholin's Gland Abscess (Bartholinitis)

Pathophysiology

Owing to their location on either side of the vaginal opening, Bartholin's glands are vulnerable to a wide variety of infectious microorganisms. The resultant edema and pus formation occlude the duct of the affected gland and form an abscess.

Etiology and Risk Factors

Various microorganisms can be transmitted from the anus, vulva, or vagina to the Bartholin's gland duct. Commonly cultured organisms include normal intestinal bacterial flora, *Staphylococcus aureus, Streptococcus, T. vaginalis, Neisseria gonorrhoeae,* and *Mycoplasma hominis.* The organisms are often introduced through improper perineal hygiene (i.e., wiping from the anus toward the vagina).

Signs and Symptoms

Perineal pain is the symptom that most commonly motivates the woman to seek medical assistance. Additional signs and symptoms include fever, labial edema, chills, malaise, and purulent discharge.

table 45-5 ***Care of Patients with Reproductive Tract Infections***

PATIENT PROBLEM	NURSING INTERVENSIONS
Denial, embarrassment related to questions about infection	Convey acceptance of patient. Use tact in eliciting information about hygiene and sexual practices. Relevant data might include the following: All products applied on or near the vulva or in the vagina: feminine hygiene products, "love potions" (i.e., flavored or scented lubricants, massage oils) Anal contact with penis, fingers, or other objects before contact with vulva or vagina Number of sexual partners; accessibility to partners if their treatment is indicated
Deficient knowledge regarding treatment and self-care	Explanation of teaching about use of creams, jellies, suppositories: Purpose Position for application or insertion Application or insertion method Position after insertion Care of equipment (i.e., applicator) Use of tampon or perineal pad to hold medication in place Instructions about perineal hygiene: Frequent washing with neutral soap Thorough rinsing No douching unless specific ordered No commercial perineal deodorants Frequent change of underpants (preferably cotton) Sitz baths to relieve pain, itching Wiping perineal-anal area from front to back; one stroke per tissue Complete full course of prescribed drug therapy

Complications

Without proper treatment, bartholinitis may progress from a local infection to a systemic infection.

Medical Diagnosis

Visual inspection reveals a swollen, often reddened mass on the affected side of the vaginal introitus. Gentle palpation causes pain, tenderness, or both. If there is drainage, a specimen may be obtained for culture and sensitivity testing. Because causative microorganisms include those responsible for transmission of STDs, the patient is usually screened for these diseases (see Chapter 47).

Medical Treatment

Conservative treatment consists of oral analgesics and moist heat in the form of frequent sitz baths or hot wet packs. The moist heat relieves pain and facilitates spontaneous rupture and drainage of the abscess. Surgical incision and drainage of the abscess may be done by the physician. More aggressive treatment with broad-spectrum antibiotics is indicated if symptoms of systemic infection are present.

NURSING CARE *of the Patient with Bartholinitis*

Basic nursing assessment and interventions are outlined in Table 45-1. Provide the appropriate instruction to help the patient comply with the prescribed treatment. Tactful instruction in basic perineal hygiene principles is in order if the evidence indicates that inappropriate or inadequate practices are being followed. Basic practices include soap-and-water cleansing at least once daily and wiping the perineal area with a clean tissue from front to back following urination or defecation.

Cervicitis

Pathophysiology

Cervicitis is inflammation of the cervix. It may be acute or chronic. Although cervicitis is usually due to an infectious process associated with STDs, the inflammation may be associated with physical or chemical trauma.

Etiology and Risk Factors

Cervicitis is caused by a variety of agents: infectious organisms, scraping of cells for diagnostic tests, cryosurgery, use of vaginal tampons or medications, childbirth, decreased estrogen levels after menopause, and use of oral contraceptives.

Signs and Symptoms

Cervicitis is usually asymptomatic, although it may cause pain, visible vaginal discharge, bleeding, or dysuria. Unsuspected cervicitis may be detected on pelvic examination or on routine Pap smears. When viewed via a speculum, the cervix appears swollen and reddened; gentle touch may precipitate bleeding. Mucopurulent discharge and vesicular or ulcerated lesions most often are associated with STDs.

Complications

Cervicitis itself is considered to be a relatively benign condition. However, if the causative agent is an infection, the infection may ascend through the reproductive tract and cause pelvic inflammatory disease. Certain microorganisms that cause cervicitis also alter the vaginal pH and exert a spermicidal effect that results in infertility.

Medical Diagnosis and Treatment

Cervicitis may be diagnosed on the basis of the pelvic examination or results of the Pap smear. Treatment depends on the causative agent(s). Infections are treated with systemic or topical antimicrobial agents. Cervicitis related to menopause is treated with topical or oral estrogen. Additional treatment options include topical application of acidic preparations in the form of douches or jellies, cauterization with silver nitrate, and cryosurgery or laser surgery. Cryosurgery is the use of a cold probe to destroy selected tissue.

NURSING CARE *of the Patient with Cervicitis*

Cervicitis usually is diagnosed and treated in outpatient settings. Treatment is administered by a physician or nurse practitioner or by the client herself. Nursing care is limited to assisting with assessment procedures, client support, and teaching the client to carry out the prescribed treatment and posttreatment procedures.

PHARMACOLOGY CAPSULE Instruct patients to complete the full course of antimicrobial therapy to treat infections.

Mastitis

Pathophysiology

Mastitis is an infection-induced inflammation of breast tissue in the lactating woman. Historically, early postpartum mastitis epidemics were common among women who delivered in hospitals and who were hospitalized for the then-usual 10 or more days. With today's short hospital stays, mastitis is associated not with hospitalization but rather with a combination of ineffective breast-feeding techniques that result in poor drainage of mammary ducts and alveoli, lowered resistance to infection due to stress and fatigue, and exposure of breast tissue to infection-causing organisms.

Etiology and Risk Factors

Staphylococcus aureus is the microorganism most commonly associated with mastitis; *Escherichia coli* and streptococci also may be the agents of infection. The nipple serves as the portal of entry for the organism. Cracked nipples are especially susceptible. A common mechanism of organism transmission is touching the nipples with unclean hands.

Signs and Symptoms

Mastitis is usually confined to one breast and may be asymptomatic except for breast tenderness and low-grade (and often unsuspected) fever. The infection therefore may be undetected if frequent breast-feeding empties breast ducts and alveoli and if the woman's natural immune response prevents spread of the infection. In symptomatic mastitis, the causative organism invades the breast connective tissue or the lobes and ducts and stimulates an inflammatory response that results in localized pain, fever, tachycardia, general malaise, and headache. The affected breast tissue feels hard and warm on palpation; the skin over the infected area is reddened.

Complications

Untreated symptomatic mastitis may result in abscess formation as the sepsis becomes localized. Enlargement of axillary lymph nodes also may result.

Medical Diagnosis and Treatment

The diagnosis is based on presenting symptoms. Symptomatic mastitis is unmistakable. If there is a purulent discharge from the nipple, a specimen can be collected for culture and sensitivity testing. However, treatment is initiated based on the symptoms alone and consists primarily of immediate and aggressive antibiotic therapy.

Symptoms are managed by frequent emptying of the breast, heat application, rest, and administration of an analgesic. The question of whether to empty the breast by breast-feeding or by artificial pumping is a controversial one. Proponents of breast-feeding contend that the infant already has been exposed to the causative organism and therefore is not likely to be further jeopardized. Others insist that breast-feeding be discontinued temporarily until antibiotic therapy is completed. There are many broad-spectrum antibiotics that are tolerated well by both mother and infant. This is significant because antibiotics taken by the mother will be present in her breast milk.

If an abscess forms, surgical excision and drainage of the abscess may be necessary, and a longer period of antibiotic therapy will be required.

NURSING CARE *of the Patient with Mastitis*

The most effective nursing intervention is the prevention of mastitis.

Assessment

Assess the breast-feeding woman's knowledge of measures to prevent mastitis. Take the patient's temperature, and assess the breasts for pain, tenderness, warmth, hardness, and purulent discharge from the nipple.

Nursing Diganoses, Goals, and Outcome Criteria: Mastitis

Nursing Diagnoses	Goals and Outcome Criteria
Risk for Injury related to possible abscess formation	Recovery without complications: absence of fever, pain, redness, and purulent drainage
Deficient Knowledge of mastitis prevention and treatment	Patient understands how to treat mastitis and prevent recurrence: patient accurately describes and demonstrates self-care measures

Interventions

Risk for Injury

If mastitis or breast abscess occurs, reinforce the prescribed treatment. If heat treatments or drug therapy are prescribed, be sure the patient understands the instructions.

Deficient Knowledge

The points commonly addressed in breast-feeding education are those that also prevent the infectious process from occurring.

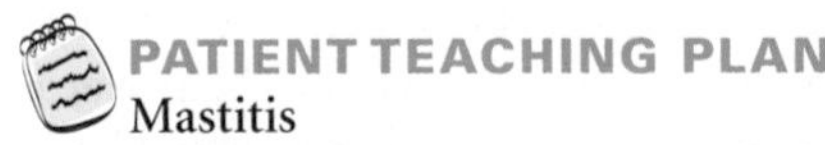

- Be sure to complete your course of antibiotics as prescribed.

- Report continued or additional symptoms.
- Pain usually can be managed with analgesics as prescribed.
- Allow for extra rest periods.
- To prevent recurrence during breast-feeding:
  - Breast-feed frequently and completely empty the breasts.
  - Wash hands thoroughly before handling breasts.
  - Avoid cracked nipples:
    - Make certain that the infant's lips and gums are around the areola and not on the nipple itself.
    - Break suction before removing the nipple from the infant's mouth.
    - Cleanse with plain water to prevent chemical trauma from soap, alcohol, and other drying agents.
    - Leave milk on nipples and expose them to the air or a heat lamp after breast-feeding.
- Wear a supportive but nonconstrictive bra.
- Get adequate rest, nutrition, and fluids.
- Promptly report early symptoms of breast infection to health care provider.

Pelvic Inflammatory Disease

Pathophysiology

Pelvic inflammatory disease (PID) is an infectious process that may affect any or all structures in the pelvic portion of the reproductive tract and peritoneal cavity. It is called an ascending infection because causative organisms migrate upward from the portal of entry, the vulva or vagina.

PID is a major female reproductive health problem and a major cause of infertility in the United States. The infectious process results in scarring and adhesions in the fallopian tubes that can cause total or partial obstruction. Total obstruction results in infertility. Partial obstruction often results in ectopic pregnancy, in which the fertilized ovum implants in a site other than the uterus, usually in the fallopian tube or the pelvic cavity. Unfortunately, the incidence of PID is particularly high in adolescent girls.

Etiology and Risk Factors

Because the majority of PID cases are caused by sexually transmitted organisms, PID is generally classified as an STD syndrome. *Neisseria gonorrhoeae, Chlamydia trachomatis,* and *Mycoplasma hominis* are recognized as the organisms most associated with PID. *Chlamydia* infection is thought to be the most commonly occurring STD and the one most often responsible for PID. As such, it is often implicated in infection of the fallopian tubes (salpingitis) and is considered to be the primary cause of ectopic pregnancy and infertility associated with tubal obstruction.

However, non-STD organisms also have been identified as causative agents. Staphylococcal, streptococcal, and other organisms have been cultured from women with PID. Sources of non–STD–associated PID include contaminated hands or instruments during gynecologic surgery, childbirth, abortion, and pelvic examinations. Women with compromised resistance to infection and women who are poorly nourished are particularly prone to developing non–STD–associated PID.

The risk of PID increases as the number of sexual partners increases. This factor is most applicable to PID caused by organisms implicated in STDs.

Vaginal douching also is considered to be a possible risk factor for PID. It is thought that the force of the fluid used in douching may propel microorganisms from the vagina through the cervical os (opening) and into the uterus, fallopian tubes, and pelvic cavity.

Signs and Symptoms

Pelvic inflammatory disease may be a silent infection with no symptoms. As a result, it may remain untreated while causing damage to pelvic structures. Symptomatic PID may appear with either the gradual onset of dull, steady, low abdominal pain or the sudden onset of severe abdominal pain, chills, and fever. Other symptoms may include dysuria, irregular bleeding, a foul-smelling vaginal discharge that may cause inflammation and skin breakdown of the vulva, and **dyspareunia** (pain during sexual intercourse).

Symptomatic PID is much more likely to be diagnosed and treated than asymptomatic PID. In many instances evidence of PID is first discovered during surgery for ectopic pregnancy, blocked fallopian tubes, ovarian abscess, or other pelvic disorders.

Complications

The risk of complications of PID increases with each repeated infection. Common effects of PID include ectopic pregnancy, infertility, and chronic abdominal discomfort. Without prompt diagnosis and aggressive treatment, infection of the entire peritoneal cavity (peritonitis) and systemic septic shock also are potential complications.

Medical Diagnosis

The diagnosis is based on the presenting symptoms (if any) and the pelvic examination. The definitive diagnosis is based on culture of the causative organism or organisms. Sonography, laparoscopy, and culdocentesis are additional diagnostic procedures that may be employed.

Medical Treatment

Treatment for PID includes rest; application of heat via warm compresses, a heating pad, or sitz baths; and a regimen of analgesics and broad-spectrum antibiotics. Depending on the severity and extent of the infection, oral and/or parenteral antibiotics are prescribed. The woman should avoid sexual intercourse for the duration of treatment. If the causative organism is thought to have been transmitted sexually, the woman's sexual partner or partners should be treated to avoid repeated infection.

NURSING CARE *of the Patient with Pelvic Inflammatory Disease*

Assessment

Nursing assessment of the woman with a disorder of the reproductive system is summarized in Table 45-1. Preparation of the patient for physical examination includes anticipatory guidance, positioning and draping, and emotional support (see Table 45-5). You need to simultaneously assist the examiner and provide support for the patient. Precautions to avoid transmission of infection to yourself and others are summarized in Table 45-6 and should be taught to the patient.

table 45-6 Precautions to Avoid Reproductive Tract Infection

Maintain optimum general health: adequate nutrition and sleep, good stress management.
Cleanse perianal area daily with neutral soap followed by thorough rinsing; apply no other products unless ordered by health care provider.
Wipe perianal area with one front-to-back swipe per tissue.
Avoid sharing of any equipment (including washcloths) used for perianal or vaginal hygiene.
Change perineal pads or tampons frequently during menses even when flow is slight. Increase soap-and-water cleansing to at least twice per day.
Inspect genitalia of partner before intercourse or other contact with perianal area. Avoid contact if any lesions or discharge are noted. The same precautions should be followed for any part of the partner's anatomy, e.g., mouth, hands, fingers, that will contact perianal area during sexual encounter.
Wash with soap and water the penis, hands, or other objects that contact anus before contact with vulva or vagina.
Use condoms with spermicidal cream or jelly for penis-vulva-vaginal contact when monogamous relationship is not well established.
Avoid intercourse during treatment for reproductive tract infection. Use condom if intercourse cannot be avoided.

Nursing Diagnoses, Goals, and Outcome Criteria: PID

Nursing Diagnoses	Goals and Outcome Criteria
Acute Pain related to inflammation	Pain relief: patient states pain relieved
Impaired Skin Integrity related to infectious drainage	Restored skin integrity: intact skin without excessive redness or edema
Deficient Knowledge of treatment and prevention of reinfection	Patient understands and carries out treatment and preventive measures: patient verbalizes instructions and states intent to follow prescribed measures

Interventions

Care of the patient with PID includes bedrest with limited activity, application of heat as ordered, administration of prescribed antibiotics, and recognizing and reporting signs and symptoms of the side effects of antibiotics.

Acute Pain

Prescribed analgesics are administered for pain control. Additional pain relief measures are discussed in Chapter 14. Monitor and record the efficacy of analgesics.

Impaired Skin Integrity

If perineal pads are needed for collection of vaginal discharge, change them frequently. Note the character, amount, color, and odor of vaginal discharge. Frequent perineal cleansing is done with mild soap and water, followed by rinsing and patting dry. Inspect the vulva for signs of inflammation or excoriation, and monitor and record the temperature.

Deficient Knowledge

Nurses play a significant role in the primary prevention of PID and in fostering early diagnosis and treatment of reproductive tract infections so that they do not result in PID. Primary prevention includes measures to reduce risk factors. All women should practice good reproductive tract hygiene habits.

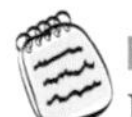

PATIENT TEACHING PLAN
Prevention of Pelvic Inflammatory Disease

When teaching prevention of PID to the sexually active woman with multiple partners or with a single partner with an unknown sexual history, include the following:

- During sexual intercourse always use protective mechanical or chemical barriers such as a condom, diaphragm, vaginal sponge, and spermicidal vaginal jelly or cream.
- Recognize signs and symptoms of common STDs.
- Seek prompt medical diagnosis and treatment of STDs or other suspected reproductive tract infections.
- Have routine yearly pelvic examination by a physician or nurse practitioner, with cultures done to detect *N. gonorrhoeae, C. trachomatis,* and other organisms.
- Routinely inspect the sexual partners' genitalia for signs of infection before each contact for sexual intercourse.

BENIGN GROWTHS

Endometriosis

Pathophysiology

Endometrial tissue that lines the uterus responds to hormonal influences during the menstrual cycle. During menstruation, small amounts of menstrual fluid are ejected through the fallopian tubes into the pelvic cavity (retrograde menstruation) rather than through the cervical os into the vagina. In some women, the endometrial cells deposited in the pelvic cavity implant on structures within the cavity. There, they continue to respond to menstrual cycle hormonal stimulation. The result is the periodically painful and potentially destructive condition called **endometriosis.** In women with endometriosis, the ectopic (out-of-place) endometrial tissue behaves in the pelvic cavity as it does in the uterus: it proliferates and then bleeds if fertilization of the ovum does not occur. As a result, more and more endometrial cells attach to pelvic structures. These cell clusters, called implants, are sometimes referred to as chocolate cysts because of their color. The implants can migrate to other areas of the body, possibly transported by blood or lymph. Bleed-

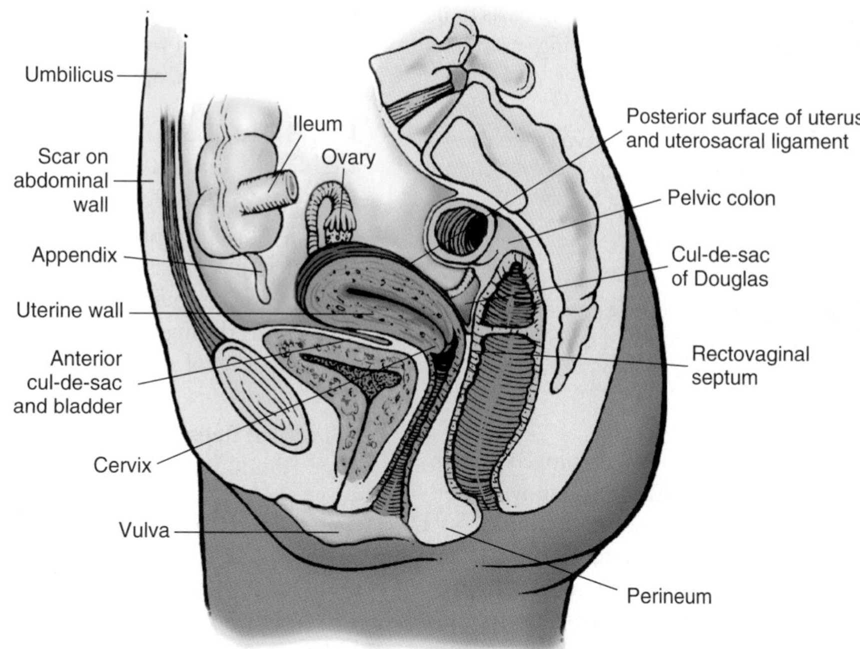

FIGURE **45-9** Common sites of endometriosis.

ing by endometrial tissue causes local inflammation and pain wherever the site of implantation may be. The number of implants gradually increases, creating multiple sites of inflammation and pain. In response to the inflammation, fibrous tissue forms that results in scarring and adhesions (Fig. 45-9).

Etiology and Risk Factors

Although it is known that almost all women experience retrograde menstruation to some degree, it is not known why some women develop endometriosis and others do not. Several theories have been explored; one is that endometriosis may be linked to a defect in the immune system of its victims. The disease is believed to occur in 10% of all women of reproductive age. The incidence and severity are greatest in women with relatives who have endometriosis.

Signs and Symptoms

As noted previously, the major symptom is pain, although some women are asymptomatic. Because the uterine endometrial tissue is bleeding simultaneously, pain appears as dysmenorrhea and may extend to a feeling of general pelvic heaviness. Additional symptoms include pain with defecation, dyspareunia, and abnormal bleeding. Emotional symptoms, including anger and depression, also are common. Infertility may be a sign of endometriosis when adhesions affect uterine position or fallopian tube patency, movement, or both.

Complications

The most common complication of endometriosis is constriction of pelvic structures by endometriosis-related adhesions. Constriction of the bowel, ureters, or both may cause partial or complete obstruction within the affected structure, creating a medical emergency.

Medical Diagnosis

Visualization and excision of endometrial implants via laparoscopy provide specimens for laboratory analysis and are the primary diagnostic procedures for endometriosis. Ultrasonography may be employed as a preliminary diagnostic tool to determine the presence of pelvic masses.

Medical Treatment

Medical management includes the use of nonsteroidal anti-inflammatory agents to relieve pain. The most commonly used drugs for pharmacologic treatment of endometriosis are gonadotropin-releasing hormone (GnRH) agonists or a synthetic androgenic steroid. GnRH agonists suppress the secretion of gonadotropin-releasing hormone, causing the estrogen level to fall, which permits endometriosis implants to shrink. There are several such drugs, including leuprolide acetate (Lupron) or goserelin acetate (Zoladex) and nafarelin acetate (Synarel). Leuprolide therapy requires monthly intramuscular injection. Goserelin is released slowly from a subdermal implant, and nafarelin is taken by nasal inhalation. Side effects are similar to those seen with danazol. Danazol (Danocrine), a synthetic androgenic steroid, inhibits gonadotropin excretion, resulting in amenorrhea and atrophy of intrauterine and ectopic endometrial tissue. Many women find the common side effects of danazol to be unacceptable: masculinizing characteristics such as voice deepening, hirsutism (excess hair growth), clitoral enlargement, and skin changes and menopausal symptoms such as hot flashes, and vaginal atrophy and dryness. Both classes of drugs are contraindicated during pregnancy, so the patient should know to use a barrier contraceptive during and for 1-3 months after the first normal menstrual period following therapy. Oral contraceptives may be prescribed on a long-term basis to inhibit endometrial proliferation, thereby relieving symptoms.

PHARMACOLOGY CAPSULE Androgens have masculinizing effects on females. The effects usually resolve when the drugs are discontinued.

PHARMACOLOGY CAPSULE Oral contraceptives are contraindicated in a woman with a history of cardiovascular disease, cerebrovascular disease, or thrombophlebitis.

Surgical management is commonly employed and includes laparoscopy for both diagnosis and removal of endometrial implants via resection, electrocauterization, or laser excision. Because it is difficult to visualize and remove all implants and because the underlying cause continues to exist, such surgery does not constitute a permanent cure and may need to be repeated at intervals. When fertility is no longer desired or complications develop, total abdominal hysterectomy with bilateral salpingo-oophorectomy (excision of the uterus, fallopian tubes, and ovaries) may be performed. Removal of the ovaries prevents the production of estrogen that would stimulate endometrial tissue. However, estrogen replacement therapy is not an option to relieve menopausal effects for these women as long as endometrial implants remain, because the implants continue to respond to the estrogen, and symptoms return.

NURSING CARE *of the Patient with Endometriosis*

Endometriosis is usually treated on an outpatient basis, so nursing care is limited unless the patient is admitted for surgery. Perhaps the most significant nursing interventions are validating that the pain is real and providing information about pain relief measures (see Chapter 14). The office or clinic nurse may be involved in patient teaching. Patient teaching is based on the treatment method selected and includes anticipatory guidance and treatment-specific instructions. Because periodic bleeding of all endometrial sites may cause anemia, teaching should include symptoms of anemia and the need for dietary or supplemental vitamin and mineral therapy. Preoperative and postoperative nursing care of the patient who has had a hysterectomy is addressed in the nursing care plan (see Nursing Care Plan: The Patient with a Hysterectomy).

CYSTS

A cyst is a closed sac-like structure that is lined with epithelium and that contains fluid, semisolid, or solid material. Cysts are classified as neoplasms and may be benign or malignant; the majority are benign. The most common ovarian and breast cysts are covered individually in Table 45-7.

For women with ovarian or breast cysts, nursing intervention focuses on teaching. Instruct the patient to keep a diary of symptoms, detailing when they occur and any factors that may be associated with the symptoms. Teaching is specific to the prescribed therapy.

FIBROID TUMORS (MYOMAS, LEIOMYOMAS)

Pathophysiology

Uterine fibroid tumors are both benign and common. It is predicted that at least 25% of all women will develop fibroid tumors during their reproductive periods. Fibroid tumors grow slowly during the reproductive years but tend to atrophy after the onset of menopause.

What Does Culture Have to do with Uterine Fibroid Tumors?

The incidence of fibroid tumors is increased among African-American women. These women should be advised to report menstrual irregularities and pain so that the condition can be diagnosed early and treatment can be initiated.

Etiology and Risk Factors

Although the exact cause is unknown, it is widely thought that fibroid tumors form and grow in response to stimulation by estrogen, primarily estradiol. Human growth hormone and human placental lactogen may also promote the tumors' development and growth.

Signs and Symptoms

Fibroid tumors may be asymptomatic, but the most common symptoms are menstrual irregularities—menorrhagia and dysmenorrhea. Discomfort from pressure on pelvic structures and dyspareunia may be associated with a large tumor. For some women, the initial hint that something is wrong is the gradual enlargement of the lower abdomen, which may be mistaken for pregnancy.

Complications

A very large fibroid tumor may compress the urethra, obstructing urine flow and causing secondary hydronephrosis. More common complications include infertility, crowding and malpositioning of the fetus during pregnancy, and degenerative changes related to interruption of blood supply.

Medical Diagnosis

On pelvic examination, the uterus is found to be enlarged and distorted. A pregnancy test, Pap smear analysis, and complete blood cell count should be done to rule out other conditions.

Medical Treatment

Many women need no treatment, and their tumors atrophy after menopause. Methods of contraception are limited by fibroid tumors: intrauterine devices are contraindicated, the estrogen in oral contraceptives may stimulate growth of the tumors, and diaphragms may be uncomfortable. For women who desire to become pregnant, some gynecologic surgeons

NURSING CARE PLAN

The Patient with a Hysterectomy

ASSESSMENT

Health History: A 42-year-old married woman has a diagnosis of uterine fibroid tumors. She has been pregnant three times and has three living children, two boys and one girl, all of whom are teenagers still living at home. Her menstrual periods have been regular, with onset every 30 days and lasting for 6 days. She describes her menstrual flow as heavy. She states that she saturates six to eight heavy day pads and six to eight super tampons per 24 hours for the first 3 days of each period, after which flow tapers off and she can manage the remainder of each period with four to six tampons per 24 hours. Her last period ended 6 days ago. She describes her health as excellent, with the exception of the uterine fibroids that were diagnosed when she was 33 years old. She is admitted for a total abdominal hysterectomy with bilateral salpingo-oophorectomy. This will be her first experience with surgery.

Physical Examination: Vital signs: temperature 97.8° F orally; pulse 72; respiration 18; blood pressure 116/74. Lungs clear on auscultation. Weight: 116 lbs. Height: 5'3". Alert. Skin color medium tan; nail beds pink with rapid capillary refill. Appears to be in good physical condition: body is firm with little evidence of adipose tissue and with excellent muscle tone; abdomen firm but protruding, appears about 5 months pregnant.

Laboratory: Urinalysis, complete blood count: All reports indicate no deviation from normal ranges except for hemoglobin (Hgb) concentration 10.4 gm/dl (normal, 11-16 gm/dl) and hematocrit 30% (normal, 31%-44%). She has been typed and cross-matched for two units of whole blood "on hold" for surgery.

Nursing Diagnosis	*Goals and Outcome Criteria*	*Interventions*
PREOPERATIVE NURSING DIAGNOSES		
Risk for situational low esteem related to perceived potential changes in femininity, effect on sexual relationship	The patient will verbalize understanding of expected changes in anatomy and physiology and of ability to resume a satisfying sexual relationship with husband after recovery from surgery.	Explain the following: 1. The only expected noticeable effects of loss of uterus and ovaries will be cessation of menstrual periods and ability to become pregnant, in addition to cessation of symptoms for which she is seeking surgery. 2. She may experience vaginal numbness for a short period of time. 3. Many women experience improved libido and sexual satisfaction after hysterectomy; sexual spontaneity may increase with lack of need for contraception. 4. Although penile or vaginal intercourse should not be resumed until at least 6 weeks following surgery, oral sex and masturbation to orgasm are safe. 5. Positions for sexual intercourse should avoid pressure on the abdominal incision for as long as incisional tenderness persists. 6. Orgasmic contractions of the uterus will no longer be present; this change of uterine sensation is noted by some but not by most women. 7. Estrogen replacement therapy (ERT) will prevent atrophy of vagina and decreased lubrication associated with removal of ovaries.
Deficient knowledge related to information or misinterpretation of effects of HRT	The patient will verbalize understanding of potential side effects of HRT and strategies to minimize side effects.	Explain the following: 1. The dosage of estrogen replacement may be adjusted for optimum therapeutic effect; she should report any concerns to her gynecologist. 2. Estrogen may increase fluid retention, which may make one "feel fat." Dietary control of sodium intake will reduce tendency for fluid retention. 3. Gradual resumption of presurgical physical activity and a well-balanced diet should maintain weight and fitness at presurgical levels.

Continued

NURSING CARE PLAN—cont'd

Nursing Diagnosis	*Goals and Outcome Criteria*	*Interventions*
POSTOPERATIVE NURSING DIAGNOSES (see Chapter 16 for general postsurgical diagnoses and care)		
Ineffective tissue perfusion related to anemia, surgical trauma, effects of anesthesia.	The patient will have adequate oxygenation of tissues, as evidenced by a pulse rate of 66-80, respiratory rate of 12-20, stable skin color, alert mental status, negative Homans' sign.	Monitor pulse, respiration, and blood pressure rates and auscultate respirations on schedule according to institutional policy. Assist patient to turn, deep breathe, cough on schedule; assist with incentive spirometer if ordered. Monitor skin color, temperature, and capillary refill, including lower extremities. Instruct and assist with foot and leg exercises while patient is confined to bed; encourage and assist with ambulation when allowed. Assess ability to answer questions appropriately. Check for Homans' sign by dorsiflexing foot; report positive sign (calf pain) to physician. If elastic hose are ordered, make sure they are applied and removed according to schedule when patient is in bed and at all times when out of bed; instruct patient about self-application. Monitor lab reports. Report to appropriate person any deviations from normal ranges. Medicate with analgesics to maximize comfort status.
Risk for deficient fluid volume related to postoperative bleeding	The patient will maintain adequate fluid volume, balanced fluid intake and output, moist mucous membranes, stable pulse and blood pressure.	Check abdominal dressing and perineal pad at least every hour for the first 12 hours; report any drainage observed on dressing, excessive vaginal bleeding. Should saturate less than one perineal pad per hour. Compare fluid intake (intravenous, oral) with urinary output (indwelling catheter collection bag or voided); report discrepancies. Monitor intravenous infusion; carry out related responsibilities according to institutional policy. Encourage fluid intake when allowed. Check mucous membranes for moisture; offer frequent mouthwashes during nothing-by-mouth status. Monitor pulse and blood pressure; compare with baseline levels; report deviations from acceptable ranges.
Urinary retention related to surgical manipulation, local tissue edema, temporary sensory or motor impairment	The patient will empty bladder at regular intervals without catheterization.	Assist patient to bathroom or commode; use bedpan only if absolutely necessary. Assist patient to assume comfortable position. Provide privacy but remain within calling distance. If patient is unable to void without assistance, employ assistive measures: run water in sink or shower; pour warm water over perineum. Teach or assist patient to perform perineal hygiene at least every 8 hours: wash vulva with warm, soapy water; rinse with warm water from irrigating apparatus; rinse perineum after every voiding. Measure and record urine ouput; note color, clarity, and odor of urine. Palpate for bladder fullness above symphysis pubis to assess for urinary retention. If patient is unable to void or is retaining urine, allow her to rest for 30 minutes and repeat attempt for spontaneous voiding. Follow order for intermittent catheterization or repeat insertion of indwelling catheter if patient is unable to void a sufficient quantity. Continue to monitor and to assist with voiding until patient consistently empties her bladder without assistance.
Constipation related to weakening of abdominal musculature, abdominal pain, decreased physical activity, dietary changes, drug side effects.	The patient will have bowel movement on or before the fourth day after surgery.	Auscultate abdomen for bowel sounds, palpate for distention. Insert rectal tube as ordered, if appropriate. When oral intake is allowed, administer antiflatulent if ordered; teach patient self-administration if allowed. Encourage early and frequent ambulation. Encourage oral intake of fluids, especially of fruit juices. Assess for nausea and vomiting; administer antiemetic if nausea and vomiting are present. Follow protocol for diet; encourage selection of high-fiber foods when patient is allowed options. Administer stool softener or laxative if ordered. Assist patient to splint abdomen while attempting to pass feces. Report inability to have a bowel movement within the allotted time period.

table 45-7 **Common Ovarian and Breast Cysts**

TYPE OF CYST	PATHOPHYSIOLOGY	SIGNS AND SYMPTOMS	DIAGNOSIS AND MANAGEMENT
Follicular ovarian cyst	Forms when a dominant follicle fails to rupture and release its ovum and thus continues to grow. Occasionally formed in response to ovarian hyperstimulation by fertility drugs. May rupture and bleed into the pelvic cavity, causing sudden, severe abdominal pain.	Usually asymptomatic unless very large, then: pelvic heaviness or congestion and an aching feeling.	Usually detected during a pelvic examination. Most disappear spontaneously in 2-3 months without treatment. If it remains on reexamination after 6 to 10 weeks, the cyst may be examined and removed via laparoscope or drained by needle aspiration.
Corpus luteum ovarian cysts	Forms after ovulation; characterized by excessive bleeding into the luteal cavity and by increased progesterone secretion. Use of fertility drugs is associated with ovarian hyperstimulation and formation of multiple cysts. Associated with more complications than follicular cysts. May rupture and hemorrhage into the pelvic cavity, causing a degree of pain related to the amount of bleeding.	Initial symptom: delayed onset of the menstrual period, followed by irregularities in menstrual amount and duration of flow. Patient may have dull, aching pelvic pain or cramping.	Is palpable as a small, tender mass on the affected ovary. If severe abdominal pain exists, ectopic pregnancy should be ruled out. May be visualized via laparoscopic or culdoscopic examination if diagnosis is questionable. Usually no treatment is indicated. Normally disappears spontaneously.
Dermoid ovarian cysts	Composed of tissue from the three embryonic germ cell layers. May contain remnants of fat, hair, teeth, cartilage, and nerve tissue. Usually arises from the ovary on a pedicle (stalk). A small number (3% to 5%) of dermoid cysts become malignant.	Aymptomatic when small. Pelvic aching or heaviness with large cyst. Moderate pain if pedicle gradually becomes twisted; extremely severe pain with sudden twisting.	Palpated as a dense, firm mass during pelvic examination. With long pedicle, the mass may be found some distance from the ovary to which it is attached. A pregnancy test is needed to rule out ectopic pregnancy. If radiographs show teeth in the mass, the diagnosis of dermoid cyst is confirmed. Any dermoid cyst should be removed surgically because of the potential for malignancy.
Breast cysts	Most commonly identified cause is ovarian estrogen secretion. Additional contributing factors may be stress and caffeine. Is an exaggerated response to hormonal influence. May enlarge during the premenstrual period and shrink from the onset of menstruation until the next ovulation. Commonly called *fibrocystic disease.* Controversial: Some fibrocystic subtypes are considered precancerous.	Most are round, freely moveable, benign cysts. May be soft or firm, depending on contents. Small cysts are numerous; breasts have lumpy "cottage cheese" consistency. Varying degrees of pain between ovulation and menstruation.	Methods of preliminary diagnosis: Palpation, mammography, and ultrasonography useful for initial study. Contents of fluid-filled cysts may be aspirated for laboratory study or just observed over time. Accurate diagnosis of solid cysts requires surgical biopsy. Treatment: Oral analgesics, heat application, and caffeine restriction. Other possible dietary measures include decreased salt intake and supplementary vitamins and fatty acids. Hormone therapy: 1. Danazol (Danocrine): Decreases secretion of estrogen. Dosage is generally low enough to avoid serious side effects. 2. Low-dose estrogen with progesterone or progestins. Most aggressive surgical treatment is mastectomy, which occasionally is an option selected by women who undergo repeated surgical biopsies.

perform myomectomy (removal of the tumor alone), usually by laser surgery. Some small tumors can be removed via laparoscopy. For tumors that are very large or that are associated with complications, hysterectomy is the usual surgery of choice. Pregnancy should be delayed for 4-6 months after myomectomy.

NURSING CARE *of the Patient with Fibroid Tumors*

Assist the physician or nurse practitioner with diagnostic procedures and provide support to the patient. Women tend to equate the word tumor with malignancy. Therefore you may need to give repeated reassurance that the fibroid tumor is benign. If the practitioner elects a conservative approach of monitoring tumor growth, the patient may need reassurance that this approach is commonly used (see Nursing Care Plan: The Patient with a Hysterectomy).

UTERINE DISPLACEMENT

Cystocele and Rectocele

Pathophysiology

Cystocele and rectocele are vaginal disorders caused by weakness of supportive structures between the vagina and bladder (cystocele) or the vagina and rectum (rectocele). They typically occur together. Bulging of the bladder and rectum through the vaginal wall is visible and palpable on vaginal examination. Although small cystoceles and rectoceles may cause no problems, larger herniations may cause problems with emptying of both bladder and bowel. Stress incontinence, incomplete bladder emptying, difficulty with expulsion of fecal matter collected in the area of herniation, and incontinence of gas or liquid feces are problems typically reported.

Etiology and Risk Factors

During pregnancy and childbirth, the muscles that support the pelvic floor may be weakened. Repeat pregnancies result in further weakening that may eventually allow the bladder and the bowel to press through the vaginal wall

Signs and Symptoms

Symptoms other than the already described common bladder and bowel problems include dyspareunia, lower back and pelvic discomfort, and recurrent bladder infections.

Medical Diagnosis and Treatment

The diagnosis is made on the basis of inspection and palpation. Treatment of small cystoceles and rectoceles may be limited to pelvic floor (Kegel) exercises, which improve muscle tone. Estrogen replacement therapy may be prescribed to improve tone and vascularity of supportive tissues. Surgical intervention via anterior colporrhaphy and posterior colporrhaphy (A & P repair) to tighten the vaginal wall has long been the treatment of choice for larger or symptomatic cystoceles and rectoceles. An anterior colporrhaphy reduces the size of the anterior vaginal wall and is used to treat a cystocele. Posterior colporrhaphy reduces the size of the posterior vaginal wall and is used to treat a rectocele. There is a risk of vaginal stenosis, which results in painful intercourse after posterior repair. These procedures usually are not done during the childbearing years because vaginal delivery would disrupt the repair.

Interestingly, nurse researchers who utilize noninvasive methods based on pelvic floor exercises report long-term success rates comparable to those found with colporrhaphy.

NURSING CARE *of the Patient with Cystocele and Rectocele*

Assessment

Assessment of the patient with a disorder of the reproductive system is outlined in Table 45-1. When a patient has uterine displacement, also record problems related to urinary and bowel function. If surgery is planned, assess the patient's understanding of the procedure, the pre- and postoperative care, and the patient's concerns.

Nursing Diagnoses, Goals, and Outcome Criteria: Cystocele and Rectocele

Nursing Diagnoses	Goals and Outcome Criteria
Stress Incontinence related to pelvic muscle weakness	Control of urine elimination: patient reports improved bladder control
Constipation related to collection of feces in herniated bowel	Normal bowel elimination: regular bowel movements without straining
Sexual Dysfunction related to painful intercourse	Satisfying sexual practices without pain: patient's statement of lack of pain during intercourse
Risk for Infection related to incomplete bladder emptying	Absence of urinary tract infections: normal body temperature; no pain on urination

After surgical intervention, additional nursing diagnoses and goals are the following:

Nursing Diagnoses	Goals and Outcome Criteria
Acute Pain related to tissue trauma	Reduced pain: patient states pain relieved, relaxed manner
Risk for Injury related to infection and stress on surgical incisions	Wound healing without disruption or infection: intact surgical incisions without increasing redness or purulent drainage
Deficient Knowledge of postoperative self-care	Patient understands surgical routines and self-care: patient accurately describes postoperative self-care

Interventions

Nursing interventions vary depending on the medical treatment.

Stress Incontinence

For conservative treatment, you can teach Kegel exercises. See Chapter 22. The exercise is viewed as a preventive measure that can be adopted in early adulthood to maintain optimum pelvic floor muscle support throughout life.

Constipation

For the patient who reports problems with expelling feces, teaching includes directions to maintain soft stool consistency and regular bowel elimination. Dietary support focuses on frequent ingestion of fluids and a wide variety of high-fiber foods such as fruits, vegetables, and grains. Regular use of bulk stool softeners may be necessary.

Sexual Dysfunction

For the patient who is treated with colporrhaphy, preoperative nursing care includes anticipatory guidance regarding the impending surgery and postsurgical period and carrying out the physician's orders. The patient may fear painful intercourse postoperatively or may be concerned about the effects of surgery on sexual function. Explain that intercourse should be delayed for a prescribed period of time for healing to occur. No permanent impairment of sexual function is expected.

Risk for Infection

Preoperative orders commonly include a vaginal douching with an antibacterial solution, a cleansing enema, and hair removal according to agency procedure. Postsurgical nursing care is directed at prevention of infection and protection of the suture line. Perineal care is provided at regular intervals. In addition to incisional infections, the patient is at risk for urinary tract infections. An indwelling urethral or suprapubic catheter commonly is left in place for several days to keep the bladder empty and thus to prevent strain on sutures and to let local edema subside. Instruct the patient to report urinary frequency, burning, or foul odor, which suggests infection of the urinary tract.

Acute Pain

Postoperative perineal care includes cleansing of the perineum at regular intervals, initial application of cold to reduce pain and swelling, and subsequent application of heat via sitz baths and heat lamps. Because postoperative pain may be severe, administer analgesics as ordered. Assess the effects of comfort measures and inform the physician if pain is not relieved.

Risk for Injury

A low-residue diet reduces fecal bulk, and stool softeners are recommended to prevent straining during defecation after surgery. Encourage adequate fluids and ambulation.

Deficient Knowledge

Discharge teaching focuses on the patient's responsibility for continued self-care as ordered by the physician. Reinforce instructions regarding diet, medications, activity restrictions, and avoidance of sexual intercourse for the time specified by the physician. Reassure the patient that loss of vaginal sensation is expected and will resolve after a few months. To minimize vaginal stenosis after posterior repair, the surgeon may instruct the patient to use dilators and vaginal lubricants and to resume intercourse 6 weeks after surgery.

Uterine Prolapse

Uterine prolapse is a condition in which the uterus descends into the vagina from its usual position in the pelvis (Fig. 45-10). Descent is rated as first degree if the cervix is above the vaginal introitus, second degree if the cervix protrudes from the introitus, and third degree if the vagina is inverted and both the cervix and the body of the uterus protrude from the introitus. If the vagina inverts, it carries with it the adjacent bladder and rectum. Although uterine prolapse can occur in women who have never been pregnant, it is most common in postmenopausal women who have had multiple pregnancies.

Etiology and Risk Factors

Cardinal ligaments support the uterus in its anatomic position. The ligaments may be congenitally weak or may become stretched during pregnancy or injured during childbirth, resulting in weakening of support. As the woman ages, other supportive structures and uterine walls tend to relax, resulting in some degree of uterine prolapse.

Signs and Symptoms

Dyspareunia, backache, and a feeling of pelvic heaviness and pressure are commonly reported symptoms. Cystocele and rectocele usually accompany uterine prolapse.

Complications

In second-degree and third-degree prolapse, the protruding uterine portion is subject to trauma and may become eroded and necrotic.

Medical Diagnosis

Second-degree and third-degree prolapse are readily detected by visual inspection. First-degree prolapse is diagnosed through pelvic examination, although early first-degree prolapse may escape detection as the uterine descent is not evident when the patient is supine.

Medical Treatment

Vaginal hysterectomy with anterior and posterior colporrhaphy is the most common surgical treatment for uterine prolapse. For the woman who desires to preserve childbearing capability, it is possible to shorten the supportive ligaments surgically and return the uterus to the correct anatomic position.

For women who are poor surgical risks or who refuse surgical treatment, pessaries may be used. Pessaries are instruments that are inserted into the vagina to apply pressure on the vaginal wall, thereby supporting the uterus in the pelvis. There are several types of pessaries, including ring ("doughnut") pessary and lever pessary. Following placement of a pessary, advise the patient to return within 24 hours for the physician to assess placement, effectiveness, and problems related to pressure on surrounding structures. Pessaries must be removed, cleaned, and replaced periodically. If they are not maintained or are fitted improperly, they may act as irritants and cause tissue erosion, malignant tissue changes, or both. Be sure to document that the patient has a pessary so that it will not be forgotten and neglected. Topical estrogen creams or vaginal tablets may improve the tone of the muscles in the pelvic floor.

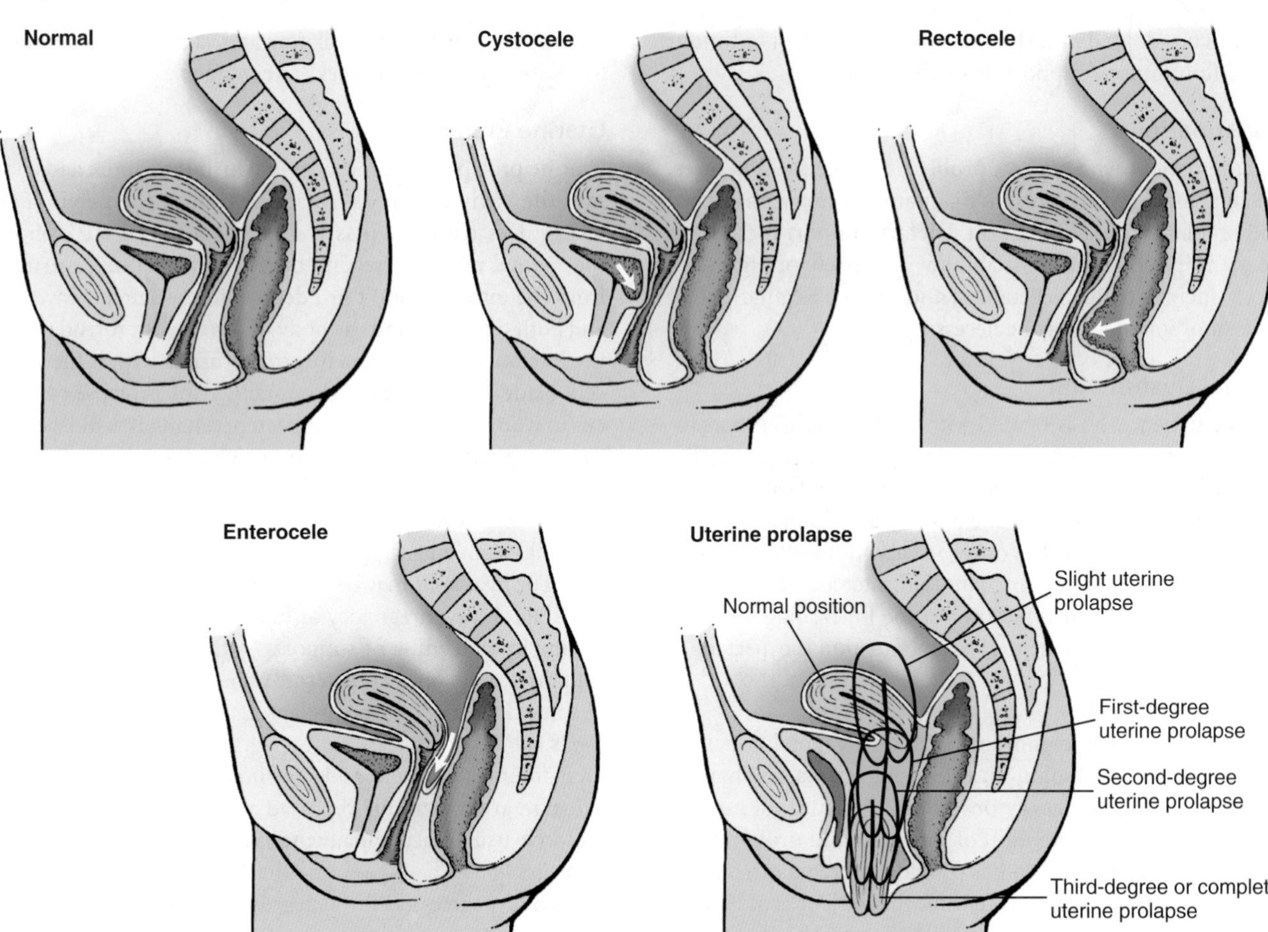

FIGURE **45-10** Types of genital prolapse.

NURSING CARE *of the Patient with Uterine Prolapse*

Assessment

Nursing assessment of the patient with a disorder of the reproductive system is outlined in Table 45-1. When the patient has uterine prolapse, record related symptoms. If the prolapsed uterus is visible, note any signs of trauma or tissue breakdown.

Nursing Diagnoses, Goals, and Outcome Criteria: Second or Third-Degree Uterine Prolapse

NURSING DIAGNOSES	GOALS AND OUTCOME CRITERIA
Disturbed Body Image related to interference with daily activities	Improved body image: positive patient remarks about self and ability to manage uterine prolapse
Sexual Dysfunction related to abnormal uterine position	Satisfying sexual function: patient states sexual activity is satisfying and without pain
Risk for Injury related to trauma of the exposed uterus	Absence of uterine trauma: no breaks in tissue integrity of uterus
Deficient Knowledge of self-care	Patient understands and practices self-care: patient accurately describes self-care, keeps follow-up appointments

Interventions

You can serve as a source of emotional support and information for the patient. Nursing care depends on the treatment selected. Proper use of a pessary can reduce the risk of uterine trauma. When a pessary is the treatment of choice, explain the importance of frequent examinations by a physician or nurse practitioner, the need to report pessary-related discomfort to the health care provider, and the need for pessary care. Although some primary health care providers prefer to remove, clean, and replace pessaries, capable patients can be taught to do this themselves.

Put on your THINKING CAP!!

A newly hired nurse in a long-term care facility is surprised to learn that some patients have pessaries. The nurse says, "Nobody uses those things any more!" How would you explain the use of pessaries in this population?

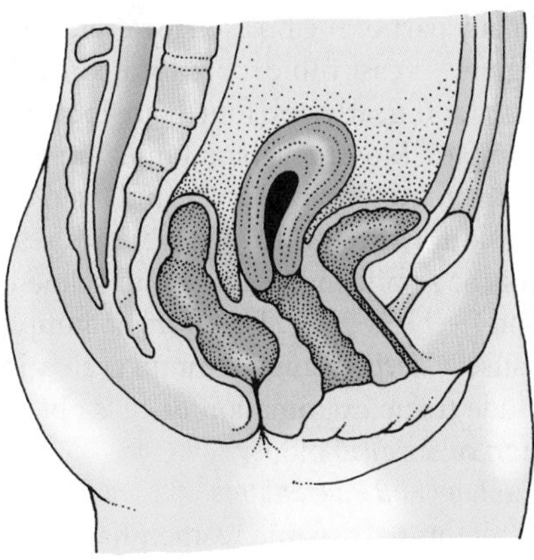

FIGURE **45-11** Normal position of the uterus.

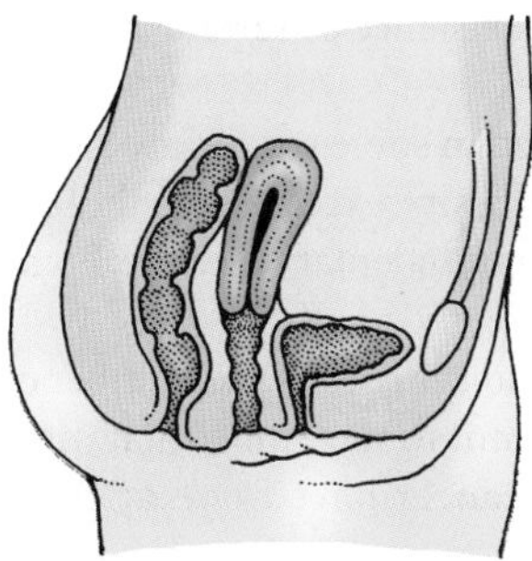

In **retroversion**, the uterus *tilts posteriorly*, and the cervix rotates anteriorly.

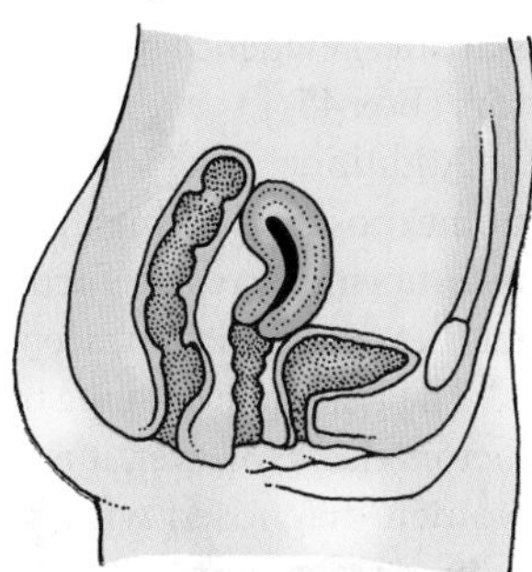

In **retroflexion**, the uterus *bends posteriorly.*

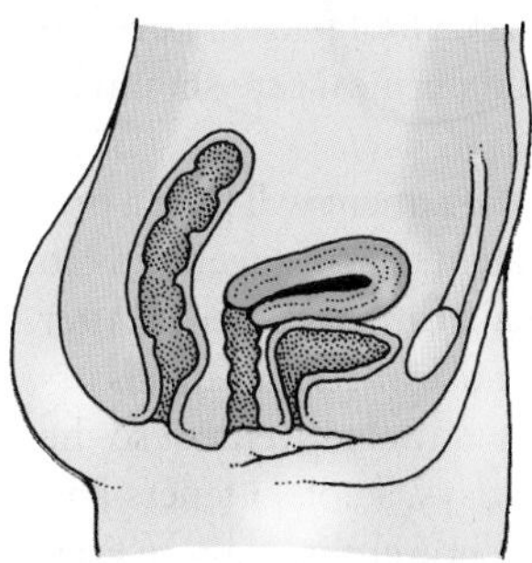

In **anteversion**, the uterus *tilts anteriorly.*

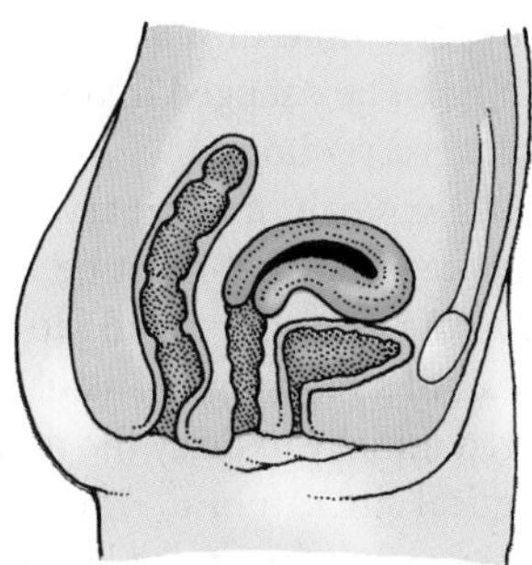

In **anteflexion**, the uterus *bends anteriorly.*

FIGURE **45-12** Types of uterine displacement.

Retroversion and Retroflexion, Anteversion and Anteflexion

The uterus is normally positioned at a 45-degree angle anterior to the vagina, with the cervix pointed downward toward the posterior vaginal wall (Fig. 45-11). Displacement from the normal position may be a normal congenital variation or may be related to a number of other factors (Fig. 45-12). Posterior displacement may be retroversion or retroflexion. Retroversion is a backward tilt of the uterus with the cervix pointed downward toward the anterior vaginal wall. With retroflexion, the body of the uterus bends backward on itself. Anterior displacement may be anteversion or anteflexion. With anteversion, the entire uterus tilts forward at a sharper angle to the vagina. With anteflexion, the uterus bends forward as if folding on itself.

Etiology and Risk Factors

Weakening and stretching of the round, broad, and uterosacral ligaments and weakened pelvic floor musculature related to childbearing are the most common causes of uterine displacement. Other causes include surgical trauma, pelvic tumors, pelvic inflammatory disease, and endometriosis.

Signs and Symptoms

Most uterine displacement is asymptomatic, although dyspareunia and low back pain may occur with retroversion.

Complications

Difficulty with conception has been associated with uterine displacement, particularly with retroversion. However, most complications are now thought to be associated with an underlying pathology (e.g., endometriosis, pelvic inflammatory disease) rather than with displacement itself.

Medical Diagnosis and Treatment

The pelvic examination reveals uterine displacement. Treatment is seldom employed, although some women find relief from backache by assuming a knee-chest position. Kegel exercises may be employed to strengthen the pelvic floor muscular support system. For patients who are not candidates for surgery, a pessary may be used (see Uterine Prolapse).

NURSING CARE *of the Patient with Retroversion and Retroflexion, Anteversion and Anteflexion*

The nurse's role is usually limited to history taking and providing information. If a pessary is inserted, provide instructions similar to those described under uterine prolapse.

VAGINAL FISTULAS

Vaginal fistulas are abnormal passageways between the vagina and other pelvic organs. A fistula between the vagina and the urinary bladder is called a vesicovaginal fistula; a urethrovaginal fistula is located between the urethra and the vagina. Both of these fistulas permit urine to flow into the vagina. A rectovaginal fistula is located between the vagina and the rectum and permits flatus and feces to pass into the vagina. Urine or fecal matter in the vagina can lead to severe vaginal and vulvar irritation and infection. Vaginal fistulas often can be diagnosed on the basis of the health history and physical examination findings. Dye may be injected into the vagina, and radiographs may be made to locate the fistula.

Surgical correction is often needed, although some small fistulas close spontaneously. Surgery may be delayed until the infection and inflammation have subsided. Preoperatively, instruct the patient in perineal hygiene and measures to control odor. Encourage fluid intake to reduce the risk of infection. The physician may prescribe sitz baths and deodorizing douches. Remember that excessive pressure during douching may force fluid through the fistula. Perineal pads are needed but must be changed frequently, and perineal care should be done every 4 hours.

After repair of a urinary fistula, the patient will have a urinary catheter that must be kept patent. Encourage fluids to promote urine output and to maintain catheter patency. After repair of a rectovaginal fistula, a liquid, low-residue diet is ordered initially to delay the need for a bowel movement so the surgical site can heal. After several days, stool softeners and laxatives may be ordered to promote bowel elimination. Enemas are contraindicated as they may disrupt the sutured area. Unfortunately, surgical correction is not always successful.

CANCER

A diagnosis of cancer of the female reproductive system can have profound psychological impact. For example, cancer implies threats to personal survival, sexual relationships, family integrity, and a woman's concept of herself as a female. You can play a potentially significant role in helping the patient cope with decision making, treatment methods and their effects, the inevitable grieving process, and the reactions of family members and friends.

Breast Cancer

Breast cancer is the most prevalent form of cancer in American women; the current prediction is that one of every eight or nine women will develop breast cancer at some point in her life. It is the second leading cause of cancer deaths in women.

Regular monthly breast self-examination and periodic mammography are important steps toward detection of breast cancer in its early stage, with prompt diagnosis and treatment producing a 5-year survival rate greater than 90%. Although it is estimated that 80% of breast lumps prove to be benign, those that are malignant must be identified and treated aggressively to prevent invasion of surrounding tissue, metastasis to distant structures, and death.

The three major types of breast cancer, according to the type of cells undergoing malignant changes, are ductal, lobular, and nipple. Malignant growths usually are singular and unilateral (affecting only one breast), and they can be found in any part of the breast. However, nearly one half of all malignant breast tumors are located in the upper outer quadrant, and nearly one fourth are located in the nipple-areolar complex. Most malignant lumps are painless and are palpated as firm, irregularly shaped, and fixed to underlying structure or skin. However, they sometimes resemble benign lumps: soft or semifirm, symmetric in shape with discrete borders, and freely movable. Therefore no lump should be ignored because it "feels" benign. Prompt evaluation is vital and may include tissue examination of cells obtained by needle aspiration or surgical biopsy.

Etiology and Risk Factors

White non-Hispanic women have the highest incidence of breast cancer. African-American women are most likely to die from it.

Although no cause has been identified for breast cancer, statistical evidence indicates the existence of several risk factors (Box 45-1).

Additional risk factors reported in some studies are radiation exposure, late menopause, obesity, excessive alcohol intake, hormone replacement therapy, sedentary lifestyle, high-fat diet, and oral contraceptives.

The risk of developing breast cancer rises as the number of factors rise. However, it is important to remember that most women diagnosed with breast cancer have none of these known risk factors.

What Does Culture Have to do with Breast Cancer?

Some genetic factors increase the risk of breast cancer. Other suspected risk factors—including high-fat diet, obesity, and sedentary lifestyle—may be culturally based. No race or culture is free of breast cancer.

Prognosis

Relative survival rates are determined by comparing survival rates among cancer patients with overall survival rates in similar groups of people who do not have cancer. When cancer is confined to the breast, the 5-year relative survival rate is 96.8%. When cancer has spread to surrounding tissue, the 5-year survival rate is 75.9%; when the disease has metastasized, the rate is 20.6%.

box 45-1 ***Established Risk Factors for Breast Cancer***

Sex: female
Family history: mother, sister, or daughter diagnosed with breast cancer
Age: 50 and older
Age at menarche: 11 years or younger
Age at first childbirth: 30 years or older
Personal medical history: benign breast biopsy, atypical hyperplasia in the breast, breast cancer
BRCA1 or BRCA2 gene mutation

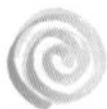

What Does Culture Have to do with Breast Cancer Survival?

Low-income African-American women more often have advanced disease when diagnosed and are more likely than white women to die from breast cancer. This population should be targeted for instruction in breast self-examination. Resources for evaluation and treatment that are available to these women must be identified.

Signs and Symptoms

Painless breast tissue thickening or lump is the initial sign, palpated during breast self-examination or visualized on a mammogram. Most late symptoms are associated with the tumor's invasion of surrounding tissues—dimpling of the skin, nipple discharge, nipple or skin retraction, edema, dilated blood vessels, ulceration, and hemorrhage. Dry, patchy nipple skin is suggestive of Paget's disease, an uncommon cancer of the nipple and areola. Chest pain may be associated with metastasis to the lung.

Complications

Infiltration of adjacent breast and axillary tissue and metastasis to distant sites are the major complications of advanced breast cancer.

Medical Diagnosis

Routine screening methods for breast cancer follow specific guidelines:

- Physical examination every 3 years until age 40, every year after age 40
- Baseline mammogram by age 40, followed by repeat mammogram every 1 to 2 years from age 40 to 49, every year beginning at age 50
- Breast ultrasound, digital mammography, or magnetic resonance imaging for questionable mammogram readings
- Biopsy of suspicious tissue for histologic analysis: fine-needle aspiration, core-needle aspiration, incisional biopsy, or excisional biopsy

Medical Treatment

If tissue examination confirms the malignancy, the patient and her physician consider surgical options based on the type, size, and extent of the cancerous growth. Women are playing increasingly active roles in the decision-making process and may "shop" for surgeons with whom they can agree on the selected surgical method. An oncologist may serve as a consultant in the decision-making process. Surgical options include lumpectomy, simple mastectomy, and radical mastectomy. Lumpectomy is removal of the tumor with a margin of surrounding healthy tissue but with preservation of most of the breast. A simple mastectomy is removal of the entire breast. Radical mastectomy is removal of all breast tissue, overlying skin, axillary lymph nodes, and underlying pectoral muscles. A variation of radical mastectomy adds removal of the internal mammary lymphatic chain. The four most commonly employed options are depicted in Figure 45-13. For treatment of early-stage cancer, there is evidence that lumpectomy plus radiotherapy offers the same long-term survival rate as more extensive surgery with radiotherapy. Additional treatment options depend on a number of factors, as outlined in Figure 45-14.

After the selected surgery is completed, the removed nodes are examined for evidence of cancer, and the cancer is staged. Breast cancer is staged according to the tumor-node-metastasis classification explained in Chapter 24. The stages are summarized in Figure 45-15.

Another critical factor is determined—whether the cancer cells are estrogen receptors (ER+) or nonreceptors (ER−). If cells are ER+, indicating that the tumor needs estrogen for growth, the drug tamoxifen citrate may be prescribed. Tamoxifen is a selective estrogen receptor modulator (SERM). SERMs block circulating estrogen from reaching the receptor cells. The use of SERMs tamoxifen and raloxifene to prevent initial malignancy in selected women who are at high risk for the development of breast cancer is under study.

Once surgery is completed, the oncologist plays an increasingly dominant role in continued management of care. Chemotherapy, hormone therapy, radiation therapy, or a combination of these may be employed before, during, or after surgery. Most physicians routinely follow lumpectomy with radiation therapy, even though evidence indicates that all malignant cells were removed. Radiation therapy is used because studies indicate that there may be small metastases without nodal involvement. See Chapter 24 for a discussion of treatment modalities.

Many women elect breast reconstruction after modified radical mastectomy or radical mastectomy. Reconstruction is performed by a plastic surgeon and may be initiated immediately after the mastectomy and before closure of the wound, or it may be delayed. Reconstruction usually begins with implantation of a tissue expander placed under the pectoralis muscle. Small amounts of normal saline are periodically injected into the expander until the expander creates a space the size of the prosthesis that will replace the expander in a future surgical procedure. Other reconstruction methods employ transfer of tissue from other areas of the patient's own body, including the abdomen and back (Table 45-8).

NURSING CARE *of the Patient with Breast Cancer*

Assessment

Nursing assessments are focused on physical manifestations of disease, physical and psychological responses to treatments, review of all body systems, presence of pain, psychosocial factors, and level of knowledge. In the immediate postoperative period, monitor the patient's vital signs, the wound dressings and drainage, and the arm on the affected side for edema.

Care of the surgical patient is covered in Chapter 16, and care of the patient who has cancer is covered in Chapter 24. Additional specific nursing diagnoses and goals for the mastectomy patient are listed in the following box.

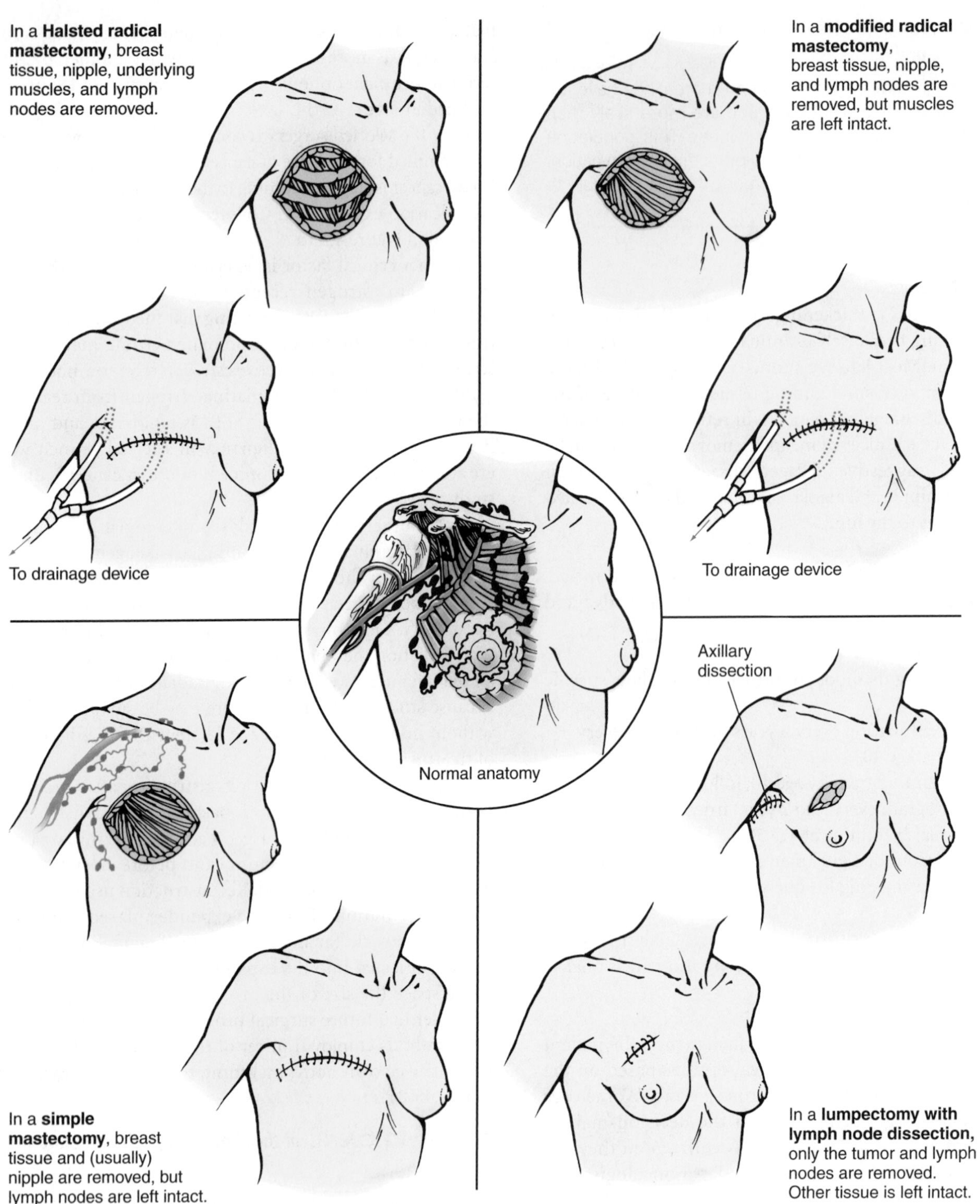

In a **Halsted radical mastectomy**, breast tissue, nipple, underlying muscles, and lymph nodes are removed.
In a **modified radical mastectomy**, breast tissue, nipple, and lymph nodes are removed, but muscles are left intact.
To drainage device
To drainage device
Normal anatomy
Axillary dissection
In a **simple mastectomy**, breast tissue and (usually) nipple are removed, but lymph nodes are left intact.
In a **lumpectomy with lymph node dissection,** only the tumor and lymph nodes are removed. Other tissue is left intact.

FIGURE **45-13** Options in the surgical management of breast cancer.

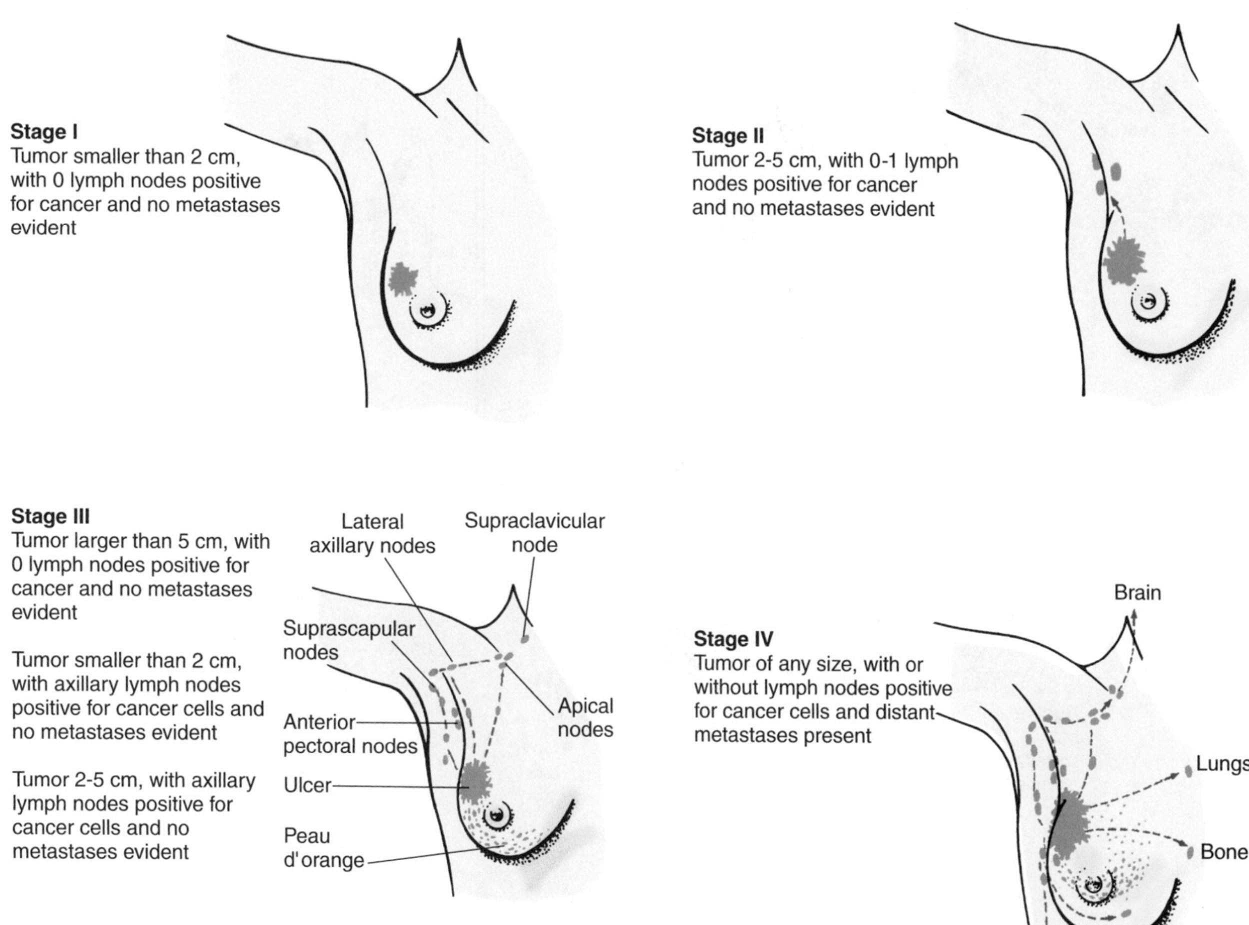
Stage I
Tumor smaller than 2 cm, with 0 lymph nodes positive for cancer and no metastases evident
Stage II
Tumor 2-5 cm, with 0-1 lymph nodes positive for cancer and no metastases evident
Stage III
Tumor larger than 5 cm, with 0 lymph nodes positive for cancer and no metastases evident
Tumor smaller than 2 cm, with axillary lymph nodes positive for cancer cells and no metastases evident
Tumor 2-5 cm, with axillary lymph nodes positive for cancer cells and no metastases evident
Lateral axillary nodes
Supraclavicular node
Suprascapular nodes
Apical nodes
Anterior pectoral nodes
Ulcer
Peau d'orange
Stage IV
Tumor of any size, with or without lymph nodes positive for cancer cells and distant metastases present
Brain
Lungs
Bone
Liver

FIGURE **45-14** Stages of breast cancer.

Nursing Diagnoses, Goals, and Outcome Criteria: Postoperative Mastectomy

Nursing Diagnoses	Goals and Outcome Criteria
Disturbed Body Image related to altered appearance, loss of breast, perceived loss of attractiveness	Improved body image: patient demonstrates comfort with the new body image
Risk for Injury related to lymphedema secondary to excision of lymph nodes	Absent or minimal lymphedema: arm circumference unchanged
Impaired Physical Mobility of affected arm related to axillary lymph node dissection	Normal mobility of affected arm: patient has full range of motion in affected arm within 6 weeks
Deficient Knowledge of self-care and resources	Patient understands self-care: patient demonstrates self-care and identifies resources

Interventions

Disturbed Body Image

The breasts are an important part of a woman's self-image. To many women, loss of a breast represents loss of femininity. Even with immediate reconstruction, the breasts do not look completely normal. The patient may see herself as sexually unattractive and fear rejection by her sexual partner. These feelings are superimposed on the fear created by a diagnosis of cancer.

Gently explore how the patient is feeling about the surgery and encourage her to express her concerns. Be accepting of the patient, whose feelings may surface in a variety of ways, including anger, denial, and depression. From the early postoperative period, encourage the patient to attend to her appearance. Provide information about breast prostheses and clothing designed for women who have had mastectomies. If the patient has had chemotherapy, hair loss also may contribute to her body image disturbance. Strategies and resources for the cancer patient with a body image disturbance are discussed in Chapter 24.

Risk for Injury

A radical mastectomy includes the removal of lymph nodes in the axilla on the affected side. Because lymph nodes normally help return tissue fluid to the bloodstream, their removal can result in lymphedema (the accumulation of fluid in the affected area). An important aspect of postoperative care after mastectomy is directed toward preventing and minimizing lymphedema in the arm on the

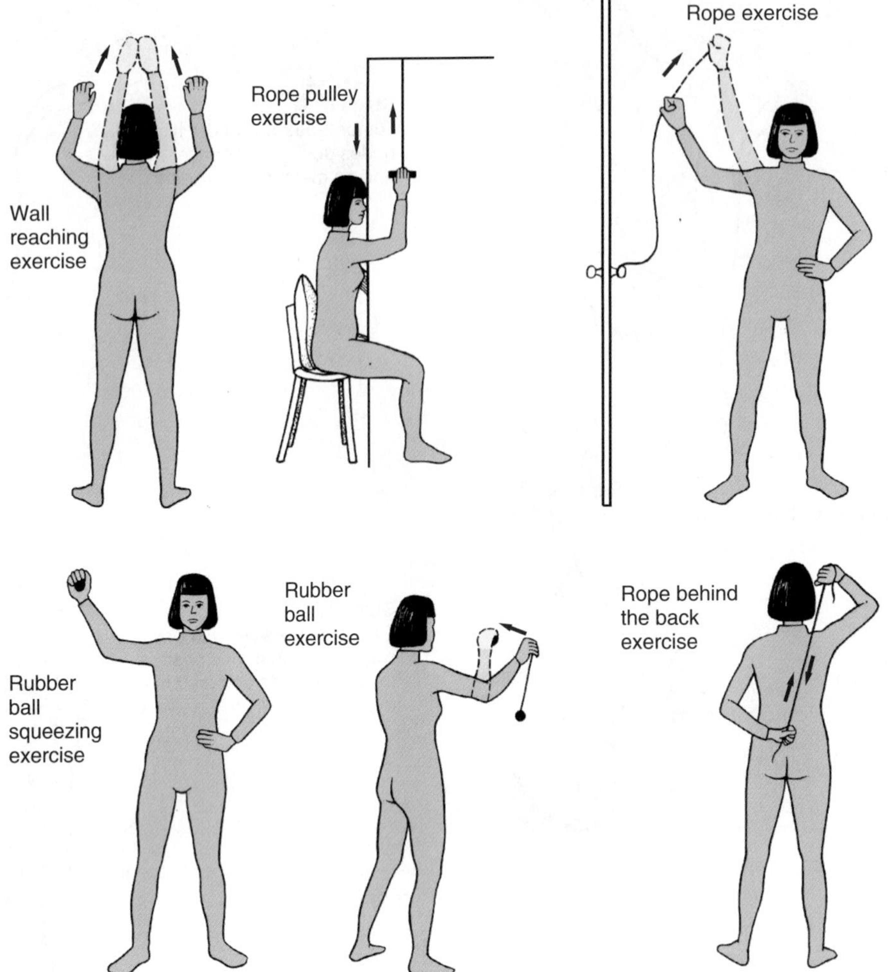

FIGURE **45-15** Arm exercises for mastectomy patients.

table 45-8 ***Examples of Breast Reconstruction Procedures***

PROCEDURE	DESCRIPTION
Implantation	An implant matching the size of the other breast is placed under the muscle of the operative side to create a breast mound.
Tissue expansion	A tissue expander is placed under the muscle and gradually expanded with saline to stretch the overlying skin and create a pocket. After several weeks, the tissue expander is exchanged for an implant.
Myocutaneous flaps	A flap of skin, fat, and muscle is transferred from the donor site to the operative area. The flap contains an appropriate amount of fat to match the other breast and is similar in appearance to breast tissue. A blood supply is established by reanastomosis of vessels from the operative area to those with the flap when possible. A new nipple may be created with tissue from the other nipple, labia, or thigh. Nipples can also be created by tattooing.

affected side. Interventions to manage lymphedema include the following:

1. Elevate the arm to a height above the level of the heart.
2. Measure blood pressures on the arm on the unaffected side, *never on the affected side.*
3. Do not use the affected arm for venipuncture, injections, or parenteral fluid administration.
4. Do not apply deodorant to or shave the axilla on the affected side.
5. Frequently measure the circumference of the affected arm; immediately report an increase.
6. Encourage frequent and progressive exercise of the arm on the affected side.
7. Encourage the patient to use the arm for as many activities of daily living as possible.

Position the patient alternately on her unaffected side and her back, observing regular postoperative care as described in Chapter 16. If the nipple has been grafted to another site for preservation for future reconstruction, it is treated as a secondary surgical site. Orders are written for specific postoperative care of the nipple. Routine assessment of the grafted nipple includes hourly observation for bleeding and signs of infection or necrosis (pallor, cyanosis, coolness).

Impaired Physical Mobility

Dissection of the lymph nodes in the axilla may or may not be indicated with a mastectomy. If the axilla is dissected, the patient is at risk for contractures unless proper positioning is maintained and exercises are begun as soon as permitted by the surgeon. Postoperatively, place the patient in semi-Fowler's position with the affected arm elevated on a pillow. Encourage her to flex and extend her fingers. Offer analgesics 30 minutes ahead of time so the exercises can be done more comfortably. The exercises should be done 3-5 times each day until full arm and shoulder range of motion is restored (see Fig. 45-15).

Deficient Knowledge

Arrangements can be made for visits from a representative of the American Cancer Society's Reach for Recovery program. The representatives are volunteers who have experienced breast cancer themselves and who have learned to cope successfully with the diagnosis, treatment, and related stressors. They assist patients by providing information, anticipatory guidance, and emotional support.

Patient teaching should have begun preoperatively but must be reinforced postoperatively. Content to cover includes signs and symptoms of infection, wound care, arm exercises, prevention of lymphedema, resources, and (if appropriate) management of the effects of chemotherapy or radiotherapy. With the patient's permission, include her significant other in the teaching process. This provides an opportunity for the partner to understand the patient's experience, to demonstrate support, and to participate in her recovery. With simple mastectomies, patients are sometimes discharged in less than 24 hours. This makes patient teaching especially challenging. Be sure to provide written information and resources along with verbal instructions.

Cervical Cancer

Cervical cancer generally grows slowly. For patients who have regular pelvic examinations and Pap smears, cervical cancer is usually diagnosed and treated in its early stage. Advanced cervical cancer may invade such surrounding structures as pelvic walls, bowel, and bladder.

Research indicates that most cervical cancer is associated with microbes such as some strains of human papillomavirus and herpes simplex virus. Thus cervical cancer is considered by many medical scientists to be an STD.

Etiology and Risk Factors

Although the exact relationship between cervical cancer and microorganisms that cause STDs is unknown, the link is strongly supported by research. Research also has revealed a relationship between intrauterine exposure to diethylstilbestrol and cervical cancer in a few women. Additional factors associated with cervical cancer are cigarette smoking, initial sexual intercourse in early adolescence, multiple sexual partners, and dietary deficiencies in folic acid and in vitamins A and C. There is no evidence that family history or the patient's menstrual history increases the risk of cervical cancer. Although cervical cancer formerly was thought to be linked to sexual intercourse with uncircumcised males, current research does not support this speculation.

What Does Culture Have to do with Cervical Cancer?

Cervical cancer is more common among Hispanic, African American, and Native American women than among Caucasions. Cultural practices including diet may explain the difference.

Signs and Symptoms

Early cervical cancer is asymptomatic. Advanced cancer also may be asymptomatic or may be associated with blood-tinged or frank bloody vaginal discharge, menstrual irregularities, or bleeding after intercourse.

Complications

Invasion of cervical cancer into adjacent structures causes site-related symptoms such as pain, backache, and bleeding. Anemia due to chronic bleeding may develop.

Medical Diagnosis

Cervical cancer often is first suspected when a positive Pap smear result reveals atypical cells. Tissue specimens obtained by multiple punch biopsy, endocervical curettage, or conization are studied for microscopic evidence of malignancy. Cervical cancer is preceded by changes in cells called dysplasia.

Cervical cancer is staged according to the extent of invasion, with stage 0 signifying limitation to the cervical epithelium and with stage IVb indicating metastasis to distant organs.

Medical Treatment

Treatment depends on the stage of the tumor and on various general health factors. Mild dysplasia may be treated with loop electrosurgical excision. This procedure, which can be done in an outpatient setting, uses electricity to destroy abnormal tissue. Localized carcinoma (in situ) may be treated with laser destruction, cryosurgery, or conization alone; total hysterectomy may be performed if childbearing is not desired.

Invasive cancer is treated with radiation, surgery, or both. Radiotherapy may be external or internal. If the therapy is internal, a sealed source is placed in the vagina for a specified period of time. Because effective treatment requires proper placement, the patient is immobilized as much as possible for the duration of the treatment. Radiotherapy and related nursing care are discussed in detail in Chapter 24.

If surgery is elected, the extent of the surgery depends on the extent of invasion. It ranges from radical hysterectomy (removal of the uterus, fallopian tubes, upper third of the vagina, and usually the ovaries) to total pelvic exenteration (removal of the uterus, ovaries, fallopian tubes, vagina, bladder, urethra, descending colon, rectum, anal canal, and pelvic lymph nodes). Nursing care of the patient with cervical cancer is discussed at the end of the section on cancer.

Ovarian Cancer

Although the incidence of ovarian cancer is relatively low compared with that of other cancers, the mortality rate from ovarian cancer is the highest of all female reproductive system cancers. The high mortality is due to the fact that ovarian cancer is asymptomatic until it is advanced, so that it usually grows for an extended period of time before it is diagnosed. In most cases, abnormal cell growth occurs in both ovaries.

More than half of ovarian cancers are diagnosed around the time of menopause, with the remaining cases divided evenly between women younger than age 40 and women older than age 60. The ovary also may be a site for metastasis from other primary cancer sites.

Because ovarian cancer rarely is found in women who have had children or who have used oral contraceptives, birth control pills often are prescribed as a preventive measure even for women for whom pregnancy is not a possibility. Prophylactic bilateral oophorectomy (surgical removal of the ovaries) is a more drastic preventive measure employed for women identified as high-risk candidates for ovarian cancer.

Etiology and Risk Factors

No specific causes have been found for ovarian cancer. However, risk factors include a family or personal history of ovarian cancer; a personal history of ovarian dysfunction or of breast, endometrial, or colorectal cancer; nulliparity (has not produced a viable offspring); and either early menarche or late menopause. Exposure to such carcinogens as asbestos and talc as well as ingestion of animal fats have been identified as possible risk factors by some researchers. However, additional studies are needed to determine whether a cause-and-effect relationship exists.

Signs and Symptoms

Ovarian cancer is asymptomatic in its early stage. Because symptoms of even advanced ovarian cancer tend to be vague and nonspecific, they usually are attributed to various other conditions before ovarian cancer is considered. Abdominal pain and bloating, gastrointestinal tract symptoms such as flatulence, and urinary tract complaints may be reported. Abnormal uterine bleeding is not common. In extremely advanced cancer, ascites may be noted.

Complications

Ovarian cancer metastasizes widely via direct invasion, peritoneal fluid, and the lymphatic and venous systems.

Medical Diagnosis

Palpable tumors are discovered on pelvic and rectal examinations. The finding of bilateral masses is particularly significant because most benign ovarian masses are unilateral. Computed tomography and ultrasound may be used as diagnostic tools. Blood may be drawn for a CA-125 serum marker test, which, if elevated above 35 units/ml, indicates the presence of an antigen associated with ovarian epithelial cancer. However, an exploratory laparotomy or laparoscopy should be done as soon as possible to directly visualize the tumor or tumors and to obtain tissue for definitive diagnosis and for staging and grading of the malignancy.

For early diagnosis, ovarian cancer should be considered as a possibility for all women, especially those women identified as high-risk candidates who present with virtually any symptoms of reproductive tract problems. Some practitioners advocate screening of blood serum for CA-125, although elevated levels can be caused by other factors in addition to ovarian cancer.

Medical Treatment

Treatment depends on the staging of the tumor or tumors. Stage 1 tumors, in which tumor growth is confined to the ovary, are surgically removed via total abdominal hysterectomy and bilateral salpingo-oophorectomy. Chemotherapy, radiotherapy, or both usually are used after surgery. Intraperitoneal chemotherapy has been used for some patients. External radiation therapy or intraperitoneal radiation may be selected depending on the stage of the cancer. More advanced tumors generally are treated palliatively with total abdominal hysterectomy and bilateral salpingo-oophorectomy. Surgical treatment is followed by chemotherapy and radiotherapy to shrink remaining tumor tissue and thus to relieve pressure and pain associated with metastases. Regardless of the stage and prognosis for survival, CA-125 levels may be monitored to assess tumor progression or regression. Nursing care of the patient with ovarian cancer is discussed at the end of the section on cancer.

Vulvar Cancer

Cancer of the vulva is the rarest but also the most visible of the cancers of the female reproductive system. It may appear as a visible and palpable lump on the vulva or as a deviation from the normally pink, moist mucosa. The lesion may be scaly; red, white, or irregularly pigmented; edematous; serosanguineous or exuding a frank bloody discharge. The most common site is the labia majora.

Malignant melanoma may be manifested in the vulva, although the vulva is a rare site for this form of cancer. Its incidence is highest in postmenopausal women. The symptoms are similar to those of the more common vulvar cancers.

Etiology and Risk Factors

The cause of vulvar cancer is unknown, but it may be related to STDs, particularly human papillomavirus.

Signs and Symptoms

The most commonly reported symptom is pruritus (itching). Pain and bleeding are additional symptoms.

Complications

Although cancer of the vulva generally remains localized, it may become invasive if not discovered and treated. It can invade adjacent structures or metastasize via the lymphatic system.

Medical Diagnosis

A preliminary diagnosis is made through palpation of a mass or by visualization of tissue that appears suspicious. Biopsy is necessary for definitive diagnosis.

Medical Treatment

Treatment depends on the extent to which the malignant cells have spread. For localized lesions, conservative removal of the malignant tissue by laser surgery may be employed. For wider, deeper, or invasive lesions, radical surgical removal through vulvectomy and bilateral dissection of groin lymph nodes or through pelvic exenteration may be necessary. Pelvic exenteration is the removal of all pelvic organs including the bladder; the descending colon and anal canal may or may not be removed. Chemotherapy, radiation therapy, or both may follow surgery. Nursing care of the patient with vulvar cancer is discussed at the end of the section on cancer.

Vaginal Cancer

The vagina seldom is the primary site for cancer; rather it is the site for the extension of cancer that originates in the vulva, cervix, or endometrium. Except for young women whose vaginal cancers are associated with intrauterine exposure to diethylstilbestrol, vaginal cancer most commonly is found in postmenopausal women.

The 5-year survival rate for women treated for *in situ* vaginal cancer approaches 100%. However, its *in situ* stage is relatively short compared with that of other reproductive tract malignancies. Invasion of adjacent tissues is common unless the cancer is detected and treated early. Because early diagnosis most often is made on the basis of a Pap smear report, a strong argument can be made for yearly Pap smears for postmenopausal women and for women who have had a hysterectomy. The presence of numerous lymph nodes in the area facilitates metastasis.

Etiology and Risk Factors

No definite cause has been identified for vaginal cancer. However, researchers have identified the following risk factors: STDs (syphilis, herpes virus type 2, human papillomavirus), a previous diagnosis of cervical or vulvar cancer, previous radiation therapy, and intrauterine exposure to diethylstilbestrol.

Signs and Symptoms

In its early and most easily treated form, vaginal cancer usually is asymptomatic. Later symptoms include a burning sensation, vaginal discharge that may have a foul odor, dyspareunia, spotting after intercourse, and vaginal bleeding. Pelvic pain usually is associated with invasion of adjacent structures.

Complications

Invasion of adjacent structures and metastasis are the most common complications of epithelial vaginal cancer. The prognosis is poor for vaginal malignant melanoma, with an extremely low 5-year survival rate.

Medical Diagnosis and Treatment

Most cases are detected during inspection of the vagina and from routine Pap smears. A definitive diagnosis is made via colposcopy and biopsy of suspicious areas followed by tissue studies. Treatment of vaginal cancer depends on the extent of invasion. In situ (localized) cancer may be treated relatively simply with local laser surgery or cryosurgery. More radical treatment is indicated if the cancer is more invasive. Possible treatments employed either singly or in combination include topical chemotherapy, internal or external radiotherapy, partial or total vaginectomy, and pelvic exenteration.

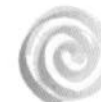

What Does Culture Have to do with Cancer of the Female Reproductive System?

The importance of reproductive capacity as a measure of a woman's value depends on cultural values. In cultures that associate the breasts with sexuality, the loss of a breast can cause a woman to feel undesirable.

NURSING CARE *of the Patient with Cancer of the Cervix, Ovaries, Vulva, or Vagina*

The patient with cancer of the cervix, ovaries, vulva, or vagina presents multiple challenges. She has been diagnosed with a life-threatening condition whose treatment very often constitutes a threat not only to her self-concept as a woman but also to her ability to function sexually. Treatments beyond local excision of affected tissue may result in disfigurement or in anatomic changes that hinder penile-vaginal intercourse, or both. The patient's psychosocial needs are as critical as her physical needs.

Assessment

Complete assessment of the patient with a disorder of the female reproductive system is summarized in Table 45-1. When the patient has or may have cancer, the health history documents signs and symptoms and possible risk factors. When reviewing the systems, describe changes or problems that may be related such as fatigue, pain, and bowel or bladder dysfunction. Explore effects of the symptoms on normal functioning. Assess the patient's concerns about the condition, which may include anxiety, fear, depression, anger, or withdrawal. The patient may express fear of the diagnosis of cancer as well as fear of the prescribed treatments. A complete physical examination should be done. The physician or nurse practitioner performs a pelvic examination that may reveal lesions, masses, and lymph node enlargement.

Nursing Diagnoses, Goals, and Outcome Criteria: Cancer of the Cervix, Ovaries, Vulva, or Vagina

Nursing Diagnoses	Goals and Outcome Criteria
Anxiety and Fear related to threat to health and lack of knowledge about the cancer and prescribed treatment	Reduced anxiety and fear: patient's statement of reduced anxiety and fear, with calm manner

Nursing Diagnoses, Goals, and Outcome Criteria: Cancer of the Cervix, Ovaries, Vulva, or Vagina—cont'd

Nursing Diagnoses	Goals and Outcome Criteria
Disturbed Body Image related to change in body appearance or function	Improved body image: positive patient statements about self and efforts to maintain or improve appearance
Altered Sexuality Patterns related to physical and emotional effects of cancer of the reproductive system	Satisfactory sexual patterns: patient's discussion of effects of disease or treatment on sexuality and coping strategies
Ineffective Family Coping related to lack of knowledge, situational crisis, role changes, or patient preoccupation with self	Appropriate family-patient interactions: family demonstration of support and positive coping
Risk for Injury (to patient and others) related to effects of radiotherapy, chemotherapy	Decreased risk of injury from treatment: maintenance of applicator position and adherence of patient and others to radiation precautions

Interventions

Anxiety and Fear

The woman needs encouragement and permission to ventilate her reaction to the diagnosis and treatment. Listen carefully to determine any knowledge deficits or misconceptions and to provide information as appropriate. Many women of all ages are computer-literate, so suggest sites that serve as reliable sources of information. Community agencies may have a lending library of books and videotapes. Anticipatory guidance is particularly important. Support groups are often helpful because patients learn from others who have had similar experiences. Many patients appreciate follow-up phone calls or the ability to call a resource person when needed.

Disturbed Body Image

The patient may be distressed if there is a change in appearance or function caused by the cancer or the treatment. Loss of reproductive capacity can be especially painful for women who still wish to bear children. You can gently explore the patient's response to the situation and encourage her to express her thoughts. Patients who are severely disturbed should be offered the benefit of a mental health professional or spiritual counselor. Encourage measures to improve the appearance, and praise the patient's positive efforts. Management of alopecia (hair loss) associated with cancer therapy is discussed in Chapter 24.

Altered Sexuality Patterns

Realistic expectations for future sexual functioning should be discussed and should focus both on sexual practices that will not be possible on a temporary or permanent basis and on alternative sexual practices that may be explored. It is critical that you show an accepting attitude toward sexuality in general and toward any specific sexual practices acceptable to the patient and her partner or partners.

Ineffective Family Coping

Include the family or identified support system in care. The family needs to understand the effects of the cancer and the treatments. They also need to appreciate the patient's need for support and for assistance during therapy and recovery. Encourage members of the household to consider ways to reduce demands on the patient. In addition, be sensitive to the needs of family members who may fear losing a loved one. Inclusion of the woman's sexual partner or partners is particularly critical if altered sexual expression is expected after treatment.

Risk for Injury

Physical care of the patient varies with the prescribed treatment and is based on physician's orders, institutional policies and procedures, and nursing diagnoses. General guidelines for the care of the patient who is having radiotherapy are covered in Chapter 24.

Internal radiation poses a nursing challenge. If a sealed radiation source is to be implanted in the vagina, an indwelling urinary catheter is inserted first. An applicator that will contain the radiation source is inserted into the vagina while the patient is in the operating room. The placement is checked on radiographs and is maintained by vaginal packing. The radiation source may be placed in the applicator before the applicator is inserted, or it may be placed in the applicator after the patient is transferred to her room and positioned in bed. The radiation dosage is determined and ordered by a radiologist; the duration of implantation is based on the total dosage but generally ranges from 24 to 72 hours.

The patient poses a source of radiation exposure to anyone within a radius of several feet, so usual radiation precautions are in force. For each nurse who is allowed to care for the patient, exposure should not exceed a total of 30 minutes per 24 hours. Visitors are screened according to protocol; those cleared to visit should be instructed to remain outside a 6-foot radius of the patient and to limit the duration of visits according to policy.

The patient is assigned a private room for the duration of internal radiotherapy. Enforce strict bedrest to prevent dislodgment of the applicator. Movement is restricted to cautious turning from side to side. The facts that radiation therapy may precipitate nausea, vomiting, and diarrhea; that movement must be restricted; and that total time for nursing care is restricted make care particularly challenging. You need to be exceptionally well organized and able to anticipate and to intervene rapidly and effectively. For example, judicious administration of antiemetics, tranquilizers, and antidiarrheal medications may moderate radiation side effects and thus facilitate patient comfort, maintenance of applicator position, and efficiency of nursing care time.

Effects on local tissue by the radioactive material produce a profuse, malodorous vaginal discharge that is largely absorbed by the packing and thus cannot be controlled with cleansing. A room deodorizer may be partially effective in making the odor tolerable. Following removal of the packing and applicator at the conclusion of therapy, administer a cleansing vaginal douche as ordered, and permit the patient to resume her normal activities. She is no longer a source of radiation exposure. Consider transfer of the patient to another room to remove her from a noxious environment and to allow housekeeping personnel to clean and air the room.

Care of the patient admitted for a pelvic exenteration is exceptionally complex and is beyond the scope of this textbook. An expert nursing staff is essential to provide the emotional support and physical care demanded for this patient.

Put on your THINKING CAP!!

A patient with pelvic cancer has had a surgical procedure that includes removal of the vagina. She tearfully says, "I will never be able to make love to my husband again." What are some things you could say or do to show acceptance of her feelings at this time?

INFERTILITY

Fertility impairment, or *infertility,* generally is defined as the inability to conceive within 1 year of regular unprotected sexual intercourse or as the ability to conceive but inability to deliver a live infant. Infertility is categorized as primary infertility if the woman has never conceived or if the man has never impregnated a woman. Secondary infertility refers to the woman who has conceived at least one time but either is not able to deliver a viable infant or is not able to conceive again. An estimated 17% of American couples want to produce children but are unable either to conceive or to deliver live infants. Of those couples, treatment enables approximately 60% to conceive and carry pregnancies to term. The remaining 40% of couples represent sterility that is not amenable to treatment.

In recent years, the entertainment and news media have provided mechanisms for the frank discussion of components of infertility: causes, psychosocial effects, and treatments. Associated problems and treatments have been described by professional health care providers and scientists, and personal accounts have been given by affected individuals. For many, the acceptance of infertility as a topic for public discussion has removed the stigma of infertility as a source of shame and embarrassment; myths have been debunked; and lay and professional people are becoming more knowledgeable about the subject. As a result, infertility has become a major subspecialty of gynecology, and infertility researchers have developed highly sophisticated and effective diagnostic techniques and treatments.

Etiology and Risk Factors

Research indicates that approximately 40% of infertility is attributable to female factors, 40% to male factors, and the remaining 20% either to a combination of male and female factors or to unknown factors. Conception depends on the interaction of a number of factors, broadly categorized as follows:

1. Timing and techniques used for sexual intercourse.
   A. Impregnation of the ovum by the sperm must occur within 24 hours after ovulation. Intercourse should be scheduled for every other day around ovulation time to optimize the potential for fertilization of the ovum.
   B. Semen should be deposited deeply in the vagina, in close proximity to the cervical os.
2. Production and release of a healthy ovum by the female and of numerous (approximately 200,000,000 per ejaculate) healthy sperm by the male.
3. Anatomically and physiologically correct female and male reproductive systems.
   A. Female: patent fallopian tubes with active fimbriated ends, uterine endometrium prepared for reception and implantation of a fertilized ovum.
   B. Male: epididymis temperature that maintains sperm viability during storage, patent seminiferous tubules, and vas deferens with enervated musculature.
4. Biochemical compatibility between female vaginal-cervical-fallopian environment and male ejaculate.

Other than faulty timing or technique for sexual intercourse, both of which are easily corrected through patient education, causes related to the remaining factors are exceptionally numerous. As has been mentioned previously, untreated or inadequately treated STDs potentially impair fertility by altering anatomy, physiology, and patency of the reproductive tracts of either or both partners.

Additional identified influences on conception include dysfunction of any part of the hypothalamic-pituitary-endocrine system, malnutrition or obesity, smoking, drug and alcohol use, exposure to toxic chemicals or radiation, nervous system disorders that affect reproductive structures that transfer ova and sperm, and male practices that maintain above-normal epididymal temperature (i.e., wearing tight underwear and pants, frequent and prolonged immersion in hot water or sauna).

Medical Diagnosis

The diagnosis is based on data obtained from exhaustive psychosocial and physical health and sexual health histories of both partners. If the histories provide clues that may explain possible detriments to fertility, such as poor timing or techniques of sexual intercourse or habitual epididymal exposure to high temperatures, further diagnostic attempts may be delayed until the couple has had time to remediate the potential problem or problems. If such simple factors are not identified, history taking is followed by systematic, comprehensive physical examinations and laboratory tests.

The male partner usually is the initial focus of diagnostic procedures because tests for diagnosis of male-associated infertility problems are generally easier, less invasive, less expensive, and (unlike a complete female fertility workup) not cycle-dependent. A semen specimen for analysis is collected by masturbation after a period of sexual abstinence that approximates the male's average frequency interval for intercourse. The specimen is then assessed for volume and for sperm count, morphology (shape), duration of viability, motility, and liquefaction. A second specimen is examined if variations from normal are found in any of the values. He may be referred to a urologist or endocrinologist for further diagnosis and possible treatment of persistent variations in the characteristics of the semen.

Evaluation of the female partner includes a battery of tests, most of them dependent on timing related to her menstrual cycle. Thus scheduling of each test is critical. Basal body temperature monitoring and recording of detailed data related to menstruation, cervical mucus characteristics, sexual intercourse, and duration of sleep are documented daily by the woman. The basal body temperature record, serum progesterone levels, and endometrial biopsy results provide data related to ovulation, cervical patency, and adequacy of the endometrium for ovum implantation.

If the basal body temperature, serum progesterone levels, and endometrial biopsy findings indicate normal hormonal functions, a postcoital test is done immediately before ovulation. The couple has intercourse the evening or morning before the scheduled test. A specimen of cervical mucus is aspirated from the cervix by the physician or nurse practitioner. The characteristics of the mucus are assessed by gross inspection and by microscopic examination. The examiner is looking for the clear, elastic mucus necessary to facilitate the progression of semen through the cervix. Abnormal consistency of the mucus may block progression of the semen beyond the cervical os. The examiner also inspects the specimens for number and motility of sperm. If a previous test of the male's semen indicated normal motility and viability of sperm but the postcoital test indicates nonviabile sperm, this suggests that the cervical mucus is not conducive to sperm survival, perhaps because of an antigen-antibody response to the semen.

Determination of uterine and fallopian tube patency and physical assessment of the peritoneal cavity are accomplished by invasive procedures: hysterosalpingography, laparoscopy, and culdoscopy. Ultrasonography may be employed for additional assessment.

Women are considered to be sterile and thus are not candidates for infertility diagnosis and treatment if they have congenital reproductive tract anomalies that cannot be corrected by surgery. Absence of one or more reproductive tract structures is also untreatable.

Medical Treatment

Treatment for infertility is related to diagnostic findings. A brief overview of specific problems and related treatments is presented in Table 45-9.

PHARMACOLOGY CAPSULE Ovulatory stimulants can cause ovarian hyperstimulation with possible rupture of the enlarged ovary.

NURSING CARE *of the Patient with an Infertility Disorder*

Assessment

Assessment of the female reproductive system is summarized in Table 45-1.

Nursing Diagnoses, Goals, and Outcome Criteria: Infertility

Nursing Diagnoses	Goals and Outcome Criteria
Situational Low Self-Esteem related to inability to conceive or feeling of failure	Improved self-esteem: positive expressions about self

table 45-9 ***Common Causes of Female Infertility and Related Medical Treatment***

ETIOLOGY	MEDICAL TREATMENT
Failure to ovulate, associated with the following:	
Delayed follicular maturation	Clomiphene citrate (Clomid)
Hypogonadotropin secretion	Menotropins (Pergonal)
Hypothalamic-pituitary dysfunction	Gonadotropin-releasing hormone
Elevated prolactin level	Bromocriptine mesylate (Parlodel)
Hypothyroidism	Thyroid-stimulating hormone
Ovarian tumors	Surgical excision
Poor-quality midcycle cervical mucus	Conjugated estrogens (Premarin) therapy
Inadequate endometrial development	Progesterone therapy
Endometriosis	Lupron therapy Gamete intrafallopian transfer
Reproductive tract infections	Antimicrobial therapy
Tubal construction	Hysterosalpingogram
Sperm-inhospitable cervical mucus	Therapeutic intrauterine insemination In vitro fertilization
Immunologic reaction to sperm	Use of condoms to reduce antibody titer, followed by unprotected intercourse at time of ovulation only In vitro fertilization

Altered Sexuality Patterns related to structured efforts to conceive or loss of spontaneity	Acknowledgment of the effects of the situation on one's sexual relationship: patient identifies ways to maintain a satisfying sexual relationship
Ineffective Coping related to unmet expectations or feelings of loss	Effective coping: patient uses healthy coping strategies
Deficient Knowledge of diagnostic and treatment procedures	Patient understands diagnostic and treatment procedures: patient verbalizes diagnostic and treatment procedures

Interventions

Fertility tests and treatments are generally done on an outpatient basis. The woman who undergoes the process usually has a prolonged relationship and frequent contacts with the nurse in the outpatient setting.

Situational Low Self-Esteem

Invasion of personal privacy is necessarily greater in fertility diagnosis and treatment than in any other condition. Gently explore the feelings of the patient and her partner about their difficulty conceiving. An open, empathetic attitude is vital if the patient is to be open. Support groups or professional counselors may help the couple maintain self-esteem.

Altered Sexuality Patterns

The most intimate details of her sexual relationship with her partner are elicited, and diagnostic and treatment procedures repeatedly violate the desire for modesty. Lovemaking becomes scheduled rather than spontaneous.

Ineffective Coping

You may be the only person with whom the woman shares her psychological reactions to the diagnosis of infertility and her subsequent emotional highs and lows throughout diagnosis and treatment. You therefore play a critical role in assisting the patient to cope with infertility. Give the patient the opportunity to discuss her thoughts and feelings about infertility and to explore coping strategies.

Deficient Knowledge

The needs of her sexual partner must be considered as well, and he should be included in patient teaching. Patient teaching includes information about diagnostic procedures, treatments, causes of infertility, and resources.

MENOPAUSE

Menopause is the cessation of menstruation that marks the end of a woman's reproductive capacity. Natural menopause is part of normal aging, but surgical menopause results from removal of the ovaries. Natural menopause occurs gradually and may permit better adaptation than surgical menopause, which suddenly eliminates the source of natural estrogen. Diminished ovarian function associated with aging causes ovulation to cease and estrogen production to decline. The onset of menopause may begin as early as age 35 but more commonly occurs between ages 40 and 55. With natural menopause, the woman's first sign may be menstrual irregularity. Menstrual periods tend to be spaced farther apart, and the amount of bleeding gradually diminishes. The entire process from earliest signs to complete cessation of menstruation usually is 2 years or less. A woman is said to be menopausal when she has not had a menstrual period for 1 year. Some women experience a surgical menopause brought on by the surgical removal of the ovaries. Unless estrogen replacement is begun promptly, the patient develops the signs and symptoms of menopause rapidly.

SIGNS AND SYMPTOMS

The signs and symptoms of menopause may include hot flashes—a warm feeling caused by vasodilation that affects the face, neck, and upper body. Hot flashes are typically accompanied by perspiration and sometimes by a feeling of faintness. Other common symptoms are vaginal dryness, insomnia, joint pain, headache, and nausea. Without estrogen, the uterus becomes smaller; the vagina shortens; and vaginal tissues become drier. Breast tissue may lose its firmness, and pubic and axillary hair become sparse. Supporting pelvic structures relax, causing some women to have stress incontinence. There may be significant loss of bone mass, thus leading to fragile bones, a condition called osteoporosis. Some women report emotional instability, irritability, and depression, but the impact of menopause on a woman is very individualized. Some grieve for the loss of reproductive capacity, and some feel a loss of femininity and sexual attractiveness. Others welcome the end of menstrual periods and no longer having to worry about the risk of pregnancy.

MEDICAL TREATMENT

Estrogen therapy decreases the risk of osteoporosis but, if taken for more than 5 years, *may* increase the risk of breast cancer. Therefore each woman's health history must be considered so that she and her physician can decide whether hormone replacement therapy will be used. Estrogens are contraindicated with estrogen-dependent cancer, undiagnosed abnormal vaginal bleeding, and current or past thromboembolic disorders.

There are many drug regimens. The patient who still has her uterus and ovaries has typically been treated with estrogen and progestins (compounds that have actions like progesterone). Because progestin decreases the risk of endometrial cancer related to estrogen therapy, they are not needed in women who no longer have a uterus. Recent findings from the Women's Health Initiative indicate the combination therapy in women with intact uteruses increases the risk of invasive breast cancer and coronary heart disease.

Oral drug therapy is most commonly used, but a transdermal form of estrogen is also available. The transdermal drug is delivered by an adhesive bandage–like patch. Estrogen creams and suppositories may be used to relieve vaginal

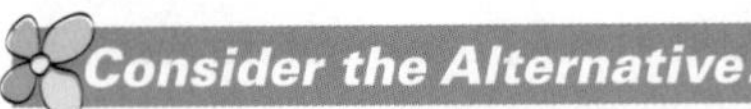

Black cohosh is sometimes used to treat menstrual cramps and as an alternative to estrogen for treatment of menopausal symptoms. Black cohosh can potentiate antihypertensive and hypoglycemic drugs. Patients are advised to limit its use to 6 months because of lack of information about long-term effects.

Consider the Alternative!

Over-the-counter options for treating hot flashes include vitamin E 400-800 IU PO daily, vitamin B complex 200 mg PO daily, and selenium per manufacturer's instructions.

Nutrition Concepts

1. Long-term dieting is associated with amenorrhea and reduced fertility.
2. Factors that may interfere with optimal nutrition for women of childbearing age include lack of resources, lack of nutrition knowledge, self-imposed dietary restrictions, and genetic idiosyncrasies.
3. High dietary fat intake has been linked to breast cancer.

dryness. Drugs used to control "hot flashes" include clonidine patches, bellergal-S, venlafaxine, and paroxetine.

NURSING CARE *of the Menopausal Patient*

Assessment

Assessment of the woman with a disorder of the reproductive system is summarized in Table 45-1. When a woman has menopausal symptoms, record them and explore how the patient is coping with this significant life change.

Nursing Diagnoses, Goals, and Outcome Criteria: Menopause

The primary nursing diagnosis for the menopausal patient is usually ineffective management of therapeutic regimen related to lack of understanding of the effects and treatment of menopause. The goal of nursing care is effective management of prescribed therapy and decreased signs and symptoms of menopause. The outcome criterion is the patient's report of reduced symptoms.

Interventions

Assess the patient's understanding of menopause and how she feels about it. The patient may need reassurance that her symptoms and responses are normal and common. If drug therapy is used, instruct the patient regarding self-medication. Caution patients on estrogen to report any signs of circulatory disorders (numbness, pain in calf, shortness of breath) to the physician immediately. Additional information about drug therapy is summarized in Table 45-3. The patient who cannot or chooses not to take hormone therapy needs additional assistance to cope with the symptoms of menopause. Women who wish to prevent "menopausal" pregnancy should utilize a reliable form of contraception for at least 1 year following cessation of menses.

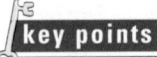

- The female reproductive system includes the external and internal genitalia and the breasts.
- Common therapeutic measures for the female reproductive system include douche, cauterization, heat application, and topical medications.
- Two common uterine bleeding disorders are metrorrhagia (bleeding or spotting between menstrual periods) and menorrhagia (menstrual periods characterized by profuse bleeding).
- The primary nursing diagnoses for the patient with a uterine bleeding disorder are deficient knowledge of condition and treatment and anxiety related to unknown cause of bleeding.
- The effects of reproductive tract infections may include infertility, changes in relationships, feelings of distrust toward sexual partners, shame, embarrassment, and diminished self-esteem.
- Because most infections are treated on an outpatient basis, the nurse's primary role is to educate the patient in preventing and treating infections.
- Benign growths of the female reproductive system include cysts of the breasts and ovaries and endometriosis.
- The primary nursing diagnoses for the patient with endometriosis, a disorder marked by the growth of endometrial tissue outside the uterus, are acute pain and deficient knowledge.
- Cysts are sac-like structures that contain fluid, semisolid, or solid material and are usually benign.
- Fibroid tumors (myomas, leiomyomas) are benign but may have to be removed because they can compress abdominal structures and lead to infertility, crowding, and malpositioning of the fetus during pregnancy and degenerative changes related to interruption of blood supply.
- Herniation of the bladder (called cystocele) or of the rectum (rectocele) into the vagina can disrupt urinary and bowel function and is often corrected surgically.
- Nursing diagnoses after surgery for correction of a cystocele or rectocele may include impaired urinary elimination, risk for injury, and acute pain.
- Uterine prolapse, the descent of the uterus into the vagina, may be treated with corrective surgery or vaginal hysterectomy.
- Abnormal uterine positions include retroversion (backward tilt), retroflexion (uterine body bends backward), anteversion (forward tilt), and anteflexion (uterine body bends forward); these conditions rarely require treatment.
- Breast cancer is the most prevalent form of cancer in American women. It has a 5-year survival rate of more than 90% when detected early.
- After mastectomy, nursing diagnoses may include risk for injury, impaired physical mobility, risk for infection, disturbed body image, and ineffective sexuality patterns.

- Cervical cancer can be detected early by regular pelvic examinations and Papanicolaou smears. Prompt treatment is usually curative.
- Ovarian cancer has the highest mortality rate of all female reproductive system cancers because it is asymptomatic in the early stages.
- Nursing diagnoses [illegible] productive syste[illegible] turbed body ima[illegible] fective family c[illegible] risk for injury.
- Infertility, the ina[illegible] sometimes be[illegible]

REVIEW QUESTIONS

1. The site of fertilization is in the:
   1. uterus.
   2. ovary.
   3. fallopian tube.
   4. vagina.
2. Which question in the health assessment provides information about the patient's menarche?
   1. At what age did you begin menstruating?
   2. Would you describe your menstrual flow as light or heavy?
   3. What was your age when you first experienced hot flashes?
   4. Do you usually have any changes in mood before your menstrual period?
3. To prepare a patient for culdoscopy, the nurse should tell her:
   1. You will be positioned as if you were having a routine pelvic examination.
   2. You will have no restrictions following the procedure.
   3. You will need to return in a week to have your sutures removed.
   4. You may have shoulder pain caused by air entering the pelvic cavity.
4. You are teaching a class on breast self-examination (BSE) to women of various ages. What should you tell women who no longer menstruate about BSE?
   1. BSE is not necessary once a woman is menopausal.
   2. Perform BSE on the same day of each month.
   3. Older women should perform BSE every day.
   4. Mammograms are only needed if you discover a lump.
5. A young woman has come to the doctor's office for a routine pelvic examination. During the health history, she tells you that her mother says douching is an essential part of feminine hygiene. What is the best response?
   1. Your body has normal processes to cleanse the vagina so douching is unnecessary.
   2. Douching is not really necessary, but it is a harmless procedure.
   3. There are no medically appropriate reasons for douching.
   4. Douching is safe if sterile solution is used.
6. Which org[illegible] pelvic infl[illegible]
   1. *Neisseria go[illegible]*
   2. *Chlamydia trachomatis*
   3. *Mycoplasma hominis*
   4. *Escherichia coli*
7. A patient completed a 6-month course of danazol (Danocrine) for treatment of endometriosis. She would like to become pregnant. You should emphasize which of the following?
   1. She will begin menstrual bleeding within one week after stopping the danazol.
   2. Her best chances of pregnancy are in the first month after completing danazol therapy.
   3. She should not become pregnant for one month because danazol can cause birth defects.
   4. She is unlikely to become pregnant for at least one year after taking danazol.
8. An elderly woman with uterine prolapse is being fitted with a pessary. What information should be included in the teaching plan?
   1. The pessary permanently corrects the uterine prolapse.
   2. Once the pessary is in place, no further care is needed.
   3. There are no complications associated with pessaries.
   4. The position of the pessary must be checked in 24 hours.
9. Which palpable breast lump is most characteristic of breast cancer?
   1. A single painless lump in the upper, upper outer quadrant of one breast
   2. A firm, painful lump that feels oval-shaped, and is freely movable
   3. Bilateral multiple small lumps that are tender just before menstruation
   4. Soft painless symmetric lumps in the lower outer quadrant of both breasts
10. Assessment of a new clinic patient provides the following data: 30-year-old female, menarche at age 10, first sexual intercourse at age 14, treated for chlamydia at age 15 and gonorrhea at age 17. You recognize that she is at increased risk for:
    1. breast cancer.
    2. uterine prolapse.
    3. cervical cancer.
    4. fibroid tumors.

ale Reproductive Disorders

objectives

1. Describe the major structures and functions of the normal male reproductive system.
2. Identify data to be collected when assessing a male patient with a reproductive system disorder.
3. Discuss commonly performed diagnostic tests and procedures and the nursing implications of each.
4. Identify common therapeutic measures used to treat disorders of the male reproductive system and the nursing implications of each.
5. For selected disorders of the male reproductive system, explain the pathophysiology, signs and symptoms, complications, medical diagnosis, and medical treatment.
6. Assist in developing a nursing care plan for a male patient with a reproductive system disorder.

key terms

Corpus (*pl.* corpora) cavernosa (KŎR-pŭs, KŎR-pō-ră, p. 970)
Ejaculation (ē-jăk-ū-LĀ-shŭn, p. 971)
Emission (ē-MĬSH-ŭn, p. 971)
Epididymitis (ĕp-ĭ-dĭd-ĕ-MĪ-tĭs, p. 978)
Erectile dysfunction (ĕ-RĔK-tīl dĭs-FŬNK-shŭn, p. 972)
Erection (ĕ-RĔK-shŭn, p. 969)
Hematocele (HĔM-ăh-tō-sēl, p. 973)
Hydrocele (HĪ-drō-sēl, p. 976)
Infertility (ĭn-fĕr-TĬL-ĭ-tē, p. 988)
Phimosis (fī-MŌ-sĭs, p. 987)
Prostatectomy (prŏs-tă-TĔK-tō-mē, p. 979)
Prostatitis (prŏs-tă-TĪ-tĭs, p. 976)
Smegma (SMĔG-mă, p. 973)
Sterile (STĔR-ĭl, p. 979)
Testis (*pl.* testes) (TĔS-tĭs, TĔS-tēz, p. 968)

ANATOMY AND PHYSIOLOGY OF THE MALE REPRODUCTIVE SYSTEM

ANATOMY

The male reproductive system consists of the scrotum, testes, epididymis, vas deferens, seminal vesicles, prostate gland, ejaculatory duct, internal urethra, and penis (Fig. 46-1).

Scrotum

The scrotum is a thin pendulous sac on the outside of the body that encloses each of the two testicles in separate compartments. The scrotum contracts into thick folds during fear, anger, arousal, or cold, drawing the testes close to the body for protection and insulation. On warm days the scrotal muscles relax and allow the scrotum to hang free of the body. Sweat glands may be activated to cool the testes and maintain a testicular temperature that is below body temperature.

Testes

The two testes (testicles) are the male reproductive organs. They lie within the scrotum, suspended from the spermatic cord (Fig. 46-2). They are composed of numerous highly coiled seminiferous tubules that produce spermatozoa and sex hormones. The testicles develop in the embryo at about the seventh week of gestation and begin producing small amounts of testosterone. Secretion of this male hormone results in the development of other male reproductive organs and causes the testes to descend into the scrotum during the last 2 months of gestation. At around 10 to 13 years of age, during puberty, the increased production of testosterone results in the production of sperm and the development of body hair, muscle mass, and other secondary sex characteristics.

Epididymis

Newly developed sperm move from each testicle through the epididymis, a coiled tubule almost 20 feet long that rests along the top and side of the testes. This passage may take several days and allows the sperm to mature and develop the capability for motility (movement) and fertilization (see Fig. 46-2).

Vas Deferens

As mature sperm leave the epididymis, they enter the vasa deferentia (*sing.*, deferens), which are tubes of secretory ducts that serve as the primary storage sites for sperm, contribute to the fluid content of semen, and contract to help propel the mature sperm into the urethra during ejaculation. The vas deferens is bundled together with the spermatic artery and veins, lymphatic vessels, and nerves by the spermatic cord; the bundle exits the scrotum and enters the pelvic cavity via the inguinal canal (see Figs. 46-1 and 46-2).

Seminal Vesicles

The seminal vesicles are hollow, twisted, tubular secretory glands located on the posterior surface of the bladder. They pro-

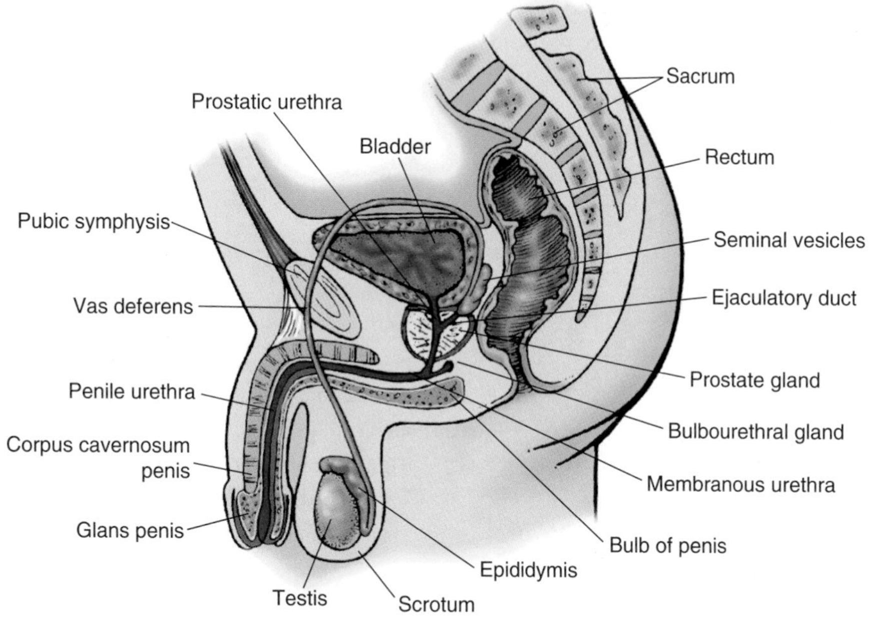

FIGURE **46-1** Male reproductive system.

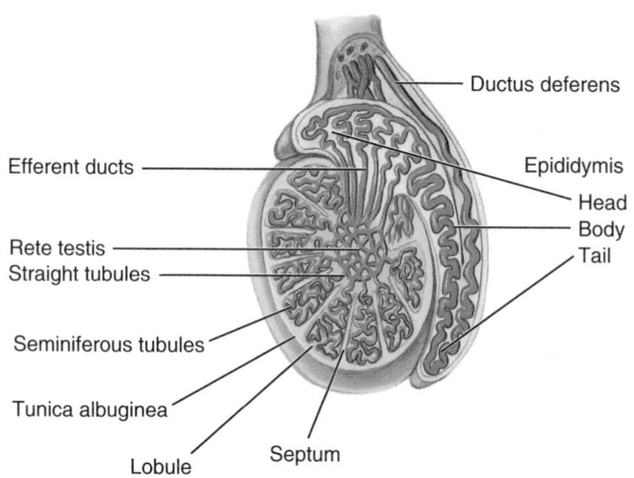

FIGURE **46-2** Basic structures of a testis.

duce a mucoid fluid that constitutes about 60% of the volume of the semen and provides nutrients and hormones important for motility and successful fertilization (Figs. 46-1 and 46-3).

Prostate Gland

The prostate is a walnut-sized fibromuscular gland that surrounds the neck of the urinary bladder and the first inch of the internal urethra. The prostate produces a thin, milky, alkaline liquid that enhances the motility and fertility of the sperm and contracts to propel semen into the urethra during ejaculation (see Fig. 46-3).

Cowper's Glands

Cowper's glands (bulbourethral glands) are pea-sized structures, located just below the prostate, that secrete a clear mucus into the urethra. The secretion contributes little to semen volume but provides lubrication during sexual arousal.

Urethra

The urethra extends from the bladder to the urinary meatus at the end of the penis. The vas deferens and the seminal vesicles come together to form the ejaculatory duct, which passes through the prostate and empties into the internal urethra. The sperm and fluids from the vasa deferentia, seminal vesicles, and prostate are propelled through the ejaculatory duct into the penile urethra during ejaculation. Although the urethra serves to empty urine from the bladder and provide outflow for semen during ejaculation, urine and semen are never in the urethra at the same time.

Penis

The external penis in its flaccid state is a soft, round cylinder of spongy tissue ending in an acorn-shaped tip known as the glans. The glans has a sensitive ridge at its base called the corona that gives rise to a hood or foreskin. In uncircumcised men, the foreskin can be rolled back to expose the glans. About one-half of the penis extends within the body toward the anus and attaches to the pelvis. Two corpora cavernosa lie on the upper side of the penis. These erectile chambers provide a huge surface area for the inflow of blood and blood storage, which results in expansion of the penis during sexual arousal, called an **erection.** The corpus spongiosum on the underside of the penis surrounds the urethra and supplies blood to the glans (Fig. 46-4).

PHYSIOLOGY

Spermatogenesis

Sperm are produced in the seminiferous tubules of the testes from about age 13 throughout the remainder of life. Testosterone is believed to set in motion the division of germinal

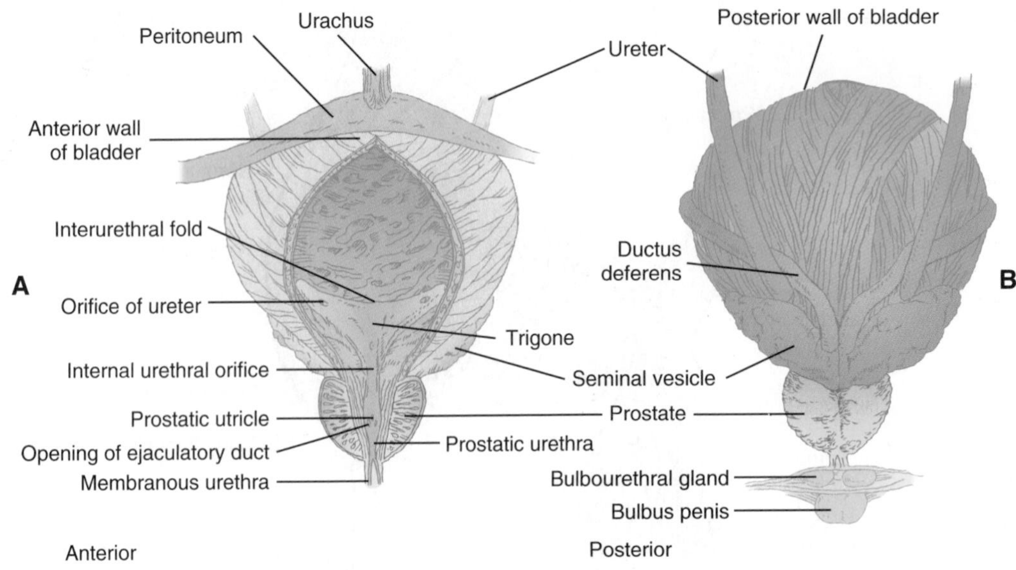

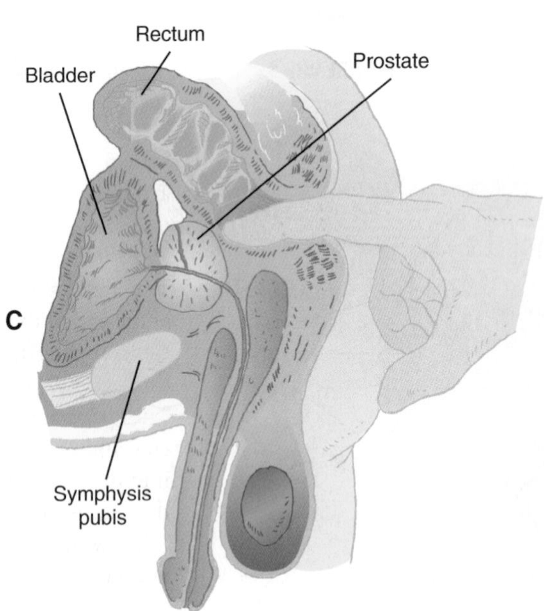

FIGURE **46-3** *A* and *B*, Anterior and posterior views of the prostate gland. *C*, Diagrammatic representation of the anatomic position of the prostate gland. It surrounds the urethra at the base of the bladder.

cells into spermatocytes, which subsequently develop into sperm. The process may take 75 days.

The cooling function of the scrotum is essential for spermatogenesis. An increase in testicular temperature may cause degeneration of some of the cells of the seminiferous tubules and may contribute to sterility.

Cryptorchidism, or failure of the testicles to descend from the abdomen into the cooler scrotum, may result in sterility. Incomplete or partial descent of the testicles may be resolved by surgical assistance before maturity, but if fetal testes are abnormally formed and do not secrete enough testosterone to cause the testicles to descend into the scrotum, surgical intervention is unlikely to be successful. The tubular epithelium of testes that remain in the warm abdomen degenerates completely and is incapable of producing sperm.

Erection

For the penis to become erect, it must have a high-pressure supply of arterial blood, a means of relaxing the smooth muscle tissue of the cavernosal arterioles, and a functioning blood storage mechanism to keep the blood in the penis long enough for sexual function. The blood pressure in the flaccid corpus cavernosa is about 6 to 8 mm Hg, very low when compared with the 120/90 mm Hg blood pressure in the arm or cavernosal artery.

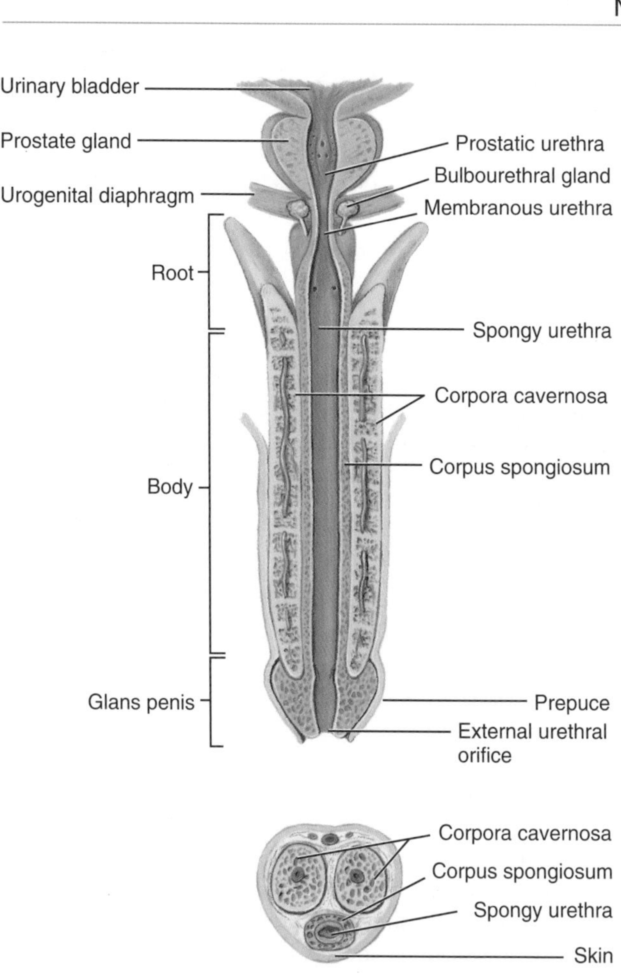

FIGURE **46-4** Cross section of the penis.

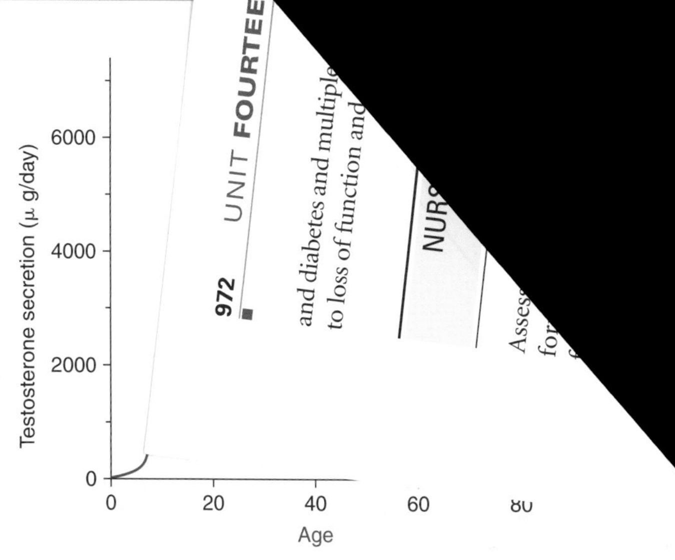

FIGURE **46-5** Testosterone secretion by age.

During sexual arousal, parasympathetic nerves release neurotransmitters that cause the cavernosal arteriole walls to relax. This allows the relatively high-pressure arterial blood to flood the sinuses of the erectile chambers, increasing the blood volume of the penis to eight to ten times the flaccid volume and raising the cavernosal blood pressure to approximately the same as arterial blood pressure.

The blood storage mechanism for the penis is unique. The cavernosal artery is buried deep in the erectile chambers, causing them to fill from the inside. The venules that drain blood from the erectile chambers are near the surface and are compressed against the outer coat of the chambers during engorgement. The elastic limitations of this covering severely decrease the drainage of blood from the chamber sinuses and maintain the erection. After stimulation ceases or ejaculation occurs, sympathetic nerves release constricting neurotransmitters that narrow the arteriole walls and decrease the inflow of blood. As the cavernosal pressure decreases, drainage increases and the penis returns to a flaccid state.

Emission and Ejaculation

The male sex act culminates in emission and ejaculation. Emission is the result of sympathetic stimulation leaving the spinal cord at L1 and L2. The pudendal nerve communicates with the spinal cord at S2 and S3 and affects motor responses for ejaculation. Physical stimulation of internal and external sex organs initiates contractions of the vasa deferentia and prostatic capsule. The contractions move sperm to the ejaculatory ducts and expel them into the internal urethra. There they mix with prostatic and seminal fluids and are propelled forward through the penile urethra. The filling of the urethra excites nerves in the sacral region of the spinal cord to initiate rhythmic muscular contractions of the internal genital organs, pelvis, and body trunk and results in ejaculation (expulsion) of semen.

Although psychic stimulation is not essential to the male sex act, it is an enhancing factor and should be considered in the physiology. Experience, culture, and self-development influence the impact of visual, fantasy, and dream stimulation on sexual sensation and nocturnal erections and emissions.

AGE-RELATED CHANGES IN THE MALE REPRODUCTIVE SYSTEM

Normal aging produces several changes in the male reproductive system. Testosterone production continues throughout life after puberty but decreases rapidly after the age of 50 (Fig. 46-5). This phenomenon has been called the male climacteric and may be associated with symptoms of hot flashes, feelings of suffocation, and psychic disorders similar to those of menopause. These symptoms may be relieved by the administration of testosterone and other androgens.

Many men believe they are too old for sex, and when this belief is supported by functional decline, they may lose interest or become depressed. Men in their late forties and early fifties may be slower to arouse and have a longer refractory period between erections, but in a healthy man, spermatogenesis and the ability to have erections last a lifetime. Changes in lifestyle related to alcohol consumption, dietary habits, exercise, and the complexities of managing chronic conditions such as hypertension

medication therapies also contribute satisfactory sexual activities.

SING ASSESSMENT OF THE MALE REPRODUCTIVE SYSTEM

sment of the male reproductive system should elicit in- mation on changes in the patient's health status, sexual unction, and sexual relationships, as well as the patient's knowledge level and ability for self-care. The extent of the nursing assessment of the male reproductive system depends on the nurse's education, experience, and role in the setting. This section describes a complete nursing assessment, although some aspects may be performed only by an examiner with advanced training.

The interview and physical assessment may be particularly difficult for some male patients because of health beliefs, the need for privacy, or defensiveness about behaviors. It is important to allow the patient to tell his own story and maintain as much control over the environment and experience as possible. Establishing a comfortable relationship with the patient is most successful if open-ended questions are used. Avoid questions beginning with "why?" Leave sensitive questions until later in the interview. It is helpful to empathize with the patient and gently pin him down about details, but it is also very important to avoid commenting on how you think he should feel or behave. Do not jump to conclusions too early or bias his story by adding your professional opinion.

HEALTH HISTORY

Present Illness

Begin the health history with a detailed description of the current problem. Complaints may include pain, weight loss, infertility, **erectile dysfunction** (impotence), alteration in self-image, scrotal masses, penile discharge, or skin lesions. If the symptoms are acute, obtain detailed information about the onset and development of the problem and about activities related to the symptoms. If the patient has pain, use descriptors such as pain scales. If the problem is a chronic one, determine what made the patient seek help at this time and what his expectations are for care.

Past Medical History

The past medical history helps to link the current problem with previous symptoms, injuries, diseases, operations, or allergies and the treatments or medications prescribed for them. Question the patient about his management of chronic health problems such as diabetes, thyroid or pituitary dysfunction, cardiovascular disease, neurologic injury or disease, and addictive behavior. Because trauma to the groin or perineum may be related to diseases of the urethra and/or penile circulation. inquire about childhood injuries or accidents. Spinal cord injuries are significant because the level of the injury dictates specific types of sexual dysfunctions.

Patients who are reluctant to discuss what many consider to be the most private part of their lives and selves also may be unwilling to do regular self-examinations or comply with recommended self-care regimens. Thoughtfully planned questioning provides clues about knowledge deficits and patient participation in health management. This information is important in developing plans for care that include the patient and his family or significant other and require their cooperation.

Family History

In the family history, note the age and health or age at death of parents, grandparents, and siblings. In addition, note any history in family members of cancer, diabetes, hypertension, stroke, and blood disorders such as sickle cell anemia and hemophilia.

Review of Systems

Review of all systems with a focus on male reproductive system disorders begins with an assessment of the patient's general health. Ask questions about changes in appetite, weight, exercise or activity level, and the management of daily self-care to reveal general changes in health status that may affect the reproductive system.

Ask the patient about changes in the skin, including lesions, drainage, bleeding, itching, or pain. If the patient has itching or pain, inquire whether it is intermittent or continuous and whether it has any relationship to specific activities or time. Encourage the patient to use descriptive terms, such as "stinging" or "aching," and ask him to indicate the intensity on a scale from 1 to 10.

Review the circulatory and pulmonary systems to obtain information about hypertension, cardiac or pulmonary disease, and exercise tolerance. Establish the relationship of these symptoms or problems to work and normal activity.

Symptoms of possible endocrine dysfunction are important because undiagnosed or poorly managed endocrine disorders may have a direct and devastating impact on sexual function, sterility, and self-image for the male patient. Ask questions about fatigue, nervousness, heat or cold intolerance, polyphagia, polydipsia, polyuria, and medications taken for pituitary or thyroid conditions.

Review of the musculoskeletal and nervous systems should include questions about weakness, paralysis, coordination problems, joint pain or stiffness, mood changes, and depression.

The health history should note medications the patient is taking because many drugs, including a number of antihypertensives, can impair sexual function.

Functional Assessment

The functional assessment elicits information about diet, usual activities, sleep and rest, medications, and the use of tobacco, alcohol, and illicit drugs. Record sources of stress and coping strategies. Once you establish a therapeutic relationship with the patient, you also should cover the interest level and satisfaction of sexual relationships. Questions may include the frequency of intercourse, the ability to have and maintain an erection, the desire and ability to have children, and the relationship of sexual function to self-image.

PHYSICAL EXAMINATION

The physical examination of the male reproductive system is accomplished by inspection and palpation. Sharing normal findings, involving the patient in the examination, proper draping, and using an unhurried manner increase the patient's comfort level. Have the patient empty the bladder before the examination and collect a urine specimen if needed. Always wear gloves to examine the genitals.

Measure the patient's height, weight, and vital signs and observe his general appearance. Inspect the skin for lesions or discolorations and the breasts for gynecomastia (enlargement). For the examination of the genitals, the patient may be standing or supine with the legs slightly spread. Inspect the distribution of the pubic hair, which is normally distributed in a diamond-shaped area across the symphysis pubis, covering the base of the penis and spreading along the inner thighs. Palpate the lower abdomen and groin for masses. The skin of the external organs and perineum should be warm, dry, and free of lesions, edema, and odor.

Penis

The normal flaccid penis is semisoft and straight. Note the size, shape, and appearance of the penis. Palpate for nodules, swelling, and lesions. If the patient is uncircumcised, retract the foreskin to observe the glans (Fig. 46-6). There may be a small amount of white, thick, odoriferous **smegma** (sebaceous secretion) between the glans and the foreskin. The urethral meatus should be at the tip of the penis. Gently squeezing the glans opens the meatus so that it can be observed for signs of irritation, infection, or discharge. If there is any discharge from lesions or the urethra, be prepared to collect a specimen for culture.

Scrotum

The skin of the scrotum should be slightly darker in color, wrinkled, and loose. Because the scrotum is close to the body and may not be well ventilated, it is important to look for irritation from heat and moisture, fungal infections, abscesses, and parasites.

Palpate the right a
and left testes, epidi
for the testes to re
touched or cooled;
warming. The left
should be oval in s
or tenderness. Old
It is important, es
there are two teste

The epididym
and extends dow
pated with the t
tender but withou
begins at the lower pole of each testicle and ex
toward the inguinal canal. It is a small cord-like structure that feels firmer than the epididymis. It should show no thickening or asymmetry.

If thickening, nodules, masses, or asymmetric conditions are discovered, they can be further investigated by shining a light through the scrotum in a darkened room, a technique called transillumination (Fig. 46-7). Hydrocele, a mass filled with serous fluid, glows red in the light. If the mass is solid (such as a **hematocele** or tumor), no light passes through it, making it appear as a dark shadow.

Examination for protrusion of the bowel through the inguinal wall or canal (hernia) should be done while the patient is standing. Inspect the lower abdomen, groin, and upper scrotal area for bulges while the patient stands quietly and again when straining as if to have a bowel movement. The practitioner with advanced training is able to palpate inguinal hernias by reaching up through the scrotum into the inguinal canal. Abnormal findings should be noted and referred to a physician.

The advanced practitioner or physician also examines the prostate gland by inserting the examining finger through the anus toward the anterior wall of the rectum. The normal prostate lies 2 to 5 cm beyond the rectal sphincter and feels smooth, rubbery, and firm. Increased firmness and enlargement of the prostate gland may indicate benign hypertrophy; a tender,

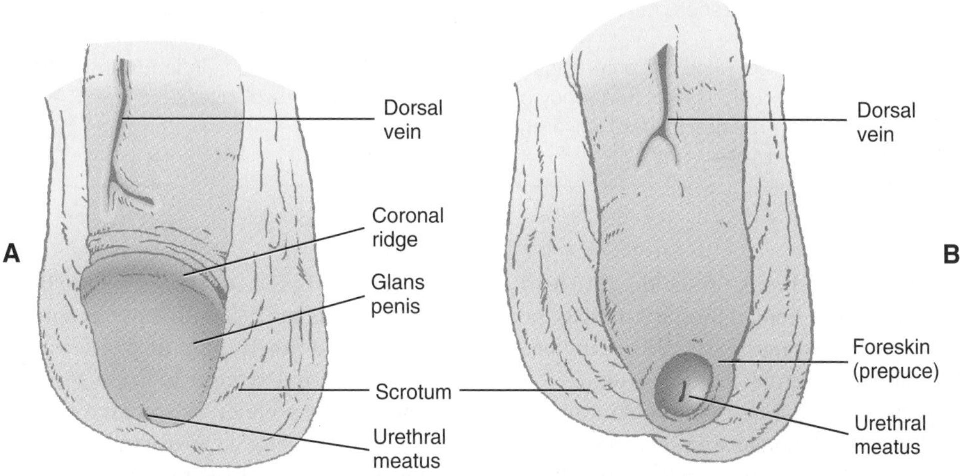

FIGURE **46-6** Appearance of the penis. *A,* Circumcised. *B,* Uncircumcised.

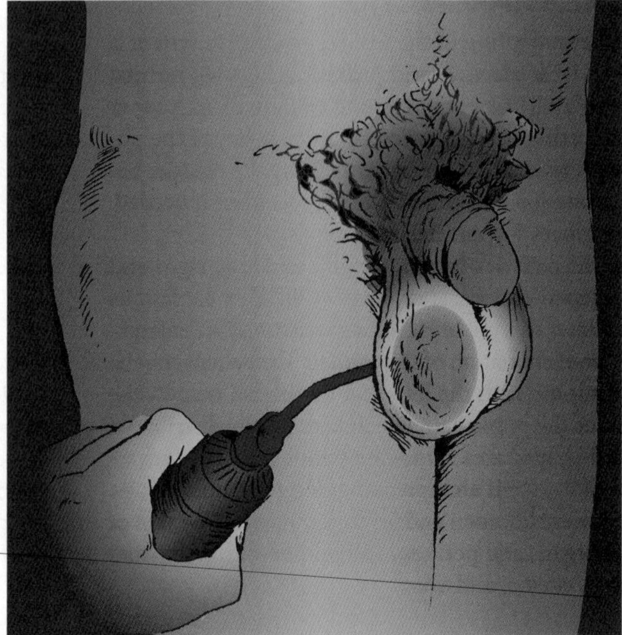

FIGURE **46-7** Transillumination of the scrotum.

table 46-1 **ASSESSMENT *of the Male Reproductive System***

HEALTH HISTORY

Present Illness: Pain, weight loss, infertility, erectile dysfunction, scrotal mass, penile discharge, lesions
Past Medical History: Previous injuries, diseases, or surgeries
Chronic Illnesses: Diabetes mellitus, cardiovascular disease, addictive behavior
Allergies
Current Medications
Family History: Diabetes, hypertension, stroke, blood disorders, cancer
Review of Systems:
General Health State: Changes in appetite, weight, activity, self-care
Skin: Lesions, drainage, bleeding, itching, pain
Cardiovascular: Edema
Respiratory: Cough, dyspnea
Endocrine: Fatigue, heat or cold intolerance, nervousness
Nervous: Paralysis
Genitourinary: Changes in urination or urine characteristics
Sexual Function: Interest in sexual relationship, frequency of intercourse, erectile dysfunction, desire to have children, effect of sexual function on self-image

HEALTH HISTORY—cont'd

Functional Assessment:
Usual Day: Occupation, home roles and responsibilities, diet, rest
Use of Tobacco and Alcohol
Stressors and Coping Strategies
Sexual Relationships

PHYSICAL EXAMINATION

Vital Signs
General Appearance of Genitalia: Skin lesions or discoloration, hair distribution
Penis: Size, shape, skin lesions, discharge, position of urinary meatus, nodules, swelling
Scrotum: Color, edema, irritation, presence of testicles, testicular tenderness or masses
Inguinal Hernia
Prostate: Size, texture, masses
Perineum: Color, lesions
Anus: Lesions, irritation, inflammation, fissures, abscesses, hemorrhoids, prolapse

boggy feeling may be the result of chronic prostatitis; and a hard prostate may harbor malignancy. Should prostatic massage be necessary, the examiner should be prepared to collect secretions from the meatus for culture or microscopic examination.

The skin of the perineum is darker than the skin on the buttocks and should be intact. The anal area has more coarse skin and is moist and without hair. Inspect the area for lesions, irritation, inflammation, fissures, abscesses, and dilated veins (hemorrhoids). Ask the patient to bear down, and reinspect the anus for rectal prolapse or internal hemorrhoids. The advanced practitioner or physician examines the anal canal with an index finger to assess for resistance, bleeding, sphincter tone, nodules, or polyps. A stool specimen may be tested for occult blood when appropriate.

The assessment of the male reproductive system is summarized in Table 46-1.

DIAGNOSTIC TESTS AND PROCEDURES

Diagnostic tests and procedures for disorders of the male reproductive system include laboratory studies and radiologic imaging procedures.

LABORATORY STUDIES

Semen Analysis

Analysis of the semen may be done to assess male fertility or to document sterilization after a vasectomy. The analysis may include gross evaluation of semen for volume, thickness, color, and pH, and microscopic evaluation of the sperm for count, motility, shape, and ability to penetrate cervical mucus. More sophisticated testing also can determine the presence of serum antibodies and genetic abnormalities. Sperm count varies from day to day and should be repeated for data to be reliable. Men with very high or very low counts are often infertile and should be evaluated for pituitary, thyroid, adrenal, or testicular dysfunctions.

Instruct the patient to abstain from sexual activity for 3 to 5 days and then collect a semen specimen in a clean container. Discourage patients from prolonged abstinence, as it may result in diminished quality and motility of the sperm. If the patient is unable to collect the specimen in the physician's office or laboratory by masturbating, it may be collected at home by using a plastic condom or coitus interruptus. Rubber condoms should not be used because the powders and lubricants used in their manufacture may be spermicidal. The specimen should be kept at room temperature, protected from heat or cold, and brought to the lab within 1 hour after collection.

Endocrinologic Studies

The endocrine system secretes hormones directly into the blood that regulate metabolism, growth, stress response, and reproduction (gonadotropins). The serum levels of these hormones can be determined from blood drawn from the patient without special preparation.

Luteinizing hormone is secreted by the anterior pituitary gland and causes stimulation of special cells (Leydig cells) in the testes to produce testosterone. As testosterone is produced, a negative feedback system reduces the amount of luteinizing hormone secreted by the pituitary. Below-normal levels of testosterone result in abnormally high levels of serum luteinizing hormone. This indicates an effort by the pituitary to stimulate Leydig cell function and return testosterone levels to normal.

Prolactin, another hormone secreted by the anterior pituitary gland, is closely related to luteinizing hormone. It has a potentiating effect on testosterone production. In some patients, when endocrine function is in question, serum prolactin levels may be tested. Secretion of prolactin is controlled by a negative feedback system. Above-normal levels of prolactin may be caused by a benign pituitary tumor and may result in gynecomastia in the male patient.

Follicle-stimulating hormone is secreted by the anterior pituitary gland and causes stimulation of cells (Sertoli cells) in the seminiferous tubules of the testes to complete the formation (spermiation) and maturation of sperm. Oversecretion of follicle-stimulating hormone is prevented and a constant level of sperm production is maintained by the negative feedback system. Below-normal levels of sperm result in increased secretion of follicle-stimulating hormone from the pituitary gland and high serum levels of follicle-stimulating hormone. Spermatogenesis results in decreased excretion of follicle-stimulating hormone and normal serum levels.

Testosterone is secreted by Leydig cells in the interstitium of the testes. Below-normal levels of testosterone may be the result of hypothalamic or pituitary dysfunction or seminiferous tubule destruction. High levels of testosterone are produced in newborn male infants, in males after puberty, and in the presence of testicular tumors that develop from Leydig cells. Lower serum levels of testosterone may be expected as the male patient ages.

Tumor Markers

Tumor markers are substances found in the serum of cancer patients. When used in conjunction with other diagnostic tools, they can be helpful in diagnosing cancer, estimating the degree of cancer development, predicting the effect of treatment, and monitoring the effect of treatment on the cancer or the return of cancer after treatment. There is no special preparation for these tests.

General Laboratory Studies

Urinalysis provides information about infection of the genitourinary tract, the presence or degree of control of diabetes, and kidney function. Samples should be clean catches unless the patient is unable to collect the urine without contamination. If appropriate instruction is given for collection, there is no need for other patient preparation. If the patient is unable to properly clean himself, cannot see well enough, or is not able to understand the instructions, it may be necessary to obtain a specimen by catheterization.

Blood studies may include a complete blood cell count to establish baseline data and provide information in forming a diagnosis when anemia or bone metastases are suspected. Alkaline phosphatase and serum calcium levels also may be measured because they increase with metastasis to bone (Table 46-2). The acid phosphatase level also may be increased with prostate cancer and with bone metastasis. Prostate-specific antigen (PSA) levels may be increased with cancer of the prostate. Thyroid function studies may be done in patients with erectile dysfunctions. Low thyroid hormone levels may result in loss of libido; high thyroid hormone levels may cause erectile dysfunction. No special preparation for these tests is usually necessary. Blood glucose levels may be determined when diabetes mellitus is a concern, and patients should be fasting for the test. The venipuncture site should be observed for bleeding and dressed with a small pressure bandage on completion of sample collection.

RADIOLOGIC IMAGING STUDIES

Computed tomography may be used in assessing metastatic testicular and prostatic tumors. Ultrasound may be used to

table 46-2 Laboratory Tests for Male Reproductive Disorders

TEST	REFERENCE VALUES	CONDITION IN WHICH LEVELS ARE ALTERED
HEMATOLOGIC TESTS (CBC)		
Hemoglobin	4-18 gm/dL	↓ In anemia; nonspecific; may indicate malignancy
Hematocrit	40%-50%	↓ In anemia; nonspecific; may indicate malignancy
Leukocytes (WBC)	4,800-11,000/mm^3	↓ In metastatic bone disease
Neutrophils	54%-62%	↓ In bone marrow depression
Lymphocytes	25%-30%	↓ In bone marrow depression
Eosinophils	1%-3%	↓ In bone marrow depression
Platelets	150,000-300,000/mm^3	↓ In bone marrow depression
BLOOD/SERUM TESTS		
Acid phosphatase	0.11-0.60 mU/ml	↑ In metastatic prostate cancer
Alkaline phosphatase	20-90 mU/ml	↑ In cancer of bone or bone metastases, liver cancer
Calcium	9.0-11.0 mg/dL	↑ In bone metastasis
TESTS FOR TUMOR MARKERS		
AFP	<10 ng/ml	↑ In nonseminomatous testicular cancer
CEA	0-2.5 ng/ml nonsmokers	↑ In prostate cancer
HCG	0.5 IU/L	↑ In germ cell testicular cancer
Prostatic acid phosphatase	0.26-0.83 U/L	↑ In metastatic prostate cancer
PSA	0-4 ng/ml	↑ In prostate cancer

Modified from Black, J. M., & Matassarin-Jacobs, E. (1993). *Luckmann and Sorensen's medical-surgical nursing: A psychophysiologic approach* (4th ed., pp. 496-497). Philadelphia: Saunders.

CBC, Complete blood cell count; *WBC*, white blood cells; *AFP*, alpha-fetoprotein; *CEA*, carcinoembryonic antigen; *hCG*, human chorionic gonadotropin; *PSA*, prostate-specific antigen.

examine scrotal masses or define prostatic lesions. Examination of the prostate is done via the rectum.

Radionuclide imaging may be done to assess testicular abnormalities such as torsion, tumors, abscesses, epididymitis, or **hydroceles**. Radioactive substances are injected intravenously or given orally. After a waiting period to allow for distribution of the substance throughout the body, scans are done to locate organs and tissues that have increased concentrations of the isotopes due to abnormal tissue metabolism.

Diagnostic tests and procedures and related nursing care are summarized in Table 46-3.

DISORDERS OF THE MALE REPRODUCTIVE SYSTEM

INFECTIONS AND INFLAMMATORY CONDITIONS

Infections of the male reproductive system may be caused by bacteria, viruses, protozoa, fungi, and ectoparasites that can be acquired through sexual contact. Sexually transmitted diseases are covered in Chapter 47. The most common inflammatory conditions are prostatitis and epididymitis. Orchitis is rare but important because it can cause sterility.

Prostatitis

Prostatitis is inflammation of the prostate gland. It may be caused by bacterial infection, but when no pathogens can be detected, the condition is classified as nonbacterial prostatitis. Bacterial prostatitis can be acute or chronic. The cause of nonbacterial prostatitis is uncertain. Diagnosis is based on the patient's complaints confirmed by laboratory studies of prostatic secretions. Signs and symptoms of acute inflammation are swelling, warmth, and tenderness. The patient also may have dysuria, frequency, hematuria, and foul-smelling urine. Patients with chronic inflammation may have minimal symptoms or malaise.

Acute and chronic bacterial prostatitis are treated with antibiotics, analgesics, and sitz baths. The current drug of choice is a 6-week course of a fluoroquinolone. The patient is advised to increase fluid intake and to rest. Stool softeners may be prescribed to prevent constipation, which is especially painful with prostatitis. Catheterization is avoided because it may cause further infection, but it may be necessary if the patient has difficulty voiding.

Nonbacterial prostatitis may be treated with a single daily dose of an alpha-adrenergic blocker to improve voiding by relaxing the bladder neck and prostate. Symptoms are managed with analgesics, anti-inflammatory agents, and sitz baths.

Most patients with prostatitis are treated as outpatients, but hospital admission may be indicated if a high fever is present or if catheterization or parenteral antibiotic therapy is needed. Assess the patient's comfort and administer analgesics and other treatments as ordered. If the patient is discharged with medications, provide instructions and information about the drugs.

table 46-3 **DIAGNOSTIC TESTS AND PROCEDURES | *Male Reproductive System***

TEST/PURPOSE	PATIENT PREPARATION	POSTPROCEDURE NURSING CARE
Mumps test Determines whether a person is susceptible or resistant to the mumps virus. An antigen is injected intradermally; the site is marked with waterproof ink and examined after 48 hr to detect an immune response.	Inform the patient that an injection will be given under the skin to determine if he has resistance to mumps. He must not wash off the marking, and he must return in 48 hr to have the results read.	To read the test, examine the site for redness and swelling after 48 hr. A red area larger than 10 mm in diameter is a positive result and indicates susceptibility to mumps. A negative result indicates resistance.
Cystoscopy Uses a lighted instrument inserted through the urethra to visualize the urethra, bladder, and prostatic urethra. May detect prostatic hypertrophy, bladder tumors.	Routine preoperative measures are indicated (signed consent form, skin scrub, food restriction). Antibiotics may be prescribed. Inform the patient the procedure is done in a special room under sterile conditions. Local anesthetic is instilled in the urethra and a sedative is given intravenously (IV).	Measure urine output for 24 hr. Urine will be pink tinged. Report excessive bleeding or inability to void promptly. Encourage fluid intake when patient is voiding well. Burning and hesitancy are common for several days. Give antibiotics as ordered.
Urethral smears and stains Prepares a small amount of material for microscopic study to detect sexually transmitted diseases and identify pathogens. The physician may massage the prostate to increase the organisms in the urethra.	Tell patient a sterile swab will be inserted into the urethra to obtain a specimen. Specimens also may be obtained from the anal canal and pharynx. Use standard precautions to handle body fluids and contaminated instruments. Collect the specimen for culture before beginning prescribed antimicrobials.	Prepare specimens and send them to the laboratory.
Cultures of organisms (obtained from a source being tested) Permits identification of pathogens and susceptibility to various antimicrobials.	Explain specimen collection process.	Prepare specimens according to laboratory protocol. Send to laboratory.
Serum acid phosphatase Detects elevations associated with metastatic prostate cancer and many other conditions. Used to assess effects of treatment for prostate cancer.	Inform patient that a venous blood sample will be drawn.	Assess venipuncture site for bleeding. Apply small dressing.
Semen analysis Examines a semen specimen to assess male fertility or to document sterilization after vasectomy.	Instruct patient to abstain from sexual activity for 3-5 days, then collect specimen in a clean container. Rubber condoms should not be used. Specimen should be kept at room temperature and brought to the lab within 1 hr.	No special care needed.
Endocrinologic studies (luteinizing hormone, prolactin, follicle-stimulating hormone, testosterone) Assess level of hormones needed for sexual development and function.	Tell the patient that a venous blood sample will be drawn.	Assess the venipuncture site for bleeding. Apply small dressing.

Continued

table 46-3 **DIAGNOSTIC TESTS AND PROCEDURES | *Male Reproductive System—cont'd***

TEST/PURPOSE	PATIENT PREPARATION	POSTPROCEDURE NURSING CARE
Tumor markers (e.g., serum prostate-specific antigen)		
Detects increases that may be associated with prostatic cancer, prostatic hypertrophy, cirrhosis, osteoporosis, and a number of other conditions.	Patient should fast for 8 hr before the test. Tell patient a venous blood sample will be drawn.	Assess the venipuncture site for oozing or hematoma. Apply small dressing.
Computed tomography		
Creates images of internal structures to locate or assess testicular and prostatic tumors.	Assess allergy to iodine or seafood if contrast dye will be injected. Report allergy to radiologist. Tell patient he will lie on a movable table while a machine moves around him. There are no sensations unless dye is injected. Some patients react to dye with nausea, vomiting, flushing, itching, or a bitter taste. Claustrophobic patients may need mild sedation.	No special postprocedure care is required. If dye is injected, the patient is encouraged to drink fluids to flush the dye from the body.
Ultrasonography		
Uses sound waves to create images of internal structures; used to study the prostate for enlargement or lesions.	Tell the patient an instrument will be inserted into the rectum to study the prostate. A full bladder is no longer required. Tell patient the procedure is uncomfortable.	No special care is needed.
Radionuclide imaging		
Uses radioactive substances injected IV or given orally followed by imaging to assess testicular abnormalities (torsion, tumors, abscesses, epididymitis, hydrocele).	Assess allergies to radioactive substance and inform radiologist if allergic. Reassure patient that radiation dose is low and does not cause cell destruction.	Fluid intake is encouraged to promote elimination of the isotope

Epididymitis

Epididymitis, inflammation of the epididymis, may be caused by infections, trauma, or the reflux of urine from the urethra through the vas deferens. Signs and symptoms are painful scrotal edema, nausea, vomiting, chills, and fever. Epididymitis is treated with bedrest, ice packs, sitz baths, analgesics, antibiotics, anti-inflammatory drugs, and scrotal support. A bridge made of tape and gauze or a rolled towel can be placed across the patient's thighs while in bed to elevate the scrotum and reduce pain. If the condition is associated with a sexually transmitted infection, the patient's sexual partner is treated with antibiotic therapy as well. Nursing care involves assessment of temperature, edema, and comfort. Carry out prescribed treatments and record their effects.

Orchitis

Orchitis is inflammation of one or both testes. It may be related to trauma or to infections such as mumps, pneumonia, or tuberculosis. Signs and symptoms of orchitis include fever, tenderness, and swelling of the affected testicle and scrotal redness. The inflammation can lead to reduced fertility or sterility. Orchitis is treated with analgesics, antipyretics, bedrest, scrotal support, and local heat to the scrotum. Nursing care includes pain management, assistance with activities of daily living, patient teaching, and anxiety reduction.

BENIGN PROSTATIC HYPERTROPHY (HYPERPLASIA)

Benign prostatic hypertrophy is enlargement of the prostate gland. It is a common age-related change. The exact cause is unknown, but researchers are trying to find links to altered hormone levels, diet, chronic inflammation, heredity, and racial factors.

Signs and Symptoms

Signs and symptoms of benign prostatic hypertrophy are described as obstructive or irritative. Obstructive symptoms include decreasing size and force of the urinary stream, urine retention, and post-void dribbling. Irritative symptoms include urgency, frequency, dysuria, nocturia, hematuria, and sometimes urge incontinence. Factors that may trigger retention are alcohol, infections, delayed voiding, bedrest, opioids, antihistamines, and chilling.

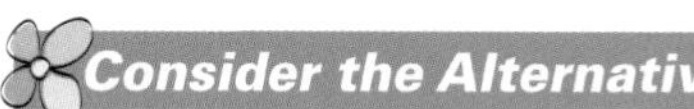

Consider the Alternative!

Saw palmetto is an extract from berries of a small tree. Like finasteride (Proscar), it effectively relieves urinary symptoms associated with benign prostatic hypertrophy (BPH) without reducing prostate size. It has few adverse effects, but does reduce serum levels of PSA, which could give a false-negative result in patients with prostate cancer.

Medical Diagnosis

A diagnosis of benign prostatic hypertrophy is based on results of the rectal examination, laboratory and radiographic studies, endoscopy, ultrasound, catheterization for residual urine, and sometimes urodynamic testing (see Chapter 38). A urine specimen and prostatic secretions are obtained and examined for evidence of infection.

Medical Treatment

Conservative measures can be taken to decrease urinary retention. Drugs that may be prescribed to treat benign prostatic hypertrophy and related symptoms include testosterone-ablating agents, testosterone-sparing agents, and alpha-adrenergic–receptor blocking agents (Table 46-4). Drugs that suppress prostatic tissue growth by decreasing testosterone levels are called testosterone-ablating agents. Examples are diethylstilbestrol and flutamide (Eulexin). Finasteride (Proscar) is a testosterone-sparing agent that reduces the size of the prostate without lowering circulating testosterone levels. Alpha-adrenergic blocking agents like tamsulosin (Flomax) and phenoxybenzamine hydrochloride (Dibenzyline) are used to relax smooth muscle in the bladder neck and prostate, thereby reducing obstruction to urinary flow.

Measures that stimulate release of prostatic fluid and reduce symptoms include sexual intercourse, hot sitz baths, and prostatic massage. If there is evidence of bacterial prostatitis, antibiotics may be prescribed.

Other conservative measures that are minimally invasive are hyperthermia, microwave therapy, needle ablation procedures, laser prostatectomy, and transurethral electrovaporization.

Surgical Treatment

Surgical intervention is usually advised if complete urinary obstruction develops, if evidence of existing or impending renal damage exists, if the patient has repeated urinary tract infections, or if significant bleeding occurs.

Types of Prostatectomy

The most widely used surgical procedure is the transurethral resection of the prostate, in which obstructing portions of the gland are cut away through a resectoscope inserted into the urethra. There is no external incision. Irrigating fluids used during and after the procedure to clear the surgical area of blood and debris may be absorbed, causing fluid volume excess. Because only part of the gland is removed, the remaining tissue can continue to grow and obstruction may recur.

A suprapubic prostatectomy is performed through the bladder by way of a low abdominal incision. It may be selected when the prostate is very large or when there are also bladder abnormalities that require surgical correction. Convalescence is longer than with a transurethral prostatectomy, and some patients develop incontinence or erectile dysfunction. A retropubic prostatectomy employs a low abdominal incision of the front of the prostate. The bladder is not cut. Although the risk is small, some men develop incontinence, erectile dysfunction, or both. A perineal prostatectomy requires an incision between the scrotum and the anus to gain access to the prostate. Radical prostatectomy is discussed in the section on prostatic cancer. New procedures employ freezing, laser incision, and the placement of stents to prevent obstruction of urine flow. Balloon dilation is controversial. Cryoablation, freezing of prostate tissue, is used mainly to treat prostate cancer. However, it is associated with a significant incidence of postoperative complications including necrosis. Transurethral laser treatment works well but is used for benign prostatic hypertrophy only, not for cancer of the prostate.

Postoperatively, the patient may have a urethral catheter or a suprapubic catheter placed or may undergo bladder irrigation.

Complications

Depending on the type of prostatectomy, the patient is at risk for urinary infection and incontinence, erectile dysfunction, hemorrhage, urinary leakage, and inflammation of the pubic bone. Retrograde ejaculation may occur, meaning that semen enters the bladder instead of being ejected through the urethra. The semen is then voided later with urine. This is not harmful to the patient but does render him sterile (infertile).

NURSING CARE *of the Patient with Benign Prostatic Hypertrophy*

Assessment

Assessment of the patient with benign prostatic hypertrophy includes a complete description of urinary symptoms: frequency, urgency, hesitancy, a change in stream size or force, and nocturia. Record the presence of pain or hematuria. Palpate the lower abdomen to detect bladder distention. If ordered, the patient may be catheterized after voiding to measure residual urine.

Nursing Diagnoses, Goals, and Outcome Criteria: Benign Prostatic Hypertrophy

NURSING DIAGNOSES	GOALS AND OUTCOME CRITERIA
Impaired Urinary Elimination related to obstruction	Normal bladder emptying: no distention on palpation, urine output approximately equal to fluid intake
Fear related to invasive diagnostic and therapeutic procedures	Reduced fear: patient states fear is reduced, appears calm
Ineffective Therapeutic Regimen Management of treatment and self-care related to lack of knowledge, limited resources	Patient understands condition, treatment, and follows prescribed plan of care: patient correctly describes condition and treatment, demonstrates self-care

table 46-4 **DRUG THERAPY | *Disorders of the Male Reproductive System***

DRUG	USE/ACTION	SIDE EFFECTS	NURSING INTERVENTIONS
TESTOSTERONE			
Methyltestosterone (Metandren) Fluoxymesterone (Halotestin) Testosterone cypionate in oil (Depo-Testosterone)	Treats hormone deficiency caused by developmental disorders, testicular diseases, or removal of testicles. Increases testosterone level.	Retention of water, sodium, potassium, and chloride. Jaundice, GI distress. Increased effects of anticoagulants and oral hypoglycemics.	Assess for hypertension and edema. Intramuscular injections should be given deeply into the gluteus muscle using the Z-track technique.
ESTROGEN PRODUCTS			
Chlorotrianisene (Tace) Estrone (Theelin Aqueous) Ethinyl estradiol (Estinyl)	Treats prostate cancer. Decreases testosterone level.	Fluid retention. Nausea and vomiting. Temporary breast enlargement (gynecomastia) and erectile dysfunction in males. Contraindicated with thrombophlebitis or clotting disorders.	Rotate vials of injectable suspension to mix. Inject into large muscle mass. Monitor blood pressure and weight.
TESTOSTERONE-ABLATING AGENTS			
Diethylstilbestrol (DES)	Palliative therapy for inoperable prostate cancer.	Anorexia, nausea, gynecomastia, hypertension.	Monitor blood pressure and weight. DES: monitor blood glucose, and be alert for signs of thrombosis.
Flutamide (Eulexin)	Decreases testosterone level. Used with LHRH to treat prostate cancer.	GI distress, hepatotoxicity, gynecomastia, erectile dysfunction, hot flashes, edema, hypertension, anxiety, confusion, mental depression.	Liver function must be monitored. Do not double up if a dose is missed. Be sure patient understands that drug must be taken with LHRH. Advise of effects on sexual function. Tell patient to report GI distress, pain in right side, dark urine, yellowish color of skin or sclera.
AGENTS USED TO TREAT ERECTILE DYSFUNCTION			
Sildenafil (Viagra)	Relaxes smooth muscle in corpus cavernosum, which increases blood flow with subsequent erection.	Headache, dizziness, abnormal vision, diarrhea, dyspepsia, priapism, urinary tract infection, flushing, rash. *MI, sudden death, cardiovascular collapse,* especially if taken with organic nitrate therapy. Numerous other contraindications including MAO inhibitors, severe hepatic or renal impairment, pregnancy or lactation (not recommended for women at this time), history of coronary artery disease, CHF, dysrhythmias, or stroke. Many interactions; see handbook.	Patient teaching: take 1 hr before sexual activity. Do not take more than once daily. *Do not take if taking organic nitrates* (nitroglycerin, etc); combination can be fatal. Drug is only effective with sexual stimulation. Patients over age 65 may be started on the lowest dose (25 mg) and increased if necessary.
Alprostadil injection (caverject) and intraurethral suppositories (MUSE)	Increases blood flow to penis.	Injection: priapism, fibrotic nodules. Suppository: urethral pain, inflammation.	Teach patient self-administration. Advise to seek treatment for persistent erection.

LHRH, Luteinizing hormone-releasing hormone; *GI,* gastrointestinal; *MI,* myocardial infarction; *CHF,* congestive heart failure.

Interventions

Impaired Urinary Elimination

Instruct the patient to void promptly when the urge is felt and to space fluid intake throughout the day rather than consuming large amounts of liquids at one time. Fluid restriction is *not* recommended because it increases the risk of urinary tract infection. The patient should avoid alcohol and antihistamines.

If the patient is unable to void and the bladder becomes distended, notify the physician. Perform catheterization as ordered, but it may be difficult to pass the catheter because of the enlarged prostate. If the catheter does not pass easily, do not force it. Inform the physician. The procedure is usually done by a urologist using special instruments.

PHARMACOLOGY CAPSULE Common nonprescription drugs, including many cold remedies, may cause urinary retention in the patient with prostatic hypertrophy.

Fear

Explore the patient's fears and provide information about anticipated procedures and effects.

Ineffective Management of Therapeutic Regimen

Because this condition requires long-term management, the patient or a caregiver must understand how to manage the condition.

PATIENT TEACHING PLAN
Prostatic Hypertrophy

- An enlarged prostate constricts the urethra, which interferes with passage of urine.
- To prevent urinary retention, drink fluids throughout the day.
- Consult your physician or pharmacist about nonprescription drugs. Common drugs such as antihistamines can cause urinary retention.
- Report signs and symptoms of infection (burning on urination, foul urine odor, cloudy urine) and obstruction (feeling of bladder fullness, inability to empty bladder, lower abdominal pain).
- Take your medications as prescribed and notify your physician of any adverse effects. (Provide the patient with information about specific drugs.)

Put on your THINKING CAP!!

Draw an illustration that you could use to teach a patient the effects of prostate enlargement.

NURSING CARE *of the Prostatectomy Patient*

Detailed care of the surgical patient is presented in Chapter 16. This section addresses the specific needs of the postoperative prostatectomy patient (see Nursing Care Plan: The Patient with a Prostatectomy).

Assessment

When the patient returns to the nursing unit, measure his vital signs and compare them with preoperative measurements. Assess and record the amount of blood in the urine and any clot formation. Drainage should be light pink in 24 hours. Bright red, thready blood may indicate arterial bleeding that requires surgical intervention. Dark blood may require traction on the urethral catheter, which puts pressure on the surgical area at the neck of the bladder. Continuous bladder irrigation prevents clot formation and subsequent obstruction that can cause bladder spasms and infection. Hang irrigating fluids and regulate flow at the prescribed rate. Monitor urine output and irrigant return to avoid overdistention of the bladder. Input and output should be balanced. Manually irrigate as ordered, using aseptic technique. Check intravenous fluids and regulate rate of flow. Assess the patient's comfort level and give analgesics as ordered.

Nursing Diagnoses, Goals, and Outcome Criteria: Prostatectomy

Nursing Diagnoses	Goals and Outcome Criteria
Risk for Deficient Fluid Volume related to hemorrhage	Normal fluid balance: balanced fluid intake and output, stable vital signs consistent with patient norms
Acute Pain related to tissue trauma and bladder spasms	Pain relief: patient states pain is relieved, relaxed expression
Risk for Infection related to invasive procedures of the urinary tract and surgical incision	Reduced risk of infection: freely flowing, clear urine
Risk for Injury related to obstructed urine flow, excessive absorption of irrigating fluids, trauma to the urinary sphincter	Absence of complications due to obstruction, water intoxication, or sphincter injury
Urge Urinary Incontinence related to poor sphincter control	Improved control of urine elimination: patient controls urine passage; has decreasing incidents of incontinence
Sexual Dysfunction related to removal of prostate, retrograde ejaculation, possible neurologic injury	Management of sexual dysfunction: patient states he understands sexual dysfunction and identifies appropriate adaptations and resources
Situational Low Self-Esteem related to anticipated alteration in sexual function	Improved self-esteem: patient makes positive statements about self
Deficient Knowledge of postoperative routines and self-care	Patient understands routines and self-care: patient correctly describes limitations and demonstrates self-care activities

Interventions

Risk for Deficient Fluid Volume

Inspect urine, dressings, and wound drainage for excess bleeding. Blood in the urine is expected for several days after a prostatectomy, but bleeding with clots can signal hemorrhage and

NURSING CARE PLAN

The Patient with a Prostatectomy

ASSESSMENT

Health History: Patient is a 77-year-old retired radio announcer who underwent a transurethral prostatectomy this morning. He returned to the nursing unit 3 hours ago. He complains of genital pain and states that he feels like he needs to empty his bladder. He appears tense and is clenching the side rails.

Physical Assessment: Vital signs: temperature, 98° F orally; pulse, 84; respiration, 18; blood pressure 122/70. Alert and oriented. Breath sounds clear on auscultation. Intravenous fluids infusing at 100 ml/hr. Three-way Foley catheter in place, taped to inner thigh, and draining freely into collection bag. Irrigation fluid set at the prescribed flow rate. Urine pink, not viscous. Several clots observed in bag.

Nursing Diagnosis	*Goals and Outcome Criteria*	*Interventions*
Risk for fluid volume deficit related to hemorrhage.	The patient will have balanced fluid intake and output without signs of hypovolemia (tachycardia, decreased urine output, hypotension, restlessness).	Monitor urine for excessive bleeding: thick, bright blood with clots. Assess for signs of hypovolemia. Be sure traction is maintained on catheter by keeping tape in place until surgeon removes it. Maintain flow of irrigating fluid as ordered. If urine flow decreases or bladder distention is detected, irrigate the catheter as ordered. Inform surgeon if unable to irrigate or urine output remains low.
Pain related to tissue trauma and bladder spasms.	The patient will verbalize relief from pain and will appear more relaxed.	Check tubing to be sure urine is draining freely. If not, reposition the tubing and milk or irrigate it as ordered or per agency policy. Notify surgeon immediately if unable to clear tubing. Administer analgesics and antispasmodics as ordered. Reposition patient. Give back rub. Use distraction. Assess effects of pain relief interventions.
Risk for infection related to invasive procedures of the urinary tract or catheterization.	The patient will remain free of infection, as evidenced by normal body temperature, normal white blood cell count, and absence of confusion or cloudy, foul urine.	Use strict aseptic techniques when handling the urinary drainage system. Keep closed system intact. Monitor temperature and urine characteristics. Report fever (greater than 101° F), confusion, cloudy or foul urine.
Risk for injury related to obstructed urine flow, excessive absorption of irrigating fluids, or trauma to urinary sphincter.	The patient will have no injuries, as evidenced by continuous urine flow and absence of signs of fluid volume excess (hypertension, bradycardia, weakness, seizures).	Maintain flow of isotonic irrigating fluid as ordered. Monitor output and assess bladder for distention. Monitor vital signs. Report signs of fluid volume excess to surgeon. Administer stool softeners as ordered to prevent constipation. Encourage fluid intake when able.
Sexual dysfunction related to removal of prostate or retrograde ejaculation.	The patient will correctly describe the physiologic effects of prostatectomy.	Be open to patient's questions about effects of surgery on sexual function. Reinforce preoperative teaching that erectile dysfunction is not common after transurethral prostate resection. Retrograde ejaculation may occur but is not harmful. Offer to include sex partner in teaching. Be sensitive to possible feelings about loss of masculinity. Patient may demonstrate some anger or sadness related to a sense of loss.
Deficient knowledge of postoperative routines or self-care.	The patient will demonstrate understanding of postoperative exercises and procedures.	Support and encourage patient to turn and deep breathe at least every 2 hr. Explain catheter and irrigation system. Tell him that some blood is normal the first few days after surgery. Encourage early ambulation as soon as permitted and explain benefits of activity to recovery. Before discharge, advise to restrict strenuous activity and heavy lifting (no more than 10-20 lb as specified by physician) for 4 to 6 weeks. If he will go home with a catheter, discuss catheter care.

must be reported immediately to the physician. Restlessness and an increasing heart rate are early signs of fluid volume deficit. Measures to control bleeding include surgical intervention and application of pressure to the prostatic area. To apply pressure, the physician may inject additional fluid into the balloon that anchors the indwelling catheter. The catheter is then pulled so that the balloon fits tightly against the neck of the bladder, and various forms of traction are used, including taping the catheter to the thigh. This traction may be maintained for several hours or more and then released by the physician.

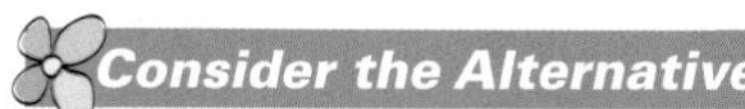

In addition to analgesics, try nonpharmacologic interventions for postoperative pain such as repositioning, back rubs, and relaxation exercises.

Acute Pain

Pain after prostatectomy may be associated with urinary obstruction, bladder spasms, and surgical trauma. If urine is not draining freely, reposition the tubing and milk or irrigate according to agency policy. Antispasmodics such as oxybutynin chloride (Ditropan), belladonna and opium suppositories, or propantheline bromide (Pro-Banthine) are usually effective in relieving bladder spasms. Administer analgesics as ordered and assess effectiveness.

Risk for Infection

To reduce the risk of infection, use strict aseptic technique when handling urinary drainage, wound drains, and dressings. Keep closed urinary drainage systems intact to prevent the introduction of pathogens. Provide wound care in accordance with the physician's orders or the agency's policy. Monitor for signs of infection, including temperature above 38.3° C (101° F), purulent wound drainage, and confusion in elderly patients.

Risk for Injury

Urinary obstruction and bladder distention can lead to renal complications (hydronephrosis), infection, and increased bleeding. Therefore, it is critical to maintain urine flow. If urine flow ceases, assess the bladder for distention. If the bladder is distended, temporarily turn off the irrigating fluid and irrigate the bladder as ordered. If you cannot clear the tubing, notify the surgeon immediately. After the catheters are removed, you must continue to monitor output because edema or scarring may occur and obstruct the urethra.

Another possible complication is water intoxication caused by absorption of irrigating fluid in addition to intravenous fluids. For that reason, isotonic fluid (normal saline) rather than pure water is used for irrigation. Manifestations of hypervolemia are hypertension, bradycardia, weakness, and seizures.

Urge Urinary Incontinence

Urinary incontinence or dribbling is common immediately after the catheter is removed. In most cases, control can be improved with perineal exercises. Instruct patients to contract and relax the perineal muscles 10 to 20 times each hour. If control does not improve, the physician may recommend biofeedback, a penile clamp, a condom catheter, or incontinence briefs. In severe cases, an artificial sphincter may be surgically implanted. Some patients never regain full control of urination. For additional information, see Chapter 22 (Incontinence).

Sexual Dysfunction and Situational Low Self-Esteem

Alterations in sexual function that may distress the patient include sterility, retrograde ejaculation, and erectile dysfunction. The patient should be encouraged to discuss these concerns with the physician before surgery. Erectile dysfunction is not common after surgical treatment of benign prostatic hypertrophy, but if it does occur, the patient may need counseling, as described later in this chapter. There is no treatment for retrograde ejaculation, but you can reassure the patient that it is not harmful. All of these alterations can threaten the patient's self-image and self-esteem. Be sensitive to the patient's feelings of loss and need to assert a masculine image. With the patient's permission, include his sex partner in teaching and counseling.

Deficient Knowledge

Teaching for postoperative care must begin in the preoperative period because patient hospitalizations are usually short and the patient may be discharged with a catheter.

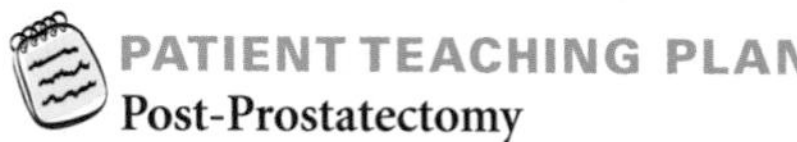

Post-Prostatectomy

- After a prostatectomy, semen may be ejaculated into the bladder (retrograde ejaculation). This is not harmful.
- Signs and symptoms of complications that should be reported include inability to pass urine, bladder distention, renewed bleeding, fever, and cloudy or foul-smelling urine.
- Practice perineal exercises as instructed to reduce the risk of incontinence.
- Walking is encouraged, but avoid strenuous activity or heavy lifting as advised by physician.
- Drink at least eight glasses of fluids each day.
- To prevent constipation and straining, which could cause bleeding, take stool softeners as prescribed and consume a high-fiber diet.
- Keep your urinary drainage system closed except when emptying it. Wash your hands before and after handling the system.
- Do not resume driving or sexual intercourse until directed by the surgeon (usually about 6 weeks).

ERECTILE DYSFUNCTION (IMPOTENCE)

The most devastating and obvious functional change for a man may be the onset of erectile dysfunction, which is the inability to produce and maintain an erection for sexual intercourse. An adequate erection requires intact neurologic capability to initiate the erection process, vigorous and unimpeded inflow of blood to fill the corpus cavernosa, and a leak-proof storage mechanism for maintaining the erection (Table 46-5).

Contributing Factors

A number of vascular, neurologic, endocrine, and psychogenic factors may cause or contribute to erectile dysfunction.

Vascular Disorders

Arteriosclerosis is the hardening of an artery due to injury to the endothelial lining of the vessel and eventual scarring. The scarring narrows the artery and may reduce blood flow through the narrowed area. Localized cavernosal artery damage

table 46-5 **Symptoms, Causes, and Treatment of Erectile Dysfunction**

TYPE OF ERECTILE DYSFUNCTION	SYMPTOMS*	CAUSES	TREATMENTS
Failure to initiate	Inability to initiate (develop) an erection.	Nerve damage due to disease or injury; stress, anxiety, or other psychological problems; hormonal disorders.	Sex therapy, hormonal therapy, vacuum constriction device, penile injections, penile implant.
Failure to fill†	Erections develop slowly and may not be sufficiently rigid for intercourse or masturbation except sometimes after extended foreplay or stimulation; sleep erections or erections on awakening may appear more rigid.	Arterial blockage(s) due to atherosclerosis, aging, or injury.	Sex therapy, vacuum constriction device, revascularization surgery (arterial bypass surgery), penile implant, sildenafil.
Failure to store†	Erections poorly maintained and not rigid enough for intercourse or masturbation.	Abnormal storage due to stress, aging, injury, or any process that causes erectile tissue to stiffen and not expand enough to compress subtunical venules.	Sex therapy, vacuum constriction device, penile injections, sildenafil, venous ligation surgery, crural plication surgery, penile implant.

Reprinted by permission of the Putnam Publishing Group from Goldstein, I., & Rothstein, L. (1990). *The potent male* (p. 39). Los Angeles: The Body Press. Copyright 1990 by Price Stern Sloan, Inc., and Irwin Goldstein and Larry Rothstein.

*Changes in erections (in rigidity or sustaining capability, or both) must occur with morning erections, during masturbation, and during intercourse for a period of 6 months to a year before the patient is considered in need of treatment for erectile dysfunction.

†Failure-to-fill erectile dysfunction and failure-to-store erectile dysfunction often occur together as the result of a disease process, atherosclerosis, or aging.

in the perineum between the scrotum and anus may result from physical injury to the pelvis, falls on the crossbar of a bicycle, horseback riding, or other blows. This type of injury may damage the artery to such an extent that scarring limits the inflow of blood, compromising ability to fill.

Atherosclerosis is the hardening or stiffening of an arterial wall due to systemic rather than localized insults. High cholesterol levels, smoking, excessive alcohol consumption, illicit drug use, and inadequate exercise contribute to disease processes that cause atherosclerosis.

Endocrine Disorders

Diabetes mellitus is a systemic disease characterized by glucose intolerance. When too little insulin is produced or the insulin produced is ineffective, the result is high blood glucose levels and disturbances of fat and protein metabolism. Patients with diabetes mellitus are at risk for erectile dysfunction due to atherosclerosis and autonomic neuropathy.

Approximately 50% of men who have diabetes, regardless of type of treatment, develop erectile dysfunction, making diabetes the most common cause of erectile dysfunction. Diabetes is believed to interfere with blood supply to the penis when arterial walls lose flexibility, or distensibility, as a result of hardening of the arteries (atherosclerosis). Atherosclerosis is a common part of the aging process but it may be accelerated by diabetes.

Autonomic neuropathy in patients with diabetes affects the ability of nerves to relax the smooth muscle surrounding the tiny sinuses (lacunar spaces) of the erectile chambers. Without relaxed muscle tone and expansion of the sinuses, adequate filling with blood for an erection may not be possible.

Effective management of diabetes mellitus is always desirable for general good health, but maintenance of strict blood glucose levels has not been shown to reduce the incidence of erectile dysfunction. Although the primary cause of erectile dysfunction related to diabetes mellitus is physiologic, the psychological reaction to the problem is an important factor. Cognitive behavioral therapy may be used to teach the patient to manage negative thinking.

Vascular surgery to clear blocked arteries is not usually recommended for people with diabetes because they often have complicating problems with nerves, cells, erectile tissue, and blood vessels throughout the penis.

Penile implants (Fig. 46-8) may be recommended for patients with problems of failure to initiate (nerve damage) or failure to fill (artery damage), which are related to diabetes. As many as one third of penile implant patients have diabetes.

Papaverine plus phentolamine self-injection is indicated as a treatment for failure to initiate or fill and has been widely accepted by patients. Patients need training in self-injection and must have hand dexterity, adequate vision, and normal weight. Alprostadil (prostaglandin E_1) is available in an injectable form and as a pellet that is inserted into the urethra. Sildenafil (Viagra) may be used.

Neurologic Disorders

Spinal cord injuries and other neurologic disorders may cause erectile dysfunction. If communication between the spinal cord and the penis remains intact, the penis becomes erect with direct stimulation. For the penis to remain erect, smooth muscle relaxation is necessary and in some way relies on com-

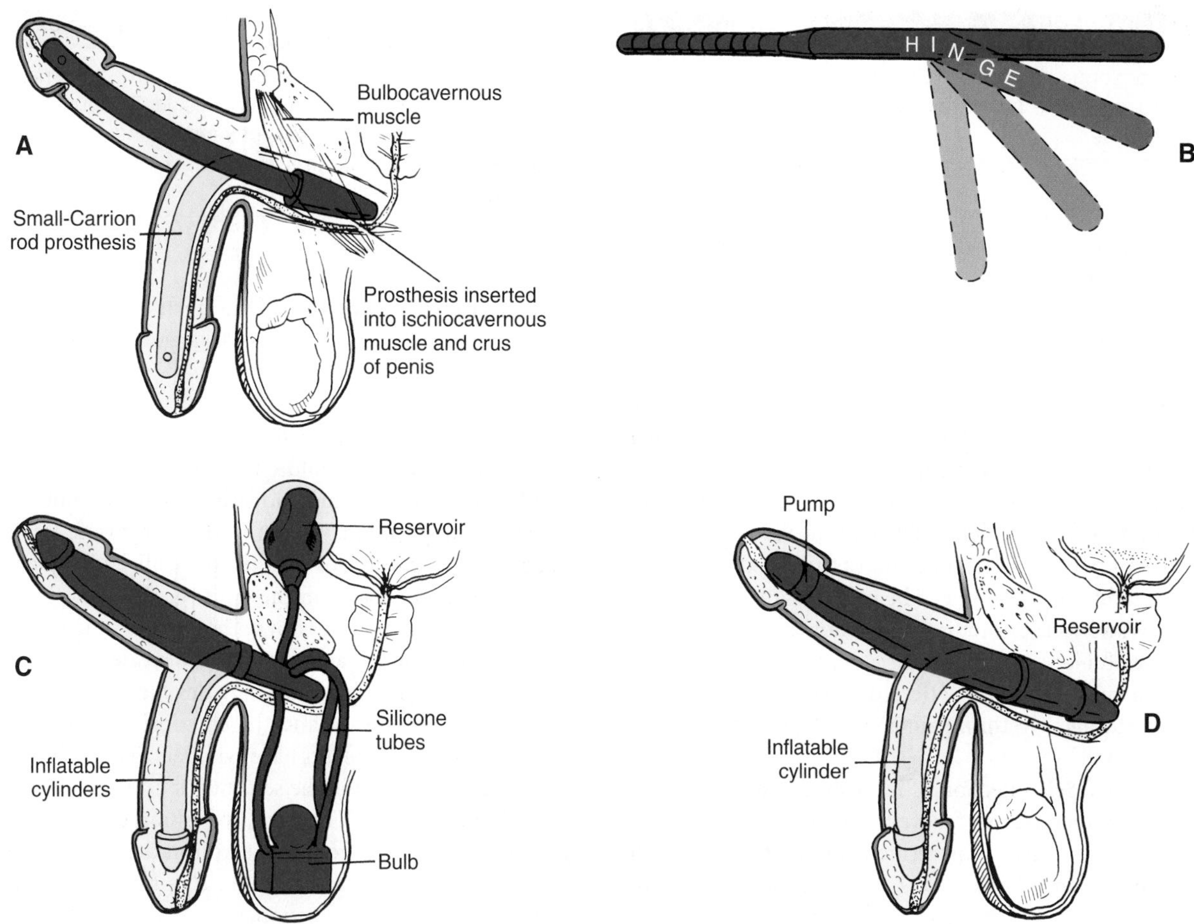

FIGURE **46-8** Penile prosthesis. *A,* Small-Carrion prosthesis. *B,* Flexi-rod semirigid implant. *C,* Inflatable prosthesis. *D,* Self-contained prosthesis.

munication between the brain and the spinal cord. The more complete the injury and the lower the injury, the more likely it is for the ability for erection to be affected, even though higher injuries tend to cause more paralysis and loss of sensation.

Treatment of erectile dysfunction related to spinal cord injuries or neurologic disorders such as multiple sclerosis may include papaverine, sildenafil, or alprostadil; vacuum constriction devices; or penile implants.

Medication Side Effects

Medications used to treat a variety of conditions may cause or contribute to erectile dysfunction. Drugs used to reduce high blood pressure (antihypertensives) are the most likely to interfere with erection. If systemic hypertension is accompanied by blockages and stiffening in the arterial walls of the penis, antihypertensives that lower the blood pressure in all the arteries of the body may reduce the blood pressure in penile arteries to the extent that failure to fill occurs. Digoxin, which is used to treat heart conditions, may increase levels of estrogen and decrease levels of testosterone; medications for stomach ulcers, such as cimetidine, may decrease libido; anticancer drugs may decrease libido; and anticholinergics and antihistamines may block neurotransmitters that cause relaxation of smooth muscle.

Treatment for erectile dysfunction related to these drugs' side effects may include changes in drugs or dosage, but such changes can be made only on a physician's order. Counseling or sex therapy, vacuum constriction devices, drug therapy, or penile implants may be appropriate for these patients.

PHARMACOLOGY CAPSULE Antihypertensive drugs are among those most likely to interfere with erection.

Psychological Factors

The psychological aspects of erectile dysfunction are extremely important and should be included in the medical history. Psychogenic erectile dysfunction is often the result of anxiety about performance. Problems may arise with aging, sexual beliefs or behavior, communication patterns or relationships with sex partners, changes in lifestyle, changes in medications, or chronic or poorly managed disease processes. The resultant anxious state may initiate the release of neurotransmitters that cause constriction of smooth muscle tissue in the penis and its arteries, reducing inflow and increasing outflow of blood from the penis, leaving it flaccid. Sex therapy

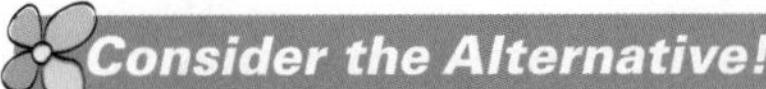

Consider the Alternative!

Siberian ginseng and *Ginkgo biloba* are herbs that some believe increase penile blood flow. Scientific validation is lacking at this time.

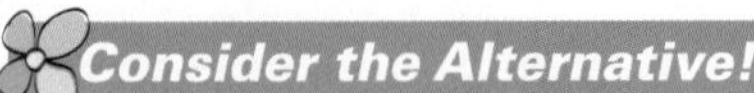

Consider the Alternative!

Therapies that may be used alone or with traditional medication to treat erectile dysfunction include acupuncture, aromatherapy (with essential oils of sandalwood, rose, jasmine, and ylang ylang), imagery, biofeedback, and progressive relaxation.

that includes behavior modification techniques may be able to restore potency.

Medical Treatment

Drug Therapy

Sildenafil. The oral vasodilator sildenafil (Viagra) may be prescribed for failure to fill or store. It must be prescribed with care in patients with cardiovascular disease because of the risk of myocardial infarction and sudden death. Sildenafil is contraindicated for patients taking nitrate vasodilators due to the risk of hypotension and cardiovascular collapse.

Alprostadil. Alprostadil can be used for intracavernosal injection (Caverject) or urethral suppositories (MUSE). It has been successful for some men. They, too, are vasodilators but produce a more localized effect on arteriole filling and improved storage. Urethral pain and urethritis are possible complications.

Papaverine. Self-injection of intracavernosal papaverine may be recommended for failure to initiate, fill, or store or for psychogenic causes. Papaverine is injected with a small needle into the erectile chambers, with relatively little pain. Erection is achieved within 10 to 15 minutes and lasts 30 to 60 minutes. Papaverine acts on smooth muscle to relax arterial walls and erectile tissue, increasing blood flow into the penis. Papaverine is often mixed with phentolamine, which blocks the constriction of erectile tissue, making it possible to sustain the erection.

Testosterone. Testosterone replacement for men with low hormone levels may be recommended for decreased desire and failure to initiate.

Vacuum Constriction Devices

Vacuum constriction devices may be prescribed for failure to initiate, fill, or store or for psychogenic causes. The flaccid penis is slipped into a cylinder, then the patient squeezes a pump that removes all of the air from the space in the cylinder around the penis, creating a vacuum that draws blood into the penis. When the erection has been achieved, a rubber ring is slipped off the bottom of the cylinder onto the penis near the base, trapping the blood safely for up to about 30 minutes. When air is again allowed into the cylinder, the cylinder can be removed.

Revascularization

Revascularization may be recommended for patients with blocked arteries. It is important to evaluate how the blockage affects both the flow of blood into the penis and the extent to which blood can be stored to maintain an erection. Arteries that block inflow are bypassed. Veins that are causing excessive drainage are removed (excision) or tied off (ligation). In addition, the tunica surrounding the erectile tissue may be tightened (plication). The increased pressure on veins caused by swelling of the erectile tissue against the tunica during erection decreases leakage and maintains the erection.

Penile Implants

Penile implants (see Fig. 46-8) may be prescribed for patients with failure to initiate, failure to fill or store (if they are not candidates for revascularization), and for some patients with psychogenic problems that are not appropriate for or responsive to counseling or sex therapy. Semirigid implants are silicon cylinders placed in the erection chambers that keep the penis firm at all times but without increasing in circumference. Some models are inflexible and create problems concealing the erection, but others are flexible enough that they can be bent downward and the erection more easily concealed. Hydraulic implants have cylinders that can be inflated by squeezing a pump in the scrotum or at the end of the penis behind the glans. The pumping action causes the cylinders to fill with fluid from a reservoir in the abdomen or the scrotum. These implants more closely duplicate the natural states of flaccidity and erection.

NURSING CARE *of the Patient with Erectile Dysfunction*

Assessment

The nursing assessment of a man with erectile dysfunction includes a health history that elicits information about the frequency of intercourse and the ability to enjoy sexual relations. Be careful not to assume that sexual activity is no longer important to older adults. Erectile dysfunction may be the first sign of diabetes mellitus, so a complete exploration of the patient's general health and family history to look for diabetes is important. Include operations, injuries, illness, cancer, and medications used regularly. Describe the patient's home life, daily activities, diet, use of alcohol and illicit drugs, exercise habits, lifestyle, health care beliefs, interpersonal relationships, capability for self-care, age, physical condition, and educational needs.

Nursing Diagnoses, Goals, and Outcome Criteria: Erectile Dysfunction

Nursing Diagnoses	Goals and Outcome Criteria
Sexual Dysfunction related to erectile dysfunction	Improved sexual function or satisfying alternatives to sexual intercourse: patient states function has improved or he is satisfied with alternatives

Situational Low Self-Esteem related to impaired sexual function	Improved self-esteem: patient makes more positive comments about self
Ineffective Therapeutic Regimen Management related to lack of knowledge of factors contributing to erectile dysfunction and measures to improve sexual function, or related to reluctance to seek help	Patient understands factors contributing to erectile dysfunction and employs measures to improve sexual function: patient states management is satisfactory

Interventions

The management of erectile dysfunction requires sensitivity and knowledge. When you have a therapeutic relationship with the patient, he may choose to share his concerns with you. Listen and be careful not to dismiss the issue as unimportant. Provide factual information and resources. If you are not well-informed about erectile dysfunction, you should refer patients to counselors with training in this area.

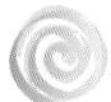

What Does Culture Have to do with Erectile Dysfunction?

Beliefs and values in relation to sexual function, as well as acceptable forms of sexual expression, are largely learned in one's culture. If a cultural belief is that older adults lose interest in sex as their abilities decline, then older adults may try to act accordingly. That is, they may accept erectile dysfunction as "normal," and not seek treatment.

PEYRONIE'S DISEASE

Peyronie's disease is the development of a hard, nonelastic, fibrous tissue (plaque) just under the skin of the penis of men between 45 and 70 years of age. The plaque develops as a result of an injury that causes inflammation and scarring of the tunica surrounding the corpora cavernosa. Loss of elasticity of the tunica results in decreased ability to fill during an erection and failure to store because of low pressure on the veins against the covering of the erectile tissue. The plaque is usually located on the dorsal midline surface of the penis and results in an upward bending of the penis during erection that may be painful and interfere with successful vaginal penetration (Fig. 46-9).

Medical Treatment

Treatment of Peyronie's disease may include topical or oral medications with vitamin E, oral para-aminobenzoic acid, tamoxifen, and colchicine. Local radiation, injections into the lesions, ultrasonography, and surgical correction are other options. The choice of treatment depends on the size of the plaque and the curvature and the resultant degree of dysfunction.

PRIAPISM

Priapism is a prolonged penile erection that is not related to sexual desire. Priapism may be caused by many factors including injury to the penis, sickle cell crisis, and neoplasms of the brain or spinal cord. Drugs that may be responsible include phenothiazines, alpha-adrenergic blockers, anticoagulants, alcohol, cocaine, marijuana, and intracavernosal injections. Prolonged priapism can interfere with blood flow to the penis. It can also obstruct urine flow, causing hydronephrosis. This erection may be very painful and constitutes an emergency situation. Failure to resolve the problem within 12 to 24 hours may result in penile ischemia, gangrene, fibrosis, and erectile dysfunction. Priapism due to a blunt blow to the groin or penis that lacerates an artery may cause bleeding into the erectile tissue, causing continuous filling until the artery is repaired or the bleeding is stopped.

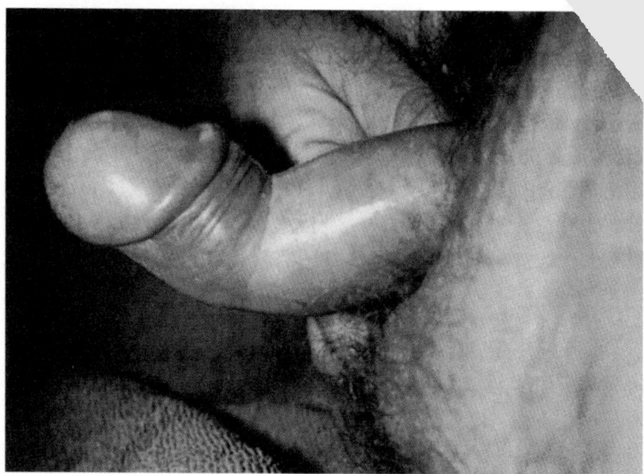

FIGURE **46-9** Peyronie's disease.

Medical Treatment

Treatment of storage priapism may include discontinuing the use of offending drugs and correcting neurologic or coagulation problems. Immediate removal of blood may be accomplished by aspirating blood from the erectile chambers or by injecting drugs that cause contraction of smooth muscle, inhibiting inflow of blood and allowing outflow. If these efforts fail, emergency surgery may be needed.

Nursing care must be particularly sensitive to the embarrassment the patient may experience. Understanding the condition and alleviating pain are important.

PHIMOSIS

Normally the penile foreskin can be retracted, exposing the glans. Inflammation under the foreskin, often associated with poor hygiene, causes edema that may prevent retraction of the foreskin. This condition, called phimosis, is treated with antimicrobials and proper cleansing. Circumcision is sometimes recommended. Uncircumcised men need to retract the foreskin for cleaning as part of daily hygiene.

INFERTILITY

Infertile is a term used to describe couples who have had unprotected intercourse over a 12-month period and have been unable to become pregnant. In approximately 30%-40% of

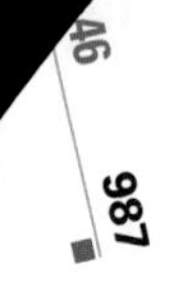

hology is found in the male alone and in f cases, a reproductive problem in the lure to conceive. It is the female partner e problem to the attention of a physi- after anxiety and apprehension have a long period of infertility increases of ultimate infertility, workup of the male partner should not be delayed.

Etiology and Risk Factors

Causes of infertility include infections, cryptorchidism, testicular torsion, varicocele, and vasectomy.

Infections

Destruction of the seminiferous tubular epithelium results in failure or reduced ability to produce sperm. Mumps in the adult man or pubescent boy may result in acute orchitis and epididymitis, accompanied by fever and debilitating pain, bilateral swelling, and redness of the testicles. If damage to seminiferous epithelium occurs, the testes will be reduced to subnormal size after recovery. Other viral infections such as tuberculosis, pneumonia, and syphilis may affect the testes, but less dramatically than mumps. Also, loss of testicular mass may appear more gradually than with mumps.

Genitourinary tract infections can cause infertility in males. *Chlamydia trachomatis* is sexually transmitted and is most prevalent in young adults with multiple sex partners. The infection is most commonly limited to the urethra and causes varying degrees of painful urination and discharge. Progressive infection may include the epididymis and prostate gland. *Neisseria gonorrhoeae* is a common urethral infection in the United States. It is sexually transmitted and may cause extremely painful urination and a purulent discharge. Infections that ascend to the epididymis may result in decreased fertility.

Cryptorchidism

Cryptorchidism is defined as any testis located in other than a dependent scrotal position. It is a common congenital condition, being found in approximately 30% of preterm male infants and in 1.0% to 3.4% of full-term male infants (Fig. 46-10). Although genetic disorders can cause cryptorchidism, the cause is usually unknown. It may be related to an endocrine or a mechanical defect, an inherent testicular disorder, or a combination of factors. Because the abdominal cavity is warmer than the scrotum, excessive warmth can damage the seminiferous epithelium of undescended testes and result in decreased spermatogenesis.

Medical treatment. Cryptorchidism must be corrected within the first 18 months of life to give the best chance for fertility. Men with undescended testes have a 10 to 30 times higher incidence of testicular cancer than men whose testes descended normally. The risk remains higher even if the condition is subsequently corrected. If the testes are within the normal path but do not descend or cannot be pulled into the scrotum, they usually do not respond to hormonal therapy, and surgery is needed. Whether medical or surgical therapy is indicated, it is performed after the first birthday and before the second birthday. Untreated bilateral cryptorchidism results in sterility. Unilateral cryptorchidism may result in a low sperm count, but spermatogenesis continues and pregnancies are sometimes initiated without difficulty.

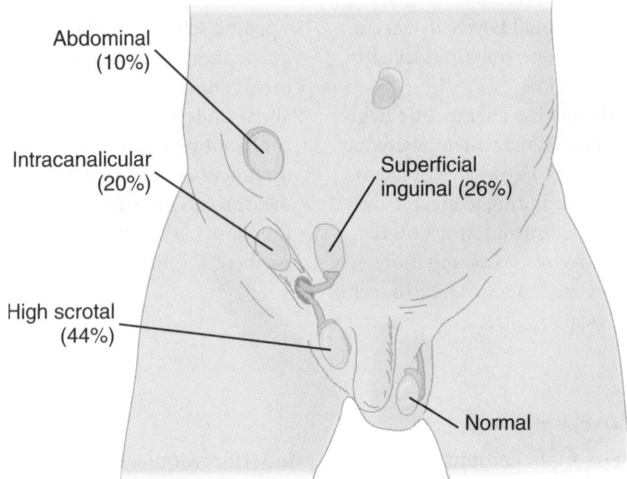

FIGURE **46-10** Common sites of undescended or mispositioned testicles.

Sometimes the testes retract as a result of overactive muscles. This usually occurs between ages 3 and 6 years. It will respond to hormonal therapy, with the testes spontaneously descending at or before puberty.

Testicular Torsion

Testicular torsion occurs unilaterally when the testicle is mobile and the spermatic cord twists, cutting off the blood supply to the testicle (Fig. 46-11). It is an acute surgical emergency requiring immediate release of the torsion or removal of the testicle. It most commonly occurs in adolescents and usually occurs when the scrotum is warm and relaxed but may occur for no apparent reason. Symptoms are intense pain, often accompanied by nausea and vomiting. After testicular torsion is corrected, lowered sperm counts and infertility may follow. There is sometimes a collateral effect on the healthy testicle. After the testicle that underwent torsion is removed, sperm counts are normal.

Varicocele

A varicocele is a lengthening and enlargement of the scrotal portion of the venous system that drains the testicle (Fig. 46-11). Varicoceles are caused by incompetent or absent valves in the spermatic venous system, which allows pooled blood and the resulting increased hydrostatic pressure to dilate the veins. The left testicle is the most common site, but bilateral or right-sided varicoceles do occur. Affected testicles may be smaller in size and may have reduced spermatogenesis. The effect of a varicocele on fertility is debated. On examination of the testes, large varicoceles may be visible through the scrotal skin as a bluish discoloration. Small varicoceles may be palpable only when the patient is asked to bear down. Treatment includes scrotal support or surgical ligation and is indicated when fertility is thought to be affected. Varicoceles may reappear after surgery, and fertility or the ability to conceive may or may not improve.

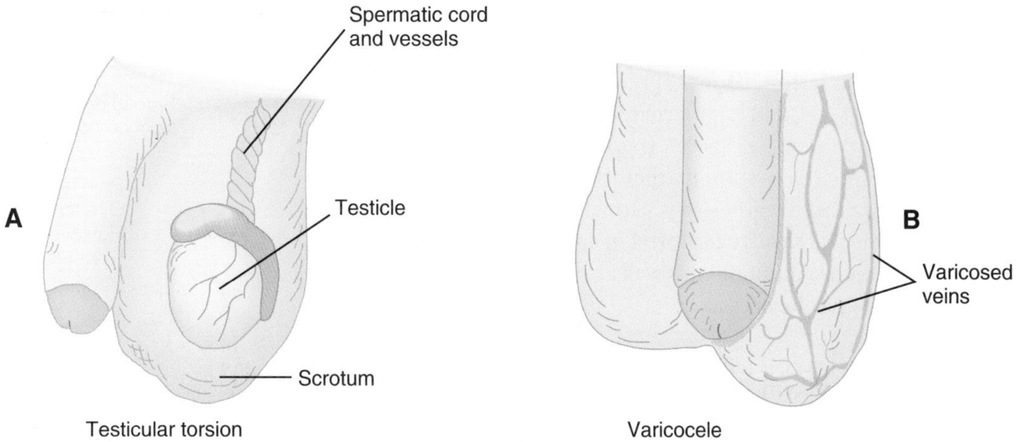

Spermatic cord and vessels
Testicle
A
Scrotum
Testicular torsion
B
Varicosed veins
Varicocele

FIGURE **46-11** Disturbances of the testes. *A,* Torsion of the testes. *B,* Varicocele.

Vasectomy

Vasectomy is the surgical removal of a portion of the vasa deferentia (Fig. 46-12). Although sperm are no longer found in the semen after the procedure, erection, ejaculation, and intercourse are unaffected. Vasectomy is usually performed as an outpatient procedure in a physician's office or outpatient clinic. Postoperative pain or swelling can be managed with application of an ice bag, mild analgesics, and scrotal support. The patient can resume intercourse as soon as he feels comfortable, but it is important that he use other methods of birth control until analysis of the semen determines that there is a complete absence of sperm. The patient can expect the analysis to be done after about 15 ejaculations following the vasectomy.

Nursing care of the vasectomy patient should include preoperative teaching about the procedure itself and the resultant infertility. Although a vasectomy can sometimes be successfully reversed, it should be considered permanent. The nurse should be sensitive to the readiness of the male patient to undergo this procedure. Fears related to postoperative loss of sexual function and the development of cancer may cause anxiety in some men, even though they desire the procedure. Acceptance and reassurance are important.

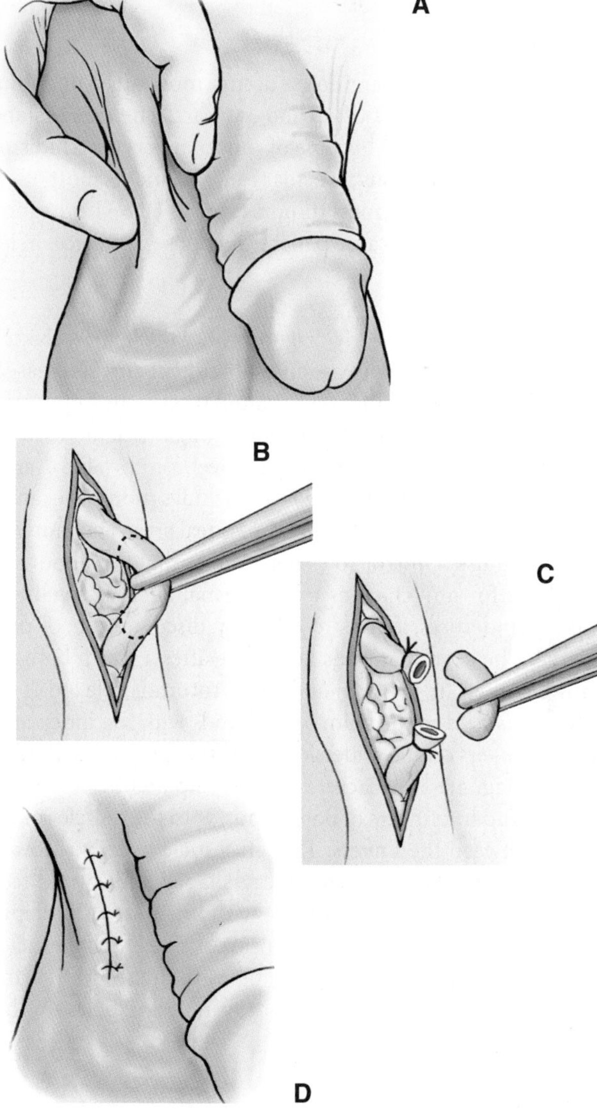

FIGURE **46-12** Vasectomy. *A,* Vas deferens located. *B,* Vas deferens exposed. *C,* Small segment of vas deferens removed and severed ends tied. *D,* Scrotal wound closed.

Put on your THINKING CAP!!

A couple visits the clinic seeking help for infertility. During the initial interview, one of them says, "My brother and his wife couldn't get pregnant either. Then he switched from briefs to boxer shorts. Within a few months, his wife was pregnant! Do you think his underwear could have had anything to do with that?" How would you reply appropriately and accurately?

PENILE CANCER

Cancer is a frightening diagnosis for any patient. Cancer of the male reproductive system may arouse the worst fears about sexual dysfunction, disfigurement, and diminished self-esteem in men, especially in young adults or adolescents.

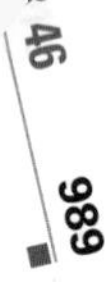

atively rare and occurs exclusively in un- have had chronic irritation and poor ctors are a history of multiple sexual mitted disease, and long-term tobacco r as a dry, wart-like, painless growth not respond to antibiotic therapy. It surgically if treated in early stages. Growths advanced stages may ulcerate and involve the foreskin and penile shaft. Extensive resection or amputation as well as resection of nearby lymph nodes may be necessary.

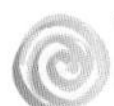

What Does Culture Have to do with Testicular Cancer?

White men, ages 10 to 34 years, are at highest risk for testicular cancer. Early detection needs to be targeted at young white males. Self-examination of the testicles should be taught to all young men, regardless of culture and ethnicity.

Tumor usually asymptomatic.
Found on testicular self-examination.
Scrotal discomfort may result from hemorrhage within tumor.
Pain is not usually elicited by squeezing. However, some men have testicular pain.
Testis does not transilluminate.
Testis may be irregular or ovoid.
Hydrocele or hematocele may develop.
Painless enlargement or heaviness of testicle.

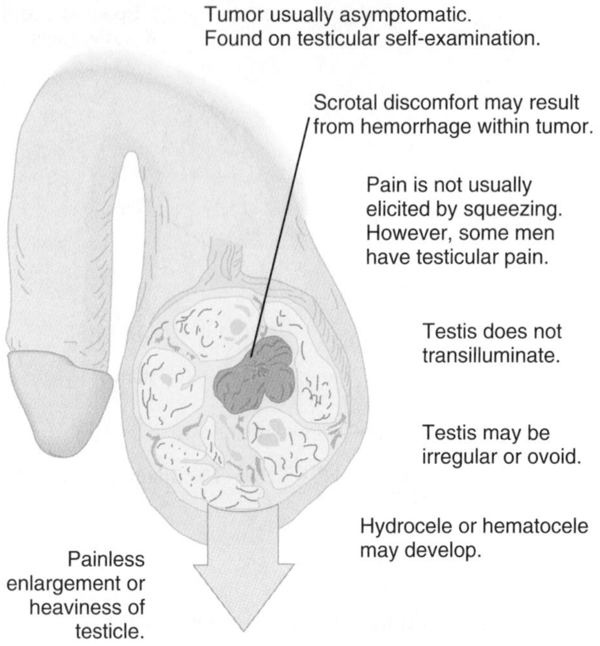

FIGURE 46-13 Characteristics of testicular tumors.

TESTICULAR CANCER

Testicular germ cell carcinoma occurs most often in young men between the ages of 18 and 34 years. The three established risk factors for this type of cancer are cryptorchidism, white race, and previous testicular cancer. Patients most often present with hard, painless tumors (Fig. 46-13). The diagnosis is often delayed because patients do not seek medical help.

Early Detection

Self-examination and early diagnosis offer the highest chance of finding early-stage disease and subsequent cure. Increased awareness of the need for self-examination is an important part of health education for men. Although men are used to touching their genitals, they may not feel comfortable examining themselves. Self-examination includes monthly examination of the penis, scrotum, and perineal area. The individual should use a mirror to visualize areas that he cannot see and look for any changes from normal such as swelling, lumps, tenderness, lesions, asymmetry, discoloration, or discharge. The examination is best done after a warm bath or shower, when he is warm and the scrotum is relaxed. The scrotum is held in the palm of his hands with the index and middle fingers on the underside of the testicle and the thumb on top (Fig. 46-14). Each testicle is palpated between the thumbs and forefingers of both hands, with the testicle rolled gently between the fingers. The left testicle usually is lower than the right. The testicles are egg-shaped and should feel firm but not hard, and smooth without lumps. The epididymis, located on the top and posterior side of each testicle, feels soft and spongy. The spermatic cords are smooth, firm, tubular structures that run upward from the testicles on the back side.

Medical Diagnosis

Diagnosis of testicular cancer is confirmed by removing the affected testis (orchiectomy) and submitting it for pathologic examination, leaving the other testicle intact and preserving

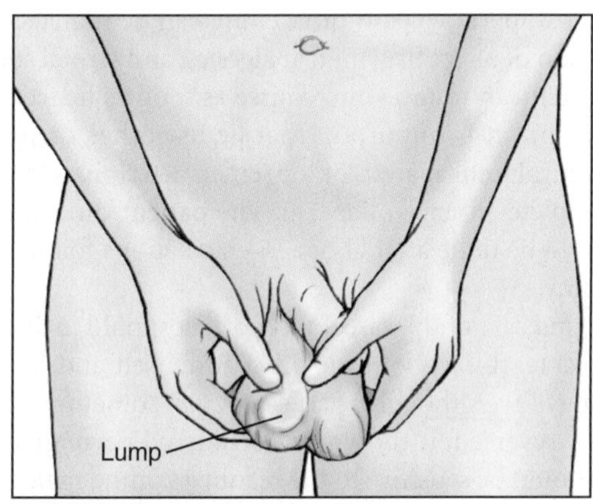
Lump

FIGURE 46-14 Testicular self-examination.

fertility when possible. The diagnosis may be supported by elevated tumor marker levels and findings on testicular ultrasound. If there is doubt about the diagnosis or if no primary site is obvious, surgical exploration is done.

Medical Treatment

Treatment for testicular cancer is designed according to the type of cancer and the stage. Seminoma is a malignant tumor of the testes that is sensitive to radiotherapy. A stage I seminoma is confined to the testes or extends into the epididymis, scrotum, or spermatic cord without lymph node involvement. After removal of the testis, radiotherapy to the pelvic region is usual and results in a 95% cure rate. If disease recurs, patients may be treated successfully with chemotherapy. Follow-up includes monitoring tumor marker levels and radiographic examinations of lymph nodes for a period of 5 years from diagnosis.

Chemotherapy usually is employed to treat non-seminiferous germ cell tumors, which are less sensitive to radiotherapy. Gastrointestinal and bone marrow complications may adversely affect any follow-up chemotherapy. Removal of retroperitoneal lymph nodes is effective but may cause erectile dysfunction, loss of ejaculation, and infertility. Chemotherapy is usually effective with relapses, and the cure rate is near 100%. Follow-up for these patients includes monitoring serum tumor markers and changes on chest radiographs.

NURSING CARE *of the Patient with Testicular Cancer*

Nursing care of the surgical patient is covered in Chapter 16, and care of the patient who has cancer is discussed in Chapter 24. Therefore, this discussion is limited to nursing care specific to the patient with testicular cancer.

Assessment

The nursing assessment of the male reproductive system is outlined in Table 46-1. When a patient has testicular cancer, also assess fears or concerns related to the effects of surgery and other treatment.

Nursing Diagnoses, Goals, and Outcome Criteria: Testicular Cancer, Postoperative

Nursing Diagnoses	Goals and Outcome Criteria
Anxiety related to the diagnosis of cancer and the anticipation of side effects of treatments	Reduced anxiety: patient states anxiety is reduced, calm manner
Acute Pain related to surgical incision	Pain relief: patient states pain relieved, relaxed manner
Impaired Urinary Elimination related to the effects of anesthesia and abdominal surgery	Normal urine elimination: no bladder distention
Risk for Injury (shock, infection, fluid and electrolyte imbalances) related to surgery	Absence of excess bleeding or infection and normal fluid balance: vital signs consistent with patient norms, oral temperature less than 38.3° C (101° F), electrolytes within normal ranges, and fluid output approximately equal to fluid intake
Constipation related to diminished or absent peristalsis caused by bowel manipulation during surgery	Normal bowel elimination: no abdominal distention, bowel sounds present, bowel movements resume
Situational Low Self-Esteem related to potential loss of reproductive capacity	Improved self-esteem: patient makes positive remarks about self
Deficient Knowledge of disease, treatment, and self-care	Patient understands disease, treatment, and self-care: patient accurately describes condition, treatment, side effects, and management of side effects; patient demonstrates self-care

Interventions

Anxiety

From the time cancer is suspected, the patient faces anxie producing threats to self-image and self-esteem. You must be sensitive to the patient's fears of altered sexual function, loss of fertility, stressful treatments, and the threat of a potentially fatal disease. You can help the patient through active listening, providing information, and referring him for counseling if needed. The patient may wish to have a significant other included in interactions with you and other health professionals.

Acute Pain

There is no pain in the early stages of testicular cancer. If the disease is advanced or if the patient has undergone surgery or radiotherapy, pain may be a problem. If so, assess the pain and take steps to treat it promptly. Analgesics may be appropriate, but you can also employ other pain control techniques such as mental imagery and relaxation exercises (see Chapter 14).

Impaired Urinary Elimination

Radical orchiectomy usually requires a short hospitalization and has few complications. Nevertheless, monitor the patient's urinary status to confirm normal function before discharge. If the patient has a radical retroperitoneal lymph node dissection, he will probably have a catheter immediately after surgery.

Risk for Injury

Some patients with testicular cancer undergo radical retroperitoneal lymph node dissection. These patients have extensive surgical incisions and usually need intensive nursing care initially. As with any major abdominal surgery, the patient is at risk for shock, infection, bowel and bladder dysfunction, and fluid and electrolyte imbalances. Shock can result from fluid loss and the effects of anesthesia during the lengthy surgery. Measure and evaluate vital signs and fluid intake and output. Monitor the patient's electrolyte levels, and administer intravenous fluids as ordered to maintain fluid and electrolyte balance. He is likely to have a urinary catheter in place and a nasogastric tube attached to suction.

Constipation

Palpate the abdomen for bowel or bladder distention, and auscultate for bowel sounds. When permitted, encourage ambulation and a diet with adequate fiber to promote bowel elimination.

Situational Low Self-Esteem

The patient may or may not be rendered sterile as a result of the treatment employed. Radical orchiectomy results in sterility but does not impair erection and orgasm. After radiotherapy, the patient's sperm count typically declines at first but usually returns to normal by 2 to 3 years after treatment is completed. The effects of chemotherapy on fertility vary with the drug used. Retroperitoneal lymph node dissection often causes erectile dysfunction and problems with ejaculation. Help the patient formulate questions for the physician

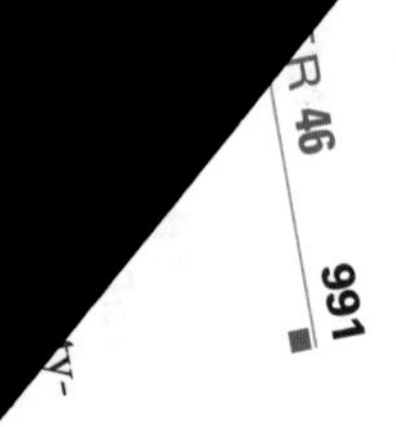

…cific treatments on sexual function and …nticipated, the patient should be coun-…out the possibility of banking sperm … this type of cancer commonly affects …l to father a child at a later date may …m.

… Knowledge

Teaching is essential to prepare the patient for treatment and to provide the tools needed for him to cope with the diagnosis. The patient teaching plan will vary greatly with the extent of the cancer and the type of treatment given. Include the type of therapy prescribed, side effects, management of side effects, and available resources.

PROSTATIC CANCER

Cancer of the prostate is found on postmortem examination in 30% of men over the age of 50, and the incidence increases steadily with each decade to 100% of men in the tenth decade. Over 300,000 new cases were diagnosed in the United States in 2000, and more than 40,000 men died of prostate cancer that year. Although the cause is unknown, genetic tendency, exposure to chemical carcinogens, viruses, gonorrhea with concurrent exposure to a virus, ingestion of a high-fat diet, late puberty, frequent intercourse, having multiple sex partners, and high fertility have all been studied in relation to cancer of the prostate.

What Does Culture Have to do with Prostate Cancer?

Rates of prostate cancer are much higher among African-American men than among white men. This group should be targeted to explain the importance of early evaluation of urinary symptoms.

Medical Diagnosis

Prostatic lesions are typically slow-growing and confined to the prostatic capsule. Younger men, however, tend to have very aggressive tumors. Prostatic tumors may go undetected until the disease is advanced and has metastasized to bone or liver. Large tumors may cause bladder outlet obstruction, rectal pressure, stool changes, painful defecation, or painful ejaculation. Because early diagnosis may improve treatment results, methods to permit early detection may be advised. The American Cancer Society recommends that all men over 40 undergo annual digital rectal examinations and that prostate-specific antigen (PSA) blood tests be done annually beginning at age 50.

The diagnosis may be based on rectal examination, transrectal ultrasound, serum tumor markers, laboratory screening tests, radiographs, radionuclide imaging, and needle aspiration/biopsy.

Medical Treatment

The treatment of prostatic cancer is controversial because of the difficulty in staging tumors and the unpredictable biologic behavior of the disease. However, the discovery of PSA as a tumor marker has allowed earlier identification and treatment of prostatic cancer. PSA is a product of prostatic tissue. It is extremely important to measure this antigen during the follow-up of patients who have undergone treatment. Persistent or rising PSA levels indicate advancing or recurrent tumor growth. Recent developments permit differentiation between PSA that is free and PSA that is bound to plasma proteins. Prostate cancer cells produce more bound than free PSA.

Localized tumors may be treated surgically or with radiation therapy. Radical prostatectomy includes removal of the prostate gland, the outer capsule, the seminal vesicles, sections of the vas deferens, and sometimes a portion of the bladder neck. Most operations include removal of the pelvic lymph nodes to check for metastasis. The surgical approach may be perineal or retropubic. The latter approach permits an autonomic nerve-sparing technique, which preserves erectile function in 70% of patients. The urinary incontinence that occurs in 10% to 15% of men who undergo radical prostatectomy subsides within 6 months in 85% to 90% of those affected.

Radiation therapy is an alternative therapy that gives equal results for about 10 years when cancer is confined to the prostate. Thereafter 20% of tumors recur. Radiation can be delivered by external beam or by implanting seeds (brachytherapy) of radioactive gold, iodine, or iridium in the prostate through hollow needles inserted under anesthesia. The seeds affect surrounding tissues less than external beam radiation. Patients often have some urinary symptoms of irritation or obstruction after the seeds are implanted.

Hormonal therapy is used to eliminate the androgenic effect, which aids tumor growth. Elimination of testosterone production also can be achieved by removing the testicles. Types of drugs used in hormonal therapy include estrogen, luteinizing hormone-releasing hormone (LHRH) analogues, and antiandrogens. Estrogen prevents the production of testosterone, but it is used less often now than in the past because of its adverse effects, including blood clots, heart failure, and breast enlargement. LHRH analogues include leuprolide (Lupron) and goserelin acetate (Zoladex). These agents inhibit the release of pituitary hormones necessary for testosterone production. Lupron is given intramuscularly and Zoladex by pellets implanted subcutaneously. Adverse effects include bone pain and urinary obstruction with initial therapy. Drugs that inhibit the action of testosterone include flutamide (Eulexin) and megestrol acetate (Megace). The adverse effects of all of these agents can include hot flashes and erectile dysfunction. When these agents are no longer effective, other drugs may be used that reduce testosterone production in the adrenals. Examples are spironolactone (Aldactone), aminoglutethimide (Cytadren), and glucocorticoids. Hormonal therapy is usually effective for a limited period of time, generally 1 to 3 years. In an effort to reduce side effects and resistance to hormonal treatment, intermittent hormonal therapy is being studied as an alternative to continuous therapy.

Chemotherapy is not commonly used for symptom relief when prostate cancer is resistant to hormones.

Sometimes "watchful waiting" is recommended for patients with a life expectancy of less than 10 years who have small cancers, or who are not good surgical risks. The patient is monitored frequently, and treatment is initiated if the tumor begins to enlarge.

NURSING CARE *of the Patient with Prostatic Cancer*

Nursing care of male patients should include a thorough investigation of the risks for cancer and an emphasis on the importance of early diagnosis. In the family history, note any type of cancer. Note any medications that the mother may have taken during pregnancy to prevent pregnancy or miscarriage, because these drugs may be related to the subsequent development of prostatic cancer. Additional details of the assessment of the male reproductive system are summarized in Table 46-1. If the patient has undergone surgery, nursing care is similar to that described earlier in this chapter for benign prostatic hypertrophy. Nursing care of the patient with cancer is presented in Chapter 24, and the care of patients who have undergone urologic surgery is covered in Chapter 38. Specific problems that may require special interventions after prostate surgery are bladder spasms, erectile dysfunction, urinary incontinence, and body image disturbances associated with changes in the reproductive system.

key points

- The male reproductive system consists of the scrotum, testes, epididymis, vas deferens, seminal vesicles, prostate gland, ejaculatory duct, Cowper's gland, internal urethra, and penis.
- Prostatitis is an inflammation of the prostate gland that is treated with antimicrobials, analgesics, and sitz baths.
- Epididymitis is an inflammation of the epididymis that is treated with bedrest, ice packs, sitz baths, analgesics, antibiotics, and scrotal support.
- Benign prostatic hypertrophy—enlargement of the prostate gland that may lead to obstruction of the urethra—may be treated with drugs or surgical intervention.
- Nursing care after prostatectomy addresses Risk for Deficient Fluid Volume, Acute Pain, Risk for Infection, Risk for Injury, Urge Urinary Incontinence, Sexual Dysfunction, Situational Low Self-Esteem, and Deficient Knowledge.
- Erectile dysfunction (impotence), the inability to achieve or maintain an erection adequate for sexual intercourse, may be treated with psychological intervention, oral drug therapy, vacuum constriction devices, self-injection therapy, intraurethral pellets, revascularization, or penile implants.
- Nursing care of the patient with erectile dysfunction may focus on Sexual Dysfunction, Situational Low Self-Esteem, and Deficient Knowledge.
- Peyronie's disease is the formation of fibrous tissue in the penis that causes it to bend upward during erection, causing pain and interfering with vaginal penetration.
- Priapism is prolonged penile erection not related to sexual desire that requires emergency treatment to prevent ischemia, gangrene, fibrosis, and erectile dysfunction.
- Infertility, the inability to impregnate despite unprotected intercourse over a 12-month period, is due to male pathology alone in approximately 30%-40% of all cases.
- Causes of infertility include infections, cryptorchidism, testicular torsion, varicocele, and vasectomy.
- Cancer of the male reproductive system may affect the penis, testicles, or prostate gland.
- Nursing care of the patient with testicular cancer focuses on Anxiety, Acute Pain, Risk for Injury, Impaired Urine Elimination, Constipation, Situational Low Self-Esteem, and Deficient Knowledge.
- Other disorders affecting the male reproductive system are hydrocele, phimosis, and paraphimosis.

REVIEW QUESTIONS

1. The hormone that is responsible for male sexual development is:
   1. luteinizing hormone.
   2. testosterone.
   3. gonadotropin.
   4. progesterone.
2. Normal age-related changes in the reproductive system of a healthy male include:
   1. steady production of testosterone from puberty to death.
   2. longer refractory period between erections.
   3. loss of ability to maintain an erection by age 70 years.
   4. decreased time needed for sexual arousal.
3. Which of the following should be included when teaching a patient about benign prostatic hypertrophy?
   1. Moderate use of alcohol will promote emptying of the bladder.
   2. Practice delaying voiding as long as you can to increase bladder capacity.
   3. Medications that contain antihistamines may cause you to retain urine.
   4. Prolonged exposure to warm temperatures promotes bladder spasms.

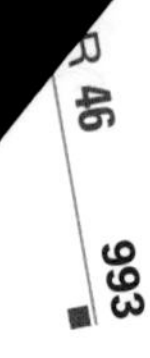

transurethral prostatectomy is
detected by inspection of the:

ssing.
ge.
istics.
n.

rug that reduces the size of the prostate without lowering circulating testosterone levels is:

1. tamsulosin (Flomax).
2. flutamide (Eulexin).
3. oxybutynin chloride (Ditropan).
4. Finasteride (Proscar).

6. Normal saline is the preferred fluid used to irrigate urinary catheters after prostatectomy because:
   1. it is isotonic and will not cause water intoxication.
   2. it is less expensive than sterile water for irrigation.
   3. it is absorbed into the bloodstream to maintain blood volume.
   4. sterile water stings when it comes in contact with the surgical sites.

7. A childhood disease that can cause infertility in males is:
   1. measles.
   2. chickenpox.
   3. mumps.
   4. diphtheria.

8. Cryptorchidism must be treated early in life to prevent:
   1. testicular torsion.
   2. varicocele.
   3. chronic infection.
   4. sterility.

9. Patient teaching related to vasectomy should include:
   1. you will be sterile immediately after the procedure.
   2. vasectomy is easily reversible if you wish to father a child later.
   3. postoperative problems with erection and ejaculation are common.
   4. you will need to have a semen analysis to determine if sperm are present.

10. Following surgery for prostate cancer, how is treatment effectiveness monitored?
    1. Measurement of the PSA level
    2. Periodic biopsies of perineal tissue
    3. Studies of urine flow rates
    4. Radiographs of the abdomen

CHAPTER

47 Sexually Transmitted Diseases

objectives

1. List infectious diseases classified as sexually transmitted diseases.
2. Explain the importance of the nurse's approach when dealing with patients who have sexually transmitted diseases.
3. Describe tests used to diagnose sexually transmitted diseases and the nursing considerations associated with each.
4. Explain why specific sexually transmitted diseases must be reported to the health department.
5. For selected sexually transmitted diseases, describe the pathophysiology, signs and symptoms, complications, and medical treatment.
6. Design a teaching plan on the prevention of sexually transmitted diseases.
7. List nursing considerations when a patient is on drug therapy for a sexually transmitted disease.
8. Identify data to be collected when assessing a patient with a sexually transmitted disease.
9. Assist in developing a nursing care plan for a patient with a sexually transmitted disease.

key terms

Chancre (SHĂNG-kĕr, p. 1001)
HIV positive (p. 1009)
Latent (LĀ-tĕnt, p. 1001)
Opportunistic infection (p. 1004)
Pelvic inflammatory disease (p. 1000)
Sexually transmitted disease (p. 996)
Vaginitis (vă-jĭ-NĪ-tĭs, p. 996)

Sexually transmitted diseases (STDs) continue to be a serious public health problem in the United States despite medical advances. These diseases spread primarily through sexual contact and may have serious and permanent consequences. Worldwide incidence of STDs increases every year. Each year, more than 100,000 women are left sterile by STDs. Eighty-five percent of the cases involve people between the ages of 15 and 30. Although STDs are more common in people of lower socioeconomic status and in those with less education and limited access to health care, all segments of the population are represented. Drug abuse and having multiple sexual partners also are risk factors. In the United States, STD rates are highest among African Americans, followed by Hispanics, and then by non-Hispanic whites.

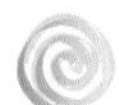

What Does Culture Have to do with Sexually Transmitted Diseases?

The incidence of STDs varies among races, but poverty, lack of education, and limited access to health care probably play a larger role than race/ethnicity. Also, cultural beliefs about sexual practices, use of condoms, and education of children about STD prevention may all affect the incidence of STDs in any given population.

Despite public education efforts, some people resist taking preventive measures. Infected people do not always inform their sexual partners, so the disease continues to be passed on. Also, symptoms are sometimes subtle; thus STDs that go undetected can spread and invade other parts of the body.

Nurses must be aware of their feelings about working with people who have STDs. There is a stigma associated with these infections, and we must assure the same quality of care to these patients that is given to patients with any other diagnoses. Judgmental behavior on the part of health care providers discourages people from seeking appropriate medical care. In this chapter, specific diseases are explained, followed by a general discussion of nursing care appropriate for all patients with STDs.

DIAGNOSTIC TESTS AND PROCEDURES

The primary measures used to diagnose STDs are serologic tests and studies of smears and cultures.

SEROLOGIC TESTS

Serologic tests may be ordered to detect infections with hepatitis A, B, C, D, and E; syphilis; human immunodeficiency virus (HIV); herpes simplex; and cytomegalovirus. These tests are designed to detect infectious diseases by measuring antigens or antibodies in the blood. Many factors can cause inaccurate results, especially with older tests. Agency laboratory procedures specify the patient preparation for specific tests.

SMEARS AND CULTURES

Patients with gonococcal, chlamydial, herpes simplex, *Trichomonas,* or yeast infections often have discharge from the vagina or penis. In addition to this discharge, exudate from lesions can be collected and studied to determine the exact infecting organism. For females, the sample may be collected from the vagina or from the cervix. The procedure varies with the type of organism suspected. To collect a sample from a male patient, a swab or a special loop may be used. The person who collects the sample wears gloves and treats the sample as a potential source of infection. The sample may be submitted for microscopic examination or for culture and sensitivity tests.

PHARMACOLOGY CAPSULE When you have an order to obtain a specimen for culture and another order to administer anti-infectives, collect the specimen before giving the first dose of the anti-infective.

DRUG THERAPY

The drugs recommended by the Centers for Disease Control (2002) are noted with the discussion of each specific infection. The CDC also recommends alternate drugs for people who are allergic to the primary drugs, pregnant women, infants and children, and people who are being treated for multiple infections. Details are available at the CDC website: http://www.cdc.gov/mmwr/preview/mmwrhtml/rr5106al.htm. Examples of drugs used to treat sexually transmitted diseases are presented in Table 47-1.

REPORTING SEXUALLY TRANSMITTED DISEASES

Confirmed cases of HIV, AIDS, gonorrhea, syphilis, chlamydia, chancroid, and viral hepatitis must be reported to the local health department. An investigator asks the patient to name sexual contacts. Those individuals are contacted and advised that they have been exposed to the disease and encouraged to seek medical evaluation. The purpose of this process is to identify and treat infected individuals so that transmission of the disease can be slowed.

SPECIFIC SEXUALLY TRANSMITTED DISEASES

CHLAMYDIAL INFECTION

Chlamydial infection is thought to be the most common STD in the United States. More than 4 million people are diagnosed with chlamydia each year. The symptoms are similar to those of gonorrhea. It was previously called *nongonococcal urethritis* or *nonspecific vaginitis.* The infecting organism is a virus-like bacterium called *Chlamydia trachomatis,* which infects both men and women. This disease is transmitted by contact with the mucous membranes in the mouth, eyes, urethra, vagina, or rectum.

Signs and Symptoms

Symptoms are more noticeable in men and include penile discharge, which is initially thin and then becomes creamy later. This symptom is generally noted 1 to 3 weeks after infection. Another common complaint among males is painful or frequent urination. Females may experience vaginal discharge and lower abdominal pain. Some patients have no symptoms.

Complications

If left untreated, chlamydial infection can result in sterility in both sexes. The sperm ducts can become inflamed and blocked. In females, pelvic inflammatory disease can block the fallopian tubes. Newborns of infected women may have eye damage or infant pneumonia. Therefore erythromycin ophthalmic ointment may be ordered for the newborn because it is effective against chlamydial infection as well as gonorrhea.

Medical Diagnosis and Treatment

The diagnosis is based on the individual's sexual history and the results of laboratory studies. A *Chlamydia* antigen test is used to screen for chlamydial infection. The most accurate test, however, is the cell tissue culture.

The infection usually is treated with a single dose of azithromycin (Zithromax) or a 7-day course of doxycycline (Vibramycin). Review the patient's complete drug profile because azithromycin (Zithromax) interacts with many other common drugs. Other antimicrobials also may be administered because patients with chlamydial infection may have gonorrhea as well. The culture should be repeated in 4 to 7 days after treatment to confirm successful treatment. The patient is advised to avoid all sexual contact (genital, oral, anal) until a cure has been achieved.

Nursing care of the patient with chlamydial infection and other STDs is discussed later in this chapter. Information about *Chlamydia* infection is summarized in Table 47-2.

GONORRHEA

Gonorrhea is one of the most commonly reported STDs in the United States. In young adults between the ages of 20 and 24, gonorrhea accounts for the highest number of cases of STDs. In children between the ages of 10 and 14, more than 10,000 cases are reported annually. Gonorrhea is transmitted most often through direct sexual contact. There have been cases of transmission to newborn infants by infected mothers and to medical personnel with skin lacerations who have come in contact with infected fluids. The infection is not picked up from toilet seats, doorknobs, or towels.

The bacterium that causes this disease is *Neisseria gonorrhoeae.* This organism lives in warm, moist areas of the body such as the cervix and the urethra. Areas affected by local gonorrhea infections may include the pharynx, rectum, urethra, prostate, epididymis, uterus, and fallopian tubes. There is a high incidence of rectal gonorrhea among homosexual and bisexual males. The presence of bacteria in the throat is common among individuals who perform oral sex (fellatio) on an infected partner. With systemic (disseminated)

table 47-1 DRUG THERAPY | *Drugs Used to Treat Sexually Transmitted Diseases*

GENERAL CONSIDERATIONS

Always assess for history of allergies before giving any anti-infective.
If patient reports being allergic to the prescribed drug, withhold it and notify the physician.
Observe all patients for possible allergic responses: rash, difficulty breathing, hypotension.
Obtain specimens for culture before administering first dose of anti-infective.
When giving intravenous anti-infectives through a secondary line, check compatibility with primary fluid.
Tell patient it is important to complete full course of treatment to prevent organisms from becoming resistant and to prevent relapse because all organisms had not been killed.
Tell patient that sexual partner(s) should be treated at the same time to prevent infection.
Assess for drug interactions.

DRUG	USE/ACTION	SIDE EFFECTS	NURSING INTERVENTIONS
ANTIBACTERIALS			
Beta-Lactams Penicillin G (Benzathine, Bicillin, Pfizerpen, Crysticillin)	Effective against organisms that cause gonorrhea and syphilis.	Nausea, vomiting, diarrhea, pain at injection site, anaphylaxis. Jarish-Herxheimer reaction: headache, fever, chills, diaphoresis, tachycardia, muscle and joint pain.	Scratch test may be ordered to assess allergy. Check drug insert for preparation of injection. Give by deep injection in large muscle. Do not pause during injection; needle may clog. Massage site. Have patient wait 30 minutes after injection in case there is allergic reaction. Tell patient Jarisch-Herxheimer reaction may occur 12 to 24 hours after injection. If allergic to cephalosporins, may also be allergic to penicillins.
Cefixime (Suprax)	Effective against gonorrhea.	Seizures, pseudomembranous colitis, diarrhea, nausea, vomiting, rash, blood, dyscrasias, pain on injection, serum sickness, superinfection.	If allergic to penicillin, may also be allergic to cephalosporins. Monitor IV injection site for pain, red streak. Monitor stools for diarrhea; notify physician if bloody mucus is present. Report vaginal or anal itching. Assess for bruising, bleeding.
Ceftriaxone sodium (Rocephin)	Effective against organism that causes gonorrhea.	Nausea, vomiting, headache, dizziness, and (rarely) bleeding. Allergic reactions, including anaphylaxis, in patients allergic to cephalosporins or penicillin. Nephrotoxicity with high doses or renal disease. Superinfections: diarrhea, candidiasis. Intravenous (IV) route: pain, thrombophlebitis. Intramuscular (IM) route: pain, induration at injection site.	
TETRACYCLINES			
Tetracycline hydrochloride (Achromycin; Panmycin, Tetracyn)	Effective against organisms that cause gonorrhea, syphilis, and chlamydial infections.	Nausea, vomiting, diarrhea, pain at injection site, allergic reactions, discoloration of developing teeth.	Contraindicated in pregnancy and lactation. Check patient's medication list for possible interactions. Oral form given with full glass of water. No milk, calcium, or antacids within an hour of tetracycline.

Continued

table 47-1 DRUG THERAPY | *Drugs Used to Treat Sexually Transmitted Diseases—cont'd*

DRUG	USE/ACTION	SIDE EFFECTS	NURSING INTERVENTIONS
TETRACYCLINES—cont'd			
Doxycycline (Vibramycin)	Effective against organisms that cause gonorrhea, granuloma inguinale, syphilis, and lymphogranuloma venereum.	Anorexia, nausea, vomting, diarrhea, dysphagia, fungal infections, anaphylaxis, increased intracranial pressure, photosensitivity. Rarely: rash, urticaria, hemolytic anemia.	Assess allergies to tetracycline and to sulfites. Monitor food intake and stools. Assess blood pressure and level of consciousness. Report genital or anal itching. Give with full glass of water.
MACROLIDES			
Erythromycin (E-Mycin, Ilosone, Erythrocin Stearate)	Effective against organisms that cause chlamydial infection, syphilis, and gonorrhea. Ophthalmic ointment used in newborn to prevent eye infection.	Nausea, vomiting, diarrhea, phlebitis at infusion site, allergic reactions, hepatitis, ototoxicity.	Report tinnitus or jaundice. Give oral drug on empty stomach with full glass of water—no fruit juice.
FLUOROQUINOLONES			
Ciprofloxacin (Cipro)	Effective against gonorrhea.	Dizziness, headache, drowsiness, seizures, hepatotoxicity, pseudomembranous colitis, tendon rupture, Stevens-Johnson syndrome, crystalluria.	Monitor liver function tests. Do not administer within 4 hours of magnesium, aluminum, zinc, or iron preparations. Can be given with food. Milk and yogurt decrease absorption.
Azithromycin (Zithromax)	Effective against chlamydia (which causes urethritis and cervicitis).	Diarrhea, nausea, vomiting, abdominal pain, vaginitis.	Caution if patient has liver impairment. Do not give with antacids. Give 1 hour before meals or 2 hours after meals.
SULFONAMIDES			
Trimethoprim-sulfamethoxazole (Bactrim, Septra)	Used to treat urinary tract infections and *Pneumocystis carinii* infections.	Rash, pruritus, nausea, vomiting, unpleasant taste, epigastric distress, crystalluria, photosensitivity, thrombocytopenia, neutropenia, anemia, leukopenia. Rarely: anaphylaxis, elevated blood urea nitrogen and creatinine levels.	Assess for itching, rash, fever, sore throat, bleeding. Tell patient to avoid excessive sun exposure. Increased fluid intake is needed to prevent crystal formation in the urine that could harm kidneys. Can be taken with food if gastrointestinal upset occurs.
MISCELLANEOUS ANTI-INFECTIVES			
Metronidazole (Flagyl)	Effective against *Trichomonas.*	Headache, dizziness, nausea, vomiting, abdominal pain, anorexia, diarrhea, skin irritation, peripheral neuropathy, leukopenia.	Give with food or milk. Instruct patient not to take a double dose if a dose is missed. Tell patient to avoid alcohol. Advise patient to follow safety precautions if dizziness occurs. Monitor fluid status because drug contains sodium. Urine may be dark. Monitor blood cell counts. Severe reaction with alcohol.
Pentamidine isethionate (Pentam 300)	An antiprotozoal used to treat infection with *Pneumocystis carinii,* an opportunistic organism that often causes infection in people with AIDS. Routes of administration include IM, IV, and inhalation.	Elevated serum creatinine levels, leukopenia, thrombocytopenia, hypoglycemia, nausea, anorexia, renal damage, bronchospasm. Pain and sterile abscess at IM injection site. Phlebitis with IV infusion.	Inhalation route contraindicated in patients with asthma or a history of anaphylactic reaction to any drug. Monitor blood pressure, pulse, blood glucose. Check IM and IV sites. Assess appetite and food intake. Watch for dyspnea.

Foscarnet sodium (Foscavir)	Treats cytomegalovirus retinitis in AIDS patients.	Fever, nausea, vomiting, diarrhea, abnormal kidney function, bone marrow suppression, changes in blood pressure, seizures, bronchospasm, urinary retention, and a number of other adverse side effects.	Monitor electrolytes. Record intake and output. Implement safety precautions if seizures occur. Monitor vital signs and blood cell counts. Encourage adequate fluid intake.
ANTIVIRALS			
Acyclovir (Zovirax)	Decreases frequency and severity of genital herpes infections. Is not curative.	Dizziness, headache, diarrhea, nausea, vomiting, renal failure, seizures.	Apply ointment with gloved finger. Do not double up if an oral dose is missed. Tell patient drug is not curative. Condoms should be used during sexual contact, and sexual contact should be avoided when lesions are present.
HAART (highly active antiretroviral therapy): a highly effective strategy to treat HIV by using various combinations of nonnucleoside reverse transcriptase inhibitors, nucleoside reverse transcriptase inhibitors, and protease inhibitors. Examples from each category are listed below.			
Nucleoside Reverse Transcriptase Inhibitors Didanosine (Videx)	Used in combination with or instead of zidovudine to treat HIV infection.	Rash, inflammation of oral mucous membranes, fever, and (rarely) pancreatitis.	Assess skin and mouth. Advise patient to practice good oral hygiene. Monitor temperature. Report nausea, vomiting, abdominal pain.
Protease Inhibitors indinavir (Crixivan), ritonavir (Norvir), saquinavir (Invirase)	Used to treat HIV infection. Are not curative.	Indinavir: gastrointestinal upset, risk of urinary calculi, agitation, headache, muscle pain, anemia, cough, body odor, skin disorders, blurred vision. Ritonavir: gastrointestinal upset, peripheral neuropathy, rash, muscle pain. Saquinavir: phototoxicity, bleeding in hemophiliacs, many other side effects when given with AZT or DDI Interferes with metabolism of many other drugs.	Monitor results of liver function studies. Check drug profile for possible interactions. Stress need to take every day as ordered. Be sure patient understands that infection can still be transmitted. Ritonavir: chocolate milk masks taste. Saquinavir: take within 2 hours of full meal, avoid direct sunlight. Indinavir: take at least 1,500 ml of fluids daily.
Nonnucleoside Reverse Transcriptase Inhibitors delavirdine (Rescriptor)	Used with other drugs to treat HIV infection. Not curative.	GI distress, fatigue, dizziness, nephrotoxicity, muscle pain, hepatitis, psychiatric symptoms. Many drug-drug interactions.	Monitor tests of liver and kidney function. Assess mental/emotional state. Help patient design schedule of multiple drugs.
Dermatologic Agents podophyllin	Topical agents used to remove genital warts.	Highly caustic; can be applied directly on warts. Excessive application can cause kidney damage, neuropathy, blood dyscrasias. Teratogenic; contraindicated during pregnancy.	Should be applied only by physician. Treated area must be washed with alcohol or soap and water within 1 to 4 hours.
imiquimod (Aldara)		Erythema, erosion, flaking. Local itching, burning, pain. No systemic effects.	Instruct patient to apply at bedtime and wash off in morning. Usual application is 3 times/week for 16 weeks or until warts are gone.
podofilox (Condylox)		Local inflammation, erosion, pain, itching, bleeding. Causes more discomfort than imiquimod but costs less, and treatment is shorter.	Instruct patient to apply twice daily for 3 consecutive days, then take 4 days off. The cycle can be repeated if needed for a maximum of 4 cycles until the warts are gone. Does not have to be washed off. Advise patient not to use more than 0.5 mg/day and apply only to warts, not to normal skin.

table 47-2 **Chlamydia *Infection***

SIGNS/SYMPTOMS	POSSIBLE COMPLICATIONS	MEDICAL TREATMENT	NURSING CONSIDERATIONS
Sometimes no signs or symptoms. *Males:* penile discharge (thin at first, then creamy); painful, frequent urination. *Females:* vaginal discharge, lower abdominal pain.	Sterility in both sexes. Transmission to newborn infants, causing eye infections or pneumonia	Azithromycin (Zithromax) or doxycycline (Vibramycin)	Counsel about importance of treatment to prevent complications. Advise of need for follow-up to be sure infection has been treated successfully. Tell patient to avoid sexual contact until cured.

table 47-3 ***Gonorrhea***

SIGNS/SYMPTOMS	POSSIBLE COMPLICATIONS	MEDICAL TREATMENT	NURSING CONSIDERATIONS
Male: Thick urethral discharge (purulent green or yellow); swelling and redness of the meatus; urinary urgency and dribbling.	Epididymitis, urethritis, infections of Cowper's and Tyson's glands.	Collect specimen for culture. Treated with ceftriaxone (Rocephin), cefixime (Suprax), followed by doxycycline (Vibramycin).	Instruct the patient that all sexual partners should also be treated. Instruct the patient to take complete prescription of the drug (if receiving ciprofloxacin [Cipro] or tetracycline for self-medication), even if symptoms have disappeared. Stress abstinence or condom use.
Female: Increased, foul-smelling vaginal discharge; dysuria (difficulty urinating); abnormal or painful menstruation; vulval soreness; peritonitis; fever; backache; lower back pain (usually involving only one side).	Infertility, urethral and labial infection, risk of tubal pregnancy, pelvic inflammatory disease, septicemia.	Same as for male patients.	Counsel about potential complications.

infection, the heart, joints, skin, and meninges may become involved.

Signs and Symptoms

Symptoms of gonorrhea typically occur 3 days to 3 weeks after exposure and are generally more apparent in males than in females. More than half of all people with gonococcal infections have no symptoms at all. Males who do have symptoms often present with whitish or greenish discharge from the penis and often complain of a burning sensation during urination. Females may experience vaginal discharge, redness and swelling of the external genitalia, a burning sensation during urination, abdominal pain, or abnormal menstruation. Symptoms generally disappear after a few weeks, but if the infection is untreated, the bacteria remain in the body and the person remains highly infectious.

Complications

If untreated, gonorrhea can cause sterility in both sexes and infections that may lead to damage to heart tissue and joints. Males may develop epididymitis and prostatitis. Females may develop pelvic inflammatory disease, which is an infection of the ovaries, fallopian tubes, and pelvic area.

Medical Diagnosis

The diagnosis is based on the individual's health history and physical examination findings as well as on laboratory analysis of exudate from infected body parts.

Medical Treatment

Treatment employs a single dose of IM ceftriaxone sodium (Rocephin), oral cefixime (Suprax), ciprofloxacin (Cipro), or ofloxacin (Floxin). If concurrent chlamydial infection has not been ruled out, the initial drug is followed with 7 days of oral doxycycline calcium (Vibramycin). One of these regimens cures most cases of gonorrhea quickly and safely. Penicillin is not used as much as it once was because many organisms have developed resistance to it. Erythromycin ophthalmic ointment may be ordered for the newborn to prevent eye infection caused by exposure to gonococci during delivery.

Be sure to instruct patients to follow up with a physician to be sure the treatment was effective. Additional information about drug therapy for gonorrhea is provided in Table 47-1.

Nursing care of the patient with gonorrhea and other STDs is covered later in this chapter. Table 47-3 summarizes information related to the signs and symptoms of gonorrhea, the possible complications, the medical treatment, and the nursing considerations.

Follow-up examination is essential after antimicrobial therapy for gonorrhea to be sure the infection has been eradicated.

SYPHILIS

Syphilis is caused by a microscopic organism, a spirochete (coiled bacterium) called *Treponema pallidum*. The organism is generally transmitted by sexual contact but also can be spread through breaks in the skin. It also can be passed through the placenta, thus causing an infant to be born with the disease (congenital syphilis).

Signs and Symptoms

Signs and symptoms change throughout the course of the disease. If untreated, syphilis progresses through four stages: primary, secondary, latent, and late.

Primary Stage

A typical lesion, called a *chancre,* is the first sign of syphilis. The chancre is generally first noticed 1 to 12 weeks after contact. During the primary stage, a reddish papule appears where the organism entered the body, usually on the genitals, anus, or mouth. Within a week, the papule becomes a painless red ulcer. Lymph nodes in the area of the chancre may be enlarged but are not tender. The chancre may last from 1 to 5 weeks. When it disappears, patients may assume they are cured when, in fact, the infecting organism has moved into the blood (Fig. 47-1).

Secondary Stage

The secondary stage occurs 1 to 6 months after contact. Symptoms may include a rash on the extremities, chest or back, palms of the hands, and soles of the feet. Pustules that contain highly contagious material often develop. Fever, sore throat, and generalized aching are also seen in this stage. The patient is contagious during the first and second stages.

Latent Stage

The latent stage, in which there are no symptoms, follows the secondary stage. Although there are no symptoms, the organisms are invading the major organs. The disease is not spread by sexual contact during the latent stage but may be transmitted by blood exposure.

Late Stage

It is generally 3 years after contact before late syphilis develops, although it may be decades. Signs and symptoms of late syphilis include arthritis, numbness of the extremities, ulcers of the skin and internal organs, and pain due to damage to the heart, blood vessels (especially the aorta), spinal cord, or brain.

Complications

The patient with untreated syphilis may develop severe, potentially fatal complications, including blindness, mental illness, paralysis, and heart disease.

Medical Diagnosis

The diagnosis is based on physical examination findings and a blood test to detect the presence of the organism. Tests for syphilis include screening and confirmation tests. Two screening tests are the Venereal Disease Research Laboratory (VDRL) test and the rapid plasma reagin (RPR) test. Both detect a protein that appears in the blood when a person has syphilis. Screening tests can be inaccurate because other factors can cause false positive reactions. Also, the tests are not effective until antibodies for *T. pallidum* are present in the blood. This may not occur until 3 to 4 weeks after exposure.

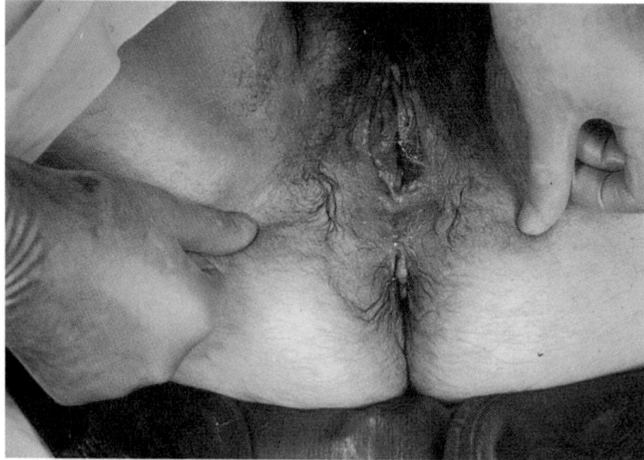

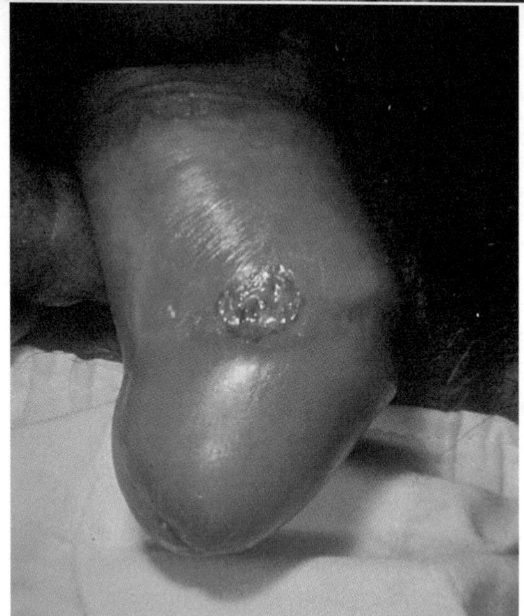

FIGURE **47-1** Chancre typical of primary syphilis.

Confirmation tests, those that specifically detect *T. pallidum,* are needed to confirm the disease. They are the fluorescent treponemal antibody absorption test (FTA-ABS) and the microhemagglutination test. Because patients with syphilis often have multiple infections, HIV testing is often recommended as well.

Medical Treatment

The treatment of choice for syphilis is parenteral penicillin G unless contraindicated. For an infection of less than 1 year's duration, a single dose is usually sufficient. For infections of

table 47-4 ***Syphilis***

SIGNS/SYMPTOMS	POSSIBLE COMPLICATIONS	MEDICAL TREATMENT	NURSING CONSIDERATIONS
PRIMARY SYPHILIS Chancre (round ulcer with well-defined margin): lesion is thickened, rubbery, and painless. If untreated, lesion persists only 3 to 6 weeks and then heals. Regional lymphadenopathy: enlarged lymph nodes only in the area of the chancre.	Prompt, effective treatment can result in complete recovery without complications. Otherwise, complications may include arthritis, bursitis, osteitis, liver enlargement, heart disease, meningitis, and central nervous system disorders.	Parenteral penicillin G given in a single dose for 8 to 12 days *Or* if patient is unable to take penicillin, PO tetracycline or doxycycline is used.	Ensure that ordered blood studies are done: VDRL, RPR, FTA-AB. Assess for transient fever, flulike symptoms, malaise. Provide rest periods. Wear gloves to assess the skin and mucous membranes. Inspect skin changes, lesions. Provide medications. After administration of parenteral antibiotics, observe patient for 30 minutes for allergic reactions such as rash, fever, or chills. Have emergency drugs on hand in the event of anaphylaxis.
SECONDARY SYPHILIS Sore throat, malaise, rash, fever, weight loss, headaches, musculoskeletal pain.			

a year's duration or longer, a longer course of therapy is indicated. Information about drug therapy for syphilis is presented in Table 47-1. Advise the patient to make a follow-up appointment with a physician to see whether the treatment was effective. Also, advise the patient not to engage in sexual activity until 1 month after completing treatment for primary or secondary syphilis.

Nursing care of the patient with syphilis and other STDs is covered later in this chapter. Table 47-4 summarizes the signs and symptoms of syphilis, possible complications, medical treatment, and nursing implications.

PHARMACOLOGY CAPSULE Patients who do not complete the prescribed course of antibiotic therapy may not be cured of the infection.

HERPES SIMPLEX

The herpesvirus has plagued humans for many centuries. Several different types of the virus are easily passed from person to person. The virus that causes cold sores (*herpes febrilis* or herpes simplex virus 1, HSV type 1) was first described in 100 AD and is transmitted through contact with open lesions, usually on the lips or inside the mouth. Prevention strategies generally focus on avoiding direct contact (kissing) and using good handwashing technique when caring for infected persons.

The incidence of genital herpes (caused by herpes simplex virus 2, or HSV type 2) has been on the rise since the 1960s. HSV type 2 is generally transmitted by sexual contact. Vaginal or anal intercourse and oral-genital contact are the primary transmission modes, but HSV type 2 can be transferred by hand contact as well.

Although herpes simplex virus types 1 and 2 are similar, type 1 is *usually* nongenital, with lesions typically above the waist. Type 2 is considered an STD because it is *most often* below the waist and is transmitted by genital contact.

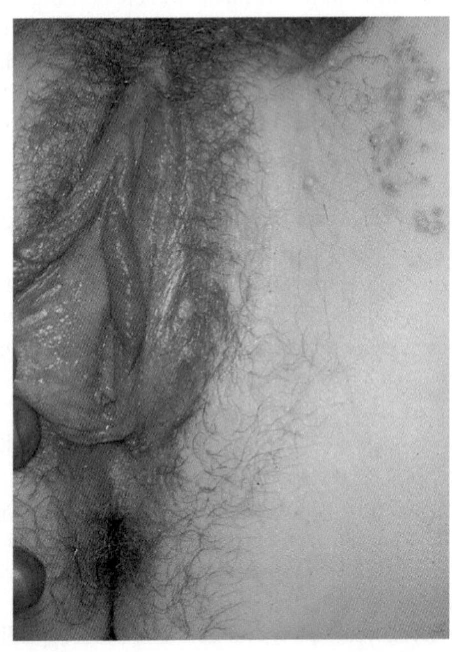

FIGURE **47-2** Genital herpes lesions on the vulva and inner thigh.

Signs and Symptoms

Symptoms of genital herpes infection include painful, itching sores on or around the genitals approximately 2 to 20 days after infection. These symptoms last about 2 to 3 weeks. A rash may appear first, followed by small blisters that eventually ulcerate. People often complain of flulike symptoms and a burning sensation during urination. Episodes of active symptoms may recur and are frequently precipitated by anxiety (Fig. 47-2).

table 47-5 ***Herpes Simplex Infections***

SIGNS/SYMPTOMS	POSSIBLE COMPLICATIONS	MEDICAL TREATMENT	NURSING CONSIDERATIONS
Painful genital lesions, burning during urination.	Localized infections; risk of infecting baby on delivery.	Treatment is basically symptomatic and includes sitz baths. Acyclovir may minimize symptoms; however, there is no cure for herpes. Recurrences may be treated with acyclovir, valacyclovir, or famciclovir.	Ensure that patient notifies sexual contacts. Inform the patient that virus can survive on objects such as towels. Assist in decreasing patient's anxiety by allowing him or her to verbalize feelings. Instruct patient to avoid sexual contact when lesions are present and to use condoms at other times.

Complications

There is an increased risk of cervical cancer in women who have genital herpes. Rates of premature births and miscarriages are high among these women. An infected woman should be taught to have a Papanicolaou's smear done annually to detect cervical cancer early. If she is pregnant, she should be supervised closely by a physician. Obstetricians recommend cesarean sections for infected women who have active lesions to decrease the risk of transmission to the baby. New diagnostic procedures allow the physician to detect active disease more accurately than in the past.

Medical Diagnosis and Treatment

A diagnosis of HSV type 2 may be suspected on the basis of the appearance of genital lesions. Laboratory tests are used to confirm the diagnosis. Exudate from lesions can be examined under a microscope and cultured to reveal the virus. An antibody test called the Herp-Check can detect active herpes. The Herp-Check results are available in 4 hours. The test is used to assess for active infections during pregnancy. If negative results are obtained near the time of delivery, the physician may permit a vaginal delivery rather than requiring a cesarean section.

There is no cure for HSV infection, but the oral antiviral drugs acyclovir (Zovirax), valacyclovir (Valtrex), or famciclovir (Famvir) help by partially controlling the signs and symptoms during initial and recurrent episodes. Patients should know to start the drug when preliminary (prodromal) symptoms of recurrence are experienced or within 1 day of the outbreak of lesions. Some patients take one of these drugs continuously to reduce the frequency of outbreaks.

Nursing care of the patient with HSV and other STDs is discussed later in this chapter. Table 47-5 summarizes the signs and symptoms of HSV infections, possible complications, medical treatment, and nursing considerations.

TRICHOMONIASIS

Trichomoniasis is a form of vaginitis that infects an estimated 1 million people each year. It is caused by the protozoan parasite *Trichomonas vaginalis* and is usually sexually transmitted. The parasite can survive for hours, however, on damp cloths and clothing.

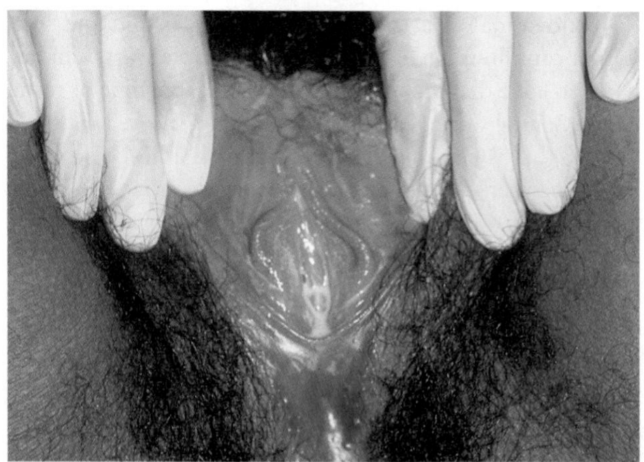

FIGURE **47-3** Trichomoniasis vaginal discharge is profuse, watery, and appears purulent.

Signs and Symptoms

Women complain of a frothy, yellowish vaginal discharge that has a foul odor. Vaginal irritation and itching may also be present. Urinary frequency and burning suggest that the infection has invaded the urethra (Fig. 47-3). If the infection becomes chronic, bladder and anal involvement are possible. Although the incidence of trichomoniasis is less common in males, it can certainly occur. Men usually have few or no symptoms.

Medical Diagnosis and Treatment

The organism may be detected by microscopic study of vaginal discharge or urine (in males). The discharge also can be cultured to reveal the organism.

Metronidazole (Flagyl) is the drug of choice for treating trichomoniasis. It is important that the patient and any sexual partners be treated at the same time to avoid reinfection.

Nursing care of the patient with trichomoniasis and other STDs is covered later in this chapter.

CONDYLOMATA ACUMINATA

Condylomata acuminata, or venereal warts, are caused by the human papillomavirus. They generally affect the genital and anal regions of both men and women. Transmission of the virus is by vaginal, anal, or genital contact with an infected person. There have been incidents of transmission from persons who had no visible signs of infection. The incubation period usually ranges from 3 weeks to 8 months.

Signs and Symptoms

Males generally present with warts on the glans, foreskin, urethral opening, penile shaft, or scrotum. These lesions may be single or multiple. In females, warts generally appear in or around the vulva, vagina, cervix, perineum, anal canal, and urethra. Less often, the lesions are seen on the labia and deep within the vaginal canal and endocervix. In homosexual and bisexual men and women who engage in anal intercourse, warts are common in the anal area. Oral, pharyngeal, and laryngeal lesions occur as well.

Condylomata warts are generally pink or red and soft, with a cauliflower-like appearance. Multiple warts can become so large that they obstruct the vaginal opening or rectal canal. Genital warts tend to grow large if they are located in an area that is kept moist by vaginal or urethral discharge. Pregnancy can stimulate venereal warts to grow very large. The reason for this rapid growth is unknown (Fig. 47-4).

Medical Diagnosis

The diagnosis is usually made on the basis of a simple observation of the warts. A biopsy of the lesions is necessary to make a definitive diagnosis.

Medical Treatment

Although there is no cure for condylomata acuminata, removal of visible warts provides symptomatic relief. Treatment provided by the physician may include cryotherapy, which uses liquid nitrogen or solid carbon dioxide to freeze the warts. Other treatments are carbon dioxide laser destruction, topical application of podophyllin or trichloroacetic acid, cautery (burning of tissue), injection of interferon into the lesions, and surgical excision. Note that podophyllin is contraindicated during pregnancy because it is teratogenic (can cause birth defects). Treatments that can be applied by the patient are podofilox 0.5% solution or gel and imiquimod 5% cream. None of these methods has proven totally effective in all cases. The recurrence rate is very high.

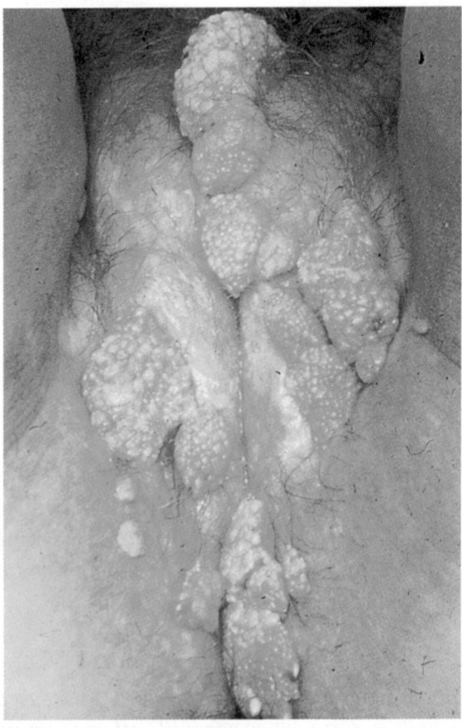

FIGURE **47-4** Condylomata acuminata in a female patient.

Nursing care of the patient with condyloma warts as well as other STDs is discussed later in this chapter.

BACTERIAL VAGINOSIS

Bacterial vaginosis caused by *Gardnerella vaginalis* was previously called nonspecific vaginitis. It can be transmitted sexually and by other modes. The signs and symptoms are genital irritation and itching, a thin gray discharge, and a fishy odor. The infection is diagnosed by microscopic examination of the discharge fluid and by culture. The condition is treated with metronidazole (Flagyl) administered orally or vaginally or clindamycin vaginal cream. The patient is advised not to consume alcohol while taking metronidazole, to avoid intercourse while being treated, and to use condoms to prevent recurrence. The combination of alcohol and metronidazole may trigger a disulfiram-like reaction, with vomiting, tachycardia, and hypotension.

HUMAN IMMUNODEFICIENCY VIRUS INFECTION

Many diseases that cause illness or death have plagued Americans, but it is likely that none of these has had the profound medical, social, economic, and psychological effects as has the human immunodeficiency virus (HIV) infection known as acquired immunodeficiency syndrome (AIDS). This syndrome is a disorder of the immune system caused by HIV. HIV gradually destroys T4 lymphocytes, which are essential for resisting pathogens. As the number of T4 lymphocytes declines, the patient becomes increasingly susceptible to **opportunistic infections.** An opportunistic infection is one that thrives when the immune system is impaired. When the immune system ceases to function effectively, the patient is said to have acquired immunodeficiency syndrome (AIDS).

Persons with AIDS are sometimes treated as outcasts because the disease is communicable and fatal and is seen more commonly in homosexuals and intravenous drug users. It is estimated that nearly 32 million people worldwide are infected. In 1999, Hispanics and African Americans accounted for 70% of newly diagnosed persons with HIV. Although there is a perception that HIV is a disease of the young, 15% of cases in the United States are in people age 50 or older.

HIV infection is discussed here because it is often transmitted sexually and requires precautions similar to those used against other STDs. Advanced AIDS is discussed with disorders of the immune system in Chapter 32.

Modes of Transmission

HIV is passed from person to person, primarily through sexual contact. Other means of transmission include sharing intravenous needles, exposure to HIV-contaminated blood products and body fluids, and transmission from mother to child before birth or through breast milk. Individuals at highest risk of infection are homosexual or bisexual men and intravenous drug users. The primary risk factors for women are injecting recreational intravenous drugs, having multiple sex partners, and having sexual contact with high-risk partners. Previously, recipients of blood and blood products, such as hemophiliacs, were at high risk for HIV infection. Blood is carefully screened today for the presence of the virus, and thus the risk of infection from transfusion of blood products has been greatly reduced.

Signs and Symptoms

It is sometimes years after exposure before any sign of illness appears. Early symptoms include fever, night sweats, anorexia, and weight loss. A variety of other symptoms that are associated with opportunistic infections acquired because of impaired immune function may eventually occur (Fig. 47-5).

Complications

Complications of HIV infection include opportunistic infections, wasting, secondary cancer, and dementia. The most common infection seen in persons with AIDS is *Pneumocystis carinii* pneumonia. For many women, vaginal candidiasis is the first symptom of HIV infection. In these patients the candidiasis is often resistant to topical antifungals but responsive to ketoconazole (Nizoral) or fluconazole (Diflucan). Skin lesions such as herpes zoster, warts, and dermatitis may also be seen. Kaposi's sarcoma is a type of skin cancer previously seen primarily in elderly men. The incidence of Kaposi's sarcoma has increased dramatically in younger people as a result of AIDS.

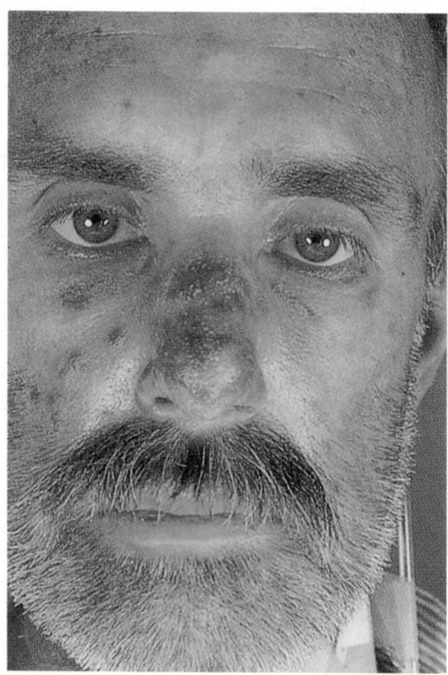

FIGURE **47-5** Kaposi's sarcoma: Advanced disease.

Medical Diagnosis

Serologic tests are most often used to detect the presence of HIV. They include a screening test known as the enzyme-linked immunosorbent assay (ELISA), the Western blot test, and the latex agglutination test. The ELISA assay detects the presence or absence of an immune response to HIV infection. If the test is positive, the ELISA is generally repeated. In the event the second ELISA is positive, a Western blot test is performed. This test is highly accurate when performed and analyzed by expert technicians. Although the Western blot test is more accurate, its tremendous cost makes the ELISA the usual examination of choice. The latex agglutination test can be done in the home and provides results in 5 minutes. New tests continue to be developed, so you may need to consult laboratory personnel about unfamiliar tests and the nursing responsibilities associated with each.

Counseling the HIV-Positive Person

People who test positive for the virus are considered to be infectious. They should be counseled to abstain from sexual activity or to use a condom. It is generally believed that infected patients will test positive within 12 months after exposure, but this area continues to be studied. The role of the nurse in counseling HIV patients merits special attention. To help reduce the liability of counseling, follow these guidelines:

1. Ensure that all available information is given to the patient.
2. Advise of the purpose of HIV testing.
3. Explain that a positive test result means a person has acquired HIV but does not mean that a person has AIDS.
4. Explain that a positive test result does not indicate that a person will develop AIDS.
5. Inform people whose test result was negative for HIV that negative results do not necessarily mean they have not been infected with HIV. The physician will probably advise retesting if the exposure occurred less than 12 weeks before the initial test.
6. People who test positive should be told that there can be false positive and false negative results.

Medical Treatment

There is no cure for HIV infection, but there are drugs that often slow the progress of the disease. These drugs include nonnucleoside reverse transcriptase inhibitors such as delavirdine (Rescriptor), protease inhibitors such as saquinavir mesylate (Invirase), and nucleoside reverse transcriptase inhibitors such as didanosine (Videx). Using combinations of drugs discourages the development of resistant strains of the virus. Information about these drugs is presented in Tables 47-1 and 32-6. Combination therapy that includes drugs from each of the above categories is referred to as HAART (highly active antiretroviral therapy). Interleukin-2 is being used experimentally to boost the immune response and may be used in combination with other drugs.

Drugs used to treat HIV infections are not curative; thus the patient must continue to take precautions to prevent transmission of the virus to others.

Prevention

The best way to prevent transmission of HIV is to abstain from sexual contact. Using condoms greatly reduces the risk of transmission of HIV during sexual contact but certainly is not 100% safe. Condoms can tear or break or may be ineffective owing to improper use. Patients should be taught to use latex condoms correctly and water-based lubricants like K-Y jelly. Efforts continue toward the development of vaccines that would protect uninfected people or prevent the progression of HIV infection to AIDS.

Infection Control Guidelines

The CDC has devised infection control guidelines that originally were meant to be used when working with persons infected with HIV. Because infected people cannot always be identified, the precautions are now required for all patients. Gloves are recommended when handling any body fluid. Masks, gowns, and goggles should be worn when the possibility of blood splattering (multiple trauma victims) is anticipated. Needleless systems are preferred but may not be available in all settings. Needles should not be bent or recapped. Puncture-proof containers are used for the disposal of all sharps, including needles. If an accidental spill of a body fluid occurs, it should be cleaned with a dilute solution of chlorine bleach. This is believed to inactivate the HIV on contact.

Patient Teaching

When a patient has an HIV infection, patient teaching is critical. The teaching responsibilities may be shared by the physician and the nurse. This chapter has addressed only general aspects of dealing with the HIV-positive patient. Chapter 32 provides a more detailed discussion of care of the patient with AIDS. Current information is available from the National AIDS Hotline (1-800-342-2437).

Put on your THINKING CAP!!

Consider this situation: A 30-year-old minister's wife is admitted after being injured in an auto accident. While hospitalized, she is diagnosed with gonorrhea. You recognize that staff are treating her differently since the gonorrhea was diagnosed. What behaviors would indicate lack of acceptance of the patient?

Do you think you would feel differently about her? What could you do to demonstrate acceptance and caring?

NURSING CARE *of the Patient with a Sexually Transmitted Disease*

Assessment

Assessment of the male and female reproductive systems is discussed in Chapters 45 and 46 and outlined in Tables 45-1 and 46-2. When a patient has an STD, certain aspects of that assessment are especially important (see Nursing Care Plan: The Patient with Gonorrhea).

Health History

Take a thorough history and identify high-risk behaviors. A discussion of sexual behavior can be awkward for you and the patient. Before nurses can deal with patients' sexuality, they must be aware of their own feelings and values. Privacy is essential for the patient interview. Address questions about sexuality in a straightforward manner. Keep in mind that many patients lack scientific knowledge about the reproductive system and sexual activity. The patient may use some words that are considered crude by professionals, but the nurse must be careful not to embarrass or shame the patient.

History of Present Illness

Begin the history by exploring the present illness that prompted the patient to seek medical care. With an STD, common reasons include pain, fever, lesions, or genital discharge. Obtain a thorough description of the signs and symptoms, including onset, duration, and severity.

Past Medical History

In the assessment of past health, be alert for serious conditions or chronic illnesses. It is especially important to document hemophilia. The obstetric history may be significant as well. If the patient is of childbearing age, record the date of the last menstrual period. Record recent and current medications and note drug allergies.

Review of Systems

The review of systems elicits potentially significant signs and symptoms, including weight change; fever; weakness; fatigue; skin rashes or lesions; oral lesions; dysuria; whether the patient is sexually active; pain, lesions, or lumps in the genitals; vaginal or penile discharge; and altered sexual functioning. A history of blood transfusions is important to document.

Functional Assessment

Relevant aspects of the functional assessment include frequency and variety of sexual behaviors, intravenous drug use, past infections with STDs, and sexual contact with a person known to have an STD. In addition, determine whether the patient may be classified as an at-risk patient because age (e.g., an adolescent experimenting with sexuality), sexual preference (male homosexual or bisexual), or habits (drug use) place him or her at a higher risk for acquiring an STD. Victims of sexual abuse (of all ages) may have been exposed to STDs. Occupation may also be significant if the patient comes into contact with potentially infected body fluids. Health care providers at risk for exposure include nursing personnel, physicians, emergency medical technicians, operating room technicians, housekeepers in health care facilities, and medical laboratory technicians.

Physical Examination

Begin the physical examination by inspecting the patient's skin for rashes and lesions. During the head and neck examination, inspect the mouth for lesions. Palpate the neck for enlarged lymph nodes. Inspect the abdomen for distention and palpate for tenderness. Depending on the setting and your specialized education, you may examine the genitals or assist the physician or nurse practitioner in the examination.

NURSING CARE PLAN

The Patient with Gonorrhea

ASSESSMENT

Health History: A 23-year-old woman comes to the physician's office because of painful urination, abdominal pain, and vaginal discharge of 3 days' duration. She has had no serious illnesses or injuries. She has had two sexual partners in the past 6 months, with her most recent contact 2 weeks ago, when a condom was not used. The patient expresses concern about sexually transmitted diseases (STDs) and HIV. She states that she cannot believe she was "so stupid" and is very embarrassed about these symptoms.

Physical Examination: The physical examination findings are all normal except the genital and pelvic examination. The vaginal tissues are red and edematous with a whitish discharge. A smear is taken for examination and reveals a gonococcal infection. Antimicrobial therapy is prescribed.

Nursing Diagnosis	*Goals and Outcome Criteria*	*Interventions*
Impaired tissue integrity and pain related to infection and inflammation.	The patient will report decreased pain, and redness and discharge will diminish.	Tell the patient that the symptoms should improve with treatment. Mild analgesics may be needed as ordered. Sitz baths may be soothing.
Risk for injury related to disease process.	The patient will report for follow-up examination and remain free of signs and symptoms of complications.	Explain that persistent infection can lead to sterility and affect the heart and joints. Emphasize the importance of returning for an examination to ensure successful treatment.
Anxiety related to possible complications of gonorrhea or stigma of STD.	The patient will express reduced anxiety and will be calm.	Provide opportunity to talk. Help her focus on the source of anxiety. For example, if she doesn't know what to expect, information is needed. If she is trying to decide how to discuss the condition with her significant others, help her solve the problem. Assure her that proper treatment is usually effective and prevents complications.
Situational low self-esteem related to diagnosis.	The patient's self-image will improve, as evidenced by positive comments about self.	Be accepting and nonjudgmental. Assure her that she has done the right thing by seeking medical attention.
Deficient knowledge of disease process, treatment, or prevention of future infections.	The patient will verbalize importance of treatment, complications of untreated infection, and measures to prevent future infections.	Explore her understanding of gonorrhea. Provide information as needed. Emphasize use of condoms in sexual contacts to reduce risk of future infections with gonorrhea or other STDs. Assess drug allergies before giving antimicrobials. Explain self-medication dosage, side effects, and adverse effects.

The examiner wears gloves to examine the genitals. A good light source is essential for thorough inspection. In the male patient, the examiner notes the general appearance of the penis, scrotum, and anal area. Any skin breaks, rashes, or redness are noted.

The nurse prepares the female patient for a pelvic examination. While the patient is on the examination table, the genitalia and the perianal area are inspected. The labia are separated and inspected for skin breaks, redness, or rashes. If a vaginal examination is to be done, ensure that the speculum and other supplies are ready. The speculum is warmed and lubricated before insertion into the vagina. Tissue and fluid specimens may be taken, including tissue scrapings for a Papanicolaou's smear. You may be responsible for preparing the specimen and sending it to the laboratory.

In cases of sexual assault, it is especially important that the examiner be specially trained to deal with such situations. Not only does the patient need a great deal of support but also the examination may produce evidence that must be preserved for legal purposes.

If a discharge is present, its color, amount, and consistency are recorded. Specimens may be collected for laboratory study. The specimen is handled as infective material, prepared according to agency procedures, labeled, and sent to the laboratory.

Assessment of the patient with an STD is outlined in Table 47-6.

Nursing Diagnoses, Goals, and Outcome Criteria: Sexually Transmitted Disease

Nursing Diagnoses	Goals and Outcome Criteria
Impaired Skin Integrity related to lesions, rash	Restored tissue integrity: healed, intact skin and mucous membranes

table 47-6 ASSESSMENT *of the Patient with a Sexually Transmitted Disease*

HEALTH HISTORY

Present Illness: Pain, fever, lesions, genital discharge
Past Medical History: Serious conditions, chronic conditions, hemophilia, obstetric history, date of last menstrual period, recent and current medications
Review of Systems: Weight change, fever, weakness, fatigue, skin rashes or lesions, oral lesions, dsyuria, whether sexually active, sexual contact with a person known to have a sexually transmitted disease, sexual dysfunction, history of blood transfusions
Functional Assessment: Frequency and variety of sexual behaviors, intravenous drug use, past sexually transmitted diseases, sexual preference, occupational exposure to infective material

PHYSICAL EXAMINATION

General Survey: Distress, lethargy
Skin: Rashes, lesions
Mouth: Lesions
Abdomen: Distention, tenderness
Genitals: General appearance; lesions; rashes; redness; color, amount, odor, and consistency of discharge

Nursing Diagnoses, Goals, and Outcome Criteria: Sexually Transmitted Disease—cont'd

Nursing Diagnoses	Goals and Outcome Criteria
Acute Pain related to lesions, inflammation	Pain relief: patient reports pain is relieved, relaxed manner
Risk for Injury related to disease process, potential adverse effects of drugs	Freedom from additional injury: absence of signs and symptoms of complications
Anxiety related to possible effects of STD, reaction of partner	Reduced anxiety: patient reports anxiety is reduced, calm manner
Situational Low Self-Esteem related to diagnosis of STD	Improved self-esteem: increased positive comments about self, confident manner
Impaired Social Interaction related to presence of communicable disease, social stigma	Resumption of satisfying social interactions: patient states is satisfied with socialization
Sexual Dysfunction related to fear of transmission, impaired skin integrity	Practices safe sexual behaviors: patient accurately describes safe behaviors, indicates will not engage in unsafe behavior
Ineffective Coping related to stigma associated with STD, shame, anger	Effective coping: patient states is better able to deal with stress of condition
Ineffective Therapeutic Regimen Management related to denial, embarrassment, lack of understanding of disease process, mode of transmission, treatment, and prevention	Effective management of therapeutic plan: patient seeks medical care and follow-up, accurately describes self-care measures, expresses intent to follow plan of care and preventive measures

Interventions

Impaired Skin Integrity

If you have daily contact with the patient, assess the patient's skin on a daily basis. Record changes in lesions. Carry out orders for treatments including topical medications and sitz baths for patients in health care settings. Monitor the temperature at regular intervals to detect fever that may accompany acute infection. Handle soiled clothing and bed linens in accordance with agency policy. Be sure that patients who will treat themselves at home understand the prescribed therapy.

Pain

Some STDs are painless, but patients may have pain associated with pelvic infection, oral lesions, or rectal lesions. The lesions of HSV are especially painful. Assess the severity of the patient's pain, and provide analgesics as ordered. Apply topical medications, ice packs, or warm compresses as ordered, or teach the patient how to do so.

Risk for Injury

Untreated STDs can lead to serious complications such as pelvic inflammatory disease and sterility. The patient with AIDS is at high risk for secondary infections (called opportunistic infections) because of impaired immune function. Infected patients also pose a threat to their sexual partners. An STD may be passed to the fetus in utero or transmitted during delivery. Therefore it is important for the patient to receive the entire course of prescribed therapy. Also stress the importance of notifying sexual contacts so that they can be tested and treated as well if necessary.

Drug therapy itself has the potential for injury. Before administering medications, assess the patient's allergies. When injections are given to an outpatient, ask the patient to remain for 30 minutes afterward in case an allergic reaction occurs. Emergency drugs, including epinephrine, corticosteroids, and diphenhydramine hydrochloride (Benadryl), must be readily available. Information about drugs commonly used to treat STDs is presented in Tables 47-1 and 32-6.

Anxiety

People may be anxious about the outcome of treatment and the potential complications of the disease. Anxiety may be heightened by the stigma associated with having contracted an STD, and the patient may feel ashamed. Encourage the patient to verbalize fears and frustrations, provide accurate information, and teach the patient how to avoid reinfection and infecting others. Patients with HIV infections also must deal with a life-threatening illness.

Situational Low Self-esteem

The patient's self-esteem may suffer because of a diagnosed STD. Provide an opportunity for the patient to talk about the effects of the disease on self-concept. Try to guide the patient to focus on his or her positive attributes. If the patient's self-esteem remains low despite nursing intervention, a referral to a mental health counselor may be suggested.

table 47-7 Comparative Safety of Various Sexual Practices to Prevent Transmission of Disease

SAFE
Mutual masturbation
Closed-mouth kissing
Body massage
Use of own sex devices or toys
POSSIBLY SAFE
Open-mouthed kissing
Vaginal or anal intercourse with properly used condom
Oral sex with properly used condom
UNSAFE
Vaginal or anal intercourse without condom
Oral sex without condom
Oral/anal contact
Insertion of hand into vagina or rectum, followed by ejaculation
Ingestion of urine or semen
Contact with blood

From Lewis, S. M., & Rickert, B. D. (1992). Altered immune response. In S. M. Lewis & I. C. Collier (Eds.), *Medical-surgical nursing* (p. 156). St. Louis: Mosby.

Impaired Social Interaction

A diagnosis of STD can be very distressing to the patient, who may fear rejection by others. The patient may be angry at the person who transmitted the infection and may be concerned about infecting others. Because STDs must be reported to public health authorities, who attempt to trace all sexual contacts, the patient may also fear reprisals. One way you can help is by demonstrating acceptance of the patient through kindness and touch.

Sexual Dysfunction

Patients with STDs may experience sexual dysfunction related to fear of transmission, the presence of lesions, or anxiety. In addition, precautions that should be taken to prevent transmission of the disease may require changes in sexual practices. In general, sexual activity should be avoided until the infection is cured. Chronic infections such as HSV and HIV require permanent alterations in sexual activity. Explore the importance of sexual activity to the patient. Accept the patient's feelings in a nonjudgmental way. Explain that emotions and sexual function are closely related and that dysfunction may be overcome by dealing with the emotional reactions to the disease. For persistent dysfunction, advise the patient to discuss the problem with the physician. Offer to make a referral to a therapist who specializes in sexual dysfunction. Encourage the patient to communicate openly with the sexual partner about the difficulties experienced. Alternative means of sexual expression (other than intercourse) may be suggested. Table 47-7 compares the relative safety of various sexual practices.

Ineffective Coping

Ineffective coping may be related to guilt, shame, anger, actual or anticipated rejection, or a combination of these. Behaviors associated with ineffective coping include failure to adhere to the prescribed treatment, failure to exercise precautions to prevent spread of the disease or reinfection, chronic anxiety or depression, and inability to cope. The patient with an HIV infection also must deal with the potential for developing AIDS, often with inadequate personal support. Show support for the patient by being sensitive, courteous, and nonjudgmental. Point out inappropriate behaviors. Encourage the patient to evaluate his or her lifestyle and to identify modifications that could reduce future risks. You may refer patients who have HSV and HIV infections to support groups. A spiritual counselor also may be contacted if the patient desires.

Ineffective Therapeutic Regimen Management

Patient teaching is essential for effective treatment and prevention of future infections. Explain to the patient what causes the infection, how it is transmitted, how it can be prevented, and why treatment and follow-up care are important. Key points to teach the patient with an STD are the following:

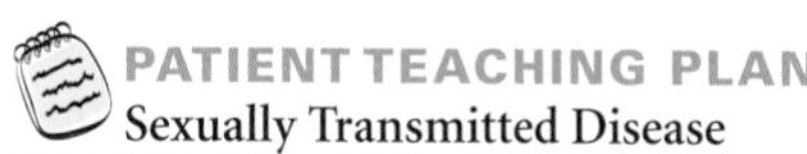

Sexually Transmitted Disease

- Be sure to complete the prescribed course of antibiotics and return so the physician can determine whether the treatment was effective.
- STDs are transmitted by sexual contact. Avoid sexual contact with high-risk individuals: people who have had multiple sex partners, prostitutes, and those with known HIV or hepatitis B infections.
- Avoid sexual activity until the condition is cured. If you engage in sexual activity, wear condoms.
- Wear condoms for all genital contact, not just intercourse.
- If you have sexual contact with high-risk individuals, people you do not know well, or persons who do not use condoms, you should have periodic medical examinations.
- Use condoms if you have condylomata.
- If you have HSV infection, you should abstain from sexual activity when lesions are present. Use condoms at other times. It is important to realize that although there are periods of remission, the condition is chronic.
- Females with HSV or condylomata are advised to have annual Papanicolaou's smears, as they are at increased risk of cervical cancer.
- If you have HIV infection, medical treatment may delay the development of AIDS. Precautions must be taken to prevent infecting sexual partners even though you may not have signs and symptoms of disease.
- Because HIV is transmitted through body fluids, you cannot donate blood if you are HIV positive.

Condom Use

Many people do not know how to use condoms correctly. At this time, only male condoms are in common use, although female condoms are available. Key points to stress about condom use are the following:

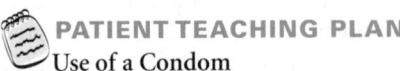

PATIENT TEACHING PLAN
Use of a Condom

- Condoms do not provide 100% protection against disease transmission.
- Latex condoms are preferred because some pathogens can pass through natural membrane condoms.
- Protect condoms from heat and sunlight to keep them from deteriorating.
- Do not use condoms that are brittle, discolored, or in damaged packages.
- Use only water-based lubricants because other lubricants can cause the condom to break. Spermicides may be used.
- To put a condom on, hold it by the tip and unroll it onto the penis. Leave a space of about 1 inch at the tip for semen.
- Withdraw the penis carefully after ejaculation to keep the condom from slipping off and spilling the contents and to avoid unprotected contact.
- Always discard used condoms for sanitary disposal.

Knowledge does not guarantee compliance, but patients cannot comply unless they understand what they need to do to care for themselves. Provide information about the disease and its treatment in terms the patient can understand. If the patient can read, include supplementary written material. Stress the importance of completing the course of therapy and returning for follow-up to reduce the risk of complications associated with untreated disease. Evaluate the patient's understanding of the material covered and explore any barriers that might prevent the patient from following the instructions.

Nutrition Concepts

1. Malnutrition is common in patients with AIDS.
2. Patients with AIDS often use alternative nutritional therapies, such as megadoses of vitamins, restrictive diets, and herbal remedies, to bolster immune function.
3. The goal of nutritional interventions in patients with AIDS is to identify and correct nutritional deficiencies.

key points

- Gonorrhea is one of the most commonly reported STDs in the United States, but it often has no symptoms even though it can lead to damage to the heart and joints as well as to pelvic inflammatory disease.
- *Chlamydia* infection is diagnosed in 4 million people in the United States each year; it can result in sterility in both sexes.
- Syphilis, if untreated, progresses through four stages, with eventual damage to the cardiovascular and nervous systems, the skin, and the joints.
- Newborns of women with gonorrhea or *Chlamydia* infection may acquire eye infections during birth.
- Herpes simplex virus (HSV) can be transmitted by sexual contact, but unlike most other STDs, it can also be transmitted by hand contact.
- Because HSV increases the risk of cervical cancer in infected women, they are advised to have annual Papanicolaou's smears.
- Condylomata acuminata, or genital warts, are caused by a virus and have a high rate of recurrence despite drug therapy, cryotherapy, cautery, and surgical or laser excision.
- Infection with HIV causes AIDS, which gradually destroys T4 lymphocytes, leaving the patient unable to resist opportunistic infections.
- Human immunodeficiency virus is transmitted through exposure to body fluids, and there is no cure for the infection although combination drug therapy can delay progress of the disease.
- Most STDs except HSV and HIV can be cured by antimicrobial agents.
- HSV infection is minimized but not cured by acyclovir sodium (Zovirax).
- Abstinence from sexual contact is the best way to prevent transmission of STDs, but use of condoms during sexual contact also reduces the risk. Standard precautions prescribe specific protective measures to be taken when working with people who have infections that can be transmitted through body fluids.
- The nursing care of patients with STDs may address impaired skin integrity, pain, risk for injury, anxiety, situational low self-esteem, impaired social interactions, ineffective sexuality patterns, ineffective coping, and ineffective therapeutic regimen management.
- Patient teaching is essential for patients with STDs and should include information about drug therapy and other treatment options, disease transmission, abstinence during treatment, and preventive measures.

REVIEW QUESTIONS

1. The purpose of reporting sexually transmitted diseases is to:
   1. prosecute the individuals who are transmitting the disease to others.
   2. emphasize to infected persons the importance of practicing safe sex.
   3. treat all infected persons to reduce transmission of the infection.
   4. teach the general public about measures to prevent STDs.
2. Erythromycin ophthalmic ointment may be ordered for the newborn because it is effective against:
   1. genital warts.
   2. chlamydial infections.
   3. human immunodeficiency virus.
   4. hepatitis B virus.
3. A patient who was diagnosed with gonorrhea did not return for treatment. When contacted, she reported that her symptoms had gone away so she thought she had recovered from the infection. The most appropriate response by the nurse would be which of the following?
   1. Symptoms often disappear after a few weeks, but without treatment, the bacteria remain in your body, and you remain highly infectious.
   2. As long as your symptoms have cleared up, there is no reason to treat you now.
   3. If you have symptoms in the future, come to the clinic immediately.
   4. Fortunately, gonorrhea has no serious complications, but I must advise you to seek treatment anyway.
4. The primary stage of syphilis is usually characterized by:
   1. a rash on the extremities, chest or back, palms of the hands, and soles of the feet.
   2. a reddish papule on the genitals, anus, or mouth that becomes a painless red ulcer.
   3. tender lymph nodes in the area of the skin lesion.
   4. fever, sore throat, and generalized aching.
5. The patient with untreated syphilis may develop:
   1. blindness, mental illness, paralysis, and heart disease.
   2. autoimmune deficiency syndrome (AIDS).
   3. cancer of the genitals.
   4. septicemia.
6. Which statement is true regarding the herpes simplex virus types 1 and 2?
   1. Type 1 is most often transmitted by genital contact.
   2. The modes of transmission of both types 1 and 2 are the same.
   3. Type 1 *only* affects the genitals, and type 2 *only* affects the mouth.
   4. Type 1 is usually nongenital, with lesions typically above the waist.
7. The teaching plan for a woman with a type 2 genital herpes simplex virus infection should include which of the following statements?
   1. You should have yearly Pap smears because you are at increased risk for cervical cancer.
   2. You should not become pregnant because the herpes virus causes fetal deformities.
   3. Once you have finished taking your medicine, you will be cured of the herpes infection.
   4. Your partner must use a condom for intercourse until you are completely cured.
8. The teaching plan for a patient with genital warts should include which of the following?
   1. This condition cannot be transmitted to a sexual partner.
   2. Genital warts are caused by poor personal hygiene.
   3. A topical medication can remove the warts but is not curative.
   4. Once the warts are removed, they are unlikely to come back.
9. Which statement is true regarding drug therapy for HIV infection?
   1. If the patient can tolerate very high doses, the chances of a cure are good.
   2. The HAART strategy uses a combination of drugs from three categories.
   3. A patient who is on drug therapy can resume sexual activity without precautions.
   4. Drugs used to treat HIV infections have very few side or adverse effects.
10. Instructions for effective use of condoms should include which of the following?
    1. Condoms provide 100% protection against disease transmission.
    2. Natural membrane condoms are preferred over latex condoms.
    3. Use only oil-based lubricants to prevent breakage of the condom.
    4. Leave a space of about 1 inch at the tip for semen.

UNIT **FIFTEEN** INTEGUMENTARY DISORDERS

48 Skin Disorders

objectives

1. Describe the structure and functions of the skin.
2. List the components of the nursing assessment of the skin.
3. Define terms used to describe the skin and skin lesions.
4. Explain the tests and procedures used to diagnose skin disorders.
5. Explain the nurse's responsibilities regarding the tests and procedures for diagnosing skin disorders.
6. Explain the therapeutic benefits and nursing considerations for patients who receive dressings, soaks and wet wraps, phototherapy, and drug therapy for skin problems.
7. For selected skin disorders, describe the pathophysiology, signs and symptoms, diagnostic tests, and medical treatment.
8. Assist in developing a nursing care plan for the patient with a skin disorder.

key terms

Acne (ĂK-nē, p. 1027)
Acrochordon (ăk-rō-KŎR-dŏn, p. 1013)
Angioma (ăn-jē-Ō-mă, p. 1013)
Débridement (dă-BRĒD-măw, p. 1037)
Dermatitis (dĕr-mă-TĪ-tĭs, p. 1022)
Intertrigo (ĭn-tĕr-TRĪ-gō, p. 1025)
Keratolytic (kĕr-ă-tō-LĬT-ĭk, p. 1019)
Lentigo (*pl.* Lentigines) (lĕn-TĪ-gō, lĕn-TĬJ-ĭ-nēz, p. 1013)
Nevus (*pl.* Nevi) (NĒ-vŭs, NĒ-vī, p. 1014)
Pemphigus (PĔM-fĭ-gŭs, p. 1029)
Pruritus (proo-RĪ-tŭs, p. 1013)
Psoriasis (sō-RĪ-ă-sĭs, p. 1024)

ANATOMY AND PHYSIOLOGY OF THE SKIN

The skin is an organ that covers the body surface. The anatomy of the skin is illustrated in Figure 48-1. It is composed of two distinct layers: the epidermis and the dermis. The epidermis is the outermost layer that covers the dermis. The base of the epidermis continually produces new cells to replace those at the surface. Epidermal cells produce melanin, a dark pigment, that helps determine the color of the skin. Strong ultraviolet light, such as in sunlight, stimulates the production of melanin.

The dermis is strong connective tissue that contains nerve endings, sweat glands, and hair roots. The dermis is well supplied with blood vessels, causing the skin to redden when surface vessels are dilated. Subcutaneous tissue lies beneath the dermis.

The hair, nails, and sebaceous glands are appendages (or derivatives) of the skin. The hair root is located in a tube in the dermis called a *hair follicle.* The arrector muscles of the hair (arrectores pilorum), located around the hair follicles, can contract, causing the hairs to stand erect and the skin to take on a gooseflesh appearance. Also around the hair follicles are sebaceous glands that secrete an oily substance called *sebum.* Sweat glands, found in most parts of the skin, secrete through the skin surface water that contains salts, ammonia, amino acids, lactic acid, ascorbic acid, uric acid, and urea.

FUNCTIONS OF THE SKIN

The functions of the skin are protection, body temperature regulation, secretion, sensation, and synthesis of vitamin D. In addition, the blood vessels of the skin can serve as a blood reservoir.

Protection

The skin performs its protective function by shielding underlying tissues from trauma and pathogens and by preventing excess loss of fluids from those tissues. A second type of protective function is fulfilled by Langerhans' cells, which initiate an immune response when foreign substances invade the epidermis.

Temperature Regulation

The skin participates in temperature regulation by altering the diameter of surface blood vessels and through sweating. To dissipate heat, the blood vessels dilate. As the blood flows close to the body surface, heat is lost through the surface. To retain heat, blood vessels constrict and heat loss is minimized. Sweating helps cool the body because heat is lost as sweat evaporates from the skin.

Secretions

Sweat is one skin secretion; sebum is another. Sebum coats the skin, creating an oily barrier that holds in water. Sweat promotes loss of body heat through evaporation, as noted previously, and plays a role in excretion of wastes.

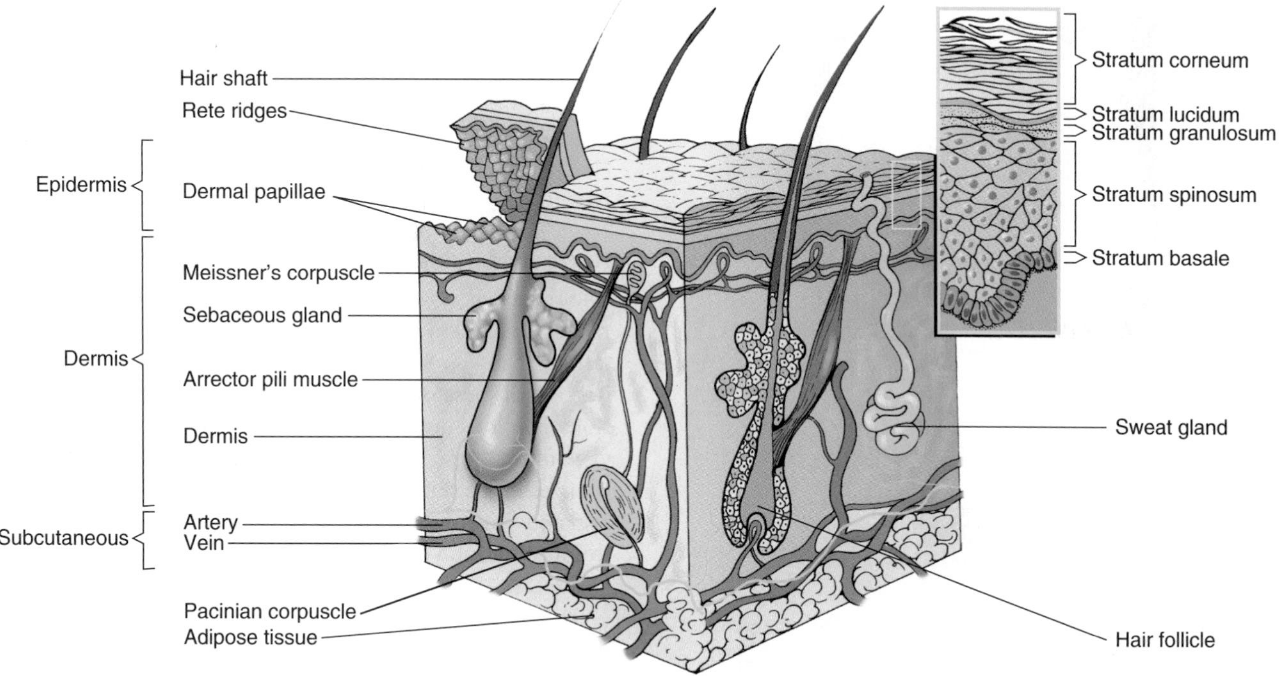

FIGURE **48-1** Anatomy of the skin.

Sensation

The skin is heavily endowed with sensory receptors for touch, pressure, pain, and temperature. When these sensory receptors are stimulated, nerves convey messages to the brain for interpretation.

Synthesis of Vitamin D

Ultraviolet rays in sunlight activate a substance in the skin that eventually is converted into vitamin D.

Blood Reservoir

The skin contains an extensive blood vessel network that can store as much as 10% of the body's total blood volume. Constriction of these superficial blood vessels shunts blood to vital organs when needed.

 ***Put on your THINKING CAP!!***

A patient who has just returned from surgery complains of being cold. Your assessment reveals pale hands and feet, weak pedal pulses, and slight shivering. Both feet and ankles are cold to the touch. Her vital signs are normal and her wound dressing is dry. Explain the basis of each of her symptoms noted.

You obtain an extra blanket and cover the patient snugly, turn up the heater in the room, and ask her to call you if she does not feel better soon. When you return in 15 minutes, her hands and feet are warm, pedal pulses palpable. She is resting quietly with no shivering. Explain how her condition changed.

AGE-RELATED CHANGES IN THE SKIN

Changes in the skin are probably the most readily recognized of all signs of physical aging. Wrinkling of the skin occurs as a result of thinning of the skin layers and degeneration of elastin fibers. There is a loss of elasticity and strength. Sweat glands decrease in size and number, although sweat production changes little until advanced age. The production of sebum by sebaceous glands decreases with age, becoming apparent earlier in women than in men. Dryness and pruritus (itching) are common. Skin often becomes paler as people age because the number of cells that produce melanin decreases. Many skin lesions are more common in the elderly. They include the following:

1. Lentigines: pigmented spots on sun-exposed areas; they are commonly called liver spots, although they have nothing to do with the liver (singular, lentigo).
2. Senile purpura: large, purplish bruises that resolve very slowly; they can result from minor trauma.
3. Senile angiomas: bright-red papules.
4. Seborrheic keratoses: waxy, raised lesions; they are flesh-colored to dark brown or black and variously sized from small and nearly flat to large and prominent.
5. Acrochordons (skin tags): small, soft, raised lesions; they are flesh-colored or pigmented.

Figure 48-2 illustrates some age-related changes in the skin.

The risk of premalignant and malignant skin lesions also increases with age. These are discussed along with other pathologic conditions later in this chapter.

By age 50 years, approximately half of all people have some gray hair. Men commonly begin to lose some hair from the

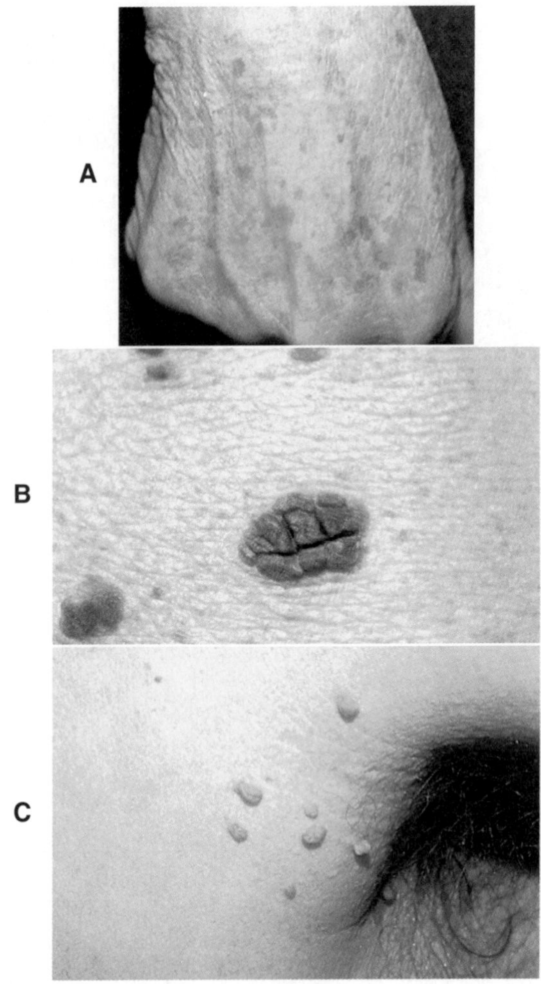

FIGURE 48-2 Common skin changes in the older adult. *A,* Lentigines. *B,* Seborrheic keratosis. *C,* Skin tags.

scalp in their fourth decade, and by the time they are 80 years of age, many men are almost bald. Scalp hair thins in women as well but usually is less obvious. Many older women and men have an increase in facial hair. Men also may have increased hair in the nares, eyebrows, or helix of the ear. In addition to aging changes in the skin and hair, the nails flatten and become dry, brittle, and discolored.

NURSING ASSESSMENT OF THE SKIN

HEALTH HISTORY

Chief Complaint and History of Present Illness

When a patient has a skin disorder, the chief complaint may be discomfort, pruritus, color changes, lesions, hair loss, or abnormal hair growth. Take a history of the present illness, describing the onset of the condition and any precipitating and alleviating factors. The progression of symptoms and changes in the distribution or appearance of lesions may be helpful in the diagnostic process.

Past Medical History

Elicit the past medical history to document previous skin diseases or problems, current and recent medications (including nonprescription drugs), and allergies. In addition to skin diseases, conditions that may have skin manifestations include diabetes mellitus, cancer, kidney failure, thyroid disease, liver disease, and anemia.

Review of Systems

The review of systems includes additional data that may be related to the skin problem: change in skin color or pigmentation, change in a mole, sores that have been slow to heal, itching, dryness or scaliness, excessive bruising, rashes, lesions, hair loss, unusual hair growth, changes in nails. The review of systems also may reveal other disorders that cause changes in the skin. Specific signs and symptoms may be associated with circulatory, respiratory, renal, hepatic, gastrointestinal, and endocrine conditions.

Put on your THINKING CAP!!

Can you think of one change in the skin that might occur with disorders of each of the following systems/organs: circulatory system, respiratory system, urinary system, and the liver?

Functional Assessment

Because the functional assessment can provide important clues to skin problems, record the patient's past and present occupations, exposure to chemicals or other irritants, skin care habits, and extent of sun exposure. Note recent changes in the work or living environment. Also inquire about current stresses and sources of anxiety.

PHYSICAL EXAMINATION

Assessment of the skin is done throughout the physical examination. Inspect the skin, noticing the color and variations in pigmentation. Sun-exposed areas are typically darker than protected areas. Note dilated blood vessels and angiomas (benign tumors composed of blood vessels). Table 48-1 describes variations in skin color and the significance of each. Carefully inspect nevi (moles) for irregularities in shape, pigmentation, and ulcerations or changes in surrounding skin. Palpate nevi for tenderness. Measure and record lesion size in centimeters. If there is a rash, describe the location, distribution, and characteristics. If there is any drainage, note the color, amount, and odor. Terms used to describe skin lesions are defined in Table 48-2 and illustrated in Figure 48-3.

Palpate the skin for temperature, moisture, texture, thickness, edema, mobility, and turgor. Assessment of mobility and turgor is illustrated in Figure 48-4.

Some skin changes are less apparent in dark-skinned people than in light-skinned people. Healthy black skin has a reddish undertone. A grayish tone may reflect cyanosis, which is best seen around the mouth, over the cheekbones, and on the

table 48-1 ***Variations in Skin Color***

COLOR CHANGE	DESCRIPTION	CAUSES
Pallor	White or pale in light-skinned people. Yellowish-brown in brown-skinned people. Ashen in black-skinned people. May be evident in mucous membranes, lips, and nail beds, as well as skin.	Vasoconstriction due to acute anxiety or fear, cold, some drugs, cigarette smoking. Edema.
Erythema	Bright red	Increased local blood flow due to inflammation, fever, or emotions such as embarrassment or anger.
Cyanosis	Bluish	Excess deoxygenated blood in the tissue due to anemia, respiratory disorders, or cardiovascular disorders.
Jaundice	Golden or greenish-yellow	Reflects increased bilirubin in the blood due to liver disease or destruction of red blood cells.

table 48-2 ***Common Skin Lesions***

LESION	CHARACTERISTICS	EXAMPLES
Macule	Distinct flat area with color different from surrounding tissue	Freckle, petechia, hypopigmentation
Papule	Any raised, solid lesion with clearly defined margins; <1 cm in diameter	Mole, wart
Vesicle	Raised, fluid-filled cavity, <1 cm in diameter	Herpes simplex, herpes zoster
Pustule	Raised, well defined cavity that contains pus	Acne, impetigo
Patch	Macule >1 cm	Vitiligo
Plaque	Combined papules that form a raised area >1 cm in diameter	Psoriasis
Nodule	Raised, solid lesion >1 cm in diameter; may be hard or soft and may extend deeper into dermis than papule	Fibroma, xanthoma
Wheal	Superficial, irregular swelling caused by fluid accumulation	Allergic response, insect bite
Tumor	Firm or soft lesion that extends deep into dermis; may be firm or soft	Lipoma, hemangioma
Bulla	Thin-walled, fluid-filled chamber >1 cm in diameter	Blister
Crust	Thick, dried exudate remaining after vesicles rupture	Impetigo, weeping eczematous dermatitis
Scale	Dry or greasy skin flakes	Psoriasis, seborrheic dermatitis, eczema
Fissure	Distinct linear crack extending into dermis	Cheilosis, tinea pedis
Erosion	Shallow, superficial depression	
Ulcer	Depression deeper than erosion, may bleed	Pressure ulcer, chancre
Excoriation	Abrasion caused by scratching	Scratching with insect bites, scabies, dermatitis
Nevus (mole)	Flat or raised, color darker than surrounding skin	
Cyst	Fluid-filled cavity in dermis or subcutaneous tissue	Sebaceous cyst

earlobes. Inflammation may be better detected by areas of abnormal warmth and firmness than by color changes. Rashes are better seen by shining a light at an angle to reveal irregularities in skin surface.

Inspect the hair for color, distribution, and oiliness and palpate to determine the texture. Inspect the scalp for scaliness, infestations, and lesions.

Inspect the shape and contour of the fingernails and toenails. Note the color of the nail bed and assess capillary refill by applying pressure to cause blanching and then releasing the pressure. The color should return to normal within 3 to 5 seconds. Assess the angle of the nail base to detect clubbing of the nails (see Fig. 28-6).

The nursing assessment of the patient with a skin disorder is outlined in Table 48-3.

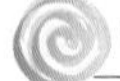

What Does Culture Have to do with Skin Assessment?

It may be more difficult to assess some skin characteristics in dark-skinned people. To inspect for cyanosis, jaundice, and pallor, check the oral mucous membranes, the conjunctivae, the palms of the hands, and the soles of the feet.

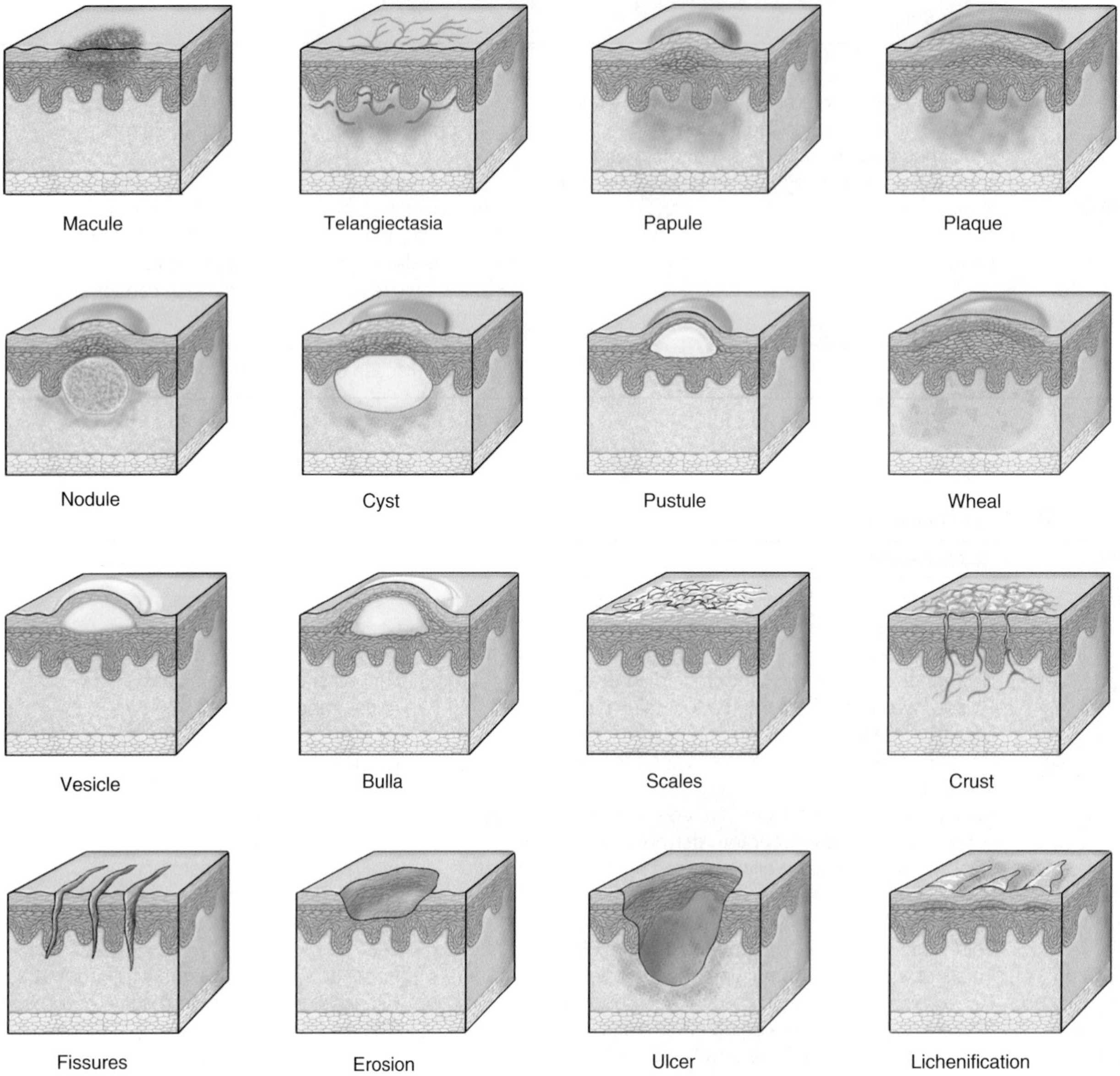

Macule Telangiectasia Papule Plaque

Nodule Cyst Pustule Wheal

Vesicle Bulla Scales Crust

Fissures Erosion Ulcer Lichenification

FIGURE **48-3** Skin lesions.

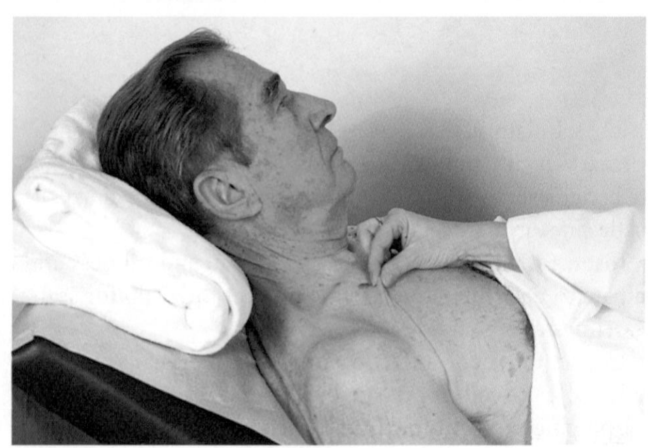

FIGURE **48-4** Skin mobility is determined by assessing how easily a large fold of skin is pinched up. Skin turgor is evaluated by observing how quickly the fold returns to the previous position.

A

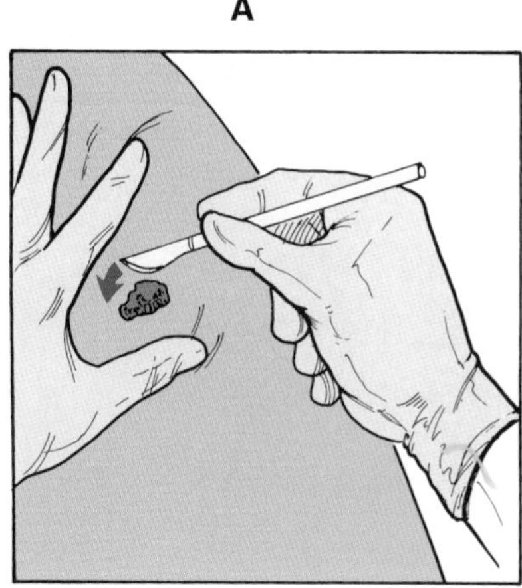

B

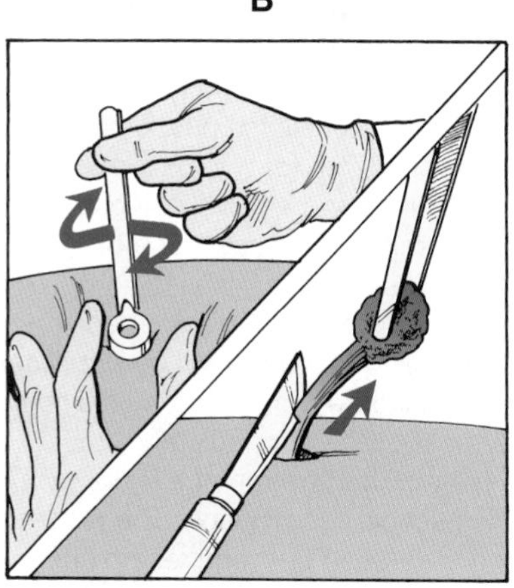

C

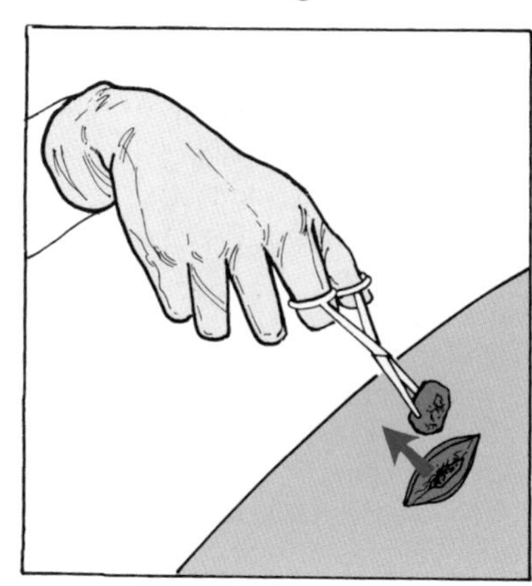

FIGURE **48-5** Types of biopsy procedures: *A,* Shave. *B,* Punch. *C,* Surgical excision.

table 48-3 **ASSESSMENT *of the Patient with a Skin Disorder***

HEALTH HISTORY	PHYSICAL EXAMINATION
Chief Complaint or History of Present Illness: Pruritus, skin color changes, lesions, hair loss, abnormal hair growth **Past Medical History:** Skin diseases or problems, drug therapy, allergies, chronic illnesses: diabetes mellitus, cancer, kidney failure, thyroid disease, liver disease, anemia **Review of Systems:** Change in skin color or pigmentation, change in a mole, sores that heal slowly, itching, dryness or scaliness, excessive bruising, changes in nails **Functional Assessment:** Occupation, exposure to chemicals or other irritants, skin care habits, extent of sun exposure, dietary habits	**Skin:** Color, pigmentation, dilated blood vessels, angiomas, nevi, lesions, rash, drainage, temperature, texture, moisture, thickness, edema, mobility, turgor, scars **Hair:** Color, distribution, oiliness, texture, nits **Scalp:** Scaliness, lesions **Nails:** Shape, contour, color of nail bed, blanching with pressure, capillary refill, angle of nail base

DIAGNOSTIC TESTS AND PROCEDURES

MICROSCOPIC EXAMINATION OF SKIN SPECIMENS

Studies of skin specimens that are used to diagnose skin conditions include:

- A potassium hydroxide (or KOH) examination to diagnose fungal infections of the skin, hair, or nails by studying a skin specimen. For a culture, the skin scraping or a nail clipping is implanted in medium.
- A Tzanck's smear is used to diagnose viral skin infections.
- A scabies scraping is used to detect scabies (mites), eggs, or feces excreted by mites.

WOOD'S LIGHT EXAMINATION

In a Wood's light examination, a black light is used to assess for pigmentation changes and superficial skin infections.

PATCH TESTING FOR ALLERGY

To identify allergens, very small amounts of common irritants are applied to the skin, covered, and later examined for allergic reactions. Assessment and treatment of allergies are explained in detail in Chapter 12.

BIOPSY

A biopsy is the removal of tissue for microscopic examination. The three types of skin biopsies (Fig. 48-5) are:

- *Shave biopsy:* a specimen no deeper than the dermis is obtained with a scalpel or other specialized instrument. Bleeding is usually minimal and controlled with pressure, cautery, or chemicals.
- *Punch biopsy:* a circular tool cuts around the lesion, which is then lifted up and severed. Pressure or chemicals usually control bleeding, but suturing may be needed to close the site. Relatively shallow excision.
- *Surgical excision:* for deep specimens, surgical excision biopsy is indicated. Sutures are required to close the defect left by the procedure.

table 48-4 **DIAGNOSTIC TESTS AND PROCEDURES | *Skin Disorders and Related Nursing Implications***

TEST/PURPOSE	PATIENT PREPARATION	POSTPROCEDURE CARE
Potassium hydroxide (KOH) examination is used along with a culture to diagnose fungal infections of the skin and nails.	Inform patient that a small scraping of skin will be taken from the affected area for microscopic examination. The skin scrapings and a nail clipping are used for cultures to determine the exact cause of the lesion. Procedure is painless.	Inform patient when results will be available.
Tzanck's smear Used to diagnose viral infections.	Tell the patient the lesion will be washed and opened to obtain a fluid sample, which will be examined microscopically. Procedure may cause mild discomfort. Results may be available immediately.	No special care.
Scabies scraping Used to assess skin lesions for the presence of scabies (mites), eggs, or feces excreted by the mites.	Inform the patient that the top of a lesion will be taken off for microscopic examination. The procedure is briefly uncomfortable but requires no anesthesia.	No special care.
Wood's light examination Uses black light to reveal superficial skin infections and changes in pigmentation.	Tell the patient the procedure is done in a dark room. The skin will be carefully inspected under black light. The procedure is noninvasive and painless.	No special care.
Patch testing Used to identify substances to which patients are allergic.	Inform the patient that various common irritants are applied to the skin and covered with special patches or tape. The patches must be left in place and examined ("read") after 48, 72, 96 hours and sometimes after 1 week. Skin reactions that indicate allergy include redness, swelling, and blisters. Patch testing is painless.	No special care.
A biopsy The removal of tissue for microscopic examination.	Tell the patient the physician will remove some tissue for diagnostic evaluation. Small shallow biopsies usually require only a dressing. Deeper biopsies require sutures. Patients are usually advised to avoid aspirin or other NSAIDs for 48 hours before the biopsy to prevent excessive bleeding.	Inspect the site for bleeding. Apply direct pressure if necessary to control bleeding. If sutures are used, instruct the patient to return on a specified date for suture removal. Tell the patient how to care for the biopsy site (protocols vary), and when results are expected.

Table 48-4 presents additional details and nursing interventions for patients undergoing diagnostic procedures.

COMMON THERAPEUTIC MEASURES

DRESSINGS

Dressings are used to protect healing wounds and to retain surface moisture to promote healing. There are many types of dressings, including wet, dry, absorptive, and occlusive dressings. Dry dressings protect wounds and absorb drainage. Wet dressings are used to decrease inflammation, soften crusts, and promote tissue granulation. Absorptive dressings are used to promote removal of excess exudate and are especially useful in wounds with necrotic tissue. Occlusive dressings protect wounds and maintain moisture to promote healing.

NEGATIVE PRESSURE WOUND THERAPY

Negative pressure wound therapy is a relatively recent development in wound care that appears to greatly reduce the time required for healing of traumatic wounds, dehisced surgical wounds, pressure ulcers, and chronic ulcers. To use this approach, the wound is first cleansed with normal saline. Then a skin preparation product is applied around the wound to receive the adhesive dressing. The wound is then filled with one of two types of sponges, depending on the wound characteristics. A tube in the sponges will be used to exert negative pressure. A transparent adhesive dressing is applied over the sponges and around the tubing so that the wound closure is airtight. The tubing is connected to suction that is set at a prescribed negative pressure. Suction may be applied intermittently or continuously as ordered. Continuous suction is less painful than intermittent suction. Notify the enterostomal therapist or physician if the pain is distressing. The pressure may have to be reduced or converted from intermittent to continuous suction. Because dressing changes are painful, give the patient an analgesic about 1 hour before the procedure. If sponges adhere to the wound surface, they can be moistened with normal saline before removal.

SOAKS AND WET WRAPS

Soaks and wet wraps are used to soothe, soften, and remove crusts, debris, and necrotic tissue. Warm water is used, and various agents may be added for specific skin conditions. A wet wrap may be applied to a single affected area or to the entire body. It is usually covered by a dry dressing and left in place for 15 to 20 minutes. Unless débridement is intended, moisten the wet dressing again before removal. Otherwise, healthy tissue may adhere to the dry material and be traumatized. After a soak, gently dry the treated area. Then apply topical medications as ordered.

PHOTOTHERAPY

Phototherapy is the use of ultraviolet light in combination with photosensitive drugs to promote shedding of the epidermis. Types of ultraviolet light are A, B, and C. Phototherapy may be used in the treatment of psoriasis, vitiligo, and chronic eczema. It is contraindicated in patients with a history of herpes simplex infection, skin cancer, cataracts, and lupus erythematosus because it aggravates these conditions. After phototherapy, the patient may have pruritus and dry skin. Assess for signs and symptoms of phototoxicity (redness, vesicles, pain).

Goeckerman Regimen

The Goeckerman regimen is a type of phototherapy specifically used to treat psoriasis and atopic dermatitis. The patient first bathes in a tar emulsion bath. Then a topical tar product is applied, and the patient is exposed to ultraviolet light.

Photochemotherapy

Photochemotherapy with a psoralen and ultraviolet A (PUVA) is a treatment that uses a combination of oral or topical 8-methoxypsoralen and ultraviolet A (long-wave ultraviolet light). It is used to treat vitiligo, psoriasis, and cutaneous T-cell lymphoma. For 8 hours before and after the treatment, the patient is instructed to wear sunscreen, protective clothing, and dark glasses to decrease exposure to other sources of ultraviolet light.

DRUG THERAPY

A number of topical and oral drugs are used to treat skin disorders and skin manifestations of other conditions. Topical drugs include **keratolytics** (capable of dissolving keratin), antipruritics, emollients, lubricants, sunscreens, tars, anti-infectives, glucocorticoids, antimetabolites, antihistamines, antiseborrheic agents, and vitamin A derivatives. Examples of selected drug classifications and their actions, side effects, and nursing interventions are presented in Table 48-5.

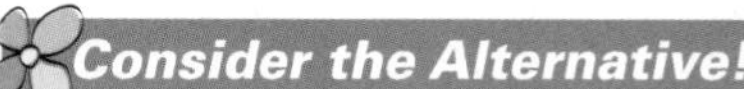

Consider the Alternative!

Topical herbal preparations that are used as emollients include balm of gilead, coltsfoot, and comfrey.

For topical application, drugs are combined with various substances in forms called *vehicles*. Topical medication vehicles include powders, lotions, aerosols, gels, creams, and ointments.

DISORDERS OF THE SKIN

PRURITUS

Pruritus is simply itching. It is a symptom rather than a disease, but is very common with many skin and systemic disorders. Therefore, an overview of pruritus is presented here.

Etiology and Risk Factors

The sensation of itching is not completely understood, but it may be triggered by touch, temperature changes, emotional stress, and chemical, mechanical, and electrical stimuli. The severity of the response to stimulation is enhanced by emotional stress, anxiety, and fear.

Pruritus is a prominent symptom with psoriasis, dermatitis, eczema, and insect bites. It may also be present with the following systemic conditions: urticaria, some cancers, renal failure, diabetes mellitus, thyroid disorders, liver disease, and anemia.

Medical Treatment

When the cause of pruritus is known, treatment is directed at correcting the cause. Measures that may help control the symptom include stress management and avoidance of known irritants, sudden temperature changes, and alcohol, tea, and coffee. Lubricants in the bath water and emollients applied after bathing also may help. Medications that often are ordered for pruritus include corticosteroids, antihistamines, and local anesthetics. In some situations, antidepressant and antiserotonin drugs may be ordered.

NURSING CARE *of the Patient with Pruritus*

Assessment

When a patient has pruritus, assess his or her symptoms and obtain a history that may help determine the cause. The history of the current illness is important because pruritus may be just one symptom of a condition that requires attention. Possible contributing factors to be documented include exposure to irritants, drug therapy, and past medical history.

Nursing Diagnoses, Goals, and Outcome Criteria: Pruritus

Nursing Diagnoses	Goals and Outcome Criteria
Impaired Skin Integrity related to scratching	Intact skin: absence of abrasions

table 48-5 **DRUG THERAPY** | ***Disorders of the Skin***

DRUG	USE/ACTION	SIDE EFFECTS	NURSING INTERVENTIONS
KERATOLYTICS			
Benzoyl peroxide Salicylic acid Sulfur Coal tar	Dissolve keratin and slow bacterial growth. Used to treat acne and psoriasis.	Excessive dryness, irritation, scaling, edema, photosensitivity.	Advise patient to avoid excessive sun exposure. Assess effects.
TOPICAL ANTIBACTERIALS			
Bacitracin Polysporin	Destroy microorganisms. Used to treat skin infections.	Contact dermatitis. Allergy (rare): itching, burning, anaphylaxis.	Assess allergies before applying. Apply as prescribed after allergy ruled out. Report itching, burning, rash, redness.
Silver sulfadiazine (Silvadene)	Bactericidal. Used to prevent and treat wound infection with serious burns.	Rash, pruritus, burning, pain. Rare: nephritis, anorexia. Can cause blood dyscrasias, hepatitis, nephrosis, hypoglycemia.	Apply to clean burn surface with gloved hand. Cover burn completely and continuously. Monitor renal and GI distress, headache, joint pain. hepatic function. Monitor vital signs, complete blood count, serum glucose.
ANTIVIRAL AGENTS			
Acyclovir (Zovirax)	Interfere with viral replication. Used to treat infections caused by herpes simplex virus types 1 and 2 and herpes zoster. Not curative but may reduce severity and duration of symptoms.	*Topical form:* burning, stinging, pruritus. *Oral form:* nausea and vomiting. *IV form:* phlebitis, rash, urticaria, hypotension, hematuria, diaphoresis. Rare: confusion, agitation, seizures. Nephrotoxicity with high IV doses.	Assess allergies. Monitor closely if patient has renal impairment. Measure intake and output. Monitor infusion site for redness. Monitor neurological status. Use gloved finger to apply ointment. Encourage adequate fluid intake.
TOPICAL ANTIFUNGAL AGENTS			
Nystatin (Mycostatin) Clotrimazole (Mycelex) Oxiconazole (Oxistat) Naftifine (Naftin) Terbinafine (Lamisil)	Effective against fungi. Used to treat fungal infections.	Irritation, erythema, burning, rash. Abdominal cramps and cystitis with vaginal preparations.	Apply as directed. Do not apply occlusive dressings without order.
ORAL ANTIFUNGAL AGENTS			
Terbinafine (Lamisil) Griseofulvin (Fulvicin P/G) Ketoconazole (Nizoral)	Used to treat fungal infections that do not respond to topicals. Common use: nail infections.	Terbinafine: hepatotoxicity, headache, diarrhea, GI distress. Griseofulvin: headache, rash, insomnia, GI distress. Ketoconazole: hepatotoxicity.	Give ketoconazole with food or milk to minimize GI effects, and 2 hours apart from any drugs that reduce gastric acidity. Monitor liver function with ketoconazole and terbinafine. Griseofulvin decreases effects of warfarin.
TOPICAL ANTI-INFLAMMATORIES			
Hydrocortisone (Cortizone, and others) Triamcinolone (Aristocort, and others) Fluocinolone (Bio-Syn, and others)	Reduce inflammation in various skin disorders.	Itching, erythema, irritation. Severe allergic reactions rare.	Do not apply occlusive dressing without order. Apply sparingly and rub in thoroughly.

VITAMIN A DERIVATIVE			
Tretinoin (Retin-A) Isotretinoin (Accutane)	Reduces formation of comedones. Increases mitosis of epithelial cells. Used to treat acne. Decreases size of sebaceous glands. Decreases sebum production. Used to treat severe acne.	Stinging, erythema, scaling expected. Allergy rare. Occasionally severe erythema, blistering. Excessive dryness of skin, nose, mouth. Conjunctivitis, vomiting, elevated serum triglycerides, bone or joint pain, muscle aches. Rare: hepatitis, inflammatory bowel disease, depression. Contraindicated during pregnancy: can cause major fetal deformities.	Tell patient not to use with keratolytics. Do not apply to eyes, mouth, angles of nose. Patient should avoid sun exposure, use sunscreen. If dryness excessive, decrease frequency of use. Tell patient to expect symptoms to worsen at first, then improve. Do not use topical acne drugs at same time. Report severe GI symptoms. Avoid sun exposure owing to photosensitivity. Explain importance of preventing pregnancy 1 mo before, during, and 1 mo after therapy. Recommend two reliable forms of contraception to be used simultaneously.
Tazarotene (Tazorac) Adapalene (Differin)	Tazarotene and adapalene both are topical agents used to treat acne. Tazarotene is also used to treat psoriasis.	Both can cause itching, burning, and stinging. More serious skin reactions sometimes occur.	Advise patients to avoid direct sunlight and use sunscreens because of photosensitivity. Acne may worsen before beneficial results occur. Instruct patient in correct application (see instructions for each drug).
PEDICULICIDES AND SCABICIDES			
Crotamiton (Eurax) Permethrin (Nix)	Kill parasites and their eggs. Used to treat pediculosis (lice) and scabies (mite) infestations.	Skin and eye irritation. Systemic effects with excessive use.	Follow directions specifically. Avoid contact with eyes. Most products are effective with one application, but a repeat treatment may be recommended. Clothing and bed linens must be treated to prevent reinfestation.
ANTIPSORIATICS			
Anthralin Tar (Estar gel)	Used to treat psoriasis.	Anthralin: erythema, inflamed eyes, staining. Tar: skin irritation, photosensitivity, staining.	Protect skin and clothing from preparations that stain. Most have unpleasant odor.
RETINOID ANTIPSORIATIC			
Acitretin (Soriatane)	Decreases proliferation of epidermal cells; anti-inflammatory, immunomodulatory. For severe psoriasis only.	Hair loss, skin peeling, dry mouth, rhinitis, gingivitis, elevated liver enzymes and triglycerides. Many other side and adverse effects.	*Contraindicated during pregnancy!* Be sure patient understands risk to fetus and uses contraception if sexually active for at least 3 years after therapy completed. Should be taken with meals. Monitor for all side effects.
PHOTOSENSITIVITY DRUG			
Methoxsalen (Oxsoralen)	Decreases proliferation of epidermal cells in psoriasis.	Nausea, headache, vertigo, rash, pruritus, burning and peeling of skin. Can cause anemia, leukopenia, thrombocytopenia, ulcerative stomatitis, bleeding, alopecia, cystitis.	Encourage patient to return for periodic blood tests as ordered and to report easy bruising or excessive bleeding.

GI, Gastrointestinal; *IV*, intravenous.

Nursing Diagnoses, Goals, and Outcome Criteria: Pruritus—cont'd

Nursing Diagnoses	Goals and Outcome Criteria
Ineffective Therapeutic Regimen Management related to lack of understanding of prevention or management of pruritus	Patient adheres to prescribed measures to prevent or treat condition: patient correctly states correct measures, demonstrates self-care

Interventions

The specific interventions vary with the cause of pruritus. If the patient has dry skin, application of lubricants or emollients may be helpful. Lotion can usually be applied to unbroken skin without a physician's order. If topical or systemic drugs are ordered, administer them or instruct the patient in their use. Inspect the skin daily to determine the effects of the treatments. Explain possible causes of pruritus and encourage the patient to avoid them.

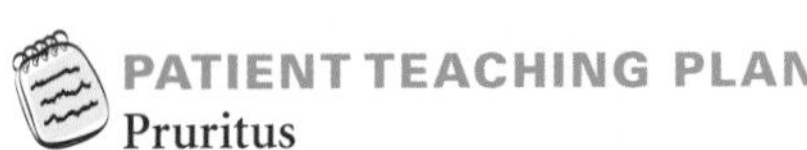

PATIENT TEACHING PLAN
Pruritus

- Avoid factors that aggravate itching such as temperature extremes, extremely dry air, irritating fabrics, chemicals, frequent hot baths, sweating, stress.
- To prevent itching, avoid extreme temperatures, humidify room air, take less frequent and cooler baths, apply emollients, avoid irritating fabrics and chemicals, and practice stress management.
- Use therapeutic measures as prescribed:
  Topical agents: lotions, creams
  Systemic agents: antihistamines—dosage, side effects
  Treatment of underlying conditions

INFLAMMATORY CONDITIONS AND INFECTIONS

Atopic Dermatitis (Eczema)

Pathophysiology

Atopic **dermatitis** is one of several disorders referred to as *eczema.* Eczema has three stages. The acute stage is characterized by a red, oozing, crusty rash and intense pruritus. Manifestations of the subacute stage include redness, excoriations, and scaling plaques or pustules. Fine scales may give the patient's skin a silvery appearance. In the chronic stage, the skin becomes dry, thickened, scaly, and brownish-gray in color (Fig. 48-6). Open lesions invite infection, and scarring may occur. Multiple stages may be present at the same time.

Etiology and Risk Factors

Most patients with atopic dermatitis have a personal or family history of asthma, hay fever, eczema, or food allergies. People with atopic dermatitis have an immune dysfunction, but it is not known whether that dysfunction is a cause or an effect of the disorder.

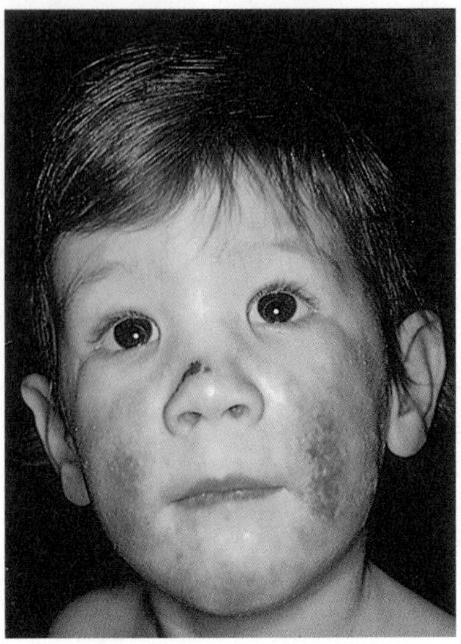

FIGURE **48-6** Atopic dermatitis.

Medical Diagnosis

A medical diagnosis of atopic dermatitis is based primarily on the health history and physical examination. Other procedures that might be done to confirm the diagnosis are skin biopsy, serum immunoglobulin E levels, and cultures to diagnose secondary infections. If allergy is suspected as a cause of dermatitis, the physician may perform allergy tests to identify allergens.

Medical Treatment

Topical corticosteroids provide the best control of inflammation. Soaks, occlusive dressings, and emollients help to keep the skin moist. Systemic antihistamines may be ordered to relieve itching and inflammation. In severe cases that do not respond to topical agents, a short course of systemic corticosteroids may be ordered. Research is in progress to determine the efficacy of the immunosuppressants tacrolimus and cyclosporine. Treatment of allergic disorders is detailed in Chapter 12.

NURSING CARE *of the Patient with Atopic Dermatitis*

Assessment

Assessment of the patient with a skin disorder is summarized in Table 48-3. When the patient has atopic dermatitis, specifically inquire about known allergies and bathing practices (frequency, water temperature, use of soaps) to identify possible contributing factors. The physical examination includes assessment of the skin for lesions, moisture and abrasions.

Nursing Diagnoses, Goals, and Outcome Criteria: Atopic Dermatitis

Nursing Diagnoses	Goals and Outcome Criteria
Impaired Skin Integrity related to excessive dryness, scratching	Improved skin integrity: intact, moist skin

Nursing Diagnoses	Goals and Outcome Criteria
Risk for Infection related to break in skin, decreased resistance to infection	Absence of infection: no fever, decreasing redness and drainage
Disturbed Body Image related to lesions	Improved body image: positive patient statements about self

Interventions

Impaired Skin Integrity

Measures that decrease itching and moisturize the skin help to maintain skin integrity. Encourage the patient to maintain the room temperature at 68° F to 75° F with 45% to 55% humidity. Advise the patient to avoid possible irritants. New clothing should be washed before wearing. Mild detergent should be used for laundry, and clothes rinsed twice. Recommend open-weave fabrics and loose clothing. Advise the use of moisturizers and sunscreens. If drugs are ordered for pruritus, administer them or instruct the patient in self-medication. Assess skin integrity and hydration on an ongoing basis.

Risk for Infection

Any break in the skin presents a portal for pathogens. Inspect the skin and report new lesions to the physician. Monitor the temperature for elevation that may reflect a systemic infection. Teach the patient the importance of protecting the skin from trauma. If scratching is a problem, the fingernails need to be cut short and kept smooth. Gloves or mittens may help prevent traumatic scratching during sleep or in the confused person. Administer antibiotics as ordered.

Disturbed Body Image

Demonstrate acceptance of the patient's appearance through attentive care and touch. Teach the patient and family that dermatitis is not contagious and is not caused by poor hygiene. Explore the patient's concerns about the skin disorder. If the patient is very stressed, the nurse can discuss coping strategies or request a referral for professional counseling.

PATIENT TEACHING PLAN
Atopic Dermatitis

- Avoid known irritants and constrictive clothing.
- Use moisturizers and sunscreens.
- Take drugs as prescribed: name, dosage or application instructions, adverse effects.
- After swimming in chlorinated water, shampoo and bathe (or shower) using a mild soap. Then apply a moisturizer.

Contact Dermatitis

Contact dermatitis is an inflammatory condition caused by contact with a substance that triggers an allergic response. Allergic and immune disorders are addressed in Chapter 12.

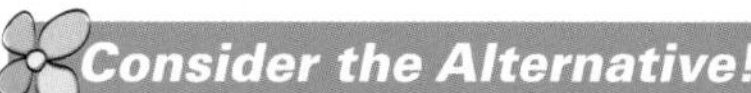

When a patient has an allergic skin reaction, be sure to assess for topical use of herbal products. For example, aloe can cause allergic dermatitis in susceptible persons, and angelica can cause a skin rash if a patient is exposed to sunlight.

Seborrheic Dermatitis

Pathophysiology

Seborrheic dermatitis is a chronic inflammatory disease of the skin. It usually affects the scalp, eyebrows, eyelids, lips, ears, sternal area, axillae, umbilicus, groin, gluteal crease, and the area under the breasts. Seborrheic dermatitis of the scalp is called dandruff. Areas affected by this condition may have fine, powdery scales, thick crusts, or oily patches. Scales may be white, yellowish, or reddish. Pruritus is common.

Etiology and Risk Factors

The cause of seborrheic dermatitis is unknown. It may be an inflammatory reaction to infection with the yeast *Malassezia.* Because the condition is aggravated by emotional stress and neurologic disease, some researchers think there may be a central nervous system influence.

Medical Diagnosis

Diagnosis of seborrheic dermatitis is based on the health history and physical examination.

Medical Treatment

Initial treatment of seborrheic dermatitis employs topical ketoconazole (Nizoral), sometimes with topical corticosteroids. Dandruff is treated with medicated shampoos used two or three times a week. Appropriate shampoos are those that contain selenium sulfide (Selsun), tar, zinc pyrithionate, or resorcin. Some corticosteroid solutions also may be prescribed.

NURSING CARE *of the Patient with Seborrheic Dermatitis*

Although seborrheic dermatitis does not require inpatient treatment, it is a common condition encountered among patients hospitalized for other reasons.

Assessment

The assessment includes determination of symptoms and identification of treatments being used. Inspect and describe the affected areas.

Nursing Diagnoses, Goals, and Outcome Criteria: Seborrheic Dermatitis

Nursing Diagnoses	Goals and Outcome Criteria
Ineffective Therapeutic Regimen Management related to lack of knowledge about treatment	Patient implements the prescribed treatment plan: correctly describes plan and self-care
Disturbed Body Image related to altered appearance (lesions)	Improved body image: decreasing signs of the condition, patient's statements reflect a positive view of self

Interventions

Explain the condition and reinforce the physician's instructions for treatment. Suggest measures to relieve pruritus, as described earlier in this chapter. Assess the patient's concerns about the condition and emphasize that seborrheic dermatitis can be controlled with treatment. Demonstrate acceptance of the patient by genuine interest and use of touch.

Psoriasis

Pathophysiology

The classic sign of psoriasis is the appearance of bright-red lesions that may be covered with silvery scales (Fig. 48-7). Although the onset is common in young adulthood, it can appear at any age. Psoriasis may affect a limited body area or may be extensive. Some people have systemic effects of the disease, such as psoriatic arthritis.

Etiology and Risk Factors

Psoriasis is a condition caused by rapid proliferation of epidermal cells. It is usually chronic with cycles of exacerbations and remissions. Multiple factors acting on a genetically predisposed person are thought to cause this disorder. Factors that aggravate psoriasis are stress, streptococcal infections, overuse of alcohol, and drugs such as lithium and beta blockers.

Medical Diagnosis

Psoriasis is diagnosed based on the health history and the physical examination.

Medical Treatment

There is no cure for psoriasis, but it can be treated topically or systemically. Patients with mild psoriasis are usually treated with topical medications: corticosteroids, coal tar derivatives alone or with UVB, and UVA with oral psoralens (PUVA). Tazarotene (Tazorac) is a topical retinoid that stays in the skin longer, leading to longer remissions. Anthralin (Anthra-Derm) may be used to remove heavy scales. With a gloved hand, it is applied only to the lesions. After a specified period of time, anthralin is removed with tissues. The patient removes the residue by showering or bathing. The medication must be handled carefully because it stains hair, skin, fingernails, furniture, and bathroom fixtures. Newer preparations such as Estar gel that do not stain are now available.

More severe psoriasis may be treated with whole-body radiation or with systemic drugs including acitretin (Soriatane), which is replacing etretinate (Tegison), methotrexate sodium, calcipotriene (Dovonex), or glucocorticoids. Patients on most forms of systemic therapy require periodic liver testing and blood studies because of the adverse effects.

PHARMACOLOGY CAPSULE Because of risks to the fetus, women should use reliable contraception during and for 3 years after therapy with Soriatane.

NURSING CARE *of the Patient with Psoriasis*

Assessment

Assessment of the patient with psoriasis includes a description of symptoms and identification of treatments being used (see Nursing Care Plan: The Patient with Psoriasis). Inspect the affected areas for lesions and scales. Document joint pain or stiffness because the condition may cause arthritis. Explore the impact of psoriasis on the patient's everyday life and the coping strategies used.

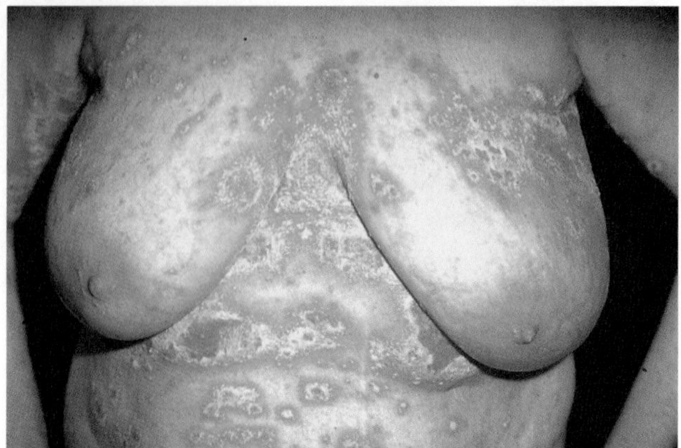

FIGURE **48-7** Psoriasis.

Nursing Diagnoses, Goals, and Outcome Criteria: Psoriasis

Nursing Diagnoses	Goals and Outcome Criteria
Ineffective Therapeutic Regimen Management related to lack of knowledge	Effective management of treatment regimen: patient correctly describes and demonstrates self-care
Disturbed Body Image related to lesions and scales on skin	Improved body image: patient's efforts to improve appearance and positive remarks about self
Social Isolation related to embarrassment about skin lesions	Decreased social isolation: patient's continued involvement in social activities

Interventions

Ineffective Therapeutic Regimen Management

The focus of nursing care for the patient with psoriasis is patient education that enables the patient to manage the prescribed regimen. The patient and family need to know that the condition is not contagious and usually responds to treatment. Teach the patient about the prescribed medications and treatments. Tell the patient to report signs of secondary infection (fever, purulent discharge, increased redness) to the physician. Also encourage adequate rest, good nutrition, and stress management.

Disturbed Body Image

Give the patient the opportunity to express feelings about psoriasis and the effects on his or her life. Demonstrate acceptance of the patient's appearance and the feelings that are expressed. Learning to manage the condition can help the patient feel more hopeful, realizing that remission will occur.

Social Isolation

Encourage the patient to maintain social contacts and plan strategies to deal with exacerbations without undue stress.

NURSING CARE PLAN

The Patient with Psoriasis

ASSESSMENT

Health History: A 45-year-old police officer came to the physician's office because of a "rash" on his trunk. He reports that he is in good health and has had no major injuries or illnesses except a left knee injury sustained in a fall as a teenager. He is taking no medications but is allergic to penicillin. He is alarmed at the rash and is afraid it might spread and that it might be something serious. The physician diagnoses psoriasis. Mr. Pickell is divorced and enjoys socializing, especially dancing. He is concerned about how people might react to his condition.

Physical Examination: Vital signs: temperature, 98.2° F orally; pulse, 84; respiration, 16; blood pressure, 144/88. Height, 5'10". Weight, 164 lb. He is alert and oriented but mildly anxious. The skin on the face and extremities is normal. Bright-red lesions with silvery scales are distributed over the anterior and posterior chest, abdomen, buttocks, and hands. Heart and breath sounds are normal. The abdomen is soft, with bowel sounds present in all four quadrants. There is full range of motion of all joints with crepitation in the left knee. Peripheral pulses are strong and symmetric. The extremities are warm and dry.

Nursing Diagnosis	*Goals and Outcome Criteria*	*Interventions*
Ineffective therapeutic regimen management related to lack of understanding of psoriasis and its treatment.	The patient will correctly describe psoriasis and prescribed treatment measures.	Explain that psoriasis typically has periods of exacerbation and remission, that it is not contagious, and that symptoms can be improved with treatment. Explain the prescribed treatment, including proper application of topical medications and side and adverse effects of drug therapy. For oral drugs, provide information about schedule as well as adverse and side effects. Tell the patient signs of secondary infection (fever, purulent drainage, increased redness) that should be reported to the physician. Encourage patient to plan for adequate rest and to eat a balanced diet. Explore stress management strategies. Refer to mental health counselor if needed. Supplement verbal teaching with written material.
Disturbed body image related to lesions and scales on skin.	The patient's body image will improve as evidenced by positive statements about self.	Demonstrate acceptance of the patient by eye contact and touch. Be aware of personal reaction to lesions. Encourage patient to share feelings about condition. Help the patient feel "in control" by providing information about management of psoriasis.
Social isolation related to embarrassment about skin lesions.	The patient will continue social activities and identify strategies to deal with social situations.	Explore how the patient thinks others will react to his condition. Role-play strategies to use in social situations. Encourage continued activity. Emphasize expected improvement.

Intertrigo

Pathophysiology

Intertrigo is inflammation of the skin where two skin surfaces touch: axillae, abdominal skinfolds, and the area under the breasts. The affected area is usually red and "weeping" with clear margins. The area may be surrounded by vesicles and pustules.

Etiology and Risk Factors

The inflammation of intertrigo results from heat, friction, and moisture between two touching body surfaces. These factors create the perfect environment for infection by *Candida albicans* (yeast) or bacteria.

Medical Diagnosis and Treatment

The medical diagnosis is based on the site and appearance of the inflamed skin, and the presence of *C. albicans* as confirmed by potassium hydroxide examination and culture of skin scrapings. If the skin is not broken, it can be washed with water twice daily. The area is then rinsed and patted dry. Talc or cellulose powder may be applied. Cornstarch is contraindicated because it supports the growth of *C. albicans.* For severe inflammation, a topical corticosteroid or combination corticosteroid, antibacterial, and antifungal (Vytone 1%) may be ordered for a short time. Wet soaks with tap water or Burow's solution are sometimes ordered to remove exudate if an infection is present.

NURSING CARE *of the Patient with Intertrigo*

Assessment

Intertrigo is fairly common among patients in long-term care facilities. Investigate complaints of pain, irritation, or redness in body folds. Monitor body temperature to detect possible infection. Inspect susceptible areas (axillae, groin, beneath breasts, abdominal skinfolds) on a daily basis.

Nursing Diagnoses, Goals, and Outcome Criteria: Intertrigo

Nursing Diagnoses	Goals and Outcome Criteria
Impaired Skin Integrity related to inflammation	Improved skin integrity: intact skin without redness
Risk for Infection related to moist environment, broken skin	Absence of infection: no fever, pain, or edema

Interventions

Areas where skin surfaces are in close contact must be kept clean and dry. Apply topical medications (antifungals and corticosteroids) as ordered. Report increasing redness and tenderness, fever, and broken skin to the physician.

Fungal Infections

Pathophysiology

Humans are susceptible to a number of fungal infections. Superficial infections of the skin and mucous membranes caused by fungi include tinea pedis (athlete's foot), tinea manus (hand), tinea cruris (groin), tinea capitis (scalp), tinea corporis (body), tinea barbae (beard), and candidiasis, which can affect the skin, mouth, vagina, gastrointestinal tract, and lungs.

Etiology and Risk Factors

The organisms that cause tinea infections take advantage of trauma in moist, warm tissue. Some organisms can be spread through direct contact or by inanimate objects. Lesions vary but may be scaly patches with raised borders. The lay term *ringworm* is sometimes used to describe these circular lesions. Pruritus is a common symptom of tinea. Tinea capitis, tinea corporis, and tinea pedis are rather easily spread by sharing contaminated objects.

Candidiasis, commonly called a yeast infection, is caused by *C. albicans.* Patients at risk for candidiasis include those who are pregnant, malnourished, immunosuppressed, or taking antibiotics or oral contraceptives. People with diabetes mellitus are also at risk for this disease. Common sites affected are the mouth, vagina, and skin. The skin around an ostomy site also is susceptible to candidiasis because of the constant moisture there. Infections of the mucous membranes are manifested as red lesions with white plaques. Skin infections with *C. albicans* are seen as moist red lesions (Fig. 48-8). The lesions often are found in folds of body tissue (see section on Intertrigo).

Medical Diagnosis

Fungal infections are usually diagnosed on the basis of the history and physical examination but may be confirmed by microscopic examination of skin scrapings using a potassium hydroxide wet mount preparation.

Medical Treatment

Fungal infections are treated with antifungal powders and creams. Wet compresses and keratolytics may be ordered to soften scales with some tinea infections. Oral candidiasis is treated with clotrimazole troches, nystatin mouthwash or lozenges, or topical amphotericin B. For AIDS patients, clotrimazole is superior to nystatin.

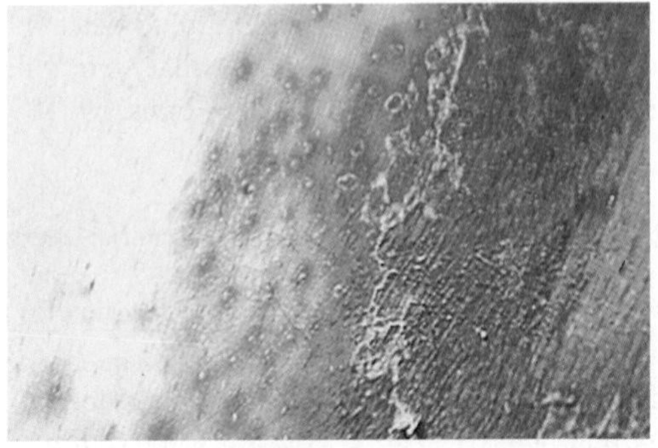

FIGURE **48-8** Candidiasis.

NURSING CARE *of the Patient with a Fungal Infection*

Assessment

The nursing assessment identifies conditions that might make a person susceptible to fungal infections: diabetes mellitus, malnutrition, and immunosuppression. Note antibiotic therapy, another risk factor. During the physical examination, inspect the skin and mucous membranes for lesions. Creamy white lesions that can be scraped off easily are characteristic of oral candidiasis.

PHARMACOLOGY CAPSULE Antibiotic therapy eliminates the microorganisms that normally control fungal growth, making the patient susceptible to fungal infections.

Nursing Diagnoses, Goals, and Outcome Criteria: Fungal Infection

Nursing Diagnoses	Goals and Outcome Criteria
Disturbed Body Image related to skin lesions	Improved body image: absence of skin lesions, patient's positive statements about appearance
Altered Oral Mucous Membrane related to oral candidiasis	Healthy oral mucous membranes: absence of oral lesions
Risk for Injury related to reinfection, spread of infection	Decreased risk of recurrent infection: patient correctly describes and demonstrates self-care

Interventions

Disturbed Body Image

Be sensitive to the patient's reaction to a skin infection. Visible lesions may be embarrassing to the patient. If the genitalia are affected, the patient may think the symptoms are due to a sexually transmitted disease. Explain the cause of the infection, how it is treated, whether it is contagious, and how transmission and reinfection can be avoided. If medication is prescribed, instruct the patient in proper use of the agent. Tell the patient to keep the affected areas of the skin as clean and dry as possible. A cool environment helps by reducing perspiration.

Eradication of candidiasis infections in bedridden patients can be especially challenging. Frequently reposition the patient to permit evaporation of moisture. The thighs can be separated by using a pillow between the knees, and a folded cloth may be placed beneath pendulous breasts.

Altered Oral Mucous Membranes

Instruct the patient with oral candidiasis in the proper use of prescribed medications. Mouthwashes may be swished to coat all oral surfaces before swallowing. Lozenges should be dissolved in the mouth. If the patient wears dentures, they should be soaked in an antifungal solution.

Risk for Injury

Advise patients with tinea infections to avoid sharing personal items such as hairbrushes and clothing. They also should dry thoroughly after bathing and wear absorbent underwear and socks.

Acne

Pathophysiology

Acne is a skin condition that affects the hair follicles and sebaceous glands. It is characterized by comedones (whiteheads and blackheads), pustules, and cysts. These lesions most often develop on the face, neck, and upper trunk. Acne commonly begins in adolescence and may last into adulthood. Most cases are mild, but serious cases with extensive inflammation can cause permanent scarring.

Etiology and Risk Factors

Acne lesions develop when androgenic hormones cause increased sebum production and bacteria *(Propionibacterium acnes)* proliferate, causing sebaceous follicles to become blocked and inflamed. Despite popular opinion, acne is not caused by fatty foods, chocolate, or poor hygiene. In addition to androgenic hormones, exacerbations of acne can be triggered by high levels of progestin in birth control pills, oil-based cosmetics, high doses of systemic corticosteroids, hormonal changes associated with the menstrual period, and some endocrine disorders.

Medical Diagnosis

Acne is diagnosed on the basis of the health history and physical examination findings.

Medical Treatment

Treatment varies with the severity of the condition. Mild cases may respond very well to topical medications, including antibiotics, keratolytics such as benzoyl peroxide, topical vitamin A preparations (tretinoin [Retin-A], tazarotene [Tazorac], and adapalene [Differin]), or azelaic acid, which suppresses growth of *P. acnes* and thins the stratum corneum. If these agents do not adequately control acne, oral antibiotics (tetracycline, azithromycin, erythromycin) may be given over a period of several months. Estrogen also may be prescribed to counteract the effects of androgenic hormones. Spironolactone may be used for its antiandrogenic effects. If acne is severe and unresponsive to all of these treatments, isotretinoin (Accutane) may be prescribed.

Nonpharmacologic treatment may include comedo extraction or cryotherapy. Dermabrasion may be used to reduce scarring.

PHARMACOLOGY CAPSULE Isotretinoin (Accutane) can cause severe fetal deformities. Therefore, females who take the drug must prevent pregnancy until at least 1 month after therapy has been completed.

NURSING CARE *of the Patient with Acne*

Assessment

Assess the patient's concerns and knowledge about acne. Document any treatments being used. Note all medical conditions and medications because some contribute to or aggravate acne. Assess the skin to determine the extent and severity of the condition.

Nursing Diagnoses, Goals, and Outcome Criteria: Acne

Nursing Diagnoses	Goals and Outcome Criteria
Disturbed Body Image related to comedones, pustules, and cysts	Improved body image: decreased lesions and patient's expression of improved body image
Ineffective Therapeutic Regimen Management related to lack of understanding of causes and treatment of acne	Effective treatment management: patient correctly describes and demonstrates prescribed skin care and self-medication

Interventions

Disturbed Body Image

When working with a person who has acne, provide support and information. Because acne almost always affects the face, most patients with moderate or severe acne suffer body image disturbances. Be sensitive to this concern and encourage the patient to see a dermatologist for treatment. This condition can be very harmful to the patient's self-esteem and should not be dismissed as a minor problem.

Ineffective Therapeutic Regimen Management

Explain the causes of acne as well as the many myths about the disease. Assure the patient that acne does not reflect poor hygiene but that cleanliness does reduce the risk of infections. Dietary interventions are no longer thought to be useful. Discourage picking or squeezing lesions because it may force infected material deeper into the follicle. Advise the patient that harsh cleansers and vigorous scrubbing have no therapeutic value.

Explain prescribed drugs, and discuss any adverse effects. Patient teaching is especially important if isotretinoin is used. Isotretinoin is an oral medication that has a drying effect on the skin. Tell the patient to expect the condition to worsen initially and then begin to improve. Advise the patient that the drug is teratogenic, meaning it is harmful to a developing fetus. Therefore, contraception must be used if the patient is sexually active while taking the drug.

Herpes Simplex

Etiology and Risk Factors

The herpes simplex virus (HSV) causes an infection that begins with itching and burning and progresses to the development of vesicles that rupture and form crusts (Fig. 48-9). Sites most often infected by the virus are the nose, lips, cheeks, ears, and genitalia. Oral HSV lesions are commonly called

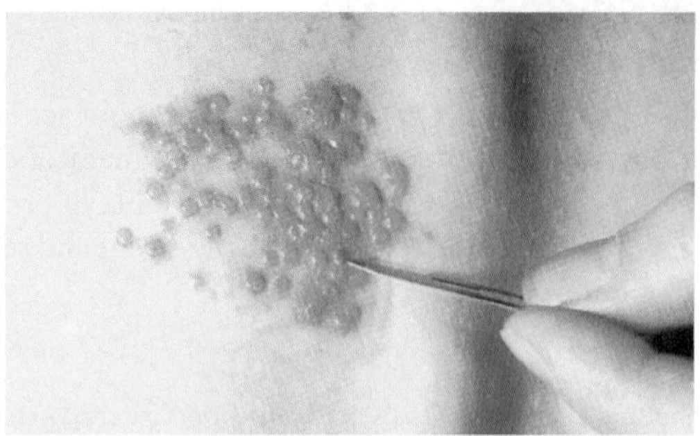

FIGURE 48-9 Herpes simplex lesions.

cold sores or fever blisters. There are two types of HSV. Infections on the face and upper body are usually caused by HSV type 1; genital infections are usually caused by HSV type 2. Patients typically have repeated outbreaks and remissions. Herpes simplex virus can be transmitted by direct contact. Genital infection is therefore considered a sexually transmitted disease and is discussed in detail in Chapter 47.

Medical Diagnosis

Diagnostic tests used to identify herpes infections include Tzanck's smear and a viral culture.

Medical Treatment

Herpes simplex infections are treated with acyclovir (Zovirax) or (for cold sores) docosanol (Abreva). Antiviral drugs are not curative but may hasten healing. Analgesics and topical anesthetics may be prescribed for pain.

NURSING CARE *of the Patient with Herpes Simplex*

Nursing care consists primarily of patient education about the nature of the herpes simplex infection and its treatment and prevention. Emphasize that the condition is contagious and tends to recur. Prevention of sexually transmitted herpes simplex is discussed in Chapter 47.

Assessment

The health history describes the development of the herpetic lesions. Document contacts with people known to be infected. Take a complete medical history with particular attention to disorders or medications that might suppress the immune response. The physical examination includes a careful inspection of the lesions. Wear gloves to avoid direct contact with lesions.

Nursing Diagnoses, Goals, and Outcome Criteria: Herpes Simplex

Nursing Diagnoses	Goals and Outcome Criteria
Acute Pain related to lesions	Pain relief: patient statement of pain relief, relaxed expression
Ineffective Coping related to anticipated recurrent lesions, embarrassment	Effective coping: patient statement of ability to cope with condition
Ineffective Therapeutic Regimen Management related to lack of understanding of cause, transmission, and treatment of HSV type 1 infections	Effective management of regimen: patient correctly describes and demonstrates self-care and identifies measures to prevent transmission to others

Interventions

Acute Pain

Document patient reports of pain. Administer analgesics and topical anesthetics as ordered, or instruct the patient in self-medication. Compresses saturated with astringent solutions such as Burow's solution are sometimes ordered.

Ineffective Coping

Explore the patient's knowledge and concerns about HSV type 1. The lesions on the face may be especially distressing because they are so obvious. Demonstrate acceptance of the patient's feelings and provide factual information to enable the patient to cope with the condition.

Ineffective Therapeutic Regimen Management

Topical and oral drugs may be ordered. Instruct the patient in use of the drugs. Stress that HSV remains in a dormant state in the body after the initial infection. Periodic recurrences are expected and may be triggered by stresses, including emotional distress, fever, trauma, sunburn, or fatigue. The patient may be able to identify personal triggers and try to avoid or minimize them. Recurrent episodes are typically less severe than the initial one.

To prevent transmission of the infection to others, advise the patient to avoid oral contact while the lesions are present. The patient should exercise good handwashing and avoid touching the lesions. Immunosuppressed patients are especially susceptible to herpes infections and must be protected from infected people.

PHARMACOLOGY CAPSULE Acyclovir (Zovirax) does not cure herpes simplex virus infections. Patients still can transmit the infection to others despite antiviral therapy.

Herpes Zoster

Etiology and Risk Factors

Herpes zoster infection is commonly called *shingles.* It is caused by the varicella-zoster virus, the same organism that causes chickenpox. In some people who have had chickenpox, the virus remains latent in nerve tissue until the infection is activated in the form of shingles. The first symptoms are pain, itching, and heightened sensitivity along a nerve pathway, followed by the formation of vesicles in the area. When the skin is affected, crusts form (Fig. 48-10). When the mucous membranes are affected, ulcers develop. The lesions typically last approximately 2 weeks. The infection is contagious to people who have not had previous exposure to the virus.

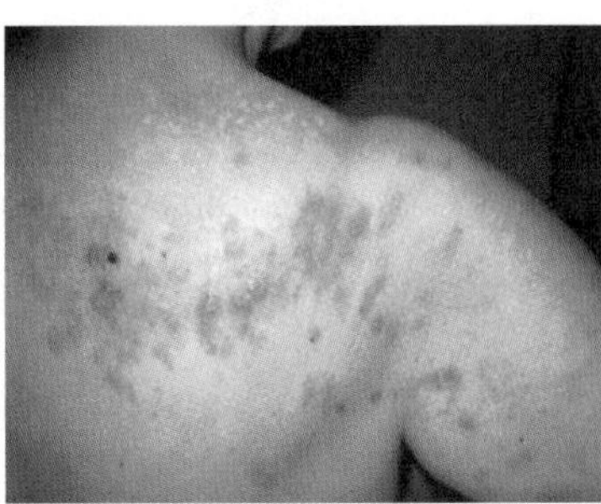

FIGURE 48-10 Herpes zoster lesions ("shingles").

The elderly are especially susceptible to complications, which include postherpetic neuralgia, trigeminal herpes zoster (affecting the facial and acoustic nerves), and ophthalmic involvement. With postherpetic neuralgia, pain and itching may persist for years. Immunosuppressed people are at greater risk for herpes zoster infections and may have very serious systemic complications.

Medical Diagnosis

A diagnosis of herpes zoster infection usually can be made on the basis of the health history and physical examination findings. The diagnosis can be confirmed by Tzanck's smear or a viral culture of material from a lesion.

Medical Treatment

Herpes zoster infection is treated with oral or intravenous acyclovir. Wet dressings soaked in Burow's solution may be ordered to loosen crusts, decrease oozing, and soothe the affected areas. Pain may be treated with analgesics and sedatives. Systemic corticosteroids also may be given to decrease the risk of herpetic neuralgia.

NURSING CARE *of the Patient with Herpes Zoster*

Assessment

Record the history of the patient's present illness. Take a complete medical history to identify conditions or treatments that might cause the patient to have a reduced immune response. Explore the extent to which the symptoms are affecting the patient's life. If this is a recurrent infection, assess the patient's understanding of the condition. In the physical examination, inspect the lesions and document distribution and appearance.

Nursing Diagnoses, Goals, and Outcome Criteria: Herpes Zoster

Nursing Diagnoses	Goals and Outcome Criteria
Impaired Skin Integrity related to lesions	Improved skin integrity: absence of vesicles and pruritus
Acute Pain related to lesions, inflammation, or postherpetic neuralgia	Pain relief: patient statement of pain relief, relaxed manner
Ineffective Coping related to long-term pain associated with postherpetic neuralgia	Effective coping: patient uses strategies to cope with acute and chronic symptoms

Interventions

Impaired Skin Integrity

Inspect the lesions each day. Apply cool medicated compresses and administer antipruritic agents as ordered.

Acute Pain

Administer prescribed analgesics and antiviral medications or instruct the patient in self-medication. Assess and document the effectiveness of the drugs in relieving pain. Inform the physician if the patient's pain persists despite medication.

Ineffective Coping

Emotional support is especially important for the patient who has chronic pain. Management of chronic pain is discussed in detail in Chapter 14. To promote healing, prevent transmission, and support coping, provide information about herpes zoster: cause, course, treatment, and communicability. Advise the patient that the condition is communicable to people who have never been exposed to chickenpox.

Necrotizing Fasciitis

Necrotizing fasciitis is an infection of the deep fascial structures under the skin. Both aerobic and anaerobic organisms may be present, including *Streptococcus, Staphylococcus, Peptostreptococcus, Bacteroides,* and *Clostridium* species. The organisms excrete enzymes that destroy tissue, including blood vessels that supply the affected area. Deprived of blood flow, tissue necrosis occurs.

Necrotizing fasciitis should be suspected when a patient has a small external wound with evidence of larger underlying inflammation. The infection may progress rapidly with loss of large amounts of tissue and can result in death. Treatment involves extensive débridement, intravenous and topical antibiotics, and eventual skin grafting.

Other Infections

A number of skin infections can occur in addition to those discussed in this chapter. Some of the more common conditions (impetigo, folliculitis, furuncles, carbuncles, erysipelas, cellulitis, and warts) are presented in Figure 48-11 and Table 48-6.

INFESTATIONS

Lice and scabies infestations are described in Table 48-7. Pediculosis is illustrated in Figure 48-12.

PEMPHIGUS

Pemphigus is a chronic autoimmune condition in which bullae (blisters) develop on the face, back, chest, groin, and umbilicus. The blisters rupture easily, releasing a foul-smelling drainage. Potassium permanganate baths may be ordered to soothe the affected areas, reduce odor, and decrease the risk of infection. Treatments may include corticosteroids, other immunosuppressants, and plasmapheresis. Patients with extensive skin loss require the same care as burn patients (see section on Nursing Care of the Patient with a Burn Injury, later in this chapter).

table 48-6 ***Additional Skin Infections***

INFECTION	CAUSE	SIGNS AND SYMPTOMS	TREATMENT
Impetigo	Group A streptococci	Vesicle or pustule that ruptures, leaving a thick crust	Antibiotic therapy: erythromycin or dicloxacillin
Folliculitis	*Staphylococcus aureus*	Inflamed hair follicles with white pustules	Warm compresses, topical antibiotics
Furuncle (boil)	*Staphylococcus aureus*	Inflamed skin and subcutaneous tissue with deep, inflamed nodules	Warm compresses, topical antibiotics
Carbuncle	*Staphylococcus aureus*	Clustered, interconnected furuncles	Systemic antibiotics, incision and drainage
Erysipelas	β-hemolytic group A streptococci	Round or oval patches that enlarge and spread; redness, swelling, tenderness, warmth	Systemic antibiotics, usually penicillin
Cellulitis	Usually *Streptococcus pyogenes*	Local tenderness and redness at first, then malaise, chills, and fever; site becomes more erythematous; nodules and vesicles may form; vesicles may rupture, releasing purulent material identified by culture	For *S. pyogenes,* penicillin, a cephalosporin, or vancomycin; other antibiotics for other organisms
Verruca (wart)	Human papillomavirus	At first, small shiny lesions; they enlarge and become rough	Electrical current to destroy lesion followed by removal with curette, cryotherapy (freezing), topical medications

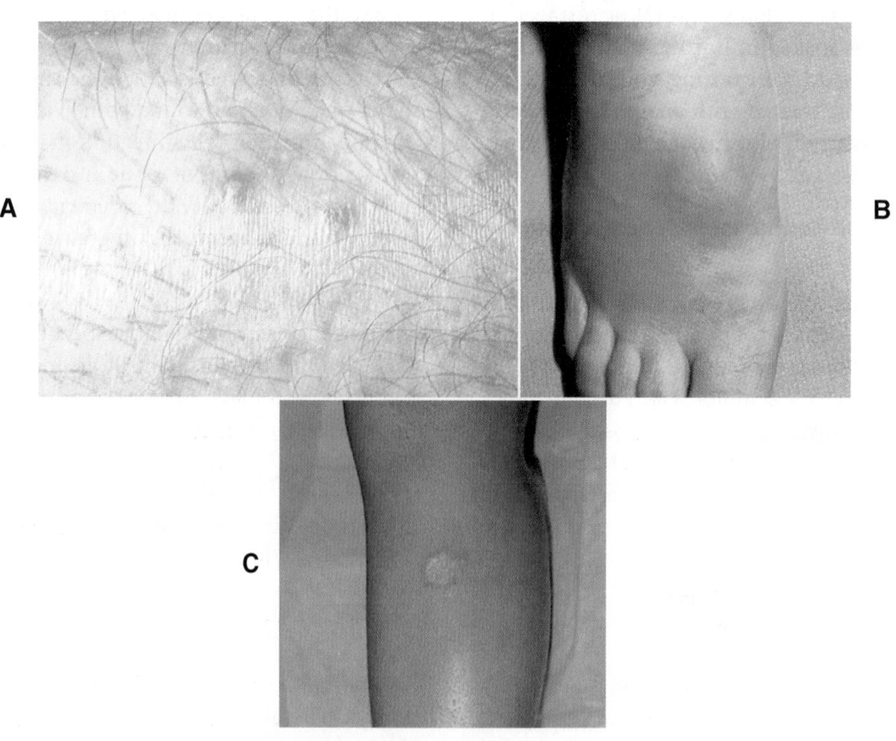

FIGURE **48-11** *A,* Folliculitis. *B,* Furuncle and abscess. *C,* Tinea corporis.

table 48-7 ***Infestations of the Skin***

INFESTATION	CAUSE	SIGNS AND SYMPTOMS	TREATMENT
Scabies	*Sarcoptes scabiei,* sometimes called "itch mite"	Thin, red lines on skin; itching	Topical scabicide applied and repeated 1 wk later; clothing and bed linens washed in hot water or dry cleaned
Lice	*Pediculus humanus* or *Phthirus pubis*	Itching of hairy areas of body (head, pubis); nits (eggs) seen as tiny white particles attached to hair shafts	Head lice: pediculicide shampoo applied to dry hair, then hair combed with fine-toothed comb to remove nits and dead lice; also treat brushes and combs Body or pubic lice: apply pediculicide lotion as directed For both sites: wash clothing and bed linens in hot water or have dry cleaned; usually need to treat all members of household Assure patient that infestations are common and not caused by unsanitary living

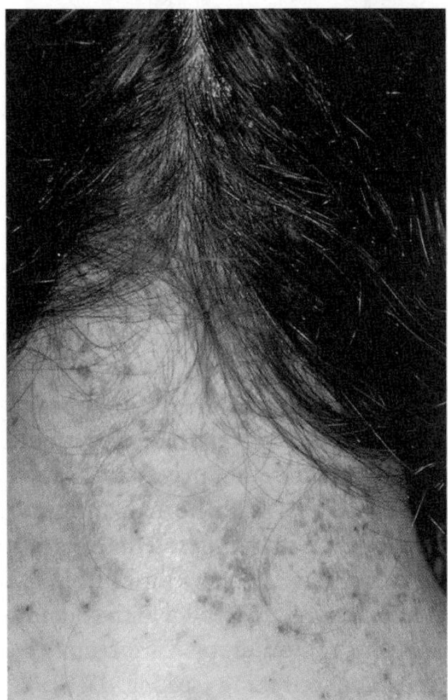

FIGURE **48-12** Pediculosis.

CANCER

Skin cancers include actinic keratosis, basal cell carcinoma, squamous cell carcinoma, melanoma, and cutaneous T-cell lymphoma (Fig. 48-13). They are most common among light-skinned people who have had repeated sun exposure. Kaposi's sarcoma is mentioned here as well because it is manifested by skin lesions. The reader is referred to Chapter 24 for detailed nursing care of the patient with cancer.

Skin cancers may be suspected because of the lesion appearance and location. The diagnosis is confirmed by microscopic examination of cells obtained from the excised lesion or a tissue sample obtained by biopsy.

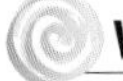

What Does Culture Have to do with Skin Cancer?

Whites have a higher incidence of skin cancer than either African Americans or Native Americans. Patients with light skin who live in sunny climates should protect themselves from excessive exposure and routinely assess for skin changes.

Actinic Keratosis

Actinic keratoses are precancerous lesions most often found on the face, neck, forearms, and backs of the hands—all areas exposed to sunlight. They may become malignant if not treated. Actinic keratoses are most common among elderly white people. They typically appear as papules or plaques of irregular shape. The hard scale on the lesion may shed and reappear (see Fig. 48-10).

A number of treatments for actinic keratosis exist, including drug therapy, cryotherapy, electrodesiccation, and surgical excision. The drug of choice for actinic keratosis is topical 5-fluorouracil. Cryotherapy is the use of liquid nitrogen to freeze and destroy the lesion. The procedure may cause a blister to form but is only slightly painful. Electrodesiccation is the use of electrical current to destroy the lesion, which is then scraped off. The patient is given a local anesthetic. Surgical excision may be done in several ways, and the patient may or may not have sutures.

Basal Cell Carcinoma

Basal cell carcinomas usually begin as painless, nodular lesions that have a pearly appearance (see Fig. 48-13). They are thought to be related to sun exposure. Basal cell carcinomas grow slowly and rarely metastasize. Nevertheless, they should be removed because they can cause local tissue destruction. Basal cell carcinomas are surgically excised or destroyed with cryotherapy or radiation.

Squamous Cell Carcinoma

Squamous cell carcinomas may appear as scaly ulcers or raised lesions. There are usually no clear lesion margins (see Fig. 48-13). Like basal cell carcinomas, they most often develop on sun-exposed areas including the lips and in the oral cavity. Squamous cell carcinomas are most often caused by overuse of tobacco and alcohol. Unlike basal cell carcinomas, they grow rapidly and metastasize. Treatment may include surgical excision, chemotherapy, and radiation therapy.

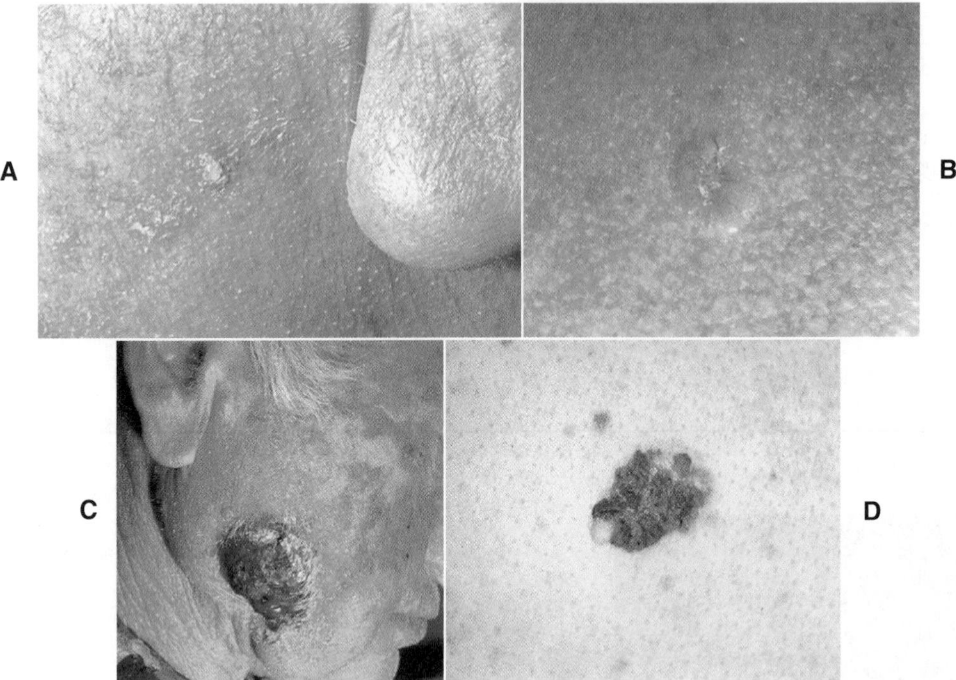

FIGURE 48-13 Skin cancers. *A,* Actinic keratosis (a premalignant lesion). *B,* Basal cell carcinoma. *C,* Squamous cell carcinoma. *D,* Malignant melanoma.

Melanoma

A malignant melanoma arises from the pigment-producing cells in the skin. It is the most serious form of skin cancer because it can be fatal if it metastasizes. Melanomas can be found anywhere on the body, not just sun-exposed areas. Typical melanomas have irregular borders and uneven coloration (see Fig. 48-13). Many are very dark, but some are light in color. They usually begin as a tan macule that enlarges. Malignant melanomas are removed surgically. A technique called Mohs' surgery is used, in which microscopic tissue samples are studied to determine the margins of the malignancy. This approach is meant to avoid leaving malignant tissue around the excised lesion. A wide area around a melanoma is usually excised.

Cutaneous T-Cell Lymphoma

Cutaneous T-cell lymphoma is characterized by the migration of malignant T cells to the skin. There are several manifestations of cutaneous T-cell lymphoma including mycosis fungoides and Sézary syndrome. At first, cutaneous T-cell lymphoma may resemble eczema, with macular lesions appearing on areas protected from the sun. They form tumors, enlarge, and can spread to distant sites. When confined to the skin, this type of lymphoma can be cured with topical chemotherapy, systemic psoralens with UVA, and/or superficial radiotherapy.

Kaposi's Sarcoma

Kaposi's sarcoma is a malignancy of the blood vessels. It is manifested by red, blue, or purple macules accompanied by pain, itching, and swelling. The lesions appear first on the legs and then on the upper body, face, and mouth. They enlarge to form large plaques that may drain. Kaposi's sarcoma may be seen in patients with human immunodeficiency virus infection, but it is not confined to this group. Local lesions may be excised or injected with intralesional chemotherapy. Systemic lesions are treated with chemotherapy, immune therapy, and radiotherapy. Unfortunately, treatment results have been discouraging (see Fig. 47-5).

DISORDERS OF THE NAILS

The two major conditions affecting the nails are infections (fungal or bacterial) and inflammation caused by ingrown nails. Infections are usually indicated by redness, swelling, and pain around the margin of the nail. They are treated with warm soaks and topical or systemic anti-infectives. Incision and drainage may be necessary.

An ingrown toenail causes painful inflammation at the distal corner of the nail. It is usually caused by trimming the nail too short at the corners or wearing shoes that are too tight on the toes. The ingrown nail should be protected from pressure as it grows out. Warm soaks may be soothing. Sometimes surgical excision of the ingrown portion of the nail is needed.

NURSING CARE *of the Patient with a Nail Disorder*

Nail disorders do not often require inpatient care unless there are complications. However, nurses may be the first to detect nail problems and often teach patients how to prevent or treat them.

Assessment

In the health history, document the diagnoses of diabetes mellitus or peripheral vascular disease. In the physical examination, include inspection of the nails for redness, swelling, or pain. Inspect the extremities for lesions and abnormal color, and palpate for warmth and peripheral pulses.

Nursing Diagnoses, Goals, and Outcome Criteria: Nail Disorder

Nursing Diagnoses	Goals and Outcome Criteria
Risk for Injury related to improper nail trimming, poor peripheral circulation	Decreased risk of injury: properly trimmed nails Absence of injury: no evidence of inflammation (redness, swelling, pain, excess warmth)
Ineffective Therapeutic Regimen Management related to lack of understanding of proper nail care and treatment of nail disorders	Effective management of therapeutic measures: patient demonstrates correct nail care and prescribed treatments

Interventions

Teach patients how to trim their nails correctly and the importance of properly fitting shoes. Toenails should be cut straight across and even with the end of the toe. Show patients with peripheral vascular disease or diabetes mellitus how to inspect their feet daily and advise them to seek medical attention for any abnormality. A seemingly minor foot infection can have drastic consequences, including amputation, for the patient with poor circulation. If the patient cannot care for the feet adequately, seek a referral to a podiatrist.

BURNS

Burns are tissue injuries caused by heat. Depending on the source of the injury, the burn is described as thermal (flame, flash, scalding liquids, hot objects), chemical, electrical, radiation, or inhalation. Burns are a leading cause of accidental death despite improved survival rates attributed to tremendous advances in the care of burn patients. Sadly, 75% of all burn injuries could have been prevented.

Emergency treatment of the burn patient is discussed in Chapter 15. Acute care of seriously burned patients is an advanced specialty that is beyond the scope of this book; therefore, this section provides a limited discussion of nursing care of the patient after reaching a medical facility.

CLASSIFICATION OF BURNS

Burns are classified by the size and depth of the tissue injury. It is important periodically to reevaluate the burn because evidence of extent of injury can change over time. Extent is often defined as the percentage of body surface area affected. To describe depth, a burn is classified as partial thickness or full thickness, depending on the layers of tissue injured.

Burn Size

Burn size may be estimated using the rule of nines or the Lund and Browder method. The rule of nines estimates the percentage of body surface area burned. Areas of the body are assigned percentage values of nine or multiples of nine (Fig. 48-14). The percentages are totaled to estimate burn size. For example, if one arm and one leg are burned, the burn size is estimated as 27%.

The Lund and Browder method also estimates the percentage of body surface burned, but the body is divided into smaller segments. Different percentages are assigned to body parts depending on the patient's age. This is more accurate than the rule of nines because it accounts for differences in body proportions. For example, the head of an infant is 19% of the total body surface area, whereas the head of an adult is only 7% of the total body surface area. Figure 48-15 is an example of the Lund and Browder chart as modified by Berkow.

Burn Depth

Partial-thickness burns are sometimes called first- or second-degree burns. A burn affecting only the epidermis is a superficial (or first-degree) burn. A burn that affects the epidermis and the dermis is a superficial or deep partial-thickness (or second-degree) burn, depending on the tissues affected. Burns that extend into even deeper tissue layers are called full-thickness (or third-degree, fourth-degree) burns (Figs. 48-16 and 48-17).

Superficial Burns. A superficial burn, like a sunburn, is pink to red and painful.

Superficial Partial-Thickness Burns. Superficial partial-thickness burns are painful and usually appear blistered or weepy and pale to red or pink. A severe sunburn can be a superficial partial-thickness burn.

Deep Partial-Thickness Burns. A deep partial-thickness burn is characterized by large, thick-walled blisters or by edema and weeping, cherry-red, exposed dermis. It is painful and sensitive to cold air.

Full-Thickness Burns. Full-thickness burns involve the epidermis, dermis, and underlying tissues, including fat, muscle, and bone. Full-thickness burns typically appear dry, feel leathery, and may be red, white, brown, or black. The burned tissue usually lacks sensation.

Burn Severity

Burn severity is based on size, depth, location, age, general health status, and mechanism of injury. There are various criteria used to define major burns. The American Burn Association criteria for a major burn in an adult are the following:

1. Burn size: 25% or more body surface area for people younger than 40 years of age; 20% or more body surface area for people older than age 40 years
2. Disfiguring or disabling injuries to the face, eyes, ears, hands, feet, or perineum

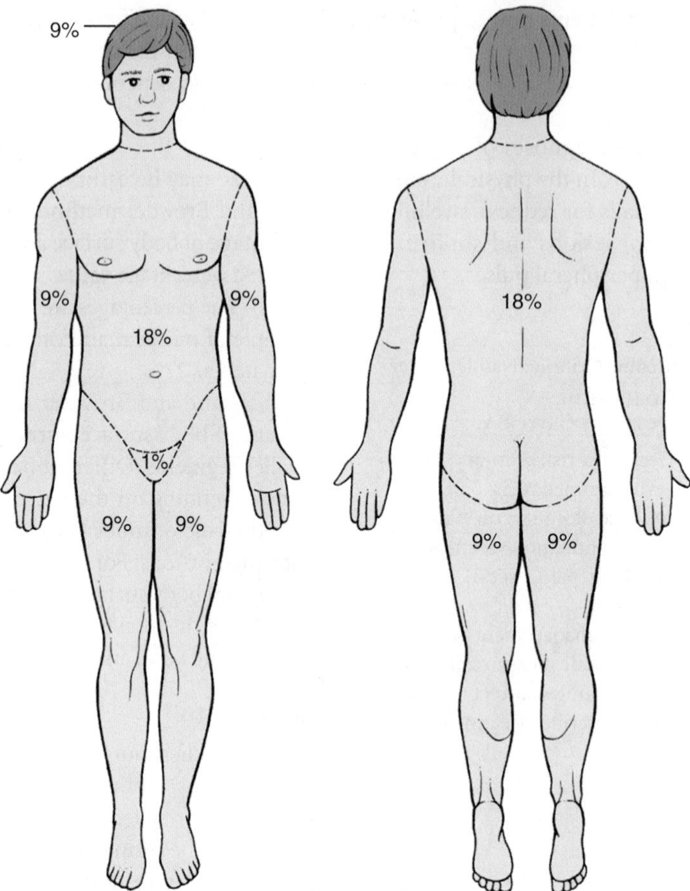

FIGURE 48-14 Rule of nines.

3. High-voltage electrical burn injury
4. Inhalation injury
5. Major trauma in addition to the burn

PATHOPHYSIOLOGY OF BURN INJURY

Local Effects

Burn-injured tissue releases chemicals that cause increased capillary permeability, which permits plasma to leak into the tissues. Injury to cell membranes permits excess sodium to enter the cell and allows potassium to escape into the extracellular compartment. These shifts in fluids and electrolytes cause local edema and a decrease in cardiac output. Fluid evaporates through the wound surface, further contributing to the declining blood volume. Eighteen to 36 hours after a burn injury, capillary permeability begins to normalize and reabsorption of edema fluid begins. Cardiac output returns to normal and then increases to meet increased metabolic demands.

Systemic Effects

Fluid Balance

The shift of plasma proteins from the capillaries may result in hypoproteinemia, which causes fluid to shift from the bloodstream to the extracellular tissue. This shift decreases blood volume and causes generalized edema in the early postburn period. Blood is shunted from the kidneys to compensate for the fluid volume deficit, and urine output falls. These fluid shifts, if not corrected, result in decreased tissue perfusion and decreased cardiac output that may lead to hypovolemic shock.

As the capillaries recover and edema fluid is reabsorbed, the patient's blood volume increases. If kidney function is adequate, urine output increases to prevent hypervolemia.

Gastrointestinal Function

Blood flow to the intestines decreases, and an ileus may develop. Some patients have stress ulcers, sometimes called Curling's ulcers, after severe burns. They are, therefore, routinely treated with antacids to neutralize gastric acid and H_2-receptor blockers to reduce gastric acid secretion.

Immune System

Because immunity is depressed after a serious burn, the patient is less able to resist infection. The loss of the protective skin barrier also puts the patient at risk for life-threatening infection.

Respiratory System

The burn patient may suffer inhalation injuries, including carbon monoxide poisoning, smoke poisoning, and thermal damage. Inhalation injury occurs with flame burns or from being trapped in an enclosed space filled with smoke. Suspect inhalation injury if the patient has facial burns, redness and swelling of the pharynx, restlessness, cough, dyspnea, or sooty sputum. Carbon monoxide displaces oxygen on hemoglobin,

Body area	0-1 Years	1-4 Years	5-9 Years	10-14 Years	15 Years	Adult
Head	19	17	13	11	9	7
Neck	2	2	2	2	2	2
Ant. trunk	13	13	13	13	13	13
Post. trunk	13	13	13	13	13	13
R. buttock	2.5	2.5	2.5	2.5	2.5	2.5
L. buttock	2.5	2.5	2.5	2.5	2.5	2.5
Genitalia	1	1	1	1	1	1
R. u. arm	4	4	4	4	4	4
L. u. arm	4	4	4	4	4	4
R. l. arm	3	3	3	3	3	3
L. l. arm	3	3	3	3	3	3
R. hand	2.5	2.5	2.5	2.5	2.5	2.5
L. hand	2.5	2.5	2.5	2.5	2.5	2.5
R. thigh	5.5	6.5	8	8.5	9	9.5
L. thigh	5.5	6.5	8	8.5	9	9.5
R. l. leg	5	5	5.5	6	6.5	7
L. l. leg	5	5	5.5	6	6.5	7
R. foot	3.5	3.5	3.5	3.5	3.5	3.5
L. foot	3.5	3.5	3.5	3.5	3.5	3.5

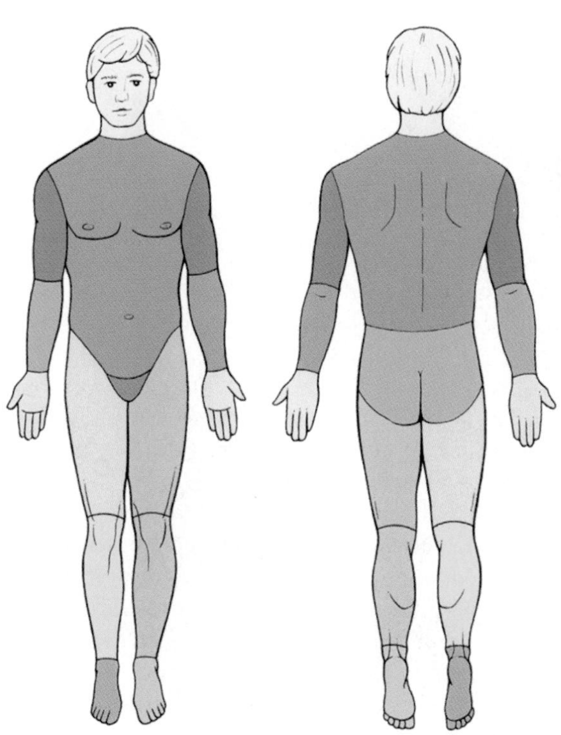

FIGURE **48-15** Berkow's adaptation of Lund and Browder method of estimating body surface area burned.

so the blood is unable to transport oxygen to the tissues. The patient will show signs of hypoxia and die if the condition is not corrected. See Chapter 15 for additional discussion of carbon monoxide poisoning. Smoke poisoning is the result of inhaling combustion byproducts. Thermal damage to the lower airway is rare but can happen if the patient was unconscious or inhaled live steam. With inhalation injury, pulmonary edema develops that may progress to adult respiratory distress syndrome.

Myocardial Depression

There is evidence of myocardial depression in the early postburn period.

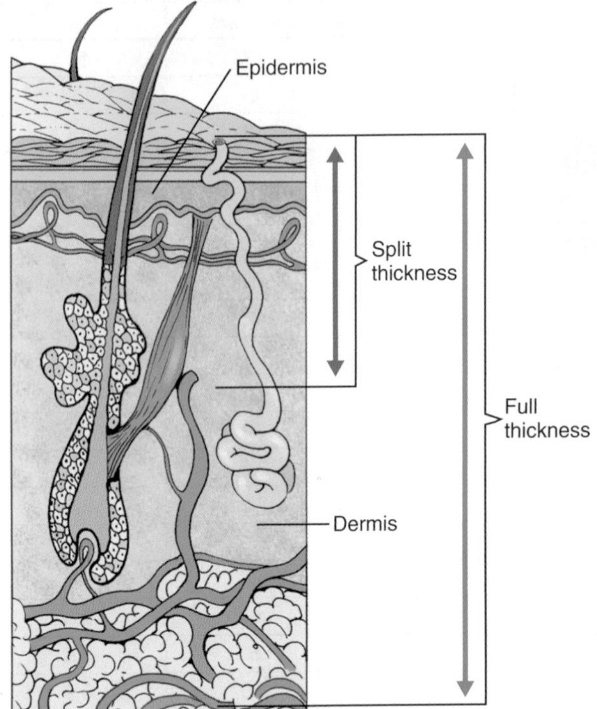

FIGURE 48-16 Burn classification by depth.

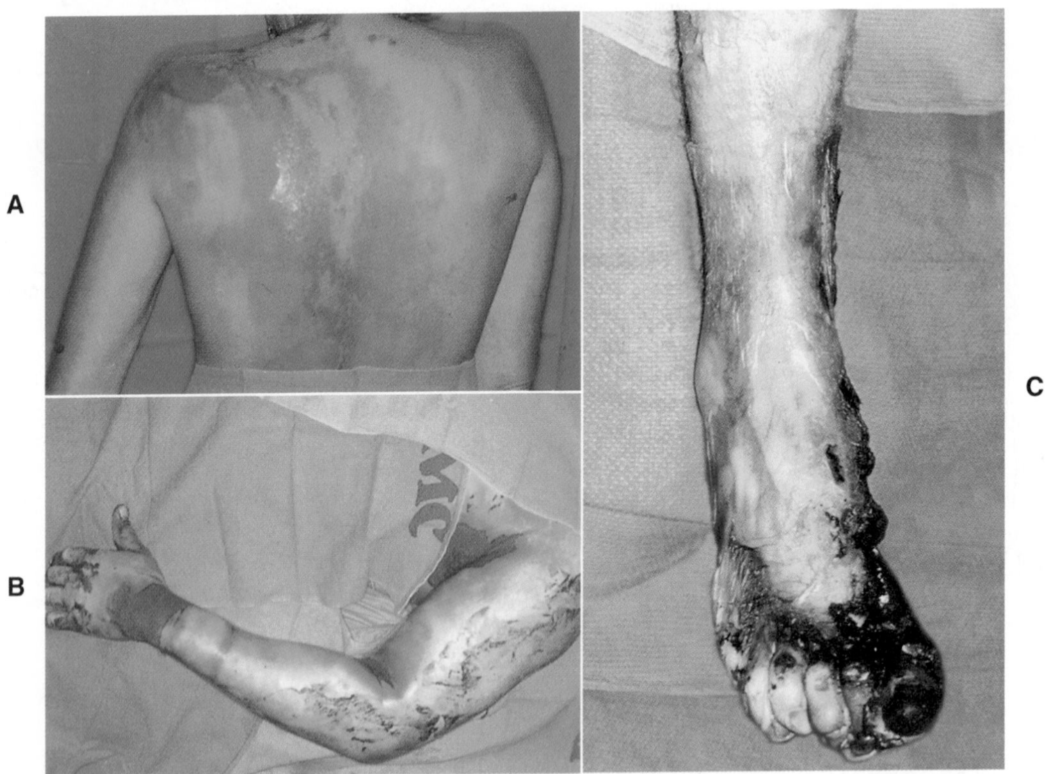

FIGURE 48-17 Burn depth. *A,* Partial thickness ("second degree"). *B,* Full thickness ("third degree") *C,* Full thickness ("fourth degree").

Psychological Effects

Psychological responses to burn injuries are highly individual. Four stages of psychological response have been identified: impact, retreat or withdrawal, acknowledgment, and reconstruction.

STAGES OF BURN INJURY

Care of the burn patient is often described in terms of three stages: emergent, acute, and rehabilitation. The emergent stage begins with the injury and ends when fluid shifts have stabilized. The acute stage begins with fluid stabilization. Some sources mark the end of the acute stage when all but 10% of the burn wounds are closed, but others define the acute stage as extending until all wounds are closed. The rehabilitation stage follows the acute stage and lasts as long as efforts continue to promote improvement or adjustment. There is some overlap between the acute and rehabilitation stages because nursing care in the acute stage can significantly affect the potential for rehabilitation.

MEDICAL TREATMENT IN THE EMERGENT STAGE

In the emergency department, the staff first assesses airway, breathing, and circulation and then determines whether the patient has injuries in addition to the burn. If inhalation injury is suspected, oxygen therapy is started. Intravenous lines are established to begin fluid resuscitation and to provide emergency vascular access. An indwelling urinary catheter and a nasogastric tube are usually inserted. Blood is drawn for baseline laboratory studies (hematocrit, electrolytes, and blood gases, if indicated). Tetanus prophylaxis may be administered. Pain is assessed and analgesics are ordered. The wound is then cleaned, débrided, and inspected.

Once the initial care is completed, the patient with serious burns is transferred to a burn specialty care unit or a critical care unit. Intravenous fluid therapy is an essential aspect of care during the first few days of burn treatment. Several formulas are used to select the volumes and solutions to be administered. Volume is based on the patient's weight and extent of injury. For the first 24 hours, intravenous fluids may consist of various combinations of electrolyte, colloid, and dextrose solutions. However, specific formulas vary among specialty care units. For example, some formulas prescribe *only* electrolyte solutions in the first 24 hours.

For the second 24 hours, volume is usually decreased based on urine output. Fluids then consist of different combinations of electrolyte, colloid, and dextrose solutions. Some formulas omit electrolyte solutions in the second 24 hours.

In addition to fluids, medical care may include mechanical ventilation, antibiotic therapy, and surgical procedures.

WOUND CARE

Wound care after a burn injury is intended to promote healing, prevent infection, control heat loss, retain function, and minimize disfigurement. Burn wounds may be treated by the open or closed method. The method of wound care is based, in part, on the state of the wound. The open method involves the use of topical antimicrobials but no dressings. Open care is less restrictive and simpler than closed care but provides greater opportunity for loss of fluid and heat through the wound surface. Closed care uses topical medications covered by dressings. Because some areas of the wound may be deeper than other areas, it is not unusual to see open care for some of the patient's wounds and closed care for others. Examples of topical medications that may be used are silver sulfadiazine (Silvadene) and mafenide acetate (Sulfamylon). To prevent tetanus, a tetanus toxoid booster is usually given if the patient has not been immunized within the past 5 years. Patients who have never been immunized are given tetanus immune globulin and the first in a series of tetanus toxoid.

For clean partial-thickness wounds that will heal without grafting, temporary wound coverings often are used. Temporary wound coverings include amniotic membranes, grafts from cadavers or pigs, and a number of synthetic materials that promote wound healing or protect donor or graft sites. Grafted areas in need of protection are often covered by temporary wound coverings as well. Donor sites also are treated with a variety of products, including fine-mesh gauze and synthetic and biosynthetic products.

Débridement

A partial-thickness burn may blister, peel, and heal with minimal long-term effects. A full-thickness burn, however, is often covered by a thick, leathery layer of burned tissue (eschar) that shelters microorganisms and inhibits healing. Eschar must be removed before healing can take place. Further, if eschar encircles a limb, it may need to be incised to permit tissue swelling without compromising circulation. **Débridement** is the removal of debris and necrotic (dead) tissue from a wound. In the case of a burn wound, débridement includes removal of eschar. Débridement may be accomplished by mechanical means (using scissors and forceps), surgical excision, or the use of enzymes. Enzymatic débridement is the use of topical medications containing enzymes capable of dissolving necrotic tissue. These substances are applied directly to the wound but should not be applied to wounds that communicate with major body cavities or to exposed nerves. Enzymatic agents may cause pain and bleeding.

Skin Grafting

A burn wound may be covered using the patient's own skin, called an *autograft.* The graft is usually taken from the thigh or buttocks using a tool called a *dermatome.* The thickness of the graft determines whether it is a split-thickness or a full-thickness graft. If a thin layer of skin is used, it is considered a split-thickness graft. A split-thickness graft may be a sheet graft (an intact section of skin) or a meshed graft. A meshed graft has multiple tiny slits that allow the skin to be stretched to cover a larger area. The slits also allow for wound exudate to be absorbed by the cover dressing. Grafts vary in size, with the smallest being pinch and postage stamp grafts. Larger grafts may be needed to cover all or part of the burn.

For very deep burns and burns of the face, neck, or hands, a full-thickness graft may be preferred. A full-thickness graft includes skin and subcutaneous tissue and provides better cosmetic results. Another type of full-thickness graft is a pedicle or flap graft, in which one end of a section or tube of donor tissue is sutured to the recipient site while another section remains attached to the donor site. This type of graft continues to receive blood from the donor site. Once the graft takes or attaches to the recipient site, the pedicle or flap is cut free from the donor site.

After grafting, the recipient site is inspected for bleeding under the graft that could interfere with survival of the graft. The area is immobilized for 3 to 7 days to permit attachment of the graft to the wound base. Splints, traction, and restraints may be used for immobilization. After an autograft, the patient's donor site requires care as well. The donor site is usually covered with fine-mesh gauze or synthetic dressings and bandages. The dressings are usually left in place until the epithelium has regenerated.

Scarring

Burn scars can be reduced by the use of pressure dressings in the early stages of care, followed by the use of custom-fitted garments that apply continuous pressure. These garments are worn 23 hours a day and may be prescribed for as long as 2 years (Fig. 48-18).

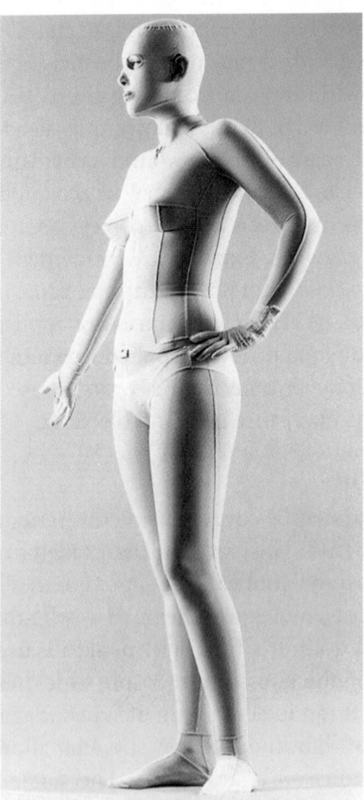

FIGURE **48-18** Antiscar pressure garment minimizes the hypertrophic scarring that is common after burn injuries.

NURSING CARE *of the Patient with Burn Injury*

Assessment

When the patient is stabilized, a complete assessment should be done. As priorities change, add relevant data.

Health History

The history of the present illness describes the circumstances surrounding the burn injury. The past medical history documents any chronic diseases, surgeries, or hospitalizations. Identify medications and allergies. Take a family history even though it is not specific to burn injuries because it may alert you to other problems. The review of systems detects current problems with each body system. In the functional assessment, describe the patient's habits and lifestyle, roles and responsibilities, stressors, and coping strategies.

Physical Examination

Begin the physical examination with vital signs. Be alert for abnormalities that suggest hypoxia (restlessness, tachypnea), excess fluid volume (bounding pulse, hypertension), deficient fluid volume (tachycardia, hypotension), hypovolemia (hypotension, tachycardia), or infection (fever, tachycardia). Measure height and weight if the patient is stable enough.

Throughout the examination, inspect the skin for burn wounds and other lesions. Note wound color and the presence of eschar. Palpate intact skin for temperature and turgor. Observe chest expansion, and auscultate the lungs for wheezing, stridor, or atelectasis. Auscultate the apical pulse for rate and rhythm. Assess the abdomen for active bowel sounds and distention. Inspect the extremities for injury and deformity. Delay range of motion assessment if an extremity is immobilized.

Nursing Diagnoses, Goals, and Outcome Criteria: Burns

Depending on the severity and type of burn, nursing diagnoses for the patient with burns may include those listed in this table. The first two are most likely to occur in the emergent stage; the remaining diagnoses may be made in the emergent, acute, or rehabilitation stage.

Nursing Diagnoses	Goals and Outcome Criteria
Decreased Cardiac Output related to hypovolemia secondary to shift of fluid from vascular to extracellular compartment	Normal cardiac output: pulse and blood pressure consistent with patient norms
Excess Fluid Volume related to changes in capillary permeability and accumulation of fluid in body tissues	Normal fluid balance: edema decreasing or absent, increased urine output
Acute Pain related to tissue trauma of burn injury	Pain relief: patient statement of pain relief, more relaxed manner
Risk for Infection related to loss of protective skin barrier	Absence of infection: normal body temperature and white blood cell count, negative wound cultures

Hypothermia related to impaired heat-regulating ability of injured skin	Normal body temperature: temperature within patient norms
Risk for Imbalanced Nutrition: Less than Body Requirements related to high metabolic demands.	Adequate nutrition: stable body weight
Impaired Physical Mobility related to contractures, therapeutic immobilization, pain	Adaptation to physical limitations: minimal contractures, clear breath sounds, bowel movements at least every 2 to 3 days
Ineffective Coping related to possible disfigurement, dysfunction, fear of death	Effective patient coping: positive patient statements about future; participates in rehabilitation efforts
Ineffective Family Coping related to uncertain outcome, fear of patient death, and altered family function	Effective family coping: positive family statements about the future; family interest in ways to help patient's recovery

Interventions

Decreased Cardiac Output

The risk of decreased cardiac output is greatest in the emergent stage when fluid has shifted from the blood to the extracellular compartment. If blood volume is not maintained, the patient's blood pressure falls and tissue perfusion is impaired. To monitor cardiac output, assess the patient's vital signs and fluid intake and output. Signs of decreased cardiac output include hypotension, tachycardia, and decreased urine output. Inadequate tissue perfusion may be manifested by cool, pale or cyanotic skin, restlessness, and confusion. Administer intravenous fluids as ordered with close, continuous monitoring of fluid status.

Fluid Volume Excess

Fluid volume excess may result from the retention of fluid in the extracellular compartment. As capillary permeability returns to normal and fluid is reabsorbed, the patient's blood volume increases. If the patient's kidneys can eliminate the excess fluid efficiently, the patient suffers no ill effects from the increasing blood volume. There is a risk, however, that the patient's circulatory system may be unable to adapt to the increased volume. This puts the patient at risk for heart failure.

Monitor the patient's vital signs for hypertension, dyspnea, and full, bounding pulse. Measure urine output and compare with fluid intake. Administer intravenous fluids as ordered and monitor closely. Document assessments.

Acute Pain

Partial-thickness wounds are typically very painful. Full-thickness burns lack sensation because of the destruction of the superficial nerves. However, burns are often uneven in depth, so patients with full-thickness burns often have pain as well. The burn patient is given opioid analgesics such as morphine as ordered. Sedatives like midazolam (Versed) may also be prescribed. Analgesics usually are given before painful wound care. If given orally, administer the medication 45 minutes before the procedure. If given intravenously, administer the drug 5 to 10 minutes ahead of time. The intramuscular route is not routinely used until fluid shifts have stabilized because absorption is less reliable. Nonsteroidal anti-inflammatory drugs also may be prescribed. Pain is aggravated by anxiety, so use measures to reduce fear and anxiety in the management of pain. Additional nursing measures for pain are described in Chapter 14. Assess and document patient response to interventions.

Risk for Infection

The burn patient, without protective skin, is at great risk for infection. Routinely monitor for signs of local infection (pus, foul odor, increased redness) and systemic infection (fever, increased white blood cell count). Infection can come from the staff, visitors, the environment, and the patient's own body. Specific infection control measures vary with the agency. Strict hand washing should be practiced by the patient and all who enter the room. Body hair around wounds is usually shaved or cut to prevent wound contamination. Do *not* shave the eyebrows because, if shaved, they tend to grow back in a disorganized pattern. Carry out wound care as ordered or according to routines of the specialty care unit.

Hypothermia

Loss of heat through the burn wound surface places the patient at risk for hypothermia (low body temperature). This is especially problematic for elderly people whose ability to maintain body temperature is already compromised because of various age-related changes.

Monitor the patient's tympanic or rectal temperature to detect declining body temperature. Keep the room warm, and use external heat sources as needed. Attempt to limit body surface area exposure during wound care. Body heat loss may be greater if the patient is on an air-fluidized bed, so carefully monitor the temperature of the bed.

Risk for Imbalanced Nutrition: Less than Body Requirements

Healing of a large burn wound requires considerable energy. It is, therefore, critical that nutrition be provided to meet the increased metabolic demands. Consult with the dietitian about the patient's nutritional needs and preferences. Calorie needs may be as much as twice the patient's baseline needs. Regular meals may need to be supplemented with between-meal feedings. Stress to the patient the need for increased intake during the recovery period. Try to create an environment conducive to eating and encourage the patient to eat all food served. Provide assistance with meals if needed. Some patients require tube feedings or total parenteral nutrition to meet their calorie needs.

Impaired Physical Mobility

Patients with burns may have restrictions on their mobility imposed by the injury or the treatment. The hazards of immobility, including pressure sores, joint contractures, pneumonia and atelectasis, constipation, and urinary infections, are covered in Chapter 20. Monitor range of motion in affected joints and perform passive or active exercises unless contraindicated. Keep injured limbs in functional positions as much as possible (Fig. 48-19). Also, exercise unaffected joints to maintain flexibility and strength. Impaired mobility may interfere with the patient's ability to participate in his or her own care. Assess self-care deficits and provide assistance as needed. As the patient moves toward recovery, the rehabilitation team helps the patient adapt self-care activities for permanent injuries.

Ineffective Coping

Severe burns can result in disfigurement and loss of function. The patient faces a long and difficult recovery period. The emotional responses of the burn patient are often like those of any grieving person: shock, disbelief, withdrawal, denial, regression, depression, and anger. Demonstrate acceptance of the patient regardless of the emotional state. Provide opportunities for the patient to express his or her thoughts and feelings. The patient may find it helpful to talk to a clinical nurse specialist, counselor, or spiritual adviser. Some patients find support groups helpful in learning to live with their injuries. Encourage the patient to identify and use coping strategies that have been effective in the past. If effective coping strategies are used, the patient eventually incorporates the physical and functional changes into a new body image.

Ineffective Family Coping

A serious burn injury that may require months or years of therapy has a tremendous impact on the family. Significant others must be included in the patient's care. When the family arrives after the injury, the physician or clinical nurse specialist advises them of the patient's injuries, what to expect when they see the patient, and what is being done for the patient. The family should be offered an opportunity to talk with a social worker, clinical nurse specialist, counselor, or spiritual adviser.

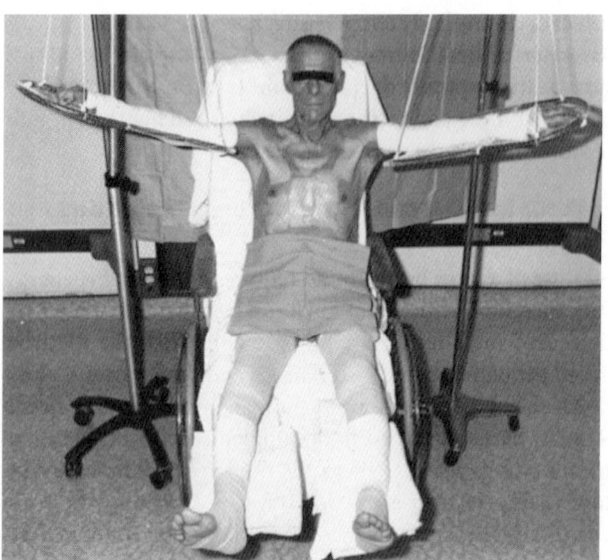

FIGURE **48-19** Therapeutic positioning. This patient's arms are extended to prevent flexion contractures. Pressure dressings on legs prevent edema and minimize scarring.

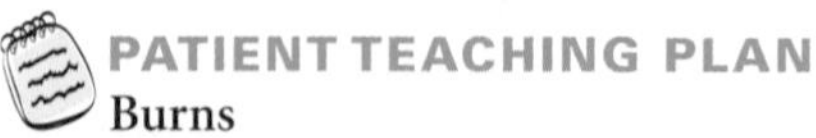

PATIENT TEACHING PLAN
Burns

When the patient is acutely ill, patient teaching consists of telling the patient what is being done, why, and what to expect. As the patient stabilizes, the teaching plan should include the following points:

- You can help prevent wound infection by practicing good hygiene and avoiding others with infections.
- Because your nutritional needs are greatly increased as a result of the healing that needs to occur, you need to eat all food provided, including meal supplements.
- Positioning, exercise, and splints help to prevent stiffening of joints, skin breakdown, and blood clots in your legs.
- Pain management is possible, so tell the nurse or the physician if your pain is not controlled.
- Protect grafts from pressure and shearing force so they can heal.
- Clothing, makeup, hairpieces, and prostheses can be used to conceal scars and improve appearance.
- Adaptive devices are available to compensate for disabilities.
- Rehabilitation resources will be provided once the acute phase has passed.

CONDITIONS TREATED WITH PLASTIC SURGERY

Plastic surgery includes aesthetic (cosmetic) and reconstructive procedures. Aesthetic surgical procedures are performed to improve appearance, whereas reconstructive procedures are done to correct abnormalities. In addition to usual surgical approaches, plastic surgery may include use of flaps and grafts, skin expansion, implants, liposuction, and microvascular surgery.

AESTHETIC SURGERY

In general, aesthetic surgery alters a body feature that is structurally normal but perceived by the patient as unattractive. Examples of aesthetic surgery are rhytidectomy, blepharoplasty, chin implants, rhinoplasty, abdominoplasty, breast augmentation, and breast reduction. A rhytidectomy, commonly called a face-lift, is done to remove facial wrinkles and tighten sagging tissue. A blepharoplasty is the removal of excess tissue around the eyes. It is usually an aesthetic procedure but may be done to improve function if droopy eyelids impair vision. Chin implants are done by placing a prosthesis to correct a receding chin. A rhinoplasty alters the shape or size, or both, of the nose. In an abdominoplasty, excess skin and adipose tissue are removed and the abdominal muscles are tightened.

Breast augmentation is breast enlargement, which may be performed to increase the size of both breasts or to improve breast symmetry. A variety of techniques have been used for breast augmentation. The most common procedure has been to implant a silicone rubber implant filled with saline. Because of possible adverse effects related to leakage of filler substances into the body, saline has replaced silicone. Breast reduction decreases breast size and may be requested to improve appearance or body proportion or to eliminate discomfort associated with excessively large breasts. Liposuction is the removal of excess adipose tissue with a suction device, most commonly used on the thighs, abdomen, arms, and buttocks.

RECONSTRUCTIVE SURGERY

A number of procedures may be classified as reconstructive. Reconstructive surgery may be done to repair disfiguring scars, restore body contours after radical surgery like mastectomy, eliminate benign lesions such as birthmarks, restore features damaged by trauma or disease, and correct developmental defects.

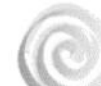

What Does Culture Have to do with Plastic Surgery?

Because attractiveness is culturally defined, people may seek various procedures that they perceive will increase their attractiveness. Be careful not to impose your views on the patient.

NURSING CARE *of the Patient Having Plastic Surgery*

When working with people who are having plastic surgery, nurses must be aware of their own biases and feelings. Nurses who view cosmetic procedures as vain or frivolous may have difficulty being supportive of patients who choose to have these procedures done. Many factors may motivate people to have aesthetic surgery. Physical appearance is a component of body image and may affect self-esteem. Some people believe that a change in appearance will benefit their personal or professional lives. A person who is very self-conscious about a physical feature can benefit immensely from aesthetic surgery. It is important not to judge the patient's motivation for seeking surgery. It is also important to be alert to the patient's unrealistic expectations for the surgical outcome.

Although each procedure may require some specific nursing interventions, this section addresses general nursing care for the patient having plastic surgery. Some specific procedures, complications, and nursing care are presented in Table 48-8.

PREOPERATIVE NURSING CARE

Many of these procedures may be done in day surgery or short-stay surgical units. Therefore, patient preparation emphasizes teaching for self-care. Initial teaching may be done by the physician, office nurse, or staff nurse.

Assessment

Health History

Document the patient's description of the problem being treated with plastic surgery and what the patient expects the procedure to accomplish. While taking the past medical history, it is especially important to note conditions that might affect wound healing, such as diabetes mellitus, circulatory disorders, and impaired blood coagulation. In the review of systems, pay special attention to the surgical area. If a blepharoplasty is being done, test and document visual acuity. The functional assessment describes the patient's lifestyle and usual activities, which may require some temporary modification after plastic surgery.

Physical Examination

The routine preoperative physical examination is performed as described in Chapter 16. Describe the condition that is being treated. Most plastic surgeons have preoperative photographs made to document the condition. If you take the photograph, be sensitive to the patient's discomfort or embarrassment.

table 48-8 *Complications of Common Plastic Surgery Procedures*

PROCEDURE	DESCRIPTION	COMPLICATIONS
Rhytidectomy (face-lift)	Removal of excess skin and tissue from face	Hematoma, hemorrhage, temporary or permanent facial nerve damage, wound infection, bruising, edema, skin necrosis, hair loss
Blepharoplasty	Removal of bulging fat and excess skin around eye	Hematoma, ectropion, corneal injury, visual loss (rare), wound infection (rare)
Rhinoplasty	Removal of excess cartilage and tissue from nose with correction of septal defects if indicated.	Hematoma, hemorrhage, temporary bruising and edema, wound infection, septal perforation, minor skin irritation
Augmentation mammaplasty	Insertion of breast-shaped synthetic implants	Hematoma, hemorrhage, wound infection, phlebitis Capsule formation and contraction
Reduction mammaplasty	Excision of excessive breast tissue and skin	Hematoma; hemorrhage; infection; fat necrosis; wound dehiscence; necrosis of nipple, areola, and skin flap

Modified from Ignatavicius, D. D., Workman, M. S., & M. A. Mishler (Eds.), *Medical-surgical nursing across the health care continuum* (3rd ed., p. 1748) Philadelphia: Saunders.

Nursing Diagnoses, Goals, and Outcome Criteria: Plastic Surgery, Preoperative

Nursing Diagnoses	Goals and Outcome Criteria
Anxiety related to uncertain outcome, anticipated change in appearance, surgical procedure	Reduced anxiety: patient's statement of less anxiety; absence of trembling or tachycardia; and relaxed expression
Deficient Knowledge related to unfamiliarity with surgical routines	Understanding of surgical routines: patient correctly describes routines, identifies any actions to be carried out prior to admission and postoperatively

Interventions

Anxiety

Assess the patient's anxiety by observing for nervousness, trembling, increased pulse, and difficulty concentrating. Share such observations and ask how the patient feels about the planned surgery. Anxiety may be reduced by encouraging the patient to express concerns, acknowledging that these feelings are normal, and providing information about what to expect.

Deficient Knowledge

Assess the patient's perception of the procedure and its outcome. Discuss surgical preoperative and postoperative procedures and self-care. Advise the patient if swelling, bruising, and scars are expected in the immediate postoperative period. Usually, patients have been told not to take drugs that prolong bleeding time, including aspirin, before surgery. Smoking is discouraged because nicotine causes vasoconstriction, which can interfere with healing. The patient may be instructed to scrub the surgical area at intervals before the procedure. Specific teaching depends on the exact procedure and the surgeon's orders or agency's protocol.

POSTOPERATIVE NURSING CARE

Routine postoperative nursing care is detailed in Chapter 16. This section emphasizes special considerations when a patient has plastic surgery.

Assessment

The patient may have had general, regional, or local anesthesia. Monitor vital signs and assess level of consciousness. Inspect dressings for drainage or bleeding but do not remove them without specific orders. Some dressings, such as those used after rhinoplasty, may serve as splints, so they must not be disturbed. Observe flaps and grafts for color and evidence of fluid accumulation, and palpate for warmth. If drains are present, inspect and measure the contents each shift. The fluid should gradually lighten from sanguineous (red) to serosanguineous (pink) to serous (pale yellow). Monitor the patient's comfort level also.

Consider the Alternative!

In addition to analgesics, recommend comfort measures, such as positioning, relaxation, and imagery, to decrease pain.

Nursing Diagnoses, Goals, and Outcome Criteria: Plastic Surgery, Postoperative

Nursing Diagnoses	Goals and Outcome Criteria
Acute Pain related to tissue trauma	Reduced pain: patient states pain relieved, relaxed manner
Risk for Infection related to surgical incision	Absence of infection: no fever or foul drainage; decreasing redness and edema
Risk for Injury related to inadequate circulation to grafted tissue, pressure created by edema or implants, nerve damage	Adequate tissue perfusion: normal tissue warmth and color; normal neuromuscular function: sensation, movement, and reflexes
Risk for Deficient Fluid Volume related to effects of liposuction	Normal fluid balance: vital signs consistent with patient norms, fluid intake equal to output
Disturbed Body Image related to altered appearance	Healthy body image: patient expresses understanding of temporary appearance; expresses satisfaction with outcome
Ineffective Therapeutic Regimen Management related to lack of information about postoperative care	Appropriate postoperative self-care: patient describes and demonstrates self-care correctly

Interventions

Acute Pain

Minor procedures such as blepharoplasty usually cause minimal pain, but major procedures such as grafting or abdominoplasty can be very painful. Pain is treated with analgesics as ordered. Aspirin usually is not ordered because it prolongs bleeding time. After surgery on the face or head, the head of the bed usually is elevated and cold compresses are ordered to decrease swelling. Assess and document the effects of interventions. Increasing pain or pain that is not responsive to treatment must be reported to the physician.

Risk for Infection

Monitor for signs and symptoms of infection, although these are unlikely to be seen during a brief hospitalization. Therefore, instruct the patient to report increasing redness, swelling, drainage, or fever. The nurse and patient must exercise good hand washing before any contact with the incisions, flaps, or grafts. Give antimicrobial drugs as ordered. Some plastic surgeons order topical antimicrobials applied to the incisions. After rhytidectomy, the patient is usually not permitted to shampoo the hair for several days to avoid contamination of the incisions.

Risk for Injury

After plastic surgery, assess the affected tissues for adequate circulation. Grafts rely on blood flow in underlying tissue to supply nutrients and oxygen and to remove wastes. Therefore, grafts must be protected from trauma and pressure. Pallor, cyanosis, and coolness in a graft suggest inadequate circulation and must be reported to the surgeon immediately. If fluid accumulates under the graft, it separates the graft from the underlying tissue, depriving it of oxygen and nutrients. Therefore, swelling or blisters must be reported to the surgeon, who may remove the accumulated fluid with a small-gauge needle and syringe.

Rhytidectomy poses a risk of injury to the facial nerve, which is manifested by facial asymmetry. If asymmetry is observed, notify the surgeon immediately. The patient may be returned to surgery in an effort to relieve the pressure on the nerve and prevent permanent damage.

After blepharoplasty, monitor the patient's visual status. Although the risk is slight, the eye could be injured during the procedure.

After abdominoplasty, the patient may be required to protect the operative site by remaining in a flexed position for a specified period of time. Familiarize yourself with specific postoperative orders of your patient's surgeon. Position the bed so that the head and knees are elevated to reduce stress on the suture line. When out of bed, the patient may be required to continue the flexed position. The patient is gradually permitted to straighten up. Again, such directions vary with different surgeons.

After breast augmentation, monitor the patient for bleeding, infection, and altered sensation. The patient is also at risk for capsule formation, in which scar tissue gradually encloses the implant, causing the breast to become hard and misshapen. The surgeon may advise the patient to massage the breast to reduce the risk of capsule formation. This procedure involves pushing each breast up, to the side, and toward the center of the chest, holding each position to the count of 10. For a period specified by the surgeon, the patient should avoid raising the arms above the head.

Risk for Deficient Fluid Volume

Patients who have liposuction are at risk for hypovolemia due to excessive fluid loss. Intravenous fluids may be ordered after surgery, and oral fluids are usually encouraged when the patient is fully alert. Monitor vital signs for tachycardia and hypotension associated with fluid volume deficit. Use caution when assisting patients out of bed. If the blood volume is low, the patient may feel dizzy or faint.

Disturbed Body Image

In the immediate postoperative period, the patient often has edema and bruising as well as visible incisions. Assure the patient that these effects will gradually resolve. You can explore measures to conceal the evidence of trauma, but no makeup should be applied to surgical incisions until they are well healed.

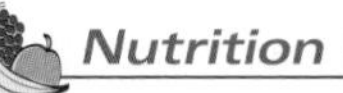

Nutrition Concepts

1. Vitamin A is essential for healthy skin.
2. Food sources of vitamin A are liver, pumpkin, sweet potatoes, carrots, spinach, broccoli, cantaloupe, and apricots.
3. Food allergies can cause atopic dermatitis.
4. Skin changes associated with malnutrition include cracked skin, dermatitis, xerosis (dry skin), purpura, and petechiae (purple or red spots).

Ineffective Therapeutic Regimen Management

In preparing for discharge, provide verbal and written instructions for self-care. The following topics must be included: drug therapy (names of drugs ordered, schedule), wound care, signs and symptoms of infection, activity restrictions, and measures to prevent complications.

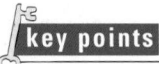

key points

- The functions of the skin are protection, body temperature regulation, secretion, sensation, synthesis of vitamin D, and blood storage.
- The skin assessment may detect skin disorders and systemic disorders that affect the skin.
- Pruritus (itching) is a symptom rather than a disease that is treated by correction or removal of the underlying cause, skin moisturizers, and drugs such as antihistamines, corticosteroids, and local anesthetics.
- Atopic dermatitis, one type of eczema, is abnormally dry, itchy skin that is treated with moisturizers, antihistamines, antibiotics, and corticosteroids.
- Seborrheic dermatitis is a chronic inflammatory disease of the skin caused by increased sebum production that is treated with medicated shampoos for the scalp and topical corticosteroids and antibiotics for other body sites.
- Psoriasis, characterized by bright-red lesions with silvery scales, may require treatment with keratolytics, radiation, and antipsoriatics.
- Fungal infections, including tinea pedis, tinea manus, tinea cruris, tinea corporis, tinea barbae, and candidiasis, are usually treated with antifungal drugs.
- Necrotizing fasciitis, a very serious infection that affects the fascia under the skin, is treated with antibiotics, débridement, and skin grafting.
- Acne, which is characterized by comedones, pustules, and cysts primarily on the face, neck, and upper trunk, may be treated with topical medications, oral antibiotics, estrogen, spironolactone, and vitamin A derivatives.
- The herpes simplex virus types 1 and 2, which cause outbreaks of vesicles that rupture and form crusts, is treated with antiviral drugs that hasten healing but are not curative.
- Herpes zoster infection (shingles) causes pain and itching along a nerve pathway and may respond to acyclovir.
- Common nursing diagnoses for the patient with an infectious or inflammatory skin disorder include

Impaired Skin Integrity, Acute Pain, Risk for (secondary) Infection, Disturbed Body Image, Social Isolation, and Ineffective Therapeutic Regimen Management.
- Lice and scabies are tiny parasites that may infest the hair and skin, causing intense itching.
- Pemphigus is a chronic autoimmune condition in which fragile bullae develop and rupture, spilling a foul drainage.
- Skin cancers include actinic keratoses, basal cell carcinomas, squamous cell carcinomas, melanomas, and cutaneous T-cell lymphoma.
- The two major conditions affecting the nails are infections and inflammation caused by ingrown nails.
- Burns are classified by size and depth of the tissue injury.
- Serious burns affect not only the skin but also fluid balance, gastrointestinal function, respiratory function, and the immune system.
- The three stages of burn injury are emergent, acute, and rehabilitation.
- Wound care after burn injury is intended to promote healing, prevent infection, control heat loss, retain function, and minimize disfigurement.
- Nursing care of the burn patient may address Decreased Cardiac Output, Excess Fluid Volume, Acute Pain, Risk for Infection, Hypothermia, Imbalanced Nutrition, Impaired Physical Mobility, Ineffective Coping, Ineffective Family Coping, and Ineffective Therapeutic Regimen Management.

REVIEW QUESTIONS

1. The skin regulates body temperature by:
   1. reacting to foreign substances that invade the epidermis.
   2. dilating and constricting surface blood vessels.
   3. secreting sebum to insulate the outer layers of skin.
   4. reacting to sunlight by producing vitamin C.
2. When assessing an older adult, you observe flat pigmented spots on the backs of both hands. You should recognize these as:
   1. lentigines.
   2. angiomas.
   3. keratoses.
   4. purpura.
3. Which interventions will help to prevent scratching and skin injury in a patient with atopic dermatitis?
   1. Maintain the room temperature around 80° F.
   2. Apply keratolytics liberally to promote healing.
   3. Wash new clothing before wearing it.
   4. Encourage hot baths.
4. Contact dermatitis is caused by:
   1. infestations of parasites.
   2. reactions to drugs.
   3. excessive skin dryness.
   4. an allergic response.
5. Patient teaching related to psoriasis should include:
   1. psoriasis usually can be cured with drug therapy.
   2. direct contact with others can transmit psoriasis.
   3. anthralin must be kept on the skin continuously.
   4. in most people, psoriasis affects only the skin.
6. An obese elderly patient in a long-term care facility has had intertrigo in body folds (axilla, beneath the breasts) on several occasions. Which measure is most appropriate to reduce the risk of a recurrence?
   1. Apply talc or cellulose powder to susceptible areas.
   2. Reduce bathing to three times each week.
   3. Liberally sprinkle cornstarch on body creases.
   4. Scrub affected areas with topical antiseptics.
7. A female patient is being treated with isotretinoin (Accutane) at the clinic for severe acne after other treatments have failed. All of the following points should be included in the teaching plan. Which is *most* important?
   1. Your skin may become very dry and peel.
   2. It may take several months to see improvement.
   3. You will sunburn very easily while on this drug.
   4. If sexually active, you must use reliable contraception.
8. A drug used to treat herpes simplex type 1 is:
   1. hydrocortisone (Cortizone).
   2. isotretinoin (Accutane).
   3. acyclovir (Zovirax).
   4. methoxsalen (Oxsoralen).
9. The best way to prevent skin cancer is to:
   1. maintain good skin hydration.
   2. avoid excessive sun exposure.
   3. take large doses of vitamin A.
   4. avoid use of tobacco products.
10. Characteristics of melanomas include:
    1. nodular lesion with a pearly appearance.
    2. irregular lesion with uneven coloration.
    3. scaly ulcer with no clear margins.
    4. painful red, blue, or purple macules.

CHAPTER 49 Eye and Vision Disorders

objectives

1. Identify the data to be collected in the nursing assessment of the eye and vision.
2. Identify the nursing responsibilities for patients having diagnostic tests or procedures to diagnose eye disorders.
3. List measures to reduce the risk of eye injuries.
4. Describe the nursing care of patients who require common therapeutic measures for eye disorders: irrigation, application of ophthalmic drugs, and surgery.
5. Describe the pathophysiology, signs and symptoms, diagnosis, and treatment of selected eye conditions.
6. Assist in developing a nursing care plan for the patient with an eye disorder.

key terms

Astigmatism (ă-STĬG-mă-tĭzm, p. 1062)
Cataract (KĂT-ă-răkt, p. 1063)
Conjunctivitis (kŏn-jŭnk-tĭ-VĪ-tĭs, p. 1060)
Cycloplegic (sī-klō-PLĒ-jĭk, p. 1053)
Ectropion (ĕk-TRŌ-pē-ŏn, p. 1060)
Entropion (ĕn-TRŌ-pē-ŏn, p. 1060)
Enucleation (ē-nū-klē-Ā-shŭn, p. 1071)
Hyperopia (hī-pĕr-Ō-pē-ă, p. 1048)
Keratitis (kĕr-ă-TĪ-tĭs, p. 1060)
Miotic (mī-ŎT-ĭk, p. 1053)
Mydriatic (mĭd-rē-ĂT-ĭk, p. 1053)
Myopia (mī-Ō-pē-ă, p. 1062)
Presbyopia (prĕz-bē-Ō-pē-ă, p. 1048)
Refraction (rē-FRĂK-shŭn, p. 1050)
Scotomata (skō-TŌ-mă-tă, p. 1048)
Tonometry (tō-NŎM-ĕ-trē, p. 1051)

It has been said that the eye is the window to the world. Indeed, vision plays an extremely important part in everyday life. It enables people to move about freely, to avoid danger, and to appreciate physical beauty. The eyes also are credited with conveying (or betraying!) one's emotions and communicating trust. Romantics speak of gazing into the eyes of a loved one.

In the United States, more than 11 million people have some vision impairment. For most people, loss of vision is perceived as a most tragic event. Nurses can play important roles in the prevention of vision loss, treatment of disorders of the eye, and rehabilitation of people with vision disturbances.

ANATOMY AND PHYSIOLOGY OF THE EYE

The eyeball is the primary structure involved in seeing. Several structures in addition to the eyeball serve to make up the visual system. The external structures of the visual system include the eyelids, eyelashes, conjunctiva, cornea, sclera, and extraocular muscles. These structures are illustrated in Figure 49-1.

EXTERNAL STRUCTURES

The external structures of the visual system serve to protect and move the eyeball. The eyelids and eyelashes protect the eye by keeping it moist and shielding it from foreign substances. The lids are lined with a mucous membrane called the palpebral conjunctiva. The membrane continues from the inner eyelid margins to form a pocket around the eye and then covers the sclera up to the margin of the iris. The portion of the membrane that covers the anterior sclera is the bulbar conjunctiva.

Lacrimal glands located above the eyes secrete tears into the eyes through lacrimal ducts in the upper eyelids. Spontaneous blinking (approximately 15 times a minute) bathes the eyeballs in tear fluid. Tear fluid provides oxygen and some nutrients to the cornea. Normally, the fluid drains from the eye through the lacrimal sac into the nose. With excessive tear production, tears run from the eyes. Increased tear production occurs with trauma, irritation, or emotional distress. Decreased tear production occurs to some extent with aging. It should be noted that the passage of tear fluid through the lacrimal sac is the route by which eye drops can be absorbed into the system. That is why eye drops can have systemic effects and explains the need to apply pressure to the lacrimal sac after instilling eye drops. Severe deficiencies in tear fluid cause dry eyes, making the cornea susceptible to injury.

Normal vision requires the eyes to move together. The simultaneous movement of both eyes in the same direction is called conjugate movement. Eye movements are coordinated by three cranial nerves and six extraocular muscles.

THE EYEBALL

The eyeball consists of three layers of tissue: the sclera, the choroid, and the retina (Fig. 49-2).

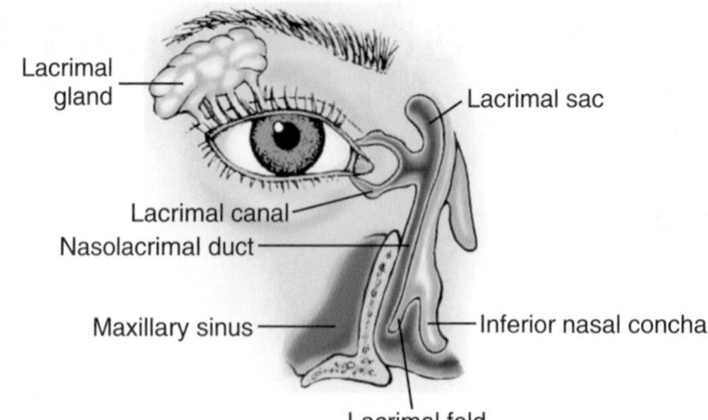

FIGURE 49-1 External parts of the visual system.

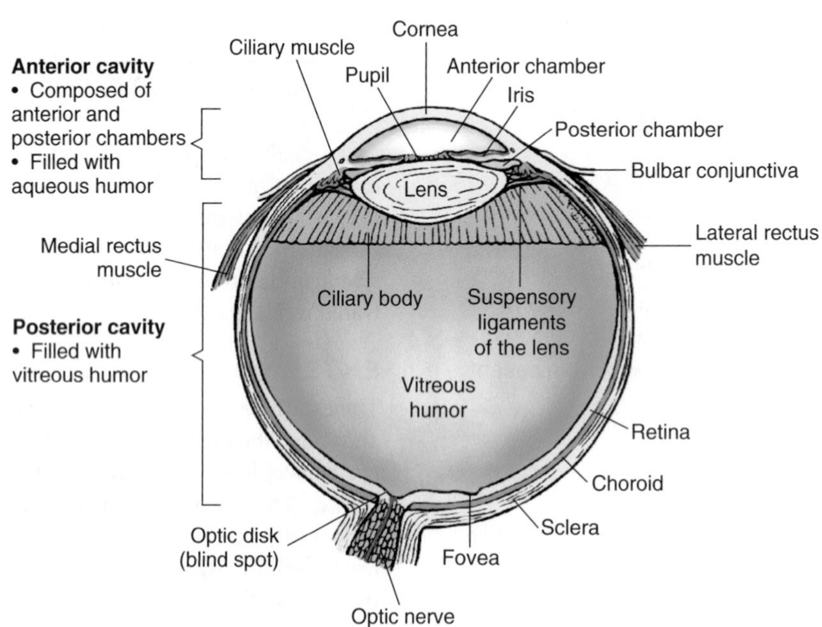

FIGURE 49-2 Internal structures of the eye.

Sclera

The sclera is the tough outer layer of the eyeball. It is mostly white except for the clear cornea over the iris. The cornea is covered by a protective membrane called the conjunctiva.

Choroid

The choroid or middle layer makes up the iris and ciliary muscle at the front of the eye. The colored part of the eye, the iris, is actually a muscle. The hole in the center of the iris is the pupil. The iris contracts and relaxes to control the amount of light entering the eye through the pupil. Dim light or severe stress causes the iris to contract. This makes the pupil dilate, or enlarge. Bright light causes the iris to relax, leaving the pupil constricted. The choroid is rich in blood vessels that deliver nourishment to the retina in the back of the eye.

Retina

The retina is the inner lining of the eyeball. It is composed of two layers. The pigmented layer is between the choroid and the sensory layer; it receives nutrients and oxygen from the choroid and supplies the sensory layer.

The area at the back of the eye contains light-sensitive receptors called rods and cones. Rods are most important for vision in dim light. Cones are used for daylight vision and color perception. The area of sharpest vision on the retina is the macula. Because the macula has no blood vessels, it depends on the choroid for nourishment.

Optic Nerve

The optic nerve enters the back of the eyeball. This nerve sends visual messages to the brain for interpretation. When the eye is examined with an ophthalmoscope, the part of the optic nerve that can be seen is referred to as the optic disk.

Fluid Chambers

Anterior Chamber

Within the eyeball are two chambers separated by the lens. The anterior chamber is located between the iris and the cornea. It is filled with aqueous humor, a clear, watery fluid. Aqueous humor is produced in the ciliary body. It flows over the lens, through the pupil, and out through the trabecular meshwork into the canal of Schlemm. The canal of Schlemm

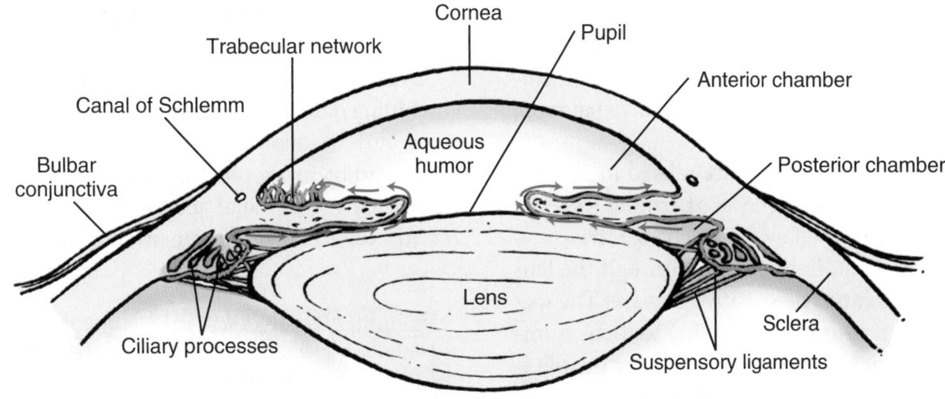

FIGURE 49-3 The flow of aqueous humor through the eye. Fluid is produced by the ciliary body. It flows through the pupil into the anterior chamber and out through the trabecular meshwork and the canal of Schlemm.

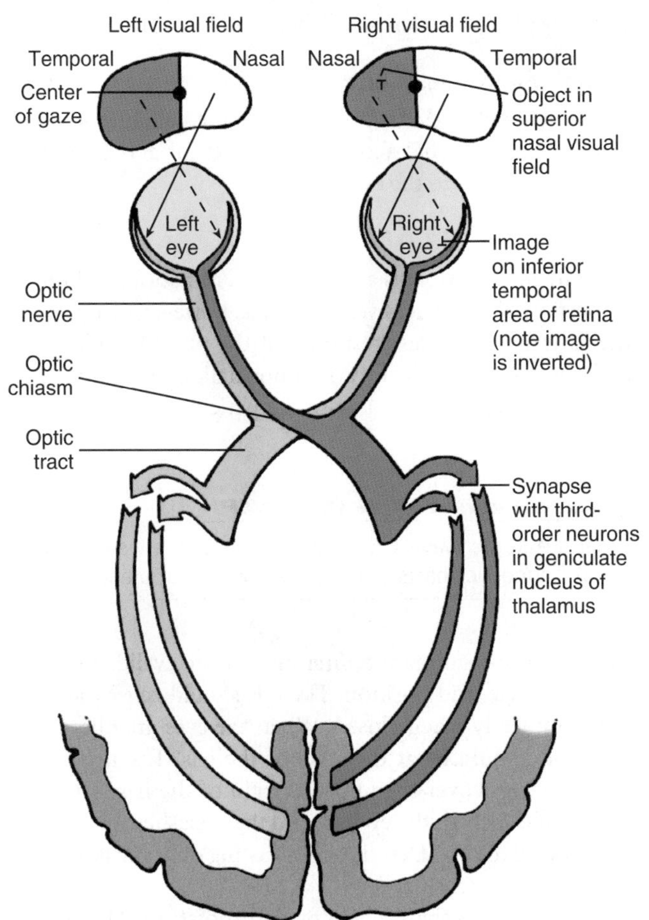

FIGURE 49-4 The visual pathway.

returns the fluid to the venous circulation. The flow of aqueous humor is illustrated in Figure 49-3.

The function of aqueous humor is to moisturize and nourish the lens and cornea. The production and drainage of the fluid from the eye must be balanced to maintain normal pressure within the eye.

Posterior Chamber

The larger posterior chamber behind the lens is filled with vitreous humor. Vitreous humor is a clear, gelatinous material that helps hold the retina in place.

Lens

The lens is a transparent structure behind the iris. It is attached to the ciliary muscle. The ciliary muscle relaxes and contracts to change the shape of the lens. This process, called *accommodation,* permits the eye to focus on objects at different distances. To focus on a near object, the ciliary muscle contracts, making the lens curve. For distance, the muscle relaxes, making the lens flatter.

VISUAL PATHWAY

As light enters the eye, it passes through the transparent cornea, aqueous humor, lens, and vitreous humor. These structures are called *refractive media.* They refract (bend) horizontal and vertical light rays so that the light rays focus on the retina.

On the retina, the light rays reflected from the image are reversed and upside down. Images are carried as impulses through the optic nerve. At the optic chiasm, fibers from the left field from each eye join to form the left optic tract. Fibers from the right field of each eye join to form the right optic tract. Images are transmitted to the brain by way of the optic tracts (Fig. 49-4).

AGE-RELATED CHANGES IN THE EYE

As people age, typical changes occur in the structures and function of the eye. The skin around the eye becomes wrinkled and looser. The eyelids usually have some excess tissue; this is not important unless it interferes with vision. The amount of fat around the eye decreases, permitting the eyeball to sink deeper into the orbit. Tear secretion diminishes, and the cornea becomes less sensitive. A grayish ring may be seen around the outer margin of the iris. This ring is called the arcus senilis. There is some disagreement about the significance of the arcus senilis. It may be related to elevated serum lipid levels; it does not affect vision. The pupil is usually smaller in the older person and responds somewhat more slowly to light.

Vision changes associated with age are related to changes in the lens and the ciliary muscle. The lens becomes less elastic, more dense, opaque, and yellow. These changes have several significant effects. First, light passing through the lens scatters, causing the patient to be sensitive to glare. The second, more important effect is that the ability to focus is impaired. This farsightedness (hyperopia) in older people is called presbyopia. This is the reason most older people have to wear glasses for reading or other close work. Some older people report seeing specks moving across the field of vision. These dark spots, called floaters, are actually bits of debris in the vitreous.

Despite the age-related changes in the eye, most older people retain adequate vision for daily activities.

NURSING ASSESSMENT OF THE EYE

HEALTH HISTORY

History of Present Illness

When assessing specific eye complaints, record changes in vision, including blurring, diplopia (double vision), spots, floaters, flashes of light, tunnel vision, altered color perception, halos around lights, blind spots (scotomata), and loss of part of the visual fields. If the patient reports pain, inquire about its location and nature (sharp, stabbing, aching). Document sensitivity to light, called photophobia. Ask the patient to describe any discharge. Drainage might be described as tears, purulent discharge, or crusting of the eyelids or eyelashes. Also note complaints that the eyes feel dry and irritated. Another complaint that might prompt the patient to seek medical attention is redness or swelling of the lids, eyes, or periorbital area (around the eyes).

Past Medical History

People tend to assume that changes in vision are caused by problems in the eye or related structures. Although this is often true, visual disturbances also can be associated with many other conditions. Therefore it is important to obtain a good history of past medical problems from the patient who reports with vision problems. Conditions to be alert for include the following:

Diabetes. Elevated blood glucose can cause temporary blurring of vision. Permanent changes in the retina associated with diabetes can cause blindness.

Neurologic disorders. Brain tumors, head injuries, and strokes are examples of conditions that may impair vision. Effects may be blurred vision, diplopia, inability to move eyes, or loss of part of the visual fields.

Thyroid disease. Hyperthyroidism may cause exophthalmos (bulging eyes).

Hypertension. Hypertension can cause changes in the blood vessels of the eye, eventually leading to vision loss.

Note any eye injury or previously diagnosed eye disease, including date of last examination and treatment.

A current medication history also is important in assessing vision problems. Some drugs can cause temporary or permanent changes in visual acuity and color vision. Others may contribute to the development of cataracts or glaucoma.

PHARMACOLOGY CAPSULE Drugs that are especially likely to be related to vision disturbances are digitalis, corticosteroids, indomethacin, and sulfisoxazole. Patients taking thioridazine, chlorpromazine, or ethambutol also should be monitored for ocular toxicity.

Family History

The family history includes any known eye diseases as well as a history of arteriosclerosis, diabetes, and thyroid disease.

Functional Assessment

The functional assessment documents the patient's occupation, roles, and usual activities. Be alert for activities that might pose a risk to the eyes.

PHYSICAL EXAMINATION

The physician performs a complete examination, including inspection of the inner eye. The nurse, however, can inspect the external eye, assess response of the pupil to light, and evaluate gross visual acuity. If abnormalities are suspected, inform the physician or advise the patient to seek medical evaluation.

Put on your THINKING CAP!!

What are some ways you could assess gross visual acuity when diagnostic charts are not available or not practical?

In the eye examination, first inspect the eyelids for redness, drainage, and position. The lids should cover the eyeball completely when closed. When the eyes are open, the lower lid should be at the level of the iris. The upper lid should barely cover the upper margin of the iris. The lids should fit closely to the eyeball, and the eyelashes should not turn toward the eye. Describe any crusting or drainage on the lids or the lashes.

Inspect the eyeball for color and moisture. The sclera should be clear white. Excessive redness may be due to irritation or inflammation. A yellow color, called icterus, is associated with liver dysfunction.

Assess the pupils for size, equality, and reaction to light. Pupils that are unequal, dilated, or do not respond to light suggest neurologic problems. Some medications also can affect pupil characteristics. Accommodation is tested by having the patient focus on your finger held at a distance and then having the patient watch the finger as it is slowly moved toward the patient's nose. The pupils should constrict, and the

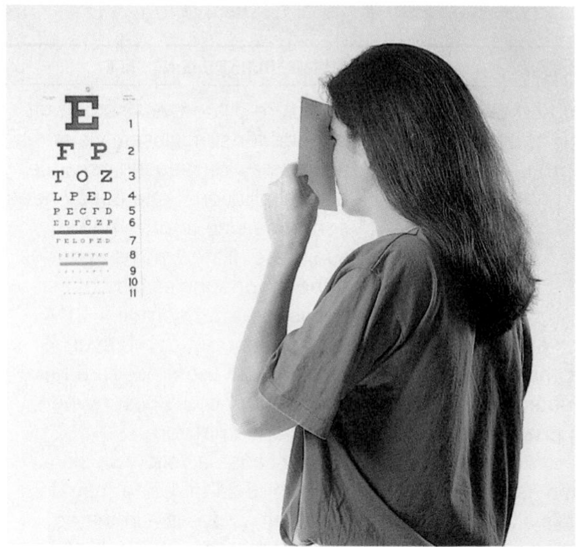

FIGURE **49-5** The Snellen chart is used to measure visual acuity.

table 49-1 ***Signs of Possible Eye Problems***

Particular trouble adjusting to a dark room
Squinting or blinking due to unusual sensitivity to light or glare
Change in color of iris
Red-rimmed and crusted or swollen eyelids
Inflamed or red eyes
Recurrent pain in or around eyes
Sudden loss of vision in one eye
Sudden hazy or blurred vision
Flashes of light or showers of black spots
Halos or rainbows around light
Curtain-like loss of vision
Loss of peripheral or side vision

Data from The Texas Society to Prevent Blindness. *Signs of possible eye trouble in adults.*

eyes converge, meaning the pupils become smaller and both eyes move to fix on the same point.

Visual acuity is commonly tested using the Snellen chart (Fig. 49-5). The Snellen chart has rows of progressively smaller letters. From a distance of 20 feet, have the patient read down the chart until more than two mistakes are made on a single line. Test each eye separately and then together. The lines are numbered 20 over 200, 100, 70, 50, 40, 30, 25, 20, and 15. The findings are reported as the last line the person could read with no more than two errors. That is, if the person read the 20/30 line with one error but made three errors on the 20/25 line, the vision would be recorded as 20/30 in the eye tested. This means that the person could read at 20 feet what a person with normal vision could read at 30 feet. The Snellen chart may be used for vision screening in clinic and office settings. In the hospital, it may be more practical simply to ask the patient to read available print. This provides some practical measure of visual acuity.

table 49-2 **ASSESSMENT *of the Patient with an Eye Disorder***

HEALTH HISTORY

Present Illness: Changes in vision, symptoms of eye disorders: pain, photophobia, drainage, dryness, irritation, redness, swelling

Past Medical History: Diabetes, neurologic disorders, thyroid disease, hypertension, previously diagnosed eye disease or injury, date of last eye examination, current medications (specifically, digitalis, corticosteroids, indomethacin, sulfonamides)

Family History: Known eye diseases, arteriosclerosis, diabetes, thyroid disease, arthritis

Functional Assessment: Occupation, roles, usual activities, changes required by eye problems

PHYSICAL EXAMINATION

Eyelids: Redness, drainage, position, closure, crusting, inversion, or eversion

Eyeball: Color, moisture

Sclera: Color, redness, jaundice

Pupils: Size, equality, reaction to light, accommodation

Visual Acuity: Measured with Snellen chart, gross acuity

Visual Fields

Extraocular Movements

Corneal Reflex

Inner Eye: Ophthalmoscopic examination of anterior chamber, lens, vitreous, and fundus (inner surface of retina)

Some nurses learn to assess visual fields, extraocular movements, and the corneal reflex. There are also several tests used to detect strabismus.

When assessing the eyes, be alert for the signs of trouble listed in Table 49-1. If any of these are present, refer the patient to the physician for evaluation. The nursing assessment of the patient with an eye disorder is summarized in Table 49-2.

DIAGNOSTIC TESTS AND PROCEDURES

Several professionals are trained to assess and treat conditions of the eye. An ophthalmologist is a physician with specialized training in diagnosing and treating eye conditions. The ophthalmologist prescribes corrective lenses for refractive errors and treats other eye conditions with medications and surgery. An optometrist is trained to diagnose errors of refraction and to prescribe corrective lenses. An optician fills prescriptions written by an ophthalmologist or optometrist and fits the prescribed lenses.

Nursing care related to diagnostic tests and procedures for disorders of the eye is described in Table 49-3.

OPHTHALMOSCOPIC EXAMINATION

The ophthalmoscopic examination involves using an ophthalmoscope (Fig. 49-6) to examine the lens, vitreous humor, retina, and optic disk. A solution such as phenylephrine ophthalmic

table 49-3 **DIAGNOSTIC TESTS AND PROCEDURES | *the Eye***

TEST/PURPOSE	PATIENT PREPARATION	POSTPROCEDURE NURSING CARE
Ophthalmologic exam Examines the inner eye through the pupil to diagnose abnormalities of retina, optic disk, and blood vessels.	Administer cycloplegic medication if ordered to dilate pupil and prevent accommodation. Room is darkened during examination.	If pupils are dilated, advise patient of need for sunglasses. Visual acuity may be reduced because of pupil dilation. Patient may need someone else to drive home.
Refraction Identifies refractive errors and corrective lens needed.	No special preparation.	If pupils are dilated, advise patient of need for sunglasses until pupils return to normal.
Tonometry One of several instruments used to measure intraocular pressure.	For procedures in which an instrument touches cornea, anesthetic drops are ordered. Inform patient of need to remain still during procedure.	Advise patient not to rub eyes for 15 min after the procedure because injury could occur when eye is anesthetized.
Fluorescein angiography Pictures of blood vessels in the eye are taken after a dye is injected into a vein in the hand or arm. Permits diagnosis of abnormalities of vessels and retina.	Signed consent required. Administer cycloplegic medication as ordered to dilate the pupil. Assess allergies to iodine, seafood. Notify physician if patient is allergic. Diphenhydramine (Benadryl) may be ordered to reduce risk of allergic reaction to dye; have emergency supplies available in case of severe allergic reaction. Tell patient a dye will be given intravenously, then photographs taken through the pupil. A blue light that will flash when photos are taken may cause temporary vision disturbance. Flashing light can trigger seizure activity in patients with epilepsy.	Dye may cause a yellowish skin color for 6-24 hr. Urine may be greenish as dye is eliminated. Visual acuity may be reduced because of pupil dilation. Advise patient to wear sunglasses. May need someone to drive patient home.
Visual fields Identifies the area a person can see while looking straight ahead. Assessed by comparing the fields the patient can see with those of an examiner with normal visual fields. Patient and examiner sit facing each other. They cover opposite eyes. Examiner moves his or her hand out of line of vision and then brings it into expected line of vision in a specific pattern. Patients states when examiner's fingers are seen.	No preparation needed.	No postprocedure care needed.

preparation may be instilled in the eye first to dilate the pupil. This permits a better view of the inner eye. A darkened room also causes the pupil to dilate.

The examiner studies the cornea, lens, and vitreous for opacities. The blood vessels at the back of the eye (called the fundus) are inspected for evidence of disease. Degenerative changes of the retina may be observed.

REFRACTION

As light enters the eye, it passes through the aqueous humor, lens, and vitreous humor. The light rays bend so that they focus on the retina. This bending is called refraction. Refractive errors occur when the light does not bend properly. This causes alterations in vision, which are discussed in more detail later. Refraction is assessed by having the patient read a chart through a series of lenses. The patient identifies which lens permits the clearest image. This enables the examiner to detect refractive errors. The procedure requires no special preparation or aftercare.

VISUAL FIELDS

Visual fields include the area a person can see while looking straight ahead without moving the head. Some conditions, such as glaucoma, retinal detachment, and certain neurologic

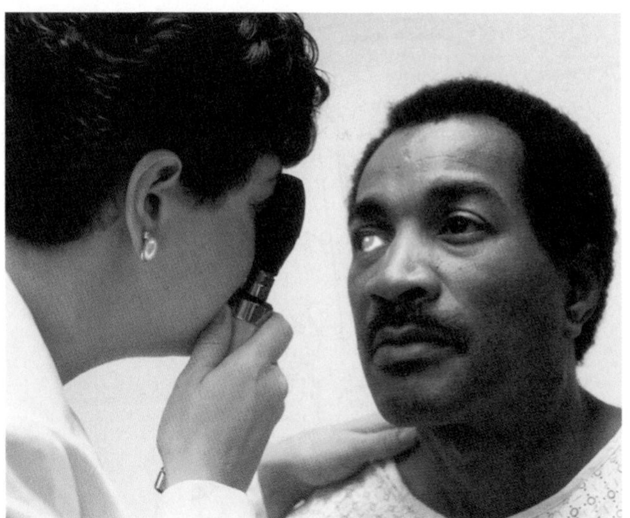

FIGURE **49-6** An ophthalmoscope is used to examine the inner structure of the eye.

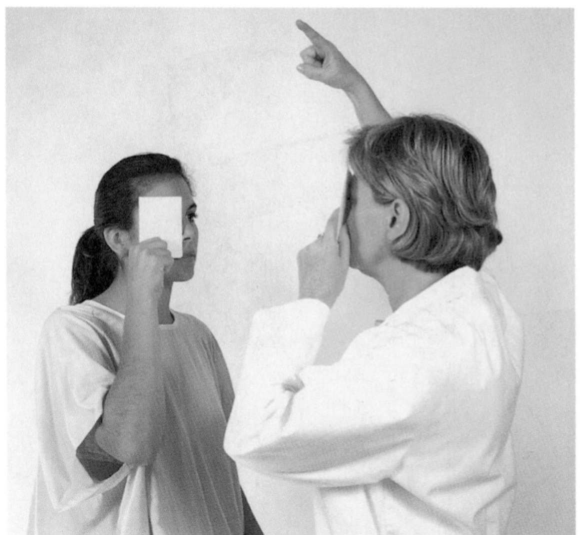

FIGURE **49-7** Assessment of visual fields.

abnormalities, cause loss of parts of the visual fields. Visual fields are assessed by comparing the patient's field of vision with that of a normal examiner (Fig. 49-7). The patient and examiner sit facing each other. The examiner moves his or her hand out of line of vision and then brings it into expected line of vision in a specific pattern. The patient states when the examiner's fingers are seen. No special preparation, equipment, or postprocedure care is needed.

TONOMETRY

Tonometry is the measurement of pressure in the anterior chamber of the eye. Normal intraocular pressure is 12 to 21 mm Hg. Routine measurement of intraocular pressure is important to detect high pressures that damage the retina if untreated.

Several procedures are used to measure intraocular pressure. The Schiotz tonometer, shown in Figure 49-8, may be used for this purpose. Another, more accurate procedure is called *applanation*. It is done with a slit-lamp microscope. A biomicroscope measures pressure even more accurately. Procedures in which the instrument touches the eye require that the cornea be anesthetized with eye drops such as proparacaine 0.5% (Ophthaine).

The pneumotonometer is a hand-held instrument that directs a puff of air to the surface of the eye. It measures intraocular pressure by measuring resistance to the air.

OPHTHALMODYNAMOMETRY

In ophthalmodynamometry, a spring plunger is used to apply pressure to the sclera while the retinal vessels are observed with an ophthalmoscope. The instrument measures the approximate pressure in the blood vessels of the eye. Both eyes are assessed. Differences in pressure from one eye to the next reflect insufficiency of the carotid artery on the side with lower pressure.

MEASURES OF ELECTRICAL POTENTIAL

Because the retina is composed of nerve tissue, it has an electrical potential that can be measured. This is useful in detecting retinal disorders, including retinitis pigmentosa, massive ischemia, widespread infection, and some chemical toxicities. Two procedures used to measure electrical potential are electroretinography and visual evoked response.

Electroretinography

In electroretinography, a contact lens is placed on the eye and exposed to a diffuse flash of light. The response of the retina is recorded. The patient must fix his or her gaze on a target and remain very still.

Visual Evoked Response

For visual evoked response, electrodes are placed on the patient's scalp, and each eye is stimulated. The electrical response is measured.

FLUORESCEIN ANGIOGRAPHY

To detect abnormal blood vessels or blood flow, fluorescein is injected intravenously, and the retina is observed and photographed as the dye circulates (Fig. 49-9).

TOPICAL DYES

Topical dyes can be applied to the eye to detect abrasions of the cornea. Fluorescein is applied and is followed by a saline rinse. The cornea is then examined. Dye permits scratches to be seen more readily.

IMAGING PROCEDURES

To obtain images of the eye for diagnostic purposes, the physician may order computed tomography scanning, ultrasonography, or magnetic resonance imaging.

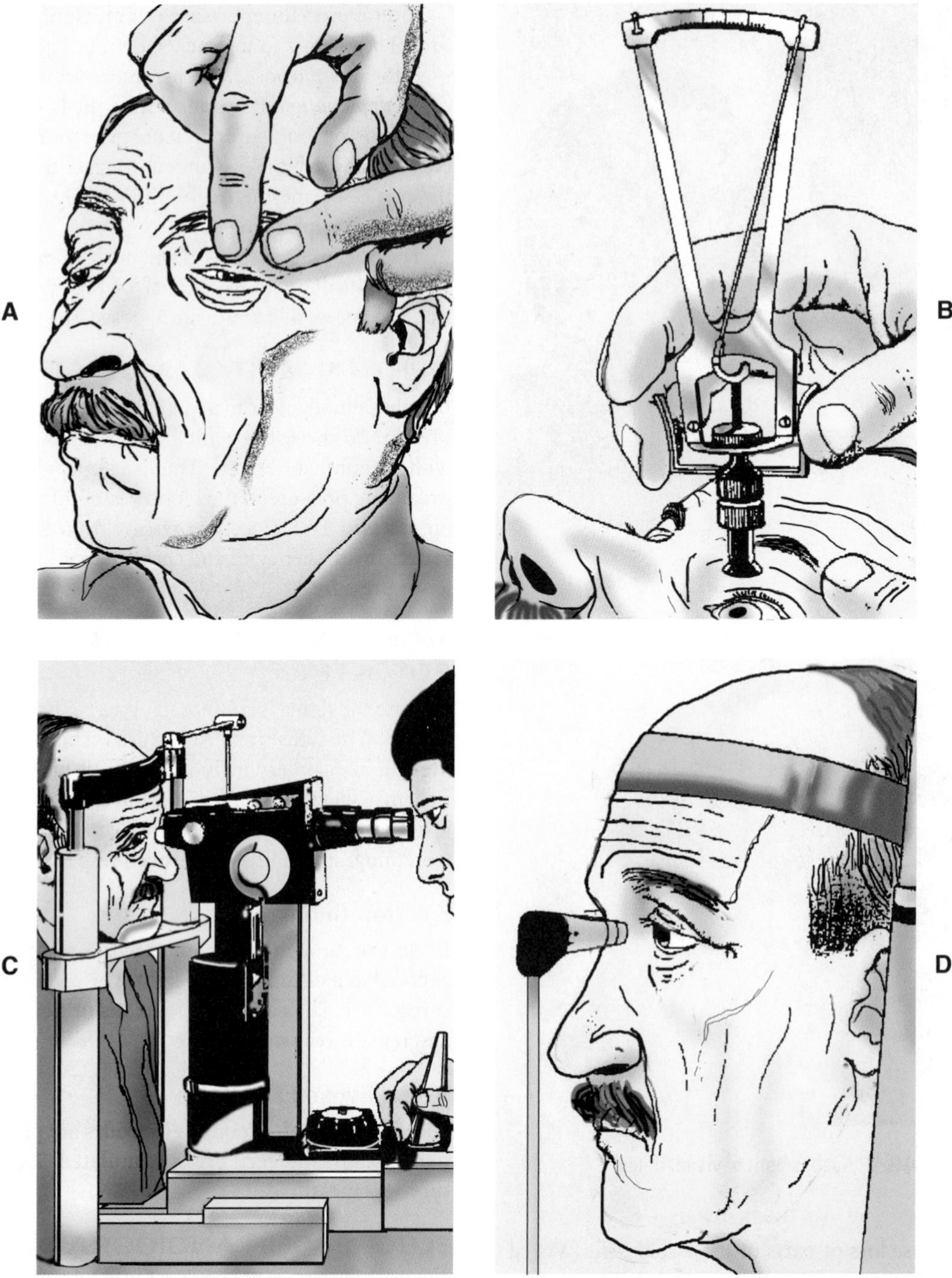

FIGURE **49-8** Techniques for measuring intraocular pressure. *A,* Palpation (only useful when pressure difference between eyes is large). *B,* Schiotz tonometry. *C,* Air puff tonometry. *D,* Goldman's applanation tonometer.

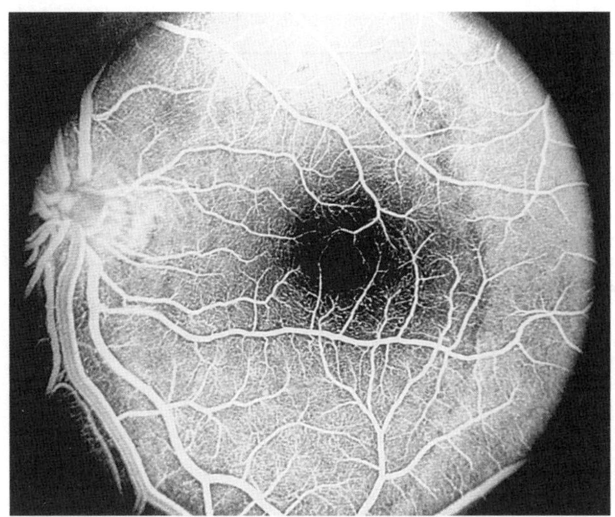

FIGURE 49-9 Fluorescein angiography permits visualization of the blood vessels of the eye to examine the inner structure of the eye.

COMMON THERAPEUTIC MEASURES

EYE IRRIGATION

Irrigations are done to remove irritating chemicals from the eye. Sterile normal saline is the best solution to use. Plain water also is acceptable, especially in emergencies. In the hospital or clinic setting, the physician sometimes orders irrigations with ophthalmic medications. Key points in irrigating the eye include the following:

1. Wearing gloves, cleanse the eyelids and eyelashes.
2. Position the patient with the affected eye down so that contaminated fluid does not run into the unaffected eye.
3. Place a basin and waterproof pad to collect the fluid.
4. Gently direct the fluid into the lower conjunctival sac from the inner canthus (corner of the eye) to the outer canthus.
5. Do not touch the eye with the tip of the irrigating syringe.
6. Have the patient blink occasionally to move particles toward the lower conjunctival sac.
7. If extended irrigation is needed, there are special irrigation systems that may be used.

TOPICAL MEDICATIONS

A number of medications can be applied directly to the eye. These include miotics, mydriatics, anesthetics, cycloplegics, antibiotics, and anti-inflammatory drugs. Mydriatics dilate the pupils; miotics constrict the pupils; and cycloplegics prevent accommodation. Some drug manufacturers color code the caps and labels of topical ophthalmic drugs to help you select the correct drug. The caps and labels of mydriatics are red; miotics are green; nonsteroidal anti-inflammatory drugs are gray; anti-infectives are brown or tan; and beta blockers are yellow or blue. Nevertheless, you must always read the drug label carefully and compare it to the physician's order. Some systemic drugs also may be ordered, such as diuretics to reduce pressure in the eye. Examples of ophthalmic drugs are included in Table 49-4.

The following are key points to remember when administering topical eye medications:

1. Be *very* careful that only medications labeled for *ophthalmic* use are put in the eye!
2. Drops should be room temperature when administered. Rolling the bottle between the palms is a good way to warm the medication.
3. Tell the patient to tilt his or her head back and look at the ceiling. The head can be turned slightly so that excess medication runs out the outer canthus of the eyes and does not contaminate the opposite eye.
4. Place your finger below the lower lid and gently pull the eyelid down to expose the conjunctival sac and create a pouch.
5. Brace the hand holding the medication and then drop the medication into the conjunctival sac without touching the eyelid with the container.
6. Tell the patient to close his or her eyes and move them as if looking around. This distributes the medication over the eye.
7. You or the patient should apply gentle pressure to the lacrimal sac at the inner canthus of the eye for approximately 1 minute. This reduces the amount of the medication entering body fluids.
8. If more than one medication is being given, wait 5 minutes between each medication.

EYE SURGERY

A number of eye conditions are treated or corrected with surgery. Eye surgery may involve surgical incisions, the use of lasers, and the application of cold probes (cryotherapy). Individualized care plans must be developed based on the specific type of procedure done. Some general considerations, however, apply to most patients having eye surgery.

PREOPERATIVE NURSING CARE

Assessment

Preoperative assessment and care are discussed in detail in Chapter 16. The preoperative assessment specifically focuses on the patient's emotional state, ability to perform self-care, and knowledge of surgical routines and outcomes. Most patients awaiting eye surgery are somewhat anxious. They may be fearful that the procedure will not be successful or that some complication will lead to further loss of vision. Determine whether there is now or will be any activity limitations. If the patient has poor vision, document the type of help needed. Also note the physician's orders for intravenous fluids or preoperative medications, or both. The patient's food and fluid intake is usually restricted from the evening before surgery to reduce the risk of nausea, vomiting, and aspiration after surgery. Because many procedures on the eye are done in day surgery facilities, be sure the patient understands the preoperative routine.

table 49-4 DRUG THERAPY | *Disorders of the Eye*

GENERAL NURSING CONSIDERATIONS

1. Advise patient to follow directions exactly.
2. If condition worsens or does not improve, notify the physician.
3. If multiple ophthalmic drugs are ordered, wait 5 minutes between them.
4. After administering ophthalmic solutions, apply gentle pressure to lacrimal sac for approximately 1 minute to decrease absorption and systemic effects.
5. Teach patient or family member correct technique for drug administration.
6. Emphasize that patients never share eye medication.

DRUG	USE/ACTION	SIDE EFFECTS	NURSING INTERVENTIONS
MIOTICS			
	Constrict the pupil; primarily used to treat glaucoma.	See Table 49-5.	See Table 49-5.
SYMPATHOMIMETICS			
Epinephrine bitartrate (Epitrate) Dipivefrin HCl (Propine) Phenylephrine (Neo-Synephrine)	Dilate pupil. Used in open-angle (chronic) glaucoma. Decrease corneal congestion. Control hemorrhage.	Cardiac stimulation, headache, brow pain, allergy, worsening of acute (narrow-angle) glaucoma.	Sunglasses needed for 6 hr. Tell patient to report eye pain immediately—may be caused by increased intraocular pressure.
ANTIMUSCARINICS			
Atrophine (Isopto Atropine) Homatropine (Isopto Homatropine) Scopolamine (Isopto Hyoscine) Cyclopentolate (Cyclogyl) Tropicamide (Mydriacyl)	Dilate pupil. Used before eye examinations and for uveitis. Decrease lacrimal gland secretion. Cyclopentolate and tropicamide preferred for eye examination because of shorter duration of action.	Photophobia, inability to accommodate, corneal dryness and irritation.	Apply at ordered time before eye examination. If eye pain occurs, may indicate undetected glaucoma. Safety measures while pupils dilated, because vision is blurred. Artificial tears may be needed.

Nursing Diagnoses, Goals, and Outcome Criteria: Eye Surgery, Preoperative

NURSING DIAGNOSES	GOALS AND OUTCOME CRITERIA
Anxiety related to uncertain outcome, lack of knowledge about surgery and surgical routines	Reduced anxiety: patient states anxiety is reduced, relaxed manner
Self-Care Deficit related to visual impairment	Achievement of activities of daily living: daily activities successfully completed

Interventions

Anxiety

Explore the patient's feelings about the surgery and provide information. Refer specific questions about the surgical procedure, risks, complications, or outcomes to the physician. Explain general surgical and postoperative routines.

Self-Care Deficit

On admission, orient the visually impaired patient to the room. Keep objects in one place, and advise the patient of any new equipment or articles in the environment. Follow agency policy for obtaining consent for surgery. Offer to read any written material to the patient.

POSTOPERATIVE NURSING CARE

Assessment

After surgery, assess the patient's vital signs and level of consciousness during recovery from anesthesia. Inspect the dressing, or the operative eye, for bleeding or drainage. Also assess patient comfort, including pain and nausea. If vision is impaired, assess the environment for safety hazards. Before dis-

table 49-4 **DRUG THERAPY | *Disorders of the Eye—cont'd***

DRUG	USE/ACTION	SIDE EFFECTS	NURSING INTERVENTIONS
ANTIBACTERIALS			
Gentamicin sulfate (Garamycin Ophthalmic) Erythromycin (Ilotycin) Polymixin B sulfate (neomycin sulfate, bacitracin) Sulfonamides (Sulamyd Ophthalmic)	Treatment or prevention of eye infections.	Allergic reaction, conjunctivitis.	Screen for previous allergic reactions. Withhold drug and notify physician if allergic. Inspect eyes and lids for increasing redness.
ANTIFUNGALS			
Natamycin (Natacyn)	Effective against some fungal infections of eye.	Rarely: allergic reaction, conjunctival edema.	Advise patient to continue treatment as prescribed (usually 14-21 days). Notify physician if symptoms continue or if edema develops.
ANTIVIRALS			
Idoxuridine (Herplex) Vidarabine (Vira-A)	Treatment of herpes simplex, keratitis.	Irritation, redness, edema, pain, itching, photophobia. Rarely: allergic reactions.	Advise sunglasses for sensitivity. Refrigerate.
TOPICAL ANESTHETICS			
Proparacaine HCl (Ophthaine, Ophthetic) Tetracaine HCl (Pontocaine)	Block sensation in external eye for tonometry, removal of sutures or foreign bodies, some surgical procedures.	Stinging, irritation. Allergic reactions rare.	Do not use discolored solution. Caution patient not to touch or rub eye or insert contact lens until sensation returns.
ANTI-INFLAMMATORY AGENTS			
Prednisolone acetate Prednisolone sodium phosphate Dexamethasone Fluorometholone	Prevent redness and swelling because of inflammation from causes other than bacterial infection.	Systemic effects possible if sufficient drug is absorbed, including fluid retention, nausea, mood swings, hypokalemia, and many others.	Apply pressure to lacrimal sac for 1-2 min after application to reduce absorption. Monitor blood studies.

charge, determine the patient's understanding of and ability to administer prescribed medications by having the patient demonstrate self-medication.

Nursing Diagnoses, Goals, and Outcome Criteria: Eye Surgery, Postoperative

NURSING DIAGNOSES	GOALS AND OUTCOME CRITERIA
Risk for Injury related to pressure or trauma	Decreased risk of injury: patient avoids potentially harmful activities (rubbing eye, bending forward, etc.)
Disturbed Sensory Perception related to vision changes caused by disease process, trauma to the eye, patching	Adaptation to impaired vision: patient makes adjustments in lifestyle to accommodate vision change
Acute Pain related to tissue trauma	Pain relief: patient states pain reduced or absent, relaxed manner
Anxiety related to temporary vision impairment	Decreased anxiety: patient states is less anxious; calm demeanor
Ineffective Therapeutic Regimen Management related to lack of understanding of self-care measures and usual postoperative course	Patient adheres to plan of care: patient demonstrates appropriate self-care

Interventions

Risk for Injury

The physician may prescribe limitations on activity or position, or both. The head of the bed is usually elevated. The patient may be wearing a bulky dressing or a small eye patch.

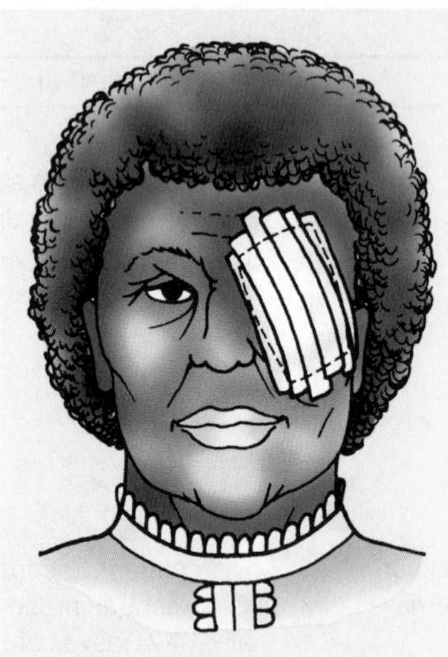

FIGURE **49-10** The shield protects the operative eye from pressure or rubbing.

Either may be covered with a lightweight metal shield (Fig. 49-10). The dressing absorbs any drainage, and the shield protects the eye from rubbing. Instruct the patient not to rub the eye. Check the physician's orders to determine whether the dressing can be changed. Eye drops or ointments may be ordered. They may be different from those used before surgery. When an eye is patched, take safety precautions to prevent injury.

An important aspect of the postoperative care of patients having eye surgery is to prevent increased intraocular pressure. Caution the patient against straining, leaning forward, lifting, and lying on the affected side. Because vomiting and retching raise intraocular pressure, treat nausea promptly.

 ***Put on your THINKING CAP!!***

After eye surgery, patients often go home the same day. Considering the usual restrictions imposed to prevent increased intraocular pressure, what are some obstacles the patient might encounter? What strategies might you suggest to the patient?

Disturbed Sensory Perception

Measures to assist the patient with visual impairment are discussed in detail in the section on Nursing Care of the Visually Impaired Patient.

Acute Pain

Although one might expect eye surgery to be painful, postoperative pain is usually mild to moderate. Give mild analgesics as ordered. If a patient reports severe pain, notify the physician.

Anxiety

To reduce anxiety, explain what is being done and why and encourage the patient to express concerns and ask questions.

Ineffective Therapeutic Regimen Management

Patients who have had eye surgery often are discharged with some medications. Provide careful directions and a written schedule for the medications. To assess the patient's ability to self-administer eye medications, have the patient demonstrate the procedure before discharge. If necessary, instruct a family member in administering the medications.

 ***Put on your THINKING CAP!!***

An 80-year-old patient is being discharged after ocular surgery. He has several topical ophthalmic drugs that must be applied twice daily. One eye is to remain patched until he sees the physician in one week. What information would you want to gather to determine whether he will be able to manage at home?

PROTECTION OF THE EYES AND VISION

Maintaining adequate vision involves the prevention of injuries and the treatment of abnormalities. Nurses must be knowledgeable about the assessment and care of the eyes.

PATIENT TEACHING

Nurses can teach people how to care for their eyes to protect vision. Adults younger than 40 years of age should have their eyes examined every 3 to 5 years. After the age of 40 years, eye examinations should be done every 2 years and should include testing for glaucoma. This permits early detection and treatment of eye disorders.

Tell patients to report sharp, stabbing eye pain or deep, throbbing eye pain. Other symptoms that should be reported to a physician are photophobia (sensitivity to light), blurred or double vision, loss of part of the visual fields, halos around lights, and floaters. Floaters are spots that appear to move across the field of vision. Some patients describe floaters as being like birds swooping past one's face. Other symptoms that require medical evaluation are burning sensations, itching, excessive tearing, and the presence of drainage from the eyes.

When there are symptoms of eye problems, patients should seek medical advice rather than trying home remedies. First aid for eye injuries is explained in Chapter 15.

Sometimes nurses have the opportunity to correct misconceptions that people have about vision. The following are some examples of *misconceptions:*

Watching too much television or sitting too close to the television injures the eyes.

Eating foods that contain large amounts of vitamin A improves vision.

Eyes need to be rinsed regularly.

Prevention of Injuries

Injuries caused by foreign objects are a major cause of vision loss. Teach young children the danger of throwing or poking objects at the faces of playmates. Assess toys for safety. Adult activities that produce sparks or cause fragments to be dispersed also cause injuries. Advise protective eyewear for such potentially dangerous activities.

Basic Eye Care

Gently cleanse the eyelids each time the face is washed. Use a clean cloth without soap. Wash the eye from the inner canthus (near the nose) toward the outer canthus. Dry crusts on the eyelids and eyelashes can usually be wiped off. If necessary, place a warm, damp cloth on the lids for several minutes to soften the crusts.

Routine eye rinses and drops are unnecessary for most people. Exceptions are people with inadequate tear production and those whose eyes do not close completely. Lubricating drops called artificial tears are available for those people. Sometimes, eye patches are applied or the lids are taped shut to prevent drying of the cornea.

IMPACT OF VISUAL IMPAIRMENT

Vision loss usually has significant impact on all areas of a person's life. Mild losses may require only some adaptations. More serious losses affect independence, mobility, employment, and interpersonal relationships. In addition, there is the loss of pleasure in seeing the people and things a person treasures.

The loss of vision triggers a grief response. People grieve for the lost function just as they might grieve after the death of a loved one. Reactions that are likely to follow loss of vision include shock, denial, anger, bargaining, and depression.

Factors that affect a person's response to this loss include personality, usual coping style, impact of vision loss on the person's life, and the circumstances of the loss. If grief is resolved in a healthy manner, adaptation and acceptance eventually occur. People who have progressive loss of vision may experience anticipatory grief. Nursing care to help the person who is grieving is discussed in Chapter 23.

NURSING CARE *of the Visually Impaired Patient*

When people hear the word *blind,* they think of someone who is unable to see. There are, however, degrees of visual impairment. Although some visually impaired people are unable to see at all, many others have partial vision. Therefore medical literature is more likely to use terms such as *visual impairment* or *visually handicapped* rather than *blind.* Also, there may be a stigma attached to the word *blind.* Some people automatically associate blindness with helplessness.

Trauma, disease, and some congenital defects account for visual handicaps throughout the life span. Some types of visual disturbances are more common in older people.

To work with the visually impaired, you need to be aware of their thoughts and feelings about visual handicaps. You should assume that people with visual impairments can be independent and productive. Pity has no place in this situation because it encourages hopelessness and helplessness. The person needs help with some tasks but should still be treated as an adult.

The extent of vision loss determines the types of assistance that might be needed. Many people have visual problems that can be corrected with eyeglasses, drug therapy, or surgical treatment. Many products are available to enable visually impaired people to function more independently. When planning care, consider whether the patient's condition is temporary, permanent, correctable, treatable, or progressive.

Assessment

The nursing assessment of the patient with an eye disorder is summarized in Table 49-2.

Nursing Diagnoses, Goals, and Outcome Criteria: Impaired Vision

Common nursing diagnoses and goals for patients with impaired vision may include the following:

Nursing Diagnoses	Goals and Outcome Criteria
Disturbed Sensory Perception related to altered reception, transmission, interpretation of visual stimuli	Adaptation to vision impairment: patient has no falls or other traumatic injuries; uses assistive devices and techniques to maintain as much independence as possible
Ineffective Coping related to decreased independence, threat to body image, denial	Effective coping: patient makes efforts to adapt, participates in self-care to maximum degree possible
Self-Care Deficit (feeding, hygiene, grooming) related to visual impairment	Appropriate self-care: patient performs activities of daily living with minimal assistance
Ineffective Therapeutic Regimen Management related to lack of understanding of treatment of vision impairment	Effective regimen management: Prescribed plan of care is managed appropriately: patient carries out plan of care; participates in rehabilitation programs if indicated

Interventions

Disturbed Sensory Perception

When a visually impaired person is admitted to the hospital, provide an orientation to the environment. The fact that the patient has visual impairment should be reflected on the nursing care plan. In addition, a sign may be posted to alert other caregivers and employees. Safety is a primary consideration for these patients. Measures to support the patient with impaired vision and to prevent injury include the following:

1. When you enter the room, announce your presence and introduce yourself to avoid startling or embarrassing the patient.
2. Speak before touching the patient to avoid startling him or her.
3. Speak in a normal tone of voice. People tend to act as if those who cannot see cannot hear, so there is a tendency to raise one's voice when talking to the visually impaired.

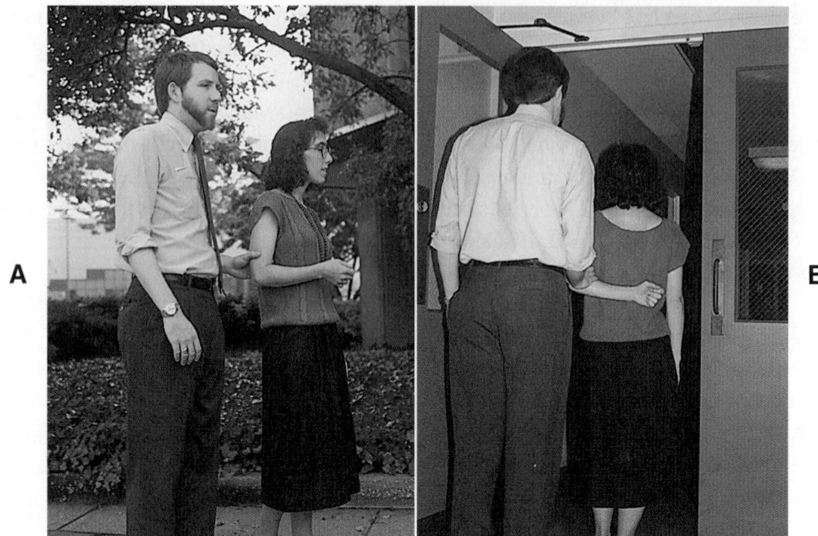

FIGURE **49-11** *A,* To escort a visually impaired person, allow the person to grasp your upper arm. *B,* To enter a narrow passage or doorway, bring your arm behind your back to alert the person.

4. Address the patient in the appropriate manner for his or her age and intellectual ability. Visual impairment is not associated with mental impairment.
5. Advise the patient what to expect during procedures.
6. Tell the patient when you leave the room.
7. Leave the bed in low position.
8. Place the call button in reach, and be sure the patient knows how to use it.
9. Keep doors either open or closed so that the ambulatory patient does not run into a partially closed door.
10. Do not rearrange the room after orienting the patient.
11. Eliminate meaningless noise from the environment as much as possible.
12. To lead a blind person, have him or her take your arm (Fig. 49-11).

The environment significantly influences the visually impaired patient's ability to function. The environment should be safe and promote maximal independence. As already mentioned, orientation to the hospital room is especially important. Make sure the patient can use the call system, locate personal items, and use the bathroom. Tell the patient if any new equipment or furniture is brought into the room. Keep pathways in the room free of clutter.

For patients who are partially sighted, lighting is very important. Glare must be reduced because it actually interferes with vision. Windows should have adjustable shades, blinds, or sheers. Floors should not be highly polished (Fig. 49-12). Color can provide important cues to enable the partially sighted person to function. This is especially true of the older person whose color perception often changes. Older people perceive warm colors (red, orange, yellow) more accurately than cool colors (blue, green). Furniture color should be distinctly different from the color of floors and walls. Light switches, handrails, and steps marked with contrasting colors are easier to locate. Dishes and cups with colored rims facilitate self-feeding and reduce spills.

Ineffective Coping

People who have lived with vision impairment usually have developed routines and strategies to cope with the situation. Ask about such routines and maintain them as much as possible. If the patient uses assistive devices such as eyeglasses or magnifying glasses, make sure they are available and encourage their use. The older person who becomes confused during hospitalization may show dramatic improvement when eyeglasses are provided.

Encourage diversional activities when appropriate. The patient with some vision may be able to enjoy reading with magnifiers or large-print reading material. Talking books are available without charge through the American Foundation for the Blind. Many bookstores stock books on tape. Braille reading material and typewriters can be used by those who have been trained in this method. Braille uses arrangements of raised dots to represent letters. The reader reads the material by moving the fingertips over the characters. Not everyone is able to master reading Braille because of the sensitive touch needed. Special telescopic lens and magnifiers can enable patients to read, write, and use a computer. Canes and guide dogs permit independent ambulation.

Self-Care Deficit

Ask the patient what assistance is required instead of assuming that help is needed. Many patients are quite independent despite impaired vision. Do not encourage dependence during hospitalization. To orient the patient to the location of foods, fluids, or other objects, think of their arrangement as a clock face (e.g., "your meat is at 3 o'clock"). A consistent en-

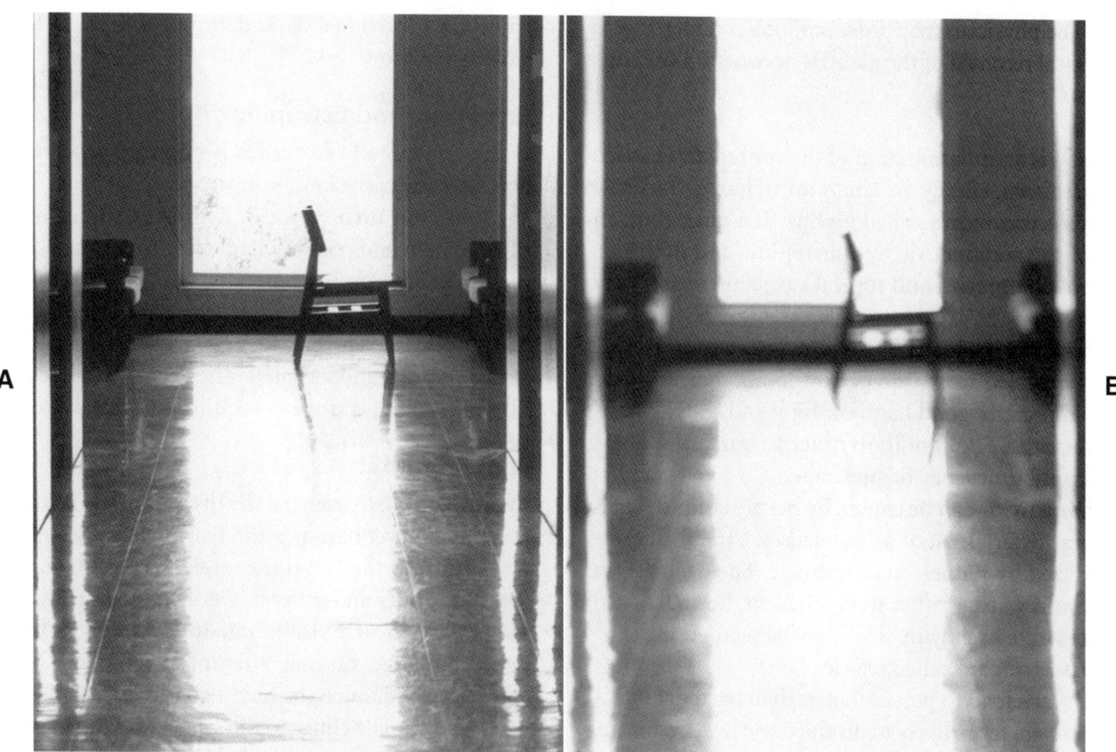

FIGURE **49-12** Glare perceived by a person with normal vision *(A)* and an older person whose eyes have undergone age-related changes *(B)*.

vironment enables the patient to be more independent with less risk of injury. Do not move furniture, personal effects, and equipment without patient consent.

Some visually impaired people have guide dogs that enable them to move about more independently. These dogs are trained to guide their owners both inside and outside the home. They usually can go anywhere their owners go. Laws that restrict pets in public places usually do not apply to guide dogs. When the dogs are wearing their harnesses, they are working and should not be distracted by friendly strangers.

Ineffective Therapeutic Regimen Management

Patients with severe impairment should be referred to specialists in rehabilitation. They need to learn self-care activities, safe mobility, and strategies to carry out usual roles such as child care and occupational skills. Teach patients with diseases of the eye any prescribed measures to cure or slow the progression of the disease.

DISORDERS AFFECTING THE EYE OR VISION

EXTERNAL EYE DISORDERS

Inflammation and Infection

The eye is a potential site for infectious and inflammatory conditions. Because of the sensitivity of the eye, such disorders can cause considerable discomfort. Some may even threaten vision if not treated.

Blepharitis

Blepharitis is an inflammation of the hair follicles along the eyelid margin. It can be caused by bacteria, most often by staphylococci. Seborrheic blepharitis is often found with seborrhea of the scalp and eyebrows.

Symptoms include itching, burning, and photophobia. Scales or crusts may be seen on the lid margins. The patient may complain that the eyelids are glued shut on awakening.

Untreated blepharitis could lead to inflammation of the cornea or hordeolum (stye). The physician may prescribe an antibiotic ointment for the condition. Be certain that any medication applied to the eye is an *ophthalmic* preparation. The eyelids also can be gently cleansed with baby shampoo solution.

Hordeolum

Hordeolum is commonly called a *stye.* It is a common acute staphylococcal infection of the eyelid margin that originates in a lash follicle. The affected area of the lid is red, swollen, and tender. The primary treatment is the application of warm, moist compresses several times a day. If a person has repeated infections, these may be related to staphylococcal infections at some other location on the body. The physician attempts to locate any other infections and may order the hordeolum treated with ophthalmic antibiotics.

Chalazion

Chalazion is an inflammation of the glands in the eyelids. Swelling prevents fluid from leaving the glands, causing them to become enlarged and tender. Warm compresses may bring some relief. The physician may order antibiotics if infection is present. Surgical removal of the gland is necessary if the condition persists.

Conjunctivitis

Conjunctivitis is an inflammation of the conjunctiva caused by microorganisms, allergy, or chemical irritants. Bacterial conjunctivitis is commonly called *pinkeye*. It is characterized by redness of the conjunctiva, mild irritation, and drainage. Warm or cool compresses and topical vasoconstrictors may be ordered.

If inflammation is caused by an infectious agent, the infection can be passed from one person to another. Infected people should practice good hand washing and should avoid sharing washcloths. The condition usually clears up spontaneously, but antibiotics may be prescribed.

Viral conjunctivitis can be caused by herpes simplex virus type 1, herpes zoster virus, or adenoviruses. Viral infections are characterized by redness and drainage. The drainage in viral infections is watery rather than purulent. Round, raised areas that are white or gray in color may be seen on the conjunctiva. These areas are called *follicles*.

Viral infections tend to persist longer than bacterial infections. They also are more likely to produce severe eye damage. The medical management varies with the causative organism. Infections caused by herpes simplex virus type 1 are treated with idoxuridine (Herpex) ointment or other topical medications. Corticosteroids are contraindicated with the herpes virus. If given in the presence of herpes simplex virus type 1, corticosteroids may contribute to deep corneal ulcers and other complications.

Other organisms that can cause conjunctivitis include chlamydia and fungi. These eye infections are more common in developing countries but are occasionally seen in the United States. They are treated with topical or systemic antimicrobial medications.

Keratitis

Keratitis is inflammation or infection, or both, of the cornea. The structure of the cornea makes it especially vulnerable to injury. The portion of the cornea in front of the pupil has no blood vessels because it must remain transparent. This means that it has no direct blood supply, making it vulnerable to infections.

Sources of infection include bacteria, viruses, and fungi. Also, chemical or mechanical injuries cause inflammation that may be followed by infection. If scar tissue forms, that portion of the cornea becomes cloudy and vision is impaired. Also, the infection can extend to the inner structures of the eye. Serious lesions can rupture if the eye is rubbed. Prompt treatment of keratitis therefore is very important to preserve vision.

Keratitis does not produce noticeable drainage, but it causes considerable pain. Medical treatment includes topical antibiotics and topical corticosteroids. Systemic antibiotics also may be ordered after culture and sensitivity results are obtained. Sometimes the physician injects antibiotics directly into the conjunctiva. Topical anesthetics are not used because the patient might accidentally cause additional injury to the anesthetized cornea. Eye pads are not used with keratitis because they provide a dark, damp environment for microorganisms to grow.

Entropion and Ectropion

Proper closure of the eyelids is important to protect the eye and keep the cornea moist. Entropion is a condition in which the lower lid turns inward. Eyelashes rub against the eye, causing pain and possibly scratching the cornea. Surgical correction usually is recommended.

Ectropion is a condition in which the lower lid droops and turns outward. The eye does not close completely, causing it to become dry and irritated. The dry cornea is easily injured. Like entropion, ectropion requires surgical correction.

Foreign Body

Everyone has experienced the discomfort of having a foreign body in the eye. Blinking and tearing usually will wash small irritants from the eye. If the foreign body remains in the eye, evert the upper and lower lids as illustrated in Figure 49-13. If the object is clearly visible and does not appear to be embedded in the eye, you may attempt to remove it. Use a sterile cotton swab to touch the object gently. If the object is not embedded, it usually clings to the swab and can be removed. Foreign bodies that are embedded in the eye should be removed only by a physician.

Chemical Spills and Splashes

Chemical spills and splashes are discussed in Chapter 15.

Corneal Opacity

A healthy cornea is clear, allowing light to enter the pupil. When the cornea is injured by infection or trauma, scar tissue

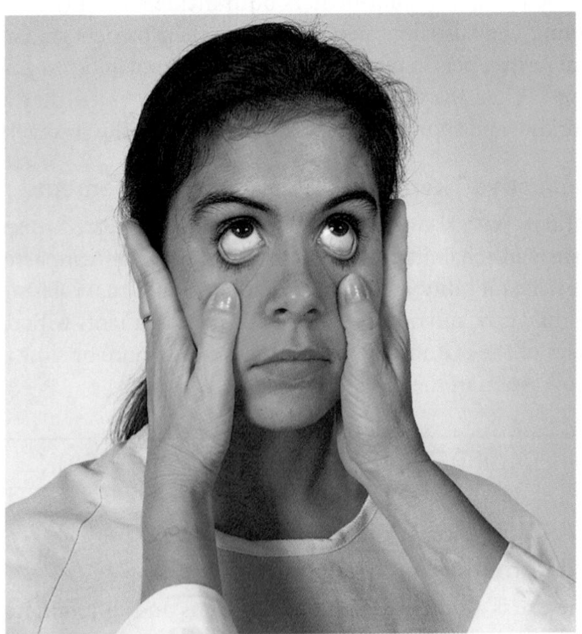

FIGURE **49-13** Eversion of the eyelid for inspection of the sclera and conjunctiva.

may form. The scar tissue is opaque, so light is unable to enter the eye. This causes varying degrees of vision impairment. The only treatment for corneal opacity is removal of the scarred cornea and replacement with a healthy cornea. The surgical procedure is called a *keratoplasty.*

Healthy corneas are obtained from donors shortly after death. This may be authorized by the donor before death or by the family. The entire donor eye is removed (enucleation) and preserved. Eye tissue is easier to preserve than other body tissues. This permits keratoplasty to be done as a scheduled procedure rather than as an emergency on-call procedure. It can be done under local anesthesia. Before surgery, eye drops may be ordered either to dilate or constrict the pupil. Usually, drops are used that constrict the pupil (miotics). Constriction of the pupil pulls the iris over the lens like a curtain and protects the lens during surgery. Sometimes, however, it is necessary to remove the lens as well as the cornea. Lens extraction is necessary if the lens is cloudy owing to injury or age-related changes. In this case, preoperative mydriatic drops are ordered to allow access to the lens.

The types of grafts used in keratoplasty are penetrating and lamellar. A penetrating graft consists of all layers of the cornea. A lamellar graft is only the superficial tissue layers of the cornea. The type of graft used depends on the extent of injury to the recipient's cornea.

During a keratoplasty, the surgeon first removes the patient's damaged cornea. An identically sized graft is then taken from the donor eye and secured to the recipient's eye with very fine sutures, as shown in Figures 49-13 and 49-14. When a penetrating keratoplasty is done, the aqueous humor is lost from the anterior chamber of the eye. The surgeon replaces the fluid with a saline solution.

NURSING CARE *of the Patient Having Keratoplasty*

Preoperative nursing care of the patient having eye surgery is discussed earlier. After surgery, the keratoplasty patient has an eye pad and a metal shield over the operative eye. Sometimes the other eye is temporarily patched as well because the eyes normally track together. This reduces eye movement until the operative eye heals.

Assessment

Assess the dressing for drainage and ask if the patient is having any pain or nausea. After the dressing is removed, inspect the eye for corneal opacity. Also evaluate the patient's visual acuity.

The normal appearance of the eye soon after keratoplasty is seen in Figure 49-15A.

In addition to routine postoperative care after eye surgery, the following specific care may apply after keratoplasty:

Nursing Diagnoses, Goals, and Outcome Criteria: Keratoplasty, Postoperative

Nursing Diagnoses	Goals and Outcome Criteria
Risk for Injury related to activities that increase intraocular pressure	Decreased risk for injury: patient avoids activities that increase intraocular pressure (bending forward, lifting, straining)
Acute Pain related to tissue trauma	Pain relief: Patient states pain relieved, relaxed manner
Disturbed Sensory Perception related to inflammation, rejection of transplanted tissue	Adaptation to temporary vision impairment: patient performs usual activities with minimal assistance. Gradual improvement in visual acuity: patient report, improved visual acuity scores
Ineffective Therapeutic Regimen Management related to lack of understanding of usual postoperative course	Effective management of prescribed plan of care: patient correctly describes and demonstrates self-care measures

Interventions

Risk for Injury

Caution the patient to avoid any activities that increase pressure in the eye, including rubbing the eye, bending forward, lifting, straining at stool, and coughing. Report and promptly treat nausea because vomiting raises intraocular pressure. Administer stool softeners as ordered to prevent constipation.

Pain

Only mild to moderate pain is expected after keratoplasty. The physician usually orders analgesics such as acetaminophen to be given as needed. Notify the physician of severe or

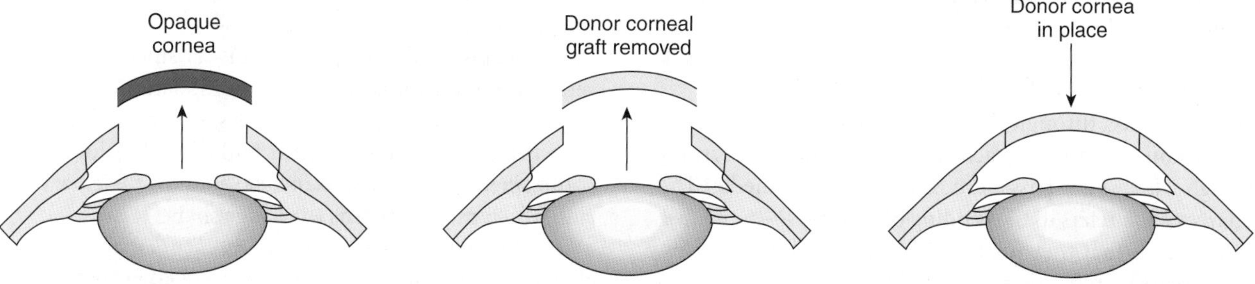

FIGURE 49-14 Keratoplasty. The damaged cornea is removed and then replaced with a corneal graft from a donor eye.

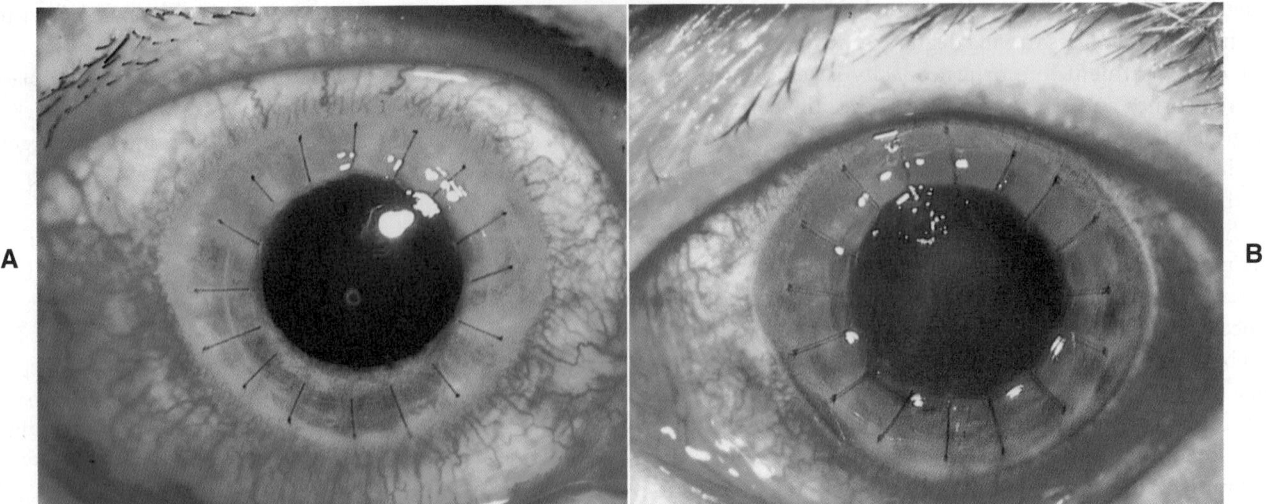

FIGURE **49-15** Keratoplasty. *A,* Appearance of the eye soon after keratoplasty. *B,* Acute corneal rejection.

increasing pain because it suggests increased intraocular pressure or infection.

Impaired Sensory Perception

Rejection of corneal grafts is not common, but it can happen. When rejection occurs, blood vessels appear in the cornea, and the cornea becomes cloudy (see Fig. 49-15B). Corticosteroid drops are ordered to reduce inflammation and the risk of rejection. Patients should know that symptoms of rejection include redness, swelling, decreased vision, and pain. Other topical medications that usually are ordered are antibiotics to prevent infection and mydriatics to dilate the pupil.

Ineffective Therapeutic Regimen Management

Nurses and patients should realize that the grafted eye must heal just like any other body part that has undergone surgery. In the movies, the physician removes the dressing dramatically. The patient blinks a few times, and the world comes into focus. In reality, it takes a while before the patient's vision clears. Reassure the patient that this is normal.

Before discharge, determine what medications the patient will be taking at home. Review the medications with the patient, demonstrate proper self-administration, and have the patient return the demonstration.

ERRORS OF REFRACTION

Light must pass through the cornea, aqueous humor, lens, and vitreous humor to reach the retina. These structures through which light passes are called refractive media. The term *refraction* refers to the bending of light rays—in the case of the eye, so that they focus on the retina. Abnormalities, called errors of refraction, occur when refractive media do not bend light rays correctly. Myopia, hyperopia, and astigmatism are common problems caused by variations in the structure of the eyeball. Figure 49-16 illustrates these variations and the type of correction required.

Types of Errors of Refraction

Myopia and Hyperopia

Myopia is the medical term for nearsightedness. In myopia, the lens is situated too far from the retina. Light rays come together to focus in front of the retina. People with myopia have difficulty seeing distant images clearly. It is often recognized in the early school years. Typically, the condition slowly progresses until adolescence. New glasses usually are needed approximately every 2 years.

When the lens is too close to the retina, light rays come together behind the retina. This condition creates *hyperopia,* commonly known as farsightedness. The hyperopic person sees clearly in the distance but has difficulty focusing on close objects. Convex corrective lenses are needed for correction.

Astigmatism

When there are irregularities in the cornea or lens, astigmatism results. Most people have some degree of astigmatism. If the condition is mild, the natural lens can correct for the abnormality. If it is severe, however, vision is distorted, and corrective lenses are needed. A person can have astigmatism with myopia or hyperopia.

Presbyopia

Presbyopia is another disorder that is classified with errors of refraction. Presbyopia is poor accommodation that is due to loss of elasticity of the ciliary muscles. Accommodation is the adjustment of the lens for near and distant vision. It is accomplished by contraction or relaxation of the ciliary muscles, which causes the lens to change shape.

Presbyopia is usually considered a normal age-related change. It most often develops after age 40 years. As it progresses, people may be observed holding reading material at arm's length. People who are already hyperopic tend to have

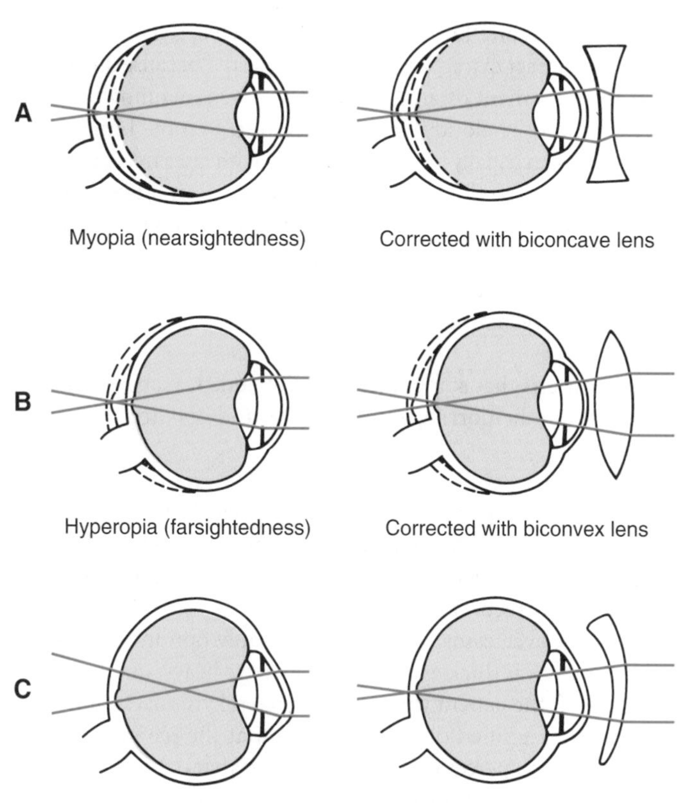

FIGURE **49-16** Refraction. *A,* Myopia: light rays converge before they reach the retina because the lens is too far from the retina. *B,* Hyperopia: light rays converge beyond the retina because the lens is too close to the retina. *C,* Astigmatism: uneven surfaces of the cornea bend light rays in a way that causes distortion of the image.

presbyopia at an earlier age than other people. Myopic people are usually able to read small print by holding it close.

Corrective lenses are needed when the visual changes become bothersome. Bifocal lenses are often prescribed. Bifocals have two different lenses. The upper part of the lens is used for distant vision, and the lower part is used for near vision. Trifocals have three lenses, for distant, closer, and near vision. Progressive lenses gradually blend the lens needed for seeing various distances. The wearer scans the lens to find the area needed for a particular task. Reading lenses must usually be changed every 2 to 3 years.

Medical Treatment

The primary treatment of errors of refraction is the prescription of corrective lenses. Eyeglasses are most often used. The obvious advantage of eyeglasses is that they require no special skills to use. Disadvantages are heavy frames and dirty lenses.

Contact lenses are tiny plastic disks made to fit over the patient's cornea. The lenses float on the tear film over the cornea. The primary advantages of contact lenses are convenience and appearance. Disadvantages include cost, the need for training and dexterity to insert and remove the lenses, and that they are easily lost. Another important disadvantage is the risk of corneal injury.

Several types of contact lenses are available. Hard lenses were developed first. They must be removed from the eye at the end of the day to prevent damage to the cornea. Soft lenses can be worn longer than hard lenses and require a shorter period of adjustment. Gas-permeable lenses are made of materials that allow oxygen and carbon dioxide to pass through them. This is important because the cornea exchanges gasses through the tear film beneath the contact lens. Extended-wear contact lenses can be worn for as long as 2 weeks. For this reason, they may be prescribed for elderly patients who have cataract surgery. Extended-wear contact lenses are more expensive than other lenses. The patient is cautioned to follow the prescribed cleaning schedule. Disposable contact lenses can be worn for up to 1 week and are then discarded.

Surgical Treatment

The past decade has seen several advancements in the surgical correction of refractive errors. *Photorefractive keratectomy* (PRK) uses an excimer laser to reshape the cornea for treatment of myopia or hyperopia. For the *laser in situ keratomileusis* (LASIK) procedure, a thin layer of the cornea is peeled back, and the laser is used to reshape the middle layer of the cornea. These procedures are done under local anesthesia in outpatient facilities. The outcomes cannot be evaluated immediately because refraction stabilizes slowly after surgery.

NURSING CARE *of the Patient with Errors of Refraction*

Nursing responsibilities for the patient with errors of refraction are limited except to encourage periodic examinations and to know if the patient uses corrective lenses. In emergency situations, the nurse may have to remove contact lenses for the patient. When caring for patients who have laser surgery, it may be your responsibility to teach postoperative care to the patient. You should include proper use of any prescribed eye drops (e.g., steroids), measures to protect the eye, and symptoms to be reported to the surgeon.

INTERNAL EYE DISORDERS

Cataract

The lens is a clear, flexible structure encased in an elastic capsule. It is located behind the iris and changes shape to focus on images of various sizes. When the lens becomes opaque (cloudy) so that it is no longer transparent, the condition is called a *cataract.*

Causes

Cataracts may be congenital, traumatic, or degenerative. Congenital cataracts are those that are present at birth. Traumatic cataracts are caused by chemical, mechanical, heat, or radiation injury. Degenerative cataracts are more common with aging, but they occur earlier in people with diabetes or Down syndrome.

Pathophysiology

The lens may become cloudy or opaque quickly or slowly. Injuries tend to cause opacity rapidly, whereas age-related opacity progresses slowly. As opacity increases, light is unable to enter the eye and vision becomes cloudy. Blindness eventually results if a cataract is untreated. With age, both eyes are usually affected, although they may not change at the same rate.

Signs and Symptoms

Signs and symptoms of cataracts include cloudy vision, seeing spots or ghost images, and floaters. The pattern of vision changes depends on the location of the developing cataract. A central cataract is located in the center of the lens. Patients with central cataracts may have fairly good peripheral vision. They may actually see better in dim light because the pupil dilates, allowing them to see around the cloudy center of the lens. Conversely, patients who have peripheral cataracts can see straight ahead but not to the side. As cataracts develop, people who initially were hyperopic may have temporary improvements in near vision. This is called "second sight."

Medical Treatment

The only curative treatment for cataract is removal of the lens, although mydriatics may be helpful in the early stages. Cataract extraction is the most frequently performed eye operation in the United States. There are several types of cataract extraction, as illustrated in Figure 49-17. If the lens and capsule are removed, it is called an intracapsular cataract extraction. For the extracapsular cataract extraction, the lens is removed, leaving the capsule in place. The most common extracapsular procedure is phacoemulsification and aspiration, in which sound waves are used to break up the lens. The lens fragments are then suctioned out of the eye. The extracapsular cataract extraction is usually preferred because it permits the placement of an artificial lens. The remaining capsule can become cloudy, causing vision to become blurred again. This can usually be corrected easily with laser treatment.

Cataract extraction is commonly done on an outpatient basis. Most patients tolerate the procedure well with just a mild sedative and local anesthesia. In some cases, general anesthesia may be preferred. Cataract surgery is usually considered safe, even for the very elderly.

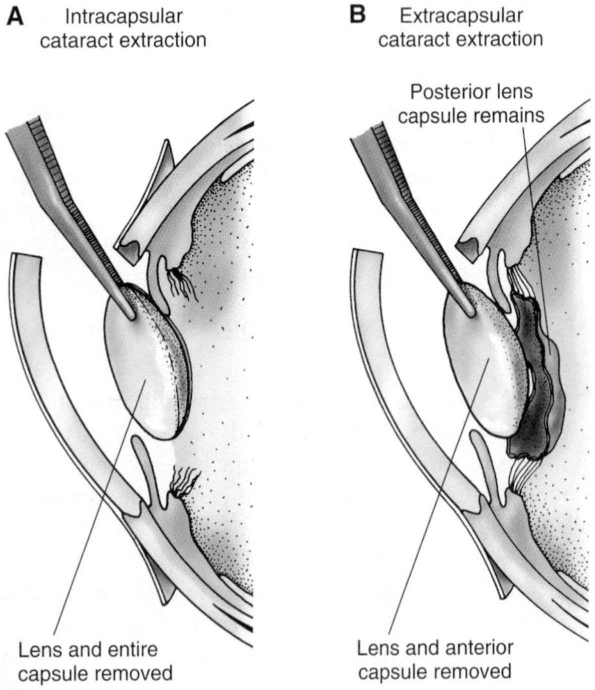

Complications

Complications that sometimes occur include leakage of vitreous humor, hemorrhage into the eye, and opening of the incision.

Lens Replacement

Once the lens has been removed, the eye is said to be aphakic. The patient is extra farsighted and unable to accommodate for changes in object size. Some type of artificial lens is needed for correction.

Cataract eyeglasses. In the past, the only option for lens replacement was thick eyeglasses. They were heavy, unattractive, and left the patient with poor peripheral vision. Cataract eyeglasses magnified objects so much that the patient also had poor depth perception. The result was that patients misjudged distances. This caused difficulty in everything from eating to driving. Another disadvantage to the use of eyeglasses was that the patient either had to have the lenses removed from both eyes or be blind in the unoperated eye. Otherwise, the strong magnification caused double vision.

Contact lenses. Contact lenses overcome many disadvantages of eyeglasses, but they have drawbacks as well. Considerable dexterity is required to insert, remove, and care for contact lenses. This makes them impractical for some older patients. The main complication of contact lens use is corneal injury.

Intraocular lenses. The invention of plastic lenses (Fig. 49-18) that can be implanted in the eye has been a tremen-

A Intracapsular cataract extraction

B Extracapsular cataract extraction

Posterior lens capsule remains

Lens and entire capsule removed

Lens and anterior capsule removed

FIGURE **49-17** Methods of cataract extraction. *A*, Intracapsular extraction. *B*, Extracapsular extraction.

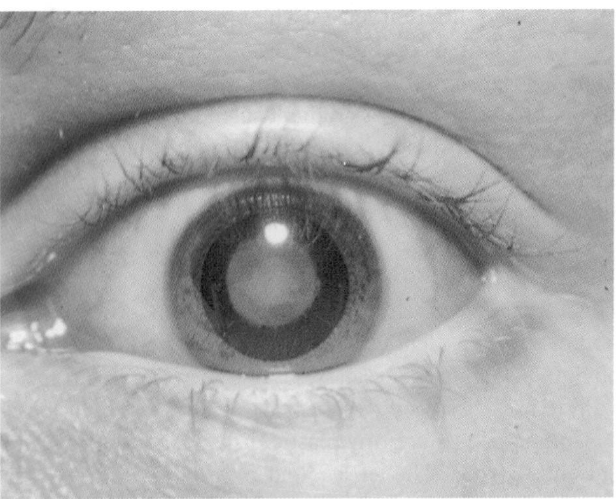

FIGURE **49-18** Intraocular lens in place after cataract extraction.

dous advance for many cataract patients. This type of lens is called an intraocular lens. The intraocular lens may be implanted immediately after removal of the natural lens, or it may be done later. Complications of insertion include corneal edema, secondary glaucoma, lens displacement, and retinal detachment.

NURSING CARE *of the Patient with Cataracts*

Cataract extractions are often are done in day-surgery clinics. You may have limited opportunity for patient and family teaching. Care of the patient having eye surgery is presented earlier in this chapter. This section emphasizes additional care specific to cataract surgery.

Preoperative care. Eye drops often are ordered at frequent intervals after cataract surgery. The orders must be followed exactly. Common drops used before cataract surgery are mydriatics, cycloplegics, and antibiotics. Mydriatics dilate the pupil, making it easier for the surgeon to access the lens. Cycloplegics temporarily paralyze the muscles of accommodation, keeping the eye still during the procedure. Antibiotics may be given to reduce the risk of infection.

POSTOPERATIVE NURSING CARE

Assessment

After cataract surgery, assess for pain and nausea. The patient is likely to return from surgery wearing a patch and shield over the operative eye. Note the presence of the patch and any apparent drainage. Also assess the patient's level of consciousness and orientation (see Nursing Care Plan: The Patient having Cataract Surgery).

NURSING CARE PLAN

The Patient having Cataract Surgery

ASSESSMENT

Health History: Mr. Gary Dickson is a 72-year-old retired welder. He complained of cloudy vision that has become increasingly worse. He reports spots moving across his field of vision. Cataracts were diagnosed, with the right lens affected more severely than the left. Mr. Dickson had a right extracapsular cataract extraction under local anesthesia this morning in the outpatient surgery department. He says he has mild pain in the eye area at this time. His record reveals a history of myocardial infarction 5 years ago and surgery for prostate enlargement 6 months ago. Although he is retired, he works every day on his small farm. He lives with his wife and an adult daughter.

Physical Examination: Mr. Dickson is alert and oriented. Vital signs: temperature, 98° F orally; pulse, 88; respiration 18; blood pressure 142/68. He is in semi-Fowler's position. An eye pad is in place over the right eye, protected with a metal shield. A small amount of clear drainage is noted seeping below the dressing.

Nursing Diagnosis	*Goals and Outcome Criteria*	*Interventions*
Risk for injury related to increased intraocular pressure (IOP), trauma.	Decreased risk for injury: patient avoids activities that increase IOP. Intraocular pressure remains 12-21 mm Hg.	Keep head of bed elevated. Instruct the patient not to impose stress on operative eye, rub the operative eye, strain, lean forward, or lie on the affected side. Administer antiemetics immediately as ordered for nausea and/or vomiting. Change damp pad as allowed. Administer eye drops (mydriatics, antimicrobials, and corticosteroids) as ordered. Encourage patient to take stool softeners as ordered to prevent constipation.
Disturbed sensory perception related to surgical trauma, lens removal, patching.	The patient will adapt to visual impairment and function in environment without injury.	Keep the bed in low position. Approach the left side. Place the call button on the left and instruct in use. Remove obstacles in the room. Assist with activities of daily living as needed.
Acute pain related to tissue trauma.	The patient will report that pain has decreased, will appear relaxed.	Assess pain. Notify the surgeon if severe (may indicate increased IOP). Administer analgesics as ordered and evaluate effects.
Anxiety related to temporary vision impairment, activity restrictions.	The patient will report decreased anxiety and will appear calm.	Explain what is being done and why. Explore feelings about surgery. Answer questions. Acknowledge fear of vision loss common with eye surgery. Respond promptly to needs.
Ineffective therapeutic regimen management related to lack of understanding of condition, self-care, and limitations.	Effective regimen management: the patient (and family member) will demonstrate instillation of medications and state activity limitations.	Explain postoperative limitations. No lifting over 5 lb, bending forward, or straining until cleared by physician. Review procedure for eye drops and have patient or family member demonstrate instillation. Supplement verbal instructions with written information.

Nursing Diagnoses, Goals, and Outcome Criteria: Cataract Surgery

Nursing Diagnoses	Goals and Outcome Criteria
Risk for Injury related to increased pressure	Reduced risk for injury: patient avoids activities that increase intraocular pressure; intraocular pressure remains 12-21 mm Hg
Disturbed Sensory Perception related to vision impairment	Adaptation to impaired vision: patient demonstrates self-care, maneuvers in environment without injury, performs activities of daily living, administers medications properly

Interventions

Risk for Injury

After cataract surgery, the most important thing is to prevent strain on the operative eye. Caution the patient not to rub the eye. Advise the patient to sleep on the unaffected side, not to lift more than 5 pounds, and to avoid bending forward. Administer stool softeners as ordered to prevent straining at stool, or instruct the patient in self-medication. If nausea occurs, it is treated promptly.

Always be aware of safety precautions after cataract surgery. When one eye is patched, the patient has limited peripheral vision. The good eye often has some degree of impairment as well. Medications may be ordered that cause blurred vision. To prevent injury, make sure that the patient is familiar with the environment and knows how to use the call button. Keep the bed in low position and the environment free of obstacles.

Impaired Sensory Perception

Confusion sometimes occurs in the postoperative period, especially in the very elderly. The confused person may fail to follow safety precautions or may place strain on the operative eye. Therefore monitor mental status and ensure that a caregiver is readily available.

Medications prescribed after cataract surgery usually include antibiotics and corticosteroids. Because the patient's vision is usually poor, you may need to teach a family member or friend how to give the medications.

A mild analgesic is usually ordered as needed. Postoperative patients with cataract surgery should not have severe pain. If a patient complains of severe pain, notify the physician. Severe pain may indicate hemorrhage or rising pressure within the eye.

Glaucoma

Glaucoma is one of the leading causes of blindness in the United States. It occurs in infants, children, and adults. It is thought to affect 1% of Americans older than 60 years of age and to account for 10% of all cases of blindness in the United States.

What Does Culture Have to do with Glaucoma?

In African Americans between 45 and 65 years of age, the prevalence of glaucoma is at least five times that of whites of the same age. Because glaucoma often has no symptoms, screening is especially important for middle-aged African Americans.

Pathophysiology

Normally, aqueous humor enters and leaves the anterior chamber so that intraocular pressure is maintained between 12 and 21 mm Hg. Glaucoma is a condition in which intraocular pressure is increased above normal. It can be caused by a number of changes that affect the flow of aqueous humor in the anterior chamber of the eye. It most often is caused by some interference with the outflow of aqueous humor. Although glaucoma may follow trauma, the exact cause is often unknown.

Excess pressure damages the back portion of the eye. It impairs blood flow to the optic nerve, resulting in vision impairment. Peripheral vision is lost first. The field of vision gradually narrows until the patient has tunnel vision. The patient who has tunnel vision can see only a small circle, as if looking through a tube or a tunnel. As the disease progresses, complete blindness eventually occurs. Vision may be restored if glaucoma is treated early; otherwise, vision loss is permanent.

Types of Glaucoma

The two types of glaucoma are open-angle glaucoma and angle-closure glaucoma. They are similar in that increased intraocular pressure is present in both, but they have some important differences. Both open-angle and angle-closure glaucoma are considered primary glaucomas. Increased intraocular pressure due to other conditions is called secondary glaucoma.

Open-angle glaucoma. Open-angle glaucoma also is called chronic glaucoma. It is more common than angle-closure glaucoma. Open-angle glaucoma results from some alteration that prevents the normal passage of aqueous humor through the trabecular meshwork. It is more common among African Americans on corticosteroid therapy, and those with a parent or sibling who has the condition.

There usually are no signs and symptoms at first. Some patients complain of tired eyes, occasional blurred vision, and halos around lights. Another clue may be the need for frequent changes in eyeglass prescriptions.

Open-angle glaucoma usually is treated first with drug therapy. The types of medications used include beta adrenergic blockers, adrenergics, cholinergics, carbonic anhydrase inhibitors, and hyperosmotic agents. Drugs work either by decreasing the production of aqueous humor or by improving the outflow of aqueous humor.

Beta blockers are relatively new in the treatment of glaucoma. Timolol maleate (Timoptic), Kerlone (betaxolol), and Betagan Liquifilm (levobunolol HCl) are examples of beta blockers used topically for glaucoma. Timolol lowers intraocular pressure, but it is not known exactly how.

Examples of adrenergic drugs used for glaucoma are epinephrine HCl (Epifrin) and dipivefrin (Propine) eye drops. Adrenergics decrease intraocular pressure by decreasing the formation of aqueous humor and increasing its outflow.

Cholinergic miotics such as pilocarpine and carbachol and cholinesterase inhibitors such as ecothiopate iodide (phospholine iodide) and physostigmine facilitate the outflow of aqueous humor. These drugs constrict the pupil, which permits fluid to flow more easily through the angle where the iris meets the cornea and into the trabecular meshwork. A disadvantage of many currently used miotics is that they must be administered frequently. Some new preparations, including ocular inserts, are effective for a longer period of time. These may eventually replace the preparations now in use.

Carbonic anhydrase inhibitors such as acetazolamide (Diamox) reduce intraocular pressure by decreasing the production of aqueous humor. Carbonic anhydrase inhibitors and osmotic diuretics are given orally or parenterally. Additional information about drugs used to treat glaucoma is provided in Table 49-4. Hyperosmotic agents, including oral glycerin and intravenous mannitol (Osmitrol), promote movement of fluid from the intraocular structures.

Surgical intervention may be recommended when drugs do not reduce pressure adequately, the patient does not use prescribed drugs properly, or adverse reactions interfere with drug therapy. Surgical procedures for glaucoma include trabeculoplasty, trabeculectomy, and cyclocryotherapy. Trabeculoplasty may be tried first because it can be done under local anesthesia in an outpatient setting. The procedure involves the use of a laser to create multiple holes in the trabecular meshwork. This is intended to improve drainage of aqueous humor from the anterior chamber. If the procedure is successful, intraocular pressure falls over a period of time. Meanwhile, the physician usually has the patient continue using glaucoma medications.

A trabeculectomy is one of several surgical procedures that creates a channel to allow aqueous humor to drain under the conjunctiva. If this procedure is not effective, cyclocryotherapy may be done. A cold probe, called a cryoprobe, is used to freeze part of the ciliary body. Freezing destroys some of the tissue, resulting in decreased production of aqueous humor.

Angle-closure glaucoma. Angle-closure glaucoma is also called acute glaucoma. It accounts for only approximately 10% of all glaucomas. With angle-closure glaucoma, the flow of aqueous humor through the pupil is blocked. Pressure forces the iris forward, causing it to block the trabecular meshwork. There is a rapid rise in intraocular pressure. Pressure is often greater than 50 mm Hg. If the pressure is not lowered promptly, permanent blindness can result. Therefore angle-closure glaucoma is considered a medical emergency. Unlike open-angle glaucoma, angle-closure glaucoma causes sudden, acute pain. Other signs and symptoms are blurred vision, halos around lights, nausea and vomiting, and headache on the affected side.

The goal of medical treatment is to reduce the intraocular pressure quickly. Drugs used initially to treat angle-closure glaucoma include cholinergics, osmotic diuretics, topical beta blockers, and carbonic anhydrase inhibitors (see Table 49-5 for details). After the pressure has been lowered, surgery is usually recommended to prevent recurrence. Iridotomy is a surgical procedure in which a window is cut in the iris to permit aqueous humor to flow through the pupil normally. The procedure may be done on both eyes because the healthy eye is likely to experience similar problems in the future. There are two types of iridotomy: peripheral and keyhole.

One other procedure is cyclodialysis, a procedure that involves opening the angle in the anterior chamber with a special instrument inserted through a small incision in the sclera.

NURSING CARE *of the Patient with Glaucoma*

Nurses who work in acute care settings are most concerned with drug therapy and patient teaching for self-care.

Assessment

General assessment of the patient with an eye disorder is outlined in Table 49-2. Nurses who work in special clinics or units may also measure intraocular pressure as indicated. When a patient has glaucoma, you must assess patient knowledge of the disease and treatment and patient ability to carry out self-care.

Nursing Diagnoses, Goals, and Outcome Criteria: Glaucoma

Nursing Diagnoses	Goals and Outcome Criteria
Risk for Injury related to increased intraocular pressure	Decreased risk for injury: adherence to prescribed measures to reduce intraocular pressure, normal intraocular pressure readings
Fear related to actual or potential loss of vision	Decreased fear: patient states feeling less fearful
Ineffective Therapeutic Regimen Management related to lack of understanding of disease, treatment, complications	Effective management of condition: patient correctly describes and adheres to prescribed drug therapy
Acute Pain related to acute increase in intraocular pressure, inflammation caused by corrective procedures	Pain relief: patient states reduced or relieved, relaxed manner

If the patient has impaired vision, additional diagnoses may be appropriate. These are discussed in detail in the section on Nursing Care of the Visually Impaired Patient. General surgical care was also addressed earlier.

Interventions

Risk for Injury

One of the most important things you can do to keep intraocular pressure within normal limits is to administer prescribed medications. Be extremely cautious in selecting and administering ophthalmic medications. Different medications are often ordered for the affected and the unaffected eye. The procedure for applying eye drops and ointments is described earlier.

Fear and Ineffective Therapeutic Regimen Management

You must be sensitive to the patient's fears about glaucoma leading to blindness. Emphasize that adherence to prescribed drug therapy can usually control intraocular pressure and

table 49-5 DRUG THERAPY | *Glaucoma*

GENERAL NURSING CONSIDERATIONS

1. Teach patient or caregivers, or both, proper way to administer eye drops.
2. Recognize that failure to control intraocular pressure can result in permanent blindness.
3. Avoid corticosteroids, succinylcholine, and anticholinergics in glaucoma patients.
4. Ophthalmic solutions should be tightly capped and protected from light.
5. Ophthalmic solutions should not be used if they change color or other characteristics.
6. Be alert for systemic effects of ophthalmic drugs.

DRUG	USE/ACTION	SIDE EFFECTS	NURSING INTERVENTIONS
BETA-ADRENERGIC BLOCKING AGENTS			
Timolol (Timoptic) Metipranolol (OptiPranolol) Carteolol (Ocupress) Levobunolol (Betagan Liquifilm) Betaxolol (Betoptic)	Treatment of chronic (open-angle) glaucoma. Decreases aqueous formation. Does not affect pupil or visual acuity. Often used in combination with other drugs. Only betaxolol is beta-1 selective, so it is preferred with asthma and COPD.	Eye irritation. Possible systemic effects: bronchospasm, heart failure. Contraindicated with asthma, heart failure.	Monitor pulse, blood pressure, and respiration. Assess for wheezing, bronchospasm, bradycardia, hypotension, dysrhythmias.
CHOLINERGICS	Increases aqueous outflow. Initial treatment of acute and chronic glaucoma.		
Pilocarpine (Isopto Carpine)		Myopia. Poor vision in dim light. Lacrimation (tearing). Systemic effects: change in pulse rate or rhythm, bronchospasm, decreased blood pressure, gastric distress, diarrhea, headache.	Advise patient to use caution for tasks requiring distant vision or vision in dim light. Antidote: atropine. Minimize side effect by applying pressure over lacrimal duct.
Pilocarpine (Ocusert ocular system)		Few side effects.	Ocusert therapeutic system lasts 1 wk. More costly.
Carbachol (Isopto Carbachol)		Carbachol at first may cause aching of the eyes, brow pain, headache, light sensitivity, and blurred vision.	
Acetylcholine (Miochol) Echothiophate iodide (Phospholine iodide)	Acetylcholine is used primarily in operating room because effect only lasts about 10 min.		Acetylcholine comes in a two-compartment vial. It is reconstituted immediately before use.
Physostigmine (Eserine)		Long-term use of Eserine causes conjunctivitis.	
ADRENERGICS	Increase aqueous outflow. For open-angle glaucoma.		
Epinephrine HCl (Epifrin) Dipivefrin (Propine)		Headache, brow ache, blurred vision, ocular irritation. Tachycardia and increased BP with systemic absorption.	Contraindicated with closed-angle glaucoma.
Apraclonidine (Iopidine)	Short-term use only.	Headache, dry mouth, conjunctivitis, ocular itching.	

table 49-5 **DRUG THERAPY | *Glaucoma—cont'd***

DRUG	USE/ACTION	SIDE EFFECTS	NURSING INTERVENTIONS
ADRENERGICS—cont'd			
Brimonidine (Alphagan)	Long-term use with open-angle glaucoma or ocular hypertension.	Hypertension with Alphagan but not with Iopidine.	Monitor BP.
PROSTAGLANDINS			
Latanoprost (Xalatan)	Increases aqueous outflow. Treats open-angle glaucoma and ocular hypertension.	Permanent darkening of green-brown, yellow-brown, and blue/gray/brown irides of the eye. Also, blurred vision, burning, headache, conjunctival hyperemia.	
CARBONIC ANHYDRASE INHIBITORS			
Acetazolamide (Diamox) Dichlorphenamide (Daranide)		Increased urinary output. Potential hypokalemia. Possible allergic response in people who are allergic to sulfonamides. Tingling of fingers and toes (paresthesia). Itching. Sore throat, skin rash, and fever may suggest serious blood disorders.	Monitor intake and output. Withhold and notify physician if patient is allergic. Assess for hypokalemia (pulse changes, mental status changes, muscle weakness, abdominal distention). Expect increased urine output. Provide access and assistance to toilet. Do not give at bedtime.
OSMOTIC DIURETICS	Treatment of acute (angle-closure) glaucoma. Preoperative preparation for glaucoma surgery.	Increased urinary output. Potential hypokalemia. Elevated blood glucose. Headache. Tissue necrosis because of infiltration of intravenous solution.	Record intake and output. Assess for hypokalemia (pulse changes, muscle weakness, mental status changes, abdominal distention). Monitor patients with diabetes for elevated glucose. Monitor IV infusion. Stop infusion if infiltration is suspected and notify RN.
Mannitol (Osmitrol)		Mannitol reserved for crisis situations because of risk of circulatory overload.	Mannitol may form crystals if cooled. If this happens, place vial in warm water until crystals dissolve. Cool to body temperature before administration.
Urea (Ureaphil)			Urea should be used within 24 hr after reconstitution.
Glycerin (Osmoglyn)			Synthetic glycerin available for people with diabetes to reduce effects on blood glucose.

IV, Intravenous.

Consider the Alternative!

Caution patients not to take over-the-counter products containing ephedra (Ma Huang) because they can raise intraocular pressure.

reduce the risk of complications. Because open-angle glaucoma is painless, the patient may not appreciate the need for ongoing treatment. Stress the importance of keeping regular appointments for evaluation of intraocular pressure. Unfortunately, nonadherence with drug therapy is a frequent nursing diagnosis with glaucoma. Remember (and teach the patient) that any drugs that dilate the pupil are contraindicated. Patients may not be aware that many nonprescription cold and allergy remedies contain chemicals that dilate the pupil. The physician or pharmacist should be consulted before taking any additional drugs.

Patients who have glaucoma should wear a bracelet to alert health care providers to the condition. They should keep their medications on hand at all times. When traveling, the patient with glaucoma should keep spare medications in separate locations in case one is lost. It is helpful to have a wallet card stating the exact medication schedule in case the patient becomes ill and is unable to give this information.

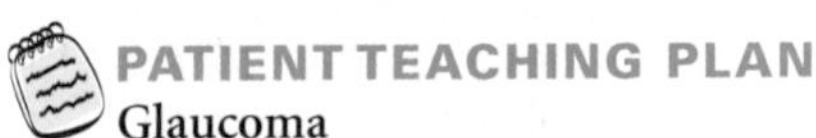

PATIENT TEACHING PLAN
Glaucoma

- Glaucoma usually responds to treatment, but it can lead to blindness if untreated.
- It is essential to have regular checkups to monitor intraocular pressure because glaucoma is usually painless.
- Consult with a pharmacist or physician before taking any new medication.
- Wear a medical alert tag.
- Take spare medication when traveling.
- Notify your physician if visual acuity or peripheral vision decreases.

Pain

Pain in acute glaucoma attacks is treated with drugs that reduce intraocular pressure. Analgesics may be given as ordered. If the patient has surgery for glaucoma, postoperative care is similar to the general care after eye surgery, described earlier. Monitoring intraocular pressure is especially important after glaucoma surgery. Postoperative pain can usually be treated with non-opioid analgesics. Report increasing or unrelieved pain to the surgeon.

Many drugs are contraindicated with glaucoma. Caution patients not to take nonprescription drugs without consulting their pharmacist or physician.

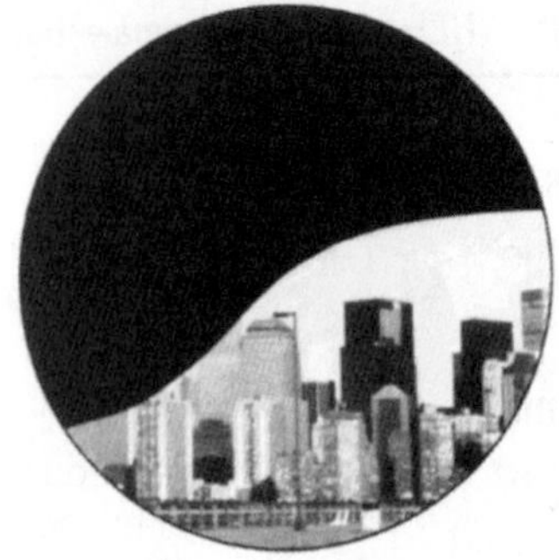

Detached retina

FIGURE **49-19** Loss of partial field of vision due to retinal detachment.

Retinal Detachment

Pathophysiology

Retinal detachment is a separation of the sensory layer of the eyeball from the pigmented layer. It begins when a tear in the retina allows fluid to collect between the sensory and the pigmented layers. The fluid causes the two layers to separate. Separation deprives the sensory layers of nutrients and oxygen that normally are supplied by the blood vessels in the choroid. This leads to damage to the nerve tissue in the sensory layer and resultant partial or complete loss of vision. Retinal tears may occur spontaneously or as a result of trauma. They are more common in older people and in people with myopia.

Signs and Symptoms

Signs and symptoms of retinal detachment depend on the location and extent of the detachment. Patients may report seeing flashes of light or floaters. Vision may be cloudy. If the area of detachment is large, vision may be lost completely. Some patients say it seems as if a curtain has come down or across the line of vision (Fig. 49-19). This is very frightening to the patient.

Medical and Surgical Treatment

Special procedures are required to repair retinal detachments. Most holes or tears must be sealed promptly. Lasers are commonly used to do this. The intense light burns the detached portion of the retina. As the area heals, scar tissue that seals the tear forms. Cryotherapy also causes scar tissue to form, but it uses a cold probe applied to the eyeball behind the tear. The cold radiates through the layers of tissue, freezing the torn tissue. Another procedure that may be employed is retinopexy in which gas is injected into the eye to apply pressure to the tear.

Scleral buckling is often done along with laser treatment or cryotherapy. The scleral buckle is a Silastic band that is secured around the eyeball under the sclera. Small pads are sutured under the band opposite the area of detachment. The band holds the pads in place. This procedure brings the layers of tissue back together by pressing from the outside. The band is left in place permanently (Fig. 49-20). The physician

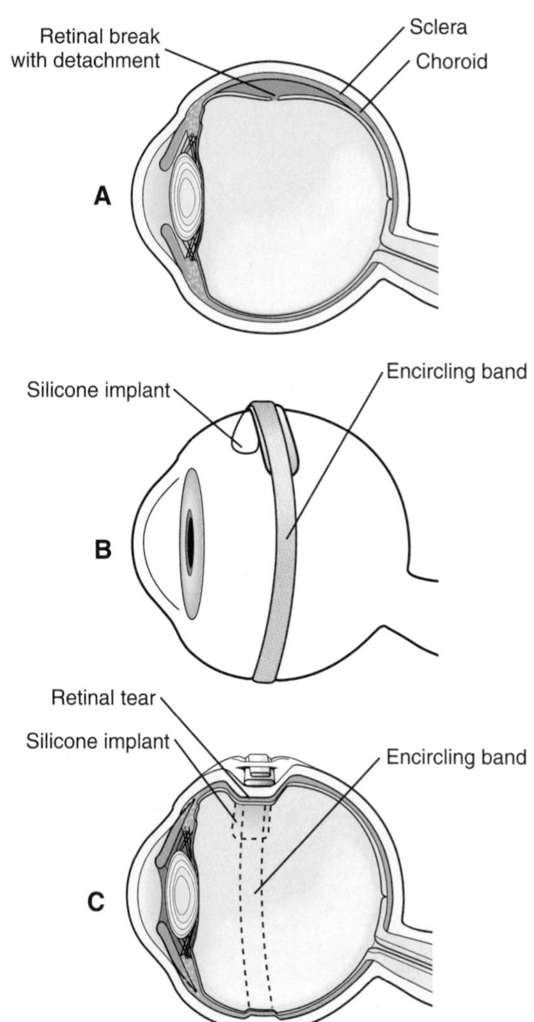

FIGURE **49-20** *A*, Retinal detachment. *B* and *C*, Scleral buckle and silicone implant in place to treat retinal detachment.

may inject an air bubble or some normal saline into the vitreous humor after the surgical procedure. The purpose of this is to apply internal pressure to the detached portion of the retina.

Sometimes tears cause bleeding into the vitreous. Significant amounts of blood in the vitreous interfere with vision. When this occurs, the physician may do a vitrectomy to remove the bloody tissue.

NURSING CARE *of the Patient with Retinal Detachment*

Before corrective measures are taken, the patient usually is placed on strict bedrest with the head elevated. In the preoperative period, many patients are very anxious. Encourage them to talk about their fears and to ask questions. Even though the procedure may be done under local anesthesia, oral intake may be restricted to reduce the risk of postoperative vomiting. Intravenous fluids may be ordered.

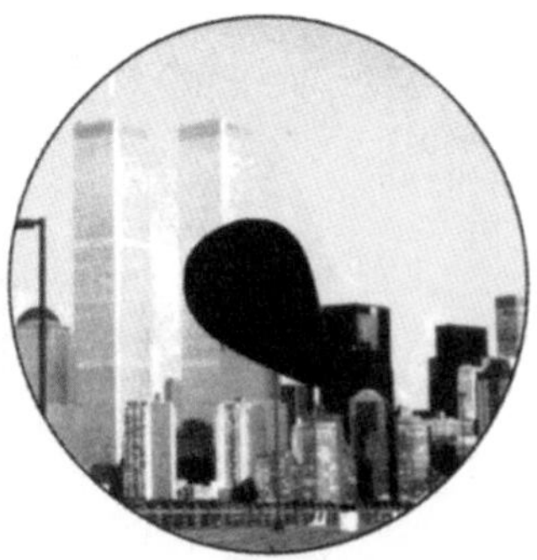

FIGURE **49-21** Vision of the patient with macular degeneration.

Consider the Alternative!

Some practitioners believe that antioxidants (vitamins C and E) may delay the onset and slow the progression of age-related macular degeneration. Additional research is needed to determine if antioxidants are effective.

Postoperative care is essentially the same as for other patients undergoing eye surgery, as described earlier in this chapter. Positioning orders may be very specific for these patients. If an air bubble has been injected, it will rise to the top of the eye. If the patient's detachment is in the back of the eye, a face-down position is necessary to keep the bubble in the right place. Saline travels down rather than up, so the same patient would need to stay face up if saline had been injected. The surgeon prescribes any activity limitations.

Senile Macular Degeneration

The macula is the part of the retina that is responsible for central vision. As people age, changes in the eye cause the macula to degenerate. Both eyes are usually affected. The condition is progressive, causing central vision to get gradually worse (Fig. 49-21). Patients often report difficulty reading or doing close work. Peripheral vision remains intact. It is usually adequate to allow mobility in familiar settings.

Regular eyeglasses do not improve vision with macular degeneration. Special telescopic lenses may be helpful. Laser treatments may offer hope to some patients with macular degeneration. The nurse needs to help the patient and family members learn to cope with declining vision. The nursing care is like that described for patients with vision impairment.

Enucleation

Some eye conditions are so serious that removal of the eyeball is the only treatment. *Enucleation* is the term used for removal of the eye. Conditions that may result in enucleation include injury, infection, sympathetic ophthalmia, and some glaucomas and malignancies.

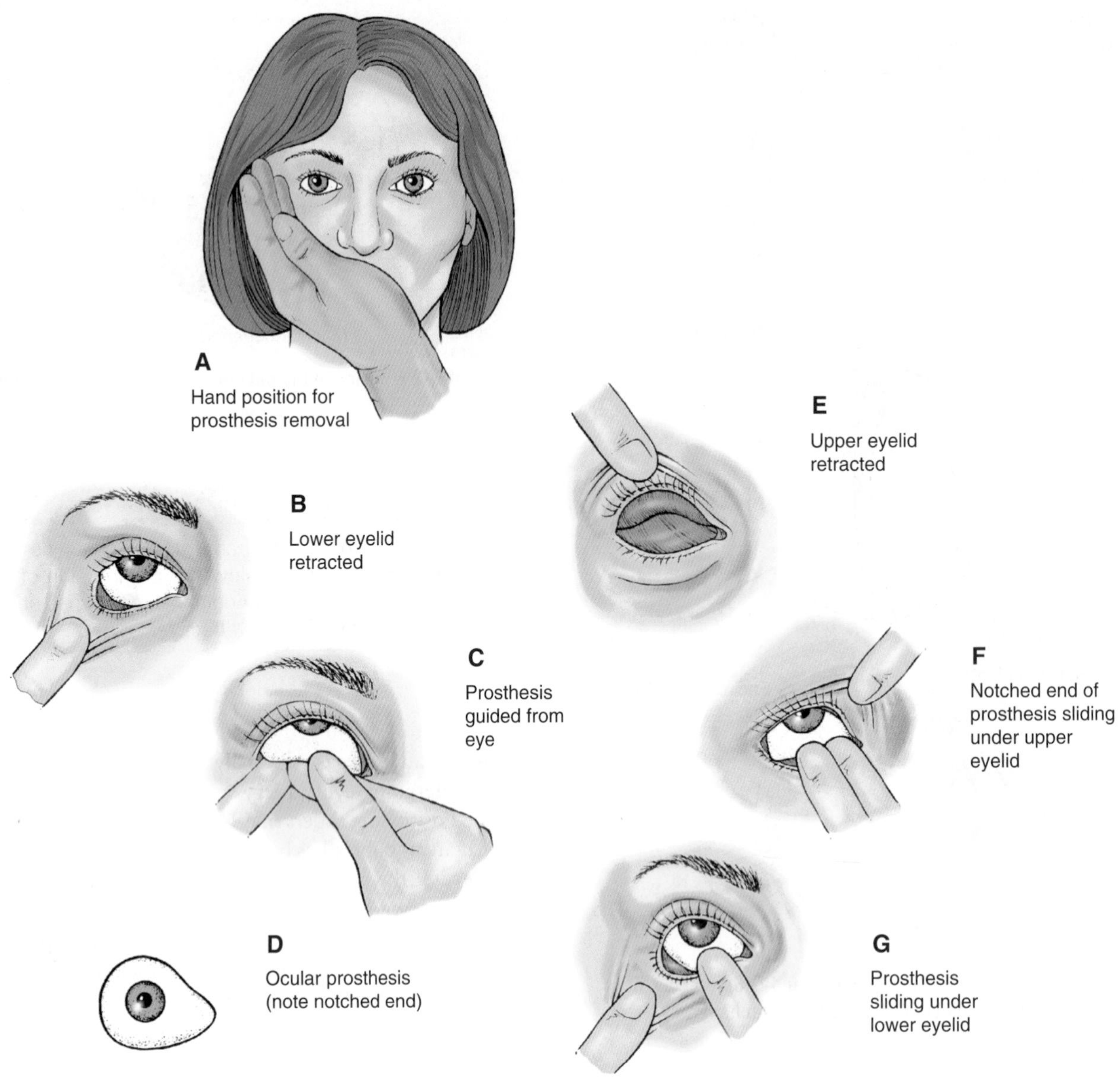

FIGURE **49-22** Removal *(A-C)* and insertion *(D-G)* of an eye prosthesis.

During the surgical procedure, the eyeball is removed. A round device is placed in the cavity, and muscles are sutured over it. The conjunctiva is then sutured over the muscle. This procedure creates a foundation for the future placement of a prosthesis. The patient returns from surgery with a temporary shell called a conformer in the prosthesis base, which is covered with a pressure dressing. Observe for excessive bleeding or increasing pain. Report any temperature elevation. After the pressure dressing is removed, the physician may order wound care and topical medications.

Approximately 1 month after the enucleation, a prosthesis can be fitted by an optician. The prosthesis is carefully made to look like the patient's natural eye. The patient must learn to insert, remove, and clean the prosthesis. Nurses also should know how to care for an eye prosthesis as illustrated in Figure 49-22. The steps to remove and clean a prosthesis are the following:

1. Wash hands thoroughly.
2. Gently depress and pull the lower lid down.
3. Allow the prosthesis to slip out over the lower lid.
4. Wash the prosthesis under running water, using the fingers to remove any debris.

If the prosthesis is to be stored, it should be placed in a container with normal saline or water. To reinsert the prosthesis do the following:

1. Raise the upper lid by pressing it up against the orbit.
2. Slip the top of the prosthesis under the orbit.
3. Pull the lower lid down so that the prosthesis can slip into place.

The patient's nursing care plan should always inform staff that the patient has a prosthesis.

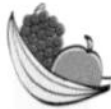

Nutrition Concepts

1. Vitamin A is essential for normal vision.
2. An early symptom of vitamin A deficiency is night blindness.
3. Severe vitamin A deficiency causes clinical eye disease that leads to blindness.

key points

- Eleven million people in the United States have some vision impairment.
- After eye surgery, nursing care addresses risk for injury, disturbed sensory perception, acute pain, anxiety, and ineffective therapeutic regimen management.
- Increased intraocular pressure must be controlled to prevent permanent vision loss.
- Vision loss affects all aspects of a person's life: independence, mobility, employment, communication, and interpersonal relationships.
- Common nursing diagnoses for patients with impaired vision include disturbed sensory perception, ineffective coping, self-care deficit, and ineffective therapeutic regimen management.
- Infectious and inflammatory conditions of the eye include blepharitis, hordeolum, chalazion, conjunctivitis, and keratitis.
- Entropion is inversion of the lower lid; ectropion is eversion of the lower lid.
- A foreign body embedded in the eye should be removed only by a physician.
- Corneal opacity is treated with removal of the scarred cornea and replacement with a healthy donor cornea in a procedure called keratoplasty.
- Errors of refraction include myopia, hyperopia, and astigmatism and are often correctable with corrective lenses.
- An opaque lens, called a cataract, can be removed and vision restored with a lens replacement in the form of eyeglasses, contact lenses, or intraocular lenses.
- Glaucoma, increased intraocular pressure, is a leading cause of blindness and is treated with drug therapy or surgery, or both.
- Nursing care of the patient with glaucoma focuses on risk for injury, fear, ineffective therapeutic regimen management, and acute pain.
- Retinal detachment is separation of the sensory layer of the eyeball from the pigmented layer and can result in partial or complete loss of vision.
- Treatments for retinal detachment include laser therapy, cryotherapy, retinopexy, scleral buckling, and vitrectomy.
- Senile macular degeneration causes progressive loss of central vision but may be improved by laser treatment.
- Enucleation is removal of the eyeball necessitated by injury, infection, sympathetic ophthalmia, and some glaucomas and malignancies.
- After enucleation, a prosthesis can be used to restore the patient's normal appearance.

REVIEW QUESTIONS

1. The fluid that fills the anterior chamber of the eye is:
   1. aqueous humor.
   2. ciliary fluid.
   3. vitreous humor.
   4. refractive fluid.
2. Your assessment of the eyes of an older adult reveals eyeballs slightly sunken in the orbits, small pupils that do not respond to light, a grayish ring around the iris, and a complaint that the eyes feel dry sometimes. Which is these would you consider *abnormal* in an older adult?
   1. Eyeballs slightly sunken
   2. Small pupils
   3. Pupils not responsive to light
   4. Eyes that feel dry sometimes
3. You are assisting with a community vision screening project. A participant says, "The nurse says my vision is 20/40 in both eyes. What does that mean?" Your response should be which of the following?
   1. You see best at 20 to 40 feet from objects.
   2. You cannot see more than 40 feet in the distance.
   3. At 40 feet, you can read what most people can read at 20 feet.
   4. At 20 feet, you can read what a person with normal vision could read at 40 feet.
4. When a patient comes to the office for an eye examination, the ophthalmologist administers phenylephrine 2.5% eye drops to:
   1. reveal any scratches on the cornea.
   2. dilate the pupil.
   3. anesthetize the cornea.
   4. dilate retinal blood vessels.
5. A patient is being discharged after cataract surgery. Discharge instructions should include:
   1. always lie on the affected side.
   2. avoid pressure on the operative eye.
   3. moderate to severe pain is expected.
   4. resume normal activities immediately.
6. To guide a visually impaired person, you should:
   1. stand side by side and hold the person's hand.
   2. let the person hold your upper arm.
   3. walk behind the patient and advise of obstacles.
   4. have the person walk behind you with hands on your shoulders.

7. Following keratoplasty, you observe that the patient's cornea is cloudy. You should:
   1. reassure the patient that cloudiness is normal for several weeks after surgery.
   2. elevate the patient's head and encourage increased fluid intake.
   3. report signs of corneal rejection to the physician.
   4. prepare the patient for emergency surgery.

8. Drugs used to treat open-angle glaucoma act by decreasing aqueous formation or:
   1. increasing aqueous outflow.
   2. dilating the canal of Schlemm.
   3. relaxing the trabecular meshwork.
   4. dilating the pupil.

9. The most serious complication of angle-closure glaucoma is:
   1. rupture of the eyeball.
   2. permanent blindness.
   3. nausea and vomiting.
   4. increased intracranial pressure.

10. Positioning after surgery for retinal detachment depends on:
    1. patient preference.
    2. intraocular pressure.
    3. location of the repaired tear.
    4. amount of bleeding.

CHAPTER

50 Ear and Hearing Disorders

objectives

1. Identify the data to be collected when assessing a patient with a disorder affecting the ear, hearing, or balance.
2. Describe the tests and procedures used to diagnose disorders of the ear, hearing, or balance.
3. Explain the nursing considerations for each of the tests and procedures.
4. Explain the nursing involvement for patients receiving common therapeutic measures for disorders of the ear, hearing, or balance.
5. For selected disorders, describe the pathophysiology, signs and symptoms, complications, and medical or surgical treatment.
6. Assist in the development of a nursing care plan for a patient with a disorder of the ear, hearing, or balance.
7. Identify measures the nurse can take to reduce the risk of hearing impairment and to detect problems early.

key terms

Cerumen (sĕ-RO͞O-mĕn, p. 1075)
Dizziness (p. 1084)
Equilibrium (ē-kwĭ-LĬB-rē-ŭm, p. 1075)
Otalgia (ō-TĂL-jē-ă, p. 1077)
Otic (Ō-tĭk, p. 1080)
Ototoxic (ō-tō-TŎK-sĭk, p. 1077)
Presbycusis (prĕz-bē-KŪ-sĭs, p. 1077)
Tinnitus (tĭ-NĪ-tĭs, p. 1077)
Tympanic membrane (tĭm-PĂN-ĭk MĔM-brān, p. 1075)
Vertigo (VĔR-tĭ-gō, p. 1084)

Approximately 1 in 1,000 infants born in the United States has some hearing impairment. No one knows exactly how many adults are hearing impaired, but approximately half of those older than age 75 years have some hearing loss. Regardless of the numbers of people affected, the impact of hearing loss is certainly significant. Health care providers can reduce disability by teaching people how to prevent hearing loss and by helping to rehabilitate those who are impaired.

ANATOMY AND PHYSIOLOGY OF THE EAR

The ears are essential organs for hearing and for position sense. Position sense enables a person to know the position of body parts without looking. It is also necessary for **equilibrium** (state of balance needed for walking, standing, and sitting).

ANATOMY

The ear has three major sections: the external ear, the middle ear, and the inner ear (Fig. 50-1).

External Ear

Auricle. The external ear includes the auricle and the external auditory canal. The auricle, also called the pinna, is the visible part of the ear.

Innervation. Many nerves innervate the ear. This is the reason pain in the ear can sometimes be traced to disorders of the nose, mouth, or neck. Of special importance is the facial nerve (the seventh cranial nerve), which lies alongside the auditory canal. The facial nerve is protected in the canal by a thin bony covering. It exits from the skull just in front of the ear and branches across the face to control muscle movement.

Lymph Drainage. Lymph nodes located in front of, behind, and below the auricle drain the ear. In the presence of ear infections, they may become enlarged.

External Auditory Canal. The external auditory canal extends from the external opening of the ear to the tympanic membrane. The **tympanic membrane** is commonly called the eardrum. The canal is lined with cells that secrete **cerumen** (earwax). The waxy secretion coats and protects the canal.

Tympanic Membrane. The tympanic membrane at the end of the external auditory canal is shiny and pearl-gray. Sound waves entering the external auditory canal cause the membrane to vibrate.

Middle Ear

Bones. The middle ear is an air-filled space in the temporal bone. It contains three small bones (ossicles): the malleus (hammer), the incus (anvil), and the stapes (stirrup). The function of these bones is to forward the sound waves transmitted by the tympanic membrane to the inner ear.

The malleus lies directly under the tympanic membrane. One portion of the malleus is attached to the membrane, and another portion is connected to the incus. The incus is connected to the stapes. The stapes has a footplate that fits into the oval window. The oval window, which opens into the vestibule, separates the middle ear from the inner ear. Sound waves are transmitted from the tympanic membrane

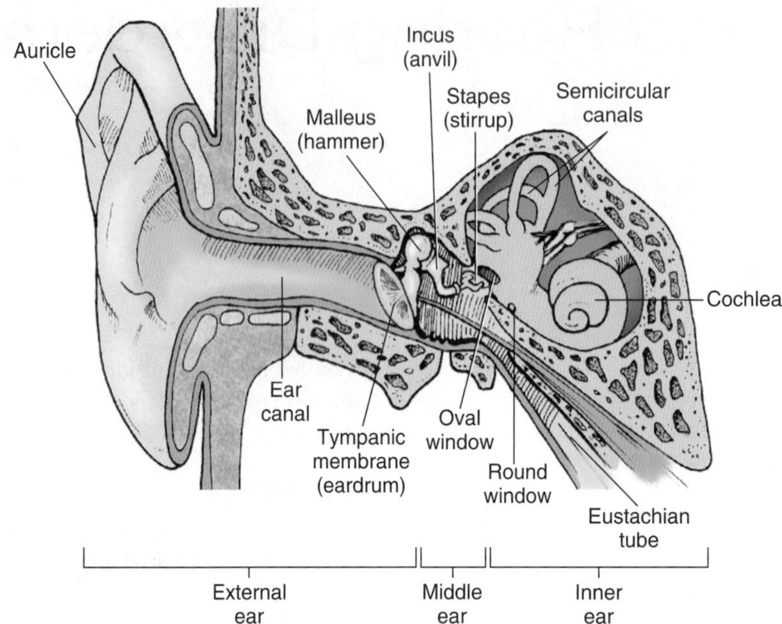

FIGURE **50-1** Anatomical structure of the ear illustrating the three major sections: the external ear, the middle ear, and the inner ear.

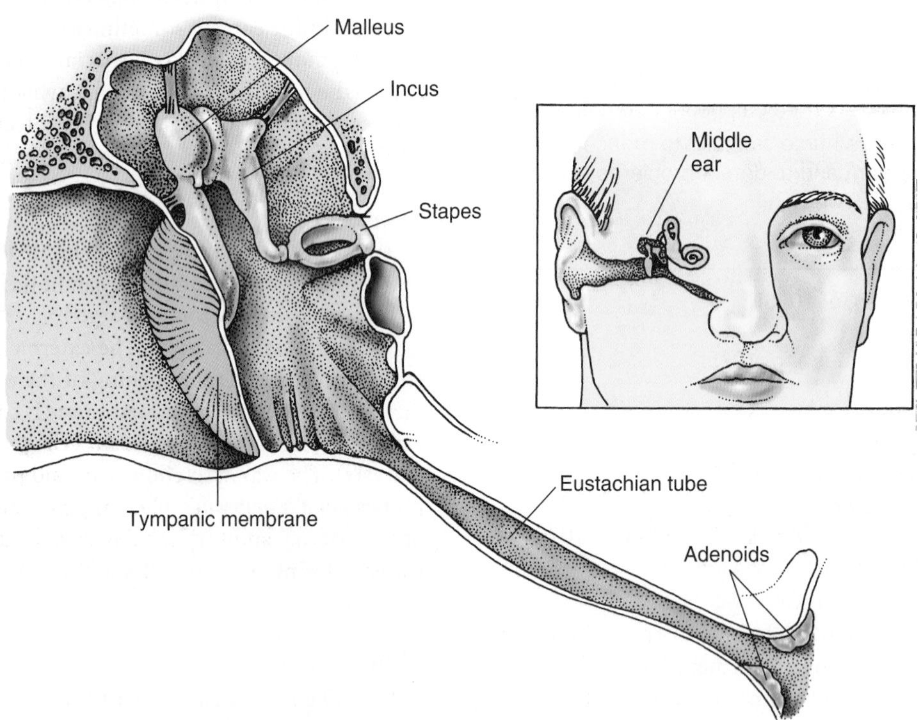

FIGURE **50-2** The eustachian tube extends from the middle ear to the nasopharynx.

to the malleus, the incus, the stapes, and then to the oval window.

Eustachian Tube. An important structure in the middle ear is the eustachian tube. The eustachian tube extends from the middle ear to the nasopharynx, as illustrated in Figure 50-2. It creates an air passage to the middle ear so that air pressure remains the same on both sides of the tympanic membrane.

Mastoid Process. The mastoid process is the bony structure behind the auricle. The interior is made up of air cells that are directly connected to the middle ear. The mastoid process is very close to the brain.

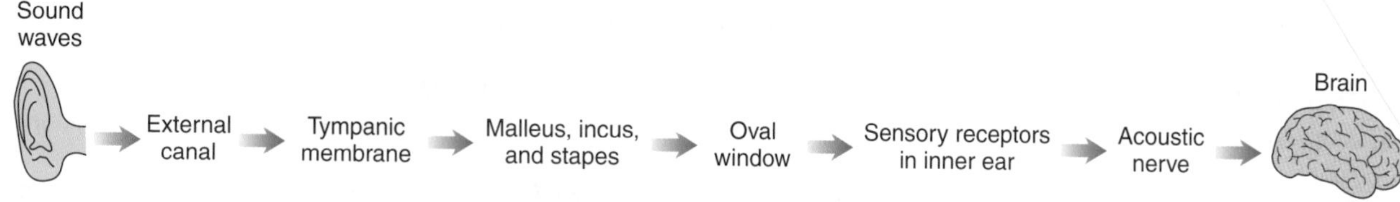

FIGURE **50-3** Physiology of hearing.

Inner Ear

The inner ear consists of the membranous labyrinth and the bony labyrinth. The membranous labyrinth contains fluid called *endolymph.* Endolymph moves with changes in body position.

The parts of the bony labyrinth are the vestibule, semicircular canals, and cochlea. The oval window opens into the vestibule. Receptors in the vestibule monitor the position of the head to maintain posture balance. Receptors in the semicircular canals monitor changes in rate or direction of movement to maintain balance during movement. The cochlea is a coiled tube that looks like a snail. It contains the organ of Corti, which is the receptor end organ of hearing. The organ of Corti transmits stimuli from the oval window to the acoustic (auditory) nerve.

PHYSIOLOGY OF HEARING

The perception and interpretation of sound depend on a complex series of steps. A malfunction at any step can result in some type of hearing impairment. Figure 50-3 illustrates the steps involved in the hearing process.

AGE-RELATED CHANGES IN THE EAR

Changes occur in the external, middle, and inner ear with aging. Some changes have no functional significance, but others can lead to serious problems with hearing or balance.

The skin of the auricle may become dry and wrinkled. Dryness of the external canal causes itching. Cerumen production declines, and the protective wax is drier. Hairs in the canal become coarser and longer, especially in men. The combination of dry cerumen and coarse hairs sometimes leads to obstruction of the canal. The eardrum thickens, and the bony joints in the middle ear degenerate somewhat. Surprisingly, these changes are not thought to impair hearing significantly.

Changes in the inner ear, however, affect sensitivity to sound, understanding of speech, and balance. Degenerative changes include atrophy of the cochlea, the cochlear nerve cells, and the organ of Corti. The result is that many older people have some degree of hearing loss, and some have problems with balance. The type of hearing loss most often associated with age is called ***presbycusis.*** Presbycusis is discussed later with other types of hearing impairments.

NURSING ASSESSMENT OF THE EXTERNAL EAR, HEARING, AND BALANCE

HEALTH HISTORY

The nursing assessment of the ear includes inspection of the external ear and evaluation of hearing and balance. If the patient's hearing impairment is severe, determine the usual means of communication. It may be necessary to call on a family member or a sign language interpreter or to use written communication during the assessment.

History of Present Illness

Obtain a full description of any symptoms that may reflect problems with the ear, including changes in hearing acuity, pain, tinnitus, dizziness, vertigo, nausea, vomiting, and problems with balance. Record changes in hearing acuity, including the kind of change that occurred and whether it was sudden or gradual. Ask the patient to describe the nature of the pain (e.g., sharp, throbbing, dull) and when it occurs. Pain in the ear is called ***otalgia.*** If **tinnitus** (ringing in the ears) is present, ask if the sound heard is continuous or intermittent. Assess the presence of dizziness, vertigo, nausea, and vomiting, and the circumstances under which they occur. Also describe any problems with balance.

Past Medical History

Ask about any previous acute or chronic ear problems. Acute conditions that may affect hearing or balance include sinus infections, dental problems, allergies, and upper respiratory infections. Chronic conditions that may be significant are hypertension, diabetes mellitus, and hypothyroidism. Note recent surgical procedures on the ear or throat, as well as a recent head injury.

Hearing impairments are often congenital (present at birth). One cause of hearing loss in an infant is rubella during the mother's pregnancy. Therefore, assess whether female patients have had rubella or have been immunized for the infection.

The medication history is important to identify any drugs taken that might be ototoxic. The term ***ototoxic*** means a drug can damage the eighth cranial nerve or the organs of hearing and balance. Examples of drugs that can have ototoxic effects are aspirin and aminoglycoside antibiotics. Ototoxicity is discussed more fully later. Also note a family history of hearing loss.

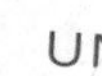

table 50-1 ASSESSMENT *of Patients with Disorders of the Ear, Hearing, and Balance*

HEALTH HISTORY	PHYSICAL EXAMINATION
Present Illness: Changes in the external ear, hearing acuity, or balance **Past Medical History:** Sinus infections, dental problems, allergies, upper respiratory infections, hypertension, diabetes mellitus, hypothyroidism, surgery on ear or throat, recent head injury, rubella and rubella immunization, recent and current medications **Family History:** Hearing impairments **Review of Systems:** Pain in ear or throat, tinnitus, dizziness, vertigo, nausea, vomiting **Functional Assessment:** Exposure to excessively loud noise, use of hearing aid	**General Survey:** Response to normal voice, gait, posture, and balance **External Ear:** Position of auricles; lesions, tenderness, or nodules **Lymph Nodes:** Enlargement of lymph nodes in front of or behind ear **Mastoid:** Tenderness **External Auditory Canal:** Obstruction, lesions, drainage **Tympanic Membrane:** Redness, bulging

PHARMACOLOGY CAPSULE Some drugs including aspirin are ototoxic. Signs and symptoms of ototoxicity are tinnitus, hearing loss, dizziness, and ataxia.

Functional Assessment

In the functional assessment, determine exposure to excessively loud noise such as amplified music, firearms being used, or noisy machinery. Record the use of any assistive hearing devices.

PHYSICAL EXAMINATION

Some general observations of the patient give important clues about hearing and balance. Observe how the patient responds to a normal voice. Patients who do not hear well use many adaptive behaviors. They may turn a good ear toward the speaker, ask people to repeat things, say "what?" frequently, or watch the speaker's mouth closely. Note the presence of a visible hearing aid. Observe the patient's posture and balance while walking and sitting.

External Ear

Assess the position of the auricles. Normally, the top of the auricle is at approximately the level of the eye. The ears should be positioned symmetrically. Inspect the auricles' shape, lesions, and nodules. The auricles and the mastoid process are palpated for tenderness. Palpation in front of, below, and behind the ear may locate enlarged lymph nodes.

External Auditory Canal

Use a penlight to inspect the outer portion of the external auditory canal. Inspect the canal for any obvious obstructions or drainage. The only normal secretion in the canal is cerumen. It should be golden to brown in color and should not block the opening to the canal. If there is any drainage, record the color, amount, and odor.

Some nurses are taught to use an otoscope to inspect the external canal and the tympanic membrane. The tympanic membrane should be shiny and pearl-gray. The nursing assessment is outlined in Table 50-1.

DIAGNOSTIC TESTS AND PROCEDURES

Several specialists handle different aspects of the diagnosis and treatment of hearing disorders. An otologist is trained to diagnose types of hearing loss. An audiologist carries out tests to determine whether a hearing aid will help a particular patient. If it is thought that a patient would benefit from a hearing aid, the audiologist also identifies the best kind of hearing aid. An otolaryngologist is a physician who specializes in diseases of the ears and throat.

Procedures and tests commonly used to diagnose disorders of the ear, hearing, and balance include the otoscopic examination, audiometry, the caloric test, electronystagmography, hearing acuity tests, and tuning fork tests. Radiographic examinations, especially the computed tomographic (CT) scan, may be used to study the mastoid bone, middle ear, and inner ear.

Diagnostic tests and procedures for patients with disorders of the ear, hearing, and balance are described in Table 50-2.

OTOSCOPIC EXAMINATION

The otoscope is the instrument used to examine the external auditory canal. The purpose of the otoscopic examination is to inspect the external auditory canal and tympanic membrane. The examination permits diagnosis of inflammatory and infectious processes as well as obstructions of the external canal.

When using an otoscope, you should:

1. Use the largest speculum that fits the ear canal easily.
2. For adult patients, pull the auricle up and back to straighten the canal, and then guide the speculum gently into the canal.
3. Steady the otoscope by resting the little finger against the patient's head, as illustrated in Figure 50-4.
4. Never force the speculum into the ear.
5. If the patient is unable to cooperate, have someone hold the head still during the examination.
6. Clean the speculum between patients and between ears on each patient.

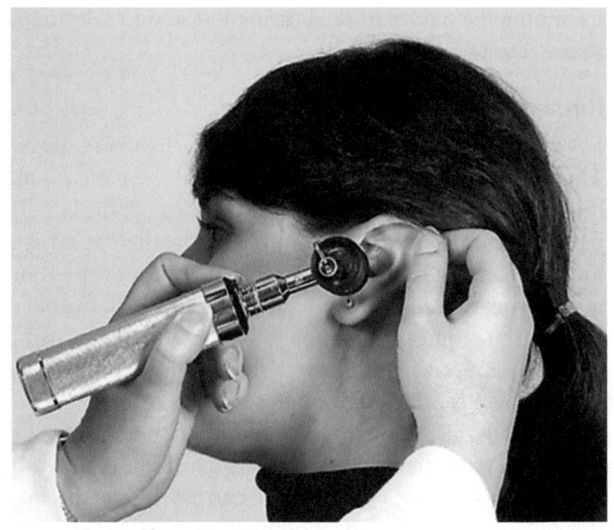

FIGURE **50-4** Correct technique for using an otoscope to examine the external auditory canal and the tympanic membrane. The adult auricle is pulled up and back; the examiner's hand is stabilized against the patient's face.

table 50-2 **DIAGNOSTIC TESTS AND PROCEDURES** | ***Disorders of the Ear, Hearing, and Balance***

TEST/PURPOSE	PATIENT PREPARATION	POSTPROCEDURE NURSING CARE
AUDIOMETRY		
Pure tone audiometry tests Detect hearing impairment by assessing the patient's ability to hear a range of sounds.	Tell the patient test will be conducted in a sound-isolated room. The examiner will place earphones on the patient and introduce tones. The patient will be asked to identify when sounds are heard and when they disappear. A tuning fork will be placed near the patient's ear, and the patient is asked when vibrating sound is heard and when it ceases. No other preparation is needed.	No special postprocedure care.
Speech audiometry Measures the ability to hear spoken words.	The patient will listen to simple words through earphones and repeat the words that are understood. No special preparation.	No special postprocedure care.
VESTIBULAR TESTS		
Caloric test The ears are irrigated with warm or cool water to assess for dizziness. Dizziness is consistent with a diagnosis of Meniere's disease.	Tell the patient that the ears will be irrigated to assess for dizziness. Tell the examiner if the patient has had central nervous system depressants, alcohol, or barbiturates because they alter test response. The examiner will then observe the patient for nystagmus, nausea, vomiting, or dizziness.	Assess for nausea. Offer small amounts of clear liquids at first. Safety measures if dizzy.
Electronystagmography Used to detect lesions in the vestibule.	Nothing by mouth for 3 hr before the test. Take eyeglasses to the test. Withhold medications as ordered. Tell the patient electrodes will be placed around the eyes, and he/she will be asked to focus on specific targets. The ears are irrigated and the patient is turned in various positions in a special chair.	Assess for nausea. Offer small amounts of clear fluids at first. Safety precautions if dizzy.

The appearance of the normal tympanic membrane is illustrated in Figure 50-5.

AUDIOMETRY

Audiometry is the assessment of the ability to hear simple sound waves. It requires a machine called an *audiometer.* Special training is needed to use the audiometer and to interpret test results. Nurses in some work settings learn to do these tests. The patient needs no special preparation for this test.

CALORIC TEST

The caloric test is used to diagnose disorders in the vestibular system or its central nervous system connections. The ear is irrigated with warm or cold water, and the patient is observed for reactions that suggest vestibular problems. A person with

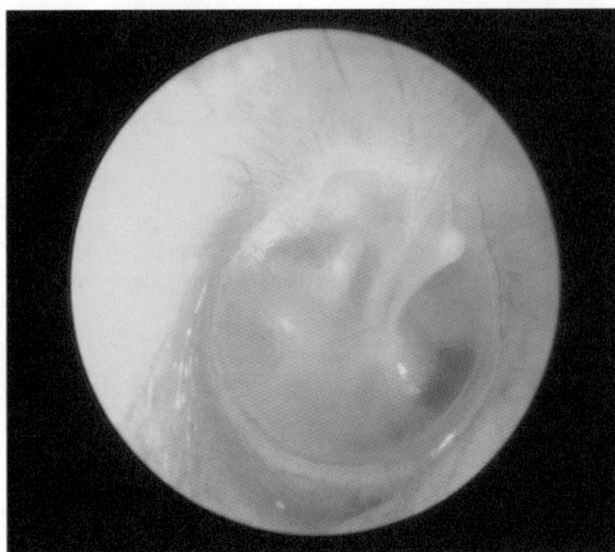

FIGURE **50-5** Normal appearance of the tympanic membrane through the otoscope.

a labyrinth disorder responds with specific abnormal eye movements (nystagmus), vertigo, and nausea and vomiting. A person with vestibular disease has a decreased or absent response to the test.

Test results are altered by central nervous system depressants, barbiturates, and alcohol. Inform the examiner if the patient has had any of these drugs before the examination.

ELECTRONYSTAGMOGRAPHY

Electronystagmography is used to detect lesions in the vestibule. Electrodes are placed around the eyes, and eye movements are measured as the patient focuses on specific targets, has the ears irrigated with warm and cool water, and is rotated and turned upside down.

The patient is usually allowed nothing by mouth for 3 hours before the test. Medications may be withheld on the physician's directions. Patients who normally wear eyeglasses are instructed to bring them to the test. After the test, the patient may report nausea and may vomit. If the patient is dizzy, take appropriate safety precautions.

HEARING ACUITY TESTS

Audiometry gives a precise measurement of hearing acuity. Other simple tests can be done by the nurse for a gross assessment of hearing. The whisper test can easily be done in any setting. Stand 1 to 2 feet from the patient, facing away from him or her. Have the patient occlude the ear on the opposite side. Exhale and then speak in a low whisper. Ask the patient to tell you what was whispered. The words can be repeated louder until the patient is able to hear them. After assessing one ear, change sides and assess the other ear. This simple test gives you an idea about the patient's general hearing ability.

TUNING FORK TESTS

Rinne's and Weber's tests use a tuning fork to assess the conduction of sound by air and by bone. These are useful in determining the nature of the hearing loss and in selecting the best treatment.

Rinne's Test

For Rinne's test, tap the tuning fork on the hand to activate it. Then place the base of the tuning fork on the patient's mastoid bone. If the vibration is conducted through the bone, the patient hears a humming sound. When the sound is no longer heard, move the fork so that the tines of the tuning fork are near but not touching the ear canal. Ask the patient if he or she can hear the sound and, if so, to report when the sound disappears. This assesses the patient's ability to hear sound waves conducted through the air.

Normally, air conduction is better than bone conduction. Therefore, the patient should be able to hear the sound transmitted through air even after it can no longer be heard through bone. This normal finding is recorded as "AC > BC" (air conduction is greater than bone conduction). If bone conduction is greater than air conduction, the patient has a conductive hearing loss.

Weber's Test

In Weber's test, place the base of an activated tuning fork on the midline of the skull. Ask the patient to identify the side in which the sound is loudest. With normal hearing in both ears, the sound is heard equally on each side. The sound is louder in an ear with conductive hearing loss and softer in an ear with sensorineural hearing loss.

COMMON THERAPEUTIC MEASURES

Problems of the ear and related structures sometimes require medications or surgery. Other therapeutic measures for problems of the ear include irrigations and the use of hearing aids. You may encounter patients who are being treated by any of these measures.

EAR DROPS

Medications intended to be placed directly into the external ear canal are called otic drops, or simply ear drops. Ear drops may be ordered to treat infection or inflammation, to reduce pain, or to soften earwax. When administering ear drops, keep the following points in mind:

1. Be sure to use an *otic* solution.
2. Warm the drops to body temperature by rolling the bottle between the palms.
3. Have the patient tilt the head so that the ear to be treated is positioned toward you.
4. Straighten the external auditory canal of an adult by pulling the auricle up and back. For a child, the auricle is pulled down and back.
5. Hold the dropper at the opening of the canal, but do not contaminate the tip by touching the skin.
6. Instruct the patient to keep the treated ear up for several minutes to keep the medication from leaking from the ear. Sometimes the physician orders a cotton ball to be placed loosely in the canal to keep the medicine in place.

Examples of commonly used otic medications are listed in Table 50-3.

PHARMACOLOGY CAPSULE Medications intended to be administered into the external ear are called otic drugs.

IRRIGATION

Irrigation is the use of a solution to cleanse the external ear canal or to remove something from the canal. A common indication for irrigation is impacted cerumen. Impacted cerumen is dried earwax that blocks the canal. The nurse may perform the irrigation, if agency policy permits, or may assist with the procedure. The following key points should be remembered when irrigating an ear:

1. Select the correct solution as ordered by the physician.
2. Warm the solution to body temperature (95° F to 105° F).
3. Have the patient sit up and hold an emesis basin under the ear to be irrigated.
4. Drape the shoulder under the basin.
5. Straighten the external canal of an adult by pulling the auricle up and back. For a child, pull the auricle down and back.
6. Select an irrigating syringe or bulb syringe with a tip that is smaller than the canal.
7. Direct the solution toward the top of the canal in a steady stream. The procedure can be repeated several times if needed.
8. Sometimes ear drops are ordered to soften impacted cerumen before irrigating.
9. Describe any substances rinsed out of the ear. If the impacted cerumen or foreign body does not wash out, inform the physician.
10. If the tympanic membrane (eardrum) is ruptured, the canal should *not* be irrigated because fluid could be forced into the middle ear.

HEARING AIDS

A hearing aid is a device that amplifies sound, that is, it makes sound louder. People with conductive hearing loss benefit the most from using a hearing aid. Those who have sensorineural or mixed losses may experience some benefit, but often not as much.

All hearing aids have four components: (1) a microphone to receive sound waves and convert them to electrical signals, (2) an amplifier to strengthen the signals, (3) a receiver to convert signals to sound waves, and (4) a battery to power the device. Various aids are designed to be worn in the ear, behind the ear, or in the middle of the chest. The device worn in the middle of the chest ("body hearing aid") is the most powerful. It consists of a wire that connects the ear speaker to an amplifier and battery worn on the body (Fig. 50-6).

The two basic types of hearing aids are bone conduction receivers and air conduction receivers. Bone conduction receivers are worn behind the ear against the skull. Air conduction receivers are worn in the external canal. An audiologist determines which type a patient needs.

Modern hearing aids use transistors, which allow the device to be very small. The hearing aid requires some care. Wash the ear mold (the part that fits into the ear) daily with soap and water and then dry it. When it is not being worn, turn the aid off and store it in a protective case with the battery compartment open. Keep extra batteries on hand.

If the hearing aid is not working, first check to be sure it is turned on. If it is on, check the ear mold to see if it needs cleaning. The next step is to check battery placement. If the battery is not inserted correctly, the hearing aid will not work. If the hearing aid has a cord, check it to see if it is broken or unplugged. If these checks fail to locate the problem, change the battery. If a new battery does not correct the problem, the cord can be changed. Should the hearing aid still not work, return it to the dealer for service.

Nurses and other health care providers need to be familiar with hearing aids and how they work. The patient's nursing care plan should indicate that the patient usually wears a hearing aid. Confusion in some older patients might be avoided if the hearing aid were kept in place. The cost of hearing aids can range from several hundred to several thousand dollars if both ears are involved. When patients are hospitalized, take care to prevent loss of these devices.

It may take considerable persuasion from family and health care providers to get a hearing-impaired person to try a hearing aid. It may be helpful to point out the benefits of improved hearing in the patient's everyday life.

Hearing aids amplify all sounds, including background noise. This is especially annoying when a person first tries to use an aid. Patients are advised to wear the aid first in quiet settings. Once they learn to adjust the volume and tone comfortably, they can try it in noisy settings. It may take several months before a hearing aid feels comfortable.

COCHLEAR IMPLANTS

A cochlear implant may be recommended for people who cannot benefit from regular hearing aids. A cochlear implant has variable results for the profoundly deaf. Some can hear well enough to understand speech on a telephone; others can hear only environmental sounds, such as sirens, doorbells, and telephones.

The cochlear implant consists of a microphone, a processor, a transmitter, and a receiver. The microphone, at ear level, picks up sounds that are amplified by the processor (Fig. 50-7). The sound, in the form of magnetic signals, is transmitted electronically to the receiver. The receiver is surgically implanted behind the ear. Electrodes attached to the receiver stimulate nerve fibers in the cochlea to produce sound. Several months of training are needed to learn to tell sounds apart. Therefore, candidates for the cochlear implant must be highly motivated and carefully screened.

TEMPORAL BONE STIMULATORS

Patients with conductive hearing loss may benefit from a temporal bone stimulator. A receiver is implanted into the skull. An external device, worn above the ear, transmits sound through the skin to the receiver. This device is not widely used.

table 50-3 **DRUG THERAPY | *Disorders of the Ear, Hearing, and Balance***

DRUG	USE/ACTION	SIDE EFFECTS	NURSING INTERVENTIONS
ANTIBIOTICS			
Chloramphenicol (Chloromycetin Otic)	Broad-spectrum antibiotic used to treat infections of lining of external auditory canal.	Hypersensitivity: redness, rash, swelling, burning, pain.	If patient shows signs of hypersensitivity, withhold drug and notify physician.
TOPICAL CORTICOSTEROIDS			
Hydrocortisone combined with neomycin sulfate and polymyxin B (Cortisporin Otic, Otocort) Polymyxin B (Otobiotic Otic) Neomycin and colistin (Coly-Mycin S Otic)	Treat inflammation, pruritus, and allergic response. Usually combined with antibacterial or antifungal drug.		Do not put in ear if tympanic membrane is perforated. Caution to avoid eye contact.
ANTIBACTERIAL AND SOFTENING AGENTS			
Carbamide peroxide with glycerin (Debrox, Murine Ear Drops)	Soften earwax. Treat aphthous ulcers.	Redness, irritation, superinfection.	Contraindications: ear surgery, perforated tympanic membrane; ear drainage, redness, pain, or tenderness. Teach patient not to clean ear with cotton swabs, which force wax deeper into ear.
DRYING AGENTS			
Boric acid in isopropyl alcohol (Ear-Dry, Swim Ear)	Dry external canal after swimming or bathing. Decrease risk of infection.	Local irritation.	Instilled in external canal immediately after swimming or bathing. Contraindicated with perforated tympanic membrane.
ANTIEMETICS			
Scopolamine (Transderm Scop) Dimenhydrinate (Dramamine) Diphenhydramine (Benadryl) Meclizine (Antivert) Chlorpromazine (Thorazine)	Prevent or treat nausea, vomiting, motion sickness	Sedation, drowsiness, tremor, fever, tachycardia, hypotension, constipation, dry mouth.	Safety precautions for drowsiness. Monitor pulse and blood pressure. Monitor stools and urinary output. Mouth care.

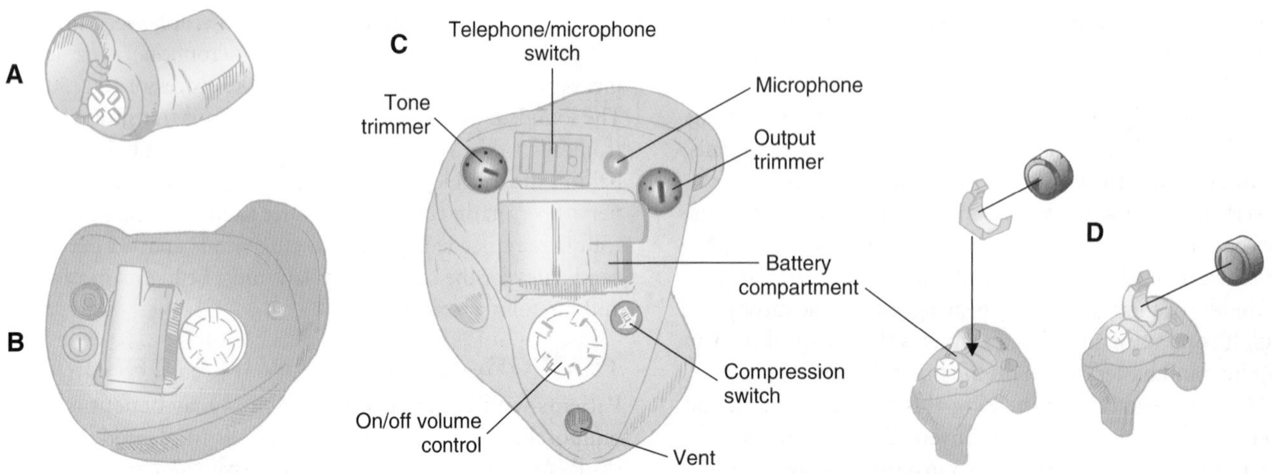

FIGURE **50-6** Types of hearing aids and components. *A,* In-the-canal aid. *B,* In-the-ear aid. *C,* Hearing aid components. *D,* Battery compartment.

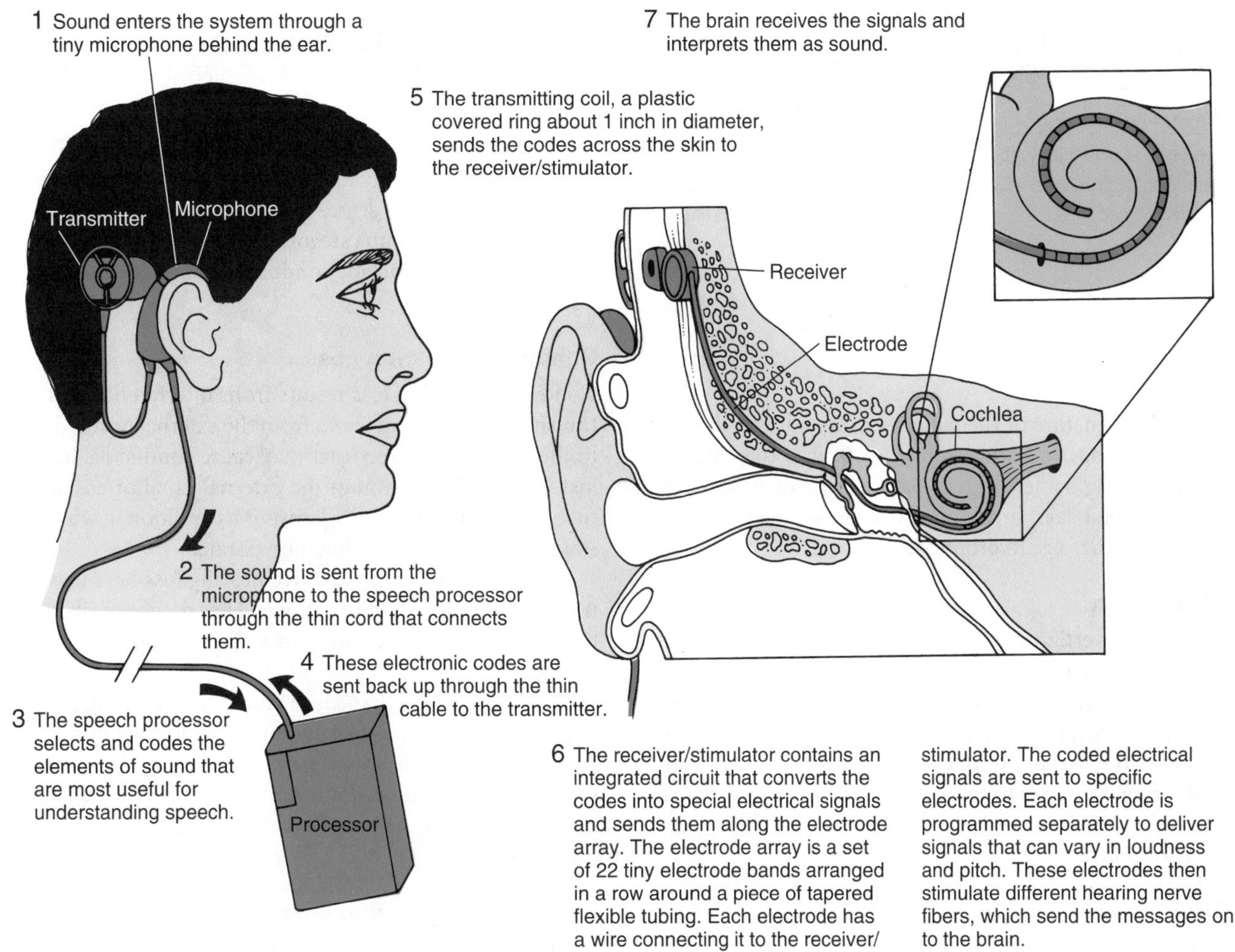

1 Sound enters the system through a tiny microphone behind the ear.
Transmitter
Microphone
2 The sound is sent from the microphone to the speech processor through the thin cord that connects them.
3 The speech processor selects and codes the elements of sound that are most useful for understanding speech.
Processor
4 These electronic codes are sent back up through the thin cable to the transmitter.
5 The transmitting coil, a plastic covered ring about 1 inch in diameter, sends the codes across the skin to the receiver/stimulator.
Receiver
Electrode
Cochlea
6 The receiver/stimulator contains an integrated circuit that converts the codes into special electrical signals and sends them along the electrode array. The electrode array is a set of 22 tiny electrode bands arranged in a row around a piece of tapered flexible tubing. Each electrode has a wire connecting it to the receiver/stimulator. The coded electrical signals are sent to specific electrodes. Each electrode is programmed separately to deliver signals that can vary in loudness and pitch. These electrodes then stimulate different hearing nerve fibers, which send the messages on to the brain.
7 The brain receives the signals and interprets them as sound.

FIGURE **50-7** Cochlear implant to restore hearing.

SURGERY ON THE EAR AND RELATED STRUCTURES

Many ear disorders are treated surgically. Nursing care of patients having specific surgical procedures is discussed with the appropriate pathophysiologic process. However, some general measures apply to most patients after surgery on the ear.

NURSING CARE *of the Patient Having Ear Surgery*

Before surgery, assess the patient's understanding of the procedure and surgical routine as well as the anxiety level. Deficient Knowledge and Anxiety are typical nursing diagnoses. Supply needed information about the preoperative and postoperative routines. If the patient is anxious, explore the specific concerns. Sometimes patient teaching and reassurance are sufficient to reduce anxiety. Notify the physician if the patient is very anxious.

Immediate preoperative care usually includes having the patient remove any articles such as eyeglasses or hearing aids. The hearing-impaired person going to surgery may feel very helpless without the hearing aid. Notify the operating room staff and ask if the patient can wear the hearing aid to the surgical suite. Place a note on the front of the chart to alert caregivers of the patient's hearing impairment and to the presence of a hearing aid.

Assessment

In the postoperative period, assess the patient for pain, nausea, dizziness, and fever. Inspect the wound dressing for drainage. Document drainage color, odor, and amount.

Nursing Diagnoses, Goals, and Outcome Criteria: Ear Surgery, Postoperative

Nursing Diagnoses	Goals and Outcome Criteria
Acute Pain related to tissue trauma or edema	Pain relief: patient states pain is relieved; relaxed manner
Risk for Injury related to dizziness or vertigo, fluid accumulation, pressure in the ear	Decreased risk for injury: maintains prescribed position, avoids behavior that increases pressure Absence of injury: patient has no falls
Risk for Infection related to surgical incision	Healing without infection: normal body temperature and white blood cell count

Nursing Diagnoses, Goals, and Outcome Criteria: Ear Surgery, Postoperative—cont'd

NURSING DIAGNOSES	GOALS AND OUTCOME CRITERIA
Disturbed Sensory Perception related to packing and edema in affected ear	Effective communication: patient and nurse use effective strategies to facilitate verbal communication

Interventions

Acute Pain

Determine the nature of the patient's pain and have the patient rate the pain on a scale from 1 to 10, with 10 being the worst pain imaginable. Surgical pain usually requires analgesics for several days. In addition, use measures such as positioning and massage to promote relaxation.

Risk for Injury

Dizziness and vertigo are common after surgery on the ear. **Dizziness** is a feeling of unsteadiness, whereas **vertigo** is the sensation that one's body or the room is spinning.

Vertigo is often triggered by sudden movements, so advise the patient to move slowly and carefully. Instruct the patient to call for help when getting up the first few times. Assist as long as dizziness is a problem. Raise siderails, and leave the bed in low position.

The ear is commonly packed and covered with a dressing. A drain may be in place. The packing is removed only by the physician. A specific position may be ordered after surgery. If drainage is being encouraged, the patient is most likely positioned on the affected side. If the procedure includes a graft on the tympanic membrane, however, the patient is usually positioned on the unaffected side.

Straining is contraindicated because it increases pressure in the ear. The patient should avoid nose blowing, coughing, and sneezing; however, if these are unavoidable, the mouth should be kept open to relieve pressure. Stool softeners may be ordered to prevent constipation and straining. Ear surgery, like any other type of surgery, creates a wound that must heal. Healing requires a balanced diet with adequate protein and vitamin C.

Risk for Infection

Take measures to reduce the risk of postoperative infection. Advise the patient to avoid crowds and people with colds for several weeks. The ear canal should be kept dry for 2 to 4 weeks as instructed by the physician. Shampooing usually is not allowed for 2 weeks, although it is restricted longer in some cases.

Disturbed Sensory Perception

While the affected ear is packed, the patient's hearing in that ear is impaired. If the patient does not hear well in the unaffected ear, you must devise appropriate means of communication. It is best to plan this with the patient before surgery.

HEARING LOSS

TYPES OF HEARING LOSS

Hearing loss covers a range from inability to hear sounds of a certain pitch to inability to hear any sounds at all. Millions of Americans have some degree of hearing impairment. Hearing losses are classified into categories. The categories of hearing loss discussed here include conductive, sensorineural, mixed, and central.

Conductive Hearing Loss

Conductive hearing loss results from interference with the transmission of sound waves from the external or middle ear to the inner ear. Factors that may cause conductive hearing loss include obstruction of the external canal or eustachian tube and otosclerosis. Otosclerosis is a condition in which the stapes in the middle ear does not vibrate.

Patients who have conductive hearing loss hear better in noisy settings than in quiet settings. They do not speak loudly because bone conduction allows them to hear their own voices.

Most conditions that cause conductive hearing loss are treatable. Obstructions usually can be removed. Otosclerosis can be treated surgically with a procedure called a stapedectomy. This condition is discussed in more detail later. Hearing aids are usually helpful for patients with conductive hearing loss.

Sensorineural Hearing Loss

Sensorineural hearing loss is sometimes called *nerve deafness.* It is a disturbance of the neural structures in the inner ear or the nerve pathways to the brain. Sensorineural hearing loss may be congenital, but it also can be caused by noise trauma, aging, Meniere's disease, ototoxicity, diabetes, and syphilis.

Patients with sensorineural hearing loss can hear sounds but have difficulty understanding speech. They often complain that speech sounds muffled. This type of hearing loss is not as easily corrected. Hearing aids may help by amplifying the sound, but it still sounds muffled.

Mixed Hearing Loss

Mixed hearing loss is a combination of conductive and sensorineural losses. Treatment of any reversible problems often results in improvement of mixed hearing loss.

Central Hearing Loss

Central hearing loss is due to some problem in the central nervous system. The patient either cannot perceive or cannot interpret sounds that are heard.

SIGNS AND SYMPTOMS

Most hearing loss progresses over time. Patients may not readily recognize the losses. They may complain that their hearing is fine but that others are mumbling. There are many behaviors that should lead the nurse to suspect hearing loss. The patient may lean toward the speaker or turn one ear toward the speaker. The patient with a hearing loss may fail to follow directions, speak while others are speaking, or turn the radio or television up very loud. Irritability and even hostility are not unusual. Some people become very suspicious of others because they cannot hear what others are saying. Hearing loss often has no other symptoms. Otalgia (ear pain), dizziness, and tinnitus (ringing in the ears) may be present with certain types of disorders.

THE IMPACT OF HEARING IMPAIRMENT

People with obvious physical disabilities usually receive some consideration and understanding from strangers. People who have hearing impairments may not be treated as well.

Those who had impairments in early childhood usually have speech difficulties. If speech is not clear, others may assume the patient is intellectually impaired. Sadly, the phrase *deaf and dumb* has been used to refer to people who neither hear nor speak. This term is understandably offensive to the hearing-impaired person. The term *deaf* is not offensive, but suggests a total inability to hear. *Hearing impairment,* on the other hand, implies a range of abilities.

It is interesting that most people accept the use of eyeglasses fairly easily, but they often are resistant to using a hearing aid. There is a tendency to deny one's hearing loss. When a person refuses to admit to a hearing loss, family members and others may stop trying to communicate. The hearing-impaired person may alienate those who would like to be close and supportive.

People with severe hearing impairment probably suffer the most severe social isolation of those with sensory disorders. Nurses can help by educating the public about hearing loss.

PATIENT TEACHING PLAN
Hearing Impaired

- Many types of hearing loss are correctable, or at least capable of being improved.
- Hearing is not related to intelligence.
- There is no reason to be ashamed of a hearing impairment.
- Some measures can be taken to reduce the risk of certain types of hearing loss.
- All women of childbearing age should be immunized for rubella to prevent one form of congenital hearing impairment.

ADAPTATIONS TO HEARING LOSS

Some hearing impairments can be corrected. If not, the patient and family need to learn to cope with the loss. For many people, hearing aids produce at least some improvement in hearing. Many patients read lips and observe body language closely to enhance understanding of spoken messages.

Sign language uses a universal set of hand signals. It provides a very effective means of communicating as long as there are others who know how to use it. Unfortunately, most nurses are not trained in this skill.

Several electronic devices are available to serve the hearing impaired. Telephones can be adapted to send and receive written messages. Earphones are readily available for use with radios, stereos, and televisions. These allow the hearing-impaired person to adjust the volume as needed. They also reduce environmental noises. Some television channels provide closed-captioned programming, in which a written script is shown on the bottom of the screen. A portable telecommunication device for the deaf makes telephone communication possible. In the home, flashing lights can be used to alert the patient to doorbells, telephone rings, and alarm clocks. For the patient who does not speak, small hand-held computers called personal communicators print out messages typed by the user.

For many years, guide dogs have been used to help people with visual impairments. A similar intervention is being used with dogs trained to assist the hearing impaired. These dogs are taught to recognize common sounds (doorbell, telephone, smoke alarm, crying baby) and to get the attention of the owner.

NURSING CARE *of the Patient with Impaired Hearing*

Assessment

Assessment of the patient with impaired hearing is summarized in Table 50-1.

Nursing Diagnoses, Goals, and Outcome Criteria: Hearing Impairments

Nursing Diagnoses	Goals and Outcome Criteria
Impaired Verbal Communication related to inability to hear	Effective communication: patient and others use alternative means of communication
Social Isolation related to inability to communicate verbally	Reduced social isolation: participation in social activities
Ineffective Coping related to change in social interaction, threat to body image, or denial	Effective coping with permanent hearing impairment: patient has satisfying social interactions, makes positive statements about self, plans realistically
Deficient Knowledge of prevention, diagnosis, and treatment of hearing impairment, and resources for adaptation	Patient knowledge of prevention and treatment: patient correctly practices preventive measures and describes treatments

Interventions

Impaired Verbal Communication

Many techniques are available to improve communication with the hearing impaired. You can use these approaches and teach others to use them as well. When working with a hearing-impaired patient, follow these guidelines:

1. Be sure the patient knows you are present. Try to move into the patient's line of vision before touching him or her.

2. Find out the patient's usual means of communication, and be sure he or she has access to any assistive devices.
3. Speak slowly and distinctly.
4. Be sure the patient can see your face clearly. Do not turn away while speaking.
5. Do not eat, smoke, or chew gum if the patient reads lips.
6. Provide adequate lighting directed *toward* your face. A strong light behind you creates a glare and makes it hard to see your features.
7. Lower your voice tone.
8. Assess the patient's ability to hear a normal voice tone. The volume can be increased a little if needed, but shouting simply distorts the message. People who wear hearing aids often complain that everyone shouts at them.
9. If the patient has a good ear, speak toward that side.
10. Amplify your voice, if necessary, by using a rolled-up sheet of paper or a stethoscope. To use the stethoscope, put the earpieces in the patient's ears and speak into the bell.
11. Help patients follow spoken messages by informing them of the topic to be addressed.
12. Use short sentences or phrases.
13. Use body language to support the verbal message.
14. Have a writing pad or magic slate available. Use it if the patient cannot understand you or if you do not understand the patient.
15. Try to validate patient understanding by encouraging feedback and assessing whether directions are followed.
16. When a hearing-impaired patient is hospitalized, be sure a call button is provided, but remind staff that the patient cannot use the intercom.

Social Isolation

The preceding guidelines may improve communication with the hearing-impaired person. The most important thing you can do, however, is to have a positive attitude toward trying to communicate with the patient. Genuine interest and attention encourage the patient to express himself or herself in whatever way is possible.

When other people seem hurried or annoyed, they discourage the patient's attempts to communicate. Some patients withdraw from social interactions. They may become isolated and depressed. Encourage the patient to learn new communication methods. Teach the patient how to use assistive devices. Information is provided about community resources for the hearing impaired. Explore the type of activities that are satisfying to the patient and encourage continued involvement. Advise the physician if the patient becomes increasingly sad or withdrawn. Counseling with a mental health professional may be suggested.

Ineffective Coping

The way people cope with hearing loss varies with the individual. Some deny the problem for as long as possible; others deliberately learn everything they can about treatments and adaptive strategies. Recognize that both of these behaviors are responses to a stressful situation. It is important to explore the patient's feelings about hearing loss. If the patient is anxious, you may use stress-reduction techniques (relaxation exercises, massage, meditation). The patient who denies hearing loss is often resistant to teaching, so he or she may not take advantage of opportunities to deal with the problem effectively.

Deficient Knowledge

Most people with hearing impairment have some hearing ability. Emphasize measures to reduce the risk of additional impairment. Advise the patient to seek prompt treatment of any symptoms of infection (fever, pain in the ear, drainage). Hearing protection is recommended in excessively noisy settings. Patients taking ototoxic drugs (e.g., aspirin) are told to contact the physician if hearing acuity worsens or tinnitus develops. If ear drops or irrigations are ordered, demonstrate the procedure and reinforce the physician's orders. Patients also need instruction in the use of hearing aids, as described in the next section.

DISORDERS AFFECTING HEARING AND BALANCE

EXTERNAL EAR AND CANAL

Foreign Bodies and Cerumen

Occasionally, foreign bodies get into the external ear canal. Most small objects can be flushed from the ear by gentle irrigation. Insects can be killed by instilling a small amount of mineral oil or alcohol. They can then be flushed from the canal. An alternative method is to hold a flashlight near the auricle. Because insects are often attracted to light, they may move out of the canal.

One of the most common causes of obstruction of the external ear canal is impacted cerumen. The patient is not always aware of the obstruction but may complain of hearing loss or tinnitus. When a large amount of hardened cerumen is present, the physician may order ear drops to soften the cerumen before irrigation. It may be necessary to repeat the procedure several times before all cerumen is removed. If the foreign body or cerumen is not removed by irrigation, the physician can use ear forceps or a cerumen spoon to remove it.

NURSING CARE *of the Patient with Impacted Cerumen*

Nurses, especially in long-term care facilities, need to inspect the ear canal routinely for impacted cerumen. The dry cerumen may be gold to dark brown. Sometimes it fills the entire canal. If both ears are affected, the patient has some degree of hearing impairment.

In this situation, the primary nursing diagnosis is **Disturbed Sensory Perception** related to obstruction of the external auditory canal. The nursing goal is restored hearing. Report the findings to the physician and carry out orders for ear drops. Irrigations may be done by the physician or the nurse if policy permits. Successful interventions are evaluated by examining the canal and documenting the absence of obstructions.

Infection and Inflammation

Infection or inflammation of the lining of the external ear canal is called *external otitis* or *swimmer's ear.* It may be caused by scratching or cleaning the ear with sharp objects. Swimming can lead to otitis by washing out protective cerumen, which leaves the lining of the external canal susceptible to injury. When infection is present, it often is caused by staphylococci or streptococci.

Signs and Symptoms

The most characteristic symptom of external otitis is pain that increases when the auricle is pulled. Other symptoms can include dizziness, fever, and drainage. Drainage may be purulent or blood tinged.

Medical Treatment

Topical antibiotics and corticosteroids are ordered to treat external otitis. If the external canal is obstructed by edema, the physician may insert an ear wick through the blocked canal. An ear wick is a long piece of gauze that extends out of the ear canal. Medication placed on the external portion of the ear wick soaks the gauze and distributes the medication in the canal. Pain is treated with aspirin or codeine. Any drainage from the ear should be treated as infected material and handled carefully.

NURSING CARE *of the Patient with External Otitis*

External otitis is typically treated on an outpatient basis, so nursing care is limited. Assessment includes inspection of the external canal and evaluation of pain. Nursing diagnoses are **Acute Pain** related to inflammation and **Deficient Knowledge** of preventive practices and treatment of external otitis. Goals of nursing care are pain relief, patient knowledge of prevention, and patient management of treatment plan.

Oral analgesics and topical corticosteroids and antibiotics are given as ordered to treat pain and to reduce inflammation and infection. Administer the prescribed drops or teach the patient to do so. Because it is awkward to put drops into one's own ear, you also may want to teach a family member how to do it. Teach patients to prevent external otitis by not using sharp instruments to clean the auditory canal and by avoiding suspected irritants such as hair spray and earphones. Advise the use of ear plugs while swimming. The physician may instruct the patient to use a drying agent (Ear-Dry) after swimming or bathing.

Criteria for effective nursing interventions are patient statement of pain relief and the patient's correct description of preventive measures and appropriate administration of prescribed medication.

Furuncle

A furuncle is an inflamed area in the external auditory canal caused by infection of a hair follicle. The area is very painful to the touch. Hearing may be impaired if swelling blocks the canal. A ruptured furuncle releases fluid that may drain from the canal. Treatment includes systemic and topical antibiotics (with an ear wick if needed). If the condition does not improve, the physician may incise and drain it. Nursing care of the patient with a furuncle is like that for external otitis.

MIDDLE EAR

Conditions of the middle ear are serious because of the risk of complications, including permanent hearing loss and involvement of the inner ear.

Otitis Media

Otitis media is an infection of the middle ear. There are several types of otitis media. Acute otitis media and chronic otitis media are sometimes called *suppurant* or *purulent otitis media* because of the presence of purulent material. In serous otitis media, sterile fluid accumulates behind the tympanic membrane. It can precede or follow acute otitis media. Adhesive otitis media may develop if fluid remains in the middle ear. It is characterized by thickening and scarring in the middle ear structures.

Acute Otitis Media

Acute otitis media usually develops with colds. Edema leads to blockage of the eustachian tubes. Fluid accumulates in the middle ear, causing painful pressure on the tympanic membrane. The tympanic membrane may rupture, resulting in scarring and subsequent hearing loss. The patient often has a fever and complains of headache. Acute otitis media is more common in children than in adults.

Medical treatment. Local and/or systemic antibiotics usually are prescribed for acute otitis media. Topical ear drops are usually combinations of antibacterials and corticosteroids given for 1 week. Prior to administering the drops, the canal should be cleared of debris. Have the patient lie on the unaffected side for a few minutes after instilling the drops to promote flow of the medication into the canal. If a wick has been placed in the canal because of swelling, apply the ear drops directly to the wick. Systemic antibacterials are necessary for generalized or severe infections. Sometimes myringotomy is performed. Myringotomy is the creation of a small opening in the tympanic membrane to reduce pressure and allow fluid to drain. If infection is eliminated, the tympanic membrane should heal without permanent damage.

Chronic Otitis Media

Chronic otitis media is characterized by hearing loss and continuous or intermittent drainage. The condition usually is not painful. On examination, the eardrum is usually perforated (ruptured) or shows signs of a healed perforation. An audiogram may detect some conductive hearing loss if the bones in the middle ear have been damaged by the chronic infection.

Possible complications of chronic otitis media include mastoiditis, meningitis, labyrinthitis, cholesteatoma, and hearing impairment.

Mastoiditis. Because the middle ear is directly connected to the air cells in the mastoid bone, infection in the middle ear can extend into the mastoid bone. And because the brain lies next to the mastoid bone, the infection can spread there as well. Signs and symptoms of mastoiditis include mastoid swelling (directly behind the ear) and soreness, headache, malaise, and an elevated white blood cell count. There may be thick, purulent drainage from the ear. Mastoiditis is very serious because it can lead to a brain abscess, meningitis (inflammation of the covering of the brain), or paralysis of the facial muscles.

Cholesteatoma. A cholesteatoma is a growth in the middle ear. When the tympanic membrane is perforated around the margin where it attaches to the ear canal, epithelial cells grow into the middle ear. The cells form a ball of tissue that grows and that may damage the facial nerve and the labyrinth. A cholesteatoma must be removed surgically.

Medical treatment. Chronic otitis media is treated with systemic antibiotics and, if the eardrum is intact, irrigations to remove debris. If the tympanic membrane does not heal, tympanoplasty may be done to repair it. The procedure may be done through the ear canal or through an incision behind the auricle. Sometimes grafts of the patient's tissue are used to repair the tear. Tissue may be taken from the external canal or the temporalis muscle. After the graft is placed, the middle ear is filled with Gelfoam, and a cotton ball is put in the external ear to hold the graft in place.

If the infection has extended to the mastoid bone, a mastoidectomy is often done at the same time. A mastoidectomy can be modified (simple) or radical. In a modified procedure, infected mastoid tissue is removed but the middle ear is left intact. In a radical mastoidectomy, all the structures in the middle ear are removed. The radical procedure is not done now as often as it was in the past.

NURSING CARE *of the Patient having Mastoidectomy*

General care of the patient having surgery on the ear is discussed earlier in this chapter. Before surgery, the emphasis is on patient teaching and reduction of anxiety. Primary considerations after surgery on the middle ear include comfort, safety, prevention of infection, and prevention of pressure on the tympanic membrane. Nursing diagnoses, goals, and interventions in relation to these problems also are described earlier. Nausea is another common problem after middle ear surgery. Keep an emesis basin nearby. The physician usually orders antiemetics to be given as needed for nausea. If the patient vomits frequently, there is a risk of deficient fluid volume. Monitor intake and output and give intravenous fluids if ordered.

The type of dressing varies. It may be small and placed over the auricle. If the surgeon entered through the mastoid bone, however, expect a large head dressing with a drain. Inspect the dressing and describe any drainage but do *not* disturb or remove the dressing.

Otosclerosis

Otosclerosis is a hereditary condition in which an abnormal growth causes the footplate of the stapes to become fixed. The fixed stapes cannot vibrate, so sound waves cannot be transmitted to the inner ear. The effect of this abnormality is a conductive hearing loss. If the disease also involves the inner ear, the patient has sensorineural hearing loss as well. The condition affects both ears but may progress faster in one ear than in the other.

Otosclerosis is most common in young white women. The onset is usually in the late teens or early twenties. During pregnancy, it progresses at a faster rate.

Signs and Symptoms

The primary symptom of otosclerosis is slowly progressive hearing loss in the absence of infection. In the early stages, the patient may report tinnitus. Rinne's test reveals bone conduction to be greater than air conduction.

Medical Treatment

Hearing aids are useful if the patient has only conductive hearing loss. The most common treatment is a surgical procedure called *stapedectomy.* The physician advises the patient of the surgical risks, including complete hearing loss, infection, prolonged vertigo, and damage to the facial nerve. Stapedectomy is done under local anesthesia. The stapes is removed and replaced with a prosthesis. A tissue graft taken from the patient is placed over the oval window. The physician puts packing in the ear canal at the completion of the stapedectomy. A small dressing is then placed over the ear. When the graft heals, hearing is restored in most patients (Fig. 50-8).

After surgery, bedrest may be ordered for several days and drugs prescribed to control nausea and vertigo. Usually, the patient is allowed to lie on the back or the unaffected side, but specific position restrictions may be ordered.

NURSING CARE *of the Patient having Stapedectomy*

Care of the patient having ear surgery is detailed earlier in this chapter. In addition to the usual preoperative teaching, tell the patient that hearing usually is worse immediately after stapedectomy but gradually improves over approximately 6 weeks.

After surgery, you should be concerned with pain relief, safety, prevention of infection, and avoidance of pressure in the ear. Nursing diagnoses, goals, and interventions related to these problems are discussed earlier. Because pressure can cause the graft to separate, it is especially important that the patient not do anything that increases pressure in the ear. After stapedectomy, nausea, vomiting, and vertigo are common.

The packing in the ear should not be disturbed. The physician removes it approximately 1 week after the surgery. After the dressing and packing are removed, the patient usually is advised to keep the ear dry for at least 2 weeks. Swimming and showering usually are not permitted for approximately 6 weeks.

The patient should avoid contact with people who have colds. A balanced diet and adequate rest are needed for tissue healing and resistance to infection. Vertigo may persist after discharge, and you must help the patient plan for assistance with activities of daily living. It is important to reinforce that hearing improvement is gradual.

INNER EAR

Labyrinthitis

Labyrinthitis is inflammation of the labyrinth. It may be acute or chronic. Acute labyrinthitis usually follows an acute upper respiratory infection, acute otitis media, pneumonia,

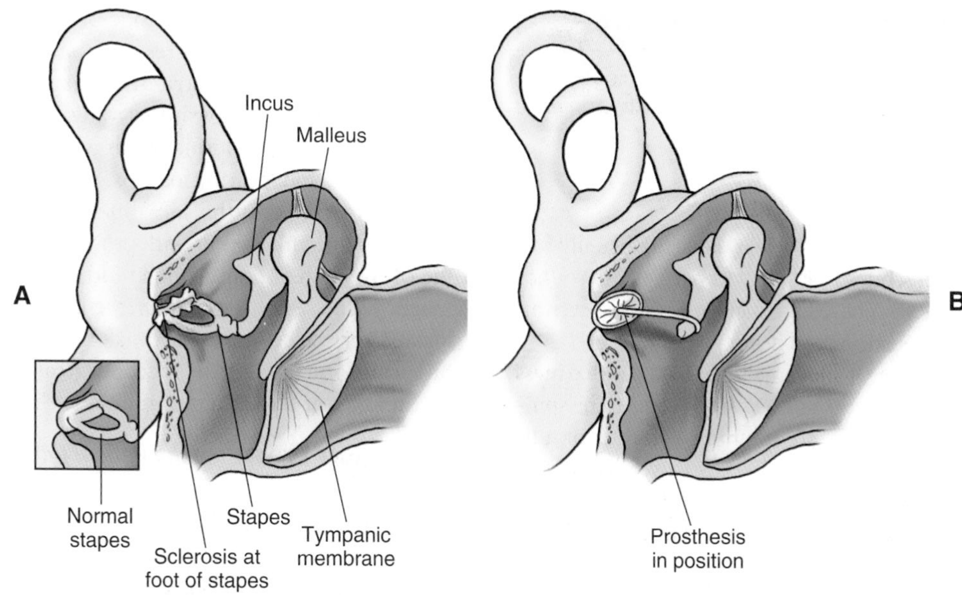

FIGURE **50-8** Otosclerosis: Before *(A)* and after *(B)* stapedectomy.

Consider the Alternative!

Caution patients who have inner ear disorders than many herbal products can cause dizziness, nausea, and vomiting. Drowsiness is another side effect of many herbals, which may enhance the sedative effects of drugs used to manage vertigo.

or influenza. It also can be an adverse effect of some drugs. One type of labyrinthitis is suppurative labyrinthitis. It is an inner ear infection that usually follows an upper respiratory infection, ear infection, or ear surgery.

Signs and Symptoms

Signs and symptoms of labyrinthitis include vertigo, nausea, vomiting, headache, and anorexia. A typical episode lasts 3 to 6 weeks. Additional symptoms of suppurative labyrinthitis are tinnitus and hearing loss.

Medical Treatment

Labyrinthitis is treated with antiemetics and supportive care until it resolves. Antibiotics are prescribed if infection is present.

NURSING CARE *of the Patient with Labyrinthitis*

During an acute episode of labyrinthitis, assess the patient's symptoms. Monitor intake and output, daily weights, and food intake if there is persistent vomiting.

Nursing Diagnoses, Goals, and Outcome Criteria: Labyrinthitis

Nursing Diagnoses	Goals and Outcome Criteria
Risk for Injury related to vertigo	Safety: absence of injury or falls
Imbalanced Nutrition: Less Than Body Requirements related to anorexia and nausea	Adequate nutrition: stable body weight
Risk for Deficient Fluid Volume related to vomiting	Adequate hydration: equal fluid intake and output, moist mucous membranes, vital signs consistent with patient norms
Anxiety related to acute illness	Reduced anxiety: patient states anxiety is reduced, calm manner

Interventions

Safety is a major concern for the patient with vertigo. Assist and supervise the patient when out of bed. Give antiemetics as prescribed for nausea and vomiting. If vomiting persists, the patient is at risk for development of fluid and electrolyte imbalances (hypokalemia, fluid volume deficit), and intravenous fluids may be needed. The patient needs reassurance that the condition resolves in time.

Meniere's Disease

Meniere's disease is a disorder of the labyrinth. More than 2 million Americans are thought to have attacks of Meniere's disease. It is most common in men older than 60 years of age. The cause is unknown, but the symptoms are related to an accumulation of fluid in the inner ear. Some things that have been found to trigger attacks include alcohol and nicotine, stress, and certain stimuli such as bright lights and sudden movements of the head.

Signs and Symptoms

Some patients with Meniere's disease have more serious symptoms than others. Acute attacks occur at regular intervals, which often can be reduced with medical treatment. During an acute attack, the classic symptoms are hearing loss and vertigo. The hearing loss is unilateral, meaning that only one ear is affected. Tinnitus accompanies acute attacks. It is heard as a low buzzing

Consider the Alternative!

Biofeedback, self-hypnosis, and relaxation techniques may be prescribed to help the patient learn to live with Meniere's disease.

sound that sometimes becomes a roar. Hearing usually improves between attacks, but some loss of low-frequency sounds may remain. Patients who have had many attacks may eventually have permanent sensorineural hearing loss.

Vertigo is a sensation of movement that causes dizziness and nausea. Patients may say that the room seems to be spinning or that they feel like they are spinning. A feeling of fullness and pressure in the ear often precedes a vertigo attack. Attacks may last several minutes to several hours. Sudden movement during an attack of vertigo can cause vomiting.

Medical Diagnosis

Diagnosis of Meniere's disease is based on the history and physical findings. The patient describes hearing and balance disturbances as described earlier. An audiogram often reveals a loss of the ability to hear low-frequency sounds. If the caloric test or electronystagmography is done, the patient with Meniere's disease has a severe attack of vertigo. A glycerol test involves audiometry testing before and after giving the patient oral glycerol (a diuretic that draws fluid from the inner ear). Improved hearing after glycerol is given suggests Meniere's disease.

Meniere's disease is actually diagnosed by ruling out other conditions that can cause similar symptoms. Therefore, the physician is likely to order a number of radiographs and other tests to detect any neurologic, allergic, or endocrine disorders.

Medical Treatment

Meniere's disease may be treated medically or surgically. Drugs prescribed during an acute attack include atropine, epinephrine, diazepam (Valium), antihistamines, antiemetics, anticholinergics, vasodilators, and diuretics. Drugs also may be prescribed between attacks in an attempt to reduce their frequency and severity.

A low-sodium diet seems to increase the length of time between attacks by reducing edema in the inner ear. If moderate sodium restriction is not effective, the patient may be put on a strict sodium-free diet. Caffeine, nicotine, and alcohol are discouraged. Vestibular rehabilitation is a series of exercises performed to help the patient develop a tolerance for vertigo. It begins with moving the eyes and the head up and down and side to side and progresses to more vigorous activity. Vestibular rehabilitation usually is taught by the physical therapist. Most patients respond positively to conservative medical treatment.

If conservative treatment fails, a procedure called *ototoxic ablation* may be done. This involves the injection through the tympanic membrane of an antibiotic that is toxic to the inner ear.

Surgical Treatment

Surgery is usually advised only when all other measures have failed. Surgical procedures work by draining excess fluid from the inner ear (endolymphatic shunt) or by cutting the part of the acoustic nerve that controls balance (vestibular nerve section). The incision may be inside or behind the ear. In general, these surgical procedures pose some risk for permanent hearing loss. More destructive surgical procedures are labyrinthotomy and labyrinthectomy.

Potential complications of surgery for Meniere's disease include infection, hearing loss, loss of cerebrospinal fluid, and damage to the seventh cranial nerve. The leakage of cerebrospinal fluid may occur with procedures that require opening of the skull. Cerebrospinal fluid is clear and thin in consistency. The seventh cranial nerve is the facial nerve that is located very close to the ear canal. It controls the movement of certain muscles of the face. Surgical procedures in and around the ear can result in trauma to the facial nerve.

NURSING CARE *of the Patient with Meniere's Disease*

Assessment

Inquire about the pattern of acute attacks (see Nursing Care Plan: The Patient with Meniere's Disease). Note substances or stimuli that trigger the episodes. Document specific symptoms including nausea, vomiting, vertigo, and tinnitus. Determine how the condition affects the patient's life, what the patient knows about the disease, and what coping mechanisms are used.

Nursing Diagnoses, Goals, and Outcome Criteria: Meniere's Disease

Nursing Diagnoses	Goals and Outcome Criteria
Risk for Injury related to vertigo	Safety: absence of falls, injuries
Risk for Deficient Fluid Volume related to vomiting	Normal hydration: equal fluid intake and output, normal vital signs, moist mucous membranes
Anxiety related to acute illness or disruption of usual lifestyle	Reduced anxiety: patient states anxiety is reduced, calm manner
Ineffective Therapeutic Regimen Management related to lack of knowledge about management of Meniere's disease	Effective therapeutic regimen management: appropriate self-care, patient correctly describes and demonstrates self-care measures

Interventions

Risk for Injury

Safety is a major concern. Attacks come on suddenly and can be dangerous in many circumstances. Fortunately, many people can recognize an aura, or peculiar feeling, that precedes an attack. They should know to seek safety promptly when an aura occurs. If driving, the patient should pull over and stop the car as soon as possible.

Risk for Deficient Fluid Volume

During an acute attack in the hospitalized patient, allow the patient to remain still because movement may trigger vomiting. Keep the room dark and quiet. Postpone nonessential care such as bathing. Promptly give medications for nausea

NURSING CARE PLAN

The Patient with Meniere's Disease

ASSESSMENT

Health History: Mr. Javier Riojas is a 62-year-old Latino who has had repeated episodes of nausea, hearing loss, and vertigo over the past year. His attacks last 2 to 3 hours, during which he is completely incapacitated. His wife brought him to the emergency department after he vomited repeatedly and seemed very weak. His health history reveals repeated urinary tract infections but no other serious illnesses or injuries. He is an accountant who has his own business.

Physical Examination: Vital signs: Oral temperature, 98° F; pulse, 88; respiration, 16; blood pressure, 136/82. Mr. Riojas appears acutely ill and unable to sit or stand. Physical findings are normal except for mild hearing loss. The physician diagnoses Meniere's disease.

Nursing Diagnosis	*Goals and Outcome Criteria*	*Interventions*
Risk for injury related to vertigo.	A safe environment will be provided: The patient will have no injuries during acute episodes.	Assist the patient to bed and allow him to remain still. Raise siderails and put the bed in low position. Place the call button in reach and caution the patient not to try to get up unassisted. Darken the room and keep it quiet. Postpone nonessential care. Provide a urinal for voiding. When the attack subsides, assist the patient out of bed until he is no longer dizzy.
Risk for deficient fluid volume related to vomiting.	The patient will be adequately hydrated as evidenced by vital signs consistent with patient's norms, moist mucous membranes, and fluid intake equal to output.	Give antiemetics and antihistamines as ordered. Provide an emesis basin. If the patient vomits, promptly empty, clean, and return the emesis basin. Administer intravenous fluids as ordered.
Anxiety related to acute illness, disruption of usual lifestyle.	The patient will state that anxiety is reduced and will appear more relaxed.	Be available, but let patient lie quietly. When the patient is able to talk, explore how the condition affects his life and how he can deal with it. Tell him that the condition can usually be improved with treatment.
Ineffective therapeutic regimen management related to lack of knowledge of condition and treatment.	The patient will describe measures to manage acute attacks and to reduce frequency of attacks.	Explain drugs to patient, including dosage, schedule, side and adverse effects, and information that should be reported to the physician. If sodium restriction is prescribed, explain that some patients benefit from the restriction. Request dietary consult if special diet ordered.

and vomiting, and keep an emesis basin close by. An intravenous infusion may be ordered to provide fluids or medications, or both. After the symptoms subside, assist the patient when getting up until dizziness goes away.

Anxiety

Patients with Meniere's disease may be anxious about the condition and the limitations it imposes. Encourage the patient to share concerns and help the patient learn how to manage the condition.

Ineffective Therapeutic Regimen Management

Interventions involve patient teaching as presented in the following box.

PATIENT TEACHING PLAN
Meniere's Disease

- You need to know prescribed medications and how to manage their side effects (provide specifics).
- Avoid alcohol and tobacco because they affect fluid in the inner ear.
- Avoid use of caffeine and decongestants.
- Avoid stimuli that tend to bring on attacks, such as noisy places and bright lights.
- Do not bend over with the head down or turn the head side to side.

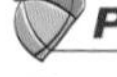

Put on your THINKING CAP!!

Think about a routine day. Consider how a person's life might be affected by frequent attacks of Meniere's disease.

POSTOPERATIVE CARE

If the patient has surgery for Meniere's disease, postoperative care depends on the exact procedure. Carefully check the physician's orders for position and activity limitations. General nursing care is concerned with safety, comfort, and detection of complications. The first few days after surgery, the patient's symptoms are usually severe. Antiemetics are ordered to control nausea and vomiting. Delay nonessential care until the patient tolerates movement. Assist patients when getting up and walking until they are able to walk steadily. The call button should always be within reach. It is not unusual for these patients to be dizzy for several days and unsteady for several weeks.

Assess for facial nerve damage by having the patient smile and show his or her teeth. If the facial nerve is damaged, the muscles on the affected side do not respond and the patient's face is not symmetric. Immediately notify the surgeon of any evidence of facial nerve damage. Nerve damage may be reversible if treated promptly.

Put on your THINKING CAP!!

Explain why patients with inner ear disorders often have problems with balance as well as with hearing.

Presbycusis

Although many older people hear very well, approximately half of those older than 75 years of age have some difficulty hearing. *Presbycusis* is the term used to describe hearing loss associated with aging. It is the result of changes in one or more parts of the cochlea. The extent of the disability depends on the location of the changes in the cochlea.

Signs and Symptoms

People with presbycusis may hear well in quiet surroundings but hear poorly in noisy places. Some patients deny that they do not hear well. They may blame others for not speaking clearly.

Medical Diagnosis and Treatment

A thorough hearing evaluation is indicated for the older person whose hearing seems to be declining. Many people have the mistaken idea that hearing loss in the elderly is inevitable and not treatable. In fact, many patients with presbycusis do benefit from hearing aids. If a hearing aid is recommended, the patient needs to learn how to use and care for it, as described earlier. Hearing aids are helpful but are not the only way to improve communication. The patient needs to be willing to tell others how they can more easily be understood. The patient also can practice and improve listening skills.

In addition to hearing aids, other electronic devices are available to improve hearing. These are described earlier and include phone amplifiers and personal earphones for radios and televisions.

NURSING CARE *of the Patient with Presbycusis*

Nursing assessment, diagnosis, goals, and interventions for the patient with impaired hearing are described earlier. In addition, nurses need to educate people about hearing loss and aging. They can also work to overcome the resistance that many people have to admitting hearing loss. Once the problem has been diagnosed, nurses can help the patient adapt and learn to use supportive devices.

Ototoxicity

Ototoxicity is damage to the ear or eighth cranial nerve caused by specific chemicals, including some drugs. Common ototoxic drugs are salicylates (aspirin) and aminoglycoside antibiotics. These and other ototoxic drugs that pose a threat to hearing are listed in Table 50-4. Ototoxicity can range from reversible tinnitus to permanent hearing loss. Hearing, balance, or both may be affected. The primary symptom of ototoxicity with salicylates is tinnitus, which disappears when the drug is discontinued. Aminoglycosides, on the other hand, can cause permanent hearing loss. The extent depends on the drug dosage and how long it was given. Patients who have poor renal function are at special risk for ototoxicity because drugs are excreted more slowly. This increases the likelihood of toxicity.

table 50-4 *Ototoxic Drugs*

ANTIBIOTICS
Aminoglycosides
Amikacin sulfate (Amikin)
Gentamicin sulfate (Garamycin)
Kanamycin sulfate (Kantrex)
Neomycin sulfate
Streptomycin sulfate
Tobramycin sulfate (Nebcin)
Erythromycin
Erythromycin estolate (Ilosone)
Erythromycin ethylsuccinate (Pediamycin)
Erythromycin stearate (Erythrocin)
Erythromycin lactobionate (Erythrocin)
Tetracycline
Minocycline (Minocin)
Miscellaneous
Vancomycin
DIURETICS
Furosemide (Lasix)
Ethacrynic acid (Edecrin)
ANTIARRHYTHMICS
Quinidine
ANTI-INFLAMMATORIES/ANALGESICS
Aspirin
Ibuprofen (Motrin)
Indomethacin (Indocin)
ANTINEOPLASTICS
Bleomycin (Blenoxane)
Cisplatin (Platinol, CDDP)
Dactinomycin (Cosmegen)
Mechlorethamine (nitrogen mustard, Mustargen)

NURSING CARE *of the Patient with Ototoxicity*

The primary nursing responsibilities are early detection and prevention of progressive hearing loss caused by ototoxic drugs. To reduce the risk of ototoxicity, be familiar with these drugs. Instruct patients to report hearing loss, tinnitus, or problems with balance. Promptly report such symptoms to the physician. Also teach patients that aspirin is not a harm-

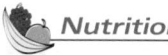

Nutrition Concepts

1. A low-salt diet is sometimes prescribed for people with Meniere's disease.

less drug. Monitor the urine output of patients on ototoxic drugs because low urine output may mean the potentially toxic drug is excreted slowly, increasing the risk of toxicity. Report low urine output to the physician. The nursing care plan should alert all staff to the potential for ototoxicity.

Disorders that impair hearing or balance can have a profound effect on a person's life and well-being. The nurse plays an important role in the prevention, early detection, and treatment of hearing and balance disturbances.

key points

- Approximately half of all adults older than 75 years of age have some hearing loss.
- Common nursing diagnoses after ear surgery include Acute Pain, Risk for Injury, Risk for Impaired Skin Integrity, Risk for Infection, and Disturbed Sensory Perception.
- Hearing losses are classified as conductive, sensorineural, mixed, or central.
- Adaptations for the hearing impaired include sign language, electronic devices, television closed captioning, personal communicators, telephones for the deaf, and trained dogs.
- Nursing care of the patient with hearing impairment addresses Impaired Verbal Communication, Social Isolation, Ineffective Coping, and Deficient Knowledge.
- Cerumen (earwax) can become impacted and obstruct the external ear canal, causing pain and hearing impairment.
- External otitis, infection and inflammation of the external ear canal, is treated with topical antibiotics and corticosteroids.
- Otitis media, infection of the middle ear, can cause permanent hearing loss and inner ear problems.
- Otosclerosis is a condition in which the stapes becomes fixed, causing a conductive and sometimes sensorineural hearing loss.
- Hearing aids are useful if the patient has only conductive hearing loss.
- The results of cochlear implants range from minimal to marked improvement.
- Labyrinthitis, which is inflammation of the labyrinth, causes vertigo and nausea and may be treated with antiemetics and antibiotics.
- Meniere's disease, characterized by attacks of hearing loss and vertigo, may be treated with drug therapy, low-sodium diet, or surgical intervention, or a combination of these.
- Nursing care of the patient with Meniere's disease may address Risk for Injury, Risk for Deficient Fluid Volume, Anxiety, and Ineffective Therapeutic Regimen Management.
- Presbycusis is hearing loss associated with aging that may be improved with a hearing aid.
- Ototoxicity is damage to the eighth cranial nerve producing effects that may range from tinnitus to permanent hearing loss.

REVIEW QUESTIONS

1. For an otoscopic examination of the external auditory canal of an adult, you should:
   1. pull the auricle straight up.
   2. pull the earlobe down.
   3. pull the auricle up and back.
   4. pull the auricle straight back.
2. During Rinne's test, a patient reports hearing the tuning fork when it is placed on the mastoid bone and when the tines are then positioned near the ear canal. How should this information be interpreted?
   1. The patient probably has an obstruction in the ear canal.
   2. The patient probably has a conductive hearing loss.
   3. The patient's response to this test is normal.
   4. The patient probably has a sensorineural hearing loss.
3. Normal age-related changes in the ears of the older adult include:
   1. increased cerumen secretion.
   2. hair in the ear canal is coarser.
   3. progressive hearing loss.
   4. increased risk of otitis media.
4. A slightly confused patient in a long-term care facility points to her ear and loudly says "I can't hear!" The patient's hearing aid appears to be positioned correctly in her ear canal. What is the *first* thing you should do?
   1. Remove the aid and clean it.
   2. Replace the battery.
   3. Turn up the volume.
   4. See if it is turned on.

5. During report it is noted that a new patient is severely hearing impaired. What is the most important question for you to ask about this patient initially?
   1. What means of communication does the patient use?
   2. Is the patient aware of the latest technology to assist the hearing impaired?
   3. Has the patient ever been hospitalized before?
   4. Why doesn't a family member stay with the patient to interpret?

6. You are preparing to administer otic drops when you notice the patient has gauze in the affected ear with a piece of narrow gauze extending from the ear. What should you do?
   1. Gently remove the packing, instill the drops, and replace the packing.
   2. Apply the drops to the narrow piece of gauze for transport into the ear.
   3. Trim the gauze so that the packing is not accidentally pulled out.
   4. Inform the registered nurse that the drops cannot be given at this time.

7. Which nursing measures are appropriate for the patient who is having an acute attack of Meniere's disease?
   1. Encourage the patient to ambulate.
   2. Advise the patient to drink additional fluids.
   3. Delay routine care until the patient is no longer dizzy.
   4. Monitor vitals every hour until stable, then every 4 hours.

8. When a patient is taking an aminoglycoside antibiotic, instructions should include:
   1. Let me know if you have any "ringing" in your ears.
   2. Check the white part of your eyes for a color change.
   3. Restrict your fluid intake to one liter each day.
   4. Change position slowly in case your blood pressure drops.

9. Stapedectomy is used to correct:
   1. sensorineural hearing loss.
   2. Meniere's disease.
   3. otosclerosis.
   4. otitis media.

10. Patients who are considering having a cochlear implant should be told:
    1. this procedure restores perfect hearing in 99% of patients.
    2. complications of cochlear implant are often disabling.
    3. results vary from minimal to excellent improvement in hearing.
    4. cochlear implants cannot enable you to discriminate speech.

CHAPTER 51

Nose, Sinus, and Throat Disorders

objectives

1. Describe the nursing assessment of the nose, sinuses, and throat.
2. Identify nursing responsibilities for patients undergoing tests or procedures to diagnose disorders of the nose, sinuses, or throat.
3. Describe the nurse's role when the following common therapeutic measures are instituted: administration of topical medications, irrigations, humidification, suctioning, tracheostomy care, and surgery.
4. Explain the pathophysiology, signs and symptoms, complications, and medical or surgical treatment of selected disorders of the nose, sinuses, and throat.
5. Assist in developing nursing care plans for patients with disorders of the nose, sinuses, or throat.

key terms

Aerosol (ĀR-ō-sŏl, p. 1099)
Allergen (ĂL-ĕr-jĕn, p. 1104)
Antihistamine (ăn-tĭ-HĪS-tă-mēn, p. 1104)
Coryza (kō-RĪ-ză, p. 1105)
Decongestant (dē-kŏn-JĔS-tănt, p. 1099)
Epistaxis (ĕp-ĭ-STĂK-sĭs, p. 1106)
Laryngectomy (lăr-ĭn-JĔK-tō-mē, p. 1112)
Laryngitis (lăr-ĭn-JĪ-tĭs, p. 1110)
Polyp (PŎL-ĭp, p. 1104)
Rhinitis (rī-NĪ-tĭs, p. 1104)
Sinusitis (sī-nŭ-SĪ-tĭs, p. 1103)
Tonsillitis (tŏn-sĭ-LĪ-tĭs, p. 1108)

The nose and throat provide passageways to the respiratory and digestive tracts. In addition, they provide routes for drainage of the sinuses and are essential for normal voice production.

Many common conditions affect the nose, sinuses, and throat. Most are not life-threatening, but they can cause considerable aggravation and loss of productivity. The most serious conditions of the nose, sinuses, and throat are hemorrhage and malignancy.

ANATOMY AND PHYSIOLOGY OF THE NOSE, SINUSES, AND THROAT

NOSE

The nose can be divided into internal and external sections. The external nose is made up of bone, cartilage, and mucous membrane. Only the upper one third of the external nose has a bony skeleton. The remainder is shaped by cartilage.

The internal nose is divided by the nasal septum, a thin wall that creates two passages. The openings on each side of the septum are the nares. The outermost portion of the internal nose, called the *vestibule,* is covered by skin that contains nasal hairs. The rest of the interior is lined with mucous membrane. The internal nose is well supplied with blood by branches of the internal and external carotids.

A layer of mucus covers the membrane. The mucus traps inspired particles and moisturizes dry air. Mucus also protects the airway because it is acidic and contains an enzyme that destroys most bacteria. Cilia sweep particles that are trapped in the mucus toward the throat to be swallowed.

Olfactory cells line the roof of the nasal cavity. These are specialized sensory cells that detect odors and relay information about odors to the brain by way of the first cranial nerve (the olfactory nerve).

The side walls of the internal nose have folds of tissue called *turbinates.* Turbinates are projections that increase the surface area that inspired air crosses. As air swirls over the turbinates, it is quickly warmed to body temperature. The turbinates also contain openings through which secretions drain from the sinuses.

SINUSES

The sinuses are spaces in the bones of the skull. They are lined with mucous membrane and filled with air. The sinuses produce mucus that drains into the nasal cavity. They also act as sound chambers for the voice, and they reduce the weight of the skull. The sinuses around the nose are called the paranasal sinuses. They include the maxillary, frontal, ethmoid, and sphenoid sinuses. There are pairs of sinuses on either side of the face (Fig. 51-1).

THROAT

The throat, or pharynx, extends from the back of the nasal cavities to the esophagus. It provides passageways from the

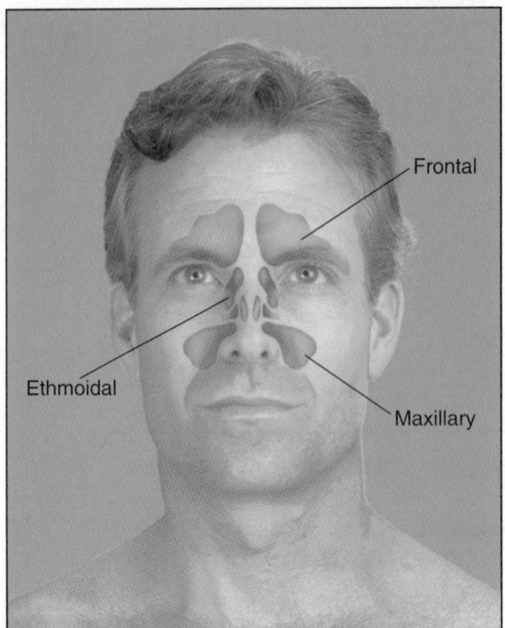

FIGURE 51-1 The paranasal sinuses.

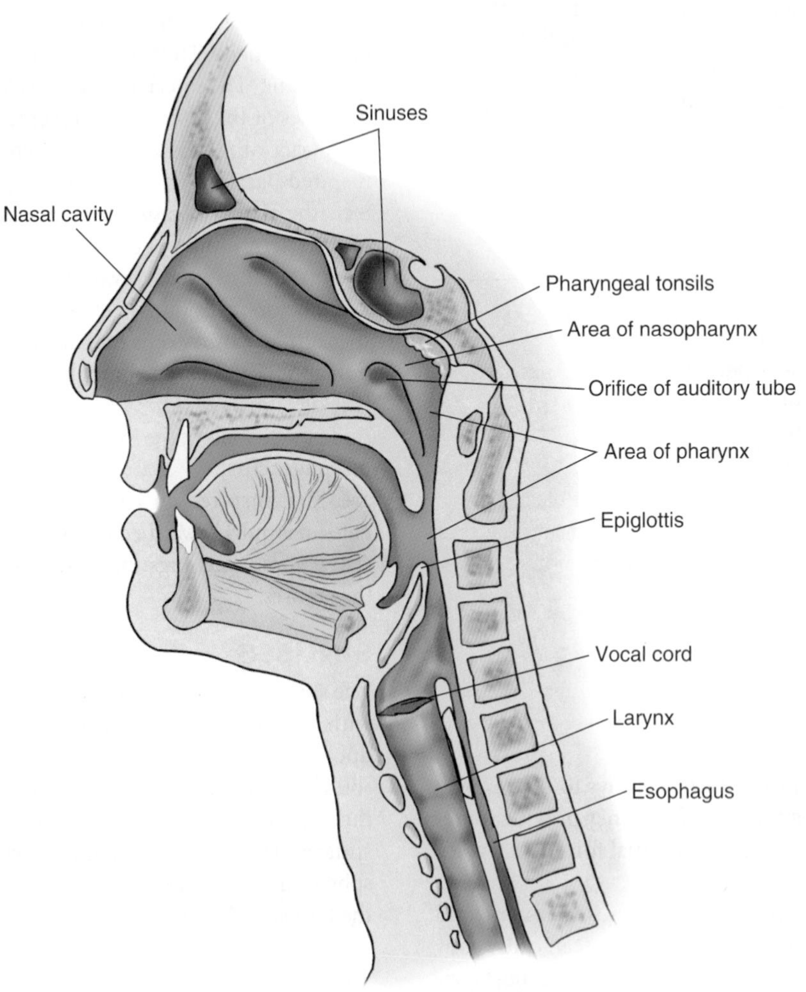

FIGURE 51-2 The nose and throat.

nose and mouth to the digestive and respiratory tracts. Figure 51-2 illustrates the structures in the throat.

The eustachian tubes that originate in the middle ear open into the nasopharynx. These tubes serve as pressure vents to prevent excessive pressure from building up in the middle ear.

Other important structures in the throat are the tonsils and adenoids. Tonsils and adenoids are masses of lymphatic tissue that guard against bacterial invasion of the respiratory and digestive tracts.

The larynx is the passageway between the throat and the trachea. The larynx is commonly referred to as the *voice box.* Two bands of tissue, the vocal cords, stretch across the interior of the larynx. The cords tighten and relax, producing different pitch sounds, as air moves through them. The sounds produced are modified and refined by the oral, nasal, and sinus cavities.

The epiglottis lies on top of the larynx. It is a flap that works like a trapdoor, closing during swallowing to prevent food and fluid from entering the airway.

NURSING ASSESSMENT OF THE NOSE, SINUSES, AND THROAT

HEALTH HISTORY

Chief Complaint and History of Present Illness

Patients often seek medical attention for symptoms that affect the nose, sinuses, and throat. Among the common complaints might be "runny nose," sore throat, hoarseness, and headache. You can aid in diagnosing and evaluating these conditions by recording a detailed description of the patient's complaints.

Past Medical History

The past medical history should assess previous streptococcal infection; sinus infections; surgery on the nose, sinuses, or throat; known allergies; and current and recent medications.

Review of Systems

The review of systems assesses for the presence of nasal discharge (amount, color), obstruction, bleeding, sneezing, snoring, throat pain or soreness, hoarseness, aphonia (loss of voice), and earache. Also note an altered sense of smell and the presence of facial pain.

PHYSICAL EXAMINATION

The nurse's examination of the nose and sinuses is usually confined to inspection of the external nose and palpation over the paranasal sinuses. Inspect the external nose for size, shape, color, and lesions. If any drainage is present, observe the amount, color, and consistency. Listen for any abnormal breath sounds and note whether the patient is breathing through the nose or the mouth. Assess patency of the nostrils by gently closing one naris at a time and instructing the patient to breathe through the other naris.

The sinuses are assessed indirectly. Palpation over the frontal and maxillary sinuses may reveal tenderness or pain. Transillumination is a procedure in which a special light is shone into the patient's mouth. The amount of light reflected through the sinuses reveals whether the cavities are filled with air, as they should be, or with fluid.

Examination of the throat is primarily an inspection of the throat at the back of the oral cavity. Inspect the mucous membranes and the tonsils for redness, swelling, drainage, and lesions. Inspection and palpation of the neck may reveal enlarged lymph nodes.

Additional physical examination may be done by the physician or a nurse with advanced preparation. A nasal speculum and a lighted scope are used to observe the mucosa of the nasal cavity. Observations should include color, drainage, and the presence of foreign bodies. The sense of smell is assessed by asking the patient to identify common scents like coffee and rubbing alcohol. Assessment of the nose, sinuses, and throat is summarized in Table 51-1.

table 51-1 ASSESSMENT *of the Nose, Sinuses, and Throat*

HEALTH HISTORY

Chief Complaint and History of Present Illness: Nasal discharge, obstruction, bleeding; upper airway symptoms: sneezing, snoring; pain or soreness in the throat or face; change in voice; earache

Past Medical History: Allergies, medications, history of streptococcal infections

Review of Systems: Amount and color of nasal discharge; nasal obstruction; blood in nasal discharge or sputum; sneezing; snoring; throat pain or soreness; hoarseness; earache; altered sense of smell; facial pain

PHYSICAL EXAMINATION

External Nose: Size, shape, lesions, drainage (color, amount, consistency)

Abnormal Breathing Sounds

Mouth Breathing

Palpation of Paranasal Sinuses: Tenderness, pain

Patency of Nares

Nasal Mucosa: Color, drainage, foreign bodies

Transillumination of Sinuses: Air, fluid

Throat: Inspection of mucous membranes and tonsils for redness, swelling, drainage, or lesions

Palpation of Neck for Enlarged Lymph Nodes

Ability to Recognize Common Odors

AGE-RELATED CHANGES IN THE NOSE, SINUSES, AND THROAT

As a person ages, the nose gets longer and tends to droop somewhat. Nasal obstruction is more common because of the softening of the cartilage of the external nose. The mucous membrane becomes thinner and produces less mucus. Some older people report having a watery or "runny" nose when eating spicy or hot foods. Drugs used to treat nasal congestion or discharge can have serious side effects for the older patient. Older people on such drugs should be monitored for

table 51-2 DIAGNOSTIC TESTS AND PROCEDURES | *for Disorders of the Nose, Sinuses, and Throat*

COMMON NURSING IMPLICATIONS
1. Confirm orders and check agency protocol.
2. Tell the patient what to expect.

TEST/PURPOSE	PATIENT PREPARATION	POSTPROCEDURE CARE
Throat culture is done to identify infective organisms.	Tell the patient a swab will be used to collect a specimen from the back of throat. Analysis of the specimen will reveal the infecting organism, if any.	No special care.
Laryngoscopy permits visualization of the larynx	NPO several hours before procedure. Administer drugs as ordered to decrease secretions and to relax the patient. Note allergies to local anesthetics on the patient's chart and identification band.	Nothing by mouth until the gag reflex returns. Monitor vital signs and respiratory status according to agency protocol. Provide lozenges or gargles as ordered for sore throat. Discourage the patient from talking, coughing, or clearing the throat for several hours after the procedure.

confusion, urinary retention, sedation, hypertension, fainting, and problems with coordination.

Epistaxis (nosebleed) is more common in older people, especially in those taking anticoagulants to slow blood clotting. If posterior nasal packing is needed to control bleeding, the older person is at greater risk for airway obstruction.

There is a decline in the sense of smell as people age. This may be due to neurologic changes but is probably aggravated by exposure to irritants such as cigarette smoke. The implications of decreased sense of smell in the elderly are significant. The older person may fail to detect smoke or gas in the home or may neglect personal hygiene owing to failure to notice body odors.

The tissues of the larynx are drier and less elastic in the older person. Some people complain of a constant tickling sensation that causes them to clear the throat frequently. Hard candies or lozenges may help by stimulating the production of saliva.

A weakened esophageal sphincter may allow gastric contents to flow back into the throat when the patient lies down. This is very irritating and may cause a burning sensation in the larynx. Elevating the head of the bed during sleep often relieves the problem.

DIAGNOSTIC TESTS AND PROCEDURES

Conditions of the nose, sinuses, and throat are diagnosed by cultures, measures of antibodies, and procedures to visualize internal structures (Table 51-2).

THROAT CULTURE

Throat cultures are done to isolate and identify infective organisms. A throat culture usually is done when streptococcal sore throat ("strep throat") is suspected. The procedure also can be used to screen for carriers of *Neisseria meningitidis* or diphtheria. Carriers harbor the organisms without showing evidence of the disease. If the physician orders the culture and antibiotics at the same time, obtain the culture specimen before starting the antibiotics.

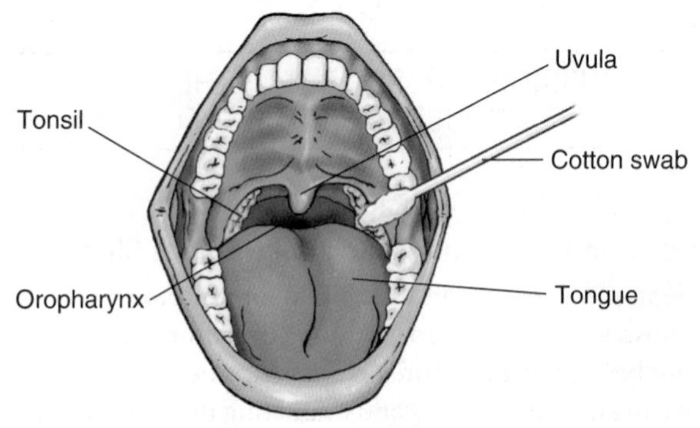

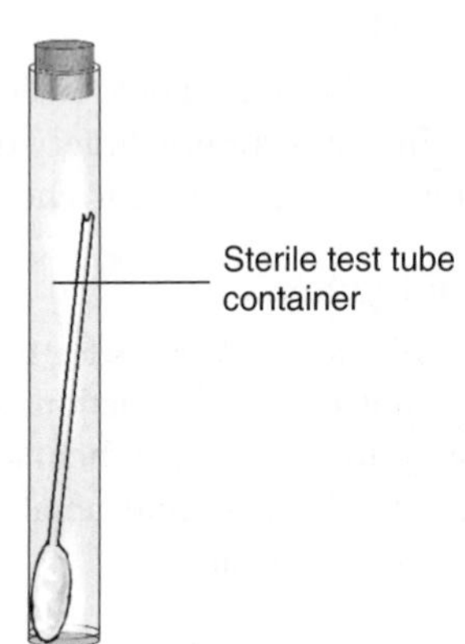

FIGURE **51-3** Throat culture technique.

Kits are available to collect and contain the specimen. The kit consists of a sterile swab or applicator and a tube of culture medium. To obtain the specimen, good lighting is essential. Tilt the patient's head back and depress the tongue with a tongue blade. Firmly but gently rotate the swab over the back of the throat, tonsils, and any obvious lesion. The swab should not touch any other area of the mouth. Because patients often gag or cough, stand to one side or wear a mask (Fig. 51-3).

Immediately place the swab in the tube of culture medium. Many commercial kits have an ampule of medium that must be broken to release the liquid. Carefully follow the directions on the kit. The results are reported in 24 to 48 hours. For results in 7 to 20 minutes, a test can be done to detect streptococcus antigens. Regardless of the results, the culture still should be done for confirmation.

LARYNGOSCOPY

Laryngoscopy is the inspection of the larynx to aid in diagnosis of abnormalities or to remove foreign bodies. A laryngoscopy may be either direct or indirect. In the direct procedure, the physician uses a fiberoptic laryngoscope (a flexible lighted tube). An indirect procedure uses mirrors to visualize the larynx. Contrast medium is sometimes instilled to outline the structures in the larynx. A tissue specimen may be taken for examination.

COMMON THERAPEUTIC MEASURES

NOSE DROPS

Some drugs are given by the nasal route—primarily to decrease nasal congestion and obstruction. Many over-the-counter nasal decongestants are available. Occasional use is not thought to be harmful, but frequent use is believed to damage the protective mechanisms in the nose. This increases the likelihood of additional obstruction and infection.

Other drugs used to treat conditions of the nose, sinuses, and throat include sympathomimetics, anticholinergics, antihistamines, antipyretics, analgesics, anesthetics, and anti-infectives. Examples of these drugs, their uses and side effects, and nursing interventions are presented in Table 51-3.

To administer nose drops, the patient may be sitting or lying down, but the head must be tilted back so that the solution flows into the back of the nose. Gently push the tip of the nose upward. Place the dropper at the opening of the nostril and squeeze to deliver the prescribed amount of medication. The dropper should not touch the nose. The patient should keep his or her head tilted back for several minutes. The patient may report feeling medication run down the throat. Provide a tissue for any nasal drainage or expectorated solution. Discard unused solution in the dropper rather than returning it to the bottle.

Put on your THINKING CAP!!

When instilling nose drops, why should the dropper *not* be allowed to touch the nose?

Some medications are available as sprays. Many sprays have pumps that administer metered doses. These require that the pump be depressed several times before using to fill the dose chamber. The drug is administered by holding the head upright, inserting the tip into the nostrils, and pumping two or three times. The patient then should inhale deeply through the nose.

PHARMACOLOGY CAPSULE Chronic use of nasal decongestant sprays may damage the protective mechanisms of the nose and cause rebound congestion.

NASAL AND THROAT IRRIGATIONS

Nasal irrigation is the washing of secretions from the nasal cavity. The procedure is not common but may be done on occasion. A throat irrigation washes out the throat. It is done to treat congestion or pain. Like nasal irrigation, it is not commonly done. See a procedure manual for details.

HUMIDIFICATION

The inspiration of dry air is uncomfortable, causes loss of body fluid, and can contribute to upper airway infections. Mouth breathing, necessitated by nasal obstruction, bypasses the turbinates that normally moisturize inspired air. A variety of devices are available to increase the humidity of inspired air.

Room humidifiers work in one of two ways: by creating an aerosol or by creating steam. Aerosols dispense tiny droplets of water into the room. Steam humidifiers increase humidity by distributing vaporized water (steam).

Because steam production requires raising water to the boiling point, there is little danger of steam humidifiers becoming contaminated. Aerosol humidifiers, however, are easily contaminated. Therefore sterile distilled water should be used with aerosol units. Plain distilled water is acceptable with steam units.

With any type of room humidifier, the fluid reservoir should be checked and refilled regularly. Daily cleaning reduces the risk of bacterial contamination. Patients who use humidifiers at home should be shown how to care for the devices. Patients who use tap water in home units can clean them with a solution of one cup of white vinegar in one gallon of water. They also are advised not to inhale aerosol directly from units that do not contain sterile water.

After nasal or sinus surgery, a bedside room humidifier may be ordered. A more effective option is a face tent or aerosol mask.

Patients who have tracheostomies inspire air directly into the trachea. Until the airway adjusts to this situation, humidification is essential to prevent excessive drying of the mucosa and secretions. If a tracheostomy tube is in place, aerosol nebulizers are used. For patients who have open stomas with tubes, tracheostomy masks with adjustable oxygen are used.

SUCTIONING

Suctioning is done to remove secretions from the upper airway. It is especially important for patients who cannot clear their upper airways effectively. Depending on the site of the secretions, you may need to suction the oral cavity, the oropharynx, the nasopharynx, and/or the trachea.

Suction *only* when there is evidence that it is necessary. Signs that indicate a need for suctioning include increased heart and respiratory rates, restlessness, and noisy expiration. Patients with tracheostomies also need suctioning when mucus is apparent in the tracheostomy tube. An indication for suctioning when a patient is on a ventilator is increased peak airway pressure.

Suctioning is not done unless indicated because it can cause complications, including hypoxia, tissue trauma, infection,

table 51-3 **DRUG THERAPY | *Nose, Sinuses, and Throat***

DRUG	USE/ACTION	SIDE EFFECTS	NURSING INTERVENTIONS
TOPICAL ANESTHETICS			
Benzocaine Cocaine Lidocaine	Anesthetic effect on skin and mucous membranes.	Allergy, sensitization, rash, burning, stinging. When sprayed on throat, can decrease gag reflex and cause dysphagia. If absorbed, lidocaine can cause drop in pulse and blood pressure. Cocaine can cause excitement and stimulation.	Inspect treated areas for side effects. Assess gag reflex before giving oral fluids or food. Monitor pulse, blood pressure, and mental status.
ANTI-INFECTIVES			
	Kill or suppress growth of microorganisms.	Nausea, vomiting, diarrhea, superinfections. Anaphylaxis if allergic.	Instruct patient to complete course of therapy as ordered. Report diarrhea or signs of new infections. Check allergies before giving drug.
ANTIPYRETICS			
Aspirin Ibuprofen	Reduce body temperature; used to treat fever. Analgesic effects.	Aspirin: high risk for allergy in patients with nasal polyps, asthma, or both; prolonged bleeding time, nephrotoxicity.	Assess for history of high risk for allergy. Watch for bleeding. Do not give with other anticoagulants. Report tinnitus, vertigo, hearing loss to physician. Tell patient not to use with possible viral infections. Ibuprofen: Assess for bleeding, tinnitus, vertigo, hearing loss, gastric discomfort. Take with full glass of water. Do not take with other drugs that prolong bleeding time.
OPIOID ANALGESICS			
	Reduce pain.	Drowsiness; decreased pulse, blood pressure, respirations; constipation; urinary retention; nausea and vomiting; pupillary constriction.	Monitor vital signs and level of consciousness. Withhold if respirations are below 12/min. Assess elimination. Safety precautions.
SYMPATHOMIMETICS			
Phenylephrine	Decongestion, vasoconstriction.	Increased pulse and blood pressure, dysrhythmias, angina, nausea, vomiting, urinary retention. Contraindicated with monoamine oxidase inhibitors.	Monitor vital signs, especially in patients with heart disease, hypertension, urinary dysfunction, diabetes, and hyperthyroidism.

vagal stimulation, and bronchospasm. The following are key points to remember when suctioning a patient:

1. Use sterile procedure. Wear a face shield if secretions may be splashed.
2. Use water-soluble, rather than oil-based, lubricant to avoid getting oil into the respiratory tract.
3. Oxygenate the patient before suctioning.
   A. If able, the patient should take three deep breaths.
   B. Other patients should be ventilated with 100% oxygen for 30 seconds to 3 minutes by manual resuscitator or by oxygen mask.
4. During insertion of the catheter, the vent should be open so that suctioning does not occur.
5. Apply suction as the catheter is withdrawn. Current thinking is that continuous suction should be applied during withdrawal of the catheter because it is less traumatic. However, some sources still recommend intermittent suction.
6. Removal of the catheter and suctioning should not take more than 10 seconds. Holding your breath while suctioning the patient helps remind you not to suction too long.
7. Rinse the catheter by suctioning normal saline through it.
8. Suction the mouth and pharynx, if needed, *after* suctioning the trachea.

table 51-3 **DRUG THERAPY | *Nose, Sinuses, and Throat—cont'd***

DRUG	USE/ACTION	SIDE EFFECTS	NURSING INTERVENTIONS
ANTICHOLINERGICS			
Atropine Scopolamine	Decrease salivary and respiratory secretions.	Side and adverse effects vary with dosage but may include dry mouth, constipation, drowsiness, blurred vision, mydriasis, urinary hesitancy, tachycardia. May cause dizziness in the elderly.	Safety precautions if dizzy or drowsy. Contraindicated in narrow-angle glaucoma and acute hemorrhage. Monitor pulse, urine output, bowel elimination. Oral hygiene.
ANTIHISTAMINES			
Diphenhydramine (Benadryl) Clemastine fumarate (Tavist)	Block effects of histamine. Used to treat allergic reactions and prevent motion sickness.	Dry mouth, anorexia, tinnitus, urinary retention or frequency, drowsiness, increased or decreased pulse. Some patients experience nervousness, stimulation, sleep disturbances.	Oral hygiene. Assess pulse, appetite, voiding. Safety precautions if drowsy. Give with food if it causes gastric distress.
GLUCOCORTICOIDS			
Nasal inhalers Beclomethasone (Beconase, Vancenase) Flunisolide (Nasalide) Oral inhalers Beclomethasone (Beclovent, Vanceril) Flunisolide (Aerobid) Triamcinolone acetonide (Azmacort)	Decrease bronchial and nasal inflammation. Decrease mucus production.	Decreased resistance to infection. Burning and dryness of nose and throat with nasal inhaler. Oral fungal infection with oral inhaler. Tachycardia, dizziness, headache, cough, unpleasant taste in mouth.	Teach patient how to use inhaler and stress prescribed frequency of use. Advise to take on schedule and not to make up missed doses. Rinse mouth after using oral inhaler.

9. Oxygenate the patient again after suctioning.
10. With a cuffed tracheostomy tube, the oropharynx and trachea are suctioned before deflating the cuff.
11. Document respiratory status before and after suctioning.

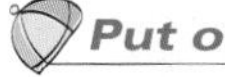
Put on your THINKING CAP!!

Why should you limit suctioning to 10 seconds?

TRACHEOSTOMY CARE

In addition to suctioning, the tracheostomy requires care to maintain cleanliness and protect the integrity of the surrounding skin. In the early postoperative phase, you will provide this care for the patient. The patient with a permanent tracheostomy should begin to participate as soon as he or she is able. Start the teaching process by placing a mirror so that the patient can see and by enlisting the patient's assistance.

A procedure manual should be consulted for details, but the following are key points to remember when doing tracheostomy care:

1. Use standard precautions.
2. Suction the tracheostomy before removing the old dressings.
3. Don sterile gloves to remove and clean the inner cannula.

4. Use a sterile solution of half hydrogen peroxide and half sterile water to clean the inner cannula.
5. Rinse and dry the inner cannula with normal saline or sterile water before reinserting it into the outer cannula.
6. Cleanse the stoma and surrounding skin with normal saline or sterile water and pat dry.
7. Be careful not to get solution into the stoma.
8. Change tracheostomy ties if soiled. If an assistant is not available, leave the old ties in place until the new ties are secure.
9. Replace the tracheostomy dressing with a precut pad or with a gauze pad folded as illustrated in Figure 51-4. Do not *cut* a pad because fibers will get into the stoma.
10. Tie the ties at the side of the neck in a square knot (not a bow).
11. Document the procedure and observations, including the appearance of the stoma, surrounding skin, and secretions.

NASAL SURGERY

Nasal surgery may be indicated for various obstructions, injuries, and chronic infections. Specific nursing care needs are discussed under individual disorders of the nose and sinuses, but general considerations are summarized here.

NURSING CARE *of the Patient having Nasal Surgery*

General care of the surgical patient is discussed in Chapter 16. Specific nursing care after nasal surgery is added here. These procedures often are done in day surgery, so your contact with the patient may be limited.

Assessment

After nasal surgery, assess for pain, pressure, anxiety, and dyspnea. Monitor the patient's vital signs to detect signs of excessive blood loss (tachycardia, restlessness, tachypnea, hypotension). Take the temperature to detect fever associated with infection. The patient with nasal packing will not be able to close the mouth for an oral temperature, so an alternate route will be necessary. Patients often have nasal packing in place with a moustache dressing to absorb drainage. Note the number of dressings saturated and the frequency of changes. Remember that bleeding from the nasal cavity may flow into the throat and be swallowed while the dressing remains dry. Therefore check the back of the throat for bleeding. Also, be alert for frequent swallowing, which may be a response to bleeding into the throat. Inspect vomitus and stool for signs of blood (bright red or "coffee ground" emesis and red, maroon, or black stools).

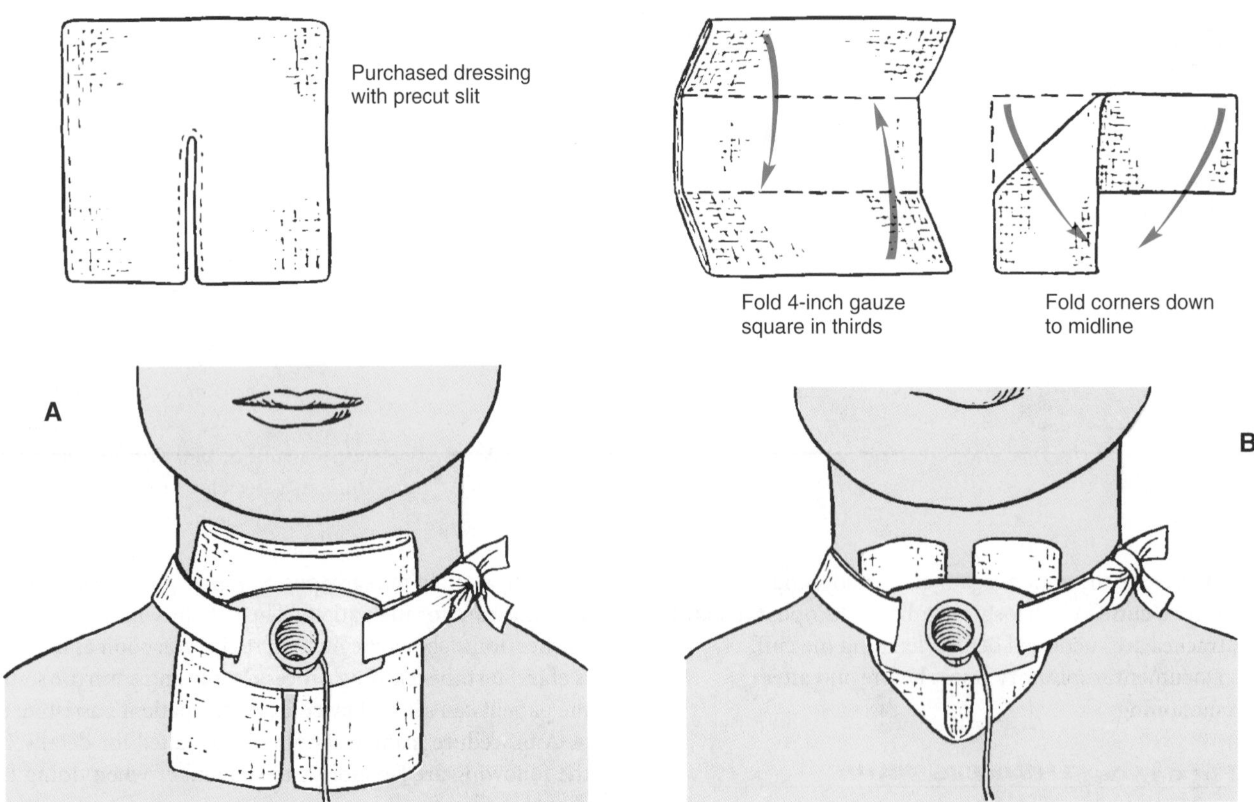

Purchased dressing with precut slit
Fold 4-inch gauze square in thirds
Fold corners down to midline
A
B

FIGURE **51-4** Tracheostomy dressings. *A,* Manufactured dressing with a precut slit has no fine threads that could enter the stoma. *B,* A 4 × 4 gauze pad folded for use as a tracheostomy dressing has no cut edges that could fray and permit fibers to enter the airway. The slit can be placed downward or upward.

Nursing Diagnoses, Goals, and Outcome Criteria: Nasal Surgery, Postoperative

Nursing Diagnoses	Goals and Outcome Criteria
Decreased Cardiac Output related to blood loss from vascular nasal passageways	Normal cardiac output: pulse and blood pressure consistent with patient norms
Acute Pain related to tissue trauma, edema, or packing	Pain relief: patient states pain reduced, appears relaxed
Impaired Gas Exchange related to airway obstruction	Adequate gas exchange: respiratory rate and effort and heart rate consistent with patient norms
Disturbed Body Image related to facial bruising	Improved body image: patient accepts temporarily altered appearance: patient acknowledges that facial discoloration is temporary, resumes normal activities

Interventions

Decreased Cardiac Output

The nasal cavity has an extensive blood supply, so there is a risk of hemorrhage after nasal surgery. To reduce the risk of bleeding, advise the patient not to do anything that increases pressure in the nose. This includes blowing the nose and straining. Laxatives or stool softeners may be ordered to prevent straining due to constipation. The patient should not take any products containing aspirin because aspirin interferes with coagulation.

Notify the physician of indications of excessive bleeding: frequent, steady saturation of dressings with blood; increased pulse and respirations; restlessness; decreased blood pressure; frequent swallowing; hematemesis (blood in vomitus); and melena (dark stools associated with blood in stool).

Acute Pain

After nasal surgery, some nasal pain is expected because of the trauma and swelling. Semi-Fowler's to high Fowler's position helps to control swelling. Administer analgesics and apply ice packs as ordered. Cold decreases pain by decreasing swelling. Other sources of discomfort after nasal surgery are dry mouth and sore throat. Frequent mouth care and, when allowed, oral fluids are soothing.

Impaired Gas Exchange

Nasal packing is often used after nasal or sinus surgery, often with a moustache dressing in place on the upper lip to absorb drainage. Only the physician removes the packing, but nurses can change the moustache dressing as needed.

Nasal packing, especially posterior packing, can interfere with breathing. Position the patient in semi-Fowler's position with the head flat against the bed.

When the nasal cavity is packed, the patient breathes through the mouth. A humidifier helps decrease dryness of the mucous membranes. Frequent oral hygiene also is comforting. Because of the nasal packing, the patient will hear a sucking sound when swallowing. Reassure him or her that this is normal. It also is common for patients to have poor appetites when the packing is present.

Disturbed Body Image

Some types of nasal surgery tend to cause "black eyes." The application of cool compresses to both eyes may reduce or prevent this effect. Reassure the patient that this effect is temporary, but be sensitive to any patient distress about it.

DISORDERS OF THE NOSE, SINUSES, THROAT, AND LARYNX

DISORDERS OF THE NOSE AND SINUSES

Sinusitis

Sinusitis is inflammation of the sinuses, most often the maxillary and frontal sinuses. The most common causative organisms are *staphylococci* and *streptococci*. The infection usually spreads from the nasal passages into the sinuses.

Sinusitis can be acute or chronic. Acute sinusitis follows obstruction of the flow of secretions from the sinus. Causes of acute sinusitis include allergic rhinitis, deviated septum, nasal polyps, tumors, airborne pollutants, and inhaled drugs such as cocaine. Chronic sinusitis is a permanent thickening of the mucous membranes in the sinuses after repeated infections.

Signs and Symptoms

Patients with sinusitis usually report pain or a feeling of heaviness over the affected area. They may report purulent drainage from the nose. When the maxillary sinuses are affected, the pain may seem like a toothache. Headache is common, especially in the morning. Fever may be present, and the white blood cell count may be elevated.

Complications

Although most patients recover without serious effects, sinus infections can be dangerous. Chronic sinusitis may follow acute sinusitis. Other potential complications are meningitis, brain abscess, osteomyelitis, and orbital cellulitis. The possibility of brain infection exists because of the location of the sinuses in the skull. Suspect neurologic complications if the patient has a high fever, vomiting, chills, seizures, or blurred vision.

Medical Diagnosis and Treatment

Sinusitis usually is based on the findings of the history and physical examination. Computed tomography provides the best confirmation. Sinus aspiration or endoscopy may be done to obtain a specimen for culture.

Antibiotics are prescribed for acute sinusitis. Other drugs that may be ordered to improve drainage or to relieve symptoms include decongestants, corticosteroids, analgesics, antipyretics, and mucolytics. The use of antihistamines is controversial because they may dry secretions, making them more difficult to clear. Warm, moist packs applied to the face can promote drainage and reduce pain. Other measures to promote drainage include increased fluid intake and use of a humidifier. Sinus irrigation is sometimes done by the physician.

Surgical Treatment

Chronic sinusitis sometimes is treated surgically. Surgery may correct the underlying problem, remove the thickened membrane, or enlarge the opening through which secretions drain. Underlying problems that might be treated surgically include deviated septum, nasal polyps, and hypertrophy of turbinates.

Two types of surgery used for sinusitis that do not respond to medical treatment are functional funduscopic sinus surgery (FESS) and the Caldwell-Luc procedure. FESS is an outpatient procedure in which specialized instruments are passed into the sinuses through the nasal cavity. Diseased tissue can be removed, and the sinus ostia (the openings that drain the sinuses) can be enlarged. Nasal packing may be done to control bleeding. The packing usually is removed after a few hours. Complications of FESS can include nasal bleeding and scarring. Although rare, CSF leakage and injury to the optic nerve are possible.

The Caldwell-Luc procedure is used to treat chronic maxillary sinusitis. The procedure involves making an incision in the upper gum line above the teeth. An opening is made between the affected sinus and the nose. This allows secretions to drain, relieving the pressure. The cavity is packed, and the packing is left in place for 48 hours. It is removed only by the physician. After the Caldwell-Luc procedure, swelling, bruising, and numbness are normal. The numbness usually lasts several weeks. Advise the patient not to blow the nose, wear dentures, or chew on the affected side until permitted by the physician (usually approximately 2 weeks).

NURSING CARE *of the Patient having Sinus Surgery*

Nursing care after sinus surgery is essentially the same as that described earlier for nasal surgery. After the Caldwell-Luc procedure, nasal packing is usually left in place until the next morning. Antral packing is left in place for 36 to 72 hours. Three to 5 days after surgery, nasal saline sprays may be ordered to moisten the nasal mucosa. Temporary numbness of the upper teeth is common after the Caldwell-Luc procedure. Sensation returns in several weeks.

Nasal Polyps

Nasal polyps are swollen masses of sinus or nasal mucosa and connective tissue that extend into the nasal passages. They tend to grow, and they eventually obstruct the nasal airway. Polyps resemble white grapes in size and shape. Most patients have multiple polyps. The exact cause is unknown, but patients often have a history of allergic rhinitis or infections. Patients who have nasal polyps, asthma, and aspirin allergy are said to have triad disease.

The size of the polyps may be reduced by removing allergens or treating the allergic response. Surgical removal under local anesthesia, however, is often necessary. Unfortunately, nasal polyps tend to recur.

NURSING CARE *of the Patient having Nasal Polyp Surgery*

Nursing care after surgery for nasal polyps is like that described earlier for nasal surgery. This procedure is often done in an outpatient surgical facility, so patient teaching before discharge is especially important. Advise the patient not to take aspirin because it increases the risk of bleeding and because some of these patients are allergic to aspirin.

Allergic Rhinitis

Allergic rhinitis, or "hay fever," is a common condition. It is classified as acute (seasonal) or chronic (perennial).

Pathophysiology

Allergic rhinitis follows exposure to a substance, called an allergen, that causes an allergic response. An allergic response is a reaction to the release of chemicals, including histamine, that cause vasodilation and increased capillary permeability. Fluid leaks from the capillaries, causing swelling of the nasal mucosa. Occasionally, these changes are triggered by overuse of decongestant nose drops or sprays.

Acute allergic rhinitis most often is due to exposure to pollens. It typically lasts several weeks, resolves, and does not return until the offending pollens reappear. The chronic form is more likely due to allergens that are continuously in the environment, such as house dust and animal dander. Symptoms may be consistent or intermittent, depending on the frequency of exposure.

Signs and Symptoms

Signs and symptoms of allergic rhinitis include nasal obstruction; sneezing; clear nasal discharge; frontal headache; and itchy, watery eyes. The nasal mucosa is often pale, but it can be red or bluish.

Medical Diagnosis

Diagnosis is made on the basis of a detailed history. With chronic symptoms, the patient may be instructed to keep a diary describing all episodes. This can help identify possible allergens.

Medical Treatment

The patient also may be referred to an allergist for further evaluation. The allergist applies solutions of common allergens to the skin. The allergens are applied in a specific pattern so that the patient's reaction to them can be assessed individually. Desensitizing injections may be advised to decrease the patient's reaction to the offending allergens. Patients often call these injections "allergy shots." The injections are composed of dilute solutions of the allergens to which the person reacts. The strength of the solution is gradually increased as the patient's tolerance grows. In a sense, this process causes the body to get used to the allergen so that it no longer reacts with an allergic response. Another outcome of allergy testing is that it identifies substances that the patient should avoid.

The drugs used to treat allergic rhinitis are primarily antihistamines and decongestants. Many such medications are available without a prescription. In general, these products should be used only on a short-term basis. Advise patients to consult with a physician or a pharmacist about the most appropriate over-the-counter drugs.

NURSING CARE *of the Patient with Allergic Rhinitis*

Patients with allergic rhinitis usually are treated as outpatients. The nurse who works in a clinic or physician's office may need to reinforce teaching about desensitization and drug therapy.

Acute Viral Coryza

Acute viral coryza, known as the common cold, can be caused by any of some 30 viruses. It is contagious and spread by droplet infection.

Signs and Symptoms

Signs and symptoms of the common cold are well known to most people. They usually consist of fever, fatigue, nasal discharge, and sore throat.

Complications

The infection usually runs its course in approximately a week. Complications that sometimes develop include otitis media, sinusitis, bronchitis, and pneumonia. Complications are more common in people with poor resistance.

Medical Treatment

Medical management of the common cold is primarily directed at relief of symptoms. Drug therapy includes antihistamines, decongestants, and antipyretics. Patients often expect to receive antibiotics. The nurse can inform them that antibiotics are not effective against infections caused by viruses. Inappropriate use of antibiotics promotes the development of resistant strains of bacteria.

Prevention

Prevention of the common cold is best accomplished by avoidance of people with colds. People with colds are most contagious during the first 2 or 3 days after symptoms appear. The very young, the very old, and those with weakened immune systems especially should be protected from exposure.

Put on your THINKING CAP!!

Design a short teaching plan on prevention of colds for first-grade children. Be creative!

NURSING CARE *of the Patient with Acute Viral Coryza*

Nursing intervention in relation to the common cold is primarily public education about prevention and about drugs prescribed for treatment. Encourage patients to rest and to drink plenty of fluids.

Consider the Alternative!

Echinacea is an herb that is widely used to boost the immune system. Only recently have these claims come under study. Early evidence is that it may decrease the severity and duration of a cold, but probably does not prevent it. Similar results have been found related to the value of vitamin C.

Tumors

Signs and Symptoms

Tumors sometimes develop in the nasal passages and sinuses. They can be benign or malignant. Sinus malignancies are more common among people in certain occupations—notably furniture makers. This suggests that the exposure to wood dust may be a factor. The primary symptom is nasal obstruction. Either one or both sides may be affected. Another sign suggestive of a tumor is a bloody discharge from one nasal passage.

Carcinomas of the external nose are more common than those of the nasopharynx. They are more common in men, usually between the ages of 50 and 70 years. The lesions typically begin as small, painless ulcers that do not heal. External nasal tumors are usually either basal cell or squamous cell carcinomas. Squamous cell carcinomas are more dangerous because they grow faster and tend to metastasize early. Basal cell carcinomas grow more slowly, but they still can be fatal if not removed.

Medical Diagnosis

A diagnosis is made by taking a biopsy sample of the tumor or removing the entire tumor for examination. The earlier a malignancy is detected and treated, the better the chances of survival. Unfortunately, carcinomas in the nasopharynx tend to metastasize to the neck, liver, and lungs fairly early. Therefore a patient with persistent nasal obstruction or bleeding should be examined by a physician.

Medical Treatment

Treatment of nasal malignancies usually consists of some combination of surgery, radiation therapy, and chemotherapy. Surgical procedures may be extensive and disfiguring, depending on the site and extent of the cancer. Reconstructive surgery or prostheses may be needed.

Benign tumors do not metastasize but are likely to be removed because they still can obstruct the nasal passages.

NURSING CARE *of the Patient with Nasal Cancer*

The general nursing care of patients undergoing nasal surgery is discussed earlier. A diagnosis of cancer has special implications for the nurse. The patient may be especially anxious and fearful of disfigurement or even death. Be supportive and encourage the patient to ask questions and express concerns. Nursing care of the patient with cancer is discussed in detail in Chapter 24.

Deviated Nasal Septum

The nose is divided into two passages by a cartilaginous wall called the septum. In most adults, the septum is slightly deviated, meaning it is off center. Minor deviations cause no symptoms and require no treatment. Major deviations, however, can obstruct the nasal passages and block sinus drainage. The patient may complain of headaches, sinusitis, and epistaxis (nosebleeds).

Surgical Treatment

Septal deviations are corrected by a surgical procedure called a submucosal resection or nasal septoplasty. The procedure usually is done under local anesthesia. An incision is made in the nasal mucosa, and the displaced bone and cartilage are removed. The mucosa is repositioned, and the nasal passage is packed with petrolatum gauze. The physician removes the packing after 24 to 48 hours.

The two major complications of submucosal resection are tears of the septum and saddle deformity. Saddle deformity is collapse of the bridge of the nose caused by removal of excessive support tissue or by contraction of the surgical scar. Nursing care of the patient having nasal surgery was described earlier.

Epistaxis

The nose has an abundant blood supply that permits it to bleed easily. The medical term for a nosebleed is ***epistaxis.*** Problems that may lead to bleeding include trauma, clotting disorders, dryness, inflammation, and hypertension.

First Aid

When epistaxis occurs, the patient should sit down and lean forward. Direct pressure should be applied for 3 to 5 minutes, as illustrated in Figure 15-7, unless the patient has had a traumatic injury to the face.

Facial trauma suggests a possible nasal fracture, and direct pressure may do more harm. An ice pack or a cold compress can be applied to the nose regardless of whether facial trauma has occurred. Once the bleeding stops, advise the patient not to blow the nose for several hours because this may trigger renewed bleeding.

Medical Treatment

If bleeding continues, medical attention is needed. The physician tries to identify the bleeding site and may treat it with silver nitrate or electric cautery. If cautery is used, the patient is given a local anesthetic.

If bleeding is not controlled, the next step is direct pressure to the nasal cavity. Two methods used to do this are placement of a nasal balloon catheter and placement of nasal packing.

Nasal balloon catheter. A nasal balloon catheter may be passed into the nasal cavity by the physician. The balloon then is inflated to apply pressure to the blood vessels. Smaller balloons anchor the catheter in place. Several different types of nasal catheters with single or double cuffs are available.

Nasal packing. The physician may pack the anterior or posterior nasal cavity, or both. Posterior nasal packing is more complicated and requires close patient monitoring. One method of packing the posterior nasal cavity is described here. Catheters are passed into the nostrils and pulled out through the mouth. Two strings are tied to the catheters and to a rolled pad. A third string is attached to the pad. As the catheters are pulled back out the nostrils, the pad is pulled into place in the posterior nasal cavity. An anterior pack is placed over the nares and secured with the two strings that are tied to the catheter. The third string remains attached to the packing. The loose end of the third string is brought out of the mouth and taped to the cheek. Figure 51-5 illustrates this procedure.

Complications. Complications related to posterior packing include infection, blockage of the eustachian tube, and airway obstruction. Posterior packing is usually left in place for 48 to 96 hours. The bulky posterior pad can depress the soft palate, causing airway obstruction. If the packing should slip out of place, it could block the airway.

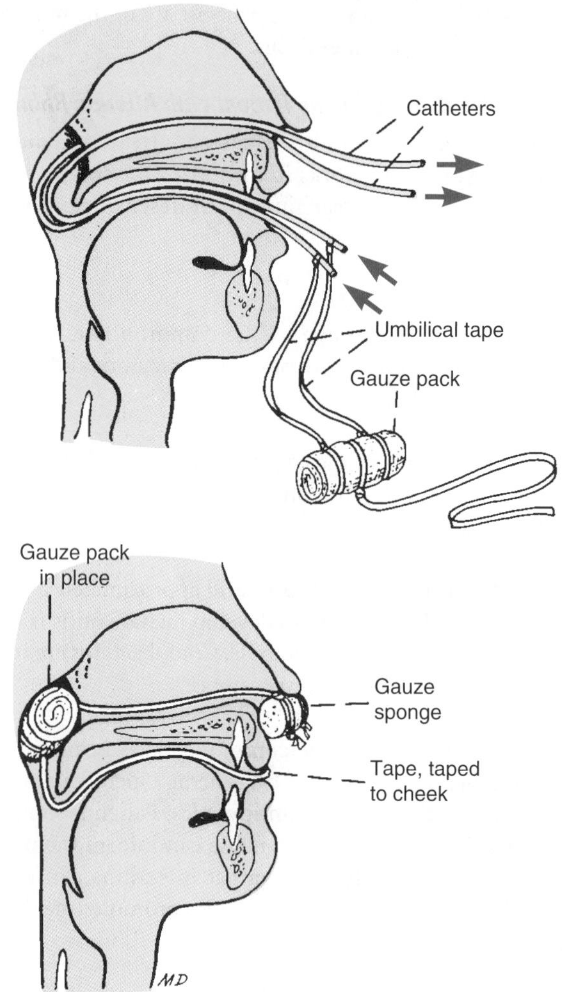

FIGURE **51-5** Placement of a posterior nasal pack used for emergency treatment of epistaxis.

NURSING CARE *of the Patient with Epistaxis*

Assessment

Severe epistaxis is an emergency, so collect only priority data until the patient is stabilized. The priority assessment when a patient has severe epistaxis is for evidence of uncontrolled bleeding and excessive blood loss. Inspect the nose and back of the throat for obvious bleeding and observe for frequent swallowing. Monitor the patient's level of consciousness and vital signs to detect signs of hypovolemia (restlessness, tachycardia, tachypnea, hypotension). Document allergies and major illnesses.

Once a nasal balloon catheter or nasal packing is in place, assess for early signs of infection and airway obstruction (dyspnea, anxiety, tachycardia). Also ask the patient about pain in the nose, pharynx, or ears.

Nursing Diagnoses, Goals, and Outcome Criteria: Epistaxis

Nursing Diagnoses	Goals and Outcome Criteria
Decreased Cardiac Output related to hypovolemia secondary to hemorrhage	Normal cardiac output: pulse and blood pressure consistent with patient's norms
Anxiety related to threat of excessive bleeding or unpleasant procedures	Reduced anxiety: patient calm, able to cooperate, states less anxious
Risk for Injury related to pressure (of packing, balloon) and possible airway obstruction	Absence of complications of balloon or packing: respiratory rate of 12 to 20 without distress
Risk for Infection related to presence or nasal packing	Absence of infection: no fever

Interventions

Decreased Cardiac Output

Throughout the period of care for epistaxis, monitor for signs of continued and excessive blood loss. Immediately report signs and symptoms of hypovolemia (increased pulse, restlessness, decreased urine output) to the physician.

PHARMACOLOGY CAPSULE Patients who are prone to bleeding usually are advised to avoid aspirin because it inhibits blood clotting.

Anxiety

When a nasal balloon or packing is used, support the patient and assist the physician during placement of the device. The patient is probably frightened by the visible blood and needs calm reassurance. Because of the discomfort and anxiety associated with posterior nasal packing, a mild sedative may be ordered.

Risk for Injury and Infection

After the catheter is inserted and the balloon inflated, it is taped in place. Because the balloon can depress the soft palate and impair breathing, check the patient's respiratory status frequently. If a catheter is used instead of packing, the catheter placement also should be checked at least every 4 hours. Deflate anchor cuffs for 10 minutes every 24 hours as ordered or according to agency policy. Be careful to deflate the correct bulb.

Patients usually are hospitalized while nasal packing is in place. Frequent mouth care is needed because the patient must breathe through the mouth. It is also important to monitor the patient's temperature for elevation, which may indicate infection of the nasopharynx. If the posterior packing slips out of place, it could block the airway. If the airway is obstructed by the packing, the strings holding the anterior pad must be cut and the packing pulled out with the third string that is taped to the cheek.

Under normal circumstances, the physician removes the packing. You can assist by supporting the patient in a sitting position and providing an emesis basin to receive the packing. Drape the patient to protect the clothing. Once the packing is removed, the patient appreciates mouth care.

DISORDERS OF THE THROAT

Pharyngitis

Pharyngitis is inflammation of the mucous membranes of the throat or pharynx. It usually occurs along with acute rhinitis or sinusitis and is more common in late fall and spring. Pharyngitis usually is caused by a virus but sometimes is caused by bacteria. It also can follow exposure to irritating substances in the environment.

Signs and Symptoms

Signs and symptoms of pharyngitis are dryness, pain, dysphagia (difficulty swallowing), and fever. The throat appears red, and the tonsils may be enlarged. Viral and bacterial pharyngitis differ in several respects. Table 51-4 shows the key features of each. Compared with viral pharyngitis, bacterial pharyngitis has a more abrupt onset and is characterized by abnormal blood cell counts, fever greater than 101° F, and muscle and joint pain. Additional signs of infection associated with beta-hemolytic streptococci are a strawberry-red tongue, vomiting, and a rash.

Complications

Patients with bacterial pharyngitis are more likely to have serious complications than those with viral pharyngitis. The most important complications are acute glomerulonephritis and rheumatic fever. If acute glomerulonephritis develops, it usually appears 7 to 10 days after the throat infection. When rheumatic fever develops, it usually appears 3 to 5 weeks after the initial infection.

Medical Diagnosis

Pharyngitis is diagnosed on the basis of the patient history and physical examination. A more specific diagnosis of viral or bacterial pharyngitis is made after the results of a throat culture and a complete blood count are obtained.

Medical Treatment

Pharyngitis is treated with rest, fluids, analgesics, and throat gargles or irrigations. Bedrest may be recommended as long as the patient has a fever. If the patient's oral intake is low, intravenous fluids may be ordered. A soft or liquid diet may be ordered because of painful swallowing. A humidifier also may be ordered to increase moisture in the room air.

The physician often orders antibiotics, usually penicillin or erythromycin, while awaiting the results of the throat culture. Obtain the culture specimen before the antibiotics are started. When the culture results are reported, the antibiotic is discontinued if there is no evidence of bacterial growth. If bacterial infection is confirmed, the antibiotic is usually continued until 48 hours after all signs and symptoms disappear. A course of antibiotic therapy may be as long as 10 days.

Prevention

To reduce the risk of pharyngitis, people with poor resistance should avoid others with upper respiratory infections. Measures that help to maintain resistance to throat infections include good nutrition, adequate rest, avoidance of chilling, and avoidance of inhaled irritants. People who have pharyngitis

table 51-4 ***Comparison of Viral and Bacterial Pharyngitis***

CHARACTERISTIC	VIRAL	BACTERIAL
Symptoms	Rhinorrhea Headache Mild hoarseness	Dysphagia Joint and muscle pain Malaise
Onset	Gradual	Abrupt
Temperature	Mild elevation	>101° F
Diagnosis	CBC: normal Culture: negative	CBC: abnormal Culture: positive
Complications	Rare	Occur in 1% to 3%; can be glomerulonephritis, rheumatic fever, otitis media, sinusitis, mastoiditis

are contagious in the early stages and should avoid contact with susceptible people.

NURSING CARE *of the Patient with Pharyngitis*

Assessment

Mild pharyngitis usually is treated on an outpatient basis, so nursing interventions are limited. Assessment should document the presence of throat pain, dysphagia, muscle and joint pain, nausea and vomiting, and rash. Take the patient's temperature, and inspect the throat for redness and enlarged tonsils.

Nursing Diagnoses, Goals, and Outcome Criteria: Pharyngitis

The primary nursing diagnosis for the patient with pharyngitis is ineffective therapeutic regimen management related to lack of understanding of treatment and importance of follow-up care. The goal of nursing care is effective management of therapeutic regimen. The criteria for goal achievement are the patient correctly describing self-care measures—including drug therapy and symptoms that should be reported—and making and keeping a follow-up appointment.

Interventions

Reinforce the physician's directions for drug therapy, if ordered. Stress the importance of completing prescribed antibiotics. Encourage patients to take 2,000 to 3,000 ml of fluids daily unless contraindicated. Fluids must be increased cautiously in the elderly because they do not adjust well to sudden changes in blood volume. Advise patients that they are contagious at first and should not be exposed to people with poor resistance. Assist the patient to schedule a follow-up appointment, and advise the patient to contact the physician if a rash or strawberry-red tongue develops within the next 2 months.

Tonsillitis

Tonsillitis is inflammation of the tonsils and other lymphatic tissue in the throat. It is most common in children but often more severe in adults. Low resistance seems to invite tonsillitis.

Causes

Tonsillitis is usually a bacterial infection, but it is sometimes caused by a virus. Common causative organisms include streptococci, staphylococci, *Haemophilus influenzae,* and pneumococci. The infection is contagious and is spread by food or airborne routes. Most cases run their course in 7 to 10 days. A person may have repeated infections that respond to treatment or may have a chronic infection.

Signs and Symptoms

A patient with tonsillitis usually reports a sore throat, difficulty swallowing, fever, chills, muscle aches, and headache. If swollen tissue blocks the eustachian tubes, there may also be pain in the ears. Offensive breath odor is often present with chronic infection.

The tonsils typically are enlarged and red. Purulent drainage or yellowish or white patches may be seen on the tonsils. Lymph nodes in the neck may be tender and enlarged.

Medical Diagnosis

To diagnose tonsillitis, the physician will probably order a complete blood count, throat culture and sensitivity, and a test for infectious mononucleosis. An elevated white blood cell count suggests a bacterial infection. The culture and sensitivity identify the pathogenic organisms present and what antibiotics are likely to be effective. A chest radiograph also may be ordered to assess for respiratory complications.

Medical Treatment

The medical treatment of tonsillitis usually includes a course of antibiotic therapy for 7 to 10 days. Analgesics and anesthetic lozenges may be prescribed for pain and antipyretics for fever. Warm saline gargles or irrigations may be ordered to decrease swelling and remove drainage. Rest and adequate fluids promote recovery and decrease the risk of complications.

Complications

A peritonsillar abscess may develop with streptococcal tonsillitis. A peritonsillar abscess is an infection of the tissue surrounding the tonsil. The affected side is very painful, and the patient has difficulty swallowing, talking, and opening the mouth. The immediate treatment is drainage of the abscess. Once the acute infection has subsided, tonsillectomy is performed.

Surgical Treatment

Tonsillectomy, removal of the tonsils, was once considered routine childhood surgery. Current thinking is that the tonsils play an important protective role as part of the immune system and should be retained if possible.

NURSING CARE PLAN

The Patient having Tonsillectomy

ASSESSMENT

Health History: Miss Janice Morgan is a 20-year-old college student who has had tonsillitis three times this year that has resulted in absences from school. Her symptoms included sore throat, dysphagia, fever and chills, muscle aches, and headache. She has had no other serious illnesses but was hospitalized overnight after an automobile accident in 1991. She takes no medications except occasional acetaminophen for headache. She was admitted for tonsillectomy, which was performed under local anesthetic this morning. She expressed hope that it will relieve her recurrent illness. She clutches her throat and complains of throat pain.

Physical Examination: Miss Morgan is drowsy but responds appropriately. Vital signs: temperature, 98° F orally; pulse, 100; respiration, 18; blood pressure 110/88. She has a small amount of sanguineous drainage. Respiratory effort and breath sounds are normal. Intravenous fluids are infusing into the antecubital space of the left arm.

Nursing Diagnosis	*Goals and Outcome Criteria*	*Interventions*
Decreased cardiac output related to excessive bleeding.	The patient will maintain normal cardiac output as evidenced by vital signs consistent with preoperative readings, minimal visible bleeding, and absence of restlessness.	Assess for signs of excessive bleeding: tachycardia and restlessness. Advise the patient not to cough or clear throat. Inspect drainage for bleeding. (Note frequent swallowing.) Report continued or excessive bleeding to surgeon. When oral fluids are permitted, have patient sip from a glass or cup rather than use a straw.
Ineffective airway clearance related to bleeding, edema, effects of anesthesia.	The patient will maintain a patent airway as evidenced by clear breath sounds and respiratory rate of 12 to 20.	Position on one side until fully alert. Elevate head of bed 45 degrees. Monitor for signs and symptoms of inadequate oxygenation: tachycardia, restlessness. Auscultate breath sounds. Have suction equipment in room.
Acute pain related to tissue trauma.	The patient will state that pain is relieved and will appear more relaxed.	Administer analgesics as ordered. Apply ice collar as ordered. Give cold or frozen liquids when permitted. Provide simple explanations and reassurance.
Deficient knowledge of postoperative care.	The patient will describe postoperative self-care.	Before discharge, teach the following: 1. Consume soft, high-protein, high-calorie diet for 10 days. Omit rough foods. 2. Drink 8 to 12 8-ounce glasses of fluids daily. No citrus juices. 3. Avoid strenuous activity or straining for 2 weeks. 4. No aspirin. 5. Earaches are common. 6. White patches naturally form over tonsillectomy sites. 7. Report any bleeding to the physician.

Tonsillectomy is usually recommended under the following conditions:

- Repeated tonsillitis in a year, especially if caused by beta-hemolytic streptococci
- Presence of a peritonsillar abscess
- Malignancy of the tonsil
- Airway obstruction by enlarged tonsils or adenoids
- Evidence that the patient is a carrier of the diphtheria organism
- Hearing loss associated with otitis media due to enlarged tonsils

If surgery is indicated, it usually is delayed until the patient's temperature returns to normal. Even though tonsillectomy is a common procedure, it should not be considered minor. The usual procedure is a tonsillectomy and an adenoidectomy. The adenoids are usually removed because they are almost always infected when the tonsils are. If only the adenoids are infected, an adenoidectomy alone may be done. In adult patients, these procedures may be done under local or general anesthesia.

NURSING CARE *of the Patient having Tonsillectomy*

Preoperative nursing care is discussed in detail in Chapter 16. Postoperative nursing care is as follows (see also Nursing Care Plan: The Patient having Tonsillectomy).

Assessment

In the immediate postoperative phase, frequently monitor the patient's responsiveness and vital signs. They usually are checked every 5 minutes until stable, then every 15 minutes for an hour, and hourly for the remainder of the first 24 postoperative hours. Inspect drainage from the mouth or vomited fluid for blood. Blood-tinged drainage is normal at first but should gradually decrease. Note excessive swallowing, which may indicate bleeding. Assess respiratory effort and skin color to evaluate oxygenation. Evaluate pain and dysphagia.

Nursing Diagnoses, Goals, and Outcome Criteria: Tonsillectomy

Nursing Diagnoses	Goals and Outcome Criteria
Decreased Cardiac Output related to excessive bleeding	Normal cardiac output and decreasing bleeding: pulse and blood pressure consistent with patient's norms, decreasing bloody drainage
Ineffective Airway Clearance related to bleeding, edema, or effects of anesthesia	Effective airway clearance and adequate oxygenation: no restlessness, normal skin color, no respiratory distress
Acute Pain related to tissue trauma	Pain relief: patient states pain relieved, relaxed manner
Ineffective Therapeutic Regimen Management related to lack of understanding	Effective management of care: patient describes and carries out self-care as prescribed

Interventions

The two major problems that may develop in the postoperative phase are hemorrhage and respiratory distress.

Decreased Cardiac Output

Continually monitor for signs of excessive bleeding. Increased pulse rate and restlessness are early signs of hypovolemia. To reduce the risk of bleeding, remind the patient not to cough or clear the throat. If suctioning is needed, do so very gently because it may cause further bleeding. Once oral fluids are permitted, the patient should not use a straw. The sucking may dislodge the clots that form at the surgical site.

Ineffective Airway Clearance

A patient who has had local anesthesia is at less risk for respiratory complications than one who had general anesthesia. After local anesthesia, position the tonsillectomy patient with the head of the bed elevated at a 45-degree angle. After general anesthesia, the bed should be flat and the patient positioned on the side or semiprone. This promotes drainage of fluid from the mouth that might otherwise be aspirated. Once the patient is fully awake, he or she may prefer a semi-Fowler's position.

Increased pulse rate, restlessness, and confusion may be early signs and symptoms of inadequate oxygenation. Cyanosis (bluish discoloration of the nail beds or lips) is a late sign of inadequate oxygenation.

Acute Pain

Analgesics are ordered for pain. Ice collars may be applied to the neck as ordered to decrease swelling and pain. Intravenous fluids usually are prescribed until the patient is able to take oral fluids well. A clear liquid diet is ordered first. Cold or frozen liquids are especially soothing after tonsillectomy.

Ineffective Therapeutic Regimen Management

Before discharge, advise the patient of measures to promote healing and prevent complications. The diet should be soft and high in protein and calories for about 10 days. Fluid intake should be 8 to 12 8-ounce glasses daily. Citrus juices are not recommended because they irritate the healing throat tissues. Earaches are common and are not cause for alarm. It is also normal for white patches to form over the tonsillectomy sites. This tissue is like a scab, and it will slough off.

If any bleeding occurs after discharge, the physician should be informed. To reduce the risk of bleeding, the patient should avoid strenuous activity or straining for 2 weeks. Aspirin should not be used because it impairs blood clotting. Smoking also is discouraged.

PATIENT TEACHING PLAN
Tonsillectomy

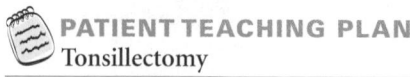

- Avoid strenuous activity for 2 weeks.
- Avoid aspirin, which interferes with blood clotting.
- Avoid smoking, which may disrupt healing.
- Drink 8 to 12 8-ounce glasses of fluid daily.
- Report bleeding to the physician.

DISORDERS OF THE LARYNX

Laryngitis

Laryngitis is inflammation of the larynx. It may occur alone, or it may accompany other upper respiratory infections. A number of factors may lead to laryngitis. Upper respiratory infections, voice strain, smoking, alcohol ingestion, and inhalation of irritating fumes are all possible factors. Some patients have chronic laryngitis caused by prolonged exposure to irritants.

Signs and Symptoms

Symptoms of laryngitis include hoarseness, cough, and scratchy or painful throat. The patient may report "losing" his or her voice. This absence of sound production is called aphonia, and it occurs in varying degrees. Changes in the voice may be permanent after long periods of chronic inflammation.

Medical Diagnosis

Diagnosis of laryngitis is based primarily on the patient's history and symptoms. The physician may use a laryngeal mirror to examine the larynx for color, edema, and growths such as polyps and tumors. With laryngitis, the vocal cords appear red and swollen. If an upper respiratory infection is suspected, a throat culture may be done to determine the pathogen and best treatment.

Medical Treatment

Treatment of acute laryngitis is primarily aimed at reducing irritation of the larynx. Voice rest is advised, meaning that the patient is to rest the larynx by not talking. An important aspect of treatment for chronic laryngitis is removal of the irritant.

NURSING CARE *of the Patient with Laryngitis*

Patients with laryngitis rarely require hospitalization, but nurses in other settings may teach people how to prevent and treat the condition.

Assessment

The assessment of the patient with laryngitis begins with a history of the problem. Document the severity of the condition, how long it has persisted, and any factors that seem to aggravate or precipitate it. Information about the patient's occupation and hobbies may provide some clues to the cause of the laryngitis. Take the patient's temperature and assess respiratory status to detect possible infection.

Nursing Diagnoses, Goals, and Outcome Criteria: Laryngitis

Nursing Diagnoses	Goals and Outcome Criteria
Impaired Verbal Communication related to aphonia or prescribed voice rest	Effective communication: patient uses nonverbal communication means
Ineffective Therapeutic Regimen Management related to lack of understanding of treatment and prevention of laryngitis	Effective management of therapeutic regimen: patient practices voice rest as ordered, avoids irritants

Interventions

When voice rest is prescribed, explain to the patient that it allows the larynx to heal. Meanwhile, an alternative means of communication must be established. Provide a pad and pencil or magic slate for written communication. For patients who cannot read or write, hand signals or pictures may be needed. A sign over the bed is needed to advise staff and visitors that the patient should not speak. It is also a good idea to put a notice on the intercom at the nurse's station that the patient cannot (or should not) speak. This alerts staff to go to the patient's room rather than asking what is needed on the intercom.

The teaching plan emphasizes measures to promote comfort and reduce future episodes of laryngitis. Discourage smoking. Advise the patient to remain in an environment with a constant temperature because sudden changes in temperature tend to aggravate laryngitis. If the air is very dry, a room humidifier reduces the discomfort of a dry nose and throat. Lozenges containing a topical anesthetic also may be ordered to soothe the irritation (see Table 51-3).

When the patient has chronic laryngitis, the primary goal of treatment is to remove the irritant. Advise the patient who smokes that stopping smoking is likely to improve the symptoms. Changes in the voice may be permanent after long periods of chronic inflammation.

Teach patients that irritants can lead to laryngitis. Patients need to recognize irritants in the home and workplace and know how to protect themselves from harm. If the patient is inclined to stop smoking, information about resources in the community can be provided. The American Cancer Society is a good source of information on how to stop smoking.

Laryngeal Nodules

Laryngeal nodules are benign masses of fibrous tissue that result primarily from overuse of the voice, but they can also follow infections. Singers and public speakers are prone to development of nodules because of the strain they put on their voices. The only symptom is hoarseness.

Nodules are surgically removed under local or general anesthesia. The removal of nodules is usually fairly simple, but they may recur if the voice is again misused. After the procedure, the patient is placed on voice rest for several days. Explain voice rest as described previously in the section on Laryngitis and emphasize the need to avoid strain on the voice.

Laryngeal Polyps

A laryngeal polyp is a swollen mass of mucous membrane attached to the vocal cord. It can cause continuous or intermittent hoarseness, depending on its location and attachment.

In heavy smokers, flabby masses of tissue may develop on both vocal cords. A procedure called stripping of the vocal cords is necessary to treat this condition. Unless the patient continues smoking, the condition usually does not return. As with other vocal cord surgery, voice rest is prescribed for patients who have polyps removed.

Cancer of the Larynx

Cancer of the larynx accounts for more than 10,000 new cancers each year. It causes more than 4,000 deaths yearly and is increasing in frequency. Cancer of the larynx is most common in men aged 50 to 65 years. The higher incidence in men is thought to be related to greater alcohol and tobacco use.

Factors believed to predispose to laryngeal cancer are exposure to smoke or other noxious fumes, alcohol consumption, vocal strain, and chronic laryngitis. People who both smoke and use alcohol are at particularly high risk.

Malignant tumors can develop at various points throughout the larynx: above the glottis, on the vocal cords, or below the vocal cords. Most malignancies of the larynx are squamous cell carcinomas.

The cure rate is highest for patients with tumors that are confined to the vocal cords. Unfortunately, malignancies in the larynx tend to spread fairly early. The most common site of metastasis is the lung. The more widespread the cancer is, the more difficult it is to treat. The death rate among men has declined slightly (−11%) over the past 20 years, but it has increased dramatically (+67%) for women.

Signs and Symptoms

Persistent hoarseness is the primary symptom of cancer of the larynx. Some patients report throat discomfort or a sensation that there is a "lump" in the throat. Other signs and symptoms of laryngeal cancer are hemoptysis (blood in sputum), difficulty swallowing or breathing, and persistent cough, sore throat, or earache. Pain and anorexia leading to weight loss are usually late symptoms of the disease.

Prevention

The most important measures to reduce the risk of cancer of the larynx are for people to stop smoking and drinking alcohol. The public also should be educated to recognize the signs and symptoms of laryngeal cancer and seek prompt medical attention. Early treatment may be able to preserve the voice.

Medical Diagnosis

A diagnosis of cancer of the larynx is confirmed by study of a tissue sample obtained during a laryngoscopy. Radiographs, computed tomographic scans, and magnetic resonance imaging are done to define the extent of the cancer. These studies give more detail about the primary site and help to locate metastases. Laboratory findings often seen with malignancies include decreased hemoglobin and hematocrit and elevated alkaline phosphatase. Remember that these changes can be due to causes other than cancer.

Medical Treatment

Treatment involves the use of surgery, radiotherapy, chemotherapy, or some combination of these. The diagnostic tests described above aid the physician in selecting the treatment of the patient with laryngeal cancer. Another important consideration is the patient's overall health state and ability to cope with the effects of specific treatments.

Radiotherapy alone can cure some small cancers that have not spread to surrounding tissues. In addition, radiation may be used before and after surgery. Brachytherapy is a form of radiotherapy that involves placing thin, hollow needles into and around the tumor. Radioactive seeds are then placed in the needles to emit continuous radiation to the area.

Chemotherapy may be administered as palliative treatment, before surgery to reduce tumor size, or postoperatively to reduce the risk of metastasis. Care of the patient undergoing radiotherapy or chemotherapy is discussed in Chapter 24.

Surgery

Surgical procedures for cancer of the larynx range from simple removal of the tumor to extensive procedures such as laryngectomy and modified or radical neck dissection (Fig. 51-6). Laser surgery may be used alone or with radiation therapy for small tumors. A laryngectomy can be total or partial. Total laryngectomy causes permanent loss of the natural voice. Figure 51-6 illustrates airflow before and after laryngectomy.

Radical neck dissection often is done at the same time as laryngectomy, especially if lymph nodes are positive for cancer. Radical neck dissection is the excision of all nonessential structures on the affected side. The sternocleidomastoid

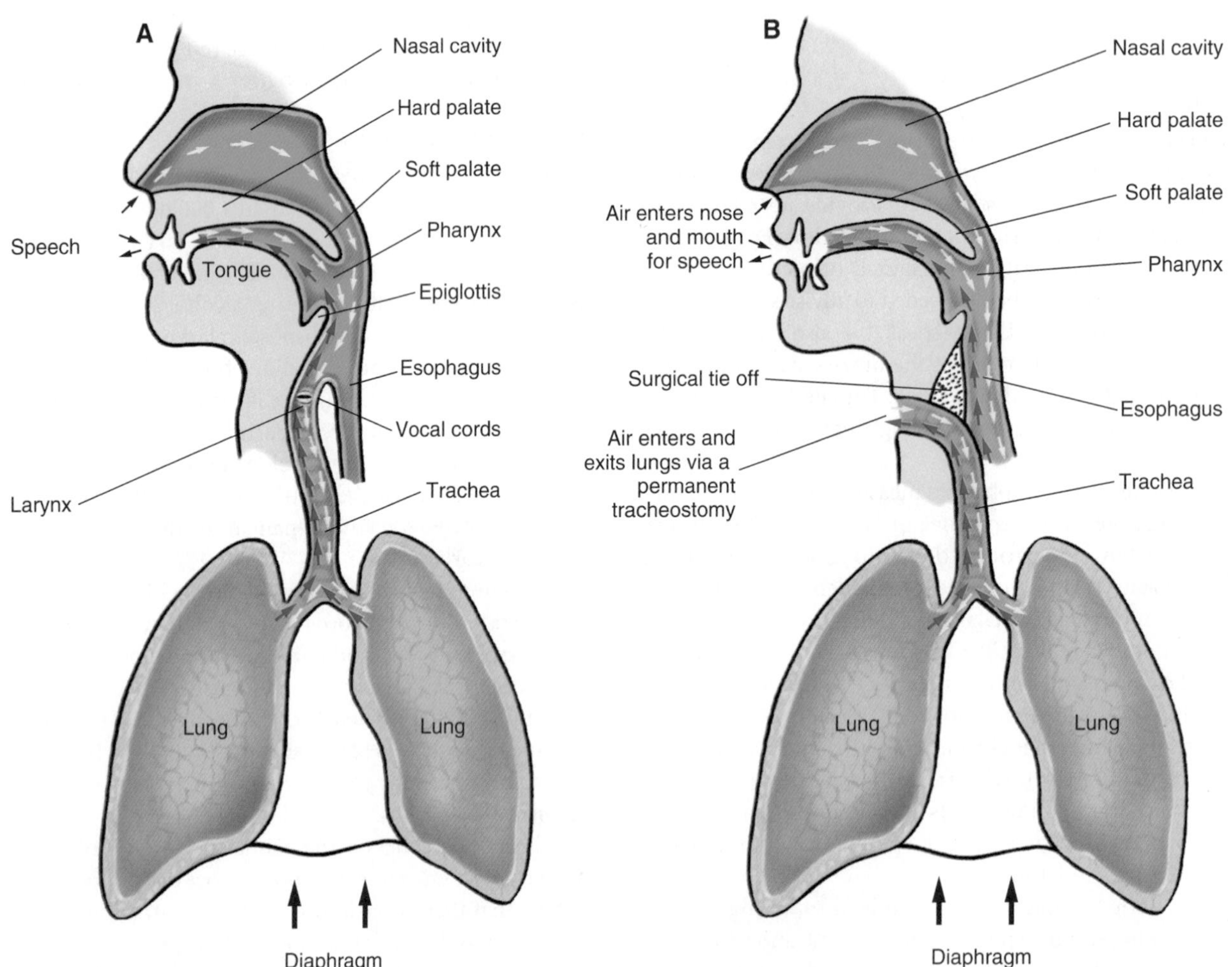

FIGURE **51-6** The throat before *(A)* and after *(B)* total laryngectomy. Arrows indicate the route of airflow.

muscle, jugular vein, submaxillary salivary gland, and surrounding soft tissue are removed. The spinal accessory nerve is cut, causing the shoulder to droop on the affected side. Figure 51-7 illustrates the appearance of the incisions after radical neck dissection. A modified radical neck dissection spares the internal jugular vein, the major cervical lymphatic vessels, and the sympathetic, vagus, and spinal accessory nerves.

NURSING CARE *of the Patient having Total Laryngectomy*

General preoperative nursing care is discussed in Chapter 16. This section addresses the specific teaching needs of the patient facing surgery for laryngeal cancer. Try to find out which procedure will be done so that preoperative teaching can be individualized.

If the patient will lose the ability to speak, information about other means of communication should be available. The physician and speech therapist can advise the patient about appropriate alternatives. The anticipated loss of the voice is very stressful to patients. The full impact may not actually hit them until later because the first concern is eliminating the cancer. Listen compassionately and accept the patient's expressions of anger or despair. Some patients benefit from meeting a volunteer from an organization for people who have had laryngectomies. Consult the patient about this before inviting a volunteer.

The patient who will have a laryngectomy and radical neck dissection can expect to go to an intensive care unit for several days. This allows close monitoring and maintenance of a patent airway with the new tracheostomy. Advise the patient in advance that this is routine and does not mean that anything has gone wrong. You can also help prepare the patient to expect intravenous lines, wound drains, a feeding tube, and, perhaps for a short time, a ventilator.

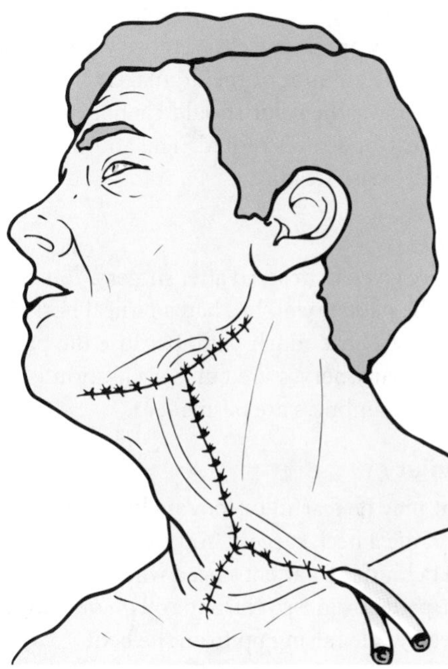

FIGURE 51-7 A radical neck dissection incision with drain tubes in place.

Postoperative care varies with the exact procedure. Procedures include partial laryngectomy, supraglottic laryngectomy, and total laryngectomy. Nursing care of the patient with a total laryngectomy is presented in detail. The unique needs of the patient with a partial or supraglottic laryngectomy are identified.

A total laryngectomy involves removal of the entire larynx, vocal cords, and epiglottis as well as supportive tissues. The opening of the pharynx to the trachea is closed, and the tracheostomy is created by bringing the trachea to the opening in the neck. The upper airway is no longer connected to the lower airway. The patient breathes through the trachea. Figure 51-6 illustrates the changes with total laryngectomy. A radical neck dissection is often done because of the high risk of metastasis to the neck.

Complications

Complications of total laryngectomy with radical neck dissection include salivary fistula, carotid artery blowout, and tracheal stenosis. A salivary fistula is a drainage pathway that forms when saliva leaks through a defect in the suture line in the pharynx. It usually closes spontaneously but sometimes requires surgical closure. Until the fistula closes, the patient must be fed through a nasogastric tube. Otherwise, whatever the patient eats leaks out the fistula.

Patients at highest risk for carotid artery blowout (rupture) are those who had radiation therapy before surgery and acquired a salivary fistula after surgery. Carotid blowout is an emergency that must be corrected surgically.

Tracheal stenosis is narrowing of the trachea that develops weeks or months after surgery. If the airway becomes obstructed, surgical correction is necessary.

The general nursing care of the postoperative patient is discussed in Chapter 16. This section addresses the special needs of the patient with total laryngectomy.

Assessment

In the immediate postoperative period, the assessment focuses on oxygenation, circulation, and comfort. Document the patient's level of consciousness. Ask about pain and observe for signs of discomfort. Measure vital signs at frequent intervals. Continuous electrocardiogram monitoring and pulse oximetry also may be used to assess oxygenation and circulation. Record fluid intake and output, and describe the characteristics of wound drainage.

Additional aspects of assessment after total laryngectomy are weight changes, ability to swallow, and effectiveness of alternate means of communication. The patient's response to the surgery, coping strategies used, and sources of support also are very important. During the rehabilitation phase, members of the health care team help the patient anticipate the effects of the surgery on everyday life and the adaptations that need to be made. Also assess the patient's readiness and ability to participate in self-care.

Nursing Diagnoses, Goals, and Outcome Criteria: Total Laryngectomy, Postoperative

Nursing Diagnoses	Goals and Outcome Criteria
Ineffective Airway Clearance related to increased pulmonary secretions or weak cough	Patent airway: respiratory rate 12 to 20 without dyspnea, breath sounds clear
Anxiety related to revised airway, uncertain outcome of cancer surgery, or threat to self-concept	Reduced anxiety: patient calm, states anxiety is reduced
Decreased Cardiac Output related to excessive blood loss	Adequate cardiac output: pulse and blood pressure consistent with patient norms, fluid intake, and output equal Minimal blood loss: decreasing bleeding, drainage lightens in color
Acute Pain related to tissue trauma	Pain relief: patient states pain reduced, relaxed manner
Risk for Injury related to excision of muscles in the neck or altered upper airway	Reduced risk for injury: patient demonstrates protection of incision during movement, avoids introduction of harmful substances into trachea
Imbalanced Nutrition: Less than Body Requirements related to dysphagia or diminished sense of smell	Adequate nutrition: stable body weight, maintenance of patient's admission weight if normal
Impaired Verbal Communication related to surgical excision of larynx	Effective communication: patient uses a means of communication that meets his or her needs
Ineffective Coping related to loss of verbal communication or altered appearance	Effective coping with body changes: patient makes realistic plans to adapt lifestyle to physical and functional changes
Risk for Infection related to altered airway or interrupted skin integrity	Absence of infection: normal body temperature and white blood cell count, no purulent drainage or secretions
Ineffective Therapeutic Regimen Management related to fear, lack of understanding of self-care	Patient assumes self-care: correctly demonstrates care of tracheostomy

Interventions

Ineffective Airway Clearance

As previously emphasized, oxygenation status must be assessed frequently. If the patient is on a ventilator, it usually is discontinued within a day after surgery. At first, the patient has a laryngectomy tube in the tracheostomy. The laryngectomy tube is shorter and wider than a tracheostomy tube, but care of the two is essentially the same.

Because the new tracheostomy bypasses the upper airway, the respiratory tract has to adjust to a dramatic change. The mucous membranes respond to the unexpected trauma and irritation by increasing secretions. Because normal humidification is absent, the secretions tend to be drier than normal, making it more difficult to remove them from the airway.

The trachea and laryngectomy tube must be kept open at all times, or else the patient would suffocate. Assess the need for suctioning (increased pulse, restlessness, audible or visible mucus) and use sterile technique to clear the airway as needed. Tracheostomy suctioning is described earlier in this chapter. Consult a procedure manual for additional details.

Factors that affect respiratory status are positioning, fluids, and humidification. Semi-Fowler's or Fowler's position permits maximal lung expansion. Turning, coughing, and deep breathing prevent pooling of secretions in the lungs. Intravenous fluids and enteral feedings maintain hydration and nutrition. Good hydration helps to thin secretions. A tracheostomy collar is used to provide oxygen and humidification of inspired air.

Anxiety

Be sensitive to the patient's anxiety. A calm approach, attentive monitoring, and simple explanations help to reduce anxiety. You must also remember to talk to the patient! There is a tendency to treat the patient who cannot speak as if he or she cannot hear either.

Decreased Cardiac Output

In the early postoperative period, the patient is at risk for excessive bleeding. Frequent monitoring of vital signs allows detection of indicators of hemorrhage, such as increasing pulse and respiratory rates and restlessness. Inspect secretions for excessive bleeding.

Drains usually are in place to remove excess fluid. Assess the color and the amount of the drainage. Over the first few postoperative days, the color should change from bright red to pink to clear or straw-colored. The amount of drainage also should decrease steadily.

Acute Pain

Analgesics are given as ordered after surgery. You may be surprised that the patient who has had a radical neck dissection may not seem to have much pain. Because the procedure is so extensive, many nerves are cut, so sensation is impaired. Some areas of numbness are permanent.

Risk for Injury

The patient may be fearful of moving his or her head, especially after radical neck surgery. You can help at first by placing a hand behind the patient's head when he or she gets out of bed. The patient can also learn to roll on one side and support the head while raising up from the bed.

The tracheostomy is open to the environment and must be protected from foreign substances. Teach the patient to avoid dusty places and to cover the tracheostomy loosely during shaving or haircuts. The patient cannot submerge the neck or allow bath water to splash into the trachea because the water would go directly into the airway.

Imbalanced Nutrition: Less than Body Requirements

Nutrition is often a problem after laryngectomy. The patient's sense of smell is impaired because inspired air no longer goes through the nose. The patient also may have some difficulty swallowing because of tissue trauma around the surgical site. Nasogastric tube feedings are given initially. Oral fluids and foods are reintroduced gradually. Nursing measures to improve appetite should be used, and the patient's weight should be monitored. Chapter 8 discusses nursing interventions for anorexia and for tube feedings.

Impaired Verbal Communication

A number of options exist for restoring some form of speech to the patient with laryngectomy. The speech therapist and the physician will recommend appropriate methods (Fig. 51-8).

Many patients are able to learn to use "esophageal speech." Air is swallowed and held in the upper esophagus. The patient then belches. The patient learns to control and use the air to produce sounds. The voice is deep but understandable. Considerable motivation and practice are needed to master esophageal speech. Patients and their families are likely to have periods of discouragement. You can help by acknowledging their feelings and demonstrating patience.

A second option is the use of an artificial larynx. Several types of electronic devices are available that produce sound. The "voice," however, has a mechanical, computerized sound that tends to attract attention.

Some patients are candidates for laryngoplasty, a procedure performed during total laryngectomy. It is done to create a connection between the pharynx and the trachea. The patient is able to speak by occluding the tracheostomy with a finger. This procedure is not an option for all patients and is not always successful.

Tracheostomy tubes and valves that facilitate speech are available. Two examples of these tubes are illustrated in Figure 51-8.

One final option for speech is the tracheoesophageal prosthesis. The surgeon creates a fistula between the trachea and the esophagus. A catheter is placed in the fistula until it heals. When the catheter is removed, a prosthesis is inserted into the fistula. Two prostheses that may be used are the Blom-Singer trapdoor prosthesis and the Panje voice button. The patient occludes the stoma with a finger during speech. A one-way valve allows air to flow only from the trachea to the esophagus.

Those patients who are unable to use any form of speech must rely on written communication, gestures, or some assistive devices. A word board is a computerized device that enables the patient to select words that are "spoken" by the computer. A personal communicator produces a printed message that the patient enters on a keyboard.

It is especially important to direct the laryngectomy patient to community resources. Organizations such as the Lost Chord Club or New Voice Club are especially useful because the members have had personal experiences with laryngectomies. The American Cancer Society can provide information about resources in the local community.

Ineffective Coping

It has been said that language separates humans from animals. The permanent loss of the ability to communicate verbally is very traumatic. Patients who require laryngectomy usually have some time to prepare for this procedure in advance, but the actual event still evokes a variety of emotional responses. Learning to live with a permanent tracheostomy and loss of the natural voice requires considerable adjustment. The patient may demonstrate behaviors typical of any loss situation: denial, anger, depression, bargaining, or acceptance. Depression may be reflected in withdrawal or refusal to learn about self-care and rehabilitative measures.

Acknowledge the patient's feelings and gently urge participation in self-care and use of alternative means of communication. The patient who learns to care for the tracheostomy and to communicate effectively feels more confident of the ability to cope. Support groups can be especially helpful because the patient sees potential role models of successful adaptation to tracheostomy. The family also requires support, encouragement, and teaching.

Risk for Infection

The tracheostomy permits unfiltered air to enter the respiratory tract. The effects are drying of the mucous membranes, increased secretions, and increased risk of infection. Use sterile technique during tracheostomy care. Protect the patient from people who have respiratory infections.

Ineffective Therapeutic Regimen Management

As soon as the patient is able, encourage participation in self-care. At first, just ask the patient to hold some supplies. Explain what is being done and why. Gradually, the patient should assume more responsibility for care of the tracheostomy. Even if the patient seems quite competent by discharge, a referral to a home health agency or visiting nurse association is recommended. The home care nurse helps the patient learn to adapt care to the home setting and to deal with various unanticipated problems. A family member or significant other should be taught tracheostomy care as well. Verbal teaching should be accompanied by written information for later use. Remember that people recall only a small percentage of what they hear.

NURSING CARE *of the Patient having Supraglottic Laryngectomy*

For patients who have cancer above the vocal cords, supraglottic laryngectomy and radical neck dissection are the usual procedures. These patients also have temporary tracheostomies. Cuffed tubes are used at first because of the danger of aspiration. These patients require oral and tracheal suctioning.

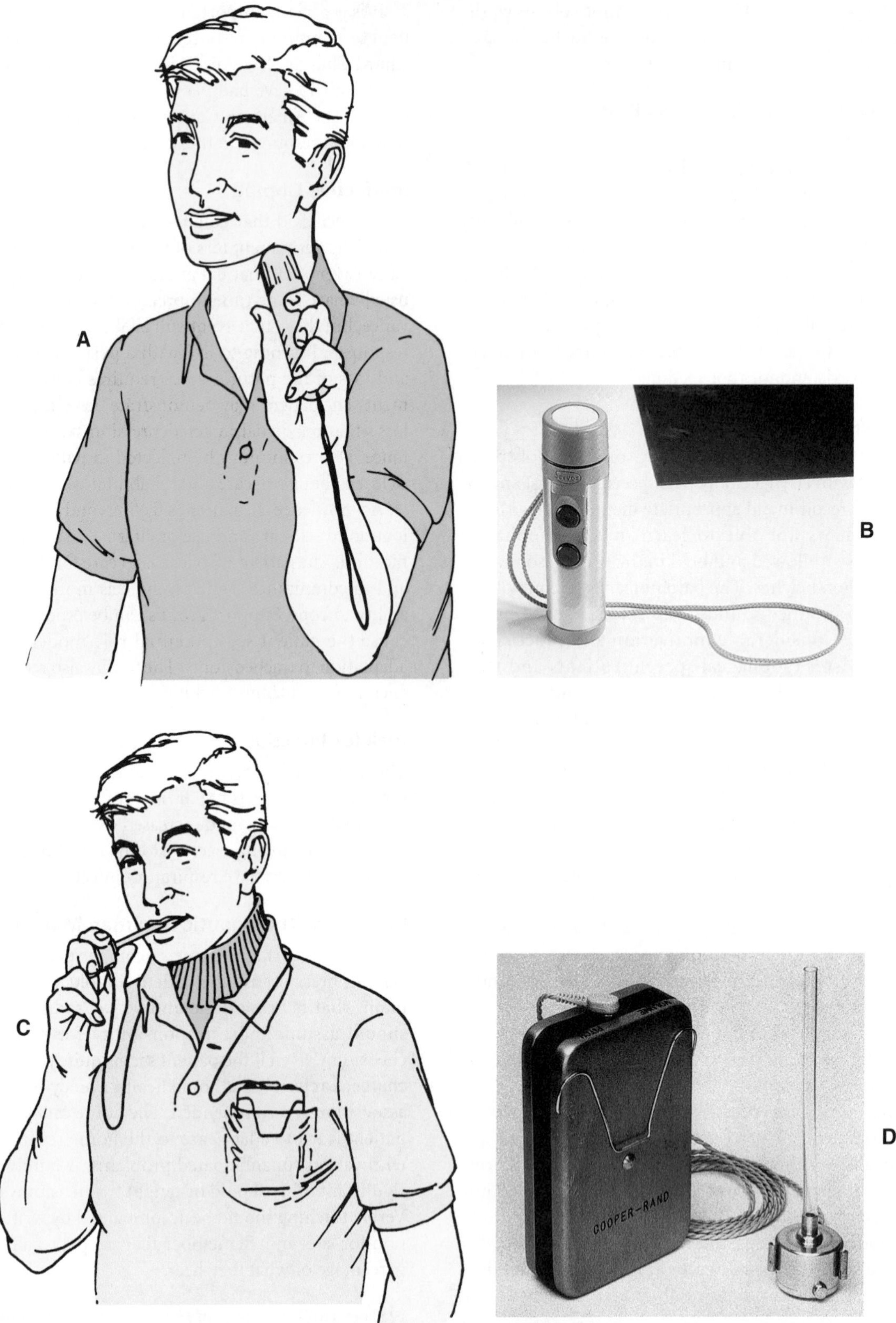

FIGURE 51-8 Postlaryngectomy speech aids. *A* and *B*, Patient using Servox Electrolarynx artificial larynx, which is held against the throat to detect vibrations from silently mouthed words and convert them to electronic sounds. *C* and *D*, The Cooper-Rand electronic speech aid allows the patient to adjust tone, pitch, and volume.

Continued

FIGURE **51-8, cont'd** *E,* Blom-Singer trapdoor tracheoesophageal prosthesis. *F,* Panje voice button.

Nursing care of the patient having supraglottic laryngectomy is in many ways like that of the patient having total laryngectomy, except that the tracheostomy is temporary, the voice is not lost, and swallowing is more problematic. Therefore additional nursing interventions are indicated to maintain good nutrition. Enteral feedings may be needed for a long time, so begin to instruct the patient in self-feeding. Some patients never regain the ability to swallow without aspirating, and total laryngectomy is recommended for them.

An example of the swallowing techniques taught to these patients is the following:

1. Assume a sitting position.
2. Take a deep breath and hold it.
3. Place food on the back of the tongue with a spoon.
4. Swallow three times while holding the breath.
5. Cough. (*Note:* When the patient has a tracheostomy, any aspirated food or fluids may be ejected through the tracheostomy.)

The patient with a supraglottic laryngectomy is also at increased risk for aspiration pneumonia. Be alert for signs and symptoms of this complication: increased pulse and respiratory rates, dyspnea, cough, crackles and rhonchi, fever, wheezing, and frothy, pink sputum. Keep a suction machine readily available.

NURSING CARE *of the Patient having Partial Laryngectomy*

If a patient has a partial laryngectomy, a temporary tracheostomy for 2 to 5 days can be expected. Intravenous fluids and enteral feedings usually are ordered at first. Like patients with supraglottic laryngectomies, these patients have considerable difficulty swallowing when oral nourishment is resumed. In general, the nursing care is similar to that of the patient having a supraglottic laryngectomy. To prevent aspiration, seat the patient upright, with the head flexed slightly forward. Semisolids are often easier to manage than thin liquids. A suction machine should be on hand in case it is needed.

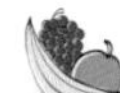

Nutrition Concepts

1. Malignancies of the upper airway often lead to inadequate nutritional intake.
2. Patients who have had partial laryngectomies are at high risk for aspiration while learning to swallow again.
3. Gastrostomy or NG tubes may be placed to maintain nutrition following partial laryngectomy.

key points

- Sinusitis is acute or chronic inflammation of the sinuses that can lead to meningitis, brain abscess, osteomyelitis, and orbital cellulitis.
- Sinusitis is treated with drug therapy or with surgery to remove obstructions and to improve drainage.
- Nasal polyps are masses of tissue that extend from the sinuses into the nasal passage; they can be surgically excised.
- Allergic rhinitis, or "hay fever," is an allergic response to a substance that produces sneezing; nasal obstruction;

clear nasal discharge; frontal headache; and itchy, watery eyes.

- Allergic rhinitis may be treated with antihistamines and decongestants or with desensitizing injections of identified allergens.
- Acute viral coryza, the common cold, is caused by a virus; is contagious; and is treated symptomatically with antihistamines, decongestants, and antipyretics.
- Tumors of the nasal passages typically cause nasal obstruction requiring surgical excision.
- Malignant tumors of the nasal passages and pharynx tend to metastasize early and may be treated with some combination of surgery, chemotherapy, and radiation therapy.
- The two kinds of carcinomas of the external nose are squamous cell carcinomas, which grow rapidly and tend to metastasize, and basal cell carcinomas, which grow more slowly and are less invasive.
- A deviated nasal septum may obstruct the nasal passages and interfere with sinus drainage.
- Surgical procedures for deviated nasal septum include nasal septoplasty and submucosal resection.
- Epistaxis (nosebleed) usually can be controlled with external pressure but sometimes requires placement of a nasal balloon catheter or packing.
- Tonsillitis is more common in children but is more often severe in adults.
- Tonsillitis may be treated with drug therapy, irrigations, or surgical excision.
- Nursing care after tonsillectomy focuses on decreased cardiac output, ineffective airway clearance, acute pain, and ineffective therapeutic regimen management.
- Cancer of the larynx may be treated with surgery, radiation therapy, chemotherapy, or a combination of these.
- After laryngectomy (removal of the larynx), the nurse addresses problems of ineffective airway clearance, anxiety, decreased cardiac output, acute pain, risk for injury, imbalanced nutrition: less than body requirements, impaired verbal communication, ineffective coping, risk for infection, and ineffective therapeutic regimen management.

REVIEW QUESTIONS

1. The function of the turbinates in the internal nose is to:

1. trap inspired particles.
2. destroy microorganisms.
3. warm inspired air
4. detect odors

2. Age-related changes in the nose, sinuses, and throat include:

1. thickening of the mucous membrane.
2. increased mucus production.
3. decreased sense of smell.
4. less risk of epistaxis.

3. The maximum time that suction should be applied during nasotracheal suctioning is:

1. 10 seconds.
2. 15 seconds.
3. 20 seconds.
4. 25 seconds

4. After nasal surgery, a patient has packing in place and a nasal drip ("moustache") dressing on the upper lip. When the moustache dressing has become saturated, you should:

1. replace the packing and the moustache dressing.
2. notify the physician.
3. reinforce the moustache dressing.
4. change the moustache dressing.

5. A patient who had nasal surgery is restless. His pulse rate has increased from 70 to 90 bpm, and his respiratory rate is 20. His nasal dressing has no fresh bleeding. What should you do *first?*

1. Order one unit of blood.
2. Take his vital signs again.
3. Inspect the back of his throat.
4. Encourage increased fluid intake.

6. The most serious complications of sinusitis include:

1. headache.
2. pain.
3. meningitis.
4. rhinitis.

7. A patient who has "triad disease" is allergic to aspirin, has asthma, and has:

1. elevated triglycerides.
2 nasal polyps.
3. tonsillitis.
4. laryngeal nodules.

8. Immediate treatment of epistaxis is to have the patient:

1. sit up, lean slightly forward, and pinch the nostrils.
2. assume a semi-Fowler's position with the head tilted back.
3. lie supine and apply a cold pack to the nose.
4. sit up and lean forward to put the head between his knees.

9. The priority nursing diagnosis after total laryngectomy is:
   1. anxiety.
   2. acute pain.
   3. ineffective airway clearance.
   4. impaired verbal communication.

10. The primary advantage of supraglottic laryngectomy over total laryngectomy is that:
    1. swallowing is easier.
    2. the voice is preserved.
    3. the tracheostomy is permanent.
    4. there is less risk of aspiration pneumonia.

CHAPTER

52 Psychological Responses to Illness

MARK D. SOUCY

objectives

1. Define mental health.
2. Discuss the concepts of stress, anxiety, adaptation, and homeostasis.
3. Discuss how age and cultural and spiritual beliefs affect an individual's ability to cope with illness.
4. Identify some basic coping strategies (defense mechanisms).
5. Discuss the concepts of anxiety, fear, stress, loss, grief, helplessness, and powerlessness in relation to illness.
6. Describe several factors that may precipitate adaptive or maladaptive coping behaviors in response to illness.
7. Discuss implementation of the nursing process to enhance a patient's mental health as the patient deals with the stresses of illness.

key terms

Adaptation (p. 1121)
Anxiety (ăng-ZĪ-ĭ-tē, p. 1124)
Conflict (p. 1121)
Coping (p. 1124)
Crisis (p. 1121)
Defense mechanism (p. 1124)
Feelings (p. 1123)
Helplessness (p. 1126)
Maladaptive coping (măl-ă-DĂP-tĭv, p. 1124)
Self-esteem (p. 1122)
Stress (p. 1121)
Stressor (p. 1121)

Part of being human is having to cope with different types of stressors at different times of life. Individual coping strategies are influenced by many factors, such as personal beliefs and values, the family, cultural practices, and community resources. Patients and their families may experience a wide range of feelings and emotions in response to illness. In order to promote adaptation to illness and to minimize maladaptive behaviors, you need to be well acquainted with the range of responses that individuals can experience during illness. The nursing process provides a systematic approach to individualized care based on careful assessment and understanding of human behavior.

DEFINITION OF MENTAL HEALTH

A person is a living being with physical, cognitive, affective, behavioral, and social dimensions who interacts with the environment to achieve a chosen life purpose. The *physical dimension* includes the biologic and physiologic aspects of a person, and it is integrated with cognitive, affective, behavioral, and social dimensions. The *cognitive dimension* involves an individual's ability to formulate thoughts, process information, and solve problems. The *affective dimension* involves an individual's ability to experience and express feelings and emotions. The *behavioral dimension* reflects a person's individuality and involves integration of the physical, cognitive, and affective dimensions. The *social dimension* involves an individual's skills in living as a member of a family and community. Together these dimensions form a holistic or total person.

Environment is everything outside a person. It includes the physical and social elements that are external to and interactive with an individual. In a health care setting, you are a part of the environment.

Mental health is a dynamic process in which a person's physical, cognitive, affective, behavioral, and social dimensions interact functionally with one another and the environment. Mentally healthy individuals are able to perceive reality accurately, manage the way that emotions are experienced and expressed, think clearly and logically, communicate effectively, anticipate events and solve problems, initiate and maintain meaningful relationships, develop a positive self-concept, and generally behave in ways that promote personal growth and development.

According to Maslow, healthy individuals possess several characteristics:

An accurate perception of reality
The ability to accept oneself and others
The ability to be spontaneous
The ability to solve problems
A need for privacy
Independence or autonomy
The ability to express the self emotionally
A frequency of "peak experiences"—happy moments that produce a sense of worth, hope, and love of life
Identification with humankind
The ability to maintain satisfactory relationships

A sense of ethics
Some sense of resistance to conformity

STRESS

Stressors can originate in any or all of the dimensions of the self. At any given moment, individuals are adapting to a variety of stressors from each of the five dimensions. Thus a person's level of health is directly related to the ability to adjust to a variety of internal and external stressors.

Stress is caused by a stressor. A stressor can be anything, positive or negative, that necessitates an adaptive response on the part of the individual. Stress is necessary for growth and development. Mild stress produces mild anxiety and enables people to use energy focused exclusively on the problem. The result can be successful problem solving, which in turn promotes self-esteem. However, stress can also be perceived as harmful. Examples of potentially harmful stressors are the loss of a job or the death of a family member.

Adaptation to stress affects the whole organism. For example, a person who is immobilized lacks the stress of exercise, so that the muscles begin to atrophy, joints become rigid and inflexible, and so on, until all the systems of the body are affected. With daily stress such as moderate exercise, muscles increase in mass, circulation improves, and joints become more flexible. So it is with mental health. The dimensions of the person—physical, cognitive, affective, behavioral, and social—are not separate entities. These dimensions interact, resulting in the development of a unique human being.

HOMEOSTASIS

Stress, response, and adaptation can be thought of as a process aimed at maintaining homeostasis or equilibrium. If stressors are relatively mild and the person is able to respond and adapt, mental health is maintained. If, however, the person is overwhelmed by many stressors or does not have sufficient coping behaviors or problem-solving strategies to maintain equilibrium, illness or crisis may ensue. A crisis results in inner tension and anxiety, which may affect an individual's ability to function.

GROWTH AND DEVELOPMENT

Growth refers to an individual's gradual process of evolution from conception until death. As human beings move through sequential stages of development, they become increasingly complex. Each individual is shaped throughout life by all of the events and perceived interactions with individuals, the community, and the environment. Growth, then, refers not only to a change in physical size and structure but also to an increasingly complex process of development.

Many theorists have attempted to explain how personality develops. Most believe that early human experiences provide the framework for all future references. Development is usually divided into stages that correspond to a specific age group. Developmental tasks are a part of the work of moving through each of these stages. In part, successful development depends on how individuals negotiate through each stage. Individual experiences influence how people respond to illness.

Infancy and early childhood are times when nurturing is critical and exploration of the world begins. As children grow and progress through school, they must learn the rules of society. Preschoolers must learn to handle joint decision-making and interpersonal conflicts. Middle childhood is a time for learning to deal with frustration and unfavorable events while also learning to celebrate good things and feeling pleasure. During adolescence, teenagers learn to develop as individuals, become independent, and begin to think for themselves. They have to learn how to delay gratification, relax, and interact with peers of both sexes. In early adulthood, people find a life partner and life work and begin a family. Adults progressing through middle age begin to look at the impact their lives have had or could have. Older age is often a time of introspection, when elders look back on their lives, accept what has been, and attempt to face increasing frailty with grace. Throughout life, individuals strive to make sense of the world by searching for meaning.

BEHAVIORAL THEORY

Behavioral theory is based on the idea that all behaviors are learned responses. Conditioning is one type of learning. An example of a conditioned response was demonstrated by Pavlov, who would ring a bell (stimulus) when feeding (reinforcement) his dog. The dog would salivate when the food was presented. The reflex response of salivation eventually occurred with the ringing of the bell only. Theorists such as B. F. Skinner, Albert Bandura, and Joseph Wople have based their theories on the idea that all behavior is learned and is a series of habitual responses to familiar stimuli.

PSYCHOLOGICAL RESPONSES TO ILLNESS

Responses to illness are as unique as the individuals who respond. Individual responses to illness are related to the individual's life experiences, self-concept, perceptions, values, cultural perspectives and spiritual beliefs, to name a few.

COPING WITH ILLNESS

Most people see illness as a distressing, abnormal state of being. This state of distress demands that individuals draw from their inner resources to cope. These resources may come from any or all of the following dimensions: physical, cognitive, affective, behavioral, social, and spiritual. For some, the inner strengths drawn from these various dimensions may be sufficient to cope effectively with illness. For others, however, attempts to cope may be ineffective or maladaptive. This is where effective nursing intervention becomes essential.

A caring attitude is basic to helping a patient cope with illness. Through the trust developed in a therapeutic nurse-patient relationship, the nurse can help the patient cope with stressors precipitated by illness.

To assess an individual's potential for coping with an illness effectively, you need to understand that the ability to cope is affected by various factors. Among these factors are age, cultural beliefs, spirituality, self-concept, family and community resources, emotions, stress, fear, anxiety, loss, grief, and mourning.

Factors that Affect Coping with Illness

Age

Age affects the coping ability of children and adults alike. The developmental process continues throughout the life span. Illness can interfere with developmental progress, and the patient's developmental stage can influence how he or she responds to illness. Much stress may be experienced when illness interferes with development. Illness can interfere with a number of adult roles. New or existing relationships, careers, family responsibilities, and a host of other roles may be affected by the onset of illness. An illness can be especially traumatic if a family breadwinner is self-employed or has insufficient health insurance.

There also are differences in the way people of different ages respond to illness. For example, young children who do not understand the gravity of an illness may not experience much stress as long as they feel well and are not separated from their parents. Among adults, it has been found that cancer patients who were younger than 50 years of age experienced more frequent and more severe psychological problems than those older than 70 (Hymovich and Hagopian, 1992).

When assessing the patient's ability to cope with illness, you need to understand that illness is a stressful, disruptive experience regardless of age. It not only disrupts the developmental process of the individual but also has a traumatic impact on spouses, children, and other loved ones. You will play an essential role in helping patients and their loved ones to cope with an illness and the changes that result.

Cultural Beliefs

Culture is a system of symbols shared by a group of humans. Culture is transmitted from each generation to the next and is influenced by other social contexts as well. Culture brings organization and security to people's lives. It provides many of the underlying values and beliefs on which behavior is based. Culture can affect attitudes toward health and illness, diet and eating practices, reaction to pain, and values concerning death and dying. Ethnicity is a broader term that denotes a group's affiliation because of a shared language, race, and cultural values.

For individuals to be seen as unique entities, their cultural and ethnic backgrounds must be considered. This becomes especially important when trying to assess whether patients need assistance in coping with the stresses of illness. Remember, however, that not all people who look as if they belong to a specific cultural or ethnic group because of language, surname, or physical characteristics necessarily identify with any specific group. Effective nursing interventions can be determined only after the patient has been assessed as a unique individual, not only as black or Latino, male or female, gay or straight.

When helping patients cope with illness, you need to recognize that your own racial and cultural background may affect your ability to intervene effectively. This is especially true if the patient's cultural values and your own values differ greatly. It is important to respect the patient, regardless of your own personal beliefs, values, and culture. A judgmental attitude on your part interferes with delivering the best nursing care possible.

Before suggesting a plan of care, you should consider whether the nursing approach being suggested is relevant to the patient's individual needs. Does the nursing care help patients deal with stress, or does it contribute to stress? Effective care is individualized according to the patient's needs, values, and beliefs.

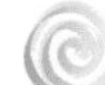

What Does Culture Have to do with Illness?

Culture shapes attitudes toward health and illness, nutrition, pain, and death and dying.

Spirituality

During the crisis of illness, patients often turn to their spiritual beliefs and values to find meaning in the experience. Patients who perhaps had not thought of themselves as being religious may suddenly have a need to visit with a spiritual counselor. Many patients experience spiritual distress when under the stress of an illness. They may feel that the illness is unfair and that God has betrayed and/or abandoned them. Sometimes people feel that the illness is a punishment from God for some transgression they believe they have made.

Spiritual distress can be characterized by the following: (1) Patients question the meaning of suffering or existence; (2) patients experience a sense of conflict between their personal beliefs (or desires) and their relationship with their God; or (3) patients experience symptoms such as nightmares, sleep disturbances, and alterations in behavior and mood.

To assess whether spirituality is an asset or a liability to the patient's ability to cope with illness, you must understand that all individuals are experts about their own spiritual needs and paths. Patients need an opportunity to express their feelings in a therapeutic and nonjudgmental environment. Simply put, your role is to listen, support, and care. Effective therapeutic nursing interventions enhance the healing process by supporting patients as they work through their spiritual distress and by shoring up their relationship with their spiritual connectedness.

Self-Concept

Self-concept refers to the notions, beliefs, and convictions persons hold about themselves. It is related to self-esteem and influences a person's relationship with others. Self-esteem develops from individuals' own evaluations of their competence and of the value others place on them. Body image refers to the combination of conscious and unconscious attitudes people have about their own bodies. Both past and present perceptions of the body and the person's feelings about their body's size, shape, function, appearance, and potential make up the body image.

Self-concept can be affected by changes in self-esteem as well as changes in body image. Patients' perception of these changes and their ability or inability to cope with the changes may result in stress, fear, and anxiety. Age and developmental levels may directly affect the patient's self-esteem and body image. Adolescents are especially vulnerable to changes in body image because they have a strong need to look like their peers. Certain changes in body image can be quite traumatic at this developmental stage. Adults also can be vulnerable.

People such as actors, models, or professional football players, who rely on their physical characteristics to make a living, may not be able to cope well with an illness or injury that affects body image. A disfiguring or disabling injury could have a devastating effect on body image and self-esteem. Their personal strengths and weaknesses would determine how well they are able to cope with the threat that illness imposes on the self-concept.

Some patients, through their life experiences, have developed coping styles that allow them to confront problems effectively. Others may require more external resources such as friends, family, and the community to cope with the stress of illness.

Family and Community Resources

The basic functions of the family include providing for physical needs, giving love, providing a sense of belonging, and strengthening the self-esteem of its members. Functional families may provide optimal support for a patient facing the stress of illness. However, the family's ability to provide support for the patient depends on many factors including the quality of relationships among family members and the family's ability to access needed resources.

Because of increasing stresses on the family unit, many families are not able to provide as much support as the patient may need. The stress of illness in a family member may overburden a family that was already only marginally coping. Illness may have precipitated such stressors as changes in family roles, economic pressures, and geographic isolation that may make it difficult to access medical and other needed resources.

Many of the functions once provided by families are increasingly being assumed by social institutions within the community. Like families, communities vary in their ability to assist their members. Some communities are well equipped to assist the family with many challenges that it may face (e.g., financial, physical, legal, spiritual, emotional). Other communities are less able to meet those same needs. This is especially true if the patient lives in an impoverished, underserved, and/or rural community. Your knowledge of available resources can be invaluable to patients and families. Throughout the hospital stay, you must anticipate the patient's needs before discharge. Providing contact information and creating links for patients in the community to help meet the needs of the patient outside the institution are essential parts of preparing the patient and his or her family for discharge. Local, state, and/or national organizations can be very helpful resources that may keep a family from succumbing to the pressures of a catastrophic illness.

Emotions

When a serious illness occurs, patients and their families must adapt to many changes. Some of these changes may involve permanent alterations in lifestyle, frequent visits to health care providers, frequent hospitalizations, financial problems, and increased social isolation. For those in crisis, coping can be difficult at best and seemingly impossible at worst.

This section discusses a broad range of feelings and emotions that people may experience. Many of these feelings are normal and to be anticipated. However, there are times when the coping methods being utilized by patients and families are maladaptive. It is important for you to differentiate adaptive from maladaptive coping mechanisms.

Stress. The term *stress* is derived from the Latin word *stringer,* which means "to draw tight." Stress is any physiologic or psychological tension that threatens a person's total equilibrium. Stress affects all dimensions of the individual. If prolonged or chronic, it poses a serious threat to physical and emotional health. As the duration or intensity of stress or the number of stressors increases, a person's ability to adapt effectively decreases.

Perceptions of stress and coping mechanisms are highly individualized. People subjected to prolonged stressors eventually became totally exhausted. Individuals who cannot cope adequately with stress may experience a threat to their emotional well-being. They may find their perceptions of reality skewed, their ability to solve problems considerably compromised, and their stress consequently increased. In other words, without effective coping strategies, individuals can be caught in a vicious cycle of ineffective coping and increased stress that will stop only at the point of total exhaustion, and may result in death.

You must learn to recognize individuals whose coping skills are ineffective and who consequently are caught in a downward spiral of debilitating exhaustion. Without effective nursing interventions to reverse this downward spiral, serious impairment will result.

Fear. The words *fear* and *anxiety* often are used interchangeably. However, fear generally denotes a response to a specific threat, and anxiety is often a response to a nonspecific threat. The body's physiologic reaction to fear is similar to its response to anxiety. The person experiencing the crisis of illness has much to fear. There may be fear of pain, fear of financial ruin, fear of disfigurement, fear of the loss of self-esteem, and fear of not being able to return to a previous lifestyle.

Fears vary according to the developmental status and age of the individual. For example, toddlers may fear separation from their mothers, whereas adolescents may fear threats to their body image. Terminally ill patients may be struggling with fears of death and dying.

You can be very helpful in assisting patients and families to cope with fear. Sometimes just allowing an opportunity to express fear helps to lessen the stress caused by fear. Providing information about tests or surgical procedures may empower clients to begin to cope with fear. However, too much information also can be very stressful. In deciding how much information to provide, you must assess the patient's current understanding of the situation and any anticipated procedures he or she may be about to face. Providing basic information and then following up by answering the patient's questions is usually best.

Anxiety. Anxiety is a vague and sometimes intense sense of impending doom or apprehension that may appear to have no clearly identifiable cause. Anxiety is often an early response to illness. The degree of anxiety may vary with the severity of the illness. Anxiety may lead to physical and psychological stress and may be caused by real or imagined fear resulting from loss. As people develop, they learn to cope with this painful emotion. The fight-or-flight response actually provides the physiologic ability for one to either fight or flee. Individuals continually regulate their behavior based on their level of perceived anxiety. When anxiety intensifies to an excessive level, the perception of reality becomes solely focused on the crisis.

Loss. Loss is an experience usually related to the involuntary separation from the self of someone or something loved or treasured. It may involve a separation from a person or object, relationship, personal attribute, hope, dream, desire, role, functional ability, or potential. Perceived loss of control, sense of worth, and loss of health are also types of loss.

Actual loss can be recognized by others as well as by the patients. Examples of actual loss include loss of a spouse or the loss of a limb. *Anticipatory loss* is a sense of loss experienced before the actual loss occurs. Families may experience anticipatory loss during the terminal stages of a loved one's illness.

Loss can be a significant stressor that precipitates feelings of fear and anxiety. The fears associated with loss can be stressful enough to compromise the ability of an individual to recover from illness. One of the first psychological steps that must be taken to begin the process of coping is to permit oneself to experience the full emotional impact of the loss. This emotional response is known as grief or mourning.

The experience of loss is related to the individual's self-concept. The extent of loss depends on how strongly the individual's sense of self was connected to that which was lost.

Grief and mourning. Grief is the subjective, emotional response that evolves from a sense of loss. Mourning is the process through which grief is faced and ultimately resolved or altered over time. Mourning occurs when a person is forced to relinquish original hopes. The process of mourning prepares the individual to reappraise values and to accept substitutions for hope.

Individuals experiencing grief may be under a great deal of stress, and stress may make them even more vulnerable to disease. They may become irritable and difficult to get along with. Sometimes they may experience a sense of guilt. Some people blame themselves for whatever they have lost. They may perceive their illness and subsequent loss as a punishment from God for not having been a better person, a better parent, or a better spouse.

To alter the loss that grief causes, the self must change. The process of change is unique to each individual and each circumstance. One individual's need for change may require only a change in exercise and dietary habits. Another person's need for change may encompass a career, a lifestyle, or the development of better strategies to cope with stress. Most changes in a person's life are stressful. The greater the change, the greater the resulting stress. To cope with stress, the individual may mobilize psychological resources known as coping mechanisms. Adaptive coping mechanisms can be effective, therapeutic ways of dealing with stress. Maladaptive coping behaviors, however, can be detrimental and decrease the ability to cope with illness. Care of the patient who has suffered a loss is detailed in Chapter 23.

COPING MECHANISMS AND STRATEGIES

Coping is the process of responding to stress or a potential stressor. Coping with stress is a self-regulatory process by which people manage their responses to stress and thus relieve the tension related to the stressor. Coping strategies can be conscious or unconscious behaviors. Unconscious coping strategies are referred to as *defense mechanisms.*

Defense Mechanisms

According to Freud, the ego may devise strategies or defense mechanisms to cope with stress or anxiety. Defense mechanisms are used in an effort to diminish anxiety; however, when used excessively or inappropriately, they can hinder the developing personality. Defense mechanisms used to protect against anxiety include the following:

Compensation—an attempt to make up for real or imagined weakness. For example, an adolescent perceived as unattractive becomes an outstanding athlete.

Denial—a refusal to acknowledge a real situation. For example, a woman who finds a suspicious lump in her breast does not keep an appointment for a breast biopsy.

Displacement—transferring the feelings associated from one source to another that is considered less threatening. For example, a boy who is angry with a teacher comes home and yells at his dog.

Identification—the emulation of admirable qualities in another to enhance one's self-esteem. For example, a child dresses and uses mannerisms similar to those of a famous rock star.

Rationalization or intellectualization—the use of logic, reasoning, and analysis to avoid unacceptable feelings. For example, a student fails to complete an assignment correctly and rationalizes subsequent feelings of incompetence by complaining about the teacher's expectations for the assignment.

Introjection—internalizing or taking on the values and beliefs of another person. For example, a child takes on the values and beliefs of a parent.

Isolation—the separation of emotion from an associated thought or memory. For example, a man appears apathetic as he discusses a fire fight in which he participated in Vietnam.

Projection—unacceptable feelings or impulses are transferred to another. For example, a partner who is jealous of her significant other accuses the partner of being jealous.

Reaction formation—avoidance of unacceptable thoughts and behaviors by expressing opposing thoughts or behaviors. For example, a patient who unconsciously hates his father continuously tells how great his father is.

Regression—withdrawing to an earlier level of development to benefit from the associated comfort levels of the previous level. For example, a child starts sucking her thumb when her new baby brother comes home from the hospital.

Repression—an unconscious defense mechanism in which unacceptable ideas, impulses, and memories are kept out of consciousness. For example, a woman cannot remember a sexual assault.

Somatization—the transfer of painful feelings to body parts, thus the persons feelings are expressed in the form of a physical symptom. For example, a woman who has experienced intolerable internal conflict develops a physical complaint of pain in the wrist that cannot be explained by diagnostic means.

Sublimation—the transformation of unacceptable impulses or drives (e.g., aggressiveness, anger, sexuality) into constructive or more acceptable behavior. For example, a person who has aggressive tendencies becomes a jack-hammer operator.

Suppression—(a conscious mechanism) a conscious or voluntary inhibition of unacceptable ideas, impulses, and memories. For example, a child who fails an algebra class puts that event out of his or her mind.

Undoing—actually or symbolically attempting to cancel out an action that was unacceptable. An example is sprinkling salt over one's left shoulder to prevent bad luck after spilling salt on the table.

Substitution—the individual replaces a highly valued, unattainable object with a less valued, attainable object. For example, the person who has a strong unconscious sexual attraction to a parent marries someone who resembles that parent.

Conversion—an emotional conflict is turned into a physical symptom, which provides the individual with some sort of benefit (secondary gain). For example, the individual who witnesses a murder then experiences sudden blindness without an organic cause.

Defense mechanisms are adapted by the individual as protective measures to allow the ego relief from anxiety. One factor that enhances the development of ego is an environment with experiences that match the child's capacity to adapt. Ideally, unhealthy defense mechanisms are shed and replaced by more realistic and efficient methods of adaptation as the individual matures.

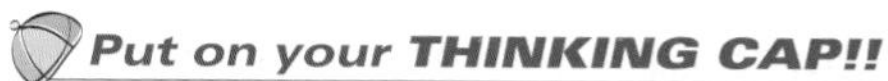
Put on your THINKING CAP!!

Recall two incidents when you recognized a defense mechanism being used to cope. Describe the behavior, label the mechanism, and indicate positive and negative outcomes of the mechanism. Share and discuss with your classmates.

Conscious Coping Strategies

Conscious coping strategies are purposeful behaviors that are used to make an unfamiliar situation into one that is perceived as more controllable and predictable. Coping strategies and mechanisms vary from individual to individual. What all these behaviors have in common is that they are attempts to help people feel less stressed and anxious about their illness. Some of these methods provide only temporary relief, whereas others provide more permanent results. It is important for you to identify and evaluate the effectiveness of coping mechanisms used by the patient.

Some techniques that can be used to help patients cope are known as *relaxation techniques.* Relaxation techniques include interventions such as imagery, relaxation strategies, therapeutic touch, and music therapy. Relaxation techniques elicit the relaxation response that reduces the effects of stress and decreases anxiety. These techniques can provide clients with self-control during moments of stress. Relaxation techniques are taught only when patients are not in acute discomfort because the exercise will be ineffective if the patient cannot concentrate. *Imagery* is the use of the imagination to develop sensory images that focus the mind away from the stressful experience and emphasize other sensory experiences and pleasant memories. *Relaxation strategies* include biofeedback, meditation, deep breathing exercises, yoga, and Zen practices. *Therapeutic touch* is a process by which the therapist acts as a channel for environmental and universal energy through the therapist's mental concentration.

Music therapy is another relaxation technique that may help the patient cope by enhancing the relaxation response and facilitating positive imagery. Musical selections should match a patient's mood and musical taste. Earphones with audio CDs or cassettes help the patient avoid annoying others and allow concentration on the music. This coping method provides only temporary relief of stress; however, use of such techniques can help to establish a therapeutic environment in which you can begin to discuss the real sources of the patient's concerns, fears, and anxieties.

Tapping into the spiritual dimension also can be a very effective way of coping with the stress of illness. You can talk with patients about their spiritual needs without relying on traditional religious language. The opportunity to discuss beliefs about a higher power or the search for meaning in suffering proves to be an effective way of coping for many patients.

MALADAPTIVE COPING MECHANISMS AND STRATEGIES

In an effort to reduce the stress and anxiety that is precipitated by the crisis of an illness, an individual may sometimes engage in thinking patterns or behaviors that are ineffective or even self-destructive. These ineffective coping mechanisms may evolve from a sense of helplessness or powerlessness.

Helplessness

Helplessness typically occurs when individuals have had repeated exposure to events they perceive as being uncontrollable. This leads to loss of motivation, feelings of despair or anxiety, and cognitive impairment. The individual may begin to express anger as a means of diminishing feelings of helplessness. This anger may take the form of a personal attack on you and other caregivers. The expression of anger is really not aimed at you but is simply an attempt to cope with feelings of loss of control. Helplessness can be prevented by allowing individuals to control as many events as possible within the constraints imposed by treatment and their energy level.

Powerlessness

Powerlessness is a feeling that one's actions cannot affect an outcome or that one lacks personal control over certain events or situations. Characteristics of powerlessness include (1) passivity; (2) nonparticipation in care and decision making; (3) dependence on others, which may lead to anger, resentment, or guilt; and (4) verbal expression of loss of control over situations or outcomes (Miller, 1992).

When people are not ready to cope with the threat of illness, unconscious defense mechanisms of avoidance, such as denial, may be used. These avoidance defense mechanisms protect individuals from having to confront and deal with the threat of illness.

Denial

Denial is the subconscious blocking out of emotional experiences. Denial can take several forms: (1) verbal denial, (2) minimizing the severity of the illness, (3) displacing symptoms onto another organ system, and (4) engaging in behaviors contrary to medical advice. The outcome of denial may be positive or negative. Denial can lead to negative consequences if people fail to engage in appropriate problem-focused behaviors. Patients who claim that they were never afraid or insist that there is nothing wrong with them are engaging in denial. Denial is maladaptive when the patient's behavior interferes significantly with obtaining appropriate care. Arguing with patients about their denial only reinforces the inappropriate behavior.

When working with people in denial, make a special effort to accept them even though it may be uncomfortable to care for individuals who deny their illnesses. You may need to allow the individual to deny the illness, while at the same time asking for cooperation. Once an effective therapeutic nurse-patient relationship has been established, patients may be better able to lower unconscious defenses and begin to discuss true feelings of fear and anxiety.

THE NURSING PROCESS IN ILLNESS

In this section the various steps of the nursing process are discussed to help you assess and plan nursing interventions that will facilitate the patient's task of dealing with the crisis of illness.

ASSESSMENT

An individual's ability to cope with an illness varies from moment to moment and from situation to situation. Therefore, assessment must be an ongoing process. To determine the effectiveness of individual coping strategies, seek answers to the following questions:

- Do individuals see themselves as effective in coping with their illness?
- What efforts have individuals made to seek information about their situation?
- How skillful are individuals in caring for themselves?
- What resources do individuals believe are available to them in dealing with their illness?
- Do individuals effectively adhere to their medical regimen?
- Do individuals feel they have been able to keep a sense of normality in their life despite their illness?
- How have individuals and their families been able to cope with any role modification that the illness has brought about?
- Have individuals been able to maintain a sense of hope in spite of the demands of the illness?
- Do individuals feel that the important relationships in their life remain intact?

After problem areas have been identified, meaningful nursing diagnoses can be formulated.

NURSING DIAGNOSIS

The purpose of a nursing diagnosis is to clearly identify and frame patient problems. The nursing diagnosis leads to the formulation of a plan of care that includes nursing interventions to help patients achieve their desired goals. Patients and their families must be included in the process so that nursing care plans are based on patients' values and perceptions of the problems. The following are a few nursing diagnoses often identified in persons with inadequate coping:

- Interrupted Family Process
- Delayed Growth and Development
- Ineffective Role Performance
- Ineffective Sexuality Patterns
- Anxiety
- Disturbed Body Image
- Caregiver Role Strain
- Defensive Coping
- Decisional Conflict
- Dysfunctional Grieving
- Fatigue
- Impaired Adjustment
- Ineffective Coping
- Compromised Family Coping
- Ineffective Denial
- Disturbed Personal Identity
- Powerlessness
- Risk for Loneliness

table 52-1 A Sample Nursing Care Plan for a Patient Ineffectively Coping with Illness

NURSING DIAGNOSIS

Ineffective Coping related to feelings of powerlessness as evidenced by patient's verbalization "I don't know if I can live through this."

GOAL AND OUTCOME CRITERIA

Patient will demonstrate more effective coping as evidenced by verbalization that he or she feels more capable of dealing with the demands of the illness.

INTERVENTIONS

1. Give patient an opportunity to verbalize feelings of powerlessness by approaching patient care in an unhurried manner.
2. Assess the patient's and family's current coping strategies and behaviors.
3. Conduct teaching sessions with the patient and family to enhance their coping skills and empower the patient to begin self-care.
4. Provide community resource information and encourage the patient to ask for help from others.
5. Implement stress reduction strategies (e.g., music therapy) to help patient cope with stressful moments.

Situational Low Self-Esteem
Disturbed Sleep Pattern
Social Isolation
Spiritual Distress

These serve only as examples of nursing diagnoses that could be identified for patients and their families. Appropriate nursing diagnoses follow a careful nursing assessment and are formulated once the patient and the family have had a chance to contribute by sharing their perception of the problem(s). Patients or family members need to agree that the identified problems are important ones if effective coping is to take place. This is especially true if a patient has a long-term or chronic illness.

NURSING GOALS, OUTCOME CRITERIA, AND INTERVENTIONS

The goal of nursing care is to help people manage and successfully cope with their illness. When effective coping strategies are used, patients can manage their illness and adapt to a new lifestyle that incorporates healthy behaviors and realistic goals. In addition, patients should emerge from the process with a positive self-concept and self-esteem.

People with chronic, debilitating illnesses may have difficulty acquiring and maintaining coping skills for long periods of time. Individuals may be able to cope with their illness today, but tomorrow may bring a whole new set of challenges. This is especially true in terminal stages of illness, when physical deterioration is on an accelerated course and every day brings new losses that need to be mourned and coped with.

Nursing interventions are based on identified nursing diagnoses. Table 52-1 provides a sample nursing care plan for a patient who is ineffectively coping with illness.

key points

- Individuals' level of health is directly related to their ability to adjust to a variety of internal and external stressors.
- Stress is necessary for growth and development.
- A stressor is anything that causes the individual stress, and adaptation to stress affects the entire organism.
- Illness or crisis may ensue if individuals are overwhelmed by many stressors or do not have the coping behaviors or problem-solving strategies necessary to maintain equilibrium.
- A crisis is the point at which the individual may move toward illness on the continuum between illness and health and can result in inner tension and anxiety, which may affect an individual's ability to function.
- Growth refers to a process of development that becomes increasingly complex.
- Anxiety is a painful emotion that results from one's perception of danger, and individuals continually regulate their behavior based on the level of perceived anxiety.
- Defense mechanisms are strategies used in an effort to diminish anxiety; however, when unconscious defense mechanisms are used excessively they can hinder the developing personality.
- Behavioral theory is based on the idea that all behavior is a learned response.
- Each person's response to illness is unique and is based on such subjective experiences as self-concept, perception of threat to body image, and spiritual and cultural values.
- Illness produces a stressful state that requires individuals to draw on their innate resources or inner strengths.
- Some people have enough inner strength to cope effectively with illness; others, however, may have ineffective or maladaptive coping abilities.
- Factors that influence an individual's ability to cope with illness are age, cultural beliefs, spirituality, self-concept, family and community resources, and emotional responses to illness.
- Specific emotional responses to illness include stress, fear, anxiety, loss, and grief and mourning.
- Coping is the process of responding to stress or a potential stressor.
- Coping strategies are conscious, purposeful behaviors that are used to make an unfamiliar situation into one that is perceived as more controllable and predictable.
- Ineffective coping mechanisms may evolve from a sense of helplessness or powerlessness.
- A nurse's caring and non-judgmental attitude is basic to helping a client cope with illness.

REVIEW QUESTIONS

1. The statement "Sometimes I feel so overwhelmed and sad" reflects which dimension of a human being?
   1. Cognitive
   2. Affective
   3. Behavioral
   4. Social

2. Which option best describes stress?
   1. Anything that requires the individual to adapt
   2. A negative or harmful experience
   3. A barrier to growth and development
   4. An emotional response to an unpleasant event

3. A developmental task of old age is to:
   1. learn how to delay gratification.
   2. find a life partner and life work.
   3. become independent.
   4. accept what has been.

4. The primary difference between fear and anxiety is that anxiety:
   1. is much more disabling than fear.
   2. indicates that the patient has poor coping skills.
   3. interferes with effective problem solving more than fear.
   4. is evoked by a nonspecific threat rather than a specific threat.

5. Which statement suggests that the patient is experiencing spiritual distress?
   1. "The medication that you gave me is not relieving my pain."
   2. "I think my cancer is punishment for the bad things I have done."
   3. "I will never be able to perform again with these terrible scars."
   4. "My family is too busy to come see me and do things for me."

6. Which data best support a nursing diagnosis of "Disturbed Body Image"?
   1. Patient states he is just glad to be alive despite some paralysis.
   2. Although burns have healed well, patient refuses to go out in public.
   3. Patient dresses every morning, brushes her hair, and applies makeup.
   4. During dressing change, patient carefully examines her incision.

7. The basic function of defense mechanisms is to:
   1. enhance self-esteem.
   2. avoid reality.
   3. disguise true feelings.
   4. reduce anxiety.

8. A 9-year-old girl likes to wear her 14-year-old sister's nail polish and tries to fix her hair like the older sister. This is an example of:
   1. regression.
   2. introjection.
   3. identification.
   4. projection.

9. The benefits of relaxation strategies include decreased anxiety and:
   1. reduced stress.
   2. improved muscle tone.
   3. increased alertness.
   4. enhanced sensation.

10. Mrs. A has been in a long-term care facility for 6 months. She has given up participation in group activities, rarely leaves her room, and is fretful and irritable. Her behavior is characteristic of:
    1. denial.
    2. isolation.
    3. helplessness.
    4. regression.

CHAPTER

53 Psychiatric Disorders

MARK D. SOUCY

objectives

1. Describe the differences between social relationships and therapeutic relationships.
2. Describe key strategies in communicating therapeutically.
3. Describe the components of the mental status examination.
4. Identify target symptoms, behaviors, and potential side effects for the following types of medications: anti-anxiety (anxiolytic), antipsychotic, and antidepressant drugs.
5. Summarize current thinking about the etiology of schizophrenia and the mood disorders.
6. Identify key features of the mental status examination and their relevance in: anxiety disorders, schizophrenia, mood disorders, cognitive disorders, and personality disorders.
7. Identify common nursing diagnoses, goals, and interventions for persons with: anxiety disorders, schizophrenia, mood disorders, cognitive disorders, and personality disorders.

key terms

Biologic approach (bī-ō-LŎJ-ĭk, p. 1129)
Denial (dĕ-NĪ-ăl, p. 1129)
Depersonalization (dē-PĔR-sŭn-ŭl-ĭ-ZĀ-shŭn, p. 1134)
Extrapyramidal side effects (EPS) (ĕks-tră-pĭ-RĂM-ĭ-dăl, p. 1136)
Interpersonal approach (p. 1129)
Parkinsonian Syndrome (SĬN-drōm, p. 1136)
Projection (p. 1129)
Psychoanalytic approach (sī-kō-ăn-ă-LĬT-ĭk, p. 1129)
Psychosis (sī-KŌ-sĭs, p. 1135)
Sensorium (sĕn-SŌ-rē-ŭm, p. 1132)
Tardive dyskinesia (TĂR-dĭv dĭs-kĭ-NĒ-zē-a, p. 1136)

How people think about and explain mental health and mental illness has varied from one geographic location and culture to another and from one time period to another. In early cultures people believed that supernatural forces were responsible for mental illness. People used rituals to appeal to these supernatural forces to cure mental illnesses. It is now understood that many factors contribute to the development of a mental illness, and many strategies are available for helping people with psychiatric disorders. Treatment settings include outpatient, intensive outpatient, partial hospitalization, and inpatient hospitalization as well as residential settings. Within these settings, treatment methods include milieu therapy, individual therapy, group or family therapy, psychoeducational groups, and treatment with medications. With the advent of new medications, treatment is increasingly handled on an outpatient basis. Nursing interventions are diverse and geared toward helping patients and families cope with the mental illness, manage their lives, and enhance quality of life. Mental illness exists and mental health exists along a continuum. People experiencing a psychiatric disorder may present with acute symptoms and require hospitalization. Others may have chronic and persistent mental illnesses. Therefore nursing interventions are delivered in many settings, including the hospital and the community.

Nurses who work with patients in other health care settings—such as medical clinics, medical and surgical inpatient units, or intensive care units—also see patients who have psychiatric difficulties along with their other health problems. Therefore the ability to provide quality nursing care to patients with mental illness in any work setting is important.

Nursing interventions are based on a number of theoretical approaches, which are described according to biologic, psychoanalytic, interpersonal, cognitive-behavioral, and other theories.

The **biologic approach** assumes that mental disorders are related to particular physiologic changes within the central nervous system. In this approach, mental illness is managed with medications, much as any other acute or chronic illness—such as diabetes—is managed. The biologic approach dominates much of the current thinking about psychiatric disorders.

The **psychoanalytic approach** is based on the theory that (1) humans function at different levels of awareness, ranging from conscious to unconscious; and (2) people use ego defense mechanisms to prevent anxiety. Some important defense mechanisms are repression, **denial,** and **projection.**

The **interpersonal approach** has three components: (1) anxiety is often communicated interpersonally; (2) the patient learns new ways of coping or maturing in a therapeutic relationship; and (3) the establishment of trust is an important first step in working with patients.

Key ideas from the cognitive-behavioral approach are that behavior is learned, that behavior increases as a result of a response to that behavior from the environment (reinforcement), and that the way a person thinks about things (their thoughts) influence emotional states and behavior.

table 53-1 Therapeutic Relationships versus Social Relationships

THERAPEUTIC	SOCIAL
1. Purpose is to benefit the patient.	1. Purpose is to benefit both participants in the relationship.
2. Relationship develops purposefully.	2. Relationship develops spontaneously.
3. Focus is on personal and emotional needs of patient.	3. Focus is on personal and emotional needs of both participants.
4. Helper has responsibility for evaluating the interaction and the changing behavior.	4. Participants are not formally responsible for evaluating their interaction.
5. Relationship has some boundaries (purpose, place, time) and a clear ending.	5. Relationship may or may not have clear boundaries and a clear ending.

Put on your THINKING CAP!!

Four patients are receiving different treatments for mental illness. An aspect of each type of treatment is listed below. Can you identify the theoretical approach behind each of them?

1. A patient is helped to develop new coping skills through a therapeutic relationship.
2. A patient is guided to recall events that could be related to her present illness.
3. A patient is helped to understand the consequences of his behavioral patterns.
4. A patient is prescribed an antianxiety (anxiolytic) drug.

ESTABLISHING THERAPEUTIC RELATIONSHIPS

In caring for a patient with a psychiatric disorder, you must first establish a therapeutic (rather than a social) relationship (Table 53-1). A range of interpersonal strategies have been found to be particularly helpful in promoting the patient's level of comfort with the nurse. They include being available, listening, clarifying, sharing observations, and accepting silence.

BEING AVAILABLE

When you are working with a patient, direct all your attention completely toward that person. Avoid involvement in any other activity, such as reading a newspaper or watching television, which might be interpreted by the patient as lack of availability. Avoid interruptions in your conversation with the patient as much as possible.

LISTENING

Use empathy when you are listening to the patient. Concentrate on what the patient is saying and remember that you are trying to hear how he or she experiences and describes his or her life. When listening therapeutically, make every effort to avoid cutting the patient off or jumping to conclusions. You are trying to get the essence of how the patient perceives his or her situation, experiences certain symptoms, and describes his or her circumstances.

To listen well, you must be aware of your own thoughts and feelings. These feelings are an important source of data for you because you may experience a wide range of feelings while interacting with patients. If you are aware of your own feelings, you will be able to manage your physical (body language) and verbal response. Listening is done by concentrating on the patient and by refraining from thinking of responses while the patient is speaking.

CLARIFYING

Clarifying is one way of validating that you understand what the patient is saying. For example, you might ask "So what you are saying is that you are feeling very sad right now?" Asking questions may also help patients clarify their thoughts. For example, if a patient says "I have problems at home," you might ask, "what is happening at home that is troubling you?" If a patient states, "my world is falling apart," You might say, "tell me more about what you mean when you say 'my world is falling apart.'" It is helpful to avoid the word "why" when asking questions. For example, instead of "why do you feel that way?," try "how is it that you came to feel that way?"

SHARING OBSERVATIONS

Patients benefit from knowing what you see and hear while listening. For example, you might say, "you are saying that your life is falling apart, and I notice that you are fidgeting and tapping your foot. It looks like this is really difficult for you." This statement provides the patient with input that he or she is heard and that you are really listening.

ACCEPTING SILENCE

Sometimes it is therapeutic to allow moments of silence between you and the patient. This is called therapeutic silence. It is important that you feel comfortable with silence since silence enables patients to consider their own thoughts as well as what you are communicating to them. While it may feel strange at first, silences allow patients to sort through their feelings and organize their thinking.

NURSING ASSESSMENT OF THE PSYCHIATRIC PATIENT

The nursing assessment of a patient with mental illness provides the foundation for nursing diagnoses and development of the plan of care. A major feature of a complete health as-

table 53-2 **Components of the Mental Status Examination**

COMPONENT	OBSERVATIONS
Appearance	Age, clothing, personal hygiene, unusual physical characteristics
Activity	Recent change in activity level, hyperactivity, agitation, psychomotor retardation, repetitive mannerisms, stereotypes
Mood and affect	Happiness, sadness, worry; constricted or expanded feelings; intensity; lability; appropriateness
Speech and language	Mutism, paucity, pressured speech, tangential speech, blocking, loose associations, word salad
Thought content	Obsessions, compulsions, phobias, delusions
Perceptual disturbances	Illusions, hallucinations
Insight and judgment	Potential for suicide
Sensorium	Orientation to time, place, person; level of consciousness
Memory and attention	Remote and recent memory; attention; calculation
General intellectual level	Vocabulary; knowledge of current events; abstract thinking

Consider the Alternative!

Be aware of any herbal supplements the patient is taking. Some can interact with drugs used for mental illness.

sessment of a psychiatric patient is the mental status examination. This examination is usually conducted as part of the admission process and is an ongoing assessment tool throughout the course of treatment. It consists of observations regarding appearance, motor function, mood and affect, speech and language, thought content, perceptual disturbances, insight and judgment, sensorium, memory, and attention (Table 53-2). Each of the areas under examination includes specific descriptors that are addressed as a part of the mental status examination.

Nursing diagnoses commonly identified in persons with major psychiatric disorders are derived from the health assessment. A partial list of these diagnoses is presented. Etiologies and/or related factors for each diagnosis are quite specific depending on the individual and his or her unique presentation. Therefore you should consult a text specific to nursing diagnoses common to psychiatric and mental health nursing.

MENTAL STATUS EXAMINATION

Appearance

The first step in a mental status examination is to observe how a person looks, specifically the following:

- Appearance in relation to stated age (does the patient look his or her stated age?)
- Appropriateness of clothing in relation to patient's particular peer group or subculture
- Personal grooming and hygiene
- Unique physical characteristics
- Motor activity

Assess any recent change in the patient's activity level (increase or decrease). Other types of activity that are observed include the following:

- Hyperactivity or activity at a level considerably above average purposeful activity
- Agitation or purposeless activity, such as wringing of hands, pacing, picking at clothing, foot tapping
- Psychomotor retardation or a decrease in movement; slowness; delayed actions, thoughts, and speech
- Repetitive movements that are part of a purposeful activity (mannerisms)
- Repetitive movements that are not part of purposeful activity (stereotypes)

Mood and Affect

Mood is a sustained feeling state or emotion that a person experiences in several aspects of life. Mood is assessed in terms of its intensity, depth, duration, and fluctuation. Words that often are used to describe mood include irritable, anxious, depressed, euphoric, labile (up and down), and despairing.

Affect describes a person's external presentation of a feeling state and emotional responsiveness. Affect ranges from blunted, flat, and constricted to euphoric, expansive, and intense. A normal affect exists when the person's body language, mannerisms, and verbal responses are consistent with the person's mood and within an average range of emotional intensity. Affect is also described according to its appropriateness and congruence. Appropriate affect exists when the person's outward emotional expression matches what he or she is saying or doing. For example, a patient who is discussing sadness and despair may be tearful and look sad. An example of an inappropriate affect is when someone is telling you that they are sad and feeling guilty about something that happened but at the same time smiling, laughing, and appearing very bright. In the latter example, the affect is considered incongruent with mood.

The intensity of feelings may be increased or decreased (diminished). Feelings also may be stable or consistent rather than labile or rapidly changing.

Speech and Language

Assessment includes observations of speech and language. Normally, speech is of normal rate, rhythm, and volume. Unusual findings in the assessment of speech include mutism (not speaking), long pauses before responding, minimal or very little speech (paucity), and pressured speech (loud and insistent). Some clues to problems of thought are evidenced in a person's speech, which is described in the following section.

Thought Content

Tangential speech may be noted, which means that a patient starts out toward a particular point but veers away and never reaches the point. Tangential speech is commonly an indicator of disorganized thinking. When the person stops speaking before reaching the point, it is called thought blocking. Loose associations—continual shifting from topic to topic—and shifting between topics to the point of incoherence ("word salad") may also be noted. Tangentiality, thought blocking, looseness of associations, and "word salad" are all noteworthy findings that are related to thought content in speech. Further assessment of thought content includes identifying the following:

Obsessions—repetitious, unwanted thoughts
Compulsions—actions repeatedly carried out in a specific manner; they typically include washing, counting, or checking
Phobias—unrealistic fears of specific objects or situations
Delusions—false ideas not based on reality and not congruent with the patient's specific religious and cultural orientation
Suicidal ideations—thoughts and/or plans of killing oneself

Obsessions and compulsions are often closely related.

This area must be assessed with clear and direct questions such as asking, "Do you have any thoughts of harming yourself or killing yourself?" Further assessment includes determining whether the patient has constructed any plans to hurt himself or herself. If the patient endorses suicidal ideations, you must ask whether the patient has made any plans to do so. If so, ask him or her to describe the plans. This information is useful in assessing the lethality of the plans. Another part of the assessment includes determining whether the patient has any means available to carry out a suicide plan. For example, if a patient has planned to shoot himself or herself, is a gun available at home? If the patient has thoughts of overdosing on medication, does the patient have available supplies of medications?

Perceptual Disturbances

Perceptual disturbances may involve any one of the senses such as vision, hearing, taste, touch, and smell. One type of perceptual disturbance is an illusion, in which a specific stimulus, such as a spot on the wall, is misinterpreted (e.g., a spot is perceived as a bug). Another is hallucination, which is a sensory experience that occurs without an external stimulus (e.g., a person sees nonexistent bugs crawling on the floor or feels nonexistent bugs crawling on the skin). Sometimes this is referred to as internal stimuli. Evidence of this may include a person sitting alone, talking as if someone were present, or looking around as if someone is talking to or calling the patient.

Insight and Judgment

Insight is the ability of a person to understand the correct cause or meaning of a situation, and judgment is the ability to assess a situation accurately and determine the appropriate course of action. Insight and judgment are often considered in relation to suicide potential.

Sensorium

Assessment of sensorium focuses on orientation in terms of time, place, person, and self. This assessment involves asking the patient direct questions (e.g., "what time is it now?," "what day is today?," "where are we now?," or "tell me your name"). The patient's level of consciousness also is assessed. The four levels of consciousness are: (1) comatose; (2) stuporous; (3) drowsy; and (4) alert.

Memory and Attention

Assess remote memory (distant past) by comparing the patient's memory of past events with what is recalled by other reliable historians. Test recent memory, or the ability to recall new information, by asking the patient to learn three unrelated words and to recall these words 5 minutes later. A quick way to determine recent memory is to ask what was eaten at the previous meal. Asking the patient to subtract 7's from 100 or 3's from 20 or to spell a word like "world" backwards can test attention as well as ability to calculate (as an aspect of general intellectual level).

General Intellectual Level

Assess general intellectual level by determining the patient's vocabulary and knowledge of current events. For example, ask the patient to name the president of the United States and the name of the previous president. Abstract thinking is another area of general intellectual level. It is assessed by asking the patient to identify the common element of two objects such as a banana and an apple (e.g., "what do a banana and an apple have in common?") or asking the patient to interpret proverbs (e.g., "What does the phrase *a rolling stone gathers no moss* mean?").

TYPES OF PSYCHIATRIC DISORDERS

ANXIETY DISORDERS

A patient with an anxiety disorder either directly experiences the highly uncomfortable feeling of anxiety or experiences a symptom like compulsive hand-washing that prevents or reduces the occurrence of anxiety. Common physical signs and symptoms of anxiety are increased heart rate, elevated blood pressure, sweaty palms, trembling, urinary frequency, diarrhea, a tight sensation in the chest, and difficulty breathing. Psychological manifestations often include irritability, restlessness, tearfulness, thought blocking, and lack of concentration.

Anxiety is experienced on various levels, ranging from mild to panic stages, depending on each person's subjective experience and ability to cope. Mild anxiety can be useful. It may motivate a person to take constructive action or focus attention on a particular task (such as concentrating on an examination). Moderate anxiety often is considered the optimal level for learning to take place. As anxiety progresses to severe or panic levels, however, an individual's ability to think clearly and to solve problems becomes progressively impaired. A person in a panic state may misperceive surrounding events altogether and may react impulsively by running or striking out. This may explain instances in which individuals jump from burning buildings despite imminent rescue.

All people experience anxiety. For most people it is episodic and does not interfere greatly with day-to-day functioning. Even normally well-adjusted people can experience anxiety of panic proportions under significant stress. If anxiety persists at a high level for an extended period and causes significant interference with daily functioning, the person usually is determined to have an anxiety disorder. Examples of anxiety disorders are panic disorder, agoraphobia, obsessive-compulsive disorder, and posttraumatic stress disorder.

Panic Disorder

In panic disorder, the person experiences recurrent panic attacks, which are episodes of intense apprehension of variable length, at times to the point of terror, and are often accompanied by feelings of impending doom. Often no triggering event can be identified. Physical symptoms of severe anxiety, such as increased pulse, elevated blood pressure, trembling, diaphoresis, shortness of breath, chest pain, and nausea also are present. This disorder tends to run in families.

Agoraphobia

The person with agoraphobia is extremely fearful of situations outside the home. This often includes fearfulness that the person may be in a place from which quick escape would be difficult (e.g., a grocery store) or a place where help may be unavailable. The person typically copes by avoiding the anxiety-producing place or situation, often becoming progressively reclusive and very dependent on family and friends. Agoraphobia may occur by itself or together with panic disorder.

Obsessive-Compulsive Disorder

Obsessive-compulsive disorder (OCD) consists of recurrent obsessions (thoughts) or compulsions (behaviors), or both, that produce distress, are time-consuming, and interfere with functioning. Obsessions frequently involve intrusive thoughts about unpleasant or even violent acts that a person cannot stop. For example, a person may be obsessed with the idea of being dirty and needing to wash. Compulsive behaviors typically evolve as a way to reduce the anxiety experienced as a result of obsessive thoughts. Examples of compulsions are hand washing, counting, and checking (e.g., repeated checking to see whether the door is locked). The person experiencing obsessions and compulsions knows these thoughts and behaviors are not "normal" and often is embarrassed by them. However, if the compulsion is resisted, the internal anxiety may become be too overwhelming to handle.

Research has found that neurophysiology plays a role in the origin of this disorder. Some studies have shown that there are changes in electroencephalography (EEG) findings in people with OCD. Many people with obsessive-compulsive disorders have considerably reduced their symptoms with therapeutic levels of particular medications such as antidepressants (tricyclics as well as selective serotonin reuptake inhibitors [SSRIs]). This phenomenon also suggests that the etiology of this disorder may be physiologic rather than a response to some unresolved unconscious conflict as was previously proposed.

Posttraumatic Stress Disorder

Posttraumatic stress disorder is a cluster of symptoms experienced following a distressing event that is outside the range of normal events (e.g., watching one's family being murdered) and one in which the person experienced intense fear, helplessness, and/or horror. Examples of symptoms include reexperiencing the trauma through repeated and intrusive recall of the event (at times as a flashback); avoiding situations that in some way remind the person of the event; feeling detached from other people; and having a heightened sense of arousal, which is experienced as difficulty falling asleep, hypervigilance, an exaggerated startle response, or a combination of these. The case of Patrick T. provides a clinical example of posttraumatic stress disorder.

> Patrick T. was admitted to the psychiatric inpatient unit with the diagnosis of posttraumatic stress disorder. Two months before admission, he and his coworker friend were in a truck accident on an overpass. Patrick watched in horror as his friend fell out of the truck, which was hanging over the edge. The fall killed his friend instantly. Patrick was able to climb out of the passenger side and sustained injuries to his back and legs. He received physical therapy for his injuries. For the past 2 weeks he has been continually preoccupied by the event, has had persistent insomnia and nightmares, repeatedly says that he should have been the one to die, becomes easily irritable, does not show feelings when with others, and jumps whenever he hears a loud noise or someone touches him unexpectedly. The nurse assigned to work with Patrick found him pacing. She remained with him as he paced. The following nursing diagnoses were immediately relevant: anxiety, altered sleep pattern, and dysfunctional grieving. Patrick and the nurse decided together that the priorities were to decrease his anxiety and to improve sleep. Patrick was willing to learn a progressive relaxation exercise (which involves relaxing one group of muscles at a time until the body is relaxed). After learning the exercise, Patrick worked on deep abdominal breathing and agreed to use this strategy when he found himself preoccupied with the accident. The nurse did not purposefully probe the details of the event, but if Patrick had brought it up, she would have listened attentively and offered support and empathy.

SOMATOFORM DISORDERS

An individual with one of the somatoform disorders experiences physical symptoms without actual physiologic dysfunction or with physical cause(s) that are affected by psychological factors in terms of onset, severity, duration, or continuance of symptoms.

Conversion Disorder

In conversion disorder, symptoms may include blindness, deafness, or paralysis of the legs without a physiologic cause.

Usually the symptoms are neurologic and occur in response to some threatening or traumatic event. The symptoms are real and not created; they can cause significant distress or impairment in social, occupational, or other important areas of functioning. In some cases a true physiologic cause for the symptoms has been discovered years later; therefore a diagnosis of conversion disorder is usually tentative and provisional.

Pain Disorder

In pain disorder, the patient experiences pain in one or more sites that causes significant distress or impairment in function. Psychological factors play a significant role in the experience of the pain; however, the pain is not intentionally produced or contrived. The pain may be related to a physiological problem; however, the psychological component is significant.

Hypochondriasis

In hypochondriasis, individuals are convinced that they have a serious medical problem in spite of the absence of any concrete medical findings. They will seek other opinions if one physician does not validate their concerns, and they often take multiple prescription medications from various health care providers. Concern about the feared illness often becomes a central part of people's lives and may impair social, occupational, or other important areas of functioning. In some cases of hypochondriasis, the person does not recognize that the concern about having a serious illness is excessive or unreasonable.

DISSOCIATIVE DISORDERS

Dissociative disorders involve a change in identity, memory, or consciousness. The change may be sudden or gradual, transient or occurring over a long period, and is thought to be an escape from anxiety. In a sense, persons unconsciously dissociate or remove themselves psychologically from anxiety-provoking situations because the situations are too much to bear. Even normal persons may experience **depersonalization** under severe stress. In this case, individuals feel they are outside of themselves or floating overhead watching what is happening, as if it were happening to someone else. Examples of dissociative disorders include amnesia or dissociative identity disorder (formerly multiple personality disorder).

Amnesia is characterized by a gap in memory, usually of a traumatic or stressful nature, that is too extensive to be explained by normal forgetfulness. There are five major types of amnesia: (1) localized amnesia, or difficulty remembering anything about the first few hours after a profoundly disturbing event; (2) selective amnesia, or the ability to remember some but not all of the events surrounding a traumatic experience; (3) generalized amnesia, or failure to remember one's entire life; (4) continuous amnesia, or inability to recall events after a specific time up to and including the present; and (5) systematized amnesia, or loss of memory for certain categories of information, such as all memories related to one's family or to a particular person.

Dissociative identity disorder is a relatively rare dissociative disorder in which two or more distinct personalities exist within the person and at least two personalities repeatedly take control of the person's behavior. Legal identity is retained by the "host personality." Other personalities within the body are called "alter personalities." Individuals with this disorder experience frequent gaps in memory for personal history, both remote and recent. Most patients with dissociative identity disorders report severe childhood abuse, including physical, sexual, or ritual cult abuse; however, these experiences are difficult to verify. Women are five times more likely to have the disorder than men are. There appears to be an inherited predisposition to the occurrence of dissociative identity disorder.

Medical Treatment

Drug Therapy

The primary anxiolytic (antianxiety) medications are the benzodiazepines (e.g., diazepam [Valium], chlordiazepoxide hydrochloride [Librium], lorazepam [Ativan], alprazolam [Xanax], and clonazepam [Klonopin]) (Table 53-3). They usually are prescribed for brief periods. Side effects are those associated with sedation, such as drowsiness, fatigue, dizziness, and confusion. Because physical and psychological dependence occurs, withdrawal from these medications must be medically supervised. Abrupt cessation of benzodiazepines may result in withdrawal symptoms including seizures.

PHARMACOLOGY CAPSULE Anxiolytic medications, which are given for anxiety disorders or as an adjunct medication for treating schizophrenia, may have side effects such as drowsiness, loss of coordination, fatigue, confusion, blurred vision, and psychological dependence.

Antidepressants now are used much more commonly to treat anxiety disorders, either alone or in combination with anxiolytics. Antidepressants, such as the SSRIs and some of the newer antidepressants (venlafaxine [Effexor] and nefazadone [Serzone]), are often very useful in reducing anxiety, decreasing distress, and improving overall functioning. This is especially true when the patient suffers from a mood disorder as well as depression.

NURSING CARE *of the Patient with an Anxiety Disorder, Somatoform Disorder, or Dissociative Disorder*

Assessment

Determine the presence of and level of anxiety (mild, moderate, severe, or panic) from the patient's self report of symptoms as well as objective observations. Particularly relevant mental status examination categories include motor activity, speech and language, and thought content.

Nursing Diagnoses, Goals, and Outcome Criteria: Anxiety, Somataform, and Dissociative Disorders

Nursing Diagnoses	Goals and Outcome Criteria
Anxiety related to severe stress as evidenced by patient's self-report, wringing and trembling of hands, and fearful appearance	Reduced anxiety: patient able to problem-solve, labels symptoms as those of anxiety

table 53-3 DRUG THERAPY | *Common Anxiolytics (Anti-Anxiety Medications) in the Benzodiazepine Class*

DRUG NAME (GENERIC/TRADE)	NURSING IMPLICATIONS	PATIENT TEACHING
Alprazolam (Xanax) Chlordiazepoxide (Librium) Clonazepam (Klonopin) Clorazepate (Tranxene) Diazepam (Valium) Halazepam (Paxipam) Lorazepam (Ativan) Oxazepam (Serax) Prazepam (Centrax)	Effective in treatment of anxiety and panic disorders Sometimes used as preoperative sedatives and to treat certain side effects of other drugs (neuroleptics) Depress the central nervous system (CNS) May potentiate other CNS depressants; administer with caution with other CNS depressants Administer with extreme caution in the elderly or frail, who may be more sensitive to the effects of these medications and be more prone to confusion or falls Abrupt cessation after prolonged or excessive use may result in withdrawal, including seizures	Avoid alcohol when taking medications in this class as alcohol will intensify their effects. Do not take more medication at one time than prescribed or use medication more frequently in a day than prescribed. Rebound anxiety may result when medication wears off, especially those with short half-lives. If this happens, report this to your practitioner. May impair driving, decrease attention and concentration, and cause drowsiness. Avoid driving or operating dangerous machinery until effects of the medicine on coordination, reaction time, motor control, and judgment are known. Do not abruptly stop taking this medication without consulting with your practitioner.

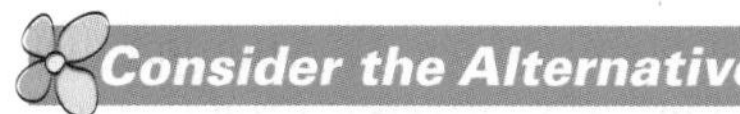

Consider the Alternative!

Useful techniques to manage anxiety include relaxation techniques, warm baths, positive self-talk, and physical exercise.

Ineffective Coping related to dissociation, amnesia in stressful situations	More effective coping with anxiety: patient recognizes ineffective ways of coping: identifies and implements new ways of coping with anxiety, stress, and their precipitants; learns and implements relaxation techniques, guided imagery, and other coping strategies

Interventions

Strategies to help patients reduce anxiety from a panic state or a severe level to a mild level center on remaining calm; speaking firmly with short, simple instructions (e.g., "sit down with me here"); and walking to a less stimulating area of the unit. Once the anxiety is reduced to a manageable level, assist patients in exploring what happened, clarifying their usual ways of relieving anxiety (e.g., anger or somatic symptoms instead of experiencing more typical anxiety symptoms), and identifying what triggered the anxiety (e.g., feelings of self-doubt regarding finding employment after discharge). You can assist clients in problem-solving decisions and can teach ways to prevent and manage heightened anxiety in the future.

SCHIZOPHRENIA

Schizophrenia is a term used to refer to a group of very serious, usually chronic, thought disorders in which the affected person's ability to interpret the world accurately is impaired by psychotic symptoms. **Psychosis** is a state in which a person has distorted perceptions of reality. Psychotic symptoms include delusions, hallucinations, and impaired speech or behavioral patterns. The symptoms are characterized as either positive or negative. Positive symptoms appear to reflect an excess or distortion of normal functions and include delusions, hallucinations, problems with communication, and bizarre behavior. Negative symptoms appear to reflect a decrease or loss of normal functions and include diminished emotional expression (flattened affect), slowed thinking and speech, and difficulty initiating goal-directed behavior.

Typically schizophrenic patients have functioned normally in early life; they often are very intelligent and well educated before the onset of the first symptoms. The symptoms usually begin in adolescence or early adulthood; however, some types of schizophrenic disorders are more often diagnosed in later life. The patient's ability to function in the areas of work, interpersonal relationships, or self-care deteriorates significantly during acute episodes and may not return to baseline after the first psychotic episode. With each subsequent episode, the ability to function independently continues to deteriorate; intelligence quotient (IQ) levels drop; and thinking becomes very concrete. Patients are unable to tolerate even the typical stressors of daily living. However, newer medications have been very successful in helping people return to their previous activities.

In one research study, the brains of persons with chronic schizophrenia were examined after death. The ventricles of the brain were found to be enlarged, whereas brain tissues that correlated with higher-level thinking had atrophied. This finding is consistent with the loss of capacity to think and function independently that is seen with most of the patients diagnosed with this disease.

Etiology and Risk Factors

The cause of schizophrenia is not certain. The model that integrates diverse potential causes states that patients who are most vulnerable to acquiring the disorder encounter factors (stress) that precipitate the disorder. The model is called the stress-diathesis model. Researchers have established that people with schizophrenia probably were genetically vulnerable to the disorder. The range of biologic factors being investigated includes (1) neurotransmitters and their receptors, including dopamine, norepinephrine, and gamma-aminobutyric acid; (2) structural abnormalities such as degeneration of the limbic system, enlargement of the lateral and third ventricles, and loss of neurons in the temporal lobe; (3) infectious agents; and (4) hormonal dysregulation.

In men, the disorder usually first occurs between 15 and 25 years of age. The usual age range for first occurrence in women is 25 to 35. There is no difference in rate by sex. The incidence worldwide is between 0.5% and 1%. Approximately 50% of all mental hospital beds are occupied by patients with schizophrenia, and 40% to 60% of people with schizophrenia are readmitted within a 2-year period after discharge from their first hospitalization. It has been estimated that two thirds of all homeless people have schizophrenia. Fifty percent of people with schizophrenia attempt suicide; 10% complete a suicide during a 20-year follow-up period.

Medical Treatment

Drug Therapy

The most commonly administered medications for people with schizophrenia are neuroleptic (antipsychotic) medications and antiparkinsonian medications, which are at times administered to prevent or relieve some of the side effects of the neuroleptics (Table 53-4). Anxiolytic medications also may be administered in conjunction with the neuroleptics to decrease agitation. There are two broad categories of neuroleptics: typical and atypical neuroleptics. The typical neuroleptics are the older neuroleptics that were very useful in treating the positive symptoms of schizophrenia such as auditory and visual hallucinations; however, they were not particularly useful in treating the negative symptoms, such as poverty of thought, delayed thinking, and decreased function. The atypical neuroleptics are known to help with both the positive and the negative symptoms and have a reduced incidence of side effects in comparison to the older, typical agents.

When working with patients who are receiving neuroleptics, you are responsible for observing and recording accurately all data relevant to the target behaviors and symptoms of the medications as well as the potential side effects. There are a variety of potential side effects, some of which have rapid onset and require immediate treatment.

One side effect that can be managed with nursing interventions and patient teaching is orthostatic hypotension (or postural hypotension), which is a drop in blood pressure when a person changes position from lying down to sitting or from sitting to standing. This problem, which creates a risk for falls, occurs most frequently in the early weeks of treatment and is more common in the morning, after the patient has been in bed during the night, as well as after a large meal. See Chapter 31 for details on the assessment and management of orthostatic hypotension.

Another group of side effects are referred to as **extrapyramidal side effects (EPS),** which stem from the impact of the antipsychotics on the extrapyramidal tracts of the central nervous system. These tracts play a role in the control of involuntary movements. Different EPS may occur at different periods in the course of medication therapy and are described as follows.

Acute dystonic reactions may occur after one dose of medication or during the first few days of treatment. The reactions consist of severe muscle contractions involving the tongue, face, neck (torticollis), and back (opisthotonos). The larynx also may be constricted (laryngospasm), which compromises the patient's airway. The reaction is reversed with benztropine mesylate (Cogentin) given intramuscularly or intravenously or with diphenhydramine hydrochloride (Benadryl), administered intravenously as ordered. Acute dystonia is a medical emergency and must be treated immediately.

After 1 to 2 weeks of treatment with antipsychotic medications, the **parkinsonian syndrome**—consisting of mask-like face, rigid posture, shuffling gait, and resting tremor—may occur. Other extrapyramidal syndromes that may occur later in treatment are akathisia, a reversible restlessness manifested as an urge to pace and difficulty sitting still.

Tardive dyskinesia is usually an irreversible syndrome that may occur after prolonged use of neuroleptic drug therapy. It consists of persistent involuntary movements of the face, jaw, and tongue that lead to grimacing; jerky movements of the upper extremities; and tonic contractions of the neck and back. Treatment includes discontinuing the causative agent; however, the symptoms most often continue.

Neuroleptic malignant syndrome occurs in 1% of people receiving neuroleptic agents (including neuroleptics and antiemetics); mortality rates reported for people with this condition range from 14% to 30%. The first symptom is usually muscular rigidity accompanied by akinesia (emotional unresponsiveness and blunted affect) and respiratory distress and may include involuntary muscle movements, but the cardinal sign is hyperthermia (101° to 103° F or higher).

Neuroleptic malignant syndrome is a medical emergency that requires immediate intervention and intensive care. Neuroleptic malignant syndrome may result in permanent impairment or even death.

One neuroleptic, clozapine [Clozaril], presents a risk for the blood disorder known as agranulocytosis, an extreme decrease in granulated white blood cells, which frequently manifests as a sore throat and fever. Patients receiving this medication require close supervision and frequent white blood cell counts. If the white cell count drops significantly or if the patient presents with sore throat, fever, and/or flu symptoms, the medication must be held, and the physician must be notified at once. Severe infection may result when the white blood cell counts drop below acceptable levels.

It is clear that in monitoring a patient for drug side effects, a wide range of data are relevant from vital signs to facial expression. Pay close attention to all patient descriptions of symptoms.

After a period of time, patients taking typical neuroleptic medications almost always experience extrapyramidal side effects such as akathisia and pseudoparkinsonism. Tardive

table 53-4 DRUG THERAPY | *Selected Neuroleptics (Antipsychotics)*

DRUG NAME (GENERIC/BRAND)	NURSING IMPLICATIONS	PATIENT TEACHING
TYPICAL NEUROLEPTICS		
Chlorpromazine (Thorazine) Thioridazine (Mellaril) Mesoridazine (Serentil) Perphenazine (Trilafon) Trifluoperazine (Stelazine) Fluphenazine (Prolixin) Thiothixene (Navane) Haloperidol (Haldol) Loxapine (Loxitane)	These agents are helpful in the treatment of positive symptoms of schizophrenia and other psychotic processes. May cause drowsiness and sedation. May cause postural hypotension, dry mouth, and blurred vision, especially in frail and elderly people. Watch for EPS such as Parkinson syndrome–like movements, muscle rigidity, dystonia, akathisia, and oculogyric crisis. Long-term administration may result in tardive dyskinesia.	Caution patient to rise slowly from a lying position to a sitting position and from sitting to standing to avoid a sudden drop in blood pressure. Caution patients to avoid driving or operating dangerous machinery until effects of the medicine on coordination, reaction time, motor control, and judgment are known. Assess the patient for abnormal, involuntary movements and report these to the prescribing practitioner. Administer medications to treat motor movement side effects as ordered. Provide the patient with hard candy or sugarless chewing gum to help with dry mouth. Provide dietary teaching to help the patient avoid or manage weight gain associated with these and other neuroleptics.
ATYPICAL NEUROLEPTICS		
Clozapine (Clozaril) Risperidone (Risperdal) Olanzapine (Zyprexa) Ziprasidone (Geodon)	These neuroleptics treat both the positive and negative symptoms of schizophrenia and other psychotic disorders. May cause drowsiness and sedation. May cause postural hypotension, dry mouth, and blurred vision, especially in frail and elderly people. Watch for EPS such as Parkinson syndrome–like movements, muscle rigidity, dystonia, akathisia, and oculogyric crisis. Although these side effects are less common in the atypical class of neuroleptics, they are still seen in patients taking these drugs. Long-term administration may also result in tardive dyskinesia, although this may be less likely.	Caution patient to rise slowly from a lying position to a sitting position and from sitting to standing to avoid a sudden drop in blood pressure. Caution patients to avoid driving or operating dangerous machinery until effects of the medicine on coordination, reaction time, motor control, and judgment are known. Assess the patient for abnormal, involuntary movements and report these to the prescribing practitioner. Administer medications to treat motor movement side effects as ordered. Provide the patient with hard candy or sugarless chewing gum to help with dry mouth. Provide dietary teaching to help the patient avoid or manage weight gain associated with these and other neuroleptics.
	In addition to the other side effects associated with atypical neuroleptics, clozapine may result in a significant drop in the white blood count. Routine blood count monitoring must be done to identify any drop in white blood cells, and the medication must be held and usually discontinued if this happens.	In addition to the above, teach the patient taking clozapine to watch for and report sore throat, fever, chills, and any other signs of infection immediately to the prescribing practitioner.

dyskinesia also is a significant risk when patients are taking the typical neuroleptic medications; thus the atypical medications are now considered first-line agents.

NURSING CARE *of the Patient with Schizophrenia*

Assessment

In completing the mental status examination, observe the following: (1) appearance: may have poor grooming and failure to bathe; (2) activity: may exhibit agitation, bizarre postures, catatonic excitement or stupor, mannerisms or stereotypes, or stiff body movements; (3) mood and affect: may have flat affect or inappropriate rage or happiness; (4) speech and language: mutism, tangential speech, blocking, or loose associations; (5) thought content: delusions that may include persecutory, grandiose, religious, or somatic; (6) perceptual disturbances: auditory hallucinations most commonly; visual hallucinations next most commonly; (7) insight and judgment: usually little insight into illness; (8) sensorium:

oriented to person, place, and time; (9) memory: usually intact, but difficulties with attention make assessment difficult.

Nursing Diagnoses, Goals, and Outcome Criteria: Schizophrenia

Nursing Diagnoses	Goals and Outcome Criteria
Disturbed Thought Processes related to delusions (false beliefs), loose associations, concrete thinking, symbolism as evidenced by patient statements such as that the president is out to get him or her	Improved thought processes: patient differentiates illusions from reality, fewer loose associations, more logical thinking
Disturbed Sensory Perception related to hallucinations, illusions, heightened response to irrelevant stimuli, as evidenced by patient's inability to tolerate group therapy, talking to herself, and looking for something when nothing is there	Improved sensory perceptual function: reduced frequency of hallucinations, less response to irrelevant environmental and other stimuli
Impaired Verbal Communication related to delayed thinking, as evidenced by very slow and delayed speech	Improved verbal communications: patient expresses thoughts clearly
Self-Care Deficit related to withdrawal and loss of motivation and judgment, as evidenced by poor hygiene, poor grooming, and avoiding others	Improved self-care: patient performs activities of daily living with maximum independence in relation to level of ability

Interventions

Disturbed Thought Processes

Nursing interventions include speaking in a gentle and nonconfronting manner, decreasing unwanted environmental stimuli, focusing on reality (real events and real people), letting the patient know that you do not share the delusion without directly confronting the delusion (do not argue or try to disprove the delusion), encouraging the patient to express feelings and anxiety, and connecting delusions with anxiety-provoking situations (see interventions for anxiety, discussed earlier).

Disturbed Sensory Perceptions

Interventions include making brief, frequent contacts with the patient (to interrupt hallucinatory experiences), encouraging the patient to pay attention to what is occurring in the environment (instead of external stimuli), encouraging involvement in quiet activities, and informing patients that hallucinations are part of the disease process.

Impaired Verbal Communication

Interventions may include seeking clarification and verbalizing the implied, which may be useful if the patient is not speaking (e.g., "it must have been difficult for you when your father didn't come after he told you he would"). You will also want to provide regular contact with the patient and use gentle encouragement, understanding that the patient's thinking may be slowed.

Self-Care Deficit

Possible interventions include providing recognition for all constructive self-care actions (e.g., "I see you've bathed and washed your hair"), demonstrating how to perform an activity if necessary, intervening to assist when necessary, offering finger foods or cans of food for the patient to open, or serving family style if the patient believes food has been poisoned.

MOOD DISORDERS

People with mood disorders experience significantly elevated or depressed moods. Some people experience cycles of elevated mood and depressed mood. An episode of depressed mood is referred to as major depression. An episode of elevated mood is called a manic episode. Alternation between significantly depressed mood and significantly elevated mood over time is termed bipolar disorder.

Major depression is one of the most common psychiatric disorders, with a lifetime prevalence of 6%. The mean age for the occurrence of depression is 40. About twice as many women as men are diagnosed with major depression. People who are single, divorced, or lacking in close relationships are more vulnerable. There is no association between major depression and race or between major depression and socioeconomic status.

For bipolar disorder, the lifetime prevalence is 1%, with the mean age at onset being 30. Rates are similar for men and women and are higher among single and divorced people than among married people. People in higher socioeconomic groups and those with lower levels of education have higher rates of bipolar disorder.

Etiology and Risk Factors

Definite causes of mood disorders have not been established. Probable causes include neurotransmitter dysregulation, neuroreceptor deficits, neuroendocrine dysfunctions, genetic factors, loss of significant others, learned helplessness, and negative thoughts about life experiences.

Medical Treatment

Drug Therapy

There are several types of antidepressant medications: tricyclic antidepressants (TCAs), selective serotonin reuptake inhibitors (SSRIs), newer agent antidepressants, and monoamine oxidase inhibitors (MAOIs) (Table 53-5).

PHARMACOLOGY CAPSULE The side effects of tricyclic antidepressant medications are drowsiness, fatigue, orthostatic hypotension, dry mouth, blurred vision, urinary retention, and constipation.

The manic phase of bipolar disease is usually treated with lithium or divalproex (Depakote) (Table 53-6). When administering medications, you are responsible for ensuring that medication has been swallowed, as opposed to being held

table 53-5 DRUG THERAPY | *Antidepressant Drugs*

DRUG (TRADE NAME)	CONSIDERATIONS
SSRIs	
Citalopram (Celexa) Fluoxetine (Prozac) Fluvoxamine (Luvox) Paroxetine (Paxil) Sertraline (Zoloft)	SSRIs can be taken once a day, making adherence to a prescribed treatment easier for the patient. SSRIs are not considered cardiotoxic; thus, an overdose is unlikely to cause life-threatening arrhythmias. Besides depression, SSRIs may be useful in panic disorder and obsessive-compulsive disorder. Some patients tolerate the medications in the AM, others in the PM.
TRICYCLICS	
Amitriptyline (Elavil) Clomipramine (Anafranil) Desipramine (Norpramin) Doxepin (Sinequan) Imipramine (Tofranil) Nortriptyline (Pamelor) Trimipramine (Surmontil)	Tricyclics affect not only serotonin but also epinephrine/norepinephrine and as such may cause cardiac complications. Severe and life-threatening dysrhythmias may result from an overdose. Side effects may be more problematic in this group of medications than with SSRIs. Many of these medicines cannot be taken once a day; bid or tid dosing must be used to reach the total daily dose.
TETRACYCLICS	
Maprotiline (Ludiomil) Mirtazapine (Remeron)	At least as potentially dangerous as tricyclics; significant sedation may occur. May be given in single or divided doses.
OTHER AGENTS	
Bupropion (Wellbutrin)	Divided doses (increase risk of seizures)
Nefazodone (Serzone)	Divided doses (sedating)
Trazodone (Desyrel)	Divided doses >100 mg (sedative)
Venlafaxine (Effexor)	Divided doses
MAOIs	
Phenelzine (Nardil)	Not first-line (first choice) drugs
Tranylcypromine (Parnate)	Strict diet restrictions. Interactions with foods containing tyramine, other antidepressants, and many other drugs can lead to life-threatening hypertensive crisis. Must be given in divided doses.

table 53-6 DRUG THERAPY | *Mood Stabilizers (Anti-Manic Agents)*

DRUG NAME (GENERIC/BRAND)	NURSING IMPLICATIONS	PATIENT TEACHING
Lithium (Lithium Carbonate, Lithobid, Lithium SR)	Used in the treatment of bipolar disorders; occasionally used as adjunct treatment for depression Narrow therapeutic range of 0.5 to 1.5 mEq/L Watch for signs of lithium toxicity (tremulousness, nausea, vomiting, diarrhea, changes in level of consciousness) Maintain adequate hydration Monitor renal function (serum creatinine and BUN) and report abnormal findings Monitor serum level of lithium Do not change from immediate release to sustained release or vice versa unless directed by prescriber because this may alter serum levels unexpectedly	Take exactly as prescribed. Drug must be taken regularly to achieve and maintain adequate blood level. Do not alter salt intake. Do not double up on doses if one is missed. Maintain adequate fluid intake, especially in hot weather. Avoid excessive use of caffeinated beverages. Keep follow-up appointments and have blood levels drawn as directed. Report signs of toxicity at once.
Valproic acid, divalproex sodium (Depakote, Depakene)	Used in the treatment of bipolar disorders Serum levels must be monitored for therapeutic range (50 to 100 μg/ml) Metabolized by the liver, thus periodic monitoring of liver enzymes is necessary May cause some sedation May cause hair loss; if moderate to severe, notify prescribing practitioner	Take medication exactly as prescribed. Drug must be taken regularly to achieve and maintain adequate blood level. Do not double up on medication if a dose is missed. Avoid driving or operating dangerous machinery until exact effects of medication are known. Keep follow-up appointments and have blood levels drawn as directed.

Consider the Alternative!

Many people use the herbal preparation St. John's wort to relieve depression. However, additional study is needed before it can be recommended as a replacement for conventional drugs used to treat major mental illnesses.

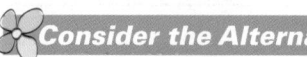

in the mouth and later discarded or saved for an overdose. As the patient responds to antidepressant medication and the energy level increases, the risk of suicide also increases.

MAOIs sometimes are prescribed for patients with a depression that is resistant to the TCAs, SSRIs, and other antidepressants. A 2-week period should elapse between ending most antidepressants and beginning an MAOI. The very serious side effect of a hypertensive crisis occurs if the patient taking an MAOI ingests tyramine-containing food or drink, such as avocados, bananas, beer, bologna, canned figs, chocolate, cheese (except cottage cheese), liver, papaya products, pâté, herring, fava beans, raisins, salami, sausage, sour cream, soy sauce, wine, and yogurt. These foods also must be avoided for 3 weeks after stopping treatment with an MAOI. Symptoms of a hypertensive crisis, which requires immediate treatment, include headache, palpitations, visual changes, neck stiffness, nausea, vomiting, sweating, sensitivity to light, pupil changes, and bradycardia or tachycardia. A "washout" period of about four weeks must elapse when discontinuing a MAOI before starting most other antidepressants.

Sexual dysfunction (anorgasmia, delayed or absent ejaculation, and decreased libido) may occur with any antidepressant but seems to be more commonly related to the SSRI antidepressants. Some antidepressants, such as nefazadone [Serzone] and bupropion [Wellbutrin], are much less likely to cause this troublesome side effect.

Put on your THINKING CAP!!

A patient with bipolar disorder is being treated for severe depression in an inpatient facility with bupropion (Wellbutrin) and divalproex sodium (Depakote). Identify the nursing implications related to these medications.

Electroconvulsive Therapy

Electroconvulsive therapy (ECT) is a form of therapy in which an electrical current is introduced to the brain through electrodes placed on the temples. The electrical current produces a grand mal seizure; however, drugs are administered to minimize the manifestations of a seizure. This type of therapy most often is prescribed when other forms of therapy have failed with people who are severely depressed. Its advantage is that it acts more quickly than medications, and in older people it may have fewer side effects.

Key nursing interventions include patient and family teaching, making certain that the patient takes nothing by mouth after midnight on the day of a treatment, asking the patient to void and to remove eyeglasses or contact lenses and dentures, administering atropine sulfate as ordered (to decrease secretions), positioning the patient on the side following the procedure to prevent aspiration, monitoring vital signs, remaining with the patient until the patient is awake, and providing orienting information as needed (e.g., "It's 10 AM Wednesday, and you just finished your treatment"). Temporary memory loss and confusion are common side effects of ECT, and instances of prolonged memory loss have occurred. You must take appropriate safety precautions and be patient with the person who has undergone this procedure.

NURSING CARE *of the Patient with Major Depression*

Assessment

In completing the mental status examination of a patient who has depression, assessment findings may include:

- Activity: patient is likely to exhibit psychomotor retardation and possibly no spontaneous movements, with a downcast gaze, although the patient may exhibit agitation (e.g., hand wringing and hair pulling), especially if elderly
- Mood and affect: may or may not have depressed feelings and may not appear depressed
- Speech and language: speech volume and rate may be decreased; response to questions may be delayed; and mutism may be present
- Thought content: patient expresses generally negative view of self and world; may ruminate about loss, guilt, suicide, and depression; if psychotic, may have delusions of guilt, failure, worthlessness, or terminal illnesses
- Insight and judgment: suicidal ideation occurs in two thirds of depressed patients, with 10% to 15% committing suicide successfully; suicide risk increases as the patient gains the energy needed to commit suicide; insight into illness may be impaired due to negative perceptions of reality
- Sensorium: patient is oriented but may not have energy to answer questions
- Memory and attention: patients commonly complain of impaired concentration and forgetfulness

Nursing Diagnoses, Goals, and Outcome Criteria: Depression

Nursing Diagnoses	Goals and Outcome Criteria
Risk for Self-Directed Violence related to hopelessness, increased energy level associated with treatment, as evidenced by patient endorsing suicidal ideations	Reduced risk of harm to self: patient seeks out staff member if an urge to harm self is experienced: develops coping skills to replace self-destructive behavior and acceptable ways of expressing anger, rage, and hostility; mobilizes social support systems

Chronic or Situational Low Self-Esteem related to negative feelings about self	Improved self-esteem: patient accepts own body, has positive feelings about self, identifies aspects of self he or she likes; identifies thoughts about self
Imbalanced Nutrition: Less than Body Requirements related to anorexia	Adequate nutrition: gains weight steadily and has more energy
Disturbed Sleep Pattern related to anxiety	Improved sleep pattern: patient sleeps within 30 minutes of retiring and remains asleep for 6 to 8 uninterrupted hours

Interventions

Risk for Self-Directed Violence

Interventions may include establishing a no-harm contract; frequently assessing a patient's suicidal potential (see questions under assessment at beginning of the chapter); taking necessary suicide precautions; removing dangerous objects such as pantyhose, belts, and any sharp objects; maintaining continuous one-to-one contact if indicated; encouraging honest expression of feelings; assisting in identifying symbols of hope in patient's life; identifying community resources for times of crisis; and communicating message that the patient is worthwhile.

Chronic or Situational Low Self-Esteem

Interventions may include helping the patient to identify positive aspects and limitations regarding his or her body; to like the body despite its imperfections; to improve hygiene, grooming, and posture, which makes positive affirmations about self; to limit self-criticism; to be aware of negative self-statements; to learn to give and receive compliments; and to develop social skills.

Imbalanced Nutrition: Less than Body Requirements

Possible interventions include involving a dietitian in planning an adequate diet for the patient; directly assisting patients to make healthy choices regarding their menu and eating choices; documenting intake; determining food preferences and attempting to satisfy those preferences; and offering small, frequent meals.

Disturbed Sleep Pattern

Interventions are discouraging sleep during the day, providing sleep-producing measures like a light small snack and warm baths, and teaching relaxation exercises to be used before retiring. The patient should avoid exercising before bedtime, refraining from watching TV in bed, or ingesting caffeine after 2 PM. The patient may be asked to keep a sleep diary.

See the Nursing Care Plan: The Patient with Major Depression.

NURSING CARE *of the Patient with Bipolar Disorder with Manic Episodes*

Assessment

The nurse may observe the following:

- Appearance: dress is often inappropriate (e.g., bright, nonmatching colors, excessive makeup and jewelry)
- Activity: hyperactive
- Mood, affect, and feelings: although frequently euphoric, the patient may also be very irritable, angry, and hostile, based on low frustration tolerance, and emotionally labile
- Speech and language: talkative, pressured speech that is difficult to interrupt; flight of ideas (continuous rapid shift from one topic to another); rate and volume increased
- Thought content: themes of self-confidence and self-aggrandizement and possibly delusions of grandeur (e.g., false belief that one has great wealth or power) or delusions of persecution
- Sensory perception: hallucinations may occur
- Insight and judgment: patient often has little insight regarding illness; judgment impaired, as evidenced by actions such as large spending sprees, sexual activities incongruent with usual behavior, suicide attempts, and homicide attempts

Nursing Diagnoses, Goals, and Outcome Criteria: Manic Episodes

NURSING DIAGNOSES	GOALS AND OUTCOME CRITERIA
Risk for Injury related to impaired judgment	Reduced risk for injury: patient does not exhibit potentially injurious activities
Risk for Violence Directed at Others related to impaired judgment, low frustration tolerance, and emotional lability	Reduced risk of violence toward others: patient does not harm others; patient verbalizes anger appropriately
Imbalanced Nutrition: Less than Body Requirements related to hyperactivity	Balanced nutrition: patient consumes necessary daily nutrients in appropriate form for manic state; maintains body weight
Disturbed Sleep Pattern related to hyperactivity	Improved sleep patterns: patient sleeps at least 6 uninterrupted hours

Interventions

Risk for Injury

Interventions include decreasing environmental stimuli (e.g., providing a quiet, simply decorated room), discouraging group activities, encouraging a few one-to-one contacts, removing hazardous objects and substances from the environment, and providing a structure that includes physical activities such as brisk walks.

NURSING CARE PLAN

The Patient with Major Depression

ASSESSMENT

Health History: A 53-year-old woman is admitted to a psychiatric hospital with a diagnosis of major depression. During the past few weeks she has become increasingly listless, apathetic, and disinterested in anyone or anything. She cries frequently, and says her life has not seemed to be worth living. She complains that she cannot sleep and has no appetite. She frequently talks about wanting to commit suicide. She was referred to a psychiatrist, who recommended that she be admitted to the hospital for treatment.

Physical Examination: Blood pressure, 110/70; pulse, 78; respiration, 22; temperature, 98.8° F orally. Height, 5'4". Weight, 120 lb. Appears apathetic, sad, and cries frequently. Somewhat disheveled. Gaunt and tired-looking.

Nursing Diagnosis	*Goals and Outcome Criteria*	*Interventions*
Risk for self-violence related to suicidal feelings.	The patient will not harm herself, as evidenced by seeking out nursing staff if she experiences the urge to harm herself, developing coping skills to replace self-destructive behavior, and developing acceptable ways to express anger, rage, and hostility.	Establish a no-harm contract; frequently assess patient's suicidal potential and take necessary suicide precautions; remove dangerous objects from the environment; maintain continuous one-to-one contact; encourage honest expression of feelings; assist in identifying symbols of hope in patient's life.
Chronic or situational low self-esteem related to depression.	The patient will maintain or enhance self-esteem, as evidenced by acceptance of own body and sense of self, identification of negative thoughts about self, and identification of aspects of self she likes.	Help patient to identify positive aspects and limitations regarding her body and to accept her body regardless of limitations. Encourage patient to improve hygiene. Assist patient to accept compliments and to limit self-criticism.
Imbalanced nutrition: less than body requirements related to anorexia or lack of interest in food.	Patient will gain weight and experience higher energy level, as evidenced by more participation and interactions in activities with others.	Involve dietitian in planning adequate diet. Determine food preferences and attempt to satisfy preferences. Offer small, frequent meals.
Disturbed sleep patterns related to depression relapse.	Patient will sleep within 30 min of retiring and remain asleep for 6 to 8 uninterrupted hr.	Provide sleep-producing measures such as small snacks, warm baths, and relaxation exercises before patient retires.

Risk for Violence Directed at Others

Interventions include decreasing environmental stimuli, observing the patient frequently, removing harmful objects, finding physical outlets, demonstrating a show of strength if necessary, administering prescribed medications, and restraining if other measures have failed to calm the patient. Restraints should be applied following an established protocol by staff who have been educated to restrain patients in a safe and humane manner. The patient in restraints should be checked at least every 15 minutes to make certain that circulation to extremities is satisfactory and to assess needs regarding nutrition and elimination.

Imbalanced Nutrition: Less than Body Requirements

Interventions include providing foods that can be consumed on the run, attempting to have the patient's favorite foods and easy-to-eat and finger foods available, and educating the patient on the importance of satisfactory nutrition.

Disturbed Sleep Pattern

Interventions may include making sure the environment has low stimuli; observing closely for signs of fatigue, such as fine tremor and puffy, dark circles below the eyes; and encouraging warm baths and soft music at bedtime.

The key medications for people with manic episodes are divalproex sodium (Depakote) or lithium carbonate. Because relief from symptoms may take up to 3 weeks, the patient also may receive an antipsychotic (neuroleptic) medication.

The therapeutic level of divalproex sodium in the blood is 50-100 μg/ml (depending on the lab). The patient may develop toxicity if the blood level exceeds the therapeutic range. Therefore a valproic acid level is done at intervals to assess blood levels. Divalproex is metabolized by the liver; thus patients with liver disorders may receive lower dosages.

Lithium is excreted by the kidneys and has a narrow therapeutic range. The therapeutic blood level for acute mania is 0.5 to 1.5 mEq/L (depending on the lab). Above 1.5 mEq/L, symptoms of toxicity occur. It is critical for the patient taking lithium to stay well hydrated. If a patient taking lithium becomes dehydrated, he or she can easily become lithium-toxic. Signs and symptoms of lithium toxicity include tremor, nausea, vomiting, diarrhea, and changes in level of consciousness.

PHARMACOLOGY CAPSULE Older adults and medically compromised patients are exceptionally vulnerable to experiencing the side effects of all psychotropic medications, especially postural hypotension, falls, and confusion.

COGNITIVE DISORDERS

The key problems for people with cognitive disorders stem from impairments in cognition or memory. The term *cognitive disorders* replaced the term *organic mental disorders* because the latter incorrectly implied that "nonorganic" mental disorders do not have a biologic basis. Delirium and dementia are two different disorders that involve deficits in orientation, memory, language comprehension, and judgment. Delirium is potentially reversible, whereas dementia is not.

Common causes of delirium are meningitis, neoplasms, drugs ranging from alcohol to steroids, endocrine dysfunction, liver abnormalities, thiamine deficiency, and postoperative states. Common types of dementia are dementia of the Alzheimer's type, vascular dementia, Pick's disease, and Parkinson's disease. Delirium and dementia are discussed in greater detail in Chapter 21.

PERSONALITY DISORDERS

Every individual exhibits particular personality traits. A person may be shy, aggressive, dependent, or manipulative. When personality traits become inflexible and dysfunctional, a person may have a personality disorder. The essential features of a personality disorder are that it is pervasive (it concerns all aspects of one's life), chronic, and maladaptive. Examples of personality disorders are as follows:

1. Paranoid Personality Disorder—a pattern of distrust and suspiciousness such that others' motives are interpreted as hostile (individual suspects that others are out to harm or deceive, doubts loyalty of friends, does not confide in others, bears grudges, feels attacked by others).
2. Schizoid Personality Disorder—a pattern of detachment from social relationships and a restricted range of emotional expression (individual does not desire or enjoy close relationships, chooses solitary activities, lacks close friends, shows emotional coldness or detachment).
3. Schizotypal Personality Disorder—a pattern of difficulties in social and interpersonal relationships in which the person suffers from acute discomfort with close relationships and therefore has a decreased capacity for such relationships. Persons with this disorder also have cognitive and perceptual distortions as well as eccentricities of behavior that make close relationships difficult.

   Note: People with paranoid, schizoid, and schizotypal personality disorders often appear odd or eccentric.
4. Antisocial Personality Disorder—a pattern of disregard for and violation of the rights of others (individual repeatedly breaks the law; lies; fails to plan ahead; shows a reckless disregard for the safety of self and others; is irresponsible; lacks remorse for having hurt, mistreated, or stolen from another).
5. Borderline Personality Disorder—a pattern of instability in interpersonal relationships, self-image, and affect and marked impulsivity (individual makes frantic efforts to avoid real or imagined abandonment; has chronic feelings of emptiness; shows inappropriate, intense anger or has difficulty controlling anger; has unstable self-image or sense of self; and exhibits recurrent suicidal behavior, gestures, or threats).
6. Histrionic Personality Disorder—a pattern of excessive emotionality and attention seeking (individual prefers to be the center of attention; is often sexually seductive or provocative; displays rapidly shifting and shallow expression of emotion; consistently uses physical appearance to draw attention to self; and shows self-dramatization, theatricality, and exaggerated expression of emotion).
7. Narcissistic Personality Disorder—a pattern of grandiosity, need for admiration, and lack of empathy (individual has an exaggerated sense of self-importance; requires excessive admiration; takes advantage of others to achieve own ends; is often envious of others; and exhibits arrogant, haughty behaviors or attitudes).

   Note: People with antisocial, borderline, histrionic, or narcissistic personality disorder often appear dramatic, emotional, or erratic.
8. Avoidant Personality Disorder—a pattern of social inhibition accompanied by feelings of inadequacy and hypersensitivity to negative evaluation (individual avoids occupational activities that involve interpersonal activities because of fear of criticism, disapproval, or rejection; is unwilling to get involved with people unless certain of being liked; is preoccupied with being criticized or rejected in social situations; views self as inferior to others; and is unusually reluctant to take personal risks).
9. Dependent Personality Disorder—a pattern of submissive and clinging behavior related to an excessive need to be taken care of (individual has difficulty making everyday decisions without an excessive amount of advice and reassurance from others, needs others to assume responsibility for most major areas in life, has difficulty initiating projects because of lack of confidence in own judgment or abilities, and urgently seeks a relationship as a source of care and support).
10. Obsessive-Compulsive Personality Disorder—a pattern of preoccupation with orderliness, perfectionism, and control (individual is preoccupied with details, rules,

lists, order, organization, or schedules to the extent that the major part of the activity is lost; shows perfectionism, rigidity, and stubbornness).

Note: Individuals with avoidant, dependent, or obsessive-compulsive personality disorder often appear anxious or fearful.

BORDERLINE PERSONALITY DISORDER

The person with borderline personality disorder has patterns involving unstable relationships, unstable self-image, and unstable mood. Two theories offer explanations for the cause of this disorder. First, because families of patients with this disorder have a greater history of alcoholism, a genetic influence is thought to exist. The second explanation is related to particular developmental experiences. Some theorists view an essential component of psychosocial development as separation-individuation. Some feel that there are problems with attachment. It is thought that between 2 and 3 years of age, the child separates from the parents as a unique self. If the parents are nonaccepting or ambivalent of the child's increasing autonomy and if the parents reinforce dependent behavior, the child does not fully experience self as separate. This problem with separation-individuation is thought to form the basis of *splitting,* a frequently utilized mechanism in borderline personality disorder. Persons who are splitting view others as all good or all bad and may shift their views of a particular other from all good to all bad. A person who has a clearly developed sense of self and who does not split views others as having a mix of good qualities and negative qualities. The case of Bonnie P. provides a clinical example of borderline personality disorder.

Nora N., a licensed vocational nurse, worked part time on a psychiatric unit. She reported to work at 11 PM one night after 5 days of not working to discover that Bonnie P. had been readmitted after opening the suture line on her wrists with a steak knife. One year ago Bonnie had cut this wrist, saying that she was trying to feel something. Bonnie told Nora that she had missed her terribly and that she hoped Nora would work with her that night. Nora said that Susan (the full-time registered nurse) would work with her that night. Bonnie swore and returned to her room. When Nora made rounds, Bonnie said she was sure something was wrong and began walking around the room with a staggering gait. Bonnie said that she had not taken anything to create this problem. Her vital signs were stable, and her pupils were normal in size and reaction to light. Nora reported the situation to Susan and reflected on her responses to Bonnie. Initially she felt anger, telling herself that Bonnie was manipulative when she did not have her way. She thought about how Bonnie manipulates others when she feels helpless (she has no idea of how to meet her own needs). She also thought about Bonnie's splitting (seeing Nora as good nurse and Susan as bad nurse). Nora felt less angry as she considered the reasons for Bonnie's behavior. When Susan entered Bonnie's bedroom, Bonnie's gait was normal. Susan contracted with Bonnie for two 10-minute periods (at the beginning and end of shift) during which Bonnie could share whatever was on her mind and discuss her goals and plans for the following day.

NURSING CARE *of the Patient with Borderline Personality Disorder*

Assessment

The most relevant aspects of the mental status examination are the following:

- Mood, affect, feelings: patient may experience mood swings or chronic feelings of emptiness and boredom or intense anger
- Insight and judgment: patient makes repeated suicidal threats and gestures and exhibits self-mutilating behavior

Nursing Diagnoses, Goals, and Outcome Criteria: Borderline Personality Disorder

Nursing Diagnoses	Goals and Outcome Criteria
Risk for Self-Directed Violence related to episodes of anger and impaired judgment	Absence of self-directed violence: patient does not harm self
Impaired Social Interaction related to unstable relationships	Improved social interaction: patient maintains relationships
Disturbed Personal Identity related to splitting	Improved sense of personal identity: patient clarifies own unique characteristics, differentiates thoughts and feelings of self and others; less splitting, clinging, and disturbing behaviors

Interventions

Risk for Self-Directed Violence

In addition to the interventions identified in the section on mood disorders, various interventions are more specific to the issues of borderline personality disorder. It is important to be aware of your own feelings in order to refrain from any automatic responses that are not helpful (such as avoiding the patient who has cut himself). If patients mutilate themselves, it is important to care for wounds without acting in a way that might reinforce the self-mutilation (such as offering sympathy). Ask patients to talk about feelings that occurred just before the self-mutilation. You can act as a role model for constructive expression of angry feelings and acknowledge the patient's positive expressions of negative feelings.

Impaired Social Interaction

Interventions include assisting patients in examining their own behaviors in relationships, communicating availability, acknowledging (reinforcing) independent behavior, and setting limits as appropriate.

Disturbed Personal Identity

Interventions include helping the patient discuss and take ownership of own thoughts and feelings; clarifying values while being cautious not to impose one's own values; and

Nutrition Concepts

1. During manic episodes, patients may not meet nutritional needs because of increased physical activity and difficulty sitting down to complete a meal.
2. Anorexia may be a problem for depressed patients.

avoiding empathetic responses that may be viewed as mind reading (such as "I know how you feel").

SUMMARY

Nurses work with patients with psychiatric disorders in a variety of settings, including psychiatric inpatient units. Treatment for psychiatric disorders is influenced by the particular culture, place, and historical time frame. You can use various strategies in communicating therapeutically with patients. The mental status examination is one aspect of the assessment of patients and is particularly relevant on a psychiatric unit. Use the mental status examination with patients systematically on admission and on an ongoing basis. For each of the major psychiatric disorders, possible observations for the relevant mental status examination categories are presented. Possible nursing diagnoses, goals, and interventions have been suggested for each disorder.

key points

- According to current thinking, mental illnesses are related to specific physiologic changes in the central nervous system.
- The psychoanalytic approach to mental illness is based on the theory that human beings function at different levels of awareness, ranging from conscious to unconscious, and that people use ego defense mechanisms to prevent anxiety.
- The interpersonal approach to mental illness has three components: (1) anxiety is often communicated interpersonally; (2) the patient learns new ways of coping or maturing in a therapeutic relationship; and (3) establishing trust is an important first step in the nurse's work with patients.
- Key ideas from the cognitive behavioral approach to mental illness are that behavior is learned, that behavior changes in response to positive consequences (positive reinforcement) or in response to the removal of negative stimuli (negative reinforcement), and that particular thoughts influence emotional states.
- In caring for a patient with a psychiatric disorder, nurses establish therapeutic (as opposed to social) relationships.
- The mental status examination consists of observations regarding appearance, mood and affect, speech and language, thought content, perceptual disturbances, insight and judgment, sensorium, and memory and attention.
- A patient with an anxiety disorder experiences either the highly uncomfortable feeling of anxiety directly or a symptom such as compulsive hand washing that prevents or reduces the occurrence of anxiety.
- In panic disorder, a patient experiences recurrent panic attacks, which are intense episodes of apprehension, at times to the point of terror, and often are accompanied by the feeling of impending doom.
- A person with agoraphobia is extremely fearful of situations outside the home from which escape may be difficult or in which help may be unavailable.
- Obsessive-compulsive disorder involves recurrent obsessions (thoughts), compulsions (behaviors), or both that produce distress and interfere with functioning.
- Posttraumatic stress disorder is a cluster of symptoms experienced following a distressing event that is outside the range of normal events (e.g., watching one's family being murdered).
- Individuals with a somatoform disorder, such as conversion disorder or hypochondriasis, are convinced that they have serious medical problems despite the absence of any concrete medical findings.
- Dissociative disorders involve a change in identity, memory, or consciousness, usually to escape from anxiety.
- Goals for the nursing care of patients with anxiety, somatoform, and dissociative disorders are to decrease anxiety to a point at which problem solving can occur and to teach methods such as relaxation techniques to interrupt anxiety as it escalates.
- The term *schizophrenia* refers to a highly problematic group of biologic disorders in which there are symptoms of psychosis, including delusions, hallucinations, marked loosening of associations, catatonia, and flat or inappropriate affect.
- People with mood disorders, such as major depression and bipolar depression, experience a significantly elevated mood, a significantly depressed mood, or both.
- Dementia is a group of disorders characterized by cognitive deficits sufficiently severe enough to impair social or occupational functioning.
- Personality disorders occur when personality traits become inflexible and dysfunctional and are pervasive (concern all aspects of one's life), chronic, and maladaptive.

REVIEW QUESTIONS

1. The primary focus of nursing care for patients with mental illness and their families is on:
   1. helping them cope with and manage mental illness.
   2. administering medications.
   3. protecting other people from the patient.
   4. controlling the patient's behavior.

2. Which of the following reflects an important characteristic of a therapeutic relationship?
   1. The relationship should benefit the patient and the nurse.
   2. The relationship has a clear purpose and ending.
   3. The relationship develops spontaneously.
   4. The relationship has no clear boundaries.

3. Which statement best illustrates the strategy of *clarifying* in a nurse-patient interaction?
   1. "When you mention your son, you look very sad."
   2. "What were you saying while I was on the telephone?"
   3. "Why do you get quiet when I ask about your husband?"
   4. "Are you saying that you are afraid of him?"

4. In the mental status exam, the nurse assesses multiple areas, including:
   1. thought content.
   2. IQ.
   3. reflexes.
   4. reaction time.

5. Mr. Brooks was hospitalized after a major automobile accident in which another person died. Mr. Brooks reports having no sensation in his legs and is unable to move them. Diagnostic studies reveal no physical basis for his symptoms. The patient's symptoms are typical of:
   1. hypochondriasis.
   2. posttraumatic stress disorder.
   3. conversion disorder.
   4. panic disorder.

6. John is a young college student who has just been diagnosed with schizophrenia. His concerned parents ask for information about his diagnosis. Which reply would be correct and appropriate?
   1. Schizophrenia is a mental illness that affects a person's thinking and distorts his view of reality.
   2. Most people with schizophrenia eventually require permanent care in a psychiatric facility.
   3. At this time there are no medications or treatments for schizophrenia.
   4. Most episodes of schizophrenia resolve with a week or two.

7. Nursing interventions to promote communication with the person who has schizophrenia include:
   1. go along with delusions to avoid upsetting the patient.
   2. provide a variety of environmental stimuli.
   3. point out the flaws in the patient's illogical statements.
   4. do not argue or try to disprove his delusions.

8. What are the nursing implications when a patient is taking phenelzine sulfate (Nardil)?
   1. Nardil is more effective if given with a tricyclic antidepressant.
   2. Patients should be taught to avoid foods that contain tyramine.
   3. Drugs that interact with Nardil can cause hypotensive crisis.
   4. Because Nardil has few interactions, it is often used in combination with other drugs.

9. People who are arrogant, need excessive admiration, and take advantage of others for their own gain may have which type of personality disorder?
   1. Borderline
   2. Obsessive-compulsive
   3. Narcissistic
   4. Histrionic

10. A patient taking divalproex (Depakote) is advised that blood samples will be taken periodically to monitor for:
    1. liver damage.
    2. dystonic reactions.
    3. kidney damage.
    4. extrapyramidal syndromes.

CHAPTER

54 Substance-Related Disorders

MARK D. SOUCY

objectives

1. Discuss the biologic, sociocultural, behavioral, and intrapersonal theories of the etiology of substance abuse or dependence.
2. Describe the components of the nursing assessment of a patient with substance abuse or dependence.
3. Describe alcohol dependence, alcohol withdrawal syndrome, medical complications of alcohol dependence, and treatment of alcohol abuse and dependence.
4. Discuss the pathophysiologic effects of frequently abused drugs.
5. Describe disorders associated with substance abuse and dependence.
6. Differentiate between drug abuse treatment and alcohol abuse treatment.
7. Describe the nursing diagnoses and interventions associated with substance abuse and dependence.
8. Discuss populations who present special problems in relation to drug abuse and dependency.

key terms

Addiction (Ă-DĬK-shŭn, p. 1150)
Co-dependent (p. 1151)
Delirium tremens (p. 1150)
Dual diagnosis (dī-ăg-NŌ-sĭs, p. 1163)
Physical dependence (p. 1157)
Psychological dependence (sī-kō-LŎJ-ĕ-kăl, p. 1154)
Substance abuse (p. 1147)
Substance dependence (p. 1147)
Tolerance (TOL-ŭr-ŭns, p. 1147)
12-Step Program (p. 1151)
Withdrawal (p. 1150)

Substance abuse and dependence have become major problems in the United States and in other parts of the world over the past 30 years. These problems have reached the point of such significance that a great deal of energy and financial resources have been targeted toward a better understanding of them. Many researchers continue to try to discover the specific causes of **substance abuse** and dependence in order to combat these disorders more effectively. It appears that many factors contribute to the development of substance abuse and dependence.

The Diagnostic and Statistical Manual (4th ed.) (DSM-IV) provides the criteria for understanding whether an individual has substance dependence, or if the disorder is less severe, substance abuse. An individual with alcohol and/or substance abuse, if not adequately treated, may progress to alcohol and/or substance dependence. **Tolerance,** a term used to describe the individual's need for more alcohol or other substance of choice in order to create the desired effect, is one of the criteria for the diagnosis of substance dependence. Other criteria include a diminished effect, resulting from using the same amount over time, the experience of physical withdrawal and/or substituting a similar substance in place of the usual one to treat discomfort associated with discontinuing the substance as well as others. In both abuse and dependence, there exists a significant degree of impairment or distress in the person's life.

ETIOLOGY AND RISK FACTORS

BIOLOGIC THEORY

The theory that is generally accepted by a majority of the experts in the field of addictionology is the biologic theory, often referred to as the medical model, which proposes that a faulty physiologic process that is not clearly understood contributes to dependence on a specific substance or substances (**substance dependence**). This theory is supported by the fact that children have been shown to be four times more likely to become alcoholic if their biologic parent or parents are alcoholic, even when the children are raised apart from the parents in homes where they are not exposed to the excessive use of alcohol. Widely publicized studies implicate a dopamine gene on human chromosome 11 for transmitting a predisposition for alcoholism from generation to generation. On the basis of these and many other studies, the medical community considers drug dependency to be a physical illness, like those that have the following characteristics: (1) incurability, (2) a genetic predisposition to develop under the right conditions, and (3) a potential to be treated effectively only by total abstinence from the substance that the body cannot handle.

SOCIOCULTURAL THEORY

Another theory suggests that sociocultural factors play a major role in the process of becoming dependent on a particular drug. Many people who live in poverty and in crime-ridden areas use drugs to relieve the stress inherent in these environments. In contrast, it can be observed that individuals with strong religious values prohibiting the excessive use of drugs have lower rates of addiction. Among select subcultures, the use of certain types of drugs can act as a rite of entry into a gang or a badge of honor proving that one has "made it." Even among middle-class Americans, it is expected that the average person will "party" on New Year's Eve, for example, often to excess. Certain cultural groups, such as the Irish, are commonly stereotyped as heavy drinkers. Country music lovers recognize that "crying in your beer" is often portrayed as the typical means of coping with loss and rejection.

BEHAVIORAL THEORY

Behavioral and learning theories look at the triggers for drinking and drug-using behaviors and how these patterns are reinforced. Substance abuse is believed to be a learned maladaptive way of coping with stress and anxiety. Family and peer group role models are studied closely for their use of substances, along with the beliefs and customs surrounding the use of drugs and alcohol. For example, if a shy teenaged girl gets more attention and feels socially more comfortable when drinking with her friends, she is more likely to continue the use of alcohol in order to be accepted by her peers.

INTRAPERSONAL THEORY

The intrapersonal or psychological theory addresses those factors innate to the personality of the individual that may predispose him or her to substance abuse. These theorists believe that the quality of intrapersonal relationships during critical developmental stages of our lives affects us profoundly. Thus, if children experience early childhood rejection, increased responsibility, unrealistic expectations, or overprotection, they may develop a dependent type of personality and consequently view themselves as inadequate or failures when attempts to get their needs met fail. Individuals may ultimately turn to alcohol or other drugs to numb the anxiety or frustration evoked by self-doubt and the daily stressors of reality.

Persons who abuse substances often have personality traits in common: many are very self-centered, have a strong need to be in control of others, seek attention, and have great difficulty delaying gratification of their needs. All of these characteristics are likely to increase the odds that they will resort to the use of drugs or alcohol to cope.

These types of intrapersonal theories originally supported the widespread acceptance of the perspective that alcoholism or drug addiction is a product of moral weakness. A more modern conclusion acknowledges that although the specific causes of misuse and addiction to various substances have not been established, they most likely involve a combination of biologic, social, cultural, behavioral, and psychological factors.

NURSING ASSESSMENT OF THE SUBSTANCE ABUSER

HEALTH HISTORY

Thorough data collection is essential to initiate the nursing process effectively when working with the substance-abusing patient. Information can be gathered from a variety of sources, including an interview with the patient, family members, significant others, a social assessment, medical records, and school or military records. Many substance abusers have sustained major losses—of jobs, relationships, property, self-esteem, and health. They may face legal charges. Often they will not seek professional help until they have "hit bottom." Even then, they may seek help only when presented with an ultimatum of some type, often from their family, employer, or a court of law.

Questioning the patient produces the most reliable data when the questioning is nonjudgmental, direct, and specific and the answers are verified by more than one source when possible. For example, if the patient reports drinking a couple of beers after work each night, you should ask exactly how many were ingested, how many ounces each contained, or how big the bottle or glass used actually was. It also is important to know when the patient ingested the drug last and how much was taken in order to predict the possibility and timing of physical withdrawal symptoms. A nonjudgmental and matter-of-fact manner is the least likely to alienate an already defensive patient. At the same time, don't be so supportive and nurturing that clients can avoid facing the negative impact substance abuse has had on their lives. Finding the most appropriate balance of support and reality-based confrontation is a highly developed skill that increases the likelihood that patients will continue in the treatment process. Many team members who work in substance abuse treatment centers are recovering from addiction themselves, which often helps the client be more honest and less defensive and feel less hopeless and alone.

Patterns and Consequences of Abuse

The patient who has been abusing one or more substances will describe typical patterns of behavior and a combination of physical or psychological withdrawal symptoms characteristic of the substances abused. A few patients may not experience any physical withdrawal symptoms despite a history of prolonged, frequent, and heavy abuse, even of some substances that usually are physically addicting. Much depends on the stage of addiction, habitual patterns of use, the patient's baseline physical status, and the combinations and interactions of the drug or drugs being misused.

Many substance abusers experience erratic and unprovoked mood swings. They may describe a lifestyle revolving almost totally around obtaining and using the substance of choice, starting early in the day, often alone, and requiring more of the substance over time to get the desired effects. Many substance abusers make efforts to hide the extent of their habit from others and, despite their best efforts to limit use of the substance, have been unsuccessful in doing so. Blackouts may have occurred when under the influence of a particular substance (especially alcohol). Blackouts are episodes of amnesia in which the individual does not remember what happened during a period of time. Patients often have significant work problems or damaged relationships as a result of being unable to meet the expectations placed on them.

Defense Mechanisms Employed

Typical defense mechanisms used by the substance abuser include denial, rationalization, intellectualization, and projection. Denial is readily apparent when patients state that they do not have a problem with drug use despite evidence to the contrary. Individuals also may initially minimize the problems they have had with using. Some deny that they need help in staying clean and sober. Some insist that they do not need to change friends or attend a 12-step program meeting such as Alcoholics Anonymous regularly.

The defense mechanism of rationalization is one in which abusers attempt to justify the reasons for their abuse of substances. This is an "excuse" for addiction. An example is the individual who insists he or she had to use heroin because there was no other way to cope with the pain of a physical injury: "The drugs my doctor gave me weren't working."

Intellectualization is closely related to rationalization but differs in that the person focuses only on objective facts as a way of avoiding dealing with unconscious conflicts and the emotions they evoke. For example, an alcoholic who killed someone while driving under the influence of alcohol would be intellectualizing if they stated that it was better that the victim die suddenly rather than have to live as a paraplegic.

Projection in substance abusers involves shifting the blame for their behavior onto someone or something else. Drug abusers using projection might insist that they became addicted to alcohol as a result of the pressure to drink at work-related social functions in order to keep colleagues from thinking they were prudes. They also may blame a spouse or loved one.

PHYSICAL EXAMINATION

On physical assessment, many substance abusers appear malnourished and poorly cared for. Evidence of physical trauma from falls, abrasions, or fights may be present. Jaundice or discolored sclera of the eyes may suggest cirrhosis or other liver problems. Hypertension is a critical sign of withdrawal and is often accompanied by the physical signs of fluid retention in the legs or a protuberant abdomen swollen by liver ascites. Confusion, memory loss, tremors, lack of coordination, and other neurologic signs are significant and may be associated with a number of causes including nutritional deficits. Be alert for needle tracks in unexpected parts of the body in an individual who is believed to have been abusing drugs intravenously. The atypical client may not have any obvious signs of physical problems, but abnormalities may be found on laboratory tests done when the client enters a treatment program.

DIAGNOSTIC TESTS

In order to assess the patient's physical status, a thorough physical examination is done on initiation of treatment, along with a basic laboratory screen chosen to identify problems in any of the major organ systems. Abnormalities are often seen on liver function tests, in electrolyte values, and on tests reflecting nutritional status and gastric function. Diseases such as hepatitis B and C that can be spread through blood and body fluids may be identified, especially among intravenous drug users. Syphilis rates are increasing, and the rapidly escalating rate of human immunodeficiency virus (HIV) infection in this population is of national concern. Infections of various kinds are common. Special neurologic, neuropsychological, and imaging studies may disclose brain damage.

BLOOD ALCOHOL STUDY

A blood alcohol study is the most accurate type of test available to measure the degree of intoxication on initiation of treatment for alcohol abuse. A blood alcohol level above 0.3% requires treatment for overdose; at concentrations of over 0.4%, death is likely. Legal intoxication definitions vary from state to state but commonly are determined when a person's blood alcohol level is above 0.05% to 0.08%.

URINE DRUG SCREENING

Urine drug screening is the preferred way of screening for the recent use of an unknown drug and is commonly done along with the initial laboratory work. Drugs that are most likely to be identified in this way include amphetamines, barbiturates, benzodiazepines, cocaine, "crack," the opiates, marijuana, PCP, LSD, opioid analgesics, sedatives, and stimulants. With this test, drug metabolites can be identified for days or weeks after use, depending on the drug used. Typically, the collection of urine samples for this type of toxicology is witnessed by a staff member of the same sex to ensure that tampering with the specimens or substitution of another person's urine has not occurred. After collection, the sample is kept under "chain of custody": each person handling the sample signs a special document that accompanies the sample until it can be analyzed. Any temporary storage of the sample is maintained under secure conditions.

HAIR ANALYSIS

Hair analysis is a recent addition to the methods for the detection of abused substances. It requires sensitive technology but may be very helpful in monitoring patients for relapse. Depending on the length of hair, substance use can be detected for up to 1 year after only 2 or 3 days of use. However, the presence of addiction or whether the person is currently under the influence of the substance cannot be implied from a positive finding. The evidence this test provides regarding long-term substance use may prove to be a valuable tool in the diagnosis and follow-up of substance abusers in the future.

ALCOHOL AND ALCOHOLISM

Alcohol is the most commonly abused drug in the United States. According to the American Society of Addiction Medicine, alcoholism is "a primary, chronic disease with psychosocial and environmental factors influencing its development and manifestations. The disease is often progressive and fatal. It is characterized by continuous or periodic impaired control over drinking, preoccupation with the drug alcohol, use of alcohol despite adverse consequences, and distortions in thinking, most notably denial." It can be noted that alcohol is referred to as a "drug" in this definition, reflecting the thinking of most health care professionals that alcohol is indeed a drug with addictive qualities similar to those of other abused drugs.

PHARMACOLOGY CAPSULE The American Society of Addiction Medicine defines alcohol as a drug because it has addictive qualities similar to those of other abused drugs.

Simple intoxication from alcohol usually lasts less than 12 hours and is followed by the unpleasant experience of a hangover beginning about 4 to 6 hours after the last drink. Typical symptoms include headache, upset stomach, vomiting, sweating, thirst, fatigue, and blurred vision or "seeing stars." The cause of these symptoms has not been pinpointed; however, it is believed to be a result of hypoglycemia, dehydration, and the buildup of acetaldehyde and lactic acid in the blood.

Chronic use involves the regular daily ingestion of large quantities of alcohol, regular heavy drinking only on weekends, or binges of heavy drinking followed by long periods of abstinence. Physical **addiction** occurs when alcohol becomes integrated into physiologic processes at the cellular level. The cell becomes dependent on the alcohol to carry on certain metabolic processes; if alcohol is no longer available, the cell goes into "shock" and is unable to compensate for the loss quickly. Thus, alcohol withdrawal syndrome begins after the individual stops or decreases the amount ingested. Heavy chronic drinkers may experience the onset of withdrawal without actually stopping drinking simply because they are no longer able to ingest enough alcohol to meet the body's demands for the substance in order to function.

Alcohol **withdrawal** syndrome involves physiologic and behavioral symptoms that begin when the individual's blood alcohol level drops. It is divided into two stages, depending on the onset and severity of symptoms. The first stage usually occurs within 6 to 12 hours after the last drink and is called *early withdrawal.* Symptoms begin with anxiety, agitation, and irritability. If the patient does not drink, tremors may be observed. Blood pressure, pulse, and temperature all begin to rise. Sweating, nausea, vomiting, and diarrhea are typical.

The second stage, *major withdrawal,* begins with the onset of seizures and hallucinations and can advance to life-threatening ***delirium tremens*** (or "DTs"). This stage usually occurs after approximately 3 days (sometimes less) without alcohol or treatment and can be predicted from extreme elevations in temperature, pulse, and blood pressure. The patient typically becomes disoriented and confused. Hallucinations are often visual and "animal" in nature. Bugs, snakes, and rats are commonly described, sometimes perceived to be crawling on the person. Familiar jokes about seeing "pink elephants" probably evolved out of this type of withdrawal experience.

Alcohol withdrawal is the *most* life-threatening withdrawal syndrome in comparison to those associated with other types of commonly abused drugs, even heroin. (Withdrawal from barbiturates and benzodiazepines also can result in delirium tremens; both types of drugs have similar central nervous system [CNS] depressant effects.) Thus, it is critical to counsel alcoholics never to attempt to withdraw on their own or "go cold turkey." They always should seek medical treatment. Most require inpatient hospitalization and administration of medications such as lorazepam (Ativan) or chlordiazepoxide (Librium) to prevent the severe consequences of withdrawal and to ensure early detection and treatment of symptoms.

MEDICAL COMPLICATIONS

Common medical complications of chronic alcoholism include cirrhosis of the liver, pancreatitis, gastrointestinal bleeding (often from esophageal varices), Wernicke's encephalopathy, Korsakoff's psychosis, and fetal alcohol syndrome.

Wernicke's Encephalopathy

Wernicke's encephalopathy is due to vitamin B_1 (thiamine) deficiency. Its symptoms include delirium, confabulation due to memory loss, unsteady gait, a sense of apprehension, and altered levels of consciousness that can proceed to coma. If it is not properly treated with vitamin supplementation, Korsakoff's psychosis may develop.

Korsakoff's Psychosis

In this disorder, both thiamine and niacin deficiencies contribute to the degeneration of the cerebrum and the peripheral nervous system. Symptoms include amnesia, confabulation, disorientation, and peripheral neuropathies. Despite treatment, some residual problems persist in both Wernicke's encephalopathy and Korsakoff's psychosis. However, dementia is permanent if the patient progresses to Korsakoff's psychosis. Both of these disorders are classified as alcohol amnesic disorders.

Fetal Alcohol Syndrome

Fetal alcohol syndrome is a medical complication that is of great concern in many countries. If a woman drinks to excess throughout pregnancy, the unborn child is at risk for symptoms such as low birth weight, mental retardation, growth deficiencies, heart defects, facial malformations, learning disabilities, and hyperactivity. Recent controversy has arisen over whether maternal alcoholism constitutes child abuse and is thus reportable under child protection statutes.

TREATMENT FOR ALCOHOL ABUSE

In recent years, active family involvement in the treatment of alcohol abuse has come to be seen as a critical factor in the effectiveness of treatment outcomes. It is accepted that the disease of alcoholism affects everyone in the family system. Alcoholism often produces predictable patterns of individual behavior or changes in roles that may significantly handicap various family members in getting their needs met. Examples of some of the labels given these atypical roles include the hero, the mascot, the lost child, and the scapegoat. Adult children of alcoholics may struggle with issues throughout their lives as a result of dysfunctional patterns of thoughts and behaviors learned in childhood through the enactment of these types of roles. Spouses of alcoholics frequently struggle with "enabling" behaviors. These are described as any behavior that "covers up" or protects alcoholics from the consequences of their drinking behaviors. For example, a woman might lie to her husband's boss as to the reasons why he will not be at work, when in reality the husband is too "hung over" to perform adequately. Those who enable are sometimes considered co-dependent in that their behavior is highly structured around managing and adapting to the substance abuser's dysfunctional behavior.

Family and peer pressure and confrontation can be critical factors in inducing the alcoholic to seek treatment. Through participation in a 12-step self-help support group for the significant others of substance abusers, called Al-Anon and Al-Ateen, spouses, children, friends, and co-workers can learn new ways of coping with issues and how to avoid enabling the alcoholic so that it becomes harder for him or her to continue the destructive pattern of drinking.

Intervention

An intervention is a planned, structured meeting by family and friends to confront the alcoholic with the effect that the person's alcohol abuse has on each member of the group. Often the alcoholic or substance abuser is brought into the meeting without prior notification about the intervention. The intervention is led by a specially trained interventionist who helps those involved in the process to prepare by writing down the ways that the person's alcohol abuse affects them personally. The interventionist offers suggestions on how to word ideas in ways less likely to evoke defensiveness and how to focus on the issues to reject the problem drinking but not the person. During the intervention, all of the participants have an opportunity to read their letters aloud to the alcohol abuser. At the end of each letter, the reader requests that the alcoholic go into treatment to get help. Usually, after hearing out a roomful of significant people confront them, the user will go unhappily, but voluntarily, directly from the intervention into a treatment program that has been arranged for in advance in the event of that outcome.

The use of this strategy has come under criticism because the user confronted in this way often feels coerced into treatment. After the intervention, they may harbor angry feelings directed at members of the family for being critical, pushy, and having "tricked" them. Ideally, for treatment to be most effective, individuals should choose to go voluntarily. Proponents of the use of intervention respond that the user may die or suffer terrible consequences of the disease before seeking help on a totally voluntary basis, and thus the ends justify the means.

Detoxification

Detoxification is usually done in an inpatient hospital. During detoxification, the patient's vital signs are monitored frequently. Initially patients do not participate in group therapy because of their physical status. Rest and nutrition are emphasized. Drugs from the anxiolytic (benzodiazepine) group most often are used in detoxification of the alcoholic; however, hypnotics like phenobarbital or chloral hydrate are used occasionally. Intravenous magnesium sulfate may be used to prevent seizures in rare cases. Scheduled anticonvulsants are prescribed if seizures occur. Fluids are encouraged to combat dehydration, and vitamin replacement therapy is instituted.

Rehabilitation

Once patients are medically stable, they are referred to either an inpatient or an outpatient treatment program, depending on individual needs and resources. The traditional inpatient program, or Minnesota model, lasts about 28 days and includes highly structured scheduling of drug education films and presentations; increasingly confrontational individual, group, and family therapy; recreational and occupational therapy; milieu therapy; and introduction to Alcoholics Anonymous (AA), a self-help support group. However, the availability of third party reimbursement for an inpatient rehabilitation stay has diminished significantly. More commonly, patients are referred to partial hospitalization programs (day treatment programs) and outpatient therapy as well as other community resources. Less common is an extended residential program that may last 1 to 2 years.

Alcoholics Anonymous

Alcoholics Anonymous is a nonprofit, worldwide organization of alcoholics who meet together anonymously in small groups at various times during the day throughout the year to assist each other in staying sober. The organization uses a strong spiritual base, which is controversial, and a 12-step program (Table 54-1) involving discussions and written exercises designed around each of the 12 steps as a means of keeping the alcoholic from relapsing. Members identify another participant of the same sex who is seasoned in the recovery process, and to whom they can relate, to act as their sponsor. The sponsor agrees to be available to the person for support and advice in staying sober. Service work in the community also is seen as integral to focusing outside oneself.

Members use regular readings from the "Big Book" of AA, written by founding members to keep themselves on track (Table 54-2 lists the 12 traditions of AA). There are no dues; the organization relies on donations. There is no political involvement or endorsements of candidates or products. Everyone involved does so on a voluntary basis. Even group leaders are volunteers and are not professional counselors. Meetings may be advertised in the community using the title "Friends of Bill W." as a means of maintaining the anonymity of participants. (Bill W. was one of the two originators of the organization.) Before discharge from an inpatient treatment program, alcoholics have the opportunity to attend various community AA meetings in order to increase the odds of continued outpatient participation and to begin the process of finding a "home group" to which they can connect.

Recently, research has begun to question what actually works in alcohol rehabilitation. Actual outcomes of the traditional types of treatment approaches have not been clearly

table 54-1 *The 12 Steps of Alcoholics Anonymous*

1. We admit we were powerless over alcohol—our lives had become unmanageable.
2. Came to believe that a Power greater than ourselves could restore us to sanity.
3. Made a decision to turn our will and lives over to the care of God, as we understood Him.
4. Made a searching and fearless moral inventory of ourselves.
5. Admitted to God, to ourselves, and to another human being the exact nature of our wrongs.
6. Were entirely ready to have God remove all these defects of character.
7. Humbly asked Him to remove our shortcomings.
8. Listed all persons we had harmed and became willing to make amends to them all.
9. Made direct amends whenever possible except when to do so would injure them or others.
10. Continued to make personal inventory and when we were wrong promptly admitted it.
11. Sought through prayer and meditation to improve our conscious contact with God, as we understood Him, praying only for knowledge of His will for us and the power to carry it out.
12. Having had a spiritual awakening as the result of these steps, we tried to carry this message to alcoholics and to practice these principles in all our affairs.

table 54-2 *The 12 Traditions of Alcoholics Anonymous*

1. Our common welfare should come first; personal recovery depends upon AA unity.
2. For our group purpose there is but one ultimate authority—a loving God as He may express Himself in our group conscience. Our leaders are but trusted servants; they do not govern.
3. The only requirement for AA membership is a desire to stop drinking.
4. Each group should be autonomous except in matters affecting other groups or AA as a whole.
5. Each group has but one primary purpose—to carry its message to the alcoholic who still suffers.
6. An AA group ought never endorse, finance, or lend the AA name to any related facility or outside enterprise, lest problems of money, property, and prestige divert us from our primary purpose.
7. Every AA group ought to be fully self-supporting, declining outside contributions.
8. Alcoholics Anonymous should remain forever nonprofessional, but our service centers may employ special workers.
9. AA, as such, ought never be organized; but we may create service boards or committees directly responsible to those they serve.
10. Alcoholics Anonymous has no opinion on outside issues; hence the AA name ought never be drawn into public controversy.
11. Our public relations policy is based on attraction rather than promotion; we need always maintain personal anonymity at the level of press, radio, and films.
12. Anonymity is the spiritual foundation of all our traditions, ever reminding us to place principles before personalities.

documented. As a result, many insurance companies no longer fund 28-day inpatient treatment. Many inpatient 28-day treatment programs have been forced to close because of a lack of clients able to afford the cost of this intensive treatment. Treatment facilities have been forced to provide brief and creative inpatient rehabilitation with rapid referral to an outpatient program and aftercare.

One trend is toward using more nontraditional treatment approaches that have produced successful outcomes. Some components of alcohol rehabilitation that have been shown to be very useful in maintaining continued sobriety are the teaching of stress management, social skills training, and behavioral approaches to marital therapy, and matching clients with a therapist who uses a style most likely to benefit their personality type. A move also is under way in which treatment programs are attempting to group patients with similar lifestyles and characteristics together rather than "lump" everyone together. Other factors being considered in developing more homogeneous small groups are styles of thinking (abstract versus concrete thinkers), sex role–related issues, ethnicity, and age. The current trend is away from a "recipe card" approach to treatment that is expected to work for anyone who is an alcoholic (see Nursing Care Plan: The Patient Abusing Alcohol).

Cost containment has stimulated the development of many new types of outpatient programs for the treatment of alcoholism. Most day treatment or partial hospitalization programs are very similar to the traditional inpatient milieu and offer similar types of therapies, but they allow patients to return to their own homes at night. In this case, the risk of relapse often requires the use of medication such as disulfiram (Antabuse) or metronidazole (Flagyl), which makes the user ill if mixed with alcohol. Usually, involvement in the program is intensive but does not last for the traditional 30 days.

Other individuals utilize active involvement in AA as the primary means for recovery by attending at least "90 meetings in 90 days." Other community programs also are avail-

NURSING CARE PLAN

The Patient Abusing Alcohol

ASSESSMENT

Health History: A 37-year-old man was admitted for alcohol detoxification. He was found lying on the floor at home, passed out, and appeared to have vomited and been incontinent of urine and feces. He has a long history of alcohol abuse but claims he does not have a problem because he only drinks beer. He recently lost his job because he was not reporting for work on time, and his wife has threatened to leave him if he does not stop drinking. His two children, ages 8 and 10, are afraid of him when he drinks. His usual intake of alcohol is two six-packs of beer a day. He has been detoxified in the hospital and is now ready for the rehabilitation phase of his treatment.

Physical Examination: Vital signs: temperature, 97.6° F orally; pulse, 80; respiration, 20; blood pressure, 128/72. Height, 5'10". Weight, 160 lb. The patient's skin and eyes have a slightly yellowish tinge. A cast is on his left arm from below the elbow to the fingers. He appears thin and wasted.

Nursing Diagnosis	*Goals and Outcome Criteria*	*Interventions*
Ineffective denial related to continued alcohol abuse.	Patient will acknowledge that he has a problem, stop ingesting alcohol, and attend Alcoholics Anonymous (AA) meetings on a regular basis.	Use confrontational techniques to help patient accept the diagnosis of alcoholism and support patient's 12-step program of rehabilitation.
Ineffective coping related to alcohol ingestion as a means of coping with stressors.	Patient will overcome his impulse to drink alcohol until intoxicated and to use alcohol as a coping mechanism, as evidenced by stopping ingestion of alcohol and substituting other coping mechanisms.	Help patient overcome cravings by introducing new coping mechanisms such as exercise and stress management skills; encourage patient to attend treatment program and AA meetings on a regular basis.
Chronic low self-esteem related to loss of control.	Patient will maintain an adequate self-concept, as evidenced by lessened self-criticism, good hygiene, and positive interactions with others.	Help patient maintain self-esteem after confrontational therapy sessions by allowing him to vent his feelings and acting as a role model for dealing with others.
Risk for injury related to excessive use of alcohol and high risk for relapse.	Patient will not injure himself or others as a result of excessive ingestion of alcohol.	Encourage patient to abstain from drinking by supporting his participation in rehabilitation activities. Intervene at the first signs of impending relapse.
Chronic low self-esteem related to guilty feelings as evidenced by expression of excessive guilt and decreased self-value.	Patient will develop a realistic sense of self, verbalize positive aspects of self and being to forgive himself, stop being self-critical, and express his true feelings.	Allow patient to vent his feelings about his illness and to explore his feelings about his past behaviors; support patient in his 12-step program of rehabilitation.

able to assist the alcoholic in the recovery process and should not be overlooked. Some are church related; some are focused on getting the recovering user back to work by providing job placement or an opportunity to return to school. One example of a community recovery program that exists in various parts of the country is the Patrician Movement. In addition, halfway houses may be available in the local area as a service of community mental health organizations.

Relapse Prevention

Relapse prevention is a key component in the treatment of persons with substance abuse or dependence. Relapse prevention involves assisting patients to identify triggers to their substance use. For example, a person may identify friends who consistently use the abused substance or places where there is drinking or using going on and recognize that allowing himself or herself to be with these friends, or in these places, sets them up to drink/use. As part of the relapse prevention strategy, the person then actively avoids these people and places. Other coping strategies also are developed that can be used if the person encounters a trigger.

Aftercare and Recovery

One of the newer aspects of the recovery process involves various types of aftercare services to assist alcoholics who have completed a treatment program successfully to make a gradual transition back into the community with the support necessary to prevent relapses. Many inpatient substance abuse programs now provide aftercare groups to discharged patients as a supplement to continued involvement in AA and other 12-step support groups such as Adult Children of Alcoholics and Codependents Anonymous.

Medications

The treatment team may recommend the use of disulfiram (Antabuse) to assist the alcoholic who is highly motivated to remain sober but recognizes that poor impulse control may increase the odds of relapse. This particular drug inhibits the metabolism of alcohol in the body, producing an uncomfortable, potentially life-threatening reaction to exposure to alcohol. Disulfiram is taken daily and lasts in the body for up to 2 weeks. Thus, if the alcoholic gets the urge to drink, the presence of the drug in the system usually provides the necessary negative reinforcement to resist the impulse. Symptoms of a disulfiram-alcohol reaction include flushing, headache, nausea, vomiting, dizziness, rapid heart rate, difficulty breathing, sweating, confusion, and hypotension that may lead to coma, convulsions, and death. The severity of the symptoms varies from person to person, and symptoms can last for 30 to 60 minutes or more.

PHARMACOLOGY CAPSULE Disulfiram (Antabuse) is sometimes used to assist a recovering alcoholic who is highly motivated to remain sober but recognizes that poor impulse control may increase odds of relapse.

The danger of giving disulfiram to a person who is poorly motivated to stop drinking is that he or she might either stop taking the medication in order to drink, or drink in spite of taking the medication and become seriously ill. As a result, careful patient teaching is essential. The patient must be taught to avoid alcohol in foods (such as salad dressings, sauces, candies, or chocolate prepared with liqueurs), in topical preparations (cologne, aftershave, or liniments), in medications (over-the-counter cold preparations or cough syrups), and in mouthwashes containing alcohol. Alcohol wipes cannot be used by the nurse to cleanse the skin in preparation for an injection without a topical reaction. Because of the risks of accidental exposure to a substance containing alcohol, patients are encouraged to wear a Medic Alert bracelet or carry a card in their wallet to alert emergency care personnel to a possible disulfiram-alcohol reaction in the event they are found unconscious. Patients also are asked to sign a consent form for the use of the drug prior to it being prescribed to document that proper instructions about diet, risks, precautions, and type of emergency care needed in the event of exposure to alcohol have been offered and are understood. It is important for the nurse to be alert for patient attempts to bypass the prohibitive effects of disulfiram by ingesting large doses of vitamin C in order to have a drink on occasion. Patients who are addicted are often very knowledgeable about drug treatment and can easily find out that massive doses of vitamin C are given intravenously for the treatment of overdose or disulfiram-alcohol reactions.

PHARMACOLOGY CAPSULE To avoid a disulfiram-alcohol reaction, patients who are taking disulfiram (Antabuse) must be instructed to avoid alcohol in foods (sauces, candies), topical preparations (cologne, aftershave), mouthwashes, and medications (over-the-counter cold preparations, cough syrup).

The use of disulfiram is contraindicated in individuals with impaired liver function, heart problems, or significant debilitation. Obviously, safe use of the drug also requires that the person have no memory impairments, self-destructive intentions, or poor judgment.

Sometimes, metronidazole (Flagyl) is used for similar purposes because it also produces an uncomfortable reaction when combined with alcohol but does not produce the severe life-threatening reactions described for disulfiram. Also, it does not remain in the system for an extended period and it still can be given in the event of many medical problems in which disulfiram is contraindicated.

Research efforts continue to attempt to identify other types of drugs that could assist alcoholics to go through withdrawal more comfortably and avoid relapse. Medications currently under scrutiny for this purpose include naltrexone hydrochloride (Trexan), antidepressants such as amitriptyline hydrochloride (Elavil), desipramine hydrochloride (Norpramin), fluoxetine hydrochloride (Prozac), and angiotensin converting enzyme (ACE) inhibitors such as enalapril maleate (Vasotec).

PHARMACOLOGY CAPSULE Do not use alcohol to cleanse injection sites if the patient is taking disulfiram.

PSYCHOACTIVE SUBSTANCES OTHER THAN ALCOHOL

Six classes of psychoactive substances other than alcohol are often associated with substance abuse or, using the term that is currently popular, chemical dependence. These are the stimulants, depressants (barbiturates and benzodiazepines), hallucinogens, narcotics (opioids), inhalants, and designer drugs (Table 54-3). Each class is different in the types of symptoms produced and the way in which patients abusing them are managed.

STIMULANTS

Stimulants include amphetamines ("speed") and similar drugs, plus cocaine or "crack."

Amphetamines

Amphetamines usually are used orally or intravenously on a daily basis or on binges. They are very psychologically addictive (producing psychological dependence)—the dose is gradually increased over time to produce the euphoria (or "high") that is extremely pleasurable. Symptoms often include hyperactivity, irritability, combativeness, and after extended use, paranoia. A person intoxicated by amphetamines may be very dangerous. There are no physical withdrawal symptoms, but the user typically experiences a profound depression and sense of exhaustion called "crashing." Tricyclic and other types of antidepressants are commonly used to treat the depression, which may persist in chronic users for up to 2 years after the last amphetamine use. Toxic psychosis may occur in approximately 90% of chronic users up to 1 year past the last use. Unfortunately, 5% to 15% of these individuals never fully recover. Neuroleptics may be used to treat toxic psychosis.

table 54-3 ***Common Mood-Altering Chemicals***

DRUG NAME	EFFECTS	SITE OF ACTION	LENGTH OF EFFECT
HALLUCINOGENS			
Mushroom (psilocybin) LSD (lysergic acid diethylamide) Mescaline (from peyote cactus) DOM (dimethoxy-methylamphetamine) STP (no chemical name) MDA, Ecstasy (methylenedioxy-amphetamine)	Altered body image Euphoria Sharpened perceptions Somatic effects: dizziness, tremors, weakness, nausea. Psychosis-like symptoms Emotional swings Suspiciousness Bizarre behavior Increased blood pressure Increased temperature Objective signs: dilated pupils, flushing, tremors	Central nervous system (CNS) Brain	Onset: 40-60 min Duration: 6-12 hr
CANNABINOIDS			
Marijuana Hashish	Failure in judgment and memory Mild intoxication Euphoria Relaxation Sexual arousal Panic states Visual hallucinations Objective signs: reddened eyes, dry mouth, incoordination; heart rate to 140/min	CNS Cardiovascular system Respiratory system	Administration and dose dependent Onset: 20-30 min Duration: 3-7 hr
OPIOIDS (OPIOIDS, SEMISYNTHETIC AND SYNTHETIC ANALGESICS)			
Codeine Morphine Heroin Hydromorphone (Dilaudid) Methadone Meperidine (Demerol) Propoxyphene (Darvon) Designer drugs	Analgesia Euphoria Escape Reduced sexual and aggressive drives Respiratory depression Sedation, sleepiness Objective signs: hypertension, pupillary constriction, constipation	Nervous tissue CNS (opioid receptors) Respiratory system	Onset: 20-30 min Duration: 4-8 hr
SEDATIVE-HYPNOTICS AND ANXIOLYTICS			
Barbiturates Secobarbital (Seconal) Phenobarbital (Nembutal) Amobarbital (Amytal) Amobarbital/Secobarbital (Tuinol) Barbiturate-like (methaqualone [Quaalude]) Benzodiazepines (alprazolam [Xanax], chlordiazepoxide [Librium], diazepam [Valium], lorazepam [Ativan])	Drowsiness, sedation Euphoria Escape Loss of aggressive and sexual drives Emotional lability Poor judgment	CNS Cardiovascular system Respiratory system	Onset: 30-40 min Duration: varies with each drug, barbiturates may have longer half-life than benzodiazepines depending on the agent

Data from Naegle, M. A. (1997). Substance-related disorders. In Haber, J., Krainovich, B., McMahon, A. L., & Price-Hoskins, P. (eds.). *Comprehensive psychiatric nursing* (5th ed., pp. 513-515). St. Louis: Mosby.

Continued

table 54-3 ***Common Mood-Altering Chemicals—cont'd***

DRUG NAME	EFFECTS	SITE OF ACTION	LENGTH OF EFFECT
STIMULANTS			
Amphetamine (methamphetamine, Dexedrine, Benzedrine) Methylphenidate (Ritalin) Cocaine, crack	Euphoria, grandiosity Wakefulness Relief of fatigue Stimulation, energy, anxiety Depression Suppression of appetite Aggressive feelings, paranoia Objective signs: sweating, dilated pupils, increased blood pressure, rapid heart and respiratory rates, tremors, seizures	CNS Peripheral nervous system Cardiovascular system	Onset: route related; 10-30 min Duration: drug related
PHENCYCLIDINES			
PCP (phencyclidine, "angel dust")	Detachment from surroundings Decreased sensory awareness Illusions of superhuman strength Acute intoxication Objective signs: flushing, fever, sweating, coma, agitation, confusion, hallucinations, paranoia, violence	CNS	Rapid onset: 2-3 min up to 45 min Duration: drug and dose related
INHALANTS			
Benzene (paint thinner, cleaning fluid, glue) Nitrites Nitrous oxide	Euphoria Giddiness, headache, fatigue, drowsiness Objective signs: dysrhythmias, damage to kidneys, liver abnormalities	CNS Cardiac effect	Onset: immediate Duration: 20-45 min
ALCOHOL			
Beverage alcohol, beer, wine	Relaxation, sedation, release of inhibitions Objective signs: incoordination, nausea, vomiting, slurred speech	CNS Respiratory system	Onset: 20 min-1 hr Duration: dose related
XANTHINES			
Caffeine	Stimulation Restlessness Anxiety Objective signs: increased heart and respiratory rates, diarrhea, gastric disorder, insomnia, tremors	CNS	Onset: 10-30 min Duration: 3-7 hr
NICOTINE			
Cigarettes Smokeless tobacco	Stimulation Enhanced performance	CNS Respiratory system Cardiovascular system Endocrine system	Onset: immediate Duration: 5-15 min

Data from Naegle, M. A. (1997). Substance-related disorders. In Haber, J., Krainovich, B., McMahon, A. L., & Price-Hoskins, P. (eds.). *Comprehensive psychiatric nursing* (5th ed., pp. 513-515). St. Louis: Mosby.

"Ice" is a new form of methamphetamine ingested by smoking, with results similar to those produced by crack (a form of cocaine that is smoked). Effects last as long as 14 hours; the user often will do anything in order to obtain the drug and also is considered at risk for being very dangerous while under the influence.

Cocaine

Cocaine is a highly addictive alkaloid of the plant *Erythroxylon coca,* which grows in Peru and Bolivia. Cocaine produces an intense feeling of euphoria that usually lasts only 30 to 60 minutes; however, the substance remains in the brain for about 10 days after use. Pure forms of cocaine are quite expensive. It is typically inhaled nasally or mixed with other drugs, like heroin, and injected intravenously ("speedballs"). It is very psychologically addicting, which is thought to be due to overstimulation of the pleasure centers of the brain. Physical withdrawal symptoms have not traditionally been thought to occur; however, a physical syndrome has been hypothesized and is currently under debate.

Symptoms of chronic inhalation include runny nose, sniffles, frequent colds, weight loss, hyperactivity, and damage to the nasal mucosa or septum that may be severe enough to require surgical repair. Psychologically, cocaine abusers lose interest in their usual activities and demonstrate abrupt mood swings, poor judgment, impatience, and ultimately suspiciousness and hallucinations. Cocaine intoxication also can occur but usually lasts only about 24 hours after the last use. Cocaine is a very dangerous drug in that strokes, seizures, and heart attacks that are sometimes fatal can occur even in first-time users.

Treatment often employs diazepam (Valium) or phenobarbital for their sedative effects. Neuroleptics may be used in the event of psychosis. Many clients are severely depressed for up to 2 years after quitting. Studies have shown that damage to the brain may impair the patient's ability to experience pleasure. Antidepressants such as imipramine (Tofranil) and cardiac drugs such as propranolol hydrochloride (Inderal) or calcium channel blockers may be helpful in this event.

Crack

Crack is a hardened form of cocaine that is smoked. It presents major problems in many urban areas of the United States because it is readily available and inexpensive compared with other drugs. It produces a tremendously addicting, short-acting psychological euphoria that is quickly followed by "crashing," which stimulates continued cravings and use. The cravings are so intense that, as with "ice," the user will do almost anything to obtain more of the drug and often resorts to violence if thwarted. Overdose of this drug is life-threatening because no drug is available to counteract the overstimulation, which results in respiratory failure.

DEPRESSANTS

Drugs misused in this category include the sedatives, hypnotics, and anxiolytics. They are obtained by prescription for anxiety or insomnia, or are purchased illegally. They are typically taken orally. Regular use results in physical dependency. Symptoms of overdose include oversedation, respiratory depression, impaired coordination, and brain damage. Intoxication with barbiturates is even more dangerous than with benzodiazepines. While benzodiazepines and barbiturates are similar to alcohol in terms of dangerous physical withdrawal reactions (delirium tremens, seizures), barbiturate overdose induces an anesthesia-like state. Symptoms of barbiturate withdrawal usually occur somewhat later, sometimes days after the last use, depending on the half-life of the particular drug. Once a person is dependent, abruptly stopping any of these drugs also may trigger psychosis.

HALLUCINOGENS

Hallucinogens include LSD (lysergic acid diethylamide or "acid"), PCP (phencyclidine or "angel dust"), MDMA (3, 4-methylenedioxymethamphetamine, known as "ecstasy" or "Adam"), and marijuana.

LSD

LSD is not physically addicting but can produce physical symptoms of altered perceptions that are dream-like, often with an altered sense of time and feelings that one has attained special insight. Emotions are intensified and labile. Individuals often experience depersonalization, in which they feel as if they are floating outside of themselves or in unreal surroundings. The drugs typically are used to enhance self-awareness and usually are taken episodically (approximately twice a week). Acute adverse reactions are most often described as a "bad trip" involving paranoia, depression, frightening hallucinations, and occasionally an acute confusional state. The person experiencing a bad trip is responsive to verbal support and reassurance. The primary danger of the use of these drugs is accidental death as a result of perceptual distortions (i.e., attempting to fly off a building) or seizures related to the cutting agent used. Cutting agents are chemicals that may be quite toxic, which are used in the manufacturing or dilution of the final drug product. Chronic long-term adverse reactions include psychosis, depression, paranoia, and flashbacks. LSD use is regaining popularity.

PCP

PCP (phencyclidine) differs from other hallucinogens in that abusers experience a psychotic state similar to that observed in schizophrenics. Brain reward areas are stimulated so that abusers can stimulate themselves mentally in a pleasurable way. Studies also suggest that this drug is strongly physically addictive, with a severe withdrawal reaction occurring after binge use. Unexpected sensory stimuli that interrupt the individual's internal experience may provoke unpredictable violence. The person may possess enormous strength and may feel no pain. The risks of use thus involve serious injury to oneself or others, in addition to severely elevated temperature, hypertensive crisis, and renal failure. Under acute intoxication, patients are best managed by reducing stimuli as much as possible, often by seclusion, even to the point of avoiding talking or performing routine treatments until the patient is stabilized. If violent, mechanical restraint is necessary.

Marijuana

Marijuana often is included in the hallucinogenic category of abused drugs because it produces an effect similar to that of LSD when smoked. The inner experience is altered so that individuals experience heightened awareness, distortion of space and time, heightened sensitivity to sound, and sometimes depersonalization. Although use may produce paranoia, the "bad trip" phenomenon of LSD is rare with marijuana. It also tends to have a sedative rather than stimulant effect and is unlikely to produce true hallucinations. Marijuana is psychologically addicting. Controversy persists about the negative effects of chronic use of this drug. It has been suggested that marijuana may produce psychosis in fragile individuals, and a lack of motivation and a reduction in fertility and sexual performance in young men. However, the studies that suggest these conclusions can be challenged by others just as convincing that present the opposite findings. Chronic smoking of marijuana irritates the lungs and may contribute to the occurrence of lung cancer.

In the medical community, marijuana shows promise for the further development of its derivatives as medication for the treatment of glaucoma, nausea and vomiting as a result of cancer chemotherapy and asthma and as an appetite stimulant.

NARCOTICS (OPIOIDS)

The narcotic drugs often misused include the opioids heroin, morphine, oxycodone (OxyContin), hydrocodone, pentazocine (Talwin), methadone, and meperidine (Demerol).

Heroin

Heroin is a highly addictive narcotic that produces a pleasant euphoria on intravenous use. The person experiences a "rush," then gradually nods off to sleep. On awakening, the person feels immune to stressors until the withdrawal symptoms begin to trigger the need to "cop a fix" again. This usually occurs 8 to 12 hours after the last use. Risks of chronic use of heroin include overdose, malnutrition, and respiratory arrest as well as hepatitis B and C and HIV infection from shared needle use.

Symptoms of withdrawal include tearing of the eyes, runny nose, gooseflesh, sweating, alternating fever and chills, muscle and joint pain, upset stomach, diarrhea, loss of appetite, restlessness, and irritability. Individuals usually are in such subjective distress that they inappropriately seek medications from the staff while in treatment. It is very challenging to work with these patients.

It is sometimes difficult to remain nonjudgmental when working with these patients. In order to support their ever-increasing habit, many people addicted to heroin resort to crime, such as stealing. Sometimes they seek detoxification only to reduce the level of the dose needed to experience the pleasurable response to the drug—a lower dose is less expensive to obtain.

INHALANTS

A very dangerous type of substance abuse is that involving inhalant misuse. Examples of chemicals often inhaled for the mind-altering response include paint, glue, aerosol sprays, "whiteout," and gasoline. They are usually placed in a plastic bag or other container that is then placed over the nose and mouth and inhaled. This also is known as "huffing." Symptoms appearing in the individual under the influence of the drug depend on the substance inhaled and include nosebleeds, bloodshot eyes, infectious lesions around the nose and mouth, and severe disorientation or unconsciousness. The risks include progressive brain damage, asphyxiation, seizures, depressed bone marrow leading to aplastic anemia, liver or kidney damage, or cardiac dysrhythmias. There is no physical withdrawal syndrome.

This particular group of drugs often is misused among teenagers because of its easy availability and low cost. The cumulative brain damage from chronic use is a very serious problem among poor and minority adolescents.

DESIGNER DRUGS

A new group of abused drugs on the illegal market includes synthetic drugs especially designed to sidestep categorization with any of the drugs identified as illegal in the United States. Although use of these drugs may not be technically illegal, their misuse presents unique hazards. "Ecstasy" is an example of a synthetic drug generally grouped with the hallucinogens; it is also called "Adam." A very similar second-generation designer drug is called "Eve." "China White" is an example of a synthetic type of heroin that acts in much the same way as heroin. Major risks are present when the abuser mixes these drugs with those from the other groups because the results are unpredictable.

DISORDERS ASSOCIATED WITH SUBSTANCE ABUSE

The risk of human immunodeficiency virus disease (HIVD), the illness that leads to acquired immunodeficiency syndrome (AIDS), continues to present the greatest danger for patients who are abusing intravenous drugs because of the common practice of sharing needles. The Centers for Disease Control and Prevention indicate an alarming number of new cases of HIV-positive diagnoses among intravenous drug users and their sexual partners. Nursing care for these patients now includes teaching them how to clean their "works" with bleach and how to use condoms correctly.

Individuals who have, or are predisposed to, a serious psychiatric illness may present with an active case of the mental disorder. By altering levels of brain chemicals that control emotions, thought processes, and behavior, misuse of these chemicals can trigger an exacerbation of an existing illness.

Another major area of concern is the effect of intrauterine exposure to these chemicals on the fetus. Fetuses carried by mothers who are physically addicted to an opioid are born addicted and also may experience developmental delays and a prolonged lack of the capacity to feel pleasure even after they have been successfully weaned from the abused drug. "Cocaine babies" are currently being studied for clues to the consequences of prenatal exposure to the drug. Findings suggest that attention deficit disorder (with or without hyperactivity) occurs more often in this population, along with dyslexia, other neurologic problems, and learning disabilities.

Clients with chronic pain disorders also are very vulnerable to the abuse of drugs, especially those of the opioid and depressant groups, because of their frequent frustration over an inability to manage their pain effectively. Also, many lack knowledge of the risks of regular use of pain medication. Many times they feel betrayed by their physician and other caregivers because these medications were prescribed for pain control, but no one ever explained the importance of temperate use along with the use of exercise and other types of supportive techniques to manage pain and avoid addiction.

TREATMENT FOR SUBSTANCE ABUSE

Substance abuse treatment is very similar to alcohol detoxification and rehabilitation. Narcotics Anonymous (NA) is structured much like AA but focuses on the abuse of drugs other than alcohol. Many times, inpatient treatment programs place recovering addicts with alcoholics for educational and therapy groups. However, the rate of relapse is much higher for most drug abuse patients, especially those who use highly addicting intravenous drugs. A booming area of research is the identification of alternative treatments and medications that will help drug abusers detoxify more comfortably from the chemicals that they are addicted to and reduce the risks of relapse. Currently, there is some support for treating drug abuse separately from alcohol abuse.

As with alcohol abuse treatment, family involvement in the process is very important. Al-Anon is the support group for family members or significant others of a substance-abusing person. It is recommended that members of the family begin attending meetings as soon as they realize that the person is using some type of drug. The intervention process described earlier may be used in an attempt to get the person into treatment.

Many patients who use drugs have legal problems, which may provide the catalyst for seeking help. Sometimes they are mandated by the courts to go into treatment; at other times their attorney recommends treatment before the case goes to court in order to influence the judge favorably prior to sentencing. In the past, many individuals were involuntarily committed to state hospital drug treatment programs for 30 days. However, many state hospital systems across the country are currently closing their drug and alcohol treatment units because of the program expense and the need to provide additional services to the seriously mentally ill, which often is judged more of a priority.

DETOXIFICATION

Detoxification from physically addicting drugs is very complex because of the likelihood of polysubstance abuse and the uncertainty of what to expect when two or more drugs are mixed together. Usually, inpatient hospitalization is recommended for safety. However, some individuals who have been using drugs that are primarily psychologically addicting may not demonstrate many physical symptoms but, rather, experience intense psychological cravings. For example, if a conversation about past drug use occurs within the recovering addict's hearing, or if something in the environment triggers memories of the "high" sensation that he or she experienced while using, the person may experience cravings that stimulate feelings of restlessness, itching, hives, flushing, and elevated blood pressure and pulse, which are believed to be psychogenic in origin. These patients need a great deal of support to help them overcome the profound urge to use. This experience puts the patient at very high risk for relapse.

MEDICATIONS

Methadone

Methadone is one drug used in the treatment of heroin addicts. There is, however, some controversy about using this medication because the drug is a synthetic opioid. The drug is a synthetic opioid analgesic that also may be prescribed appropriately for chronic severe pain. Given orally (in diskette or liquid form), it is absorbed slowly and does not produce the "rush" normally experienced with the intravenous use of heroin. It also alleviates the cravings for more opioids for a short period of time, depending on the dose given. In detoxification, the dose of the drug is gradually reduced without telling patients exactly what dose they are getting. Although this process is one of substituting another addictive drug for the one misused by the client, some believe it to be justified in that withdrawal from methadone is less uncomfortable for the patient. The patient also risks severe respiratory depression in the event that heroin is injected while methadone is in the system. The most typical problematic side effects of methadone include severe constipation and profound sweating.

PHARMACOLOGY CAPSULE Methadone is a synthetic opioid analgesic that may be used in the detoxification of heroin-related opioid addiction.

Clonidine

Clonidine hydrochloride (Catapres) has become a more popular means of assisting the substance abuser through detoxification. It is a non-opiate antihypertensive drug that partially blocks withdrawal symptoms. Clonidine does not completely remove the unpleasant feelings accompanied by heroin withdrawal. Unfortunately, some may leave treatment because of the inherent discomfort and unrealistic expectations that they should not feel sick at all while using the drug to withdraw.

Naloxone

Naloxone hydrochloride (Narcan) is an opioid antagonist that counteracts the dangerous respiratory depressant effects of heroin or other opiate overdose. When Narcan is given to a person who is addicted and under the influence of an opiate, the person may experience acute withdrawal symptoms.

Put on your THINKING CAP!!

Can you explain why Narcan would cause a person who is addicted to opioids to experience acute withdrawal symptoms?

Many other drugs are currently under investigation to determine whether they could assist the substance abuser by reducing the cravings for the drug abused or by counteracting the long-term psychological consequences of use of certain drugs. Examples of these include some of the antidepressants, anticonvulsants, and various herbal agents.

Still other medications may be used in the supportive treatment of those undergoing opiate withdrawal to control symptoms such as diarrhea, abdominal cramping, and generalized, diffuse pain.

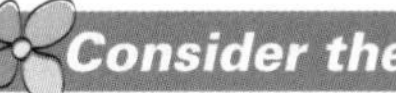
Consider the Alternative!

Some herbal remedies are being studied for use as agents to reduce withdrawal symptoms.

REHABILITATION

In most cases, the process of rehabilitation for drug abuse is very similar to that for alcohol abuse. Instead of attendance at AA meetings, the client often participates in NA at least some of the time. This support group is based on the 12 steps of AA, except that the word "alcohol" is replaced by "drugs" in all of the literature, and the case histories used for reading assignments are about other addicts in recovery related specifically to the use of drugs other than alcohol in an attempt to help the client identify with people with similar struggles. Relapse rates for individuals abusing drugs other than alcohol alone are much higher and present unique issues. Trends suggest that future treatment programs will be more likely to separate clients into small groups of people facing similar issues and having similar characteristics in order to individualize the recovery process much more than is typically done in the majority of settings at present. Although most current settings may advertise more than one "track" for substance abuse treatment, in reality clients share the same facilities and participate in most of the traditional programming mixed together despite different learning styles and other issues. It has been suggested that this practice may actually place clients who do not fit the traditional mold at higher risk for relapse.

On an outpatient basis, these clients are encouraged to participate in NA on a regular basis (90 meetings in the first 90 days), just as those recovering from alcoholism do. Attempts are usually made to allow the client to experience different group locations and times prior to discharge from the inpatient setting in order to increase the likelihood that the client will participate as recommended. Various other community programs may be available, such as the Patrician Movement, which provides outpatient treatment on an ongoing basis for those who cannot afford more costly inpatient rehabilitation. Many private health care systems are opening day treatment programs for substance abusers as insurance reimbursement for long-term inpatient programs becomes less available.

AFTERCARE AND RECOVERY

Recovering substance abusers may be offered an opportunity to participate in a support group provided by the hospital at which they received treatment. Many of the same people who went through treatment at the same time participate together. Because the relationships built during this time of crisis are often intense, the groups can be very helpful in preventing relapse. Hopefully, clients also will continue regular participation in NA groups on an ongoing basis. Some individuals do well in halfway houses, which allow for a new living environment surrounded by other recovering addicts during the difficult transition back into the community. Sometimes it is recommended that patients do not return to work until their ability to cope with stress is more developed.

METHADONE MAINTENANCE

Some patients who have experienced multiple relapses into heroin abuse after treatment may have sustained permanent damage to chemical receptor sites in the brain, which decreases their ability to resist relapse. As a result, methadone maintenance is not uncommon. In this process, the person goes to a methadone clinic on a daily or three times a week basis to receive a dose or doses of the medication to cover the next 24 to 72 hours. A single dose may be administered in liquid form or in a diskette dissolved in juice, and the person is carefully observed by clinic staff members to ensure that the medication is actually taken and not hoarded in any way. The patient may continue this process indefinitely, often for many years. Sometimes the dose of the methadone is maintained at the same level without attempts to reduce the dose, while at other times gradual titration is attempted.

Methadone maintenance programs have been criticized highly across the United States because the process is often viewed as exchanging one addiction for another without attempts to detoxify the patient. In addition, clinic records and security have been lax in many instances, resulting in clinic methadone thefts and illegal sales on the street. Supporters of the programs counter these arguments by pointing out that criteria for involvement in these programs require that patients have been unsuccessful in remaining "clean" after detoxification on more than one occasion and that they no longer are "forced" into crime to support their habit. In addition, methadone is administered in such a way that no rush is experienced, allowing the person to return to school or work and reintegrate into society without the risk of losing everything to relapse. Methadone maintenance programs also are more cost-effective than residential treatment or jail time.

The controversy over methadone maintenance has resulted in the frequent use of naltrexone (Trexan) as an alternative. This drug is related to naloxone (Narcan) and is a pure opioid antagonist. This means that the drug reduces or completely blocks the effects of any intravenous opioids in the patient's system. The detoxified patient is placed on this drug to help prevent use of heroin. If the patient takes small doses of heroin while on naltrexone, no effect is experienced; however, if the patient injects large doses, he or she will become very physically ill and may die or sustain serious injury such as a coma. An addicted person taking naltrexone soon after regular use of heroin will experience withdrawal symptoms due to the antagonist actions of the drug.

Currently, research is under way to evaluate the use of various types of other psychotropic medications to stabilize altered neurochemical and neurophysiologic alterations in the brains of addicted persons. This may eventually provide an answer to the problem of the high rates of relapse in opioid abusers.

PHARMACOLOGY CAPSULE Methadone maintenance is used for patients who have experienced multiple relapses into heroin abuse following standard treatment and rehabilitation efforts.

NURSING CARE *of the Person with a Substance Disorder*

Assessment

The initial step in developing a nursing plan of care for the substance abuser is always a thorough assessment. On the basis of the initial assessment on admission or first contact with the patient, you can identify and prioritize problems that must be addressed in order to maximize the likelihood that the patient will remain sober. Examples of the types of problems often seen in substance abusers of any kind include denial, poor impulse control, high risk for injury, high risk for relapse, guilt, and low self-esteem. Detailed assessment of the person with a substance disorder is detailed at the beginning of this chapter.

Nursing Diagnoses, Goals, and Outcome Criteria: Substance Abuse

Nursing Diagnoses	Goals and Outcome Criteria
Ineffective Coping related to substance use evidenced by using substances to deal with anxiety, emotional discomfort, and stress	Improved coping: identifies and uses healthy alternative coping strategies to deal with anxiety, emotional discomfort, and stress; patient verbalizes strategies to prevent relapse
Ineffective Denial related to substance use and refusal to acknowledge actual consequences of substance use	Verbalizes an internalized sense that the substance use is unhealthy, out of control, and that the treatment is required
Risk for Injury related to excessive use of the drug and high risk for relapse, manifested by a history of falls; driving while under the influence and combining the substance abused with other substances; being aggressive while under the influence; reduced attendance at AA or NA meetings; frequent dreams of drug use; returning to places where one used drugs; not seeking relief for high stress.	Decreased risk for injury to self and others: patient does not engage in dangerous activities when under drug influence

Interventions

Nursing interventions for substance abusers in detoxification involve regular physical assessment (with the frequency determined by the severity of symptoms), administration of appropriate medications, and teaching the patients about their actions and consequences. Providing adequate nutrition is critical, as the patient may have been eating very irregularly and also may be quite dehydrated. High levels of anxiety during detoxification also require a great deal of reassurance and support, providing the opportunity to help the patient begin to process the impending decision to continue in rehabilitation.

Once the patient has agreed to participate in rehabilitation, the focus of nursing care changes from one of primarily attending to the physical concerns of the patient to assisting the client in processing the meaning of his or her substance abuse and planning for a future without continued use of that substance. The biggest issue to be addressed at first is the heavily entrenched denial that most substance abusers possess. Often they minimize the severity of the abuse, perhaps lying outright about how much they actually were using. You must work toward penetrating this denial without further damaging the individual's self-esteem. This has traditionally demanded more confrontational techniques than appropriate in other types of psychiatric treatment. In many "substance use only" treatment programs, the style of confrontation used was often overly hostile and critical. This approach is no longer seen as the most helpful to the patient. Studies now show that patients who were treated in this way were far more likely to leave treatment early to return to their "drugging and drinking." This is of great concern because the person may never return to treatment and may die or be seriously injured as a result of the continued substance abuse.

You also can be very helpful in assisting the patient to work through the 12-step process. After intense, educational AA or NA meetings and group therapy sessions during most of the day, patients often want to ventilate feelings and process thoughts about what they are learning. Conflicts with family members, bosses, friends, or parents often are overwhelming. Patients usually lack the skills to handle these types of interpersonal stressors because of habitual avoidance of issues through past substance abuse. You can act as an ally in helping patients cope and begin to practice new ways of reacting. Teaching stress management and practicing these new skills with patients can greatly increase the odds that they will not relapse after discharge.

Relapse prevention is a critical area to attend to in dealing with each patient. The patient must be taught to recognize symptoms that often lead to relapse. Examples of these include overtiredness or poor health, being unnecessarily dishonest with others, impatience, argumentativeness, depression, self-pity, cockiness, forgetting or minimizing the risk of relapse, unreasonable expectations of self and others, decreased or irregular participation in AA or NA meetings or daily meditation and self-inventory, use of a chemical other than those previously abused, forgetting to be thankful that their lives are better, and feeling all-powerful.

Another means of intervention that is very effective is to act as a good role model in handling feelings, participating appropriately in meetings, and communicating to the patient in a way that supports the program. For example, telling patients that participation in AA meetings is not necessary for recovery could undermine their struggle to initiate the profound changes in lifestyle necessary to stay drug free.

POPULATIONS OF SUBSTANCE ABUSERS WITH SPECIAL PROBLEMS

The unique characteristics of many groups of individuals influence the process of recovery and contribute to a high risk for relapse into chronic use of whatever substance the person has abused. Recent research in addressing these problems has proved very promising to date. As mentioned earlier, the trend is to provide specially designed treatment approaches for groups of individuals who have common traits and problems that may contribute to their dependency on alcohol or other drugs.

THE ELDERLY

Although elderly people use approximately 25% of the medications used in the United States, only about 2% to 5% of men and less than 1% of women over the age of 65 years abuse alcohol. Elderly people are more likely to abuse over-the-counter and prescription sleeping pills, pain medications, or tranquilizers than illegal drugs such as cocaine. Misuse is seldom for recreational purposes among this age group.

Because of a decreased ability to metabolize and eliminate alcohol or drugs from the body, elderly individuals who do abuse drugs over extended periods of time may experience significant medical problems as a result. The most typical physical consequences of chronic alcohol abuse among the elderly include malnutrition, cirrhosis of the liver, bone thinning, gastritis, poor memory, and decreased cognitive ability to process new information. If the person combines alcohol with any other medication that has central nervous system depressant effects, the danger of oversedation, impaired responses, or respiratory depression is very great.

Most of the elderly who abuse alcohol have maintained a regular pattern of use over many years without obvious problems. As their bodies age, their ability to tolerate the same quantities decreases, putting them at risk for falls or other injuries as a result of intoxication. Others turn to first-time or heavier patterns of use to cope with anxiety produced by the typical stressors of aging such as retirement, losses of significant others, family conflict, health problems, social isolation, and loss of self-worth. Among the elderly who move to more affluent retirement communities, a rise in alcoholism has been noted. This may be due to involvement in cocktail parties, regular drinking with meals, and peer pressure to participate in order to be accepted.

Problems of abuse in the elderly population are usually diagnosed by the family physician as a result of complaints related to the psychological or physical effects of alcohol abuse, such as memory impairment or insomnia. Elderly people often deny that they have a substance abuse problem and may resist treatment without the support and pressure of their family.

Treatment of alcoholism in the elderly is similar to that of younger individuals except that the period of withdrawal must be more closely monitored and occur more slowly because of the elderly person's physical fragility. Rehabilitation groups and educational programs should ideally be structured to permit processing information more slowly to allow for the cognitive slowing that is normal for this age group. Also, cognitive changes may be more pronounced because of the neurologic effects of chronic use of alcohol or other drugs, or both. Involvement in AA is critical and can be difficult if patients do not have easy access to a "home group" with other elderly people who can relate to their problems and issues.

ADOLESCENTS

Substance abuse among adolescents has received much attention in recent years. It is estimated that one in four adolescents becomes involved in substance abuse. It also has become apparent that children are experimenting with drugs at younger ages than ever before. The younger the age at onset of drug use, the greater is the risk for significant interference in the physical and psychological development of the individual.

The developmental issues of this age group also contribute to the adolescent's vulnerability. This is a stage of establishing one's identity, experimenting with newly developed abilities to think abstractly, egocentricity, limited impulse control, and poor judgment. Identification with one's peer group is an important aspect of feeling accepted. Average adolescents view themselves as omnipotent and deny the likelihood of negative consequences of their behaviors. This is the age of rebellion.

Substance abuse in this population also is viewed as a symptom of family issues. The family is often dysfunctional—patterns of communication may be ineffective, and children in the family may be emotionally or physically neglected, abused, or subject to rigid, unrealistic expectations for their behavior. There may be a family history of substance abuse, or the adolescent may fall in with the "wrong crowd" of other young people who are already involved in the drug culture.

The progression of physical consequences of substance abuse in the adolescent population is correlated with the risks related to the substance abused and the likelihood of polysubstance abuse. The risks of accidental overdose or suicide are significant. Intravenous drug use and the likelihood of sexual activity without the use of precautions have been linked to an increased risk of HIV infection among adolescents.

Entry into treatment usually occurs as a result of a crisis situation revealing the severity of drug use and parental insistence. Breaking through adolescents' denial is the most difficult aspect of treatment, especially because they seldom want to be in treatment and do not see the potential negative consequences of their behaviors. It also may be difficult to distinguish the abuser from the adolescent who is still in the early stages of experimentation and unlikely to persist in chronic substance abuse. Most adolescents do not reach the point of believing it when saying, "Hi, I'm an alcoholic" (or drug abuser), at the beginning of each AA or NA meeting.

Rehabilitation of the adolescent substance abuser requires that the approach to treatment be modified to meet the needs of this age group more effectively. It remains very controversial to mix adolescents with adults in treatment programs because of adolescents' vulnerability to being influenced by the more experienced and usually charismatic adult substance user. Obviously, careful supervision is necessary if mixing age groups for treatment is the only option. In addition, many of the abstract concepts addressed in the 12 steps of AA may need to be adapted to the level of understanding of the individual adolescent.

Successful rehabilitation usually involves regular involvement in an AA group made up of younger people whom the adolescent can relate to; successful development of a new, non–drug-using peer group; and reentry into school with the support of other recovering classmates. AA group meetings may be held at high schools in some cities.

THE DUALLY DIAGNOSED

Patients who already have been diagnosed with a serious psychiatric illness and also have a substance abuse problem (dual diagnosis) have special concerns for rehabilitation. Dually diagnosed patients usually have psychiatric illnesses of depression, schizophrenia, or bipolar illness. Often, mental retardation and organic brain disease also are included in the group of medical problems identified as presenting special concerns in the event of a concurrent substance abuse problem. (Many times, substance abusers have a personality disorder, although this group of psychiatric disorders is generally not considered to be the result of some physiologic process and usually is not included under dual diagnosis.)

In some individuals, chronic drug or alcohol abuse may exacerbate an already fragile neurophysiology, producing psychiatric symptoms. This is seen in cases of young adolescents who use marijuana or some other type of drug prior to their first psychotic break in schizophrenia. Toxic psychosis may occur more frequently with the use of cocaine or amphetamines mixed with alcohol. In other cases, people may use a mind-altering drug to treat psychiatric symptoms without understanding the reason. They just know that they feel better.

People with chronic psychiatric problems require special teaching and supervision in the event of substance relapse. Antipsychotic medications do not mix with alcohol. If a bipolar patient is on lithium, the fluid losses as a result of drinking alcohol could precipitate lithium toxicity. Patients taking anxiolytic or antidepressant agents with alcohol could risk accidental overdose as a result of additive effects on the central nervous system or could be deliberately attempting to harm themselves.

The approach to rehabilitation must be modified to adapt to this special population. Each patient's ability to comprehend the abstract ideas from the 12-step process of AA will vary. In addition, traditionalists in the recovery process often frown upon the use of any mind-altering chemical and may subtly pressure dually diagnosed clients to stop their prescribed medications. This lack of knowledge and rigid approach to recovery could contribute to exacerbation of the underlying psychiatric illness.

PEER ASSISTANCE PROGRAMS

Substance abuse is expected to be one of the most widespread problems of the next 20 years. People from all walks of life are at risk, including health care professionals who are at high risk because of easier access to addictive drugs. As a result, many professional groups have developed peer assistance programs. These programs are designed to offer a supportive alternative to health professionals (physicians, dentists, nurses, and others) who become addicted to a substance instead of taking immediate disciplinary action against their licenses.

Peer assistance programs for nurses exist in every state. Referrals are made by the individuals themselves or by their employers and peers who have reason to believe an individual's practice is impaired by the use of a substance. With the help of representatives of the program, usually volunteers, information is gathered to support an intervention in hopes of getting the nurse into treatment and recovery.

The goals of an intervention for a nurse whose practice is impaired are as follows:

- Assist the nurse whose practice is impaired to receive treatment.
- Protect the public from an untreated nurse.
- Help the recovering nurse reenter nursing in a systematic, planned, and safe way.
- Assist in monitoring the continued recovery of the nurse for a period of time.

Usually there is also at least a 2-year time period after diagnosis and onset of treatment in which the nurse is required to attend AA or NA groups regularly, to participate in peer support groups, to meet routinely with an identified support person representing the peer assistance program, and to undergo random urine drug screens to ensure that he or she has not relapsed. If nurses are unable to comply with the process, then information regarding their substance use and how that has impaired their practice can be turned over to the Board of Nurse Examiners for that state. Until that point, however, the information regarding each nurse involved is kept confidential and, if they successfully complete the requirements of the program, will never become part of the licensing board's records. Many peer assistance programs also work with nurses whose practices have become impaired as a result of mental illness.

Substance abuse will continue to be a major health care problem in the future. Nurses who work in this field are presented with difficult challenges and must be able to be nonjudgmental and supportive of the patients with whom they work. The knowledge base for this specialty area is growing quickly as a result of the widespread research currently being done. No matter where nurses work, they will come in contact with patients whose health status is compromised by substance abuse. The opportunity to play a powerful role in promoting healthier lifestyles is one that can be very fulfilling.

Nutrition Concepts

1. Heavy drug or alcohol intake has a negative effect on nutrition because it displaces foods in the diet that are more nutritious and impairs absorption and metabolism of nutrients in the body.
2. The nutritional goals for persons with alcoholism are to support them in avoiding alcohol and to correct nutritional deficits.
3. Individuals with chronic alcoholism may receive supplements of folate and vitamin B_6.
4. Stimulants may induce anorexia; however, as the effects of the stimulants subside, hunger develops.

key points

- The majority of experts in substance abuse subscribe to the biologic theory, which proposes that faulty physiologic processes contribute to dependence on a specific substance and that drug dependency is a physical illness.
- Some theorists contend that sociocultural factors contribute to the development of substance abuse.
- According to behavioral and learning theories, substance abuse is a learned maladaptive way of coping with stress and anxiety.
- The interpersonal or psychological theory states that innate personality factors may predispose individuals to substance abuse. Substance abusers have many common personality traits, including self-centeredness, a need to be in control of others, attention seeking, and difficulty delaying gratification of their needs.
- Although the specific causes of substance abuse have not been established, it is most likely that the true cause involves a combination of biologic, cultural, behavioral, and psychological factors.
- To obtain reliable data when questioning a person about substance abuse, the nurse must be nonjudgmental, direct, and specific. The information obtained should be verified by more than one person when possible.
- The lifestyle of substance abusers may focus entirely on obtaining and using the substance of choice, with an increasing need for more and more in order to get the desired effects.
- Substance abusers often have erratic and unprovoked mood swings, blackouts, significant work problems, and damaged relationships.
- Typical defense mechanisms used by substance abusers include denial, rationalization, intellectualization, and projection.
- Most alcohol abusers appear malnourished and poorly cared for, have evidence of physical trauma from falls or violence, appear jaundiced, and when in withdrawal, may be hypertensive with signs of fluid retention.
- Tests for detecting substance abuse include a blood alcohol study, a urine drug screen, and hair analysis.
- Chronic alcoholism involves the regular daily ingestion of large amounts of alcohol, regular heavy drinking only on weekends, or binges of heavy drinking followed by long periods of abstinence.
- Physical addiction occurs when the cells of the body are dependent on alcohol to carry out certain metabolic processes; without the alcohol, the cells go into shock.
- Alcohol withdrawal syndrome begins after an individual stops or decreases the amount of alcohol ingested and involves physiologic and behavioral symptoms that begin when the individual's blood alcohol level drops.
- Alcoholism has an impact on the entire family. Family and peer pressure can be critical factors in inducing an alcoholic to seek treatment.
- Strategies that have been successful in alcohol rehabilitation are 12-step programs, stress management, social skills training, behavioral approaches to marital therapy, and matching clients with therapists who use a style most likely to benefit their personality type.
- The six classes of psychoactive substances other than alcohol that are often associated with substance abuse are stimulants, depressants, hallucinogens, narcotics (opioids), inhalants, and designer drugs.
- Drug abuse treatment is similar to alcohol detoxification and rehabilitation; however, relapse rates are higher and treatment may need to be more individualized.
- Methadone maintenance may be used for long-term heroin abusers who have sustained permanent damage to chemical receptor sites in the brain and therefore have a decreased ability to resist relapses or who fail multiple attempts at rehabilitation.

REVIEW QUESTIONS

1. The theory that substance dependence is caused by faulty physiologic processes is the:
   1. biologic theory.
   2. behavioral theory.
   3. sociocultural theory.
   4. intrapersonal theory.

2. Mr. White was arrested for public intoxication and was advised by his attorney to enroll in an alcohol treatment program. A nurse interviews him when he comes to a mental health center. He tells the nurse he really doesn't have a problem with alcohol, he just had a few too many while celebrating with a friend. This is an example of which defense mechanism?
   1. Rationalization
   2. Projection
   3. Denial
   4. Intellectualization

3. What is the chief advantage of using hair analysis to detect drug use?
   1. Hair samples can be taken without patient permission.
   2. Hair samples will reveal drug use as long as a year later.
   3. It is not possible for a patient to substitute someone else's hair.
   4. The chain of custody is unnecessary with hair samples.

4. An alcoholic patient was injured in an automobile accident. She said she had her last drink 2 hours before the accident. About 8 hours after admission, she developed symptoms of early alcohol withdrawal. You should anticipate delirium tremens by:
   1. 12 hours after her last drink.
   2. 24 hours after her last drink.
   3. 48 hours after her last drink.
   4. 72 hours after her last drink.

5. Mr. Jones calls the hospital to report that his wife, a dietitian, cannot come to work because she has the "flu." In reality, she consumed a large amount of alcohol the previous evening and has a hang-over. This has happened several times in the past. Mr. Jones behavior is an example of:
   1. providing support.
   2. enabling behavior.
   3. rationalization.
   4. compensation

6. When a patient who is taking disulfiram (Antabuse) consumes alcohol, expected outcomes include:
   1. hypertensive crisis.
   2. cardiac depression.
   3. nausea and vomiting.
   4. abdominal pain and diarrhea.

7. Young people should be warned that inhalants can cause:
   1. progressive brain damage.
   2. sexual dysfunction.
   3. schizophrenia.
   4. aggressive behavior.

8. A patient being treated for an overdose of opioids is given Narcan. Narcan is given to:
   1. stimulate the heart.
   2. raise the blood pressure.
   3. treat respiratory depression.
   4. sedate the patient and prevent seizures.

9. The primary drug abused by older adults is/are:
   1. cocaine.
   2. amphetamines.
   3. sedatives/sleeping aids.
   4. alcohol.

10. Which statement most accurately describes drug use among adolescents?
    1. Only 1 in 10 adolescents has problems with substance abuse.
    2. Adolescents tend to deny any possible negative outcomes of drug use.
    3. Most adolescents seek treatment for substance abuse on their own.
    4. Adolescents should be treated with adults who can model mature behavior.

APPENDIX

A Abbreviations

ACTH Adrenocorticotropic hormone
AD Autonomic dysreflexia
ADH Antidiuretic hormone
ADL Activities of daily living
AICD Automatic implantable cardioverter-defibrillator
AIDS Acquired immunodeficiency syndrome
ALL Acute lymphocytic leukemia
ALS Amyotrophic lateral sclerosis
AMI Acute myocardial infarction
AML Acute myelogenous leukemia
ARDS Adult respiratory distress syndrome
ATC Around the clock
bid Twice a day
BMR Basal metabolic rate
BPH Benign prostatic hypertrophy
BRM Biologic response modifier
BSE Breast self-examination
BUN Blood urea nitrogen
CAD Coronary artery disease
CAL Chronic airflow limitation
CBC Complete blood count
CHF Congestive heart failure
CLL Chronic lymphocytic leukemia
CML Chronic myelogenous leukemia
CNS Central nervous system
CO Cardiac output
COLD Chronic obstructive lung disease
COPD Chronic obstructive pulmonary disease
CP Cerebral palsy
CPK Creatine phosphokinase
CSF Cerebrospinal fluid
CT Computed tomography
CVA Cerebrovascular accident
CVP Central venous pressure
DC Dilated cardiomyopathy
D & C Dilation and curettage
DES Diethylstilbestrol
DI Diabetes insipidus
DM Diabetes mellitus
DRG Diagnosis-related group
ECF Extracellular fluid
ECG Electrocardiogram
EEG Electroencephalogram
ESR Erythrocyte sedimentation rate
ET Enterostomal therapist
ETT Exercise tolerance test
FEV Forced expiratory volume
FFP Fresh frozen plasma
FRC Functional residual capacity
FVC Forced vital capacity
GBS Guillain-Barré syndrome
GI Gastrointestinal
HCT Hematocrit
HDL High-density lipoprotein
Hgb Hemoglobin
HIV Human immunodeficiency virus
IADL Instrumental activities of daily living
IBD Inflammatory bowel disease
IC Inspiratory capacity
ICP Intracranial pressure
IDDM Insulin-dependent diabetes mellitus (outdated term)
IE Infective endocarditis
IM Intramuscular, intramuscularly
IV Intravenous
LA Left atrium
LDH Lactic dehydrogenase
LDL Low-density lipoprotein
LES Lower esophageal sphincter
LOC Level of consciousness
LSD Lysergic acid diethylamide (a hallucinogenic drug)
LV Left ventricle
MG Myasthenia gravis
MI Myocardial infarction
MRI Magnetic resonance imaging
MS Multiple sclerosis
MV Minute volume
NG Nasogastric
NIDDM Non–insulin-dependent diabetes mellitus (outdated term)
NPO Nothing by mouth
NSAID Nonsteroidal anti-inflammatory drug
NTG Nitroglycerin
OA Osteoarthritis
OBRA Omnibus Reconciliation Act (included nursing home regulations)
OOB Out of bed
PACU Postanesthesia care unit (recovery room)
PCA Patient-controlled analgesia
PCP Phencyclidine
PE Pulmonary embolism

PET	Positron emission tomography
PIC	Peripherally inserted catheter
PID	Pelvic inflammatory disease
PO	By mouth
PRN	As needed
PTT	Partial thromboplastin time
PVD	Peripheral vascular disease
q	Every
RA	Rheumatoid arthritis
RA	Right atrium
RAP	Right atrial pressure
RBC	Red blood (cell) count
RMR	Resting metabolic rate
ROM	Range of motion
RV	Right ventricle
SC	Subcutaneous
SCD	Sudden cardiac death
SLE	Systemic lupus erythematosus
STD	Sexually transmitted disease
SVR	Systemic vascular resistance
TENS	Transcutaneous electrical nerve stimulation
V_{TG}	Thoracic gas volume
TIA	Transient ischemic attack
TLC	Total lung capacity
TPN	Total parenteral nutrition
UTI	Urinary tract infection
VAS	Visual analog scale
VC	Vital capacity
VLVD	Very low density lipoprotein
WBC	White blood (cell) count

Complete Bibliography & Reader References

Chapter 1

Agency for Healthcare Research and Quality. (2001). *Hospitalization in the United States, 1997.* Retrieved April 28, 2001 from http://www.ahcpr.gov/data/hcup/factbk1/index.htm.

Boon, T. (1998). Don't forget the hospice option. *RN, 61*(2), 30-33.

Davis, S. M. (1997). Subacute care: Yesterday's med/surg. *RN, 60*(11), 57-58.

Dentzer, S. (1998, January-February). A guide to managed health care. *Modern Maturity,* 35-41.

Elder, K. N., et al. (1998). Managed care: The value you bring. *American Journal of Nursing, 98*(6), 34-40.

Ellis, J., & Hartley, C. (1995). *Nursing in today's world: Challenges, issues, and trends* (5th ed., Chaps. 8 & 10). Philadelphia: Lippincott.

Goldsmith, C. (1998). Speak up! Managed care is not the enemy. *RN, 61*(1), 68.

Health Care Financing Administration. (2001). *National health expenditures projections: 2000-2010.* Retrieved April 28, 2001 from http://www.hcfa.gov/stats/NHE-Proj/proj2000/default.htm.

Health Care Financing Administration. (2001). *Highlights—National health expenditures, 1999.* Retrieved April 28, 2001 from http://www.hcfa.gov/stats/NHE-oact/hilites.htm.

Hill, S., & Howlett, H. (1997). *Success in practical nursing: Personal and vocational issues* (3rd ed.). Philadelphia: WB Saunders.

Long, C. O., & Jones, A. M. (2000). Community-based nursing and home health care. In S.M. Lewis, M. M. Heitkemper, & S. R. Dirksen (Eds.), *Medical-surgical nursing: Assessment and management of clinical problems* (5th ed., pp. 16-28). St. Louis: Mosby.

Medicare information (2001). Available at Nursing Home Information Site: Medicare summary http://www.members.tripod.com/~volfangary/Medicare.html. February 24, 2001.

Monahan, F. D., Drake, T., & Neighbors, M. (1998). *Medical-surgical nursing: Foundations for clinical practice.* Philadelphia: WB Saunders.

Perkins, E. M. (1998). Speak up! Death can be a caring choice. *RN, 60*(3), 72.

Tellis-Nayak, M. (1998). Understanding your patient's options. *American Journal of Nursing, 98*(8), 44-49.

Zerwekh, J., & Claborn, J. (1997). *Nursing today: Transition and trends* (Chaps. 11-13). Philadelphia: WB Saunders.

ADDITIONAL RESOURCES

American Association for Ambulatory Care Nursing: 1-800-262-6877/http://www.inurse.com/~AAACN

Center for Patient Care Advocacy: http://www.patient advocacy.org

Home Health Care Nurse's Association: http://www.junior.apk.net/~nurse/

Hospice Foundation of America: 1-800-854-3402; http://www.hospicefoundation.org

Hospice Hands: http://hospice-cares.com

National Committee for Quality Assurance: http://www.ncqa.org

Chapter 2

Benefield, L. (1996). Making the transition to home care nursing. *American Journal of Nursing, 96*(10), 47-49.

Matteson, M. A., McConnell, E. S., & Linton, A. D. (1997). *Gerontological nursing* (2nd ed.). Philadelphia: WB Saunders.

Monks, K. M. (2000). *Pocket guide to home health care.* Philadelphia: WB Saunders.

Stanhope, M., & Lancaster, J. (1997). *Community health nursing: Process and practice for promoting health* (4th ed.). St. Louis: Mosby.

Chapter 3

Anderson, M. A. (1997). *Nursing leadership, management, and professional practice for the LPN/LVN* (Chaps. 5 & 11). Philadelphia: FA Davis.

Boucher, M. A. (1998). Delegation alert. *American Journal of Nursing, 98*(2), 26-33.

Entry level competencies of graduates of educational programs in practical nursing. (1994). New York: NLN Council of Practical Nursing Programs.

Hill, S., & Howlett, H. (1997). *Success in practical nursing: Personal and vocational issues* (Chaps. 16, 18, & 19). Philadelphia: WB Saunders.

Yoder-Wise, P. S. (1999). *Leading and managing in nursing* (Chaps. 17 & 19). St. Louis: Mosby.

Zerwekh, J., & Claborn, J. (Eds.). (2000). *Nursing today: Transition and trends* (3rd ed., Chap. 8). Philadelphia: WB Saunders.

Chapter 4

Anderson, M. A. (1997). *Nursing leadership, management, and professional practice for the LPN/LVN* (Chaps. 5 & 11). Philadelphia: FA Davis.

Boucher, M. A. (1998). Delegation alert. *American Journal of Nursing, 98*(2), 26-33.

Entry level competencies of graduates of educational programs in practical nursing. (1994). New York: NLN Council of Practical Nursing Programs.

Hill, S., & Howlett, H. (1997). *Success in practical nursing: Personal and vocational issues* (Chaps. 16, 18, & 19). Philadelphia: WB Saunders.

Yoder-Wise, P. S. (1999). *Leading and managing in nursing* (Chaps. 17 & 19). St. Louis: Mosby.

Zerwekh, J., & Claborn, J. (Eds.). (2000). *Nursing today: Transition and trends* (3rd ed., Chap. 8). Philadelphia: WB Saunders.

Chapter 5

American Nurses Association. (1998, January-February). ANA addressing cultural diversity in the profession. *American Nurse, 30*(1), 25.

Andrews, M. M., & Boyle, J. S. (Eds.). (1995). *Transcultural concepts in nursing care* (2nd ed.). Philadelphia: Lippincott.

Black, J. M., & Matassarin-Jacobs, E. (2001). *Medical-surgical nursing: Clinical management for continuity of care* (6th ed., Chaps. 3, 4, 9). Philadelphia: WB Saunders.

Ellis, J. R. (1998). Cultural competence in nursing care. In F. D. Monahan, D. T. Drake, & M. Neighbors (Eds.). *Medical-surgical nursing: Foundations for clinical practice* (pp. 1230-1231). Philadelphia: WB Saunders.

Evans, B. M. (1999). Complementary therapies and HIV infection. *American Journal of Nursing, 99*(2), 42-45.

Federwisch, A. (1998). Missing pieces: The puzzle of diversity in health care. *Health Week, 3*(16), 1.

Geissler, E. M. (1998). *Cultural assessment* (2nd ed.). St. Louis: Mosby.

Hill, S. S., & Howlett, H. A. (1997). *Success in practical nursing* (3rd ed., Chaps. 14 & 15). Philadelphia: WB Saunders.

Ignatavicius, D. D., Workman, M. L., & Mishler, M. (1999). *Medical-surgical nursing: A nursing process approach* (3rd ed.). Philadelphia: WB Saunders.

Jarvis, C. (1996). *Physical examination and health assessment* (2nd ed., pp. 8-10, 50-57, 95-96, 217). Philadelphia: WB Saunders.

Keegan, L. (1998). Alternative and complementary therapies. *Nursing 98, 28*(4), 50-53.

Kudzma, E. C. (1999). Culturally competent: drug administration. *American Journal of Nursing, 99*(8), 46-52.

Leininger, M. M. (1988). Transcultural eating patterns and nutrition: Transcultural nursing and anthropological perspectives. *Holistic Nursing Practice, 3*(1), 16-25.

Leininger, M. M. (1991). Transcultural nursing: The study and practice field. *Imprint, 38*(2), 55.

Lester, N. (1998). Cultural competence: A nursing dialogue. *American Journal of Nursing, 98*(8), 26-34.

Lester, N. (1998). Cultural competence: A nursing dialogue, Part 2. *American Journal of Nursing, 98*(9), 36-44.

Luckmann, J. (1997). *Saunders manual of nursing care* (Chap. 2). Philadelphia: WB Saunders.

Meleis, A. I. (1996). Culturally competent scholarship: Substance and rigor. *Advances in Nursing Science, 19*(2), 1-16.

Spector, R. (1995). *Cultural diversity in health and illness* (4th ed., pp. 137-142). Norwalk, Conn: Appleton & Lange.

White, L., & Duncan, G. (1998). *Medical-surgical nursing: An integrated approach* (Chaps. 6 & 7). Albany, NY: Delmar.

Chapter 6

Curtis, B. (1996). Managing a multitude: Whether you have two kids or a bunch, this mom offers tips to help keep your family life under control. *Vibrant Life, 12*(5), 20-21.

De Montigny, F., Beaudet, L., & Dumas, L. (1996). The impact of a child's death on the family. *Canadian Nurse, 92*(10), 39-42.

Friedman, M. M. (1992). *Family nursing: Theory and practice* (3rd ed.). Norwalk, Conn: Appleton & Lange.

Friedman, M. M. (1997). *Family nursing: Theory, research, and practice* (4th ed.). Stamford, Conn: Appleton & Lange.

Hanson, S. M. H., & Boyd, S. T. (1996). *Family health care nursing: Theory, practice, and research.* Philadelphia: FA Davis.

Holicky, R. (1996). Caring for the caregivers: The hidden victims of illness and disability. *Rehabilitation Nursing, 21*(5), 247-252.

Hooper, J. I. (1996). The family receiving home care: Functional health pattern assessment. *Home Care Provider, 1*(5), 238-245.

Kahana, E., Biegel, D. E., & Wykle, M. L. (1994). *Family caregiving across the lifespan.* Thousand Oaks, Calif: Sage Publications.

Kasahara, M., Shemon, K. A., & Holzschuh, L. A. (1994). A biopsychosocial model for comprehensive care of the elderly. *Caring, 13*(9), 4.

Leahey, M., & Harper-Jaques, S. (1996). Family-nurse relationships: Core assumptions and clinical implications. *Journal of Family Nursing, 2*(2), 133-151.

Leonard, K. M., Enzle, S. S., McTavish, J., Cumming, C. E., & Cumming, D. C. (1995). Prolonged cancer death—A family affair. *Cancer Nursing, 18*(3), 222-227.

Meckler, L. (2001). Traditional family seems to be making a comeback. *San Antonio Express News,* p. 10A, April 13, 2001.

Chapter 7

American heritage dictionary (3rd ed.). New York: Houghton Mifflin, 1992.

Black, J. M., Hawks, J. H., & Keene, A. M. (2001). *Medical-surgical nursing: Clinical management for continuity of care* (6th ed., Chaps. 1, 2, & 20). Philadelphia: WB Saunders.

Evans, B. M. (1999). Complementary therapies and HIV infection. *American Journal of Nursing, 99*(2), 42-45.

Henderson, V. (1964). The nature of nursing. *American Journal of Nursing, 64,* 64.

Ignatavicius, D. D., Workman, M. L., & Mishler, M. (1999). *Medical-surgical nursing: A nursing process approach* (3rd ed., Chaps. 1 & 8). Philadelphia: WB Saunders.

Institute of Medicine. (1999). *Leading health indicators for healthy people 2010. Second interim report.* Washington, DC: National Academy Press.

Keegan, L. (1998). Alternative and complementary therapies. *Nursing 98, 28*(4), 50-53.

Lewis, S. M., Heitkemper, M. M., & Dirksen, S. R. (2000). *Medical-surgical nursing: assessment and management of clinical problems* (5th ed., Chap. 7). St. Louis: Mosby.

Potter, P., & Perry, A. (1997). *Fundamentals of nursing* (4th ed.). St. Louis: Mosby.

U.S. Department of Health and Human Services, Public Health Service. (2000). *Healthy people 2010.* Available at http://www.health.gov/healthypeople/ on March 6, 2001.

INTERNET RESOURCE

Office of Alternative Medicine: http://www.altmed.od.nih.gov

Chapter 8

Bell, M. L. (1997). Nutritional considerations. In M. A. Matteson, et al. (Eds.), *Gerontological nursing* (2nd ed., pp. 765-789). Philadelphia: WB Saunders.

Cammon, S. A., & Hackshaw, H. S. (2000). Are we starving our patients? *American Journal of Nursing, 100*(5), 43-47.

Dudek, S. G. (2000). Malnutrition in hospitals: who's assessing what patients eat? *American Journal of Nursing, 100*(4), 36-43.

Hankins, J., Lonsway, R.A.W., Hedrick, C., & Perdue, M. B. (2001). *Infusion therapy in clinical practice* (2nd ed.). Philadelphia: WB Saunders.

Heitz, U. E., & Horne, M. M. (2001). *Fluid, electrolyte, and acid-base balance.* St. Louis: Mosby.

Krupp, K. B. (1998). Going with the flow. How to prevent feeding tubes from clogging. *Nursing 98, 28*(4), 54-55.

Mahan, L. K., & Escott-Stump, S. (2000). *Krause's food, nutrition, and diet therapy* (10th ed.). Philadelphia: WB Saunders.

Metheny, N., Wehrle, M. A., & Wiersema, L. (1998). Testing feeding tube placement: Auscultation vs. pH method. *American Journal of Nursing, 98*(5), 37-42.

Orbanic, S. (2001). Understanding bulimia. *American Journal of Nursing, 101*(3), 35-42.

Chapter 9

Erikson, E. (1963). *Childhood and society* (2nd ed.). New York: Norton.

Ignatavicius, D. D., Workman, M. L., & Mishler, M. (1999). *Medical-surgical nursing: A nursing process approach* (3rd ed., Chaps. 5 & 6). Philadelphia: WB Saunders.

Murray, R. B., & Zentner, J. P. (1996). *Nursing assessment and health promotion strategies through the life span* (6th ed.). East Norwalk, Conn: Appleton & Lange.

Rosdahl, C. (1995). *Textbook of basic nursing* (Chap. 11). Philadelphia: Lippincott.

Sheehy, G. (1995). *New passages.* New York: Random House.

U.S. Department of Health and Human Services, Public Health Service. (2000). *Healthy people 2010.* Available at http://www.health.gov/healthypeople/document/html/volume1/toc.htm on March 6, 2001.

Chapter 10

Alzheimer's Association. (2001). *General statistics/demographics.* Available on http://www.alz.org/hc/overview/stats.htm on February 6, 2001.

Erikson, E. (1963). *Childhood and society.* New York: Norton.

Gunter, L., & Estes, C. (1979). *Education for gerontologic nursing.* New York: Springer.

Kee, J. L., & Hayes, E. R. (2000). *Pharmacology: A nursing process approach* (3rd ed.). Philadelphia: WB Saunders.

Lehne, R. A. (2001). *Pharmacology for nursing care.* Philadelphia: WB Saunders.

Masters, W. H., & Johnson, V. E. (1966). *Human sexual response* (p. 233). Boston: Little, Brown.

Matteson, M. A., McConnell, E., & Linton, A. D. (1997). *Gerontological nursing: Concepts and practice* (2nd ed.). Philadelphia: WB Saunders.

Chapter 11

Aquilino, M. L., & Keenan, G. (2000). Having our say: Nursing's standardized nomenclatures. *American Journal of Nursing, 100*(7), 33-38.

Alfaro-LeFevre, R. (1998). *Applying nursing process: A step by step guide* (4th ed.). Philadelphia: Lippincott.

Carpenito, L. (1997). *Nursing diagnosis: Application to clinical practice* (7th ed.). Philadelphia: Lippincott-Raven.

Cirone, N. (1998, April). Charting tips: Correcting charting errors. *Nursing, 28*(4), 65.

Ennis, R. (1985). A logical basis for measuring critical thinking skills. *Educational Leadership, 43*(2), 44-48. Cited in P. R. Cook (1995). Using critical thinking skills to improve medication administration. *MEDSURG Nursing 4*(4), 309-313.

Facione, N. C., & Facione, P. A. (1996). Externalizing the critical thinking in knowledge development and clinical judgment. *Nursing Outlook, 44,* 129-136.

Hill, S. S., & Howlett, H. A. (1997). *Success in practical nursing: Personal and vocational issues* (3rd ed., Chap. 2). Philadelphia: WB Saunders.

Ignatavicius, D., & Hausman, K. A. (1995). *Clinical pathways for collaborative practice.* Philadelphia: WB Saunders.

Ignatavicius, D., Workman, M., & Mishler, M. (1999). *Medical-surgical nursing: A nursing process approach* (3rd ed., Chaps. 1 & 3). Philadelphia: WB Saunders.

Jarvis, C. (1999). *Physical examination and health assessment* (3rd. ed.). Philadelphia: WB Saunders.

Johnson, M., Bulechek, G., Dochterman, J.M., Maas, M., & Moorhead, S. (Eds.). (2001). *Nursing diagnoses, outcomes, and interventions: NANDA, NOC, and NIC linkages.* St. Louis: Mosby.

Luckmann, J. (Ed.). (1997). *Saunders manual of nursing care* (Chaps, 1, 4, & 5). Philadelphia: WB Saunders.

North American Nursing Diagnosis Association. (2001). *Nursing diagnoses:* Definitions and classification 2001. Philadelphia: NANDA.

INTERNET RESOURCE

NurseCom: http://www.nursecominc.com

Chapter 12

Black, J. M., Hawks, J. H., & Keene, A. M. (2001). *Medical-surgical nursing: Clinical management for continuity of care* (6th ed., Chaps. 16 & 17). Philadelphia: WB Saunders.

Guyton, A. C., & Hall, J. E. (1996). *Textbook of medical physiology* (9th ed., Chap. 34). Philadelphia: WB Saunders.

Herlihy, B., & Maebius, N. K. (2000). *The human body in health and illness.* Philadelphia: WB Saunders.

Ignatavicius, D. D., Workman, M. L., & Mishler, M. A. (1999). *Medical-surgical nursing: A nursing process approach* (3rd ed.). Philadelphia: WB Saunders.

Jones, L., Hannum, D. (1998). Playing it safe with a particulate respirator. *Nursing 98, 28*(1), 50-51.

Lehne, R. A. (2001). *Pharmacology for nursing care* (4th ed.). Philadelphia: WB Saunders.

Monahan, F. D., & Neighbors, M. (1998). *Medical-surgical nursing* (Chap. 12). Philadelphia: WB Saunders.

Potter, P., & Perry, A. (2001). *Fundamentals of nursing: Concepts, process and practice* (5th ed., Chap. 33). St. Louis: Mosby.

Sheff, B. (1998). VRE and MRSA: Putting bad bugs out of business. *Nursing 98, (March) 28,* 40-44.

INTERNET RESOURCES

The Centers for Disease Control can be accessed on the World Wide Web at http://www.cdc.gov

Information about infectious diseases and immunization can be accessed on the World Wide Web at http://www.healthtouch.com

The Agency on Health Care Policy and Research Clinical Practice Guidelines can be accessed at http://www.ahcpr.gov

Chapter 13

Abrams, A. C. (2001). *Clinical drug therapy: Rationales for nursing practice* (6th ed.), Philadelphia: Lippincott.

Black, J. M., Hawks, J. H., &. Keene, A. M. (2001). *Medical-surgical nursing: Clinical management for continuity of care* (6th ed.). Philadelphia: WB Saunders.

DeJong, M. J. (1998). Emergency! Hyponatremia. *American Journal of Nursing, 98*(12), 36.

Guyton, A. C., & Hall, J. E. (1996). *Textbook of medical physiology* (9th ed.). Philadelphia: WB Saunders.

Heitz, U. E., & Horne, M. M. (2001). *Fluid, electrolyte, and acid-base balance.* St. Louis: Mosby.

Herlihy, B., & Maebius, N. K. (2000). *The human body in health and illness.* Philadelphia: WB Saunders.

Horne, C., & Derrico, D. (1999). Mastering ABGs. *American Journal of Nursing, 99*(8), 26-33.

Ignatavicius, D. D., Workman, M. L., & Mishler, M. A. (1999). *Medical-surgical nursing: A nursing process approach* (3rd ed.). Philadelphia: WB Saunders.

Jacobs, D.S., DeMott, W. R., Grady, H. J., Horvat, R. T., Huestis, D. W., & Kasten, B. L. (1996). *Laboratory Test Handbook.* Hudson (Cleveland): Lexi-Comp, Inc.

Jaffe, H. S., & McVan, B. F. (1997). *Davis's laboratory and diagnostic test handbook.* Philadelphia: FA Davis.

Jarvis, C. (1999). *Physical examination and health assessment* (3rd ed.). Philadelphia: WB Saunders.

Luckmann, J. (1997). *Saunders manual of nursing care.* Philadelphia: WB Saunders.

Phillips, L. D. (1997). *Manual of I.V. therapeutics* (2nd ed.). Philadelphia: FA Davis.

Wong, F. W. H. (1999). A new approach to ABG interpretation. *American Journal of Nursing, 99*(8), 34-36.

Chapter 14

Acute Pain Management Guidelines Panel. (1992). *Acute pain management: Operative and medical procedures and trauma. Clinical practice guidelines* (AHCPR Publication No. 92-0032). Rockville, Md: Agency for Health Care Policy and Research, Public Health Service, U.S. Department of Health and Human Services.

American Pain Society. (1999). *Principles of analgesic use in the treatment of acute pain and chronic cancer pain* (4th ed.). Skokie, Ill: Author.

Delgin, J., & Vallerand, A. (2000). *Davis' drug guide for nurses* (7th ed.). Philadelphia: FA Davis.

Dossey, B. (1995). Using imagery to help your patient heal. *American Journal of Nursing, 95*(6), 40-47.

Jacox, A., Carr, C. B., Payne, R., et al. (1994, March). *Management of cancer pain: Clinical practice guideline No. 9* (AHCPR Publication No. 94-0592). Rockville, Md: Agency for Health Care Policy and Research, U.S. Department of Health and Human Services, Public Health Service.

Joint Commission on Accreditation of Healthcare Organizations. (2000). *Pain assessment and management.* Illinois: Joint Commission.

Loeb, J. (1999). Pain management in long-term care. *American Journal of Nursing, 99*(2) 48-52.

Loeser, J.D. (Ed.) (2000). *Bonica's management of pain* (3rd ed.). Philadelphia: Lippincott, Williams & Wilkins.

McCaffery, M., & Pasero, C. (1999). *Pain: Clinical manual.* St. Louis: Mosby.

Pasero, C (1998). Teaching patients how to use PCA. *American Journal of Nursing, 98*(9), 14-15.

Strevy, S. (1998). Myths and facts about pain. *RN, 61*(2), 42-47.

Waitman, J. & McCaffery, M. (2000). Meperidine—liability. *American Journal of Nursing, 100*(2), 57-58.

INTERNET RESOURCES

Joint Commission on Accreditation of Healthcare Organizations: http://www.jcaho.org

Agency for Healthcare Research and Quality: http://www.ahrq.org

American Pain Society: http://www.ampainsoc.org

American Cancer Society: http://www.cancer.org

Arthritis Foundation: http://www.arthritis.org

Hospice Foundation of America: http://www.hospicefoundation.org

North American Chronic Pain Association: http://www.chronicpaincanada.org

Chapter 15

Adam, R. D., & Sullivan, J. B. (2000). Venomous snake bites. In L. Goldman & J. C., Benett (Eds.), *Cecil textbook of medicine* (21st ed., pp. 2001-2003). Philadelphia: WB Saunders.

American Heart Association. (2000). *International CPR and ECC guidelines 2000: Major changes and revisions.* Retrieved on April 21, 2002 from http://www.cpr-exx.org/Whats_new/Whats_menu.htm.

Asselin, M. E., & Cullen, H. A. (2001). New BLS guidelines. *Nursing 2001, 31*(3), 48-50.

Bennett (Eds.), *Cecil textbook of medicine* (21st ed., pp. 2001-2003). Philadelphia: WB Saunders.

American Heart Association. (1994). *Instructor's manual for basic life support.* Dallas: Author.

Barbarito, C. (1998). Emergency! Hypertension-induced epistaxis. *American Journal of Nursing, 98*(2), 48.

Black, J. M., & Matassarin-Jacobs, E. (1997). *Medical-surgical nursing: Clinical management for continuity of care* (5th ed.). Philadelphia: WB Saunders.

Huston, C. J. (1998). Emergency! Cervical spine injury. *American Journal of Nursing, 98*(6), 33.

Ignatavicius, D. D., Workman, M. L., & Mishler, M. A. (1999). *Medical-surgical nursing: A nursing process approach* (3rd ed.). Philadelphia: WB Saunders.

Monahan, F. D., & Neighbors, M. (1998). *Medical-surgical nursing foundations for clinical practice* (2nd ed.). Philadelphia: WB Saunders.

Wade, C. F. (2000). Keeping Lyme disease at bay. *American Journal of Nursing, 100*(7), 26-32.

Chapter 16

Abrams, A. C. (2001). *Clinical drug therapy* (6th ed.). Philadelphia: Lippincott.

Black, J. M., Hawks, J. H., & Keene, A. M. (2001). *Medical-surgical nursing: Clinical management for continuity of care* (6th ed.). Philadelphia: WB Saunders.

Faries, J. (1998). Easing your patient's postoperative pain. *Nursing 98, 28*(6), 58-60.

Hodge, D. (Ed.). (1999). *Day surgery: A nursing approach.* Edinburgh: Churchill Livingstone.

Ignatavicius, D. D., Workman, M. L., & Mishler, M. A. (1999). *Medical-surgical nursing: A nursing process approach* (3rd ed.). Philadelphia: WB Saunders.

Jarvis, C. (1999). *Physical examination and health assessment* (3rd ed.). Philadelphia: WB Saunders.

King, M. E., & Kinney, A. Y. (2001). Tissue adhesives: A sticky solution to wound repair. *Nursing 2001, 31*(3), 52-53.

Kingsley, C. (2001). Epidural analgesia: your role. *RN, 64*(3), 53-58.

Mahan, L. K., & Escott-Stump, S. (2000). *Krause's food, nutrition, and diet therapy* (10th ed.). Philadelphia: WB Saunders.

Messinger, J. A., Hoffman, L. A., O'Donnell, J. M., & Dunworth, B. A. (1999). Getting conscious sedation right. *American Journal of Nursing, 99*(12), 44-50.

Phillips, J. K. (1998). Actionstat: Wound dehiscence. *Nursing 98, 28*(3), 33.

Walton, J. (2001). Helping high-risk surgical patients beat the odds. *Nursing 2001, 31*(3), 54-60.

Chapter 17

Ignatavicius, D. D., Workman, M. L., & Mishler, M. A. (1999). *Medical-surgical nursing: A nursing process approach* (3rd ed.). Philadelphia: WB Saunders.

Love, G. (1998). Controlling pain: Easing the discomfort of venipuncture. *Nursing 98, 28*(3), 30.

Masoorli, S. (1998). Removing a PICC? Proceed with caution. *Nursing 98, 28*(3), 56-57.

Perucca, R. (2001). Changing and discontinuing infusion therapy. In J. Hankins, R. A. W. Lonsway, C. Hedrick, & M. B. Perdue. *Infusion therapy in clinical practice* (2nd ed., pp. 398-403). Philadelphia: WB Saunders.

Perucca, R. (2001). Infusion monitoring and catheter care. In J. Hankins, R. A. W. Lonsway, C. Hedrick, & M. B. Perdue, *Infusion therapy in clinical practice* (2nd ed., pp. 389-397). Philadelphia: WB Saunders.

Perucca, R. (2001). Infusion therapy equipment: Types of infusion therapy equipment. In J. Hankins, R. A. W. Lonsway, C. Hedrick, & M. B. Perdue, *Infusion therapy in clinical practice* (2nd ed., pp. 300-333). Philadelphia: WB Saunders.

Perucca, R. (2001). Obtaining vascular access. In J. Hankins, R. A. W. Lonsway, C. Hedrick, & M. B. Perdue, *Infusion therapy in clinical practice* (2nd ed., pp. 375-388). Philadelphia: WB Saunders.

Walther, K. (2001). Intravenous therapy in the older adult. In J. Hankins, R. A. W. Lonsway, C. Hedrick, & M. B. Perdue, *Infusion therapy in clinical practice* (2nd ed., pp. 592-603). Philadelphia: WB Saunders.

INTERNET RESOURCES

Intravenous Nurses Society: http://www.ins1.org

SpringNet: http://www.springnet.com

Chapter 18

Abrams, A. C. (2001). *Clinical drug therapy* (6th ed.). Philadelphia: Lippincott.

Atassi, K. A., & Harris, M. L. (2001). Disseminated intravascular coagulation. *Nursing 2001, 31*(3), 64.

Dax, J. M., & Hermey, C. L. (2000). Nursing management: shock and multiple organ dysfunction syndrome. In S. M. Lewis, M. M Heitkemper, & S. R Dirksen (Eds.), *Medical-surgical nursing: Assessment and management of clinical problems* (5th ed., pp. 1865-1894). St. Louis: Mosby.

Geissler, E. M. (1998). *Pocket guide to cultural assessment* (2nd ed.). St. Louis: Mosby.

LaFramboise, L. N. (2001). Management of clients with shock and multisystem disorders. In J. M. Black, J. H. Hawks, & A. M. Keene (Eds.), *Medical-surgical nursing: Clinical management for positive outcomes* (6th ed., pp. 2231-2259). Philadelphia: WB Saunders.

Melander, S., & Bucher, L. (1999). *Pocket companion for critical care nursing.* Philadelphia: WB Saunders.

Monahan, F. D., & Neighbors, M. A. (1998). *Medical-surgical nursing: Foundations for clinical practice* (2nd ed.). Philadelphia: WB Saunders.

Chapter 19

Capazuti, E., Talerico, K. A., Cochran, I., Becker, H., Strumpf, N., & Evans, L. (1999). Individualized interventions to prevent bed-related falls and reduce siderail use. *Journal of Gerontological Nursing, 25*(11), 26-33.

Matteson, M. A., McConnell, E. S., & Linton, A. D. (1997). *Gerontological nursing.* Philadelphia: WB Saunders.

Meiner, S. E., & Miceli, D. G. (2000). Safety. In A.G. Lueckenotte (Ed.), Gerontologic nursing (2nd ed., pp. 232-255), St. Louis: Mosby.

Rogers, P. D., & Bocchino, N. L. (1999). Restraint-free care: Is it possible? *American Journal of Nursing, 99*(10), 26-33.

Stone, J. T., & Wyman, J. F. (1999). Falls. In J. T. Stone, J. F. Wyman, & S. A. Salisbury (Eds.), *Clinical gerontological nursing* (2nd ed., pp. 341-366). Philadelphia: WB Saunders.

Walker, B. L. (1998). Preventing falls. *RN, 61*(5), 40-43.

Chapter 20

Agency for Health Care Policy and Research. (1992). *How to predict and prevent pressure ulcers . . . clinical practice guidelines released by the Agency for Health Care Policy and Research.* Retrieved from http://www.ahcpr.gov on May 28, 2001.

Agency for Health Care Policy and Research. (1994). *Pressure ulcer treatment . . . clinical practice guidelines released by the Agency for Health Care Policy and Research.* Retrieved from http://www.ahcpr.gov on May 28, 2001.

Lueckenotte, A.G. (2000). *Gerontologic nursing* (2nd ed.). St. Louis: Mosby

Matteson, M. A., McConnell, E. S., & Linton, A. D. (1997). *Gerontological nursing* (2nd. ed.). Philadelphia: WB Saunders.

National Pressure Ulcer Advisory Panel. (1996). Pressure ulcer research: Etiology, assessment, and early intervention. *Dermatology Nursing, 8*(1), 41-47.

Stone, J. T., Wyman, J. F., & Salisbury, S. A. (1999). *Clinical gerontological nursing: A guide to advanced practice* (2nd ed.). Philadelphia: WB Saunders.

Chapter 21

Adams, T., & Clarke, C. L. (1999). *Dementia care.* London: Bailliere Tindall.

Lancaster, M. M., Abusamra, L. C., & Clark, W. G. (1998). Management of difficult behaviors. In R. C. Hamdy, J. M. Turnbull, J. Edwards, & M. M. Lancaster (Eds.), *Alzheimer's disease: a handbook for caregivers* (3rd ed., pp. 150-170). St. Louis: Mosby.

Matteson, M. A., Linton, A. D., & Barnes, S. J. (1996). Cognitive developmental approach to dementia. *Image: Journal of Nursing Scholarship, 28*(3), 233-240.

Matteson, M. A., Linton, A. D., Barnes, S. J., Cleary, B. L., & Lichtenstein, M. J. (1996). The relationship between Piaget and cognitive levels in persons with Alzheimer's disease and related disorders. *Aging: Clinical and Experimental Research, 8*(1), 61-69.

Matteson, M. A., McConnell, E. S., & Linton, A. D. (1997). *Gerontological nursing: Concepts and practice* (2nd ed.). Philadelphia: WB Saunders.

Chapter 22

Ahronheim, J. C. (2000). Special problems in the geriatric patient. In L. Goldman & J. C. Bennett (Eds.), *Cecil textbook of medicine* (21st ed., pp. 22-25). Philadelphia: WB Saunders.

American Society of Colon and Rectal Surgeons. (2000). *Bowel incontinence.* Retrieved from http://www.fascrs.org/brochures/bowel-incontinence.html on September 21, 2000.

Bates, P. (2000). Nursing management: Renal and urologic problems. In S. M. Lewis, M. J. Heitkemper, & S. R. Dirksen (Eds.), *Medical-surgical nursing: Assessment and management of clinical problems* (5th ed., pp. 1261-1298). Philadelphia: WB Saunders.

Engelberg, S. J. H., McDowell, B. J., & Lovell, A. (2000). In A. G. Lueckenotte, *Gerontologic nursing* (2nd ed., pp. 586-614). St. Louis: Mosby.

Fantl, J.A., Newman, D. K., Colling, J., et al. (January 1996). Managing acute and chronic urinary incontinence. In Clinical Practice Guideline. Quick Reference Guide for Clinicians, No. 2, 1996 Update (AHCPR Pub. No. 96-0686). Rockville, Md: U.S. DHHS, Public Health Service, Agency for Health Care Policy and Research.

Fillingham, S., & Douglas, J. (1997). *Urological nursing* (2nd ed.). London: Bailliere Tindall.

Gray, M. (2000). Urinary retention: Management in the acute care setting, Part 1. *American Journal of Nursing, 100*(7), 40-48.

Gray, M. (2000). Urinary retention: Management in the acute care setting, Part 2. *American Journal of Nursing, 100*(8), 36-44.

Johnson, S. T. (2000). From incontinence to confidence. *American Journal of Nursing, 100*(2), 69-76.

Ouslander, J. G. (2000). Urinary incontinence. In L. Goldman & J. C. Bennett (Eds.), *Cecil textbook of medicine* (21st ed., pp. 640-642). Philadelphia: WB Saunders.

Roberts, R. G. (2001). Current management strategies for overactive bladder. *A Supplement to Patient Care for the Nurse Practitioner, Spring 2001,* 22-33.

Smith, M. (1998). Gynecologic disorders. In E. H. Duthie & P. R. Katz (Eds.), *Practice of geriatrics* (3rd ed., pp. 524-534). Philadelphia: WB Saunders.

Potter, P. A., & Perry, A. G. (2001). *Fundamentals of nursing* (5th ed.). St. Louis: Mosby.

U.S. Department of Health and Human Services. (1992). *Urinary incontinence in adults* (AHCPR Pub. No. 92-0038). Rockville, Md: Author.

Chapter 23

Ad Hoc Committee of the Harvard Medical School to Examine the Definition of Brain Death. (1968). A definition of irreversible coma. *Journal of the American Medical Association, 205*(6), 337-340.

American Medical Association's Institute for Ethics, EPEC (Education for Physicians on End of Life Care). (1999). *Trainer's and participant's handbooks.*

Banks, G. (2000). Verifying a death. *Nursing Standard, 14*(33), 22-23.

Capron, A. M. (2001). Brain death—Well settled yet still unresolved. *New England Journal of Medicine, 344,* 1244-1246.

Carpenito, L. J. (1999). *Nursing diagnoses: Application to clinical nursing practice* (8th ed.). Philadelphia: Lippincott.

Davitz, L., Sameshima, Y., Davitz, J., et al. (1976). Suffering as viewed in six different cultures. *American Journal of Nursing, 76*(8), 1296-1297.

Ebersole, P., & Hess, P. (1998). *Toward healthy aging* (5th ed.). St. Louis: Mosby.

Geissler, E. M. (1998). *Mosby's pocket guide: Cultural assessment.* St. Louis: Mosby.

Kübler-Ross, E. (1974). *Questions and answers on death and dying.* New York: Macmillan.

Kübler-Ross, E. (1975). *Death, the final stage of growth.* Englewood Cliffs, NJ: Prentice-Hall.

Kübler-Ross, E. (1978). *To live until we say goodbye.* Englewood Cliffs, NJ: Prentice-Hall.

Kübler-Ross, E. (1981). *Living with death and dying.* New York: Macmillan.

Kübler-Ross, E. (1983). *On children and death.* New York: Macmillan.

Lynn, J. & Harrold, J. (1999). *Handbook for mortals: Guidance for people facing serious illness.* New York: Oxford University Press.

Lynn, J., Schuster, J. L., & Kabcenell, A. (2000). *Improving care for the end of life.* New York: Oxford University Press.

Lugton, J., & Kindlin, M. (Eds.). (1999). *Palliative care: The nursing role.* Edinburgh: Churchill Livingstone.

Martocchio, B. C. (1985). Grief and bereavement: Healing through hurt. *Nursing Clinics of North America, 20*(6), 327-341.

Matteson, M. A., McConnell, E. S., & Linton, A. D. (1997). *Gerontological nursing: Concepts and practice* (2nd ed.). Philadelphia: WB Saunders.

National Council of Hospice Professionals. (1997). *Guidelines for curriculum development on end-of-life and palliative care in nursing education.* Arlington, Va: National Council.

Omnibus Reconciliation Act. (1990). Title IV. Section 4206. Congressional Record. October 26, 1990, 12638.

The Quality Standards Subcommittee of the American Academy of Neurology. (1995). Practice parameters for determining brain death in adults (summary statement). *Neurology, 45,* 275-287.

Rando, T. A. (1993). *Treatment of complicated mourning.* Champaign, Ill: Research Press.

Roark, D. C. (2000) Overhauling the organ donation system. *American Journal of Nursing, 200*(6), 44-49.

Schonwetter, R. S., Hawke, W., Knight, C. F. (Eds.). (1999). *Hospice and palliative medicine core: Curriculum and review syllabus,* American Academy of Hospice and Palliative Medicine. Dubuque, Iowa: Kendall/Hunt Publishing Co.

Strauss, A. L., & Glaser, B. G. (1970). Awareness of dying. In B. Schoenberg, et al. (Eds.), *Loss and grief: Psychosocial management in medical practice.* New York: Columbia University Press.

Wijdicks, E. F. M. (2001). Current concepts: The diagnosis of brain death. *New England Journal of Medicine, 344,* 1215-1221.

INTERNET RESOURCES

Association for Death Education and Counseling: http://www.adec.org

Last Acts—a national coalition to improve care at end of life: http://www.lastacts.org

Online Information on Palliative and End-of-Life Care: http://www.palliativecarenursing.net

Partnership for Caring: http://www.partnershipforcaring.org

Coalition of Donation: http://www.shareyourlife.org

Chapter 24

Abrams, A. C. (2001). *Clinical drug therapy* (6th ed.). Philadelphia: Lippincott, Williams & Wilkins.

Agency for Health Care Policy and Research. (1994). *Management of cancer pain: Adults* (AHCPR Publication No. 94-0593). Rockville, Md: U.S. Department of Health and Human Services.

American Cancer Society. (2001). *Cancer in Minorities.* Retrieved from http://www.americancancersociety.org on June 7, 2001.

American Cancer Society. (2001). *Complementary and alternative methods.* Retrieved from http://www.cancer.org/alt_therapy/index.htm on June 7, 2001.

American Cancer Society. (2001). *Statistics.* Retrieved from http://www3.cancer.org on June 9, 2001.

American Cancer Society. (2000). *Complementary and alternative cancer methods.* Atlanta, Ga: Author.

Black, J. M., Hawks, J., & Keene, A. M. (2001). *Medical-surgical nursing: Clinical management for continuity of care* (6th ed.). Philadelphia: WB Saunders.

Boon, T. (1998). Don't forget the hospice option. *RN, 61*(2), 30-33.

Brenner, M. K. (2000). Stem cell transplantation. In L. Goldman & J. C. Bennett (Eds.), *Cecil textbook of medicine* (21st ed., pp. 987-991) Philadelphia: WB Saunders.

Chernecky, C. C., & Berger, B. J. (2001). *Laboratory tests and diagnostic procedures.* (3rd ed.). Philadelphia: WB Saunders.

Concus, A. P., & Singer, M. I. (2000). Head and neck cancer. In L. Goldman & J. C. Bennett (Eds.), *Cecil textbook of medicine* (21st ed., 2257-2262). Philadelphia: WB Saunders.

Held-Warmkessel, J. (1998). Chemotherapy complications. *Nursing 98, 28*(4), 41-45.

Ignatavicius, D. D., Workman, M. L., & Mishler, M. A. (1999). *Medical-surgical nursing: A nursing process approach* (3rd ed.). Philadelphia: WB Saunders.

Keegan, L. (1998). Alternative and complementary therapies. *Nursing 98, 28*(4), 50-53.

Lewis, S. M., Heitkemper, M. M., & Dirksen, S. R. (Eds.). (2000). *Medical-surgical nursing: Assessment and management of clinical problems.* (5th ed.). St. Louis: Mosby.

Mahan, L. K., & Escott-Stump, S. (2000). *Krause's food, nutrition, and diet therapy* (10th ed.). Philadelphia: WB Saunders.

Meyers, J. S. (2000). Chemotherapy-induced hypersensitivity reaction. *American Journal of Nursing, 100*(4), 53-54.

Moldawer, N., & Carr, E. (2000). The promise of recombinant interleukin-2. *American Journal of Nursing, 100*(5), 35-40.

INTERNET RESOURCES

American Cancer Society: http://www.cancer.org

National Cancer Institute—International Cancer Information Center: http://www.nci.nih.gov

Oncology Nursing Society: http://www.ons.org

ADDITIONAL RESOURCES

The following resources are old, but offer many good, practical tips for the patient:

American Cancer Society. (1997). *A cancer source book for nurses* (7th ed.). Atlanta, Ga: Author.

National Cancer Institute. (1987). *Chemotherapy and you* (NIH Publication No. 88-1136). Bethesda, Md: National Institutes of Health.

National Cancer Institute. (1987). *Radiation therapy and you.* Bethesda, Md: Author.

National Cancer Institute. (1992). *Eating hints: Recipes and tips for better nutrition during cancer treatment.* Bethesda, Md: Author.

Chapter 25

Black, J. M., Hawks, J. H., & Keene, A. M. (2001). *Medical-surgical nursing: Clinical management for continuity of care* (6th ed.). Philadelphia: WB Saunders.

Erwin-Toth, P. (2001). Caring for a stoma is more than skin deep. *Nursing 2001, 31*(5), 36-41.

Ignatavicius, D. D., Workman, M. L., & Mishler, M. A. (1999). *Medical-surgical nursing: A nursing process approach* (3rd ed.). Philadelphia: WB Saunders.

Lewis, S. M., Heitkemper, M. M., & Dirksen, S. R. (2000). *Medical-surgical nursing: Assessment and management of clinical problems* (5th ed.). St. Louis: Mosby.

INTERNET RESOURCES

American Cancer Society: http://www.acs.org

United Ostomy Association: http://www.uoa.org

Crohn's & Colitis Foundation of America: http://www.ccfa.org
Wound, Ostomy and Continence Nurses Society: http://www.wocn.org

ADDITIONAL RESOURCE

Ostomy Quarterly lists mail order houses that sell discount ostomy supplies: 1-800-826-0826.

Chapter 26

Barker, E. (2002). *Neuroscience nursing: A spectrum of care.* St. Louis: Mosby.

Chasen, E. R., & Umlauf, M. G. (2000). Post-polio syndrome. *American Journal of Nursing, 100*(12), 60-63.

Crigger, N., & Forbes, W. (1997). Assessing neurologic function in older patients. *American Journal of Nursing, 97*(3), 37-40.

Goetz, C., & Pappert, E. (1999). *Textbook of clinical neurology.* Philadelphia: WB Saunders.

Goldsmith, C. (1999). Parkinson's disease. *American Journal of Nursing, 99*(2), 46-47.

Halper, J., & Holland, N. (1998). New strategies, new hope: Meeting the challenge of multiple sclerosis. *American Journal of Nursing, 98*(11), 39-45.

Hock, N. H. (1999). Brain attack: the stroke continuum. *Nursing Clinics of North America, 34*(3), 689-723.

Karch, A. M. (2001). *Lippincott's nursing drug guide.* Philadelphia: Lippincott.

Lewis, A. M. (1999). Neurologic emergencies! *Nursing, 29*(10), 54-56.

Luckmann, J. (1997). *Saunders manual of nursing care.* Philadelphia: WB Saunders.

O'Neill, L. J., & Carter, D. E. (1998). The implications of head injury for family relationships. *British Journal of Nursing, 7*(14), 842-846.

Schulman-Green, D. J. (1999). Communicating with the facially inexpressive older adult. *Journal of Gerontological Nursing, 25*(11), 40-43.

Shafer, P. O. (1999). New therapies in the management of acute or cluster seizures and seizure emergencies. *Journal of Neuroscience Nursing, 31*(4), 224-230.

Stewart-Amidei, C., & Kunkel, J. A. (2001). *AANN's neuroscience nursing: Human responses to neurologic dysfunction* (2nd ed.), Philadelphia, WB Saunders.

Worsham, T. L. (2000). Easing the course of Guillain-Barré syndrome. *RN, 63*(3), 46-50.

Chapter 27

American Heart Association. (2000). *Heart and stroke statistical update,* Dallas, Tx: American Heart Association.

American Association of Neuroscience Nurses. (1998). Recommendations for the nursing management of the hyperacute ischemic stroke patient. *AANN Clinical Guideline Series,* Chicago.

Brass, L. M. (2001). Advances in long-term stroke prevention with antiplatelet therapy. *Journal of Stroke and Cerebrovascular Diseases, 10*(2), Suppl. 1, 18-23.

Brillhart, B. (2000). Nursing management: Patient with a stroke. In S. M. Lewis, M. M. Heitkemper, & S. D. Dirksen (Eds.), *Medical-surgical nursing: Assessment and management of clinical problems* (5th ed., pp. 1645-1671). St. Louis: Mosby.

Brockington, C. D., & Lyden, P. (2000). Stroke prevention and acute intervention: Review of recent advances. *Formulary, 35,* 328-342.

Chung, C-S., & Caplan, L. R. (1999). Neurovascular disorders. In C. Goetz & E. Pappert (Eds.), *Textbook of clinical neurology* (Chap. 45). Philadelphia: WB Saunders.

Guyton, A. C., & Hall, J. E. (1996). *Textbook of medical physiology* (9th ed.). Philadelphia: WB Saunders.

Hydo, B. (1995). Designing an effective clinical pathway for stroke. *American Journal of Nursing, 95*(3), 44-51.

Jarvis, C. (2000). *Physical examination and health assessment* (3rd ed.). Philadelphia: WB Saunders.

Lehne, R. A. (2001). *Pharmacology for nursing care* (4th ed.). Philadelphia: WB Saunders.

Monahan, F. D., & Neighbors, M. (1998). *Medical-surgical nursing foundations for clinical practice* (2nd ed.). Philadelphia: WB Saunders.

Pulsinelli, P. A. (2000). Ischemic cerebrovascular disease. In J. C. Bennett & F. Plum (Eds.), *Cecil textbook of medicine* (21st ed., pp. 2099-2109). Philadelphia: WB Saunders.

Senelick, R.C., Rossi, P. W., & Dougherty, K. (1999). Living with stroke: A guide for families. HealthSouth Press.

Weinsier, R. L. (2000). Diet. In L. Goldman & J. C. Bennett (Eds.), *Cecil textbook of medicine* (21st ed., pp. 29-31). Philadelphia: WB Saunders.

INTERNET RESOURCE

National Stroke Association: http://www.stroke.org

Chapter 28

Barker, E. (2002). *Neuroscience nursing: A spectrum of care.* St. Louis: Mosby.

Bruegge, M. V. (1997). Assessment of clients with neurologic disorders. In J. M. Black & E. Matassarin-Jacobs (Eds.), *Medical-surgical nursing: Clinical management for continuity of care* (5th ed., pp. 709-742). Philadelphia: WB Saunders.

Carson, P. (1997). Nursing care of clients with disorders of the spinal cord, peripheral nerves, and cranial nerves. In J. M. Black & E. Matassarin-Jacob (Eds.), *Medical-surgical nursing: Clinical management for continuity of care* (5th ed., pp. 890-932). Philadelphia: WB Saunders.

French, J. K., & Phillips, J. A. (1991). Shattered images: Recovery for the SCI client. *Rehabilitation Nursing, 16*(13), 134-136.

Hodgson, B. B., & Kizior, R. J. (1999). *Nurse's drug handbook.* Philadelphia: WB Saunders.

Huston, C. J. (1998). Cervical spine injury. *American Journal of Nursing, 98*(6), 33.

Ignatavicius, D. D., Workman, M. L., & Mishler, M. A. (1995). *Medical-surgical nursing: A nursing process approach* (2nd ed.). Philadelphia: WB Saunders.

Jarvis, C. (1996). *Physical examination and health assessment* (2nd ed.). Philadelphia: WB Saunders.

Kanacki, L. (1997). How to guide ventilator-dependent patients from hospital to home. *American Journal of Nursing, 97*(2), 37-39.

Luckmann, J. (1997). *Saunders manual of nursing care.* Philadelphia: WB Saunders.

Zejdlik, C. P. (1992). *Management of spinal cord injury* (2nd ed.). Boston: Jones & Bartlett.

Chapter 29

Abrams, A. C. (2001). *Clinical drug therapy* (6th ed.). Philadelphia: Lippincott-Raven.

Bache, J., Armitt, C., & Gadd, C. (1998). *Practical procedures in the emergency department.* London: Mosby.

Black, J. M., Hawks, J. H., & Keene, A. M. (2001). *Medical-surgical nursing: Clinical management for positive outcomes* (6th ed.). Philadelphia: WB Saunders.

Carroll, P. (1998). Closing in on safer suctioning. *RN, 61*(5), 22-27.

Gibbar-Clements, T., Shirrell, D., Dooley, R., & Smiley, B. (2000). The challenge of warfarin therapy. *American Journal of Nursing, 100*(3), 38-40.

Horne, C., & Derrico, D. (1999). Mastering ABGs. *American Journal of Nursing, 99*(8), 26-33.

Jarvis, C. (2000). *Physical examination and health assessment* (3rd ed.). Philadelphia: WB Saunders.

Lehne, R. A. (2001). *Pharmacology for nursing care* (4th ed.). Philadelphia: WB Saunders.

Owen, A. (1998). Respiratory assessment revisited. *Nursing 98, 28*(4), 48-49.

Skidmore-Roth, L. (2002). *Mosby's nursing drug reference.* St. Louis: Mosby.

Turkoski, B. B., Lance, B. R., & Bonfiglio, M. F. (1999). *Drug information handbook for nursing* (2nd ed.). Hudson (Cleveland): Lexi-Comp Inc.

Wong, F. W. H. (1999). A new approach to ABG interpretation. *American Journal of Nursing, 99*(8), 34-36.

Chapter 30

Ambrose, M. S. (1998). Chronic dyspnea. *Nursing 98, 28*(5), 41-47.

American Cancer Society. (2001). *Cancer facts and figures 2000.* Atlanta, Ga: Author.

Benowitz, N. L. (2000). Tobacco. In L. Goldman & J. C. Bennett (Eds.), *Cecil textbook of medicine* (21st ed., pp. 33-37). Philadelphia: WB Saunders.

Carroll, P. (2001). How to intervene before asthma turns deadly. *RN, 64*(5), 52-58.

Chiramannil, A. (1998). Lung cancer. *American Journal of Nursing, 98*(4), 46-47.

Drazen, J. M. (2000). Asthma. In L. Goldman & J. C. Bennett (Eds.), *Cecil textbook of medicine* (21st ed., pp. 387-393. Philadelphia: WB Saunders.

Heuther, S. E., & McCance, K. L. (2000). *Understanding pathophysiology.* St. Louis: Mosby.

Ignatavicius, D. D., & Hausman, K. A. (1995). *Clinical pathways for collaborative practice.* Philadelphia: WB Saunders.

Jones, L., & Hannum, D. (1998). Playing it safe with a particulate respirator. *Nursing 98, 28*(1), 50-51.

Lehne, R. A. (2001). *Pharmacology for nursing care* (4th ed.). Philadelphia: WB Saunders.

Lewis, S. M., Heitkemper, M. M., & Dirksen, S. R. (Eds.). (2000). *Medical-surgical nursing: assessment and management of clinical problems* (5th ed., Chaps. 24, 26, 27). St. Louis: Mosby.

Miller, Y. E. (2000). Pulmonary neoplasms. In L. Goldman & J. C. Bennett (Eds.), *Cecil textbook of medicine* (21st ed., pp. 449-454). Philadelphia: WB Saunders.

Monahans, F. D., & Neighbors, M. (1998). *Medical-surgical nursing foundations for clinical practice* (2nd ed.). Philadelphia: WB Saunders.

Owen, C. L. (1999). New directions in asthma management. *American Journal of Nursing, 99*(3), 26-33.

Reilly, J.J., & Mentzer, S. J. (2000). Surgical approach to lung disease. In L. Goldman & J. C. Bennett (Eds.), *Cecil textbook of medicine* (21st ed., pp. 475-479). Philadelphia: WB Saunders.

Rodarte, J. R. (2000). Chronic bronchitis and emphysema. In L. Goldman & J. C. Bennett (Eds.), *Cecil textbook of medicine* (21st ed., pp. 393-401). Philadelphia: WB Saunders.

Skidmore-Roth, L. (2002). *Mosby's nursing drug reference.* St. Louis: Mosby.

Ward-Collins, D. (1998). Noncompliance: Isn't there a better way to say it? *American Journal of Nursing, 98*(5), 26-32.

Weinberger, S. E. (2000). Sarcoidosis. In L. Goldman & J. C. Bennett (Eds.), *Cecil textbook of medicine* (21st ed., pp. 433-436). Philadelphia: WB Saunders.

Welsh, M. J. (2000). Cystic fibrosis. In L. Goldman & J. C. Bennett (Eds.), *Cecil textbook of medicine* (21st ed., pp. 401-405). Philadelphia: WB Saunders.

Chapter 31

American Association of Blood Banks, America's Blood Centers, & American Red Cross. (2000). *Circular of information for the use of human blood and blood components* (Stock number 003011OL01). Available on the American Association of Blood Banks web site, http://www.aabb.org/all_about_blood/coi/aabb_coi.htm.

Braunwald, E., Fauci, A. S., Kasper, D. L., Hauser, S. L., Longo, D. L., & Jameson, J. L. (2001). *Harrison's principles of internal medicine* (15th ed.). New York: McGraw-Hill.

DeVita, V. T., Jr., Hellman, S., & Rosenberg, S. A. (2001). *Cancer: principles and practice of oncology* (6th ed.). Philadelphia: Lippincott-Raven.

Eliopoulos, C. (1999). *Integrating conventional and alternative therapies.* St. Louis: Mosby.

Fischbach, F. (2000). *A manual of laboratory and diagnostic tests* (6th ed.). Philadelphia: Lippincott.

Phipps, W. J., Sands, J. K., & Marek, J. F. (1999). *Medical-surgical nursing: Concepts and clinical practice* (6th ed.). St. Louis: Mosby.

Shannon, M. T., Wilson, B. A., & Stang, C. L. (2002). *Health professional's drug guide 2002.* Upper Saddle River, NJ: Prentice Hall.

Yarbro, C. H., Frogge, M. H., Goodman, M., & Groenwald, S. L. (2000). *Cancer nursing: Principles and practice* (5th ed.). Philadelphia: WB Saunders.

Young-McCaughan, S., & Jennings, B. M. (1998). Hematologic and immunologic systems. In J. G. Alspach (Ed.), *Core curriculum for critical care nursing* (5th ed., pp. 601-646). Philadelphia: WB Saunders.

Chapter 32

American Cancer Society. (2001). *Cancer facts and figures—2001.* Atlanta, Ga: Author.

Braunwald, E., Fauci, A. S., Kasper, D. L., Hauser, S. L., Longo, D. L., & Jameson, J. L. (2001). *Harrison's principles of internal medicine* (15th ed.). New York: McGraw-Hill.

Bush, M. (2000). Nursing management: arthritis and connective tissue disorders. In S. M. Lewis, M. M. Heitkemper, & S. R. Dirksen (Eds.), *Medical-surgical nursing: Assessment and management of clinical problems* (5th ed., pp. 1819-1861). St. Louis: Mosby.

Casciato, D. A., & Lowitz, B. B. (2000). *Manual of clinical oncology* (4th ed.). Boston: Little, Brown.

DeVita, V. T., Jr., Hellman, S., & Rosenberg, S. A. (2001). *Cancer: Principles and practice of oncology* (6th ed.). Philadelphia: Lippincott-Raven.

Eliopoulos, C. (1999). *Integrating conventional and alternative therapies.* St. Louis: Mosby.

Fischbach, F. (2000). *A manual of laboratory and diagnostic tests* (6th ed.). Philadelphia: Lippincott.

Fischer, D. S., Knobf, M. T., & Durivage, H. J. (1997). *Cancer chemotherapy handbook* (5th ed.). St. Louis: Mosby.

Janeway, C. A., Travers, P., Walport, M., & Shlomchik, M. (2001). *Immunobiology: The immune system in health and disease* (5th ed.). London, UK: Current Biology Limited & Garland Publishing.

Lehne, R. A. (2001). *Pharmacology and nursing care* (4th ed.). Philadelphia: WB Saunders.

Miaskowski, C., & Buchsel P. (1999). *Mosby's comprehensive clinical manual of oncology nursing.* St Louis: Mosby.

Phipps, W. J., Sands, J. K., & Marek, J. F. (1999). *Medical-surgical nursing: Concepts and clinical practice* (6th ed.). St. Louis: Mosby.

Shannon, M. T., Wilson, B. A., & Stang, C. L. (2002). *Health professional's drug guide 2002.* Upper Saddle River, NJ: Prentice Hall.

Stites, D. P., Terr, A. I., Parslow, T. G. (1997). *Medical immunology* (9th ed.). Norwalk, Conn: Appleton & Lange.

Yarbro, C. H., Frogge, M. H., Goodman, M., & Groenwald, S. L. (2000). *Cancer nursing: Principles and practice* (5th ed.). Philadelphia: WB Saunders.

Young-McCaughan, S., & Jennings, B. M. (1998). Hematologic and immunologic systems. In J. G. Alspach (Ed.), *Core curriculum for critical care nursing* (5th ed., pp. 601-646). Philadelphia: WB Saunders.

Chapter 33

American Heart Association. (2001). *ACLS provider manual.* The Association.

American Heart Association website: http://www.americanheart.org.

Ballard, J. C., Wood, L. L., & Lansing, A. M. (1997). Transmyocardial revascularization: Criteria for selecting patients, treatment, and nursing care. *Critical Care Nurse, 17*(1), 42-49.

Bernstein A. D., & Parsonnet, V. (1995). Pacemaker and defibrillator codes. In K. A. Ellenbogen, G. N. Kay, & B. L. Wilkoff. *Clinical cardiac pacing* (pp. 279-283). Philadelphia: WB Saunders.

DeJong, M. J. (1998). Clinical snapshot: Infective endocarditis. *American Journal of Nursing, 98*(5), 34-35.

Dugan, K. J. (1998). Caring for patients with pericarditis. *Nursing 98, 28*(3), 50-51.

Edgar, W. F., Ebersole, N., & Mayfield, M. G. (1999). MIDCAB. *American Journal of Nursing, 99*(7), 40-46.

Gulanick, M. (1998). Cardiac rehabilitation nursing: Changing needs, roles, and direction. *American Journal of Nursing, 98*(2), 49-51.

Halm, M. A., & Penque, S. (1999). Heart disease in women. *American Journal of Nursing, 99*(4), 26-32.

Hodge, P., & Ullrich, S. (1999). Does your assessment include alternative therapies? *RN, 62*(6), 47-49.

House-Fancher, M. A., & Martinez, L. G. (2000). Congestive heart failures and cardiac surgery. In S. M. Lewis, M. M. Heitkemper, & S. R. Ruff (Eds.), *Medical-surgical nursing* (5th ed., pp. 793-816). St. Louis: Mosby.

Ignatavicius, D. D., Workman, M. L., & Mishler, M. A. (1999). *Medical-surgical nursing across the health care continuum* (3rd ed.). Philadelphia: WB Saunders.

Lehne, R. A. (2001). *Pharmacology for nursing care* (4th ed.). Philadelphia: WB Saunders.

Lezon, K. (1998). Code blue: Defibrillate. *Nursing 98, 28*(4), 58-60.

Martinez, L. G., & House-Fancher, M. A. (2000). Coronary artery disease. In S. M. Lewis, M. M. Heitkemper, & S. R. Ruff (Eds.), *Medical-surgical nursing* (5th ed., pp. 841-886). St. Louis: Mosby.

Matteson, M. A., McConnell, E. S., & Linton, A. D. (1996). *Gerontological nursing* (2nd ed.). Philadelphia: WB Saunders.

Mizell, J. L., Maglish, B. L., & Mathery, R. G. (1997). Minimally invasive direct coronary artery bypass graft surgery. *Critical Care Nurse, 17*(3), 46-55.

O'Brien, L. (1998). Clinical snapshot: Angina pectoris. *American Journal of Nursing, 98*(1), 48-49.

Platek, Y. M., & Atzori, M. (1999). PTMR. *American Journal of Nursing, 9*(7), 64-66.

Ralstin, A. M. (2000). Cardiovascular system. In S. M. Lewis, M. M. Heitkemper, & S. R. Ruff (Eds.), *Medical-surgical nursing* (5th ed., pp. 793-816). St. Louis: Mosby.

Rockwell, J. M. (1999). Heart failure (Critical Care Extra). *American Journal of Nursing, 99*(10), 24 BB, 24 DD, 24 FF, 24 HH.

Siomko, A. J. (2000). Demystifying cardiac markers. *American Journal of Nursing, 100*(1), 36-41.

Wilson, D. E., & Tracy, M. F. (2000). CABG and the elderly (Critical Care Extra). *American Journal of Nursing, 100*(5), 24 AA, 24 DD, 24FF, 24 HH, 24

Chapter 34

Benowitz, N. L. (2000). Tobacco. In L. Goldman & J. C. Bennett (Eds.), *Cecil textbook of medicine* (21st ed., pp. 33-37). Philadelphia: WB Saunders.

Chernecky, C. C., & Berger, B. J. (2001). *Laboratory tests and diagnostic procedures.* (3rd ed.). Philadelphia: WB Saunders.

Daugherty, J. (2000). Vascular disorders: Nursing management. In Lewis, S. M., Heitkemper, M. M., & Dirksen, S. D. (Eds.), *Medical-surgical nursing: Assessment and management of clinical problems* (5th ed., pp. 378-1009). St. Louis: Mosby.

Deglin, J. H., & Vallerand, A. H. (2001). *Davis's drug guide for nurses* (7th ed.). Philadelphia: FA Davis.

Herlihy, B., & Maebius, N. K. (2000). *The human body in health and illness.* Philadelphia: WB Saunders.

Hiatt, W. R. (2000). Atherosclerotic peripheral arterial disease. In L. Goldman & J. C. Bennett (Eds.), *Cecil textbook of medicine* (21st ed., pp. 357-362). Philadelphia: WB Saunders.

Hull, R. D. (2000). Peripheral venous disease. In L. Goldman & J. C. Bennett (Eds.), *Cecil textbook of medicine* (21st ed., pp. 367-372). Philadelphia: WB Saunders.

Ignatavicius, D. D., Workman, M. L., & Mishler, M. A. (1999). *Medical-surgical nursing across the health care continuum* (3rd ed.). Philadelphia: WB Saunders.

Lehne, R. A. (2001). *Pharmacology for nursing care* (4th ed.). Philadelphia: WB Saunders.

Leifer, G. (2001). Hyperbaric oxygen therapy. *American Journal of Nursing, 101*(8), 26-35.

Matteson, M. A., McConnell, E. S., & Linton, A. D. (Eds.). (1997). *Gerontological nursing* (2nd ed.). Philadelphia: WB Saunders.

Olin, J. W. (2000). Other peripheral arterial diseases. In L. Goldman & J. C. Bennett (Eds.), *Cecil textbook of medicine* (21st ed., pp. 362-367). Philadelphia: WB Saunders.

Skidmore-Roth, L. (2002). *Mosby's nursing drug reference 2002.* St. Louis: Mosby.

Chapter 35

Abrams, A. C. (2001). *Clinical drug therapy* (6th ed.). Philadelphia: Lippincott.

Hurley, M. L. (1998). New hypertension guidelines. *RN, 61*(3), 25-28.

Lehne, R. A. (2001). *Pharmacology for nursing care.* Philadelphia: WB Saunders.

Matteson, M. A., McConnell, E. S., & Linton, A. D. (1997). *Gerontological nursing* (2nd ed.), Philadelphia: WB Saunders.

National High Blood Pressure Education Program. (1999). *Statement from the national high blood pressure education program.* Retrieved from http://www.nhlbi.nih.gov/health/prof/heart/hbp/salt_up2.htm. on July 9, 2001.

National Institutes of Health. (1997). *The sixth report of the Joint National Committee on Prevention, Detection, Evaluation, and Treatment of High Blood Pressure* (NIH Pub. No. 98-4080). Bethesda, Md: Author.

Skidmore-Roth, L. (2002). *Mosby's nursing drug reference.* St. Louis: Mosby.

Ward-Collins, D. (1998). Noncompliance: Isn't there a better way to say it? *American Journal of Nursing, 98*(5), 26-32.

Chapter 36

Black, J. M., Hawks, J. H., & Keene, A. M. (2001). *Medical-surgical nursing: Clinical management for continuity of care* (6th ed.). Philadelphia: WB Saunders.

Chernecky, C. C., & Berger, B. J. (2001). *Laboratory tests and diagnostic procedures* (3rd ed.). Philadelphia: WB Saunders.

Cohen, S., & Parkman, H. P. (2000). Diseases of the esophagus. In L. Goldman & J. C. Bennett (Eds.), *Cecil textbook of medicine* (21st ed., pp. 658-668). Philadelphia: WB Saunders.

Deglin, J. H., & Vallerand, A. H. (1999). *Davis's drug guide for nurses* (7th ed.). Philadelphia: FA Davis.

Eliopoulos, C. (1999). *Integrating conventional and alternative therapies.* St. Louis: Mosby.

Graham, D. Y. (2000). Peptic therapy: Medical therapy. In L. Goldman & J. C. Bennett (Eds.), *Cecil textbook of medicine* (21st ed., pp. 675-678). Philadelphia: WB Saunders.

Ignatavicius, D. D., Workman, M. L., & Mishler, M. A. (1999). *Medical-surgical nursing across the health care continuum* (3rd ed.). Philadelphia: WB Saunders.

Jarvis, C. (2000). *Physical examination and health assessment* (3rd ed.). Philadelphia: WB Saunders.

Lehne, R. A. (2001). *Pharmacology for nursing care* (4th ed.). Philadelphia: WB Saunders.

Matteson, M. A., McConnell, E. S., & Linton, A. D. (1997). *Gerontological nursing* (2nd ed.). Philadelphia: WB Saunders.

Rustgi, A. K. (2000). Neoplasms of the stomach. In L. Goldman & J. C. Bennett (Eds.), *Cecil textbook of medicine* (21st ed., pp. 738-741). Philadelphia: WB Saunders.

Semrad, C. E., & Chang, E. B. (2000). Malabsorption syndromes. In L. Goldman & J. C. Bennett (Eds.), *Cecil textbook of medicine* (21st ed., pp. 712-722). Philadelphia: WB Saunders.

Snape, W. J. (2000). Disorders of gastrointestinal motility. In L. Goldman & J. C. Bennett (Eds.), *Cecil textbook of medicine* (21st ed., pp. 694-702). Philadelphia: WB Saunders.

Soll, A. H. (2000). Gastritis and Helicobacter pylori. In L. Goldman & J. C. Bennett (Eds.), *Cecil textbook of medicine* (21st ed., pp. 694-702). Philadelphia: WB Saunders.

Soll, A. H. (2000). Peptic ulcer disease: epidemiology, pathophysiology, clinical manifestations, and diagnosis. In L. Goldman & J. C. Bennett (Eds.), *Cecil textbook of medicine* (21st ed., pp. 671-675). Philadelphia: WB Saunders.

Stenson, W. F. (2000). Inflammatory bowel disease. In L. Goldman & J. C. Bennett (Eds.), *Cecil textbook of medicine* (21st ed., pp. 722-729). Philadelphia: WB Saunders.

Wilcox, C. M. (2000). Miscellaneous inflammatory diseases of the intestine. In L. Goldman & J. C. Bennett (Eds.), *Cecil textbook of medicine* (21st ed., pp. 729-732). Philadelphia: WB Saunders.

Chapter 37

Chernecky, C. C., & Berger, B. J. (2001). *Laboratory tests and diagnostic procedures* (3rd ed.). Philadelphia: WB Saunders.

Diehl, A. M. (2000). Acute and chronic failure and hepatic encephalopathy. In L. Goldman & J. C. Bennett (Eds.), *Cecil textbook of medicine* (21st ed., pp. 813-816). Philadelphia: WB Saunders.

DiMagno, E. P. (2000). Carcinoma of the pancreas. In L. Goldman & J. C. Bennett (Eds.), *Cecil textbook of medicine* (21st ed., pp. 750-752). Philadelphia: WB Saunders.

Eliopoulos, C. (1999). *Integrating conventional and alternative therapies.* St. Louis: Mosby.

Elrod, R. (2000). Nursing management: Liver, biliary tract, and pancreas problems. In S. M. Lewis, M. M. Heitkemper, & S. R. Dirksen (Eds.), *Medical-surgical nursing: Assessment and management of clinical problems* (5th ed., pp. 1191-1237). Philadelphia: WB Saunders.

Fallon, M. (2000). Hepatic tumors. In L. Goldman & J. C. Bennett (Eds.), *Cecil textbook of medicine* (21st ed., pp. 819-821). Philadelphia: WB Saunders.

Friedman, S. L. (2000). Alcoholic liver disease, cirrhosis, and its major sequelae. In L. Goldman and J. C. Bennett (Eds.), *Cecil textbook of medicine* (21st ed., pp. 804-812). Philadelphia: WB Saunders.

Guyton, A. C., & Hall, J. E. (1996). *Textbook of medical physiology* (9th ed.). Philadelphia: WB Saunders.

Hoofnagle, J. H., & Lindsay, K. L. (2000). Acute viral hepatitis. In L. Goldman & J. C. Bennett (Eds.), *Cecil textbook of medicine* (21st ed., pp. 783-790). Philadelphia: WB Saunders.

Ignatavicius, D. D., Workman, M. L., & Mishler, M. A. (1999). *Medical-surgical nursing across the health care continuum* (3rd ed.). Philadelphia: WB Saunders.

Jarvis, C. (2000). *Physical examination and health assessment* (3rd ed.). Philadelphia: WB Saunders.

Lehne, R. A. (2001). *Pharmacology for nursing care* (4th ed.). Philadelphia: WB Saunders.

Mahan, L. K., & Escott-Stump, S. (2000). *Krause's food, nutrition, and diet therapy* (10th ed.). Philadelphia: WB Saunders.

Roberts, J. P. (2000). Liver transplantation. In L. Goldman & J. C. Bennett (Eds.), *Cecil textbook of medicine* (21st ed., pp. 816-817). Philadelphia: WB Saunders

Schmid, R. E. (September 2, 2001). Hispanics get cirrhosis alert. *San Antonio Express News.* Page 10A.

Soergel, K. H. (2000). Pancreatitis. In L. Goldman & J. C. Bennett (Eds.), *Cecil textbook of medicine* (21st ed., pp. 752-759). Philadelphia: WB Saunders

INTERNET RESOURCE

Division of Gastroenterology at the University of California, San Francisco: http://www.sadieo.ucsf.edu

Chapter 38

Bates, P. (2000). Nursing management: Renal and urologic problems. In S. M. Lewis, M. M. Heitkemper, & S. R. Dirksen (Eds.), *Medical-surgical nursing: Assessment and management of clinical problems* (5th ed., pp. 1261-1298). Philadelphia: WB Saunders.

Brunier, G., & Bartucci, M. (2000). Nursing management: Acute and chronic renal failure. In S. M. Lewis, M. M. Heitkemper, & S. R. Dirksen (Eds.), *Medical-surgical nursing: Assessment and management of clinical problems* (5th ed., pp. 1299-1341). Philadelphia: WB Saunders.

Curtis, J. J. (2000). Treatment of irreversible renal failure. In L. Goldman & J. C. Bennett (Eds.), *Cecil textbook of medicine* (21st ed., pp. 578-586). Philadelphia: WB Saunders.

Eliopoulos, C. (1999). *Integrating conventional and alternative therapies.* St. Louis: Mosby.

Ignatavicius, D. D., Workman, M. L., & Mishler, M. A. (1999). *Medical-surgical nursing across the health care continuum* (3rd ed.). Philadelphia: WB Saunders.

Jarvis, C. (2000). *Physical examination and health assessment* (3rd ed.). Philadelphia: WB Saunders.

Lehne, R. A. (2001). *Pharmacology for nursing care* (4th ed.). Philadelphia: WB Saunders.

Luke, R. G. (2000). Chronic renal failure. In L. Goldman & J. C. Bennett (Eds.), *Cecil textbook of medicine* (21st ed., pp. 571-578). Philadelphia: WB Saunders.

Mitch, W. E. (2000). Acute renal failure. In L. Goldman & J. C. Bennett (Eds.), *Cecil textbook of medicine* (21st ed., pp. 567-571). Philadelphia: WB Saunders.

Shapiro, C. L., Garnick, M. B., & Kantoff, P. W. (2000). Tumors of the kidneys, ureter, and bladder. In L. Goldman & J. C. Bennett (Eds.), *Cecil textbook of medicine* (21st ed., pp. 631-635). Philadelphia: WB Saunders.

Chapter 39

Arnett, F. C. (2001). Rheumatoid arthritis. In L. Goldman & J. C. Bennett (Eds.), *Cecil textbook of medicine* (21st ed., pp. 1492-1499). Philadelphia: WB Saunders.

Ball, E. V. (2001). Behçet's disease. In L. Goldman & J. C. Bennett (Eds.), *Cecil textbook of medicine* (21st ed., pp. 1540-1541). Philadelphia: WB Saunders.

Ball, E. V. (2001). Nonarticular rheumatism. In L. Goldman & J. C. Bennett (Eds.), *Cecil textbook of medicine* (21st ed., pp. 1559-1560). Philadelphia: WB Saunders.

Black, J. M., Hawks, J. H., & Keene, A. M., (2001). *Medical-surgical nursing: Clinical management for positive outcomes* (6th ed.). Philadelphia: WB Saunders.

Calkins, E., & Vladutiu, A. O. (1998). Musculoskeletal disorders. In E. H. Duthie & P. R. Katz (Eds.), *Practice of geriatrics* (3rd ed., pp. 421-435). Philadelphia: WB Saunders.

Chernecky, C. C., & Berger, B. J. (2001). *Laboratory tests and diagnostic procedures* (3rd ed.). Philadelphia: WB Saunders.

Cush, J. J., & Lipsky, P. E. (2001). The spondyloarthropathies. In L. Goldman & J. C. Bennett (Eds.), *Cecil textbook of medicine* (21st ed., pp. 1499-1507). Philadelphia: WB Saunders.

Geissler, E. (1998). *Mosby's pocket guide to cultural assessment* (2nd ed.). St. Louis: Mosby.

Goldman, L., & Bennett, J. C., (2001). *Cecil textbook of medicine* (21st ed.). Philadelphia: WB Saunders.

Hershfield, M. S. (2001). Gout and uric acid metabolism. In L. Goldman & J. C. Bennett (Eds.), *Cecil textbook of medicine* (21st ed., pp. 1541-1548). Philadelphia: WB Saunders.

Hochberg, M. C. (2001). Sjögren's syndrome. In L. Goldman & J. C. Bennett (Eds.), *Cecil textbook of medicine* (21st ed., pp. 1522-1524). Philadelphia: WB Saunders.

Hodgson, B. B., & Kizior, R. J. (2000). *Saunders nursing drug handbook 2000.* Philadelphia: WB Saunders.

Jacob, S. W., & Francone, C. A. (1989). *Elements of anatomy and physiology* (2nd ed.). Philadelphia: WB Saunders.

Jarvis, C. (2000). *Health assessment and physical examination* (3rd ed.). Philadelphia: WB Saunders.

Lehne, R. A. (2001). *Pharmacology for nursing care* (4th ed.). Philadelphia: WB Saunders.

Mahan, L. K., & Escott-Stump, S. (2000). *Krause's food, nutrition and diet therapy* (10th ed.). Philadelphia: WB Saunders.

Monahan, F. D., & Neighbors, M. (1998). *Medical-surgical nursing* (2nd ed.). Philadelphia: WB Saunders.

Ruddy, S., Harris, E. D., Jr., & Sledge, C. B. (2001) *Kelley's textbook of rheumatology* (6th ed.). Philadelphia: WB Saunders.

Schnitzer, T. J. (2001). Osteoarthritis (degenerative bone disease). In L. Goldman & J. C. Bennett (Eds.), *Cecil textbook of medicine* (21st ed., pp. 1550-1554). Philadelphia: WB Saunders.

Sculco, T. P. (1998). Orthopedic disorders. In E. H. Duthie & P. R. Katz (Eds.), *Practice of geriatrics* (3rd ed., pp. 436-447). Philadelphia: WB Saunders.

Seton. (2001). New applications of technology relieve back pain without surgery. *Good Health* (pp. 28-29). Austin Tx: Author.

Wortman, R. L. (2001). Idiopathic inflammatory myopathies. In L. Goldman & J. C. Bennett (Eds.), *Cecil textbook of medicine* (21st ed., pp. 1534-1538). Philadelphia: WB Saunders.

Chapter 40

Maher, A. B., Salmond, S. W., & Pellino, T. A. (1998). *Orthopaedic nursing* (2nd ed.). Philadelphia: WB Saunders.

Monahan, F. D., & Neighbors, M. (1998). *Medical-surgical nursing* (2nd ed.). Philadelphia: WB Saunders.

Ruda, S. C. (2000). Nursing management of musculoskeletal disorders. In S. M. Lewis, M. M. Heitkemper, & S. D. Dirksen (Eds.) *Medical-surgical nursing: Assessment and management of clinical problems* (5th ed., pp. 1762-1818). Philadelphia: WB Saunders.

Sculco, T. P. (1998). Orthopedic disorders. In E. H. Guthrie & P. R. Katz (Eds.), *Practice of geriatrics* (3rd ed., pp. 436-447). Philadelphia: WB Saunders.

Tapson, V. F. (2000). Pulmonary embolism. In L. Goldman & J. C. Bennett (Eds.), *Cecil textbook of medicine* (21st ed., p. 441-448). Philadelphia: WB Saunders.

Chapter 41

Chernecky, C. C., & Berger, B. J. (2001). *Laboratory tests and diagnostic procedures* (3rd ed.). Philadelphia: WB Saunders.

Monahan, F. D., & Neighbors, M. A. (1998). *Medical-surgical nursing: Foundations for clinical practice* (2nd ed., pp. 837-886). Philadelphia: WB Saunders.

Nunnelee, J. D. (2001). Management of clients with vascular disorders. In J. M. Black, J. H. Hawks, & A. M. Keene (Eds.), *Medical-surgical nursing: Clinical management for positive outcomes* (6th ed., pp. 1399-1432). Philadelphia: WB Saunders.

Ruda, S. C. (2000). Nursing management: Musculoskeletal problems. In S. M. Lewis, M. M. Heitkemper, & S. R. Dirksen (Eds.). *Medical-surgical nursing: Assessment and management of clinical problems* (5th ed., pp. 1762-1818). St. Louis: Mosby

Williamson, V. (1998). Amputation. In A. B. Maher, S. W. Salmond, & T. A. Pellino (Eds.), *Orthopaedic nursing* (2nd ed., pp. 718-745). Philadelphia: WB Saunders.

Chapter 42

Black, J. M., & Matassarin-Jacobs, E. (1997). *Medical-surgical nursing: Clinical management for continuity of care* (5th ed.). Philadelphia: WB Saunders.

Clayton, L. H., & Dilley, K. B. (1998). Clinical snapshot: Cushing's syndrome. *American Journal of Nursing, (98)*7, 40-41.

Deglin, J. H., & Vallerand, A. H. (2001). *Davis's drug guide for nurses* (7th ed.). Philadelphia: FA Davis.

Eliopoulos, C. (1999). *Integrating conventional and alternative therapies.* St. Louis: Mosby.

Ignatavicius, D. D., Workman, M. L., & Mishler, M. (1999). *Medical-surgical nursing across the health continuum* (3rd ed.). Philadelphia: WB Saunders.

Kokko, J. P. (2000). Fluids and electrolytes. In L. Goldman & J. C. Bennett (Eds.), *Cecil textbook of medicine* (21st ed., pp. 540-567). Philadelphia: WB Saunders.

Lehne, R. A. (2001). *Pharmacology and nursing care* (6th ed.). Philadelphia: WB Saunders.

Loriaux, D. L. (2000). The adrenal cortex. In L. Goldman & J. C. Bennett (Eds.), *Cecil textbook of medicine* (21st ed., pp. 1250-1257). Philadelphia: WB Saunders.

Jarvis, C. (1996). *Physical examination and health assessment* (2nd ed., pp. 1205-1221). Philadelphia: WB Saunders.

Matteson, M. A., McConnell, E. S., & Linton, A. D. (Eds.). (1997). *Gerontological nursing* (2nd ed.). Philadelphia: WB Saunders.

Molitch, M. E. (2000). Anterior pituitary. In L. Goldman & J. C. Bennett (Eds.), *Cecil textbook of medicine* (21st ed., pp. 1208-1225). Philadelphia: WB Saunders.

O'Connor, D. T. (2000). The adrenal medulla, catecholamines, and pheochromocytoma. In L. Goldman & J. C. Bennett (Eds.), *Cecil textbook of medicine* (21st ed., pp. 1257-1262). Philadelphia: WB Saunders.

Chapter 43

Black, J. M., & Matassarin-Jacobs, E. (1997). *Medical-surgical nursing: Clinical management for continuity of care* (5th ed.). Philadelphia: WB Saunders.

Dillman, W. H. (2000). The thyroid. In L. Goldman & J. C. Bennett (Eds.), *Cecil textbook of medicine* (21st ed., pp. 1231-1250). Philadelphia: WB Saunders.

Ignatavicius, D. D., Workman, M. L., & Mishler, M. A. (1995). *Medical-surgical nursing: A nursing process approach* (2nd ed.). Philadelphia: WB Saunders.

Lehne, R. A. (1994). *Pharmacology for nursing care* (2nd ed.). Philadelphia: WB Saunders.

Matteson, M. A., McConnell, E. S., & Linton, A. D. (1997). *Gerontological nursing* (2nd ed.). Philadelphia: WB Saunders.

Skidmore, L. (2002). *Mosby's nursing drug reference.* St. Louis: Mosby.

Spiegel, A. M. (2000). The parathyroid glands, hypercalcemia, and hypocalcemia. In L. Goldman & J. C. Bennett (Eds.), *Cecil textbook of medicine* (21st ed., pp. 1398-1406). Philadelphia: WB Saunders.

Chapter 44

Abrams, A. C. (2001). *Clinical drug therapy* (6th ed.). Philadelphia: Lippincott.

Black, J. M., Hawks, J. H., & Keene, A. M. (2001). *Medical-surgical nursing: Clinical management for continuity of care* (6th ed.). Philadelphia: WB Saunders.

Cypress, M. (2001). Diabetes update: Acute complications. *RN, 64*(4), 26-32.

Davidson, M. B. (1998). *Diabetes mellitus diagnosis and treatment* (4th ed.). Philadelphia: WB Saunders.

Deglin, J. H., & Vallerand, A. H. (2001). *Davis's drug guide for nurses* (7th ed.). Philadelphia: FA Davis.

Fain, J. A. (2001). Management of clients with diabetes mellitus. In J. M. Black, J. H. Hawks, & A. M. Keene (Eds.), *Medical-surgical nursing: Clinical management for positive outcomes* (6th ed., pp. 1149-1191). Philadelphia: WB Saunders.

Flier, J. S. (1996). Hypoglycemia/pancreatic islet cell disorders. In J. C. Bennett & F. Plum (Eds.), *Cecil textbook of medicine* (20th ed., pp. 1278-1282). Philadelphia: WB Saunders.

Goldberg, J. M. (2001). Nutrition and exercise. *RN, 64*(7), 34-40.

Halpin-Landry, J. E., & Goldsmith, S. (1999). Feet first: Diabetes care. *American Journal of Nursing, 99*(2), 26-34.

Hernandez, D. (1998). Microvascular complications of diabetes. *American Journal of Nursing, 98*(6), 26-31.

Knight, J. (1998). Inserting an insulin catheter. *Nursing 98, 28*(2), 58-60.

Plummer, E. S. (2001). Diabetes update: Chronic complications. *RN, 64*(5), 34-42.

Robertson, C. (2001). Diabetes update: The untold story of disease progression. *RN, 64*(3), 60-65.

Sammer, C. E. (2001). How should you respond to hypoglycemia? *Nursing 2001, 31*(7), 48-50.

Sherwin, R. S. (2000). Diabetes mellitus. In L. Goldman & J. C. Bennett (Eds.), *Cecil textbook of medicine* (21st ed., pp. 1263-1285). Philadelphia: WB Saunders.

Valentine, V. (2000). Nursing management: Patient with diabetes mellitus. In S. M. Lewis, M. M. Heitkemper, & S. R. Dirksen (Eds.), *Medical-surgical nursing: Assessment and management of clinical problems* (5th ed., pp. 1367-1405). St. Louis: Mosby.

Chapter 45

American Cancer Society. *Cancer facts and figures—2000.* Atlanta, Ga: Author.

Dell, D. (2001). Regaining range of motion after breast surgery. *Nursing 2001, 31*(10), 50-52.

Duthie, E. H., & Katz, P. R. (1998). *Practice of geriatrics* (3rd ed.). Philadelphia: WB Saunders.

Eliopoulos, C. (1999). *Conventional and alternative therapies.* St. Louis: Mosby.

Hoskins, C. N., & Haber, J. (2000). Adjusting to breast cancer. *The American Journal of Nursing, 100*(4), 26-33.

Ignatavicius, D. D., Workman, M. L., & Mishler, M. A. (1999). *Medical-surgical nursing: A nursing process approach* (3rd ed.). Philadelphia: WB Saunders.

Jones, H. W. (2000). Ovarian carcinoma. In L. Goldman & J. C. Bennett (Eds.), *Cecil textbook of medicine* (21st ed., pp. 1381-1382). Philadelphia: WB Saunders.

Lehne, R. A. (2001). *Pharmacology for nursing care* (4th ed.). Philadelphia: WB Saunders.

Machia, J. (2001). Breast cancer: Risk prevention, and tamoxifen. *American Journal of Nursing, 101*(4), 26-35.

Monahan, F. D., & Neighbors, M. (1998). *Medical-surgical nursing* (2nd ed.). Philadelphia: WB Saunders.

Muss, H. B. (2000). Breast cancer and differential diagnosis of benign nodules. In L. Goldman & J. C. Bennett (Eds.), *Cecil textbook of medicine* (21st ed., pp. 1373-1380). Philadelphia: WB Saunders.

Rebar, R. W. (2000). Menstrual cycle and fertility. In L. Goldman & J. C. Bennett (Eds.), *Cecil textbook of medicine* (21st ed., pp. 1327-1340). Philadelphia: WB Saunders.

Risks and benefits of estrogen plus progestin in healthy postmenopausal women. Obtained August 6, 2002 from http://www.jama.ama-assn.org/issuesv288n3/joc21036.html.

Writing group for the Women's Health Initiative investigators. *JAMA* (online) *288*(3), July 17, 2002.

Youngkin, E. Q., & Davis, M. S. (1998). *Women's health: A primary care clinical guide.* Stamford, Conn: Appleton & Lange.

Chapter 46

American Cancer Society. (2000). *Cancer facts and figures—2000.* Atlanta, Ga: Author.

Bates, P. M. (2001). Management of men with reproductive disorders. In Black, J. M., Hawks, J. H., & Keene, A. M. (Eds.), *Medical-surgical nursing: Clinical management for positive outcomes* (6th ed., pp. 945-977). Philadelphia: WB Saunders.

Eliopoulos, C. (1999). *Integrating conventional and alternative therapies.* St. Louis: Mosby.

Meredith, C. (2000). Nursing management: Male genitourinary problems. In S. M. Lewis, M. M. Heitkemper, & S. R. Dirksen (Eds.), *Medical-surgical nursing: Assessment and management of clinical problems* (5th ed., pp. 1553-1578). St. Louis: Mosby.

Partin, A. W. (2000). Diseases of the prostate. In L. Goldman & J. C. Bennett (Eds.), *Cecil textbook of medicine* (21st ed., pp. 635-642). Philadelphia: WB Saunders.

Swerdloff, R. S., & Wang, C. (2000). The testis and male sexual function. In L. Goldman & J. C. Bennett (Eds.), *Cecil textbook of medicine* (21st ed., pp. 1306-1317). Philadelphia: WB Saunders.

Chapter 47

Blair, M. (2001). Management of clients with sexually transmitted diseases. In J. M. Black, J. H. Hawks, & A M. Keene (6th ed., pp. 1041-1057. Philadelphia: WB Saunders.

Bradley-Springer, L. (2001). HIV prevention: What works? *American Journal of Nursing, 101*(6), 45-50.

Bursaw, M., Keenan, K., & Ehrhart, M. (2001). HIV update. *Nursing 2001, 31*(2), 62-63.

Esch, J. F., & Frank, S. V. (2001). Drug resistance and nursing practice. *American Journal of Nursing, 101*(6), 30-35.

Jones, S. G. (2001). Taking HAART: How to support patients with HIV/AIDS. *Nursing 2001, 31*(2), 36-41.

Lehne, R. A. (2001). Pharmacology for nursing care (4th ed.). Philadelphia: WB Saunders.

Luft, J. (2000). Nursing management: sexually transmitted diseases. In S. M. Lewis, M. M. Heitkemper, & S. R. Dirksen (Eds.), *Medical-surgical nursing: Assessment and management of clinical problems* (5th ed., pp. 1495-1510). St. Louis: Mosby.

Trzcianowska, H., & Mortensen, E. (2001). HIV and AIDS: Separating fact from fiction. *American Journal of Nursing, 101*(6), 53-59.

Unvarski, P. J. (2001). The past 20 years of AIDS. 26-29. *American Journal of Nursing, 101*(6), 26-36.

Williams, A. B. (2001). Adherence to HIV regimens: 10 vital lessons. *American Journal of Nursing, 101*(6), 37-43.

Workowski, K. A., Levine, W. C. (2002). Sexually transmitted diseases treatment guidelines. Retrieved from http://www.cdc/mmwr/preview/mmwrhtml/rr5106al.htm on May 9, 2002.

INTERNET RESOURCES

University of California, San Francisco Library: http://www.library.ucsf.edu
AIDSLINE, National Library of Medicine: http://www.healthgate.com/AMA/search.html
Centers for Disease Control and Prevention: http://www.cdc.gov

Chapter 48

Black, J. M., Hawks, J. A., & Keene, A. M. (2001). *Medical-surgical nursing: Clinical management for continuity of care* (6th ed.). Philadelphia: WB Saunders.

Cornwell, P. (2001). Management of clients with burn injury. In J. M. Black, J. H. Hawks, & A. M. Keene (Eds.), *Medical-surgical nursing: Clinical management for positive outcomes* (6th ed., pp. 1331-1359). Philadelphia: WB Saunders.

Deglin, J. H., & Vallerand, A. P. (2001). *Davis's drug guide for nurses* (7th ed.). Philadelphia: FA Davis.

Dirksen, S. R. (1999). Nursing assessment: Integumentary system. In S. M. Lewis, M. M. Heitkemper, & S. R. Dirksen (Eds.), *Medical-surgical nursing: Assessment and management of clinical problems* (5th ed., pp. 482-492). St. Louis: Mosby.

Dismukes, W. E. (2000). Candidiasis. In L. Goldman & J. C. Bennett (Eds.), *Cecil textbook of medicine* (21st ed., pp. 1871-1875). Philadelphia: WB Saunders.

Eliopoulos, C. (1999). *Integrating conventional and alternative therapies.* St. Louis: Mosby.

Goodman, M., & Mellon-Reppen, S. (2001). Management of clients with breast disorders. In J. M. Black, J. H. Hawks, & A. M. Keene (Eds.), *Medical-surgical nursing: Clinical management for positive outcomes* (6th ed., pp. 1011-1040). Philadelphia: WB Saunders.

Ignatavicius, D. D., Workman, M. L., & Mishler, M. A. (1999). *Medical-surgical nursing across the health care continuum* (3rd ed.). Philadelphia: WB Saunders.

Lehne, R. A. (2001). *Pharmacology for nursing care* (4th ed.). Philadelphia: WB Saunders.

Nicol, N. H., & Black, J. M. (2001). Management of clients with integumentary disorders. In J. M. Black, J. H. Hawks, & A. M. Keene (Eds.), *Medical-surgical nursing: Clinical management for positive outcomes* (6th ed., pp. 1279-1330). Philadelphia: WB Saunders.

Parker, F. (2000). Skin diseases of general importance. In L. Goldman & J. C. Bennett (Eds.), *Cecil textbook of medicine* (21st ed., pp. 2276-2298). Philadelphia: WB Saunders.

Shipp, M. A., & Harris, N. L. (2000). Non-Hodgkin's lymphomas. In L. Goldman & J. C. Bennett (Eds.), *Cecil textbook of medicine* (21st ed., pp. 962-969). Philadelphia: WB Saunders.

United States Army Institute of Surgical Research. (1996). *Critical path: Major burns.* Fort Sam Houston, Tx: Author.

Chapter 49

Black, J. M., & Matassarin-Jacobs, E. (2001). *Medical-surgical nursing: Clinical management for continuity of care* (5th ed.). Philadelphia: WB Saunders.

Deglin, J. H., & Vallerand, A. H. (2001). *Davis's drug guide for nurses* (7th ed.). Philadelphia: FA Davis.

Eliopoulos, C. (1999). *Integrating conventional and alternative therapies.* St. Louis: Mosby.

Fay, A., & Jakobiec, F. A. (2000). Diseases of the visual system. In L. Goldman & J. C. Bennett (Eds.), *Cecil textbook of medicine* (21st ed., pp. 2224-2235). Philadelphia: WB Saunders.

Ignatavicius, D. D., Workman, M. L., & Mishler, M. A. (1999). *Medical-surgical nursing across the health care continuum* (3rd ed.). Philadelphia: WB Saunders.

Jarvis, C. (2000). *Physical examination and health assessment* (3rd ed.). Philadelphia: WB Saunders.

Lehne, R. A. (2001). *Pharmacology for nursing care* (4th ed.). Philadelphia: WB Saunders.

Mahan, L. K., & Escott-Stump, S. (2000). *Krause's food, nutrition, & diet therapy.* Philadelphia: WB Saunders.

INTERNET RESOURCES

American Foundation for the Blind: http://www.igc.apc.org/afb/index.html
Guide Dogs for the Blind: http://www.guidedogs.com
Talking Books: National Library Service for the Blind and Visually Handicapped: http://www.lcweb.loc.gov/nls.html

Chapter 50

Baloh, R. W. (2000). Hearing and equilibrium. In L. Goldman & J. C. Bennett (Eds.), *Cecil textbook of medicine* (21st ed., pp. 2250-2257). Philadelphia: WB Saunders.

Deglin, J. H., & Vallerand, A. H. (2001). *Davis's drug guide for nurses* (7th ed.). Philadelphia: FA Davis.

Ignatavicius, D. D., Workman, M. L., & Mishler, M. (1999). *Medical-surgical nursing across the health continuum* (3rd ed.). Philadelphia: WB Saunders.

Jarvis, C. (1999). *Physical examination and health assessment* (3rd ed.). Philadelphia: WB Saunders.

Smith, S. C., & Wilbur, M. E. (2000). Nursing management: visual and auditory problems. In S. M. Lewis, M. M. Heitkemper, & S. R. Dirksen (Eds.), *Medical-surgical nursing: Assessment and management of clinical problems* (5th ed., pp. 442-481). St. Louis: Mosby.

Chapter 51

Carroll, P. (1998). Closing in on safer suctioning. *RN, 61*(5), 22-27.

Chernecky, C. C., & Berger, B. J. (2001). *Laboratory tests and diagnostic procedures* (3rd ed.). Philadelphia: WB Saunders.

Clark, L. K. (2001). Management of clients with upper airway disorders. In J. M. Black, J. H. Hawks, & A. M. Keene (Eds.), *Medical-surgical nursing: Clinical management for positive outcomes* (6th ed., pp. 1651-1684). Philadelphia: WB Saunders.

Deglin, J. H., & Vallerand, A. H. (2001). *Davis's drug guide for nurses* (7th ed.). Philadelphia: FA Davis.

Jarvis, C. (2001). *Physical examination and health assessment* (3rd ed.). Philadelphia: WB Saunders.

Lehne, R. A. (2001). *Pharmacology for nursing care* (4th ed.). Philadelphia: WB Saunders.

Potter, P. A., & Perry, A. G. (2001). *Fundamentals of nursing* (5th ed.). St. Louis: Mosby.

Skidmore-Roth, L. (2002). *Mosby's nursing drug reference* (7th ed.). St. Louis: Mosby.

Strohl, K. P. (2000). Upper airway diseases. In L. Goldman & J. C. Bennett (Eds.), *Cecil textbook of medicine* (21st ed., pp. 2246-2249). Philadelphia: WB Saunders.

Chapter 52

Caunt, H. (1992). Preoperative nursing intervention to relieve stress. *British Journal of Nursing, 1*(4), 171-172.

Dossey, B. M., Guzzetta, C. E., & Kenner, C. V. (1992). *Critical care nursing: Body-mind-spirit.* Philadelphia: Lippincott.

Fortinash, K. M., & Holoday-Worret, P. A. (2000). *Psychiatric mental health nursing.* St. Louis: Mosby.

Fortinash, K. M., & Holoday-Worret, P. A. (1999). *Psychiatric nursing care plans.* St. Louis: Mosby.

Houldin, A. D., & Hogan-Quigley, B. (1995). Psychological intervention for older hip fracture patients. *Journal of Gerontological Nursing, 21*(12), 20-26, 48-49.

Hymovich, D. P., & Hagopian, G. A. (1992). *Chronic illness in children and adults: A psychosocial approach.* Philadelphia: WB Saunders.

Keltner, N. L., Schwecke, L. H., & Bostrom, C. E. (Eds.) (1999). *Psychiatric nursing* (3rd ed.). St. Louis: Mosby.

Maslow, A. H. (1968). *Toward a psychology of being.* New York: Van Nostrand Reinhold.

Miller, J. F. (2000). *Coping with chronic illness: Overcoming powerlessness* (3rd ed.). Philadelphia: FA Davis.

Milliken, M. E. (1998). *Understanding human behavior: A guide for health care providers.* Albany, NY: Delmar Publishers.

Oakland, S., Ostell, A., Herrmann, M., Britz, A., Bartels, C., & Wallesch, C. (1995). The impact of aphasia on the patient and family in the first year poststroke. *Topics in Stroke Rehabilitation, 2*(3), 5-19.

Pennock, B. E., Crawshaw, L., Maher, T., Price, T., & Kaplan, P. D. (1994). Distressful events in the ICU as perceived by patients recovering from coronary artery bypass surgery. *Heart & Lung: Journal of Critical Care, 23*(4), 323-327.

Selye, H. (1978). *The stress of life* (2nd ed.). New York: McGraw-Hill.

Stuart, G. W., & Laraia, M.T. (2001). *Principles and practice of psychiatric nursing.* St. Louis: Mosby.

Swan, B. A. (1996). Assessing symptom distress in ambulatory surgery patients. *MEDSURG Nursing, 5*(5), 348-354.

Townsend, M. C. (2000). *Psychiatric mental health nursing: Concepts of care* (3rd ed.). Philadelphia: FA Davis.

Varcarolis, E. M. (2002). *Foundations of psychiatric mental health nursing: A clinical approach.* Philadelphia: WB Saunders.

Chapter 53

Abrams, A. C. (1998). *Clinical drug therapy: Rationales for nursing practice* (5th ed.). Philadelphia: Lippincott-Raven Publishers.

American Psychiatric Association. (1994). *Diagnostic and statistical manual of mental disorders* (4th ed.). Washington, DC: Author.

Bendik, M. F. (2000). The Schizophrenias. In K. M. Fortinash & P. A. Holoday-Worret, *Psychiatric-mental health nursing.* St. Louis: Mosby.

Benjamin, L. S. (1996). *Interpersonal diagnosis and treatment of personality disorders* (2nd ed.). New York: Guilford Press.

Brandt, B., & Ugarriza, D. N. (1996). Electroconvulsive therapy and the elderly client. *Journal of Gerontological Nursing, 22*(12), 14-20.

Dawber, N. (1997). Current approaches and interventions for schizophrenia. *Nursing Standard, 11*(49), 49-56.

Haber, J., Krainovich-Miller, B., McMahon, A. L., & Price-Hoskins, P. (1997). *Comprehensive psychiatric nursing.* St. Louis: Mosby.

Lee, F. (1997). Understanding schizophrenia. *Nursing Standard, 11*(36), 26-27.

Legge, A. (1997). Care of the older person. Depression: It's not inevitable and it is treatable. *Community Nurse, 2*(11), 16-17.

Linton, A. D., & Harris, J. A. (2000). *Pharmacology companion for introductory nursing care of adults.* Philadelphia: WB Saunders.

Marston, T. (1997). Mental health: In search of the right balance—schizophrenia. *Nursing Times, 93*(22), 30.

Montgomery, S. A. (1995). Managing depression in the community. *Professional Nurse, 10*(12), 805-807.

Stuart, G. W., & Laraia, M. T. (2001). *Principles and practice of psychiatric nursing* (7th ed.). St. Louis: Mosby

Tinklenberg, M. (1997). Healthwatch: Options for treatment of schizophrenia expanding. *Nurseweek* (California Statewide Edition), *10*(7), 19.

Chapter 54

Campbell, J. (1995). Making sense of the effects of alcohol. *Nursing Times, 91*(5), 38-39.

Castledine, G. (1995). Don't drink and nurse: Alcohol abuse in nursing. *British Journal of Nursing, 4*(2), 102.

Catanzarite, A. M. (1992). *Managing the chemically dependent nurse: A guide to identification, intervention, and retention.* Chicago: American Hospital Publishing.

Clement, M. (1995). Continuing education: Recognizing dependence on alcohol in the elderly. *Nurseweek* (California Statewide Edition), *8*(20), 8.

Cook, J. S. (1991). Drug abuse. In J. S. Cook & K. L. Fontaine (Eds.), *Essentials of mental health nursing* (2nd ed., pp. 484-528). Redwood City, Calif: Addison-Wesley Nursing.

Cooper, D. B. (1994). Problem drinking. *Nursing Times, 90*(14), 36-39.

Cooper, D. B. (1994). Use of chlormethiazole in alcohol home detoxification. *Professional Nurse, 10*(3), 146.

Cooper, D. B. (1993). Withdrawing gracefully detoxification. *Nursing Times, 89*(17), 42-44.

Dryfoos, J. G. (1993). Preventing substance use: Rethinking strategies. *American Journal of Public Health, 83*(6), 793-795.

Fishbain, D. A., Rosomoff, H. L., & Rosomoff, R. S. (1992). Drug abuse, dependence, and addiction in chronic pain patients. *The Clinical Journal of Pain, 8*(2), 77-85.

Gorman, M. (1996). Substance abuse: Alcoholic patients: keeping hope alive. *American Journal of Nursing, 96*(1), 20.

Gorman, M. (1996). Substance abuse: Starting recovery. *American Journal of Nursing, 96*(9), 15.

Hepple, J. (1996). Alcohol and older people. *Elderly Care, 8*(6), 34-35.

Knowlton, L. (1995). Dual diagnosis: The challenge. *Journal of the American Psychiatric Nurses Association, 1*(3), 102-104.

Kupkowski, M. J., & Robinette, A. L. (1996). Intervention for a homeless alcoholic—PCLNs: Who are they? How can they help you? *American Journal of Nursing, 96*(11), 15.

Merritt, P. (1997). Guilt and shame in recovering addicts: A personal account. *Journal of Psychosocial Nursing and Mental Health Services, 35*(7), 46.

Moos, R. H., King, M. J., & Patterson, M. A. (1996). Outcomes of residential treatment of substance abuse in hospital- and community-based programs. *Psychiatric Services, 47*(1), 68-74.

Navarra, T. (1995). Enabling behavior: The tender trap. *American Journal of Nursing, 95*(1), 50-52.

Pizzi, C. L., & Mion, L. C. (1993). Alcoholism in the elderly: Implications for hospital nurses. *MEDSURG Nursing, 2*(6), 453-458.

Riggin, O. Z., & Redding, B. A. (2000). Substance related disorders. In K. M. Fortinash & P. A. Holoday-Worret (Eds.), *Psychiatric-mental health nursing.* St. Louis: Mosby.

Watson, H. E. (1996). Minimal interventions for problem drinkers. *Journal of Substance Misuse for Nursing, Health and Social Care, 1*(2), 107-110.

Wilson, S. (1994). Can you spot an alcoholic patient? *RN, 57*(1), 46-51.

Illustration Credits

Chapter 1

Figure 1-1 from Monahan, F. D., & Neighbors, M. (1998). *Medical-surgical nursing: Foundations for clinical practice* (2nd ed.). Philadelphia: WB Saunders. Figures 1-2, 1-3 from Potter, P. A., & Perry, A. G. (2001). *Fundamentals of nursing* (5th ed.). St. Louis: Mosby. Figure 1-4 from Ignatavicius, D. D., Workman, M. L., & Mishler, M. A. (1999). *Medical-surgical nursing across the health care continuum* (3rd ed.). Philadelphia: WB Saunders.

Chapter 2

Figure 2-1 courtesy of Edwards Lifesciences, Irvine, Calif. Figure 2-2 from Potter, P. A., & Perry, A. G. (2001). *Fundamentals of nursing* (5th ed.). St. Louis: Mosby. Figure 2-3 from Lindeman, C. A., & McAthie, M. (1999). *Fundamentals of contemporary nursing practice.* Philadelphia: WB Saunders.

Chapter 3

Figure 3-1 from Potter, P. A., & Perry, A. G. (2001). *Fundamentals of nursing* (5th ed.). St. Louis: Mosby. Figure 3-2 modified from Tappen, R. M. (1989). *Nursing leadership and management: Concepts and practice* (2nd ed.). Philadelphia: FA Davis.

Chapter 4

Figures 4-2, 4-3 from Potter, P. A., & Perry, A. G. (2001). *Fundamentals of nursing* (5th ed.). St. Louis: Mosby.

Chapter 5

Figure 5-1 from Monahan, F. D., & Neighbors, M. (1998). *Medical-surgical nursing: Foundations for clinical practice* (2nd ed.). Philadelphia: WB Saunders. Figure 5-2 from Potter, P. A., & Perry, A. G. (2001). *Fundamentals of nursing* (5th ed.). St. Louis: Mosby.

Chapter 6

Figure 6-1 from Potter, P. A., & Perry, A. G. (2001). *Fundamentals of nursing* (5th ed.). St. Louis: Mosby.

Chapter 7

Figure 7-1 from Ignatavicius, D. D., Workman, M. L., & Mishler, M. A. (1999). *Medical-surgical nursing across the health care continuum* (3rd ed.). Philadelphia: WB Saunders. Figure 7-2 redrawn from Maslow, A. H. (1970). *Motivation and personality* (3rd ed.), reprinted by permission of Pearson Education, Inc., Upper Saddle River, NJ.

Chapter 8

Figure 8-1 from U. S. Department of Agriculture (1993). *Human nutrition information service: Making healthy food choices.* Washington, DC: USDA; redrawn from Mahan, L. K., & Arlin, M. (1992). *Krause's food, nutrition, and diet therapy* (4th ed.). Philadelphia: WB Saunders. Figure 8-2 from Food and Drug Administration. (1995). *Daily values for food labels.* Washington, DC: U. S. Government Printing Office. Figure 8-3 from Monahan, F. D., & Neighbors, M. (1998). *Medical-surgical nursing: Foundations for clinical practice* (2nd ed.). Philadelphia: WB Saunders. Figure 8-4 from Mahan, L. K., & Escott-Stump, S. (2000). *Krause's food, nutrition, and diet therapy* (10th ed.). Philadelphia: WB Saunders.

Chapter 9

Figure 9-1 from Ignatavicius, D. D., Workman, M. L., & Mishler, M. A. (1999). *Medical-surgical nursing across the health care continuum* (3rd ed.). Philadelphia: WB Saunders.

Chapter 10

Figure 10-1 from Ignatavicius, D. D., Workman, M. L., & Mishler, M. A. (1999). *Medical-surgical nursing across the health care continuum* (3rd ed.). Philadelphia: WB Saunders. Figure 10-2 CLG Photographics, St. Louis.

Chapter 11

Figures 11-1, 11-2, 11-3, 11-4, 11-5 from Jarvis, C. (2000). *Physical examination and health assessment* (3rd ed.). Philadelphia: WB Saunders.

Chapter 12

Figures 12-1, 12-2 from Monahan, F. D., & Neighbors, M. (1998). *Medical-surgical nursing: Foundations for clinical practice* (2nd ed.). Philadelphia: WB Saunders. Figure 12-3 from Elkin, M. K., Perry, A. G., & Potter, P. A. (2000). *Nursing interventions and clinical skills* (2nd ed.). St. Louis: Mosby. Figure 12-4 from Black, J. M., Hawks, J. H., & Keene, A. M. (2001). *Medical-surgical nursing: Clinical management for positive outcomes* (6th ed.). Philadelphia: WB Saunders.

Chapter 13

Figure 13-1 from Black, J. M., Hawks, J. H., & Keene, A.M. (2001). *Medical-surgical nursing: Clinical management for positive outcomes* (6th ed.). Philadelphia: WB Saunders.

Chapter 14

Figures 14-1, 14-4, 14-6 from Ignatavicius, D. D., Workman, M. L., & Mishler, M. A. (1999). *Medical-surgical nursing across the health care continuum* (3rd ed.). Philadelphia: WB Saunders. Figure 14-5 from Acute Pain Management Guidelines Panel. (1992). *Acute pain management* (DHHS Publication No. 92-0052). Rockville, Md: Agency for Health Care Policy and Research, Public Health Service, US Department of Health and Human Services. Figure 14-7 from Lewis, S. M., Heitkemper, M. M., & Dirksen, S. R. (Eds.). (2000). *Medical-surgical nursing: Assessment and management of clinical problems* (5th ed.). St. Louis: Mosby.

Chapter 15

Figures 15-1, 15-3, 15-5 from Lewis, S. M., Heitkemper, M. M., & Dirksen, S. R. (Eds.). (2001). *Medical-surgical nursing: Assessment and management of clinical problems* (5th ed.). St. Louis: Mosby. Figure 15-2 from Potter, P. A., & Perry, A. G. (2001). *Fundamentals of nursing* (5th ed.). St. Louis: Mosby. Figure 15-8A and B from Jarvis, C. (2000). *Physical examination and health assessment* (3rd ed.). Philadelphia: WB Saunders. Figure 15-9 from Monahan, F. D., & Neighbors, M. (1998). *Medical-surgical nursing: Foundations for clinical practice* (2nd ed.). Philadelphia: WB Saunders.

Chapter 16

Figures 16-1, 16-2, 16-6, photographs by Stephen Matteson, Jr. Figures 16-3, 16-5 courtesy of Northwest Hospital Center, Randallstown, Md. Figures 16-4, 16-7, 16-8, 16-9, 16-10, 16-12A and B, 16-15 from Ignatavicius, D. D., Workman, M. L., & Mishler, M. A. (1999). *Medical-surgical nursing across the health care continuum* (3rd ed.). Philadelphia: WB Saunders. Figures 16-11, 16-13 from Monahan, F. D., Neighbors, M. (1998). *Medical-surgical nursing: Foundations for clinical practice* (2nd ed.). Philadelphia: WB Saunders. Figures 16-12C and D courtesy of C. R. Bard, Inc., Covington, Ga. Figure 16-14 courtesy of DHD Healthcare, Wampsville, NY.

Chapter 17

Figure 17-1B from Potter, P. A., & Perry, A. G. (2001). *Fundamentals of nursing* (5th ed.). St. Louis: Mosby. Figure 17-3 redrawn from Winters, B. (1984). Implantable vascular access devices, *Oncology Nursing Forum, 11*(6), 25-30. Figure 17-4A courtesy of B. Braun Medical, Inc., Bethlehem, Pa. Figure 17-4B courtesy of ICU Medical, Inc., San Clemente, Calif. Figure 17-5 from Lewis, S. M., Heitkemper, M. M., & Dirksen, S. R. (Eds.). (2000). *Medical-surgical nursing: Assessment and management of clinical problems* (5th ed.). St. Louis: Mosby. Figure 17-7A from 3M Co., St. Paul, Minn. Figure 17-7B from Bolander, V. B. (1994). *Sorenson and Luckmann's basic nursing: A psychophysiologic approach* (3rd ed.). Philadelphia: WB Saunders.

Chapter 18

Figures 18-1, 18-2 from Black, J. M., Hawks, J. H., & Keene, A. M. (2001). *Medical-surgical nursing: Clinical management for positive outcomes* (6th ed.). Philadelphia: WB Saunders. Figure 18-3 from Ignatavicius, D. D., Workman, M. L., & Mishler, M. A. (1999). *Medical-surgical nursing across the health care continuum* (3rd ed.). Philadelphia: WB Saunders.

Chapter 20

Figure 20-2 from Ignatavicius, D. D., Workman, M. L., & Mishler, M. A. (1999). *Medical-surgical nursing across the health care continuum* (3rd ed.). Philadelphia: WB Saunders. Figure 20-3 from Norton, D., McLaren, R., & Eston-Smith, A. N. (1962). *An investigation of geriatric nursing problems in the hospital.* London: National Corporation for the Care of Old People (now the Centre for Policy on Ageing). Figure 20-4 courtesy of Support Systems International, Inc., Charleston, SC. Figure 20-5 from Black, J. M., Hawks, J. H., & Keene, A. M. (2001). *Medical-surgical nursing: Clinical management for positive outcomes* (6th ed.). Philadelphia: WB Saunders.

Chapter 21

Figures 21-1, 21-3, photograph by Stephen Matteson, Jr. Figure 21-2 from Leahy, J. M., & Kizilay, P. E. (1998). *Foundations of nursing practice: A nursing process approach.* Philadelphia: WB Saunders.

Chapter 22

Figure 22-1 modified from Jacob, S. W., & Francone, C. A. (1982). *Structure and function in man* (5th ed.). Philadelphia: WB Saunders. Figure 22-2 from Black, J. M., Hawks, J. H., & Keene, A. M. (2001). *Medical-surgical nursing: Clinical management for positive outcomes* (6th ed.). Philadelphia: WB Saunders. Figure 22-3 from Monahan, F. D., & Neighbors, M. (1998). *Medical-surgical nursing: Foundations for clinical practice* (2nd ed.). Philadelphia: WB Saunders. Figure 22-4 from Greengold, B. A., & Ouslander, J. (1986). Bladder retraining. *Journal of Gerontological Nursing, 12*(6), 31-35. Figure 22-5 from Thibodeau, G. A., & Patton, K. P. (1999). *Anatomy & physiology* (4th ed.). St. Louis: Mosby.

Chapter 23

Figures 23-1, 23-2 reprinted by permission of Partnership for Caring, 1620 Eye Street, NW; Suite 202, Washington, DC 20006 (1-800-989-9455).

Chapter 24

Figure 24-1 from American Cancer Society. (1991). *Cancer facts and figures—1997.* Atlanta, Ga: Author; used by permission; 1997 Cancer Facts and Figures—1997; American Cancer Society, Inc. Figure 24-2 from Seeram, E. (1994). *Computed tomography.* Philadelphia: WB Saunders. Figure 24-3 from Monahan, F. D., & Neighbors, M. (1998). *Medical-surgical nursing: Foundations for clinical practice* (2nd ed.). Philadelphia: WB Saunders. Figure 24-4, photograph by Stephen Matteson, Jr. Figure 24-5 from Lindeman, C. A., & McAthie, M. (1999). *Fundamentals of contemporary nursing practice.* Philadelphia: WB Saunders.

Chapter 25

Figure 25-1A from Potter, P. A., & Perry, A. G. (2001). *Fundamentals of nursing* (5th ed.). St. Louis: Mosby. Figure 25-1B, permission to use and/or reproduce this copyrighted material has been granted by the owner, Hollister, Inc., Libertyville, Ill. Figures 25-2, 25-3, 25-5 from Monahan, F. D., & Neighbors, M. (1998). *Medical-surgical nursing: Foundations for clinical practice* (2nd ed.). Philadelphia: WB Saunders. Figure 25-4 from Ignatavicius, D. D., Workman, M. L., & Mishler, M. A. (1999). *Medical-surgical nursing across the health care continuum* (3rd ed.). Philadelphia: WB Saunders. Figure 25-6 from Black, J. M., & Matassarin-Jacobs, E. (1997). *Medical-surgical nursing: Clinical management for continuity of care* (5th ed.). Philadelphia: WB Saunders.

Chapter 26

Figures 26-1, 26-3, 26-4, 26-8, 26-12, 26-15, 26-17, 26-18 from Monahan, F. D., & Neighbors, M. (1998). *Medical-surgical nursing: Foundations for clinical practice* (2nd ed.). Philadelphia: WB Saunders. Figures 26-2, 26-7, 26-9, 26-10, 26-13, 26-14, 26-19 from Black, J. M., Hawks, J. H., & Keene, A. M. (2001). *Medical-surgical nursing: Clinical management for positive outcomes* (6th ed.). Philadelphia: WB Saunders. Figure 26-5 courtesy of Linda R. Littlejohn, RN, BSN, CCRN, CNRN, Neuro Clinician, and Mission Hospital Regional Medical Center, Mission Viejo, Calif. Figure 26-6 from Thibodeau, G. A., & Patton, K. P. (1999). *Anatomy & physiology* (4th ed.). St. Louis: Mosby. Figure 26-11 from Black, J. M., & Matassarin-Jacobs, E. (1993). *Luckmann and Sorensen's medical-surgical nursing: A psychophysiologic approach* (4th ed.). Philadelphia: WB Saunders. Figure 26-15 from Black, J. M., & Matassarin-Jacobs, E. (1997). *Medical-surgical nursing: Clinical management for continuity of care* (5th ed.). Philadelphia: WB Saunders. Figure 26-20 from Ignatavicius, D. D., Workman, M. L., & Mishler, M. A. (1999). *Medical-surgical nursing across the health care continuum* (3rd ed.). Philadelphia: WB Saunders.

Chapter 27

Figures 27-1, 27-5 from Monahan, F. D., & Neighbors, M. (1998). *Medical-surgical nursing: Foundations for clinical practice* (2nd ed.). Philadelphia: WB Saunders. Figures 27-2, 27-4 from Ignatavicius, D. D., Workman, M. L., & Mishler, M. A. (1999). *Medical-surgical nursing across the health care continuum* (3rd ed.). Philadelphia: WB Saunders. Figures 27-3, 27-8 from Black, J. M., Hawks, J. H., & Keene, A. M. (2001). *Medical-surgical nursing: Clinical management for positive outcomes* (6th ed.). Philadelphia: WB Saunders. Figures 27-6, 27-9 from Potter, P. A., & Perry, A. G. (2001). *Fundamentals of nursing* (5th ed.). St. Louis: Mosby. Figures 27-7A, B, and C Sammons Preston. Figure 27-7D from Lewis, S. M., Heitkemper, M. M., & Dirksen, S. R. (2000). *Medical-surgical nursing: Assessment and management of clinical problems* (5th ed.). St. Louis: Mosby.

Chapter 28

Figures 28-1, 28-2 redrawn from Jarvis, C. (1996). *Physical examination and health assessment* (2nd ed.). Philadelphia: WB Saunders. Figure 28-3 adapted from Jacob, W. W., & Francone, C. A. (1989). *Elements of anatomy and physiology* (2nd ed.). Philadelphia: WB Saunders. Figures 28-4, 28-10 from Monahan, F. D., & Neighbors, M. (1998). *Medical-surgical nursing: Foundations for clinical practice* (2nd ed.). Philadelphia: WB Saunders. Figures 28-5, 28-6, 28-7 from Ignatavicius, D. D., Workman, M. L., & Mishler, M. A. (1999). *Medical-surgical nursing across the health care continuum* (3rd ed.). Philadelphia: WB Saunders. Figures 28-8, 28-9 from Black, J. M., & Matassarin-Jacobs, E. (1993). *Luckmann and Sorensen's medical-surgical nursing: A psychophysiologic approach* (4th ed.). Philadelphia: WB Saunders.

Chapter 29

Figures 29-1, 29-2 from Monahan, F. D., & Neighbors, M. (1998). *Medical-surgical nursing: Foundations for clinical practice* (2nd ed.). Philadelphia: WB Saunders. Figures 29-3, 29-4, 29-5, 29-7, 29-8, 29-13, 29-14, 29-15 from Black, J. M., Hawks, J. H., & Keene, A. M. (2001). *Medical-surgical nursing: Clinical management for positive outcomes* (6th ed.). Philadelphia: WB Saunders. Figure 29-6 from Black, J. M., & Matassarin-Jacobs, E. (1997). *Medical-surgical nursing: Clinical management for continuity of care* (5th ed.). Philadelphia: WB Saunders. Figure 29-9 from Potter, P. A., & Perry, A. G. (2001). *Fundamentals of nursing* (5th ed.). St. Louis: Mosby. Figures 29-10, 29-11, 29-12B from Ignatavicius, D. D., Workman, M. L., & Mishler, M. A. (1999). *Medical-surgical nursing across the health care continuum* (3rd ed.). Philadelphia: WB Saunders. Figure 29-12A courtesy of Genzyme Biosurgery, Fall River, Mass.

Chapter 30

Figures 30-1, 30-3, 30-4, 30-10 from Black, J. M., & Matassarin-Jacobs, E. (1993). *Luckmann and Sorensen's medical-surgical nursing: A psychophysiologic approach* (4th ed.). Philadelphia: WB Saunders. Figure 30-2 from Monahan, F. D., & Neighbors, M. (1998). *Medical-surgical nursing: Foundations for clinical practice* (2nd ed.). Philadelphia: WB Saunders. Figures 30-5, 30-6, 30-7, 30-9 from Black, J. M., Hawks, J. H., & Keene, A. M. (2001). *Medical-surgical nursing: Clinical management for positive outcomes* (6th ed.). Philadelphia: WB Saunders. Figure 30-8 from Ignatavicius, D. D., Workman, M. L., & Mishler, M. A. (1999). *Medical-surgical nursing across the health care continuum* (3rd ed.). Philadelphia: WB Saunders.

Chapter 31

Figure 31-1A from Thibodeau, G. A., & Patton, K. P. (1999). *Anatomy & physiology* (4th ed.). St. Louis: Mosby. Figures 31-1B, 31-2 from Rodak, B. F. (1995). *Diagnostic hematology,* Philadelphia: WB Saunders.

Chapter 32

Figure 32-1 from Monahan, F. D., & Neighbors, M. (1998). *Medical-surgical nursing: Foundations for clinical practice* (2nd ed.). Philadelphia: WB Saunders. Figures 32-2, 32-3 from Young-McCaughan, S., & Jennings, B. M. (1998). Hematologic and immunologic systems. In J. G. Alspach (Ed.), *Core curriculum for critical care nursing* (5th ed.). Philadelphia: WB Saunders.

Chapter 33

Figures 33-1, 33-2, 33-3, 33-4, 33-5, 33-9, 33-10, 33-12, 33-15 from Monahan, F. D., & Neighbors, M. (1998). *Medical-surgical nursing: Foundations for clinical practice* (2nd ed.). Philadelphia: WB Saunders. Figures 33-7, 33-13, 33-16 from Ignatavicius, D. D., Workman, M. L., & Mishler, M. A. (1999). *Medical-surgical nursing across the health care continuum* (3rd ed.). Philadelphia: WB Saunders. Figure 33-11 from Ballard, J. C., Wood, L. L., & Lansing, A. (1997). Transmyocardial revascularization: Criteria for selecting patients, treatment, and nursing care, reprinted with permission. *Critical Care Nurse, 17*(1):42-49. Figure 33-14A, E, and F copyright Medtronic, Inc., Minneapolis, Minn. Figure 33-14B copyright St. Jude Medical, Inc., 2002; this image is provided courtesy of St. Jude Medical, Inc. All rights reserved. St. Jude Medical is a registered trademark of St. Jude Medical, Inc. Figure 33-14C courtesy of Alliance Medical Products. Irvine, Calif. Figure 33-14D and G courtesy of Edwards Lifesciences, Irvine, Calif. Figure 33-17 from Ignatavicius, D. D., Workman, M. L., & Mishler, M. A. (1995). *Medical-surgical nursing: A nursing process approach* (2nd ed.). Philadelphia: WB Saunders. Figures 33-18, 33-19, 33-20, 33-21, 33-22, 33-23, 33-25, 33-26, 33-27, 33-28, 33-29, 33-30 from Ignatavicius, D. D., & Bayne, M. V. (1991). *Medical-surgical nursing: A nursing process approach.* Philadelphia: WB Saunders. Figure 33-24 from Black, J. M., & Matassarin-Jacobs, E. (1993). *Luckmann and Sorensen's medical-surgical nursing: A psychophysiologic approach* (4th ed.). Philadelphia: WB Saunders.

Chapter 34

Figures 34-1, 34-2, 34-3, 34-4, 34-5, 34-8 from Monahan, F. D., & Neighbors, M. (1998). *Medical-surgical nursing: Foundations for clinical practice* (2nd ed.). Philadelphia: WB Saunders. Figure 34-7 from Ignatavicius, D. D., Workman, M. L., & Mishler, M. A. (1999). *Medical-surgical nursing across the health care continuum* (3rd ed.). Philadelphia: WB Saunders.

Chapter 35

Figure 35-2 from Monahan, F. D., & Neighbors, M. (1998). *Medical-surgical nursing: Foundations for clinical practice* (2nd ed.). Philadelphia: WB Saunders.

Chapter 36

Figures 36-1, 36-5, 36-8, 36-9, 36-11B, 36-13, 36-14, 36-16, 36-17, 36-18, 36-19 from Monahan, F. D., & Neighbors, M. (1998). *Medical-surgical nursing: Foundations for clinical practice* (2nd ed.). Philadelphia: WB Saunders. Figures 36-2, 36-15 from Black, J. M., Hawks, J. H., & Keene, A. M. (2001). *Medical-surgical nursing: Clinical management for positive outcomes* (6th ed.). Philadelphia: WB Saunders. Figure 36-3 from Laufer, I., & Levine, M. C. (1992). *Double contrast gastrointestinal radiology* (2nd ed.). Philadelphia: WB Saunders. Figure 36-4 from Jacob, S. W., & Francone, C. A. (1998). *Elements of anatomy and physiology* (2nd ed.). Philadelphia: WB Saunders. Figures 36-6, 36-20, 36-21, 36-22 from Lewis, S. M., Heitkemper, M. M., & Dirksen, S. R. (2000). *Medical-surgical nursing: Assessment and management of clinical problems* (5th ed.). St. Louis: Mosby. Figures 36-7, 36-11A, 36-12 from Ignatavicius, D. D., Workman, M. L., & Mishler, M. A. (1999). *Medical-surgical nursing across the health care continuum* (3rd ed.). Philadelphia: WB Saunders. Figure 36-10 from Shafer, W. G., Hine, M. K., & Levy, B. M. (1983). *A textbook of oral pathology* (4th ed.). Philadelphia: WB Saunders.

Chapter 37

Figures 37-1, 37-7, 37-10, 37-12 from Monahan, F. D., & Neighbors, M. (1998). *Medical-surgical nursing: Foundations for clinical practice* (2nd ed.). Philadelphia: WB Saunders. Figure 37-5 from Lewis, S. M., Heitkemper, M. M., & Dirksen, S. R. (2000). *Medical-surgical nursing: Assessment and management of clinical problems* (5th ed.). St. Louis: Mosby. Figures 37-6, 37-8, 37-9 from Ignatavicius, D. D., Workman, M. L., & Mishler, M. A. (1999). *Medical-surgical nursing across the health care continuum* (3rd ed.). Philadelphia: WB Saunders. Figures 37-11, 37-13 from Black, J. M., Hawks, J. H., & Keene, & A. M. (2001). *Medical-surgical nursing: Clinical management for positive outcomes* (6th ed.). Philadelphia: WB Saunders.

Chapter 38

Figures 38-1, 38-2, 38-3, 38-4, 38-5, 38-8, 38-10, 38-11, 38-14, 38-15 from Monahan, F. D., & Neighbors, M. (1998). *Medical-surgical nursing: Foundations for clinical practice* (2nd ed.). Philadelphia: WB Saunders. Figure 38-6 from Jacob, S. W., & Francone, C. A. (1998). *Elements of anatomy and physiology* (2nd ed.). Philadelphia: WB Saunders. Figures 38-7, 38-9, 38-12, 38-13 from Black, J. M., Hawks, J. H., & Keene, A. M. (2001). *Medical-surgical nursing: Clinical management for positive outcomes* (6th ed.). Philadelphia: WB Saunders.

Chapter 39

Figures 39-1, 39-4, 39-8, 39-9A from Ignatavicius, D. D., Workman, M. L., & Mishler, M. A. (1999). *Medical-surgical nursing across the health care continuum* (3rd ed.). Philadelphia: WB Saunders. Figures 39-2, 39-9B from the AHPA Arthritis Teaching Slide Collection, 1980; used with permission of the American College of Rheumatology. Figure 39-3 from Black, J. M., & Matassarin-Jacobs, E. (1993). *Luckmann and Sorensen's medical-surgical nursing: A psychophysiologic approach* (4th ed.). Philadelphia: WB Saunders. Figure 39-5 courtesy of the Chattanooga Group, Hixson, Tenn. Figure 39-6 from Black, J. M., & Matassarin-Jacobs, E. (1997). *Luckmann and Sorensen's medical-surgical nursing: Clinical management for continuity of care* (5th ed.). Philadelphia: WB Saunders. Figure 39-7 from Black, J. M., Hawks, J. H., & Keene, A. M. (2001). *Medical-surgical nursing: Clinical management for positive outcomes* (6th ed.). Philadelphia: WB Saunders.

Chapter 40

Figure 40-1 from Lewis, S. M., Heitkemper, M. M., & Dirksen, S. R. (Eds.). (2000). *Medical-surgical nursing: Assessment and management of clinical problems* (5th ed.). St. Louis: Mosby. Figure 40-2 from Ignatavicius, D. D., Workman, M. L., & Mishler, M. A. (1999). *Medical-surgical nursing across the health care continuum* (3rd ed.). Philadelphia: WB Saunders. Figures 40-3, 40-4, 40-10 from Black, J. M., Hawks, J. H., & Keene, A. M. (2001). *Medical-surgical nursing: Clinical management for positive outcomes* (6th ed.). Philadelphia: WB Saunders. Figure 40-5 courtesy of Stryker, Howmedica Osteonics, Inc. 40-6 courtesy of Smith & Nephew, Inc., Orthopaedic Division, Memphis, Tenn. Figure 40-7 redrawn from Polaski, A. K., & Tatro., S. E. (1996). *Luckmann's core principles and practice of medical-surgical nursing,* Philadelphia: WB Saunders. Figures 40-8, 40-9 from Potter, P. A., & Perry, A. G. (2001). *Fundamentals of nursing* (5th ed.). St. Louis: Mosby.

Chapter 41

Figure 41-1 from Monahan, F. D., & Neighbors, M. (1998). *Medical-surgical nursing: Foundations for clinical practice* (2nd ed.). Philadelphia: WB Saunders. Figures 41-2, 41-3 courtesy of Otto Bock Orthopedic Industry, Inc., Minneapolis, Minn. Figure 41-4 from Black, J. M., Hawks, J. H., & Keene, A. M. (2001). *Medical-surgical nursing: Clinical management for positive outcomes* (6th ed.). Philadelphia: WB Saunders.

Chapter 42

Figures 42-1, 42-2, 42-5, 42-6 from Ignatavicius, D. D., Workman, M. L., & Mishler, M. A. (1999). *Medical-surgical nursing across the health care continuum* (3rd ed.). Philadelphia: WB Saunders. Figure 42-3 courtesy of C. M. Charles & C. M. MacBryde. Figure 42-4 from Mendeloff, A., & Smith, D. E. (Eds.). (1956). Acromegaly, diabetes, hypermetabolism, proteinuria and heart failure, Clinical Pathological Conference, *American Journal of Medicine, 20,* 133. Figure 42-7 from Bondy, P. K., & Rosenberg, L. E. (1980). *Metabolic control and disease* (8th ed.). Philadelphia: WB Saunders.

Chapter 43

Figures 43-1, 43-7 from Monahan, F. D., & Neighbors, M. (1998). *Medical-surgical nursing: Foundations for clinical practice* (2nd ed.). Philadelphia: WB Saunders. Figure 43-2 from Seidel, H. S., Ball, J. W., Dains, J. E., & Benedict, G.W. (1999). *Mosby's guide to physical examination* (4th ed.). St. Louis: Mosby. Figure 43-3 from Ignatavicius, D. D., Workman, M. L., & Mishler, M. A. (1999). *Medical-surgical nursing across the health care continuum* (3rd ed.). Philadelphia: WB Saunders. Figure 43-4 from Ignatavicius, D. D., & Bayne, M. V. (1991). *Medical-surgical nursing: A nursing process approach.* Philadelphia: WB Saunders. Figure 43-5 from Jacob, S. W., & Francone, C. A. (1989). *Elements of anatomy and physiology* (2nd ed.). Philadelphia: WB Saunders. Figure 43-6 from Wilson, J., & Foster, D. (1985). *Williams textbook of endocrinology* (7th ed.). Philadelphia: WB Saunders.

Chapter 44

Figure 44-2 adapted from American Diabetes Association. (1992). *Teaching standards for diabetes mellitus* (5th ed.). Austin, Tx: American Diabetes Association, Texas Affiliate, Inc. Figure 44-3 from Black, J. M., Hawks, J. H., & Keene, A. M. (2001). *Medical-surgical nursing: Clinical management for positive outcomes* (6th ed.). Philadelphia: WB Saunders. Figure 44-4A and B courtesy of Medtronic MiniMed, Northridge, Calif.

Chapter 45

Figures 45-1, 45-2, 45-3, 45-4, 45-5, 45-7, 45-9, 45-10, 45-15 from Monahan, F. D., & Neighbors, M. (1998). *Medical-surgical nursing: Foundations for clinical practice* (2nd ed.) Philadelphia: WB Saunders. Figure 45-6 from Ignatavicius, D. D., Workman, M. L., & Mishler, M. A. (1995). *Medical-surgical nursing: A nursing process approach* (2nd ed.). Philadelphia: WB Saunders. Figures 45-8, 45-11, 45-12, 45-13, 45-14 from Ignatavicius, D. D., Workman, M. L., & Mishler, M. A. *Medical-surgical nursing across the health care continuum* (3rd ed.). Philadelphia: WB Saunders.

Chapter 46

Figures 46-1, 46-12, 46-14 from Monahan, F. D., & Neighbors, M. (1998). *Medical-surgical nursing: Foundations for clinical practice* (2nd ed.). Philadelphia: WB Saunders. Figures 46-2, 46-4 from Applegate, E. J. (2000). *The anatomy and physiology learning system textbook* (2nd ed.). Philadelphia: WB Saunders. Figures 46-3, 46-6, 46-7, 46-10, 46-11, 46-13 from Black, J. M., Hawks, J. H., & Keene, A. M. (2001). *Medical-surgical nursing: Clinical management for positive outcomes* (6th ed.). Philadelphia: WB Saunders. Figure 46-5 from Guyton, A. C., & Hall, J. C. (1996). *Textbook of medical physiology* (9th ed.). Philadelphia: WB Saunders. Figure 46-8 from Black, J. M., Matassarin-Jacobs, E. (1997). *Medical-surgical nursing: Clinical management for continuity of care* (5th ed.). Philadelphia: WB Saunders. Figure 46-9 courtesy of Dr. Hans Stricker, Department of Urology, Henry Ford Hospital, Detroit, Mich.

Chapter 47

Figures 47-1A, 47-2, 47-3 courtesy of Leonard Wolf, MD, New York, NY. Figures 47-1B, 47-4 courtesy of New York City Health Department. Figure 47-5 from Friedman-Kien, A. E. (1989). *Color atlas of AIDS.* Philadelphia: WB Saunders.

Chapter 48

Figures 48-1, 48-3, 48-14, 48-15, 48-16 from Monahan, F. D., & Neighbors, M. (1998). *Medical-surgical nursing: Foundations for clinical practice* (2nd ed.). Philadelphia: WB Saunders. Figures 48-2, 48-8, 48-9, 48-10, 48-11, 48-13A, B, and C from Lookingbill, D. P., & Marks, J. G., Jr. (1993). *Principles of dermatology* (2nd ed.). Philadelphia: WB Saunders. Figures 48-4, 48-13D from Jarvis, C. (2000). *Physical examination and health assessment* (3rd ed.). Philadelphia: WB Saunders. Figures 48-5, 48-19 from Black, J. M., & Matassarin-Jacobs, E. (1993). *Luckmann and Sorensen's medical-surgical nursing* (4th ed.). Philadelphia: WB Saunders. Figure 48-6 from Hurwitz, S. (1993). *Clinical pediatric dermatology: A textbook of skin disorders of childhood and adolescence* (2nd ed.). Philadelphia: WB Saunders. Figure 48-7 courtesy of Columbia-Presbyterian Dermatology Associates, New York, NY. Figure 48-12 from Callen, J. P., Greer, K. E., Hood, A. F., et al. (1993). *Color atlas of dermatology.* Philadelphia: WB Saunders. Figure 48-17 from Black, J. M., Hawks, J. H., & Keene, A. M. (2001). *Medical-surgical nursing: Clinical management for positive outcomes* (6th ed.). Philadelphia: WB Saunders. Figure 48-18 courtesy of Smith & Nephew, Inc., San Antonio, Tx.

Chapter 49

Figures 49-1, 49-2, 49-3, 49-4, 49-22 from Monahan, F. D., & Neighbors, M. (1998). *Medical-surgical nursing: Foundations for clinical practice* (2nd ed.). Philadelphia: WB Saunders. Figures 49-5, 49-7, 49-13 from Jarvis, C. (2000). *Physical examination and health assessment* (3rd ed.). Philadelphia: WB Saunders. Figures 49-6, 49-8, 49-10, 49-17 from Ignatavicius, D. D., Workman, M. L., & Mishler, M. A. (1999). *Medical-surgical nursing across the health care continuum* (3rd ed.). Philadelphia: WB Saunders. Figures 49-9, 49-16 from Black, J. M., Hawks, J. H., & Keene, A. M. (2001). *Medical-surgical nursing: Clinical management for positive outcomes* (6th ed.). Philadelphia: WB Saunders. Figure 49-11 courtesy of Cleveland Society for the Blind. Figure 49-12 from Matteson, M. A., McConnell, E. S., & Linton, A. D. ({AU: Please provide year.}) *Gerontological nursing* (2nd ed.). Philadelphia: WB Saunders. Figures 49-15A and B, 49-18 courtesy of Ophthalmic Photography at the University of Michigan W. K. Kellogg Eye Center, Ann Arbor, Mich. Figures 49-19, 49-21 courtesy of the National Industries for the Blind, Wayne, NJ. Figure 49-20 from Lewis, S. M., Hietkemper, M. M., & Dirksen, S. D. (2000). *Medical-surgical nursing: Assessment and management of clinical problems* (5th ed.). St. Louis: Mosby.

Chapter 50

Figures 50-1, 50-8 from Monahan, F. D., & Neighbors, M. (1998). *Medical-surgical nursing: Foundations for clinical practice* (2nd ed.). Philadelphia: WB Saunders. Figures 50-2, 50-5 from Ignatavicius, D. D., Workman, M. L., & Mishler, M. A. (1999). *Medical-surgical nursing across the health care continuum* (3rd ed.). Philadelphia: WB Saunders. Figure 50-4 from Seidel, H. M., Ball, J. W., Dains, J. E., & Benedict, G. W. (1999). *Mosby's guide to physical examination* (4th ed.). St. Louis: Mosby. Figure 50-6 courtesy of Arnold G. Schuring, MD. Figure 50-7 from Black, J. M., Hawks, J. H., & Keene, A. M. (2001). *Medical-surgical nursing: Clinical management for positive outcomes* (6th ed.). Philadelphia: WB Saunders.

Chapter 51

Figures 51-1, 51-2, 51-3, 51-6 from Monahan, F. D., & Neighbors, M. (1998). *Medical-surgical nursing: Foundations for clinical practice* (2nd ed.). Philadelphia: WB Saunders. Figures 51-4, 51-5, 51-8A and C from Black, J. M., Hawks, J. H., & Keene, A. M. (2001). *Medical-surgical nursing: Clinical management for positive outcomes* (6th ed.). Philadelphia: WB Saunders. Figures 51-7, 51-8E from Lewis, S. M., Heitkemper, M. M., & Dirksen, S. R. (Eds.). (2000). *Medical-surgical nursing: Assessment and management of clinical problems* (5th ed.). St. Louis: Mosby. Figure 51-8B courtesy of Servox AG, Germany. Figure 51-8D courtesy of Luminaud, Inc. Mentor, Ohio. Figure 51-8F from Ignatavicius, D. D., Workman, M. L., & Mishler, M. A. (1999). *Medical-surgical nursing across the health care continuum* (3rd ed.). Philadelphia: WB Saunders.

Glossary

A

Acid A solution containing a high number of hydrogen ions.

Acid–base balance The homeostasis of the hydrogen ion (H^+) concentration in body fluids.

Acidosis Abnormal pH of body fluids caused by excess acid in relation to bicarbonate.

Acne Inflammatory skin disorder characterized by comedones, pustules, and cysts.

Acquired immunity Antibody-mediated or cell-mediated response that is specific to a particular pathogen and is activated when needed.

Acrochordon Small, soft, raised lesion (skin tag).

Acromegaly Disease of middle-aged adults resulting from overproduction of growth hormone by the anterior pituitary.

Action Ability to respond to others with genuineness, compassion, sensitivity, and self-disclosure to promote their well-being.

Active acquired immunity Immunity developed after direct contact with an antigen through illness or vaccination.

Active exercise Exercise carried out by the patient.

Active transport Movement of solutes across membranes; requires the expenditure of energy.

Acute illness Illness or disease that has a relatively rapid onset and a short duration.

Acute pain Pain that occurs after injury to tissues from surgery, trauma, or disease. It is usually sudden in onset, temporary, easily localized, and decreases as healing takes place.

Adaptation The organism's attempts to return to homeostasis.

Addiction Behavioral pattern of compulsive drug use characterized by craving for an opioid and obtaining and using the drug for effects other than pain relief.

Addison's disease Disease resulting from a deficiency of adrenocorticotropic hormone caused by destruction or dysfunction of the adrenal glands.

Adrenaline Epinephrine; a powerful vasoactive substance produced by the adrenal medulla in times of stress or danger.

Adrenocorticotropic hormone (ACTH) A pituitary hormone that stimulates the cortex of the adrenal glands to produce adrenal hormones.

Advance directive Written statement of a person's wishes regarding medical treatment.

Advanced cardiac life support Use of drugs and equipment to provide continuing care for a person who has suffered cardiac or respiratory arrest.

Aerosol Solid or liquid particles suspended in a gas.

Affect Feelings such as happiness, sadness, or worry. Inappropriate affect is incongruence between the thought and the feeling expressed.

Afterload The amount of resistance the left ventricle must overcome to open the aortic valve.

Ageism A process of systematic stereotyping and discrimination against people because of their age; usually directed against older people.

Aging The process of growing older or more mature.

Agoraphobia Fear of situations outside the home.

Akathisia A reversible condition of restlessness manifested as an urge to pace.

Algor mortis Cooling of the body after death.

Alkaline (base) A solution containing a low number of hydrogen ions.

Alkalosis Abnormal pH of body fluids caused by excess bicarbonate in relation to acid.

Allergen An antigen that causes a hypersensitive reaction.

Alopecia Loss of hair.

Amino acids A group of 22 substances that can be bonded in different ways to make a variety of proteins. The body can manufacture sufficient amounts of these if the nine essential amino acids are provided in the diet.

Amputation Removal of a limb, part of a limb, or an organ; may be done by surgical means or through an accident.

Amputee Individual who has undergone an amputation.

Amyopathy (amyotonia) Loss of muscle tone.

Analgesia A state of not feeling pain.

Analgesic Drug that acts on the nervous system to relieve or reduce the suffering or intensity of pain.

Anaphylactic shock A severe, potentially fatal, allergic reaction characterized by hypotension and bronchial constriction.

Anastomosis Communication or connection between two organs or parts of organs.

Androgens Hormones produced by the adrenal cortex, the testes, and the ovaries that stimulate the development of male characteristics.

Anemia A reduction in the number of red blood cells or in the quantity of hemoglobin in the blood.

Anesthesia Partial or complete loss of sensation with or without loss of consciousness.

Anesthesiologist A physician who specializes in the administration of anesthetics and monitors the patient while the patient is under anesthesia.

Anesthetic An agent that abolishes the pain sensation.

Angioma Benign tumor composed of blood vessels.

Ankylosis Joint immobility.

Anorectal incontinence Fecal incontinence caused by weak perineal muscles, loss of anal reflexes, loss of anal sphincter tone, or rectal prolapse.

Anorexia Loss of appetite for food.

Anteflexion Bending forward of the top of an organ.

Anteversion Bending forward of an entire organ.

Antibody A protein that is created in response to a specific antigen.

Antibody-mediated acquired immunity Defensive response by B cells assisted by T_H cells, aimed at invading microorganisms such as bacteria.

Antidiuretic hormone (ADH) A hormone released by the posterior pituitary gland that causes the reabsorption of water in the distal tubules and collecting ducts of the kidney.
Antigen A substance, usually a protein, that is capable of stimulating a response from the immune system.
Antihistamine Drug that blocks the effects of histamine, which is a body chemical that causes allergic symptoms.
Antineoplastic An agent that inhibits the maturation or reproduction of malignant cells.
Antithrombotic Capable of preventing the formation of blood clots.
Anuria Absence of urine production.
Anxiety A vague sense of impending doom or apprehension that appears to have no clearly identifiable cause.
Aphasia Inability to understand words or to respond with words, or both.
Apical Referring to the pointed end of a structure.
Apnea Cessation of breathing.
Arteriosclerosis Abnormal thickening, hardening, and loss of elasticity of the arterial walls.
Arthralgia Pain in a joint.
Arthritis Inflammation of a joint.
Arthroplasty Plastic repair of a joint.
Asbestosis Interstitial fibrosis of the lungs caused by inhalation of asbestos fibers.
Ascites Accumulation of excess fluid in the peritoneal cavity.
Assessment Collection of data about the health status of a patient or client.
Assignment Identification and delegation of specific tasks to a specific person who is hired and paid to perform these tasks.
Assimilation Process of replacing or giving up values, beliefs, and practices for those of another culture.
Asthma A condition characterized by episodes of bronchospasm that causes wheezing and dyspnea.
Astigmatism Error of refraction caused by uneven curvature of the cornea or lens; causes visual distortion.
Atelectasis Collapsed lung or part of a lung.
Atherosclerosis Abnormal thickening and hardening of the arterial walls caused by fat and fibrin deposits.
Aura A peculiar sensation that precedes a set of symptoms.
Auscultation Listening to sounds produced by the body, such as heart, lung, and intestinal sounds.
Autocratic leadership Authoritative, directive, or bureaucratic type of leadership.
Autoimmunity A condition in which the body is unable to distinguish self from nonself, causing the immune system to react and destroy its own tissues.
Automaticity Ability of a cell to generate an impulse without external stimulation.
Automatism Aimless behavior performed without conscious control or knowledge.
Autonomic dysreflexia Abnormally exaggerated response of the autonomic nervous system to a stimulus.
Autopsy Examination of a body after death to determine or confirm the cause of death.
Avulsion Tearing away of tissue.
Azotemia Accumulation of nitrogenous compounds in the blood.

B

Bacteria Several classifications of one-celled microorganisms that are capable of multiplying rapidly and causing illness.
Basal metabolic rate Energy expended in the resting state; measured with the body at complete mental and physical rest, but not asleep.
Basic life support Immediate care given to prevent cardiac or respiratory arrest or to support circulation and respiration of a victim of cardiac arrest until advanced medical support is available.
Behçet's disease Chronic syndrome with oral, gastrointestinal, and genital ulcerations and uveitis; arthritis, vasculitis, synovitis, meningitis, and phlebitis.
Benign Not malignant.
Biologic age The functional capabilities of various organ systems in the body.
Biologic approach Assumes that mental disorders are related to physiologic changes within the central nervous system.
Biopsy Excision of a small piece of tissue for microscopic examination; usually done to determine a specific diagnosis.
Bipolar disorder Disorder characterized by alternating periods of elevated mood (manic episodes) and depression.
Blepharitis Inflammation of the hair follicles and glands on the margins of the eyelids.
Body image One's physical and psychological experiences that influence the perception of one's own body.
Bone marrow Spongy center of bones where the white blood cells, red blood cells, and platelets are made.
Bone remodeling Process in which immature bone cells are gradually replaced by mature bone cells.
Borderline personality disorder Disorder characterized by exhibition of unstable relationships, unstable self-image, and unstable mood.
Botulism Food poisoning caused by *Clostridium botulinum.*
Bouchard's nodes Enlarged proximal interphalangeal joints of the fingers.
Brachytherapy Placement of a radiation source in the body to treat a malignancy.
Bradycardia Slow heart rate, usually defined as fewer than 60 beats per minute.
Bronchiectasis Permanent dilation of a portion of the bronchi or bronchioles.
Bronchitis Bronchial inflammation.
Bruit A murmur detected by auscultation.
Bulla Blister.

C

Cachexia Profound wasting, loss of body mass, usually related to malnutrition.
Calculus (*pl.* calculi) Abnormal concentration, commonly called a stone, that is formed of mineral salts and is found in hollow organs or their passages.
Calorie Standard unit for measuring energy; the amount of heat needed to raise the temperature of 1 gm of water at a standard temperature by 1° C.
Cannula A tube that can be inserted into a body cavity or duct; needle or catheter employed for intravenous therapy.

Capitation Accepting a fixed amount of money to provide health care services to all health care plan members with no additional billing.
Carcinogen A substance that can cause cancer.
Cardiac output Liters of blood ejected by either ventricle per minute.
Cardiac tamponade The presence of blood in the pericardial sac that causes decreased cardiac output.
Cardiopulmonary arrest Absence of heartbeat and breathing.
Cardioversion Delivery of an electrical shock to the myocardium to restore normal sinus rhythm.
Caries Destructive process of tooth decay.
Caring A process characterized by understanding, action, and concern.
Cataract Clouding or opacity of the normally transparent lens within the eye; causes blurred vision and objects to take on a yellowish hue.
Catecholamines Chemicals (dopamine, epinephrine, norepinephrine) released at sympathetic nerve endings in response to stress.
Cathartic Agent that stimulates bowel evacuation; usually rapid in effect and producing a watery stool.
Cell-mediated acquired immunity Defensive response by T_c cells aimed at intracellular defects such as viruses and cancer.
Cerebral death Absence of cerebral cortex functioning.
Cerumen Waxy secretion in the external auditory canal; earwax.
Cervicitis Inflammation of the cervix (narrow, lower end of the uterus).
Chalazion An inflamed, enlarged meibomian gland on the eyelid.
Chancre A papule that breaks down into a painless ulcer at the site of entry of the organism that causes syphilis.
Cheilitis Inflammation of the lips.
Cheilosis Cracking of the lips and corners of the mouth.
Chemical restraints Psychotropic medications given to subdue agitated or confused patients.
Chemotherapy Use of chemicals to treat illness.
Choking Airway obstruction caused by a foreign body in the airway.
Cholangitis Inflammation of the biliary ducts.
Cholecystectomy Removal of the gallbladder.
Cholecystitis Inflammation of the gallbladder.
Choledocholithiasis Obstruction of the common bile duct by a gallstone.
Cholelithiasis Presence of gallstones in the gallbladder.
Chronic illness Permanent impairment or disability that requires long-term rehabilitation and medical or nursing treatment.
Chronic pain Pain that lasts longer than 3 to 6 months and is associated with nerve or tissue damage. It usually continues after the normal time for healing or it may occur spontaneously. It is difficult to localize, may not be detectable with current diagnostic techniques, and may not respond to usual treatments.
Chvostek's sign Spasm of the facial muscles when the facial nerve is tapped; indicative of hypocalcemia.
Cirrhosis Chronic, progressive liver disease.
Client Recipient of nursing care in situations; denotes a feeling of partnership or working with someone.
Closed amputation Amputation in which a limb or part of a limb is removed and the wound is surgically closed.
Closed or simple fracture Fracture in which the broken bone does not break through the skin.
Closed reduction or manipulation Nonsurgical realignment of the bones to their previous anatomic position using traction, angulation, or rotation or a combination of these.
Clotting factors Substances in the blood that help the blood to clot, numbered I through XII.
Co-dependency Exaggerated dependent pattern of self-defeating behaviors, beliefs, and feelings learned as a result of pathologic relationship to a chemically dependent, or otherwise dysfunctional, person.
Cognition Workings of the mind; language, memory, intellect, and reasoning.
Cognitive behavioral approach Approach to therapy that uses behavior modification (positive and negative reinforcement) and recognizes that particular thoughts influence emotional states.
Cognitive developmental approach Approach to management of behavioral symptoms of dementia in which the environment and interactions are adapted to the patient's cognitive abilities.
Collateral Accessory; side branch.
Colostomy Surgically created opening in the colon.
Colporrhaphy Operative technique that narrows the vagina by suturing the vaginal wall.
Comminuted fracture Fracture in which the bone is broken or crushed into small pieces.
Communicable disease Illness, caused by infectious organisms or their toxins, that can be transmitted, either directly or indirectly, from one person to another.
Community-acquired infections Infections that are acquired in day-to-day contact with the public.
Compartment syndrome Serious complication of a fracture caused by internal or external pressure on the affected area, resulting in decreased blood flow, pain, and tissue damage.
Compensation Adaptations made by the heart and circulation to maintain normal cardiac output.
Complement One of a series of proteins that enhance the inflammatory process and immune response.
Complementary proteins Combination of incomplete proteins that provide all nine essential amino acids when consumed together.
Complete fracture Fracture in which the break extends across the entire bone, dividing it into two separate pieces.
Complete protein Protein containing all nine essential amino acids; usually of animal origin (e.g., meat, eggs).
Compliance Elasticity.
Compromised host precautions Actions taken to help protect patients with low white blood cell counts from infection.
Compulsions Incessant behaviors such as hand washing that interfere with normal functioning.
Conduction deafness A hearing impairment due to a blockage of the ear canal caused by excessive wax buildup, abnormal structures, or infection.
Conductivity Ability of the cell to transmit electrical impulses rapidly and efficiently to distant regions of the heart.

Conflict Psychological struggle that results when two incompatible possibilities occur at the same time.
Confusion Disordered consciousness; lack of orientation in relation to person, place, and/or time.
Congenital amputation Deformity or absence of a limb or limbs occurring during fetal development.
Conjunctivitis Inflammation of the membrane lining the eyelids and the eyeball.
Constipation Condition characterized by infrequent bowel movements with hard stools that are passed with difficulty.
Contamination Presence of an infectious organism on a body surface or an object.
Continent Capable of controlling natural impulses; in relation to an ostomy, able to retain feces or urine.
Contractility Capacity for shortening in response to stimuli.
Contracture Shortening of the muscles and tendons.
Contralateral Opposite side.
Conversion disorder Loss of body function (such as paralysis) without physiologic cause.
Coping Any behavioral or cognitive activity used to deal with stress.
Coping strategy An adaptive or maladaptive mental attitude, behavior, or both that is consciously or unconsciously perceived as helping to reduce stress, anxiety, or fear.
Cor pulmonale Right-sided heart failure associated with pulmonary disease.
Corpus (*pl.* corpora) cavernosa Erectile chamber of the penis.
Coryza Discharge from the nasal mucous membranes.
Crackles Abnormal lung sounds heard on auscultation; discrete single sounds heard on inspiration, occur in brief bursts; may be fine (high pitched and soft) or coarse (low pitched and loud); "rales."
Crede's technique Expression of urine from the bladder by applying pressure over the lower abdomen.
Crepitus Crackling sound or sensation.
Crest syndrome A form of a systemic scleroderma less severe than other forms, consisting of calcinosis cutis, Raynaud's phenomenon, esophageal dysfunction, sclerodactyly, and telangiectasia.
Cretinism Permanent mental and physical retardation caused by congenital deficiency of thyroid hormones.
Crisis The point at which the individual moves toward illness and disequilibrium.
Cultural diversity The existence of many cultures in a society.
Culture Integrated system of learned values, beliefs, and practices that is characteristic of a society and that guides individual behavior.
Cushing's disease Disease caused by the hypersecretion of glucocorticoids due to excessive release of adrenocorticotropic hormone by the pituitary.
Cushing's syndrome Disorder resulting from excessive glucocorticoids in the body as a result of tumor or hypersecretion of the pituitary or by prolonged administration of large doses of exogenous steroids.
Cusp Cup-shaped structure; semilunar heart valves have three cusps.
Cycloplegic Agent that paralyzes the ciliary muscle so that the eye does not accommodate.
Cystectomy Removal or resection of the urinary bladder or of a cyst.
Cystocele Herniation of the urinary bladder into the vagina.
Cystotomy Creation of a surgical opening into the bladder.
Cytologic Related to cells or the study of cells.

D

Débride To remove debris, including necrotic tissue.
Decerebrate posturing Abnormal extension of the upper extremities with extension of the lower extremities; accompanies increased pressure on the entire cerebrum and the motor tract structures of the brain stem.
Decongestant Agent that reduces swelling, especially of the nasal mucous membranes
Decorticate posturing Abnormal flexion of the upper extremities with extension of the lower extremities; accompanies increased pressure on the frontal lobes.
Deep partial thickness burn A burn that involves the epidermis and the dermis.
Defense mechanism A mechanism, usually unconscious, used to relieve or diminish anxiety.
Defibrillation Termination of cardiac fibrillation, usually by electric shock.
Dehiscence Separation of previously joined edges; reopening of a surgical wound.
Delayed union Fracture healing that does not occur in the normally expected time.
Delegation Turning over part of one person's responsibility to another person, with that person's consent.
Delirium A disturbance of consciousness and a change in cognition that develop over a short period of time.
Dementia A clinical syndrome or collection of symptoms that is chronic in nature and is characterized by impairment of intellectual function, problem-solving ability, judgment, memory, orientation, and appropriate behavior.
Democratic leadership Achievement of goals through participation by all group members.
Denial A defense mechanism in which the individual thinks and behaves as if not aware of an unpleasant reality.
Depersonalization A state of feeling outside of oneself, watching what is happening as if it were happening to someone else.
Depression A mood of sadness; a withdrawal from usual commitments.
Dermatitis Inflammation of the skin.
Dermatome Area of skin supplied by sensory nerve fibers from a single posterior spinal root.
Dermatomyositis An acute, subacute, or chronic disease marked by nonsuppurative inflammation of the skin, subcutaneous tissue, and muscles, with necrosis of muscle fibers.
Diabetes insipidus Disease caused by inadequate secretion of antidiuretic hormone by the posterior portion of the pituitary.
Diagnosis-related group (DRG) System of reimbursement standards for care in hospitals. The reimbursement is based on a fixed fee for a diagnostic category, regardless of cost.

Dialysis Passage of molecules through a semipermeable membrane into a special solution.
Diaphoresis Excessive perspiration.
Diaphoretic Wet with excessive perspiration.
Diarrhea The passage of frequent watery stools.
Diffusion The random movement of particles in all directions through a solution.
Diplopia Double vision.
Disability Measurable loss of function, usually delineated to indicate a diminished capacity for work (*see* Handicap).
Discoid lupus Circular, scaly lesions with erythematous raised rims; occurs over scalp, ears, face, and areas exposed to sun.
Disorder A term used when a definite organic cause is established for behaviors and symptoms (*see* Syndrome).
Dissociative disorder Change in identity, memory, or consciousness that allows persons to remove themselves from anxiety-provoking situations, for example, multiple personality disorder and amnesias.
Distress Stress that is perceived as harmful.
Diuresis Increased production of urine.
Dizziness Feeling of unsteadiness.
Dual diagnosis Simultaneous existence of a major psychiatric condition and a medical condition.
Dysarthria Inability to speak clearly because of neurologic damage that impairs normal muscle control.
Dysfunctional communication An unclear transmission of a message or information that prohibits the receiver from understanding the intent or meaning of what the sender transmits.
Dysmenorrhea Painful menstruation.
Dyspareunia Difficult or painful sexual intercourse in women.
Dyspepsia Epigastric discomfort after meals, caused by impaired digestion.
Dysphagia Difficulty swallowing.
Dysphasia Difficulty speaking.
Dysplasia Abnormal cells.
Dyspnea Difficulty breathing.
Dyspraxia Partial inability to initiate coordinated voluntary motor acts.
Dysreflexia Disordered response to stimuli; NANDA diagnosis for person with spinal cord injury at or above the seventh thoracic vertebra who experiences or is at risk for experiencing autonomic dysreflexia.
Dysrhythmia Disturbance of rhythm; arrhythmia.
Dysuria Difficult or painful urination.

E

Ecchymosis Purplish skin lesions resulting from blood leaking out of the blood vessels.
Ectropion In relation to the eyelid, outward turning of the lid.
Ego In psychoanalytic theory, the "rational self" or "reality" principle of personality; mediates between id and superego.
Egocentric Belief that one is the center of the universe.
Eicosanoid A class of fatty acids that regulate blood vessel vasodilation, temperature elevation, white blood cell activation, and other physiologic processes involved in immunity.
Ejaculation Reflexive expulsion of semen from the male urethra.
Ejection fraction Percentage of ventricular end-diastolic volume ejected with each contraction of the left ventricle.
Electroconvulsive therapy Controversial therapy that uses electrical current to the brain to evoke a grand mal seizure.
Electrolyte A substance that develops an electrical charge when dissolved in water.
Electromyography Diagnostic procedure in which needle electrodes are used to detect electrical impulses in muscle tissue; impulses are recorded and provide information about function of the nerves that supply muscles.
Embolism Sudden obstruction of an artery by a floating clot or foreign material.
Embolus (*pl.* emboli) An unattached blood clot or other substance in the circulatory system.
Emesis Vomiting.
Emission Delivery of semen into the internal urethra by rhythmic smooth muscle contractions of the epididymis, vas deferens, seminal vesicles, and prostate.
Emotional lability Instability; episodes of unexplained and uncontrollable happiness and sadness.
Empathy The ability to identify with and understand another person's situation, feelings, and motives.
Emphysema Abnormal accumulation of air in body tissue; in the lung, a disorder characterized by loss of lung elasticity with trapping of air, retained carbon dioxide, and dyspnea.
Empowerment Giving patients the information they need to be active participants in their care.
Encephalitis Inflammation of brain tissue.
Enculturation The process of learning to be part of a culture.
Endocrine gland Gland that secretes a substance directly into the blood.
Endogenous Internally produced or caused by internal factors.
Endometriosis A condition in which endometrial tissue is located outside the uterus.
Energy Capacity to do work; the way the body uses nutrients received through food consumption.
Entropion In relation to the eyelid, inward turning of the lid.
Enucleation Removal of an intact organ, such as the eyeball.
Enuresis Involuntary passage of urine, usually during sleep.
Epididymitis Inflammation of the epididymis.
Epidural Situated within the spinal canal or on the outside of the dura mater; opioids may be administered epidurally for pain relief.
Epistaxis Nosebleed.
Equianalgesic Having approximately the same degree of pain relief effect.
Equilibrium State of balance needed for walking, standing, and sitting.
Erection Swelling and rigidity of the penis.
Eructation Expulsion of gas from the stomach through the mouth; belching.
Erythema Redness of the skin; usually a sign that capillaries have become congested because of impaired blood flow.

Estrogens Hormones produced by the ovaries, adrenal glands, and fetoplacental unit in women that are responsible for the sexual development and maturation of women.
Ethics Values, codes, and principles related to what is right that influence decisions in nursing practice.
Ethnic group Group of individuals with a unique identity based on shared traditions, national origin, physical characteristics, and customs.
Euglycemia Normal blood glucose level.
Eustress Stress that is perceived as helpful (e.g., graduation, vacation).
Evisceration Protrusion of internal organs through a wound.
Excitability Ability of a cell to respond to an electrochemical stimulus.
Exocrine gland Gland that secretes substances externally through ducts.
Exogenous Developed outside the organism.
Exophthalmos Protrusion of the eyeballs associated with hyperthyroidism.
Expressive aphasia Difficulty speaking, reading, and writing; characterized as nonfluent; caused by lesion in Broca's area.
External fixation Use of rods, pins, nails, screws, or metal plates to align bone fragments and keep them in place for healing; similar to internal fixation, but the devices in the bone are attached to an external frame.
Extracellular fluid Fluid outside the cell.
Extrapyramidal effects Side effects of antipsychotic drugs on the portion of the central nervous system controlling involuntary movements.
Extravasation Escape of fluid or blood from a blood vessel into body tissue.
Extrinsic factors Factors in the environment.

F

Fall Circumstance in which one unintentionally falls to the ground or hits an object such as a chair or stair.
Family Two or more persons who are joined together by bonds of sharing and emotional closeness and who identify themselves as being part of a family.
Fasciculation Small involuntary muscle contraction.
Fat embolism Condition in which fat globules are released from the marrow of the broken bone into the bloodstream, migrate to the lungs, and cause pulmonary hypertension.
Fat-soluble vitamins Vitamins that are soluble in fat solvents, are absorbed into the body with other lipids, and build up in fat cells; includes vitamins A, D, E, and K.
Fear Analogous to anxiety, but related to dread of a specific or real occurrence.
Fecal incontinence The inability to control the passage of feces.
Fee for service An established fee set by physicians or health care providers for services or procedures actually provided.
Feelings All emotional and physical responses and sensations.
Filtration Transfer of water and solutes through a membrane from a region of high pressure to a region of low pressure.
Fixation Procedure done during the open reduction surgical procedure to attach the fragments of the broken bone together when reduction alone is not feasible.
Flaccid Soft; in relation to muscles, lacking tone.
Flaccidity Diminished muscle tone.
Flail chest Loss of support in the chest wall where several adjacent ribs are broken in more than one place.
Flatulence Formation of excessive gas in the stomach or intestines.
Flatus Gas in the digestive tract that is expelled through the rectum.
Fluent aphasia Ability to speak clearly but without meaning.
Fluid Any liquid or gas.
Fluid volume deficit An abnormally decreased volume of extracellular fluid.
Fluid volume excess An abnormally increased volume of extracellular water and electrolytes or intracellular water.
Fracture Break or disruption in the continuity of a bone.
Frostbite Serious tissue damage caused by cold.
Frostnip Mild tissue damage caused by cold.
Full thickness burn Burn involving the epidermis, dermis, and underlying tissues such as fat, muscle, and bone.
Functional communication The clear transmission of a message or information that enables the receiver to understand the intent or meaning of what the sender transmits.
Functional incontinence Inappropriate voiding in the presence of normal bladder and urethral function.
Fungi Vegetable-like organisms that feed on organic matter and are capable of producing disease.

G

Gangrene Necrosis or death of tissue, usually due to a deficient or absent blood supply; may result from inflammatory processes, injury, arteriosclerosis, frostbite, or diabetes mellitus.
Gastrectomy Removal of all or part of the stomach.
Gastritis Inflammation of the stomach.
Gastrostomy A surgically created opening in the stomach.
Gerontological nurses Professional nurses and advanced level practitioners such as nurse practitioners, clinical specialists, and nurses holding national certification in the specialty of gerontological nursing.
Gerontology The study of aging.
Gigantism Disease caused by excessive growth hormone in children and young adolescents resulting in excessive proportional growth.
Gingivitis Inflammation of the gums.
Gland Organ or structure that secretes substances used in other areas of the body.
Glaucoma Condition in which high pressure of the fluid in the eye causes damage to the optic nerve.
Glucocorticoid Class of adrenocortical hormones that affect protein and carbohydrate metabolism and help protect the body against stress.
Glucometer Electronic device used to measure blood glucose.
Gluconeogenesis Synthesis of glucose from sources other than carbohydrates.
Glycogenesis Formation of glycogen from glucose.
Glycogenolysis Splitting of glycogen into glucose.

Glycosuria Presence of glucose in the urine.
Goiter Enlargement of the thyroid gland.
Goitrogen Substance that suppresses thyroid function.
Goniometer Instrument used to measure joint range of motion.
Granuloma A collection of inflammatory cells commonly surrounded by fibrotic tissue that represents a chronic inflammatory response to infectious or noninfectious agents.
Gratification Sense of comfort and satisfaction derived from the fulfillment of one's needs.
Gravidity Describes state of a woman with respect to the total number of pregnancies.
Greenstick fracture Fracture in which the bone is broken on one side but only bent on the other; most common in children.
Grief An emotional response to a loss.
Growth and development Physical, cognitive, and psychological development that is predictable and sequential.
Guillotine amputation Type of amputation in which a limb or portion of a limb is severed from the body and the wound is left open; a type of open amputation.

H

Handicap Inability to perform one or more normal daily activities because of mental or physical disability (*see* Disability).
Health maintenance organization (HMO) Health care organization responsible for both financing and delivering comprehensive health services to an enrolled population for a prepaid fixed fee.
Heartburn (pyrosis) Burning or tight sensation rising from the lower sternum to the throat.
Heat stroke Body core temperature of 106° F or more.
Heberden's nodes Protrusions of the distal interphalangeal finger joints associated with osteoarthritis.
Heimlich maneuver Technique for ejecting a foreign body from the airway by using abdominal thrusts.
Helminths Worms that are parasites found in the soil and water and are transmitted to humans from hand to mouth.
Hematocele Accumulation of blood in the scrotum, usually as a result of blunt trauma.
Hematocrit Percentage of red blood cells in whole blood.
Hematuria Blood in the urine.
Hemiparesis Weakness on one side of the body.
Hemiplegia Paralysis on one side of the body.
Hemoconcentration Concentration of the blood.
Hemodynamics Study of the movement of blood and the forces that affect it.
Hemoglobin Protein of the red blood cell that carries oxygen.
Hemorrhage Loss of a large amount of blood.
Hemostasis The control of bleeding.
Hemothorax Presence of blood in the pleural cavity causing the lung on the affected side to collapse.
Hepatic Pertaining to the liver.
Hepatitis Inflammation of the liver.
Hepatomegaly Enlargement of the liver.
HIV Human immunodeficiency virus.
HIV positive A condition in which the blood has antibodies for the human immunodeficiency virus (HIV), meaning the individual has been infected with this virus.
Holism A way of viewing people as whole individuals.
Homeostasis A tendency of the biologic system to maintain stability of the internal environment while continuously adjusting to changes necessary for survival.
Homonymous hemianopsia Loss of half the field of vision; loss is on the side opposite the brain lesion.
Hopelessness A condition of lack of hope, which may hinder action.
Hordeolum Inflammation of a sebaceous gland of the eyelid; commonly called a "sty."
Humoral immunity An immediate response to specific antigens involving B lymphocytes and the production of antibodies.
Hydrocele Accumulation of clear fluid in the tunica vaginalis of the testicle or along the spermatic cord.
Hypercalcemia Abnormally high serum calcium.
Hypercapnia Excess carbon dioxide in the blood.
Hyperglycemia Abnormally high serum glucose.
Hyperkalemia Abnormally high serum potassium.
Hyperlipidemia Excess insoluble fats in the blood.
Hypernatremia Abnormally high serum sodium.
Hyperopia Farsightedness; ability to see distant objects better than near objects.
Hypertension Persistent elevation of arterial blood pressure of 140/90 mm Hg or greater.
Hyperthermia Elevation of body core temperature above 99° F.
Hypertonic solution A solution that has a higher concentration of electrolytes than normal body fluids.
Hypertrophy Enlargement of existing cells resulting in increased size of an organ or tissue.
Hyperuricemia Elevated level of uric acid in the blood.
Hyperventilation Abnormally prolonged and deep breathing.
Hypervolemia Increased circulating blood volume.
Hypocalcemia Abnormally low serum calcium.
Hypochondriasis Belief that a serious medical condition exists when medical findings are absent.
Hypoglycemia Abnormally low level of glucose in the blood.
Hypokalemia Abnormally low serum potassium.
Hyponatremia Abnormally low serum sodium.
Hypophysectomy Surgical removal of all or part of the pituitary gland.
Hypotension Abnormally low blood pressure.
Hypothermia Decrease in body core temperature below 95° F.
Hypotonic solution A solution that has a lower concentration of electrolytes than normal body fluids.
Hypovolemia Reduced circulating blood volume.
Hypoxemia Low level of oxygen in the blood.
Hypoventilation Reduced movement of air into the alveoli.
Hypoxia Low oxygen level; decreased availability of oxygen to body tissues.
Hysterectomy Surgical removal of the uterus.

I

Iatrogenic infections Infections transmitted in the caregiving process.

Icterus Jaundice; golden yellow skin color caused by deposition of bile pigments.
Id In psychoanalytic theory, the "pleasure principle" of the personality.
Ileostomy Surgically created opening in the ileum.
Immobility The inability to move; imposed restriction on entire body.
Immunity Resistance to or protection from a disease.
Immunodeficiency A condition in which the immune system is unable to defend the body against a foreign invasion of antigens.
Immunoglobulin Membrane-bound, Y-shaped binding proteins produced by B lymphocytes; when immunoglobulins are released from the cell membrane, they are called antibodies.
Immunosuppressant Agent that reduces immune response.
Impaction (fecal) Accumulation of stool in the intestines that is not readily eliminated.
Impairment Physical or psychological disturbance in functioning.
Impotence (erectile dysfunction) Inability to achieve and maintain an erection for sexual intercourse.
Incomplete fracture Fracture in which the bone breaks only part way across, leaving some portion of the bone intact.
Incomplete protein Protein lacking one or more essential amino acids.
Incontinence Inability to hold urine.
Infarct An area of ischemic necrosis caused by disruption of circulation.
Infection Condition in which the body is invaded by infectious organisms that multiply, causing injury and a local inflammatory response that may progress to a systemic response.
Infertility Inability to conceive and produce viable offspring.
Infiltration A collection of infused fluid in tissues surrounding a cannula inserted for intravenous therapy.
Inflammation Nonspecific immune response that occurs in response to bodily injury.
Innate immunity Defensive system that is operational at all times, consisting of anatomic and physiologic barriers, the inflammatory response, and the ability of certain cells to phagocytose invaders.
Insoluble fiber Indigestible roughage found in plant cells; aids in stool formation and elimination.
Isotonic A solution that has the same concentration of electrolytes as normal body fluids.
Inspection Purposeful observation or scrutiny of the person as a whole and then of each body system.
Inspissated Thickened and dried; often used to describe pulmonary secretions.
Instinct Inborn source of bodily need or impulse.
Interferon A substance produced in viral infections that inhibits the replication of viruses.
Intermediate care facility Nursing homes that provide custodial care for people who are unable to care for themselves because of mental or physical infirmity.
Internal fixation Use of rods, pins, nails, screws, or metal plates to align bone fragments and keep them in place for healing.
Interpersonal approach Approach to therapy whereby the patient learns new ways to behave in a therapeutic relationship built on trust.
Intertrigo Skin inflammation where two skin surfaces touch.
Intracellular fluid Fluid within the cell.
Intracerebral Within the cerebrum.
Intracranial Within the skull.
Intracranial pressure Pressure within the cranium/skull.
Intrinsic factors Factors related to the internal functioning of an individual, such as the aging process or physical illness.
Ipsilateral Same side.
Ischemia Deficient blood flow due to obstruction or constriction of blood vessels.
Isolation technique Isolation of infected patients from other patients and health care workers.
Isometric exercise Muscle contraction without movement used to maintain muscle tone.
Isotonic solution A term used to describe a solution that has the same concentration of electrolytes as normal body fluids.

J

Jaundice Golden yellow color of the skin, sclerae, and mucous membranes caused by deposition of bile pigments; associated with liver dysfunction or bile obstruction causing hyperbilirubinemia.

K

Keratitis Inflammation of the cornea.
Keratolytic Capable of dissolving keratin, the outer surface of the epidermis.
Ketoacidosis Metabolic acidosis related to accumulated ketone bodies in the blood.
Ketone bodies Products of fatty acid metabolism.
Kyphosis Abnormal curvature of the thoracic spine as viewed from the side.

L

Laissez-faire leadership Nondirective type of leadership.
Laryngectomy Surgical removal of the larynx.
Laryngitis Inflammation of the larynx.
Laryngospasm Spasmodic closure of the larynx.
Latent Dormant; during the latency period of a disease, there are no signs or symptoms of the disease.
Lavage Irrigation.
Laxative Agent that softens stool and promotes bowel evacuation.
Leadership Guidance or showing the way to others.
Lentigo (*pl.* lentigines) Pigmented spot on sun-exposed skin.
Leukemia Cancer of the white blood cells in which the bone marrow produces too many immature white blood cells.
Leukocytes White blood cells that play a key role in immune responses to infectious organisms and other antigens.
Leukocytosis Part of the inflammatory process that causes an increase in white blood cells.
Leukopenia Reduced number of leukocytes (white blood cells) in the blood.

Leukoplakia Hard white patches on the gums, oral mucosa, or tongue that tend to become malignant.
Libido In psychoanalytic theory, psychic energy used to operate the id, ego, and superego.
Lipids Fats in solid or liquid form; store energy, carry fat-soluble vitamins, maintain healthy skin and hair; supply essential fatty acids; and promote a feeling of fullness (satiety).
Lipoatrophy Decreased subcutaneous fat mass.
Lipohypertrophy Increased subcutaneous fat mass.
Lipoproteins Lipid-wrapped proteins carried into the bloodstream; they include high-density and low-density lipoproteins, which carry cholesterol.
Lithotomy Removal of calculi through an incision in a duct or organ.
Lithotripsy Crushing or disintegration of calculi.
Livor mortis Discoloration of the body after death.
Long-term care facility Nursing home that provides intermediate and nonskilled or custodial care for people who are unable to care for themselves because of mental or physical disabilities.
Loss A real or potential absence of someone or something that is valued.
Lymphocytopenia Reduced number of lymphocytes in the blood; also called lymphopenia.
Lymphoma Cancer of the lymph system.
Lymphopenia Lymphocytopenia; reduced number of lymphocytes in the blood.

M

Macrovascular Pertaining to the large blood vessels.
Macule A flat, colored lesion such as a freckle.
Maladaptive Attempts to cope using strategies that ultimately do not return the individual to homeostasis.
Malaise Vague feeling of discomfort.
Malignant Tending to progress in virulence; has the characteristics of becoming increasingly undifferentiated, invasive of surrounding tissues, and colonizing distant sites.
Managed health care The provision of comprehensive health care at a reasonable cost through enrollment in an HMO, PPO, or similar plan with incentives to save costs.
Management Effective use of selected methods to achieve desired outcomes.
Metastasis Process by which cancer spreads to distant sites.
Mastitis Inflammation of breast tissue.
Matrix Intercellular substance of a tissue.
Medicaid Program that provides health care services for needy, lower-income, and disabled individuals through funds distributed at the state level.
Medical asepsis Limiting the spread of microorganisms; often called clean technique.
Medicare Health insurance program administered by the federal government that is funded by Social Security payments.
Menarche Age at first menstruation.
Menopause Cessation of menstruation.
Menorrhagia Menstrual periods characterized by profuse or prolonged bleeding.
Menstruation Vaginal discharge of a mixture of blood and other fluids and tissue that is formed in the uterus to receive a fertilized ovum.
Mental health continuum A model used to demonstrate the range of mental health on a line between health at one end and illness at the opposite extreme.
Mental status examination Observations and descriptions regarding appearance, mood and affect, speech and language, thought content, perceptual disturbances, insight and judgment, sensorium and memory, and attention.
Metastasis Process by which cancer spreads to distant sites.
Metrorrhagia Bleeding or spotting between menstrual periods.
Microvascular Pertaining to the small blood vessels (i.e., arterioles, capillaries, and venules).
Micturition Urination.
Mineralocorticoid Type of hormone secreted by the adrenal cortex and involved in the regulation of fluid and electrolyte levels in the body.
Minerals Small amounts of metals (calcium, sodium, potassium) and nonmetals (chloride, phosphate) that are essential to the body; can build up.
Miotic agent Agent that causes the pupil to constrict.
Monoamine oxidase inhibitor (MAOI) Class of antidepressant drugs; patients on MAO inhibitors must be carefully monitored to avoid life-threatening food and drug interactions.
Mood Feeling state experienced by the patient over a period of time; can be constricted (not experiencing a variety of feelings) or expanded (experiencing more than usual feelings).
Morals Ethical habits of a person.
Multiple personality disorder Exhibition by one person of two or more distinct personalities.
Murmur A sound heard on auscultation of the heart that usually indicates turbulent blood flow across heart valves.
Myalgia Muscle pain.
Mycoplasmas Gram-negative organisms usually causing infections in the respiratory tract.
Mydriatic agent Agent that causes the pupil to dilate.
Myelinated Surrounded with a sheath.
Myopathy Muscle disease; *adj.* myopathic.
Myopia Nearsightedness; ability to see near objects better than distant objects.
Myxedema Facial edema that develops with severe, long-term hypothyroidism; sometimes used as a synonym for hypothyroidism.

N

Natural immunity Immunity that is present at birth.
Necrotizing vasculitis Any of a group of disorders characterized by inflammation and necrosis of blood vessels occurring in a broad spectrum of cutaneous and systemic disorders.
Neoplasm Tumor; may be benign or malignant.
Nephropathy Kidney disease.
Nephrostomy Surgically created opening in the kidney to drain urine.
Nephrotoxic Having a harmful effect on kidney tissue.
Neuralgia Pain in a nerve or along the course of a nerve.
Neurogenic bladder Condition in which the bladder does not function normally because of some disorder affecting the nerves of the bladder.

Neurogenic (bowel) incontinence Reflexive uncontrolled bowel movement, usually seen with dementia.
Neurohypophysis Posterior portion of the pituitary gland.
Neuroleptic malignant syndrome Effect of medication that can develop after one dose or after years of drug therapy; the first symptoms usually are muscular rigidity, accompanied by akinesia and respiratory distress; the cardinal sign is hyperthermia (body temperature 101–103° F or higher).
Neuropathic pain Pain that arises from a damaged nerve.
Neuropathy Pathologic changes in the peripheral nervous system.
Neurotoxin Substance that poisons or impairs nerve tissue.
Neurotransmitter Biochemical messenger at nerve endings that stimulates an excitatory or inhibitory response.
Nevus (*pl.* nevi) Mole.
Nociception Process of pain transmission; usually related to pain sensation resulting from stimulation of pain receptors and transmission of stimuli to the pain fibers, spinal cord, and brain.
Nocturia Urination during the night.
Nodule Small mass of tissue that can be palpated.
Nonfluent aphasia Difficulty initiating speech.
Nonsteroidal anti-inflammatory drug (NSAID) Nonopioid drug that reduces pain and inflammation.
Nonunion Failure of a fracture to heal.
Nosocomial infections Hospital-acquired infections that were not present at the time of admission.
Nurse anesthetist A registered nurse who specializes in the administration of anesthetics and monitors the condition of patients receiving anesthetics.
Nursing diagnosis Actual or potential health problems derived from data gathered during the assessment of a patient or client.
Nursing process Systematic, problem-solving approach to providing nursing care in an organized, scientific manner.

O

Object permanence Idea that an object or person continues to exist even though no longer in sight; object permanence does not develop until about 2 years of age, according to Piaget.
Objective data Information about the patient that can be detected with the senses.
Obsessions Recurrent intrusive thoughts that interfere with normal functioning.
Obsessive-compulsive disorder Recurrent obsessions, compulsions, or both that produce distress and interfere with daily functions.
Oedipus complex Occurs during the phallic stage in psychoanalytic theory; the child unconsciously desires the parent of the opposite sex; this conflict is resolved when the child identifies with the parent of the same sex.
Older Americans Act Act passed in 1965 to ensure that elderly persons have an adequate income and suitable housing, physical and mental health services, community services, and the opportunity to pursue meaningful activities.
Oliguria Decreased urine output.
Omnibus Reconciliation Act (OBRA) Law enacted in 1987 to protect patients in long-term care facilities.
Oncofetal antigen A gene product that normally is suppressed in adult tissues but reappears in the presence of some types of cancer.
Open amputation Amputation that is left open; usually done in cases of infection or necrosis.
Open or compound fracture Fracture in which the fragments of the broken bone break through the skin.
Open reduction Surgical procedure in which an incision is made at the fracture site, usually on patients with open (compound) or comminuted fractures, to cleanse the area of fragments and debris.
Opioid agonist Any morphine-like drug that produces bodily effects including pain relief.
Opportunistic infection An infection caused by an organism that usually does not cause a disease but becomes pathogenic when body defenses are impaired.
Orthopnea Difficulty breathing when lying down.
Orthostatic hypotension Sudden drop in systolic blood pressure when changing from a lying or sitting position to a standing position.
Orthostatic vital sign changes Changes in the vital signs as a person moves from lying to sitting to standing positions in which the pulse increases by 20 points and the blood pressure decreases by 20 points, indicating that the patient is hypovolemic.
Osmolality The concentration of a solution; measured as the number of dissolved particles per kilogram of water.
Osmolarity The concentration of a solution; measured as the number of dissolved particles per liter of solution.
Osmosis Movement of water across a membrane from a less concentrated solution to a more concentrated solution.
Osteoarthritis A noninflammatory degenerative joint disease marked by degeneration of the articular cartilage, hypertrophy of bone at the margins, and changes in the synovial membrane.
Osteomyelitis Infection of the bone.
Osteoporosis Decreased bone mass.
Ostomy Surgical procedure that creates an opening into a body structure.
Otalgia Pain in the ear.
Otic Pertaining to the ear.
Ototoxic Capable of injuring the eighth cranial (acoustic) nerve or other structures involved in hearing and balance.
Overflow incontinence (fecal) Uncontrolled passage of stool associated with constipation.
Overflow incontinence (urine) Involuntary loss of urine associated with a full bladder.
Oximeter A device that uses a photoelectric sensor to measure the oxygen saturation of the blood.
Oxygenation The transport of oxygen from the lungs to the tissues.

P

Pain Unpleasant sensory and emotional experience associated with actual or potential tissue damage existing whenever the person says it does; a unique, private experience involving the whole person in a time dimension of past, present, and future and influenced by internal and external environments.
Pain threshold Level of intensity that causes the sensation or feeling of pain.

Pain tolerance Amount of pain a person is willing to endure before taking action to relieve pain.
Palliative Relieves symptoms or improves function without correcting the basic problem.
Palpation Method of physical examination that uses touch to assess various parts of the body.
Palpitation A heartbeat that is strong, rapid, or irregular enough that the person is aware of it.
Pancreatitis Inflammation of the pancreas.
Panic disorder Experience of intense episodes of apprehension to the point of terror.
Papule A raised area on the skin that is less than 1 cm in diameter.
Paracentesis Removal of ascitic fluid from the peritoneal cavity.
Paraphimosis Retraction of phimotic foreskin, causing painful swelling of the glans.
Paraplegia Loss of motor and sensory function due to damage to the spinal cord that spares the upper extremities but, depending on the level of the damage, affects the trunk, pelvis, and lower extremities.
Paresthesia An abnormal sensation.
Parity Describes state of a woman with respect to the number of pregnancies carried 20 or more weeks.
Parkinsonian syndrome Adverse effect of long-term antipsychotic drug therapy; patient exhibits mask-like face, shuffling gait, resting tremor, and rigid posture.
Parotiditis Inflammation of the parotid (salivary) gland; most commonly called parotitis.
Parotitis Inflammation of the parotid gland.
Paroxysmal nocturnal dyspnea Sudden difficulty breathing when asleep.
Participative leadership A mixture of autocratic and democratic leadership; feedback from group members is used by the leader to make a final decision.
Passive acquired immunity Temporary immunity acquired after receiving antibodies or lymphocytes produced by another individual.
Passive exercise Exercise of the patient that is carried out by the therapist or nurse without the assistance of the patient.
Pathogen Disease-causing microorganism.
Pathologic fracture Fracture that occurs because of a pathologic condition in the bone, such as a tumor or disease process, that causes a spontaneous break.
Patient A person for whom the nurse provides care; denotes a feeling of doing to or for.
Patient-controlled analgesia Self-administration of an analgesic by a patient instructed in doing so; usually refers to self-dosing with intravenous opioids through a programmable pump.
Patient's Bill of Rights Document issued by the American Hospital Association in 1973 that addresses the quality of care for patients.
Peer group Group of people with which the individual identifies and derives a sense of belonging.
Pelvic inflammatory disease An infection of the ovaries, fallopian tubes, and pelvic area.
Pemphigus Chronic autoimmune condition characterized by blisters on the face, back, chest, groin, and umbilicus.
Percussion Tapping on the skin to assess the underlying tissues.
Perforation Hole or break in a structure.
Perfusion Passage of blood through the vessels of an organ.
Periarteritis nodosa An inflammatory disease of the outer coats of small and medium-sized arteries, marked by a variety of systemic symptoms.
Periarticular Around the joint.
Periorbital edema Accumulation of excess fluid around the eye.
Peritoneum Membrane that lines the walls of the abdominal and pelvic cavities.
Peritonitis Inflammation of the peritoneum.
Personality Deeply ingrained patterns of behavior that include the way one relates to, perceives, and thinks about the environment and self.
Personality disorders Pervasive, chronic, and maladaptive personality characteristics that interfere with normal functioning; examples are paranoid, schizoid, antisocial, borderline, avoidant, obsessive-compulsive, and passive-aggressive.
Pessary A device inserted into the vagina to support the uterus.
Petechia Small (1 to 3 mm) red or reddish purple spots on the skin resulting from capillaries breaking and leaking small amounts of blood into the tissues.
pH The symbol used to indicate hydrogen ion concentration. A solution with a low pH (<7) is an acid; a solution with a high pH (>7) is alkaline or base. A pH of 7 is neutral. The normal pH of body fluids is between 7.35 and 7.45.
Phagocytes Certain white blood cells (neutrophils, monocytes, and macrophages) that engulf and destroy invading pathogens, dead cells, and cellular debris.
Phantom limb Sensation that a limb still exists following amputation; the perception that pain exists in a removed limb is called phantom limb pain.
Phimosis Constriction of the opening in the prepuce so the prepuce cannot be retracted back over the glans.
Phlebitis Inflammation of a vein.
Phlebothrombosis Development of venous thrombi without venous inflammation.
Photophobia Excessive sensitivity to light.
Physical assessment Physical examination that is a systematic, thorough way of obtaining objective data.
Physical dependence Physical need for the substance on which one is dependent in order to avoid unpleasant physical withdrawal symptoms.
Physical restraint Anything that restricts movement, and cannot be removed by the individual.
Plasma Clear, straw-colored fluid that carries the red blood cells, white blood cells, and platelets through the circulatory system.
Platelet Small, disk-shaped blood component responsible for activating the blood clotting system.
Pneumoconiosis One of many occupational diseases caused by inhalation of particles of industrial substances.
Pneumonitis Inflammation of the lung.
Pneumothorax Presence of air in the pleural cavity that causes the lung on the affected side to collapse.
Poikilothermy Coolness in an area of the body due to decreased blood flow.

Poison Any substance that, in small quantities, is capable of causing harm following ingestion, inhalation, injection, or contact with the skin.
Polydipsia Excessive thirst.
Polymyalgia rheumatica A connective tissue disorder characterized by stiffness and pain in the shoulders and hips.
Polymyositis A chronic, progressive inflammatory disease of skeletal muscle.
Polyp Growth that protrudes from a mucous membrane.
Polyphagia Excessive hunger, food ingestion.
Polyuria Excessive urine output.
Postictal After a seizure.
Posttraumatic stress disorder Symptoms experienced following a traumatic event; examples are flashbacks, detachment, and sleep difficulties.
Powerlessness Feeling that one's action will not affect an outcome or that one lacks personal control over certain events or situations.
Preferred provider organization (PPO) System that uses a network of independent physicians, hospitals, and other providers who provide services to a pool of patients for a discounted fee.
Preload The amount of blood in the left ventricle at the end of diastole; the pressure generated at the end of diastole.
Presbycusis The term for hearing loss associated with old age.
Presbyopia A visual impairment associated with older age in which the lens becomes more rigid and less able to change shape, resulting in a decreased ability to focus on near objects.
Pressure ulcer An open wound caused by pressure on a bony prominence; also called a "pressure sore."
Primary prevention The first level of prevention; includes steps taken to improve health and prevent disease and injury.
Problem-oriented medical record Method of record keeping that focuses on patient problems rather than on medical diagnoses.
Progressive systemic sclerosis (PSS) Scleroderma; multisystem autoimmune disorder characterized by hardening of the skin and affecting blood vessels, gastrointestinal tract, lungs, heart, and kidneys.
Projection A defense mechanism in which one sees others as a source of one's own unacceptable thoughts, feelings, or impulses.
Prolapse Downward displacement.
Prostatectomy Removal of all or part of the prostate gland.
Prostatitis Inflammation of the prostate gland.
Prostatodynia Prostatic and pelvic pain in the absence of infection or inflammation.
Proteins Large organic compounds made of various combinations of amino acids; found in meat, milk, fish, and eggs.
Protozoa One-celled organisms capable of producing disease that usually is spread by contaminated food and water.
Pruritus Itching.
Psoriasis Skin condition characterized by scaly lesions and caused by rapid proliferation of epidermal cells.
Psychoanalytic approach Based on the theory that people function at different levels of awareness (conscious to unconscious) and that ego defense mechanisms such as denial and repression are used to prevent anxiety.
Psychological age The behavioral capacity of a person to adapt to changing environmental demands.
Psychological dependence Intense craving for the substance on which one is dependent without physical withdrawal symptoms.
Psychosis A state in which a person's perception of reality is impaired, thereby interfering with the capacity to function and to relate to others.
Ptosis Drooping of the upper eyelid.
Public Health Service Branch of the Department of Health and Human Services of the U.S. government whose chief purpose is to provide better health services for the American people.
Purpura Red or reddish purple skin lesions 3 mm or more in size, resulting from blood leaking outside the blood vessels.
Pyrogen A substance released in inflammation that causes body temperature to increase.

Q

Quadriplegia Loss of motor and sensory function in all four extremities due to damage to the spinal cord.

R

Radiotherapy The use of radiation in the treatment of cancer and other diseases.
Range-of-motion exercise Exercise in which each joint is moved in various directions to the farthest possible extreme without producing pain.
Receptive aphasia Inability to comprehend words; characterized as fluent; lesion in Wernicke's area.
Recovery Lifelong process of maintaining abstinence from the substance to which one is addicted; a return to moderate substance use is never the end result of recovery.
Rectocele Herniation of part of the rectum into the vagina.
Red blood cell Biconcave, disk-shaped blood component responsible for carrying oxygen to the tissues and removing waste carbon dioxide from the tissues.
Red blood cell count Total number of red blood cells found in one cubic millimeter of blood.
Reduction Process of bringing the ends of the broken bone into proper alignment.
Reflex training Technique to stimulate defecation using the Valsalva maneuver and rectal stretching.
Reflux Backward flow.
Refraction Bending of light rays.
Regeneration Replacement of damaged cells by cells of their own kind during the wound healing process.
Regurgitation Backward flow (cardiovascular system); gentle ejection of the stomach contents into the mouth without nausea or retching (digestive tract).
Rehabilitation Process of restoring individuals to best possible health and functioning following physical or mental impairment.
Reiter's syndrome A connective tissue disease characterized by a triad of arthritis, urethritis, and conjunctivitis.

Relaxation State of decreased anxiety and muscle tension.
Repair Replacement of damaged cells by connective tissue and then eventually by scar tissue during the wound healing process.
Replantation Surgical reattachment of a limb to its original site.
Residual limb Stump; partial limb remaining after amputation.
Resources Persons, items, concepts, or organizations that can be drawn on for a sense of support (e.g., family, money, skills, beliefs).
Respiration Exchange of oxygen and carbon dioxide in the alveoli (external respiration) and in the tissues and cells (internal respiration).
Respiratory arrest Absence of breathing.
Resting metabolic rate Measurement of energy expenditure made at any time of the day and 3 to 4 hours after the last meal.
Retinopathy Disease of the retina of the eye.
Retroflexion Bending backward of the upper portion of an organ.
Retroversion Bending backward of an entire organ.
Reverse isolation Protection of severely compromised clients from other patients and health care workers.
Reversible ischemic neurologic deficit Neurologic deficit that lasts more then 24 hours but resolves completely; caused by diminished cerebral blood flow.
Rheumatoid arthritis A chronic systemic disease characterized by inflammatory changes occurring throughout the body's connective tissues; most apparent in diarthroses (synovial joints).
Rhinitis Inflammation of the nasal mucous membrane.
Rhonchus (*pl.* rhonchi) Dry, rattling sound caused by partial bronchial obstruction.
Rickettsiae Microorganisms that usually are transmitted to humans through flea and tick bites.
Rigor mortis Stiffening of the body after death.
Role How a person is expected to behave in a situation or what is expected of a person in a certain position.

S

Salpingo-oophorectomy Surgical excision of a fallopian tube and ovary.
Sanguineous Bloody.
Saturated fatty acids Compounds that come chiefly from animal sources and are usually solid at room temperature; also coconut and palm oils.
Scheduled toileting Encouraging patients to use the toilet at specific times based on their usual patterns.
Schizophrenia Very serious group of usually chronic thought disorders in which patients' ability to interpret the world around them is severely impaired; symptoms include impaired thinking patterns, hallucinations, bizarre behavior, delusions, and emotional responses that do not coincide with events.
Sclerodactyly Hardening and shrinking of connective tissue of fingers and toes; scleroderma of fingers and toes.
Scleroderma Chronic multisystem autoimmune disease characterized by hardening of the skin and affecting the blood vessels, gastrointestinal tract, lungs, heart, and kidneys.
Sclerotherapy Injection of hardening agents into blood vessels.
Scotoma Blind spots.
Secondary prevention The second level of prevention; includes steps taken to detect disease early and begin treatment as soon as possible.
Seizure Convulsion; series of involuntary contractions of voluntary muscles.
Selectively permeable membranes Membranes that separate fluid compartments of the body and regulate movement of water and certain solutes from one compartment to another.
Self A term to describe one's personhood.
Self-concept One's mental image or picture of oneself.
Self-esteem The perception of self as having worth.
Sensorineural deafness A hearing impairment resulting from damage to the nerve centers within the brain as a result of exposure to loud noises, disease, and certain drugs.
Sensorium Level of consciousness and orientation to time, place, person, and self.
Septum A wall that divides a body cavity.
Serosanguineous Made up of blood and serum.
Serous Containing serum.
Sexually transmitted disease A disease that can be transmitted by intimate genital, oral, or rectal contact.
Shearing forces Caused by two contacting parts sliding on each other.
Shock Acute circulatory failure that can lead to death; caused by blood loss, heart failure, overwhelming infection, severe allergic reactions, or extreme pain or fright.
Shroud A wrap in which the body is placed after death for transport to the morgue or mortuary.
Sinusitis Inflammation of the paranasal sinuses.
Sjögren's syndrome A symptom complex of unknown etiology marked by the triad of keratoconjunctivitis, xerostomia, and the presence of a connective tissue disease.
Skilled nursing facility Type of long-term care facility that provides rehabilitative care for people who need nursing care that consists of observation during illness, administration of medications and treatments, bowel or bladder retraining, and changing of sterile dressings.
Skilled observation and assessment Used to determine adequacy of home environment, knowledge level of the patient and family regarding care procedures, side effects of treatment, and family's level of comfort in performing specific procedures.
Skilled procedures Certain nursing procedures, such as dressing changes, Foley catheter insertions, and venipuncture.
Smegma Sebaceous secretion found beneath the foreskin.
Social age The roles and habits of a person in relation to other members of society.
Soluble fiber Partially digestible roughage found in plant cells; aids in stool softening and works chemically to reduce absorption of certain substances in the bloodstream.
Solution A liquid containing one or more dissolved substances.

Somatoform disorder Characterized by vague, multiple, recurring physical complaints that are not caused by real physical illness.
Somogyi effect Rebound response to excess insulin, causing hyperglycemia.
Spastic Increased muscle tone, characterized by sudden, involuntary muscle spasms.
Spasticity Abnormally increased muscle tone.
Spermatocele A cystic mass on the epididymis.
Sprain An injury to a ligament.
Sputum Mucus secretion from the respiratory tract.
Staged amputation Amputation that is done over the course of several operations, usually to control the spread of infection or necrosis.
Steatorrhea Excess fat in the stools.
Stenosis Narrowing of a passage or opening.
Sterile Free of microorganisms; infertile.
Sterility State of being free of microorganisms; unable to reproduce.
Stoma Opening created to drain contents of an organ.
Stomatitis Inflammation of the oral mucosa.
Strain An injury to muscle tissues or the tendons that attach them to bones, or both.
Stress A physical and emotional state always present in individuals that is intensified when an internal or external environmental change or threat occurs to which they must respond.
Stress fracture Fracture caused by either sudden force or prolonged stress.
Stress incontinence Involuntary loss of urine during physical exertion.
Stressor A factor that causes stress.
Stump The distal portion of an amputated limb.
Subarachnoid Between the arachnoid and pia mater layers of the membranes covering the brain.
Subculture A group of individuals within a culture whose members share different beliefs, values, and attitudes from those of the dominant culture.
Subjective data Information reported by patients or family members.
Substance abuse Maladaptive pattern of substance use that differs from generally accepted cultural norms; sometimes referred to as chemical abuse or drug abuse.
Substance dependence Ingestion of substances in gradually increasing amounts due to a physical need; used interchangeably with the terms chemical dependence and drug dependence.
Superficial partial thickness burn Burn that affects the epidermis.
Support system Resources that are used to cope with stress.
Surgical asepsis Elimination of microorganisms from any object that comes in contact with the patient; often called sterile technique.
Symptomatic incontinence Fecal incontinence associated with colorectal disease.
Syncope Fainting.
Syndrome Refers to behaviors and symptoms.
Syndrome of inappropriate antidiuretic hormone Disorder caused by excess antidiuretic hormone production; symptoms include decreased urination, edema, and fluid overload.
Systemic Related to the body as a whole.
Systole Contraction phase of the cardiac cycle.

T

Tachycardia Rapid heart rate, usually defined as greater than 100 beats per minute.
Tachypnea Rapid respiratory rate.
Tardive dyskinesia Frequently irreversible side effect of antipsychotic medication that develops after years of use; symptoms include involuntary movements of face, jaw, and tongue, leading to grimacing, jerky movements of upper extremities, and tonic contractions of neck and back.
Telangiectasis Vascular lesion created by dilation of a group of small blood vessels.
Tertiary prevention The third level of prevention; includes steps taken to prevent disease recurrence or complications of diagnosed disease or injury.
Testis (*pl.* testes) The male reproductive organs.
Tetany Steady muscle contraction; caused by hypocalcemia.
Theory X Management by autocratic rule with little participation in decision making by workers.
Theory Y Democratic style of management with some participation in decision making by workers.
Theory Z Management with full participation in decision making by workers.
Thoracentesis Insertion of a needle through the chest wall into the pleural space to remove fluid, blood, or air or to instill medication.
Thoracotomy Surgical opening of the chest wall.
Thrombocytopenia Abnormally reduced number of platelets in the blood.
Thromboembolism Obstruction of a blood vessel with a blood clot transported through the bloodstream.
Thrombophlebitis Development of venous thrombi in the presence of venous inflammation.
Thrombosis Development or presence of a thrombus.
Thrombus (*pl.* thrombi) Stationary blood clot.
Thyroiditis Inflammation of the thyroid gland.
Thyrotoxicosis Excessive metabolic stimulation caused by elevated thyroid hormone level.
Tinnitus Ringing, buzzing, or roaring noise in the ears.
Tissue perfusion Blood flow through the blood vessels of tissue.
Tolerance Physiologic result of repeated doses of an opioid where the same dose is no longer effective in achieving the same analgesic effect; a larger dose of the opioid is required to achieve the same analgesic effect.
Tonicity A measure of the concentration of electrolytes in a fluid.
Tonometry Measurement of pressure such as intraocular pressure.
Tonsillitis Inflammation of the tonsils.
Tophus (*pl.* tophi) Deposit of sodium urate crystals under the skin.
Transcultural nursing Integration of cultural considerations into all aspects of nursing care.
Transcutaneous electrical nerve stimulation (TENS) Method of producing analgesia through electrical impulses applied to the skin.

Transient incontinence Temporary loss of control over voiding.
Transient ischemic attack Diminished cerebral blood flow producing neurologic deficits that last less than 24 hours.
Triglycerides Lipids composed of three fatty acid chains and a glycerol molecule.
Trousseau's sign Carpopedal spasm after compression of the nerves in the upper arm; a sign of hypocalcemia.
12-Step Program Self-help support process outlining 12 steps to overcoming a physical or psychological dependence on something outside oneself that has a destructive impact on one's life.
Tympanic membrane Eardrum; the membrane that separates the external and middle portions of the ear.

U

Understanding Ability to listen to and relate to others in order to perceive their feelings and the meaning of their words.
Unipolar depression Depressed mood.
Universal donor Person with type O-negative blood who can donate blood to anyone because the person does not have any of the common antigens present in the blood.
Universal recipient Person with type AB-positive blood who can receive transfusions with any type of blood because the person has all the common antigens (A, B, and Rh) present in the blood.
Unsaturated fatty acids Compounds that come from plants or fish and are generally liquid at room temperature; can be monounsaturated (olive, peanut, canola, and avocado oils) or polyunsaturated (corn, safflower, and sesame oils).
Uremia Azotemia; the signs and symptoms typical of chronic renal failure.
Ureterostomy Surgically created opening in the ureter.
Urethritis Inflammation of the urethra.
Urge incontinence Involuntary loss of urine, usually shortly after a strong urge to void.
Urinary incontinence The inability to control the passage of urine.
Uveitis Usually refers to inflammation of the iris, ciliary body, and/or choroid of the eye; also used to indicate inflammation of sclera, cornea, and/or retina.

V

Vaginitis Inflammation of the vagina.
Values Principles or standards that determine the worth you give to an idea or action.
Value system Personal standards for decision making.
Varices Enlarged, tortuous blood or lymphatic vessels.
Vasculitis Inflammation of blood vessels.
Vasoconstriction Decrease in blood vessel diameter.
Vasodilation Increase in blood vessel diameter.
Ventilation Movement of air in and out of the lungs.
Vertigo Sensation that one's body or one's surroundings are rotating.
Vesicle Small fluid-filled bladder or sac; blister.
Vesicostomy Surgically created opening into the urinary bladder.
Viruses Infectious microorganisms that can live and reproduce only within living cells; capable of causing illness, inflammation, and cell destruction.
Viscosity Resistance to flow related to the friction between two components; thickness.
Vitamins Organic compounds supplied by food that the body needs for normal growth and development.
Void Urinate.
Vulvitis Inflammation of the vulva.

W

Water-soluble vitamins Vitamins that are soluble in water; not as potentially toxic as fat-soluble vitamins and readily excreted by the body; includes vitamins *except* A, D, E, and K.
Wheeze High-pitched sound heard as air passes through constricted airways.
Withdrawal Unpleasant and sometimes life-threatening physical substance-specific syndrome occurring after stopping or reducing the habitual dose or frequency of an abused drug.

X

Xerostomia Dry mouth caused by inadequate production of saliva.

Index

A

t, Table; *f*, figure.

C

D

E

J

M

Q

R

S

W

X

Y

Z

Answers to **REVIEW** QUESTIONS

Chapter 1

1. 4
2. 3
3. 1
4. 2
5. 3

Chapter 2

1. 2
2. 2
3. 1
4. 3
5. 3
6. 4
7. 1

Chapter 3

1. 4
2. 3
3. 3
4. 1
5. 4
6. 2

Chapter 4

1. 4
2. 4
3. 1
4. 3
5. 4
6. 2
7. 3

Chapter 5

1. 2
2. 1
3. 2
4. 4
5. 3

Chapter 6

1. 2
2. 3
3. 1
4. 4
5. 3

Chapter 7

1. 3
2. 2
3. 3
4. 4
5. 1
6. 4
7. 3
8. 2

Chapter 8

1. 2
2. 4
3. 1
4. 3
5. 4
6. 3
7. 3
8. 2
9. 4
10. 2
11. 1

Chapter 9

1. 3
2. 4
3. 2
4. 1
5. 2
6. 2

Chapter 10

1. 1
2. 1
3. 3
4. 3
5. 2
6. 2
7. 4
8. 3
9. 1
10. 4

Chapter 11

1. 4
2. 2
3. 1
4. 1
5. 1
6. 3
7. 4
8. 2
9. 1

Chapter 12

1. 3
2. 2
3. 1
4. 3
5. 4
6. 3
7. 1
8. 4
9. 2
10. 1
11. 2
12. 2
13. 3
14. 3
15. 4

Chapter 13

1. 4
2. 1
3. 3
4. 2
5. 4
6. 2
7. 2
8. 3
9. 1
10. 3
11. 2
12. 4

Chapter 14

1. 1
2. 2
3. 3
4. 4
5. 4
6. 2
7. 1
8. 4
9. 3
10. 3

Chapter 15

1. 1
2. 4
3. 2
4. 2
5. 1
6. 4
7. 3
8. 2
9. 4
10. 1

Chapter 16

1. 2
2. 2
3. 3
4. 3
5. 4
6. 4
7. 1
8. 2

Chapter 17

1. 1
2. 2
3. 4
4. 3
5. 1

Chapter 18

1. 4
2. 2
3. 1
4. 3
5. 3
6. 2
7. 2
8. 4
9. 2
10. 4

Chapter 19

1. 1
2. 4
3. 1
4. 3

Chapter 20

1. 3
2. 1
3. 2
4. 1
5. 4
6. 1
7. 2

Chapter 21

1. 1
2. 3
3. 1
4. 2
5. 3
6. 4

Chapter 22

1. 4
2. 2
3. 4
4. 1
5. 2
6. 1
7. 3
8. 3
9. 1
10. 2
11. 3

Chapter 23

1. 2
2. 4
3. 2
4. 3
5. 4
6. 4
7. 1
8. 2
9. 3
10. 1
11. 4

Chapter 24

1. 1
2. 3
3. 2
4. 3
5. 4
6. 4
7. 1
8. 3
9. 2
10. 4

Chapter 25

1. 2
2. 4
3. 1
4. 3
5. 4
6. 1
7. 3
8. 3
9. 3
10. 1

Chapter 26

1. 1
2. 3
3. 4
4. 4
5. 3
6. 2
7. 1
8. 4
9. 3

Chapter 27

1. 2
2. 3
3. 4
4. 4
5. 1
6. 2
7. 2
8. 4
9. 3
10. 2

Chapter 28

1. 2
2. 1
3. 2
4. 3
5. 4
6. 4
7. 1
8. 3
9. 3
10. 1

Chapter 29

1. 3
2. 4
3. 1
4. 2
5. 2
6. 3
7. 4
8. 4
9. 1
10. 2

Chapter 30

1. 4
2. 1
3. 2
4. 3
5. 2
6. 4
7. 1
8. 2
9. 4
10. 2

Chapter 31

1. 4
2. 3
3. 3
4. 4
5. 2
6. 1
7. 3
8. 1
9. 1
10. 3

Chapter 32

1. 1
2. 3
3. 2
4. 4
5. 1
6. 3
7. 1
8. 2
9. 4
10. 3

Chapter 33

1. 4
2. 1
3. 3
4. 2
5. 4
6. 1
7. 4
8. 3
9. 2
10. 4
11. 2
12. 3
13. 3
14. 1